SAUNDERS
Comprehensive Review
for the NCLEX-RN® EXAMINATION

SAUNDERS
Comprehensive Review
for the
NCLEX-RN®
EXAMINATION

5 EDITION

LINDA ANNE SILVESTRI, PhD, RN

Instructor of Nursing
Salve Regina University
Newport, Rhode Island
President
Nursing Reviews, Inc.
and
Professional Nursing Seminars, Inc.
Charlestown, Rhode Island
Instructor: NCLEX-RN® and NCLEX-PN® Review Courses

ELSEVIER
SAUNDERS

ELSEVIER
SAUNDERS

3251 Riverport Lane
St. Louis, Missouri 63043

SAUNDERS COMPREHENSIVE REVIEW FOR THE NCLEX-RN®
EXAMINATION

ISBN: 978-1-4377-0825-7

Notices

Knowledge and best practice in this field are constantly changing. As new research and experience
broaden our understanding, changes in research methods, professional practices, or medical
treatment may become necessary.

Practitioners and researchers must always rely on their own experience and knowledge in
evaluating and using any information, methods, compounds, or experiments described herein. In
using such information or methods they should be mindful of their own safety and the safety of
others, including parties for whom they have a professional responsibility.

With respect to any drug or pharmaceutical products identified, readers are advised to check the
most current information provided (i) on procedures featured or (ii) by the manufacturer of each
product to be administered, to verify the recommended dose or formula, the method and duration
of administration, and contraindications. It is the responsibility of practitioners, relying on their
own experience and knowledge of their patients, to make diagnoses, to determine dosages and the
best treatment for each individual patient, and to take all appropriate safety precautions.
To the fullest extent of the law, neither the Publisher nor the authors, contributors, or editors,
assume any liability for any injury and/or damage to persons or property as a matter of products
liability, negligence or otherwise, or from any use or operation of any methods, products,
instructions, or ideas contained in the material herein.

ISBN: 978-1-4377-0825-7

Vice President and Publisher: Loren Wilson
Senior Editor: Kristin Geen
Acquisitions Editor: Nancy O'Brien
Developmental Editor: Todd McKenzie
Publishing Services Managers: Anne Altepeter, Jeff Patterson
Senior Project Managers: Doug Turner, Clay Broeker
Multimedia Producer: Sarah Spalding-Eichorn
Designer: Margaret Reid

Printed in the United States of America

Last digit is the print number: 9 8 7 6 5 4 3

To my parents—
To my mother, **Frances Mary,**
and in loving memory of my father, **Arnold Lawrence,**
who taught me to always love, care, and be the best that I could be.

And
in loving memory of my sweet and loyal West Highland terrier **Pynsea,**
who was always by my side as I created this publication.

To All Future Registered Nurses,

Congratulations to you!

You should be very proud and pleased with yourself on your most recent well-deserved accomplishment of completing your nursing program to become a registered nurse. I know that you have worked very hard to become successful and that you have proven to yourself that indeed you can achieve your goals.

In my opinion, you are about to enter the most wonderful and rewarding profession that exists. Your willingness, desire, and ability to assist those who need nursing care will bring great satisfaction to your life. In the profession of nursing, your learning will be a lifelong process. This aspect of the profession makes it stimulating and dynamic. Your learning process will continue to expand and grow as the profession continues to evolve. Your next very important endeavor will be the learning process involved to achieve success in your examination to become a registered nurse.

I am excited and pleased to be able to provide you with the *Saunders Pyramid to Success* products, which will help you prepare for your next important professional goal, becoming a registered nurse. I want to thank all of my former nursing students whom I have assisted in their studies for the NCLEX-RN exam for their willingness to offer ideas regarding their needs in preparing for licensure. Student ideas have certainly added a special uniqueness to all of the products available in the *Saunders Pyramid to Success*.

Saunders Pyramid to Success products provide you with everything that you need to ready yourself for the NCLEX-RN exam. These products include material that is required for the NCLEX-RN exam for all nursing students regardless of educational background, specific strengths, areas in need of improvement, or clinical experience during the nursing program.

So let's get started and begin our journey through the *Saunders Pyramid to Success*, and welcome to the wonderful profession of nursing!

Sincerely,

Linda Anne Silvestri

Linda Anne Silvestri

About the Author

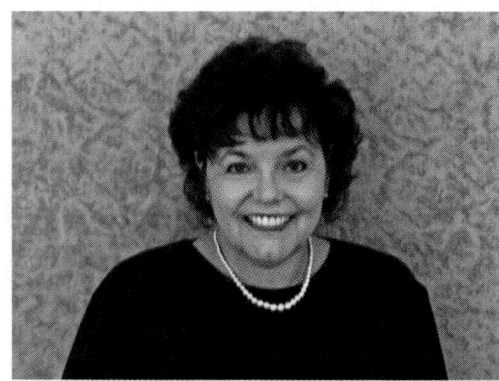

Linda Anne Silvestri. (Photo by Laurent W. Valliere.)

As a child, I always dreamed of becoming either a nurse or a teacher. Initially I chose to become a nurse because I really wanted to help others, especially those who were ill. Then I realized that both of my dreams could come true; I could be both a nurse and a teacher. So I pursued my dreams.

I received my diploma in nursing at Cooley Dickinson Hospital School of Nursing in Northampton, Massachusetts. Afterward, I worked at Baystate Medical Center in Springfield, Massachusetts, where I cared for clients in acute medical-surgical units, the intensive care unit, the emergency department, pediatric units, and other acute care units. Later I received an associate degree from Holyoke Community College in Holyoke, Massachusetts, my BSN from American International College in Springfield, Massachusetts, and my MSN from Anna Maria College in Paxton, Massachusetts, with a dual major in Nursing Management and Patient Education. I received my PhD in Nursing from the University of Nevada, Las Vegas, and conducted research on self-efficacy and the predictors of NCLEX success. I am also a member of the Honor Society of Nursing, Sigma Theta Tau International, Phi Kappa Phi, the Western Institute of Nursing, the Eastern Nursing Research Society, National League for Nursing, and the Golden Key International Honour Society.

As a native of Springfield, Massachusetts, I began my teaching career as an instructor of medical-surgical nursing and leadership-management nursing in 1981 at Baystate Medical Center School of Nursing. In 1989, I relocated to Rhode Island and began teaching advanced medical-surgical nursing and psychiatric nursing to RN and LPN students at the Community College of Rhode Island. While teaching there, a group of students approached me for assistance in preparing for the NCLEX examination. I have always had a very special interest in test success for nursing students because of my own personal experiences with testing. Taking tests was never easy for me, and as a student I needed to find methods and strategies that would bring success. My own difficult experiences, desire, and dedication to assist nursing students to overcome the obstacles associated with testing inspired me to develop and write the many products that would foster success with testing. My experiences as a student, nursing educator, and item writer for the NCLEX exams aided me as I developed a comprehensive review course to prepare nursing graduates for the NCLEX examination.

Later, in 1994, I began teaching medical-surgical nursing at Salve Regina University in Newport, Rhode Island, and remain there as an adjunct faculty member. I also prepare nursing students at Salve Regina University for the NCLEX-RN examination.

I established Professional Nursing Seminars, Inc., in 1991 and Nursing Reviews, Inc, in 2000. Both companies are dedicated to conducting review courses for the NCLEX-RN and the NCLEX-PN examinations and helping nursing graduates achieve their goals of becoming registered nurses, licensed practical/vocational nurses, or both.

Today, I conduct review courses for the NCLEX examinations throughout New England and am the successful author of numerous review products. I am so pleased that you have decided to join me on your journey to success in testing for nursing examinations and for the NCLEX-RN examination!

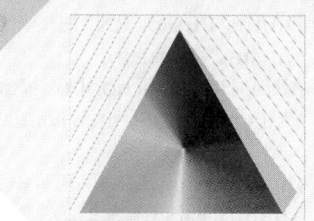

Contributors

CONTRIBUTORS

Sarah Hollenberg, RN
Nursing Graduate
College of Nursing
University of Missouri—St. Louis
St. Louis, Missouri
Chapter 4: The NCLEX-RN® Examination:
From a Graduate's Perspective

Bethany Hawes Sykes, EdD, RN, CEN, CCRN
Adjunct Faculty
Department of Nursing
Salve Regina University
Newport, Rhode Island
Chapter 34: Health and Physical Assessment
of the Adult Client

Laurent W. Valliere, BS
Vice President
Professional Nursing Seminars, Inc.
Charlestown, Rhode Island
Chapter 3: Pathways to Success

ANCILLARY CO-AUTHOR

Jacqueline B. Arnett, BSN, CPN
Registered Nurse and Staff Development Coordinator
Nursing Administration
Life Care Centers of America
Tucson, Arizona

ITEM WRITERS

Jacqueline B. Arnett, BSN, CPN
Registered Nurse and Staff Development Coordinator
Nursing Administration
Life Care Centers of America
Tucson, Arizona

Mary C. Carrico, MS, RN
Associate Professor of Nursing
West Kentucky Community and Technical College
Paducah, Kentucky

Patricia Delmoe, RN, MN
Nursing Faculty Maricopa
Nursing Banner Boswell/Mesa
Mesa Community College
Mesa, Arizona

Christine R. Durbin, PhD, JD, RN
Assistant Professor
School of Nursing
Southern Illinois University Edwardsville
Edwardsville, Illinois

Tamara Gailey, MSN, RN
Nursing Instructor
Great Basin College
Elko, Nevada

Miki Goodwin, PhD, RN, PHN
Fast Track Program Coordinator
Idaho State University
Pocatello, Idaho

Wendy Greenspan, MSN, RN, CCRN
Nursing Instructor
Department of Nursing
Rockland Community College
Suffern, New York

Marilyn Johnessee Greer, MS, RN
Associate Professor of Nursing
Rockford College
Rockford, Illinois

Kimberly Little, PhD, RN, CNE
Assistant Professor of Nursing
Cabarrus College of Health Sciences
Concord, North Carolina

Donna Russo, RN, MSN, CCRN, CNE
Nursing Instructor
ARIA Health School of Nursing
Philadelphia, Pennsylvania

Julie Snyder, MSN, RN-BC
Adjunct Faculty
School of Nursing
Old Dominican University
Norfolk, Virginia

Sharon Souter, PhD, RN, CNE
Dean and Associate Professor
Scott and White College of Nursing
University of Mary Hardin-Baylor
Belton, Texas

Linda Turchin, MSN, RN, CNE
Assistant Professor
Department of Nursing
Fairmont State University
Fairmount, West Virginia

The author and publisher would also like to acknowledge the following individuals for contributions to the previous editions of this book:

JoAnn Acierno, BSN, RN
Omaha, Nebraska

Marion G. Anema, PhD, RN
Nashville, Tennessee

Marianne P. Barba, MS, RN, CPC
Coventry, Rhode Island

Carol A. Baxter, EdD, RN
Lancaster, Pennsylvania

Eloise M. Brotzman, MSEd, MSN, RNC
Bethlehem, Pennsylvania

Reitha Cabaniss, MSN, RN
Sumiton, Alabama

Janice Almon Call, MSN, RN, C
Gainesville, Texas

Darlene Nebel Cantu, MSN, RNC
San Antonio, Texas

Heather Carlson, RN
Newport, Rhode Island

Elizabeth M. Carson, EdD, RN
Rockford, Illinois

Shannon Chase, RN
Newport, Rhode Island

Jane Anne Claffy, MSN, RNC
Germantown, New York

Alice D. Coomes, MSN, RN
Owensboro, Kentucky

Barbara Cornett, PhD, CNS, RN, CHES
Westerville, Ohio

Gloria Coschigano, MSN, RN, CS
Valhalla, New York

Nancy Wilson Darland, MSN, RNC, CNS
Ruston, Louisiana

Jean W. Davis, EdD, RN, CS
Miami Shores, Florida

Jean DeCoffe, MSN, RN
Milton, Massachusetts

Carole A. Devine, MSN, RN
Kingston, Rhode Island

Katherine H. Dimmock, JD, EdD, MSN, RN
Milwaukee, Wisconsin

Mary L. Dowell, PhD, RN, BC
Belton, Texas

Julie Eggert, PhD, GNP-C, AOCN
Clemson, South Carolina

Kerry H. Fater, PhD, RN, CS
North Dartmouth, Massachusetts

Ginette G. Ferszt, PhD, RN, CS
Kingston, Rhode Island

Katherine A. Fletcher, PhD, RN, CS
Kansas City, Kansas

Cathy Fortenbaugh, MSN, RN, AOCN, CNS-C
Philadelphia, Pennsylvania

Jane H. Freeman, EdD, RN
Jacksonville, Alabama

Cynthia A. Gaudet, MSN, RN
Springfield, Massachusetts

Rita S. Glazebrook, PhD, RN, CNP
Northfield, Minnesota

Kimberly Green, RN
Newport, Rhode Island

Karen Clark Griffith, PhD, RN
Iowa City, Iowa

Sheila C. Grossman, PhD, APRN-BC
Fairfield, Connecticut

Joyce Hammer, MSN, RN
Detroit, Michigan

Jacqueline Lynne Harris, MNSc, RN, ONC
Searcy, Arkansas

Amy Zlomek Hedden, RN, MS, NP
Bakersfield, California

Beverly K. Hogan, APRN, BC
Birmingham, Alabama

Mary Ann Hogan, MSN, RN, CS
Amherst, Massachusetts

Mary Kathleen Jackson, BSN, RN, CPN
Whiteville, North Carolina

Gail M. Johnson, EdD, MSN, RN, CNAA, BC
Trenton, New Jersey

Juanita F. Johnson, PhD, RN
Shawnee, Oklahoma

Katherine Theresa Jorgensen, MSN, RN, MA
Vermillion, South Dakota

Katje A. Koning, RN
Storrs, Connecticut

Elisa Mangosing Lemmon, MSN, RN, C
Newport News, Virginia

Teresa Leonard, MSN, RN, CCRN
Florence, Alabama

Carol O. Long, PhD, RN
Tempe, Arizona

Marilyn Lusk, MSN, MS, RN
Kingman, Arizona

Lois S. Marshall, PhD, RN
Miami, Florida

Linda Ann Martin, MSN, RN, APN-C
Trenton, New Jersey

Dorothy Mae Mathers, MSN, RN
Williamsport, Pennsylvania

Ellyn E. Matthews, PhD, RN, AOCN, CRNI
Denver, Colorado

Ellen C. McElroy, DSN, RN
Birmingham, Alabama

Susan A. Moore, PhD, RN
Memphis, TN

Jo Ann Barnes Mullaney, PhD, RN, CS
Newport, Rhode Island

Betsy J. Nield, MS, RNC
Warwick, Rhode Island

Tina Nink, MSN, RN, FNP
Oglesby, Illinois

Lolita T. O'Donnell, PhD, MSN, RN
Fairfax, Virginia

Kathleen A. Ohman, EdD, MS, RN, CCRN
St. Cloud, Minnesota

Patricia A. Parsons, MSN, MS, RN
Austin, Minnesota

Elizabeth Phillip, MSN, RN
Bethlehem, Pennsylvania

Tommie Wright Pniewski, MSN, RN, CNAA
Hopkinsville, Kentucky

Emily Porterfield, RN, LDN
Greenville, North Carolina

Ethel Pruden, MSN, RN
Savannah, Georgia

Marion Sawyier, MSN, RN
Albuquerque, New Mexico

Nancy Schlapman, PhD, RN
Kokomo, Indiana

Jane Schlickau, MN, RN, ARNP, CTN
Winfield, Kansas

Joan Schmitke, DSN, APRN, FNP, BC
Richmond, Kentucky

Bruce Austin Scott, MSN, APRN, BC
Stockton, California

Geneva Scott, MSN, RN, BSS
Weatherford, Texas

Shirley Sherrick-Escamilla, PhD(c), MSN, RNC
Detroit, Michigan

Shellie Simons, MS, RN
Boston, Massachusetts

Mary M. Smith, MSN, RN
Charlotte, North Carolina

Fran Soukup, RN, MSN, EdS
Albany, New York

Marian I. Stewart, MSN, RN
Lynchburg, Tennessee

Linda D. Taylor, PhD(c), RN, OCN
Rockford, Illinois

Lynn Tesh, MSN, RN
Asheboro, North Carolina

Vicki L. Vann, MS, ARNP
Tampa, Florida

Cheryl J. Vitacco-Grab, MSN, RNC
Lancaster, Pennsylvania

Loretta A. Wack, MSN, PNP, FNP
Weyers Cave, Virginia

Mary Hauser Whitaker, MSN, RN
Richmond, Kentucky

Cheryle I. Whitney, MSN, RN
The Woodlands, Texas

Chris Winkelman, RN, PhD, CNP, CCRN
Cleveland, Ohio

Danette Wood, EdD, MSN, RN, CCRN
Statesboro, Georgia

Terry Yoesting, MS, RN
Denison, Texas

CONSULTANTS

Nicole Marie Valliere, BSN, RN
Professional Nurse I—Pediatrics
Hasbro Children's Hospital
Providence, Rhode Island

Dianne E. Ventrice
Reference Consultant
Nursing Reviews, Inc.
Charlestown, Rhode Island

Reviewers

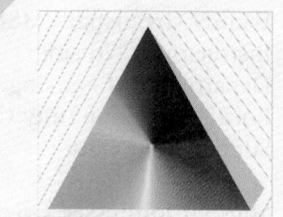

Jacqueline B. Arnett, BSN, CPN
Registered Nurse and Staff Development Coordinator
Nursing Administration
Life Care Centers of America
Tucson, Arizona

Cynthia Elnora Ashby, MS, RN
Adjunct Faculty
Ashby Educational Assessment Program
The University of Houston Victoria at Cinco Ranch
Houston, Texas

Marilee Aufdenkamp, MS, RN
Assistant Professor
School of Nursing
Creighton University
Omaha, Nebraska

Susan F. Beasley, MSN, RN, CNE
Nursing Faculty
Department of Nursing
Technical College of the Lowcountry
Beaufort, South Carolina

Mary C. Carrico, MS, RN
Associate Professor of Nursing
West Kentucky Community and Technical College
Paducah, Kentucky

Olivia Catolico, PhD, CNL, RN, BC
Associate Professor
Department of Nursing
Dominican University of California
San Rafael, California

Claire Cottrell, RN, MSN
Nursing Instructor
Associate Degree Nursing Division
Mississippi Gulf Coast Community College
Perkinston, Mississippi

Paula Cox-North, MN, NP-C
Pacific Medical Centers
Department of Gastroenterology
School of Nursing
University of Washington
Seattle, Washington

Christine R. Durbin, PhD, JD, RN
Assistant Professor
School of Nursing
Southern Illinois University Edwardsville
Edwardsville, Illinois

Susan C. Engle, MSN, RN
Professor
Department of Health Occupation
Napa Valley College
Napa, California

Douglas A. Fabick, BS, RN, CEN
Tennessee ACLS Regional Faculty
Chair of Northeast Tennessee ECC
Volunteer Department
American Heart Association
Kingsport, Tennessee

Tamara Gailey, MSN, RN
Nursing Instructor
Great Basin College
Elko, Nevada

Susan Johnson Garbutt, DNP, RN, CIC
RN Program Director
Galen School of Nursing
St. Petersburg, Florida

Cené L. Gibson, MSN, ARNP
Family Nurse Practitioner
Regional Clinical Coordinator
Frontier School of Midwifery and Family Nursing,
Oklahoma City, Oklahoma

Wendy Greenspan, MSN, RN, CCRN
Instructor of Nursing
Department of Nursing
Rockland Community College
Suffern, New York

Marilyn Johnessee Greer, MS, RN
Associate Professor of Nursing
Department of Nursing
Rockford College
Rockford, Illinois

Sheila Grossman, PhD, FNP, APRN-BC
Professor and Coordinator
FNP Track
School of Nursing
Fairfield University
Fairfield, Connecticut

Deborah Hamolsky, MS, RN, AOCNS
Clinical Nurse
Carol Franc Buck Breast Care Center
Helen Diller Family Comprehensive Cancer Center
University of California, San Francisco
San Francisco, California

Sarah M. Howell, MSN, RN
Assistant Professor of Nursing
Department of Nursing
Mississippi University of Women
Columbus, Mississippi

Cheryl A. Lehman, PhD, RN, CRRN, CNS
Associate Professor/Clinical
Acute Nursing Department
School of Nursing
University of Texas Health Science Center
  at San Antonio
San Antonio, Texas

Sue Ann McCann, MSN, RN, DCN
CTCL and Research Coordinator
Department of Dermatology and Nursing
University of Pittsburg Medical Center
Pittsburg, Pennsylvania

Mariann Montgomery, MSN, RN, CNE
Assistant Professor
Department of Nursing
Kent State University Tuscarawas
New Philadelphia, Ohio

Sherry Neely, MSN, RN, CRNP
Associate Professor
Department of Nursing
Butler County Community College
Butler, Pennsylvania

Joshua J. Neumiller, PharmD, CDE, CGP, FASCP
Assistant Professor of Pharmacotherapy
Department of Pharmacotherapy
Washington State University
Spokane, Washington

Deborah Palada, MSN, APRN, CPNP
Pediatric Nurse Practitioner
Department of Pediatrics
St. Mary's Hospital
Jefferson City, Missouri

Brenda Pavill, PhD, RN, FNP, IBCLC
Associate Professor
School of Nursing
University of North Carolina, Wilmington
Wilmington, North Carolina

Suzanne Pellar, MS, RN, CNS-BC
Assistant Professor of Nursing
Purdue University North Central
Westville, Indiana

Barbara D. Powe, PhD, RN
Director
Underserved Population Research
Behavioral Research Center
American Cancer Society
Atlanta, Georgia

Catherine Napoli Rice, EdD, RN
Associate Professor
Department of Nursing
Western Connecticut State University
Danbury, Connecticut

Dottie Roberts, MSN, MACI, RN, CMSRN, OCNS-C
Nursing Instructor
South University
Columbia, South Carolina

Katherine Roberts, MSN, RN
Assistant Professor of Nursing
Department of Nursing
Lamar University
Beaumont, Texas

Jana C. Saunders, PhD, RN, CNS
Professor
Health Sciences Center
Anita Thigpen Perry School of Nursing
Texas Tech University
Lubbock, Texas

Angela E. Silvestri, RN
Nursing Graduate
Salve Regina University
Newport, Rhode Island

Susan E. Sitter, MSN, RN
Professor of Nursing
Department of Nursing
Edinboro University of Pennsylvania
Edinboro, Pennsylvania

Beryl Stetson, MSN, RNBC, LCCE, CLC
Assistant Professor
Department of Nursing
Raritan Valley Community College
Somerville, New Jersey

E. Bradley Strecker, MA, BSN, RN, CCRN
Nursing Faculty
Department of Science
Columbia College
Columbia, Missouri

Darlene M. Thomay, RN, BA, DNC
Staff Nurse
Infusion Room
Medical Specialties Clinic
MetroHealth
Cleveland, Ohio

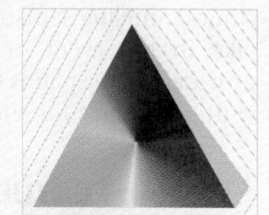

Preface

"To laugh often and much, to appreciate beauty, to find the best in others, to leave the world a bit better, to know that even one life has breathed easier because you have lived, this is to have succeeded."

Ralph Waldo Emerson

Welcome to Saunders *Pyramid to Success*!

AN ESSENTIAL RESOURCE FOR TEST SUCCESS

Saunders Comprehensive Review for the NCLEX-RN® Examination is one in a series of products designed to assist you in achieving your goal of becoming a registered nurse. This text will provide you with a comprehensive review of all of the nursing content areas specifically related to the new 2010 test plan for the NCLEX-RN examination, which is implemented by the National Council of State Boards of Nursing. This resource will help you achieve success on your nursing examinations during nursing school and on the NCLEX-RN examination.

ORGANIZATION

This book contains 20 units and 77 chapters. The chapters are designed to identify specific components of nursing content, and they contain practice questions, both multiple choice and alternate item formats, that reflect the chapter content and the 2010 test plan for the NCLEX-RN exam. The final unit contains a 75-question Comprehensive Test.

The new test plan identifies a framework based on *Client Needs*. These Client Needs categories include Safe and Effective Care Environment, Health Promotion and Maintenance, Psychosocial Integrity, and Physiological Integrity. *Integrated Processes* are also identified as a component of the test plan. These include Caring, Communication and Documentation, Nursing Process, and Teaching and Learning. All the chapters address the components of the test plan framework.

SPECIAL FEATURES OF THE BOOK

PYRAMID TERMS

Each content area, discussed in either a chapter or a unit, begins with *Pyramid Terms* and their definitions. These *Pyramid Terms* terms are important to the discussion of the content. Therefore they are in bold magenta type throughout the content section.

PYRAMID TO SUCCESS

The *Pyramid to Success*, a feature part of the chapter or unit introduction, provides you with an overview, guidance, and direction regarding the focus of review in the particular content area, as well as the content area's relative importance to the 2010 test plan for the NCLEX-RN exam. Specific nursing content areas, as specified in the test plan, are identified. The *Pyramid to Success* reviews the Client Needs as they pertain to the content in that unit or chapter. These points identify the specific components to keep in mind as you review the chapter.

PYRAMID POINTS

Pyramid Points are the little icons that are placed next to specific content throughout the chapters. The *Pyramid Points* highlight content that is important for preparing for the NCLEX-RN examination and identify content that typically appears on the NCLEX-RN examination.

PYRAMID ALERTS

Pyramid Alerts are the red text found throughout the chapters that alert you to important information about nursing concepts. These alerts identify content that typically appears on the NCLEX-RN examination.

PRIORITY NURSING ACTIONS

Numerous *Priority Nursing Actions* boxes have been placed throughout the chapters. These boxes present a clinical nursing situation and the priority actions to take in the event of its occurrence. A rationale is provided that explains the correct order of action, along with a reference for additional research.

SPECIAL FEATURES FOUND ON THE COMPANION CD

HEART, LUNG, AND BOWEL SOUND QUESTIONS

The accompanying software contains *Audio Questions* representative of content addressed in the 2010 test plan for the NCLEX-RN exam. These questions are in NCLEX-style format, and each question presents an audio sound as a component of the question.

VIDEO QUESTIONS

The accompanying software also contains new *Video Questions* representative of content addressed in the 2010 test plan for the NCLEX-RN exam. These questions are in NCLEX-style format, and each question presents a video clip as a component of the question.

AUDIO REVIEW SUMMARIES

The companion CD now includes three *Audio Review Summaries* that cover challenging subject areas under the 2010 NCLEX-RN test plan, including *Pharmacology*, *Acid-Base Balance*, and *Fluids and Electrolytes*. These audio reviews are downloadable in mp3 format, and you can listen to them at your convenience any time on your computer, iPod, or portable mp3 player of choice.

PRACTICE QUESTIONS

While preparing for the NCLEX-RN examination, it is crucial for students to practice taking test questions. This book contains 1032 NCLEX-style multiple-choice and alternate item format questions. The accompanying software includes all the questions from the book, plus an additional 3478 questions for a total of 4510 questions.

MULTIPLE-CHOICE AND ALTERNATE ITEM FORMAT QUESTIONS

Starting with Unit II, each chapter is followed by a practice test. Each practice test contains several multiple-choice questions and an alternate item format question. The alternate item format questions at the end of the chapters and on the accompanying CD may be presented as one of the following:
- Fill-in-the-blank question
- Multiple response question

- Prioritizing (ordered response) question, also known as a drag-and-drop question
- Figure/illustration question, also known as a hot spot question
- Graphic options question, in which each option contains a figure or illustration
- Chart/exhibit question
- Audio question that include a heart, lung, or bowel sound
- Video question

These questions provide you with practice in prioritizing, decision-making, and critical thinking skills.

ANSWER SECTION

The answer sections include the correct answer, rationale, test-taking strategy, question categories, and a reference. The structure for the answer section is unique and provides the following information:
- *Rationale:* The rationale provides you with the significant information regarding both correct and incorrect options.
- *Test-Taking Strategy:* The test-taking strategy provides a logical path for selecting the correct option and helps you select an answer to a question on which you might have to guess. Specific suggestions for review are identified in the test-taking strategy.
- *Question Categories:* Each question is tagged with categories based on the 2010 NCLEX-RN test plan. Additional content categories are provided with each question to assist you in identifying areas in need of review. The categories identified with each practice question include Level of Cognitive Ability, Client Needs, Integrated Process, and the specific nursing Content Area. All categories are identified by their full names so that you do not need to memorize codes or abbreviations. Additionally, every question on the companion CD is organized by these question codes, so you can customize your study session to be as specific or as generic as you need.
- *Reference:* A reference, including a page number, is provided so you can easily find the information that you need to review in your undergraduate nursing textbooks.

PHARMACOLOGY AND MEDICATION CALCULATIONS REVIEW

Students consistently state that pharmacology is an area with which they need assistance. The 2010 NCLEX-RN test plan continues to incorporate pharmacology in the examination as it has in the past. Therefore pharmacology chapters have been included for your review and practice. This book includes 13 pharmacology chapters, a medication and intravenous calculation chapter, and a pediatric medication calculation chapter. Each of these chapters is followed by a practice test that uses the same question format described earlier. This book contains numerous pharmacology questions. Additionally, more than 700 pharmacology questions can be found on the accompanying software.

NCLEX-RN® REVIEW CD

Packaged in this book is a CD containing more than 4500 practice questions. This CD contains all the multiple choice questions; the alternate item format questions; the heart, lung, and bowel sound questions; and the video questions. This CD also includes a 75-question pretest that provides you with feedback on your strengths and weaknesses. The results of your pretest will generate an individualized study calendar to guide you in your preparation for the NCLEX examination. This Windows- and Mac-compatible program offers three testing modes for review: study, quiz, and exam. In addition, the companion CD includes three mp3-downloadable *Audio Review Summaries* that discuss pharmacology, acid-base balance, and fluids and electrolytes to help you study these difficult subjects on the go.

HOW TO USE THIS BOOK

Saunders Comprehensive Review for the NCLEX-RN® Examination is especially designed to help you with your successful journey to the peak of the Saunders *Pyramid to Success*, becoming a registered nurse. As you begin your journey through this book, you will be introduced to all the important points regarding the 2010 NCLEX-RN examination, the process of testing, and unique and special tips regarding how to prepare yourself for this very important examination.

You should begin your process through the Saunders *Pyramid to Success* by reading all of Unit I in this book and becoming familiar with the central points regarding the NCLEX-RN examination. Read Chapter 4, written by a nursing graduate who recently passed the examination and note what she has to say about the testing experience. Chapter 5, "Test-Taking Strategies," will provide you with the critical testing strategies that will guide you in selecting the correct option or assist you in selecting an answer to a question if you must guess. Keep these strategies in mind as you proceed through this book. Continue by studying the specific content areas addressed in Units II through XIX. Review the *Pyramid Terms* and *Pyramid to Success* notes, and identify the Client Needs specific to the test plan in each area. Read through the chapters and focus on the *Pyramid Points* and *Pyramid Alerts* that identify the areas most likely to be tested on the NCLEX-RN examination. Pay particular attention to the Priority Nursing Actions boxes because they provide information about

the steps that you will take in clinical situations requiring prioritization.

As you read each chapter, identify your areas of strength and those in need of further review. Highlight these areas and test your abilities by taking all the practice tests provided at the end of the chapters. Be sure to review all the rationales and the test-taking strategies. The rationale provides you with information regarding both the correct and incorrect options. The test-taking strategy offers a logical path to selecting the correct option. Use the references to easily find any information you need to review.

After reviewing all the chapters in the book, turn to Unit XX, the Comprehensive Test. Take this examination and then review each question, answer, and rationale. Identify any areas requiring further review; then take the time to review those areas again in both the book and the companion CD.

CLIMBING THE *PYRAMID TO SUCCESS*

The purpose of this book is to provide a **comprehensive review** of the nursing content you will be tested on during the NCLEX-RN examination. However, *Saunders Comprehensive Review for the NCLEX-RN® Examination* is intended to do more than simply prepare you for the rigors of the NCLEX; this book is also meant to serve as a valuable study tool that you can refer to throughout your nursing program, with customizable software to help identify and reinforce key content areas.

After using this book for comprehensive content review, your next step on the *Pyramid to Success* is to get additional practice with a **Q&A review** product. *Saunders Q&A Review for the NCLEX-RN® Examination* offers more than 5200 unique practice questions in the book and on the companion CD. The questions are focused on the Client Needs and Integrated Processes of the NCLEX test plan, making it easy to access

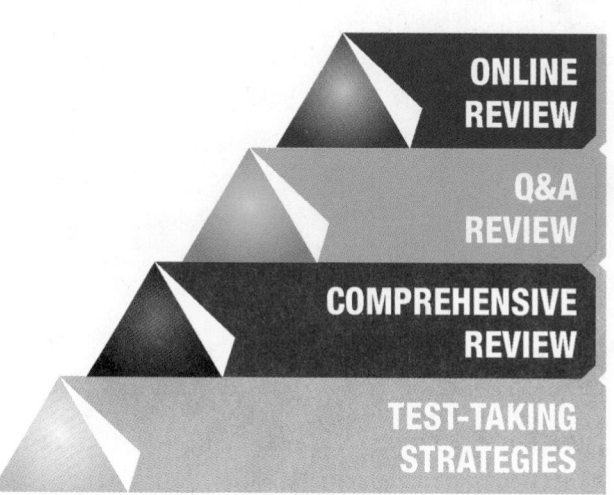

your study area of choice. For on-the-go Q&A review, you can pick up *Saunders Q&A Review Cards for the NCLEX-RN® Examination*, or, if you own an iPhone or iPod Touch, you can search for "Saunders Q&A Review" in Apple's App Store.

Your final step on the *Pyramid to Success* is to master the **online review**. *Saunders Online Review for the NCLEX-RN® Examination* provides an interactive and individualized platform to get you ready for your final licensure exam. This online course provides a high-level content overview, supplemented with instructional videos, animations, audio, illustrations, case studies, and several subject matter exams. In addition, you can assess your progress with a pre-test and post-test cumulative exam in a computerized environment that prepares you for the actual NCLEX-RN exam.

At the base of the *Pyramid to Success* are my **test-taking strategies**, which provide a foundation for understanding and unpacking the complexities of NCLEX exam questions, including alternate item formats. *Saunders Strategies for Test Success: Passing Nursing School and the NCLEX® Exam* takes a detailed look at all the test-taking strategies you will need to know in order to pass any nursing examination, including the NCLEX. Special tips are integrated for beginning nursing students, and there are 500 practice questions included so you can apply the testing strategies.

Good Luck with your journey through the Saunders *Pyramid to Success*. I wish you continued success throughout your new career as a registered nurse!

Linda Anne Silvestri, PhD, RN

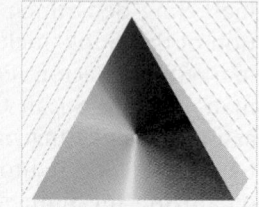

Acknowledgments

Sincere appreciation and warmest thanks are extended to the many individuals who in their own ways have contributed to the publication of this book.

First, I want to thank all my nursing students at the Community College of Rhode Island in Warwick who approached me in 1991 and persuaded me to help them prepare to take the NCLEX-RN examination. Their enthusiasm and inspiration led to the commencement of my professional endeavors in conducting review courses for the NCLEX-RN exam for nursing students. I also thank the numerous nursing students who have attended my review courses for their willingness to share their needs and ideas. Their input has certainly added a special uniqueness to this publication.

I wish to acknowledge all the nursing faculty who taught in my review courses for the NCLEX-RN exam. Their commitment, dedication, and expertise have certainly helped nursing students achieve success with the NCLEX-RN exam. Additionally, I want to acknowledge and sincerely thank Laurent W. Valliere, or Larry, for his contribution to this publication, for teaching in my review courses for the NCLEX-RN exam, and for his commitment and dedication in helping my nursing students prepare for the NCLEX-RN exam from a non-academic point of view. Larry has supported my many professional endeavors and was so loyal and loving to me each and every moment as I worked to achieve my professional goals. Larry, thank you so much! A special thank you also goes to Sarah Hollenberg, RN, for writing a chapter for this book about her experiences preparing for and taking the NCLEX-RN examination. I would like to acknowledge Jackie Arnett, a registered nurse and staff development coordinator for Life Care Centers of America in Tucson, Arizona, for her impeccable revisions to the Instructor's Evolve Resources accompanying this text, as well as for all her help reviewing and writing practice items for this book and companion CD. I also wish to acknowledge Lois Marshall for her useful contributions to the previous edition of the Instructor's Evolve Resources. Thank you Lois and Jackie for making this an invaluable resource!

I want to thank Nancy O'Brien, my former managing editor, for her creativity and all of her assistance in the initial planning of this edition of the book. I also sincerely acknowledge and thank two very important individuals from Elsevier Health Sciences: my senior editor, Kristin Geen, and my developmental editor, Todd McKenzie. Thank you, Kristin, for your continuous enthusiasm, tremendous support, and expert professional guidance throughout the preparation of this publication. And, Todd, well, I could not have completed this without him! Todd was with me during the initial planning of this publication and throughout its entire process of preparation and publication. So a very special and sincere thank you extends to Todd. Todd provided me with a tremendous amount of support during the many personal obstacles that I faced during the preparation of this publication. Additionally, his creativity, planning, and capable organizational and prioritizing skills kept me on track. He was an expert at maintaining the enormous amount of order needed to submit my manuscript into production. Thank you, Todd!

A special thank you and acknowledgment goes to two important individuals, Dianne Elodia Ventrice, and Lawrence Fiorentino. They provided continuous support and dedication to my work in both the NCLEX exam review courses and preparing this publication. Dianne was so dedicated to my work, and she helped maintain its excellent quality by providing expert reference support and expert secretarial responsibilities for the fifth edition of this book.

I want to acknowledge all of the staff at Elsevier for their tremendous assistance throughout the preparation and production of this publication. A special thank you to all of them. I thank all the important people in the production department, including Doug Turner, my longtime senior project manager; Clay Broeker, senior project manager; Anne Altepeter and Jeff Patterson, publishing services managers; Sarah Spalding-Eichorn, multimedia producer; David Rushing, multimedia team lead; and Margaret Reid, designer, who all played such significant roles in finalizing this publication. I sincerely thank those in the marketing department who helped with the promotion of this book, including Bob Boehringer, executive marketing director; Pat Crowe, executive marketing manager; and Susan Copeland and Jamie Heberlein, associate marketing managers. I would like to thank Jennifer Palada, editorial assistant, for all her help organizing the numerous contributors and reviewers involved in this project. I also sincerely thank Lauren Harms, developmental editor, for assisting me in completing this project. And a special thank you to Loren Wilson, vice president and publisher, for her years of expert guidance and continuous support for all the products in the *Pyramid to Success*.

I would also like to acknowledge Patricia Mieg, former educational sales representative, who encouraged me to submit my ideas and initial work for the first edition of this book to the W.B. Saunders Company.

I want to acknowledge my parents who opened my door of opportunity in education. I thank my mother, Frances Mary, for all of her love, support, and assistance as I continuously worked to achieve my professional goals. I thank my father, Arnold Lawrence, who always provided insightful words of encouragement. My memories of his love and support will always remain in my heart. I am certain that he would be very proud of my professional accomplishments.

I also thank my sister, Dianne Elodia Ventrice, and my brother, Lawrence Peter Silvestri, as well as all my nieces and nephews who were continuously supportive, giving, and helpful during my research and preparation of this publication.

I want to acknowledge all the individuals who reviewed content and practice questions and the item writers who updated and provided many of the practice questions. I also thank Dr. Bethany Sykes for her work in organizing Chapter 34, "Health and Physical Assessment of the Adult Client." I also thank the many faculty and student reviewers for their thoughts and ideas. A very special thank you to all of you!

I also need to thank Salve Regina University for the opportunity to educate nursing students in the baccalaureate nursing program and for its support during my research and writing of this publication. I would like to especially acknowledge my colleagues, Dr. Peggy Matteson, Dr. Ellen McCarty, Dr. JoAnn Mullaney, and Dr. Bethany Sykes for all their encouragement and support.

I wish to acknowledge the Community College of Rhode Island, which provided me the opportunity to educate nursing students in the Associate Degree of Nursing Program, and a special thank you to Patricia Miller, MSN, RN, and Michelina McClellan, MS, RN, from Baystate Medical Center, School of Nursing, in Springfield, Massachusetts, who were my first mentors in nursing education.

Lastly, a very special thank you to all my nursing students, past, present and future. All of you light up my life! Your love and dedication to the profession of nursing and your commitment to provide health care will bring never ending rewards!

Linda Anne Silvestri, PhD, RN

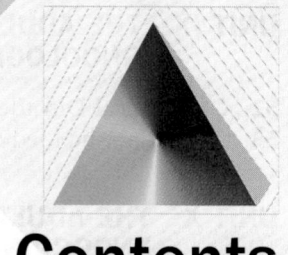

Contents

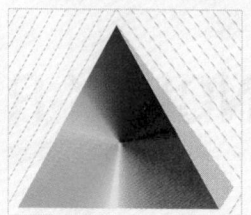

NCLEX-RN® Exam Preparation

The NCLEX-RN® Examination

Welcome to the Pyramid to Success

Saunders Comprehensive Review for the NCLEX-RN® Examination is specially designed to help you begin your successful journey to the peak of the pyramid, becoming a registered nurse. As you begin your journey, you will be introduced to all the important points regarding the NCLEX-RN examination and the process of testing, and to the unique and special tips regarding how to prepare yourself for this important examination. You will read what a nursing graduate who recently passed the NCLEX-RN examination has to say about the test. Important test-taking strategies are detailed. These details will guide you in selecting the correct option or assist you in selecting an answer to a question at which you must guess.

Each of the content areas in this book begins with the Pyramid to Success. The Pyramid to Success addresses specific points related to the NCLEX-RN examination, including the Pyramid Terms, and the Client Needs and Integrated Processes as identified in the test plan framework for the examination. Pyramid Terms are key words that are defined and are set in **boldface** throughout each chapter to direct your attention to significant points for the examination. The Client Needs specific to the content of the chapter are identified.

Throughout each chapter, you will find Pyramid Point bullets that identify areas most likely to be tested on the NCLEX-RN examination. Read each chapter, and identify your strengths and areas that are in need of further review. Test your strengths and abilities by taking all the practice tests provided in this book and on the accompanying software. Be sure to read all the rationales and test-taking strategies. The rationale provides you with significant information regarding the correct and incorrect options. The test-taking strategy provides you with the logical path to selecting the correct option. The test-taking strategy also identifies the content area to review, if required. The reference source and page number are provided so that you can

find the information easily that you need to review. Each question is coded based on the level of cognitive ability, the Client Needs category, the Integrated Process, and the nursing content area.

Following the completion of your comprehensive review in this book, continue on your journey through the Pyramid to Success with the companion book, *Saunders Q&A Review for the NCLEX-RN® Examination,* which provides you with more than 5200 practice questions based on the NCLEX-RN examination test plan framework, with a specific focus on Client Needs and Integrated Processes. Then, you will be ready for *Saunders Online Review for the NCLEX-RN® Examination.* Additional products in Saunders Pyramid to Success include *Saunders Strategies for Test Success: Passing Nursing School and the NCLEX® Exam* and *Saunders Q&A Review Cards for the NCLEX-RN® Exam.* These products are described next.

Saunders Online Review for the NCLEX-RN® Examination addresses all areas of the test plan identified by the National Council of State Boards of Nursing (NCSBN). The course contains a pretest that provides feedback regarding your strengths and weaknesses and generates an individualized study schedule in a calendar format. Content review is in an outline format and includes self-check practice questions and case studies, figures and illustrations, a glossary, and animations and videos. Numerous online exams are included. There are more than 2000 practice questions; the types of questions in this course include multiple-choice and alternate item formats.

Saunders Strategies for Test Success: Passing Nursing School and the NCLEX® Exam focuses on the test-taking strategies that will help you pass your nursing examinations while in nursing school and will prepare you for the NCLEX-RN examination. The chapters describe various test-taking strategies and include sample questions that illustrate how to use the strategies; 500 practice questions accompany this book. The practice questions reflect the framework and the content identified in the current NCLEX-RN test plan and include multiple-choice and alternate item format questions. Several appendices are included that provide a review of test-taking strategies, cultural characteristics and practices, pharmacology strategies, medication and intravenous calculations, laboratory values, positioning guidelines, and therapeutic diets.

Saunders Q&A Review Cards for the NCLEX-RN® Exam is organized specifically by the test plan framework of the current NCLEX-RN test plan. This product provides you with 1000 unique practice test questions on portable and easy-to-use cards. The question is on the front of the card, and the answer, rationale, test-taking strategy, and Integrated Process code are on the back of the card. This product includes multiple-choice questions and alternate item format questions, including fill-in-the-blank, multiple-response, prioritizing (ordered response), image (hot-spot questions), and chart/exhibit questions.

All the products in Saunders Pyramid to Success can be obtained online by visiting http://elsevierhealth.com or by calling 800-545-2522.

Let's begin our journey through the Pyramid to Success.

EXAMINATION PROCESS

An important step in the Pyramid to Success is to become as familiar as possible with the examination process. Candidates facing the challenge of this examination can experience significant anxiety. Knowing what the examination is all about and knowing what you will encounter during the process of testing will assist in alleviating fear and anxiety. The information contained in this chapter addresses the procedures related to the development of the NCLEX-RN examination test plan, the components of the test plan, and the answers to the questions most commonly asked by nursing students and graduates preparing to take the NCLEX-RN examination. The information contained in this chapter related to the test plan was obtained from the NCSBN Web site (http://www.ncsbn.org) and from the NCSBN test plan for the NCLEX-RN Examination (effective date, April 2010). You can obtain additional information regarding the test and its development by accessing the NCSBN Web site or by writing to the National Council of State Boards of Nursing, 111 East Wacker Drive, Suite 2900, Chicago, IL 60601. You are encouraged to access the NCSBN Web site because this site provides you with valuable information about the NCLEX and other resources available to an NCLEX candidate.

COMPUTER ADAPTIVE TESTING

The acronym *CAT* stands for computer adaptive test, which means that the examination is created as the test-taker answers each question. All the test questions are categorized based on the test plan structure and the level of difficulty of the question. As you answer a question, the computer determines your competency based on the answer you selected. If you selected a correct answer to a question, the computer scans the question bank and selects a more difficult question. If you selected an incorrect answer, the computer scans the question bank and selects an easier question. This process continues until the test plan requirements are met and a reliable pass-or-fail decision is made.

When a test question is presented on the computer screen, you must answer it or the test will not move on. This means that you will not be able to skip questions, go back and review questions, or go back and change answers. In a CAT examination, once an answer is recorded, all subsequent questions administered depend, to an extent, on the answer selected for that question. Skipping and returning to earlier questions are not compatible with the logical methodology of a CAT. The inability to skip questions or go back to change previous answers will not be a disadvantage to you; you will not fall into that "trap" of changing a correct answer to an incorrect one with the CAT system.

If you are faced with a question that contains unfamiliar content, you may need to guess at the answer. There is no penalty for guessing on this examination. With most of the questions, the answer will be right there in front of you. If you need to guess, use your nursing knowledge and clinical experiences to their fullest extent and all the test-taking strategies that you have practiced in this review program.

You do not need any computer experience to take this examination. A keyboard tutorial is provided and administered to all test-takers at the start of the examination. The tutorial will instruct you on the use of the on-screen optional calculator, the use of the mouse, and how to record an answer. In addition to the traditional four-option, multiple-choice question, the tutorial provides instructions on how to respond to alternate item format questions. This tutorial is provided on the NCSBN Web site, and you are encouraged to view the tutorial when you are preparing for the NCLEX examination. Additionally, at the testing site, a proctor is present to assist in explaining the use of the computer to ensure your full understanding of how to proceed.

DEVELOPMENT OF THE TEST PLAN

The test plan for the NCLEX-RN examination is developed by the NCSBN. The NCLEX examination is a national examination; the NCSBN considers the legal scope of nursing practice as governed by state laws and regulations, including the nurse practice act, and uses these laws to define the areas on the examination that will assess the competence of the test-taker for licensure.

The NCSBN also conducts an important study every 3 years, known as a practice analysis study, to determine the framework for the test plan for the examination. The participants in this study include newly licensed registered nurses from all types of basic nursing education programs. From a list provided, the participants select the nursing activities that they perform, the frequency of performing these specific activities, the impact of the activities on maintaining client safety, and the setting where the activities were performed. A panel of content experts at the NCSBN analyzes the results of the study and makes decisions regarding the test plan framework. The results of this study, most recently conducted in 2008, provided the structure for the test plan implemented in April 2010.

ITEM WRITERS

The NCSBN selects question (item) writers after an extensive application process. The writers are registered nurses who hold a master's degree or a higher degree. Many of the writers are nursing educators; a nurse currently employed in clinical nursing practice and working directly with nurses who have entered practice within the past 12 months also may be selected to participate in this process. Question writers voluntarily submit an application to become a writer and must meet specific criteria established by the council to be accepted as participants in the process.

TEST PLAN

The content of the NCLEX-RN examination reflects the activities identified in the practice analysis study conducted by the NCSBN. The questions are written to address Level of Cognitive Ability, Client Needs, and Integrated Processes as identified in the test plan developed by the NCSBN (Box 1-1).

Level of Cognitive Ability

The practice of nursing requires critical thinking in decision making. Most questions on the NCLEX examination are written at the application level or higher levels of cognitive ability, such as the analysis level. Box 1-2 presents an example of a question that requires you to apply data.

Box 1-1 Examination Questions

Each examination question addresses the following:
- A Level of Cognitive Ability
- A Client Needs category
- An Integrated Process

Client Needs

In the test plan implemented in April 2010, the NCSBN has identified a test plan framework based on Client Needs. The NCSBN identifies four major categories of Client Needs. Some of these categories are divided further into subcategories. The Client Needs categories include Safe and Effective Care Environment, Health Promotion and Maintenance, Psychosocial Integrity, and Physiological Integrity (Table 1-1).

Safe and Effective Care Environment

The Safe and Effective Care Environment category includes two subcategories, Management of Care and Safety and Infection Control. According to the NCSBN, Management of Care (16% to 22% of questions) addresses content that tests the nurse's knowledge, skills, and ability required to ensure a safe care delivery setting to protect clients, families, significant others,

Box 1-2 Level of Cognitive Ability: Applying

A nurse notes blanching, coolness, and edema at the peripheral intravenous (IV) site. Based on these findings, the nurse implements which action?
1. Discontinues the IV
2. Applies a warm compress
3. Checks for a blood return
4. Measures the area of infiltration

Answer: 1
This question requires that you focus on the data identified in the question and determine that the client is experiencing an infiltration. Next you need to consider the harmful effects of infiltration and determine the action to implement. Because infiltration can be damaging to the surrounding tissue, the most appropriate action is to discontinue the IV to prevent any further damage.

TABLE 1-1 Client Needs Categories and Percentage of Questions on the NCLEX-RN® Examination

Client Needs Category	Percentage of Questions
Safe and Effective Care Environment	
Management of Care	16-22
Safety and Infection Control	8-14
Health Promotion and Maintenance	6-12
Psychosocial Integrity	6-12
Physiological Integrity	
Basic Care and Comfort	6-12
Pharmacological and Parenteral Therapies	13-19
Reduction of Risk Potential	10-16
Physiological Adaptation	11-17

visitors, and health care personnel. The NCSBN indicates that Safety and Infection Control (8% to 14% of questions) addresses content that tests the nurse's knowledge, skills, and ability required to protect clients, families, significant others, visitors, and health care personnel from health and environmental hazards. Box 1-3 presents examples of questions that address these two subcategories.

Health Promotion and Maintenance

The Health Promotion and Maintenance category (6% to 12% of questions) addresses the principles related to growth and development. According to the NCSBN, this Client Needs category also addresses content that tests the nurse's knowledge, skills, and ability required to assist the client, family members, and significant others to prevent health problems; to recognize alterations in health; and to develop health practices that promote and support wellness. See Box 1-4 for an example of a question in this Client Needs category.

Psychosocial Integrity

The Psychosocial Integrity category (6% to 12% of questions) addresses content that tests the nurse's knowledge, skills, and ability required to promote and support the ability of the client, client's family, and client's significant other to cope, adapt, and problem solve during

stressful events. The NCSBN also indicates that this Client Needs category addresses the emotional, mental, and social well-being of the client, family, or significant other, and the knowledge, skills, and ability required to care for the client with an acute or chronic mental illness. See Box 1-5 for an example of a question in this Client Needs category.

Box 1-4 Health Promotion and Maintenance

The nurse is choosing age-appropriate toys for a toddler. Which of the following would be the best toy?
1. Puzzle
2. Toy soldiers
3. Large stacking blocks
4. A card game with large pictures

Answer: 3

This question addresses the Client Needs category, Health Promotion and Maintenance, and specifically relates to the principles of growth and development of a toddler. Toddlers like to master activities independently, such as stacking blocks. Because toddlers do not have the developmental ability to determine what could be harmful, toys that are safe need to be provided. A puzzle and toy soldiers provide objects that can be placed in the mouth and may be harmful for a toddler. A card game with large pictures may require cooperative play, which is more appropriate for a school-age child.

Box 1-3 Safe and Effective Care Environment

Management of Care

A nurse has received the client assignment for the day. Which client should the nurse assess first?
1. The client who has a nasogastric tube attached to intermittent suction
2. The client who needs to receive subcutaneous insulin before breakfast
3. The client who is 2 days postoperative and is complaining of incisional pain
4. The client who has a blood glucose level of 50 mg/dL and complaints of blurred vision

Answer: 4

This question addresses the subcategory, Management of Care, in the Client Needs category, Safe and Effective Care Environment. It requires you to establish priorities by comparing the needs of each client and deciding which need is urgent. The client described in option 4 has a blood glucose level and symptoms reflective of hypoglycemia. This client should be assessed first so that treatment can be implemented. Although the clients in options 1, 2, and 3 have needs that require assessment, they are not a priority and can wait until the client in option 4 is stabilized.

Safety and Infection Control

A nurse prepares to care for a client on contact precautions who has a hospital-acquired infection caused by methicillin-resistant *Staphylococcus aureus* (MRSA). The client has an abdominal wound that requires irrigation and has a tracheostomy attached to a mechanical ventilator, which requires frequent suctioning. The nurse assembles which of the following necessary protective items before entering the client's room?
1. Gloves and a gown
2. Gloves, mask, and goggles
3. Gloves, mask, gown, and goggles
4. Gloves, gown, and shoe protectors

Answer: 3

This question addresses the subcategory, Safety and Infection Control, in the Client Needs category, Safe and Effective Care Environment. It addresses content related to protecting oneself from contracting an infection and requires that you consider the methods of possible transmission of infection, based on the client's condition. Because splashes of infective material can occur during the wound irrigation or suctioning of the tracheostomy, option 3 is correct.

Physiological Integrity

The Physiological Integrity category includes four sub-categories, Basic Care and Comfort, Pharmacological and Parenteral Therapies, Reduction of Risk Potential, and Physiological Adaptation. The NCSBN describes these subcategories as follows. Basic Care and Comfort (6% to 12% of questions) addresses content

---

Box 1-5 Psychosocial Integrity

A client with coronary artery disease has selected guided imagery to help cope with psychological stress. Which of the following statements indicates the client's understanding of this stress reduction measure?
1. "This will work for me only if I am alone in a quiet area."
2. "This will help only if I play music at the same time."
3. "I need to do this only when I lie down in case I fall asleep."
4. "The best thing about this is that I can use it anywhere, anytime."

Answer: 4

This question addresses the Client Needs category, Psychosocial Integrity, and the content addresses coping mechanisms. Guided imagery involves the client's creation of an image in the mind, concentrating on the image, and gradually becoming less aware of the offending stimulus. It can be done anytime and anywhere; some clients may use other relaxation techniques or play music with it.

---

that tests the nurse's knowledge, skills, and ability required to provide comfort and assistance to the client in the performance of activities of daily living. Pharmacological and Parenteral Therapies (13% to 19% of questions) addresses content that tests the nurse's knowledge, skills, and ability required to administer medications and parenteral therapies such as intravenous therapies and the administration of blood and blood products. Reduction of Risk Potential (10% to 16% of questions) addresses content that tests the nurse's knowledge, skills, and ability required to prevent complications or health problems related to the client's condition or any prescribed treatments or procedures. Physiological Adaptation (11% to 17% of questions) addresses content that tests the nurse's knowledge, skills, and ability required to provide care to clients with acute, chronic, or life-threatening conditions. See Box 1-6 for examples of questions in this Client Needs category.

Integrated Processes

The NCSBN identifies four processes that are fundamental to the practice of nursing. These processes are a component of the test plan and are incorporated throughout the major categories of Client Needs. The Integrated Process subcategories include Caring, Communication and Documentation, Nursing Process (Assessment, Analysis, Planning, Implementation, and Evaluation), and Teaching and Learning. See Box 1-7

Box 1-6 Physiological Integrity

Basic Care and Comfort

A client with Parkinson's disease develops akinesia while ambulating, increasing the risk for falls. Which suggestion should the nurse provide to the client to alleviate this problem?
1. Use a wheelchair to move around.
2. Stand erect and use a cane to ambulate.
3. Keep the feet close together while ambulating and use a walker.
4. Consciously think about walking over imaginary lines on the floor.

Answer: 4

This question addresses the subcategory, Basic Care and Comfort, in the Client Needs category, Physiological Integrity, and addresses client mobility and promoting assistance in an activity of daily living to maintain safety. Clients with Parkinson's disease can develop bradykinesia (slow movement) or akinesia (freezing or no movement). Having these clients imagine lines on the floor to step over can keep them moving forward while remaining safe.

Pharmacological and Parenteral Therapies

The nurse monitors a client receiving digoxin (Lanoxin) for which early manifestation of digoxin toxicity?
1. Anorexia
2. Facial pain
3. Photophobia
4. Yellow color perception

Answer: 1

This question addresses the subcategory, Pharmacological and Parenteral Therapies, in the Client Needs category, Physiological Integrity. Digoxin is a cardiac glycoside that is used to manage and treat heart failure and to control ventricular rates in clients with atrial fibrillation. The most common early manifestations of toxicity include gastrointestinal disturbances such as anorexia, nausea, and vomiting. Neurological abnormalities can also occur early and include fatigue, headache, depression, weakness, drowsiness, confusion, and nightmares. Facial pain, personality changes, and ocular disturbances (photophobia, light flashes, halos around bright objects, yellow or green color perception) are also signs of toxicity, but are not early signs.

for an example of a question that incorporates the Integrated Process of caring.

TYPES OF QUESTIONS ON THE EXAMINATION

The types of questions that may be administered on the examination include multiple-choice; fill-in-the-blank; multiple-response; prioritizing (ordered response), also known as drag and drop; questions that contain a picture or graphic (hot spot), chart/exhibit, or graphic option item; and audio or video item formats. Some questions may require you to use the mouse and cursor on the computer. For example, you may be presented with a picture that displays the arterial vessels of an adult client. In this picture, you may be asked to "point and click" (using the mouse) on the area (hot spot) where the dorsalis pedis pulse could be felt. In all types of questions, the answer is scored as either right or wrong. Credit is not given for a partially correct answer. Additionally, all question types may include pictures, graphics, tables, charts, sound, or video. The NCSBN provides specific directions for you to follow with all question types to guide you in your process of testing. Be sure to read these directions as they appear on the computer screen. Examples of some of these types of questions are noted in this chapter. All question types are provided in this book and on the accompanying software.

Multiple-Choice Questions

Most of the questions that you will be asked to answer will be in the multiple-choice format. These questions provide you with data about a client situation and four answers or options.

Box 1-7 Integrated Processes

A client is scheduled for angioplasty. The client says to the nurse, "I'm so afraid that it will hurt and will make me worse off than I am." Which response by the nurse is therapeutic?
1. "Can you tell me what you understand about the procedure?"
2. "Your fears are a sign that you really should have this procedure."
3. "Try not to worry. This is a well-known and easy procedure for the doctor."
4. "Those are very normal fears, but please be assured that everything will be okay."

Answer: 1

This question addresses the subcategory, Caring, in the category, Integrated Processes. Option 1 is a therapeutic communication technique that explores the client's feelings, determines the level of client understanding about the procedure, and displays caring. Option 2 demeans the client and does not encourage further sharing by the client. Option 3 diminishes the client's feelings by directing attention away from the client and to the physician's importance. Option 4 does not address the client's fears and puts the client's feelings on hold.

Box 1-6 Physiological Integrity—cont'd

Reduction of Risk Potential
A magnetic resonance imaging (MRI) study is prescribed for a client with a suspected brain tumor. The nurse implements which action to prepare the client for this test?
1. Keeps the client NPO for 6 hours before the test
2. Shaves the groin for insertion of a femoral catheter
3. Removes all metal-containing objects from the client
4. Instructs the client in inhalation techniques for the administration of the radioisotope

Answer: 3

This question addresses the subcategory, Reduction of Risk Potential, in the Client Needs category, Physiological Integrity, and the nurse's responsibilities in preparing the client for the diagnostic test. In an MRI study, radiofrequency pulses in a magnetic field are converted into pictures. All metal objects, such as rings, bracelets, hairpins, and watches, should be removed. In addition, a history should be taken to ascertain whether the client has any internal metallic devices, such as orthopedic hardware, pacemakers, or shrapnel. For an abdominal MRI study, the client is usually NPO. NPO status is not necessary for an MRI study of the head. The groin may be shaved for an angiogram, and inhalation of the radioisotope may be prescribed with a positron emission tomography (PET) scan or ventilation/perfusion lung scan.

Physiological Adaptation
A client with renal insufficiency has a magnesium level of 3.6 mg/dL. Based on this laboratory result, the nurse interprets which of the following signs as significant?
1. Hyperpnea
2. Drowsiness
3. Hypertension
4. Physical hyperactivity

Answer: 2

This question addresses the subcategory, Physiological Adaptation, in the Client Needs category, Physiological Integrity. It addresses an alteration in body systems. The normal magnesium level is 1.6 to 2.6 mg/dL. A magnesium level of 3.6 mg/dL indicates hypermagnesemia. Neurological manifestations begin to occur when magnesium levels are elevated and are noted as symptoms of neurological depression, such as drowsiness, sedation, lethargy, respiratory depression, muscle weakness, and areflexia. Bradycardia and hypotension also occur.

Box 1-8 Fill-in-the-Blank Question

A prescription reads: acetaminophen (Tylenol Extra Strength) liquid, 650 mg orally every 4 hours PRN for pain. The medication label reads: 500 mg/15 mL. The nurse prepares how many milliliters to administer one dose?

Answer: $\boxed{19.5}$ mL

Formula:

$$\frac{\text{Desired}}{\text{Available}} \times \text{Volume} = \text{mL}$$

$$\frac{650\ \text{mg}}{500\ \text{mg}} \times 15\ \text{mL} = 19.5\ \text{mL}$$

In this question, you need to use the formula for calculating a medication dose. When the dose is determined, you will need to type your numeric answer in the answer box. Always follow the specific directions noted on the computer screen when answering the question. Also, remember that there will be an on-screen calculator on the computer for your use if needed.

Box 1-9 Multiple-Response Question

An emergency department nurse is caring for a child suspected of acute epiglottitis. Which interventions apply in the care of the child? **Select all that apply.**

- ☐ **1.** Obtain a throat culture.
- ☑ **2.** Ensure a patent airway.
- ☑ **3.** Prepare the child for a chest x-ray.
- ☐ **4.** Maintain the child in a supine position.
- ☑ **5.** Obtain a pediatric-size tracheostomy tray.
- ☑ **6.** Place the child on an oxygen saturation monitor.

In a multiple-response question, you will be asked to select or check all the options, such as interventions, that relate to the information in the question. To answer this question, recall that acute epiglottitis is a serious obstructive inflammatory process that requires immediate intervention. To reduce respiratory distress, the child should sit upright. Examination of the throat with a tongue depressor or attempting to obtain a throat culture is contraindicated because the examination can precipitate further obstruction. The child is placed on an oxygen saturation monitor to monitor oxygenation status. A lateral neck and chest x-ray is obtained to determine the degree of obstruction, if present. Tracheostomy and intubation may be necessary if respiratory distress is severe. Remember to follow the specific directions given on the computer screen.

Fill-in-the-Blank Questions

Fill-in-the-blank questions may ask you to perform a medication calculation, determine an intravenous flow rate, or calculate an intake or output record on a client. You will need to type only a number (your answer) in the answer box. If the question requires rounding the answer, this needs to be performed at the end of the calculation. The rules for rounding an answer are provided in the tutorial provided by the NCSBN, and are also provided in the specific question. Additionally, you must type in a decimal point if necessary; however, it is not necessary to type a "0" before the decimal point. See Box 1-8 for an example.

Multiple-Response Questions

For a multiple-response question, you will be asked to select or check all the options, such as nursing interventions, that relate to the information in the question. No partial credit is given for correct selections. You need to do exactly as the question asks, which will be to select all the options that apply. See Box 1-9 for an example.

Prioritizing (Ordered Response) or Drag and Drop Questions

In this type of question, you will be asked to use the computer mouse to drag and drop your nursing actions in order of priority. Information will be presented in a question, and, based on the data, you

need to determine what you will do first, second, third, and so forth. The unordered options will be located in boxes on the left side of the screen, and you need to move all options in order of priority to ordered response boxes on the right side of the screen. Specific directions for moving the options are provided with the question. See Box 1-10 for an example.

Picture or Graphic (Hot Spot) Questions

A question with a picture or graphic will ask you to answer the question based on the picture or graphic. The question could contain a chart, a table, or a figure or illustration. You also may be asked to use the computer mouse to point and click on a specific area in the visual. A figure or illustration may appear in any type of question, including a multiple-choice question. See Box 1-11 for an example.

Chart/Exhibit Questions

In this type of question, you will be presented with a problem and a chart or exhibit. You will be provided with tabs or buttons that you need to click to obtain the information needed to answer the question. A prompt or message will appear that will indicate the need to click on a tab or button. See Box 1-12 for an example.

Box 1-10 Prioritizing (Ordered Response), or Drag and Drop Question

A nurse is preparing to suction a client who has a tracheostomy tube and gathers the supplies needed for the procedure. Arrange in order of priority the actions that the nurse takes to perform this procedure. All options must be used.

Unordered Options	Ordered Response
Hyperoxygenate the client.	Place the client in a semi-Fowler's position.
Place the client in a semi-Fowler's position.	Turn on the suction device and set the regulator at 80 mm Hg.
Turn on the suction device and set the regulator at 80 mm Hg.	Apply gloves and attach the suction tubing to the suction catheter.
Apply gloves and attach the suction tubing to the suction catheter.	Hyperoxygenate the client.
Apply intermittent suction and slowly withdraw the catheter while rotating it back and forth.	Insert the catheter into the tracheostomy until resistance is met and then pull back 1 cm.
Insert the catheter into the tracheostomy until resistance is met and then pull back 1 cm.	Apply intermittent suction and slowly withdraw the catheter while rotating it back and forth.

　　This question requires you to arrange in order of priority the nursing actions that should be taken to suction a client who has a tracheostomy tube. The nurse positions the client first, and then turns the suction device on and sets the regulator. The nurse then dons gloves and attaches the suction tubing to the suction catheter. The nurse hyperoxygenates the client before and after suctioning. The nurse then inserts the catheter into the tracheostomy until resistance is met and pulls back 1 cm, applies intermittent suction, and slowly withdraws the catheter while rotating it back and forth. Remember that the client and equipment are prepared before performing the procedure. Also, remember that on the NCLEX examination, you will use the computer mouse to place the unordered options in an ordered response.

Box 1-11 Picture or Graphic (Hot Spot) Question

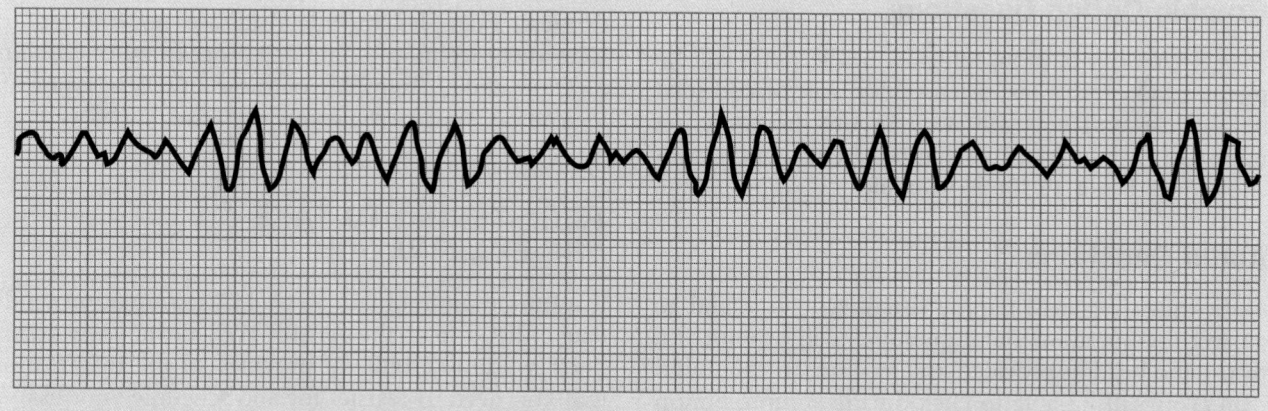

Rhythm strip. (From Ignatavicius, D., & Workman, M. [2010]. *Medical-surgical nursing: Patient-centered collaborative care* [6th ed.]. St. Louis: Saunders.)

A client who experienced a myocardial infarction is being monitored via cardiac telemetry. The nurse notes the sudden onset of this cardiac rhythm on the monitor and immediately takes which action?
1. Takes the client's blood pressure
2. Initiates cardiopulmonary resuscitation (CPR)
3. Places a nitroglycerin tablet under the client's tongue
4. Continues to monitor the client and then contacts the physician

Answer: 2
This question requires you to identify the cardiac rhythm, and then determine the priority nursing action. This cardiac rhythm identifies a coarse ventricular fibrillation (VF). The goals of treatment are to terminate VF promptly and to convert it to an organized rhythm. The physician or an advanced cardiac life support (ACLS)–qualified nurse or other health care provider must immediately defibrillate the client. If a defibrillator is not readily available, CPR is initiated until the defibrillator arrives. Options 1, 3, and 4 are incorrect actions and delay life-saving treatment.

Box 1-12 Chart/Exhibit Question

CLIENT'S CHART		
History and Physical	**Medications**	**Diagnostic Results**
Item 1: Has renal calculi *Item 2:* Had thrombophlebitis 1 year ago	*Item 3:* Multivitamin orally daily	*Item 4:* Electrocardiogram: normal

The nurse reviews the history and physical examination documented in the medical record of a client requesting a prescription for oral contraceptives. The nurse determines that oral contraceptives are contraindicated because of which documented item?

Answer: 2

This chart/exhibit question provides you with data from the client's medical record and asks you to identify the item that is a contraindication to the use of oral contraceptives. Oral contraceptives are contraindicated in women with a history of any of the following: thrombophlebitis and thromboembolic disorders, cardiovascular or cerebrovascular diseases (including stroke), any estrogen-dependent cancer or breast cancer, benign or malignant liver tumors, impaired liver function, hypertension, and diabetes mellitus with vascular involvement. Adverse effects of oral contraceptives include increased risk of superficial and deep venous thrombosis, pulmonary embolism, thrombotic stroke (or other types of strokes), myocardial infarction, and accelerations of preexisting breast tumors.

Box 1-13 Graphic Options Question

The nurse places the client in which position to administer a soapsuds enema?

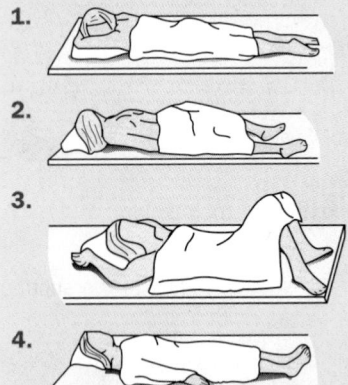

1.
2.
3.
4.

Answer: 2

This question requires you to select the picture that represents your answer choice. To administer an enema, the nurse assists the client into the left side-lying (Sims) position with the right knee flexed. This position allows the enema solution to flow downward by gravity along the natural curve of the sigmoid colon and rectum, improving the retention of solution. Option 1 is a prone position. Option 3 is a dorsal recumbent position. Option 4 is a supine position.

Reference: Potter, P., & Perry, A. (2009). *Fundamentals of nursing* (7th ed.). St. Louis: Mosby.

Graphic Option Questions

In this type of question, the option selections will be pictures rather than text. Each option will be preceded by a circle, and you will need to use the computer mouse to click in the circle that represents your answer choice. See Box 1-13 for an example.

Audio Questions

Audio questions will require listening to a sound to answer the question. These questions will prompt you to use the headset provided and to click on the sound icon. You will be able to click on the volume button to adjust the volume to your comfort level, and you will be able to listen to the sound as many times as necessary. Content examples include, but are not limited to, various lung sounds, heart sounds, or bowel sounds. Examples of these question types are located on the accompanying software.

Video Questions

Video questions will require viewing an animation or video clip to answer the question. These questions will prompt you to click on the video icon. There may be sound associated with the animation and video, in which you will be prompted to use the headset.

Content examples include, but are not limited to, assessment techniques, nursing procedures, or communication skills. Examples of these question types are located on the accompanying software.

REGISTERING TO TAKE THE EXAMINATION

It is important to obtain an NCLEX examination candidate bulletin from the NCSBN Web site at www.ncsbn.org because this bulletin provides all the information that you need to register for and schedule your examination. It also provides you with Web site and telephone information for NCLEX examination contacts. The initial step in the registration process is to submit an application to the state board of nursing in the state in which you intend to obtain licensure. You need to obtain information from the board of nursing regarding the specific registration process because the process may vary from state to state. When you receive confirmation from the board of nursing that you have met all of the state requirements, you can register to take the NCLEX examination with Pearson Vue. You may register for the examination through the Internet, by U.S. mail, or by telephone. The NCLEX candidate Web site is http://www.pearsonvue.com/nclex.

Following the registration instructions and completing the registration forms precisely and accurately are important. Registration forms not properly completed or not accompanied by the proper fees in the required method of payment will be returned to you and will delay testing. You must pay a fee for taking the examination; you also may have to pay additional fees to the board of nursing in the state in which you are applying. You will then be made eligible by the licensure board and will receive an Authorization to Test (ATT) form. If you do not receive an ATT form within two weeks of registration, you should contact the candidate services at 1-866-496-2539 (U.S. candidates).

AUTHORIZATION TO TEST FORM AND SCHEDULING AN APPOINTMENT

You cannot make an appointment until the board of nursing declares eligibility and you receive an ATT form. Note the validity dates on the ATT form, and schedule a date and time when you receive the ATT. The examination will take place at a Pearson Professional Center; U.S. candidates can make an appointment through the Internet (http://www.pearsonvue.com/nclex) or by telephone (1-866-496-2539). You can schedule an appointment at any Pearson Professional Center. You do not have to take the examination in the same state in which you are seeking licensure. A confirmation of your appointment with the appointment date and time and the directions to the testing center will be sent to you.

The ATT form contains important information, including your test authorization number, candidate identification number, and validity date. You need to take your ATT form to the test center on the day of your examination. You will not be admitted to the examination if you do not have it.

CANCELING OR RESCHEDULING THE APPOINTMENT

If for any reason you need to cancel or reschedule your appointment to test, you can make the change on the candidate Web site (http://www.pearsonvue.com/nclex) or by calling candidate services. The change needs to be made one full business day (24 hours) before your scheduled appointment. If you fail to arrive for the examination or fail to cancel your appointment to test without providing appropriate notice, you will forfeit your examination fee and your ATT form will be invalidated. This information will be reported to the board of nursing in the state in which you have applied for licensure, and you will be required to register and pay the testing fees again.

DAY OF THE EXAMINATION

It is important that you arrive at the testing center at least 30 minutes before the test is scheduled. If you arrive late for the scheduled testing appointment, you may be required to forfeit your examination appointment. If it is necessary to forfeit your appointment, you will need to reregister for the examination and pay an additional fee. The board of nursing will be notified that you did not take the test. A few days before your scheduled date of testing, take the time to drive to the testing center to determine its exact location, the length of time required to arrive to that destination, and any potential obstacles that might delay you, such as road construction, traffic, or parking sites.

You must have the ATT and proper identification (ID) to be admitted to take the examination. Acceptable identification includes U.S. driver's license, passport, U.S. state ID, or U.S. military ID. All acceptable identification must be valid and not expired and contain a photograph and signature (in English). Additionally, the first and last names on the ID must match the ATT form. According to the NCSBN guidelines, any name discrepancies require legal documentation, such as a marriage license, divorce decree, or court action legal name change.

SPECIAL TESTING CIRCUMSTANCES

If you require special testing accommodations, you should contact the board of nursing before submitting a registration form. The board of nursing will provide the procedures for the request. The board of nursing must authorize special testing accommodations. Following board of nursing approval, the NCSBN reviews the requested accommodations and must approve the request. If the request is approved, the candidate will be notified and provided the procedure for registering for and scheduling the examination.

TESTING CENTER

The test center is designed to ensure complete security of the testing process. Strict candidate identification requirements have been established. You must bring the ATT form and required forms of identification. You will be asked to read the rules related to testing. A digital fingerprint and palm vein print will be taken, and this procedure is usually done twice. A digital signature and photograph will also be taken at the test center. These identity confirmations will accompany the NCLEX exam results. Additionally, if you leave the testing room for any reason, you may be required to perform these identity confirmation procedures again to be readmitted to the room.

Personal belongings are not allowed in the testing room. Secure storage, such as a locker and locker key, will be provided for you; however, storage space is limited, so you must plan accordingly. In addition, the testing center will not assume responsibility for your personal belongings. The testing waiting areas are generally small; friends or family members who accompany you are not permitted to wait in the testing center while you are taking the examination.

Once you have completed the admission process, the proctor will escort you to the assigned computer. You will be seated at an individual work space area that includes computer equipment, appropriate lighting, and erasable note board or white board and a marker. No items, including unauthorized scratch paper, are allowed into the testing room. Electronic devices, such as watches, beepers, or cell phones, are not allowed in the testing room. Eating, drinking, or the use of tobacco is not allowed in the testing room. You will be observed at all times by the test proctor while taking the examination. Additionally, video and audio recordings of all test sessions are made. Pearson Professional Centers has no control over the sounds made by typing on the computer by others. If these sounds are distracting, raise your hand to summon the proctor. Earplugs are available on request.

You must follow the directions given by the test center staff and must remain seated during the test except when authorized to leave. If you think that you have a problem with the computer, need an additional erasable or white board, need to take a break, or need the test proctor for any reason, you must raise your hand. You are also encouraged to access the candidate Web site (http://www.pearsonvue.com/nclex) to obtain additional information about the physical environment of the test center.

TESTING TIME

The maximum testing time is 6 hours; this period includes the tutorial, the sample items, all breaks, and the examination. All breaks are optional. The first optional break will be offered after 2 hours of testing. The second optional break is offered after 3½ hours of testing. Remember that all breaks count against testing time. If you take a break, you must leave the testing room and, when you return, you may be required to perform identity confirmation procedures to be readmitted.

LENGTH OF THE EXAMINATION

The minimum number of questions that you will need to answer is 75. Of these 75 questions, 60 will be operational (scored) questions and 15 will be pretest (unscored) questions. The maximum number of questions in the test is 265. Fifteen of the total number of questions that you need to answer will be pretest (unscored) questions.

The pretest questions are questions that may be presented as scored questions on future examinations.

These pretest questions are not identified as such. In other words, you do not know which questions are the pretest (unscored) questions.

PASS-OR-FAIL DECISIONS

All the examination questions are categorized by test plan area and level of difficulty. This is an important point to keep in mind when you consider how the computer makes a pass-or-fail decision because a pass-or-fail decision is not based on a percentage of correctly answered questions.

After the minimum number of questions have been answered (75 questions; 60 operational and 15 pretest questions), the computer compares the test-taker's ability level with the standard required for passing. The standard required for passing is based on the expert judgment of several individuals appointed by the NCSBN. If the test-taker is clearly above the passing standard, the examination ends, and the test-taker passes the examination. If the test-taker is clearly below the passing standard, the examination ends, and the test-taker fails the examination. If the computer is unable to determine clearly whether the test-taker has passed or failed because the test-taker's ability is close to the passing standard, the computer continues asking questions until the outcome is determined.

If the examination ends because you have run out of time, the computer may not have enough information to make a clear pass-or-fail decision. If this is the case, the computer will review the test-taker's performance during testing. If the test-taker's ability was consistently above the passing standard on the last 60 questions, the test-taker passes. If the test-taker's ability falls to or below the passing standard, even once, the test-taker fails.

COMPLETING THE EXAMINATION

When the examination has ended, you will complete a brief computer-delivered questionnaire about your testing experience. After you complete this questionnaire, you need to raise your hand to summon the test proctor. The test proctor will collect and inventory all erasable or white boards and then permit you to leave.

PROCESSING RESULTS

Every computerized examination is scored twice, once by the computer at the testing center and again after the examination is transmitted to Pearson Professional Centers. No results are released at the test center. The board of nursing receives your result within 12 to 24 hours, and your result will be mailed to you 2 days to 2 weeks after you take the examination. In some states, an unofficial result can be obtained via the Quick Results Service 2 business days after taking the examination. This can be done through the Internet or telephone, and there is a fee for this service. Information about obtaining your NCLEX result by this method can be obtained on the NCSBN Web site under candidate services.

CANDIDATE PERFORMANCE REPORT

'A candidate performance report is provided to a test-taker who failed the examination. This report provides the test-taker with information about her or his strengths and weaknesses in relation to the test plan framework and provides a guide for studying and retaking the examination. If a retake is necessary, most states require 45 days between examination administration. Test-takers should refer to the state board of nursing in the state in which licensure is sought for procedures regarding when the examination can be taken again.

INTERSTATE ENDORSEMENT

Because the NCLEX-RN examination is a national examination, you can apply to take the examination in any state. When licensure is received, you can apply for interstate endorsement, which is obtaining another license in another state to practice nursing in that state. The procedures and requirements for interstate endorsement may vary from state to state, and these procedures can be obtained from the state board of nursing in the state in which endorsement is sought. You may also be allowed to practice nursing in another state if the state has enacted a Nurse Licensure Compact. The state boards of nursing can be accessed via the NCSBN Web site at http://www.ncsbn.org. States that participate in the Nurse Licensure Compact can also be located on this Web site.

NURSE LICENSURE COMPACT

It may be possible to hold one license from the state of residency and practice nursing in another state under the mutual recognition model of nursing licensure if the state has enacted a Nurse Licensure Compact. To obtain information about the Nurse Licensure Compact and the states that are part of this interstate compact, access the NCSBN Web site at http://www.ncsbn.org.

ADDITIONAL INFORMATION ABOUT THE EXAMINATION

Additional information regarding the NCLEX-RN examination can be obtained through the NCLEX examination candidate bulletin located on the NCSBN Web site and from the NCSBN, 111 East Wacker Drive, Suite 2900, Chicago, IL 60601. The telephone number for the NCLEX examinations department is 866-293-9600. The Web site is http://www.ncsbn.org.

2

Preparation for the NCLEX-RN® Examination: Transitional Issues for Foreign-Educated Nurses

You have taken an important first step—seeking the information that you need to know to become a registered nurse (RN) in the United States. The challenge that is presented to you is one that requires great patience and endurance. The positive result of your endeavor will reward you professionally, however, and give you the personal satisfaction of knowing that you have become part of a family of highly skilled professionals, registered nurses.

NATIONAL COUNCIL OF STATE BOARDS OF NURSING

The National Council of State Boards of Nursing (NCSBN) is the agency that develops and administers the NCLEX-RN examination, the examination that you need to pass to become licensed as a registered nurse in the United States. Guidelines and procedures must be followed and documents must be sought and submitted to become eligible to take this examination. This chapter provides general information regarding the process you need to pursue to become a registered nurse in the United States. An important first step in the process of obtaining information about becoming a registered nurse in the United States is to access the NCSBN Web site at http://www.ncsbn.org and obtain information provided for international nurses in the NCLEX Web site link. The NCSBN provides information about some of the documents you need to obtain as an international nurse seeking licensure as a registered nurse in the United States and about credentialing agencies. The NCSBN also provides a resource manual for international nurses that contains all of the necessary licensure information regarding the requirements for education, English proficiency, and immigration requirements such as visas and VisaScreens. You are encouraged to access the NCSBN Web site to obtain the most current information about seeking licensure as a registered nurse in the United States.

⚠ A first step is to access the NCSBN Web site at http://www.ncsbn.org and obtain information provided for international nurses in the NCLEX Web site link.

STATE REQUIREMENTS FOR LICENSURE

An important factor to consider as you pursue this process is that some requirements may vary from state to state. You need to contact the board of nursing in the state in which you are planning to obtain licensure to determine the specific requirements and documents that you need to submit. Boards of nursing can decide either to use a credentialing agency to evaluate your documents or to review your documents at the specific state board, known as in-house evaluation. When you contact the board of nursing in the state in which you intend to work as a nurse, inform them that you were educated outside of the United States and ask that they send you an application to apply for licensure by examination. Be sure to specify that you are applying for registered nurse (RN) licensure. You should also ask about the specific documents needed to become eligible to take the NCLEX exam. You can obtain contact information for each state board of nursing through the NCSBN Web site at http://www.ncsbn.org. When you have accessed the NCSBN Web site, select the link titled "Boards of Nursing." Additionally, you can write to the NCSBN regarding the NCLEX exam. The address is 111 East Wacker Drive, Suite 2900, Chicago, IL 60601. The telephone number for the NCSBN is (866) 293-9600; the fax number is (312) 279-1036.

⚠ Contact the board of nursing in the state in which you are planning to obtain licensure to determine the specific requirements and documents that you need to submit. Documents that you need to submit vary state by state.

CREDENTIALING AGENCIES

The state board of nursing in the state in which you are seeking licensure may choose to use a credentialing agency to review your documents. It is necessary that you seek this information from the state board and use the credentialing agency that the state requires. The state board of nursing will provide you with the name and contact information of the credentialing agency. Seeking this information is important because you need to know where to send your required documents. Additionally, the NCSBN Web site (http://www.ncsbn.org) can provide information about credentialing agencies.

GENERAL LICENSURE REQUIREMENTS

Required documents may vary depending on the state requirements. These documents must be sent to either the state board of nursing or the credentialing agency specified by the state. Neither the credentialing agency nor the state board of nursing will accept these documents if they are sent directly from you. These documents must be official documents sent directly from the licensing authority or other agency in your home country to verify validity. Some of the general documents required are listed in Box 2-1; however, remember that the documents you need to submit vary state by state. Use the list provided in Box 2-1 as a checklist for yourself after you have found out about the documents you are required to submit.

When all of your documents have been submitted, they will be reviewed. If you have met the eligibility requirements to take the NCLEX examination, you will be notified that you are eligible. Then you need to obtain an application to take the NCLEX exam from the state in which you intend to seek licensure and submit the required fees. Your application will be reviewed and processed, and you will be notified that you can make an appointment to take the NCLEX exam. Additional information about the application process for the NCLEX exam can be obtained at the NCSBN Web site at www.ncsbn.org. Box 2-2 provides a brief guide of the general steps to take in the licensure process.

⚠ Official documents must be sent directly from the licensing authority or other agency in your home country.

WORK VISA

A foreign-educated nurse who wants to work in the United States needs to obtain the proper work visa or visas. Obtaining the work visa is a U.S. federal government requirement. To obtain information about the work visa and the application process, contact the Department of Homeland Security (DHS), Office of

Box 2-1 Some Documents Needed to Obtain Licensure

1. Proof of citizenship or lawful alien status
2. Work visa
3. VisaScreen certificate
4. Commission on Graduates of Foreign Nursing Schools (CGFNS) certificate
5. Criminal background check documents
6. Official transcripts of educational credentials sent directly to credentialing agency or board of nursing from home country school of nursing
7. Validation of a comparable nursing education as that provided in U.S. nursing programs; this may include theoretical instruction and clinical practice in a variety of nursing areas, including, but not limited to, medical nursing, surgical nursing, pediatric nursing, maternity and newborn nursing, community and public health nursing, and mental health nursing
8. Validation of safe professional nursing practice in home country
9. Copy of nursing license or diploma or both
10. Proof of proficiency in the English language
11. Photograph(s)
12. Social security number
13. Application and fees

Box 2-2 General Steps in the Licensure Process

1. Access the NCSBN Web site at http://www.ncsbn.org and read the literature provided for international nurses.
2. Contact the board of nursing in the state in which you are planning to obtain licensure to determine the specific requirements and documents that you need to submit.
3. Have the required documents sent from the appropriate agency in your home country.
4. When you are notified about eligibility to take the NCLEX exam, obtain the application form from the state in which you intend to obtain licensure, complete the form, and submit it with required fees.
5. Schedule an appointment to take the NCLEX exam when you receive your Authorization to Test (ATT) form.
6. Take the NCLEX exam.
7. Become a registered nurse in the United States.

U.S. Citizenship and Immigration Services (USCIS). The Web site is http://uscis.gov/graphics/howdoi/Health_Cert.htm.

VISASCREEN

U.S. immigration law requires certain health care professionals to complete a screening program successfully before receiving an occupational (work) visa

(Section §343 of the Illegal Immigration Reform and Immigration Responsibility Act of 1996). To become a registered nurse in the United States, you are required to obtain a VisaScreen certificate. You can ask about the VisaScreen certificate when you make your initial contact with the state board of nursing in which you are seeking licensure. The VisaScreen is a federal screening program, and the certificate needs to be obtained through an organization that offers this program.

⚠ Obtaining the work visa and the VisaScreen is a U.S. federal government requirement.

The Commission on Graduates of Foreign Nursing Schools (CGFNS) is an organization that offers this federal screening program. The VisaScreen components of this program include an educational analysis, license verification, assessment of proficiency in the English language, and an examination that tests nursing knowledge. When the applicant successfully achieves each component, the applicant is presented with a VisaScreen certificate. You can obtain information related to the VisaScreen through the CGFNS Web site at http://www.cgfns.org. The CGFNS Web site also provides you with specific information about the components of this program.

The Commission on Graduates of Foreign Nursing Schools (CGFNS) is also a credentialing agency and awards a CGFNS certificate to the applicant when all eligibility requirements are met. Some state boards of nursing use the CGFNS as a credentialing agency and require a CGFNS certificate, whereas others do not. Check with the state board of nursing regarding this certificate. The CGFNS certification program contains three parts, and you must complete all parts successfully to be awarded a CGFNS certificate. The three parts include a credentials review, a qualifying examination that tests nursing knowledge, and an English language proficiency examination. These components are similar to those needed to obtain the VisaScreen certificate. You can obtain information related to the CGFNS certificate through the CGFNS Web site at http://www.cgfns.org.

⚠ The NCLEX examination is administered in English only.

REGISTERING TO TAKE THE NCLEX® EXAM

When you have completed all state and federal requirements and received documentation that you are eligible to take the NCLEX examination, you can register for the exam. You need to obtain information from the state board of nursing in the state in which you are seeking licensure regarding the specific registration process because the process may vary from state to state. The NCLEX candidate Web site is http://www.pearsonvue.com/nclex, and you are encouraged to access this site for additional information. Following the registration instructions and completing the registration forms precisely and accurately are important. You must pay a fee for taking the examination, and you may have to pay additional fees to the board of nursing in the state in which you are applying. When your eligibility is determined by the state licensure board, you will receive an Authorization to Test (ATT) form. You cannot make an appointment to test until the board of nursing declares eligibility and you receive an ATT form.

⚠ Registration forms for taking the NCLEX exam that are not properly completed or not accompanied by the proper fees in the required method of payment will be returned to you and will delay testing.

The examination takes place at a Pearson Professional Center, and you can make an appointment through the Internet or by telephone. You can schedule an appointment at any Pearson Professional Center. You do not have to take the exam in the state in which you are seeking licensure. NCLEX exam testing abroad is also available in some countries, and it is recommended that you visit the NCLEX Web site for current information about international testing sites. Chapter 1 contains additional information regarding the NCLEX exam and testing procedures. You can also obtain information about the registration process and testing procedures from the NCSBN Web site at http://www.ncsbn.org.

PREPARING TO TAKE THE NCLEX® EXAM

When you have successfully completed the requirements to become eligible to take the NCLEX exam, you have one more important goal to achieve: to pass the NCLEX exam.

⚠ Begin preparing for the NCLEX exam as soon as possible; start preparing even before you begin the licensure process.

I highly recommend adequate preparation for the NCLEX exam because the examination is difficult. An important step that you have taken in preparing is that you are using this book, *Saunders Comprehensive Review for the NCLEX-RN® Examination*. After you have reviewed the content and answered the practice questions, the next step in your journey to success is to use the companion book, *Saunders Q&A Review for the NCLEX-RN® Examination*; this book provides you with more than 5200 practice questions based on the NCLEX-RN examination test plan framework, with a specific focus on Client Needs and Integrated Processes. Then you will be ready for *Saunders Online Review for the NCLEX-RN® Examination*. Additional products in Saunders Pyramid to Success include *Saunders Strategies for Test Success: Passing Nursing School and the NCLEX® Exam* and *Saunders Q&A Review Cards for the NCLEX-RN® Exam*. These additional products are described next.

Saunders Online Review for the NCLEX-RN® Examination addresses all areas of the test plan identified by the NCSBN. The course contains a pretest that provides feedback regarding your strengths and weaknesses and that generates an individualized study schedule in a calendar format. Content review is in an outline format and includes self-check practice questions and case studies, figures and illustrations, a glossary, and animations and videos. Numerous practice exams are included. There are more than 2000 practice questions, and the types of questions in this course include multiple-choice and alternate item formats.

Saunders Strategies for Test Success: Passing Nursing School and the NCLEX® Exam focuses on the test-taking strategies that will prepare you for the NCLEX-RN exam. The chapters describe all the test-taking strategies and include several sample questions that illustrate how to use the test-taking strategy. This book has 500 practice questions. All the practice questions reflect the framework and the content identified in the current NCLEX-RN test plan and include multiple-choice and alternate item format questions. Several appendices

are included that provide a review of test-taking strategies, cultural characteristics and practices, pharmacology strategies, medication and intravenous calculations, laboratory values, positioning guidelines, and therapeutic diets.

Saunders Q&A Review Cards for the NCLEX-RN® Exam is organized specifically by the test plan framework of the current NCLEX-RN test plan. This product provides 1000 practice test questions on portable and easy to use cards. The question is on the front of the card, and the answer, rationale, test-taking strategy, and Integrated Process code are on the back of the card. This product includes multiple-choice questions and alternate item format questions including fill-in-the-blank, multiple-response, prioritizing (ordered response), image (hot spot questions), and chart/exhibit questions.

All the products in Saunders Pyramid to Success can be obtained online by visiting http://elsevierhealth. com or by calling 800-545-2522.

⚠ Stay positive and confident, and believe that you can achieve your goal.

Finally, never lose sight of your goal. Patience and dedication contribute significantly to your achieving the status of registered nurse. Remember, success is climbing a mountain, facing the challenge of obstacles, and reaching the top of the mountain. I wish you the best success in your journey and beginning your career as a registered nurse in the United States.

3

Pathways to Success

Laurent W. Valliere, BS

THE PYRAMID TO SUCCESS

Preparing to take the NCLEX-RN examination can produce a great deal of anxiety. You may be thinking that the NCLEX-RN exam is the most important examination you will ever have to take and that it reflects the culmination of everything that you have worked so hard for. The NCLEX-RN exam is an important examination because receiving your nursing license means that you can begin your career as a registered nurse. Your success on the NCLEX-RN exam involves getting rid of all your thoughts that allow this examination to appear overwhelming and intimidating. Such thoughts can take complete control over your destiny. A strong positive attitude, a structured plan for preparation, and maintaining control in your pathway to success ensure achievement in reaching the peak of the Pyramid to Success (Fig. 3-1).

PATHWAYS TO SUCCESS (Box 3-1)

Foundation

The foundation of pathways to success begins with a strong positive attitude, the belief that you will achieve success, and developing control. It also includes developing a list of your personal short-term and long-term goals and a plan for preparation. A strong positive attitude, belief in yourself, control, and a list of personal goals will help lead you to becoming a registered nurse. Without these components, your pathway to success leads to nowhere and has no endpoint. You will expend energy and valuable time in your journey, lack control over where you are heading, and experience exhaustion without any accomplishment. It is imperative that you take the time to develop a positive attitude and establish your short-term and long-term goals.

Where do you start? To begin this process, find a location that offers solitude. Sit or lie in a comfortable position, close your eyes, relax, inhale deeply, hold your breath to a count of four, exhale slowly, and, again, relax. Repeat this breathing exercise several times until you begin to feel relaxed, free from anxiety, and in control of your destiny. Allow your mind to become void of all the mind chatter; now you are in control

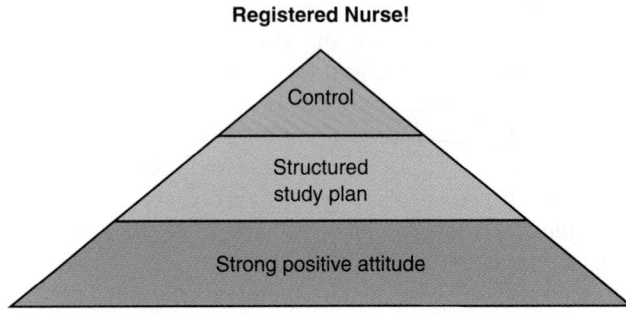

Registered Nurse!

- Control
- Structured study plan
- Strong positive attitude

▲ **FIGURE 3-1** Pyramid to Success.

and your mind's eye can see for miles. Your highway of life has a multitude of destinations to which you may travel. Next, reflect on all that you have accomplished and the path that brought you to where you are today. Keep a journal of your reflections as you plan the order of your journey through the Pyramid to Success.

List

It is time to create the "List." The List is your set of short-term and long-term goals. At this time, you may or may not have a scheduled date for taking the NCLEX-RN examination. Begin by developing the goals that you wish to accomplish today, tomorrow, over the next month, and in the future. Allow yourself the opportunity to list all that is flowing from your mind. Write your goals in your personal journal. When the List is complete, put it away for 2 or 3 days. After that time, retrieve and review the List and begin the process of planning to prepare for the NCLEX-RN exam.

Plan for Preparation

Now that you have the List in order, look at the goals that relate to studying for the licensing exam. The first task is to decide what study pattern works best for you. Think about what has worked most successfully for you in the past. Questions that must be

Box 3-1 Pathways to Success

Foundation
Maintaining a strong positive attitude
Thinking about short-term and long-term realistic goals
Developing a plan for preparation
Maintaining control

List
Writing short-term and long-term realistic goals in a journal

Plan for Preparation
Developing a study plan and schedule
Deciding on the place to study
Balancing personal and work obligations with the study schedule
Sharing the study schedule and personal needs with others
Implementing the study plan

Positive Pampering
Planning time for exercise and fun activities
Establishing healthy eating habits
Including activities in the schedule that provide positive mental stimulation

Final Preparation
Reviewing goals
Identifying goals achieved
Remaining focused to complete the plan of study
Writing down the date and time of the examination and posting it next to your name with the letters "RN" following, and the word "yes!"
Planning a test drive to the testing center
Relaxing activities on the day before the examination

Day of the Examination
Grooming yourself for success
Eating a nutritious breakfast
Maintaining a confident and positive attitude
Maintaining control—breath and focus
Meeting the challenges of the day
Reaching the peak of the Pyramid to Success

Box 3-2 Developing a Plan for Study

Do I work better alone or in a group study environment?
If I work best in a group, does the group consist of one, two, or more study partners?
Who are these study partners?
How long should my study sessions last?
Does the time of day that I study make a difference for me?
Do I retain more if I study in the morning?
How does my work schedule affect my study pattern?
How do I balance my family obligations with my need to study?
Do I have a comfortable study area at home or do I need to find another environment that is conducive to my study needs?

The length of the study session depends on you and your ability to focus and concentrate. You need to think about quality rather than quantity when you are deciding on a realistic amount of time for each session. Plan to schedule at least 2 hours of quality time daily. If you can spend more than 2 hours, by all means do so.

You may be asking yourself, "What do you mean by quality time?" Quality time means spending uninterrupted quiet time at your study session. This may mean that you will have to isolate yourself for these study sessions. Think again about what has worked for you during nursing school when you studied for examinations; select a study place now that has worked for you in the past. If you have a special study room at home that you have always used, plan your study sessions in that special room. If you have always studied at a library, plan your study sessions at the library. If you plan to study at home, make the time spent studying uninterrupted and quiet. Sometimes it is difficult to balance your study time with your family obligations and possibly a work schedule, but, if you can, plan your study time when you know that you will be at home alone. Try to eliminate anything that may be distracting during your study time. Unplug your telephone or shut off your cell phone so that you will not be disturbed. If you have small children, plan your study time during their nap time or during their school hours.

Your plan must include how you will manage your study needs and the demands of your work, family, and friends. Take time to think about how you will balance your everyday commitments with your plan for study. Your family and friends are key players in your life and are going to become part of your Pyramid to Success. After you have established your study needs, communicate your needs and the importance of your study plan in achieving your goal of becoming a registered nurse to your family and friends.

A difficult part of the plan may be how to deal with family members and friends who choose not to participate in your plan for success. What if an individual

addressed to develop your plan for study are listed in Box 3-2.

The plan must include a schedule. Use a calendar to plan and document the times and nursing content areas for your study sessions. Establish a realistic schedule that includes your daily, weekly, and future goals, and adhere to it. This consistency will provide advantages to you and the people supporting you. A daily schedule allows you to plan your content areas for study more carefully. Stick to your plan of study. Adherence to the plan helps you develop a rhythm that can enhance your retention and positive momentum. The people who are supporting you will share this rhythm and will be able to schedule their activities and lives better when you are consistent with your study schedule. You are moving forward, and you are in control.

chooses not to be part of your plan? For example, what do you do if a friend asks you to go to a movie and it is your scheduled study time? Your friend may say, "Come on. Take some time off. You have plenty of time to study. Study later when we get back!" You are faced with a decision. You must weigh all the factors carefully. You must keep your goals in mind and remember that your need for positive momentum is critical. Your decision may not be an easy one, but it must be one that will help ensure your goal of becoming a registered nurse is achieved. A positive momentum and meeting your goals are most important.

POSITIVE PAMPERING

Positive pampering means that you must continue to care for yourself holistically. Positive momentum can be maintained only if you are properly balanced. Proper exercise, diet, and positive mental stimulation are crucial to achieving your goal of becoming a registered nurse. Just as you have developed a schedule for study, you should have a schedule that includes some fun and some form of physical activity. It is your choice—aerobics, running, walking, weight lifting, bowling, or whatever makes you feel good about yourself. Time spent away from the hard study schedule and devoted to some form of fun and physical exercise pays you back a hundred fold. You will feel alive and more energetic with a schedule that includes these activities.

Establish healthy eating habits. Stay away from fatty foods because they slow you down. Eat lighter meals and eat more frequently. Include complex carbohydrates in your diet for energy, and be careful not to include too much caffeine in your daily diet. Continue to feel good about yourself because you are in control.

Take the time to pamper yourself with activities that make you feel even better about who you are. Make dinner reservations at your favorite restaurant with someone who is special and is supporting your goal to become a registered nurse. Take walks in a place that has a particular tranquility that enables you to reflect on the positive momentum that you have achieved and maintained. Whatever it is, wherever it takes you, allow yourself the time to do some positive pampering.

FINAL PREPARATION

You have established the foundation of your Pyramid to Success. You have developed your list of goals and your study plan, and you have maintained your positive momentum. You are moving forward, and you are in control. When you receive your date and time for the NCLEX-RN examination, you may immediately think, "I am not ready!" Stop! Reflect on all that you have achieved. Think about your goal achievement and the organization of the positive life momentum with which you have surrounded yourself. Think about all the people who love and support your effort to become a registered nurse. Believe that the challenge that awaits you is one that you have successfully prepared for and will lead you to your goal of becoming a registered nurse.

Take a deep breath and organize the remaining days so that they support your educational and personal needs. Support your positive momentum with a visual technique. Write your name in large letters, and write the letters "RN" after it. Post one or more of these visual reinforcements in areas that you frequent. This form of visual motivational technique works for many nursing graduates preparing for this examination.

Through all that you have accomplished so far, it is imperative that you not fall into the trap of expecting too much of yourself. The idea of perfection must not drive you to a point that causes your positive momentum to hesitate. You must believe in who you are, as you are, and stay focused on your goal. Allow yourself the opportunity to continue to carry out your plan in a manner that is most conducive to who you are, not someone else. The date and time are at hand. Write down the date and time, and underneath write the word "yes!" Post this next to your name plus "RN"

You must ensure that you have command over how to get to the testing center. A test run is a must. Time the drive, and allow for road construction or whatever might occur to slow traffic down. On the test run, when you arrive at the test facility, you may want to walk into it. Go in and become familiar with the lobby and the surroundings. This may help alleviate some of the peripheral nervousness associated with entering an unknown building. Remember that you must do whatever it takes to keep yourself in control. If familiarizing yourself with the facility will help you maintain positive momentum, by all means be sure to do so. Who is in control? You are!

It is time to check your study plan and make the necessary adjustments now that a firm date and time are set. Adjust your review so that it flows to your needs and that your study plan ends 2 days before the examination. The mind is like a muscle. If it is overworked, it has no strength or stamina. Your strategy is to rest the body and mind on the day before the examination. Your strategy is to stay in control and allow yourself the opportunity to be absolutely fresh and attentive on the day of the examination. This strategy will help you control the nervousness that is natural, achieve the clear thought processes required, and feel confident that you have done all that is necessary to prepare and conquer this challenge. The day before the examination is to be one of pleasure. Treat yourself to what you enjoy the most.

Relax! Take a deep breath, hold to a count of four, and exhale slowly. You have prepared yourself well for the challenge of tomorrow. Allow yourself a restful night's sleep, and wake up on the day of the examination knowing that you are absolutely prepared to succeed. Look at your name with "RN" after it and the word "yes!"

DAY OF THE EXAMINATION (Box 3-3)

Wake up believing in yourself and that all you have accomplished is about to propel you to the professional level of registered nurse. Allow yourself plenty of time, eat a nutritious breakfast, and groom yourself for success. You are ready to meet the challenges of the day and overcome any obstacle that may face you. Today will soon be history, and tomorrow will bring you the envelope on which you read your name with the words "Registered Nurse" after it.

Be proud and confident of your achievements. You have worked hard to achieve your goal of becoming a registered nurse. If you believe in yourself and your goals, no one person or obstacle can move you off the pathway that leads to success, to the peak of the Pyramid! Congratulations, and I wish you the very best in your career as a registered nurse!

Box 3-3 Day of the Examination

Breathe: Inhale deeply, hold your breath to a count of four, exhale slowly
Believe: Have positive thoughts today and always about your achievements
Control: You are in command
Believe: This is your day
Visualize: R.N. with your name

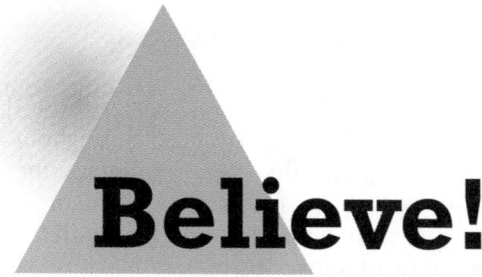

4

The NCLEX-RN® Examination: From a Graduate's Perspective

Sarah Hollenberg, RN

The NCLEX exam was always one of those daunting topics that loomed over my head throughout nursing school. During my first three semesters, the NCLEX exam seemed so far away that I put it on the "back burner" to deal with my current hurdles. As every nursing student knows, there is so much on your plate while in nursing school that you just don't have time to "wrap your head around it all." Although all along I knew I needed to face the NCLEX exam, as my last semester approached I realized that the NCLEX exam had managed to creep up on me. It was time to start formulating a plan of action. Initially, the panic set in. I had viewed the NCLEX exam as a compilation of all the stresses that I experienced before each test in nursing school, and that's a lot of stress! I had to calm down and look at this rationally. People do pass this test. I needed to realize that this goal was absolutely attainable. I just needed to use the knowledge I had gained over the years and continue to prepare myself for this exam after graduation.

My school conducted a review class during the last semester that was dedicated to reviewing areas of the NCLEX exam, test strategies, and question formats. We used *Saunders Comprehensive Review for the NCLEX-RN® Examination*, the book that you are currently reading, for this class. It worked out great because it made me very familiar with the book and the CD accompanying it. Our tests for the class came directly from the CD. Answering practice questions repeatedly until the grade I wanted was achieved provided great practice on its own. I really liked the breakdown of the outline of the book, which made it easy to focus on specific body systems and topics. Each week we focused on a content area included in the book. This review and the pretest on the CD helped to identify my areas of strengths and weaknesses. The amount of information to know is massive, and being able to narrow your focus to what you need to do to prepare is a huge time saver. I kept track of my weak areas so that I could spend more time on those areas and incorporate them into my study plan after graduation.

Making a study plan was crucial to ensure that I used my time and resources effectively to increase my chance of passing. First things first post-graduation, celebrate! Take a break, let yourself breathe, and give yourself the kudos you deserve. Graduating from nursing school is a major accomplishment, and it needs to be celebrated. I graduated near the end of December and decided to go ahead and enjoy the holidays. I took this time off to relax, let loose, and feel the happiness about how far I had come. After I basked in the glory of getting through countless tests, skills test outs, and the stress, it was time to study and tackle the NCLEX exam. Just taking that time helped to boost my confidence about the NCLEX exam because I reflected back on the times in school when I thought I may not make it, but I did. I read and asked friends about different ideas for setting up a study plan; however, in the end I just did what worked best for me.

I set goals on how many review questions to do and the minimum amount of time to study each day. I set up study periods of 1 hour in the morning and 1 hour at night. I tried to do at least 100 to 200 questions a day. Even though I thought I had developed a pretty decent study plan, sticking to it was difficult. Life, as it usually does, gets in the way. One thing I made sure of was not to beat myself up if I missed a day to study or didn't get in quite as much as I would have liked.

One thing I found to be important was to have practice questions available at all times. Whenever I would find myself somewhere waiting around and with nothing to do, I would regret not having practice questions with me. These were perfect opportunities to get in some additional study time. After being caught in that situation, I decided to bring practice questions with me everywhere, stuffed away in my book bag or purse, so that at anytime I could grab them and look them over. I can remember going to the doctor's office and being in the waiting room answering practice questions. I even reviewed practice questions as I was waiting to be interviewed for nursing jobs and fellowships. I used flashcards and a test-taking strategies book by Linda Silvestri. These were easy to transport from place to place because they are small in size. Have practice questions on hand at all times for those spur-of-the-moment study opportunities.

When it came to my "sit down planned study sessions," initially I tried to review chapters of the book. I didn't read each chapter, but I would skim and look over information that was more difficult for me or that I found to be confusing. So to start with I really did try to review each area to some extent. I focused on my weaknesses and devoted extra time to those areas to strengthen my knowledge and feel more confident.

Another technique that helped me was to split the practice questions and topics up and not to take on too much at a time. Also, I would limit the amount of time I spent studying at each session; otherwise I would get to a point at which everything began to jumble in my brain. Just as in nursing school, I found that I could retain information better this way. It took me some time to go through the practice questions during study sessions because I would make sure to read the rationales for all of the options. I thought it was important to read the rationale for every practice question, even those that I got correct to make sure that my thought process was accurate. Reading the rationales is such a great way to see how your mind should be thinking to select the correct option, which is crucial on the actual test day.

When I studied, I made sure that I was comfortable and without distractions. I chose to study on my own and with a group of nursing classmates. When I studied on my own, it worked well because it was easier to focus and get through more practice questions. In a group, when going over specific topics and questions, others may be stronger in your weak areas and bring up ways of answering practice questions that you weren't thinking of at the time. Another great thing about studying with a group is that you have the opportunity to relax and talk with your friends when you take breaks during the study session. It is also nice to have people around you who understand what you're going through and share a lot of the same feelings that you have about taking the NCLEX exam.

Another important concern was when exactly to take the test. When I received my Authorization to Test (ATT) form, I debated between signing up for the first available test spot and taking my time to schedule an appointment. I decided to take my time and schedule the exam for a month or two after graduation. I wanted to make sure I felt fully prepared and didn't want to be rushing into it. I think this decision helped me cut down on some of the stress I was feeling. Also, once I set the date it made me crack down on my studying even more because I knew the date was approaching.

When studying, my main tactic was to do numerous practice questions. I would go through a few practice questions, check my answers, and read the rationales. Then if I needed more information about that topic, I would refer to the book chapters and read about the topic, such as a specific medication, disease process, or nursing considerations. With this strategy, I noticed that after doing more and more questions I would get better and better with thinking through the information and answering correctly. Additionally, using the test-taking strategies, I found myself able to answer the really difficult practice questions accurately. I really felt my confidence increasing. I wrote the test-taking strategies on a note pad so that as I first began doing practice questions I could refer to them. Having the test-taking strategies visually in front of me helped me learn to apply them to every practice question; soon I didn't need them visually in front of me.

When it came to a week before the test, I continued to study as I had been. A few days before my scheduled date, I met with those left in my study group who hadn't tested yet for some studying and for getting my fears off my chest. Every time I'd heard that another classmate had passed the NCLEX exam, it made me feel better about testing. The day before the test I decided to take everyone's advice and to try to relax and not study. Originally I decided to go ahead and pamper myself for the day, although I did sneak in a few practice questions here and there. At this point, doing practice questions was practically a habit. I also took a break to spend time with friends and family.

My test was scheduled bright and early at 8:00 A.M. The night before, I made sure that I had all the proper paperwork and necessary items to test, such as my ID, packed and ready to go. I didn't want to do any rushing around in the early morning. It was early to bed for me. I woke up and made sure to eat breakfast, but nothing too heavy. I didn't want to have any reason to be uncomfortable while taking this test. I also made sure to wear comfortable clothes and decided to wear a few layers so that I could adjust for whatever temperature the testing center would be. I left my house plenty early so that I would not have to worry about traffic or other possible delays. I remember pulling up and even sitting in my car relaxing and listening to music to calm my nerves. I checked in early and made sure to smile brightly for that inopportune photo required of each test participant.

Once inside, I remembered a friend's recommendation to take advantage of the ear plugs provided. I thought this was a good idea, especially considering how easily I can be distracted. There is also something provided to you to write on at your computer station. The very first thing that I did was write ABC's, Maslow's hierarchy, and my lab values. I wrote these down just as reminders to have by my side as a comfort, even though I had them memorized. Once I began my test, I realized that the ear plugs were uncomfortable probably because I have never used any; they were actually a distraction for me. I felt much better without them and it was plenty quiet; honestly, I was so focused on the questions I didn't need them.

One reminder is to read the questions carefully and each option fully; remember, you cannot skip questions. That was one thing that was difficult for me because through nursing school I was definitely one to change my answers. Another important point besides reading very carefully is not taking too much time on each question. There will be questions on the test in which you do not know the answer. You have to apply the best strategy and select the best option available. Just remember to think positively and be confident. This test is passable and you are prepared.

When I left, I tried to think confidently, but I was worried. It was a difficult test to judge. I figured it was over and I can't change it now, so thinking optimistically was my best option. I did feel confident, but waiting for the test results felt just as difficult as the test. They give you information at the testing center regarding how to check your results. I opted for the online option and checked it the minute I could. It shows your name and across the way "passed" in small letters on the screen. I was practically in tears I was so excited. I felt so proud the first time I was able to write "RN" behind my name instead of "GN" Even to this day I feel the pride and satisfaction of writing those letters behind my name.

Just remember to stay calm, prepare the best you can, and be confident and optimistic!

Test-Taking Strategies

I. PYRAMID TO SUCCESS (Box 5-1)

II. HOW TO AVOID READING INTO THE QUESTION (Box 5-2)

A. Pyramid points

1. Avoid asking yourself, "Well, what if ...?" because this will lead you right into the "forbidden" area, reading into the question.
2. Focus only on the information in the question, read every word, and make a decision about what the question is asking.
3. Look for the strategic words in the question, such as *immediate*, *initial*, *first*, *priority*, *side effect*, or *toxic effect*; strategic words make a difference with regard to what the question is asking.
4. In multiple-choice questions, multiple-response questions, or questions that require you to number in order of priority, read every choice or option presented before selecting answers.
5. Always use the process of elimination when choices or options are presented; after you have eliminated options, reread the question before selecting your final choice or choices.

6. With questions that require you to fill in the blank, focus on the information in the question and determine what the question is asking; if the question requires you to calculate a medication dose, an intravenous flow rate, or intake and output amounts, recheck your work in calculating and always use the on-screen calculator to verify the answer.
7. Avoid asking yourself the "forbidden" words, "Well, what if ...?," when deciding on an answer to a question.

Box 5-2 Practice Question: Avoiding the "What if ..." Syndrome and Reading into the Question

A nurse is caring for a hospitalized client with a diagnosis of congestive heart failure who suddenly complains of shortness of breath and dyspnea. The nurse takes which *immediate* action?

1. Calls the physician
2. Administers oxygen to the client
3. Elevates the head of the client's bed
4. Prepares to administer furosemide (Lasix)

Answer: 3

Test-Taking Strategy: Now you may immediately think the client has developed pulmonary edema, a complication of congestive heart failure, and needs a diuretic. Although pulmonary edema is a complication of congestive heart failure, there is no information in the question that indicates the presence of pulmonary edema. The question simply states that the client suddenly complains of shortness of breath and dyspnea. Read the question carefully. Note the strategic word *immediate* and focus on the subject: the client's complaints. Although the physician may need to be notified, this is not the immediate action. A physician's prescription is needed to administer oxygen. Furosemide is a diuretic and may or may not be prescribed for the client. Because there is no information in the question that indicates the presence of pulmonary edema, option 3 is correct. The question is asking you for a nursing action, so that is what you need to look for as you eliminate the incorrect options. Use nursing knowledge and test-taking strategies to assist in answering the question. Remember to avoid the "What if...?" syndrome and reading into the question.

Box 5-1 Pyramid to Success

- Avoid asking yourself, "Well, what if ...?" because this will lead you right into reading into the question.
- Focus only on the information in the question, read every word, and make a decision regarding what the question is asking.
- Look for the strategic words in the question; strategic words make a difference with regard to what the question is asking about.
- Always use the process of elimination when choices or options are presented; when you have eliminated options, reread the question before selecting your final choice or choices.
- Determine if the question is a positive or negative event query.
- Use all your nursing knowledge, your clinical experiences, and your test-taking skills and strategies to answer the question.

B. Ingredients of a question (Box 5-3)

1. The ingredients of a question include the event, which is a client or clinical situation; the event query; and the options or answers.
2. The event provides you with the content about the client or clinical situation that you need to think about when answering the question.
3. The event query asks something specific about the content of the event.
4. The options are all the answers provided with the question.
5. In a multiple-choice question, there will be four options and you must select one; read every option carefully and think about the event and the event query as you use the process of elimination.
6. In a multiple-response question, there will be several options and you must select all options that apply to the event in the question; visualize the event and use your nursing knowledge and your clinical experiences to answer the question.
7. In a prioritizing (ordered response)/drag and drop question, you will be required to list in order of priority nursing interventions or other data; visualize the event and use your nursing knowledge and clinical experiences to answer the question.

8. A fill-in-the-blank question will not contain options, and some picture or graphic (hot spot) questions and audio or video item formats may or may not contain options. A graphic option item will contain options in the form of a picture or graphic.
9. A chart exhibit question will most likely contain options; read the question carefully and all of the information in the chart or exhibit before selecting an answer.

III. STRATEGIC WORDS (Boxes 5-4 and 5-5)

A. Strategic words focus your attention on a critical point to consider when answering the question and will assist you in eliminating the incorrect options.
B. Some strategic words may indicate that all the options are correct and that it will be necessary to prioritize to select the correct option (Box 5-6).
C. As you read the question, look for the strategic words; strategic words make a difference with regard to the focus of the question.

Box 5-3 Ingredients of a Question: Event, Event Query, and Options

Event: A nurse is caring for a client with terminal cancer.
Event Query: The nurse considers which of the following when planning opioid pain relief?
Options:
1. Not all pain is real.
2. Opioid analgesics are highly addictive.
3. Opioid analgesics can cause tachycardia.
4. Around-the-clock dosing gives better pain relief than PRN dosing.

Answer: 4
Test-Taking Strategy: Focus on the client's diagnosis. Administering around-the-clock dosing provides increased pain relief and decreases stressors associated with pain, such as anxiety and fear. Option 1 is not of concern here. Opioid analgesics may be addictive, but this is not a concern for a client with terminal cancer. Not all opioid analgesics cause tachycardia.

Box 5-4 Common Strategic Words

Best	Initial
Early or late	Most appropriate or least
First	appropriate
Immediately	Most likely or least likely

Box 5-5 Practice Question: Strategic Words

A nurse is caring for a client who just returned from the recovery room after undergoing abdominal surgery. The nurse monitors for which *early sign* of hypovolemic shock?
1. Sleepiness
2. Increased pulse rate
3. Increased depth of respiration
4. Increased orientation to surroundings

Answer: 2
Test-Taking Strategy: Note the strategic words *early sign*. Focusing on these strategic words, recall that cardiovascular changes occur early in hypovolemic shock. Sleepiness is expected in a client who just returned from surgery. Increased orientation to surroundings is expected and will occur as the effects of anesthesia resolve. Although increased depth of respirations occurs in hypovolemic shock, it is not an early sign. Rather, it occurs as the shock progresses. Remember to look for strategic words.

Box 5-6 Common Strategic Words That Indicate the Need to Prioritize

Best	Most appropriate or least
Essential	appropriate
First	Most important
Highest priority	Most likely or least likely
Immediate	Primary
Initial	Vital
Next	

IV. SUBJECT OF THE QUESTION (Box 5-7)

A. The subject of the question is the specific topic that the question is asking about.

B. Identifying the subject of the question will assist in eliminating the incorrect options and direct you to selecting the correct option.

V. POSITIVE AND NEGATIVE EVENT QUERIES (Boxes 5-8 and 5-9)

A. A positive event query uses strategic words that ask you to select an option that is correct; for example, the event query may read, "Which statement by a client *indicates an understanding* of the side effects of the prescribed medication?"

B. A negative event query uses strategic words that ask you to select an option that is an incorrect item or statement; for example, the event query may read, "Which statement by a client *indicates a need for further teaching* about the side effects of the prescribed medication?"

VI. QUESTIONS THAT REQUIRE PRIORITIZING

A. Many questions in the examination will require you to use the skill of prioritizing nursing actions.

B. Look for the strategic words in the question that indicate the need to prioritize (see Box 5-6).

C. Remember that when a question requires prioritization, all options may be correct and you need to determine the correct order of action.

D. Strategies to use to prioritize include the ABCs (airway, breathing, and circulation), Maslow's Hierarchy of Needs theory, and the steps of the nursing process.

E. The ABCs (Box 5-10)
1. Use the ABCs—airway, breathing, and circulation—when selecting an answer or determining the order of priority.
2. Remember the order of priority—airway, breathing, and circulation.
3. Airway is always the first priority.

F. Maslow's Hierarchy of Needs theory (Box 5-11; Fig. 5-1)

Box 5-7 Subject of the Question

A nurse is teaching a client in skeletal leg traction about measures to increase bed mobility. Which item would be *most helpful* for this client?
1. Television
2. Fracture bedpan
3. Overhead trapeze
4. Reading materials

Answer: 3
Test-Taking Strategy: Focus on the subject: to increase bed mobility. Also note the strategic words *most helpful*. The use of an overhead trapeze is extremely helpful in assisting a client to move about in bed and to get on and off the bedpan. Television and reading materials are helpful in reducing boredom and providing distraction. A fracture bedpan is useful in reducing discomfort with elimination. Remember to focus on the subject.

Box 5-8 Practice Question: Positive Event Query

A child with hemophilia is brought into the emergency department after being hit on the neck with a baseball. *A nurse should immediately check the child for:*
1. Airway obstruction
2. Factor VIII deficiency
3. Spontaneous hematuria
4. Headache and slurred speech

Answer: 1
Test-Taking Strategy: This question is an example of a positive event query question. Trauma to the neck may cause bleeding into the tissues of the neck, which may compromise the airway. Factor VIII deficiency is not a symptom of hemophilia, but rather a common form of the disease. Hematuria is a symptom of hemophilia, but it is not associated with neck injury. Headache and slurred speech are associated with head trauma and are not the priority in this situation. Use the ABCs—airway, breathing, and circulation—to answer this question. Remember that airway assessment is always a first priority.

Box 5-9 Practice Question: Negative Event Query

A nurse has reinforced discharge instructions to a client who has undergone a right mastectomy with axillary lymph node dissection. Which statement by the client indicates a *need for further instruction* regarding home care measures?
1. "It is all right to use a straight razor to shave under my arms."
2. "I need to be sure that I do not have blood pressures or blood drawn from my right arm."
3. "I should inform all of my other health care providers that I have had this surgical procedure."
4. "I need to be sure to wear thick mitt hand covers or use thick pot holders when I am cooking and touching hot pans."

Answer: 1
Test-Taking Strategy: This question is an example of a negative event query question. Note the strategic words *need for further instruction*. These strategic words indicate that you need to select an option that identifies an incorrect client statement. Recalling that edema and infection are the concerns with this client and that the client needs to be instructed in the measures that will avoid trauma to the affected arm will direct you to the correct option. Remember to watch for negative event queries.

1. According to Maslow's Hierarchy of Needs theory, physiological needs are the priority, followed by safety and security needs, love and belonging needs, self-esteem needs, and, finally, self-actualization needs; select the option or determine the order of priority by addressing physiological needs first.

2. When a physiological need is not addressed in the question or noted in one of the options, continue to use Maslow's Hierarchy of Needs theory as a guide and look for the option that addresses safety.

Box 5-10 Practice Question: Use of the ABCs

A client with a diagnosis of cancer is receiving morphine sulfate for pain. A nurse employs which priority action in the care of the client?
1. Monitors stools
2. Encourages fluid intake
3. Monitors the urine output
4. Encourages the client to cough and breathe deeply

Answer: 4
Test-Taking Strategy: Use the ABCs—airway, breathing, and circulation—as a guide to direct you to the correct option. Recall that morphine sulfate suppresses the cough reflex and the respiratory reflex. Although options 1, 2, and 3 are components of the plan of care, the correct option addresses airway. Remember to use the ABCs—airway, breathing, and circulation—to prioritize.

Box 5-11 Practice Question: Maslow's Hierarchy of Needs Theory

A nurse caring for a client experiencing dystocia determines that the *highest priority* is frequent:
1. Position changes and providing comfort measures
2. Explanations to family members about what is happening to the client
3. Monitoring for changes in the physical condition of the mother and fetus
4. Reinforcement of breathing techniques learned in childbirth preparatory classes

Answer: 3
Test-Taking Strategy: All the options are correct and would be implemented during the care of this client. Note the strategic words *highest priority,* however, and use Maslow's Hierarchy of Needs theory to prioritize, remembering that physiological needs come first. Doing so will direct you to option 3. Also, option 3 is the only option that addresses both the mother and the fetus. Remember to use Maslow's Hierarchy of Needs theory to prioritize.

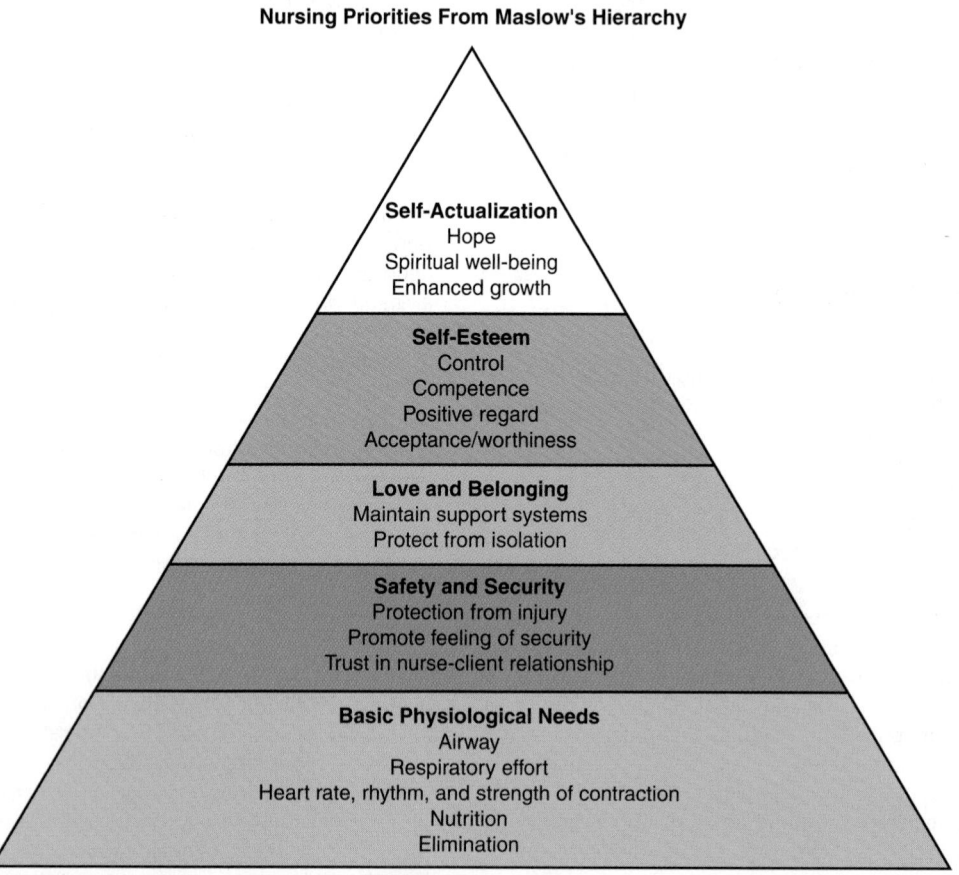

Nursing Priorities From Maslow's Hierarchy

Self-Actualization
Hope
Spiritual well-being
Enhanced growth

Self-Esteem
Control
Competence
Positive regard
Acceptance/worthiness

Love and Belonging
Maintain support systems
Protect from isolation

Safety and Security
Protection from injury
Promote feeling of security
Trust in nurse-client relationship

Basic Physiological Needs
Airway
Respiratory effort
Heart rate, rhythm, and strength of contraction
Nutrition
Elimination

▲ **FIGURE 5-1** Use Maslow's hierarchy to establish priorities. (From Harkreader, H., Hogan, M.A., & Thobaben, M. [2007]. *Fundamentals of nursing: Caring and clinical judgment* [3rd ed.]. St. Louis: Saunders.)

G. Steps of the nursing process
  1. Use the steps of the nursing process to prioritize.
  2. The steps include assessment, analysis, planning, implementation, and evaluation and are followed in this order.
  3. Assessment
    a. Assessment questions address the process of gathering subjective and objective data relative to the client, confirming the data, and communicating and documenting the data.
    b. Remember that assessment is the first step in the nursing process.
    c. When you are asked to select your first, immediate, or initial nursing action, follow the steps of the nursing process to prioritize when selecting the correct option.
    d. Look for strategic words in the options that reflect assessment (Box 5-12).
    e. If an option contains the concept of assessment or the collection of client data, the best choice is to select that option (Box 5-13).

    f. If an assessment action is not one of the options, follow the steps of the nursing process as your guide to select your first, immediate, or initial action.
    g. Possible exception to the guideline—if the question presents an emergency situation, read carefully; in an emergency situation, an intervention may be the priority.
  4. Analysis (Box 5-14)
    a. Analysis questions are the most difficult questions because they require understanding of the principles of physiological responses and require interpretation of the data based on assessment.
    b. Analysis questions require critical thinking and determining the rationale for therapeutic prescriptions or interventions that may be addressed in the question.
    c. Analysis questions may address the formulation of a nursing diagnosis and the communication and documentation of the results of the process of analysis.
  5. Planning (Box 5-15)
    a. Planning questions require prioritizing nursing diagnoses, determining goals and outcome criteria for goals of care, developing the plan of care, and communicating and documenting the plan of care.

Box 5-12 Assessment: Strategic Words

Ascertain	Gather
Assess	Identify
Check	Monitor
Collect	Observe
Determine	Obtain information
Find out	Recognize

Box 5-13 Practice Question: The Nursing Process—Assessment

A client who has had an application of a right long arm cast complains of pain at the wrist when the arm is passively moved. A nurse should *first*:
1. Elevate the arm.
2. Document the findings.
3. Medicate with an additional dose of an opioid.
4. Check for paresthesias and paralysis of the right arm.

Answer: 4
Test-Taking Strategy: Note the strategic word *first*. Use the steps of the nursing process to answer the question, remembering that assessment is the first step. The only option that addresses assessment is option 4. Options 1, 2, and 3 address the implementation step of the nursing process. Also, these options are inaccurate first actions. The arm in a cast should have already been elevated (option 1). The client may be experiencing compartment syndrome, a complication following trauma to the extremities and application of a cast. Additional data need to be collected to determine if this complication is present. Remember that assessment is the first step in the nursing process.

Box 5-14 Practice Question: The Nursing Process—Analysis

A nurse reviews the arterial blood gas results of a client and notes the following: pH 7.45, Pco_2 30 mm Hg, and HCO_3^- 22 mEq/L. The nurse analyzes these results as indicating which condition?
1. Metabolic acidosis, compensated
2. Respiratory alkalosis, compensated
3. Metabolic alkalosis, uncompensated
4. Respiratory acidosis, uncompensated

Answer: 2
Test-Taking Strategy: The normal pH is 7.35 to 7.45. In a respiratory condition, an opposite effect will be seen between the pH and the Pco_2. In this situation, the pH is at the high end of the normal value and the Pco_2 is low. In an alkalotic condition, the pH is elevated. The values identified in the question indicate a respiratory alkalosis. Compensation occurs when the pH returns to a normal value. Because the pH is in the normal range at the high end, compensation has occurred.

   In a case of respiratory imbalance, you will find an opposite response between the pH and the Pco_2 as indicated in the question. You can eliminate options 1 and 3. Also, remember that the pH increases in an alkalotic condition and compensation occurs, as evidenced by a normal pH. Remember that analysis is the second step in the nursing process.

b. Regarding nursing diagnoses, remember that actual client problems rather than at-risk for client problems will most likely be the priority.

6. Implementation (Box 5-16)

a. Implementation questions address the process of organizing and managing care, counseling and teaching, providing care to achieve established goals, supervising and coordinating care, and communicating and documenting nursing interventions.

Box 5-15 Practice Question: The Nursing Process—Planning

A nurse develops a plan of care for a client with a cataract. Which nursing diagnosis is the priority?
1. *Fear* related to loss of eyesight
2. *Risk for injury* related to decreased vision
3. *Disturbed sensory perception* (visual) related to ocular lens opacity
4. *Social isolation* related to decreased ability to mobilize in the community

Answer: 3

Test-Taking Strategy: This question relates to planning nursing care and asks you to identify the priority nursing diagnosis. Use Maslow's Hierarchy of Needs theory to answer the question. Remembering that physiological needs are the priority will direct you to option 3. Although *Risk for injury* is an at-risk rather than an actual problem, according to Maslow's Hierarchy of Needs theory, safety is the second priority. *Fear* and *Social isolation* are psychosocial needs and would be the last priorities in this situation. Remember that planning is the third step of the nursing process.

Box 5-16 Practice Question: The Nursing Process—Implementation

A nurse is caring for a hospitalized client with angina pectoris who begins to experience chest pain. The nurse administers a nitroglycerin (Nitrostat) tablet sublingually as prescribed, but the pain is unrelieved. The nurse should take which action *next*?
1. Reposition the client.
2. Contact the physician.
3. Call the client's family.
4. Administer another nitroglycerin tablet.

Answer: 4

Test-Taking Strategy: Implementation questions address the process of organizing and managing care. This question also requires that you prioritize the nursing actions. Note the strategic word *next* and that the client is hospitalized. Recalling that the nurse would administer three nitroglycerin tablets 5 minutes apart from each other to relieve chest pain will assist in directing you to option 4. Remember that implementation is the fourth step of the nursing process.

---

b. Focus on a nursing action rather than on a medical action when you are answering a question, unless the question is asking you what prescribed medical action is anticipated.

c. On the NCLEX-RN exam, the only client that you need to be concerned about is the client in the question that you are answering; avoid the "What if …?" syndrome and remember that the client in the question on the computer screen is your only assigned client.

d. Answer the question from a textbook and ideal point of view; remember that the nurse has all the time and all of the equipment needed to care for the client readily available at the bedside.

e. Avoid the "What if …?" syndrome and remember that you do not need to run to the treatment room to obtain, for example, sterile gloves because the sterile gloves will be at the client's bedside.

7. Evaluation (Box 5-17)

a. Evaluation questions focus on comparing the actual outcomes of care with the expected outcomes and communicating and documenting findings.

b. These questions focus on assisting in determining the client's response to care and identifying factors that may interfere with achieving expected outcomes.

c. In an evaluation question, watch for negative event queries because they are frequently used in evaluation-type questions.

Box 5-17 Practice Question: The Nursing Process—Evaluation

A nurse is monitoring the function of a client's chest tube drainage system. The nurse notes that the fluid in the water seal chamber is below the 2-cm mark. The nurse interprets that:
1. There is a leak in the system.
2. The client has a pneumothorax.
3. Suction should be added to the system.
4. Water should be added to the chamber.

Answer: 4

Test-Taking Strategy: Focus on the data in the question. It makes sense to add water to the chamber if the water level is too low. The water seal chamber should be filled to the 2-cm mark to provide an adequate water seal between the external environment and the client's pleural cavity. The water seal prevents air from reentering the pleural cavity. Because evaporation of water can occur, the nurse should remedy this problem by adding water until the level is again at the 2-cm mark. Options 1, 2, and 3 are incorrect interpretations. Remember that evaluation is the fifth step of the nursing process.

VII. CLIENT NEEDS

A. Safe and effective care environment
   1. According to the National Council of State Boards of Nursing (NCSBN), these questions test the concepts that the nurse provides nursing care; collaborates with other health care team members to facilitate effective client care; and protects clients, significant others, and health care personnel from environmental hazards.
   2. Focus on safety with these types of questions, and remember the importance of hand washing, call bells, bed positioning, appropriate use of side rails, asepsis, and use of standard and other precautions.

B. Physiological integrity
   1. The NCSBN indicates that these questions test the concepts that the nurse provides comfort and assistance in the performance of activities of daily living and provides care related to the administration of medications and parenteral therapies.
   2. These questions also address the nurse's ability to reduce the client's potential for developing complications or health problems related to treatments, procedures, or existing conditions and providing care to clients with acute, chronic, or life-threatening physical health conditions.
   3. Focus on Maslow's Hierarchy of Needs theory in these types of questions and remember that physiological needs are a priority and are addressed first.
   4. Use the ABCs—airway, breathing, and circulation—and the steps of the nursing process when selecting an option addressing physiological integrity.

C. Psychosocial integrity
   1. The NCSBN notes that these questions test the concepts that the nurse provides nursing care that promotes and supports the emotional, mental, and social well-being of the client and significant others.
   2. Content addressed in these questions relates to supporting and promoting the client's or significant others' ability to cope, adapt, or problem-solve in situations such as illnesses; disabilities; or stressful events such as abuse, neglect, or violence.
   3. In this Client Needs category, you may be asked communication-type questions that relate to how you would respond to a client, a client's family member or significant other, or other health care team members.
   4. Use therapeutic communication techniques to answer communication questions because of their effectiveness in the communication process.
   5. Remember to select the option that focuses on the thoughts, feelings, concerns, anxieties, or fears of the client, client's family member, or significant other (Box 5-18).

Box 5-18 Practice Question: Communication

A client scheduled for bowel surgery states to a nurse, "I'm not sure if I should have this surgery." Which response by the nurse is appropriate?
1. "It's your decision."
2. "Don't worry. Everything will be fine."
3. "Why don't you want to have this surgery?"
4. "Tell me what concerns you have about the surgery."

Answer: 4
Test-Taking Strategy: Use therapeutic communication techniques to answer communication questions and remember to focus on the client's thoughts, feelings, concerns, anxieties, and fears. Option 4 is the only option that addresses the client's concern. Option 1 is a blunt response and does not address the client's concern. Option 2 provides false reassurance. Option 3 can make the client feel defensive. Remember to use therapeutic communication techniques and focus on the client.

D. Health promotion and maintenance
   1. According to the NCSBN, these questions test the concepts that the nurse provides and assists in directing nursing care to promote and maintain health.
   2. Content addressed in these questions relates to assisting the client and significant others during the normal expected stages of growth and development, and providing client care related to the prevention and early detection of health problems.
   3. Use the Teaching and Learning theory if the question addresses client teaching, remembering that the client's willingness, desire, and readiness to learn is the first priority.
   4. Watch for negative event queries because they are frequently used in questions that address Health Promotion and Maintenance and client education.

VIII. ELIMINATING COMPARABLE OR ALIKE OPTIONS (Box 5-19)

A. When reading the options, look for options that are comparable or alike.
B. Comparable or alike options can be eliminated as possible answers.

IX. ELIMINATE OPTIONS CONTAINING CLOSE-ENDED WORDS (Box 5-20)

A. Some close-ended words include *all*, *always*, *every*, *must*, *none*, *never*, and *only*.
B. Eliminate options that contain close-ended words because these words infer a fixed or extreme meaning; these types of options are usually incorrect.

Box 5-19 Practice Question: Eliminate Comparable or Alike Options

A nurse is caring for a group of clients. On review of the clients' medical records, the nurse determines that which client is at risk for excess fluid volume?
1. The client on diuretics
2. The client with renal failure
3. The client with an ileostomy
4. The client on gastrointestinal suctioning

Answer: 2
Test-Taking Strategy: Focus on the subject of the question, the client at risk for excess fluid volume. Think about the pathophysiology associated with each condition identified in the options. The only client who retains fluid is the client with renal failure. The client on diuretics, the client with an ileostomy, and the client on gastrointestinal suctioning all lose fluid. Remember to eliminate comparable or alike options.

Box 5-20 Practice Question: Eliminate Options That Contain Close-Ended Words

A client is to undergo a barium swallow and the nurse provides preprocedure instructions to the client. The nurse instructs the client to:
1. Avoid eating or drinking after midnight before the test.
2. Limit self to *only* two cigarettes on the morning of the test.
3. Have a clear liquid breakfast *only* on the morning of the test.
4. Take *all* routine medications with a glass of water on the morning of the test.

Answer: 1
Test-Taking Strategy: Note the close-ended words *only* in options 2 and 3 and *all* in option 4. Remember to eliminate options that contain close-ended words because these options are usually incorrect. Also, note that options 2, 3, and 4 are comparable or alike options in that they all involve taking in something on the morning of the test. Remember to eliminate options that contain close-ended words.

Box 5-21 Practice Question: Look for the Umbrella Option

A client who is admitted to the hospital is diagnosed with urethritis caused by chlamydial infection. A nurse implements which of the following precautions to prevent contraction of the infection during care?
1. Enteric precautions
2. Contact precautions
3. Standard precautions
4. Wearing gloves and a mask

Answer: 3
Test-Taking Strategy: Focus on the client's diagnosis and recall that this infection is sexually transmitted. Also, note that option 3 is the umbrella option. Remember that the umbrella option is a broad or universal option that includes the concepts of the other options in it.

Box 5-22 Practice Question: Use the Guidelines for Delegating and Assignment-Making

A nurse in charge of a long-term care facility is planning the client assignments for the day and *most appropriately* assigns which client to the nursing assistant?
1. A client on strict bedrest
2. A client with dyspnea who is receiving oxygen therapy
3. A client scheduled for transfer to the hospital for surgery
4. A client with a gastrostomy tube who requires tube feedings every 4 hours

Answer: 1
Test-Taking Strategy: Note that the question asks for the assignment to be delegated to the nursing assistant. When asked questions related to delegation, think about the role description of the employee and the needs of the client. A client with dyspnea who is receiving oxygen therapy, a client scheduled for transfer to the hospital for surgery, or a client with a gastrostomy tube who requires tube feedings every 4 hours has both physiological and psychosocial needs that require care by a licensed nurse. The nursing assistant has been trained to care for a client on bedrest. Remember to match the client's needs with the scope of practice of the health care provider.

C. Options that contain open-ended words, such as *may, usually, normally, commonly,* or *generally,* should be considered as possible correct options.

X. LOOK FOR THE UMBRELLA OPTION (Box 5-21)

A. When answering a question, look for the umbrella option.
B. The umbrella option is one that is a broad or universal statement and that usually contains the concepts of the other options within it.
C. The umbrella option will be the correct answer.

XI. USE THE GUIDELINES FOR DELEGATING AND MAKING ASSIGNMENTS (Box 5-22)

A. You may be asked a question that will require you to decide how you will delegate a task or assign clients to other health care providers.
B. Focus on the information in the question and what task or assignment is to be delegated.
C. When you have determined what task or assignment is to be delegated, consider the client's needs and match the client's needs with the scope of practice of the health care providers identified in the question.

D. The nurse practice act and any practice limitations define which aspects of care can be delegated and which must be performed by a registered nurse.

E. Generally, noninvasive interventions, such as skin care, range-of-motion exercises, ambulation, grooming, and hygiene measures, can be assigned to a nursing assistant.

F. A licensed practical nurse can perform the tasks that a nursing assistant can perform and can usually perform certain invasive tasks, such as dressings, suctioning, urinary catheterization, and administering medications orally or by the subcutaneous or intramuscular route; some piggyback intravenous medications may also be administered.

G. A registered nurse can perform the tasks that a licensed practical nurse can perform and is responsible for assessment and planning care, analyzing client data, implementing and evaluating client care, supervising care, initiating teaching, and administering medications intravenously.

XII. ANSWERING PHARMACOLOGY QUESTIONS (Box 5-23)

A. If you are familiar with the medication, use nursing knowledge to answer the question.

B. Remember that the question will identify the generic name and the trade name of the medication.

Box 5-23 Practice Question: Answering Pharmacology Questions

Quinapril hydrochloride (Accupril) is prescribed as adjunctive therapy in the treatment of heart failure. After administering the first dose, a nurse monitors which of the following *most closely*?
1. Weight
2. Urine output
3. Lung sounds
4. Blood pressure

Answer: 4
Test-Taking Strategy: Focus on the name of the medication and note the strategic words *most closely*. This tells you that all the options may be correct and that you must prioritize. Recall that the medication names of most angiotensin-converting enzyme (ACE) inhibitors end with "*-pril*" and that these medications are used to treat hypertension. Excessive hypotension ("first-dose syncope") can occur in clients with heart failure or in clients who are severely salt-depleted or volume-depleted. Although weight, urine output, and lung sounds would be monitored, the nurse would *most closely* monitor the client's blood pressure. Remember to use pharmacology guidelines to assist in answering questions about medications.

C. If the question identifies a medical diagnosis, try to form a relationship between the medication and the diagnosis; for example, you can determine that cyclophosphamide (Cytoxan) is an antineoplastic medication if the question refers to a client with breast cancer who is taking this medication.

D. Try to determine the classification of the medication being addressed to assist in answering the question. Identifying the classification will assist in determining a medication's action or side effects or both; for example, diltiazem (*Cardizem*) is a cardiac medication.

E. Recognize the common side effects associated with each medication classification and relate the appropriate nursing interventions to each side effect; for example, if a side effect is hypertension, the associated nursing intervention would be to monitor the blood pressure.

F. Learn medications that belong to a classification by commonalities in their medication names; for example, medications that are xanthine bronchodilators end with "*-line*" (e.g., theophyl*line*).

G. Look at the medication name and use medical terminology to assist in determining the medication action; for example, *Lopressor* lowers (*lo*) the blood pressure (*pressor*).

H. If the question requires a medication calculation, remember that a calculator is available on the computer; talk yourself through each step to be sure the answer makes sense, and recheck the calculation before answering the question, particularly if the answer seems like an unusual dosage.

I. Pharmacology: Pyramid Points to remember
1. Generally, the client should not take an antacid with medication because the antacid will affect the absorption of the medication.
2. Enteric-coated and sustained-release tablets should not be crushed; also, capsules should not be opened.
3. The client should never adjust or change a medication dose or abruptly stop taking a medication.
4. The nurse never adjusts or changes the client's medication dosage and never discontinues a medication.
5. The client needs to avoid taking any over-the-counter medications or any other medications, such as herbal preparations, unless they are approved for use by the health care provider.
6. The client needs to avoid consuming alcohol.
7. Medications are never administered if the order is difficult to read, is unclear, or identifies a medication dose that is not a normal one.

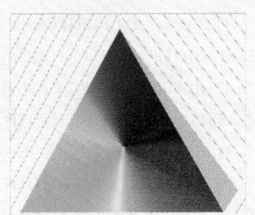

UNIT II

Issues in Nursing

Cultural Diversity and Health Practices

PYRAMID TERMS

acculturatione Process of learning norms, beliefs, and behavioral expectations of a group other than one's own group.

belief A theory accepted as true by a culture.

cultural assimilation Process in which individuals from a minority group are absorbed by the dominant culture and take on the characteristics of the dominant culture.

cultural competence Acquisition of knowledge, understanding, and appreciation of a culture that facilitates provision of culturally appropriate health care.

cultural diversity Differences among groups of people that result from ethnic, racial, and cultural variables.

cultural imposition Tendency to impose one's own beliefs, values, and patterns of behavior on individuals from another culture.

culture Dynamic network of knowledge, beliefs, patterns of behavior, ideas, attitudes, values, and norms that are unique to a particular group of people.

dominant culture Group whose values prevail within a society.

ethnic group People within a culture who share characteristics based on race, religion, color, national origin, or language.

ethnicity An individual's identification of self as part of an ethnic group.

ethnocentrism An assumption of cultural superiority and an inability to accept the ways of another culture.

minority group Ethnic, cultural, racial, or religious group that constitutes less than a numerical majority of the population.

race A grouping of people based on biological similarities; members of a racial group have similar physical characteristics, such as blood group; facial features; and color of skin, hair, and eyes.

racism Discrimination directed toward individuals or groups who are perceived to be inferior.

stereotyping Expectation that all people within the same racial, ethnic, or cultural group act alike and share the same beliefs and attitudes.

subculture Social group within a culture that has distinctive characteristics, such as patterns of behavior or beliefs.

values Principles and standards that have meaning and worth to an individual, family, group, community, or culture.

PYRAMID TO SUCCESS

Nurses often care for clients who come from ethnic, cultural, or religious backgrounds that are different from their own. Awareness of and sensitivity to the unique health and illness beliefs and practices of people of different backgrounds are essential for the delivery of safe and effective care. Acknowledgment and acceptance of cultural differences with a nonjudgmental attitude are essential to providing culturally sensitive care. The NCLEX-RN exam test plan is unique and individualized to the client's culture and beliefs. The nurse needs to avoid stereotyping and needs to be aware that there are several subcultures within cultures and there are several dialects within languages. In nursing practice, the nurse needs to assess the client's perceived needs before planning and implementing a plan of care. See Figure 6-1 for Giger and Davidhizar's Transcultural Assessment Model.

CLIENT NEEDS

Safe and Effective Care Environment

Acting as a client advocate

Ensuring ethical practices

Ensuring legal rights and responsibilities

Establishing priorities

Maintaining confidentiality

Providing continuity of care

Respecting the client's control of personal environment and property

Upholding client rights

Health Promotion and Maintenance

Considering cultural issues related to family systems and family planning

Respecting cultural preferences and lifestyle choices

Promoting health and wellness

Preventing disease

Providing health screening

Identifying changes related to the aging process

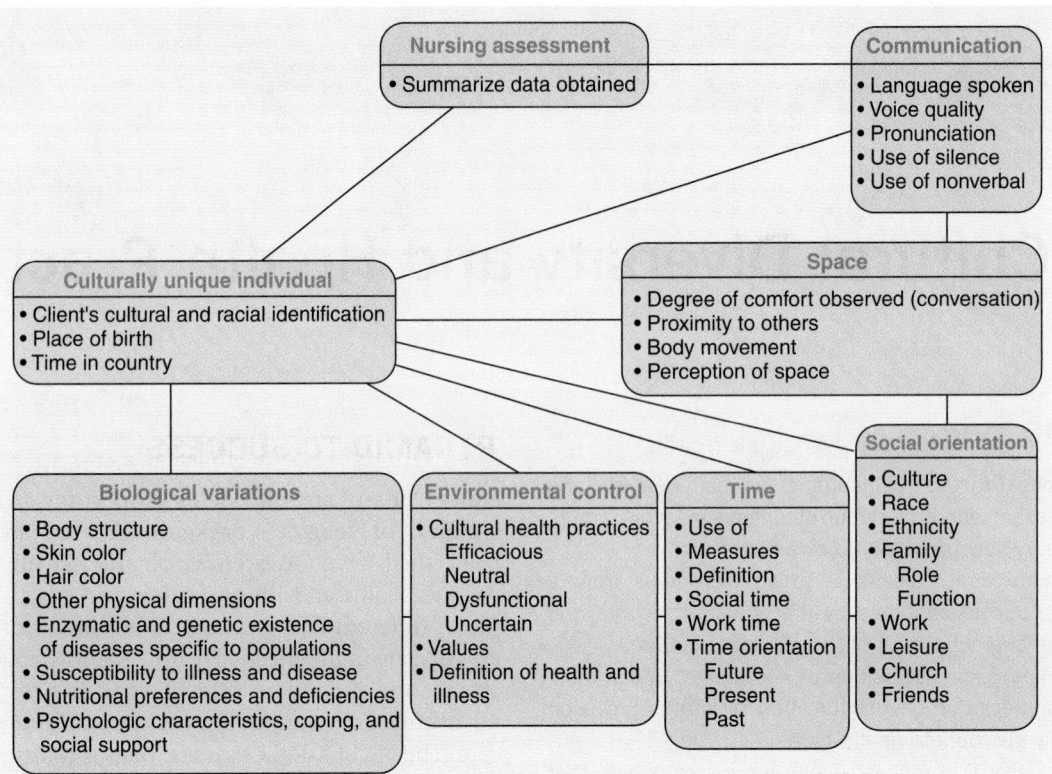

▲ **FIGURE 6-1** Giger and Davidhizar's Transcultural Assessment Model. (From Giger, J., & Davidhizar, R. [2008]. *Transcultural nursing: Assessment and intervention* [5th ed.]. St. Louis: Mosby.)

Psychosocial Integrity

Providing a therapeutic environment

Identifying clients who do not speak or understand English and determining how language needs will be met.

Assessing culture preferences and incorporating these preferences when planning and implementing care.

Respecting religious and spiritual influences on health (Box 6-1)

Identifying support systems

Identifying family dynamics as they relate to the client's culture

Assessing the use of effective coping mechanisms

Identifying end-of-life care issues

Physiological Integrity

Identifying cultural differences for providing holistic client care

Identifying cultural issues related to alternative and complementary therapies

Identifying cultural issues related to receiving blood and blood products

Implementing therapeutic procedures considering cultural preferences

Providing nonpharmacological comfort interventions

Providing nutrition and oral hydration (see Box 6-1)

Providing palliative care

I. AFRICAN AMERICANS

A. Description: Citizens or residents of the United States who may have origins in any of the black populations in Africa.

B. Communication
   1. Members are competent in standard English.
   2. Head nodding does not always mean agreement.
   3. Prolonged eye contact may be interpreted as rudeness or aggressive behavior.
   4. Nonverbal communication may be important.
   5. Personal questions asked on initial contact with a person may be viewed as intrusive.

C. Time orientation and personal space preferences
   1. Time orientation varies according to age, socioeconomics, and **subcultures** and may include past, present, or future orientation.
   2. Members may be late for an appointment because relationships and events that are occurring may be deemed more important than being on time.
   3. Members are comfortable with close personal space when interacting with family and friends.

D. Social roles
   1. Large extended family networks are important; older adults are respected.
   2. Many households may be headed by a single-parent woman.
   3. Religious **beliefs** and church affiliation are sources of strength.

Box 6-1 Religions and Dietary Preferences

Seventh Day Adventist (Church of God)
Alcohol and caffeinated beverages are usually prohibited.
Many are lacto-ovovegetarians; those who eat meat avoid pork.
Overeating is prohibited; 5 to 6 hours between meals without snacking is practiced.

Buddhism
Alcohol is usually prohibited.
Many are lacto-ovovegetarians.
Some eat fish, and some avoid only beef.

Roman Catholicism
They avoid meat on Ash Wednesday and Fridays of Lent.
They practice optional fasting during Lent season.
Children, pregnant women, and ill individuals are exempt from fasting.

Church of Jesus Christ of Latter-Day Saints (Mormon)
Alcohol, coffee, and tea are usually prohibited.
Consumption of meat is limited.
The first Sunday of the month is optional for fasting.

Hinduism
Many are vegetarians; those who eat meat do not eat beef or pork.
Fasting rituals vary.
Children are not allowed to participate in fasting.

Islam
Pork, birds of prey, alcohol, and any meat product not ritually slaughtered are prohibited.

During the month of Ramadan, fasting occurs during the daytime.

Jehovah's Witness
Any foods to which blood has been added are prohibited.
They can eat animal flesh that has been drained.

Judaism
Orthodox believers need to adhere to dietary kosher laws:
- Meats allowed include animals that are vegetable eaters, cloven-hoofed animals, and animals that are ritually slaughtered.
- Fish that have scales and fins are allowed.
- Any combination of meat and milk is prohibited.

During Yom Kippur, 24-hour fasting is observed.
Pregnant women and seriously ill individuals are exempt from fasting.
During Passover, only unleavened bread is eaten.

Pentecostal (Assembly of God)
Alcohol is usually prohibited.
Members avoid consumption of anything to which blood has been added.
Some individuals avoid pork.

Eastern Orthodox
During Lent, all animal products, including dairy products, are forbidden.
Fasting occurs during Advent.
Exceptions from fasting include illness and pregnancy.

E. Health and illness
   1. Religious **beliefs** profoundly affect ideas about health and illness.
   2. Food preferences include such items as fried foods, chicken, pork, greens, and rice; some pregnant African-American women engage in pica.

F. Health risks
   1. Sickle cell anemia
   2. Hypertension
   3. Heart disease
   4. Cancer
   5. Lactose intolerance
   6. Diabetes mellitus
   7. Obesity

G. Interventions
   1. Assess each individual for cultural preferences because there are many individual and **subculture** variations.
   2. Build a relationship based on trust.
   3. Assess the meaning of the client's verbal and nonverbal behavior.
   4. Be flexible and avoid rigidity in scheduling care.
   5. Encourage family involvement.
   6. Alternative modes of healing include herbs, prayer, and laying on of hands practices.

⚠ Learn about the cultures of clients with whom you will be working; also, ask clients about their health care practices and preferences.

II. AMISH

A. Description: The Amish are known for simple living, plain dress, and reluctance to adopt modern convenience and can be considered a distinct **ethnic group**; the various Amish church fellowships are Christian religious denominations that form a very traditional subgrouping of Mennonite churches. (See Box 6-2 for Amish communities.)

B. Cultural **beliefs** and preferences (Box 6-3)

⚠ Cultural beliefs and preferences vary depending on specific Amish community membership.

C. Interventions
   1. Assess each individual for cultural preferences because there may be individual and group variations.
   2. Speak to both the husband and the wife regarding health care decisions because they consider themselves partners in family life.

3. Health instructions must be given in simple, clear language.
4. Most Amish need to have church (bishop and community) permission to be hospitalized because the community will come together to help pay the costs.
5. Usually, Amish do not have health insurance because it is a "worldly product" and may show a lack of faith in God.

6. Barriers to modern health care include distance, lack of transportation, cost, and language (most do not understand scientific jargon).

⚠ Be alert to cues regarding eye contact, personal space, time concepts, and understanding of the recommended plan of care.

III. ASIAN AMERICANS

A. Description: Americans of Asian descent; can include **ethnic groups** such as Chinese Americans, Filipino Americans, Indian Americans, Vietnamese Americans, Korean Americans, Japanese Americans and others whose national origin is from the Asian continent.
B. Communication
   1. Languages include Chinese, Japanese, Korean, Filipino, Vietnamese, and English.
   2. Silence is valued.
   3. Eye contact may be considered inappropriate or disrespectful.
   4. Criticism or disagreement is not expressed verbally.
   5. Head nodding does not always mean agreement.
   6. The word "no" may be interpreted as disrespect for others.
C. Time orientation and personal space preferences
   1. Time orientation reflects respect for the past, but includes emphasis on the present and future.

Box 6-2 Amish Communities

Old Order Amish
Members live in rural communities in North America and are known for their plain dress and limited use of technology.

Amish Mennonites
This broad term is used for churches that split from the Old Order Amish; some have a lifestyle similar to the Old Order Amish, whereas others do not.

Beachy Amish
Members have fewer limits on the use of technology and do not shun those who join Mennonite churches.

New Order Amish
This is the least restrictive Amish group; the use of electricity in the home is permitted, and shunning is not practiced.

Box 6-3 Amish Cultural Beliefs and Preferences

Amish maintain a culture distinct and separate from the non-Amish.
They usually speak a German dialect called Pennsylvania Dutch.
German language is usually used during worship; English is usually learned in school.
Men follow the laws of the Hebrew Scriptures with regard to beards (mustaches are not grown because of the long-perceived association of mustaches with the military).
Men usually dress in a plain, dark-colored suit; women usually wear a plain dress with long sleeves, bonnet, and apron.
Women are not allowed to hold positions of power in the congregational organization.
Marriage outside the faith is usually not allowed.
Family life has a patriarchal structure.
Although the roles of women are considered equally important to those of men, they are very unequal in terms of authority.
Unmarried women remain under the authority of their fathers.
Wives are submissive to their husbands.
Amish generally remain separate from the rest of the world, physically and socially.
They reject materialism and worldliness.

Some Amish prefer not to be photographed.
They value living simply and may choose to avoid technology, such as electricity and cars.
Amish highly value responsibility, generosity, and helping others.
They often work as farmers, builders, quilters, and homemakers.
Some Amish use traditional health care and alternative health care measures and practices, such as healers, herbs, and massage.
They believe that health is a gift from God, but that clean living and a balanced diet help maintain it.
Amish have lower risk factors for disease than the general population because of their work in manual labor, consumption of fresh foods, and rare consumption of tobacco and alcohol.
Many choose not to have health insurance and maintain mutual aid funds for Amish members to help with medical costs.
Funerals are conducted in the home without a eulogy, flower decorations, or any other display; caskets are plain and simple without adornment.
At death, a woman is usually buried in her bridal dress.
One is believed to live on after death, either with eternal reward in heaven or punished in hell.

2. Formal personal space is preferred except with family and close friends.
3. Members usually do not touch others during conversation.
4. For some **cultures**, touching is unacceptable between members of the opposite gender.
5. The head is considered to be sacred in some **cultures**; touching someone on the head may be disrespectful.

D. Social roles
1. Members are devoted to tradition.
2. Large extended-family networks are common.
3. Loyalty to immediate and extended family and honor are valued.
4. Family unit is structured and hierarchical.
5. Men have the power and authority, and women are expected to be obedient.
6. Education is viewed as important.
7. Religions include Taoism, Buddhism, Confucianism, Shintoism, Hinduism, Islam, and Christianity.
8. Social organizations are strong within the community.

E. Health and illness
1. Health is a state of physical and spiritual harmony with nature and a balance between positive and negative energy forces (yin and yang).
2. A healthy body may be viewed as a gift from the ancestors.
3. Illness may be viewed as an imbalance between yin and yang.
4. Yin foods are cold and yang foods are hot; one eats cold foods when one has a hot illness, and one eats hot foods when one has a cold illness.
5. Illness may also be attributed to prolonged sitting or lying or to overexertion.
6. Food preferences include raw fish, rice, and vegetables.

F. Health risks
1. Hypertension
2. Heart disease
3. Cancer
4. Lactose intolerance
5. Thalassemia

G. Interventions
1. Assess each individual for cultural preferences because there are many individual and **subculture** variations.
2. Be aware of and respect physical boundaries; request permission to touch the client before doing so.
3. Limit eye contact.
4. Avoid gesturing with hands.
5. If possible, a female client prefers a female health care provider.
6. Clarify responses to questions and expectations of the health care provider.

7. Be flexible and avoid rigidity in scheduling care.
8. Encourage family involvement.
9. Alternative modes of healing include herbs, acupuncture, restoration of balance with foods, massage, and offering of prayers and incense.

⚠ If health care recommendations, interventions, or treatments do not fit within the client's cultural values, they will not be followed.

IV. HISPANIC AND LATINO AMERICANS

A. Description: Americans of origins in Latin countries; Mexican Americans, Cuban Americans, Colombian Americans, Dominican Americans, Puerto Rican Americans, Spanish Americans, and Salvadoran Americans are some Hispanic and Latino American subgroups.

B. Communication
1. Languages include primarily English and Spanish.
2. Members tend to be verbally expressive, yet confidentiality is important.
3. Avoiding eye contact with a person in authority may indicate respect and attentiveness.
4. Direct confrontation is usually disrespectful and the expression of negative feelings may be impolite.
5. Dramatic body language, such as gestures or facial expressions, may be used to express emotion or pain.

C. Time orientation and personal space preferences
1. Members are usually oriented more to the present.
2. Members may be late for an appointment because relationships and events that are occurring are valued more than being on time.
3. Members are comfortable in close proximity with family, friends, and acquaintances.
4. Members are very tactile and use embraces and handshakes.
5. Members value the physical presence of others.
6. Politeness and modesty are important.

D. Social roles
1. The nuclear family is the basic unit; also, large, extended-family networks are common.
2. The extended family is highly regarded.
3. Needs of the family take precedence over the needs of an individual family member.
4. Depending on age and **acculturation** factors, men are usually the decision makers and wage earners, and women are the caretakers and homemakers.
5. Religion usually is Catholicism, but may vary depending on origin.
6. Members usually have strong church affiliations.
7. Social organizations are strong within the community.

E. Health and illness
  1. Health may be viewed as a reward from God or a result of good luck.
  2. Some members believe that health results from a state of physical and emotional balance.
  3. Illness may be viewed by some members to be a result of God's punishment for sins.
  4. Some members may adhere to nontraditional health measures such as folk medicine.

F. Health risks
  1. Hypertension
  2. Heart disease
  3. Diabetes mellitus
  4. Obesity
  5. Lactose intolerance
  6. Parasites

G. Interventions
  1. Assess each individual for cultural preferences because there are many individual and **subculture** variations.
  2. Allow time for the client to discuss treatment options with family members.
  3. Protect privacy.
  4. Offer to call clergy because of the significance of religious preferences related to illnesses.
  5. Ask permission before touching a child when planning to examine or care for him or her.
  6. Be flexible regarding time of arrival for appointments and avoid rigidity in scheduling care.
  7. Alternative modes of healing include herbs, consultation with lay healers, restoration of balance with hot or cold foods, prayer, and religious medals.

  ⚠ Treat each client and individuals accompanying the client with respect and appreciate the differences and diversity of beliefs about health, illness, and treatment modalities.

V. NATIVE AMERICANS

A. Description: term that the U.S. government uses to describe indigenous peoples from the regions of North America encompassed by the continental United States, including parts of Alaska and the island state of Hawaii; comprise a large number of distinct tribes, states, and **ethnic groups**, many of which survive as intact political communities.

B. Communication
  1. There is much linguistic diversity, depending on origin.
  2. Silence indicates respect for the speaker for some groups.
  3. Some members may speak in a low tone of voice and expect others to be attentive.
  4. Eye contact may be viewed as a sign of disrespect.
  5. Body language is important.

C. Time orientation and personal space preferences
  1. Members are oriented primarily to the present.
  2. Personal space is important.
  3. Members may lightly touch another person's hand during greetings.
  4. Massage may be used for newborn to promote bonding between the infant and mother.
  5. Some groups may prohibit touching of a dead body.

D. Social roles
  1. Members are family oriented.
  2. Basic family unit is the extended family, which often includes persons from several households.
  3. In some groups, grandparents are viewed as family leaders.
  4. Elders are honored.
  5. Children are taught to respect traditions.
  6. The father usually does all the work outside the home, and the mother assumes responsibility for domestic duties.
  7. Sacred myths and legends provide spiritual guidance for some groups.
  8. Most members adhere to some form of Christianity, and religion and healing practices are usually integrated.
  9. Community social organizations are important.

E. Health and illness
  1. Health is usually considered a state of harmony between the individual, family, and environment.
  2. Some groups believe that illness is caused by supernatural forces and disequilibrium between the person and environment.
  3. Traditional health and illness **beliefs** may continue to be observed by some groups, including natural and religious folk medicine tradition.
  4. For some groups, food preferences include cornmeal, fish, game, fruits, and berries.

F. Health risks
  1. Alcohol abuse
  2. Obesity
  3. Heart disease
  4. Diabetes mellitus
  5. Tuberculosis
  6. Arthritis
  7. Lactose intolerance
  8. Gallbladder disease

G. Interventions
  1. Assess each individual for cultural preferences because there may be individual variations.
  2. Clarify communication.
  3. Understand that the client may be attentive, even when eye contact is absent.
  4. Be attentive to your own use of body language.
  5. Obtain input from members of the extended family.
  6. Encourage the client to personalize space in which health care is delivered; for example, encourage the client to bring personal items or objects to the hospital.

7. In the home, assess for the availability of running water, and modify infection control and hygiene practices as necessary.

8. Alternative modes of healing include herbs, restoration of balance between the person and the universe, and consultation with traditional healers.

⚠ If language barriers pose a problem, seek a qualified medical interpreter; avoid using ancillary staff or family members as interpreters.

VI. WHITE AMERICANS

A. Description: term used to include U.S. citizens or residents having origins in any of the original people of Europe, the Middle East, or North Africa; the term is interchangeable with Caucasian American.

B. Communication
1. Languages include language of origin (e.g., Italian, Polish, French, Russian) and English.
2. Silence can be used to show respect or disrespect for another, depending on the situation.
3. Eye contact is usually viewed as indicating trustworthiness in most origins.

C. Time orientation and personal space preferences
1. Members are usually future oriented.
2. Time is valued; members tend to be on time and to be impatient with people who are not on time.
3. Some members may tend to avoid close physical contact.
4. Handshakes are usually used for formal greetings.

D. Social roles
1. The nuclear family is the basic unit; the extended family is also important.
2. The man is usually the dominant figure, but a variation of gender roles exists within families and relationships.
3. Religions are varied, depending on origin.
4. Community social organizations are important.

E. Health and illness
1. Health is usually viewed as an absence of disease or illness.
2. Many members usually have a tendency to be stoical when expressing physical concerns.
3. Members usually rely primarily on the modern Western health care delivery system.
4. Food preferences are based on origin; many members prefer items containing carbohydrates and red meat items.

F. Health risks
1. Cancer
2. Heart disease
3. Diabetes mellitus
4. Obesity
5. Hypertension

G. Interventions
1. Assess each individual for cultural preferences based on origin.
2. Build a relationship based on trust.
3. Assess the meaning of the client's verbal and nonverbal behavior.
4. Respect the client's personal space and time.
5. Be flexible and avoid rigidity in scheduling care.
6. Encourage family involvement.

VII. END-OF-LIFE CARE (Box 6-4)

A. Christian Science religion is unlikely to use medical means to prolong life.

B. People in the Jewish faith generally oppose prolonging life after irreversible brain damage.

C. Eastern Orthodox religions, Muslims, and Orthodox Jews may prohibit, oppose, or discourage autopsy.

D. Muslims prohibit organ donation.

E. Amish permit organ donation with the exception of heart transplants (the heart is the soul of the body).

F. Buddhists in the United States encourage organ donation and consider it an act of mercy.

G. Mormon, Eastern Orthodox, Islamic, and Jewish (Conservative and Orthodox) faiths discourage, oppose, or prohibit cremation.

H. Hindus prefer cremation and cast the ashes in a holy river.

I. Hispanic and Latino groups
1. The family generally makes decisions and may request to withhold the diagnosis or prognosis from the client.
2. Extended-family members often are involved in end-of-life care (pregnant women may be prohibited from caring for dying clients or attending funerals).
3. Several family members may be at the dying client's bedside.
4. Vocal expression of grief and mourning are acceptable and expected.
5. Members refuse procedures that alter the body, such as organ donation or autopsy.
6. Dying at home may be considered bad luck.

J. African Americans
1. Members discuss issues with the spouse or older family member (elders are held in high respect).
2. Family is highly valued and is central to the care of terminally ill members.
3. Open displays of emotion are common and accepted.
4. Organ and blood donation usually are not allowed.
5. Members prefer to die at home.

K. Asian Americans
1. Family members may make decisions about care and often do not tell the client the diagnosis or prognosis.

Box 6-4 Religion and End-of-Life Care

Christianity

Catholic and Orthodox
A priest anoints the sick.
Other sacraments before death include reconciliation and holy communion.

Protestant
No last rites are provided (anointing of the sick is accepted by some groups).
Prayers are given to offer comfort and support.

Church of Jesus Christ of Latter-Day Saints (Mormons)
A sacrament may be administered if the client requests.

Jehovah's Witness
Members do not believe in sacraments.
Members are excommunicated if they receive a blood transfusion.

Amish
Funerals are conducted in the home without a eulogy, flower decorations, or any other display; caskets are plain and simple, without adornment.
At death, a woman is usually buried in her bridal dress.
One is believed to live on after death, either with eternal reward in heaven or punished in hell.

Islam
Second-degree male relatives such as cousins or uncles should be the contact person and determine whether the client or family should be given information about the client.

The client may choose to face Mecca (west or southwest in the United States).
The head should be elevated above the body.
Discussions about death usually are not welcomed.
Stopping medical treatment is against the will of Allah (Arabic word for God).
Grief may be expressed through slapping or hitting the body.
If possible, only a same-gender Muslim should handle the body after death; if not possible, non-Muslims should wear gloves so as not to touch the body.

Judaism
Prolongation of life is important (a client on life support must remain so until death).
A dying person should not be left alone (a rabbi's presence is desired).
Autopsy and cremation are forbidden.

Hinduism
Rituals include tying a thread around the neck or wrist of the dying person, sprinkling the person with special water, and placing a leaf of basil on their tongue.
After death, the sacred threads are not removed, and the body is not washed.

Buddhism
A shrine to Buddha may be placed in the client's room.
Time for meditation at the shrine is important and should be respected.
Clients may refuse medications that may alter their awareness (e.g., opioids).
After death, a monk may recite prayers for 1 hour (need not be done in the presence of the body).

---

2. Dying at home may be considered bad luck.
3. Organ donation is usually not allowed.
L. Native Americans
1. Family meetings may be held to make decisions about end-of-life and the type of treatments that should be pursued.
2. Some groups avoid contact with the dying (may prefer to die in the hospital).

⚠ Provide individualized end-of-life care to client and families.

VIII. COMPLEMENTARY AND ALTERNATIVE MEDICINE (CAM)

A. Description
1. Therapies are used in addition to conventional treatment to provide healing resources and focus on the mind-body connection.
2. High-risk therapies (therapies that are invasive) and low-risk therapies (those that are noninvasive) are included in CAM.
3. The National Center for Complementary and Alternative Medicine (NCCAM) has proposed

Box 6-5 Categories of Complementary and Alternative Medicine (CAM)

Whole medical systems
Mind-body medicine
Biologically based practices
Manipulative and body-based practices
Energy medicine

a classification system that includes five categories of complementary and alternative types of therapy (Box 6-5).
B. Whole medical systems
1. Traditional Chinese medicine (TCM): Focuses on restoring and maintaining a balanced flow of vital energy; interventions include acupressure, acupuncture, herbal therapies, diet, meditation, tai chi, and qi gong (exercise that focuses on breathing, visualization, and movement).
2. Ayurveda: Focuses on the balance of mind, body, and spirit; interventions include diet, medicinal herbs, detoxification, massage, breathing exercises, meditation, and yoga.

Box 6-6 Biologically Based Practices

Aromatherapy
The use of topical or inhaled oils (plant extracts) that promote and maintain health

Herbal Therapies
The use of herbs derived mostly from plant sources that maintain and restore balance and health

Macrobiotic Diet
Diet high in whole-grain cereals, vegetables, beans, sea vegetables, and vegetarian soups
Elimination of meat, animal fat, eggs, poultry, dairy products, sugars, and artificially produced food from the diet

Orthomolecular Therapy
Focus on nutritional balance, including use of vitamins, essential amino acids, essential fats, and minerals

Box 6-7 Commonly Used Herbs and Health Products

Aloe: Anti-inflammatory and antimicrobial effect; accelerates wound healing
Angelica: Antispasmodic and vasodilator; balances the effects of estrogen
Bilberry: Improves microcirculation in the eyes
Black cohosh: Produces estrogen-like effects
Cat's claw: Antioxidant; stimulates the immune system, lowers blood pressure
Chamomile: Antispasmodic and anti-inflammatory; produces mild sedative effect
Dehydroepiandrosterone (DHEA): Converts to androgens and estrogen; slows the effects of aging; used for erectile dysfunction
Echinacea: Stimulates immune system
Evening primrose: Assists with metabolism of fatty acid
Feverfew: Anti-inflammatory; used for migraine headaches, arthritis, and fever
Garlic: Antioxidant; used to lower cholesterol levels
Ginger: Antiemetic; used for nausea and vomiting
Ginkgo biloba: Antioxidant; used to improve memory
Ginseng: Increases physical endurance and stamina; used for stress and fatigue
Glucosamine: Amino acid that assists in the synthesis of cartilage
Goldenseal: Anti-inflammatory and antimicrobial used to stimulate the immune system; has an anticoagulant effect and may increase blood pressure
Kava: Antianxiety and skeletal muscle relaxant; produces a sedative effect
Melatonin: A hormone that regulates sleep; used for insomnia
Milk thistle: Antioxidant; stimulates the production of new liver cells, reduces liver inflammation; used for liver and gallbladder disease
Peppermint oil: Antispasmodic; used for irritable bowel syndrome
St. John's wort: Antibacterial, antiviral, antidepressant
Saw palmetto: Antiestrogen activity; used for urinary tract infections and benign prostatic hypertrophy
Valerian: Used to treat nervous disorders such as anxiety, restlessness, and insomnia
Zinc: Antiviral; stimulates the immune system

3. Homeopathy: Focuses on healing and interventions consisting of small doses of specially prepared plant and mineral extracts that assist in the innate healing process of the body.
4. Naturopathy: Focuses on enhancing the natural healing responses of the body; interventions include nutrition, herbology, hydrotherapy, acupuncture, physical therapies, and counseling.

C. Mind-body medicine
1. Mind-body medicine focuses on the interactions among the brain, mind, body, and behavior and on the powerful ways in which emotional, mental, social, spiritual, and behavioral factors can directly affect health.
2. Interventions include biofeedback, hypnosis, relaxation therapy, meditation, visual imagery, yoga, tai chi, qi gong, cognitive-behavioral therapies, group supports, autogenic training, and spirituality.

D. Biologically based practices (Box 6-6)
1. Biologically based therapies in CAM use substances found in nature, such as herbs, foods, and vitamins.
2. Therapies include botanicals, prebiotics and probiotics, whole-food diets, functional foods, animal-derived extracts, vitamins, minerals, fatty acids, amino acids, and proteins.

E. Manipulative and body-based practices
1. Interventions involve manipulation and movement of the body by a therapist.
2. Interventions include practices such as chiropractic and osteopathic manipulation, massage therapy, and reflexology.

F. Energy medicine
1. Energy therapies focus on energy originating within the body or on energy from other sources.
2. Interventions include sound energy therapy, light therapy, acupuncture, qi gong, reiki and johre, therapeutic touch, intercessory prayer, whole medical systems, and magnetic therapy.

IX. HERBAL THERAPIES (Box 6-7)

A. Herbal therapy is the use of herbs (plant or a plant part) for the therapeutic value on health.
B. Some herbs have been determined to be safe, but some herbs, even in small amounts, can be toxic.
C. If the client is taking prescription medications, the client should consult with the health care provider regarding the use of herbs because serious herb-medication interactions can occur.
D. Client teaching points
1. Discuss herbal therapies with the health care provider before use.

2. Contact the physician if any side effects of the herbal substance occur.
3. Contact the health care provider before stopping the use of a prescription medication.
4. Avoid using herbs to treat a serious medical condition such as heart disease.
5. Avoid taking herbs if pregnant or attempting to get pregnant or if nursing.
6. Do not give herbs to infants or young children.
7. Purchase herbal supplements only from a reputable manufacturer; the label should contain the scientific name of the herb, name and address of the manufacturer, batch or lot number, date of manufacture, and expiration date.
8. Adhere to the recommended dose; if herbal preparations are taken in high doses, they can be toxic.
9. Moisture, sunlight, and heat may alter the components of herbal preparations.
10. If surgery is planned, the herbal therapy may need to be discontinued 2 to 3 weeks before surgery.

⚠ Some herbs have been determined to be safe, but some herbs, even in small amounts, can be toxic. Inform the client to discuss herbal therapies with the health care provider before use.

X. LOW-RISK THERAPIES

A. Low-risk therapies are therapies that have no adverse effects and, when implementing care, can be used by the nurse who has training and experience in their use.
B. Common low-risk therapies
1. Meditation
2. Relaxation techniques
3. Imagery
4. Music therapy
5. Massage
6. Touch
7. Laughter and humor
8. Spiritual measures, such as prayer

💿 MORE QUESTIONS ON THE CD!

Practice Questions

1. An ambulatory care nurse is discussing preoperative procedures with a Japanese American client who is scheduled for surgery the following week. During the discussion, the client continually smiles and nods the head. The nurse interprets this nonverbal behavior as:
   1. Reflecting a cultural value
   2. An acceptance of the treatment
   3. The client is agreeable to the required procedures.
   4. The client understands the preoperative procedures.

2. When communicating with a client who speaks a different language, the best practice for a nurse is to:
   1. Speak loudly and slowly.
   2. Stand close to the client and speak loudly.
   3. Arrange for an interpreter when communicating with the client.
   4. Speak to the client and family together to increase the chances that the topic will be understood.

3. A nurse educator is providing in-service education to the nursing staff regarding transcultural nursing care; a staff member asks the nurse educator to describe the concept of acculturation. Which of the following is the appropriate response?
   1. "It is a subjective perspective of the person's heritage and a sense of belonging to a group."
   2. "It is a process of learning a different culture to adapt to a new or changing environment."
   3. "It is a group of individuals in a society who are culturally distinct and have a unique identity."
   4. "It is a group that shares some of the characteristics of the larger population group of which it is a part."

4. A nurse is providing discharge instructions to a Chinese-American client regarding prescribed dietary modifications. During the teaching session, the client continuously turns away from the nurse. The nurse should implement which appropriate action?
   1. Continue with the instructions, verifying client understanding.
   2. Walk around the client so that the nurse constantly faces the client.
   3. Give the client a dietary booklet and return later to continue with the instructions.
   4. Tell the client about the importance of the instructions for the maintenance of health care.

5. A nurse educator asks a student to list the five categories of complementary and alternative medicine (CAM), developed by the National Center for Complementary and Alternative Medicine (NCCAM). Which of the following, if stated by the nursing student, would indicate an understanding of the five categories of CAM?
   1. Herbology, hydrotherapy, acupuncture, nutrition, and chiropractic care
   2. Mind-body medicine, traditional Chinese medicine, homeopathy, naturopathy, and healing touch
   3. Biologically based practices, body-based practices, magnetic therapy, massage therapy, and aromatherapy
   4. Whole medical systems, mind-body medicine, biologically based practices, manipulative and body-based practices, and energy medicine

6. Which of the following clients has the lowest risk of obesity and diabetes mellitus?
   1. A 45-year-old Native-American man
   2. A 23-year-old Asian-American woman
   3. A 35-year-old Hispanic-American man
   4. A 40-year-old African-American woman

7. A nurse is preparing a plan of care for a client who is a Jehovah's Witness. The client has been told that surgery is necessary. The nurse considers the client's religious preferences in developing the plan of care and documents that:
   1. Religious sacraments are important.
   2. Medication administration is not allowed.
   3. Surgery is prohibited in this religious group.
   4. The administration of blood and blood products is forbidden.

8. Which of the following meal trays would be appropriate for a nurse to deliver to a client of Orthodox Judaism faith who follows a kosher diet?
   1. Pork roast, rice, vegetables, mixed fruit, milk
   2. Crab salad on a croissant, vegetables with dip, potato salad, milk
   3. Sweet and sour chicken with rice and vegetables, mixed fruit, juice
   4. Fettuccini Alfredo with shrimp and vegetables, salad, mixed fruit, iced tea

9. An Asian-American client is experiencing a fever. A nurse recognizes that the client is likely to self-treat the disorder with:
   1. Magnetic therapy
   2. Intercessory prayer
   3. Foods considered to be yin
   4. Foods considered to be yang

10. The role of a nurse regarding complementary and alternative medicine (CAM) should include:

   1. Advising the client about "good" versus "bad" therapies
   2. Recommending herbal remedies that the client should use
   3. Discouraging the client from using any alternative therapies
   4. Educating the client about therapies that he or she is using or is interested in using

11. An antihypertensive medication has been prescribed for a client with hypertension. The client tells a clinic nurse that she would like to take an herbal substance to help lower her blood pressure. The nurse should take which appropriate action?
   1. Tell the client that herbal substances are not safe and should never be used.
   2. Encourage the client to discuss the use of an herbal substance with the physician.
   3. Teach the client how to take her blood pressure so that it can be monitored closely.
   4. Tell the client that if she takes the herbal substance she will need to have her blood pressure checked frequently.

Alternate Item Format: Multiple Response

12. A nurse describes low-risk therapies to a client and includes which of the following in the discussion? **Select all that apply.**
    ❑ 1. Herbs
    ❑ 2. Prayer
    ❑ 3. Touch
    ❑ 4. Massage
    ❑ 5. Relaxation
    ❑ 6. Acupuncture

ANSWERS
1. 1
Rationale: Nodding or smiling by a Japanese-American client may reflect only the cultural value of interpersonal harmony. This nonverbal behavior may not be an indication of agreement with the speaker, an acceptance of the treatment, or an understanding of the procedure.
Test-Taking Strategy: Use the process of elimination. Eliminate options 2 and 3 first because they are comparable or alike. From the remaining options, select option 1 because it is characteristic of Asian-American cultures. In addition, option 4 is an incorrect interpretation of the client's nonverbal behavior. Review the cultural characteristics of the Japanese-American population if you had difficulty with this question.
Level of Cognitive Ability: Understanding
Client Needs: Psychosocial Integrity

Integrated Process: Nursing Process—Evaluation
Content Area: Fundamental Skills—Cultural Diversity
Reference: Giger, J., & Davidhizar, R. (2008). *Transcultural nursing assessment and intervention* (5th ed., p. 15). St. Louis: Mosby.

2. 3
Rationale: Arranging for an interpreter would be the best practice when communicating with a client who speaks a different language. Options 1 and 2 are inappropriate and are ineffective ways in which to communicate. Option 4 is inappropriate because it violates privacy and does not ensure correct translation.
Test-Taking Strategy: Note the strategic words *best practice* in the question. Eliminate option 4 first because it violates the client's right to privacy. Next, eliminate options 1 and 2 noting the word *loudly* in these options and because they are

nontherapeutic actions. Review the best communication techniques for a client who speaks a different language if you had difficulty with this question.
Level of Cognitive Ability: Applying
Client Needs: Psychosocial Integrity
Integrated Process: Communication and Documentation
Content Area: Fundamental Skills—Cultural Diversity
References: Jarvis, C. (2008). *Physical examination and health assessment* (5th ed., pp. 71–72). St. Louis: Saunders.

Lewis, S., Heitkemper, M., Dirksen, S., & Bucher, L. (2007). *Medical-surgical nursing: Assessment and management of clinical problems* (7th ed., p. 36). St. Louis: Mosby.

3. 2
Rationale: Acculturation is a process of learning a different culture to adapt to a new or changing environment. Option 1 describes ethnic identity. Option 3 describes an ethnic group. Option 4 describes a subculture.
Test-Taking Strategy: Focus on the subject, acculturation. Think about the definition of acculturation to help direct you to option 2. Review the definition of acculturation if you had difficulty with this question.
Level of Cognitive Ability: Applying
Client Needs: Psychosocial Integrity
Integrated Process: Teaching and Learning
Content Area: Fundamental Skills—Cultural Diversity
Reference: Jarvis, C. (2008). *Physical examination and health assessment* (5th ed., p. 40). St. Louis: Saunders.

4. 1
Rationale: Most Chinese Americans maintain a formal distance with others, which is a form of respect. Many Chinese Americans are uncomfortable with face-to-face communications, especially when eye contact is direct. If the client turns away from the nurse during a conversation, the most appropriate action is to continue with the conversation. Walking around to the client so that the nurse faces the client is in direct conflict with the cultural practice. The client may consider it a rude gesture if the nurse returns later to continue with the explanation. Telling the client about the importance of the instructions for the maintenance of health care may be viewed as degrading.
Test-Taking Strategy: Eliminate options 3 and 4 first because these actions are nontherapeutic. To select from the remaining options, think about the cultural practices of Chinese Americans and recall that direct eye contact is uncomfortable for the client. Option 1 is the appropriate action. If you had difficulty with this question, review the communication practices of this cultural group.
Level of Cognitive Ability: Applying
Client Needs: Psychosocial Integrity
Integrated Process: Nursing Process—Implementation
Content Area: Fundamental Skills—Cultural Diversity
Reference: Jarvis, C. (2008). *Physical examination and health assessment* (5th ed., p. 73). St. Louis: Saunders.

5. 4
Rationale: The five categories of complementary and alternative medicine (CAM) include whole medical systems, mind-body medicine, biologically based practices, manipulative and body-based practices, and energy medicine. The other options contain therapies within each category of CAM.

Test-Taking Strategy: Focus on the subject of the question. Noting that the question asks about categories, not therapies, will assist in directing you to option 4. Review the categories of CAM if you had difficulty with this question.
Level of Cognitive Ability: Understanding
Client Needs: Physiological Integrity
Integrated Process: Teaching and Learning
Content Area: Fundamental Skills—Cultural Diversity
Reference: Potter, P., & Perry, A. (2009). *Fundamentals of nursing* (7th ed., p. 774). St. Louis: Mosby.

6. 2
Rationale: From the options provided, Asian Americans have the lowest risk of obesity and diabetes mellitus. Because of their health and dietary practices, Native Americans, African Americans, and Hispanic Americans have a high risk of obesity and diabetes mellitus.
Test-Taking Strategy: Note the strategic words *lowest risk, obesity,* and *diabetes mellitus.* Think about the health and dietary practices of each cultural group to direct you to option 2. If you had difficulty with this question, review the characteristics of the Asian-American culture.
Level of Cognitive Ability: Understanding
Client Needs: Health Promotion and Maintenance
Integrated Process: Nursing Process—Assessment
Content Area: Fundamental Skills—Cultural Diversity
Reference: Lewis, S., Heitkemper, M., Dirksen, S., & Bucher, L. (2007). *Medical-surgical nursing: Assessment and management of clinical problems* (7th ed., p. 972). St. Louis: Mosby.

7. 4
Rationale: Among Jehovah's Witnesses, surgery is not prohibited, but the administration of blood and blood products is forbidden. This religious group does not believe in sacraments. Administration of medication is an acceptable practice except if the medication is derived from blood products.
Test-Taking Strategy: Focus on the religious group addressed in the question. Remember that the administration of blood and any associated blood products is forbidden in Jehovah's Witnesses. Review the characteristics of this religious group if you had difficulty with this question.
Level of Cognitive Ability: Applying
Client Needs: Psychosocial Integrity
Integrated Process: Communication and Documentation
Content Area: Fundamental Skills—Cultural Diversity
Reference: Lewis, S., Heitkemper, M., Dirksen, S., & Bucher, L. (2007). *Medical-surgical nursing: Assessment and management of clinical problems* (7th ed., p. 32). St. Louis: Mosby.

8. 3
Rationale: Orthodox Judaism believers adhere to dietary kosher laws. In this religion, the dairy-meat combination is unacceptable. Only fish that have scales and fins are allowed; meats that are allowed include animals that are vegetable eaters, cloven-hoofed, and ritually slaughtered.
Test-Taking Strategy: Use the process of elimination, recalling that the dairy-meat combination is unacceptable in this religious group. Eliminate option 1 because this option contains pork roast and milk. Next eliminate options 2 and 4 because both options contain shell fish. Review the dietary rules of this religious group if you had difficulty with this question.

Level of Cognitive Ability: Applying
Client Needs: Psychosocial Integrity
Integrated Process: Nursing Process—Implementation
Content Area: Fundamental Skills—Cultural Diversity
References: Giger, J., & Davidhizar, R. (2008). *Transcultural nursing assessment and intervention* (5th ed., p. 609). St. Louis: Mosby.

Potter, P., & Perry, A. (2009). *Fundamentals of nursing* (7th ed., p. 457). St. Louis: Mosby.

9. 3

Rationale: In the Asian-American culture, health is believed to be a state of physical and spiritual harmony with nature and a balance between positive and negative energy forces (yin and yang). Yin foods are cold and yang foods are hot. Cold foods are eaten when one has a hot illness (fever), and hot foods are eaten when one has a cold illness. Options 1 and 2 are not health practices specifically associated with the Asian-American culture or the yin and yang theory.
Test-Taking Strategy: Focus on the client's culture and the client's diagnosis, fever. Remember that cold foods (yin foods) are eaten when one has a hot illness, and hot foods (yang foods) are eaten when one has a cold illness. If you are unfamiliar with the yin and yang theory and the health practices of the Asian-American culture, review this information.
Level of Cognitive Ability: Understanding
Client Needs: Psychosocial Integrity
Integrated Process: Nursing Process—Evaluation
Content Area: Fundamental Skills—Cultural Diversity
References: Giger, J., & Davidhizar, R. (2008). *Transcultural nursing assessment and intervention* (5th ed., p. 460). St. Louis: Mosby.

Jarvis, C. (2008). *Physical examination and health assessment* (5th ed., p. 45). St. Louis: Saunders.

10. 4

Rationale: Complementary (alternative) therapies include a wide variety of treatment modalities that are used in addition to conventional therapy to treat a disease or illness. Educating the client about therapies that he or she uses or is interested in using is the nurse's role. Options 1, 2, and 3 are inappropriate actions for the nurse to take.
Test-Taking Strategy: Use therapeutic communication techniques. Eliminate options 1, 2, and 3 because they are nontherapeutic. Recommending an herbal remedy or discouraging a client from doing something is not within the role practices of the nurse. Additionally, it is nontherapeutic to advise a client to do something. Option 4 is the only option that is appropriate and therapeutic. Review therapeutic communication techniques and the nurse's role in educating clients about alternative therapies if you had difficulty with this question.
Level of Cognitive Ability: Applying
Client Needs: Physiological Integrity
Integrated Process: Nursing Process—Implementation
Content Area: Fundamental Skills—Cultural Diversity

Reference: Potter, P., & Perry, A. (2009). *Fundamentals of nursing* (7th ed., p. 772). St. Louis: Mosby.

11. 2

Rationale: Although herbal substances may have some beneficial effects, not all herbs are safe to use. Clients who are being treated with conventional medication therapy should be encouraged to avoid herbal substances with similar pharmacological effects because the combination may lead to an excessive reaction or to unknown interaction effects. The nurse would advise the client to discuss the use of the herbal substance with the physician. Options 1, 3, and 4 are inappropriate nursing actions.
Test-Taking Strategy: Use the process of elimination. Eliminate option 1 first because of the close-ended word *never*. Next, eliminate options 3 and 4 because they are comparable or alike and relate to blood pressure monitoring. Review the limitations associated with the use of herbal substances if you had difficulty with this question.
Level of Cognitive Ability: Applying
Client Needs: Physiological Integrity
Integrated Process: Nursing Process—Implementation
Content Area: Fundamental Skills—Cultural Diversity
References: Lewis, S., Heitkemper, M., Dirksen, S., & Bucher, L. (2007). *Medical-surgical nursing: Assessment and management of clinical problems* (7th ed., p. 101). St. Louis: Mosby.

Potter, P., & Perry, A. (2009). *Fundamentals of nursing* (7th ed., pp. 781–783). St. Louis: Mosby.

ALTERNATE ITEM FORMAT: MULTIPLE RESPONSE

12. 2, 3, 4, 5

Rationale: Low-risk therapies are therapies that have no adverse effects and, when implementing care, can be used by a nurse who has training and experience in their use. Low-risk therapies include meditation, relaxation techniques, imagery, music therapy, massage, touch, laughter and humor, and spiritual measures, such as prayer. The other options are not considered low-risk therapies.
Test-Taking Strategy: Focus on the strategic words *low-risk*. Recalling that low-risk therapies are therapies that are noninvasive and that have no adverse effects and can be used by a nurse who has training and experience will direct you to the correct options. Review complementary and alternative medicine (CAM) and low-risk therapies if you had difficulty with this question.
Level of Cognitive Ability: Understanding
Client Needs: Physiological Integrity
Integrated Process: Nursing Process—Implementation
Content Area: Fundamental Skills—Cultural Diversity
References: Lewis, S., Heitkemper, M., Dirksen, S., & Bucher, L. (2007). *Medical-surgical nursing: Assessment and management of clinical problems* (7th ed., pp. 97–98). St. Louis: Mosby.

Potter, P., & Perry, A. (2009). *Fundamentals of nursing* (7th ed., p. 774). St. Louis: Mosby.

Ethical and Legal Issues

PYRAMID TERMS

advance directive Written document recognized by state law that provides directions concerning the provision of care when a client is unable to make his or her own treatment choices; the two basic types of advance directives include living wills and durable powers of attorney.

advocacy Acting on the behalf of the client and protecting the client's rights to make his or her own decisions.

confidentiality/information security In the health care system, refers to the protection of privacy of the client's personal health information.

consent Voluntary act whereby a person agrees to allow someone else to do something.

ethics The ideals of right and wrong; guiding principles that individuals may use to make decisions.

HIPAA (Health Insurance Portability and Accountability Act) Federal law that establishes standards for the privacy and security of health information and a standard for electronic data interchange of health information.

informed consent A client's understanding of the reason for the proposed intervention, with its benefits and risks, and agreement with the treatment by signing a consent form.

law A system composed of general rules governing conduct and the procedures for resolving disputes when rules are not followed.

malpractice Type of negligence; failure to meet the standards of acceptable care, which results in harm to another person.

negligence Conduct that falls below a standard of care; failure to meet a client's needs either willfully or by omission or failure to act.

Patient's Bill of Rights The rights and responsibilities of clients receiving care.

values Beliefs and attitudes that may influence behavior and the process of decision making.

PYRAMID TO SUCCESS

Across all settings in the practice of nursing, nurses frequently are confronted with ethical and legal issues related to client care. The professional nurse has the responsibility to be aware of the ethical principles, laws, and guidelines related to providing safe and quality care to clients. In the Pyramid to Success, focus on ethical practices; the nurse practice act and client's rights, particularly confidentiality, information security, and informed consent; advocacy, documentation, and advance directives; and cultural, religious, and spiritual issues. Knowledgeable use of information technology, such as an electronic health record, is also an important role of the nurse.

CLIENT NEEDS

Safe and Effective Care Environment

Acting as an advocate
Advance directives documents
Confidentiality and information security issues related to the client's health care
Ensuring client rights
Establishing priorities
Ethical practice in health care
Issues surrounding informed consent
Legal responsibilities and information technology related to client care
Quality improvement procedures
Resource management
Use of information technology

Health Promotion and Maintenance

Developmental stages and transitions
High-risk behaviors of the client
Lifestyle choices of the client

Psychosocial Integrity

Abuse and neglect issues
Available support systems
Chemical or other dependencies
Coping mechanisms
Cultural, spiritual, and religious issues
End-of-life care and grief and loss

Physiological Integrity

Alterations in body systems
Palliative and comfort care for the client
Unexpected responses to therapies

I. ETHICS

A. Description: The branch of philosophy concerned with the distinction between right and wrong based on a body of knowledge, not based only on opinions
B. Morality: Behavior in accordance with customs or tradition, usually reflecting personal or religious beliefs
C. Ethical principles: Codes that direct or govern nursing actions (Box 7-1)
D. **Values**: Beliefs and attitudes that may influence behavior and the process of decision making
E. **Values** clarification: Process of analyzing one's own **values** to understand oneself more completely regarding what is truly important
F. Ethical codes
   1. Ethical codes provide broad principles for determining and evaluating client care.
   2. These codes are not legally binding, but the board of nursing has authority in most states to reprimand nurses for unprofessional conduct that results from violation of the ethical codes.
   3. Specific ethical codes are as follows:
      a. The Code for Nurses developed by the International Council of Nurses
      b. American Nurses Association Code of Ethics (Box 7-2)
G. Ethical dilemma
   1. An ethical dilemma occurs when there is a conflict between two or more ethical principles.
   2. No correct decision exists, and the nurse must make a choice between two alternatives that are equally unsatisfactory.
   3. Such dilemmas may occur as a result of differences in cultural or religious beliefs.
   4. Ethical reasoning is the process of thinking through what one should do in an orderly and systematic manner to provide justification for actions based on principles; the nurse should gather all information to determine if an ethical dilemma exists, examine his or her own values, verbalize the problem, consider possible courses of action, negotiate the outcome, and evaluate the action taken.
H. Advocate
   1. An advocate is a person who speaks up for or acts on the behalf of the client, protects the client's right to make his or her own decisions, and upholds the principle of fidelity.

Box 7-1 Ethical Principles

Autonomy	Respect for an individual's right to self-determination
Nonmaleficence	The obligation to do or cause no harm to another
Beneficence	The duty to do good to others and to maintain a balance between benefits and harms; paternalism is an undesirable outcome of beneficence, in which the health care provider decides what is best for the client and encourages the client to act against his or her own choices
Justice	The equitable distribution of potential benefits and tasks determining the order in which clients should be cared for
Veracity	The obligation to tell the truth
Fidelity	The duty to do what one has promised

Box 7-2 American Nurses Association Code of Ethics

The nurse, in all professional relationships, practices with compassion and respect for the inherent dignity, worth, and uniqueness of every individual, unrestricted by considerations of social or economic status, personal attributes, or the nature of health problems.

The nurse's primary commitment is to the client, whether an individual, family, group, or community.

The nurse promotes, advocates for, and strives to protect the health, safety, and rights of the client.

The nurse is responsible and accountable for individual nursing practice and determines the appropriate delegation of tasks consistent with the nurse's obligation to provide optimum client care.

The nurse owes the same duties to self as to others, including the responsibility to preserve integrity and safety, to maintain competence, and to continue personal and professional growth.

The nurse participates in establishing, maintaining, and improving health care environments and conditions of employment conducive to the provision of quality health care and consistent with the values of the profession through individual and collective action.

The nurse participates in the advancement of the profession through contributions to practice, education, administration, and knowledge development.

The nurse collaborates with other health professionals and the public in promoting community, national, and international efforts to meet health needs.

The profession of nursing, as represented by associations and their members, is responsible for articulating nursing values, for maintaining the integrity of the profession and its practice, and for shaping social policy.

2. An advocate represents the client's viewpoint to others.
3. An advocate avoids letting personal **values** influence **advocacy** for the client and supports the client's decision, even when it conflicts with the advocate's own preferences or choices.

I. **Ethics** committees
   1. **Ethics** committees take a multidisciplinary approach to facilitate dialogue regarding ethical dilemmas.
   2. These committees develop and establish policies and procedures to facilitate the prevention and resolution of dilemmas.

⚠ An important nursing responsibility is to act as a client advocate and protect the client's rights.

II. REGULATION OF NURSING PRACTICE

A. Nurse practice act
   1. A nurse practice act is a series of statutes that have been enacted by each state legislature to regulate the practice of nursing in that state.
   2. Nurse practice acts set educational requirements for the nurse, distinguish between nursing practice and medical practice, and define the scope of nursing practice.
   3. Additional issues covered by nurse practice acts include licensure requirements for protection of the public, grounds for disciplinary action, rights of the nurse licensee if a disciplinary action is taken, and related topics.
   4. All nurses are responsible for knowing the provisions of the act of the state or province in which they work.

B. Standards of care
   1. Standards of care are guidelines that identify what the client can expect to receive in terms of nursing care.
   2. The guidelines determine whether nurses have performed duties in an appropriate manner.
   3. If a nurse does not perform duties within accepted standards of care, the nurse places himself or herself in jeopardy of legal action.
   4. If a nurse is named as a defendant in a **malpractice** lawsuit and proceedings show that the nurse followed neither the accepted standards of care outlined by the state or province nurse practice act nor the policies of the employing institution, the nurse's legal liability is clear; he or she is liable.

C. Employee guidelines
   1. Respondent superior: The employer is held liable for any negligent acts of an employee if the alleged negligent act occurred during the employment relationship and was within the scope of the employee's responsibilities.
   2. Contracts
      a. Nurses are responsible for carrying out the terms of a contractual agreement with the employing agency and the client.
      b. The nurse-employee relationship is governed by established employee handbooks and client care policies and procedures that create obligations, rights, and duties between those parties.
   3. Institutional policies
      a. Written policies and procedures of the employing institution detail how nurses are to perform their duties.
      b. Policies and procedures are usually specific and describe the expected behavior on the part of the nurse.
      c. Although policies are not **laws**, courts generally rule against nurses who violate policies.
      d. If the nurse practices nursing according to client care policies and procedures established by the employer, functions within the job responsibility, and provides care consistently in a non-negligent manner, the nurse minimizes the potential for liability.

⚠ The nurse must follow the guidelines identified in the nurse practice act and agency policies and procedures when delivering client care.

D. Hospital staffing
   1. Charges of abandonment may be made against nurses who "walk out" when staffing is inadequate.
   2. Nurses in short staffing situations are obligated to make a report to the nursing administration.

E. Floating
   1. Floating is an acceptable, legal practice used by health care facilities to alleviate understaffing and overstaffing.
   2. Legally, a nurse cannot refuse to float unless a union contract guarantees that nurses can work only in a specified area or the nurse can prove lack of knowledge for the performance of assigned tasks.
   3. Nurses in a floating situation must not assume responsibility beyond their level of experience or qualification.
   4. Nurses who float should inform the supervisor of any lack of experience in caring for the type of clients on the new nursing unit.
   5. The nurse should request and be given orientation to the new unit.

F. Disciplinary action
   1. Boards of nursing may deny, revoke, or suspend any license to practice as a registered nurse, according to their statutory authority.
   2. Some causes for disciplinary action are as follows:

a. Unprofessional conduct

b. Conduct that could affect the health and welfare of the public adversely

c. Breach of client **confidentiality**

d. Failure to use sufficient knowledge, skills, or nursing judgment

e. Physically or verbally abusing a client

f. Assuming duties without sufficient preparation

g. Knowingly delegating to unlicensed personnel nursing care that places the client at risk for injury

h. Failure to maintain an accurate record for each client

i. Falsifying a client's record

j. Leaving a nursing assignment without properly notifying appropriate personnel

III. LEGAL LIABILITY

A. Laws

1. Nurses are governed by civil and criminal **law** in roles as providers of services, employees of institutions, and private citizens.

2. A nurse has a personal and legal obligation to provide a standard of client care expected of a reasonably competent professional nurse.

3. Professional nurses are held responsible (liable) for harm resulting from their negligent acts or their failure to act.

B. Types of **laws** (Box 7-3; Fig. 7-1)

C. Negligence and **malpractice** (Box 7-4)

1. **Negligence** is conduct that falls below the standard of care.

2. **Negligence** can include acts of commission and acts of omission.

3. A nurse who does not meet appropriate standards of care may be held liable.

4. **Malpractice** is **negligence** on the part of a nurse.

5. **Malpractice** is determined if the nurse owed a duty to the client and did not carry out the duty and the client was injured because the nurse failed to perform the duty.

Box 7-3 Types of Law

Contract Law

Contract law is concerned with enforcement of agreements among private individuals.

Civil Law

Civil law is concerned with relationships among persons and the protection of a person's rights. Violation may cause harm to an individual or property, but no grave threat to society exists.

Criminal Law

Criminal law is concerned with relationships between individuals and governments, and with acts that threaten society and its order; a crime is an offense against society that violates a law and is defined as a misdemeanor (less serious nature) or felony (serious nature).

Tort Law

A tort is a civil wrong, other than a breach in contract, in which the law allows an injured person to seek damages from a person who caused the injury.

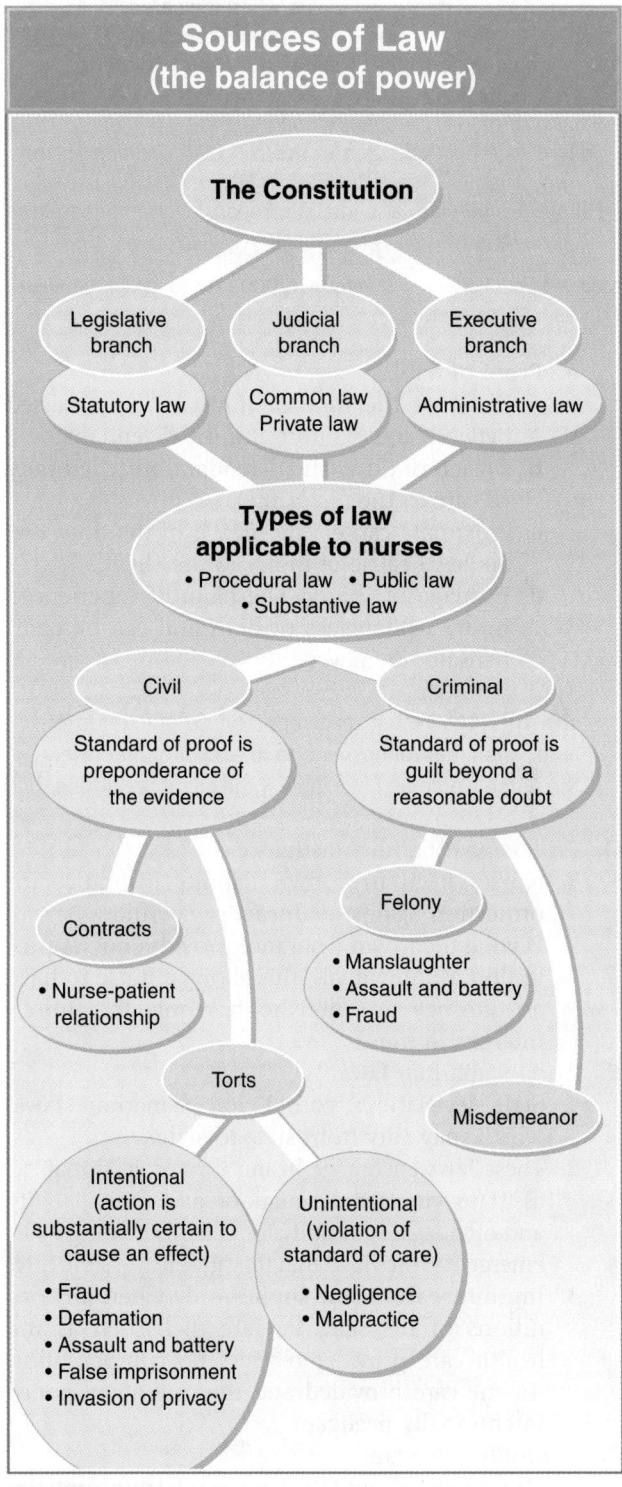

▲ **FIGURE 7-1** Sources of law for nursing practice. (From Harkreader, H., & Hogan, M.A. [2007]. *Fundamentals of nursing: Caring and clinical judgment.* [3rd ed.]. St. Louis: Saunders.)

Box 7-4 Negligent Acts

Medication errors that result in injury to the client
Intravenous administration errors such as incorrect flow rates or failure to monitor a flow rate that results in injury to the client
Falls that occur as a result of failure to provide safety to the client
Failure to use sterile technique when indicated
Failure to check equipment for proper functioning
Burns sustained by the client as a result of failure to monitor bath temperature or equipment
Failure to monitor a client's condition
Failure to report changes in the client's condition to the physician
Failure to provide a complete report to the oncoming nursing staff

Modified from Potter, P., & Perry, A. (2009). *Fundamentals of nursing* (7th ed.). St. Louis: Mosby.

6. Proof of liability
   a. Duty: At the time of injury, a duty existed between the plaintiff and the defendant.
   b. Breach of duty: The defendant breached duty of care to the plaintiff.
   c. Proximate cause: The breach of the duty was the legal cause of injury to the client.
   d. Damage or injury: The plaintiff experienced injury or damages or both and can be compensated by **law**.

⚠ The nurse must meet appropriate standards of care when delivering care to the client; otherwise the nurse would be held liable if the client is harmed.

D. Professional liability insurance
   1. Nurses need their own liability insurance for protection against **malpractice** lawsuits.
   2. Having their own insurance provides nurses protection as individuals; this allows a nurse to have an attorney present who has only the nurse's interests in mind.
E. Good Samaritan **laws**
   1. State legislatures pass Good Samaritan **laws**, which may vary from state to state.
   2. These **laws** encourage health care professionals to assist in emergency situations and limit liability and offer legal immunity for persons helping in an emergency, provided that they give reasonable care.
   3. Immunity from suit applies only when all conditions of the state **law** are met, such as the health care provider receives no compensation for the care provided and the care given is not intentionally negligent.
F. Controlled substances
   1. The nurse should adhere to facility policies and procedures concerning administration of controlled substances, which are governed by federal and state **laws**.

2. Controlled substances must be kept locked securely, and only authorized personnel should have access to them.

IV. COLLECTIVE BARGAINING

A. Collective bargaining is a formalized decision-making process between representatives of management and representatives of labor to negotiate wages and conditions of employment.
B. When collective bargaining breaks down because the parties cannot reach an agreement, the employees usually call a strike.
C. Striking presents a moral dilemma to many nurses because nursing practice is a service to people.
D. The United American Nurses (UAN) is an affiliate of the American Federation of Labor and Congress of Industrial Organizations (AFL-CIO) and the American Nurses Association. UAN staff nurses set the standard for RNs in organizing, collective bargaining, and contracts. Additional information can be obtained at http://www.uannurse.org.

V. LEGAL RISK AREAS

A. Assault
   1. Assault occurs when a person puts another person in fear of a harmful or offensive contact.
   2. The victim fears and believes that harm will result because of the threat.
B. Battery is an intentional touching of another's body without the other's **consent**.
C. Invasion of privacy includes violating **confidentiality**, intruding on private client or family matters, and sharing client information with unauthorized persons.
D. False imprisonment
   1. False imprisonment occurs when a client is not allowed to leave a health care facility when there is no legal justification to detain the client.
   2. False imprisonment occurs when restraining devices are used without an appropriate clinical need.
   3. A client can sign an Against Medical Advice form when the client refuses care and is competent to make decisions.
   4. The nurse should document circumstances in the medical record to avoid allegations by the client that cannot be defended.
E. Defamation is a false communication that causes damage to someone's reputation, either in writing (libel) or verbally (slander).
F. Fraud results from a deliberate deception intended to produce unlawful gains.

VI. CLIENT'S RIGHTS

A. Description
   1. The client's rights document, also called the **Patient's Bill of Rights**, reflects acknowledgment

Box 7-5 Patient's Rights When Hospitalized

Right to considerate and respectful care

Right to be informed about diagnosis, possible treatments, likely outcome, and to discuss this information with the physician

Right to know the names and roles of the persons who are involved in care

Right to consent or refuse a treatment

Right to have an advance directive

Right to privacy

Right to expect that medical records are confidential

Right to review the medical record and to have information explained

Right to expect that the hospital will provide necessary health services

Right to know if the hospital has relationships with outside parties that may influence treatment or care

Right to consent or refuse to take part in research

Right to be told of realistic care alternatives when hospital care is no longer appropriate

Right to know about hospital rules that affect treatment, and about charges and payment methods

From Christensen, B., & Kockrow, E. (2006). *Foundations of nursing* (5th ed.). St. Louis: Mosby; and modified from American Hospital Association (1992). *A patient's bill of rights*. http://www.patienttalk.info/AHA-Patient_Bill_of_Rights.htm.

Box 7-6 Laws and Standards

American Hospital Association
Issued Patient's Bill of Rights

American Nurses Association
Developed the Code for Nurses, which defines the nurse's responsibility for upholding the client's rights

Mental Health Systems Act
Developed rights for mentally ill clients

The Joint Commission
Developed policy statements on the rights of mentally ill individuals

Box 7-7 Rights for the Mentally Ill

Right to be treated with dignity and respect

Right to communicate with persons outside the hospital

Right to keep clothing and personal effects with them

Right to religious freedom

Right to be employed

Right to manage property

Right to execute wills

Right to enter into contractual agreements

Right to make purchases

Right to education

Right to habeas corpus (written request for release from the hospital)

Right to an independent psychiatric examination

Right to civil service status, including the right to vote

Right to retain licenses, privileges, or permits

Right to sue or be sued

Right to marry or divorce

Right to treatment in the least restrictive setting

Right not to be subject to unnecessary restraints

Right to privacy and confidentiality

Right to informed consent

Right to treatment and to refuse treatment

Right to refuse participation in experimental treatments or research

Modified from Stuart, G., & Laraia, M. (2009). *Principles and practice of psychiatric nursing* (9th ed.). St. Louis: Mosby.

of a client's right to participate in her or his health care with an emphasis on client autonomy.

2. The document provides a list of the rights of the client and responsibilities that the hospital cannot violate (Box 7-5).

3. The client's rights protect the client's ability to determine the level and type of care received; all health care agencies are required to have a Client's Bill of Rights posted in a visible area.

4. Several **laws** and standards pertain to client's rights (Box 7-6).

B. Rights for the mentally ill (Box 7-7)

1. The Mental Health Systems Act created rights for mentally ill people.

2. The Joint Commission has developed policy statements on the rights of mentally ill people.

3. Psychiatric facilities are required to have a client's bill of rights posted in a visible area.

C. Organ donation and transplantation

1. A client has the right to decide to become an organ donor and a right to refuse organ transplantation as a treatment option.

2. An individual who is at least 18 years old may indicate a wish to become a donor on his or her driver's license (state-specific) or in an **advance directive**.

3. The Uniform Anatomical Gift Act provides a list of individuals who can provide **informed consent** for the donation of a deceased individual's organs.

4. The United Network for Organ Sharing sets the criteria for organ donations.

5. Some organs, such as the heart, lungs, and liver, can be obtained only from a person who is on mechanical ventilation and has suffered brain death, whereas other organs or tissues can be removed several hours after death.

6. A donor must be free of infectious disease and cancer.

7. Requests to the deceased's family for organ donation usually are done by the physician or nurse specially trained for making such requests.

8. Donation of organs does not delay funeral arrangements, no obvious evidence that the organs were removed from the body shows when the body is dressed, and the family incurs no cost for removal of the organs donated.

D. Religious beliefs: Organ donation and transplantation
  1. Catholic Church: Organ donation and transplants are acceptable.
  2. Orthodox Church: Church discourages organ donation.
  3. Islam (Muslim) beliefs: Body parts may not be removed or donated for transplantation.
  4. Jehovah's Witness: An organ transplant may be accepted, but the organ must be cleansed with a nonblood solution before transplantation.
  5. Orthodox Judaism
     a. All body parts removed during autopsy must be buried with the body because it is believed that the entire body must be returned to the earth; organ donation may not be considered by family members.
     b. Organ transplantation may be allowed with the rabbi's approval.
  6. Refer to Chapter 6 for additional information regarding end-of-life-care.

VII. INFORMED CONSENT

A. Description
  1. **Informed consent** is the client's approval (or that of the client's legal representative) to have his or her body touched by a specific individual.
  2. **Consents**, or releases, are legal documents that indicate the client's permission to perform surgery, perform a treatment or procedure, or give information to a third party.
  3. There are different types of **consents** (Box 7-8).
  4. **Informed consent** indicates the client's participation in the decision regarding health care.
  5. The client must be informed, in understandable terms, of the risks and benefits of the surgery or treatment, what the consequences are for not having the surgery or procedure performed, treatment options, and the name of the health care provider performing the surgery or procedure.
  6. A client's questions about the surgery or procedure must be answered before signing the **consent**.
  7. A **consent** must be signed freely by the client without threat or pressure and must be witnessed (witness must be an adult).
  8. A client who has been medicated with sedating medications or any other medications that can affect the client's cognitive abilities should not be asked to sign a **consent**.
  9. Legally, the client must be mentally and emotionally competent to give **consent**.
  10. If a client is declared mentally or emotionally incompetent, the next of kin, appointed guardian (appointed by the court), or durable power of attorney has legal authority to give **consent** (Box 7-9).

Box 7-8 Types of Consents

Admission Agreement
Admission agreements are obtained at the time of admission and identify the health care agency's responsibility to the client.

Immunization Consent
An immunization consent may be required before the administration of certain immunizations; the consent indicates that the client was informed of the benefits and risks of the immunization.

Blood Transfusion Consent
A blood transfusion consent indicates that the client was informed of the benefits and risks of the transfusion. Some clients hold religious beliefs that would prohibit them from receiving a blood transfusion, even in a life-threatening situation.

Surgical Consent
Surgical consent is obtained for all surgical or invasive procedures or diagnostic tests that are invasive. The physician, surgeon, or anesthesiologist who performs the operative or other procedure is responsible for explaining the procedure, its risks and benefits, and possible alternative options.

Research Consent
The research consent obtains permission from the client regarding participation in a research study. The consent informs the client about the possible risks, consequences, and benefits of the research.

Special Consents
Special consents are required for the use of restraints, photographing the client, disposal of body parts during surgery, donating organs after death, or performing an autopsy.

Box 7-9 Mentally or Emotionally Incompetent Clients

Declared incompetent
Unconscious
Under the influence of chemical agents such as alcohol or drugs
Chronic dementia or other mental deficiency that impairs thought processes and ability to make decisions

  11. A competent client older than 18 years of age must sign the **consent**.
  12. In most states, when a nurse is involved in the **informed consent** process, the nurse is witnessing only the signature of the client on the **informed consent** form.
  13. An **informed consent** can be waived for urgent medical or surgical intervention as long as institutional policy so indicates.

14. A client has the right to refuse information and waive the **informed consent** and undergo treatment, but this decision must be documented in the medical record.
15. A client may withdraw **consent** at any time.

⚠️ An informed consent is a legal document, and the client must be informed, in understandable terms, of the risks and benefits of surgery, treatments, procedures, and plan of care. The client needs to be a participant in decisions regarding health care.

B. Minors
1. A minor is a client under legal age as defined by state statute (usually younger than 18 years).
2. A minor may not give legal **consent**, and **consent** must be obtained from a parent or the legal guardian.
3. Parental or guardian **consent** should be obtained before treatment is initiated for a minor except in the following cases: in an emergency; in situations in which the **consent** of the minor is sufficient, including treatment related to substance abuse, treatment of a sexually transmitted infection, human immunodeficiency virus (HIV) testing and acquired immunodeficiency syndrome (AIDS) treatment, birth control services, pregnancy, or psychiatric services; the minor is an emancipated minor; or a court order or other legal authorization has been obtained.

C. Emancipated minor
1. An emancipated minor has established independence from his or her parents through marriage, pregnancy, service in the armed forces, or by a court order.
2. An emancipated minor is considered legally capable of signing an **informed consent**.

VIII. HEALTH INSURANCE PORTABILITY AND ACCOUNTABILITY ACT

A. Description
1. The **Health Insurance Portability and Accountability Act (HIPAA)** describes how personal health information (PHI) may be used and how the client can obtain access to the information.
2. PHI includes individually identifiable information that relates to the client's past, present, or future health; treatment; and payment for health care services.
3. The act requires health care agencies to keep PHI private, provides information to the client about the legal responsibilities regarding privacy, and explains the client's rights with respect to PHI.
4. The client has various rights as a consumer of health care under **HIPAA**, and any client requests may need to be placed in writing; a fee may be attached to certain client requests.

5. The client may file a complaint if the client believes that privacy rights have been violated.
B. Client's rights include the right to do the following:
1. Inspect a copy of PHI.
2. Ask the health care agency to amend the PHI that is contained in a record if the PHI is inaccurate.
3. Request a list of disclosures made regarding the PHI as specified by **HIPAA**.
4. Request to restrict how the health care agency uses or discloses PHI regarding treatment, payment, or health care services, unless information is needed to provide emergency treatment.
5. Request that the health care agency communicates with the client in a certain way or at a certain location; the request must specify how or where the client wishes to be contacted.
6. Request a paper copy of the **HIPAA** notice.
C. Health care agency use and disclosure of PHI
1. The health care agency obtains PHI in the course of providing or administering health insurance benefits.
2. Use or disclosure of PHI may be done for the following:
   a. Health care payment purposes
   b. Health care operations purposes
   c. Treatment purposes
   d. Providing information about health care services
   e. Data aggregation purposes to make health care benefit decisions
   f. Administering health care benefits
3. There are additional uses or disclosures of PHI (Box 7-10)

IX. CONFIDENTIALITY AND INFORMATION SECURITY

A. Description
1. In the health care system, confidentiality refers to the protection of privacy of the client's PHI.
2. Clients have a right to privacy in the health care system.
3. A special relationship exists between the client and nurse, in which information discussed is not shared with a third party who is not directly involved in the client's care.
4. Violations of privacy occur in various ways (Box 7-11).
B. Nurse's responsibility
1. Nurses are bound to protect client **confidentiality** by most nurse practice acts, by ethical principles and standards, and by institutional and agency policies and procedures.
2. Disclosure of confidential information exposes the nurse to liability for invasion of the client's privacy.
3. The nurse needs to protect the client from indiscriminate disclosure of health care information that may cause harm (Box 7-12).

Box 7-10 Uses or Disclosures of Personal Health Information

Compliance with legal proceedings or for limited law enforcement purposes

To a family member or significant other in a medical emergency

To a personal representative appointed by the client or designated by law

For research purposes in limited circumstances

To a coroner, medical examiner, or funeral director about a deceased person

To an organ procurement organization in limited circumstances

To avert a serious threat to the client's health or safety or the health or safety of others

To a governmental agency authorized to oversee the health care system or government programs

To the Department of Health and Human Services for the investigation of compliance with the Health Insurance Portability and Accountability Act or to fulfill another lawful request

To federal officials for lawful intelligence or national security purposes

To protect health authorities for public health purposes

To appropriate military authorities if a client is a member of the armed forces

In accordance with a valid authorization signed by the client

Modified from U.S. Department of Health and Human Services Office for Civil Rights. http://www.hhs.gov/ocr/privacy/hipaa/understanding/consumers/index.html.

Box 7-11 Violations and Invasion of Client Privacy

Taking photographs of the client

Release of medical information to an unauthorized person, such as a member of the press, family, friend, or neighbor of the client, without the client's permission

Use of the client's name or picture for the health care agency's sole advantage

Intrusion by the health care agency regarding the client's affairs

Publication of information about the client

Publication of embarrassing facts

Public disclosure of private information

Leaving the curtains or room door open while a treatment or procedure is being performed

Allowing individuals to observe a treatment or procedure without the client's consent

Leaving a confused or agitated client sitting in the nursing unit hallway

Interviewing a client in a room with only a curtain between clients or where conversation can be overheard

Accessing medical records when unauthorized to do so

Box 7-12 Maintenance of Confidentiality

Not discussing client issues with other clients or staff uninvolved in the client's care

Not sharing health care information with others without the client's consent (includes family members or friends of the client)

Keeping all information about a client private, and not revealing it to someone not directly involved in care

Discussing client information only in private and secluded areas

Protecting the medical record from all unauthorized readers

C. Medical records
   1. Medical records are confidential.
   2. The client has the right to read the medical record and have copies of the record.
   3. Only staff members directly involved in care have legitimate access to a client's record; these may include physicians and nurses caring for the client, technicians, therapists, social workers, unit secretaries, client advocates, administrators (e.g., for statistical analysis, staffing, quality care review). Others must ask permission from the client to review a record.
   4. The medical record is sent to the records or the health information department after discharge of the client from the health care facility.
D. Information technology/computerized medical records
   1. Health care employees should have access only to the client's records in the nursing unit or work area.
   2. **Confidentiality/information security** can be protected by the use of special computer access codes to limit what employees have access to in computer systems.
   3. The use of a password or identification code is needed to enter and sign off a computer system.
   4. A password or identification code should never be shared with another person.
   5. Personal passwords should be changed periodically to prevent unauthorized computer access.
E. When conducting research, any information provided by the client is not to be reported in any manner that identifies the client and is not to be made accessible to anyone outside the research team.

▲ The nurse must always protect client confidentiality.

X. LEGAL SAFEGUARDS

A. Risk management
   1. Risk management is a planned method to identify, analyze, and evaluate risks, followed by a plan for reducing the frequency of accidents and injuries.
   2. Programs are based on a systematic reporting system for incidents or unusual occurrences.

Box 7-13 Incidents That Need to Be Reported

Accidental omission of prescribed therapies
Circumstances that led to injury or a risk for client injury
Client falls
Medication administration errors
Needle-stick injuries
Procedure-related or equipment-related accidents
A visitor injury that occurred in the health care agency premises
A visitor who exhibits symptoms of a communicable disease

Box 7-14 Telephone Prescriptions (Orders)

Date and time the entry.
Repeat the order to the physician, and record the order.
Sign the order; begin with "t.o." (telephone order), write the physician's name, and sign the order.
If another nurse witnessed the order, that nurse's signature follows.
The physician needs to countersign the order within a timeframe according to agency policy.

Box 7-15 Components of a Medication Prescription (Order)

Date and time order was written
Medication name
Medication dosage
Route of administration
Frequency of administration
Physician's or health care provider's signature

Box 7-16 Documentation Guidelines: Narrative and Information Technology

Use a black-colored ink pen for narrative documentation.
Date and time entries.
Provide objective, factual, and complete documentation.
Document care, medications, treatments, and procedures as soon as possible after completion.
Document client responses to interventions.
Document consent for or refusal of treatments.
Document calls made to other health care providers.
Do not document for others or change documentation for other individuals.
Sign and title each entry.
Use quotes as appropriate for subjective data.
Use correct spelling, grammar, and punctuation.
Avoid unacceptable abbreviations.
Avoid judgmental or evaluative statements, such as "uncooperative client."
Do not leave blank spaces on documentation forms.
Follow agency policies when an error is made (draw one line through the error, initial, and date).
Follow agency guidelines regarding late entries.
Use only the user identification code, name, or password for computerized documentation.
Never lend access identification computer codes to another person; change password at regular intervals.
Maintain privacy and confidentiality of documented information printed from the computer.

B. Incident reports (Box 7-13)
   1. The incident report is used as a means of identifying risk situations and improving client care.
   2. Follow specific documentation guidelines.
   3. Fill out the report completely, accurately, and factually.
   4. The report form should not be copied or placed in the client's record.
   5. Make no reference to the incident report form in the client's record.
   6. The report is not a substitute for a complete entry in the client's record regarding the incident.
   7. If a client injury or error in care occurred, assess the client frequently.
C. Safeguarding valuables
   1. Client's valuables should be given to a family member or secured for safekeeping in a stored and locked designated location, such as the agency's safe; the location of the client's valuables should be documented per agency policy.
   2. Many health care agencies require a client to sign a release to free the agency of the responsibility for lost valuables.
   3. A client's wedding band can be taped in place unless a risk exists for swelling of the hands or fingers.
   4. Religious items, such as medals or scapulars, may be pinned to the client's gown if allowed by agency policy.
D. Physicians' prescriptions
   1. A nurse is obligated to carry out a physician's prescription (order) except when the nurse believes a prescription to be inappropriate or inaccurate.
   2. A nurse carrying out an inaccurate prescription may be legally responsible for any harm suffered by the client.
   3. The nurse should clarify with the physician an unclear or inappropriate prescription.
   4. If no resolution occurs regarding the prescription in question, the nurse should contact the nurse manager or supervisor.
   5. The nurse should follow specific guidelines for telephone prescriptions (Box 7-14).
   6. The nurse should ensure that all components of a medication prescription are documented (Box 7-15).
E. Documentation
   1. Documentation is legally required by accrediting agencies, state licensing **laws**, and state nurse and medical practice acts.
   2. The nurse should follow agency guidelines and procedures (Box 7-16).

F. Client and family teaching
   1. Provide complete instructions in a language that the client or family can understand.
   2. Document client and family teaching, what was taught, evaluation of understanding, and who was present during the teaching.
   3. Inform the client of what could happen if information shared during teaching is not followed.

⚠ The nurse should never carry out a prescription (order) if it is unclear or inappropriate. The physician should be contacted immediately.

XI. ADVANCE DIRECTIVES

A. Patient Self-Determination Act
   1. The Patient Self-Determination Act is a **law** that indicates clients must be provided with information about their rights to identify written directions about the care that they wish to receive in the event that they become incapacitated and are unable to make health care decisions.
   2. On admission to a health care facility, the client is asked about the existence of an **advance directive**, and if one exists, it must be documented and included as part of the medical record; if the client signs an **advance directive** at the time of admission, it must be documented in the client's medical record.
   3. The two basic types of **advance directives** include living wills and durable powers of attorney.
      a. Living will: lists the medical treatment that a client chooses to omit or refuse if the client becomes unable to make decisions and is terminally ill.
      b. Durable powers of attorney: appoints a person (health care proxy) chosen by the client to make health care decisions on the client's behalf when the client can no longer make decisions.

B. Do not resuscitate (DNR) orders
   1. The DNR is an order written by a physician when a client has indicated a desire to be allowed to die if the client suffers cardiac or respiratory arrest.
   2. The client or his or her legal representative must provide **informed consent** for the DNR status.
   3. The DNR order must be defined clearly so that other treatment, not refused by the client, will be continued.
   4. The DNR order must be reviewed regularly according to agency policy.
   5. All health care personnel must know whether a client has a DNR order.
   6. If a client does not have a DNR order, health care personnel need to make every effort to revive the client.
   7. DNR protocols may vary state to state, and it is important for the nurse to know his or her state's protocols.

C. The nurse's role
   1. Discussing **advance directives** with the client opens the communication channel to establish what is important to the client and what the client may view as promoting life versus prolonging dying.
   2. The nurse needs to ensure that the client has been provided with information about the right to identify written directions about the care that the client wishes to receive.
   3. On admission to a health care facility, the nurse determines whether an **advance directive** exists and ensures that it is part of the medical record.
   4. The nurse ensures that the physician is aware of the presence of an **advance directive**.
   5. All health care workers need to follow the directions of an **advance directive** to be safe from liability.
   6. Some agencies have specific policies that prohibit a nurse from signing as a witness to a legal document, such as a living will.
   7. If allowed by the agency, when a nurse acts as a witness to a legal document, the nurse must document the event and the factual circumstances surrounding the signing in the medical record; documentation as a witness should include who was present, any significant comments by the client, and the nurse's observations of the client's conduct during this process.

XII. REPORTING RESPONSIBILITIES

A. Nurses are required to report certain communicable diseases or criminal activities such as child or elder abuse or domestic violence; dog bite, gunshot, or stab wounds, assaults, and homicides; and suicides to the appropriate authorities.

B. Impaired nurse
   1. If a nurse suspects that a co-worker is abusing chemicals and potentially jeopardizing a client's safety, the nurse must report the individual to the nursing administration in a confidential manner. (Client safety is always the first priority.)
   2. Nursing administration notifies the board of nursing regarding the nurse's behavior.

C. Occupational Safety and Health Act (OSHA)
   1. OSHA requires that an employer provide a safe workplace for employees according to regulations.
   2. Employees can confidentially report working conditions that violate regulations.
   3. An employee who reports unsafe working conditions cannot be retaliated against by the employer.

D. Sexual harassment
   1. Sexual harassment is prohibited by state and federal **laws**.
   2. Sexual harassment includes unwelcome conduct of a sexual nature.
   3. Follow agency policies and procedures to handle reporting a concern or complaint.

🔘 **MORE QUESTIONS ON THE CD!**

Practice Questions

13. A nurse hears a client calling out for help, hurries down the hallway to the client's room, and finds the client lying on the floor. The nurse performs a thorough assessment, assists the client back to bed, notifies the physician of the incident, and completes an incident report. Which of the following should the nurse document on the incident report?
1. The client fell out of bed.
2. The client climbed over the side rails.
3. The client was found lying on the floor.
4. The client became restless and tried to get out of bed.

14. A client is brought to the emergency department by emergency medical services (EMS) after being hit by a car. The name of the client is unknown, and the client has sustained a severe head injury and multiple fractures and is unconscious. An emergency craniotomy is required. Regarding informed consent for the surgical procedure, which of the following is the best action?
1. Obtain a court order for the surgical procedure.
2. Ask the EMS team to sign the informed consent.
3. Transport the victim to the operating room for surgery.
4. Call the police to identify the client and locate the family.

15. A nurse has just assisted a client back to bed after a fall. The nurse and physician have assessed the client and have determined that the client is not injured. After completing the incident report, the nurse implements which action next?
1. Reassess the client.
2. Conduct a staff meeting to describe the fall.
3. Document in the nurse's notes that an incident report was completed.
4. Contact the nursing supervisor to update information regarding the fall.

16. A registered nurse arrives at work and is told to report (float) to the intensive care unit (ICU) for the day because the ICU is understaffed and needs additional nurses to care for the clients. The nurse has never worked in the ICU. The nurse should take which action first?
1. Call the hospital lawyer.
2. Refuse to float to the ICU.
3. Call the nursing supervisor.
4. Report to the ICU and identify tasks that can be performed safely.

17. A nurse who works on the night shift enters the medication room and finds a co-worker with a tourniquet wrapped around the upper arm. The co-worker is about to insert a needle, attached to a syringe containing a clear liquid, into the antecubital area. The appropriate initial action by the nurse is which of the following?
1. Call security.
2. Call the police.
3. Call the nursing supervisor.
4. Lock the co-worker in the medication room until help is obtained.

18. A hospitalized client tells the nurse that a living will is being prepared and that the lawyer will be bringing the will to the hospital today for witness signatures. The client asks the nurse for assistance in obtaining a witness to the will. The appropriate response to the client is which of the following?
1. "I will sign as a witness to your signature."
2. "You will need to find a witness on your own."
3. "Whoever is available at the time will sign as a witness for you."
4. "I will call the nursing supervisor to seek assistance regarding your request."

19. A nurse has made an error in a narrative documentation of an assessment finding on a client and obtains the client's record to correct the error. The nurse corrects the error by:
1. Documenting a late entry into the client's record
2. Trying to erase the error for space to write in the correct data
3. Using whiteout to delete the error to write in the correct data
4. Drawing one line through the error, initialing and dating the line, and then documenting the correct information

20. A nurse employed in a hospital is waiting to receive a report from the laboratory via the facsimile (fax) machine. The fax machine activates and the nurse expects the report, but instead receives a sexually oriented photograph. The appropriate initial nursing action is to:
1. Call the police.
2. Cut up the photograph and throw it away.
3. Call the nursing supervisor and report the incident.
4. Call the laboratory and ask for the individual's name who sent the photograph.

21. A nursing instructor delivers a lecture to nursing students regarding the issue of client's rights and asks a nursing student to identify a situation that represents an example of invasion of client privacy. Which of the following, if identified by the student, indicates an understanding of a violation of this client right?

1. Performing a procedure without consent
2. Threatening to give a client a medication
3. Telling the client that he or she cannot leave the hospital
4. Observing care provided to the client without the client's permission

22. Nursing staff members are sitting in the lounge taking their morning break. A nursing assistant tells the group that she thinks that the unit secretary has acquired immunodeficiency syndrome (AIDS) and proceeds to tell the nursing staff that the secretary probably contracted the disease from her husband, who is supposedly a drug addict. Which legal tort has the nursing assistant violated?

1. Libel
2. Slander
3. Assault
4. Negligence

23. An 87-year-old woman is brought to the emergency department for treatment of a fractured arm. On physical assessment, the nurse notes old and new ecchymotic areas on the client's chest and legs and asks the client how the bruises were sustained. The client, although reluctant, tells the nurse in confidence that her son frequently hits her if supper is not prepared on time when he arrives home from work. Which of the following is the appropriate nursing response?

1. "Oh, really. I will discuss this situation with your son."
2. "This is a legal issue, and I must tell you that I will need to report it."
3. "Let's talk about the ways you can manage your time to prevent this from happening."
4. "Do you have any friends that can help you out until you resolve these important issues with your son?"

24. A nurse calls the physician regarding a new medication prescription because the dosage prescribed is higher than the recommended dosage. The nurse is unable to locate the physician, and the medication is due to be administered. Which action should the nurse implement?

1. Contact the nursing supervisor.
2. Administer the dose prescribed.
3. Hold the medication until the physician can be contacted.
4. Administer the recommended dose until the physician can be located.

Alternate Item Format: Prioritizing (Ordered Response)

25. A client involved in a head-on automobile crash has awakened from a coma and asks for her husband, who was killed in the same accident. The family does not want the client to know at this time that her husband has died. The family wants all nursing staff to tell the client that the husband was taken by helicopter to another hospital, has a head injury, and is in the intensive care unit (ICU). Because the American Nurses Association Code of Ethics requires the nurse to preserve integrity, but the nurse wants to follow the family's instruction, the nurse faces an ethical dilemma. Number in order the steps for systematic processing of the ethical dilemma. (Number 1 is the first step, and number 6 is the last step.)

___ Evaluate the action.
___ Verbalize the problem.
___ Negotiate the outcome.
___ Consider possible courses of action.
___ Gather all of the information relevant to the case.
___ Examine and determine one's own values on the issues.

ANSWERS

13. 3

Rationale: The incident report should contain the client's name, age, and diagnosis. The report should contain a factual description of the incident, any injuries experienced by those involved, and the outcome of the situation. Option 3 is the only option that describes the facts as observed by the nurse. Options 1, 2, and 4 are interpretations of the situation and are not factual information as observed by the nurse.

Test-Taking Strategy: Use the process of elimination and read the information contained in the question to select the correct option. Remember to focus on factual information when

documenting, and avoid including interpretations. This will direct you to option 3. Review documentation principles related to incident reports if you had difficulty with this question.

Level of Cognitive Ability: Applying
Client Needs: Safe and Effective Care Environment
Integrated Process: Communication and Documentation
Content Area: Leadership and Management—Ethical/Legal
References: Cherry, B., & Jacob, S. (2008). *Contemporary nursing: Issues, trends & management* (4th ed., pp. 171–172). St. Louis: Mosby.

Potter, P., & Perry, A. (2009) *Fundamentals of nursing* (7th ed., pp. 336–337). St. Louis: Mosby.

14. 3
Rationale: Generally, there are two situations in which informed consent of an adult client is not needed. One is when an emergency is present and delaying treatment for the purpose of obtaining informed consent would result in injury or death to the client. The second is when the client waives the right to give informed consent. Option 1 will delay emergency treatment, and option 2 is inappropriate. Although option 4 may be pursued, it is not the best action.
Test-Taking Strategy: Use the process of elimination. Recalling that when an emergency is present and a delay in treatment for the purpose of obtaining informed consent could result in injury or death will direct you to option 3. Review the issues surrounding informed consent if you had difficulty with this question.
Level of Cognitive Ability: Applying
Client Needs: Safe and Effective Care Environment
Integrated Process: Nursing Process—Implementation
Content Area: Leadership and Management—Ethical/Legal
Reference: Black, J., & Hawks, J. (2009). *Medical-surgical nursing: Clinical management for positive outcomes* (8th ed., p. 2191). St. Louis: Saunders.

15. 1
Rationale: After a client's fall, the nurse must frequently reassess the client because potential complications do not always appear immediately after the fall. The client's fall should be treated as private information and shared on a "need to know" basis. Communication regarding the event should involve only the individuals participating in the client's care. An incident report is a problem-solving document; however, its completion is not documented in the nurse's notes. If the nursing supervisor has been made aware of the incident, the supervisor will contact the nurse if status update is desired.
Test-Taking Strategy: Focus on the data in the question and the strategic word *next*. Using the steps of the nursing process will direct you to option 1. Remember that assessment is the first step. Review guidelines related to incident reports and care to the client after sustaining a fall if you had difficulty with this question.
Level of Cognitive Ability: Applying
Client Needs: Safe and Effective Care Environment
Integrated Process: Nursing Process—Implementation
Content Area: Leadership and Management—Ethical/Legal
References: Ackley, B., Ladwig, G., Swan, B., & Tucker, S. (2008). *Evidence-based nursing care guidelines: Medical-surgical interventions* (pp. 340–341). St. Louis: Mosby.
Potter, P., & Perry, A. (2009). *Fundamentals of nursing* (7th ed., pp. 336–337, 403). St. Louis: Mosby.
Zerwekh, J., & Claborn, J. (2009). *Nursing today: Transition and trends* (6th ed., pp. 459–460). St. Louis: Saunders.

16. 4
Rationale: Floating is an acceptable legal practice used by hospitals to solve understaffing problems. Legally, a nurse cannot refuse to float unless a union contract guarantees that nurses can work only in a specified area or the nurse can prove the lack of knowledge for the performance of assigned tasks. When encountering this situation, the nurse should set priorities and identify potential areas of harm to the client. The nursing supervisor is called if the nurse is expected to perform tasks that he or she cannot safely perform. Calling the hospital lawyer is a premature action.

Test-Taking Strategy: Use the process of elimination, noting the strategic word *first*. Eliminate option 2 first because of the word *refuse*. Next, eliminate options 1 and 3 because they are premature actions. Review nursing responsibilities related to floating if you had difficulty with this question.
Level of Cognitive Ability: Applying
Client Needs: Safe and Effective Care Environment
Integrated Process: Nursing Process—Implementation
Content Area: Leadership and Management—Ethical/Legal
Reference: Potter, P., & Perry, A. (2009). *Fundamentals of nursing* (7th ed., pp. 335–336). St. Louis: Mosby.

17. 3
Rationale: Nurse practice acts require reporting impaired nurses. The board of nursing has jurisdiction over the practice of nursing and may develop plans for treatment and supervision of the impaired nurse. This incident needs to be reported to the nursing supervisor, who will then report to the board of nursing and other authorities, such as the police, as required. The nurse may call security if a disturbance occurs, but no information in the question supports this need, and so this is not the initial action. Option 4 is an inappropriate and unsafe action.
Test-Taking Strategy: Note the strategic words *initial action*. Eliminate option 4 first because this is an inappropriate and unsafe action. Recall the lines of organizational structure to assist in directing you to option 3. If you had difficulty with this question, review the nurse's responsibilities when substance abuse is suspected or occurs in the workplace.
Level of Cognitive Ability: Applying
Client Needs: Safe and Effective Care Environment
Integrated Process: Nursing Process—Implementation
Content Area: Leadership and Management—Ethical/Legal
References: Potter, P., & Perry, A. (2009). *Fundamentals of nursing* (7th ed., pp. 8–9). St. Louis: Mosby.
Zerwekh, J., & Claborn, J. (2009). *Nursing today: Transition and trends* (6th ed., pp. 430–431). St. Louis: Saunders.

18. 4
Rationale: Living wills are required to be in writing and signed by the client. The client's signature must be witnessed by specified individuals or notarized. Laws and guidelines regarding living wills vary from state to state, and it is the responsibility of the nurse to know the laws. Many states prohibit any employee, including a nurse of a facility where the client is receiving care, from being a witness. Option 2 is nontherapeutic and not a helpful response. The nurse should seek the assistance of the nursing supervisor.
Test-Taking Strategy: Note the strategic word *appropriate*. Options 1 and 3 are comparable or alike and should be eliminated first. Option 2 is eliminated because it is a nontherapeutic response. Review legal implications associated with living wills if you had difficulty with this question.
Level of Cognitive Ability: Applying
Client Needs: Safe and Effective Care Environment
Integrated Process: Nursing Process—Implementation
Content Area: Leadership and Management—Ethical/Legal
References: Cherry, B., & Jacob, S. (2008). *Contemporary nursing issues: Trends and management* (4th ed., pp. 176–177). St. Louis: Mosby.
Tomey, A. (2009). *Guide to nursing management and leadership* (8th ed., p. 497). St. Louis: Mosby.

19. 4
Rationale: If the nurse makes an error in narrative documentation in the client's record, the nurse should follow agency policies to correct the error. This includes drawing one line through the error, initialing and dating the line, and then documenting the correct information. A late entry is used to document additional information not remembered at the initial time of documentation. Erasing data from the client's record and the use of whiteout are prohibited.
Test-Taking Strategy: Use the process of elimination and principles related to documentation. Recalling that alterations to a client's record are to be avoided will assist in eliminating options 2 and 3. From the remaining options, focusing on the subject of the question and using knowledge regarding the principles related to documentation will direct you to option 4. Review the principles and guidelines related to documentation if you had difficulty with this question.
Level of Cognitive Ability: Applying
Client Needs: Safe and Effective Care Environment
Integrated Process: Communication and Documentation
Content Area: Leadership and Management—Ethical/Legal
Reference: Potter, P., & Perry, A. (2009). *Fundamentals of nursing* (7th ed., p. 388). St. Louis: Mosby.

20. 3
Rationale: Sexual harassment in the workplace is prohibited by state and federal laws. Sexually suggestive jokes, touching, pressuring a co-worker for a date, and open displays of or transmitting sexually oriented photographs or posters are examples of conduct that could be considered sexual harassment by another worker. If the nurse believes that he or she is being subjected to unwelcome sexual conduct, these concerns should be reported to the nursing supervisor immediately. Option 1 is unnecessary at this time. Options 2 and 4 are inappropriate initial actions.
Test-Taking Strategy: Note the strategic word *initial*. Remember that using the organizational channels of communication is best. This will assist in directing you to option 3. Review nursing responsibilities when sexual harassment occurs in the workplace if you had difficulty with this question.
Level of Cognitive Ability: Applying
Client Needs: Safe and Effective Care Environment
Integrated Process: Nursing Process—Implementation
Content Area: Leadership and Management—Ethical/Legal
Reference: Tomey, A. (2009). *Guide to nursing management and leadership* (8th ed., pp. 164–166). St. Louis: Mosby.

21. 4
Rationale: Invasion of privacy occurs with unreasonable intrusion into an individual's private affairs. Performing a procedure without consent is an example of battery. Threatening to give a client a medication constitutes assault. Telling the client that the client cannot leave the hospital constitutes false imprisonment.
Test-Taking Strategy: The strategic words in the question are *invasion of client privacy*. Focus on these strategic words to direct you to option 4. If you had difficulty with this question, review the situations that include invasion of privacy.
Level of Cognitive Ability: Understanding
Client Needs: Safe and Effective Care Environment
Integrated Process: Caring
Content Area: Leadership and Management—Ethical/Legal

References: Cherry, B., & Jacob, S. (2008). *Contemporary nursing issues: Trends and management* (4th ed., pp. 175–176). St. Louis: Mosby.
Zerwekh, J., & Claborn, J. (2009). *Nursing today: Transition and trends* (6th ed., p. 424). St. Louis: Saunders.

22. 2
Rationale: Defamation is a false communication or a careless disregard for the truth that causes damage to someone's reputation, either in writing (libel) or verbally (slander). An assault occurs when a person puts another person in fear of a harmful or an offensive contact. Negligence involves the actions of professionals that fall below the standard of care for a specific professional group.
Test-Taking Strategy: Focus on the data in the question and eliminate options 3 and 4 first because their definitions are unrelated to the data. Recalling that slander constitutes verbal defamation will direct you to option 2 from the remaining options. Review the definitions of libel, slander, assault, and negligence if you had difficulty with this question.
Level of Cognitive Ability: Understanding
Client Needs: Safe and Effective Care Environment
Integrated Process: Nursing Process—Implementation
Content Area: Leadership and Management—Ethical/Legal
Reference: Cherry, B., & Jacob, S. (2008). *Contemporary nursing issues: Trends and management* (4th ed., p. 174). St. Louis: Mosby.

23. 2
Rationale: The nurse must report situations related to child or elder abuse, gunshot wounds and other criminal acts, and certain infectious diseases. Confidential issues are not to be discussed with nonmedical personnel or the client's family or friends without the client's permission. Clients should be assured that information is kept confidential, unless it places the nurse under a legal obligation. Options 1, 3, and 4 do not address the legal implications of the situation and do not ensure a safe environment for the client.
Test-Taking Strategy: Focus on the data in the question and note that an 87-year-old woman is receiving physical abuse by her son. Recall the nursing responsibilities related to client safety and reporting obligations. Options 1, 3, and 4 should be eliminated because they are comparable or alike in that they do not protect the client from injury. Review the nursing responsibilities related to reporting obligations if you had difficulty with this question.
Level of Cognitive Ability: Applying
Client Needs: Safe and Effective Care Environment
Integrated Process: Nursing Process—Implementation
Content Area: Leadership and Management—Ethical/Legal
Reference: Potter, P., & Perry, A. (2009). *Fundamentals of nursing* (7th ed., pp. 562–563). St. Louis: Mosby.

24. 1
Rationale: If the physician writes a prescription that requires clarification, the nurse's responsibility is to contact the physician. If there is no resolution regarding the prescription because the physician cannot be located or because the prescription remains as it was written after talking with the physician, the nurse should contact the nurse manager or nursing supervisor for further clarification as to what the next step should be. Under no circumstances should the nurse proceed to carry out the prescription until obtaining clarification.

Test-Taking Strategy: Use the process of elimination and eliminate options 2 and 4 first because they are comparable or alike and are unsafe actions. Holding the medication can result in client injury. The nurse needs to take action. Option 1 clearly identifies the required action in this situation. Review nursing responsibilities related to the physician's prescriptions if you had difficulty with this question.
Level of Cognitive Ability: Applying
Client Needs: Safe and Effective Care Environment
Integrated Process: Nursing Process—Implementation
Content Area: Leadership and Management—Ethical/Legal
Reference: Potter, P., & Perry, A. (2009). *Fundamentals of nursing* (7th ed., p. 336). St. Louis: Mosby.

ALTERNATE ITEM FORMAT: PRIORITIZING (ORDERED RESPONSE)
25. 6, 3, 5, 4, 1, 2
Rationale: Ethical reasoning is the process of thinking through what one ought to do in an orderly and systematic manner to provide justification for actions based on principles. First, the nurse determines whether or not the issue involves an ethical dilemma and gathers information that is relevant to the case. Next, the nurse undertakes personal value clarification and identifies his or her own values regarding the issue. Third, the nurse verbalizes the problem in a simple sentence. Fourth, the nurse considers possible courses of action. In this case, the nurse may choose to seek the counsel of the agency's ethicist regarding the issue. Fifth, the nurse negotiates the outcome by developing a confidence in her or his own point of view with deep respect for the opinions of others. In this case, the nurse may negotiate with the family to determine a course of action that would allow the nurse to preserve integrity and yet allow the family to determine when the client should be informed of the tragic loss. Finally, the nurse evaluates the action.
Test-Taking Strategy: Use the steps of the nursing process to assist in answering the question. Assessment is the first step; the nurse gathers information about the case and examines this information in terms of his or her own values. Next, the nurse analyzes the data and defines the problem. This is followed by planning and determining possible courses of action. Then the nurse negotiates the course of action with the family, and afterward implements it. Finally the nurse evaluates the action. Review the procedure for the systematic processing of an ethical dilemma if you had difficulty with this question.
Level of Cognitive Ability: Applying
Client Needs: Psychosocial Integrity
Integrated Process: Nursing Process—Implementation
Content Area: Leadership and Management—Ethical/Legal
Reference: Cherry, B., & Jacob, S. (2008). *Contemporary nursing issues: Trends and management* (4th ed., pp. 188–189). St. Louis: Mosby.

Leadership, Delegating, and Prioritizing Client Care

PYRAMID TERMS

accountability Moral concept that involves acceptance by a professional nurse of the consequences of a decision or action.

authority Legitimate power or official right to act.

case management Health care delivery strategy that supports managed care; it is an interdisciplinary health care delivery approach that provides comprehensive client care using available resources to promote quality and cost-effective care.

critical pathway Clinical management care plan for providing client-centered care and for planning and monitoring the client's progress within an established time frame; multidisciplinary collaboration and teamwork ensure shared decision making and quality client care.

delegation Process of transferring a selected nursing task in a situation to an individual who is competent to perform that specific task.

disaster Any human-made or natural event that causes destruction and devastation that cannot be alleviated without assistance; internal disasters are events that occur within a health care agency, whereas external disasters are events that occur outside the health care agency.

emergency response plan A health care agency's preparedness and response plan in the event of a disaster.

evidence-based practice Approach to client care in which the nurse integrates the client's preferences, clinical expertise, and the best research evidence to deliver quality care.

leadership Interpersonal process that involves influencing others (followers) to achieve goals.

management Accomplishment of tasks or goals by oneself or by directing others.

prioritizing Deciding which needs or problems require immediate action and which ones could tolerate a delay in action until a later time because they are not urgent.

quality improvement Also known as performance improvement, focuses on processes or systems that significantly contribute to client safety and effective client care outcomes; criteria are used to monitor outcomes of care and to determine the need for change to improve the quality of care.

triage Classifying procedure that ranks clients according to their need for medical care.

PYRAMID TO SUCCESS

A professional nurse is a leader and a manager. As described in the NCLEX-RN exam test plan, a professional nurse needs to provide integrated, cost-effective care to clients by coordinating, supervising, and collaborating or consulting with members of the multidisciplinary health care team. A primary Pyramid Point focuses on the skills required to prioritize client care activities. Pyramid Points also focus on concepts of management, case management, quality improvement, the process of delegation, an emergency response plan, and triaging clients.

CLIENT NEEDS

Safe and Effective Care Environment

Case management concepts
Consulting or collaborating with members of the health care team
Delegating client care activities and providing continuity of care
Emergency response plan
Establishing priorities related to client care activities
Leadership and management skills
Quality improvement
Supervising the delivery of client care
Triaging clients

Health Promotion and Maintenance

Client's ability to perform self-care
Disease prevention measures and health and wellness
Health promotion programs
Health screening
Performing physical assessment techniques

Psychosocial Integrity

Available support systems
Cultural, spiritual, and religious issues
Therapeutic interactions with others

Physiological Integrity

Ensuring that palliative and comfort care is provided to the client

Ensuring that emergencies are handled using a prioritization procedure

Potential for alterations in body systems

Unexpected responses to therapy

I. HEALTH CARE DELIVERY SYSTEMS

A. Managed care
1. Managed care is a broad term used to describe strategies used in the health care delivery system that reduce the costs of health care.
2. Client care is outcome driven and is managed by a **case management** process.
3. Managed care emphasizes the promotion of health, client education and responsible self-care, early identification of disease, and the use of health care resources.

B. Case management
1. **Case management** is a health care delivery strategy that supports managed care; it uses an interdisciplinary health care delivery approach that provides comprehensive client care throughout the client's illness using available resources to promote high-quality and cost-effective care.
2. **Case management** includes assessment and development of a plan of care, coordination of all services, referral, and follow-up.
3. **Critical pathways** are used, and variation analysis is conducted.

⚠ Case management involves consultation and collaboration with an interdisciplinary health care team.

C. Case manager
1. A case manager is a professional nurse who assumes responsibility for coordinating the client's care at admission and after discharge.
2. The case manager establishes a plan of care with the client, coordinates any consultations and referrals, and facilitates discharge.

D. Critical pathway
1. A **critical pathway** is a clinical **management** care plan for providing client-centered care and for planning and monitoring the client's progress within an established time frame; multidisciplinary collaboration and teamwork ensure shared decision making and quality client care.
2. All members of the health care team work with one plan to achieve the same client outcomes.
3. The goal of a **critical pathway** is to anticipate and recognize negative variance (i.e., problematic differences) early so that appropriate action can be taken and positive client outcomes can result.
4. Variation analysis
   a. Actual deviations or detours from a **critical pathway** are variances.
   b. Positive variance occurs when a client achieves maximum benefit and is discharged earlier than anticipated on the **critical pathway**.
   c. Negative variance occurs when untoward events prevent a timely discharge and the length of hospital stay is longer than planned for a client on a specific **critical pathway**.
   d. Variation analysis is a continuous process that the case manager and other caregivers conduct by comparing the specific client outcomes with the expected outcomes described on the **critical pathway**.
   e. Accurate monitoring of the **critical pathway** with variation analysis can estimate the financial impact of actual client outcomes on the health care facility, especially when the client is not achieving expected outcomes.
   f. If the variance is predictable, negotiation with health care insurers for cost coverage of an additional length of health care facility stay can maximize client care revenues.
   g. If the variance is not predicted and additional cost coverage is not negotiated with health care insurers, the hospital may not be reimbursed for a longer period of client care.

E. CareMaps
1. A CareMap is a model for a **critical pathway**.
2. The CareMap incorporates day-to-day expected client outcomes and outcomes anticipated at discharge or at the end of a treatment phase.
3. The CareMap outlines clinical assessments, treatments and procedures, dietary interventions, activity and exercise therapies, client education, and discharge planning.

F. Nursing care plan
1. A nursing care plan is a written guideline and communication tool that identifies the client's pertinent assessment data, problems and nursing diagnoses, goals, interventions, and expected outcomes.
2. The plan enhances continuity of care by identifying specific nursing actions necessary to achieve the goals of care.
3. The client and family are involved in developing the plan of care, and the plan identifies short-term and long-term goals.
4. Client problems, goals, interventions, and expected outcomes are documented in the care plan, which provides a framework for evaluation of the client's response to nursing actions.

II. NURSING DELIVERY SYSTEMS

A. Functional nursing
1. Functional nursing involves a task approach to client care, with tasks being delegated by the charge nurse to individual members of the team.
2. This type of system is task-oriented, and the team member focuses on the delegated task rather than the total client; this results in fragmentation of care and lack of **accountability** by the team member.

B. Team nursing
1. The team generally is led by a registered nurse (team leader) who is responsible for assessing, developing nursing diagnoses, planning, and evaluating each client's plan of care.
2. The team leader determines the work assignment; each staff member works fully within the realm of his or her educational and clinical expertise and job description.
3. Each staff member is accountable for client care and outcomes of care delivered in accordance with the licensing and practice scope as determined by health care agency policy and state law.
4. Modular nursing is similar to team nursing, but takes into account the structure of the unit; the unit is divided into modules allowing nurses to care for a group of clients who are geographically close by.

C. Relationship-based practice (primary nursing)
1. Relationship-based practice (primary nursing) is concerned with keeping a nurse at the bedside, actively involved in client care, while planning goal-directed, individualized care.
2. One (primary) nurse is responsible for managing and coordinating the client's care while in the hospital and for discharge, and an associate nurse cares for the client when the primary nurse is off-duty.

D. Client-focused care
1. This is also known as the total care or case method; a registered nurse assumes total responsibility for planning and delivering care to a client.
2. The client may have different nurses assigned during a 24-hour period; however, the nurse provides all necessary care needed for the assigned time period.

III. PROFESSIONAL RESPONSIBILITIES

A. Accountability
1. The process in which individuals have an obligation (or duty) to act and are answerable for their actions
2. Involves assuming only the responsibilities that are within one's scope of practice and not assuming responsibility for activities in which competence has not been achieved

3. Involves admitting mistakes rather than blaming others and evaluating the outcomes of one's own actions
4. Includes a responsibility to the client to be competent, providing nursing care in accordance with standards of nursing practice and adhering to the professional ethics codes

⚠ Accountability is accepting responsibility for one's actions. A nurse is always responsible for his or her actions when providing care to a client.

B. Leadership and **management**
1. **Leadership** is the interpersonal process that involves influencing others (followers) to achieve goals.
2. **Management** is the accomplishment of tasks or goals by oneself or by directing others.

C. Theories of **leadership** and **management** (Box 8-1)

D. Leader and manager approaches
1. Autocratic
   a. The leader or manager is focused and maintains strong control, makes decisions, and addresses all problems.
   b. The leader or manager dominates the group and commands rather than seeks suggestions or input.
2. Democratic
   a. This is also called participative.
   b. It is based on the belief that every group member should have input into the development of goals and problem solving.
   c. A democratic leader or manager acts primarily as a facilitator and resource person and is concerned for each member of the group.
   d. The democratic style is a more "talk with the members" style and much less authoritarian than the autocratic style.

Box 8-1 Theories of Leadership and Management

Charismatic: Based on personal beliefs and characteristics
Quantum: Based on the concepts of chaos theory; maintaining a balance between tension and order prevents an unstable environment and promotes creativity
Relational: Based on collaboration and teamwork
Servant: Based on a desire to serve others; the leader emerges when another's needs assume priority
Shared: Based on the belief that several individuals share the responsibility for achieving the health care agency's goals
Transactional: Based on the principles of social-exchange theory
Transformational: Based on the individual's commitment to the health care agency's vision and focuses on promoting change

3. Laissez-faire
   a. A laissez-faire leader or manager assumes a passive, nondirective, and inactive approach and relinquishes part or all of the responsibilities to the members of the group.
   b. Decision making is left to the group, with the laissez-faire leader or manager providing little, if any, guidance, support, or feedback.
4. Situational
   a. Situational style uses a combination of styles based on the current circumstances and events.
   b. Situational styles are assumed according to the needs of the group and the tasks to be achieved.
5. Bureaucratic
   a. The leader or manager believes that individuals are motivated by external forces.
   b. The leader/manager relies on organizational policies and procedures for decision making.
E. Effective leader and manager behaviors (Box 8-2)
F. Effective leader and manager qualities (Box 8-3)
G. Functions of **management** (Box 8-4)

Box 8-2 Effective Leader and Manager Behaviors

Treats employees as unique individuals
Inspires employees and stimulates critical thinking
Shows employees how to think about old problems in new ways
Is visible to employees; is flexible; and provides guidance, assistance, and feedback
Communicates a vision, establishes trust, and empowers employees
Motivates employees to achieve goals

Modified from Huber, D. (2010). *Leadership and nursing care management* (4th ed.). St. Louis: Saunders.

Box 8-3 Effective Leader and Manager Qualities

Effective communicator
Credible
Critical thinker
Initiator of action
Risk taker
Is persuasive and influences employees

Box 8-4 Functions of Management

Planning: Determining objectives and identifying methods that lead to achievement of objectives
Organizing: Using resources (human and material) to achieve predetermined outcomes
Directing: Guiding and motivating others to meet expected outcomes
Controlling: Using performance standards as criteria for measuring success and taking corrective action

H. Problem-solving process and decision making
   1. Problem solving involves obtaining information and using it to reach an acceptable solution to a problem.
   2. Decision making involves identifying a problem and deciding which alternatives can best achieve objectives.
   3. Steps of the problem-solving process are similar to the steps of the nursing process (Table 8-1).
I. Types of managers
   1. Frontline manager
      a. Frontline managers function in supervisory roles closely identified with the actual delivery of client care.
      b. Frontline roles include charge nurse, team leader, and client care coordinator.
      c. Frontline managers coordinate the activity of all staff who provide client care and supervise team members during the manager's period of **accountability**.
   2. Middle manager
      a. Middle manager roles include unit manager and supervisor.
      b. A middle manager's responsibilities include supervising staff, preparing budgets, preparing work schedules, writing and implementing policies that guide client care and unit operations, and maintaining the quality of client services.
   3. Nurse executive
      a. A nurse executive is a top-level nurse manager and may be the director of nursing services or the vice-president for client care services.
      b. The nurse executive supervises numerous departments and works closely with the administrative team of the organization.
      c. The nurse executive ensures that all client care provided by nurses is consistent with the objectives of the health care organization.

IV. POWER

A. Power is the ability to do or act to achieve desired results.

TABLE 8-1 Similarities of the Problem-Solving Process and the Nursing Process

Problem-Solving Process	Nursing Process
Identifying a problem and collecting data about the problem	Assessment
Determining the exact nature of the problem	Analysis
Deciding on a plan of action	Planning
Carrying out the plan	Implementation
Evaluating the plan	Evaluation

Box 8-5 Types of Power

Reward: Ability to provide incentives
Coercive: Ability to punish
Referent: Based on attraction
Expert: Based on having an expert knowledge base and skill level
Legitimate: Based on a position in society
Personal: Derived from a high degree of self-confidence
Informational: When one person provides explanations why another should behave in a certain way

B. Powerful people are able to modify behavior and influence others to change, even when others are resistant to change.

C. Effective nurse leaders use power to improve the delivery of care and to enhance the profession.

D. Power that is effective is power that is shared.

E. There are different types of power (Box 8-5).

V. EMPOWERMENT

A. Empowerment is an interpersonal process of enabling others to do for themselves.

B. Empowerment occurs when individuals are able to influence what happens to them more effectively.

C. Empowerment involves open communication, mutual goal setting, and decision making.

D. Nurses can empower clients through teaching and advocacy.

VI. FORMAL ORGANIZATIONS

A. An organization's mission statement communicates in broad terms its reason for existence; the geographic area that the organization serves; and attitudes, beliefs, and values from which the organization functions.

B. Goals and objectives are measurable activities specific to the development of designated services and programs of an organization.

C. The organizational chart depicts and communicates how activities are arranged, how **authority** relationships are defined, and how communication channels are established.

D. Policies, procedures, and protocols
  1. Policies are guidelines that define the organization's standpoint on courses of action.
  2. Procedures are based on policy and define methods for tasks.
  3. Protocols prescribe a specific course of action for a specific type of client or problem.

E. Centralization is the making of decisions by a few individuals at the top of the organization or by managers of a department or unit, and decisions are communicated thereafter to the employees.

F. Decentralization is the distribution of **authority** throughout the organization to allow for increased responsibility and **delegation** in decision making.

⚠️ A nurse must follow policies, procedures, and protocols of the health care agency in which he or she is employed.

VII. EVIDENCE-BASED PRACTICE

A. **Evidence-based practice** is an approach to client care in which the nurse integrates the client's preferences, clinical expertise, and the best research evidence to deliver quality care.

B. Determining the client's personal, social, cultural, and religious preferences ensures individualization and is a component of implementing evidence-based practice.

C. A nurse needs to be an observer and identify and question situations that require change or result in a less than desirable outcome.

D. Use of information technology such as online resources, including research publications, provides current research findings related to areas of practice.

E. The nurse needs to follow **evidence-based practice** protocols developed by the institution and question the rationale for nursing approaches identified in the protocols as necessary.

⚠️ Evidence-based practice requires that a nurse base nursing practice on evidence from clinical research studies. The nurse should also be alert to clinical issues that warrant investigation and develop a researchable problem about the issue.

VIII. QUALITY IMPROVEMENT

A. Also known as performance improvement, **quality improvement** focuses on processes or systems that significantly contribute to client safety and effective client care outcomes; criteria are used to monitor outcomes of care and to determine the need for change to improve the quality of care.

B. **Quality improvement** processes or systems may be named quality assurance, continuous quality **management**, or continuous **quality improvement**.

C. When **quality improvement** is part of the philosophy of a health care agency, every staff member becomes involved in ways to improve client care and outcomes.

D. A retrospective ("looking back") audit is an evaluation method used to inspect the medical record after the client's discharge for documentation of compliance with the standards.

E. A concurrent ("at the same time") audit is an evaluation method used to inspect compliance of nurses with predetermined standards and criteria

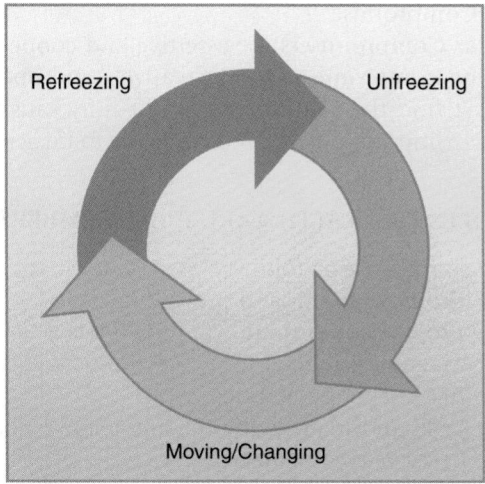

▲ **FIGURE 8-1** Elements of a successful change. (From Huber, D. [2010]. *Leadership and nursing care management* [4th ed.]. St. Louis: Saunders.)

while the nurses are providing care during the client's stay.

F. Peer review is a process in which nurses employed in an organization evaluate the quality of nursing care delivered to the client.

G. The **quality improvement** process is similar to the nursing process and involves a multidisciplinary approach.

H. An outcome describes the most positive response to care; comparison of client responses to the expected outcomes indicates whether the interventions are effective, whether the client has progressed, how well standards are met, and whether changes are necessary.

I. A nurse is responsible for recognizing trends in nursing practice, identifying recurrent problems, and initiating opportunities to improve the quality of care.

⚠ Quality improvement processes improve the quality of care delivery to clients and the safety of health care agencies.

IX. CHANGE PROCESS

A. Change is a dynamic process that leads to an alteration in behavior.

1. Lewin's basic concept of the change process includes three elements for successful change: unfreezing, moving and changing, and refreezing (Fig. 8-1).

   a. Unfreezing is the first phase of the process, during which the problem is identified and individuals involved gather facts and evidence supporting a basis for change.

   b. During the moving and changing phase, change is planned and implemented.

   c. Refreezing is the last phase of the process, during which the change becomes stabilized.

■■■■ **PRIORITY NURSING ACTIONS!** ■■■■

Order of Priority in Assessing a Group of Clients

A nurse is assigned to the following clients. The order of priority in assessing the clients is as follows:

1. A client with heart failure who has a 4-lb weight gain since yesterday and is experiencing shortness of breath

2. A 24-hour postoperative client who had a wedge resection of the lung and has a closed chest tube drainage system

3. A client admitted to the hospital for observation who has absent bowel sounds

4. A client who is undergoing surgery for a hysterectomy on the following day

The nurse determines the order of priority by considering the needs of the client. The nurse also uses guidelines for prioritizing, such as the ABCs (airway, breathing, and circulation), Maslow's Hierarchy of Needs theory, and the steps of the nursing process. Clients 1 and 2 have conditions that relate to the respiratory system or cardiac system (client 1). These clients are the high priorities. Client 1 is the first priority because this client is experiencing shortness of breath (life-threatening). There is no indication that client 2 is experiencing any difficulty. Because client 4 is scheduled for surgery on the following day, this client would be the last priority (low priority), and the nurse would assess this client and prepare this client for surgery after other clients are assessed. Because absent bowel sounds could be an indication of a bowel obstruction (intermediate priority), this client would be priority 3.

Reference: Potter, P., & Perry, A. (2009). *Fundamentals of nursing* (7th ed., p. 307). St. Louis: Mosby.

2. **Leadership** style influences the approach to initiating the change process. (See Priority Nursing Actions.)

B. Types of change

1. Planned change: A deliberate effort to improve a situation

2. Unplanned change: Change that is unpredictable but is beneficial and may go unnoticed

C. Resistance to change (Box 8-6)

1. Resistance to change occurs when an individual rejects proposed new ideas without critically thinking about the proposal.

2. Change requires energy.

3. The change process does not guarantee positive outcomes.

D. Overcoming barriers

1. Create a flexible and adaptable environment.

2. Encourage the people involved to plan and set goals for change.

3. Include all involved in the plan for change.

4. Focus on the benefits of the change in relation to improvement of client care.

Box 8-6 Reasons for Resisting Change

Conformity
One goes along with others to avoid conflict.

Dissimilar Beliefs and Values
Differences can impede positive change.

Habit
Routine, set behaviors are often hard to change.

Secondary Gains
Benefits or payoff are present, so there is no incentive to change.

Threats to Satisfying Basic Needs
Change may be perceived as a threat to self-esteem, security, or survival.

Fear
One fears failure or has fear of the unknown.

5. Delineate the drawbacks from failing to make the change in relation to client care.
6. Evaluate the change process on an ongoing basis, and keep everyone informed of the progress.
7. Provide positive feedback to all involved.
8. Commit to the time it takes to change.

X. CONFLICT

A. Conflict arises from a perception of incompatibility or difference in beliefs, attitudes, values, goals, priorities, or decisions.
B. Types of conflict
   1. Intrapersonal: Occurs within a person
   2. Interpersonal: Occurs between and among clients, nurses, or other staff members
   3. Organizational: Occurs when an employee confronts the policies and procedures of the organization
C. Modes of conflict resolution
   1. Avoidance
      a. Avoiders are unassertive and uncooperative.
      b. Avoiders do not pursue their own needs, goals, or concerns, and they do not assist others to pursue theirs.
      c. Avoiders postpone dealing with the issue.
   2. Accommodation
      a. Accommodators neglect their own needs, goals, or concerns (unassertive) while trying to satisfy those of others.
      b. Accommodators obey and serve others and often feel resentment and disappointment because they "get nothing in return."
   3. Competition
      a. Competitors pursue their own needs and goals at the expense of others.
      b. Competitors also may stand up for rights and defend important principles.

4. Compromise
   a. Compromisers are assertive and cooperative.
   b. Compromisers work creatively and openly to find the solution that most fully satisfies all important goals and concerns to be achieved.

XI. ROLES OF HEALTH CARE TEAM MEMBERS

A. Nurse roles are as follows:
   1. Promote health and prevent disease
   2. Provide comfort and care to clients
   3. Make decisions
   4. Act as client advocate
   5. Lead and manage the nursing team
   6. Serve as case manager
   7. Function as a rehabilitator
   8. Communicate effectively
   9. Educate clients, families, and communities and health care team members
   10. Act as a resource person
   11. Allocate resources in a cost-effective manner
B. Physician: A physician diagnoses and treats disease.
C. Physician assistant
   1. A physician assistant acts to a limited extent in the role of the physician during the physician's absence
   2. The physician assistant conducts physical examinations, performs diagnostic procedures, assists in the operating room and emergency department, and performs treatments.
   3. Certified and licensed physician assistants in some states have prescriptive powers.
D. Physical therapist: A physical therapist assists in examining, testing, and treating physically disabled clients.
E. Occupational therapist: An occupational therapist develops adaptive devices that help chronically ill or handicapped clients perform activities of daily living.
F. Respiratory therapist: A respiratory therapist delivers treatments designed to improve the client's ventilation and oxygenation status.
G. Nutritionist: A nutritionist or dietitian assists in planning dietary measures to improve or maintain a client's nutritional status.
H. Continuing care nurse: This nurse coordinates discharge plans for the client.
I. Assistive personnel, including nursing assistants, unlicensed personnel, and client care technicians, help a registered nurse with specified tasks and functions.
J. Pharmacist: A pharmacist formulates and dispenses medications.
K. Social worker: A social worker counsels clients and families about home care services and assists the continuing care nurse with planning discharge.
L. Chaplain: A chaplain offers spiritual support and guidance to clients and families.

M. Administrative staff: Administrative or support staff members organize and schedule diagnostic tests and procedures and arrange for services needed by the client and family.

XII. HEALTH CARE TEAM COLLABORATION

A. Client care planning can be accomplished through referrals to or consultations or collaborations with other health care specialists and through client care conferences, which involve members from all health care disciplines. This approach helps ensure continuity of care.

B. Reports
1. Reports should be factual, accurate, current, complete, and organized.
2. Reports should include essential background information, subjective data, objective data, any changes in the client's status, nursing diagnoses, treatments and procedures, medication administration, client teaching, discharge planning, family information, the client's response to treatments and procedures, and the client's priority needs.
3. Change of shift report
   a. The report facilitates continuity of care among nurses who are responsible for a client.
   b. The report may be written, oral, audiotaped, or provided during walking rounds at the client's bedside.
   c. The report describes the client's health status and informs the nurse on the next shift about the client's needs and priorities for care.
4. Telephone reports
   a. Purposes include informing a physician of a client's change in status, communicating information about a client's transfer to or from another unit or facility, and obtaining results of laboratory or diagnostic tests.
   b. The telephone report should be documented and should include when the call was made, who made the call, who was called, to whom information was given, what information was given, and what information was received.
5. Transfer reports
   a. Transferring nurse reports provide continuity of care and may be given by telephone or in person (Box 8-7).
   b. Receiving nurse should repeat transfer information to ensure client safety and ask questions to clarify information about the client's status.

XIII. CONSULTATION WITH THE HEALTH CARE TEAM

A. Consultation is a process in which a specialist is sought to identify methods of care or treatment plans to meet the needs of a client.

Box 8-7 Transfer Reports

Client's name, age, physician, and diagnoses
Current health status and plan of care
Client's needs and priorities for care
Any assessments or interventions that need to be performed after transfer, such as laboratory tests, medication administration, or dressing changes
Need for any special equipment
Additional considerations such as allergies, resuscitation status, precautionary considerations, or family issues

---

Box 8-8 Discharge Teaching

How to administer prescribed medications
Side effects of medications that need to be reported to the physician
Prescribed dietary and activity measures
Complications of the medical condition that need to be reported to the physician
How to perform prescribed treatments
How to use special equipment prescribed for the client
Schedule for home care services that are planned
How to access available community resources
When to obtain follow-up care

B. Consultation is needed when a nurse encounters a problem that cannot be solved using nursing knowledge, skills, and available resources.
C. Consultation also is needed when the exact problem remains unclear; a consultant can objectively and more clearly assess and identify the exact nature of the problem.
D. Rapid response teams are being developed within hospitals to provide nursing staff with internal consultative services provided by expert clinicians.
E. Rapid response teams are used to assist nursing staff with early detection and resolution of client problems.

XIV. DISCHARGE PLANNING

A. Discharge planning begins when the client is admitted to the hospital or health care facility.
B. Discharge planning is a multidisciplinary process that ensures that the client has a plan for continuing care after leaving the health care facility and assists in the client's transition from one environment to another.
C. All caregivers need to be involved in discharge planning, and referrals to other health care professionals or agencies may be needed. A physician's prescription may be needed for the referral, and the referral needs to be approved by the client's health care insurer.
D. A nurse should anticipate the client's discharge needs and make the referral as soon as possible (involving the client and family in the referral process).
E. The nurse needs to educate the client and family regarding care at home (Box 8-8).

XV. DELEGATION AND ASSIGNMENTS

A. Delegation

1. **Delegation** is a process of transferring performance of a selected nursing task in a situation to an individual who is competent to perform that specific task.
2. **Delegation** involves achieving outcomes and sharing activities with other individuals who have the **authority** to accomplish the task.
3. The nurse practice act and any practice limitations define which aspects of care can be delegated and which must be performed by a registered nurse.
4. Even though a task may be delegated to someone, the nurse who delegates maintains **accountability** for the task.
5. Only the task, not the ultimate **accountability**, may be delegated to another.
6. The five rights of delegation include the right task, right circumstances, right person, right direction/communication, and right supervision/evaluation.

⚠ Delegate only tasks for which you are responsible. A nurse who delegates is accountable for the task; the person who assumes responsibility for the task is also accountable.

B. Principles and guidelines of delegating (Box 8-9)
C. Assignments
1. Assignment is transferring performance of client care activities to specific staff members.
2. Guidelines for client care assignments
   a. Always ensure client safety.
   b. Be aware of individual variations in work abilities.
   c. Determine which tasks can be delegated and to whom.
   d. Match the task to the delegatee based on the nurse practice act and appropriate position descriptions.
   e. Provide directions that are clear, concise, accurate, and complete.

f. Validate the delegatee's understanding of the directions.
g. Communicate a feeling of confidence to the delegatee, and provide feedback promptly after the task is performed.
h. Maintain continuity of care as much as possible when assigning client care.

XVI. TIME MANAGEMENT

A. Description
1. Time **management** is a technique designed to assist in completing tasks within a definite time period.
2. Learning how, when, and where to use one's time and establishing personal goals and time frames are part of time **management**.
3. Time **management** requires an ability to anticipate the day's activities, to combine activities when possible, and not to be interrupted by nonessential activities.
4. Time **management** involves efficiency in completing tasks as quickly as possible and effectiveness in deciding on the most important task to do (i.e., **prioritizing**) and doing it correctly.

B. Principles and guidelines
1. Identify tasks, obligations, and activities and write them down.
2. Organize the work day; identify which tasks must be completed in specified time frames.
3. Prioritize client needs according to importance.
4. Anticipate the needs of the day and provide time for unexpected and unplanned tasks that may arise.
5. Focus on beginning the daily tasks, working on the most important first while keeping goals in mind; look at the final goal for the day, which helps in the breakdown of tasks into manageable parts.
6. Begin client rounds at the beginning of the shift, collecting data on each assigned client.
7. Delegate tasks when appropriate.
8. Keep a daily hour-by-hour log to assist in providing structure to the tasks that must be

---

Box 8-9 Principles and Guidelines of Delegating

- Delegate the right task to the right delegatee. Be familiar with the experience of the delegatees, their scopes of practice, their job descriptions, agency policy and procedures, and the state nurse practice act.
- Provide clear directions about the task and ensure that the delegatee understands the expectations.
- Determine the degree of supervision that may be required.
- Provide the delegatee with the authority to complete the task; provide a deadline for completion of the task.
- Evaluate the outcome of care that has been delegated.
- Provide feedback to the delegatee regarding his or her performance.

- *Generally*, noninvasive interventions, such as skin care, range-of-motion exercises, ambulation, grooming, and hygiene measures, can be assigned to a nursing assistant.
- *Generally*, a licensed practical nurse (LPN) or licensed vocational nurse (LVN) can perform not only the tasks that a nursing assistant can perform, but also certain invasive tasks, such as dressing changes, suctioning, urinary catheterization, and medication administration (oral, subcutaneous, and intramuscular), according to the education and job description of the LPN or LVN.
- A registered nurse can perform the tasks that an LPN or LVN can perform and is responsible for assessment and planning care, initiating teaching, and administering medications intravenously.

accomplished, and cross tasks off the list as they are accomplished.

9. Use health care agency resources wisely, anticipating resource needs, and gather the necessary supplies before beginning the task.

10. Organize paperwork and continuously document task completion and necessary client data throughout the day (i.e., documentation should be concurrent with completion of a task or observation of pertinent client data).

11. At the end of the day, evaluate the effectiveness of time **management**.

 XVII. PRIORITIZING CARE

A. Prioritizing is deciding which needs or problems require immediate action and which ones could tolerate a delay in response until a later time because they are not urgent.

B. Guidelines for **prioritizing** (Box 8-10)

C. Setting priorities for client teaching
1. Determine client's immediate learning needs.
2. Review the learning objectives established for the client.
3. Determine what the client perceives as important.
4. Assess the client's anxiety level and the time available to teach.

D. Prioritizing when caring for a group of clients
1. Identify the problems of each client.
2. Review nursing diagnoses.
3. Determine which client problems are most urgent based on basic needs, the client's changing or unstable status, and complexity of the client's problems.
4. Anticipate the time that it may take to care for the priority needs of the clients.
5. Combine activities, if possible, to resolve more than one problem at a time.
6. Involve the client in his or her care as much as possible. (See Priority Nursing Actions.)

Box 8-10 Guidelines for Prioritizing

- The nurse and the client mutually rank the client's needs in order of importance based on the client's preferences and expectations, safety, and physical and psychological needs; what the client sees as his or her priority needs may be different from what the nurse sees as the priority needs.
- Priorities are classified as high, intermediate, or low.
- Client needs that are life-threatening or that could result in harm to the client if they are left untreated are high priorities.
- Nonemergency and non–life-threatening client needs are intermediate priorities.
- Client needs that are not related directly to the client's illness or prognosis are low priorities.
- When providing care, the nurse needs to decide which needs or problems require immediate action and which ones could be delayed until a later time because they are not urgent.
- The nurse considers client problems that involve actual or life-threatening concerns before potential health-threatening concerns.
- When prioritizing care, the nurse must consider time constraints and available resources.
- Problems identified as important by the client must be given high priority.
- The nurse can use the ABCs—airway, breathing, and circulation—as a guide when determining priorities; client needs related to maintaining a patent airway are always the priority.
- The nurse can use Maslow's Hierarchy of Needs theory as a guide to determine priorities and to identify the levels of physiological needs, safety, love and belonging, self-esteem, and self-actualization (basic needs are met before moving to other needs in the hierarchy).
- The nurse can use the steps of the nursing process as a guide to determine priorities, remembering that assessment is the first step of the nursing process.

■ PRIORITY NURSING ACTIONS! ■

Triaging Clients at the Site of an Accident

A nurse is the first responder at the scene of a school bus accident. The nurse triages the victims from highest to lowest priority as follows:

1. Confused child with bright red blood pulsating from a leg wound
2. Child with a closed head wound and multiple compound fractures of the arms and legs
3. Child with a simple fracture of the arm complaining of abdominal pain
4. Sobbing child with several minor lacerations on the face, arms, and legs

Triage systems identify which victims are the priority and should be treated first. Rankings are based on immediacy of needs, including victims with immediate threat to life requiring immediate treatment (emergent), victims whose injuries are not life-threatening provided that they are treated within 1 to 2 hours (urgent), and victims with sustained local injuries who do not have immediate complications and can wait several hours for medical treatment (nonurgent). Victim 1 has a wound that is pulsating bright red blood; this indicates arterial puncture. The child is also confused, which indicates the presence of hypoxia and shock (emergent). Victim 2 has sustained multiple trauma, so this victim is also classified as emergent and would require immediate treatment; however, victim 1 is the higher priority because of the arterial puncture. Victim 3 sustained injuries that are not life-threatening provided that the injuries can be treated in 1 to 2 hours (urgent). Victim 4 sustained minor injuries that can wait several hours for treatment (nonurgent).

References: McKinney, E., James, S., Murray, S., & Ashwill, J. (2009). *Maternal-child nursing* (3rd ed., pp. 854, 849). St. Louis: Saunders.

Stanhope, M., & Lancaster, J. (2008). *Public health nursing: population-centered health care in the community* (7th ed., p. 468). St. Louis: Mosby.

Use the ABCs (airway, breathing, and circulation), Maslow's Hierarchy of Needs theory, and the steps of the nursing process (assessment is first) to prioritize.

XVIII. DISASTERS AND EMERGENCY RESPONSE PLAN

A. Description
1. A **disaster** is any human-made or natural event that causes destruction and devastation that cannot be alleviated without assistance (Box 8-11).
2. Internal **disasters** are **disasters** that occur within a health care agency (e.g., health care agency fire, structural collapse, radiation spill), whereas external **disasters** are **disasters** that occur outside the health care agency (e.g., mass transit accident that could send hundreds of victims to emergency departments).
3. An **emergency response plan** is a formal plan of action for coordinating the response of the health care agency staff in the event of a **disaster** in the health care agency or surrounding community.

B. American Red Cross (ARC)
1. The ARC has been given **authority** by the federal government to provide **disaster** relief.
2. All ARC **disaster** relief assistance is free, and local offices are located across the United States.

Box 8-11 Types of Disasters

Human-Made Disasters
Dam failures resulting in flooding
Hazardous substance accidents such as pollution, chemical spills, or toxic gas leaks
Accidents involving release of radioactive material
Resource shortages such as food, water, and electricity
Structural collapse, fire, or explosions
Terrorist attacks such as bombing, riots, and bioterrorism
Mass transportation accidents

Natural Disasters
Blizzards
Communicable disease epidemics
Cyclones
Droughts
Earthquakes
Floods
Forest fires
Hailstorms
Hurricanes
Landslides
Mudslides
Tidal waves
Tornadoes
Volcanic eruptions

---

3. The ARC participates with the government in developing and testing community **disaster** plans.
4. The ARC identifies and trains personnel for emergency response.
5. The ARC works with businesses and labor organizations to identify resources and individuals for **disaster** work.
6. The ARC educates the public about ways to prepare for a **disaster**.
7. The ARC operates shelters, provides assistance to meet immediate emergency needs, and provides **disaster** health services, including crisis counseling.
8. The ARC handles inquiries from family members.
9. The ARC coordinates relief activities with other agencies.
10. Nurses are involved directly with the ARC and assume functions such as managers, supervisors, and educators of first aid; they also participate in **emergency response plans** and **disaster** relief programs and provide services, such as blood collection drives and immunization programs.

C. Phases of **disaster** management
1. The Federal Emergency Management Agency (FEMA) identifies four **disaster management** phases: mitigation, preparedness, response, and recovery (Box 8-12).
2. Mitigation encompasses the following:
   a. Actions or measures that can prevent the occurrence of a **disaster** or reduce the damaging effects of a **disaster**
   b. Determination of the community hazards and community risks (actual and potential threats) before a **disaster** occurs
   c. Awareness of available community resources and community health personnel to facilitate mobilization of activities and minimize chaos and confusion if a **disaster** occurs
   d. Determination of the resources available for care to infants, older adults, disabled individuals, and individuals with chronic health problems
3. Preparedness encompasses the following:
   a. Plans for rescue, evacuation, and caring for **disaster** victims

---

Box 8-12 Federal Emergency Management Agency (FEMA): Four Disaster Management Phases

Mitigation
Preparedness
Response
Recovery

b. Plans for training **disaster** personnel and gathering resources, equipment, and other materials needed for dealing with the **disaster**

c. Identification of specific responsibilities for various emergency response personnel

d. Establishment of a community **emergency response plan** and an effective public communication system

e. Development of an emergency medical system and a plan for activation

f. Verification of proper functioning of emergency equipment

g. Collection of anticipatory provisions and creation of a location for providing food, water, clothing, shelter, other supplies, and needed medicine

h. Inventory of supplies on a regular basis and replenishment of outdated supplies

i. Practice of community **emergency response plans** (mock **disaster** drills)

4. Response encompasses the following:
   a. Putting **disaster** planning services into action and the actions taken to save lives and prevent further damage
   b. Primary concerns include safety, physical health, and mental health of victims and members of the **disaster** response team

5. Recovery encompasses the following:
   a. Actions taken to return to a normal situation after the **disaster**
   b. Preventing debilitating effects and restoring personal, economic, and environmental health and stability to the community

D. Levels of **disaster**
   1. FEMA identifies three levels of **disaster** with FEMA response (Box 8-13).

2. When a federal emergency has been declared, the federal response plan may take effect and activate emergency support functions.

3. The emergency support functions of the ARC include performing emergency first aid, sheltering, feeding, providing a **disaster** welfare information system, and coordinating bulk distribution of emergency relief supplies.

4. **Disaster** medical assistant teams (teams of specially trained personnel) can be activated and sent to a **disaster** site to provide **triage** and medical care to victims until they can be evacuated to a hospital.

E. Nurse's role in **disaster** planning
   1. Personal and professional preparedness
      a. Make personal and family preparations (Box 8-14).
      b. Be aware of the **disaster** plan at the place of employment and in the community.
      c. Maintain certification in **disaster** training and in cardiopulmonary resuscitation.
      d. Participate in mock **disaster** drills, including a bomb threat drill.
      e. Prepare professional emergency response items, such as a copy of nursing license, personal health care equipment such as a stethoscope, cash, warm clothing, record-keeping materials, and other nursing care supplies.

Box 8-13 Federal Emergency Management Agency (FEMA) Levels of Disaster

Level III Disaster
Minor disaster that involves a minimal level of damage, but could result in a presidential declaration of an emergency

Level II Disaster
Moderate disaster that is likely to result in a presidential declaration of an emergency, with moderate federal assistance

Level I Disaster
Massive disaster that involves significant damage and results in a presidential disaster declaration, with major federal involvement and full engagement of federal, regional, and national resources

---

Box 8-14 Emergency Plans and Supplies

Plan a meeting place for family members.
Identify where to go if an evacuation is necessary.
Determine when and how to turn off water, gas, and electricity at main switches.
Locate the safe spots in the home for each type of disaster.
Replace water supply every 3 months and food supply every 6 months.
Include the following supplies:
■ A 3-day supply of water (1 gallon per person per day)
■ A 3-day supply of nonperishable food
■ Clothing and blankets
■ First-aid kit
■ Adequate supply of prescription medication
■ Battery-operated radio
■ Flashlight and batteries
■ Credit card, cash, or traveler's checks
■ Extra set of car keys and a full tank of gas in the car
■ Sanitation supplies for washing, toileting, and disposing of trash
■ Extra pair of eyeglasses
■ Special items for infants, older adults, or disabled individuals
■ Items needed for a pet such as food, water, and leash
■ Important documents in a waterproof case

2. **Disaster** response
   a. In the heath care agency setting, if a **disaster** occurs, the agency **disaster** preparedness plan (**emergency response plan**) is activated immediately, and a nurse responds by following the directions identified in the plan.
   b. In the community setting, if a nurse is the first responder to a **disaster**, the nurse cares for the victims by attending to the victims with life-threatening problems first; when rescue workers arrive at the scene, immediate plans for **triage** should begin.

⚠ In the event of a disaster, activate the emergency response plan immediately.

F. Triage
   1. In a **disaster** or war, **triage** consists of brief assessment of victims that allows a nurse to classify victims according to the severity of the injury, urgency of treatment, and place for treatment.
   2. In an emergency department, **triage** consists of brief assessment of clients that allows a nurse to classify clients according to their need for care and establishing priorities of care; the type of illness or injury, the severity of the problem, and the resources available govern the process.
G. Three-tier system (commonly used in health care agencies) (Box 8-15).
H. Emergency department **triage** system
   1. A commonly used rating system in an emergency department is a three-tier system that uses the categories of emergent, urgent, and nonurgent; these categories may be identified by color coding or numbers (Box 8-16).
   2. A nurse needs to be familiar with the **triage** system of the health care agency.
   3. When caring for a client who has died, the nurse needs to recognize the importance of family and religious rituals and provide support to loved ones.
   4. Organ donation procedures of the health care agency need to be addressed if appropriate.

⚠ Think survivability. If you are the first responder to a scene of a disaster, such as a train crash, the priority victim is the one whose life can be saved.

I. Client assessment in the emergency department
   1. Primary assessment
      a. The purpose of primary assessment is to identify any client problem that poses an immediate or potential threat to life.
      b. A nurse gathers information primarily through objective data and, on finding any abnormalities, immediately initiates interventions.
      c. The nurse uses the ABCs—airway, breathing, and circulation—as a guide in assessing a client's needs and assesses a client who has sustained a traumatic injury for signs of a head injury or cervical spine injury.
   2. Secondary assessment
      a. A nurse performs secondary assessment after the primary assessment and after treatment for any primary problems identified.
      b. Secondary assessment identifies any other life-threatening problems that a client might be experiencing.
      c. The nurse obtains subjective and objective data, including a history, general overview, vital sign measurements, neurological assessment, pain assessment, and complete or focused physical assessment.

Box 8-16 Emergency Department Triage

Emergent (Red): Priority 1 (Highest)
This classification is assigned to clients who have life-threatening injuries and need immediate attention and continuous evaluation, but have a high probability for survival when stabilized.

Such clients include trauma victims, clients with chest pain, clients with severe respiratory distress or cardiac arrest, clients with limb amputation, clients with acute neurological deficits, and clients who have sustained chemical splashes to the eyes.

Urgent (Yellow): Priority 2
This classification is assigned to clients who require treatment and whose injuries have complications that are not life-threatening, provided that they are treated within 1 to 2 hours; these clients require continuous evaluation every 30 to 60 minutes thereafter.

Such clients include clients with a simple fracture, asthma without respiratory distress, fever, hypertension, abdominal pain, or a renal stone.

Nonurgent (Green): Priority 3
This classification is assigned to clients with local injuries who do not have immediate complications and who can wait several hours for medical treatment; these clients require evaluation every 1 to 2 hours thereafter.

Such clients include clients with conditions such as a minor laceration, sprain, or cold symptoms.

Box 8-15 Three-Tier System (Commonly Used in Health Care Agencies)

1. Life-threatening (emergent): Victim has life-threatening injuries, but they are readily correctable.
2. Urgent: Victim must be treated within 1 to 2 hours.
3. Delayed (nonurgent): Victim has no injury, is noncritical, or is ambulatory.

MORE QUESTIONS ON THE CD!

Practice Questions

26. A nurse is assigned to care for four clients. In planning client rounds, which client should the nurse assess first?
1. A client scheduled for a chest x-ray
2. A client requiring daily dressing changes
3. A postoperative client preparing for discharge
4. A client receiving nasal oxygen who had difficulty breathing during the previous shift

27. A nurse employed in an emergency department is assigned to triage clients coming to the emergency department for treatment on the evening shift. The nurse should assign highest priority to which of the following clients?
1. A client complaining of muscle aches, a headache, and malaise
2. A client who twisted her ankle when she fell while rollerblading
3. A client with a minor laceration on the index finger sustained while cutting an eggplant
4. A client with chest pain who states that he just ate pizza that was made with a very spicy sauce

28. A new nursing graduate is attending an agency orientation regarding the nursing model of practice implemented in the health care facility. The nurse is told that the nursing model is a team nursing approach. The nurse understands that planning care delivery will be based on which characteristic of this type of nursing model of practice?
1. A task approach method is used to provide care to clients.
2. Managed care concepts and tools are used in providing client care.
3. A single registered nurse is responsible for providing care to a group of clients.
4. A registered nurse leads nursing personnel in providing care to a group of clients.

29. A registered nurse has received the assignment for the day shift. After making initial rounds and checking all of the assigned clients, which client will the registered nurse plan to care for first?
1. A client who is ambulatory
2. A client scheduled for physical therapy at 1 PM
3. A client with a fever who is diaphoretic and restless
4. A postoperative client who has just received pain medication

30. A nurse is giving a bed bath to an assigned client when a nursing assistant enters the client's room and tells the nurse that another assigned client is in pain and needs pain medication. The appropriate nursing action is which of the following?
1. Finish the bed bath and then administer the pain medication to the other client.
2. Ask the nursing assistant to find out when the last pain medication was given to the client.
3. Ask the nursing assistant to tell the client in pain that medication will be administered as soon as the bed bath is complete.
4. Cover the client, raise the side rails, tell the client that you will return shortly, and administer the pain medication to the other client.

31. A nurse manager has implemented a change in the method of the nursing delivery system from functional to team nursing. A nursing assistant is resistant to the change and is not taking an active part in facilitating the process of change. Which of the following is the best approach in dealing with the nursing assistant?
1. Ignore the resistance.
2. Exert coercion with the nursing assistant.
3. Provide a positive reward system for the nursing assistant.
4. Confront the nursing assistant to encourage verbalization of feelings regarding the change.

32. A registered nurse is planning the client assignments for the day. Which of the following is the most appropriate assignment for a nursing assistant?
1. A client requiring a colostomy irrigation
2. A client receiving continuous tube feedings
3. A client who requires urine specimen collections
4. A client with difficulty swallowing food and fluids

33. A new unit nurse manager is holding her first staff meeting. The manager greets the staff and comments that she has been employed to bring about quality improvement. The manager provides a plan that she developed and a list of tasks and activities for which each staff member must volunteer to perform. In addition, she instructs staff members to report any problems directly to her. What type of leadership style do the new manager's characteristics suggest?
1. Autocratic
2. Situational
3. Democratic
4. Laissez-faire

34. A registered nurse employed in a long-term care facility is planning assignments for the clients on a nursing unit. The registered nurse needs to assign four clients and has a licensed practical (vocational) nurse and three nursing assistants on a

nursing team. Which of the following clients would the registered nurse most appropriately assign to the licensed practical (vocational) nurse?
1. A client who requires a bed bath
2. An older client requiring frequent ambulation
3. A client who requires a 24-hour urine collection
4. A client requiring abdominal wound irrigations and dressing changes every 3 hours

Alternate Item Format: Chart/Exhibit and Prioritizing (Ordered Response)

35. A home health care nurse is planning client visits and nursing activities for the day. The nurse begins the visits at 9 AM. All clients live within a 5-mile radius. List in order of priority how the nurse should plan the order of the assignments for the day. (Number 1 is the first client or nursing activity for the day and number 6 is the last.)

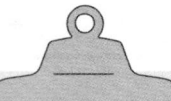

CHART/EXHIBIT

CLIENT ASSIGNMENT AND NURSING ACTIVITIES
___ A client requiring admission
___ A client being visited by the home health aide at 10:30 AM
___ A client requiring supervision of the dressing change
___ The first dressing change for a client requiring twice-daily dressing changes
___ A client with diabetes mellitus who needs a fasting blood glucose level drawn
___ The second dressing change for a client requiring twice-daily dressing changes

ANSWERS

26. 4

Rationale: Airway is always the highest priority, and the nurse would attend to the client who has been experiencing an airway problem first. The clients described in options 1, 2, and 3 have needs that would be identified as intermediate priorities.

Test-Taking Strategy: Use Maslow's Hierarchy of Needs theory and the ABCs—airway, breathing, and circulation—to answer the question. Remember that airway is always the highest priority. This will direct you to option 4. Review principles related to prioritizing if you had difficulty with this question.

Level of Cognitive Ability: Applying

Client Needs: Safe and Effective Care Environment

Integrated Process: Nursing Process—Planning

Content Area: Leadership and Management—Delegating/Prioritizing

References: Jarvis, C. (2008). *Physical examination and health assessment* (5th ed., p. 6). St. Louis: Saunders.

Potter, P., & Perry, A. (2009). *Fundamentals of nursing* (7th ed., p. 307). St. Louis: Mosby.

27. 4

Rationale: In an emergency department, triage involves brief client assessment to classify clients according to their need for care and includes establishing priorities of care. The type of illness or injury, the severity of the problem, and the resources available govern the process. Clients with trauma, chest pain, severe respiratory distress or cardiac arrest, limb amputation, and acute neurological deficits, or who have sustained chemical splashes to the eyes are classified as emergent and are the number 1 priority. Clients with conditions such as a simple fracture, asthma without respiratory distress, fever, hypertension, abdominal pain, or a renal stone have urgent needs and are classified as a number 2 priority. Clients with conditions such as a minor laceration, sprain, or cold symptoms are classified as nonurgent and are a number 3 priority.

Test-Taking Strategy: Note the strategic words *highest priority*. Use the ABCs—airway, breathing, and circulation—to direct you to option 4. A client experiencing chest pain is always classified as priority number 1 until a myocardial infarction has been ruled out. Review the triage classification system commonly used in a hospital emergency department if you had difficulty with this question.

Level of Cognitive Ability: Applying

Client Needs: Safe and Effective Care Environment

Integrated Process: Nursing Process—Implementation

Content Area: Leadership and Management—Delegating/Prioritizing

References: Black, J., & Hawks, J. (2009). *Medical-surgical nursing: Clinical management for positive outcomes* (8th ed., p. 2194). St. Louis: Saunders.

Zerwekh, J., & Claborn, J. (2009). *Nursing today: Transition and trends* (6th ed., pp. 577–579). St. Louis: Saunders.

28. 4

Rationale: In team nursing, nursing personnel are led by a registered nurse leader in providing care to a group of clients. Option 1 identifies functional nursing. Option 2 identifies a component of case management. Option 3 identifies primary nursing (relationship-based practice).

Test-Taking Strategy: The subject of the question relates to team nursing. Keep this subject in mind and use the process of elimination. Option 4 is the only option that identifies the concept of a team approach. Review the various types of nursing delivery systems if you had difficulty with this question.

Level of Cognitive Ability: Understanding

Client Needs: Safe and Effective Care Environment

Integrated Process: Nursing Process—Planning

Content Area: Leadership and Management—Delegating/Prioritizing

Reference: Zerwekh, J., & Claborn, J. (2009). *Nursing today: Transition and trends* (6th ed., pp. 323–324). St. Louis: Saunders.

29. 3

Rationale: The registered nurse would plan to care for the client who has a fever and is diaphoretic and restless first because this client's needs are the priority. Waiting for pain medication to take effect before providing care to the postoperative client is best. The client who is ambulatory and the client scheduled for physical therapy later in the day do not have priority needs related to care.

Test-Taking Strategy: Note the strategic words *care for first* and use principles related to prioritizing. Noting the words *diaphoretic* and *restless* will assist in directing you to this option. Review the principles related to prioritizing if you had difficulty with this question.
Level of Cognitive Ability: Applying
Client Needs: Safe and Effective Care Environment
Integrated Process: Nursing Process—Planning
Content Area: Leadership and Management—Delegating/Prioritizing
References: Cherry, B., & Jacob, S. (2008). *Contemporary nursing issues: Trends and management* (4th ed., p. 498). St. Louis: Mosby.
    Zerwekh, J., & Claborn, J. (2009). *Nursing today: Transition and trends* (6th ed., pp. 32–33). St. Louis: Saunders.

30. 4

Rationale: The nurse is responsible for the care provided to assigned clients. The appropriate action in this situation is to provide safety to the client who is receiving the bed bath and prepare to administer the pain medication. Options 1 and 3 delay the administration of medication to the client in pain. Option 2 is not a responsibility of the nursing assistant.

Test-Taking Strategy: Use the process of elimination and principles related to priorities of care. Options 1 and 3 delay the administration of pain medication, and option 2 is not a responsibility of the nursing assistant. The appropriate action is to plan to administer the medication. Review principles related to priorities of care if you had difficulty with this question.
Level of Cognitive Ability: Applying
Client Needs: Safe and Effective Care Environment
Integrated Process: Nursing Process—Implementation
Content Area: Leadership and Management—Delegating/Prioritizing
Reference: Zerwekh, J., & Claborn, J. (2009). *Nursing today: Transition and trends* (6th ed., p. 317). St. Louis: Saunders.

31. 4

Rationale: Confrontation is an important strategy to meet resistance head on. Face-to-face meetings to confront the issue at hand will allow verbalization of feelings, identification of problems and issues, and development of strategies to solve the problem. Option 1 will not address the problem. Option 2 may produce additional resistance. Option 3 may provide a temporary solution to the resistance, but will not address the concern specifically.

Test-Taking Strategy: Use the process of elimination. Options 1 and 2 can be eliminated first because of the words *ignore* in option 1 and *coercion* in option 2. From the remaining options, select option 4 over option 3 because this option specifically addresses the subject and would provide problem-solving

measures. If you had difficulty with this question, review the strategies associated with dealing with resistance to change.
Level of Cognitive Ability: Applying
Client Needs: Safe and Effective Care Environment
Integrated Process: Nursing Process—Implementation
Content Area: Leadership and Management—Delegating/Prioritizing
References: Marriner-Tomey, A. (2009). *Guide to nursing management and leadership* (8th ed., pp. 326–327). St. Louis: Mosby.
    Zerwekh, J., & Claborn, J. (2009). *Nursing today: Transition and trends* (6th ed., pp. 213, 218). St. Louis: Saunders.

32. 3

Rationale: The nurse must determine the most appropriate assignment based on the skills of the staff member and the needs of the client. In this case, the most appropriate assignment for a nursing assistant would be to care for the client who requires urine specimen collections. The nursing assistant is skilled in this procedure. Colostomy irrigations and tube feedings are not performed by unlicensed personnel. The client with difficulty swallowing food and fluids is at risk for aspiration.

Test-Taking Strategy: Note the strategic words *most appropriate,* and note the subject, an assignment to a nursing assistant. Eliminate option 4 first because of the words *difficulty swallowing.* Next, eliminate options 1 and 2 because they are comparable or alike and are both invasive procedures. Review the principles of delegation and tasks and activities that can be assigned to a nursing assistant if you had difficulty with this question.
Level of Cognitive Ability: Applying
Client Needs: Safe and Effective Care Environment
Integrated Process: Nursing Process—Planning
Content Area: Leadership and Management—Delegating/Prioritizing
References: Cherry, B., & Jacob, S. (2008). *Contemporary nursing issues: Trends and management* (4th ed., p. 80). St. Louis: Mosby.
    Marriner-Tomey, A. (2009). *Guide to nursing management and leadership* (8th ed., p. 54). St. Louis: Mosby.

33. 1

Rationale: The autocratic leader is focused, maintains strong control, makes decisions, and addresses all problems. The autocrat dominates the group and commands, rather than seeks suggestions or input. In this situation, the manager addresses a problem (quality improvement) with the staff, designs a plan without input, and wants all problems reported directly back to her. A situational leader will use a combination of styles, depending on the needs of the group and the tasks to be achieved. The situational leader would work with the group to validate that the information that the leader gained as a new employee was accurate and that a problem existed. Then, the leader would take the time to get to know the group and determine which approach to change (if needed) would work best according to the needs of the group and the nature and substance of the change that was required. A democratic leader is participative and would likely meet with each staff person individually to determine the staff member's perception of the problem. The democratic leader would also speak with the staff about any issues and ask the staff for input with developing a plan. A laissez-faire leader is passive and nondirective. The laissez-faire leader would state what the problem was and inform the staff that the staff needed to come up with a plan to "fix it."

Test-Taking Strategy: Focus on the data in the question and note the strategic words *provides a plan that she developed, each staff member must volunteer to perform,* and *instructs staff members to report any problems directly to her.* Remember that autocratic managers take control and dominate. Review the various types of leadership styles if you had difficulty with this question.

Level of Cognitive Ability: Understanding
Client Needs: Safe and Effective Care Environment
Integrated Process: Nursing Process—Planning
Content Area: Leadership and Management—Delegating/Prioritizing
References: Cherry, B., & Jacob, S. (2008). *Contemporary nursing issues: Trends and management* (4th ed., p. 336). St. Louis: Mosby.

   Marriner-Tomey, A. (2009). *Guide to nursing management and leadership* (8th ed., p. 183). St. Louis: Mosby.

34. 4

Rationale: When delegating nursing assignments, the nurse needs to consider the skills and educational level of the nursing staff. Collecting a 24-hour urine sample, giving a bed bath, and assisting with frequent ambulation can be provided most appropriately by the nursing assistant. The licensed practical (vocational) nurse is skilled in wound irrigations and dressing changes and most appropriately would be assigned to the client who needs this care.

Test-Taking Strategy: Focus on the subject, assignment to a licensed practical/vocational nurse. Recall that education and job position as described by the nurse practice act and employee guidelines need to be considered when delegating activities and making assignments. Options 1, 2, and 3 can be eliminated because they are noninvasive tasks that a nursing assistant can perform. If you had difficulty with this question, review the principles of delegation and assignment making and the tasks and activities that can be assigned to licensed and unlicensed personnel.

Level of Cognitive Ability: Applying
Client Needs: Safe and Effective Care Environment
Integrated Process: Nursing Process—Planning
Content Area: Leadership and Management—Delegating/Prioritizing

Reference: Cherry, B., & Jacob, S. (2008). *Contemporary nursing issues: Trends and management* (4th ed., pp. 406–407). St. Louis: Mosby.

ALTERNATE ITEM FORMAT: CHART/EXHIBIT AND PRIORITIZING (ORDERED RESPONSE)

35. 5, 3, 4, 2, 1, 6

Rationale: The nurse would plan to visit the client with diabetes mellitus first and draw the fasting blood glucose level because this client needs to remain NPO until the blood is drawn. This client also would be unable to take any medication, such as insulin, until the blood is drawn. The nurse would plan to see the client requiring twice-daily dressing changes next because the dressing changes should be spaced as far apart as possible. The nurse then would plan to see the client being visited by the home health aide and provide instructions and directions to the home health aide regarding care to the client. The nurse then would visit the client requiring supervision of the dressing change and would perform the admission next because that may take more time than the other clients. The nurse then would return to the client requiring the second twice-daily dressing change.

Test-Taking Strategy: Note the needs of the clients and the role of the nurse in caring for each of the clients. Noting that the client with diabetes mellitus needs to remain NPO until the blood is drawn will assist in determining that this client needs to be visited first. Noting that the client requiring twice-daily dressing changes will need to be visited twice will assist in determining the next and last client visit of the day, because dressing changes should be spaced as far apart as possible. Next, note that the home health aide will be with the client at 10:30 AM; this client will be seen next. From the remaining clients, select the client requiring a supervised dressing change to be seen next because the client admission may take time. If you had difficulty with this question, review the process of planning care and time management.

Level of Cognitive Ability: Applying
Client Needs: Safe and Effective Care Environment
Integrated Process: Nursing Process—Planning
Content Area: Leadership and Management—Delegating/Prioritizing

Reference: Marriner-Tomey, A. (2009). *Guide to nursing management and leadership* (8th ed., pp. 37, 46). St. Louis: Mosby.

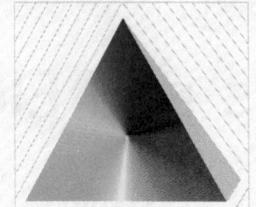

UNIT III

Nursing Sciences

Fluids and Electrolytes

PYRAMID TERMS

calcium A mineral element needed for the process of bone formation, coagulation of blood, excitation of cardiac and skeletal muscle, maintenance of muscle tone, conduction of neuromuscular impulses, and the synthesis and regulation of the endocrine and exocrine glands. The normal adult level is 8.6 to 10 mg/dL.

fluid volume deficit Dehydration in which the fluid intake of the body is not sufficient to meet the fluid needs of the body.

fluid volume excess Fluid intake or fluid retention that exceeds the fluid needs of the body. Also called *overhydration* or *fluid overload*.

homeostasis The tendency of biological systems to maintain relatively constant conditions in the internal environment while continuously interacting with and adjusting to changes originating within or outside the system.

hypercalcemia A serum calcium level that exceeds 10 mg/dL.

hypocalcemia A serum calcium level less than 8.6 mg/dL.

hyperkalemia A serum potassium level that exceeds 5.1 mEq/L.

hypokalemia A serum potassium level less than 3.5 mEq/L.

hypermagnesemia A serum magnesium level that exceeds 2.6 mg/dL.

hypomagnesemia A serum magnesium level less than 1.6 mg/dL.

hypernatremia A serum sodium level that exceeds 145 mEq/L.

hyponatremia A serum sodium level less than 135 mEq/L.

hyperphosphatemia A serum phosphorus level that exceeds 4.5 mg/dL.

hypophosphatemia A serum phosphorus level less than 2.7 mg/dL.

magnesium Concentrated in the bone, cartilage, and within the cell itself; required for the use of adenosine triphosphate as a source of energy. It is necessary for the action of numerous enzyme systems such as carbohydrate metabolism, protein synthesis, nucleic acid synthesis, and contraction of muscular tissue. It also regulates neuromuscular activity and the clotting mechanism. The normal adult level is 1.6 to 2.6 mg/dL.

potassium A principal electrolyte of intracellular fluid and the primary buffer within the cell itself. It is needed for nerve conduction, muscle function, acid-base balance, and osmotic pressure. Along with calcium and magnesium, potassium controls the rate and force of contraction of the heart and thus cardiac output. The normal adult level is 3.5 to 5.1 mEq/L.

phosphorus Needed for generation of bony tissue. It functions in the metabolism of glucose and lipids, in the maintenance of acid-base balance, and in the storage and transfer of energy from one site in the body to another. Phosphorus levels are evaluated in relation to calcium levels because of their inverse relationship; when calcium levels are decreased, phosphorus levels are increased, and when phosphorus levels are decreased, calcium levels are increased. The normal adult level is 2.7 to 4.5 mg/dL.

sodium An abundant electrolyte that maintains osmotic pressure and acid-base balance and transmits nerve impulses. The normal adult level is 135 to 145 mEq/L.

THE PYRAMID TO SUCCESS

Pyramid Points focus primarily on the assessment of a fluid and electrolyte imbalance, interventions, and evaluating the expected outcomes. Fluids and electrolytes constitute a content area that is sometimes complex and difficult to understand. The nurse must understand cell functions and properties and the concepts related to body fluids as outlined in this chapter. Pyramid Points focus on the common fluid and electrolyte disturbances. As you review this content, focus on the Pyramid Points related to the causes, assessment findings, and related treatments. In any fluid or electrolyte imbalance, nursing interventions include monitoring significant laboratory results and monitoring the client's cardiovascular, respiratory, gastrointestinal, neuromuscular, renal, integumentary, and central nervous system status.

CLIENT NEEDS

Safe and Effective Care Environment

Consulting with members of the health care team
Establishing priorities for care

Maintaining standard, transmission-based, and other precautions to prevent transmission of infection to self and others

Handling hazardous and infectious materials to prevent injury to health care personnel and others

Maintaining medical and surgical asepsis and preventing infection in the client when samples for laboratory studies are obtained or when intravenous (IV) solutions are administered

Preventing accidents and ensuring safety of the client when an imbalance exists, particularly when changes in cardiovascular, respiratory, gastrointestinal, neuromuscular, renal, or central nervous systems occur, or when the client is at risk for complications such as seizures, respiratory depression, or dysrhythmias

Health Promotion and Maintenance

Implementing health screening and monitoring for the potential risk for a fluid and electrolyte imbalance

Performing physical assessment techniques

Providing education related to medication and diet management

Providing education related to the potential risk for a fluid and electrolyte imbalance, measures to prevent an imbalance, signs and symptoms of an imbalance, and actions to take if signs and symptoms develop

Psychosocial Integrity

Providing reassurance to the client who is experiencing a fluid or electrolyte imbalance

Providing support and continuously informing the client of the purposes for prescribed interventions

Physiological Integrity

Identifying clients who are at risk for a fluid or electrolyte imbalance

Monitoring laboratory values

Assisting in managing emergencies

Monitoring for complications related to the imbalance

Assessing for expected and unexpected responses to therapeutic interventions and documenting findings

I. CONCEPTS OF FLUID AND ELECTROLYTE BALANCE

A. Electrolytes
1. Description: A substance that is dissolved in solution and some of its molecules split or dissociate into electrically charged atoms or ions (Box 9-1)
2. Measurement
   a. The metric system is used to measure volumes of fluids—liters (L) or milliliters (mL).
   b. The unit of measure that expresses the combining activity of an electrolyte is the milliequivalent (mEq).

Box 9-1 Properties of Electrolytes and Their Components

Atom

An atom is the smallest part of an element that still has the properties of the element.

The atom is composed of particles known as the *proton* (positive charge), *neutron* (neutral), and *electron* (negative charge).

Protons and neutrons are in the nucleus of the atom; therefore the nucleus is positively charged.

Electrons carry a negative charge and revolve around the nucleus.

As long as the number of electrons is the same as the number of protons, the atom has no net charge; that is, it is neither positive nor negative.

Atoms that gain, lose, or share electrons are no longer neutral.

Molecule

A molecule is two or more atoms that combine to form a substance.

Ion

An ion is an atom that carries an electrical charge because it has gained or lost electrons.

Some ions carry a negative electrical charge and some carry a positive charge.

Cation

A cation is an ion that carries a positive charge and has given away or lost electrons.

The result is fewer electrons than protons, and the result is a positive charge.

Anion

An anion is an ion that has gained electrons and therefore carries a negative charge.

When an ion has gained or taken on electrons, it assumes a negative charge and the result is a negatively charged ion.

---

c. One milliequivalent (1 mEq) of any cation always reacts chemically with 1 mEq of an anion.

d. Milliequivalents provide information about the number of anions or cations available to combine with other anions or cations.

B. Body fluid compartments (Fig. 9-1)
1. Description
   a. Fluid in each of the body compartments contains electrolytes.
   b. Each compartment has a particular composition of electrolytes, which differs from that of other compartments.
   c. To function normally, body cells must have fluids and electrolytes in the right compartments and in the right amounts.
   d. Whenever an electrolyte moves out of a cell, another electrolyte moves in to take its place.

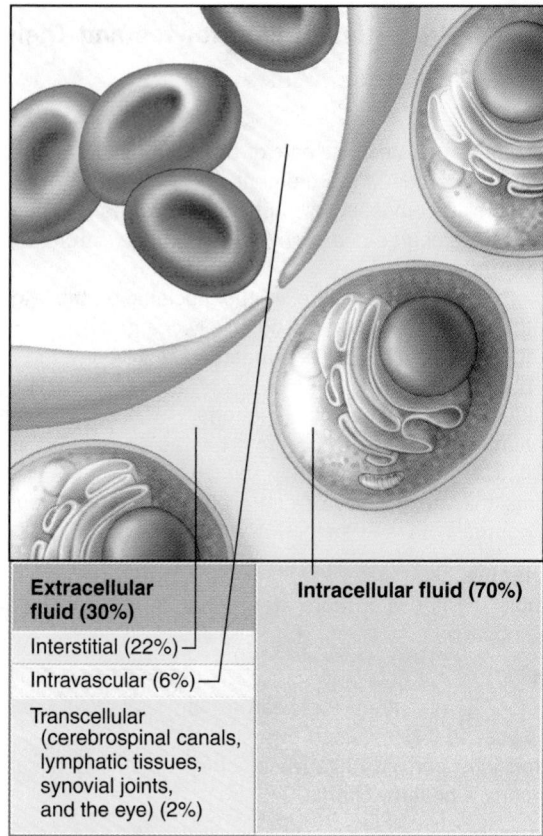

▲ FIGURE 9-1 Distribution of fluid by compartments in the average adult. (From Harkreader, H., Hogan, M.A., & Thobaben, M. [2007]. *Fundamentals of nursing: Caring and clinical judgment* [3rd ed., p. 615]. St. Louis: Saunders.)

Extracellular fluid (30%)
Interstitial (22%)
Intravascular (6%)
Transcellular (cerebrospinal canals, lymphatic tissues, synovial joints, and the eye) (2%)

Intracellular fluid (70%)

   e. The numbers of cations and anions must be the same for **homeostasis** to exist.

   f. Compartments are separated by semipermeable membranes.

  2. Intravascular compartment: Refers to fluid inside a blood vessel

  3. Intracellular compartment

   a. The intracellular compartment refers to all fluid inside the cell.

   b. Most bodily fluids are inside the cell.

  4. The extracellular compartment

   a. Refers to fluid outside the cell.

   b. The extracellular compartment includes the interstitial fluid, which is fluid between cells (sometimes called the *third space*), blood, lymph, bone, connective tissue, water, and transcellular fluid.

C. Third-spacing

  1. Third-spacing is the accumulation and sequestration of trapped extracellular fluid in an actual or potential body space as a result of disease or injury.

  2. The trapped fluid represents a volume loss and is unavailable for normal physiological processes.

  3. Fluid may be trapped in body spaces such as the pericardial, pleural, peritoneal, or joint cavities;

the bowel; or the abdomen, or within soft tissues after trauma or burns.

  4. Assessing the intravascular fluid loss caused by third-spacing is difficult. The loss may not be reflected in weight changes or intake and output records, and may not become apparent until after organ malfunction occurs.

D. Edema

  1. Edema is an excess accumulation of fluid in the interstitial space.

  2. Localized edema occurs as a result of traumatic injury from accidents or surgery, local inflammatory processes, or burns.

  3. Generalized edema, also called *anasarca*, is an excessive accumulation of fluid in the interstitial space throughout the body and occurs as a result of conditions such as cardiac, renal, or liver failure.

E. Body fluid

  1. Description

   a. Body fluids transport nutrients to the cells and carry waste products from the cells.

   b. Total body fluid (intracellular and extracellular) amounts to about 60% of body weight in the adult, 55% in the older adult, and 80% in the infant.

   c. Thus infants and older adults are at a higher risk for fluid-related problems than younger adults; children have a greater proportion of body water than adults and the older adult has the least proportion of body water.

  2. Constituents of body fluids

   a. Body fluids consist of water and dissolved substances.

   b. The largest single fluid constituent of the body is water.

   c. Some substances, such as glucose, urea, and creatinine, do not dissociate in solution; that is, they do not separate from their complex forms into simpler substances when they are in solution.

   d. Other substances do dissociate; for example, when **sodium** chloride is in a solution, it dissociates, or separates, into two parts or elements.

⚠ Infants and older adults need to be monitored closely for fluid imbalances.

F. Body fluid transport

  1. Diffusion

   a. Diffusion is the process whereby a solute (substance that is dissolved) may spread through a solution or solvent (solution in which the solute is dissolved).

   b. Diffusion of a solute spreads the molecules from an area of higher concentration to an area of lower concentration.

c. A permeable membrane allows substances to pass through it without restriction.

d. A selectively permeable membrane allows some solutes to pass through without restriction but prevents other solutes from passing freely.

e. Diffusion occurs within fluid compartments and from one compartment to another if the barrier between the compartments is permeable to the diffusing substances.

2. Osmosis

a. Osmotic pressure is the force that draws the solvent from a less concentrated solute through a selectively permeable membrane into a more concentrated solute, thus tending to equalize the concentration of the solvent.

b. If a membrane is permeable to water but not to all the solutes present, the membrane is a selective or semipermeable membrane.

c. Osmosis is the movement of solvent molecules across a membrane in response to a concentration gradient, usually from a solution of lower to one of higher solute concentration.

d. When a more concentrated solution is on one side of a selectively permeable membrane and a less concentrated solution is on the other side, a pull called *osmotic pressure* draws the water through the membrane to the more concentrated side, or the side with more solute.

3. Filtration

a. Filtration is the movement of solutes and solvents by hydrostatic pressure.

b. The movement is from an area of higher pressure to an area of lower pressure.

4. Hydrostatic pressure

a. Hydrostatic pressure is the force exerted by the weight of a solution.

b. When a difference exists in the hydrostatic pressure on two sides of a membrane, water and diffusible solutes move out of the solution that has the higher hydrostatic pressure by the process of filtration.

c. At the arterial end of the capillary, the hydrostatic pressure is higher than the osmotic pressure; therefore fluids and diffusible solutes move out of the capillary.

d. At the venous end, the osmotic pressure, or pull, is higher than the hydrostatic pressure, and fluids and some solutes move into the capillary.

e. The excess fluid and solutes remaining in the interstitial spaces are returned to the intravascular compartment by the lymph channels.

5. Osmolality

a. Osmolality refers to the number of osmotically active particles per kilogram of water; it is the concentration of a solution.

b. In the body, osmotic pressure is measured in milliosmoles (mOsm).

c. The normal osmolality of plasma is 270 to 300 milliosmoles/kilogram (mOsm/kg) water.

G. Movement of body fluid

1. Description

a. Cell membranes separate the interstitial fluid from the intravascular fluid.

b. Cell membranes are selectively permeable; that is, the cell membrane and the capillary wall allow water and some solutes free passage through them.

c. Several forces affect the movement of water and solutes through the walls of cells and capillaries.

d. The greater the number of particles within the cell, the more pressure exists to force the water through the cell membrane.

e. If the body loses more electrolytes than fluids, as can happen in diarrhea, then the extracellular fluid contains fewer electrolytes or less solute than the intracellular fluid.

f. Fluids and electrolytes must be kept in balance for health; when they remain out of balance, death can occur.

2. Isotonic solutions

a. When the solutions on both sides of a selectively permeable membrane have established equilibrium or are equal in concentration, they are isotonic.

b. Isotonic solutions are isotonic to human cells, and thus very little osmosis occurs; isotonic solutions have the same osmolality as body fluids.

c. Refer to Table 14-1 for a list of isotonic solutions.

3. Hypotonic solutions

a. When a solution contains a lower concentration of salt or solute than another more concentrated solution, it is considered hypotonic.

b. A hypotonic solution has less salt or more water than an isotonic solution; these solutions have lower osmolality than body fluids.

c. Hypotonic solutions are hypotonic to the cells; therefore osmosis would continue in an attempt to bring about balance or equality.

d. Refer to Table 14-1 for a list of hypotonic solutions.

4. Hypertonic solutions

a. A solution that has a higher concentration of solutes than another less concentrated solution is hypertonic; these solutions have a higher osmolality than body fluids.

b. Refer to Table 14-1 for a list of hypertonic solutions.

5. Osmotic pressure
   a. The amount of osmotic pressure is determined by the concentration of solutes in solution.
   b. When the solutions on each side of a selectively permeable membrane are equal in concentration, they are isotonic.
   c. A hypotonic solution has less solute than an isotonic solution, whereas a hypertonic solution contains more solute.
   d. A solvent moves from the less concentrated solute side to the more concentrated solute side to equalize concentration.
6. Active transport
   a. If an ion is to move through a membrane from an area of lower concentration to an area of higher concentration, an active transport system is necessary.
   b. An active transport system moves molecules or ions against concentration and osmotic pressure.
   c. Metabolic processes in the cell supply the energy for active transport.
   d. Substances that are transported actively through the cell membrane include ions of **sodium**, **potassium**, **calcium**, iron, and hydrogen, some of the sugars, and the amino acids.
H. Body fluid intake and output (Fig. 9-2)
   1. Body fluid intake
      a. Water enters the body through three sources—orally ingested liquids, water in foods, and water formed by oxidation of foods.
      b. About 10 mL of water is released by the metabolism of each 100 calories of fat, carbohydrates, or proteins.

Fluid intake		Fluid output	
Ingested water	1200-1500 mL	Kidneys	1500 mL
Ingested food	800-1100 mL	Insensible loss	
Metabolic oxidation	300 mL	through skin	600-800 mL
		Insensible loss	
TOTAL	2300-2900 mL	through lungs	400-600 mL
		Gastrointestinal tract	100 mL
		TOTAL	2600-3000 mL

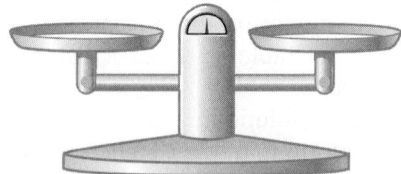

▲ **FIGURE 9-2** Sources of fluid intake and fluid output. (From Harkreader, H., Hogan, M.A., & Thobaben, M. [2007]. *Fundamentals of nursing: Caring and clinical judgment* [3rd ed., p. 626]. St. Louis: Saunders.)

2. Body fluid output
   a. Water lost through the skin is called *insensible loss* (the individual is unaware of losing that water).
   b. The amount of water lost by perspiration varies according to the temperature of the environment and of the body, but the average amount of loss by perspiration alone is 100 mL/day.
   c. Water lost from the lungs is called *insensible loss* and is lost through expired air that is saturated with water vapor.
   d. The amount of water lost from the lungs varies with the rate and the depth of respiration.
   e. Large quantities of water are secreted into the gastrointestinal tract, but almost all this fluid is reabsorbed.
   f. A large volume of electrolyte-containing liquids moves into the gastrointestinal tract and then returns again into the extracellular fluid.
   g. Severe diarrhea results in the loss of large quantities of fluids and electrolytes.
   h. The kidneys play a major role in regulating fluid and electrolyte balance and excrete the largest quantity of fluid.
   i. Normal kidneys can adjust the amount of water and electrolytes leaving the body.
   j. The quantity of fluid excreted by the kidneys is determined by the amount of water ingested and the amount of waste and solutes excreted.
   k. As long as all organs are functioning normally, the body is able to maintain balance in its fluid content.

⚠ The client with diarrhea is at high risk for a fluid and electrolyte imbalance.

I. Maintaining fluid and electrolyte balance
   1. Description
      a. **Homeostasis** is a term that indicates the relative stability of the internal environment.
      b. Concentration and composition of body fluids must be nearly constant.
      c. When one of the substances in a client is deficient—either fluids or electrolytes—the substance must be replaced normally by the intake of food and water or by therapy such as IV solutions and medications.
      d. When the client has an excess of fluid or electrolytes, therapy is directed toward assisting the body to eliminate the excess.
   2. The kidneys play a major role in controlling balance in fluid and electrolytes.
   3. The adrenal glands, through the secretion of aldosterone, also aid in controlling extracellular fluid volume by regulating the amount of **sodium** reabsorbed by the kidneys.

4. Antidiuretic hormone from the pituitary gland regulates the osmotic pressure of extracellular fluid by regulating the amount of water reabsorbed by the kidney.

II. FLUID VOLUME DEFICIT

A. Description
1. Dehydration occurs when the fluid intake of the body is not sufficient to meet the fluid needs of the body.
2. The goal of treatment is to restore fluid volume, replace electrolytes as needed, and eliminate the cause of the **fluid volume deficit**.

B. Types of **fluid volume deficits**
1. Isotonic dehydration
   a. Water and dissolved electrolytes are lost in equal proportions.
   b. Known as *hypovolemia*, isotonic dehydration is the most common type of dehydration.
   c. Isotonic dehydration results in decreased circulating blood volume and inadequate tissue perfusion.
2. Hypertonic dehydration
   a. Water loss exceeds electrolyte loss.
   b. The clinical problems that occur result from alterations in the concentrations of specific plasma electrolytes.
   c. Fluid moves from the intracellular compartment into the plasma and interstitial fluid spaces, causing cellular dehydration and shrinkage.
3. Hypotonic dehydration
   a. Electrolyte loss exceeds water loss.
   b. The clinical problems that occur result from fluid shifts between compartments, causing a decrease in plasma volume.
   c. Fluid moves from the plasma and interstitial fluid spaces into the cells, causing a plasma volume deficit and causing the cells to swell.

C. Causes of **fluid volume deficits**
1. Isotonic dehydration
   a. Inadequate intake of fluids and solutes
   b. Fluid shifts between compartments
   c. Excessive losses of isotonic body fluids
2. Hypertonic dehydration—conditions that increase fluid loss, such as excessive perspiration, hyperventilation, ketoacidosis, prolonged fevers, diarrhea, early-stage renal failure, and diabetes insipidus
3. Hypotonic dehydration
   a. Chronic illness
   b. Excessive fluid replacement (hypotonic)
   c. Renal failure
   d. Chronic malnutrition

D. Assessment (Table 9-1)

E. Interventions

1. Monitor cardiovascular, respiratory, neuromuscular, renal, integumentary, and gastrointestinal status.
2. Prevent further fluid losses and increase fluid compartment volumes to normal ranges.

TABLE 9-1 Assessment Findings: Fluid Volume Deficit and Fluid Volume Excess

Fluid Volume Deficit	Fluid Volume Excess
CARDIOVASCULAR	
• Thready, increased pulse rate • Decreased blood pressure and orthostatic (postural) hypotension • Flat neck and hand veins in dependent positions • Diminished peripheral pulses • Decreased central venous pressure • Dysrhythmias	• Bounding, increased pulse rate • Elevated blood pressure • Distended neck and hand veins • Elevated central venous pressure • Dysrhythmias
RESPIRATORY	
• Increased rate and depth of respirations • Dyspnea	• Increased respiratory rate (shallow respirations) • Dyspnea • Moist crackles on auscultation
NEUROMUSCULAR	
• Decreased central nervous system activity, from lethargy to coma • Fever, depending on the amount of fluid loss • Skeletal muscle weakness	• Altered level of consciousness • Headache • Visual disturbances • Skeletal muscle weakness • Paresthesias
RENAL	
• Decreased urine output	• Increased urine output if kidneys can compensate; decreased urine output if kidney damage is the cause
INTEGUMENTARY	
• Dry skin • Poor turgor, tenting • Dry mouth	• Pitting edema in dependent areas • Pale, cool skin
GASTROINTESTINAL	
• Decreased motility and diminished bowel sounds • Constipation • Thirst • Decreased body weight	• Increased motility in the gastrointestinal tract • Diarrhea • Increased body weight • Liver enlargement • Ascites
LABORATORY FINDINGS	
• Increased serum osmolality • Increased hematocrit • Increased blood urea nitrogen (BUN) level • Increased serum sodium level • Increased urinary specific gravity	• Decreased serum osmolality • Decreased hematocrit • Decreased BUN level • Decreased serum sodium level • Decreased urine specific gravity

3. Provide oral rehydration therapy if possible and IV fluid replacement if the dehydration is severe; monitor intake and output.
4. Generally, isotonic dehydration is treated with isotonic fluid solutions, hypertonic dehydration with hypotonic fluid solutions, and hypotonic dehydration with hypertonic fluid solutions.
5. Administer medications as prescribed, such as antidiarrheal, antimicrobial, antiemetic, and antipyretic medications, to correct the cause and treat any symptoms.
6. Administer oxygen as prescribed.
7. Monitor electrolyte values and prepare to administer medication to treat an imbalance, if present.

III. FLUID VOLUME EXCESS

A. Description
1. Fluid intake or fluid retention exceeds the fluid needs of the body.
2. **Fluid volume excess** is also called *overhydration* or *fluid overload.*
3. The goal of treatment is to restore fluid balance, correct electrolyte imbalances if present, and eliminate or control the underlying cause of the overload.

B. Types
1. Isotonic overhydration
    a. Known as *hypervolemia*, isotonic overhydration results from excessive fluid in the extracellular fluid compartment.
    b. Only the extracellular fluid compartment is expanded, and fluid does not shift between the extracellular and intracellular compartments.
    c. Isotonic overhydration causes circulatory overload and interstitial edema; when severe or when it occurs in a client with poor cardiac function, congestive heart failure and pulmonary edema can result.
2. Hypertonic overhydration
    a. Occurrence of hypertonic overhydration is rare and is caused by an excessive **sodium** intake.
    b. Fluid is drawn from the intracellular fluid compartment; the extracellular fluid volume expands, and the intracellular fluid volume contracts.
3. Hypotonic overhydration
    a. Hypotonic overhydration is known as *water intoxication.*
    b. The excessive fluid moves into the intracellular space, and all body fluid compartments expand.
    c. Electrolyte imbalances occur as a result of dilution.

C. Causes
1. Isotonic overhydration
    a. Inadequately controlled IV therapy
    b. Renal failure
    c. Long-term corticosteroid therapy

2. Hypertonic overhydration
    a. Excessive **sodium** ingestion
    b. Rapid infusion of hypertonic saline
    c. Excessive **sodium** bicarbonate therapy
3. Hypotonic overhydration
    a. Early renal failure
    b. Congestive heart failure
    c. Syndrome of inappropriate antidiuretic hormone secretion
    d. Inadequately controlled IV therapy
    e. Replacement of isotonic fluid loss with hypotonic fluids
    f. Irrigation of wounds and body cavities with hypotonic fluids

D. Assessment (see Table 9-1)
E. Interventions
1. Monitor cardiovascular, respiratory, neuromuscular, renal, integumentary, and gastrointestinal status.
2. Prevent further fluid overload and restore normal fluid balance.
3. Administer diuretics; osmotic diuretics typically are prescribed first to prevent severe electrolyte imbalances.
4. Restrict fluid and **sodium** intake as prescribed.
5. Monitor intake and output; monitor weight.
6. Monitor electrolyte values, and prepare to administer medication to treat an imbalance if present.

⚠ A client with renal failure is at high risk for fluid volume excess.

IV. HYPONATREMIA

A. Description
1. **Hyponatremia** is a serum **sodium** level lower than 135 mEq/L (Box 9-2).
2. **Sodium** imbalances usually are associated with fluid volume imbalances.
B. Causes
1. Increased **sodium** excretion
    a. Excessive diaphoresis
    b. Diuretics

Box 9-2 Sodium

Normal Value
135 to 145 mEq/L

Common Food Sources

Bacon	Milk
Butter	Mustard
Canned food	Processed food
Cheese, such as American or cottage cheese	Snack food
	Soy sauce
Frankfurters	Table salt
Ketchup	White and whole-wheat
Lunch meat	bread

c. Vomiting

d. Diarrhea

e. Wound drainage, especially gastrointestinal

f. Renal disease

g. Decreased secretion of aldosterone

2. Inadequate **sodium** intake

a. Nothing by mouth

b. Low-salt diet

3. Dilution of serum **sodium**

a. Excessive ingestion of hypotonic fluids or irrigation with hypotonic fluids

b. Renal failure

c. Freshwater drowning

d. Syndrome of inappropriate antidiuretic hormone secretion

e. Hyperglycemia

f. Congestive heart failure

C. Assessment (Table 9-2)

D. Interventions

1. Monitor cardiovascular, respiratory, neuromuscular, cerebral, renal, and gastrointestinal status.

2. If **hyponatremia** is accompanied by a **fluid volume deficit** (hypovolemia), IV **sodium** chloride infusions are administered to restore **sodium** content and fluid volume.

3. If **hyponatremia** is accompanied by **fluid volume excess** (hypervolemia), osmotic diuretics are administered to promote the excretion of water rather than **sodium**.

4. If caused by inappropriate or excessive secretion of antidiuretic hormone, medications that antagonize antidiuretic hormone may be administered.

5. Instruct the client to increase oral **sodium** intake and inform the client about the foods to include in the diet (see Box 9-2).

6. If the client is taking lithium (Lithobid), monitor the lithium level, because **hyponatremia** can cause diminished lithium excretion, resulting in toxicity.

⚠ Hyponatremia precipitates lithium toxicity in a client taking lithium (Lithobid).

TABLE 9-2 Assessment Findings: Hyponatremia and Hypernatremia

Hyponatremia	Hypernatremia
CARDIOVASCULAR	
• Symptoms vary with changes in vascular volume • Normovolemic: rapid pulse rate; normal blood pressure • Hypovolemic: thready, weak, rapid pulse rate; hypotension; flat neck veins; normal or low central venous pressure • Hypervolemic: rapid, bounding pulse; blood pressure normal or elevated; normal or elevated central venous pressure	• Heart rate and blood pressure responds to vascular volume status
RESPIRATORY	
• Shallow, ineffective respiratory movement is a late manifestation related to skeletal muscle weakness	• Pulmonary edema if hypervolemia is present
NEUROMUSCULAR	
• Generalized skeletal muscle weakness that is worse in the extremities • Diminished deep tendon reflexes	• Early: spontaneous muscle twitches; irregular muscle contractions • Late: skeletal muscle weakness; deep tendon reflexes diminished or absent
CENTRAL NERVOUS SYSTEM	
• Headache • Personality changes • Confusion • Seizures • Coma	• Altered cerebral function is the most common manifestation of hypernatremia • Normovolemia or hypovolemia: agitation, confusion, seizures • Hypervolemia: lethargy, stupor, coma
GASTROINTESTINAL	
• Increased motility and hyperactive bowel sounds • Nausea • Abdominal cramping and diarrhea	• Extreme thirst
RENAL	
• Increased urinary output	• Decreased urinary output
INTEGUMENTARY	
• Dry mucous membranes	• Dry and flushed skin • Dry and sticky tongue and mucous membranes • Presence or absence of edema, depending on fluid volume changes
LABORATORY FINDINGS	
• Serum sodium level less than 135 mEq/L • Decreased urinary specific gravity	• Serum sodium level that exceeds 145 mEq/L • Increased urinary specific gravity

V. HYPERNATREMIA

A. Description: **Hypernatremia** is a serum **sodium** level that exceeds 145 mEq/L (see Box 9-2).

B. Causes
1. Decreased **sodium** excretion
    a. Corticosteroids
    b. Cushing's syndrome
    c. Renal failure
    d. Hyperaldosteronism
2. Increased **sodium** intake: excessive oral **sodium** ingestion or excessive administration of **sodium**-containing IV fluids
3. Decreased water intake: nothing by mouth
4. Increased water loss: increased rate of metabolism, fever, hyperventilation, infection, excessive diaphoresis, watery diarrhea, diabetes insipidus

C. Assessment (see Table 9-2)

D. Interventions
1. Monitor cardiovascular, respiratory, neuromuscular, cerebral, renal, and integumentary status.
2. If the cause is fluid loss, prepare to administer IV infusions.
3. If the cause is inadequate renal excretion of **sodium**, prepare to administer diuretics that promote **sodium** loss.
4. Restrict **sodium** and fluid intake as prescribed (see Box 9-2).

⚠ Monitor the client closely for signs of a potassium imbalance. A potassium imbalance can cause cardiac dysrhythmias that can be life-threatening!

VI. HYPOKALEMIA

A. Description
1. **Hypokalemia** is a serum **potassium** level lower than 3.5 mEq/L (Box 9-3).
2. **Potassium** deficit is potentially life-threatening because every body system is affected.

B. Causes
1. Actual total body **potassium** loss
    a. Excessive use of medications such as diuretics or corticosteroids
    b. Increased secretion of aldosterone, such as in Cushing's syndrome
    c. Vomiting, diarrhea
    d. Wound drainage, particularly gastrointestinal
    e. Prolonged nasogastric suction
    f. Excessive diaphoresis
    g. Renal disease impairing reabsorption of **potassium**
2. Inadequate **potassium** intake: nothing by mouth
3. Movement of **potassium** from the extracellular fluid to the intracellular fluid
    a. Alkalosis
    b. Hyperinsulinism

Box 9-3 Potassium

Normal Value
3.5 to 5.1 mEq/L

Common Food Sources

Avocado	Potatoes
Bananas	Pork, beef, veal
Cantaloupe	Raisins
Carrots	Spinach
Fish	Strawberries
Mushrooms	Tomatoes
Oranges	

4. Dilution of serum **potassium**
    a. Water intoxication
    b. IV therapy with **potassium**-poor solutions

C. Assessment (Tables 9-3 and 9-4)

D. Interventions
1. Monitor cardiovascular, respiratory, neuromuscular, gastrointestinal, and renal status, and place the client on a cardiac monitor.
2. Monitor electrolyte values.
3. Administer **potassium** supplements orally or intravenously, as prescribed.
4. Oral **potassium** supplements
    a. Oral **potassium** supplements may cause nausea and vomiting and they should not be taken on an empty stomach; if the client complains of abdominal pain, distention, nausea, vomiting, diarrhea, or gastrointestinal bleeding, the supplement may need to be discontinued.
    b. Liquid **potassium** chloride has an unpleasant taste and should be taken with juice or another liquid.
5. Intravenously administered **potassium** (Box 9-4)
6. Institute safety measures for the client experiencing muscle weakness.
7. If the client is taking a **potassium**-losing diuretic, it may be discontinued; a **potassium**-sparing diuretic may be prescribed.
8. Instruct the client about foods that are high in **potassium** content (see Box 9-3).

⚠ Potassium is never administered by IV push, intramuscular, or subcutaneous routes. IV potassium is always diluted and administered using an infusion device!

VII. HYPERKALEMIA

A. Description: **Hyperkalemia** is a serum **potassium** level that exceeds 5.1 mEq/L (see Box 9-3).

TABLE 9-3 Assessment Findings: Hypokalemia and Hyperkalemia

Hypokalemia	Hyperkalemia
CARDIOVASCULAR	
• Thready, weak, irregular pulse • Weak peripheral pulses • Orthostatic hypotension	• Slow, weak, irregular heart rate • Decreased blood pressure
RESPIRATORY	
• Shallow, ineffective respirations that result from profound weakness of the skeletal muscles of respiration • Diminished breath sounds	• Profound weakness of the skeletal muscles leading to respiratory failure
NEUROMUSCULAR	
• Anxiety, lethargy, confusion, coma • Skeletal muscle weakness, eventual flaccid paralysis • Loss of tactile discrimination • Paresthesias • Deep tendon hyporeflexia	• Early: muscle twitches, cramps, paresthesias (tingling and burning followed by numbness in the hands and feet and around the mouth) • Late: profound weakness, ascending flaccid paralysis in the arms and legs (trunk, head, and respiratory muscles become affected when the serum potassium level reaches a lethal level)
GASTROINTESTINAL	
• Decreased motility, hypoactive to absent bowel sounds • Nausea, vomiting, constipation, abdominal distention • Paralytic ileus	• Increased motility, hyperactive bowel sounds • Diarrhea
LABORATORY FINDINGS	
• Serum potassium level lower than 3.5 mEq/L • Electrocardiogram changes: ST depression, shallow, flat or inverted T wave, and prominent U wave	• Serum potassium level that exceeds 5.1 mEq/L • Electrocardiographic changes: tall peaked T waves, flat P waves, widened QRS complexes, and prolonged PR intervals

TABLE 9-4 Electrocardiographic Changes in Electrolyte Imbalances

Electrolyte Imbalance	Electrocardiographic Changes
Hypocalcemia	Prolonged ST interval Prolonged QT interval
Hypercalcemia	Shortened ST segment Widened T wave
Hypokalemia	ST depression Shallow, flat, or inverted T wave Prominent U wave
Hyperkalemia	Tall peaked T waves Flat P waves Widened QRS complex Prolonged PR interval
Hypomagnesemia	Tall T waves Depressed ST segment
Hypermagnesemia	Prolonged PR interval Widened QRS complexes

Box 9-4 Precautions with Intravenously Administered Potassium

Potassium is never given by intravenous (IV) push or by the intramuscular or subcutaneous route.

A dilution of no more than 1 mEq/10 mL of solution is recommended.

After adding potassium to an IV solution, rotate and invert the bag to ensure that the potassium is distributed evenly throughout the IV solution.

Ensure that the IV bag containing potassium is properly labeled.

The maximum recommended infusion rate is 5 to 10 mEq/hr, never to exceed 20 mEq/hr under any circumstances.

A client receiving more than 10 mEq/hr should be placed on a cardiac monitor and monitored for cardiac changes, and the infusion should be controlled by an infusion device.

Potassium infusion can cause phlebitis; therefore the nurse should assess the IV site frequently for signs of phlebitis or infiltration. If either occurs, the infusion should be stopped immediately.

The nurse should assess renal function before administering potassium, and monitor intake and output during administration.

B. Causes
  1. Excessive **potassium** intake
     a. Overingestion of **potassium**-containing foods or medications, such as **potassium** chloride or salt substitutes
     b. Rapid infusion of **potassium**-containing IV solutions
  2. Decreased **potassium** excretion
     a. **Potassium**-sparing diuretics
     b. Renal failure
     c. Adrenal insufficiency, such as in Addison's disease
  3. Movement of **potassium** from the intracellular fluid to the extracellular fluid
     a. Tissue damage
     b. Acidosis

   c. Hyperuricemia
   d. Hypercatabolism
C. Assessment (see Tables 9-3 and 9-4)
D. Interventions
   1. Monitor cardiovascular, respiratory, neuromuscular, renal, and gastrointestinal status; place the client on a cardiac monitor.
   2. Discontinue IV **potassium** (keep the IV catheter patent), and hold oral **potassium** supplements.
   3. Initiate a **potassium**-restricted diet.
   4. Prepare to administer **potassium**-excreting diuretics if renal function is not impaired.
   5. If renal function is impaired, prepare to administer **sodium** polystyrene sulfonate (Kayexalate), a cation exchange resin that promotes gastrointestinal **sodium** absorption and **potassium** excretion.
   6. Prepare the client for dialysis if **potassium** levels are critically high.
   7. Prepare for the IV administration of hypertonic glucose with regular insulin to move excess **potassium** into the cells.
   8. Monitor renal function.
   9. When blood transfusions are prescribed for a client with a **potassium** imbalance, the client should receive fresh blood, if possible; transfusions of stored blood may elevate the **potassium** level because the breakdown of older blood cells releases **potassium**.
   10. Teach the client to avoid foods high in **potassium** (see Box 9-3).
   11. Instruct the client to avoid the use of salt substitutes or other **potassium**-containing substances.

⚠ Monitor the serum potassium level closely when a client is receiving a potassium-sparing diuretic!

VIII. HYPOCALCEMIA

A. Description: **Hypocalcemia** is a serum **calcium** level lower than 8.6 mg/dL (Box 9-5).
B. Causes
   1. Inhibition of **calcium** absorption from the gastrointestinal tract
      a. Inadequate oral intake of **calcium**
      b. Lactose intolerance
      c. Malabsorption syndromes such as celiac sprue or Crohn's disease
      d. Inadequate intake of vitamin D
      e. End-stage renal disease
   2. Increased **calcium** excretion
      a. Renal failure, polyuric phase
      b. Diarrhea

Box 9-5 Calcium

Normal Value
8.6 to 10 mg/dL

Common Food Sources

Cheese	Sardines
Collard greens	Spinach
Milk and soy milk	Tofu
Rhubarb	Yogurt

---

   c. Steatorrhea
   d. Wound drainage, especially gastrointestinal
   3. Conditions that decrease the ionized fraction of **calcium**
      a. Hyperproteinemia
      b. Alkalosis
      c. Medications such as **calcium** chelators or binders
      d. Acute pancreatitis
      e. **Hyperphosphatemia**
      f. Immobility
      g. Removal or destruction of the parathyroid glands
C. Assessment (Table 9-5; Fig. 9-3; see Table 9-4)
D. Interventions
   1. Monitor cardiovascular, respiratory, neuromuscular, and gastrointestinal status; place the client on a cardiac monitor.
   2. Administer **calcium** supplements orally or **calcium** intravenously.
   3. When administering **calcium** intravenously, warm the injection solution to body temperature before administration and administer slowly; monitor for electrocardiographic changes, observe for infiltration, and monitor for **hypercalcemia**.
   4. Administer medications that increase **calcium** absorption.
      a. Aluminum hydroxide reduces serum **phosphorus** levels, causing the countereffect of increasing **calcium** levels.
      b. Vitamin D aids in the absorption of **calcium** from the intestinal tract.
   5. Provide a quiet environment to reduce environmental stimuli.
   6. Initiate seizure precautions.
   7. Move the client carefully, and monitor for signs of a pathological fracture.
   8. Keep 10% **calcium** gluconate available for treatment of acute **calcium** deficit.
   9. Instruct the client to consume foods high in **calcium** (see Box 9-5).

TABLE 9-5 Assessment Findings: Hypocalcemia and Hypercalcemia

Hypocalcemia	Hypercalcemia
CARDIOVASCULAR • Decreased heart rate • Hypotension • Diminished peripheral pulses	• Increased heart rate in the early phase; bradycardia that can lead to cardiac arrest in late phases • Increased blood pressure • Bounding, full peripheral pulses
RESPIRATORY • Not directly affected; however, respiratory failure or arrest can result from decreased respiratory movement because of muscle tetany or seizures	• Ineffective respiratory movement as a result of profound skeletal muscle weakness
NEUROMUSCULAR • Irritable skeletal muscles: twitches, cramps, tetany, seizures • Painful muscle spasms in the calf or foot during periods of inactivity • Paresthesias followed by numbness that may affect the lips, nose, and ears in addition to the limbs • Positive Trousseau's and Chvostek's signs • Hyperactive deep tendon reflexes • Anxiety, irritability	• Profound muscle weakness • Diminished or absent deep tendon reflexes • Disorientation, lethargy, coma
RENAL • Urinary output varies depending on the cause	• Urinary output varies depending on the cause • Formation of renal calculi; flank pain
GASTROINTESTINAL • Increased gastric motility; hyperactive bowel sounds • Cramping, diarrhea	• Decreased motility and hypoactive bowel sounds • Anorexia, nausea, abdominal distention, constipation
LABORATORY FINDINGS • Serum calcium level less than 8.6 mg/dL • Electrocardiographic changes: prolonged ST interval, prolonged QT interval	• Serum calcium level that exceeds 10 mg/dL • Electrocardiographic changes: shortened ST segment, widened T wave

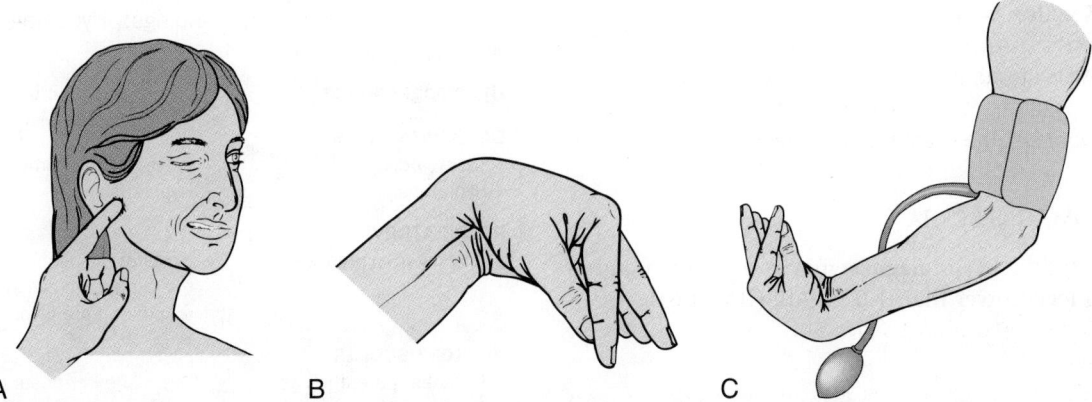

▲ **FIGURE 9-3** Tests for hypocalcemia. **A,** Chvostek's sign is contraction of facial muscles in response to a light tap over the facial nerve in front of the ear. **B,** Trousseau's sign is a carpal spasm induced by inflating a blood pressure cuff (**C**) above the systolic pressure for a few minutes. (From Lewis, S., Heitkemper, M., & Dirksen, S. [2007]. *Medical-surgical nursing* [7th ed.]. St. Louis: Mosby.)

IX. HYPERCALCEMIA

A. Description: **Hypercalcemia** is a serum **calcium** level that exceeds 10 mg/dL (see Box 9-5).

B. Causes
    1. Increased **calcium** absorption
        a. Excessive oral intake of **calcium**
        b. Excessive oral intake of vitamin D

    2. Decreased **calcium** excretion
        a. Renal failure
        b. Use of thiazide diuretics
    3. Increased bone resorption of **calcium**
        a. Hyperparathyroidism
        b. Hyperthyroidism

c. Malignancy (bone destruction from metastatic tumors)
d. Immobility
e. Use of glucocorticoids
4. Hemoconcentration
   a. Dehydration
   b. Use of lithium
   c. Adrenal insufficiency
C. Assessment (see Tables 9-4 and 9-5)
D. Interventions
1. Monitor cardiovascular, respiratory, neuromuscular, renal, and gastrointestinal status; place the client on a cardiac monitor.
2. Discontinue IV infusions of solutions containing **calcium** and oral medications containing **calcium** or vitamin D.
3. Discontinue thiazide diuretics and replace with diuretics that enhance the excretion of **calcium**.
4. Administer medications as prescribed that inhibit **calcium** resorption from the bone, such as **phosphorus**, calcitonin (Calcimar), bisphosphonates, and prostaglandin synthesis inhibitors (aspirin, nonsteroidal anti-inflammatory drugs).
5. Prepare the client with severe **hypercalcemia** for dialysis if medications fail to reduce the serum **calcium** level.
6. Move the client carefully and monitor for signs of a pathological fracture.
7. Monitor for flank or abdominal pain, and strain the urine to check for the presence of urinary stones.
8. Instruct the client to avoid foods high in **calcium** (see Box 9-5).

⚠ A client with a calcium imbalance is at risk for a pathological fracture. Move the client carefully and slowly; assist the client with ambulation.

X. HYPOMAGNESEMIA

A. Description: **Hypomagnesemia** is a serum **magnesium** level lower than 1.6 mg/dL (Box 9-6).

Box 9-6 Magnesium

Normal Value
1.6 to 2.6 mg/dL

Common Food Sources
Avocado	Oatmeal
Canned white tuna	Peanut butter
Cauliflower	Peas
Green leafy vegetables, such as spinach and broccoli	Pork, beef, chicken
	Potatoes
	Raisins
Milk	Yogurt

B. Causes
1. Insufficient **magnesium** intake
   a. Malnutrition and starvation
   b. Vomiting or diarrhea
   c. Malabsorption syndrome
   d. Celiac disease
   e. Crohn's disease
2. Increased **magnesium** secretion
   a. Medications such as diuretics
   b. Chronic alcoholism
3. Intracellular movement of **magnesium**
   a. Hyperglycemia
   b. Insulin administration
   c. Sepsis
C. Assessment (Table 9-6; see Table 9-4)
D. Interventions
1. Monitor cardiovascular, respiratory, gastrointestinal, neuromuscular, and central nervous system status; place the client on a cardiac monitor.
2. Because **hypocalcemia** frequently accompanies **hypomagnesemia**, interventions also aim to restore normal serum **calcium** levels.
3. Administer **magnesium** sulfate by the IV route in severe cases (intramuscular injections cause pain and tissue damage); monitor serum **magnesium** levels frequently.
4. Initiate seizure precautions.
5. Monitor for diminished deep tendon reflexes, suggesting **hypermagnesemia**, during the administration of **magnesium**.

TABLE 9-6 Assessment Findings: Hypomagnesemia and Hypermagnesemia

Hypomagnesemia	Hypermagnesemia
CARDIOVASCULAR	
• Tachycardia	• Bradycardia, dysrhythmias
• Hypertension	• Hypotension
RESPIRATORY	
• Shallow respirations	• Respiratory insufficiency when the skeletal muscles of respiration are involved
NEUROMUSCULAR	
• Twitches; paresthesias	• Diminished or absent deep tendon reflexes
• Positive Trousseau's and Chvostek's signs	• Skeletal muscle weakness
• Hyperreflexia	
• Tetany, seizures	
CENTRAL NERVOUS SYSTEM	
• Irritability	• Drowsiness and lethargy that progresses to coma
• Confusion	
LABORATORY FINDINGS	
• Serum magnesium level less than 1.6 mg/dL	• Serum magnesium level that exceeds 2.6 mg/dL
• Electrocardiographic changes: tall T waves, depressed ST segments	• Electrocardiographic changes: prolonged PR interval, widened QRS complexes

6. Oral preparations of **magnesium** may cause diarrhea and increase **magnesium** loss.
7. Instruct the client to increase the intake of foods that contain **magnesium** (see Box 9-6).

XI. HYPERMAGNESEMIA

A. Description: **Hypermagnesemia** is a serum **magnesium** level that exceeds 2.6 mg/dL (see Box 9-6).
B. Causes
   1. Increased **magnesium** intake
      a. **Magnesium**-containing antacids and laxatives
      b. Excessive administration of **magnesium** intravenously
   2. Decreased renal excretion of **magnesium** as a result of renal insufficiency
C. Assessment (see Tables 9-4 and 9-6)
D. Interventions
   1. Monitor cardiovascular, respiratory, neuromuscular, and central nervous system status; place the client on a cardiac monitor.
   2. Diuretics are prescribed to increase renal excretion of **magnesium**.
   3. Intravenously administered **calcium** chloride or **calcium** gluconate may be prescribed to reverse the effects of **magnesium** on cardiac muscle.
   4. Instruct the client to restrict dietary intake of **magnesium**-containing foods (see Box 9-6).
   5. Instruct the client to avoid the use of laxatives and antacids containing **magnesium**.

⚠ Calcium gluconate is the antidote for magnesium overdose!

XII. HYPOPHOSPHATEMIA

A. Description
   1. **Hypophosphatemia** is a serum **phosphorus** level lower than 2.7 mg/dL (Box 9-7).
   2. A decrease in the serum **phosphorus** level is accompanied by an increase in the serum **calcium** level.

Box 9-7 Phosphorus

Normal Value
2.7 to 4.5 mg/dL

Common Food Sources
Fish
Organ meats
Nuts
Pork, beef, chicken
Whole-grain breads and cereals

B. Causes
   1. Insufficient **phosphorus** intake: malnutrition and starvation
   2. Increased **phosphorus** excretion
      a. Hyperparathyroidism
      b. Malignancy
      c. Use of **magnesium**-based or aluminum hydroxide–based antacids
   3. Intracellular shift
      a. Hyperglycemia
      b. Respiratory alkalosis
C. Assessment
   1. Cardiovascular
      a. Decreased contractility and cardiac output
      b. Slowed peripheral pulses
   2. Respiratory: shallow respirations
   3. Neuromuscular
      a. Weakness
      b. Decreased deep tendon reflexes
      c. Decreased bone density that can cause fractures and alterations in bone shape
      d. Rhabdomyolysis
   4. Central nervous system
      a. Irritability
      b. Confusion
      c. Seizures
   5. Hematological
      a. Decreased platelet aggregation and increased bleeding
      b. Immunosuppression
D. Interventions
   1. Monitor cardiovascular, respiratory, neuromuscular, central nervous system, and hematological status.
   2. Discontinue medications that contribute to **hypophosphatemia**.
   3. Administer **phosphorus** orally along with a vitamin D supplement.
   4. Prepare to administer **phosphorus** intravenously when serum **phosphorus** levels fall below 1 mg/dL and when the client experiences critical clinical manifestations.
   5. Administer IV **phosphorus** slowly because of the risks associated with **hyperphosphatemia**.
   6. Assess the renal system before administering **phosphorus**.
   7. Move the client carefully, and monitor for signs of a pathological fracture.
   8. Instruct the client to increase the intake of the **phosphorus**-containing foods while decreasing the intake of any **calcium**-containing foods (Box 9-7; see Box 9-5).

⚠ A decrease in the serum phosphorus level is accompanied by an increase in the serum calcium level and an increase in the serum phosphorus level is accompanied by a decrease in the serum calcium level.

XIII. HYPERPHOSPHATEMIA

A. Description
1. **Hyperphosphatemia** is a serum **phosphorus** level that exceeds 4.5 mg/dL (see Box 9-7).
2. Most body systems tolerate elevated serum **phosphorus** levels well.
3. An increase in the serum **phosphorus** level is accompanied by a decrease in the serum **calcium** level.
4. The problems that occur in **hyperphosphatemia** center on the **hypocalcemia** that results when serum **phosphorus** levels increase.

B. Causes
1. Decreased renal excretion resulting from renal insufficiency
2. Tumor lysis syndrome
3. Increased intake of **phosphorus**, including dietary intake or overuse of phosphate-containing laxatives or enemas
4. Hypoparathyroidism

C. Assessment: Refer to assessment of **hypocalcemia**.

D. Interventions
1. Interventions entail the management of **hypocalcemia**.
2. Administer phosphate-binding medications that increase fecal excretion of **phosphorus** by binding **phosphorus** from food in the gastrointestinal tract.
3. Instruct the client to avoid phosphate-containing medications, including laxatives and enemas.
4. Instruct the client to decrease the intake of food that is high in **phosphorus** (see Box 9-7).
5. Instruct the client in medication administration: take phosphate-binding medications, emphasizing that they should be taken with meals or immediately after meals.

⊙ MORE QUESTIONS ON THE CD!

Practice Questions

36. The nurse is caring for a client with congestive heart failure. On assessment, the nurse notes that the client is dyspneic and that crackles are audible on auscultation. The nurse suspects excess fluid volume. What additional signs would the nurse expect to note in this client if excess fluid volume is present?
1. Weight loss
2. Flat neck and hand veins
3. An increase in blood pressure
4. A decreased central venous pressure (CVP)

37. A nurse is preparing to care for a client with a potassium deficit. The nurse reviews the client's record and determines that the client was at risk for developing the potassium deficit because the client:

1. Sustained tissue damage
2. Requires nasogastric suction
3. Has a history of Addison's disease
4. Is taking a potassium-sparing diuretic

38. A nurse reviews a client's electrolyte laboratory report and notes that the potassium level is 3.2 mEq/L. Which of the following would the nurse note on the electrocardiogram as a result of the laboratory value?
1. U waves
2. Absent P waves
3. Elevated T waves
4. Elevated ST segment

39. A nursing student needs to administer potassium chloride intravenously as prescribed to a client with hypokalemia. The nursing instructor determines that the student is unprepared for this procedure if the student states that which of the following is part of the plan for preparation and administration of the potassium?
1. Obtaining a controlled intravenous (IV) infusion pump
2. Monitoring urine output during administration
3. Preparing the medication for bolus administration
4. Diluting the medication in appropriate amount of normal saline

40. A nurse caring for a group of clients reviews the electrolyte laboratory results and notes a potassium level of 5.5 mEq/L on one client's laboratory report. The nurse understands that which client is at highest risk for the development of a potassium value at this level?
1. The client with colitis
2. The client with Cushing's syndrome
3. The client who has been overusing laxatives
4. The client who has sustained a traumatic burn

41. A nurse is reviewing laboratory results and notes that a client's serum sodium level is 150 mEq/L. The nurse reports the serum sodium level to the physician and the physician prescribes dietary instructions based on the sodium level. Which food item does the nurse instruct the client to avoid?
1. Peas
2. Nuts
3. Cauliflower
4. Processed oat cereals

42. A nurse is assessing a client with a suspected diagnosis of hypocalcemia. Which of the following clinical manifestations would the nurse expect to note in the client?

1. Twitching
2. Hypoactive bowel sounds
3. Negative Trousseau's sign
4. Hypoactive deep tendon reflexes

43. A nurse caring for a client with hypocalcemia would expect to note which of the following changes on the electrocardiogram?
1. Widened T wave
2. Prominent U wave
3. Prolonged QT interval
4. Shortened ST segment

44. A nurse reviews the electrolyte results of an assigned client and notes that the potassium level is 5.4 mEq/L. Which of the following would the nurse expect to note on the electrocardiogram as a result of the laboratory value?
1. ST depression
2. Inverted T wave
3. Prominent U wave
4. Tall peaked T waves

45. A nurse caring for a group of clients reviews the electrolyte laboratory results and notes a sodium level of 130 mEq/L on one client's laboratory report. The nurse understands that which client is at highest risk for the development of a sodium value at this level?
1. The client with Cushing's syndrome
2. The client who is taking diuretics
3. The client with hyperaldosteronism
4. The client who is taking corticosteroids

46. A nurse is caring for a client with acute congestive heart failure who is receiving high doses of a diuretic. On assessment, the nurse notes that the client has flat neck veins, generalized muscle weakness, and diminished deep tendon reflexes. The nurse suspects hyponatremia. What additional signs would the nurse expect to note in a client with hyponatremia?
1. Extreme thirst
2. Decreased urinary output
3. Hyperactive bowel sounds
4. Increased specific gravity of the urine

47. A nurse reviews a client's laboratory report and notes that the client's serum phosphorus level is 2 mg/dL. Which condition most likely caused this serum phosphorus level?
1. Alcoholism
2. Renal insufficiency
3. Hypoparathyroidism
4. Tumor lysis syndrome

48. A nurse is reading a physician's progress notes in the client's record and reads that the physician has documented "insensible fluid loss of approximately 800 mL daily." The nurse interprets that this type of fluid loss can occur through:
1. The skin
2. Urinary output
3. Wound drainage
4. The gastrointestinal tract

49. A nurse is assigned to care for a group of clients. On review of the clients' medical records, the nurse determines that which client is at risk for a fluid volume deficit?
1. A client with a colostomy
2. A client with congestive heart failure
3. A client on long-term corticosteroid therapy
4. A client receiving frequent wound irrigations

50. A nurse caring for a client who has been receiving IV diuretics suspects that the client is experiencing a fluid volume deficit. Which assessment finding would the nurse note in a client with this condition?
1. Lung congestion
2. Decreased hematocrit
3. Increased blood pressure
4. Decreased central venous pressure (CVP)

51. A nurse is assigned to care for a group of clients. On review of the clients' medical records, the nurse determines that which client is at risk for fluid volume excess?
1. The client taking diuretics
2. The client with renal failure
3. The client with an ileostomy
4. The client who requires gastrointestinal suctioning

Alternate Item Format: Multiple Response

52. The nurse provides instructions to a client with a low potassium level about the foods that are high in potassium and tells the client to consume which foods? **Select all that apply.**
❑ 1. Peas
❑ 2. Raisins
❑ 3. Potatoes
❑ 4. Cauliflower
❑ 5. Cantaloupe
❑ 6. Strawberries

ANSWERS

36. 3

Rationale: A fluid volume excess is also known as overhydration or fluid overload and occurs when fluid intake or fluid retention exceeds the fluid needs of the body. Assessment findings associated with fluid volume excess include cough, dyspnea, crackles, tachypnea, tachycardia, elevated blood pressure, bounding pulse, elevated CVP, weight gain, edema, neck and hand vein distention, altered level of consciousness, and decreased hematocrit. Options 1, 2, and 4 identify signs noted in fluid volume deficit.

Test-Taking Strategy: Use the process of elimination and focus on the subject, fluid volume excess. Note that options 1, 2, and 4 are comparable or alike in that each of these signs reflects a decrease. Option 3 reflects an increase. If you had difficulty with this question, review the assessment findings noted in fluid volume excess.

Level of Cognitive Ability: Analyzing
Client Needs: Physiological Integrity
Integrated Process: Nursing Process—Assessment
Content Area: Fundamental Skills—Fluids & Electrolytes/Acid-Base
Reference: Black, J., & Hawks, J. (2009). *Medical-surgical nursing: Clinical management for positive outcomes* (8th ed., p. 1441–1443). St. Louis: Saunders.

37. 2

Rationale: The normal serum potassium level is 3.5 mEq/L to 5.1 mEq/L. A potassium deficit is known as *hypokalemia*. Potassium-rich gastrointestinal fluids are lost through gastrointestinal suction, placing the client at risk for hypokalemia. The client with tissue damage or Addison's disease and the client taking a potassium-sparing diuretic are at risk for hyperkalemia.

Test-Taking Strategy: Use the process of elimination. Note that the subject of the question is potassium deficit. Option 2 is the only option that identifies a loss of body fluid. If you had difficulty with this question, review the causes of hypokalemia.

Level of Cognitive Ability: Understanding
Client Needs: Physiological Integrity
Integrated Process: Nursing Process—Assessment
Content Area: Fundamental Skills—Fluids & Electrolytes/Acid-Base
Reference: Ackley, B., Ladwig, G., Swan, B., & Tucker, S. (2008). *Evidence-based nursing care guidelines: Medical-surgical interventions* (p. 291). St. Louis: Mosby.

38. 1

Rationale: A serum potassium level lower than 3.5 mEq/L indicates hypokalemia. Potassium deficit is a common electrolyte imbalance and is potentially life-threatening. Electrocardiographic changes include inverted T waves, ST segment depression, and prominent U waves. Absent P waves are not a characteristic of hypokalemia but may be noted in a client with atrial fibrillation.

Test-Taking Strategy: From the information in the question, you need to determine that the client is experiencing hypokalemia. From this point, you must know the electrocardiographic changes that are expected when hypokalemia

exists. Remember that a prominent U wave is indicative of hypokalemia. If you had difficulty with this question, review the electrocardiographic changes that occur in hypokalemia.

Level of Cognitive Ability: Analyzing
Client Needs: Physiological Integrity
Integrated Process: Nursing Process—Assessment
Content Area: Fundamental Skills—Fluids & Electrolytes/Acid-Base
Reference: Ackley, B., Ladwig, G., Swan, B., & Tucker, S. (2008). *Evidence-based nursing care guidelines: Medical-surgical interventions* (p. 293). St. Louis: Mosby.

39. 3

Rationale: Potassium chloride administered intravenously must always be diluted in IV fluid and infused via an infusion pump or controller. Potassium chloride is never given by bolus (IV push). Giving potassium chloride by IV push can result in cardiac arrest. Dilution in normal saline is recommended, and dextrose solution is avoided because this type of solution increases intracellular potassium shifting. The IV bag containing the potassium chloride is always gently agitated before hanging. The IV site is monitored closely because potassium chloride is irritating to the veins and there is risk of phlebitis. The nurse monitors urinary output during administration and contacts the physician if the urinary output is less than 30 mL/hr.

Test-Taking Strategy: Focus on the subject, the administration of potassium chloride intravenously. Note the strategic word *unprepared*. This word indicates a negative event query and the need to select the incorrect action. Noting the word *bolus* in option 3 will direct you to the correct option. Review the procedure for the administration of IV potassium chloride if you had difficulty with this question.

Level of Cognitive Ability: Understanding
Client Needs: Physiological Integrity
Integrated Process: Teaching and Learning
Content Area: Pharmacology
Reference: Gahart, B., & Nazareno, A. (2009). *Intravenous medications* (25th ed., p. 1086). St. Louis: Mosby.

40. 4

Rationale: A serum potassium level higher than 5.1 mEq/L indicates hyperkalemia. Clients who experience cellular shifting of potassium in the early stages of massive cell destruction, such as with trauma, burns, sepsis, or metabolic or respiratory acidosis, are at risk for hyperkalemia. The client with Cushing's syndrome or colitis and the client who has been overusing laxatives are at risk for hypokalemia.

Test-Taking Strategy: Use the process of elimination. Eliminate options 1 and 3 first because they are comparable or alike, with both reflecting a gastrointestinal loss. From the remaining options, recalling that cell destruction causes potassium shifts will assist in directing you to the correct option. Also, remember that Cushing's syndrome presents a risk for hypokalemia and that Addison's disease presents a risk for hyperkalemia. If you had difficulty with this question, review the risk factors associated with hyperkalemia.

Level of Cognitive Ability: Analyzing
Client Needs: Physiological Integrity
Integrated Process: Nursing Process—Assessment

9 Fluids and Electrolytes

99

Content Area: Fundamental Skills—Fluids & Electrolytes/Acid-Base
Reference: Potter, P., & Perry, A. (2009). *Fundamentals of nursing* (7th ed., p. 973). St. Louis: Mosby.

41. 4
Rationale: The normal serum sodium level is 135 to 145 mEq/L. A serum sodium level of 150 mEq/L indicates hypernatremia. Based on this finding, the nurse would instruct the client to avoid foods high in sodium. Nuts, cauliflower, and peas are good food sources of phosphorus. Processed foods are high in sodium content.
Test-Taking Strategy: First, you must determine that the client has hypernatremia. Next, note the strategic word *avoid* in the question. Eliminate options 1 and 3 first because these are vegetables. From the remaining options, note the word *processed* in option 4. Processed foods tend to be higher in sodium content. Review foods high in sodium content if you had difficulty with this question.
Level of Cognitive Ability: Applying
Client Needs: Physiological Integrity
Integrated Process: Teaching and Learning
Content Area: Fundamental Skills—Fluids & Electrolytes/Acid-Base
Reference: Nix, S. (2009). *Williams' basic nutrition and diet therapy* (13th ed., p. 486). St. Louis: Mosby.

42. 1
Rationale: The normal serum calcium level is 8.6 to 10 mg/dL. A serum calcium level lower than 8.6 mg/dL indicates hypocalcemia. Signs of hypocalcemia include paresthesias followed by numbness, hyperactive deep tendon reflexes, and a positive Trousseau's or Chvostek's sign. Additional signs of hypocalcemia include increased neuromuscular excitability, muscle cramps, twitching, tetany, seizures, irritability, and anxiety. Gastrointestinal symptoms include increased gastric motility, hyperactive bowel sounds, abdominal cramping, and diarrhea.
Test-Taking Strategy: Use the process of elimination, noting that options 2, 3, and 4 are comparable or alike in that they reflect a hypoactivity. The option that is different is option 1. Review the assessment signs and symptoms noted in hypocalcemia if you had difficulty with this question.
Level of Cognitive Ability: Analyzing
Client Needs: Physiological Integrity
Integrated Process: Nursing Process—Assessment
Content Area: Fundamental Skills—Fluids & Electrolytes/Acid-Base
Reference: Potter, P., & Perry, A. (2009). *Fundamentals of nursing* (7th ed., p. 973). St. Louis: Mosby.

43. 3
Rationale: The normal serum calcium level is 8.6 to 10 mg/dL. A serum calcium level lower than 8.6 mg/dL indicates hypocalcemia. Electrocardiographic changes that occur in a client with hypocalcemia include a prolonged ST or QT interval. A shortened ST segment and a widened T wave occur with hypercalcemia. Prominent U waves occur with hypokalemia.

Test-Taking Strategy: Use knowledge regarding the electrocardiographic changes that occur in a calcium imbalance to answer the question. Remember that hypocalcemia causes a prolonged ST or QT interval. If you had difficulty with this question, review the electrocardiographic changes that occur in these conditions.
Level of Cognitive Ability: Analyzing
Client Needs: Physiological Integrity
Integrated Process: Nursing Process—Assessment
Content Area: Fundamental Skills—Fluids & Electrolytes/Acid-Base
Reference: Black, J., & Hawks, J. (2009). *Medical-surgical nursing: Clinical management for positive outcomes* (8th ed., p. 158). St. Louis: Saunders.

44. 4
Rationale: A serum potassium level greater than 5.1 mEq/L indicates hyperkalemia. Electrocardiographic changes associated with hyperkalemia include flat P waves, prolonged PR intervals, widened QRS complexes, and tall peaked T waves.
Test-Taking Strategy: From the information in the question, you need to determine that this condition is a hyperkalemic one. From this point, you must know the electrocardiographic changes that are expected when hyperkalemia exists. Remember that tall peaked T waves are associated with hyperkalemia. If you had difficulty with this question, review the normal serum potassium level and the electrocardiographic changes that occur in hyperkalemia.
Level of Cognitive Ability: Analyzing
Client Needs: Physiological Integrity
Integrated Process: Nursing Process—Assessment
Content Area: Fundamental Skills—Fluids & Electrolytes/Acid-Base
Reference: Ackley, B., Ladwig, G., Swan, B., & Tucker, S. (2008). *Evidence-based nursing care guidelines: Medical-surgical interventions* (p. 287). St. Louis: Mosby.

45. 2
Rationale: Hyponatremia is evidenced by a serum sodium level less than 135 mEq/L. Hyponatremia can occur in the client taking diuretics. The client taking corticosteroids and the client with Cushing's syndrome or hyperaldosteronism are at risk for hypernatremia.
Test-Taking Strategy: First, determine that the client is experiencing hyponatremia. Next, you must know the causes of hyponatremia to direct you to option 2. Also recall that when a client takes a diuretic, the client loses fluid and electrolytes. Review the normal serum sodium level and the causes of hyponatremia if you had difficulty with this question.
Level of Cognitive Ability: Analyzing
Client Needs: Physiological Integrity
Integrated Process: Nursing Process—Assessment
Content Area: Fundamental Skills—Fluids & Electrolytes/Acid-Base
References: Ackley, B., Ladwig, G., Swan, B., & Tucker, S. (2008). *Evidence-based nursing care guidelines: Medical-surgical interventions* (p. 299). St. Louis: Mosby.
   Potter, P., & Perry, A. (2009). *Fundamentals of nursing* (7th ed., p. 973). St. Louis: Mosby.

46. 3

Rationale: Hyponatremia is evidenced by a serum sodium level lower than 135 mEq/L. Hyperactive bowel sounds indicate hyponatremia. Options 1, 2, and 4 are signs of hypernatremia. In hyponatremia, increased urinary output and decreased specific gravity of the urine would be noted.

Test-Taking Strategy: Focus on the data in the question and the subject of the question. Recalling the signs of hyponatremia will direct you to option 3. Remember that increased bowel motility and hyperactive bowel sounds indicate hyponatremia. If you had difficulty with this question, review the assessment signs associated with hyponatremia and hypernatremia.

Level of Cognitive Ability: Analyzing
Client Needs: Physiological Integrity
Integrated Process: Nursing Process—Assessment
Content Area: Fundamental Skills—Fluids & Electrolytes/Acid-Base
References: Black, J., & Hawks, J. (2009). *Medical-surgical nursing: Clinical management for positive outcomes* (8th ed., p. 144). St. Louis: Saunders.
   Potter, P., & Perry, A. (2009). *Fundamentals of nursing* (7th ed., p. 973). St. Louis: Mosby.

47. 1

Rationale: The normal serum phosphorus level is 2.7 to 4.5 mg/dL. The client is experiencing hypophosphatemia. Causative factors relate to malnutrition or starvation and the use of aluminum hydroxide–based or magnesium-based antacids. Malnutrition is associated with alcoholism. Renal insufficiency, hypoparathyroidism, and tumor lysis syndrome are causative factors of hyperphosphatemia.

Test-Taking Strategy: First you must determine that the client is experiencing hypophosphatemia. From this point, you must know the causes of hypophosphatemia in order to answer correctly. If you had difficulty with this question, review the causative factors associated with hypophosphatemia.

Level of Cognitive Ability: Analyzing
Client Needs: Physiological Integrity
Integrated Process: Nursing Process—Assessment
Content Area: Fundamental Skills—Fluids & Electrolytes/Acid-Base
Reference: Black, J., & Hawks, J. (2009). *Medical-surgical nursing: Clinical management for positive outcomes* (8th ed., p.164). St. Louis: Saunders.

48. 1

Rationale: Sensible losses are those of which the person is aware, such as through wound drainage, gastrointestinal tract losses, and urination. Insensible losses may occur without the person's awareness. Insensible losses occur daily through the skin and the lungs.

Test-Taking Strategy: Note that the subject of the question is insensible fluid loss. Use the process of elimination, noting that options 2, 3, and 4 are comparable or alike. The types of losses in options 2, 3, and 4 can be measured for accurate output. Fluid loss through the skin cannot be measured accurately; it can only be approximated. If you had difficulty with this question, review the difference between sensible and insensible fluid loss.

Level of Cognitive Ability: Understanding
Client Needs: Physiological Integrity

Integrated Process: Communication and Documentation
Content Area: Fundamental Skills—Fluids & Electrolytes/Acid-Base
Reference: Black, J., & Hawks, J. (2009). *Medical-surgical nursing: Clinical management for positive outcomes* (8th ed., p. 133). St. Louis: Saunders.

49. 1

Rationale: A fluid volume deficit occurs when the fluid intake is not sufficient to meet the fluid needs of the body. Causes of a fluid volume deficit include vomiting, diarrhea, conditions that cause increased respirations or increased urinary output, insufficient intravenous fluid replacement, draining fistulas, and the presence of an ileostomy or colostomy. A client with congestive heart failure or on long-term corticosteroid therapy, or a client receiving frequent wound irrigations, is at risk for fluid volume excess.

Test-Taking Strategy: Read the question carefully, noting that it asks for the client at risk for a deficit. Read each option and think about the fluid imbalance that can occur in each. The clients presented in options 2, 3, and 4 retain fluid. The only condition that can cause a deficit is the condition noted in option 1. If you had difficulty with this question, review the causes of a fluid volume deficit.

Level of Cognitive Ability: Analyzing
Client Needs: Physiological Integrity
Integrated Process: Nursing Process—Assessment
Content Area: Fundamental Skills—Fluids & Electrolytes/Acid-Base
Reference: Black, J., & Hawks, J. (2009). *Medical-surgical nursing: Clinical management for positive outcomes* (8th ed., p. 697). St. Louis: Saunders.

50. 4

Rationale: A fluid volume deficit occurs when the fluid intake is not sufficient to meet the fluid needs of the body. Assessment findings in a client with a fluid volume deficit include increased respirations and heart rate, decreased CVP, weight loss, poor skin turgor, dry mucous membranes, decreased urine volume, increased specific gravity of the urine, increased hematocrit, and altered level of consciousness. The normal CVP is between 4 and 11 cm H_2O. A client with dehydration (fluid volume deficit) has a low CVP. The assessment findings in options 1, 2, and 3 are seen in a client with fluid volume excess.

Test-Taking Strategy: Use the process of elimination and focus on the subject, fluid volume deficit. Eliminate options 1 and 3 first. Lung congestion is noted in fluid volume excess, as is increased blood pressure. From the remaining options, recall that CVP reflects the pressure under which blood is returned to the superior vena cava and right atrium. Therefore pressure (volume) would be decreased in a deficient fluid volume. If you had difficulty with this question, review the assessment findings noted in fluid volume deficit.

Level of Cognitive Ability: Analyzing
Client Needs: Physiological Integrity
Integrated Process: Nursing Process—Assessment
Content Area: Fundamental Skills—Fluids & Electrolytes/Acid-Base
Reference: Potter, P., & Perry, A. (2009). *Fundamentals of nursing* (7th ed., p. 973). St. Louis: Mosby.

51. 2

Rationale: A fluid volume excess is also known as *overhydration* or *fluid overload* and occurs when fluid intake or fluid retention exceeds the fluid needs of the body. The causes of fluid volume excess include decreased kidney function, congestive heart failure, use of hypotonic fluids to replace isotonic fluid losses, excessive irrigation of wounds and body cavities, and excessive ingestion of sodium. The client taking diuretics, the client with an ileostomy, and the client who requires gastrointestinal suctioning are at risk for fluid volume deficit.

Test-Taking Strategy: Use the process of elimination and focus on the subject, fluid volume excess. Read each option and think about the fluid imbalance that can occur in each. The clients presented in options 1, 3, and 4 lose fluid. The only condition that can cause an excess is the condition noted in option 2. If you had difficulty with this question, review the causes of fluid volume excess.

Level of Cognitive Ability: Analyzing
Client Needs: Physiological Integrity
Integrated Process: Nursing Process—Assessment
Content Area: Fundamental Skills—Fluids & Electrolytes/ Acid-Base
References: Black, J., & Hawks, J. (2009). *Medical-surgical nursing: Clinical management for positive outcomes* (8th ed., p. 811). St. Louis: Saunders.
   Potter, P., & Perry, A. (2009). *Fundamentals of nursing* (7th ed., p. 973). St. Louis: Mosby.

ALTERNATE ITEM FORMAT: MULTIPLE RESPONSE

52. 2, 3, 5, 6

Rationale: The normal potassium level is 3.5 to 5.1 mEq/L. Common food sources of potassium include avocado, bananas, cantaloupe, carrots, fish, mushrooms, oranges, potatoes, pork, beef, veal, raisins, spinach, strawberries, and tomatoes. Peas and cauliflower are high in magnesium.

Test-Taking Strategy: Focus on the subject: foods high in potassium. Read each food item and recall that peas and cauliflower are high in magnesium. Review the food items high in potassium if you had difficulty with this question.

Level of Cognitive Ability: Applying
Client Needs: Physiological Integrity
Integrated Process: Teaching and Learning
Content Area: Fundamental Skills—Fluids & Electrolytes/ Acid-Base
Reference: Nix, S. (2009). *Williams' basic nutrition and diet therapy* (13th ed., p. 136). St. Louis: Mosby.

10

Acid-Base Balance

PYRAMID TERMS

Allen's test A test to assess for collateral circulation to the hand by evaluating the patency of the radial and ulnar arteries.

compensation Compensation refers to the body processes that occur to counterbalance an acid-base disturbance. When compensation has occurred, the pH will be within normal limits.

metabolic acidosis A total concentration of buffer base that is lower than normal, with a relative increase in the hydrogen ion concentration. This results from loss of buffer bases or retention of too many acids without sufficient bases, and occurs in conditions such as renal failure and diabetic ketoacidosis, from the production of lactic acid, and from the ingestion of toxins, such as acetylsalicylic acid (aspirin).

metabolic alkalosis A deficit or loss of hydrogen ions or acids or an excess of base (bicarbonate) that results from the accumulation of base or from a loss of acid without a comparable loss of base in the body fluids. This occurs in conditions resulting in hypovolemia, the loss of gastric fluid, excessive bicarbonate intake, the massive transfusion of whole blood, and hyperaldosteronism.

respiratory acidosis A total concentration of buffer base that is lower than normal, with a relative increase in hydrogen ion concentration; thus a greater number of hydrogen ions is circulating in the blood than the buffer system can absorb. This is caused by primary defects in the function of the lungs or by changes in normal respiratory patterns as a result of secondary problems. Any condition that causes an obstruction of the airway or depresses respiratory status can cause respiratory acidosis.

respiratory alkalosis A deficit of carbonic acid or a decrease in hydrogen ion concentration that results from the accumulation of base or from a loss of acid without a comparable loss of base in the body fluids. This occurs in conditions that cause overstimulation of the respiratory system.

THE PYRAMID TO SUCCESS

Acid-base imbalance is a content area that sometimes is viewed as complex and difficult to understand. You must understand the description of each imbalance and then review the causes of each disorder, correlating the pathophysiology with each cause. From this point, note the assessment signs related to each disorder and the treatment associated with the clinical manifestations. Maintenance of a patent airway is a priority. The nurse also needs to monitor vital signs, cardiovascular status, neurological status, intake and output, laboratory values, and arterial blood gas values. Remember that safety precautions should always be initiated. Seizure precautions may also be needed.

CLIENT NEEDS

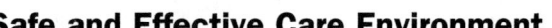

Safe and Effective Care Environment

Establishing priorities
Maintaining standard and transmission-based precautions and surgical asepsis
Obtaining informed consent for invasive procedures
Preventing accidents
Providing safety for the client during implementation of various treatments for the acid-base imbalance

Health Promotion and Maintenance

Identifying clients at risk for an acid-base imbalance
Performing physical assessment techniques
Preventing disease
Promoting health and wellness
Teaching the client and family about prevention, early detection, and treatment measures for health disorders

Psychosocial Integrity

Identifying support systems
Monitoring for sensory and perceptual alterations
Providing emotional support to the client and family

Physiological Integrity

Administering and monitoring medications, intravenous fluids, and other therapeutic interventions
Assisting with diagnostic tests
Monitoring for alterations in body systems

Monitoring for changes in status and for complications

Monitoring for expected effects of pharmacological and parenteral therapies

Monitoring laboratory values

Obtaining an arterial blood gas specimen and analyzing the results

Providing basic care and comfort

Providing wound care when blood is obtained for an arterial blood gas study

Reducing the likelihood that an acid-base imbalance will occur

I. HYDROGEN IONS, ACIDS, AND BASES

A. Hydrogen ions
   1. Vital to life
   2. Expressed as pH
   3. Circulate in the body in two forms:
      a. Volatile hydrogen of carbonic acid
      b. Nonvolatile form of hydrogen and organic acids
B. Acids
   1. Acids are produced as end products of metabolism.
   2. Acids contain hydrogen ions and are hydrogen ion donors, which means that acids give up hydrogen ions to neutralize or decrease the strength of an acid or to form a weaker base.
   3. The strength of an acid is determined by the number of hydrogen ions it contains.
   4. The number of hydrogen ions in body fluid determines its acidity, alkalinity, or neutrality.
   5. The lungs excrete 13,000 to 30,000 mEq/day of volatile hydrogen in the form of carbonic acid as carbon dioxide (CO_2).
   6. The kidneys excrete 50 mEq/day of nonvolatile acids.
C. Bases
   1. Contain no hydrogen ions.
   2. Are hydrogen ion acceptors; they accept hydrogen ions from acids to neutralize or decrease the strength of a base or to form a weaker acid.

II. REGULATORY SYSTEMS FOR HYDROGEN ION CONCENTRATION IN THE BLOOD (Box 10-1)

A. Buffers
   1. Buffers are the fastest acting regulatory system.

Box 10-1 Regulatory Systems for Hydrogen Ion Concentration in the Blood

Buffers
   Primary buffer systems in extracellular fluid: hemoglobin system; plasma protein system; carbonic acid–bicarbonate system; phosphate buffer system
Lungs
Kidneys
Potassium exchange

   2. Provide immediate protection against changes in hydrogen ion concentration in the extracellular fluid.
   3. Buffers are reactors that function only to keep the pH within the narrow limits of stability when too much acid or base is released into the system, and buffers absorb or release hydrogen ions as needed.
   4. Buffers serve as a transport mechanism that carries excess hydrogen ions to the lungs.
   5. Once the primary buffer systems react, they are consumed, leaving the body less able to withstand further stress until the buffers are replaced.
B. Primary buffer systems in extracellular fluid
   1. Hemoglobin system
      a. Red blood cells contain hemoglobin.
      b. System maintains acid-base balance by a process called chloride shift.
      c. Chloride shifts in and out of the cells in response to the level of O_2 in the blood.
      d. For each chloride ion that leaves a red blood cell, a bicarbonate ion enters.
      e. For each chloride ion that enters a red blood cell, a bicarbonate ion leaves.
   2. Plasma protein system
      a. The system functions along with the liver to vary the amount of hydrogen ions in the chemical structure of plasma proteins.
      b. Plasma proteins have the ability to attract or release hydrogen ions.
   3. Carbonic acid–bicarbonate system
      a. Primary buffer system in the body.
      b. The system maintains a pH of 7.4 with a ratio of 20 parts bicarbonate (HCO_3^-) to 1 part carbonic acid (H_2CO_3) (Fig. 10-1).
      c. This ratio (20:1) determines the hydrogen ion concentration of body fluid.

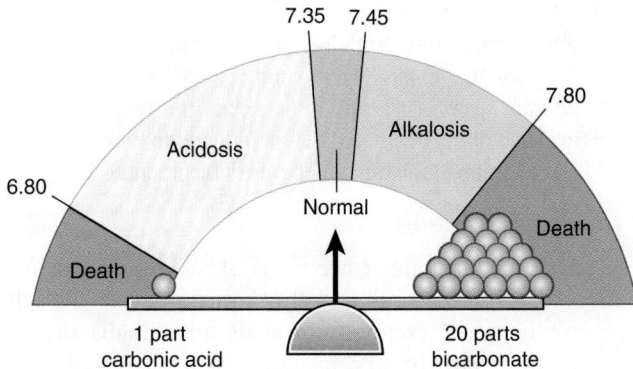

▲ **FIGURE 10-1** Acid-base balance. In the healthy state, a ratio of 1 part carbonic acid to 20 parts bicarbonate provides a normal serum pH between 7.35 and 7.45. Any deviation to the left of 7.35 results in an acidotic state. Any deviation to the right of 7.45 results in an alkalotic state. (From Harkreader, H., Hogan, M.A., & Thobaben, M. [2007]. *Fundamentals of nursing: caring and clinical judgment* [3rd ed., p. 624, Figure 25-5]. St. Louis: Saunders.)

d. Carbonic acid concentration is controlled by the excretion of CO_2 by the lungs; the rate and depth of respiration change in response to changes in the CO_2.

e. The kidneys control the bicarbonate concentration and selectively retain or excrete bicarbonate in response to bodily needs.

4. Phosphate buffer system
   a. System is present in the cells and body fluids and is especially active in the kidneys.
   b. System acts like bicarbonate and neutralizes excess hydrogen ions.

C. Lungs
   1. The lungs are the second defense of the body and interact with the buffer system to maintain acid-base balance.
   2. In acidosis, the pH decreases and the respiratory rate and depth increase in an attempt to exhale acids. The carbonic acid created by the neutralizing action of bicarbonate can be carried to the lungs, where it is reduced to CO_2 and water and is exhaled; thus hydrogen ions are inactivated and exhaled.
   3. In alkalosis, the pH increases and the respiratory rate and depth decrease; CO_2 is retained and carbonic acid increases to neutralize and decrease the strength of excess bicarbonate.
   4. The action of the lungs is reversible in controlling an excess or deficit.
   5. The lungs can hold hydrogen ions until the deficit is corrected or can inactivate hydrogen ions, changing the ions to water molecules to be exhaled along with CO_2, thus correcting the excess.
   6. The process of correcting a deficit or excess takes 10 to 30 seconds to complete.
   7. The lungs are capable of inactivating only hydrogen ions carried by carbonic acid; excess hydrogen ions created by other mechanisms must be excreted by the kidneys.

⚠ Monitor the client's respiratory status closely. In acidosis, the respiratory rate and depth increase in an attempt to exhale acids. In alkalosis, the respiratory rate and depth decrease; CO_2 is retained to neutralize and decrease the strength of excess bicarbonate.

D. Kidneys
   1. The ultimate correction of acid-base disturbances depends on the kidneys, even though the renal excretion of acids and alkalis occurs more slowly.
   2. **Compensation** requires a few hours to several days; however, the **compensation** is more thorough and selective than that of other regulators, such as the buffer systems and lungs.
   3. In acidosis, the pH decreases and excess hydrogen ions are secreted into the tubules and combine with buffers for excretion in the urine.

4. In alkalosis, the pH increases and excess bicarbonate ions move into the tubules, combine with sodium, and are excreted in the urine.
5. Selective regulation of bicarbonate occurs in the kidneys.
   a. The kidneys restore bicarbonate by excreting hydrogen ions and retaining bicarbonate ions.
   b. Excess hydrogen ions are excreted in the urine in the form of phosphoric acid.
   c. The alteration of certain amino acids in the renal tubules results in a diffusion of ammonia into the kidneys; the ammonia combines with excess hydrogen ions and is excreted in the urine.

E. Potassium (K^+)
   1. Potassium plays an exchange role in maintaining acid-base balance.
   2. The body changes the potassium level by drawing hydrogen ions into the cell or by pushing them out of the cell.
   3. The potassium level changes to compensate for hydrogen ion level changes (Fig. 10-2).
      a. In acidosis, the body protects itself from the acidic state by moving hydrogen ions into the cell. Therefore potassium moves out to make room for hydrogen ions and the serum potassium level increases.
      b. In alkalosis, the cells release hydrogen ions into the blood in an attempt to increase the acidity of the blood; this forces the serum potassium into the cell and potassium levels decrease.

⚠ When the client experiences an acid-base imbalance, monitor the potassium level closely because the potassium moves in or out of the cells in an attempt to maintain acid-base balance.

III. **RESPIRATORY ACIDOSIS**

A. Description: The total concentration of buffer base is lower than normal, with a relative increase in hydrogen ion concentration; thus a greater number of hydrogen ions is circulating in the blood than can be absorbed by the buffer system.

B. Causes (Box 10-2)
   1. **Respiratory acidosis** is caused by primary defects in the function of the lungs or changes in normal respiratory patterns.
   2. Any condition that causes an obstruction of the airway or depresses the respiratory system can cause **respiratory acidosis**.
   3. Asthma: Spasms resulting from allergens, irritants, or emotions cause the smooth muscles of the bronchioles to constrict, resulting in ineffective gas exchange.
   4. Atelectasis: Excessive mucus collection, with the collapse of alveolar sacs caused by mucous plugs, infectious drainage, or anesthetic medications, results in ineffective gas exchange.

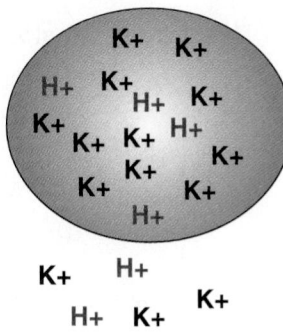

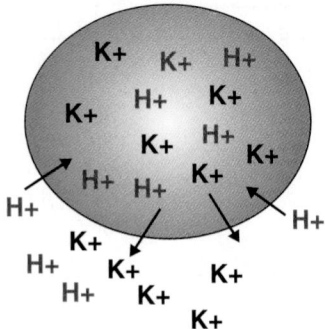

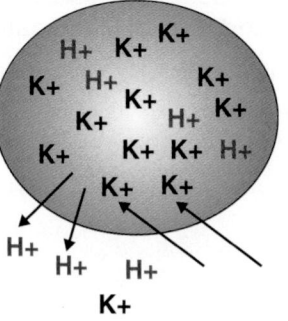

Under normal conditions, the intracellular potassium content is much greater than that of the extracellular fluid. The concentration of hydrogen ions is low in both compartments.

In acidosis, the extracellular hydrogen ion content increases, and the hydrogen ions move into the intracellular fluid. To keep the intracellular fluid electrically neutral, an equal number of potassium ions leave the cell, creating a relative hyperkalemia.

In alkalosis, more hydrogen ions are present in the intracellular fluid than in the extracellular fluid. Hydrogen ions move from the intracellular fluid into the extracellular fluid. To keep the intracellular fluid electrically neutral, potassium ions move from the extracellular fluid into the intracellular fluid, creating a relative hypokalemia.

▲ **FIGURE 10-2** Movement of potassium in response to changes in the extracellular fluid hydrogen ion concentration. (From Ignatavicius, D., & Workman, M. [2010]. *Medical-surgical nursing: Patient-centered collaborative care* [6th ed.]. St. Louis: Saunders. Courtesy of M. Linda Workman.)

Box 10-2 Causes of Respiratory Acidosis

Asthma
Atelectasis
Brain trauma
Bronchiectasis
Bronchitis
Central nervous system depressants
Emphysema
Hypoventilation
Pulmonary edema
Pneumonia
Pulmonary emboli

---

5. Brain trauma: Excessive pressure on the respiratory center or medulla oblongata depresses respirations.
6. Bronchiectasis: Bronchi become dilated as a result of inflammation, and destructive changes and weakness in the walls of the bronchi occur.
7. Bronchitis: Inflammation causes airway obstruction, resulting in inadequate gas exchange.
8. Central nervous system (CNS) depressants such as sedatives, opioids, and anesthetics depress the respiratory center, leading to hypoventilation; carbon dioxide is retained and the hydrogen ion concentration increases.
9. Emphysema: Loss of elasticity of alveolar sacs restricts air flow in and out, primarily out, leading to an increased CO_2 level.
10. Hypoventilation: Carbon dioxide is retained and the hydrogen ion concentration increases, leading to the acidic state; carbonic acid is retained and the pH decreases.

11. Pulmonary edema: Extracellular accumulation of fluid in pulmonary tissue causes disturbances in alveolar diffusion and perfusion.
12. Pneumonia: Excess mucus production and lung congestion cause airway obstruction, resulting in inadequate gas exchange.
13. Pulmonary emboli: Emboli cause a pulmonary artery and airway obstruction, resulting in inadequate gas exchange.

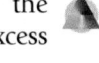 If the client has a condition that causes an obstruction of the airway or depresses the respiratory system, monitor the client for respiratory acidosis.

C. Assessment: In an attempt to compensate, the kidneys retain bicarbonate and excrete excess hydrogen ions into the urine (Table 10-1).
D. Interventions
 1. Monitor for signs of respiratory distress.
 2. Administer oxygen as prescribed.
 3. Place the client in a semi-Fowler's position, unless contraindicated.
 4. Encourage and assist the client to turn, cough, and deep-breathe.
 5. Prepare to administer respiratory treatments as prescribed.
 6. Encourage hydration to thin secretions, unless excess fluid intake is contraindicated.
 7. Suction the client's airway, if necessary and if not contraindicated.
 8. Reduce restlessness by improving ventilation rather than by administering tranquilizers, sedatives, or opioids because these medications further depress respirations.

TABLE 10-1 Clinical Manifestations of Acidosis

Respiratory ($\uparrow$ Pco$_2$)	Metabolic ($\downarrow$ HCO$_3^-$)
NEUROLOGICAL	
Drowsiness	Drowsiness
Disorientation	Confusion
Dizziness	Headache
Headache	Coma
Coma	
CARDIOVASCULAR	
Decreased blood pressure	Decreased blood pressure
Ventricular fibrillation (related to hyperkalemia from compensation)	Dysrhythmias (related to hyperkalemia from compensation)
Warm, flushed skin (related to peripheral vasodilation)	Warm, flushed skin (related to peripheral vasodilation)
GASTROINTESTINAL	
No significant findings	Nausea, vomiting, diarrhea, abdominal pain
NEUROMUSCULAR	
Seizures	No significant findings
RESPIRATORY	
Hypoventilation with hypoxia (lungs are unable to compensate when there is a respiratory problem)	Deep, rapid respirations (compensatory action by the lungs)

From Lewis, S., Heitkemper, M., & Dirksen, S. (2007). *Medical-surgical nursing: Assessment and management of clinical problems* (7th ed.). St. Louis: Mosby.

9. Monitor electrolyte values, particularly the potassium level.
10. Administer antibiotics for respiratory infection or other medications as prescribed.
11. Prepare for endotracheal intubation and mechanical ventilation if CO$_2$ levels rise above 50 mm Hg and if signs of acute respiratory distress are present.

IV. RESPIRATORY ALKALOSIS

A. Description: A deficit of carbonic acid and a decrease in hydrogen ion concentration that results from the accumulation of base or from a loss of acid without a comparable loss of base in the body fluids.
B. Causes (Box 10-3)
   1. **Respiratory alkalosis** results from conditions that cause overstimulation of the respiratory system.
   2. Fever: Causes increased metabolism, resulting in overstimulation of the respiratory system.
   3. Hyperventilation: Rapid respirations cause the blowing off of CO$_2$, leading to a decrease in carbonic acid.
   4. Hypoxia: Stimulates the respiratory center in the brainstem, which causes an increase in the respiratory rate in order to increase oxygen; this

Box 10-3 Causes of Respiratory Alkalosis

Fever
Hyperventilation
Hypoxia
Hysteria
Overventilation by mechanical ventilators
Pain

causes hyperventilation, which results in a decrease in the CO$_2$ level.
   5. Hysteria: Hysteria often is neurogenic and related to a psychoneurosis; however, this condition leads to vigorous breathing and excessive exhaling of CO$_2$.
   6. Overventilation by mechanical ventilators: The administration of O$_2$ and the depletion of CO$_2$ can occur from mechanical ventilation, causing the client to be hyperventilated.
   7. Pain: Overstimulation of the respiratory center in the brainstem results in a carbonic acid deficit.

⚠ If the client has a condition that causes overstimulation of the respiratory system, monitor the client for respiratory alkalosis.

C. Assessment: Initially the hyperventilation and respiratory stimulation cause abnormal rapid respirations (tachypnea); in an attempt to compensate, the kidneys excrete excess circulating bicarbonate into the urine (Table 10-2)
D. Interventions
   1. Monitor for signs of respiratory distress.
   2. Provide emotional support and reassurance to the client.
   3. Encourage appropriate breathing patterns.
   4. Assist with breathing techniques and breathing aids as prescribed.
      a. Encourage voluntary holding of the breath if appropriate
      b. Provide use of a rebreathing mask as prescribed
      c. Provide carbon dioxide breaths as prescribed (rebreathing into a paper bag)
   5. Provide cautious care with ventilator clients so that they are not forced to take breaths too deeply or rapidly.
   6. Monitor electrolyte values, particularly potassium and calcium levels.
   7. Administer medications as prescribed.
   8. Prepare to administer calcium gluconate for tetany as prescribed.

V. METABOLIC ACIDOSIS

A. Description: A total concentration of buffer base that is lower than normal, with a relative increase in the hydrogen ion concentration, resulting from loss of too much base and/or retention of too much acid.

TABLE 10-2 Clinical Manifestations of Alkalosis

Respiratory ($\downarrow$ Pco_2)	Metabolic ($\uparrow$ HCO$_3^-$)
NEUROLOGICAL	
Lethargy	Drowsiness
Lightheadedness	Dizziness
Confusion	Nervousness
	Confusion
CARDIOVASCULAR	
Tachycardia	Tachycardia
Dysrhythmias (related to hypokalemia from compensation)	Dysrhythmias (related to hypokalemia from compensation)
GASTROINTESTINAL	
Nausea	Anorexia
Vomiting	Nausea
Epigastric pain	Vomiting
NEUROMUSCULAR	
Tetany	Tremors
Numbness	Hypertonic muscles
Tingling of extremities	Muscle cramps
Hyperreflexia	Tetany
Seizures	Tingling of extremities
	Seizures
RESPIRATORY	
Hyperventilation (lungs are unable to compensate when there is a respiratory problem)	Hypoventilation (compensatory action by the lungs)

Modified from Lewis, S., Heitkemper, M., & Dirksen, S. (2007). *Medical-surgical nursing: Assessment and management of clinical problems* (7th ed.). St. Louis: Mosby.

Box 10-4 Causes of Metabolic Acidosis

Diabetes mellitus or diabetic ketoacidosis
Excessive ingestion of acetylsalicylic acid (aspirin)
High-fat diet
Insufficient metabolism of carbohydrates
Malnutrition
Renal insufficiency or renal failure
Severe diarrhea

B. Causes (Box 10-4)
  1. Diabetes mellitus or diabetic ketoacidosis: An insufficient supply of insulin causes increased fat metabolism, leading to an excess accumulation of ketones or other acids; the bicarbonate then ends up being depleted.
  2. Excessive ingestion of acetylsalicylic acid (aspirin) causes an increase in the hydrogen ion concentration.
  3. High-fat diet: A high intake of fat causes a much too rapid accumulation of the waste products of fat metabolism, leading to a buildup of ketones and acids.
  4. Insufficient metabolism of carbohydrates: When the O_2 supply is not sufficient for the

metabolism of carbohydrates, lactic acid is produced and lactic acidosis results.
  5. Malnutrition: Improper metabolism of nutrients causes fat catabolism, leading to an excess buildup of ketones and acids.
  6. Renal insufficiency or renal failure results in the following:
    a. Increased waste products of protein metabolism are retained.
    b. Acids increase, and bicarbonate is unable to maintain acid-base balance.
  7. Severe diarrhea: Intestinal and pancreatic secretions are normally alkaline; therefore excessive loss of base leads to acidosis.

⚠ An insufficient supply of insulin in a client with diabetes mellitus can result in metabolic acidosis known as *diabetic ketoacidosis.*

C. Assessment: To compensate for the acidosis, hyperpnea with Kussmaul's respiration occurs as the lungs attempt to exhale the excess CO_2 (see Table 10-1).
D. Interventions
  1. Monitor for signs of respiratory distress.
  2. Assess level of consciousness for central nervous system depression.
  3. Monitor intake and output and assist with fluid and electrolyte replacement as prescribed.
  4. Prepare to administer solutions intravenously as prescribed to increase the buffer base.
  5. Initiate safety and seizure precautions.
  6. Monitor the serum potassium level closely; as **metabolic acidosis** resolves, potassium moves back into the cell and the serum potassium level decreases.
E. Interventions in diabetes mellitus and diabetic ketoacidosis
  1. Give insulin as prescribed to hasten the movement of serum glucose into the cell, thereby decreasing the concurrent ketosis.
  2. When glucose is being properly metabolized, the body will stop converting fats to glucose.
  3. Monitor for circulatory collapse caused by polyuria, which may result from the hyperglycemic state; osmotic diuresis may lead to extracellular volume deficit.

⚠ Monitor the client experiencing severe diarrhea for manifestations of metabolic acidosis.

F. Interventions in renal failure
  1. In renal failure, dialysis may be used to remove protein and waste products, thereby lessening the acidotic state.
  2. A diet low in protein and high in calories decreases the amount of protein waste products, which in turn lessens the acidosis.

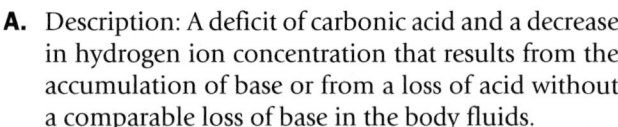

Box 10-5 Causes of Metabolic Alkalosis

Diuretics
Excessive vomiting or gastrointestinal suctioning
Hyperaldosteronism
Ingestion of and/or infusion of excess sodium bicarbonate
Massive transfusion of whole blood

Box 10-6 Normal Arterial Blood Gas Values

pH	7.35-7.45
P_{CO_2}	35-45 mm Hg
HCO_3^-	22-27 mEq/L
P_{O_2}	80-100 mm Hg

VI. METABOLIC ALKALOSIS

A. Description: A deficit of carbonic acid and a decrease in hydrogen ion concentration that results from the accumulation of base or from a loss of acid without a comparable loss of base in the body fluids.

B. Causes (Box 10-5)
1. **Metabolic alkalosis** results from a dysfunction of metabolism that causes an increased amount of available base solution in the blood or a decrease in available acids in the blood.
2. Diuretics: The loss of hydrogen ions and chloride from diuresis causes a compensatory increase in the amount of bicarbonate in the blood.
3. Excessive vomiting or gastrointestinal suctioning leads to an excessive loss of hydrochloric acid.
4. Hyperaldosteronism: Increased renal tubular reabsorption of sodium occurs, with the resultant loss of hydrogen ions.
5. Ingestion of and/or infusion of excess sodium bicarbonate causes an increase in the amount of base in the blood.
6. Massive transfusion of whole blood: The citrate anticoagulant used for the storage of blood is metabolized to bicarbonate.

C. Assessment: To compensate, respiratory rate and depth decrease to conserve CO_2 (see Table 10-2).

⚠ Monitor the client experiencing excessive vomiting or the client with gastrointestinal suctioning for manifestations of metabolic alkalosis.

D. Interventions
1. Monitor for signs of respiratory distress.
2. Monitor potassium and calcium serum levels.
3. Institute safety precautions.
4. Prepare to administer medications as prescribed to promote the kidney excretion of bicarbonate.
5. Prepare to replace potassium chloride as prescribed.
6. Treat the underlying cause of the alkalosis.

VII. ARTERIAL BLOOD GASES (Box 10-6)

A. Collection of an arterial blood gas specimen
1. Obtain vital signs.
2. Determine whether the client has an arterial line in place.
3. Perform the **Allen's test** to determine the presence of collateral circulation (see Priority Nursing Actions).

▬▬▬▬▬ Priority Nursing Actions! ▬▬▬▬▬

Actions to Take When Performing the Allen's Test
1. Explain the procedure to the client.
2. Apply pressure over the ulnar and radial arteries simultaneously.
3. Ask the client to open and close the hand repeatedly.
4. Release pressure from the ulnar artery while compressing the radial artery.
5. Assess the color of the extremity distal to the pressure point.
6. Document the findings.

The Allen's test is performed before obtaining an arterial blood specimen from the radial artery to determine the presence of collateral circulation and the adequacy of the ulnar artery. Failure to determine the presence of adequate collateral circulation could result in severe ischemic injury to the hand if damage to the radial artery occurs with arterial puncture. The nurse first would explain the procedure to the client. To perform the test, the nurse applies direct pressure over the client's ulnar and radial arteries simultaneously. While applying pressure, the nurse asks the client to open and close the hand repeatedly; the hand should blanch. The nurse then releases pressure from the ulnar artery while compressing the radial artery and assesses the color of the extremity distal to the pressure point. If pinkness fails to return within 6 seconds, the ulnar artery is insufficient, indicating that the radial artery should not be used for obtaining a blood specimen. Finally, the nurse documents the findings.

Reference: Pagana, K., & Pagana, T. (2009). *Mosby's diagnostic and laboratory test reference* (9th ed., pp. 118-119). St. Louis: Mosby.

4. Assess factors that may affect the accuracy of the results, such as changes in the O_2 settings, suctioning within the past 20 minutes, and client's activities.
5. Provide emotional support to the client.
6. Assist with the specimen draw by preparing a heparinized syringe.
7. Apply pressure immediately to the puncture site following the blood draw; maintain pressure for 5 minutes, or for 10 minutes if the client is taking anticoagulants.
8. Appropriately label the specimen and transport it on ice to the laboratory.
9. On the laboratory form, record the client's temperature and the type of supplemental oxygen that the client is receiving.

TABLE 10-3 Acid-Base Imbalances: Usual Laboratory Value Changes

Imbalance	pH	HCO$_3^-$	Pao$_2$	Paco$_2$	K$^+$
Respiratory acidosis	U: Decreased PC: Decreased C: Normal	U: Normal PC: Increased C: Increased	Usually decreased	U: Increased PC: Increased C: Increased	Increased
Respiratory alkalosis	U: Increased PC: Increased C: Normal	U: Normal PC: Decreased C: Decreased	Usually normal but depends on other accompanying conditions	U: Decreased PC: Decreased C: Decreased	Decreased
Metabolic acidosis	U: Decreased PC: Decreased C: Normal	U: Decreased PC: Decreased C: Decreased	Usually normal but depends on other accompanying conditions	U: Normal PC: Decreased C: Decreased	Increased
Metabolic alkalosis	U: Increased PC: Increased C: Normal	U: Increased PC: Increased C: Increased	Usually normal but depends on other accompanying conditions	U: Normal PC: Increased C: Increased	Decreased

C, Compensated; *PC*, partially compensated; *U*, uncompensated.

Box 10-7 Analyzing Arterial Blood Gas Results

If you can remember the following Pyramid Points and Pyramid Steps, you will be able to analyze any blood gas report.

Pyramid Points

In acidosis, the pH is decreased.
In alkalosis, the pH is elevated.
The respiratory function indicator is the Pco$_2$.
The metabolic function indicator is the bicarbonate ion (HCO$_3^-$).

Pyramid Steps

Pyramid Step 1
Look at the blood gas report. Look at the pH. Is the pH elevated or decreased? If the pH is elevated, it reflects alkalosis. If the pH is decreased, it reflects acidosis.

Pyramid Step 2
Look at the Pco$_2$. Is the Pco$_2$ elevated or decreased? If the Pco$_2$ reflects an opposite relationship to the pH, then the condition is a respiratory imbalance. If the Pco$_2$ does not reflect an opposite relationship to the pH, go to Pyramid Step 3.

Pyramid Step 3
Look at the HCO$_3^-$. Does the HCO$_3^-$ reflect a corresponding relationship with the pH? If it does, then the condition is a metabolic imbalance.

Pyramid Step 4
Compensation has occurred if the pH is in a normal range of 7.35 to 7.45. If the pH is not within normal range, look at the respiratory or metabolic function indicators.
   If the condition is a respiratory imbalance, look at the HCO$_3^-$ to determine the state of compensation.
   If the condition is a metabolic imbalance, look at the Pco$_2$ to determine the state of compensation.

B. Respiratory acid-base imbalances (Table 10-3)
   1. Remember that the respiratory function indicator is the Pco$_2$.
   2. In a respiratory imbalance, you will find an opposite relationship between the pH and the Pco$_2$; in

other words, the pH will be elevated with a decreased Pco$_2$ (alkalosis) or the pH will be decreased with an elevated Pco$_2$ (acidosis).
   3. Look at the pH and the Pco$_2$ to determine whether the condition is a respiratory problem.
   4. **Respiratory acidosis**: The pH is decreased; the Pco$_2$ is elevated.
   5. **Respiratory alkalosis**: The pH is elevated; the Pco$_2$ is decreased.
C. Metabolic acid-base imbalances (see Table 10-3)
   1. Remember, the metabolic function indicator is the bicarbonate ion (HCO$_3^-$).
   2. In a metabolic imbalance, there is a corresponding relationship between the pH and the HCO$_3^-$; in other words, the pH will be elevated and the HCO$_3^-$ will be elevated (alkalosis), or the pH will be decreased and the HCO$_3^-$ will be decreased (acidosis).
   3. Look at the pH and the HCO$_3^-$ to determine whether the condition is a metabolic problem.
   4. **Metabolic acidosis**: The pH is decreased; the HCO$_3^-$ is decreased.
   5. **Metabolic alkalosis**: The pH is elevated; the HCO$_3^-$ is elevated.

⚠ In a respiratory imbalance, the ABG result indicates an opposite relationship between the pH and the Pco$_2$.
In a metabolic imbalance, the ABG result indicates a corresponding relationship between the pH and the HCO$_3^-$.

D. **Compensation** (see Table 10-3)
   1. **Compensation** refers to the body processes that occur to counterbalance the acid-base disturbance.
   2. When **compensation** has occurred, the pH is within normal limits.
E. Steps for analyzing arterial blood gas results (Box 10-7)

MORE QUESTIONS ON THE CD!

Practice Questions

53. A nurse reviews the arterial blood gas results of a client and notes the following: pH 7.45, P_{CO_2} of 30 mm Hg, and HCO_3^- of 22 mEq/L. The nurse analyzes these results as indicating which condition?
1. Metabolic acidosis, compensated
2. Respiratory alkalosis, compensated
3. Metabolic alkalosis, uncompensated
4. Respiratory acidosis, uncompensated

54. A nurse is caring for a client with a nasogastric tube that is attached to low suction. The nurse monitors the client, knowing that the client is at risk for which acid-base disorder?
1. Metabolic acidosis
2. Metabolic alkalosis
3. Respiratory acidosis
4. Respiratory alkalosis

55. A client with a 3-day history of nausea and vomiting presents to the emergency department. The client is hypoventilating and has a respiratory rate of 10 breaths/min. The electrocardiogram (ECG) monitor displays tachycardia, with a heart rate of 120 beats/min. Arterial blood gases are drawn and the nurse reviews the results, expecting to note which of the following?
1. A decreased pH and an increased CO_2
2. An increased pH and a decreased CO_2
3. A decreased pH and a decreased HCO_3^-
4. An increased pH with an increased HCO_3^-

56. A nurse caring for a client with an ileostomy understands that the client is most at risk for developing which acid-base disorder?
1. Metabolic acidosis
2. Metabolic alkalosis
3. Respiratory acidosis
4. Respiratory alkalosis

57. A nurse is caring for a client with diabetic ketoacidosis and documents that the client is experiencing Kussmaul's respirations. Based on this documentation, which of the following did the nurse observe?
1. Respirations that cease for several seconds
2. Respirations that are regular but abnormally slow
3. Respirations that are labored and increased in depth and rate
4. Respirations that are abnormally deep, regular, and increased in rate

58. A client who is found unresponsive has arterial blood gases drawn and the results indicate the following: pH is 7.12, P_{CO_2} is 90 mm Hg, and HCO_3^- is 22 mEq/L. The nurse interprets the results as indicating which condition?
1. Metabolic acidosis with compensation
2. Respiratory acidosis with compensation
3. Metabolic acidosis without compensation
4. Respiratory acidosis without compensation

59. A nurse plans care for a client with chronic obstructive pulmonary disease (COPD), understanding that the client is most likely to experience what type of acid-base imbalance?
1. Metabolic acidosis
2. Metabolic alkalosis
3. Respiratory acidosis
4. Respiratory alkalosis

60. A nurse reviews the blood gas results of a client with atelectasis. The nurse analyzes the results and determines that the client is experiencing respiratory acidosis. Which of the following validates the nurse's findings?
1. pH 7.25, P_{CO_2} 50 mm Hg
2. pH 7.35, P_{CO_2} 40 mm Hg
3. pH 7.50, P_{CO_2} 52 mm Hg
4. pH 7.52, P_{CO_2} 28 mm Hg

61. A nurse is caring for a client who is on a mechanical ventilator. Blood gas results indicate a pH of 7.50 and a P_{CO_2} of 30 mm Hg. The nurse has determined that the client is experiencing respiratory alkalosis. Which laboratory value would most likely be noted in this condition?
1. Sodium level of 145 mEq/L
2. Potassium level of 3 mEq/L
3. Magnesium level of 2 mg/dL
4. Phosphorus level of 4 mg/dL

Alternate Item Format: Multiple Response

62. A nurse notes that a client's arterial blood gas results reveal a pH of 7.50 and a P_{CO_2} of 30 mm Hg. The nurse monitors the client for which clinical manifestations associated with these arterial blood gas results? **Select all that apply.**
❑ 1. Nausea
❑ 2. Confusion
❑ 3. Bradypnea
❑ 4. Tachycardia
❑ 5. Hyperkalemia
❑ 6. Lightheadedness

ANSWERS

53. 2

Rationale: The normal pH is 7.35 to 7.45. In a respiratory condition, an opposite effect will be seen between the pH and the P_{CO_2}. In this situation, the pH is at the high end of the normal value and the P_{CO_2} is low. In an alkalotic condition, the pH is elevated. Therefore the values identified in the question indicate a respiratory alkalosis. When the pH returns to a normal value, compensation has occurred.

Test-Taking Strategy: Remember that in a respiratory imbalance you will find an opposite response between the pH and the P_{CO_2} as indicated in the question. Therefore you can eliminate options 1 and 3. Also, remember that the pH increases in an alkalotic condition and compensation can be evidenced by a normal pH. Option 2 reflects a respiratory alkalotic condition and compensation and describes the blood gas values as indicated in the question. Review the steps related to reading blood gas values and the findings noted in respiratory alkalosis if you had difficulty with this question.

Level of Cognitive Ability: Analyzing
Client Needs: Physiological Integrity
Integrated Process: Nursing Process—Analysis
Content Area: Fundamental Skills—Fluids & Electrolytes/Acid-Base
References: Black, J., & Hawks, J. (2009). *Medical-surgical nursing: Clinical management for positive outcomes* (8th ed., p. 173). St. Louis: Saunders.
    Potter, P., & Perry, A. (2009). *Fundamentals of nursing* (7th ed., p. 977). St. Louis: Mosby.

54. 2

Rationale: Metabolic alkalosis is defined as a deficit or loss of hydrogen ions or acids or an excess of base (bicarbonate) that results from the accumulation of base or from a loss of acid without a comparable loss of base in the body fluids. This occurs in conditions resulting in hypovolemia, the loss of gastric fluid, excessive bicarbonate intake, the massive transfusion of whole blood, and hyperaldosteronism. Loss of gastric fluid via nasogastric suction or vomiting causes metabolic alkalosis as a result of the loss of hydrochloric acid. Options 1, 3, and 4 are incorrect interpretations.

Test-Taking Strategy: Remembering that a client receiving nasogastric suction loses hydrochloric acid will direct you to the option identifying an alkalotic condition. Because the question addresses a situation other than a respiratory one, the acid-base disorder would be a metabolic condition. If you had difficulty with this question, review the causes of metabolic alkalosis.

Level of Cognitive Ability: Understanding
Client Needs: Physiological Integrity
Integrated Process: Nursing Process—Analysis
Content Area: Fundamental Skills—Fluids & Electrolytes/Acid-Base
Reference: Black, J., & Hawks, J. (2009). *Medical-surgical nursing: Clinical management for positive outcomes* (8th ed., p. 625). St. Louis: Saunders.

55. 4

Rationale: Clients experiencing nausea and vomiting would most likely present with metabolic alkalosis resulting from loss of gastric acid, thus causing the pH and HCO_3^- to increase. Symptoms experienced by the client would include hypoventilation and tachycardia. Option 1 reflects a respiratory acidotic condition. Option 2 reflects a respiratory alkalotic condition. Option 3 reflects a metabolic acidotic condition.

Test-Taking Strategy: Focus on the data in the question and note that the client is vomiting. Recalling that vomiting most likely causes metabolic alkalosis will assist in directing you to option 4. Review the causes of metabolic alkalosis if you had difficulty with this question.

Level of Cognitive Ability: Analyzing
Client Needs: Physiological Integrity
Integrated Process: Nursing Process—Analysis
Content Area: Fundamental Skills—Fluids & Electrolytes/Acid-Base
Reference: Black, J., & Hawks, J. (2009). *Medical-surgical nursing: Clinical management for positive outcomes* (8th ed., pp. 175–176). St. Louis: Saunders.

56. 1

Rationale: Metabolic acidosis is defined as total concentration of buffer base that is lower than normal, with a relative increase in the hydrogen ion concentration. This results from loss of buffer bases or retention of too many acids without sufficient bases, and occurs in conditions such as renal failure; diabetic ketoacidosis; from the production of lactic acid; from the ingestion of toxins, such as acetylsalicylic acid (aspirin); malnutrition; or severe diarrhea. Intestinal secretions are high in bicarbonate and may be lost through enteric drainage tubes or an ileostomy, or with diarrhea. These conditions result in metabolic acidosis. Options 2, 3, and 4 are incorrect interpretations and do not occur in the client with an ileostomy.

Test-Taking Strategy: Note that the client's condition described in the question is a gastrointestinal disorder. This will direct you toward a metabolic disorder. Remembering that intestinal fluids are primarily alkaline will assist you in selecting the correct option. When excess bicarbonate is lost, acidosis will result. If you had difficulty with this question, review the causes of metabolic acidosis.

Level of Cognitive Ability: Understanding
Client Needs: Physiological Integrity
Integrated Process: Nursing Process—Analysis
Content Area: Fundamental Skills—Fluids & Electrolytes/Acid-Base
Reference: Black, J., & Hawks, J. (2009). *Medical-surgical nursing: Clinical management for positive outcomes* (8th ed., pp. 176–177). St. Louis: Saunders.

57. 4

Rationale: Kussmaul's respirations are abnormally deep, regular, and increased in rate. Apnea is described as respirations that cease for several seconds. In bradypnea, respirations are regular but abnormally slow. In hyperpnea, respirations are labored and increased in depth and rate.

Test-Taking Strategy: Use knowledge of the description of Kussmaul's respirations. Recalling that this type of respiration occurs in diabetic ketoacidosis will direct you to option 4. Review the characteristics of this type of respiration if you had difficulty with this question.

Level of Cognitive Ability: Understanding

Client Needs: Physiological Integrity
Integrated Process: Nursing Process—Assessment
Content Area: Fundamental Skills—Fluids & Electrolytes/Acid-Base
Reference: Potter, P., & Perry, A. (2009). *Fundamentals of nursing* (7th ed., p. 532). St. Louis: Mosby.

58. 4
Rationale: The acid-base disturbance is respiratory acidosis without compensation. The normal pH is 7.35 to 7.45. The normal Pco_2 is 35 to 45 mm Hg. In respiratory acidosis the pH is decreased and the Pco_2 is elevated. The normal bicarbonate (HCO_3^-) level is 22 to 27 mEq/L. Because the bicarbonate is still within normal limits, the kidneys have not had time to adjust for this acid-base disturbance. Additionally, the pH is not within normal limits. Therefore the condition is without compensation. Options 1, 2, and 3 are incorrect interpretations.
Test-Taking Strategy: Remember that in a respiratory imbalance you will find an opposite response between the pH and the Pco_2. Also, remember that the pH is decreased in an acidotic condition and that compensation is reflected by a normal pH. Review the interpretation of arterial blood gas values if you had difficulty with this question.
Level of Cognitive Ability: Analyzing
Client Needs: Physiological Integrity
Integrated Process: Nursing Process—Analysis
Content Area: Fundamental Skills—Fluids & Electrolytes/Acid-Base
Reference: Black, J., & Hawks, J. (2009). *Medical-surgical nursing: Clinical management for positive outcomes* (8th ed., p. 173). St. Louis: Saunders.

59. 3
Rationale: Respiratory acidosis is most often caused by hypoventilation in a client with COPD. Other acid-base disturbances can occur in a client with COPD during exacerbation of the disease but the most likely imbalance is respiratory acidosis. Options 1, 2, and 4 are incorrect options.
Test-Taking Strategy: Note the strategic words *most likely* and *chronic*. Remembering that hypoventilation results in respiratory acidosis will direct you to option 3. Review the causes of respiratory acidosis if you had difficulty with this question.
Level of Cognitive Ability: Understanding
Client Needs: Physiological Integrity
Integrated Process: Nursing Process—Planning
Content Area: Fundamental Skills—Fluids & Electrolytes/Acid-Base
Reference: Black, J., & Hawks, J. (2009). *Medical-surgical nursing: Clinical management for positive outcomes* (8th ed., pp. 175-176). St. Louis: Saunders.

60. 1
Rationale: Atelectasis is a condition characterized by the collapse of alveoli, preventing the respiratory exchange of oxygen and carbon dioxide in a part of the lungs. The normal pH is 7.35 to 7.45. The normal Pco_2 is 35 to 45 mm Hg. In respiratory acidosis, the pH is decreased and the Pco_2 is elevated. Option 2 identifies normal values. Option 3 identifies an alkalotic condition. Option 4 identifies respiratory alkalosis.

Test-Taking Strategy: Remember that in a respiratory imbalance you will find an opposite response between the pH and the Pco_2. Also, remember that the pH is decreased in an acidotic condition. Option 2 reflects a normal blood gas result. Options 3 and 4 reflect an elevated pH, which indicates an alkalotic condition. Option 1 is the only option that reflects an acidotic condition. Review blood gas findings in respiratory acidosis if you had difficulty with this question.
Level of Cognitive Ability: Analyzing
Client Needs: Physiological Integrity
Integrated Process: Nursing Process—Analysis
Content Area: Fundamental Skills—Fluids & Electrolytes/Acid-Base
References: Black, J., & Hawks, J. (2009). *Medical-surgical nursing: Clinical management for positive outcomes* (8th ed., p. 1915). St. Louis: Saunders.
Pagana, K., & Pagana, T. (2009). *Mosby's diagnostic and laboratory test reference* (9th ed., pp. 113, 115). St. Louis: Mosby.

61. 2
Rationale: Respiratory alkalosis is defined as a deficit of carbonic acid or a decrease in hydrogen ion concentration that results from the accumulation of base or from a loss of acid without a comparable loss of base in the body fluids. This occurs in conditions that cause overstimulation of the respiratory system. Clinical manifestations of respiratory alkalosis include headache, tachypnea, paresthesias, tetany, vertigo, convulsions, hypokalemia, and hypocalcemia. Options 1, 3, and 4 identify normal laboratory values. Option 2 identifies the presence of hypokalemia.
Test-Taking Strategy: Focus on the data in the question and use knowledge about the interpretation of arterial blood gas values to determine that the client is experiencing respiratory alkalosis. Next recall the manifestations that occur in this condition and the normal laboratory values. The only abnormal laboratory value is the potassium level, option 2. Review the clinical manifestations of respiratory alkalosis and normal laboratory values if you had difficulty with this question.
Level of Cognitive Ability: Understanding
Client Needs: Physiological Integrity
Integrated Process: Nursing Process—Analysis
Content Area: Fundamental Skills—Fluids & Electrolytes/Acid-Base
References: Black, J., & Hawks, J. (2009). *Medical-surgical nursing: Clinical management for positive outcomes* (8th ed., pp. 174-175). St. Louis: Saunders.
Potter, P., & Perry, A. (2009). *Fundamentals of nursing* (7th ed., p. 976). St. Louis: Mosby.

ALTERNATE ITEM FORMAT: MULTIPLE RESPONSE
62. 1, 2, 4, 6
Rationale: Respiratory alkalosis is defined as a deficit of carbonic acid or a decrease in hydrogen ion concentration that results from the accumulation of base or from a loss of acid without a comparable loss of base in the body fluids. This occurs in conditions that cause overstimulation of the respiratory system. Clinical manifestations of respiratory alkalosis include lethargy, lightheadedness, confusion, tachycardia,

dysrhythmias related to hypokalemia, nausea, vomiting, epigastric pain, and numbness and tingling of the extremities. Hyperventilation (tachypnea) occurs.

Test-Taking Strategy: Focus on the data in the question and use knowledge about the interpretation of arterial blood gas values to determine that the client is experiencing respiratory alkalosis. Next it is necessary to think about the pathophysiology that occurs in this condition and recall the manifestations that occur. Review the clinical manifestations of respiratory alkalosis if you had difficulty with this question.

Level of Cognitive Ability: Analyzing
Client Needs: Physiological Integrity
Integrated Process: Nursing Process—Analysis
Content Area: Fundamental Skills—Fluids & Electrolytes/Acid-Base

References: Black, J., & Hawks, J. (2009). *Medical-surgical nursing: Clinical management for positive outcomes* (8th ed., pp. 174–175). St. Louis: Saunders.

Potter, P., & Perry, A. (2009). *Fundamentals of nursing* (7th ed., p. 976). St. Louis: Mosby.

Laboratory Values

PYRAMID TERMS

blood The liquid pumped by the heart through the arteries, veins, and capillaries. Blood is composed of a clear yellow fluid (plasma), formed elements, and cell types with different functions (Fig. 11-1).

blood cell Any of the formed elements of the blood, including red cells (erythrocytes), white cells (leukocytes), and platelets (thrombocytes).

plasma The watery, straw-colored, fluid part of lymph and the blood in which the formed elements (blood cells) are suspended. Plasma is made up of water, electrolytes, protein, glucose, fats, bilirubin, and gases and is essential for carrying the cellular elements of the blood through the circulation.

serum The clear and thin fluid part of blood that remains after coagulation. Serum contains no blood cells, platelets, or fibrinogen.

venipuncture Puncture into a vein to obtain a blood specimen for testing; the antecubital veins are the veins of choice because of ease of access.

a result of the disorder. This process will assist you in determining the correct answer. For example, if the question asks about the immune status of a client receiving chemotherapy, assessment of laboratory values will focus on the white blood cell (WBC) count and the neutrophils. You will need to analyze these results as possibly being low and determine the specific client need, which in this case would be the risk for infection. In the client receiving chemotherapy who has a low WBC count, your plan centers on the immune system and protecting the client from infection. Implementation focuses on preventive interventions related to infection, perhaps protective isolation measures. Evaluation may focus on maintenance of a normal temperature in the client. Box 11-1 lists some of the common abbreviations found in laboratory values. The Priority Nursing Actions box lists the steps needed for obtaining a blood sample.

 ## THE PYRAMID TO SUCCESS

This chapter identifies the normal adult values for the most common laboratory tests. It is important to remember that normal laboratory values may vary slightly, depending on the laboratory setting and equipment used in testing. If you are familiar with the normal values, you will be able to determine whether an abnormality exists when a laboratory value is presented in a question. The questions on the NCLEX-RN examination related to laboratory values will require you to identify whether the laboratory value is normal or abnormal, and then you are required to think critically about the effects of the laboratory value in terms of the client. Pyramid Points focus on knowledge of the normal values for the most common laboratory tests, therapeutic serum medication levels of commonly prescribed medications, and determination of the need to implement specific actions based on the findings. When a question is presented on the NCLEX-RN examination regarding a specific laboratory value, note the disorder presented in the question and the associated body organ affected as

CLIENT NEEDS

Safe and Effective Care Environment

Applying principles of infection control
Ensuring surgical asepsis when obtaining a specimen
Implementing procedures for handling hazardous and infectious materials
Maintaining standard, transmission-based, and surgical asepsis
Obtaining informed consent for specific procedures
Verifying the identity of the client

Health Promotion and Maintenance

Preparing the client for the laboratory test
Discussing the importance of follow-up laboratory studies
Identifying community resources available for the follow-up
Implementing posttest procedures
Describing specific interventions or home care measures required based on the results

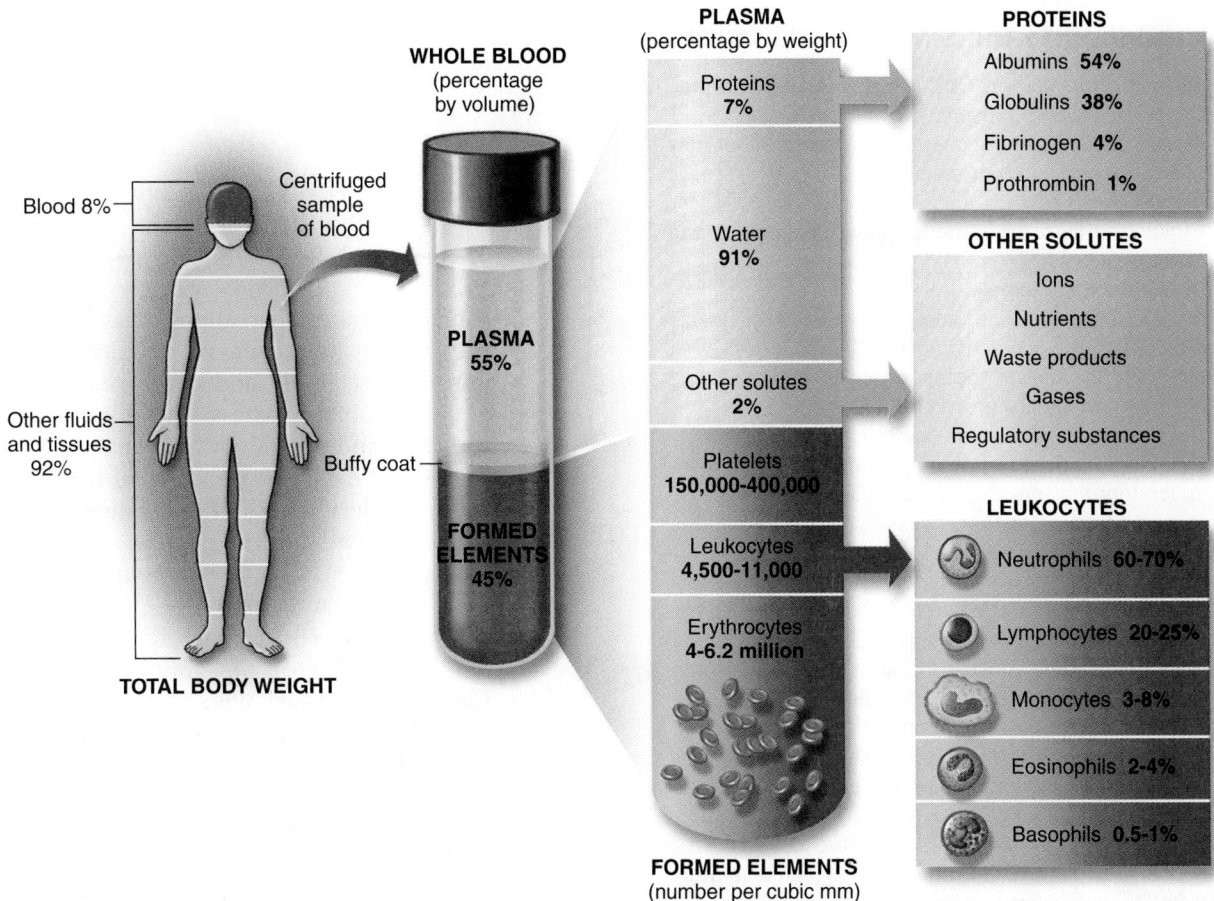

▲ **FIGURE 11-1** Approximate values for the components of blood in a normal adult. (Modified from Thibodeau, G.A., & Patton, K.T. [2010]. *The human body in health and disease* [5th ed.]. St. Louis: Mosby.)

Box 11-1 Pyramid Abbreviations

Abbreviation	Definition
g/dL	grams per deciliter
IU/L	International units per liter
mcg/dL	micrograms per deciliter
mcg/mL	micrograms per milliliter
mEq/L	milliequivalents per liter
mg/dL	milligrams per deciliter
microunits/mL	microunits per milliliter
mL/kg	milliliters per kilogram
mm³	millimeters cubed
mm/hr	millimeters per hour
ng/mL	nanograms per milliliter
pg/mL	picogram per milliliter
units/L	units per liter
μL	microliters

Monitoring for signs and symptoms that indicate the need to notify the health care provider

Psychosocial Integrity

Communicating the purpose of the laboratory test to the client

Communicating with the client regarding the laboratory results

Providing emotional support during testing

Physiological Integrity

Identifying normal values for the most common laboratory tests

Identifying therapeutic serum medication levels of commonly prescribed medications

Monitoring for clinical manifestations associated with an abnormal laboratory value

Providing comfort measures

Reporting significant laboratory values

Determining the significance of an abnormal laboratory value and the need to implement specific actions based on the laboratory results

Monitoring for potential complications related to a test

⚠ Drawing blood specimens from an extremity in which an intravenous solution is infusing can produce an inaccurate result. Prolonged use of a tourniquet and clenching and unclenching the hand before venous sampling can increase the blood level of potassium, producing an inaccurate result.

Actions to Take When Obtaining a Blood Sample
1. Check physician's prescription.
2. Identify foods, medications, or other factors that may affect the procedure or results.
3. Identify the client.
4. Explain the purpose of the test and procedure to the client.
5. Draw the blood sample.
6. Provide pressure and apply a Band-Aid or gauze dressing to the venipuncture site.
7. Maintain and deliver the specimen to the laboratory according to agency procedure.
8. Document specifics about the procedure.

The nurse should check the physician's prescription for the laboratory test prescribed and then ensure that the client is prepared for the test; for example, that NPO status has been maintained if needed. The nurse would also identify any foods, medications, or other factors that may affect test results. For example, a diet high in fat or leafy vegetables may shorten the prothrombin time. Additionally, there are many medications that can increase or decrease some test results. The nurse then identifies the client and makes sure that the test has been explained to the client. The nurse (or appropriate person as indicated by agency procedure) draws the blood sample, provides pressure, and applies a Band-Aid or gauze dressing to the venipuncture site. Once the client is comfortable, the nurse maintains and delivers the specimen to the laboratory according to agency procedure. The nurse always follows standard and transmission-based precautions as necessary in performing this procedure. The nurse should also check agency guidelines and laboratory manuals regarding the procedure for obtaining the specific blood sample. The nurse then documents the specifics about the procedure.

Reference: Pagana, K., & Pagana, T. (2009). *Mosby's diagnostic and laboratory test reference* (9th ed.). St. Louis: Mosby.

I. ELECTROLYTES (Table 11-1)

A. Serum sodium
   1. Description
      a. A major cation of extracellular fluid
      b. Maintains osmotic pressure and acid-base balance, and assists in the transmission of nerve impulses
      c. Is absorbed from the small intestine and excreted in the urine in amounts dependent on dietary intake
      d. Minimum daily requirement of sodium is approximately 15 mEq.
   2. Nursing consideration: Drawing **blood** samples in the extremity in which an intravenous (IV) solution of sodium chloride is infusing increases the level, producing an inaccurate result.
B. Serum potassium
   1. Description

TABLE 11-1 Normal Adult Electrolyte Values

Electrolyte	Value
Sodium	135-145 mEq/L
Potassium	3.5-5.1 mEq/L
Chloride	98-107 mEq/L
Bicarbonate (venous)	22-29 mEq/L

      a. A major intracellular cation, potassium regulates cellular water balance, electrical conduction in muscle cells, and acid-base balance.
      b. The body obtains potassium through dietary ingestion and the kidneys preserve or excrete potassium, depending on cellular need.
      c. Potassium levels are used to evaluate cardiac function, renal function, gastrointestinal function, and the need for IV replacement therapy.
   2. Nursing considerations
      a. Note that the client is receiving potassium supplementation on the laboratory form.
      b. Clients with elevated WBC counts and platelet counts may have falsely elevated potassium levels.
C. Serum chloride
   1. Description
      a. A hydrochloric acid salt that is the most abundant body anion in the extracellular fluid
      b. Functions to counterbalance cations, such as sodium, and acts as a buffer during oxygen and carbon dioxide exchange in red **blood cells** (RBCs)
      c. Aids in digestion and maintaining osmotic pressure and water balance
   2. Nursing consideration: Any condition accompanied by prolonged vomiting, diarrhea, or both will alter chloride levels.
D. Serum bicarbonate
   1. Description: Part of the bicarbonate-carbonic acid buffering system and mainly responsible for regulating the pH of body fluids
   2. Nursing consideration: Ingestion of acidic or alkaline solutions may cause increased or decreased results, respectively.

II. COAGULATION STUDIES

A. Activated partial thromboplastin time (aPTT)
   1. Description
      a. The aPTT evaluates how well the coagulation sequence is functioning by measuring the amount of time it takes in seconds for recalcified citrated **plasma** to clot after partial thromboplastin is added to it.
      b. The test screens for deficiencies and inhibitors of all factors, except VII and XIII.
      c. Usually, the aPTT is used to monitor heparin therapy and screen for coagulation disorders.

2. Value: 20 to 36 seconds, depending on the type of activator used
3. Nursing considerations
   a. If the client is receiving intermittent heparin therapy, draw the **blood** sample 1 hour before the next scheduled dose.
   b. Do not draw samples from an arm into which heparin is infusing.
   c. Transport specimen to the laboratory immediately.
   d. Provide direct pressure to the **venipuncture** site for 3 to 5 minutes.
   e. The aPTT should be between 1.5 and 2.5 times normal when the client is receiving heparin therapy; if the value is prolonged (longer than 90 seconds), the client is at risk for bleeding.

🔺 If the aPTT value is prolonged (longer than 90 seconds) in a client receiving IV heparin therapy, initiate bleeding precautions.

B. Prothrombin time (PT) and international normalized ratio (INR)
   1. Description
      a. Prothrombin is a vitamin K–dependent glycoprotein produced by the liver that is necessary for fibrin clot formation.
      b. Each laboratory establishes a normal or control value based on the method used to perform the PT test.
      c. The PT measures the amount of time it takes in seconds for clot formation and is used to monitor response to warfarin sodium (Coumadin) therapy or to screen for dysfunction of the extrinsic clotting system resulting from liver disease, vitamin K deficiency, or disseminated intravascular coagulation.
      d. A PT value within 2 seconds (plus or minus) of the control is considered normal.
      e. The INR is a frequently used test to measure the effects of oral anticoagulants.
      f. The INR standardized the PT ratio and is calculated in the laboratory setting by raising the observed PT ratio to the power of the international sensitivity index specific to the thromboplastin reagent used.
   2. Values
      a. PT: 9.6 to 11.8 seconds (male adult); 9.5 to 11.3 seconds (female adult)
      b. INR: 2 to 3 for standard warfarin therapy
      c. INR: 3 to 4.5 for high-dose warfarin therapy
   3. Nursing considerations
      a. A baseline PT should be drawn before anticoagulation therapy is started; note the time of collection on the laboratory form.
      b. Provide direct pressure to the **venipuncture** site for 3 to 5 minutes.

   c. Concurrent warfarin therapy with heparin therapy can lengthen the PT for up to 5 hours after dosing.
   d. Diets high in green leafy vegetables can increase the absorption of vitamin K, which shortens the PT.
   e. Orally administered anticoagulation therapy usually maintains the PT at 1.5 to 2 times the laboratory control value.
   f. A PT longer than 30 seconds places the client at risk for bleeding.

🔺 If the PT value is longer than 30 seconds in a client receiving warfarin therapy, initiate bleeding precautions.

C. Clotting time
   1. Description: The time required for the interaction of all factors involved in the clotting process
   2. Value: 8 to 15 minutes
   3. Nursing considerations
      a. The client should not receive heparin therapy for 3 hours before specimen collection because the heparin therapy will affect the results.
      b. The test result is falsely prolonged by anticoagulant therapy, test tube agitation, or exposure of the specimen to high temperatures.

D. Platelet count
   1. Description
      a. Platelets function in hemostatic plug formation, clot retraction, and coagulation factor activation.
      b. Platelets are produced by the bone marrow to function in hemostasis.
   2. Value: 150,000 to 400,000 cells/mm^3
   3. Nursing considerations
      a. Monitor the **venipuncture** site for bleeding in clients with known thrombocytopenia.
      b. High altitudes, chronic cold weather, and exercise increase platelet counts.
      c. Bleeding precautions should be instituted in clients with a low platelet count.

🔺 Monitor the platelet count closely in clients receiving chemotherapy because of the risk for thrombocytopenia.

III. ERYTHROCYTE STUDIES

A. Erythrocyte sedimentation rate
   1. Description
      a. Rate at which erythrocytes settle out of anticoagulated **blood** in 1 hour
      b. A nonspecific test used to detect illnesses associated with acute and chronic infection, inflammation, advanced neoplasm, and tissue necrosis or infarction

2. Value: 0 to 30 mm/hr, depending on age of client
3. Nursing consideration: Fasting is not necessary, but a fatty meal may cause **plasma** alterations.

B. Hemoglobin and hematocrit
  1. Description
     a. Hemoglobin is the main component of erythrocytes and serves as the vehicle for transporting oxygen and carbon dioxide.
     b. Hemoglobin determinations are important in identifying anemia.
     c. Hematocrit represents RBC mass and is an important measurement in the identification of anemia or polycythemia (Table 11-2).
  2. Nursing consideration: Fasting is not required.

C. **Serum** iron
  1. Description
     a. Iron is found predominantly in hemoglobin.
     b. Iron acts as a carrier of oxygen from the lungs to the tissues and indirectly aids in the return of carbon dioxide to the lungs.
     c. Iron aids in diagnosing anemias and hemolytic disorders.
  2. Normal values
     a. Male adult: 65 to 175 mcg/dL
     b. Female adult: 50 to 170 mcg/dL
  3. Nursing consideration: Level of iron will be increased if the client has ingested iron before the test.

D. RBC count (erythrocytes)
  1. Description
     a. RBCs function in hemoglobin transport, which results in delivery of oxygen to the body tissues.
     b. RBCs are formed by red bone marrow, have a life span of 120 days, and are removed from the **blood** via the liver, spleen, and bone marrow.
     c. The RBC count aids in diagnosing anemias and **blood** dyscrasias.
     d. The RBC count evaluates the ability of the body to produce RBCs in sufficient numbers.

2. Values
   a. Female adult: 4 to 5.5 million cells/μL
   b. Male adult: 4.5 to 6.2 million cells/μL
3. Nursing consideration: Fasting is not required.

IV. SERUM ENZYMES AND CARDIAC MARKERS (Table 11-3)

A. Creatine kinase (CK)
  1. Description
     a. Creatine kinase is an enzyme found in muscle and brain tissue that reflects tissue catabolism resulting from cell trauma.
     b. The CK level begins to rise within 6 hours of muscle damage, peaks at 18 hours, and returns to normal in 2 to 3 days.
     c. The test for CK is performed to detect myocardial or skeletal muscle damage or central nervous system damage; a normal CK value is 26 to 174 units/L.
     d. Isoenzymes include CK-MB (cardiac), CK-BB (brain), and CK-MM (muscles).
     e. Isoenzyme CK-MB is found mainly in cardiac muscle, CK-BB is found mainly in brain tissue, and CK-MM is found mainly is skeletal muscle.

TABLE 11-2 Normal Adult Blood Components

Blood Component	Normal Value
HEMOGLOBIN	
Male adult	14-16.5 g/dL
Female adult	12-15 g/dL
HEMATOCRIT	
Male adult	42%-52%
Female adult	35%-47%
IRON	
Male adult	65-175 mcg/dL
Female adult	50-170 mcg/dL
RED BLOOD CELLS	
Male adult	4.5-6.2 million/μL
Female adult	4-5.5 million/μL

TABLE 11-3 Normal Adult Serum Enzymes/Cardiac Markers

Serum Enzyme	Normal Value
Creatine kinase (CK)	26-174 units/L
CK isoenzymes	
CK-MB	0%-5% of total
CK-MM	95%-100% of total
CK-BB	0%
Lactate dehydrogenase	140-280 units/L
Lactate dehydrogenase isoenzymes	
LDH1	14%-26%
LDH2	29%-39%
LDH3	20%-26%
LDH4	8%-16%
LDH5	6%-16%
Troponin I	<0.6 ng/mL; >1.5 ng/mL indicates myocardial infarction
Troponin T	>0.1-0.2 ng/mL indicates myocardial infarction
Myoglobin	<90 mcg/L; elevation could indicate myocardial infarction
Atrial natriuretic peptides (ANP)	22 to 27 pg/mL
Brain natriuretic peptides (BNP)	Less than 100 pg/mL
C-type natriuretic peptides (CNP)	Not yet determined; reference range provided with results and should be reviewed

2. Values
   a. CK-MB: 0% to 5% of total
   b. CK-MM: 95% to 100% of total
   c. CK-BB: 0%
3. Nursing considerations
   a. If the test is to evaluate skeletal muscle, instruct the client to avoid strenuous physical activity for 24 hours before the test.
   b. Also instruct the client to avoid ingestion of alcohol for 24 hours before the test.
   c. Invasive procedures and intramuscular injections may falsely elevate CK levels.

B. Lactate dehydrogenase (LDH)
   1. Description
      a. The LDH isoenzymes affected by acute myocardial infarction are LDH1 and LDH2.
      b. The LDH level begins to rise about 24 hours after myocardial infarction and peaks in 48 to 72 hours; thereafter, it returns to normal, usually within 7 to 14 days.
      c. The presence of an LDH flip (when LDH1 is higher than LDH2) is helpful in diagnosing a myocardial infarction.
   2. Nursing considerations
      a. The LDH isoenzyme levels should be interpreted in view of the clinical findings.
      b. Testing should be repeated on 3 consecutive days.

C. Troponins
   1. Description
      a. Troponin is a regulatory protein found in striated muscle (skeletal and myocardial).
      b. Increased amounts of troponins are released into the bloodstream when an infarction causes damage to the myocardium.
      c. Levels elevate as early as 3 hours after myocardial injury. Troponin I levels may remain elevated for 7 to 10 days and troponin T levels may remain elevated for as long as 10 to 14 days.
      d. Serial measurements are important to compare with a baseline test.
   2. Values
      a. Troponin I: Value usually is lower than 0.6 ng/mL; value higher than 1.5 ng/mL is consistent with a myocardial infarction.
      b. Troponin T: Higher than 0.1 to 0.2 ng/mL is consistent with a myocardial infarction.
   3. Nursing considerations
      a. Testing is repeated in 12 hours, followed by daily testing for 3 to 5 days.
      b. Rotate **venipuncture** sites.

D. Myoglobin
   1. Description
      a. Myoglobin is an oxygen-binding protein that is found in striated (cardiac and skeletal) muscle that releases oxygen at very low tensions.

   b. Any injury to skeletal muscle will cause a release of myoglobin into the **blood**.
   2. Values: Normal value is lower than 90 mcg/L; an elevation could indicate myocardial infarction.
   3. Nursing considerations
      a. The level can rise as early as 2 hours after a myocardial infarction, with a rapid decline in the level after 7 hours.
      b. Because the myoglobin level is not cardiac-specific and rises and falls so rapidly, its use in diagnosing myocardial infarction may be limited.

E. Natriuretic peptides
   1. Description
      a. Natriuretic peptides are neuroendocrine peptides that are used to identify clients with congestive heart failure (CHF).
      b. There are three major peptides: atrial natriuretic peptides (ANP) synthesized in cardiac atrial muscle, brain natriuretic peptides (BNP) synthesized in cardiac ventricle muscle, and C-type natriuretic peptides (CNP) synthesized by endothelial cells
      c. BNP is the primary marker for identifying CHF as the cause of dyspnea.
   2. Values:
      a. ANP: 22 to 27 pg/mL
      b. BNP: less than 100 pg/mL
      c. CNP: not yet determined
   3. Nursing consideration: Fasting is not required.

⚠ The higher the BNP level, the more severe the CHF. If the BNP is elevated the dyspnea is due to CHF; if it is normal the dyspnea is due to a pulmonary problem.

V. SERUM GASTROINTESTINAL STUDIES

A. Albumin
   1. Description
      a. A main **plasma** protein of **blood**
      b. Maintains oncotic pressure and transports bilirubin, fatty acids, medications, hormones, and other substances that are insoluble in water
      c. Increased in conditions such as dehydration, diarrhea, and metastatic carcinoma; decreased in conditions such as acute infection, ascites, and alcoholism
      d. Presence of detectable albumin, or protein, in the urine is indicative of abnormal renal function
   2. Value: 3.4 to 5 g/dL
   3. Nursing consideration: Fasting is not required.

B. Alkaline phosphatase
   1. Description
      a. Alkaline phosphatase is an enzyme normally found in bone, liver, intestine, and placenta.

   b. The level rises during periods of bone growth, liver disease, and bile duct obstruction.
   2. Value: 4.5 to 13 King-Armstrong units/dL
   3. Nursing considerations
      a. The client may need to fast 12 hours before the test.
      b. Hepatotoxic medications administered within 12 hours before specimen collection can cause a falsely elevated value.
      c. Transport the specimen to the laboratory immediately.

C. Ammonia
   1. Description
      a. Ammonia is a byproduct of protein catabolism; most of it is created by bacteria acting on proteins present in the gut.
      b. Ammonia is metabolized by the liver and excreted by the kidneys as urea.
      c. Elevated levels resulting from hepatic dysfunction may lead to encephalopathy.
      d. Venous ammonia levels are not a reliable indicator of hepatic coma.
   2. Value: 10 to 80 mcg/dL
   3. Nursing considerations
      a. Instruct the client to fast, except for water, and to refrain from smoking for 8 to 10 hours before the test; smoking increases ammonia levels.
      b. Place the specimen on ice and transport to the laboratory immediately.

D. Alanine aminotransferase (ALT)
   1. Description: Used to identify hepatocellular disease of the liver and to monitor improvement or worsening of the disease.
   2. Value: 4 to 6 international units/L
   3. Nursing considerations
      a. Previous intramuscular injections may cause elevated levels.
      b. No fasting is required.

E. Aspartate aminotransferase (AST)
   1. Description: Used to evaluate a client with suspected hepatocellular disease (may also be used along with other cardiac markers to evaluate coronary artery occlusive disease)
   2. Value: 0 to 35 units/L
   3. Nursing considerations
      a. Previous intramuscular injections may cause elevated levels
      b. No fasting is required.

F. Amylase
   1. Description
      a. This enzyme, produced by the pancreas and salivary glands, aids in the digestion of complex carbohydrates and is excreted by the kidneys.
      b. In acute pancreatitis, the amylase level is greatly increased; the level starts rising 3 to

6 hours after the onset of pain, peaks at about 24 hours, and returns to normal in 2 to 3 days after the onset of pain.
   2. Value: 25 to 151 units/L
   3. Nursing considerations
      a. On the laboratory form, list the medications that the client has taken during the previous 24 hours before the test.
      b. Note that many medications may cause false-positive or false-negative results.
      c. Results are invalidated if the specimen was obtained less than 72 hours after cholecystography with radiopaque dyes.

G. Lipase
   1. Description
      a. This pancreatic enzyme converts fats and triglycerides into fatty acids and glycerol.
      b. Elevated lipase levels occur in pancreatic disorders; elevations may not occur until 24 to 36 hours after the onset of illness and may remain elevated for up to 14 days.
   2. Value: 10 to 140 units/L
   3. Nursing considerations: Endoscopic retrograde cholangiopancreatography (ERCP) may increase lipase activity.

H. Bilirubin
   1. Description
      a. Bilirubin is produced by the liver, spleen, and bone marrow and is also a byproduct of hemoglobin breakdown.
      b. Total bilirubin levels can be broken down into direct bilirubin, which is excreted primarily via the intestinal tract, and indirect bilirubin, which circulates primarily in the bloodstream.
      c. Total bilirubin levels increase with any type of jaundice; direct and indirect bilirubin levels help differentiate the cause of the jaundice.
   2. Values
      a. Bilirubin, direct (conjugated): 0 to 0.3 mg/dL
      b. Bilirubin, indirect (unconjugated): 0.1 to 1 mg/dL
      c. Bilirubin, total: Lower than 1.5 mg/dL
   3. Nursing considerations
      a. Instruct the client to eat a diet low in yellow foods, avoiding foods such as carrots, yams, yellow beans, and pumpkins, for 3 to 4 days before the **blood** is drawn.
      b. Instruct the client to fast for 4 hours before the **blood** is drawn.
      c. Note that results will be elevated with the ingestion of alcohol or the administration of morphine sulfate, theophylline, ascorbic acid (vitamin C), or acetylsalicylic acid (aspirin).
      d. Note that results are invalidated if the client has received a radioactive scan within 24 hours before the test.

4off

I. Lipids
  1. Description
     a. **Blood** lipids consist primarily of cholesterol, triglycerides, and phospholipids.
     b. Lipid assessment includes total cholesterol, high-density lipoprotein (HDL), low-density lipoprotein (LDL), and triglycerides.
     c. Cholesterol is present in all body tissues and is a major component of LDLs, brain and nerve cells, cell membranes, and some gallbladder stones.
     d. Triglycerides constitute a major part of very low-density lipoproteins and a small part of LDLs.
     e. Triglycerides are synthesized in the liver from fatty acids, protein, and glucose, and are obtained from the diet.
     f. Increased cholesterol levels, LDL levels, and triglyceride levels place the client at risk for coronary artery disease.
     g. HDL helps protect against the risk of coronary artery disease
  2. Values:
     a. Cholesterol: 140 to 199 mg/dL
     b. Low-density lipoproteins: Lower than 130 mg/dL
     c. HDLs: 30 to 70 mg/dL
     d. Triglycerides: Lower than 200 mg/dL
  3. Nursing considerations
     a. Oral contraceptives may increase the lipid level.
     b. Instruct the client to abstain from foods and fluid, except for water, for 12 to 14 hours and from alcohol for 24 hours before the test.
     c. Instruct the client to completely avoid high-cholesterol foods with the evening meal before the test.

J. Protein
  1. Description
     a. Protein reflects the total amount of albumin and globulins in the **plasma**.
     b. Protein regulates osmotic pressure and is necessary for the formation of many hormones, enzymes, and antibodies; it is a major source of building material for blood, skin, hair, nails, and internal organs.
     c. Increased in conditions such as Addison's disease, autoimmune collagen disorders, chronic infection, and Crohn's disease.
     d. Decreased in conditions such as burns, cirrhosis, edema, and severe hepatic disease.
  2. Value: 6 to 8 g/dL
  3. Nursing considerations: Instruct the client to avoid a high-fat diet for 8 hours before the test.

K. Uric acid
  1. Description
     a. Uric acid is formed as the purines adenine and guanine are metabolized continuously during the formation and degradation of DNA and RNA. It is also formed from the metabolism of dietary purines.
     b. Elevated amounts of uric acid deposit in joints and soft tissue and cause gout.
     c. Conditions of increased cellular turnover, as well as slowed renal excretion of uric acid, may cause hyperuricemia.
     d. Elevated levels of urinary uric acid precipitate into urate stones in the kidneys.
  2. Values
     a. Male adult: 4.5 to 8 mg/dL
     b. Female adult: 2.5 to 6.2 mg/dL
  3. Nursing considerations
     a. Instruct the client to fast for 8 hours before the test.
     b. Theophylline, caffeine, and vitamin C may cause falsely elevated results.

Clients with liver disease often have prolonged clotting times; therefore, provide prolonged pressure at the venipuncture site and monitor the site closely for bleeding.

VI. GLUCOSE STUDIES

A. Fasting **blood** glucose
  1. Description
     a. Glucose is a monosaccharide found in fruits and is formed from the digestion of carbohydrates and the conversion of glycogen by the liver.
     b. Glucose is the main source of cellular energy for the body and is essential for brain and erythrocyte function.
     c. Fasting **blood** glucose levels are used to help diagnose diabetes mellitus and hypoglycemia (Table 11-4).
  2. Nursing considerations
     a. Instruct the client to fast for 8 to 12 hours before the test.
     b. Instruct a client with diabetes mellitus to withhold morning insulin or oral hypoglycemic medication until after the **blood** is drawn.

TABLE 11-4 Normal Adult Glucose Values

Measurement Setting	Normal Value
Glucose, fasting	70-110 mg/dL
Glucose monitoring (capillary blood)	60-110 mg/dL
Glucose tolerance test, oral	
Baseline fasting	70-110 mg/dL
30-min fasting	110-170 mg/dL
60-min fasting	120-170 mg/dL
90-min fasting	100-140 mg/dL
120-min fasting	70-120 mg/dL
Glucose, 2-hr postprandial	<140 mg/dL

B. Glucose tolerance test (see Table 11-4)
  1. Description
    a. The glucose tolerance test aids in the diagnosis of diabetes mellitus.
    b. If the glucose levels peak at higher than normal at 1 and 2 hours after injection or ingestion of glucose and are slower than normal to return to fasting levels, then diabetes mellitus is confirmed.
  2. Nursing considerations
    a. Instruct the client to eat a high-carbohydrate (200- to 300-g) diet for 3 days before the test.
    b. Instruct the client to avoid alcohol, coffee, and smoking for 36 hours before the test.
    c. Instruct the client to fast for 10 to 16 hours before the test.
    d. Instruct the client to avoid strenuous exercise for 8 hours before and after the test.
    e. Instruct the client with diabetes mellitus to withhold morning insulin or oral hypoglycemic medication.
    f. Instruct the client that the test may take 3 to 5 hours, requires IV or oral administration of glucose, and multiple **blood** samples.
C. Glycosylated hemoglobin
  1. Description
    a. Glycosylated hemoglobin is **blood** glucose bound to hemoglobin.
    b. Hemoglobin A_{1c} (glycosylated hemoglobin A; HbA_{1c}) is a reflection of how well **blood** glucose levels have been controlled for the past 3 to 4 months.
    c. Hyperglycemia in clients with diabetes is usually a cause of an increase in the HbA_{1c}.
  2. Values
    a. Values are expressed as a percentage of the total hemoglobin.
    b. Good control of diabetes: 7% or lower
    c. Fair control of diabetes: 7% to 8%
    d. Poor control of diabetes: Higher than 8%
  3. Nursing consideration: Fasting is not required before the test.
D. Glycosylated **serum** albumin (fructosamine)
  1. Description
    a. Reflects average **serum** glucose levels over a period of 2 to 3 weeks
    b. More sensitive to recent changes than the HbA_{1c}
  2. Values: Normal ranges vary according to method of testing used; nondiabetic client, 1.5 to 2.7 mmol/L; diabetic client, 2 to 5 mmol/L.
  3. Nursing consideration: The client needs to fast for 12 hours before the test.
E. Diabetes mellitus autoantibody panel
  1. Description: Used to evaluate insulin resistance and to identify type 1 diabetes and clients with a suspected allergy to insulin
  2. Value: Less than 1:4 titer with no antibody detected

  3. Nursing considerations
    a. Radioactive scans within 7 days before the test may interfere with test results.
    b. No fasting is required.

VII. RENAL FUNCTION STUDIES

A. Serum creatinine
  1. Description
    a. Creatinine is a specific indicator of renal function.
    b. Increased levels of creatinine indicate a slowing of the glomerular filtration rate.
  2. Value: 0.6 to 1.3 mg/dL
  3. Nursing consideration: Instruct the client to avoid excessive exercise for 8 hours and excessive red meat intake for 24 hours before the test.
B. Blood urea nitrogen
  1. Description
    a. Urea nitrogen is the nitrogen portion of urea, a substance formed in the liver through an enzymatic protein breakdown process.
    b. Urea is normally freely filtered through the renal glomeruli, with a small amount reabsorbed in the tubules and the remainder excreted in the urine.
    c. Elevated levels indicate a slowing of the glomerular filtration rate.
  2. Value: 8 to 25 mg/dL
  3. Nursing consideration: Creatinine and urea nitrogen levels should be analyzed when renal function is evaluated.

VIII. ELEMENTS

A. Calcium
  1. Description
    a. Calcium is a cation absorbed into the bloodstream from dietary sources and functions in bone formation, nerve impulse transmission, and contraction of myocardial and skeletal muscles.
    b. Calcium aids in **blood** clotting by converting prothrombin to thrombin.
  2. Value: 8.6 to 10 mg/dL
  3. Nursing considerations
    a. Instruct the client to eat a diet with a normal calcium level (800 mg/day) for 3 days before the test.
    b. Instruct the client that fasting may be required for 8 hours before the test.
B. Magnesium
  1. Description
    a. Magnesium is used as an index to determine metabolic activity and renal function.
    b. Magnesium is needed in the **blood**-clotting mechanism, regulates neuromuscular activity, acts as a cofactor that modifies the activity of many enzymes, and has an effect on the metabolism of calcium.

2. Value: 1.6 to 2.6 mg/dL
3. Nursing considerations
   a. Prolonged use of magnesium products causes increased **serum** levels.
   b. Long-term parenteral nutrition therapy or excessive loss of body fluids may decrease **serum** levels.
C. Phosphorus
   1. Description
      a. Phosphorus is important in bone formation, energy storage and release, urinary acid-base buffering, and carbohydrate metabolism.
      b. Phosphorus is absorbed from food and is excreted by the kidneys.
      c. High concentrations of phosphorus are stored in bone and skeletal muscle.
   2. Value: 2.7 to 4.5 mg/dL
   3. Nursing considerations: Instruct the client to fast before the test.

IX. THYROID STUDIES

A. Description
   1. Thyroid studies are performed if a thyroid disorder is suspected.
   2. Thyroid studies help differentiate primary thyroid disease from secondary causes and from abnormalities in thyroxine-binding globulin levels.
B. Values
   1. Thyroid-stimulating hormone (also called thyrotropin): 0.2 to 5.4 microunits/mL
   2. Thyroxine (T_4): 5 to 12 mcg/dL
   3. Thyroxine, free (FT_4): 0.8 to 2.4 ng/dL
   4. Triiodothyronine (T_3): 80 to 230 ng/dL
C. Nursing consideration: Test results may be invalid if the client has undergone a radionuclide scan within 7 days before the test.

X. WHITE BLOOD CELL COUNT

A. Description
   1. WBCs function in the immune defense system of the body.
   2. The WBC count assesses leukocyte distribution.
B. Value: 4500 to 11,000 cells/mm^3 (Table 11-5)

TABLE 11-5 Normal Adult White Blood Cell Differential Count

Cell Type	Count
Neutrophils	1800-7800 cells/mm^3
Bands	0-700 cells/mm^3
Eosinophils	0-450 cells/mm^3
Basophils	0-200 cells/mm^3
Lymphocytes	1000-4800 cells/mm^3
Monocytes	0-800 cells/mm^3

C. Nursing considerations
   1. A "shift to the left" means that an increased number of immature neutrophils is present in the **blood**.
   2. A low total WBC count with a left shift indicates a recovery from bone marrow depression or an infection of such intensity that the demand for neutrophils in the tissue is higher than the capacity of the bone marrow to release them into the circulation.
   3. A high total WBC count with a left shift indicates an increased release of neutrophils by the bone marrow in response to an overwhelming infection or inflammation.
   4. A "shift to the right" means that cells have more than the usual number of nuclear segments; found in liver disease, Down syndrome, and megaloblastic and pernicious anemia.

⚠ Monitor the WBC count closely in clients receiving chemotherapy because of the risk for neutropenia.

XI. HEPATITIS TESTING

A. Description
   1. Tests include radioimmunoassay, enzyme-linked immunosorbent assay (ELISA), and microparticle enzyme immunoassay.
   2. Serological tests for specific hepatitis virus markers assist in defining the specific type of hepatitis.
B. Values
   1. The presence of immunoglobulin M (IgM) antibody to hepatitis A virus and the presence of the total antibody to hepatitis A virus identify the disease.
   2. Detection of hepatitis B core antigen (HBcAg), envelope antigen (HBeAg), and surface antigen (HBsAg), or their corresponding antibodies, constitutes hepatitis B assessment.
   3. Hepatitis C is confirmed by the presence of antibodies to hepatitis C virus.
   4. Serological hepatitis D virus determination is made by detection of the hepatitis D antigen (HDAg) early in the course of the infection and by detection of anti–hepatitis D virus antibody in the later disease stages.
   5. Specific serological tests for hepatitis E virus include detection of IgM and IgG antibodies to hepatitis E.
   6. Hepatitis G virus has been found in some **blood** donors (donated **blood**), IV drug users, hemodialysis clients, and clients with hemophilia; however, hepatitis G virus does not appear to cause significant liver disease.
C. Nursing consideration: If the radioimmunoassay technique is being used, the injection of radionuclides within 1 week before the **blood** test is performed may cause falsely elevated results.

XII. HUMAN IMMUNODEFICIENCY VIRUS (HIV) AND ACQUIRED IMMUNODEFICIENCY SYNDROME (AIDS) TESTING

A. Description
1. Testing detects HIV, which is the cause of AIDS.
2. Common tests used to determine the presence of antibodies to HIV include ELISA, Western blot, and immunofluorescence assay (IFA).
3. A single reactive ELISA test by itself cannot be used to diagnose HIV and should be repeated in duplicate with the same **blood** sample; if the result is repeatedly reactive, follow-up tests using Western blot or IFA should be performed.
4. A positive Western blot or IFA result is considered confirmatory for HIV.
5. A positive ELISA result that fails to be confirmed by Western blot or IFA should not be considered negative, and repeat testing should take place in 3 to 6 months.

B. CD4$^+$ T-cell counts
1. Monitors the progression of HIV
2. As the disease progresses, usually the number of CD4$^+$ T-cells decreases, with a resultant decrease in immunity.
3. Normal CD4$^+$ T-cell count is between 500 and 1600 cells/L.
4. Generally, the immune system remains healthy with CD4$^+$ T-cell counts higher than 500 cells/L.
5. Immune system problems occur when the CD4$^+$ T-cell count is between 200 and 499 cells/L.
6. Severe immune system problems occur when the CD4$^+$ T-cell count is lower than 200 cells/L.

C. CD4-to-CD8 ratio
1. Monitors progression of disease.
2. Normal ratio is approximately 2:1.

D. Viral culture involves placing the infected client's **blood cells** in a culture medium and measuring the amount of reverse transcriptase activity over a specified period of time.

E. Viral load testing measures the presence of HIV viral genetic material (RNA) or another viral protein in the client's **blood**.

F. The p24 antigen assay quantifies the amount of HIV viral core protein in the client's **serum**.

G. Oral testing for HIV
1. Uses a device that is placed against the gum and cheek for 2 minutes
2. Fluid (not saliva) is drawn into an absorbable pad, which, in an HIV-positive individual, contains antibodies.
3. The pad is placed in a solution and a specified observable change is noted if the test result is positive.

4. If the result is positive, a **blood** test is needed to confirm the results.

H. Home test kits for HIV
1. In one at-home test kit, a drop of **blood** is placed on a test card with a special code number; the card is mailed to a laboratory for testing for HIV antibodies.
2. The individual receives the results by calling a special telephone number and entering the special code number; test results are then given.

I. Nursing considerations
1. Maintain issues of confidentiality surrounding HIV and AIDS testing.
2. Follow prescribed state regulations and protocols related to reporting positive test results.

XIII. URINE TESTS (Table 11-6)

XIV. THERAPEUTIC SERUM MEDICATION LEVELS (Table 11-7)

TABLE 11-6 Normal Adult Values: Urine Tests

Name of Test	Value
Color	Pale yellow
Odor	Specific aromatic odor, similar to ammonia
Turbidity	Clear
pH	4.5-7.8
Specific gravity	1.016 to 1.022
Glucose	<0.5 g/day
Ketones	None
Protein	None
Bilirubin	None
Casts	None to few
Crystals	None
Bacteria	None or <1000/mL
Red blood cells	<3 cells/HPF
White blood cells	≤4 cells/HPF
Chloride	110-250 mEq/24 hr
Magnesium	7.3-12.2 mg/dL
Potassium	25-125 mEq/24 hr
Sodium	40-220 mEq/24 hr
Uric acid	250-750 mg/24 hr

HPF, High-powered field.

TABLE 11-7 Therapeutic Serum Medication Levels

Medication	Therapeutic Range
Acetaminophen (Tylenol)	10-20 mcg/mL
Amikacin (Amikin)	25-30 mcg/mL
Amitriptyline	120-150 ng/mL
Carbamazepine (Tegretol)	5-12 mcg/mL
Chloramphenicol (Chloromycetin)	10-20 mcg/mL
Desipramine (Norpramin)	150-300 ng/mL
Digoxin (Lanoxin)	0.5-2 ng/mL
Disopyramide (Norpace)	2-5 mcg/mL
Ethosuximide (Zarontin)	40-100 mcg/mL
Gentamicin	5-10 mcg/mL
Imipramine (Tofranil)	150-300 ng/mL
Lidocaine (Xylocaine)	1.5-5 mcg/mL
Lithium (Lithobid)	0.5-1.2 mEq/L
Magnesium sulfate	4-7 mg/dL
Phenobarbital (Luminal)	10-30 mcg/mL
Phenytoin (Dilantin)	10-20 mcg/mL
Propranolol (Inderal)	50-100 ng/mL
Salicylate	100-250 mcg/mL
Theophylline	10-20 mcg/mL
Tobramycin (Nebcin)	5-10 mcg/mL
Valproic acid (Depakene)	50-100 mcg/mL

 MORE QUESTIONS ON THE CD!

Practice Questions

63. A client with atrial fibrillation who is receiving maintenance therapy of warfarin sodium (Coumadin) has a prothrombin time (PT) of 35 seconds. Based on the prothrombin time, the nurse anticipates which of the following prescriptions?
1. Adding a dose of heparin sodium
2. Holding the next dose of warfarin
3. Increasing the next dose of warfarin
4. Administering the next dose of warfarin

64. The nurse checks the laboratory result for a serum digoxin level that was prescribed for a client earlier in the day and notes that the result is 2.4 ng/mL. The nurse should take which immediate action?

1. Notify the physician.
2. Check the client's last pulse rate.
3. Record the normal value on the client's flow sheet.
4. Administer the next dose of the medication as scheduled.

65. A client has been admitted to the hospital for urinary tract infection and dehydration. The nurse determines that the client has received adequate volume replacement if the blood urea nitrogen level drops to:
1. 3 mg/dL
2. 15 mg/dL
3. 29 mg/dL
4. 35 mg/dL

66. A client arrives in the emergency room complaining of chest pain that began 4 hours ago. A troponin T blood specimen is obtained, and the results indicate a level of 0.6 ng/mL. The nurse determines that this result indicates:
1. A normal level
2. A low value that indicates possible gastritis
3. A level that indicates a myocardial infarction
4. A level that indicates the presence of possible angina

67. A client is receiving a continuous intravenous infusion of heparin sodium to treat deep vein thrombosis. The client's activated partial thromboplastin (aPTT) time is 65 seconds. The nurse anticipates that which action is needed?
1. Discontinuing the heparin infusion
2. Increasing the rate of the heparin infusion
3. Decreasing the rate of the heparin infusion
4. Leaving the rate of the heparin infusion as is

68. A client with a history of cardiac disease is due for a morning dose of furosemide (Lasix). Which serum potassium level, if noted in the client's laboratory report, should be reported before administering the dose of furosemide?
1. 3.2 mEq/L
2. 3.8 mEq/L
3. 4.2 mEq/L
4. 4.8 mEq/L

69. A client with a history of gastrointestinal bleeding has a platelet count of 300,000 cells/mm^3. The nurse should take which action after seeing the laboratory results?

1. Report the abnormally low count.
2. Report the abnormally high count.
3. Place the client on bleeding precautions.
4. Place the normal report in the client's medical record.

70. An adult client with cirrhosis has been following a diet with optimal amounts of protein because neither an excess nor a deficiency of protein has been helpful. The nurse evaluates the client's status as being most satisfactory if the total protein level is which of the following values?
1. 0.4 g/dL
2. 3.7 g/dL
3. 6.4 g/dL
4. 9.8 g/dL

71. A client with diabetes mellitus has a glycosylated hemoglobin A_{1c} level of 9%. Based on this test result, the nurse plans to teach the client about the need to:
1. Avoid infection.
2. Take in adequate fluids.
3. Prevent and recognize hypoglycemia.
4. Prevent and recognize hyperglycemia.

72. The nurse is caring for a client with a diagnosis of cancer who is immunosuppressed. The nurse would consider implementing neutropenic precautions if the client's white blood cell count was which of the following?
1. 2000 cells/mm^3
2. 5800 cells/mm^3
3. 8400 cells/mm^3
4. 11,500 cells/mm^3

73. A client brought to the emergency department states that he has accidentally been taking two times his prescribed dose of warfarin (Coumadin) for the past week. After noting that the client has no evidence of obvious bleeding, the nurse plans to do which of the following?

1. Prepare to administer an antidote.
2. Draw a sample for type and crossmatch and transfuse the client.
3. Draw a sample for an activated partial thromboplastin time (aPTT) level.
4. Draw a sample for prothrombin time (PT) and international normalized ratio (INR).

74. The nurse is assigned to a 40-year-old client who has a diagnosis of chronic pancreatitis. The nurse anticipates the client's serum amylase level to be which of the following?
1. 45 units/L
2. 100 units/L
3. 300 units/L
4. 500 units/L

75. An adult female client has a hemoglobin level of 10.8 g/dL. The nurse interprets that this result is most likely caused by which of the following conditions noted in the client's history?
1. Dehydration
2. Heart failure
3. Iron deficiency anemia
4. Chronic obstructive pulmonary disease

Alternate Item Format: Multiple Response

76. Several laboratory tests are prescribed for a client, and the nurse reviews the results of the tests. Select the abnormal laboratory test results that the nurse should report. **Select all that apply.**
❑ 1. Calcium, 7 mg/dL
❑ 2. Magnesium, 1 mg/dL
❑ 3. Phosphorus, 3.6 mg/dL
❑ 4. Neutrophils, 1000/mm^3
❑ 5. Serum creatinine, 1 mg/dL
❑ 6. White blood cells, 3000/mm^3

ANSWERS

63. 2

Rationale: The normal PT is 9.6 to 11.8 seconds (male adult) or 9.5 to 11.3 seconds (female adult). A therapeutic PT level is 1.5 to 2 times higher than the normal level. Because the value of 35 seconds is high (and perhaps near the critical range), the nurse should anticipate that the client would not receive further doses at this time. Therefore the prescriptions noted in options 1, 3, and 4 are incorrect.

Test-Taking Strategy: Recall that the normal PT is 9.6 to 11.8 seconds (male adult) or 9.5 to 11.3 seconds (female adult) and that a therapeutic PT level is 1.5 to 2 times higher than the normal level. Remember that a PT level greater than 30 seconds places the client at risk for bleeding; this will direct you to the correct option. If this question was difficult, review the normal PT level and the expected level if the client is receiving warfarin sodium.

Level of Cognitive Ability: Analyzing
Client Needs: Physiological Integrity
Integrated Process: Nursing Process—Analysis
Content Area: Fundamental Skills—Laboratory Values
References: Kee, J., Hayes, E., & McCuistion, L. (2009). *Pharmacology: A nursing process approach* (6th ed., p. 680). St. Louis: Saunders.

Pagana, K., & Pagana, T. (2009). *Mosby's diagnostic and laboratory test reference* (9th ed., p. 779). St. Louis: Mosby.

64. 1

Rationale: The normal therapeutic range for digoxin is 0.5 to 2 ng/mL. A level of 2.4 ng/mL exceeds the therapeutic range and indicates toxicity. The nurse should notify the physician, who may give further prescriptions about holding further doses of digoxin. Option 3 is incorrect because the level is not normal. The next dose should not be administered because the serum digoxin level exceeds the therapeutic range. Checking the client's last pulse rate may have limited value in this situation. Depending on the time that has elapsed since the last assessment, a current assessment of the client's status may be more useful.

Test-Taking Strategy: Note the strategic word *immediate*. To choose correctly, you must be familiar with the therapeutic range for this medication and note that the level of 2.4 ng/mL is a toxic one. This will direct you to option 1. If this question was difficult, review the immediate nursing interventions if the client has a toxic digoxin level.

Level of Cognitive Ability: Applying
Client Needs: Physiological Integrity
Integrated Process: Nursing Process—Implementation
Content Area: Fundamental Skills—Laboratory Values
Reference: Pagana, K., & Pagana, T. (2009). *Mosby's diagnostic and laboratory test reference* (9th ed., p. 354). St. Louis: Mosby.

65. 2

Rationale: The normal blood urea nitrogen level is 8 to 25 mg/dL. Values such as those in options 3 and 4 reflect continued dehydration. Option 1 reflects a lower than normal value, which may occur with fluid volume overload, among other conditions.

Test-Taking Strategy: Use the process of elimination and knowledge of the normal blood urea nitrogen level to answer the question. Option 2 is the only option that identifies a normal value. Review the normal blood urea nitrogen level if you had difficulty with this question.

Level of Cognitive Ability: Understanding
Client Needs: Physiological Integrity
Integrated Process: Nursing Process—Evaluation
Content Area: Fundamental Skills—Laboratory Values
Reference: Pagana, K., & Pagana, T. (2009). *Mosby's diagnostic and laboratory test reference* (9th ed., p. 954). St. Louis: Mosby.

66. 3

Rationale: Troponin is a regulatory protein found in striated muscle. The troponins function together in the contractile apparatus for striated muscle in skeletal muscle and in the myocardium. Increased amounts of troponins are released into the bloodstream when an infarction causes damage to the myocardium. A troponin T value that is higher than 0.1 to 0.2 ng/mL is consistent with a myocardial infarction. A normal troponin I level is lower than 0.6 ng/mL.

Test-Taking Strategy: Note that the subject of the question relates to the troponin T. Knowing that a level higher than 0.1 to 0.2 ng/mL is consistent with a myocardial infarction will direct you to option 3. Review the normal troponin T and the normal troponin I level if you had difficulty with this question

Level of Cognitive Ability: Analyzing

Client Needs: Physiological Integrity
Integrated Process: Nursing Process—Analysis
Content Area: Fundamental Skills—Laboratory Values
Reference: Chernecky, C., & Berger, B. (2008). *Laboratory tests and diagnostic procedures* (5th ed., p. 1116). St. Louis: Saunders.

67. 4

Rationale: The normal aPTT varies between 20 and 36 seconds, depending on the type of activator used in testing. The therapeutic dose of heparin for treatment of deep vein thrombosis is to keep the aPTT between 1.5 and 2.5 times normal. This means that the client's value should not be less than 30 seconds or greater than 90 seconds. Thus the client's aPTT is within the therapeutic range and the dose should remain unchanged.

Test-Taking Strategy: Remember that the normal range is 20 to 36 seconds and that the aPTT should be between 1.5 and 2.5 times normal when the client is receiving heparin therapy. Simple multiplication of 1.5 and 2.5 by 20 and 30 will yield a range of 30 to 90 seconds. This client's value is 65 seconds. If this question was difficult, review the aPTT level and the expected level if the client is receiving heparin.

Level of Cognitive Ability: Analyzing
Client Needs: Physiological Integrity
Integrated Process: Nursing Process—Analysis
Content Area: Fundamental Skills—Laboratory Values
Reference: Gahart, B., & Nazareno, A. (2009). *Intravenous medications* (25th ed., p. 670). St. Louis: Mosby.

68. 1

Rationale: The normal serum potassium level in the adult is 3.5 to 5.1 mEq/L. Option 1 is the only value that falls below the therapeutic range. Administering furosemide to a client with a low potassium level and a history of cardiac problems could precipitate ventricular dysrhythmias. Options 2, 3, and 4 are within the normal range.

Test-Taking Strategy: Note the subject of the question, the level that should be reported. This indicates that you are looking for an abnormal level. Remember, the normal serum potassium level in the adult is 3.5 to 5.1 mEq/L. This will direct you to option 1. If this question was difficult, memorize the normal serum potassium level.

Level of Cognitive Ability: Applying
Client Needs: Physiological Integrity
Integrated Process: Nursing Process—Implementation
Content Area: Fundamental Skills—Laboratory Values
Reference: Chernecky, C., & Berger, B. (2008). *Laboratory tests and diagnostic procedures* (5th ed., p. 891). St. Louis: Saunders.

69. 4

Rationale: A normal platelet count ranges from 150,000 to 400,000 cells/mm^3. The nurse should place the report containing the normal laboratory value in the client's medical record. A platelet count of 300,000 cells/mm^3 is not an elevated count. The count also is not low; therefore bleeding precautions are not needed.

Test-Taking Strategy: Use the process of elimination. Remember that options that are comparable or alike are not likely to be correct. With this in mind, eliminate options 1 and 3 first. From the remaining options, recalling the normal range for this laboratory test will direct you to option 4. Review the normal platelet count if you had difficulty with this question.

Level of Cognitive Ability: Applying
Client Needs: Physiological Integrity
Integrated Process: Nursing Process—Implementation
Content Area: Fundamental Skills—Laboratory Values
Reference: Pagana, K., & Pagana, T. (2009). *Mosby's diagnostic and laboratory test reference* (9th ed., p. 731). St. Louis: Mosby.

70. 3
Rationale: The normal range for total serum protein level in the adult client is 6 to 8 g/dL. The client with cirrhosis often has low total protein levels as a result of inadequate nutrition. Excess protein is not helpful, though, because a function of the liver is to metabolize protein. A diseased liver may not metabolize protein well. Options 1 and 2 identify low values, and option 4 identifies a high protein value.
Test-Taking Strategy: Note the strategic words *most satisfactory*. Recalling the normal total protein level will direct you to option 3. Review total serum protein level if you had difficulty with this question.
Level of Cognitive Ability: Understanding
Client Needs: Physiological Integrity
Integrated Process: Nursing Process—Evaluation
Content Area: Fundamental Skills—Laboratory Values
Reference: Pagana, K., & Pagana, T. (2009). *Mosby's diagnostic and laboratory test reference* (9th ed., p. 769). St. Louis: Mosby.

71. 4
Rationale: In the test result for glycosylated hemoglobin A_{1c}, 7% or less indicates good control, 7% to 8% indicates fair control, and 8% or higher indicates poor control. This test measures the amount of glucose that has become permanently bound to the red blood cells from circulating glucose. Elevations in the blood glucose level will cause elevations in the amount of glycosylation. Thus the test is useful in identifying clients who have periods of hyperglycemia that are undetected in other ways. Elevations indicate continued need for teaching related to the prevention of hyperglycemic episodes.
Test-Taking Strategy: Use the process of elimination and knowledge regarding the values for glycosylated hemoglobin A_{1c} and their significance to answer the question. Focusing on the level identified in the question will assist in directing you to option 4. If you had difficulty with this question or are unfamiliar with the glycosylated hemoglobin A_{1c}, review this content.
Level of Cognitive Ability: Applying
Client Needs: Health Promotion and Maintenance
Integrated Process: Teaching and Learning
Content Area: Fundamental Skills—Laboratory Values
Reference: Pagana, K., & Pagana, T. (2009). *Mosby's diagnostic and laboratory test reference* (9th ed., p. 492). St. Louis: Mosby.

72. 1
Rationale: The normal white blood cell count ranges from 4500 to 11,000/mm³. The client who has a decrease in the

number of circulating white blood cells is immunosuppressed. The nurse implements neutropenic precautions when the client's values fall sufficiently below the normal level. The specific value for implementing neutropenic precautions usually is determined by agency policy. Options 2, 3, and 4 are normal values.
Test-Taking Strategy: Use the process of elimination and focus on the subject, the need to implement neutropenic precautions. Recalling that the normal white blood cell count is 4500 to 11,000/mm³ will direct you to option 1. Review the normal white blood cell counts if you had difficulty with this question.
Level of Cognitive Ability: Understanding
Client Needs: Physiological Integrity
Integrated Process: Nursing Process—Planning
Content Area: Fundamental Skills—Laboratory Values
References: Pagana, K., & Pagana, T. (2009). *Mosby's diagnostic and laboratory test reference* (9th ed., p. 998). St. Louis: Mosby.
  Swearingen, P. (2008). *All-in-one care planning resource: Medical-surgical, pediatric, maternity, & psychiatric nursing care plans* (2nd ed., p. 15). St. Louis: Mosby.

73. 4
Rationale: The next action is to draw a sample for PT and INR level to determine the client's anticoagulation status and risk for bleeding. These results will provide information as to how to best treat this client (e.g., if an antidote such as vitamin K or a blood transfusion is needed). The aPTT monitors the effects of heparin therapy.
Test-Taking Strategy: Use a process of elimination. Eliminate option 3 because it is unrelated to warfarin therapy and relates to heparin therapy. Next, eliminate options 1 and 2 because these therapies would not be implemented unless the PT and INR levels are known. Review care to the client receiving warfarin therapy and the purpose of the PT and INR if you had difficulty with this question.
Level of Cognitive Ability: Applying
Client Needs: Physiological Integrity
Integrated Process: Nursing Process—Planning
Content Area: Fundamental Skills—Laboratory Values
Reference: Kee, J., Hayes, E., & McCuistion, L. (2009). *Pharmacology: A nursing process approach* (6th ed., pp. 682–683). St. Louis: Saunders.

74. 3
Rationale: The normal serum amylase level is 25 to 151 units/L. With chronic cases of pancreatitis, the rise in serum amylase levels usually does not exceed three times the normal value. In acute pancreatitis, the value may exceed five times the normal value. Options 1 and 2 are within normal limits. Option 4 is an extremely elevated level seen in acute pancreatitis.
Test-Taking Strategy: Note the strategic word *chronic* in the question. Recalling the normal amylase level and focusing on the strategic word will direct you to option 3. Review the normal serum amylase level and the findings in chronic pancreatitis if you had difficulty with this question.
Level of Cognitive Ability: Analyzing
Client Needs: Physiological Integrity
Integrated Process: Nursing Process—Analysis
Content Area: Fundamental Skills—Laboratory Values

Reference: Swearingen, P. (2008). *All-in-one care planning resource: Medical-surgical, pediatric, maternity, & psychiatric nursing care plans* (2nd ed., p. 470). St. Louis: Mosby.

75. 3

Rationale: The normal hemoglobin level for an adult female client is 12 to 15 g/dL. Iron deficiency anemia can result in lower hemoglobin levels. Dehydration may increase the hemoglobin level by hemoconcentration. Heart failure and chronic obstructive pulmonary disease may increase the hemoglobin level as a result of the body's need for more oxygen-carrying capacity.

Test-Taking Strategy: Use the process of elimination. Evaluate each of the options in terms of whether each is likely to raise or lower the hemoglobin level. Also, note the relationship between hemoglobin level in the question and option 3. Review the normal hemoglobin level if you had difficulty with this question.

Level of Cognitive Ability: Analyzing

Client Needs: Physiological Integrity

Integrated Process: Nursing Process—Analysis

Content Area: Fundamental Skills—Laboratory Values

References: Black, J., & Hawks, J. (2009). *Medical-surgical nursing: Clinical management for positive outcomes* (8th ed., pp. 2004–2005). St. Louis: Saunders.

Chernecky, C., & Berger, B. (2008). *Laboratory tests and diagnostic procedures* (5th ed., p. 617). St. Louis: Saunders.

ALTERNATE ITEM FORMAT: MULTIPLE RESPONSE

76. 1, 2, 4, 6

Rationale: The normal values include the following: calcium, 8.6 to 10 mg/dL; magnesium, 1.6 to 2.6 mg/dL; phosphorus, 2.7 to 4.5 mg/dL; neutrophils, 1800 to 7800/mm^3; serum creatinine, 0.6 to 1.3 mg/dL; and white blood cells, 4500 to 11,000/mm^3. The calcium level noted is low; the magnesium level noted is low; the phosphorus level noted is normal; the neutrophil level noted is low; the serum creatinine level noted is normal; and the white blood cell level is low.

Test-Taking Strategy: Note the strategic word *abnormal* in the question. Recalling the normal laboratory values for the blood studies identified in the options will assist in answering this question. Review these normal values if you had difficulty with this question.

Level of Cognitive Ability: Understanding

Client Needs: Physiological Integrity

Integrated Process: Nursing Process—Implementation

Content Area: Fundamental Skills—Laboratory Values

Reference: Chernecky, C., & Berger, B. (2008). *Laboratory tests and diagnostic procedures* (5th ed., pp. 278, 369, 744). St. Louis: Saunders.

12

Nutrition

PYRAMID TERMS

absorption Passage of digested nutrients through the wall of the stomach or small intestine into the blood or lymph system.

enteral nutrition Administration of nutrition with liquefied foods into the gastrointestinal tract via a tube.

malnutrition Deficiency of the nutrients required for development and maintenance of the human body.

metabolism Ongoing chemical process within the body that converts digested nutrients into energy for the functioning of body cells.

nutrients Carbohydrates, fats or lipids, proteins, vitamins, minerals, electrolytes, and water that must be supplied in adequate amounts to provide energy, growth, development, and maintenance of the human body.

 ## THE PYRAMID TO SUCCESS

Nutrition is a basic need that must be met for all clients. Nurses must have the knowledge required to educate and care for healthy clients and for clients with nutritional needs or disorders requiring alterations in dietary measures. The NCLEX-RN examination addresses the dietary measures required for basic needs and for particular body system alterations. When presented with a question related to nutrition, consider the client's diagnosis and the particular requirement or restriction necessary for treatment of the disorder. Pyramid Points focus on the common types of therapeutic diets, nutrients contained in food items, and supplemental or enteral feedings.

CLIENT NEEDS

Safe and Effective Care Environment

Consulting with members of the health care team such as a dietitian regarding dietary needs

Obtaining informed consent for invasive procedures

Maintaining standard and transmission-based and asepsis

Providing information to the client about community classes for nutrition education

Health Promotion and Maintenance

Initiating health promotion programs
Performing physical assessment
Preventing disease
Promoting health and wellness
Providing dietary teaching

Psychosocial Integrity

Considering cultural preferences related to nutritional patterns and lifestyle choices
Identifying coping mechanisms
Identifying religious and spiritual influences on health

Physiological Integrity

Assessing elimination patterns
Monitoring for alterations in body systems
Monitoring of enteral feedings and the client's ability to tolerate feedings
Monitoring of fluid and electrolyte balance
Monitoring of laboratory values
Monitoring of nutritional intake and oral hydration

I. NUTRIENTS

A. Carbohydrates (Box 12-1)
   1. Carbohydrates are the preferred source of energy.
   2. Sugars, starches, and cellulose provide 4 cal/g.
   3. Carbohydrates promote normal fat **metabolism**, spare protein, and enhance lower gastrointestinal function.
   4. Major food sources of carbohydrates include milk, grains, fruits, and vegetables.
   5. Inadequate carbohydrate intake affects **metabolism**.
B. Fats (Box 12-2)
   1. Fats provide a concentrated source and a stored form of energy.
   2. Fats protect internal organs and maintain body temperature.
   3. Fats enhance **absorption** of the fat-soluble vitamins.
   4. Fats provide 9 cal/g.

5. Inadequate fat intake leads to clinical manifestations of sensitivity to cold, skin lesions, increased risk of infection, and amenorrhea in women.
6. Diets high in fat can lead to obesity and increase the risk of cardiovascular disease and some cancers.

C. Proteins (Box 12-3)
   1. Amino acids, which make up proteins, are critical to all aspects of growth and development of body tissues, and provide 4 cal/g.
   2. Proteins build and repair body tissues, regulate fluid balance, maintain acid-base balance, produce antibodies, provide energy, and produce enzymes and hormones.
   3. Essential amino acids are required in the diet because the body cannot manufacture them.
   4. High-quality proteins or complete proteins such as eggs, dairy products, meat, fish, and poultry contain adequate amounts of essential amino acids.
   5. Foods that do not contain the essential amino acids in sufficient amounts are lower quality or incomplete proteins.
   6. Inadequate protein can cause protein energy **malnutrition** and severe wasting of fat and muscle tissue.

D. Vitamins (Box 12-4)
   1. Vitamins facilitate **metabolism** of proteins, fats, and carbohydrates and act as catalysts for metabolic functions.
   2. Vitamins promote life and growth processes, and maintain and regulate body functions.
   3. Fat-soluble vitamins A, D, E, and K can be stored in the body, so an excess can cause toxicity.
   4. The B vitamins and vitamin C are water-soluble vitamins, are not stored in the body, and can be excreted in the urine.

Box 12-1 Food Sources of Carbohydrates

Cellulose
Apples
Beans
Bran
Cabbage

Fructose
Fruits
Honey

Glucose
Carrots
Corn
Dates
Grapes
Oranges

Lactose
Milk

Starch
Barley
Beets, carrots, and peas
Corn
Oats
Potatoes and pasta
Rye
Wheat

Sucrose
Apricots
Granulated table sugar
Honeydew and cantaloupe
Molasses
Peaches
Peas and corn
Plums

Box 12-2 Food Sources of Fats

Cholesterol
Animal products
Egg yolks
Liver and organ meats
Shellfish

Monounsaturated Fats
Duck and goose
Eggs
Olive and peanut oils

Polyunsaturated Fats
Corn oil
Safflower oil
Sunflower oil

Saturated Fats
Beef
Butter
Hard yellow cheeses
Luncheon meats

Box 12-3 Food Sources of Protein

Bread and cereal products
Dairy products
Dried beans
Eggs
Meats, fish, and poultry

Box 12-4 Food Sources of Vitamins

Water-Soluble Vitamins
Folic acid: Green, leafy vegetables; liver, beef, and fish; legumes; grapefruit and oranges
Niacin: Meats, poultry, fish, beans, peanuts, grains
Vitamin B_1 (thiamine): Pork and nuts, whole-grain cereals, and legumes
Vitamin B_2 (riboflavin): Milk, lean meats, fish, grains
Vitamin B_6 (pyridoxine): Yeast, corn, meat, poultry, fish
Vitamin B_{12} (cobalamin): Meat, liver
Vitamin C (ascorbic acid): Citrus fruits, tomatoes, broccoli, cabbage

Fat-Soluble Vitamins
Vitamin A: Liver, egg yolk, whole milk, green or orange vegetables, fruits
Vitamin D: Fortified milk, fish oils, cereals
Vitamin E: Vegetable oils; green, leafy vegetables; cereals; apricots, apples, and peaches
Vitamin K: Green leafy vegetables; cauliflower and cabbage

5. Vitamin K acts as a catalyst for facilitating blood-clotting factors, especially prothrombin.

6. Vitamin C functions in the production of collagen, a vital component in wound healing.

7. Vitamin A maintains eyesight and epithelial linings.

E. Minerals (Box 12-5)

1. Minerals are components of hormones, cells, tissues, and bones.

2. Minerals act as catalysts for chemical reactions and enhancers of cell function.

3. Almost all foods contain some form of minerals.

4. A deficiency of minerals can occur in chronically ill or hospitalized clients.

5. Electrolytes play a major role in osmolality and body water regulation, acid-base balance, enzyme reactions, and neuromuscular activity (see Chapter 9 for additional information regarding electrolytes).

⚠ Always assess the client's ability to eat and swallow and promote independence in eating as much as is possible.

II. FOOD GUIDE PYRAMID (Fig. 12-1)

A. The food guide pyramid (MyPyramid)

1. MyPyramid provides individualized guidance to healthy eating and physical activity.

2. Activity, which is illustrated by the person climbing the steps in Figure 12-1, symbolizes the importance of finding a balance between food and physical activity.

3. Food groups, illustrated by the bands on the pyramid in Figure 12-1, include grains, vegetables, fruits, milk, and meat and beans.

4. ChooseMyPlate: provides a balanced diet that includes grains, vegetables, fruits, dairy products, and protein foods (refer to: http://www.choosemyplate.gov/)

B. Shape of the pyramid

1. The wide base of each food group band on the pyramid indicates foods with little or no solid fats or added sugars; these are foods that should be eaten most often.

2. The narrower part of the food group band indicates foods containing more added sugars and solid fats; these foods should be eaten less often (increased activity is needed when these foods are eaten).

⚠ Always consider the client's cultural and personal choices when planning nutritional intake.

III. THERAPEUTIC DIETS

A. Clear liquid diet

1. Indications

a. Clear liquid diet provides fluids and some electrolytes to prevent dehydration.

Box 12-5 Food Sources of Minerals

Calcium
Broccoli
Carrots
Cheese
Collard greens
Green beans
Milk
Rhubarb
Spinach
Tofu
Yogurt

Chloride
Salt

Magnesium
Avocado
Canned white tuna
Cauliflower
Cooked rolled oats
Green leafy vegetables
Milk
Peanut butter
Peas
Pork, beef, chicken
Potatoes
Raisins
Yogurt

Phosphorus
Fish
Nuts
Organ meats
Pork, beef, chicken
Whole-grain breads and cereals

Potassium
Avocado
Bananas
Cantaloupe
Carrots

Fish
Mushrooms
Oranges
Pork, beef, veal
Potatoes
Raisins
Spinach
Strawberries
Tomatoes

Sodium
American cheese
Bacon
Butter
Canned food
Cottage cheese
Cured pork
Hot dogs
Ketchup
Lunch meat
Milk
Mustard
Processed food
Snack food
Soy sauce
Table salt
White and whole-wheat bread

Iron
Breads and cereals
Dark green vegetables
Egg yolk
Liver
Meats

Zinc
Eggs
Leafy vegetables
Meats
Protein-rich foods

b. Clear liquid diet is used as an initial feeding after complete bowel rest.

c. Clear liquid diet is used initially to feed a malnourished person or a person who has not had any oral intake for some time.

d. Clear liquid diet is used for bowel preparation for surgery or tests, as well as postoperatively and in clients with fever, vomiting, or diarrhea.

e. Clear liquid diet is used in gastroenteritis or pancreatitis.

2. Nursing considerations

a. Clear liquid diet is deficient in energy (calories) and many **nutrients**.

b. Clear liquid diet is easily digested and absorbed.

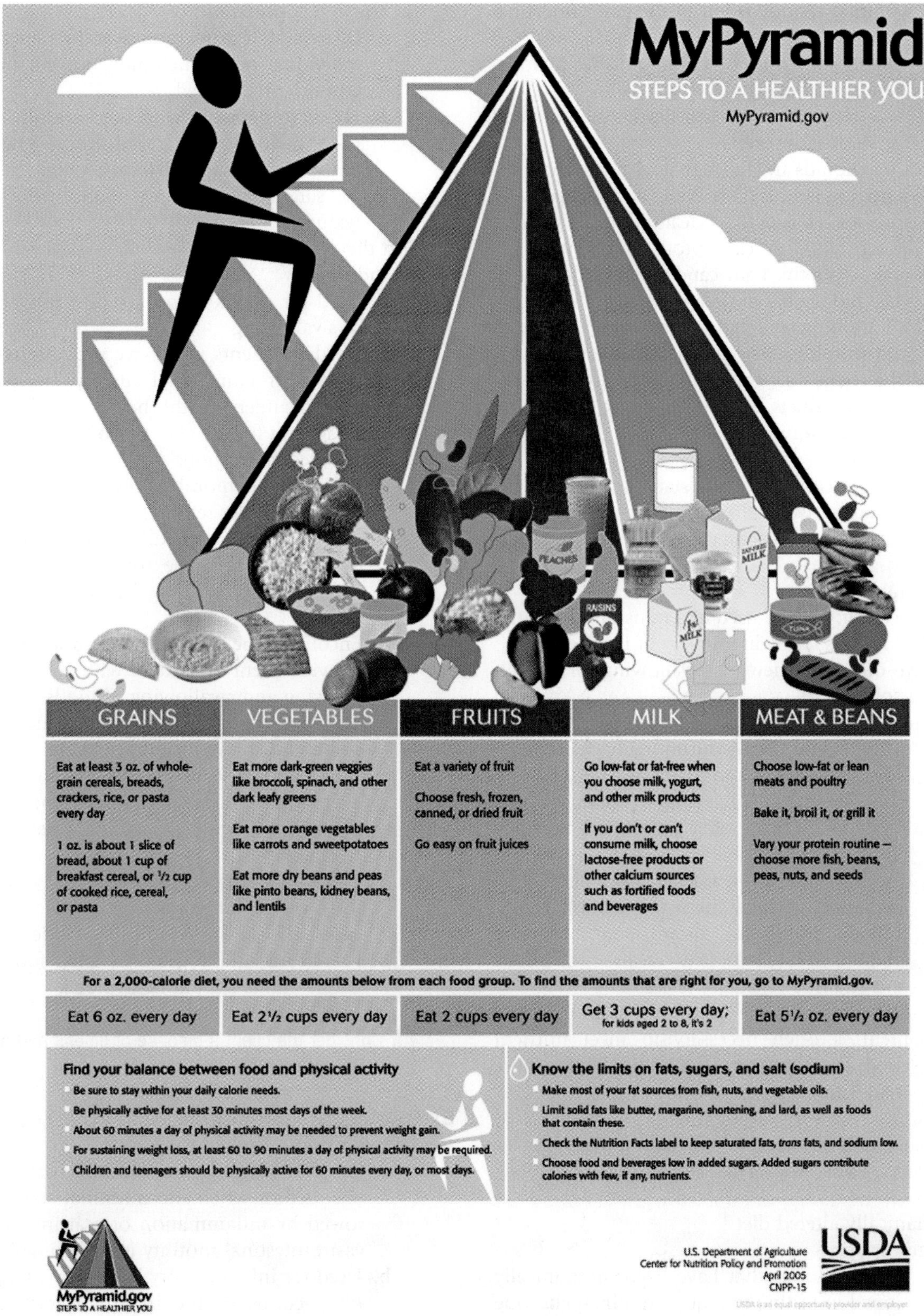

MyPyramid
STEPS TO A HEALTHIER YOU
MyPyramid.gov

GRAINS	VEGETABLES	FRUITS	MILK	MEAT & BEANS
Eat at least 3 oz. of whole-grain cereals, breads, crackers, rice, or pasta every day	Eat more dark-green veggies like broccoli, spinach, and other dark leafy greens	Eat a variety of fruit	Go low-fat or fat-free when you choose milk, yogurt, and other milk products	Choose low-fat or lean meats and poultry
1 oz. is about 1 slice of bread, about 1 cup of breakfast cereal, or ½ cup of cooked rice, cereal, or pasta	Eat more orange vegetables like carrots and sweetpotatoes	Choose fresh, frozen, canned, or dried fruit	If you don't or can't consume milk, choose lactose-free products or other calcium sources such as fortified foods and beverages	Bake it, broil it, or grill it
	Eat more dry beans and peas like pinto beans, kidney beans, and lentils	Go easy on fruit juices		Vary your protein routine — choose more fish, beans, peas, nuts, and seeds

For a 2,000-calorie diet, you need the amounts below from each food group. To find the amounts that are right for you, go to MyPyramid.gov.

Eat 6 oz. every day	Eat 2½ cups every day	Eat 2 cups every day	Get 3 cups every day; for kids aged 2 to 8, it's 2	Eat 5½ oz. every day

Find your balance between food and physical activity
- Be sure to stay within your daily calorie needs.
- Be physically active for at least 30 minutes most days of the week.
- About 60 minutes a day of physical activity may be needed to prevent weight gain.
- For sustaining weight loss, at least 60 to 90 minutes a day of physical activity may be required.
- Children and teenagers should be physically active for 60 minutes every day, or most days.

Know the limits on fats, sugars, and salt (sodium)
- Make most of your fat sources from fish, nuts, and vegetable oils.
- Limit solid fats like butter, margarine, shortening, and lard, as well as foods that contain these.
- Check the Nutrition Facts label to keep saturated fats, *trans* fats, and sodium low.
- Choose food and beverages low in added sugars. Added sugars contribute calories with few, if any, nutrients.

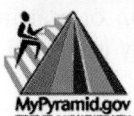

MyPyramid.gov
STEPS TO A HEALTHIER YOU

U.S. Department of Agriculture
Center for Nutrition Policy and Promotion
April 2005
CNPP-15

USDA is an equal opportunity provider and employer

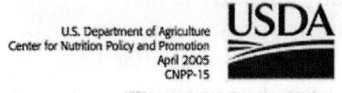

USDA

▲ **FIGURE 12-1** MyPyramid. (From U.S. Department of Agriculture. http://www.mypyramid.gov.)

c. Minimal residue is left in the gastrointestinal tract.

d. Clients may find a clear liquid diet unappetizing and boring.

e. As a transition diet, clear liquids are intended for short-term use.

f. Clear liquids and foods that are relatively transparent to light and are liquid at body temperature are considered "clear liquids," such as water, bouillon, clear broth, carbonated beverages, gelatin, hard candy, lemonade, Popsicles, and regular or decaffeinated coffee or tea.

g. By limiting caffeine intake, upset stomach and sleeplessness may be prevented.

h. The client may consume salt and sugar.

i. Dairy products and fruit juices with pulp are not clear liquids.

⚠ Monitor the client's hydration status by assessing intake and output, weight, monitoring for edema, and monitoring for signs of dehydration.

B. Full liquid diet
1. Indication: may be used as a transition diet after clear liquids following surgery or for clients who have difficulty chewing, swallowing, or tolerating solid foods
2. Nursing considerations
   a. A full liquid diet is nutritionally deficient in energy (calories) and many **nutrients**.
   b. The diet includes clear and opaque liquid foods, and those that are liquid at body temperature.
   c. Foods include all clear liquids and items such as plain ice cream, sherbet, breakfast drinks, milk, pudding and custard, soups that are strained, refined cooked cereals, fruit juices, and strained vegetable juices.
   d. Use of a complete nutritional liquid supplement is often necessary to meet nutrient needs for clients on a full liquid diet for more than 3 days.

⚠ Provide nutritional supplements such as those high in protein, as prescribed for the client on a liquid diet.

C. Mechanically altered diet
1. Indications
   a. Provides foods that have been mechanically altered in texture to require minimal chewing
   b. Used for clients who have difficulty chewing but can tolerate more variety in texture than a liquid diet offers
   c. Used for clients who have dental problems, surgery of the head or neck, or dysphagia (requires swallowing evaluation and may require thickened liquids)

2. Nursing considerations
   a. Degree of texture modification depends on individual need, including pureed, mashed, ground, or chopped.
   b. Foods to be avoided in mechanically altered diets include nuts; dried fruits; raw fruits and vegetables; fried foods; tough, smoked, or salted meats; and foods with coarse textures.

D. Soft diet
1. Indications
   a. Used for clients who have difficulty chewing or swallowing
   b. Used for clients who have ulcerations of the mouth or gums, oral surgery, broken jaw, plastic surgery of the head or neck, or dysphagia, or for the client who has had a stroke
2. Nursing considerations
   a. Clients with mouth sores should be served foods at cooler temperatures.
   b. Clients who have difficulty chewing and swallowing because of dry mouth can increase salivary flow by sucking on sour candy.
   c. Encourage the client to eat a variety of foods.
   d. Provide plenty of fluids with meals to ease chewing and swallowing of foods.
   e. Drinking fluids through a straw may be easier than drinking from a cup or glass.
   f. All foods and seasonings are permitted; however, liquid, chopped, or pureed foods or regular foods with a soft consistency are tolerated best.
   g. Foods that contain nuts or seeds, which easily can become trapped in the mouth and cause discomfort, should be avoided.
   h. Raw fruits and vegetables, fried foods, and whole grains should be avoided.

⚠ Consider the client's disease or illness and how it may impact on nutritional status.

E. Low-residue, low-fiber diet
1. Indications
   a. Supplies foods that are least likely to form an obstruction when the intestinal tract is narrowed by inflammation or scarring or when gastrointestinal motility is slowed
   b. Used for inflammatory bowel disease, partial obstructions of the intestinal tract, gastroenteritis, diarrhea, or other gastrointestinal disorders
2. Nursing considerations
   a. Foods that are low in residue include white bread, refined cooked cereals, cooked potatoes without skins, white rice, and refined pasta.

b. Foods to limit or avoid are raw fruits (except bananas), vegetables, nuts and seeds, plant fiber, and whole grains.

c. Dairy products should be limited to two servings a day.

F. High-residue, high-fiber diet
1. Indication: Used for constipation, irritable bowel syndrome when the primary symptom is alternating constipation and diarrhea, and asymptomatic diverticular disease
2. Nursing considerations
   a. High-residue diet provides 20 to 35 g of dietary fiber daily.
   b. Volume and weight are added to the stool, speeding the movement of undigested materials through the intestine.
   c. High-residue foods are fruits and vegetables and whole-grain products.
   d. Increase fiber gradually and provide adequate fluids to reduce possible undesirable side effects such as abdominal cramps, bloating, diarrhea, and dehydration.
   e. Gas-forming foods should be limited (Box 12-6)

G. Cardiac diet (Box 12-7; see Box 12-2)
1. Indications
   a. Indicated for atherosclerosis, diabetes mellitus, hyperlipidemia, hypertension, myocardial infarction, nephrotic syndrome, and renal failure
   b. Reduces the risk of heart disease
2. Nursing consideration: Restricts total amounts of fat, including saturated, trans, polyunsaturated, and monounsaturated; cholesterol; and sodium

Box 12-6 Gas-Forming Foods

Apples	Figs
Artichokes	Honey
Barley	Melons
Beans	Milk
Bran	Molasses
Broccoli	Nuts
Brussels sprouts	Onions
Cabbage	Radishes
Celery	Soybeans
Cherries	Wheat
Coconuts	Yeast
Eggplant	

Box 12-7 Sodium-Free Spices and Flavorings

Allspice	Ginger
Almond extract	Lemon extract
Bay leaves	Maple extract
Caraway seeds	Marjoram
Cinnamon	Mustard powder
Curry powder	Nutmeg
Garlic powder or garlic	

H. Fat-restricted diet
1. Indications
   a. Used to reduce symptoms of abdominal pain, steatorrhea, flatulence, and diarrhea associated with high intakes of dietary fat, and to decrease nutrient losses caused by ingestion of dietary fat in individuals with malabsorptive disorders
   b. Used for clients with malabsorption disorders, pancreatitis, gallbladder disease, and gastroesophageal reflux
2. Nursing considerations
   a. Restricts total amount of fat, including saturated, trans, polyunsaturated, and monounsaturated
   b. Clients with malabsorption may also have difficulty tolerating fiber and lactose.
   c. Vitamin and mineral deficiencies may occur in clients with diarrhea or steatorrhea.
   d. A fecal fat test indicates fat malabsorption with excretion of more than 6 to 8 g fat (or more than 10% of fat consumed) per day during the 3 days of specimen collection.

I. High-calorie, high-protein diet
1. Indication: Used for severe stress, burns, wound healing, cancer, human immunodeficiency virus, acquired immunodeficiency syndrome, chronic obstructive pulmonary disease, respiratory failure, or any other type of debilitating disease
2. Nursing considerations
   a. Encourage nutrient-dense, high-calorie, high-protein foods such as whole milk and milk products, peanut butter, nuts and seeds, beef, chicken, fish, pork, and eggs.
   b. Some high-calorie foods include sugar, cream, gravy, oil, butter, mayonnaise, dried fruit, avocado, and honey.
   c. Encourage snacks between meals, such as milkshakes, instant breakfasts, and nutritional supplements.

⚠ Calorie counts assist in determining the client's total nutritional intake and can identify a deficit or excess intake.

J. Carbohydrate-consistent diet
1. Indication: Used for clients with diabetes mellitus, hypoglycemia, hyperglycemia, and obesity
2. Nursing considerations
   a. The Exchange System for Meal Planning, developed by the American Dietetic Association and the American Diabetes Association, is a food guide that may be recommended.
   b. The Exchange System groups foods according to the amounts of carbohydrates, fats, and proteins they contain.

c. Major food groups include the carbohydrate, meat and meat substitute, and fat groups.
d. The MyPyramid diet may also be recommended.

K. Sodium-restricted diet (see Box 12-7)
1. Indication: Used for hypertension, heart failure, renal disease, cardiac disease, and liver disease
2. Nursing considerations
    a. Individualized; can include 4 g of sodium daily (no-added salt diet), 2 to 3 g of sodium daily (moderate restriction), 1 g of sodium daily (strict restriction), or 500 mg of sodium daily (severe restriction and seldom prescribed)
    b. Encourage intake of fresh foods, rather than processed foods, which contain higher amounts of sodium.
    c. Canned, frozen, instant, smoked, pickled, and boxed foods usually contain higher amounts of sodium. Lunch meats, soy sauce, salad dressings, fast foods, soups, and snacks such as potato chips and pretzels also contain large amounts of sodium.
    d. Certain medications contain significant amounts of sodium.
    e. Salt substitutes may be used to improve palatability; most salt substitutes contain large amounts of potassium and should not be used by clients with renal disease.

L. Protein-restricted diet
1. Indication: Used for renal disease and liver disease
2. Nursing considerations
    a. Provide enough protein to maintain nutritional status but not an amount that will allow the buildup of waste products from protein **metabolism** (40 to 60 g of protein daily).
    b. The less protein allowed, the more important it becomes that all protein in the diet be of high biological value (contain all essential amino acids in recommended proportions).
    c. An adequate total energy intake from foods is critical for clients on protein-restricted diets (protein will be used for energy, rather than for protein synthesis).
    d. Special low-protein products, such as pastas, bread, cookies, wafers, and gelatin made with wheat starch, can improve energy intake and add variety to the diet.
    e. Carbohydrates in powdered or liquid forms can provide additional energy.
    f. Vegetables and fruits contain some protein and, for very low-protein diets, these foods must be calculated into the diet.
    g. Foods are limited from the milk, meat, bread, and starch exchange.

M. Renal diet (see Boxes 12-3 and 12-5)
1. Indication: Used for the client with acute or chronic renal failure and those requiring hemodialysis or peritoneal dialysis

2. Nursing considerations
    a. Controlled amounts of protein, sodium, phosphorus, calcium, potassium, and fluids may be prescribed; may also need modification in fiber, cholesterol, and fat based on individual requirements
    b. Most clients receiving dialysis need to restrict fluids (Box 12-8).

⚠ An initial assessment includes identifying food and medication interactions.

N. Potassium-modified diet (see Box 12-5)
1. Indications
    a. Low-potassium diet is indicated for hyperkalemia, which may be caused by impaired renal function, hypoaldosteronism, Addison's disease, angiotensin-converting enzyme inhibitor medications, immunosuppressive medications, potassium-sparing diuretics, and chronic hyperkalemia.
    b. High-potassium diet is indicated for hypokalemia, which may be caused by renal tubular acidosis, gastrointestinal losses (diarrhea, vomiting), intracellular shifts, potassium-wasting diuretics, antibiotics, mineralocorticoid or glucocorticoid excess resulting from primary or secondary aldosteronism, Cushing's syndrome, or exogenous corticosteroid use.
2. Nursing considerations
    a. Foods that are low in potassium include applesauce, green beans, cabbage, lettuce, peppers, grapes, blueberries, cooked summer squash, cooked turnip greens, pineapple, and raspberries.
    b. Box 12-5 lists foods that are high in potassium.

O. High-calcium diet
1. Indication: Calcium is needed during bone growth and in adulthood to prevent osteoporosis and to facilitate vascular contraction, vasodilation, muscle contraction, and nerve transmission.
2. Nursing considerations
    a. Primary dietary sources of calcium are dairy products (see Box 9-5 for food items high in calcium).

Box 12-8 Measures to Relieve Thirst

Chew gum or suck hard candy.
Freeze fluids so they take longer to consume.
Add lemon juice to water to make it more refreshing.
Gargle with refrigerated mouthwash.

b. Lactose-intolerant clients should incorporate nondairy sources of calcium into their diet regularly.

P. Low-purine diet
1. Indication: Used for gout, kidney stones, and elevated uric acid levels
2. Nursing considerations
   a. Purine is a precursor for uric acid, which forms stones and crystals.
   b. Foods to restrict include anchovies, herring, mackerel, sardines, scallops, glandular meats, gravies, meat extracts, wild game, goose, and sweetbreads.

Q. High-iron diet
1. Indication: Used for clients with anemia
2. Nursing considerations
   a. The high-iron diet replaces iron deficit from inadequate intake or loss.
   b. The diet includes organ meats, meat, egg yolks, whole-wheat products, dark green leafy vegetables, dried fruit, and legumes.

R. Miscellaneous diets: See Boxes 9-2, 9-3, 9-6, and 9-7, for foods high in sodium, potassium, magnesium, and phosphorus, respectively.

IV. VEGETARIAN DIETS

A. Types (Box 12-9)

B. Nursing considerations
1. Ensure that the client eats a sufficient amount of varied foods to meet nutrient and energy needs.
2. Clients should be educated about consuming complementary proteins over the course of each day to ensure that all essential amino acids are provided.
3. Potential deficiencies in vegetarian diets include energy, protein, vitamin B_{12}, zinc, iron, calcium, omega-3 fatty acids, and vitamin D (if limited exposure to sunlight).
4. To enhance **absorption** of iron, vegetarians should consume a good source of iron and vitamin C with each meal.

Box 12-9 Types of Vegetarian Diets

Lacto-Ovo Vegetarian
Consumes eggs and dairy products, but excludes meat, poultry, and seafood

Lacto Vegetarian
Consumes dairy products, but excludes eggs, meat, poultry, and seafood

Vegan
Excludes animal products

Pesco Vegetarian
Consumes seafood, but excludes meat, poultry, eggs, and dairy products

---

5. Foods commonly eaten include tofu, tempeh, soy milk and soy products, meat analogues, legumes, nuts and seeds, sprouts, and a variety of fruits and vegetables.
6. Soy protein is considered equivalent in quality to animal protein.

⚠ Body mass index (BMI) can be calculated by dividing the client's weight in kilograms by height in meters squared. For example, a client who weighs 75 kg (165 pounds) and is 1.8 m^2 (5 feet 9 inches) tall has a BMI of 23.15 (75 divided by 1.8 = 23.15).

V. ENTERAL NUTRITION

A. Description: Provides liquefied foods into the gastrointestinal tract via a tube

B. Indications
1. When the gastrointestinal tract is functional but oral intake is not meeting estimated nutrient needs
2. Used for clients with swallowing problems, burns, major trauma, liver or other organ failure, or severe **malnutrition**

C. Nursing considerations
1. Clients with lactose intolerance need to be placed on lactose-free formulas.
2. See Chapter 21 for information regarding the administration of gastrointestinal tube feedings and associated complications.

💿 MORE QUESTIONS ON THE CD!

Practice Questions

77. The nurse is teaching a client who has iron deficiency anemia about foods she should include in her diet. The nurse determines that the client understands the dietary modifications if she selects which of the following from her menu?
    1. Nuts and milk
    2. Coffee and tea
    3. Cooked rolled oats and fish
    4. Oranges and dark green leafy vegetables

78. A nurse is planning to teach a client with malabsorption syndrome about the necessity of following a low-fat diet. The nurse develops a list of high-fat foods to avoid and includes which food item on the list?
    1. Oranges
    2. Broccoli
    3. Cream cheese
    4. Broiled haddock

79. The nurse instructs a client with renal failure who is receiving hemodialysis about dietary modifications. The nurse determines that the client understands these dietary modifications if the client selects which items from the dietary menu?
    1. Cream of wheat, blueberries, coffee
    2. Sausage and eggs, banana, orange juice
    3. Bacon, cantaloupe melon, tomato juice
    4. Cured pork, grits, strawberries, orange juice

80. The nurse is conducting a dietary assessment on a client who is on a vegan diet. The nurse provides dietary teaching focusing on foods high in which vitamin that may be lacking in a vegan diet?
    1. Vitamin A
    2. Vitamin B_{12}
    3. Vitamin C
    4. Vitamin E

81. A client with hypertension has been told to maintain a diet low in sodium. A nurse who is teaching this client about foods that are allowed includes which food item in a list provided to the client?
    1. Tomato soup
    2. Boiled shrimp
    3. Instant oatmeal
    4. Summer squash

82. A nurse is caring for a client with cirrhosis of the liver. To minimize the effects of the disorder, the nurse teaches the client about foods that are high in thiamine. The nurse determines that the client has the best understanding of the dietary measures to follow if the client states an intention to increase the intake of:
    1. Pork
    2. Milk
    3. Chicken
    4. Broccoli

83. The nurse is instructing a client with hypertension on the importance of choosing foods low in sodium. The nurse should teach the client to limit which of the following foods?
    1. Apples
    2. Bananas
    3. Smoked sausage
    4. Steamed vegetables

84. A client who is recovering from surgery has been advanced from a clear liquid diet to a full liquid diet. The client is looking forward to the diet change because he has been "bored" with the clear liquid diet. The nurse would offer which full liquid item to the client?
    1. Tea
    2. Gelatin
    3. Custard
    4. Popsicle

85. A client is recovering from abdominal surgery and has a large abdominal wound. A nurse encourages the client to eat which food item that is naturally high in vitamin C to promote wound healing?
    1. Milk
    2. Oranges
    3. Bananas
    4. Chicken

Alternate Item Format: Multiple Response

86. A postoperative client has been placed on a clear liquid diet. The nurse provides the client with which items that are allowed to be consumed on this diet. **Select all that apply.**
    ❑ 1. Broth
    ❑ 2. Coffee
    ❑ 3. Gelatin
    ❑ 4. Pudding
    ❑ 5. Vegetable juice
    ❑ 6. Pureed vegetables

ANSWERS
77. 4
Rationale: Dark green leafy vegetables are a good source of iron and oranges are a good source of vitamin C, which enhances iron absorption. All other options are not food sources that are high in iron and vitamin C.
Test-Taking Strategy: Use knowledge of foods high in iron and vitamin C and recall that vitamin C enhances iron absorption. Use the process of elimination to eliminate options 1, 2, and 3 because they do not contain sources of iron and vitamin C. Review food sources of vitamins and minerals if you had difficulty with this question.

Level of Cognitive Ability: Understanding
Client Needs: Physiological Integrity
Integrated Process: Nursing Process—Evaluation
Content Area: Fundamental Skills—Nutrition
Reference: Nix, S. (2009). *Williams' basic nutrition and diet therapy* (13th ed., pp. 139–140). St. Louis: Mosby.

78. 3
Rationale: Fruits and vegetables tend to be lower in fat because they do not come from animal sources. Broiled haddock is also naturally lower in fat. Cream cheese is a high-fat food.
Test-Taking Strategy: Use the process of elimination and focus on the subject of the question, the high-fat food.

Options 1 and 2 (fruit and vegetable) can be eliminated first. From the remaining options, remember that cheese is high in fat content. Review foods that are high in fat content if you had difficulty with this question.
Level of Cognitive Ability: Applying
Client Needs: Physiological Integrity
Integrated Process: Teaching and Learning
Content Area: Fundamental Skills—Nutrition
Reference: Nix, S. (2009). *Williams' basic nutrition and diet therapy* (13th ed., p.38). St. Louis: Mosby.

79. 1
Rationale: The diet for a client with renal failure who is receiving hemodialysis should include controlled amounts of sodium, phosphorus, calcium, potassium, and fluids. The food items in options 2, 3, and 4 are high in sodium, phosphorus, or potassium.
Test-Taking Strategy: Focus on the client's diagnosis to recall that sodium needs to be limited. Noting the items sausage (option 2), bacon (option 3), and cured pork (option 4) will assist in eliminating these options. Review dietary guidelines for the client with renal failure if you had difficulty with this question.
Level of Cognitive Ability: Understanding
Client Needs: Physiological Integrity
Integrated Process: Nursing Process—Evaluation
Content Area: Fundamental Skills—Nutrition
References: Ignatavicius, D., & Workman, M. (2010). *Medical-surgical nursing: Patient-centered collaborative care* (6th ed., p. 1617). St. Louis: Saunders.
  Nix, S. (2009). *Williams' basic nutrition and diet therapy* (13th ed., p. 419). St. Louis: Mosby.

80. 2
Rationale: Vegans do not consume any animal products. Vitamin B_{12} is found in animal products and therefore would most likely be lacking in a vegan diet. Vitamins A, C, and E are found in fresh fruits and vegetables, which are consumed in a vegan diet.
Test-Taking Strategy: Focus on the subject, a vegan diet. Recalling the food items eaten and restricted in this diet will direct you to the correct option. Remember that vegans do not consume any animal products. Review vegan diets and sources of vitamins if you had difficulty with this question.
Level of Cognitive Ability: Applying
Client Needs: Physiological Integrity
Integrated Process: Teaching and Learning
Content Area: Fundamental Skills—Nutrition
Reference: Nix, S. (2009). *Williams' basic nutrition and diet therapy* (13th ed., p. 53). St. Louis: Mosby.

81. 4
Rationale: Foods that are lower in sodium include fruits and vegetables (option 4), because they do not contain physiological saline. Highly processed or refined foods (options 1 and 3) are higher in sodium unless their food labels specifically state "low sodium." Saltwater fish and shellfish are high in sodium.
Test-Taking Strategy: Use the process of elimination. Begin to answer this question by eliminating option 2, recalling that saltwater fish and shellfish are high in sodium. Next, eliminate options 1 and 3 because they are processed foods. Review the foods that are high in sodium if you had difficulty with this question.
Level of Cognitive Ability: Applying
Client Needs: Physiological Integrity
Integrated Process: Teaching and Learning
Content Area: Fundamental Skills—Nutrition
Reference: Black, J., & Hawks, J. (2009). *Medical-surgical nursing: Clinical management for positive outcomes* (8th ed., pp. 138, 1439). St. Louis: Saunders.

82. 1
Rationale: The client with cirrhosis needs to consume foods high in thiamine. Thiamine is present in a variety of foods of plant and animal origin. Pork products are especially rich in this vitamin. Other good food sources include nuts, whole grain cereals, and legumes. Milk contains vitamins A, D, and B_2. Poultry contains niacin. Broccoli contains vitamins C, E, and K and folic acid.
Test-Taking Strategy: Note the strategic words *best understanding*. This may indicate that more than one option may be a food that contains thiamine. Remembering that pork products are especially rich in thiamine will direct you to option 1. Review food items high in thiamine if you had difficulty with this question.
Level of Cognitive Ability: Understanding
Client Needs: Physiological Integrity
Integrated Process: Nursing Process—Evaluation
Content Area: Fundamental Skills—Nutrition
Reference: Nix, S. (2009). *Williams' basic nutrition and diet therapy* (13th ed., p. 106). St. Louis: Mosby.

83. 3
Rationale: Smoked foods are high in sodium. Options 1, 2, and 4 are fruits and vegetables that are low in sodium.
Test-Taking Strategy: Note the strategic word *limit* and use the process of elimination, recalling the food items that are high in sodium. Remember that smoked foods are high in sodium. If you had difficulty with this question, review the foods high in sodium.
Level of Cognitive Ability: Applying
Client Needs: Physiological Integrity
Integrated Process: Teaching and Learning
Content Area: Fundamental Skills—Nutrition
Reference: Nix, S. (2009). *Williams' basic nutrition and diet therapy* (13th ed., pp. 132–133). St. Louis: Mosby.

84. 3
Rationale: Full liquid food items include items such as plain ice cream, sherbet, breakfast drinks, milk, pudding and custard, soups that are strained, refined cooked cereals, and strained vegetable juices. A clear liquid diet consists of foods that are relatively transparent. The food items in options 1, 2, and 4 are clear liquids.
Test-Taking Strategy: Focus on the subject, a full liquid item. Remember that a clear liquid diet consists of foods that are relatively transparent. This will assist you in eliminating options 1, 2, and 4. Review food items allowed on a clear liquid diet and a full liquid diet if you had difficulty with this question.
Level of Cognitive Ability: Applying
Client Needs: Physiological Integrity
Integrated Process: Nursing Process—Implementation

Content Area: Fundamental Skills—Nutrition
Reference: Nix, S. (2009). *Williams' basic nutrition and diet therapy* (13th ed., p. 330). St. Louis: Mosby.

85. 2

Rationale: Citrus fruits and juices are especially high in vitamin C. Bananas are high in potassium. Meats and dairy products are two food groups that are high in the B vitamins.

Test-Taking Strategy: Note the strategic words *naturally high* in the question. Use the process of elimination, recalling that citrus fruits and juices are high in vitamin C. Review the foods high in vitamin C if you are unfamiliar with them.

Level of Cognitive Ability: Applying
Client Needs: Physiological Integrity
Integrated Process: Nursing Process—Implementation
Content Area: Fundamental Skills—Nutrition
Reference: Nix, S. (2009). *Williams' basic nutrition and diet therapy* (13th ed., pp. 105, 437). St. Louis: Mosby.

ALTERNATE ITEM FORMAT: MULTIPLE RESPONSE
86. 1, 2, 3

Rationale: A clear liquid diet consists of foods that are relatively transparent to light and are clear and liquid at room and body temperature. These foods include items such as water, bouillon, clear broth, carbonated beverages, gelatin, hard candy, lemonade, Popsicles, and regular or decaffeinated coffee or tea. The incorrect food items are items that are allowed on a full liquid diet.

Test-Taking Strategy: Focus on the subject, a clear liquid diet. Recalling that a clear liquid diet consists of foods that are relatively transparent to light and are clear will assist in answering the question. Review foods allowed on a clear and full liquid diet if you had difficulty with this question.

Level of Cognitive Ability: Applying
Client Needs: Physiological Integrity
Integrated Process: Nursing Process—Implementation
Content Area: Fundamental Skills—Nutrition
Reference: Nix, S. (2009). *Williams' basic nutrition and diet therapy* (13th ed., p. 330). St. Louis: Mosby.

Parenteral Nutrition

PYRAMID TERMS

fat emulsion (lipids) A white, opaque solution administered intravenously during parenteral nutrition therapy to prevent fatty acid deficiency.

parenteral nutrition (PN) Administration of a nutritionally complete formula through a central or peripheral intravenous (IV) catheter. In the clinical setting, the term *PN* may be used interchangeably with the term *total parenteral nutrition (TPN)* or *hyperalimentation*.

peripheral parenteral nutrition (PPN) Parenteral nutrition administered through a peripheral vein in an extremity. PN solutions administered peripherally are not as calorically dense as those administered though a central vein.

▲ THE PYRAMID TO SUCCESS

The NCLEX-RN examination test plan addresses parenteral nutrition (PN) as related content in the Client Needs area of Physiological Integrity, Pharmacological and Parenteral Therapies. Pyramid Points focus on the administration, maintenance, and discontinuation of PN and fat emulsions; nursing interventions; the interventions required in monitoring for side effects or adverse effects; and the actions to take if a complication arises. Pyramid Points also focus on home care instructions for the client receiving **PN** at home.

▲ CLIENT NEEDS

Safe and Effective Care Environment

Consulting with members of the health care team, including the dietitian

Handling hazardous and infectious materials

Initiating home health care referrals

Maintaining standard, transmission-based, and surgical asepsis to prevent infection

Obtaining informed consent for venous access and placement of the catheter

Health Promotion and Maintenance

Promoting health and wellness related to nutrition

Providing client and family education regarding the administration of PN at home

Providing client and family education regarding monitoring for side or adverse effects and actions to take if a complication arises

Psychosocial Integrity

Discussing role changes related to the client's need to receive PN

Identifying support systems in the home to assist with the administration of PN

Physiological Integrity

Assessing the central venous access device for administering PN

Monitoring for expected effects

Monitoring laboratory values

Monitoring nutritional needs

Monitoring for potential side or adverse effects and actions to take if a complication arises

Providing comfort and assistance in the performance of activities of daily living

Promoting rest and sleep

I. PARENTERAL NUTRITION (PN)

A. Description
1. Supplies nutrients via the veins
2. Supplies carbohydrates in the form of dextrose, fats in an emulsified form, proteins in the form of amino acids, vitamins, minerals, electrolytes, and water
3. Prevents subcutaneous fat and muscle protein from being catabolized by the body for energy

B. Indications
1. Clients with severely dysfunctional or nonfunctional gastrointestinal tracts who are unable to process nutrients may benefit from **PN**.
2. Clients who can take some oral nutrition, but not enough to meet their nutrient requirements, may benefit from **PN**.

3. Clients with multiple gastrointestinal surgeries, gastrointestinal trauma, severe intolerance to enteral feedings, or intestinal obstructions, or who need to rest the bowel for healing, may benefit from **PN**.
4. Clients with severe nutritionally deficient conditions such as acquired immunodeficiency syndrome, cancer, burn injuries, malnutrition, or clients receiving chemotherapy may benefit from **PN**.

⚠ PN is the least desirable form of nutrition and is used when there is no other nutritional alternative. Other forms of administering nutrition such as orally or via a gastrointestinal tube are initiated first.

C. Administration of **PN** (Fig. 13-1)
1. Central vein
    a. **PN** is administered through a central vein when the client requires a larger concentration of carbohydrates (greater than 10% glucose concentration).
    b. The subclavian or internal jugular vein is the central vein normally used when **PN** is a short-term intervention (less than 4 weeks).
    c. When **PN** is anticipated for an extended period (longer than 4 weeks), a more permanent catheter, such as a peripherally inserted central catheter (PICC) line, a tunneled catheter, or an implanted vascular access device, is used.
2. Peripheral vein (**PN**)
    a. **PN** can be administered through a peripheral vein, typically in the arm, via a PICC line.

b. **PN** administered through a peripheral vein delivers isotonic or mildly hypertonic solutions.

⚠ The delivery of hypertonic solutions into peripheral veins can cause sclerosis, phlebitis, or swelling. Monitor closely for these complications.

II. COMPONENTS OF PARENTERAL NUTRITION

A. Carbohydrates
1. Concentrations of dextrose (glucose) range from 5% to 70%.
2. The strength of the dextrose solution depends on the client's nutritional needs, the route of administration (central or peripheral), and agency protocols.
3. Carbohydrates typically provide 60% to 70% of calorie (energy) needs.
4. Dextrose provides 3.4 kcal/g.

B. Amino acids (protein)
1. Concentrations range from 3.5% to 20%; lower concentrations are most commonly used for peripheral vein administration and higher concentrations are most often administered through a central vein.
2. Amino acid solutions provide approximately 4 kcal/g of protein.
3. About 15% to 20% of total energy needs should come from protein.

C. Fat emulsion (lipids)
1. Lipids provide up to 30% of calorie (energy) needs.
2. Lipids provide nonprotein calories and prevent or correct fatty acid deficiency.

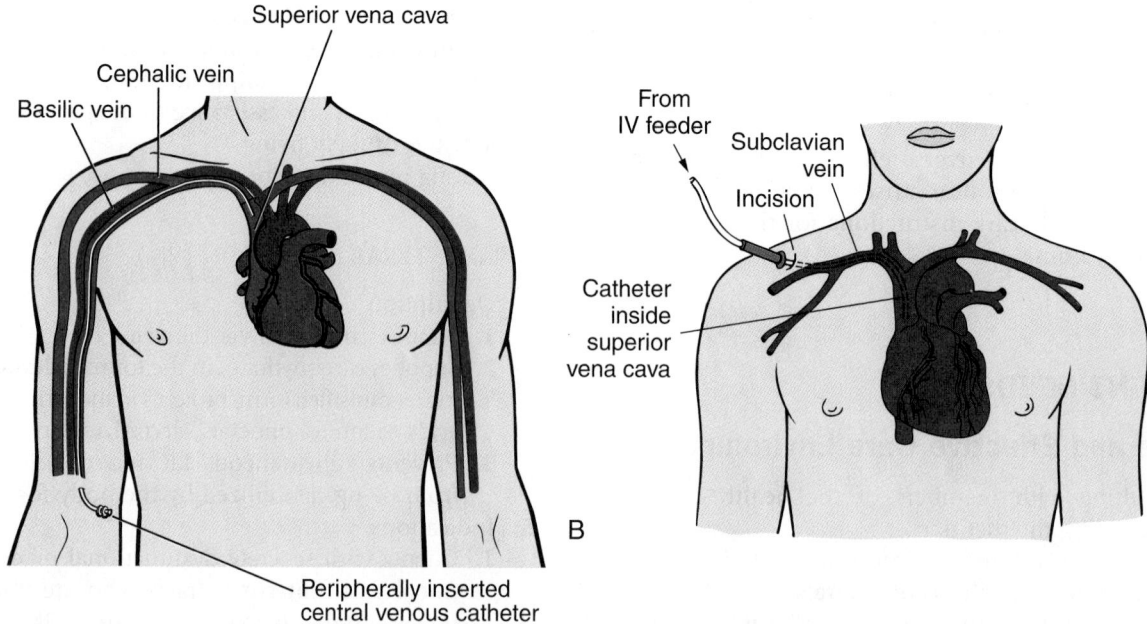

▲ **FIGURE 13-1 A,** Placement of peripherally inserted central catheter through antecubital fossa. (Modified from Lewis, S., Heitkemper, M., Dirksen, S., O'Brien P., & Bucher, L. [2007]. *Medical-surgical nursing: Assessment and management of clinical problems* [7th ed.]. St. Louis: Mosby.) **B,** Placement of central venous catheter inserted into subclavian vein. (From Elkin, M., Perry, A., & Potter, P. [2008]. *Nursing interventions and clinical skills* [4th ed., p. 787]. St. Louis: Mosby.)

3. Available concentrations are 10%, 20%, and 30%, providing 1.1, 2, and 3 kcal/mL, respectively
4. Lipid solutions are isotonic and therefore can be administered through a peripheral or central vein; the solution may be administered through a separate IV line below the filter of the main IV administration set by a Y-connector or as an admixture to the **PN** solution (3-in-1 admixture consisting of dextrose, amino acids, lipids).
5. Most **fat emulsions** are prepared from soybean or safflower oil, with egg yolk to provide emulsification; the primary components are linoleic, oleic, palmitic, linolenic, and stearic acids.
6. Glucose-intolerant clients or clients with diabetes mellitus may benefit from receiving a larger percentage of their **PN** from lipids, which helps control blood glucose levels and lower insulin requirements caused by infused dextrose.
7. Examine the bottle for separation of emulsion into layers or fat globules or for the accumulation of froth; if observed, do not use and return the solution to the pharmacy.
8. Additives should not be put into the **fat emulsion** solution.
9. Follow agency policy regarding the filter size that should be used; usually a 1.2-μm filter or larger should be used because the lipid particles are too large to pass through a 0.22-μm filter.
10. Infuse solution at the flow rate prescribed—usually slowly at 1 mL/min initially—monitor vital signs every 10 minutes, and observe for adverse reactions for the first 30 minutes of the infusion. If signs of an adverse reaction occur, stop the infusion and notify the physician (Box 13-1).
11. If no adverse reaction occurs, adjust the flow rate to the prescribed rate.
12. Monitor serum lipids 4 hours after discontinuing the infusion.

⚠ Fat emulsions (lipids) contain egg yolk phospholipids and should not be given to clients with egg allergies.

D. Vitamins
1. **PN** solutions usually contain a standard multivitamin preparation to meet most vitamin needs and prevent deficiencies.

Box 13-1 Signs of an Adverse Reaction to Lipids

Chest and back pain	Flushing
Chills	Headache
Cyanosis	Nausea and vomiting
Diaphoresis	Pressure over the eyes
Dyspnea	Thrombophlebitis
Fever	Vertigo

2. Individual vitamin preparations can be added, as needed and as prescribed.
E. Minerals and trace elements: Commercial mineral and trace element preparations are available in different concentrations to promote normal metabolism.
F. Electrolytes: Electrolyte requirements for individuals receiving **PN** therapy vary, depending on body weight, presence of malnutrition or catabolism, degree of electrolyte depletion, changes in organ function, ongoing electrolyte losses, and the disease process.
G. Water: The amount of water needed in a **PN** solution is determined by electrolyte balance and fluid requirements.
H. Insulin: May be added to control the blood glucose level because of the high concentration of glucose in the **PN** solution.
I. Heparin: May be added to reduce the buildup of a fibrinous clot at the catheter tip.

III. ADMINISTRATION AND DISCONTINUATION

A. Types of administration
1. Continuous **PN**
   a. Infused continuously over 24 hours
   b. Most commonly used in a hospital setting
   c. Less risk of complications when administered continuously
2. Intermittent **PN**
   a. Generally 12-hour infusions that are usually given at night
   b. Allows client requiring **PN** on long-term basis to participate in activities of daily living during the day without the inconvenience of an IV bag and pump set
   c. Monitor glucose levels closely.
   d. Preferable for use in home settings
B. Discontinuing **PN** therapy
1. Gradually decrease the flow rate for 1 to 2 hours while increasing oral intake (this assists in preventing hypoglycemia).
2. After removing the IV catheter, change the dressing daily until the insertion site heals.
3. Encourage oral nourishment.
4. Record oral intake, body weight, and laboratory results of serum electrolyte and glucose levels.

⚠ Abrupt discontinuation of a PN solution can result in hypoglycemia. The flow rate should be decreased gradually when the PN is discontinued.

IV. COMPLICATIONS (Table 13-1)

A. Description
1. Pneumothorax and air embolism are associated with central line placement; air embolism is also associated with tubing changes.

TABLE 13-1 Complications of Parenteral Nutrition

Complication	Possible Cause	Signs or Symptoms	Intervention	Prevention
Air embolism	• Catheter system opened or IV tubing disconnected • Air entry on IV tubing changes	• Apprehension • Chest pain • Dyspnea • Hypotension • Loud churning sound heard over pericardium on auscultation • Rapid and weak pulse • Respiratory distress	• Clamp the catheter. • Place the client in a left side-lying position with the head lower than the feet. • Notify the physician. • Administer oxygen.	• Make sure all catheter connections are secure. • Clamp the catheter when not in use (follow agency protocol for flushing and clamping the catheter). • Instruct the client in the Valsalva maneuver for tubing and cap changes. • For tubing and cap changes, place the client in the Trendelenburg position (if not contraindicated), with the head turned in the opposite direction of the insertion site; client should hold breath and bear down.
Hyperglycemia	• Client receiving solution too quickly • Not enough insulin • Infection	• Restlessness • Weakness • Confusion • Diaphoresis • Elevated blood glucose level (>200 mg/dL) • Excessive thirst • Fatigue • Kussmaul's respirations • Coma (when severe)	• Notify the physician. • The infusion rate may need to be slowed. • Administer regular insulin as prescribed. • Monitor blood glucose levels.	• Assess the client for a history of glucose intolerance. • Assess the client's medication history. • Begin infusion at a slow rate as prescribed. • Monitor blood glucose levels. • Use strict aseptic technique.
Hypervolemia	• Excessive fluid administration or administration of fluid too rapidly • Renal dysfunction • Heart failure • Hepatic failure	• Bounding pulse • Crackles on lung auscultation • Headache • Increased blood pressure • Jugular vein distention • Weight gain greater than desired	• Slow or stop IV infusion. • Restrict fluids. • Administer diuretics. • Use dialysis (in extreme cases).	• Assess client's history for risk for hypervolemia. • Administer solution via an electronic infusion device. • Monitor intake and output. • Monitor weight daily.
Hypoglycemia	• PN abruptly discontinued • Too much insulin being administered	• Anxiety • Diaphoresis • Hunger • Low blood glucose level (<70 mg/dL) • Shakiness • Weakness	• Administer IV dextrose. • Notify the physician. • Monitor blood glucose level.	• Gradually decrease PN solution when discontinued. • Infuse 10% dextrose at same rate as the PN to prevent hypoglycemia when the PN solution is discontinued. • Monitor glucose levels when insulin is being given.
Infection	• Poor aseptic technique • Catheter contamination • Contamination of solution	• Chills • Fever • Elevated white blood cell count • Redness or drainage at insertion site	• Notify the physician • Remove catheter. • Send catheter tip to the laboratory for culture. • Prepare to obtain blood cultures. • Prepare for antibiotic administration.	• Use strict aseptic techniques. • Monitor temperature. • Assess IV site for signs of infection. • Change site dressing, solution, and tubing as specified by agency policy. • Do not disconnect tubing unnecessarily.
Pneumothorax	• Inexact catheter placement	• Chest or shoulder pain • Sudden shortness of breath • Cyanosis • Tachycardia • Absence of breath sounds on affected side	• Notify the physician • Prepare to obtain a chest x-ray • Small pneumothorax may resolve. • Larger pneumothorax may require chest tube.	• Monitor for signs of pneumothorax. • Obtain a chest x-ray after insertion of the catheter to ensure proper catheter placement. • PN is not initiated until correct catheter placement is verified and the absence of pneumothorax is confirmed.

IV, Intravenous; *PN,* parenteral nutrition.

Modified from Ignatavicius, D., & Workman, M. (2010). *Medical-surgical nursing: Patient-centered collaborative care* (6th ed). St. Louis: Saunders.

2. Other complications include infection (catheter-related), hypervolemia, and metabolic alterations such as hyperglycemia and hypoglycemia; these complications are usually caused by the **PN** solution itself.

B. Air embolism
1. Air embolism occurs because of the entry of air into the catheter system.
2. Instruct the client in the Valsalva maneuver for IV tubing and cap changes.
3. For tubing and cap changes, place the client in the Trendelenburg position (if not contraindicated) with the head turned in the opposite direction of the insertion site (increases intrathoracic venous pressure); also, ask the client to take a deep breath, hold it, and bear down.
4. Check all catheter connections and secure (use tape per agency protocol) tubing connections.
5. If an air embolism is suspected, do the following:
   a. Clamp the IV catheter.
   b. Place the client in a left side-lying position with the head lower than the feet (to trap air in right side of the heart).
   c. Notify the physician.
   d. Administer oxygen as prescribed.

C. Hyperglycemia
1. Hyperglycemia occurs because of the high concentration of dextrose (glucose) in the solution. If the client receives the solution too rapidly, does not receive enough insulin, or contracts an infection, hyperglycemia can occur.
2. Assess the client for a history of glucose intolerance.
3. Assess the client's medication history (corticosteroids may increase the blood glucose level).
4. Begin infusion at a slow rate (usually 40 to 60 mL/hr) as prescribed.
5. Monitor blood glucose levels every 4 to 6 hours or according to agency protocol.
6. Administer regular insulin as prescribed.

D. Hypervolemia
1. Hypervolemia occurs if the client receives the IV solution too rapidly; the client with cardiac, renal, or hepatic dysfunction is at high risk.
2. **PN** is always delivered via an electronic infusion device.
3. Never increase the infusion rate to "catch up" if the IV infusion gets behind.
4. Monitor intake and output.
5. Weigh the client daily (ideal weight gain is 1 to 2 lb/week).

E. Hypoglycemia
1. Hypoglycemia occurs when the **PN** is abruptly discontinued or when too much insulin is administered.
2. Monitor the blood glucose level.
3. Gradually decrease the infusion rate when discontinuing **PN**.

4. When an infusion of hypertonic glucose is stopped, an infusion of 10% dextrose should be instituted and maintained for 1 to 2 hours to prevent hypoglycemia.
5. Assess the blood glucose level 1 hour after discontinuing **PN**.
6. Prepare for the administration of glucose or IV dextrose if hypoglycemia occurs.

F. Infection
1. Infection can occur as a result of poor aseptic technique or via catheter or solution contamination.
2. Use strict aseptic technique. Because the **PN** solution has a high concentration of glucose, it is a medium for bacterial growth.
3. Monitor temperature. If the client has a fever, suspect sepsis.
4. Assess the IV site for redness, swelling, tenderness, or drainage.
5. Change the **PN** solution every 12 to 24 hours as prescribed or according to agency protocol.
6. Change the IV tubing every 24 hours or according to agency protocol.
7. Change the dressing at the IV site every 48 hours or according to agency protocol (see Priority Nursing Actions).

■■■■■ **PRIORITY NURSING ACTIONS!** ■■■■■

Actions to Take If an Infection Is Suspected at a Central Venous Catheter Site
1. Notify the physician.
2. Remove the catheter and prepare for possible restart at a different location.
3. Remove the tip of the catheter and send it to the laboratory for culture.
4. Prepare the client for obtaining blood cultures.
5. Prepare for antibiotic administration.
6. Document the occurrence, the actions taken, and the client's response.

Signs of infection at the catheter site include redness or drainage. The client will also exhibit chills, fever, and an elevated white blood cell count. If the nurse suspects infection, the physician is notified because of the risk for sepsis. The catheter is removed and the client is prepared for a possible restart at a different location as prescribed. Also, intravenous (IV) antibiotics may be prescribed and an IV site will be needed for administration. The catheter tip is sent to the laboratory for culture to identify the bacteria present so that the effective antibiotic is prescribed. Blood cultures are also performed to determine the presence of bacteria in the blood. Antibiotics are not started until blood cultures are obtained; otherwise the results of the cultures may not be accurate. Finally the nurse documents the occurrence, actions taken, and the client's response.

Reference: Ignatavicius, D., & Workman, M. (2010). *Medical-surgical nursing: Patient-centered collaborative care.* (6th ed. p. 228.) St. Louis: Saunders.

Box 13-2 Home Care Instructions

Teach the client and caregiver how to obtain, administer, and maintain parenteral nutrition fluids.

Teach the client and caregiver how to change a sterile dressing.

Obtain a daily weight at the same time of day in the same clothes.

Stress that if a weight gain of more than 3 lb/week is noted, this may indicate excessive fluid intake and should be reported.

Monitor the blood glucose level and report abnormalities immediately.

Teach the client and caregiver about the signs and symptoms of side or adverse effects such as infection, thrombosis, air embolism, and catheter displacement.

Teach the client and caregiver the actions to take if a complication arises and about the importance of reporting complications to the health care provider.

For symptoms of thrombosis, the client should report edema of the arm or at the catheter insertion site, neck pain, and jugular vein distention.

Leaking of fluid from the insertion site or pain or discomfort as the fluids are infused may indicate displacement of the catheter; this must be reported immediately.

Encourage the client and caregiver to contact the health care provider if they have questions about administration or any other questions.

Inform the client and caregiver about the importance of follow-up care.

G. Pneumothorax

1. Pneumothorax can occur as a result of inexact catheter placement that results in puncture of the pleural space.
2. After insertion of the catheter, obtain a portable chest x-ray film to confirm correct catheter placement and to detect the presence of a pneumothorax. **PN** is not initiated until correct catheter placement is verified and the absence of pneumothorax is confirmed.

V. ADDITIONAL NURSING CONSIDERATIONS

A. Check the **PN** solution with the physician's prescription to ensure that the prescribed components are contained in the solution.

B. To prevent infection and solution incompatibility, IV medications and blood are not given through the **PN** line.

C. Monitor partial thromboplastin time and prothrombin time for clients receiving anticoagulants.

D. Monitor electrolyte and albumin levels and liver and renal function studies, as well as any other prescribed laboratory studies.

E. In severely dehydrated clients, the albumin level may drop initially after initiating **PN**, because the treatment restores hydration.

F. With severely malnourished clients, monitor for "refeeding syndrome" (a rapid drop in potassium, magnesium, and phosphate serum levels).

G. Abnormal liver function values may indicate intolerance to or an excess of **fat emulsion** or problems with metabolism with glucose and protein.

H. Abnormal renal function tests may indicate an excess of amino acids.

I. **PN** solutions should be stored under refrigeration and administered within 24 hours from the time they are prepared (remove from refrigerator 0.5 to 1 hour before use).

J. **PN** solutions that are cloudy or darkened should not be used and should be returned to the pharmacy.

K. Additions of substances such as nutrients to **PN** solutions should be made in the pharmacy and not on the nursing unit.

VI. HOME CARE INSTRUCTIONS (Box 13-2)

MORE QUESTIONS ON THE CD!

Practice Questions

87. A client is being weaned from parenteral nutrition (PN) and is expected to begin taking solid food today. The ongoing solution rate has been 100 mL/hr. A nurse anticipates that which of the following prescriptions regarding the PN solution will accompany the diet order?
1. Discontinue the PN.
2. Decrease PN rate to 50 mL/hr.
3. Start 0.9% normal saline at 25 mL/hr.
4. Continue current infusion rate orders for PN.

88. A nurse is preparing to change the parenteral nutrition (PN) solution bag and tubing. The client's central venous line is located in the right subclavian vein. The nurse asks the client to take which essential action during the tubing change?
1. Breathe normally.
2. Turn the head to the right.
3. Exhale slowly and evenly.
4. Take a deep breath, hold it, and bear down.

89. A client with parenteral nutrition (PN) infusing has disconnected the tubing from the central line catheter. A nurse assesses the client and suspects an air embolism. The nurse should immediately place the client in which position?
1. On the left side, with the head lower than the feet
2. On the left side, with the head higher than the feet

3. On the right side, with the head lower than the feet
4. On the right side, with the head higher than the feet

90. A client receiving parenteral nutrition (PN) complains of a headache. A nurse notes that the client has an increased blood pressure, bounding pulse, jugular vein distention, and crackles bilaterally. The nurse determines that the client is experiencing which complication of PN therapy?
1. Sepsis
2. Air embolism
3. Hypervolemia
4. Hyperglycemia

91. A client is receiving nutrition by means of parenteral nutrition (PN). A nurse monitors the client for complications of the therapy and assesses the client for which of the following signs of hyperglycemia?
1. Fever, weak pulse, and thirst
2. Nausea, vomiting, and oliguria
3. Sweating, chills, and abdominal pain
4. Weakness, thirst, and increased urine output

92. A nurse is changing the central line dressing of a client receiving parenteral nutrition (PN) and notes that the catheter insertion site appears reddened. The nurse next assesses which of the following items?
1. Client's temperature
2. Expiration date on the bag
3. Time of last dressing change
4. Tightness of tubing connections

93. A nurse is preparing to hang fat emulsion (lipids) and notes that fat globules are visible at the top of the solution. The nurse takes which of the following actions?
1. Rolls the bottle of solution gently
2. Obtains a different bottle of solution
3. Shakes the bottle of solution vigorously
4. Runs the bottle of solution under warm water

94. A client receiving parenteral nutrition (PN) suddenly spikes a fever. A nurse notifies the physician, and the physician initially prescribes that the solution and tubing be changed. The nurse should do which of the following with the discontinued materials?
1. Discard them in the unit trash.
2. Return them to the hospital pharmacy.
3. Send them to the laboratory for culture.
4. Save them for return to the manufacturer.

95. A client has been discharged to home on parenteral nutrition (PN). With each visit, a home care nurse assesses which of the following parameters most closely in monitoring this therapy?
1. Pulse and weight
2. Temperature and weight
3. Pulse and blood pressure
4. Temperature and blood pressure

96. A nurse is caring for a group of adult clients on an acute care medical-surgical nursing unit. The nurse understands that which of the following clients would be the least likely candidate for parenteral nutrition (PN)?
1. A 66-year-old client with extensive burns
2. A 42-year-old client who has had an open cholecystectomy
3. A 27-year-old client with severe exacerbation of Crohn's disease
4. A 35-year-old client with persistent nausea and vomiting from chemotherapy

97. A nurse is preparing to hang the first bag of parenteral nutrition (PN) solution via the central line of an assigned client. The nurse obtains which most essential piece of equipment before hanging the solution?
1. Urine test strips
2. Blood glucose meter
3. Electronic infusion pump
4. Noninvasive blood pressure monitor

98. A nurse is making initial rounds at the beginning of the shift and notes that the parenteral nutrition (PN) bag of an assigned client is empty. Which of the following solutions readily available on the nursing unit should the nurse hang until another PN solution is mixed and delivered to the nursing unit?
1. 5% dextrose in water
2. 10% dextrose in water
3. 5% dextrose in Ringer's lactate
4. 5% dextrose in 0.9% sodium chloride

99. A nurse is monitoring the status of a client's fat emulsion (lipid) infusion and notes that the infusion is 1 hour behind. Which of the following actions by the nurse is appropriate?
1. Adjust the infusion rate to catch up over the next hour.
2. Increase the infusion rate to catch up over the next 2 hours.
3. Ensure that the fat emulsion infusion rate is infusing at the prescribed rate.
4. Adjust the infusion rate to run wide open until the solution is back on time.

100. A client receiving parenteral nutrition (PN) in the home setting has a weight gain of 5 lb in 1 week. The nurse next assesses the client to detect the presence of which of the following?
1. Thirst
2. Polyuria
3. Decreased blood pressure
4. Crackles on auscultation of the lungs

101. A nurse is caring for a restless client who is beginning nutritional therapy with parenteral nutrition (PN). The nurse should plan to ensure that which of the following is done to prevent the client from injury?
1. Calculate daily intake and output.
2. Monitor the temperature once daily.
3. Secure all connections in the PN system.
4. Monitor blood glucose levels every 12 hours.

Alternate Item Format: Prioritizing (Ordered Response)

102. A nurse is monitoring a client receiving parenteral nutrition (PN). The client suddenly develops respiratory distress, dyspnea, and chest pain, and the nurse suspects air embolism. Number the actions that the nurse would take in order of priority. (Number 1 is the first action and number 6 is the last action.)

_4_ Administer oxygen.
_5_ Contact the physician.
_6_ Document the occurrence.
_1_ Take the client's vital signs.
_2_ Clamp the intravenous (IV) catheter.
_3_ Position the client in left Trendelenburg's position.

ANSWERS

87. 2

Rationale: When a client begins eating a regular diet after a period of receiving PN, the PN is decreased gradually. PN that is discontinued abruptly can cause hypoglycemia. Clients often have anorexia after being without food for some time, and the digestive tract also is not used to producing the digestive enzymes that will be needed. Gradually decreasing the infusion rate allows the client to remain adequately nourished during the transition to a normal diet and prevents the occurrence of hypoglycemia. Even before clients are started on a solid diet, they are given clear liquids followed by full liquids to further ease the transition. A solution of normal saline does not provide the glucose needed during the transition of discontinuing the PN and could cause the client to experience hypoglycemia.
Test-Taking Strategy: Use the process of elimination and note the strategic word *weaned* in the question. Recalling the effects of PN and the complications that occur will direct you to option 2. Remember that hypoglycemia can occur if the PN is discontinued abruptly. If you had difficulty with this question, review the procedures related to discontinuing PN solution.
Level of Cognitive Ability: Analyzing
Client Needs: Physiological Integrity
Integrated Process: Nursing Process—Planning
Content Area: Fundamental Skills—Safety/Infection Control
References: Black, J., & Hawks, J. (2009). *Medical-surgical nursing: Clinical management for positive outcomes* (8th ed., p. 583). St. Louis: Saunders.
Gahart, B., & Nazareno, A. (2009). *Intravenous medications* (25th ed., p. 1125). St. Louis: Mosby.
Nix, S. (2009). *Williams' basic nutrition and diet therapy* (13th ed., p. 446). St. Louis: Mosby.

88. 4

Rationale: The client should be asked to perform the Valsalva maneuver during tubing changes. This helps avoid air embolism during tubing changes. The nurse asks the client to take a deep breath, hold it, and bear down. If the intravenous line is on the right, the client turns his or her head to the left. This position increases intrathoracic pressure. Options 1 and 3 are inappropriate and could cause the potential for an air embolism during the tubing change.
Test-Taking Strategy: Note the strategic word *essential*. Use the process of elimination, recalling that air embolism is a complication that can occur during tubing changes. This will direct you to option 4. Review the procedure for PN bag and tubing change if you had difficulty with this question.
Level of Cognitive Ability: Applying
Client Needs: Physiological Integrity
Integrated Process: Nursing Process—Implementation
Content Area: Fundamental Skills—Safety/Infection Control
References: Ignatavicius, D., & Workman, M. (2010). *Medical-surgical nursing: Patient-centered collaborative care* (6th ed., p. 224). St. Louis: Saunders.
Kee, J., Hayes, E., & McCuistion, L. (2009). *Pharmacology: A nursing process approach* (6th ed., p. 261). St. Louis: Saunders.

89. 1

Rationale: Air embolism occurs when air enters the catheter system, such as when the system is opened for intravenous (IV) tubing changes or when the IV tubing disconnects. Air embolism is a critical situation; if it is suspected, the client should be placed in a left side-lying position. The head should be lower than the feet. This position is used to minimize the effect of the air traveling as a bolus to the lungs by trapping it in the right side of the heart. Options 2, 3, and 4 are incorrect positions if an air embolism is suspected.
Test-Taking Strategy: Use the process of elimination and recall that the goal in this emergency situation is to trap air in the right side of the heart. Think about the position that will achieve this goal; this will direct you to option 1. If you had difficulty with this question, review the immediate interventions when air embolism is suspected.

Level of Cognitive Ability: Applying
Client Needs: Physiological Integrity
Integrated Process: Nursing Process—Implementation
Content Area: Critical Care
References: Ignatavicius, D., & Workman, M. (2010). *Medical-surgical nursing: Patient-centered collaborative care* (6th ed., p. 231). St. Louis: Saunders.

Perry, A., & Potter, P. (2010). *Clinical nursing skills & techniques* (7th ed., p. 850). St. Louis: Mosby.

90. 3

Rationale: Hypervolemia is a critical situation and occurs from excessive fluid administration or administration of fluid too rapidly. Clients with cardiac, renal, or hepatic dysfunction are also at increased risk. The client's signs and symptoms presented in the question are consistent with hypervolemia. The increased intravascular volume increases the blood pressure, whereas the pulse rate increases as the heart tries to pump the extra fluid volume. The increased volume also causes neck vein distention and shifting of fluid into the alveoli, resulting in lung crackles. The signs and symptoms presented in the question do not indicate hyperglycemia, air embolism, or sepsis.
Test-Taking Strategy: Use the process of elimination, focusing on the signs and symptoms presented in the question. Recalling the signs of hypervolemia will direct you to option 3. If you had difficulty with this question, review the signs of hypervolemia.
Level of Cognitive Ability: Analyzing
Client Needs: Physiological Integrity
Integrated Process: Nursing Process—Analysis
Content Area: Critical Care
Reference: Swearingen, P. (2008). *All-in-one care planning resource: Medical-surgical, pediatric, maternity, & psychiatric nursing care plans* (2nd ed., p. 575). St. Louis: Mosby.

91. 4

Rationale: The high glucose concentration in PN places the client at risk for hyperglycemia. Signs of hyperglycemia include excessive thirst, fatigue, restlessness, confusion, weakness, Kussmaul's respirations, diuresis, and coma when hyperglycemia is severe. If the client has these symptoms, the blood glucose level should be checked immediately. Options 1, 2, and 3 do not identify signs specific to hyperglycemia.
Test-Taking Strategy: For an option to be correct, all of the parts of that option must be correct. Begin to answer this question by eliminating options 1 and 3 because fever and chills are indicative of infection. Choose option 4 over option 2 because the client with hyperglycemia has increased urine output rather than decreased urine output. Review the signs of hyperglycemia if you had difficulty with this question.
Level of Cognitive Ability: Applying
Client Needs: Physiological Integrity
Integrated Process: Nursing Process—Assessment
Content Area: Fundamental Skills—Nutrition
References: Perry, A., & Potter, P. (2010). *Clinical nursing skills & techniques* (7th ed., p. 850). St. Louis: Mosby.

Swearingen, P. (2008). *All-in-one care planning resource: Medical-surgical, pediatric, maternity, & psychiatric nursing care plans* (2nd ed., p. 576). St. Louis: Mosby.

92. 1

Rationale: Redness at the catheter insertion site is a possible indication of infection. The nurse would next assess for other signs of infection. Of the options given, the temperature is the next item to assess. The tightness of tubing connections should be assessed each time the PN is checked; loose connections would result in leakage, not skin redness. The expiration date on the bag is a viable option, but this also should be checked at the time the solution is hung and with each shift change. The time of the last dressing change should be checked with each shift change.
Test-Taking Strategy: Note the strategic word *next*. This question requires that you prioritize based on the information provided in the question. Also note the relationship between *site appears reddened* in the question and the word *temperature* in the correct option. Focusing on the subject of infection will direct you to option 1. Review the signs of infection in the client receiving PN if you had difficulty with this question.
Level of Cognitive Ability: Applying
Client Needs: Physiological Integrity
Integrated Process: Nursing Process—Assessment
Content Area: Fundamental Skills—Safety/Infection Control
References: Perry, A., & Potter, P. (2010). *Clinical nursing skills & techniques* (7th ed., p. 850, 855). St. Louis: Mosby.

Swearingen, P. (2008). *All-in-one care planning resource: Medical-surgical, pediatric, maternity, & psychiatric nursing care plans* (2nd ed., p. 575). St. Louis: Mosby.

93. 2

Rationale: Fat emulsion (lipids) is a white, opaque solution administered intravenously during parenteral nutrition therapy to prevent fatty acid deficiency. The nurse should examine the bottle of fat emulsion for separation of emulsion into layers or fat globules or for the accumulation of froth. The nurse should not hang a fat emulsion if any of these are observed and should return the solution to the pharmacy. Therefore options 1, 3, and 4 are inappropriate actions.
Test-Taking Strategy: Remember that options that are comparable or alike are not likely to be correct. With this in mind, eliminate options 1 and 3 first. Select between the remaining options by recalling the significance of fat globules in the solution. Also, think about the potential adverse effect of fat globules entering the client's bloodstream. Review the procedure for administering fat emulsion if you had difficulty with this question.
Level of Cognitive Ability: Applying
Client Needs: Physiological Integrity
Integrated Process: Nursing Process—Implementation
Content Area: Fundamental Skills—Safety/Infection Control
References: Perry, A., & Potter, P. (2010). *Clinical nursing skills & techniques* (7th ed., p. 853). St. Louis: Mosby.

Skidmore-Roth, L. (2009). *Mosby's drug guide for nurses* (8th ed., pp. 396–397). St. Louis: Mosby.

94. 3

Rationale: When the client who is receiving PN spikes a temperature, a catheter-related infection should be suspected. The solution and tubing should be changed, and the discontinued materials should be cultured for infectious organisms. The other options are incorrect. Because culture for infectious organisms is necessary, the discontinued materials are not discarded or returned to the pharmacy or manufacturer.

Test-Taking Strategy: Use the process of elimination. Identifying the subject of the question, infection, and correlating the fever with infection associated with the intravenous line should direct you to option 3. Remember that the discontinued materials need to be cultured. Review the procedure when infection is suspected in the client receiving PN if you had difficulty with this question.

Level of Cognitive Ability: Applying
Client Needs: Physiological Integrity
Integrated Process: Nursing Process—Implementation
Content Area: Fundamental Skills—Safety/Infection Control
Reference: Ignatavicius, D., & Workman, M. (2010). *Medical-surgical nursing: Patient-centered collaborative care* (6th ed., p. 234). St. Louis: Saunders.

95. 2
Rationale: The client receiving PN at home should have her or his temperature monitored as a means of detecting infection, which is a potential complication of this therapy. An infection also could result in sepsis because the catheter is in a blood vessel. The client's weight is monitored as a measure of the effectiveness of this nutritional therapy and to detect hypervolemia. The pulse and blood pressure are important parameters to assess, but they do not relate specifically to the effects of PN.

Test-Taking Strategy: Note the strategic words *most closely*, which tell you that more than one or all the options may be partially or totally correct. Remember also that when there are multiple parts to an option, all the parts must be correct for that option to be correct. Recalling that infection and hypervolemia are complications of PN and that weight is monitored as a measure of the effectiveness of this nutritional therapy will direct you to option 2. Review the priority assessments of a client receiving PN if you had difficulty with this question.

Level of Cognitive Ability: Applying
Client Needs: Physiological Integrity
Integrated Process: Nursing Process—Assessment
Content Area: Fundamental Skills—Nutrition
Reference: Perry, A., & Potter, P. (2010). *Clinical nursing skills & techniques* (7th ed., pp. 856–857). St. Louis: Mosby.

96. 2
Rationale: Parenteral nutrition is indicated in clients whose gastrointestinal tracts are not functional or who cannot take in a diet enterally for extended periods. Examples of these conditions include those of the clients identified in options 1, 3, and 4. Other clients would be those who have had extensive surgery, have multiple fractures, are septic, or have advanced cancer or acquired immunodeficiency syndrome. The client with the open cholecystectomy is not a candidate because this client would resume a regular diet within a few days following surgery.

Test-Taking Strategy: Note the strategic words *least likely*, which tell you that the correct option is the client who does not require this type of nutritional support. Use nursing knowledge of these various conditions and baseline knowledge of the purposes of PN to make your selection.

Review the indications for PN if you had difficulty with this question.

Level of Cognitive Ability: Analyzing
Client Needs: Physiological Integrity
Integrated Process: Nursing Process—Assessment
Content Area: Fundamental Skills—Nutrition
Reference: Ignatavicius, D., & Workman, M. (2010). *Medical-surgical nursing: Patient-centered collaborative care* (6th ed., p. 1396). St. Louis: Saunders.

97. 3
Rationale: The nurse obtains an electronic infusion pump before hanging a PN solution. Because of the high glucose content, use of an infusion pump is necessary to ensure that the solution does not infuse too rapidly or fall behind. Because the client's blood glucose level is monitored every 4 to 6 hours during administration of PN, a blood glucose meter also will be needed, but this is not the most essential item needed before hanging the solution. Urine test strips (to measure glucose) rarely are used because of the advent of blood glucose monitoring. Although the blood pressure will be monitored, a noninvasive blood pressure monitor is not the most essential piece of equipment needed for this procedure.

Test-Taking Strategy: Note the strategic words *most essential*. They tell you that the correct option identifies the item needed to start the infusion. Visualizing the procedure for initiating PN will direct you to option 3. Review the procedure for initiating PN if you had difficulty with this question.

Level of Cognitive Ability: Applying
Client Needs: Physiological Integrity
Integrated Process: Nursing Process—Planning
Content Area: Fundamental Skills—Medications/Blood & IV Therapy
Reference: Perry, A., & Potter, P. (2010). *Clinical nursing skills & techniques* (7th ed., p. 852). St. Louis: Mosby.

98. 2
Rationale: The client is at risk for hypoglycemia; therefore the solution containing the highest amount of glucose should be hung until the new PN solution becomes available. Because PN solutions contain high glucose concentrations, the 10% dextrose in water solution is the best of the choices presented. The solution selected should be one that minimizes the risk of hypoglycemia. Options 1, 3, and 4 will not be as effective in minimizing the risk of hypoglycemia.

Test-Taking Strategy: Use the process of elimination, recalling that this particular client is at risk for hypoglycemia. With this in mind, you would then select the solution that minimizes this risk to the client. Also, remember that options that are comparable or alike are not likely to be correct. Each of the incorrect options represents a solution that contains 5% dextrose. Review the nursing actions to prevent hypoglycemia in the client receiving PN if you had difficulty with this question.

Level of Cognitive Ability: Applying
Client Needs: Physiological Integrity
Integrated Process: Nursing Process—Implementation
Content Area: Fundamental Skills—Nutrition

Reference: Perry, A., & Potter, P. (2010). *Clinical nursing skills & techniques* (7th ed., p. 850). St. Louis: Mosby.

99. 3
Rationale: The nurse should not increase the rate of a fat emulsion to make up the difference if the infusion timing falls behind. Doing so could place the client at risk for fat overload. Additionally, increasing the rate suddenly can cause fluid overload. The same principle (not increasing the rate) applies to PN or any intravenous (IV) infusion. Therefore options 1, 2, and 4 are incorrect.
Test-Taking Strategy: Focus on the data in the question and note the strategic word *appropriate*. Remember also that options that are comparable or alike are not likely to be correct. This guides you to eliminate options 1 and 2 first. Choose option 3 over option 4, recalling that the nurse never increases the infusion rate or adjusts an infusion rate to run wide open if an infusion is behind. Review these safety principles related to IV therapy if you had difficulty with this question.
Level of Cognitive Ability: Applying
Client Needs: Physiological Integrity
Integrated Process: Nursing Process—Implementation
Content Area: Fundamental Skills—Medications/Blood & IV Therapy
References: Perry, A., & Potter, P. (2010). *Clinical nursing skills & techniques* (7th ed., p. 858). St. Louis: Mosby.
Swearingen, P. (2008). *All-in-one care planning resource: Medical-surgical, pediatric, maternity, & psychiatric nursing care plans* (2nd ed., p. 575). St. Louis: Mosby.

100. 4
Rationale: Optimal weight gain when the client is receiving PN is 1 to 2 lb/week. The client who has a weight gain of 5 lb/week while receiving PN is likely to have fluid retention. This can result in hypervolemia. Signs of hypervolemia include increased blood pressure, crackles on lung auscultation, a bounding pulse, jugular vein distention, headache, and weight gain more than desired. Options 1 and 2 are associated with hyperglycemia. Option 3 is likely to be noted in deficient fluid volume.
Test-Taking Strategy: Focus on the subject of the question, a weight gain of 5 lb in 1 week. This should direct your thinking to the potential for hypervolemia. With this in mind, use the process of elimination, selecting the option that identifies the signs of hypervolemia. If you had difficulty with this question, review the signs and symptoms of hypervolemia associated with the administration of PN.
Level of Cognitive Ability: Analyzing
Client Needs: Physiological Integrity
Integrated Process: Nursing Process—Assessment
Content Area: Critical Care
Reference: Perry, A., & Potter, P. (2010). *Clinical nursing skills & techniques* (7th ed., p. 853). St. Louis: Mosby.

101. 3
Rationale: The nurse should plan to secure all connections in the tubing (tape is used per agency protocol). This helps prevent the restless client from pulling the connections apart

accidentally. The nurse should also monitor intake and output, but this does not relate specifically to a risk for injury as presented in the question. Also, options 2 and 4 do not relate to a risk for injury as presented in the question. In addition, the client's temperature and blood glucose levels are monitored more frequently than the timeframes identified in the options to detect signs of infection and hyperglycemia, respectively.
Test-Taking Strategy: Note the strategic words *restless, ensure, prevent*, and *injury*. Focus on the subject of the question, which is safety. This will direct you to option 3. Review the precautions related to PN if you had difficulty with this question.
Level of Cognitive Ability: Applying
Client Needs: Safe and Effective Care Environment
Integrated Process: Nursing Process—Planning
Content Area: Fundamental Skills—Safety/Infection Control
Reference: Perry, A., & Potter, P. (2010). *Clinical nursing skills & techniques* (7th ed., p. 852). St. Louis: Mosby.

ALTERNATE ITEM FORMAT: PRIORITIZING (ORDERED RESPONSE)
102. 4, 3, 6, 5, 1, 2
Rationale: Air embolism occurs when air enters the catheter system during IV tubing changes or when the IV tubing disconnects. Air embolism is a critical situation. If air embolism is suspected, the nurse would first clamp the IV catheter to prevent further introduction of air and the air embolism from traveling through the heart to the pulmonary system. The nurse would next place the client in a left side-lying position with the head lower than the feet (to trap air in right side of the heart). The nurse would notify the physician and administer oxygen as prescribed. The nurse would monitor the client closely and take the client's vital signs. Finally, the nurse documents the occurrence.
Test-Taking Strategy: Think about the pathophysiology and effects of an air embolism. Recalling that a primary concern is that the embolism will travel to the pulmonary system will assist in determining that the catheter needs to be clamped first and that the client needs to be positioned to trap the air in the right side of the heart. Because this event is an emergency, the nurse notifies the physician next and the physician will provide a prescription for oxygen, if necessary. The nurse monitors the client and takes the client's vital signs frequently. Review the immediate nursing interventions for a client experiencing air embolism if you had difficulty with this question.
Level of Cognitive Ability: Applying
Client Needs: Physiological Integrity
Integrated Process: Nursing Process—Implementation
Content Area: Leadership and Management—Delegating/Prioritizing
References: Ignatavicius, D., & Workman, M. (2010). *Medical-surgical nursing: Patient-centered collaborative care* (6th ed., p. 231). St. Louis: Saunders.
Perry, A., & Potter, P. (2010). *Clinical nursing skills & techniques* (7th ed., p. 850, 858). St. Louis: Mosby.

Intravenous Therapy

PYRAMID TERMS

air embolism An obstruction caused by a bolus of air that enters the vein through an inadequately primed intravenous (IV) line, from a loose connection, during a tubing change, or during removal of an IV line.

catheter embolism An obstruction caused by breakage of the catheter tip during IV line insertion or removal.

hypertonic Solutions that are more concentrated or have a higher osmolality than body fluids.

hypotonic Solutions that are more dilute or have a lower osmolality than body fluids.

infiltration Seepage of IV fluid out of the vein and into the surrounding interstitial spaces.

isotonic Solutions that have the same osmolality as body fluids.

phlebitis An inflammation of the vein that can occur from mechanical or chemical (medication) trauma or from a local infection.

THE PYRAMID TO SUCCESS

Professional nurses are responsible for managing and providing care to clients receiving IV therapy. Pyramid Points focus on the safety measures required to initiate, maintain, and remove an IV line, including a peripherally inserted central catheter (PICC). Assessment of the client for allergies, including latex sensitivity, before initiation of an IV line is a critical nursing responsibility. Additional nursing responsibilities include monitoring for complications related to the IV line and initiating the measures required when an IV complication occurs. Pyramid Points focus on the signs and symptoms of infection, infiltration, phlebitis, circulatory overload, and air embolism, as well as the treatment measures associated with each. Maintaining an epidural infusion is also a Pyramid Point.

CLIENT NEEDS

Safe and Effective Care Environment

Applying principles of infection control
Consulting with members of the health care team
Establishing priorities

Handling hazardous or infectious materials safely
Maintaining standard precautions, transmission-based precautions, and surgical asepsis during handling of equipment and supplies
Obtaining informed consent for invasive procedures
Preventing errors in administering IV fluids
Using equipment such as electronic IV infusion devices safely

Health Promotion and Maintenance

Assessing the client's ability to perform self-care
Considering lifestyle choices related to home care of the IV line
Evaluating the client's home environment for self-care modifications
Promoting health and wellness
Teaching the client and family about care of the IV line
Performing physical assessment techniques

Psychosocial Integrity

Assessing coping mechanisms
Assessing the client's emotional response to treatment
Identifying support systems in the home for caring for the IV line

Physiological Integrity

Assessing and caring for central venous access devices
Initiating immediate interventions if a complication occurs
Maintaining IV therapy
Monitoring for complications of IV therapy
Monitoring for expected effects of IV therapy
Monitoring laboratory values for fluid and electrolyte imbalances

I. INTRAVENOUS THERAPY

A. Purpose and uses
   1. Used to sustain clients who are unable to take substances orally
   2. Replaces water, electrolytes, and nutrients more rapidly than oral administration

3. Provides immediate access to the vascular system for the rapid delivery of specific solutions without the time required for gastrointestinal tract absorption
4. Provides a vascular route for the administration of medication or blood components

B. Types of solutions (Table 14-1)
  1. **Isotonic** solutions
    a. Have the same osmolality as body fluids
    b. Increase extracellular fluid volume
    c. Do not enter the cells because no osmotic force exists to shift the fluids
  2. **Hypotonic** solutions
    a. Are more dilute solutions and have a lower osmolality than body fluids
    b. Cause the movement of water into cells by osmosis
    c. Should be administered slowly to prevent cellular edema
  3. **Hypertonic** solutions
    a. Are more concentrated solutions and have a higher osmolality than body fluids
    b. Concentrate extracellular fluid and cause movement of water from cells into the extracellular fluid by osmosis
  4. Colloids
    a. Also called plasma expanders
    b. Pull fluid from the interstitial compartment into the vascular compartment
    c. Used to increase the vascular volume rapidly, such as in hemorrhage or severe hypovolemia

TABLE 14-1 Types of Intravenous Solutions

Solution	Tonicity
0.9% sodium chloride (normal saline); (0.9% NS)	Isotonic
5% dextrose in water (D_5W)	Isotonic
5% dextrose in 0.225% saline (D_5W/¼ NS)	Isotonic
Lactated Ringer's (LR)	Isotonic
0.45% sodium chloride (normal saline); (½ NS)	Hypotonic
0.225% sodium chloride (normal saline); (¼ NS)	Hypotonic
0.33% sodium chloride (normal saline); (⅓ NS)	Hypotonic
3% sodium chloride (normal saline); (3% NS)	Hypertonic
5% sodium chloride (normal saline); (5% NS)	Hypertonic
10% dextrose in water ($D_{10}W$)	Hypertonic
5% dextrose in 0.9% sodium chloride (normal saline); D_5W/NS	Hypertonic
5% dextrose in 0.45% sodium chloride (normal saline); (D_5W/½ NS)	Hypertonic
5% dextrose in lactated Ringer's (D_5LR)	Hypertonic
Dextran	Colloid
Albumin	Colloid

⚠ Administration of an IV solution or medication provides immediate access to the vascular system. This is a benefit of administering solutions or medications via this route but can also present a risk. Therefore, it is critical to ensure that physician's prescriptions are checked carefully and the correct solution or medication is administered as prescribed. Always follow the six rights for medication administration.

II. INTRAVENOUS DEVICES

A. IV cannulas
  1. Steel needles or butterfly sets
    a. The set is a wing-tip needle with a metal cannula, plastic or rubber wings, and a plastic catheter or hub.
    b. The needle is 0.5 to 1.5 inches in length, with needle gauge sizes from 16 to 26.
    c. **Infiltration** is more common with these devices.
    d. The butterfly infusion set commonly is used in children and older clients, whose veins are likely to be small or fragile.
  2. Plastic cannulas
    a. Plastic cannulas may be an over-the-needle device or an in-needle catheter and are used primarily for short-term therapy.
    b. The over-the-needle device is preferred for rapid infusion and is more comfortable for the client.
    c. The in-needle catheter can cause **catheter embolism** if the tip of the cannula breaks.

B. IV gauges
  1. The gauge refers to the diameter of the lumen of the needle or cannula.
  2. The smaller the gauge number, the larger the diameter of the lumen; the larger the gauge number, the smaller the diameter of the lumen.
  3. The size of the gauge used depends on the solution to be administered and the diameter of the available vein.
  4. Large-diameter lumens (smaller gauge numbers) allow a higher fluid rate than smaller diameter lumens and allow the administration of higher concentrations of solutions.
  5. For rapid emergency fluid administration, blood products, or anesthetics, large-diameter lumen needles or cannulas are used, such as a 14-, 16-, 18-, or 19-gauge.
  6. For peripheral fat infusions (lipids), a 20- or 21-gauge lumen or cannula is used.
  7. For standard IV fluid and clear liquid IV medications, a 22- or 24-gauge lumen or cannula is used.
  8. If the client has very small veins, a 24- to 25-gauge lumen or cannula is used.

C. IV containers
1. Container may be glass or plastic.
2. Squeeze the plastic bag to ensure intactness and assess the glass bottle for any cracks before hanging.

⚠ Do not write on a plastic IV bag with a marking pen because the ink may be absorbed through the plastic into the solution. Use a label and a ballpoint pen for marking the bag, placing the label onto the bag.

D. IV tubing (Fig. 14-1)
1. IV tubing contains a spike end for the bag or bottle, drip chamber, roller clamp, Y site, and adapter end for attachment to the cannula or needle that is inserted into the client's vein.
2. Shorter secondary tubing is used for piggyback solutions, connecting them to the injection sites nearest to the drip chamber (Fig. 14-2).
3. Special tubing is used for medication that absorbs into plastic (check specific medication administration guidelines when administering IV medications).
4. Vented and nonvented tubing are available.
    a. A vent allows air to enter the IV container as the fluid leaves.
    b. A vented adapter can be used to add a vent to a nonvented IV tubing system.
    c. Use nonvented tubing for flexible containers.
    d. Use vented tubing for glass or rigid plastic containers to allow air to enter and displace the fluid as it leaves; fluid will not flow from a rigid IV container unless it is vented.

⚠ Extension tubing can be added to an IV tubing set to provide extra length to the tubing. Add extension tubing to the IV tubing set for children, clients who are restless, or clients who have special mobility needs.

E. Drip chambers (Fig. 14-3)
1. Macrodrip chamber
    a. The chamber is used if the solution is thick or is to be infused rapidly.

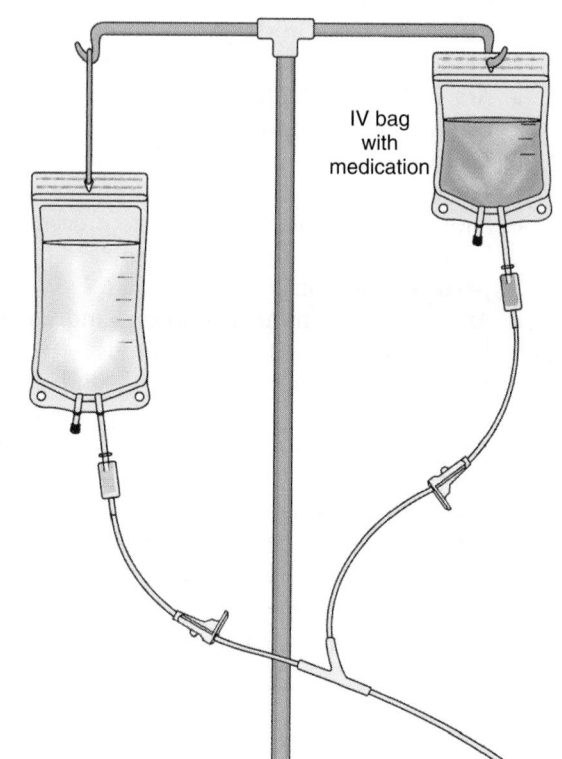

IV bag with medication

▲ **FIGURE 14-2** Secondary bag with medication. (Modified from Kee, J., & Marshall, S. [2009]. *Clinical calculations: With applications to general and specialty areas* [6th ed.]. St. Louis: Saunders.)

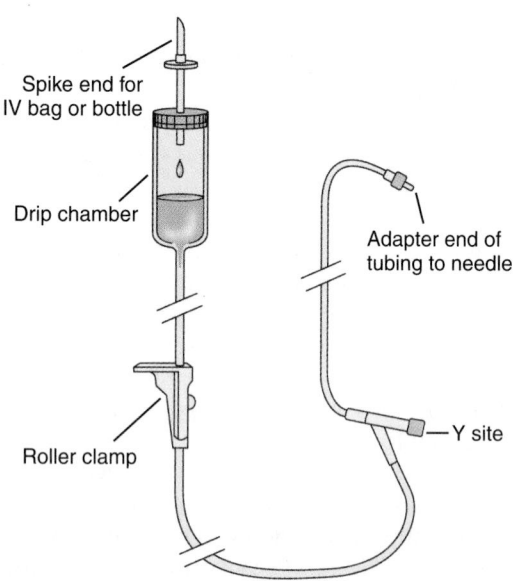

Spike end for IV bag or bottle

Drip chamber

Adapter end of tubing to needle

Roller clamp

Y site

▲ **FIGURE 14-1** Intravenous tubing. (From Kee, J. & Marshall, S. [2009]. *Clinical calculations: With applications to general and specialty areas* [6th ed.]. St. Louis: Saunders.)

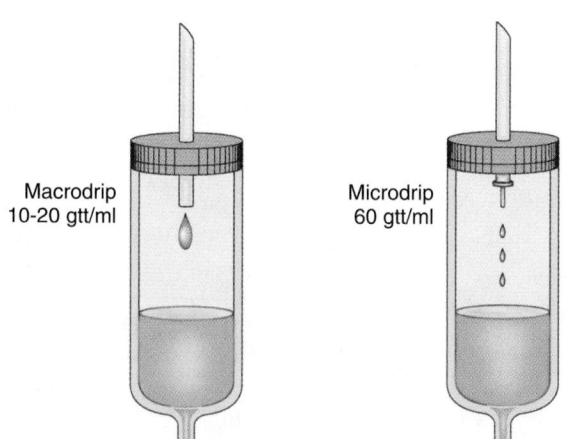

Macrodrip 10-20 gtt/ml

Microdrip 60 gtt/ml

▲ **FIGURE 14-3** Macrodrip and microdrip sizes. (From Kee, J., & Marshall, S. [2009]. *Clinical calculations: With applications to general and specialty areas* [6th ed.]. St. Louis: Saunders.)

b. The drop factor varies from 10 to 20 gtt/mL, depending on the manufacturer.

c. Read the tubing package to determine how many drops per milliliter are delivered (drop factor).

2. Microdrip chamber

a. Normally, the chamber has a short vertical metal piece (stylet) where the drop forms.

b. The chamber delivers about 60 gtt/mL.

c. Read the tubing package to determine the drop factor (gtt/mL).

d. Microdrip chambers are used if fluid will be infused at a slow rate (less than 50 mL/hr) or if the solution contains potent medication that needs to be titrated, such as in a critical care setting or in pediatric clients.

F. Filters

1. Filters provide protection by preventing particles from entering the client's veins.

2. They are used in IV lines to trap small particles such as undissolved antibiotics or salt, or medications that have precipitated in solution.

3. Assess the agency policy regarding the use of filters.

4. A 0.22-μm filter is used for most solutions, a 1.2-μm filter is used for solutions containing lipids or albumin, and a special filter is used for blood components.

5. Change filters every 24 to 72 hours (depending on agency policy) to prevent bacterial growth.

G. Needleless infusion devices

1. Needleless infusion devices include recessed needles, plastic cannulas, and one-way valves; these systems decrease the exposure to contaminated needles.

2. Do not administer parenteral nutrition or blood products through a one-way valve.

H. Intermittent infusion devices

1. Intermittent infusion devices are used when intravascular accessibility is desired for intermittent administration of medications by IV push or IV piggyback.

2. Patency is maintained by periodic flushing with normal saline solution (sodium chloride and normal saline are interchangeable names).

3. Depending on agency policy, when administering medication, flush with 1 to 2 mL of normal saline to confirm placement of the IV cannula; administer the prescribed medication and then flush the cannula again with 1 to 2 mL of normal saline to maintain patency.

I. Electronic IV infusion devices

1. IV infusion pumps control the amount of fluid infusing and should be used with central venous lines, arterial lines, solutions containing medication, and parenteral nutrition infusions.

2. A syringe pump is used when a small volume of medication is administered; the syringe that contains the medication and solution fits into a pump and is set to deliver the medication at a controlled rate.

3. Patient controlled analgesia (PCA) is a device that allows the client to self-administer IV medication, such as an analgesic; the client can administer bolus doses at set intervals and the pump can be set to lock out bolus doses that are not within the preset time frame to prevent overdose.

⚠ Check electronic IV infusion devices frequently. Although these devices are electronic, this does not ensure that they are infusing solutions and medications accurately.

III. LATEX ALLERGY

A. Assess the client for an allergy to latex.

B. IV supplies, including IV catheters, IV tubing, IV ports (particularly IV rubber injection ports), rubber stoppers on multidose vials, and adhesive tape, may contain latex.

C. Latex-safe IV supplies need to be used for clients with a latex allergy.

D. A three-way stopcock, rather than a rubber injection port, needs to be used on plastic tubing.

E. See Chapter 70 for additional information regarding latex allergy.

IV. SELECTION OF A PERIPHERAL IV SITE

A. Veins in the hand, forearm, and antecubital fossa are suitable sites (Fig. 14-4).

B. Veins in the lower extremities (legs and feet) are not suitable for an adult client because of the risk of thrombus formation and the possible pooling of medication in areas of decreased venous return (Box 14-1).

C. Veins in the scalp and feet may be suitable sites for infants (see Fig. 14-4).

D. Assess the veins of both arms closely before selecting a site.

E. Start the IV infusion distally to provide the option of proceeding up the extremity if the vein is ruptured or **infiltration** occurs; if **infiltration** occurs from the antecubital vein, the lower veins in the same arm usually cannot be used for further puncture sites.

F. Determine the client's dominant side, and select the opposite side for a venipuncture site.

G. Bending the elbow on the arm with an IV may easily obstruct the flow of solution, causing **infiltration** that could lead to thrombophlebitis.

H. Avoid checking the blood pressure on the arm receiving the IV infusion if possible.

I. Do not place restraints over the venipuncture site.

J. Use an armboard as needed when the venipuncture site is located in an area of flexion.

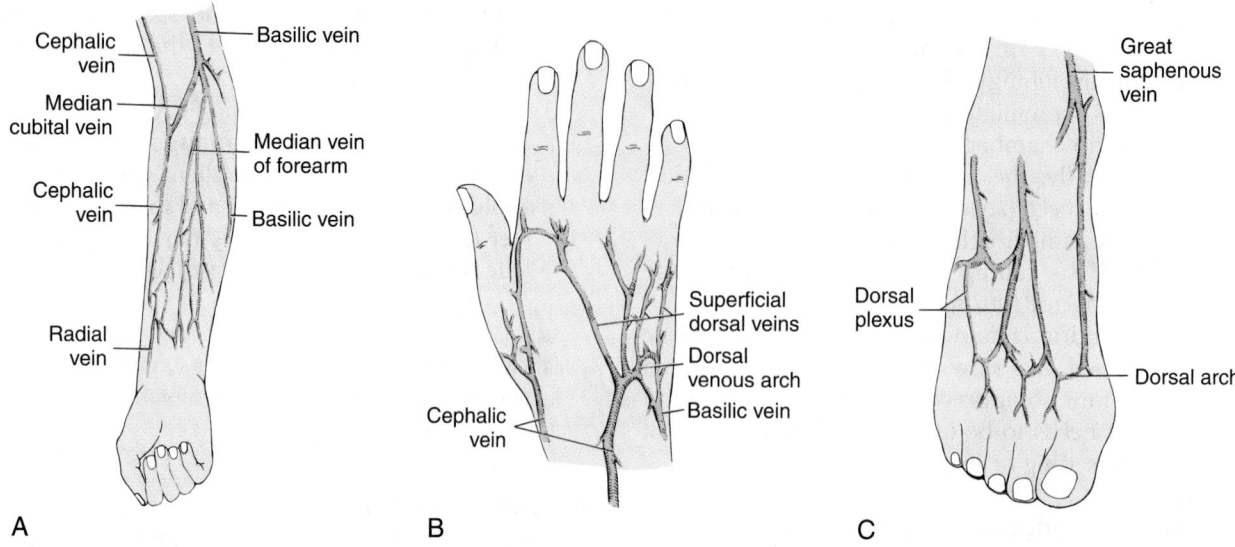

▲ **FIGURE 14-4** Common intravenous sites. **A,** Inner arm. **B,** Dorsal surface of hand. **C,** Dorsal surface of the foot (children only). (From Potter, P., & Perry, A. [2009]. *Fundamentals of nursing* [7th ed.]. St. Louis: Mosby.)

Box 14-1 Peripheral Intravenous Sites to Avoid

Edematous extremity
An arm that is weak, traumatized, or paralyzed
The arm on the same side as a mastectomy
An arm that has an arteriovenous fistula or shunt for dialysis
A skin area that is infected

 In an adult, the most frequently used sites for inserting an IV cannula/needle are the veins of the forearm because the bones of the forearm act as a natural support and splint.

V. ADDITION OF MEDICATION TO AN IV SOLUTION

A. Assess for compatibility of medication and solution.
B. When adding medication to the IV bag, mix the bag end to end several times before hanging it to disperse the medication.
C. Manufacturer-prepared IV medication systems are available; these systems are similar to a secondary IV with medication or a piggyback system.
D. Ensure that the medication can be mixed in soft plastic because some medications absorb into the soft plastic and should be mixed only in glass.

VI. INITIATION AND ADMINISTRATION OF IV SOLUTIONS

A. Check the IV solution against the physician's prescription for the type, amount, percentage of solution, and rate of flow; follow the six rights for medication administration.
B. Assess the health status and medical disorders of the client and identify client conditions that contraindicate use of a particular IV solution or IV equipment such as an allergy to cleansing solution, adhesive materials, or latex.
C. Check client's identification and explain the procedure to the client; assess client's previous experience with IV therapy and preference for insertion site.
D. Wash hands thoroughly before inserting an IV line and before working with an IV line; wear gloves.
E. Use sterile technique when inserting an IV line and when changing the dressing over the IV site.
F. Change the venipuncture site every 48 to 72 hours, depending on agency policy.
G. Change the IV dressing every 72 hours, when the dressing is wet or contaminated, or as specified by the agency policy.
H. Change the IV tubing every 24 to 72 hours, depending on agency policy.
I. Do not let an IV bag or bottle of solution hang for more than 24 hours to diminish the potential for bacterial contamination and possibly sepsis.
J. Do not allow the IV tubing to touch the floor to prevent potential bacterial contamination.
K. Before adding medications to solutions, swab access ports with 70% alcohol, an equally effective solution, or as specified by the agency policy.
L. Refer to the Priority Nursing Actions box for instructions on inserting an IV.
M. Refer to the Priority Nursing Actions box for instructions on removing an IV.

▬▬▬ PRIORITY NURSING ACTIONS! ▬▬▬

Actions for Inserting a Peripheral Intravenous Line

Refer to VI, Initiation and Administration of IV Solutions, for additional preprocedure and postprocedure interventions.

1. Check the physician's prescription and determine the type and size of infusion device and prepare intravenous (IV) tubing and solution; prime the IV tubing to remove air from the system; explain procedure to the client.
2. Select the vein for insertion; apply tourniquet and palpate the vein for resilience (see Fig. 14-4)
3. Clean the skin with an antimicrobial solution, using an inner to outer circular motion, or as specified by the agency policy
4. Stabilize the vein below the insertion site and puncture the skin and vein observing for blood in the flashback chamber; when observed, advance the catheter into the vein (if unsuccessful, a new sterile device is used for the next attempt at insertion).
5. Apply pressure above the insertion site with the middle finger of the nondominant hand and retract the stylet from the catheter; connect the end of the IV tubing to the catheter tubing, secure it, and begin IV flow.
6. Tape and secure insertion site with a dressing as specified by agency procedure; label the tubing, dressing, and solution bags clearly, indicating the date and time.
7. Document the specifics about the procedure such as number of attempts at insertion; the insertion site, type and size of device, solution and flow rate and time; and the client's response; additionally follow agency procedure for documentation of procedure.

The nurse checks the physician's prescription for the IV line and then determines the type and size of infusion device. The type and size is important to ensure adequate flow of the prescribed solution. For example, if a blood product is prescribed then the nurse would need to insert an appropriate catheter gauge size for blood delivery. The nurse also considers the client's size, age, mobility and other factors in selecting the type and size of the infusion device. The nurse prepares the appropriate IV tubing and primes the IV tubing to remove air from the system. The appropriate vein is selected, the tourniquet is applied, and the vein is checked and palpated for resilience. Strict surgical asepsis is employed and the skin is cleaned with an antimicrobial solution (as specified by the agency policy) using an inner to outer circular motion. The vein is stabilized to prevent its movement and the skin is punctured. Blood in the flashback chamber indicates that the device is in the vein and when noted the catheter is carefully advanced to avoid puncture of the back wall of the vein. The stylet is removed from the catheter device, the IV tubing is connected, and the IV flow is started. The nurse tapes and secures the site and labels the tubing, dressing, and solution bag appropriately and according to agency policy. The nurse checks the site and ensures that the solution is flowing. Finally the nurse documents the specifics about the procedure.

Reference: Potter, P., & Perry, A. (2009). *Fundamentals of nursing* (7th ed., pp. 994–1004). St. Louis: Mosby.

▬▬▬ PRIORITY NURSING ACTIONS! ▬▬▬

Actions for Removing a Peripheral Intravenous Line

1. Check the physician's prescription and explain the procedure to the client; ask the client to hold the extremity still during cannula/needle removal.
2. Turn off the intravenous (IV) tubing clamp and remove the dressing and tape covering the site, while stabilizing the catheter.
3. Apply light pressure with sterile gauze or other material as specified by agency procedure over the site and withdraw the catheter using a slow, steady movement, keeping the hub parallel to the skin.
4. Apply pressure for 2 to 3 minutes using dry sterile gauze (apply pressure for a longer period of time if the client has a bleeding disorder or is taking anticoagulant medication).
5. Inspect the site for redness, drainage, or swelling; check the catheter for intactness.
6. Document the procedure and the client's response.

The nurse checks for a physician's prescription to remove the IV line and then explains the procedure to the client. The nurse asks the client to hold the extremity still during removal. The IV tubing clamp is placed in the *off* position and the dressing and tape is removed. The nurse is careful to stabilize the catheter so that it is not pulled, resulting in vein trauma. Light pressure is applied over the site to stabilize the catheter and it is removed using a slow, steady movement, keeping the hub parallel to the skin. Pressure is applied until hemostasis occurs. The site is inspected for redness, drainage, or swelling and the catheter is checked for intactness to ensure that any part of it has not broken off. Finally the nurse documents the procedure and the client's response.

Reference: Elkin, M., Perry, A., & Potter, P. (2007). *Nursing interventions & clinical skills* (4th ed., pp. 620–621).St. Louis: Mosby.

VII. PRECAUTIONS FOR IV LINES

A. On insertion, an IV line can cause initial pain and discomfort for the client.
B. An IV puncture provides a route of entry for microorganisms into the body.
C. Medications administered by the IV route enter the blood immediately, and any adverse reactions or allergic responses can occur immediately.
D. Fluid (circulatory) overload or electrolyte imbalances can occur from excessive or too rapid infusion of IV fluids.
E. Incompatibilities between certain solutions and medications can occur.

⚠ A client with congestive heart failure usually is not given a solution containing saline because this type of fluid promotes the retention of water and would therefore exacerbate heart failure by increasing the fluid overload.

VIII. COMPLICATIONS (Table 14-2)

A. Air embolism
1. Description: A bolus of air enters the vein through an inadequately primed IV line, from a loose connection, during tubing change, or during removal of the IV.
2. Prevention and interventions
   a. Prime tubing with fluid before use, and monitor for any air bubbles in the tubing.
   b. Secure all connections.
   c. Replace the IV fluid before the bag or bottle is empty.
   d. Monitor for signs of **air embolism**; if suspected, clamp the tubing, turn the client on the left side with the head of the bed lowered (Trendelenburg's position) to trap the air in the right atrium, and notify the physician.

B. Catheter embolism
1. Description: An obstruction that results from breakage of the catheter tip during IV line insertion or removal
2. Prevention and interventions
   a. Remove the catheter carefully.
   b. Inspect the catheter when removed.
   c. If the catheter tip has broken off, place a tourniquet as proximally as possible to the IV site on the affected limb, notify the physician immediately, prepare to obtain a radiograph, and prepare the client for surgery to remove the catheter piece(s), if necessary.

C. Circulatory overload
1. Description: Also known as *fluid overload*; results from the administration of fluids too rapidly especially in a client at risk for fluid overload
2. Prevention and interventions
   a. Identify clients at risk for circulatory overload.
   b. Calculate and monitor the drip (flow) rate frequently.
   c. Use an electronic IV infusion device and frequently check the drip rate or setting (at least every hour for an adult).
   d. Add a time tape (label) to the IV bag or bottle (Fig. 14-5).
   e. Monitor for signs of circulatory overload. If circulatory overload occurs, decrease the flow rate to a minimum, at a keep-vein-open rate; elevate the head of the bed; keep the client warm; assess lung sounds; assess for edema; and notify the physician.

TABLE 14-2 Signs of Complications of Intravenous Therapy

Complication	Signs
Air embolism	Tachycardia Dyspnea Hypotension Cyanosis Decreased level of consciousness
Catheter embolism	Decrease in blood pressure Pain along the vein Weak, rapid pulse Cyanosis of the nail beds Loss of consciousness
Circulatory overload	Increased blood pressure Distended jugular veins Rapid breathing Dyspnea Moist cough and crackles
Electrolyte overload	Signs depend on the specific electrolyte overload imbalance
Hematoma	Ecchymosis, immediate swelling and leakage of blood at the site, and hard and painful lumps at the site
Infection	Local—redness, swelling, and drainage at the site Systemic—chills, fever, malaise, headache, nausea, vomiting, backache, tachycardia
Infiltration	Edema, pain, and coolness at the site; may or may not have a blood return
Phlebitis	Heat, redness, tenderness at the site Not swollen or hard Intravenous infusion sluggish
Thrombophlebitis	Hard and cordlike vein Heat, redness, tenderness at site Intravenous infusion sluggish
Tissue damage	Skin color changes, sloughing of the skin, discomfort at the site

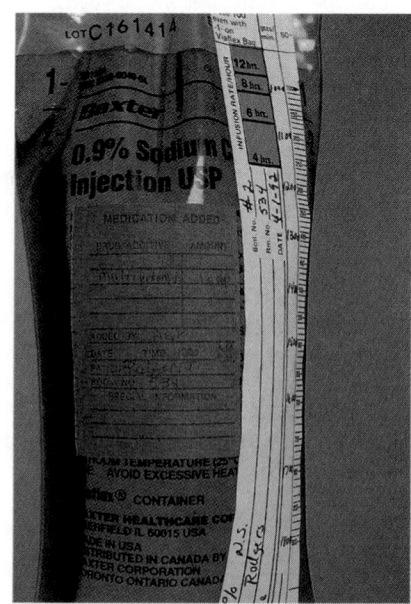

▲ **FIGURE 14-5** Intravenous fluid bag with medication label and time tape. (Modified from Potter, P., & Perry, A. [2009]. *Fundamentals of nursing* [7th ed.]. St. Louis: Mosby.)

⚠ Clients with respiratory, cardiac, renal, or liver disease, older clients, and very young persons are at risk for circulatory overload and cannot tolerate an excessive fluid volume.

D. Electrolyte overload
1. Description: An electrolyte imbalance caused by too rapid or excessive infusion or by use of an inappropriate IV solution
2. Prevention and interventions
   a. Assess laboratory value reports.
   b. Verify the correct solution.
   c. Calculate and monitor the flow rate.
   d. Use an electronic IV infusion device and frequently check the drip rate or setting (at least every hour for an adult).
   e. Add a time tape (label) to the IV bag or bottle (see Fig. 14-5).
   f. Place a red medication sticker on the bag or bottle if a medication, such as potassium chloride, has been added to the IV solution (see Fig. 14-5).
   g. Monitor for signs of an electrolyte imbalance, and notify the physician if they occur.

⚠ Lactated Ringer's solution contains potassium and should not be administered to clients with renal failure.

E. Hematoma
1. Description: The collection of blood in the tissues after an unsuccessful venipuncture or after the venipuncture site is discontinued and blood continues to ooze into the tissue
2. Prevention and interventions
   a. When starting an IV, avoid piercing the posterior wall of the vein.
   b. Do not apply a tourniquet to the extremity immediately after an unsuccessful venipuncture.
   c. When discontinuing an IV, apply pressure to the site for 2 to 3 minutes and elevate the extremity; apply pressure longer for clients with a bleeding disorder or who are taking anticoagulants.
   d. If a hematoma develops, elevate the extremity and apply pressure and ice as prescribed.
F. Infection
1. Description
   a. Infection occurs from the entry of microorganisms into the body through the venipuncture site.
   b. Venipuncture interrupts the integrity of the skin, the first line of defense against infection.
   c. The longer the therapy continues, the greater the risk for infection.
   d. Infection can occur locally at the IV insertion site or systemically from the entry of microorganisms into the body.

2. At-risk clients
   a. Immunocompromised clients with diseases such as cancer, human immunodeficiency virus, or acquired immunodeficiency syndrome are at risk for infection.
   b. Clients receiving treatments such as chemotherapy who have an altered or lowered white blood cell count are at risk for infection.
   c. Older clients, because aging alters the effectiveness of the immune system, are at risk for infection.
   d. Clients with diabetes mellitus are at risk for infection.
3. Prevention and interventions
   a. Assess the client for predisposition to or risk for infection.
   b. Maintain strict asepsis when caring for the IV site.
   c. Monitor for signs of local or systemic infection.
   d. Monitor white blood cell counts.
   e. Check fluid containers for cracks, leaks, cloudiness, or other evidence of contamination.
   f. Change tubing and site dressing every 24 to 72 hours according to agency policy.
   g. Use antimicrobial ointment at the IV site.
   h. Label the IV site, bag or bottle, and tubing with the date and time to ensure that these are changed on time according to agency policy.
   i. Ensure that the IV solution is not hanging for more than 24 hours.
   j. If infection occurs, the physician is notified; discontinue the IV, and place the venipuncture device in a sterile container for possible culture.
   k. Prepare to obtain blood cultures as prescribed if infection occurs.
   l. Restart an IV in the opposite arm to differentiate sepsis (systemic infection) from local infection at the IV site.

⚠ A client with diabetes mellitus usually does not receive dextrose (glucose) solutions because the solution can increase the blood glucose level.

G. Infiltration
1. Description
   a. **Infiltration** is a form of tissue damage; it may also called *extravasation*.
   b. **Infiltration** is seepage of the IV fluid out of the vein and into the surrounding interstitial spaces.
   c. **Infiltration** occurs when an access device has become dislodged or perforates the wall of the vein or when venous backpressure occurs because of a clot or venospasm.
2. Prevention and interventions
   a. Avoid venipuncture over an area of flexion.

b. Anchor the cannula and a loop of tubing securely with tape.

c. Use an armboard or splint as needed if the client is restless or active.

d. Monitor the IV rate for a decrease or a cessation of flow.

e. Evaluate the IV site for **infiltration** by occluding the vein proximal to the IV site. If the IV fluid continues to flow, the cannula is probably outside the vein (infiltrated); if the IV flow stops after occlusion of the vein, the IV device is still in the vein.

f. Lower the IV fluid container below the IV site, and monitor for the appearance of blood in the IV tubing; if blood appears, the IV device is most likely in the vein.

g. If **infiltration** has occurred, remove the IV device immediately; elevate the extremity and apply compresses (warm or cool, depending on the IV solution that was infusing and the physician's prescription) over the affected area.

h. Do not rub an infiltrated area, which can cause hematoma.

H. Phlebitis and thrombophlebitis
1. Description
   a. **Phlebitis** is an inflammation of the vein that can occur from mechanical or chemical (medication) trauma or from a local infection.
   b. **Phlebitis** can cause the development of a clot (thrombophlebitis).
2. Prevention and interventions
   a. Use an IV cannula smaller than the vein, and avoid using very small veins when administering irritating solutions.
   b. Avoid using the lower extremities (legs and feet) as an access area for the IV.
   c. Avoid venipuncture over an area of flexion.
   d. Anchor the cannula and a loop of tubing securely with tape.
   e. Use an armboard or splint as needed if the client is restless or active.
   f. Change the venipuncture site every 48 to 72 hours, depending on agency policy.
   g. If **phlebitis** occurs, remove the IV device immediately and restart it in the opposite extremity; notify the physician if **phlebitis** is suspected, and apply warm, moist compresses, as prescribed.
   h. If thrombophlebitis occurs, do not irrigate the IV catheter; remove the IV, notify the physician, and restart the IV in the opposite extremity.

I. Tissue damage
1. Description
   a. Tissues most commonly damaged include the skin, veins, and subcutaneous tissue.
   b. Tissue damage can be uncomfortable and can cause permanent negative effects.

2. Prevention and interventions
   a. Use a careful and gentle approach when applying a tourniquet.
   b. Avoid tapping the skin over the vein when starting an IV.
   c. Monitor for ecchymosis when penetrating the skin with the cannula.
   d. Assess for allergies to tape or dressing adhesives.
   e. Monitor for skin color changes, sloughing of the skin, or discomfort at the IV site.
   f. Notify the physician if tissue damage is suspected.

⚠ Always document the occurrence of a complication, assessment findings, actions taken, and the client's response.

IX. CENTRAL VENOUS CATHETERS

A. Description
1. Central venous catheters (Fig. 14-6) are used to deliver hyperosmolar solutions, measure central venous pressure, infuse parenteral nutrition, or infuse multiple IV solutions or medications.
2. Catheter position is determined by radiography after insertion.
3. The catheter may have a single, double, or triple lumen.
4. The catheter may be inserted peripherally and threaded through the basilic or cephalic vein into the superior vena cava, inserted centrally through the internal jugular or subclavian veins, or surgically tunneled through subcutaneous tissue.
5. With multilumen catheters, more than one medication can be administered at the same time without incompatibility problems, and only one insertion site is present.

⚠ For central line insertion, tubing change, and line removal, place the client in the Trendelenburg's position if not contraindicated or in the supine position, and instruct the client to perform the Valsalva maneuver to increase pressure in the central veins when the IV system is open.

B. Tunneled central venous catheters
1. A more permanent type of catheter, such as the Hickman, Broviac, or Groshong catheter, is used for long-term IV therapy.
2. The catheter may be single lumen or multilumen.
3. The catheter is inserted in the operating room, and the catheter is threaded into the lower part of the vena cava at the entrance of the right atrium.
4. The catheter is fitted with an intermittent infusion device to allow access as needed and to keep the system closed and intact.

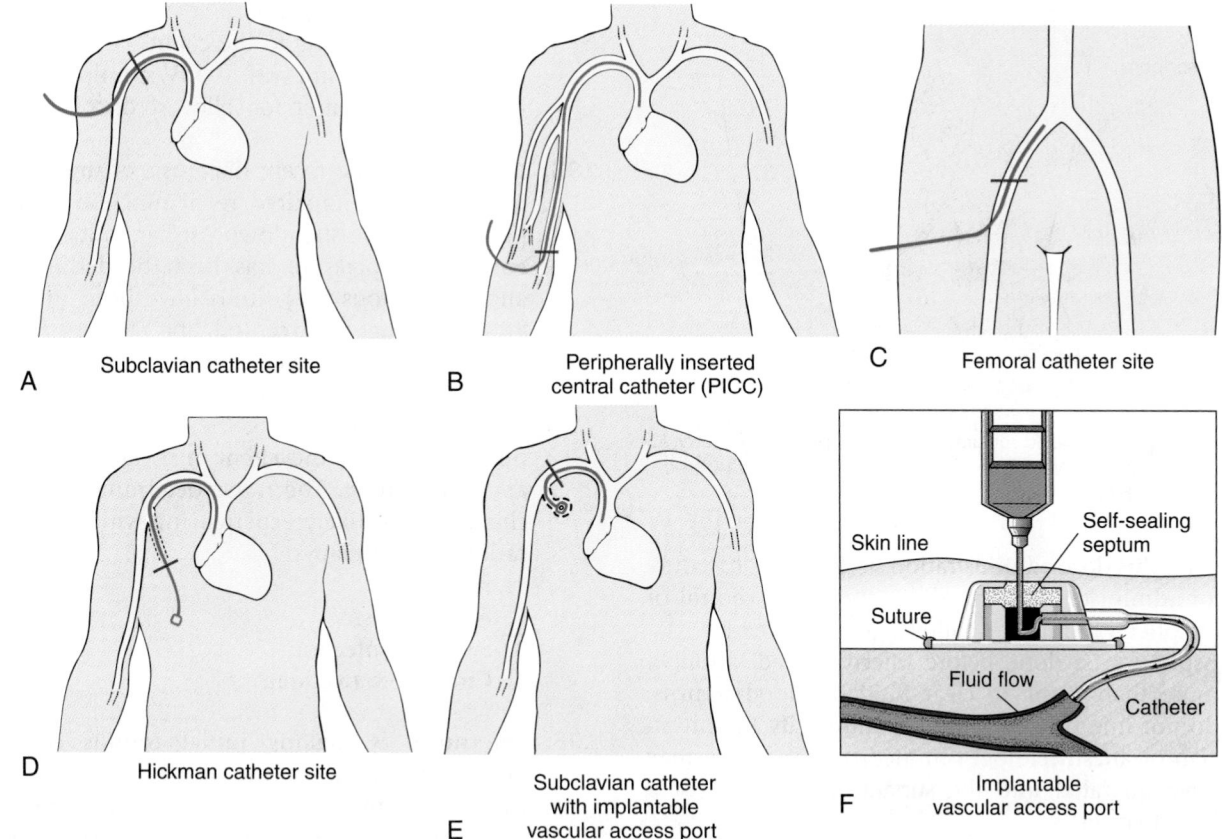

A Subclavian catheter site

B Peripherally inserted central catheter (PICC)

C Femoral catheter site

Skin line

Self-sealing septum

Suture

Fluid flow

Catheter

D Hickman catheter site

E Subclavian catheter with implantable vascular access port

F Implantable vascular access port

▲ **FIGURE 14-6** Central venous access sites. **A,** Subclavian catheter. **B,** Peripherally inserted central catheter (PICC). **C,** Femoral catheter. **D,** Hickman catheter. **E,** Subclavian catheter with implantable vascular access port. **F,** Implantable vascular access port. (From Kee, J. & Marshall, S. [2009]. *Clinical calculations: With applications to general and specialty areas* [6th ed.]. St. Louis: Saunders; **F** redrawn from Winters, B. [1984]. Implantable vascular access devices. *Oncology Nursing Forum*, 11, 25-30.)

5. Patency is maintained by flushing with a diluted heparin solution or normal saline solution, depending on the type of catheter, per agency policy.

C. Vascular access ports (implantable port)

1. Surgically implanted under the skin, ports such as a Port-a-Cath, Mediport, or Infusaport are used for long-term administration of repeated IV therapy.

2. For access, the port requires palpation and injection through the skin into the self-sealing port with a noncoring needle, such as a Huber-point needle.

3. Patency is maintained by periodic flushing with a diluted heparin solution as prescribed and as per agency policy.

D. PICC line

1. The catheter is used for long-term IV therapy, frequently in the home.

2. The basilic vein usually is used, but the median cubital and cephalic veins in the antecubital area also can be used.

3. The catheter is threaded so that the catheter tip may terminate in the subclavian vein or superior vena cava.

4. A small amount of bleeding may occur at the time of insertion and may continue for 24 hours, but bleeding thereafter is not expected.

5. **Phlebitis** is a common complication.

6. Insertion is below the heart level; therefore **air embolism** is not common.

X. EPIDURAL CATHETER (Fig. 14-7)

A. Catheter is placed in the epidural space for the administration of analgesics; this method of administration reduces the amount needed to control pain; therefore, the client experiences fewer side effects.

B. Assess client's vital signs, level of consciousness, and motor and sensory function.

C. Monitor insertion site for signs of infection and be sure that the catheter is secured to the client's skin and that all connections are taped to prevent disconnection.

D. Check physician's prescription regarding solution and medication administration.

E. For continuous infusion, monitor the electronic infusion device for proper rate of flow.

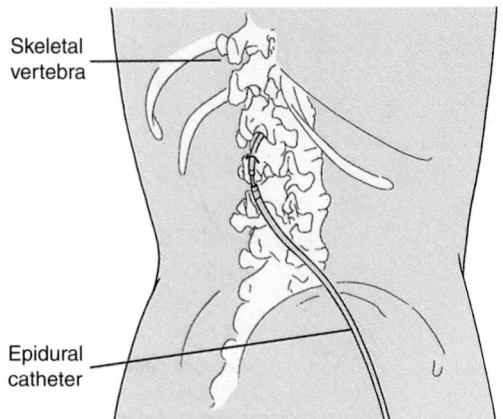

Skeletal vertebra

Epidural catheter

▲ **FIGURE 14-7** Tunneled epidural catheter. (From Elkin, M., Perry, A., & Potter, P. (2007). *Nursing interventions & clinical skills* [4th ed.]. St. Louis: Mosby.)

F. For bolus dose administration, follow the procedure for administering bolus doses through a central or peripheral IV line and follow agency procedure.

G. Aspiration is done before injecting medication; if more than 1 mL of clear fluid or blood returns, do not inject the medication and notify the physician or anesthesiologist immediately (catheter may have migrated into the subarachnoid space or a blood vessel).

 Contraindications to an epidural catheter and administration of epidural analgesia include skeletal and spinal abnormalities, bleeding disorders, use of anticoagulants, history of multiple abscesses, and sepsis.

🔘 MORE QUESTIONS ON THE CD!

Practice Questions

103. A client had a 1000-mL bag of 5% dextrose in 0.9% sodium chloride hung at 3 PM. The nurse making rounds at 3:45 PM finds that the client is complaining of a pounding headache and is dyspneic, is experiencing chills, and is apprehensive, with an increased pulse rate. The intravenous (IV) bag has 400 mL remaining. The nurse should take which action first?
1. Call the physician.
2. Slow the IV infusion.
3. Sit the client up in bed.
4. Remove the IV catheter.

104. The nurse has a prescription to hang an intravenous (IV) bag of 1000 mL 5% dextrose in water with 20 mEq potassium chloride. The nurse should plan to do which of the following immediately after injecting the potassium chloride into the port of the IV bag?

1. Rotate the bag gently.
2. Attach the tubing to the client.
3. Prime the tubing with the IV solution.
4. Check the solution for yellowish discoloration.

105. A client with the recent diagnosis of myocardial infarction and impaired renal function is recuperating on the step-down cardiac unit. The client's blood pressure has been borderline low and intravenous (IV) fluids have been infusing at 100 mL/hr via a central line catheter in the right internal jugular for approximately 24 hours to increase renal output and maintain the blood pressure. Upon entering the client's room, the nurse notes that the client is breathing rapidly and is coughing. The nurse determines that the client is most likely experiencing which complication of IV therapy?
1. Hematoma
2. Air embolism
3. Systemic infection
4. Circulatory overload

106. The nurse is making initial rounds on the nursing unit to assess the condition of assigned clients. The nurse notes that a client's intravenous (IV) site is cool, pale, and swollen, and the solution is not infusing. The nurse concludes that which of the following complications has occurred?
1. Infection
2. Phlebitis
3. Infiltration
4. Thrombosis

107. The nurse is inserting an intravenous line into a client's vein. After the initial stick, the nurse continues to advance the catheter if:
1. The catheter advances easily.
2. The vein is distended under the needle.
3. The client does not complain of discomfort.
4. Blood return shows in the backflash chamber of the catheter.

108. The nurse notes that the site of a client's peripheral intravenous (IV) catheter is reddened, warm, painful, and slightly edematous proximal to the insertion point of the IV catheter. After taking appropriate steps to care for the client, the nurse documents in the medical record that the client experienced:
1. Phlebitis of the vein
2. Infiltration of the IV line
3. Hypersensitivity to the IV solution
4. Allergic reaction to the IV catheter material

109. The nurse is preparing a continuous intravenous (IV) infusion at the medication cart. As the nurse goes to attach the distal end of the IV tubing to a needleless device, the exposed tubing drops and hits the top of the medication cart. Which of the following is the appropriate action by the nurse?
1. Obtain new IV tubing.
2. Attach a new needleless device.
3. Wipe the distal end of the tubing with Betadine.
4. Scrub the needleless device with an alcohol swab.

110. A physician has written a prescription to discontinue an intravenous (IV) line. The nurse obtains which of the following supplies from the unit supply area for applying pressure to the site after removing the IV catheter?
1. Elastic wrap
2. Betadine swab
3. Adhesive bandage
4. Sterile 2 × 2 gauze

111. A client has just undergone insertion of a central venous catheter at the bedside. The nurse would be sure to check the results of which of the following before initiating the flow rate of the client's intravenous (IV) solution at 100 mL/hr?
1. Serum osmolality
2. Serum electrolyte levels
3. Portable chest x-ray film
4. Intake and output record

112. A client involved in a motor vehicle crash presents to the emergency department with severe internal bleeding. The client is severely hypotensive and unresponsive. The nurse anticipates that which intravenous (IV) solution will most likely be prescribed to increase intravascular volume, replace immediate blood loss volume, and increase blood pressure?
1. 5% dextrose in lactated Ringer's
2. 0.33% sodium chloride (⅓ normal saline)
3. 0.225% sodium chloride (¼ normal saline)
4. 0.45% sodium chloride (½ normal saline)

113. The nurse provides a list of instructions to a client being discharged to home with a peripherally inserted central catheter (PICC). The nurse determines that the client needs further instructions if the client made which statement?
1. "I need to wear a Medic-Alert tag or bracelet."
2. "I need to have a repair kit available in the home for use if needed."
3. "I need to keep the insertion site protected when in the shower or bath."
4. "I need to keep my activity level to a minimum while this catheter is in place."

Alternate Item Format: Multiple Response
114. A client rings the call bell and complains of pain at the site of an intravenous (IV) infusion. The nurse assesses the site and determines that phlebitis has developed. The nurse should take which actions in the care of this client? **Select all that apply.**
❑ 1. Notifies the physician.
❑ 2. Removes the IV catheter at that site.
❑ 3. Applies warm moist packs to the site.
❑ 4. Starts a new IV line in a proximal portion of the same vein.
❑ 5. Documents the occurrence, actions taken, and the client's response

Alternate Item Format: Fill-In-The-Blank
115. The nurse is completing a time tape for a 1000-mL IV bag that is scheduled to infuse over 8 hours. The nurse has just placed the 11:00 AM marking at the 500-mL level. The nurse would place the mark for noon at which numerical level (mL) on the time tape?
_____ mL

ANSWERS
103. 2
Rationale: The client's symptoms are compatible with circulatory overload. This may be verified by noting that 600 mL has infused in the course of 45 minutes. The first action of the nurse is to slow the infusion. Other actions may follow in rapid sequence. The nurse may elevate the head of the bed to aid the client's breathing, if necessary. The nurse also notifies the physician. The IV catheter is not removed; it may be needed once the complication has been resolved.
Test-Taking Strategy: Use the process of elimination and note the strategic word *first*. This tells you that more than one or all of the options are likely to be correct actions and that the nurse needs to prioritize them according to a time sequence. You must be able to recognize the signs of circulatory overload. From this point, select the option that provides the intervention specific to circulatory overload. Review the immediate nursing actions in the event of circulatory overload if you had difficulty with this question.
Level of Cognitive Ability: Applying
Client Needs: Physiological Integrity
Integrated Process: Nursing Process—Implementation
Content Area: Leadership and Management—Delegating/Prioritizing

References: Ignatavicius, D., & Workman, M. (2010). *Medical-surgical nursing: Patient-centered collaborative care* (6th ed., p.230). Philadelphia: Saunders.

Potter, P., & Perry, A. (2009) *Fundamentals of nursing* (7th ed., p 1024). St Louis: Mosby.

104. 1
Rationale: After adding a medication to a bag of IV solution, the nurse should agitate or rotate the bag gently to mix the medication evenly in the solution. The nurse should then attach a completed medication label. The nurse can then prime the tubing. The IV solution should have been checked for discoloration before the medication was added to the solution. The tubing is attached to the client last.
Test-Taking Strategy: Note the strategic words *immediately after injecting*. They imply a correct time sequence, and you need to prioritize. Visualize and think through the steps of adding medication to an IV bag, and make your choice accordingly. Review the procedure for adding potassium chloride to an IV bag if you had difficulty with this question.
Level of Cognitive Ability: Applying
Client Needs: Physiological Integrity
Integrated Process: Nursing Process—Implementation
Content Area: Fundamental Skills—Medications/Blood & IV Therapy
References: Edmunds, M. (2010). *Introduction to clinical pharmacology* (6th ed., p. 119). St. Louis: Mosby.

Potter, P., & Perry, A. (2009). *Fundamentals of nursing* (7th ed., p. 756). St. Louis: Mosby.

105. 4
Rationale: Circulatory (fluid) overload is a complication of intravenous therapy. Signs include rapid breathing, dyspnea, a moist cough, and crackles. When circulatory overload is present, the client's blood pressure also increases. Hematoma is characterized by ecchymosis, swelling, and leakage at the IV insertion site, as well as hard and painful lumps at the site. Air embolism is characterized by tachycardia, dyspnea, hypotension, cyanosis, and decreased level of consciousness. Systemic infection is characterized by chills, fever, malaise, headache, nausea, vomiting, backache, and tachycardia.
Test-Taking Strategy: Focus on the data in the question. Noting that the client is experiencing rapid breathing and is coughing will assist in directing you to the correct option. Review the signs of circulatory overload if you had difficulty with this question.
Level of Cognitive Ability: Analyzing
Client Needs: Physiological Integrity
Integrated Process: Nursing Process—Analysis
Content Area: Critical Care
References: Ignatavicius, D., & Workman, M. (2010). *Medical-surgical nursing: Patient-centered collaborative care* (6th ed., p. 230). St. Louis: Saunders.

Potter, P., & Perry, A. (2009). *Fundamentals of nursing* (7th ed., p 1024). St Louis: Mosby.

106. 3
Rationale: An infiltrated IV is one that has dislodged from the vein and is lying in subcutaneous tissue. Pallor, coolness, and swelling are the results of IV fluid being deposited in the subcutaneous tissue. When the pressure in the tissues exceeds the pressure in the tubing, the flow of the IV solution will stop. The corrective action is to remove the catheter and start a new IV line at another site. Infection, phlebitis, and thrombosis are likely to be accompanied by warmth at the site, not coolness.
Test-Taking Strategy: Focus on the clinical manifestations identified in the question. Noting the strategic word *cool* in the question will direct you to option 3. Remember that pallor, coolness, and swelling are signs of infiltration. Review the signs of infiltration if you had difficulty with this question.
Level of Cognitive Ability: Analyzing
Client Needs: Physiological Integrity
Integrated Process: Nursing Process—Assessment
Content Area: Fundamental Skills—Medications/Blood & IV Therapy
References: Perry, A., & Potter, P. (2010). *Clinical nursing skills & techniques* (7th ed., p. 755). St. Louis: Mosby.

Potter, P., & Perry, A. (2009). *Fundamentals of nursing* (7th ed., p 1012). St Louis: Mosby.

107. 4
Rationale: The IV catheter has entered the lumen of the vein successfully when blood backflash shows in the IV catheter. The vein should have been distended by the tourniquet before the vein was cannulated. Client discomfort varies with the client, the site, and the nurse's insertion technique and is not a reliable measure of catheter placement. The nurse should not advance the catheter until placement in the vein is verified by blood return.
Test-Taking Strategy: Use the process of elimination, focusing on the subject of the question: correct placement of an IV catheter. Noting the strategic words *blood return* in option 4 will direct you to this option because a blood return is expected if the catheter is in a vein. Review the steps for inserting an IV catheter if you had difficulty with this question.
Level of Cognitive Ability: Applying
Client Needs: Physiological Integrity
Integrated Process: Nursing Process—Implementation
Content Area: Fundamental Skills—Medications/Blood & IV Therapy
Reference: Potter, P., & Perry, A. (2009). *Fundamentals of nursing* (7th ed., p 1000). St Louis: Mosby.

108. 1
Rationale: Phlebitis at an IV site can be distinguished by client discomfort at the site and by redness, warmth, and swelling proximal to the catheter. If phlebitis occurs, the nurse should discontinue the IV line and insert a new IV line at a different site. Coolness at the site would be noted if the IV catheter was infiltrated. An allergic reaction produces a rash, redness, and itching. A major reaction, such as hypersensitivity, can cause dyspnea, a swollen tongue, and cyanosis.
Test-Taking Strategy: Use the process of elimination. Options 3 and 4 are comparable or alike and therefore are eliminated first. Choose option 1 over option 2 after recalling that warmth is noted with phlebitis and coolness is noted with infiltration. Review the signs and symptoms of phlebitis if you had difficulty with this question.
Level of Cognitive Ability: Analyzing
Client Needs: Physiological Integrity

Integrated Process: Communication and Documentation
Content Area: Fundamental Skills—Medications/Blood & IV Therapy
Reference: Perry, A., & Potter, P. (2010). *Clinical nursing skills & techniques* (7th ed., p. 755). St. Louis: Mosby.

109. 1

Rationale: The nurse should obtain a new IV tubing because contamination has occurred and could cause systemic infection to the client. Wiping with Betadine is insufficient and is contraindicated because the tubing will be attached directly to a catheter in the client's vein. The needleless device has not been contaminated and does not need replacement or cleaning.
Test-Taking Strategy: Use the process of elimination and knowledge of basic infection control measures and IV therapy concepts to answer this question. Clearly, only one option is correct. Remember that if an item is contaminated, discard it and obtain a new sterile item. Review surgical aseptic technique if you had difficulty with this question.
Level of Cognitive Ability: Applying
Client Needs: Safe and Effective Care Environment
Integrated Process: Nursing Process—Implementation
Content Area: Fundamental Skills—Medications/Blood & IV Therapy
Reference: Perry, A., & Potter, P. (2010). *Clinical nursing skills & techniques* (7th ed., pp. 188, 742). St. Louis: Mosby.

110. 4

Rationale: A dry sterile dressing such as a sterile 2 × 2 is used to apply pressure to the discontinued IV site. This material is absorbent, sterile, and nonirritating. A Betadine swab would irritate the opened puncture site and would not stop the blood flow. An adhesive bandage or elastic wrap may be used to cover the site once hemostasis has occurred.
Test-Taking Strategy: Use the process of elimination and note the strategic words *applying pressure*. Visualize this procedure, thinking about each of the items identified in the options to direct you to option 4. Review the procedure for removing an IV catheter if you had difficulty with this question.
Level of Cognitive Ability: Applying
Client Needs: Physiological Integrity
Integrated Process: Nursing Process—Implementation
Content Area: Fundamental Skills—Medications/Blood & IV Therapy
Reference: Perry, A., & Potter, P. (2010). *Clinical nursing skills & techniques* (7th ed., p. 770). St. Louis: Mosby.

111. 3

Rationale: Before beginning administration of IV solution, the nurse should assess whether the chest radiograph reveals that the central catheter is in the proper place. This is necessary to prevent infusion of IV fluid into pulmonary or subcutaneous tissues. The other options represent items that are useful for the nurse to be aware of in the general care of this client, but they do not relate to this procedure.
Test-Taking Strategy: Use the process of elimination and note the words *central venous catheter at the bedside*. Recalling the potential complications associated with the insertion of central venous catheters will direct you to option 3. Review the principles of care for a central venous catheter after insertion if you had difficulty with this question.
Level of Cognitive Ability: Applying
Client Needs: Physiological Integrity
Integrated Process: Nursing Process—Assessment
Content Area: Fundamental Skills—Medications/Blood & IV Therapy
References: Ignatavicius, D., & Workman, M. (2010). *Medical-surgical nursing: Patient-centered collaborative care* (6th ed., pp. 217, 222). St. Louis: Saunders.
  Perry, A., & Potter, P. (2010). *Clinical nursing skills & techniques* (7th ed., p. 780). St. Louis: Mosby.

112. 1

Rationale: The goal of therapy with this client is to expand intravascular volume as quickly as possible. The 5% dextrose in lactated Ringer's (hypertonic solution) would increase intravascular volume and immediately replace lost fluid volume until a transfusion could be administered, resulting in an increase in the client's blood pressure. The solutions in options 2, 3, and 4 would not be given to this client because they are hypotonic solutions and, instead of increasing intravascular space, the solutions would move into the cells via osmosis.
Test-Taking Strategy: Focus on the data in the question, noting that the client requires increased intravascular volume. Recalling IV fluid types and how hypotonic and hypertonic solutions function within the intravascular space will direct you to the correct option. Review these types of IV fluids if you had difficulty with this question.
Level of Cognitive Ability: Understanding
Client Needs: Physiological Integrity
Integrated Process: Nursing Process—Planning
Content Area: Critical Care
Reference: Perry, A., & Potter, P. (2010). *Clinical nursing skills & techniques* (7th ed., pp. 741–742). St. Louis: Mosby.

113. 4

Rationale: The client should be taught that only minor activity restrictions apply with this type of catheter. The client should protect the site during bathing and should carry or wear a Medic-Alert identification. The client should have a repair kit in the home for use as needed because the catheter is for long-term use.
Test-Taking Strategy: Note the strategic words *needs further instructions*. These words indicate a negative event query and the need to select the incorrect client statement. Recalling that the PICC is for long-term use will assist in directing you to option 4. To keep activity to a minimum with such a catheter is unreasonable. Review home care instructions for a client with a PICC if you had difficulty with this question.
Level of Cognitive Ability: Evaluating
Client Needs: Physiological Integrity
Integrated Process: Teaching and Learning
Content Area: Fundamental Skills—Medications/Blood & IV Therapy
Reference: Perry, A., & Potter, P. (2010). *Clinical nursing skills & techniques* (7th ed., pp. 756, 765). St. Louis: Mosby.

ALTERNATE ITEM FORMAT: MULTIPLE RESPONSE

114. 1, 2, 3, 5

Rationale: Phlebitis is an inflammation of the vein that can occur from mechanical or chemical (medication) trauma or from a local infection and can cause the development of a clot (thrombophlebitis). The nurse should remove the IV at the phlebitic site and apply warm moist compresses to the area to speed resolution of the inflammation. Because phlebitis has occurred, the nurse also notifies the physician about the IV complication. The nurse should restart the IV in a vein other than the one that has developed phlebitis. Finally, the nurse documents the occurrence, actions taken, and the client's response

Test-Taking Strategy: Focus on the subject: actions to take if phlebitis occurs. Recall that phlebitis is an inflammation of the vein. This will assist in eliminating option 4 because an IV should be restarted in a vein other than the one that has developed phlebitis. Review nursing interventions related to the occurrence of phlebitis if you had difficulty with this question.

Level of Cognitive Ability: Applying
Client Needs: Physiological Integrity
Integrated Process: Nursing Process—Implementation
Content Area: Fundamental Skills—Medications/Blood & IV Therapy

Reference: Perry, A., & Potter, P. (2010). *Clinical nursing skills & techniques* (7th ed., p. 755). St. Louis: Mosby.

ALTERNATE ITEM FORMAT: FILL-IN-THE-BLANK

115. 375

Rationale: If the IV is scheduled to run over 8 hours, then the hourly rate is 125 mL/hr. Using 500 mL as the reference point, the next hourly marking would be at 375 mL, which is 125 mL less than 500.

Test-Taking Strategy: Use basic principles related to pharmacology math and IV administration to answer this question. Subtract 125 from 500 to yield 375. If this question was difficult, review the procedure for marking an IV solution by using a time tape.

Level of Cognitive Ability: Applying
Client Needs: Physiological Integrity
Integrated Process: Nursing Process—Implementation
Content Area: Fundamental Skills—Medications/Blood & IV Therapy

References: Edmunds, M. (2010). *Introduction to clinical pharmacology* (6th ed., p. 119). St. Louis: Mosby.

Potter, P., & Perry, A. (2009). *Fundamentals of nursing* (7th ed., p. 756). St. Louis: Mosby.

Administration of Blood Products

PYRAMID TERMS

ABO A type of antigen system. The ABO type of the donor should be compatible with the recipient's. Type A can match with type A or O; type B can match with type B or O; type O can match only with type O; type AB can match with type A, B, AB, or O.

autologous donation A donation of the client's own blood before a scheduled procedure.

blood salvage An autologous donation that involves suctioning blood from body cavities, joint spaces, or other closed body sites during a procedure.

circulatory overload A complication resulting from the infusion of blood at a rate too rapid for the size, age, cardiac status, or clinical condition of the recipient.

compatibility Matching of blood from two persons by two different types of antigen systems, ABO and Rh, present on the membrane surface of the red blood cells, to prevent a transfusion reaction.

crossmatching The testing of the donor's blood and the recipient's blood for compatibility.

designated donor A compatible donor who has been selected by the recipient.

fresh-frozen plasma A blood product administered to increase the level of clotting factors in clients with such a deficiency.

iron overload A delayed transfusion complication that occurs in clients who receive multiple blood transfusions, such as clients with anemia or thrombocytopenia.

platelets A blood product administered to clients with low platelet counts and to thrombocytopenic clients who are bleeding actively or are scheduled for an invasive procedure.

red blood cells A blood product used to replace erythrocytes lost as a result of trauma or surgical interventions or in clients with bone marrow suppression.

Rh factor Rh stands for *rhesus factor*. A person having the factor is Rh positive; a person lacking the factor is Rh negative. The presence or absence of Rh antigens on the surface of red blood cells determines the classification as Rh positive or Rh negative.

septicemia The presence of infective agents or their toxins in the bloodstream. Septicemia is a serious infection and must be treated promptly; otherwise, the infection leads to circulatory collapse, profound shock, and death.

transfusion reaction A hemolytic reaction caused by blood type or Rh incompatibility. An allergic transfusion reaction most often occurs in clients with a history of allergy. A febrile transfusion reaction most commonly occurs in clients with antibodies directed against the transfused white blood cells. A bacterial transfusion reaction occurs after transfusion of contaminated blood products.

THE PYRAMID TO SUCCESS

Pyramid Points focus on the safe administration of blood components, managing and providing care related to the procedure for administering blood components, and monitoring for complications. Focus is on the safe procedure for administering blood products and on the signs and symptoms of transfusion reaction. Pyramid Points also focus on the immediate interventions if a transfusion reaction occurs, and evaluation and documentation of expected and unexpected effects of the therapy.

CLIENT NEEDS

Safe and Effective Care Environment

Establishing priorities of care
Ensuring ethical practice and legal responsibilities
Handling of hazardous and infectious materials
Identifying the client prior to the administration of the blood product
Implementing standard, transmission-based precautions, and surgical asepsis
Maintaining continuity of care and providing close supervision during a blood transfusion
Obtaining informed consent for the administration of blood products
Upholding client rights

Health Promotion and Maintenance

Identifying lifestyle choices related to receiving a blood transfusion
Providing client education about the procedure and the signs of a transfusion reaction

Psychosocial Integrity

Ensuring therapeutic interactions with the client regarding the procedure for blood administration

Identifying religious, spiritual, and cultural considerations related to blood administration

Physiological Integrity

Administering blood products safely

Assessing venous access devices for blood administration

Managing medical emergencies if a transfusion reaction or other complication occurs

Monitoring for complications related to blood administration

Monitoring laboratory values and documenting the client's response to receiving the blood product

I. TYPES OF BLOOD COMPONENTS

A. Packed **red blood cells** (PRBCs)
1. **Red blood cells** are a blood product used to replace erythrocytes; infusion time for 1 unit is usually between 2 and 4 hours.
2. Each unit increases the hemoglobin level by 1 g/dL and hematocrit by 2% to 3%; the change in laboratory values takes 4 to 6 hours after completion of the blood transfusion.
3. Evaluation of an effective response is based on the resolution of the symptoms of anemia and an increase in the erythrocyte count.

⚠ Washed red blood cells (depleted of plasma, platelets, and leukocykos) may be prescribed for a client with a history of allergic transfusion reactions or those who underwent hematopoietic stem cell transplant.

B. Platelets
1. **Platelets** are used to treat thrombocytopenia and platelet dysfunctions.
2. **Crossmatching** is not required but usually is done (platelet concentrates contain few **red blood cells**).
3. The volume in a unit of **platelets** may vary; always check the bag for the volume of the blood component (in milliliters).
4. **Platelets** are administered immediately upon receipt from the blood bank and are given rapidly, usually over 15 to 30 minutes.
5. Evaluation of an effective response is based on improvement in the platelet count, and platelet counts normally are evaluated 1 hour and 18 to 24 hours after the transfusion.

C. Fresh-frozen plasma
1. **Fresh-frozen plasma** may be used to provide clotting factors or volume expansion; it contains no **platelets**.
2. **Fresh-frozen plasma** is infused within 2 hours of thawing while clotting factors are still viable and is infused over a period of 15 to 30 minutes.

3. Rh **compatibility** and **ABO compatibility** are required for the transfusion of plasma products.
4. Evaluation of an effective response is assessed by monitoring coagulation studies, particularly the prothrombin time and the partial thromboplastin time, and resolution of hypovolemia.

D. Cryoprecipitates
1. Prepared from **fresh-frozen plasma,** cryoprecipitates can be stored for 1 year. Once thawed, the product must be used; 1 unit is administered over 15 to 30 minutes.
2. Used to replace clotting factors, especially factor VIII and fibrinogen
3. Evaluation of an effective response is assessed by monitoring coagulation studies and fibrinogen levels.

E. White blood cells (WBCs)
1. Used to treat a client with sepsis or a neutropenic client with an infection that is unresponsive to antibiotics
2. One unit—approximately 400 mL—is administered over 1 hour.
3. Evaluation of an effective response is assessed by monitoring the white blood cell count and differential counts.

⚠ Document the necessary information about the blood transfusion in the client's medical record (follow agency guidelines). Include the client's tolerance and response to the transfusion and the effectiveness of the transfusion.

II. TYPES OF BLOOD DONATIONS

A. Autologous
1. A donation of the client's own blood before a scheduled procedure is autologous; it reduces the risk of disease transmission and potential transfusion complications.
2. **Autologous donation** is not an option for a client with leukemia or bacteremia.
3. A donation can be made every 3 days as long as the hemoglobin remains within a safe range.
4. Donations should begin within 5 weeks of the transfusion date and end at least 3 days before the date of transfusion.

B. Blood salvage
1. **Blood salvage** is an autologous donation that involves suctioning blood from body cavities, joint spaces, or other closed body sites.
2. Blood may need to be "washed," a special process that removes tissue debris before reinfusion.

C. Designated donor
1. Designated donation occurs when recipients select their own compatible donors.
2. Donation does not reduce the risk of contracting infections transmitted by the blood; however, recipients feel more comfortable identifying their donors.

TABLE 15-1 Compatibility Chart for Red Blood Cell Transfusions

		Recipient			
		A	B	AB	O
D o n o r	A	X		X	
	B		X	X	
	AB			X	
	O	X	X	X	X

The ABO type of the donor should be compatible with the recipient's. Type A can receive from type A or O; type B from type B or O; type AB can receive from type A, B, AB, or O; type O only from type O.
From Ignatavicius, D., & Workman, M. (2010). *Medical-surgical nursing: Patient-centered collaborative care* (6th ed.). St. Louis: Saunders.

III. COMPATIBILITY (Table 15-1)

A. Client (the recipient) blood samples are drawn and labeled at the client's bedside at the time the blood sample is drawn; the client is asked to state his or her name, which is compared with the name on the client's identification band or bracelet.

B. The recipient's **ABO** type and Rh type are identified.

C. An antibody screen is done to determine the presence of antibodies other than anti-A and anti-B.

D. **Crossmatching** is done, in which donor **red blood cells** are combined with the recipient's serum and Coombs' serum; the crossmatch is compatible if no red blood cell agglutination occurs.

E. The universal red blood cell donor is O negative; the universal recipient is AB positive.

⚠ The donor's blood and the recipient's blood must be tested for compatibility. If the blood is not compatible, a life-threatening transfusion reaction can occur.

IV. INFUSION CONTROLLERS AND PUMPS

A. Infusion controllers and pumps may be used to administer blood products if they are designed to function with opaque solutions; special intravenous tubing is used specifically for blood products to prevent hemolysis of **red blood cells**.

B. Always consult manufacturer guidelines for how to use the controller or pump.

C. Special manual pressure cuffs designed specifically for blood product administration may be used to increase the flow rate, but it should not exceed 300 mm Hg.

D. Standard sphygmomanometer cuffs are not to be used to increase the flow rate because they do not exert uniform pressure against all parts of the bag.

V. BLOOD WARMERS

A. Blood warmers may be used to prevent hypothermia and adverse reactions when several units of blood are being administered.

B. Special warmers have been designed for this purpose, and only devices specifically approved for this use can be used.

⚠ If blood warming is necessary use only warming devices specifically designed and approved for warming blood products. Do not warm blood products in a microwave oven or in hot water.

VI. PRECAUTIONS AND NURSING RESPONSIBILITIES (Box 15-1)

⚠ Check the client's identity before administering a blood product. Be sure to check the physician's prescription, that the client has an appropriate venous access site, that crossmatching procedures have been completed, that an informed consent has been obtained, and that the correct client is receiving the correct type of blood.

VII. COMPLICATIONS (Box 15-2)

A. Transfusion reactions

1. Description
   a. A **transfusion reaction** is an adverse reaction that happens as a result of receiving a blood transfusion
   b. Types of transfusion reactions include hemolytic, allergic, febrile or bacterial reactions (**septicemia**), or transfusion-associated graft-versus-host disease (GVHD).

2. Signs of an immediate **transfusion reaction**
   a. Chills and diaphoresis
   b. Muscle aches, back pain, or chest pain
   c. Rashes, hives, itching, and swelling
   d. Rapid, thready pulse
   e. Dyspnea, cough, or wheezing
   f. Pallor and cyanosis
   g. Apprehension
   h. Tingling and numbness
   i. Headache
   j. Nausea, vomiting, abdominal cramping, and diarrhea

3. Signs of a **transfusion reaction** in an unconscious client
   a. Weak pulse
   b. Fever
   c. Tachycardia or bradycardia
   d. Hypotension
   e. Visible hemoglobinuria
   f. Oliguria or anuria

4. Delayed transfusion reactions
   a. Reactions can occur days to years after a transfusion.
   b. Signs include fever, mild jaundice, and a decreased hematocrit level.

⚠ Stay with the client for the first 15 minutes of the infusion of the blood and monitor the client for signs and symptoms of a transfusion reaction; the first 15 minutes of the transfusion are the most critical, and the nurse must stay with the client.

Box 15-1 Precautions and Nursing Responsibilities

General Precautions

A large volume of refrigerated blood infused rapidly through a central venous catheter into the ventricle of the heart can cause cardiac dysrhythmias.

No solution other than normal saline should be added to blood components.

Medications are never added to blood components or piggybacked into a blood transfusion.

To avoid the risk of septicemia, infusions (1 unit) should not exceed prescribed time for administration (2 to 4 hours for packed red blood cells); follow evidence-based practice guidelines and agency procedure.

The blood administration set should be changed with each unit of blood, or according to agency policy, to reduce the risk of septicemia.

Check the blood bag for the date of expiration; components expire at midnight on the day marked on the bag unless otherwise specified.

Inspect the blood bag for leaks, abnormal color, clots, and bubbles.

Blood must be administered as soon as possible (within 20 to 30 minutes) from its being received from the blood bank, because this is the maximal allowable time out of monitored storage.

Never refrigerate blood in refrigerators other than those used in blood banks; if the blood is not administered within 20 to 30 minutes, return it to the blood bank.

The recommended rate of infusion varies with the blood component being transfused and depends on the client's condition; generally blood is infused as quickly as the client's condition allows.

Components containing few red blood cells and platelets may be infused rapidly, but caution should be taken to avoid circulatory overload.

The nurse should measure vital signs and assess lung sounds before the transfusion and again after the first 15 minutes and every hour until 1 hour after the transfusion is completed.

Blood Bank Precautions

Blood will be released from the blood bank only to personnel specified by agency policy.

The name and identification number of the intended recipient must be provided to the blood bank, and a documented permanent record of this information must be maintained.

Blood should be transported from the blood bank to only one client at a time to prevent blood delivery to the wrong client.

Client Identity and Compatibility

Check the physician's prescription for the administration of the blood product.

The most critical phase of the transfusion is confirming product compatibility and verifying client identity.

Two licensed nurses need to check the physician's prescription, the client's identity, and the client's identification band or bracelet and number, verifying that the name

and number are identical to those on the blood component tag.

At the bedside, the nurse asks the client to state his or her name, and the nurse compares the name with the name on the identification band or bracelet.

The nurse checks the blood bag tag, label, and blood requisition form to ensure that ABO and Rh types are compatible.

If the nurse notes any inconsistencies when verifying client identity and compatibility, the nurse notifies the blood bank immediately.

Client Assessment

Assess for any cultural or religious beliefs regarding blood transfusions.

A Jehovah's Witness cannot receive blood or blood products; this group believes that blood transfusions have eternal consequences.

Ensure that an informed consent has been obtained.

Explain the procedure to the client and determine whether the client has ever received a blood transfusion or experienced any previous reactions to blood transfusions.

Check the client's vital signs; assess renal, circulatory, and respiratory status and the client's ability to tolerate intravenously administered fluids.

If the client's temperature is elevated, notify the physician before beginning the transfusion; a fever may be a cause for delaying the transfusion in addition to masking a possible symptom of an acute transfusion reaction.

Administration of the Transfusion

Maintain standard and transmission-based precautions and surgical asepsis as necessary.

Insert an intravenous (IV) line and infuse normal saline; maintain the infusion at a keep-vein-open rate.

An 18- or 19-gauge IV needle will be needed to achieve a maximum flow rate of blood products and prevent damage to red blood cells; if a smaller gauge needle must be used, red blood cells may be diluted with normal saline (check agency procedure).

A central venous catheter is an acceptable venous access option for blood transfusions; for a multilumen catheter, use the largest catheter port available or check the port size to ensure that it is adequate for blood administration.

Always check the bag for the volume of the blood component.

Blood products should be infused through administration sets designed specifically for blood; use a Y-tubing or straight tubing blood administration set that contains a filter designed to trap fibrin clots and other debris that accumulate during blood storage (Fig. 15-1).

Premedicate the client with acetaminophen (Tylenol) or diphenhydramine (Benadryl), as prescribed, if the client has a history of adverse reactions; if prescribed, oral medications should be administered 30 minutes before the transfusion is started, and intravenously administered medications may be given immediately before the transfusion is started.

Box 15-1 Precautions and Nursing Responsibilities—cont'd

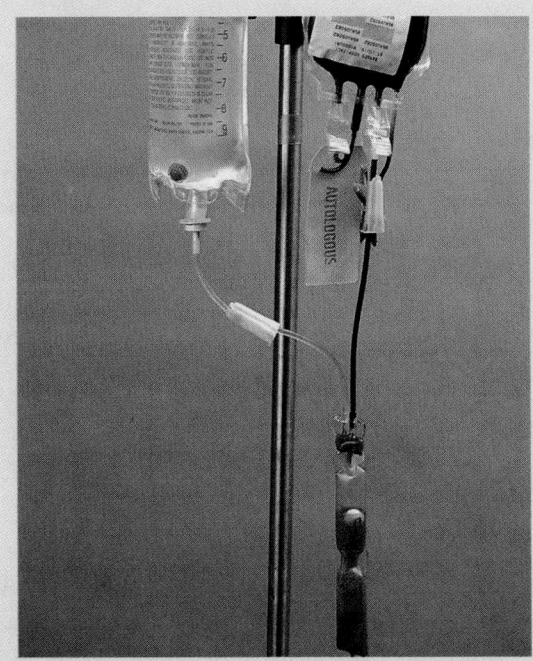

▲ **FIGURE 15-1** Tubing for blood administration has an in-line filter. (From Potter, P., & Perry, A. [2009]. *Fundamentals of nursing* [7th ed.]. St. Louis: Mosby.

Instruct the client to report anything unusual immediately.

Determine the rate of infusion by the physician's prescription or, if not specified, by agency policy.

Begin the transfusion slowly under close supervision; if no reaction is noted within the first 15 minutes, the flow can be increased to the prescribed rate.

During the transfusion, monitor the client for signs and symptoms of a transfusion reaction; the first 15 minutes of the transfusion are the most critical, and the nurse must stay with the client.

If a major ABO incompatibility exists or a severe allergic reaction occurs, the reaction is usually evident within the first 50 mL of the transfusion.

Document the client's tolerance to the administration of the blood product.

Monitor appropriate laboratory values and document effectiveness of treatment related to the specific type of blood product.

Reactions to the Transfusion

If a transfusion reaction occurs, stop the transfusion, change the IV tubing down to the IV site, keep the IV line open with normal saline, notify the physician and blood bank, and return the blood bag and tubing to the blood bank.

Do not leave the client alone, and monitor the client for any life-threatening symptoms.

Obtain appropriate laboratory samples according to agency policies, such as blood and urine samples (free hemoglobin indicates that red blood cells were hemolyzed).

Box 15-2 Complications of a Blood Transfusion

Transfusion reactions	Disease transmission
Circulatory overload	Hypocalcemia
Septicemia	Hyperkalemia
Iron overload	

▰▰▰ PRIORITY NURSING ACTIONS ▰▰▰

Actions to Take in the Care of a Client Experiencing a Transfusion Reaction

1. Stop the transfusion.
2. Change the intravenous (IV) tubing down to the IV site and keep the IV line open with normal saline.
3. Notify the physician and blood bank.
4. Stay with the client, observing signs and symptoms and monitoring vital signs as often as every 5 minutes.
5. Prepare to administer emergency medications as prescribed.
6. Obtain a urine specimen for laboratory studies (perform any other laboratory studies as prescribed).
7. Return blood bag, tubing, attached labels, and transfusion record to the blood bank.
8. Document the occurrence, actions taken, and the client's response.

If the client exhibits signs of a transfusion reaction, the nurse immediately stops the transfusion and changes the IV tubing down to the IV site to prevent the entrance of additional blood solution into the client. Normal saline solution is hung and infused to keep the IV line open in the event that emergency medications need to be administered. The physician is notified and the nurse also notifies the blood bank of the occurrence. The nurse stays with the client and monitors the client closely while other personnel obtain needed supplies to treat the client. As prescribed by the physician, the nurse administers emergency medications. The nurse then obtains a urine specimen for laboratory studies and any other laboratory studies as prescribed to check for free hemoglobin indicating that red blood cells were hemolyzed. The blood bag, tubing, attached labels, and transfusion record are returned to the blood bank so that the blood bank can check the items to determine the reason that the reaction occurred. Finally the nurse documents the occurrence, actions taken, and the client's response.

Reference: Potter, P., & Perry, A. (2009). *Fundamentals of nursing* (7th ed.). St. Louis: Mosby.

5. Interventions (see Priority Nursing Actions above)
   a. Stop the transfusion.
   b. Keep the intravenous line open with 0.9% (normal) saline.
   c. Notify the physician and blood bank.
   d. Remain with the client, observing signs and symptoms and monitoring vital signs as often as every 5 minutes.

e. Prepare to administer emergency medications such as antihistamines, vasopressors, fluids, and corticosteroids, as prescribed.

f. Obtain a urine specimen for laboratory studies (perform any other laboratory studies as prescribed).

g. Return blood bag, tubing, attached labels, and transfusion record to the blood bank.

⚠ Stop the transfusion immediately if a blood transfusion reaction is suspected.

B. Circulatory overload

1. Description: Caused by the infusion of blood at a rate too rapid for the client to tolerate

2. Assessment
   a. Cough, dyspnea, chest pain, and wheezing on auscultation of the lungs
   b. Headache
   c. Hypertension
   d. Tachycardia and a bounding pulse
   e. Distended neck veins

3. Interventions
   a. Slow the rate of infusion.
   b. Place the client in an upright position, with the feet in a dependent position.
   c. Notify the physician.
   d. Administer oxygen, diuretics, and morphine sulfate, as prescribed.
   e. Monitor for dysrhythmias.
   f. Phlebotomy also may be a method of prescribed treatment in a severe case.

⚠ Immediately slow the rate of infusion and place the client in an upright position, with the feet in a dependent position, if circulatory overload is suspected.

C. Septicemia

1. Description: Occurs with the transfusion of blood that is contaminated with microorganisms

2. Assessment
   a. Rapid onset of chills and a high fever
   b. Vomiting
   c. Diarrhea
   d. Hypotension
   e. Shock

3. Interventions
   a. Notify the physician.
   b. Obtain blood cultures and cultures of the blood bag.
   c. Administer oxygen, intravenous fluids, antibiotics, vasopressors, and corticosteroids prescribed.

D. Iron overload

1. Description: A delayed transfusion complication that occurs in clients who receive multiple blood

transfusions, such as clients with anemia or thrombocytopenia

2. Assessment
   a. Vomiting
   b. Diarrhea
   c. Hypotension
   d. Altered hematological values

3. Interventions
   a. Deferoxamine (Desferal), administered intravenously or subcutaneously, removes accumulated iron via the kidneys.
   b. Urine turns red as iron is excreted after the administration of deferoxamine; treatment is discontinued when serum iron levels return to normal.

⚠ Contact the physician immediately if a transfusion reaction or a complication of blood administration arises.

E. Disease transmission

1. A disease most commonly transmitted is hepatitis C, which is manifested by anorexia, nausea, vomiting, dark urine, and jaundice; the symptoms usually occur within 4 to 6 weeks after the transfusion.

2. Other infectious agents and diseases transmitted by blood transfusion include hepatitis B virus, human immunodeficiency virus, human herpesvirus type 6, Epstein-Barr virus, human T-cell leukemia, cytomegalovirus, and malaria.

3. Donor screening has greatly reduced the risk of transmission of infectious agents; additionally, antibody testing of donors for human immunodeficiency virus has greatly reduced the risk of transmission.

F. Hypocalcemia

1. Citrate in transfused blood binds with calcium and is excreted.

2. Assess serum calcium level before and after the transfusion.

3. Monitor for signs of hypocalcemia (hyperactive reflexes, paresthesias, tetany, muscle cramps, positive Trousseau's sign, positive Chvostek's sign).

4. Slow the transfusion and notify the physician if signs of hypocalcemia occur.

G. Hyperkalemia

1. Stored blood liberates potassium through hemolysis.

2. The older the blood, the greater the risk of hyperkalemia; therefore clients at risk for hyperkalemia, such as those with renal insufficiency or renal failure, should receive fresh blood.

3. Assess the date on the blood and the serum potassium level before and after the transfusion.

4. Monitor the potassium level and for signs of hyperkalemia (paresthesias, weakness, abdominal cramps, diarrhea, and dysrhythmias).

5. Slow the transfusion and notify the physician if signs of hyperkalemia occur.

 MORE QUESTIONS ON THE CD!

Practice Questions

116. Packed red blood cells have been prescribed for a client with low hemoglobin and hematocrit levels. The nurse takes the client's temperature before hanging the blood transfusion and records 100.6° F orally. Which of the following is the appropriate nursing action?
1. Begin the transfusion as prescribed.
2. Delay hanging the blood and notify the physician.
3. Administer an antihistamine and begin the transfusion.
4. Administer two tablets of acetaminophen (Tylenol) and begin the transfusion.

117. The nurse has received a prescription to transfuse a client with a unit of packed red blood cells. Before explaining the procedure to the client, the nurse asks which initial question?
1. "Have you ever had a transfusion before?"
2. "Why do you think that you need the transfusion?"
3. "Have you ever gone into shock for any reason in the past?"
4. "Do you know the complications and risks of a transfusion?"

118. A client receiving a transfusion of packed red blood cells (PRBCs) begins to vomit. The client's blood pressure is 90/50 mm Hg from a baseline of 125/78 mm Hg. The client's temperature is 100.8° F orally from a baseline of 99.2° F orally. The nurse determines that the client may be experiencing which complication of a blood transfusion?
1. Septicemia
2. Hyperkalemia
3. Circulatory overload
4. Delayed transfusion reaction

119. The nurse determines that a client is having a transfusion reaction. After the nurse stops the transfusion, which action should immediately be taken next?
1. Remove the intravenous (IV) line.
2. Run a solution of 5% dextrose in water.
3. Run normal saline at a keep-vein-open rate.
4. Obtain a culture of the tip of the catheter device removed from the client.

120. The nurse has just received a unit of packed red blood cells from the blood bank for transfusion to an assigned client. The nurse is careful to select tubing especially made for blood products, knowing that this tubing is manufactured with:
1. An air vent.
2. An in-line filter.
3. A microdrip chamber.
4. Tinted tubing to protect the blood from light.

121. A client has received a transfusion of platelets. The nurse evaluates that the client is benefiting most from this therapy if the client exhibits which of the following?
1. Increased hematocrit level
2. Increased hemoglobin level
3. Decline of elevated temperature to normal
4. Decreased oozing of blood from puncture sites and gums

122. The nurse has obtained a unit of blood from the blood bank and has checked the blood bag properly with another nurse. Just before beginning the transfusion, the nurse assesses which priority item?
1. Vital signs
2. Skin color
3. Urine output
4. Latest hematocrit level

123. The nurse has just received a prescription to transfuse a unit of packed red blood cells for an assigned client. Approximately how long will the nurse need to stay with the client to ensure that a transfusion reaction is not occurring?
1. 5 minutes
2. 15 minutes
3. 30 minutes
4. 45 minutes

124. A client has a prescription to receive a unit of packed red blood cells. The nurse should obtain which of the following intravenous (IV) solutions from the IV storage area to hang with the blood product at the client's bedside?
1. Lactated Ringer's
2. 0.9% sodium chloride
3. 5% dextrose in 0.9% sodium chloride
4. 5% dextrose in 0.45% sodium chloride

125. The nurse listening to morning report learns that an assigned client received a unit of granulocytes the previous evening. The nurse makes a note to assess the results of which of the following daily serum laboratory studies to assess the effectiveness of the transfusion?
1. Hematocrit level
2. Erythrocyte count
3. Hemoglobin level
4. White blood cell count

126. A client is brought to the emergency department having experienced blood loss related to an arterial laceration. Fresh-frozen plasma is prescribed and transfused to replace fluid and blood loss. The nurse understands that the rationale for transfusing fresh-frozen plasma in this client is:
1. To treat the loss of platelets
2. To promote rapid volume expansion
3. That the transfusion must be done slowly
4. That it will increase the hemoglobin and hematocrit levels

127. The nurse who is about to begin a blood transfusion knows that blood cells start to deteriorate after a certain period of time. Which of the following items is important to check regarding the age of blood cells before the transfusion is begun?
1. Expiration date
2. Presence of clots
3. Blood group and type
4. Blood identification number

128. A client requiring surgery is anxious about the possible need for a blood transfusion during or after the procedure. The nurse suggests to the client to do which of the following to reduce the risk of possible transfusion complications?
1. Give an autologous blood donation before the surgery.
2. Ask a friend or family member to donate blood ahead of time.
3. Take iron supplements before surgery to boost hemoglobin levels.
4. Request that any donated blood be screened twice by the blood bank.

129. A client with severe blood loss resulting from multiple trauma requires rapid transfusion of several units of blood. The nurse asks another health team member to obtain which device for use during the transfusion procedure to help reduce the risk of cardiac dysrhythmias?
1. Pulse oximetry
2. Cardiac monitor
3. Infusion controller
4. Blood-warming device

Alternate Item Format: Prioritizing (Ordered Response)

130. A unit of packed red blood cells has been prescribed for a client with low hemoglobin and hematocrit levels. The nurse notifies the blood bank of the prescription, and a blood specimen is drawn from the client for typing and cross-matching. The nurse receives a telephone call from the blood bank and is informed that the unit of blood is ready for administration. Number the actions in order of priority that the nurse should take to administer the blood. (Number 1 is the first action and number 6 is the last action.)
_____ Hang the bag of blood.
_____ Obtain the unit of blood from the blood bank.
_____ Ensure that an informed consent has been signed.
_____ Insert an 18- or 19- gauge intravenous catheter into the client.
_____ Verify the physician's prescription for the blood transfusion.
_____ Ask a licensed nurse to assist in confirming blood compatibility and verifying client identity.

ANSWERS
116. 2
Rationale: If the client has a temperature higher than 100° F, the unit of blood should not be hung until the physician is notified and has the opportunity to give further prescriptions. The physician likely will prescribe that the blood be administered regardless of the temperature, but the decision is not within the nurse's scope of practice to make. The nurse needs a physician's prescription to administer medications to the client.
Test-Taking Strategy: Use the process of elimination. Eliminate options 1, 3, and 4 because they all indicate beginning the transfusion. Additionally, options 3 and 4 indicate administering medication to the client, which is not done without a physician's prescription. Review the nursing responsibilities before administering a blood transfusion if you had difficulty with this question.
Level of Cognitive Ability: Applying
Client Needs: Physiological Integrity
Integrated Process: Nursing Process—Implementation

Content Area: Fundamental Skills—Medications/Blood & IV Therapy
Reference: Perry, A., & Potter, P. (2010). *Clinical nursing skills & techniques* (7th ed., pp. 788, 791). St. Louis: Mosby.

117. 1
Rationale: Asking the client about personal experience with transfusion therapy provides a good starting point for client teaching about this procedure. Options 3 and 4 are not helpful because they may elicit a fearful response from the client. Although determining whether the client knows the reason for the transfusion is important, option 2 is not an appropriate statement in terms of eliciting information from the client regarding an understanding of the need for the transfusion.
Test-Taking Strategy: Use the process of elimination and note that the strategic words in the question are *initial question*. This tells you that the correct option is the best starting point for discussion about the transfusion therapy. Options 3 and 4 have emotionally laden trigger words, including *gone into shock*

and *risks*, respectively, which make them incorrect. From the remaining options, focus on the strategic words and use therapeutic communication techniques to direct you to option 1. Review pretransfusion assessment procedures if you had difficulty with this question.
Level of Cognitive Ability: Applying
Client Needs: Physiological Integrity
Integrated Process: Nursing Process—Assessment
Content Area: Fundamental Skills—Medications/Blood & IV Therapy
Reference: Perry, A., & Potter, P. (2010). *Clinical nursing skills & techniques* (7th ed., p. 788). St. Louis: Mosby.

118. 1
Rationale: Septicemia occurs with the transfusion of blood contaminated with microorganisms. Signs include chills, fever, vomiting, diarrhea, hypotension, and the development of shock. Hyperkalemia causes weakness, paresthesias, abdominal cramps, diarrhea, and dysrhythmias. Circulatory overload causes cough, dyspnea, chest pain, wheezing, tachycardia, and hypertension. A delayed transfusion reaction can occur days to years after a transfusion. Signs include fever, mild jaundice, and a decreased hematocrit level.
Test-Taking Strategy: Focus on the data in the question. Noting that the client's temperature is elevated will direct you to option 1. Review the signs of complications of a blood transfusion and the indications of septicemia if you had difficulty with this question.
Level of Cognitive Ability: Analyzing
Client Needs: Physiological Integrity
Integrated Process: Nursing Process—Analysis
Content Area: Fundamental Skills—Medications/Blood & IV Therapy
Reference: Black, J., & Hawks, J. (2009). *Medical-surgical nursing: Clinical management for positive outcomes* (8th ed., pp. 2013, 2015). St. Louis: Saunders.

119. 3
Rationale: If the nurse suspects a transfusion reaction, the nurse stops the transfusion and infuses normal saline at a keep-vein-open rate pending further physician prescriptions. This maintains a patent IV access line and aids in maintaining the client's intravascular volume. The nurse would not remove the IV line because then there would be no IV access route. Obtaining a culture of the tip of the catheter device removed from the client is incorrect. First, the catheter should not be removed. Second, cultures are performed when infection, not transfusion reaction, is suspected. Normal saline is the solution of choice over solutions containing dextrose because saline does not cause red blood cells to clump.
Test-Taking Strategy: Note the strategic word *next*. Knowing that the IV should not be removed assists in eliminating options 1 and 4. Recalling that normal saline, not dextrose, is used when administering a unit of blood will direct you to option 3. Review care for the client experiencing a transfusion reaction if you had difficulty with this question.
Level of Cognitive Ability: Applying
Client Needs: Physiological Integrity
Integrated Process: Nursing Process—Implementation
Content Area: Leadership and Management—Delegating/Prioritizing
Reference: Perry, A., & Potter, P. (2010). *Clinical nursing skills & techniques* (7th ed., pp. 795–796). St. Louis: Mosby.

120. 2
Rationale: The tubing used for blood administration has an in-line filter. The filter helps ensure that any particles larger than the size of the filter are caught in the filter and are not infused into the client. The tubing should be macrodrip, not microdrip, to allow blood to flow freely through the drip chamber. An air vent is unnecessary because the blood bag is not made of glass. Option 4 is incorrect because blood does not need to be protected from light.
Test-Taking Strategy: Use the process of elimination. Read each option carefully and visualize the process of blood administration. Remember that tubing used for blood administration has an in-line filter. Review concepts related to tubing used for blood administration if you had difficulty with this question.
Level of Cognitive Ability: Applying
Client Needs: Physiological Integrity
Integrated Process: Nursing Process—Implementation
Content Area: Fundamental Skills—Medications/Blood & IV Therapy
References: Ignatavicius, D., & Workman, M. (2010). *Medical-surgical nursing: Patient-centered collaborative care* (6th ed., p. 918). St Louis: Saunders.
 Potter, P., & Perry, A. (2009). *Fundamentals of nursing* (7th ed., p. 1022). St Louis: Mosby.

121. 4
Rationale: Platelets are necessary for proper blood clotting. The client with insufficient platelets may exhibit frank bleeding or oozing of blood from puncture sites, wounds, and mucous membranes. Increased hemoglobin and hematocrit levels would occur when the client has received a transfusion of red blood cells. An elevated temperature would decline to normal after infusion of granulocytes if those cells were instrumental in fighting infection in the body.
Test-Taking Strategy: Use knowledge regarding the potential uses and benefits of the various types of blood product transfusions. Eliminate options 1 and 2 first because they are comparable or alike. From the remaining options, recalling that platelets are necessary for proper blood clotting will direct you to option 4. If this question was difficult, review the types of blood products available for transfusion and their indications for use.
Level of Cognitive Ability: Evaluating
Client Needs: Physiological Integrity
Integrated Process: Nursing Process—Evaluation
Content Area: Fundamental Skills—Medications/Blood & IV Therapy
Reference: Ignatavicius, D., & Workman, M. (2010). *Medical-surgical nursing: Patient-centered collaborative care* (6th ed., p. 920). St Louis: Saunders.

122. 1
Rationale: A change in vital signs during the transfusion from baseline may indicate that a transfusion reaction is occurring. This is why the nurse assesses vital signs before the procedure and again after the first 15 minutes. The other options do not identify assessments that are a priority just before beginning a transfusion.
Test-Taking Strategy: Note the strategic words *just before beginning the transfusion* and *priority*. This tells you that more than one of the options may be partially or totally correct

and that the correct option needs to be assessed for possible comparison during the transfusion. Use the ABCs—airway, breathing, and circulation—to direct you to option 1. Review the nursing interventions for preparing to administer a blood transfusion if you had difficulty with this question.
Level of Cognitive Ability: Applying
Client Needs: Physiological Integrity
Integrated Process: Nursing Process—Assessment
Content Area: Fundamental Skills—Medications/Blood & IV Therapy
Reference: Perry, A., & Potter, P. (2010). *Clinical nursing skills & techniques* (7th ed., p. 787). St. Louis: Mosby.

123. 2
Rationale: The nurse must remain with the client for the first 15 minutes of a transfusion, which is usually when a transfusion reaction may occur. This enables the nurse to detect a reaction and intervene quickly. The nurse engages in safe nursing practice by obtaining coverage for the other assigned clients during this time. Therefore options 1, 3, and 4 are incorrect time frames.
Test-Taking Strategy: Use knowledge regarding blood transfusion procedures to answer this question. Remember that the client must be monitored directly for the first 15 minutes of the transfusion. Review the nursing responsibilities involved in beginning a blood transfusion if you had difficulty with this question.
Level of Cognitive Ability: Applying
Client Needs: Physiological Integrity
Integrated Process: Nursing Process—Planning
Content Area: Fundamental Skills—Medications/Blood & IV Therapy
Reference: Ignatavicius, D., & Workman, M. (2010). *Medical-surgical nursing: Patient-centered collaborative care* (6th ed., p. 918). St Louis: Saunders.

124. 2
Rationale: Sodium chloride 0.9% (normal saline) is a standard isotonic solution used to precede and follow infusion of blood products. Dextrose is not used because it could result in clumping and subsequent hemolysis of red blood cells. Lactated Ringer's is not the solution of choice with this procedure.
Test-Taking Strategy: Use the process of elimination and eliminate options 3 and 4 first because they are comparable or alike in that both solutions contain dextrose. From the remaining options, remember that normal saline is the solution compatible with red blood cells. If this question was difficult, review the procedures related to the administration of blood.
Level of Cognitive Ability: Applying
Client Needs: Physiological Integrity
Integrated Process: Nursing Process—Implementation
Content Area: Fundamental Skills—Medications/Blood & IV Therapy
Reference: Perry, A., & Potter, P. (2010). *Clinical nursing skills & techniques* (7th ed., p. 796). St. Louis: Mosby.

125. 4
Rationale: The client who has neutropenia may receive a transfusion of granulocytes, or white blood cells. These clients

often have severe infections and are unresponsive to antibiotic therapy. The nurse notes the results of follow-up white blood cell counts to evaluate the effectiveness of the therapy. The nurse also continues to monitor the client for signs and symptoms of infection. Erythrocyte count and hemoglobin and hematocrit levels are determined after transfusion of packed red blood cells.
Test-Taking Strategy: Use the process of elimination. Recalling that granulocytes are a component of white blood cells will assist in directing you to option 4. In addition, note that options 1, 2, and 3 are comparable or alike in that these options all refer to erythrocytes. Review the types of blood products and their indications for use if you had difficulty with this question.
Level of Cognitive Ability: Evaluating
Client Needs: Physiological Integrity
Integrated Process: Nursing Process—Evaluation
Content Area: Fundamental Skills—Medications/Blood & IV Therapy
Reference: Ignatavicius, D., & Workman, M. (2010). *Medical-surgical nursing: Patient-centered collaborative care* (6th ed., p. 920). St Louis: Saunders.

126. 2
Rationale: Fresh-frozen plasma is often used for volume expansion as a result of fluid and blood loss. It does not contain platelets, so it is not used to treat any type of low platelet count disorder. It is rich in clotting factors and can be thawed quickly and transfused quickly. It will not specifically increase the hemoglobin and hematocrit level.
Test-Taking Strategy: Focus on the data in the question. Note the relationship between the words *experienced blood loss* and option 2. Review the purpose and use for fresh-frozen plasma if you had difficulty with this question.
Level of Cognitive Ability: Understanding
Client Needs: Physiological Integrity
Integrated Process: Nursing Process—Planning
Content Area: Fundamental Skills—Medications/Blood & IV Therapy
References: Ignatavicius, D., & Workman, M. (2010). *Medical-surgical nursing: Patient-centered collaborative care* (6th ed., p. 917). St Louis: Saunders.
Perry, A., & Potter, P. (2010). *Clinical nursing skills & techniques* (7th ed., p. 790). St. Louis: Mosby.

127. 1
Rationale: The nurse notes the expiration date on the unit of blood to ensure that the blood is fresh. Blood cells begin to deteriorate over time, so safe storage usually is limited to 35 days. Careful notation of the expiration date by the nurse is an essential part of the verification process before hanging a unit of blood. The nurse also notes the blood identification (unit) number, blood group and type, and client's name. The nurse also inspects the unit of blood for leaks, abnormal color, clots, and bubbles and returns the unit to the blood bank if clots are noted.
Test-Taking Strategy: Use the process of elimination and note that the strategic word in this question is *deteriorate*. To answer this question correctly, you must know which part of the pretransfusion verification procedure relates to the

freshness of the unit of blood. Keeping this in mind should direct you to option 1. Review the procedure for checking blood if you had difficulty with this question.
Level of Cognitive Ability: Applying
Client Needs: Physiological Integrity
Integrated Process: Nursing Process—Implementation
Content Area: Fundamental Skills—Medications/Blood & IV Therapy
Reference: Ignatavicius, D., & Workman, M. (2010). *Medical-surgical nursing: Patient-centered collaborative care* (6th ed., p. 919). St Louis: Saunders.

128. 1
Rationale: A donation of the client's own blood before a scheduled procedure is autologous. Donating autologous blood to be reinfused as needed during or after surgery reduces the risk of disease transmission and potential transfusion complications. The next most effective way is to ask a family member to donate blood before surgery. Blood banks do not provide extra screening on request. Preoperative iron supplements are helpful for iron deficiency anemia but are not helpful in replacing blood lost during the surgery.
Test-Taking Strategy: Use the process of elimination and focus on the subject, reducing the risk of possible transfusion complications. Recalling that an autologous transfusion is the collection of the client's own blood will direct you to option 1. Review the information related to disease transmission and blood donation procedures if you had difficulty with this question.
Level of Cognitive Ability: Applying
Client Needs: Physiological Integrity
Integrated Process: Nursing Process—Implementation
Content Area: Fundamental Skills—Medications/Blood & IV Therapy
Reference: Perry, A., & Potter, P. (2010). *Clinical nursing skills & techniques* (7th ed., p. 786). St. Louis: Mosby.

129. 4
Rationale: If several units of blood are to be administered, a blood warmer should be used. Rapid transfusion of cool blood places the client at risk for cardiac dysrhythmias. To prevent this, the nurse warms the blood using a blood-warming device. Pulse oximetry and cardiac monitoring equipment are useful for the early assessment of complications but do not reduce the occurrence of cardiac dysrhythmias. Electronic infusion devices are not helpful in this case because the infusion must be rapid, and infusion devices generally are used to control the flow rate. In addition, not all infusion devices are made to handle blood or blood products.
Test-Taking Strategy: Use the process of elimination and note the strategic words *rapid* and *reduce the risk*. These words tell you that the infusions will infuse quickly and that the correct option is the one that will minimize the risk of cardiac dysrhythmias. Eliminate options 1 and 2 first because these items are used to assess for rather than reduce the risk of complications. From the remaining options, use knowledge related to the complications of transfusion therapy and note the relationship between the words *several units of blood* in

the question and *blood warming device* in the correct option. Review the concepts related to the use of a blood warmer if you had difficulty with this question.
Level of Cognitive Ability: Applying
Client Needs: Physiological Integrity
Integrated Process: Nursing Process—Planning
Content Area: Fundamental Skills—Medications/Blood & IV Therapy
References: Ackley, B., Ladwig, G., Swan, B., & Tucker, S. (2008). *Evidence-based nursing care guidelines: Medical-surgical interventions* (p. 110). St. Louis: Mosby.
Potter, P., & Perry, A. (2009). *Fundamentals of nursing* (7th ed., p. 1023). St Louis: Mosby.

ALTERNATE ITEM FORMAT: PRIORITIZING (ORDERED RESPONSE)
130. 6, 4, 2, 3, 1, 5
Rationale: The nurse would first verify the physician's prescription for the blood transfusion and ensure that the client has been informed about the procedure and has signed an informed consent. Once this has been done, the nurse would ensure that at least an 18- or 19-gauge intravenous needle is inserted into the client. Blood has a thicker and stickier consistency than intravenous solutions, and using an 18- or 19-gauge catheter ensures that the bore of the catheter is large enough to prevent damage to the blood cells. Next, the blood is obtained from the blood bank, once the nurse is sure that the client has been informed and has an adequate access for administering the blood. Once the blood has been obtained, two registered nurses, or one registered and a licensed practical nurse (depending on agency policy), must together check the label on the blood product against the client's identification number, blood group, and complete name. This minimizes the risk of error in checking information on the blood bag and thereby minimizes the risk of harm or injury to the client. The nurse should measure vital signs and assess lung sounds and then hang the transfusion.
Test-Taking Strategy: Remember that a physician's prescription is needed for treatments and procedures. This will direct you to the first nursing action. Recalling that the client needs to be informed about a procedure will assist in determining that the next action would be to ensure that the client has signed a consent form. Next, remember that client preparation for the procedure is important. You would not obtain the blood from the blood bank unless the client was prepared; therefore the nurse would ensure that the client had an adequate intravenous access. Once blood is obtained, remember that verifying compatibility and client identity is critical before hanging the blood. Review the procedure for administering blood if you had difficulty with this question.
Level of Cognitive Ability: Applying
Client Needs: Physiological Integrity
Integrated Process: Nursing Process—Implementation
Content Area: Leadership and Management—Delegating/Prioritizing
Reference: Perry, A., & Potter, P. (2010). *Clinical nursing skills & techniques* (7th ed., p. 791). St. Louis: Mosby.

UNIT IV

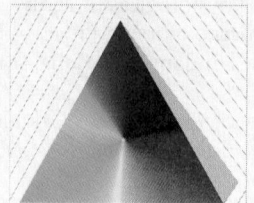

Fundamental Skills

Provision of a Safe Environment

PYRAMID TERMS

home safety Removing items from the home environment and avoiding situations or events that place the client at risk for accident or injury.

health care–associated (nosocomial) infections Infections acquired in the hospital or other health care facility that were not present or incubating at the time of the client's admission; also referred to as hospital-acquired infections.

physical hazards Any situation or event that places the client at risk for accident, injury, or death.

restraints (safety devices) Physical devices (that the client is unable to remove) applied to restrict a client's movement are known as *physical restraints*. Medications given to inhibit a specific behavior or movement are known as *chemical restraints*.

poison Any substance that impairs health or destroys life when ingested, inhaled, or otherwise absorbed by the body.

standard precautions Guidelines used by all health care providers for all clients to reduce the risk of infection for clients and caregivers.

transmission-based precautions Guidelines used in addition to standard precautions for specific syndromes that are highly suggestive of infections until a diagnosis is confirmed.

warfare agent Biological or chemical substance that can cause mass destruction or fatality.

THE PYRAMID TO SUCCESS

Safety and Infection Control is a subcategory of the Client Needs component, Safe and Effective Care Environment, of the NCLEX-RN examination test plan. Pyramid Points focus on safety measures, maintaining environmental safety in the home, preventing accidents, using safety devices, emergency response plans, priority nursing actions in the event of a disaster, and biological and chemical warfare agents. Pyramid Points also focus on standard and transmission-based precautions and the measures required to handle hazardous or infectious materials.

CLIENT NEEDS

Safe and Effective Care Environment

Emergency response plan and biological and chemical warfare agents

Ensuring that client's rights are upheld, including informed consent

Establishing priorities

Following guidelines regarding the use of safety devices

Handling hazardous and infectious materials safely

Maintaining precautions to prevent errors, accidents, and injury

Using ergonomic principles

Using standard and transmission-based precautions and surgical asepsis procedures

Health Promotion and Maintenance

Assisting clients and families to identify environmental hazards in the home

Performing home safety assessments

Teaching clients and families about accident prevention

Teaching clients and families about measures to be implemented in an emergency or disaster

Teaching clients and families about preventing the spread of infection

Psychosocial Integrity

Assessing the client for sensory and perceptual alterations

Identifying cultural and religious lifestyles

Identifying support systems

Physiological Integrity

Assisting the client with activities of daily living

Implementing priority nursing actions in an emergency or disaster

Managing and providing care to clients with infectious diseases

Providing comfort and assistance to the client

Using assistive devices to prevent injury

Actions to Take in the Event of a Fire
1. Rescue clients who are in immediate danger.
2. Activate the fire alarm.
3. Confine the fire.
4. Extinguish the fire: obtain the fire extinguisher.
5. Pull the pin on the fire extinguisher.
6. Aim at the base of the fire.
7. Squeeze the extinguisher handle.
8. Sweep extinguisher from side to side to coat the area of the fire evenly.

Remember the mnemonic *RACE* to prioritize in the event of a fire. *R* is rescue clients in immediate danger, *A* is alarm (sound the alarm), *C* is confine the fire by closing all doors, and *E* is extinguish. To properly use the fire extinguisher, remember the mnemonic *PASS* to prioritize in the use of a fire extinguisher. *P* is pull the pin, *A* is aim at the base of the fire, *S* is squeeze the handle, and *SS* is sweep from side to side to coat the area evenly.

Reference: Potter, P., & Perry, A. (2009). *Fundamentals of nursing* (7th ed., pp. 839-841). St. Louis: Mosby.

I. ENVIRONMENTAL SAFETY

A. Fire safety (see Priority Nursing Actions)
  1. Keep open spaces free of clutter.
  2. Clearly mark fire exits.
  3. Know the locations of all fire alarms, exits, and extinguishers (Table 16-1; also see Priority Nursing Actions).
  4. Know the telephone number for reporting fires.
  5. Know the fire drill and evacuation plan of the agency.
  6. Never use the elevator in the event of a fire.
  7. Turn off oxygen and appliances in the vicinity of the fire.
  8. In the event of a fire, if a client is on life support, maintain respiratory status manually with an Ambu bag (resuscitation bag) until the client is moved away from the threat of the fire and can be placed back on life support.
  9. In the event of a fire, ambulatory clients can be directed to walk by themselves to a safe area and, in some cases, may be able to assist in moving clients in wheelchairs.
  10. Bedridden clients generally are moved from the scene of a fire by stretcher, their bed, or wheelchair.
  11. If a client must be carried from the area of a fire, appropriate transfer techniques need to be used.
  12. If fire department personnel are at the scene of the fire, they will help evacuate clients.

⚠ Remember the mnemonic *RACE* to set priorities in the event of a fire and the mnemonic *PASS* to use a fire extinguisher.

TABLE 16-1 Types of Fire Extinguishers

Type	Class of Fire
A	Wood, cloth, upholstery, paper, rubbish, plastic
B	Flammable liquids or gases, grease, tar, oil-based paint
C	Electrical equipment

B. Electrical safety
  1. Electrical equipment must be maintained in good working order and should be grounded; otherwise it presents a **physical hazard**
  2. Use a three-pronged electrical cord.
  3. In a three-pronged electrical cord, the third longer prong of the cord is the ground; the other two prongs carry the power to the piece of electrical equipment.
  4. Check electrical cords and outlets for exposed, frayed, or damaged wires.
  5. Avoid overloading any circuit.
  6. Read warning labels on all equipment; never operate unfamiliar equipment.
  7. Use safety extension cords only when absolutely necessary, and tape them to the floor with electrical tape.
  8. Never run electrical wiring under carpets.
  9. Never pull a plug by using the cord; always grasp the plug itself.
  10. Never use electrical appliances near sinks, bathtubs, or other water sources.
  11. Always disconnect a plug from the outlet before cleaning equipment or appliances.
  12. If a client receives an electrical shock, turn off the electricity before touching the client.

⚠ Any electrical equipment that the client brings into the health care facility must be inspected for safety before use.

C. Radiation safety
  1. Know the protocols and guidelines of the health care agency.
  2. Label potentially radioactive material.
  3. To reduce exposure to radiation, do the following:
     a. Limit the time spent near the source.
     b. Make the distance from the source as great as possible.
     c. Use a shielding device such as a lead apron.
  4. Monitor radiation exposure with a film (dosimeter) badge.
  5. Place the client who has a radiation implant in a private room.
  6. Never touch dislodged radiation implants.
  7. Keep all linens in the client's room until the implant is removed.

Box 16-1 Physiological Changes in Older Clients That Increase Risk of Accidents

Musculoskeletal Changes
Strength and function of muscles decrease.
Joints become less mobile and bones become brittle.
Postural changes and limited range of motion occur.

Nervous System Changes
Voluntary and autonomic reflexes become slower.
Decreased ability to respond to multiple stimuli occurs.
Decreased sensitivity to touch occurs.

Sensory Changes
Decreased vision and lens accommodation and cataracts develop.
Delayed transmission of hot and cold impulses occurs.
Impaired hearing develops, with high-frequency tones less perceptible.

Genitourinary Changes
Increased nocturia and occurrences of incontinence may occur.

Modified from Potter A, & Perry, P. (2009). *Fundamentals of nursing* (7th ed., p. 816). St. Louis: Mosby. (Modified from Ebersole, P., Hess, P., & Luggen, A. [2004] *Toward healthy aging* [6th ed.]. St. Louis: Mosby.)

D. Disposal of infectious wastes
  1. Handle all infectious materials as a hazard.
  2. Dispose of waste in designated areas only, using proper containers for disposal.
  3. Ensure that infectious material is labeled properly.
  4. Dispose of all sharps immediately after use in closed, puncture-resistant disposal containers that are leakproof and labeled or color-coded.

⚠ Needles (sharps) should not be recapped, bent, or broken because of the risk of accidental injury (needle stick).

E. Physiological changes in the older client that increase the risk of accidents (Box 16-1)
F. Measures to prevent falls (Box 16-2)
G. Restraints (safety devices)
  1. **Restraints (safety devices)** are protective devices used to limit the physical activity of a client or to immobilize a client or an extremity for safety purposes.
  2. Physical **restraints** restrict client movement through the application of a device.
  3. Chemical **restraints** are medications given to inhibit a specific behavior or movement.
  4. Interventions
     a. Use alternative devices whenever possible, such as pressure-sensitive beds or chair pads with alarms or other types of bed or chair alarms.

Box 16-2 Measures to Prevent Falls

Assess the client's risk for falling.
Assign the client at risk for falling to a room near the nurses' station.
Alert all personnel to the client's risk for falling.
Assess the client frequently.
Orient the client to physical surroundings.
Instruct the client to seek assistance when getting up.
Explain the use of the call bell system.
Use safety devices such as bed or chair alarms that alert health care personnel.
Keep the bed in the low position with side rails adjusted to a safe position (follow agency policy).
Lock all beds, wheelchairs, and stretchers.
Keep clients' personal items within their reach.
Eliminate clutter and obstacles in the client's room.
Provide adequate lighting.
Reduce bathroom hazards.
Maintain the client's toileting schedule throughout the day.

  b. If safety devices are necessary, the physician's prescriptions should state the type of restraint, identify specific client behaviors for which **restraints** are to be used, and identify a limited time frame for use.
  c. Physicians' prescriptions for safety devices should be renewed within a specific time frame according to the policy of the agency.
  d. Safety devices are not to be prescribed PRN, that is, as needed.
  e. The reason for the safety device should be given to the client and the family, and their permission should be sought.
  f. Safety devices should not interfere with any treatments or affect the client's health problem.
  g. Use a half-bow or safety knot (quick release tie) to secure the device to the bed frame or chair, not to the side rails.
  h. Ensure that enough slack is on the straps to allow some movement of the body part.
  i. Assess skin integrity and neurovascular and circulatory status every 30 minutes and remove the safety device at least every 2 hours to permit muscle exercise and to promote circulation (follow agency policies).
  j. Continually assess and document the need for safety devices (Box 16-3).

⚠ A physician's prescription for use of a safety device is needed. Alternative measures for safety devices should always be used first.

  5. Alternatives to safety devices
     a. Orient the client and family to the surroundings.

Box 16-3 Documentation Points With Use of a Safety Device

Reason for safety device
Method of use for safety device
Date and time of application of safety device
Duration of use of safety device and client's response
Release from safety device with periodic exercise and cir-
culatory, neurovascular, and skin assessment
Assessment of continued need for safety device
Evaluation of client's response

b. Explain all procedures and treatments to the client and family.
c. Encourage family and friends to stay with the client, and use sitters for clients who need supervision.
d. Assign confused and disoriented clients to rooms near the nurses' station.
e. Provide appropriate visual and auditory sti-muli to the client, such as clocks, calendars, television, and a radio.
f. Place familiar items, such as family pictures, near the client's bedside.
g. Maintain toileting routines.
h. Eliminate bothersome treatments, such as tube feedings, as soon as possible.
i. Evaluate all medications that the client is receiving.
j. Use relaxation techniques with the client.
k. Institute exercise and ambulation schedules as the client's condition allows.

H. Poisons
1. A **poison** is any substance that impairs health or destroys life when ingested, inhaled, or other-wise absorbed by the body.
2. Specific antidotes or treatments are available only for some types of **poisons**.
3. The capacity of body tissue to recover from a **poison** determines the reversibility of the effect.
4. **Poison** can impair the respiratory, circulatory, central nervous, hepatic, gastrointestinal, and renal systems of the body.
5. The toddler, the preschooler, and the young school-age child must be protected from acci-dental poisoning.
6. In older adults, diminished eyesight and impaired memory may result in accidental ingestion of poisonous substances or an over-dose of prescribed medications.
7. A Poison Control Center phone number should be visible on the telephone in homes with small children; in all cases of suspected poisoning, the number should be called immediately.
8. Interventions
   a. Remove any obvious materials from the mouth, eyes, or body area immediately.

Box 16-4 Common Drug-Resistant Health-Care Associated Infections

Vancomycin-resistant enterococci
Methicillin-resistant *Staphylococcus aureus*
Multidrug-resistant tuberculosis

b. Identify the type and amount of substance ingested.
c. Call the Poison Control Center before attempting an intervention.
d. If the victim vomits or vomiting is induced, save the vomitus if requested to do so, and deliver it to the Poison Control Center.
e. If instructed by the Poison Control Center to take the person to the emergency depart-ment, call an ambulance.
f. Never induce vomiting following ingestion of lye, household cleaners, grease, or petroleum products.
g. Never induce vomiting in an unconscious victim.

⚠ The Poison Control Center should be called first before attempting an intervention.

II. HEALTH CARE–ASSOCIATED (NOSOCOMIAL) INFECTIONS (Box 16-4)

A. **Health care–associated (nosocomial) infections** also are referred to as *hospital-acquired infections*.
B. Such infections are infections acquired in a hospital or other health care facility that were not present or incubating at the time of a client's admission.
C. Illness impairs the normal defense mechanisms of the body.
D. The hospital environment provides exposure to a variety of virulent organisms that the client has not been exposed to in the past; therefore the client has not developed resistance to these organisms.
E. Infections can be transmitted by health care personnel who fail to practice proper handwashing procedures or fail to change gloves between client contacts.
F. At many health care agencies, dispensers containing an alcohol-based solution for hand rubs are mounted at the entrance to each client's room.

III. STANDARD PRECAUTIONS

A. Description
1. Nurses must practice **standard precautions** with all clients in any setting, regardless of the diag-nosis or presumed infectiousness.
2. **Standard precautions** include handwashing and the use of gloves, masks, eye protection, and gowns, when appropriate, for client contact.

3. These precautions apply to blood, all body fluids (whether or not they contain blood), secretions and excretions, nonintact skin, and mucous membranes.

B. Interventions

1. Wash hands between client contacts; after contact with blood, body fluids, secretions or excretions, nonintact skin, or mucous membranes; after contact with equipment or contaminated articles; and immediately after removing gloves.

2. Wear gloves when touching blood, body fluids, secretions, excretions, nonintact skin, mucous membranes, or contaminated items; remove gloves and wash hands between client care contacts.

3. Wear masks, eye protection, or face shields if client care activities may generate splashes or sprays of blood or body fluid.

4. Wear gowns if soiling of clothing is likely from blood or body fluid; wash hands after removing a gown.

5. Clean and reprocess client care equipment properly and discard single-use items.

6. Place contaminated linen in leak-proof bags and handle to prevent skin and mucous membrane exposure.

7. Use needleless devices or special needle safety devices whenever possible to reduce the risk of needle sticks and sharps injuries to health care workers.

8. Discard all sharp instruments and needles in a puncture-resistant container; dispose of needles uncapped or use a mechanical device for recapping the needle, if necessary and available.

9. Clean spills of blood or body fluids with a solution of bleach and water (diluted 1:10) or agency-approved disinfectant.

⚠ Handle all blood and body fluids from all clients as if they were contaminated.

IV. TRANSMISSION-BASED PRECAUTIONS

A. Transmission-based precautions include airborne, droplet, and contact precautions

B. Airborne precautions
1. Diseases
   a. Measles
   b. Chickenpox (varicella)
   c. Disseminated varicella zoster
   d. Tuberculosis
2. Barrier protection
   a. Single room is maintained under negative pressure; door remains closed except upon entering and exiting.
   b. Negative airflow pressure is used in the room, with a minimum of 6 to 12 air exchanges per hour depending on health care agency protocol.
   c. Ultraviolet germicide irradiation or high-efficiency particulate air filter is used in the room
   d. Health care workers wear mask or personal respiratory protection device.
   e. Mask placed on client when client is out of the room; client leaves the room only if necessary.

C. Droplet precautions
1. Diseases
   a. Adenovirus
   b. Diphtheria (pharyngeal)
   c. Epiglottitis
   d. Influenza, including H1N1 influenza
   e. Meningitis
   f. Mumps
   g. Mycoplasmal pneumonia or meningococcal pneumonia
   h. Parvovirus B19
   i. Pertussis
   j. Pneumonia
   k. Rubella
   l. Scarlet fever
   m. Sepsis
   n. Streptococcal pharyngitis
2. Barrier protection
   a. Private room or cohort client
   b. Use of a mask
   c. Mask placed on client when client is out of the room; client leaves the room only if necessary.

D. Contact precautions
1. Diseases
   a. Colonization or infection with a multidrug-resistant organism
   b. Enteric infections, such as *Clostridium difficile*
   c. Respiratory infections, such as respiratory syncytial virus
   d. H1N1 influenza: Infection can occur by touching something with flu viruses on it and then touching the mouth or nose.
   e. Wound infections
   f. Skin infections, such as cutaneous diphtheria, herpes simplex, impetigo, pediculosis, scabies, staphylococci, and varicella zoster
   g. Eye infection such as conjunctivitis
2. Barrier protection
   a. Private room or cohort client
   b. Use of gloves and a gown when in contact with the client

V. EMERGENCY RESPONSE PLAN AND DISASTERS

A. Know the emergency response plan of the agency.
B. *Internal disasters* are those in which the agency is in danger.
C. *External disasters* occur in the community, and victims are brought to the health care facility for care.

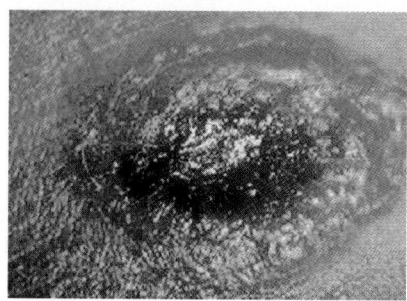

▲ **FIGURE 16-1** Anthrax. (From *Mosby's dictionary of medicine, nursing, & health professions* [8th ed.]. [2009]. St. Louis: Mosby.)

 D. When the health care agency is notified of a disaster, the nurse would follow the guidelines specified in the emergency response plan of the agency.

E. See Chapter 8 for additional information on disaster planning.

⚠ In the event of a disaster, the emergency response plan is immediately activated.

VI. BIOLOGICAL WARFARE AGENTS

A. A **warfare agent** is a biological or chemical substance that can cause mass destruction or fatality.

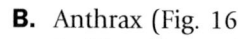 **B.** Anthrax (Fig. 16-1)

1. The disease is caused by *Bacillus anthracis* and can be contracted through the digestive system, abrasions in the skin, or inhalation through the lungs.

2. Anthrax is transmitted by direct contact with bacteria and spores; spores are dormant encapsulated bacteria that become active when they enter a living host (no person-to-person spread) (Box 16-5).

3. The infection is carried to the lymph nodes and then spreads to the rest of the body by way of the blood and lymph; high levels of toxins lead to shock and death.

4. In the lungs, anthrax can cause buildup of fluid, tissue decay, and death (fatal if untreated).

5. A blood test is available to detect anthrax (magnifies DNA from the blood sample and matches it to anthrax DNA).

6. Anthrax is usually treated with antibiotics such as ciprofloxacin (Cipro), doxycycline, or penicillin.

7. The vaccine has limited availability.

C. Smallpox (Fig. 16-2)

1. Smallpox is transmitted in air droplets and by handling contaminated materials and is highly contagious.

2. Symptoms begin 7 to 17 days after exposure and include fever, back pain, vomiting, malaise, and headache.

Box 16-5 Anthrax: Transmission and Symptoms

Skin

Spores enter the skin through cuts and abrasions and are contracted by handling contaminated animal skin products.

Infection starts with an itchy bump like a mosquito bite that progresses to a small liquid-filled sac.

The sac becomes a painless ulcer with an area of black, dead tissue in the middle.

Toxins destroy surrounding tissue.

Gastrointestinal

Infection occurs following the ingestion of contaminated undercooked meat.

Symptoms begin with nausea, loss of appetite, and vomiting.

The disease progresses to severe abdominal pain, vomiting of blood, and severe diarrhea.

Inhalation

Infection is caused by the inhalation of bacterial spores, which multiply in the alveoli.

The disease begins with the same symptoms as the flu, including fever, muscle aches, and fatigue.

Symptoms suddenly become more severe with the development of breathing problems and shock.

Toxins cause hemorrhage and destruction of lung tissue.

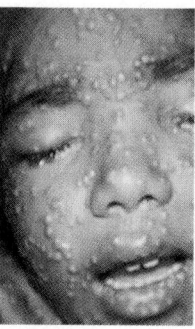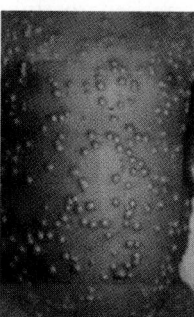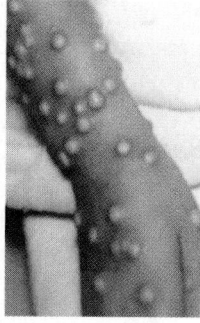

▲ **FIGURE 16-2** Smallpox. (From McKinney, E., James, S., Murray, S., & Ashwill, J. [2009]. *Maternal-child nursing* [3rd ed.]. St. Louis: Saunders. Courtesy of Centers for Disease Control and Prevention. [2002]. *Evaluating patients for smallpox.* Atlanta: Author.)

3. Papules develop 2 days after symptoms develop and progress to pustular vesicles that are abundant on the face and extremities initially.

4. A vaccine is available to those at risk for exposure to smallpox.

D. Botulism

1. Botulism is a serious paralytic illness caused by a nerve toxin produced by the bacterium *Clostridium botulinum* (death can occur within 24 hours).

2. Its spores are found in the soil and can spread through the air or food (improperly canned food) or via a contaminated wound.

3. Botulism cannot be spread from person to person.
4. Symptoms include abdominal cramps, diarrhea, nausea and vomiting, double vision, blurred vision, drooping eyelids, difficulty swallowing or speaking, dry mouth, and muscle weakness.
5. Neurological symptoms begin 12 to 36 hours after ingestion of foodborne botulism and 24 to 72 hours after inhalation and can progress to paralysis of the arms, legs, trunk, or respiratory muscles (mechanical ventilation is necessary).
6. If diagnosed early, foodborne and wound botulism can be treated with an antitoxin that blocks the action of toxin circulating in the blood.
7. Other treatments include induction of vomiting, enemas, and penicillin.
8. No vaccine is available.

E. Plague
1. Plague is caused by *Yersinia pestis*, a bacteria found in rodents and fleas.
2. Plague is contracted by being bitten by a rodent or flea that is carrying the plague bacterium, by the ingestion of contaminated meat, or by handling an animal infected with the bacteria.
3. Transmission is by direct person-to-person spread.
4. Forms include bubonic (most common), pneumonic, and septicemic (most deadly).
5. Symptoms usually begin within 1 to 3 days and include fever, chest pain, lymph node swelling, and a productive cough (hemoptysis).
6. The disease rapidly progresses to dyspnea, stridor, and cyanosis; death occurs from respiratory failure, shock, and bleeding.
7. Antibiotics are only effective if administered immediately; the usual medications of choice include streptomycin or gentamicin.
8. A vaccine is available.

F. Tularemia
1. Tularemia (also called *deer fly fever* or *rabbit fever*) is an infectious disease of animals caused by the bacillus *Francisella tularensis*.
2. The disease is transmitted by ticks, deer flies, or contact with an infected animal.
3. Symptoms include fever, headache, an ulcerated skin lesion with localized lymph node enlargement, eye infections, gastrointestinal ulcerations, or pneumonia.
4. Treatment is with antibiotics.
5. Recovery produces lifelong immunity (a vaccine is available).

G. Hemorrhagic fever
1. Hemorrhagic fever is caused by several viruses, including Marburg, Lassa, Junin, and Ebola.
2. The virus is carried by rodents and mosquitoes.

3. The disease can be transmitted directly by person-to-person spread via body fluids.
4. Symptoms include fever, headache, malaise, conjunctivitis, nausea, vomiting, hypotension, hemorrhage of tissues and organs, and organ failure.
5. No known specific treatment is available; treatment is symptomatic.

⚠ Anthrax is transmitted by direct contact with bacteria and spores and can be contracted through the digestive system, abrasions in the skin, or inhalation through the lungs.

VII. CHEMICAL WARFARE AGENTS

A. Sarin
1. Sarin is a highly toxic nerve gas that can cause death within minutes of exposure.
2. It enters the body through the eyes and skin and acts by paralyzing the respiratory muscles.
B. Phosgene is a colorless gas normally used in chemical manufacturing that if inhaled at high concentrations for a long enough period will lead to severe respiratory distress, pulmonary edema, and death.
C. Mustard gas is yellow to brown and has a garlic-like odor that irritates the eyes and causes skin burns and blisters.
D. Ionizing radiation
1. Acute radiation exposure develops after a substantial exposure to radiation.
2. Exposure can occur from external radiation or internal absorption.
3. Symptoms depend on the amount of exposure to the radiation and range from nausea and vomiting, diarrhea, fever, electrolyte imbalances, and neurological and cardiovascular impairment to leukopenia, purpura, hemorrhage, and death.

VIII. NURSE'S ROLE FOR EXPOSURE TO WARFARE AGENTS

A. Be aware that initially, a bioterrorism attack may resemble a naturally occurring outbreak of an infectious disease.
B. Nurses and other health care workers must be prepared to assess and determine what type of event occurred, the number of clients who may be affected, and how and when clients will be expected to arrive to the health care agency.
C. It is essential to determine any changes in the microorganism that may increase its virulence or make it resistant to conventional antibiotics or vaccines.
D. See Chapter 8 for additional information on disasters and emergency response planning.

MORE QUESTIONS ON THE CD!

Practice Questions

131. A nurse is preparing to initiate an intravenous line containing a high dose of potassium chloride and plans to use an intravenous infusion pump. The nurse brings the pump to the bedside, prepares to plug the pump cord into the wall, and notes that no receptacle is available in the wall socket. Which of the following is the appropriate nursing action?
1. Initiate the intravenous line without the use of a pump.
2. Contact the electrical maintenance department for assistance.
3. Plug in the pump cord in the available plug above the room sink.
4. Use an extension cord from the nurses' lounge for the pump plug.

132. A nurse obtains a prescription from a physician to restrain a client by using a jacket safety device and instructs a nursing assistant to apply the safety device to the client. Which observation by the nurse indicates unsafe application of the safety device by the nursing assistant?
1. A safety knot in the safety device straps
2. Safety device straps that are safely secured to the side rails
3. Safety device straps that do not tighten when force is applied against them
4. Safety device secured so that two fingers can slide easily between the safety device and the client's skin

133. The nurse is caring for a client with meningitis and implements which transmission-based precautions for this client?
1. Private room or cohort client
2. Personal respiratory protection device
3. Private room with negative airflow pressure
4. Mask worn by staff when the client needs to leave the room

134. A nurse is giving a report to a nursing assistant who will be caring for a client who has hand restraints (safety devices). The nurse instructs the nursing assistant to check the skin integrity of the restrained hands:
1. Every 2 hours
2. Every 3 hours
3. Every 4 hours
4. Every 30 minutes

135. A nurse is planning care for a client with an internal radiation implant. Which of the following is an incorrect component to include in the plan of care?
1. Wearing gloves when emptying the client's bedpan
2. Keeping all linens in the room until the implant is removed
3. Wearing a lead apron when providing direct care to the client
4. Placing the client in a semiprivate room at the end of the hallway

136. Contact precautions are initiated for a client with a health care–associated (nosocomial) infection caused by methicillin-resistant *Staphylococcus aureus*. The nurse prepares to provide colostomy care and obtains which of the following protective items needed to perform this procedure?
1. Gloves and gown
2. Gloves and goggles
3. Gloves, gown, and shoe protectors
4. Gloves, gown, goggles, and face shield

137. A nurse enters a client's room and finds that the wastebasket is on fire. The nurse immediately assists the client out of the room. What is the next nursing action?
1. Call for help.
2. Extinguish the fire.
3. Activate the fire alarm.
4. Confine the fire by closing the room door.

138. A mother calls a neighbor who is a nurse and tells the nurse that her 3-year-old child has just ingested liquid furniture polish. The nurse would direct the mother immediately to:
1. Induce vomiting.
2. Call an ambulance.
3. Call the Poison Control Center.
4. Bring the child to the emergency department.

139. An emergency department nurse receives a telephone call and is informed that a tornado has hit a local residential area and that numerous casualties have occurred. The victims will be brought to the emergency department. The initial nursing action is which of the following?
1. Prepare the triage rooms.
2. Activate the emergency response plan.
3. Obtain additional supplies from the central supply department.
4. Obtain additional nursing staff to assist in treating the casualties.

Alternate Item Format: Multiple Response

140. A community health nurse is providing a teaching session about terrorism to members of the community and is discussing information regarding anthrax. The nurse tells those attending that anthrax can be transmitted by which route(s)? **Select all that apply**.

☐ 1. Bites from ticks or deer flies
☐ 2. Inhalation of bacterial spores
☐ 3. Through a cut or abrasion in the skin
☐ 4. Direct contact with an infected individual
☐ 5. Sexual contact with an infected individual
☐ 6. Ingestion of contaminated undercooked meat

ANSWERS

131. 2

Rationale: Electrical equipment must be maintained in good working order and should be grounded; otherwise it presents a physical hazard. An intravenous line that contains a high dose of potassium chloride should be administered by pump. The nurse needs to use hospital resources for assistance. A regular extension cord should not be used because it poses a risk for fire. Use of electrical appliances near a sink also presents a hazard.

Test-Taking Strategy: Use the process of elimination. Noting the strategic words *high dose* in the question will assist in eliminating option 1. Recalling safety issues related to electrical hazards will assist in eliminating options 3 and 4. If you had difficulty with this question, review the interventions related to electrical safety.

Level of Cognitive Ability: Applying
Client Needs: Safe and Effective Care Environment
Integrated Process: Nursing Process—Implementation
Content Area: Fundamental Skills—Safety/Infection Control
Reference: Perry, A., & Potter, P. (2010). *Clinical nursing skills & techniques* (7th ed., p. 323). St. Louis: Mosby.

132. 2

Rationale: The safety device straps are secured to the bed frame and never to the side rail to avoid accidental injury in the event that the side rail is released. A half-bow or safety knot should be used for applying a safety device because it does not tighten when force is applied against it and it allows quick and easy removal of the safety device in case of an emergency. The jacket safety device should be secure, and one to two fingers should slide easily between the safety device and the client's skin.

Test-Taking Strategy: Note the strategic words *indicates unsafe application*. These words indicate a negative event query and ask you to select an option that is an incorrect observation. Read each option carefully. The words *secured to the side rails* in option 2 should direct your attention to this as an incorrect and unsafe action. Review guidelines related to the application of safety devices if you had difficulty with this question.

Level of Cognitive Ability: Understanding
Client Needs: Safe and Effective Care Environment
Integrated Process: Teaching and Learning
Content Area: Fundamental Skills—Safety/Infection Control
Reference: Potter, P., & Perry, A. (2009). *Fundamentals of nursing* (7th ed., p. 838). St. Louis: Mosby.

133. 1

Rationale: Meningitis is transmitted by droplet infection. Precautions for this disease include a private room or cohort client and use of a standard precaution mask. Private negative airflow pressure rooms and personal respiratory protection devices are required for clients with airborne disease such as tuberculosis. When appropriate, a mask must be worn by the client and not the staff when the client leaves the room.

Test-Taking Strategy: Use the process of elimination to determine the correct precaution needs for this client. Focusing on the client's diagnosis and recalling that meningitis is transmitted by droplets will direct you to option 1. Review transmission-based categories including precaution criteria for the client with meningitis if you had difficulty with this question.

Level of Cognitive Ability: Applying
Client Needs: Safe and Effective Care Environment
Integrated Process: Nursing Process—Implementation
Content Area: Fundamental Skills—Safety/Infection Control
Reference: Potter, P., & Perry, A. (2009). *Fundamentals of nursing* (7th ed., p. 663). St. Louis: Mosby.

134. 4

Rationale: The nurse should instruct the nursing assistant to check safety devices and skin integrity every 30 minutes. The neurovascular and circulatory status of the extremity should also be checked every 30 minutes. Additionally, the safety device should be removed at least every 2 hours to permit muscle exercise and to promote circulation. Agency guidelines regarding the use of safety devices should always be followed.

Test-Taking Strategy: Use the process of elimination. In this situation, selecting the option that identifies the most frequent time frame is best. Review the guidelines related to the use of safety devices if you had difficulty with this question.

Level of Cognitive Ability: Applying
Client Needs: Safe and Effective Care Environment
Integrated Process: Teaching and Learning
Content Area: Leadership and Management—Delegating/Prioritizing
Reference: Potter, P., & Perry, A. (2009). *Fundamentals of nursing* (7th ed., pp. 837–838). St. Louis: Mosby.

135. 4

Rationale: A private room with a private bath is essential if a client has an internal radiation implant. This is necessary to prevent accidental exposure of other clients to radiation. Options 1, 2, and 3 are accurate interventions for a client with a radiation implant.

Test-Taking Strategy: Use the process of elimination and note the strategic word *incorrect*. This word indicates a negative event query and the need to select the incorrect nursing intervention. Option 1 can be eliminated first because this is a component of standard precautions for all clients. Options 2 and 3 can be eliminated next because they directly relate to radiation safety.

Remember that the client with an internal radiation implant needs to be placed in a private room. Review radiation safety principles if you had difficulty with this question.
Level of Cognitive Ability: Applying
Client Needs: Safe and Effective Care Environment
Integrated Process: Nursing Process—Planning
Content Area: Fundamental Skills—Safety/Infection Control
Reference: Black, J., & Hawks, J. (2009). *Medical-surgical nursing: Clinical management for positive outcomes* (8th ed., p. 274). St. Louis: Saunders.

136. 4

Rationale: Splashes of body secretions can occur when providing colostomy care. Goggles and a face shield are worn to protect the mucous membranes of the eyes during interventions that may produce splashes of blood, body fluids, secretions, or excretions. In addition, contact precautions require the use of gloves, and a gown should be worn if direct client contact is anticipated. Shoe protectors are not necessary.
Test-Taking Strategy: Note the strategic words *contact precautions* and *colostomy*. Use the process of elimination and visualize care for this client to determine the necessary items required in caring for this client. This will direct you to option 4. If you had difficulty with this question, review transmission-based precautions and care to the client requiring colostomy care.
Level of Cognitive Ability: Applying
Client Needs: Safe and Effective Care Environment
Integrated Process: Nursing Process—Implementation
Content Area: Fundamental Skills—Safety/Infection Control
Reference: Potter, P., & Perry, A. (2009). *Fundamentals of nursing* (7th ed., p. 663). St. Louis: Mosby.

137. 3

Rationale: The order of priority in the event of a fire is to rescue the clients who are in immediate danger. The next step is to activate the fire alarm. The fire then is confined by closing all doors and, finally, the fire is extinguished.
Test-Taking Strategy: Remember the mnemonic *RACE* to prioritize in the event of a fire. *R* is rescue clients in immediate danger, *A* is alarm (sound the alarm), *C* is confine the fire by closing all doors, and *E* is extinguish or evacuate. If you had difficulty with this question, review the principles related to fire safety.
Level of Cognitive Ability: Applying
Client Needs: Safe and Effective Care Environment
Integrated Process: Nursing Process—Implementation
Content Area: Fundamental Skills—Safety/Infection Control
Reference: Potter, P., & Perry, A. (2009). *Fundamentals of nursing* (7th ed., pp. 839–840). St. Louis: Mosby.

138. 3

Rationale: If a poisoning occurs, the Poison Control Center should be contacted immediately. Vomiting should not be induced if the victim is unconscious or if the substance ingested is a strong corrosive or petroleum product. Bringing the child to the emergency department or calling an ambulance would not be the initial action because this would delay treatment. The Poison Control Center may advise the mother to bring the child to the emergency department and, if this is the case, the mother should call an ambulance.
Test-Taking Strategy: Use the process of elimination and note the strategic word *immediately*. Eliminate options 2 and 4 because these options will delay treatment. Recalling that vomiting should not be induced if a corrosive substance was ingested will assist in eliminating option 1. Review poison control measures if you had difficulty with this question.
Level of Cognitive Ability: Applying
Client Needs: Safe and Effective Care Environment
Integrated Process: Nursing Process—Implementation
Content Area: Fundamental Skills—Safety/Infection Control
Reference: Potter, P., & Perry, A. (2009). *Fundamentals of nursing* (7th ed., p. 842). St. Louis: Mosby.

139. 2

Rationale: In an external disaster (a disaster that occurs outside of the institution or agency), many victims may be brought to the emergency department for treatment. Although options 1, 3, and 4 may be components of preparing for the casualties, the initial nursing action must be to activate the emergency response plan.
Test-Taking Strategy: Note the strategic word *initial* and determine the priority action. Note that option 2 is the umbrella option. If the emergency response plan is activated then options 1, 3, and 4 will occur. Review procedures related to management of an external disaster if you had difficulty with this question.
Level of Cognitive Ability: Applying
Client Needs: Safe and Effective Care Environment
Integrated Process: Nursing Process—Implementation
Content Area: Fundamental Skills—Safety/Infection Control
Reference: Black, J., & Hawks, J. (2009). *Medical-surgical nursing: Clinical management for positive outcomes* (8th ed., pp. 2213–2214). St. Louis: Saunders.

ALTERNATE ITEM FORMAT: MULTIPLE RESPONSE

140. 2, 3, 6

Rationale: Anthrax is caused by *Bacillus anthracis* and can be contracted through the digestive system or abrasions in the skin, or inhaled through the lungs. It cannot be spread from person to person or animal to person, and it is not contracted via bites from ticks or deer flies.
Test-Taking Strategy: Knowledge regarding the methods of contracting anthrax is needed to answer this question. Remember that it is not spread by person-to-person contact or contracted via tick or deer fly bites. Review information related to this infection if you had difficulty with this question.
Level of Cognitive Ability: Applying
Client Needs: Safe and Effective Care Environment
Integrated Process: Teaching and Learning
Content Area: Fundamental Skills—Safety/Infection Control
References: Black, J., & Hawks, J. (2009). *Medical-surgical nursing: Clinical management for positive outcomes* (8th ed., p. 338). St. Louis: Saunders.

Ignatavicius, D., & Workman, M. (2010). *Medical-surgical nursing: Patient-centered collaborative care* (6th ed., pp. 672–673). St. Louis: Saunders.

Administration of Medication and Intravenous Solutions

PYRAMID TERMS

conversion The first step in the calculation of a medication problem.

generic name Also known as the nonproprietary name of a medication, or the U.S. adopted name; each medication has only one generic name.

medication reconciliation An organized process to avoid medication errors by comparing the client's medication prescriptions to all the medications that the client was previously taking.

milliequivalent An expression of the number of grams of a medication contained in 1 mL of a solution; abbreviated mEq.

parenteral Given by injection, such as by the intravenous, intramuscular, subcutaneous, or intradermal route.

percentage solution The number of grams of a medication per 100 mL of solution.

ratio solution The number of grams of a medication per total milliliters of solution.

reconstitution Dissolving a powder in a sterile diluent before use, usually in sterile water or normal saline.

trade name Also known as the proprietary or brand name of a medication. The trade name is the name under which a medication is marketed. A medication can have many trade names; therefore trade names must be approved by the U.S. Food and Drug Administration (FDA) to ensure that no two trade names are alike.

unit A measurement of a medication in terms of its action, not its physical weight.

THE PYRAMID TO SUCCESS

When a medication or intravenous calculation question is presented, a nurse should always use the appropriate formula to solve the problem. The nurse should not use shortcuts to make these calculations. The problem and answer should be expressed in the correct units of measure. Be careful with decimal points. Correct placement of the decimal point is important or the answer will be incorrect. When solving a medication calculation problem, the nurse determines whether the answer is within reason and makes sense. In the clinical setting, the nurse should always seek assistance if unsure of the accuracy of a calculation.

On the NCLEX-RN examination, the fill-in-the-blank questions may require that you calculate a medication dose or an intravenous (IV) flow rate. You will be provided with a computer on-screen calculator for these medication and IV problems. Even if you use the calculator to calculate dosages and flow rates, you need to check the calculation before selecting an option or typing the answer. Follow the formula, place the decimal point in the correct place, and check the accuracy of the calculation. Remember that practice makes perfect.

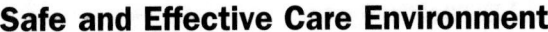

CLIENT NEEDS

Safe and Effective Care Environment

Handling hazardous and infectious materials
Maintaining client's rights
Maintaining surgical asepsis
Maintaining standard and transmission-based precautions
Preventing errors
Using equipment safely

Health Promotion and Maintenance

Performing a physical assessment of a client
Preventing diseases
Respecting lifestyle choices
Teaching the client about prescribed medication(s) or IV therapy

Psychosocial Integrity

Identifying support systems
Identifying the cultural, religious, and spiritual factors influencing health
Interacting therapeutically with the client and family
Identifying the use of coping mechanisms

Physiological Integrity

Administering medications and IV therapy
Assessing for expected and unexpected effects of pharmacological therapy

Box 17-1 Medication Administration

Assess the medication prescription.

Compare the client's medication prescription with all the medications that the client was previously taking (medication reconciliation).

Ask the client about a history of allergies.

Assess the client's current condition and the purpose for the medication or intravenous solution.

Determine the client's understanding regarding the purpose of the prescribed medication or need for intravenous solution.

Teach the client about the medication and about self-administration at home.

Identify and address concerns (social, cultural, religious) that the client may have about taking the medication.

Assess the need for conversion when preparing a dose of medication for administration to the client.

Assess the six rights of medication administration: right medication, right dose, right client, right route, right time, and right documentation.

Assess the vital signs, check significant laboratory results, and identify any potential interactions (food or medication interactions) before administering medication, when appropriate.

Document the administration of the prescribed therapy and client's response to the therapy.

Box 17-2 Metric System

Abbreviations	Equivalents
meter: m	1 mcg = 0.000001 g
liter: L	1 mg = 1000 mcg or 0.001 g
milliliter: mL	1 g = 1000 mg
kilogram: kg	1 kg = 1000 g
gram: g	1 kg = 2.2 lb
milligram: mg	1 mL = 0.001 L
microgram: mcg	

Box 17-3 Apothecary and Household Systems

Abbreviations	Equivalents
Apothecary (Weight)	1 gr = 60 or 65 mg
grain: gr	5 gr = 300 or 325 mg
ounce: oz	15 gr = 1000 mg or 1 g
	$\frac{1}{150}$ gr = 0.4 mg
Household (Volume)	1 fl oz = 30 mL
drops: gtt	1 T = 15 mL or 3 tsp
teaspoon: t or tsp	1 t or tsp = 5 mL
tablespoon: T or tbs	1 C = 8 fl oz
fluid ounce: fl oz	1 qt = 946 mL or 0.946 L
cup: C	1 qt = 2 pt or 32 fl oz
pint: pt	1 pt = 16 fl oz
quart: qt	16 oz = 1 lb
	2.2 lb = 1 kg
Household (Weight)	
pound: lb	

Box 17-4 Conversion Between Metric Units

Problem 1

Convert 2 g to milligrams.

Solution

Change a larger unit to a smaller unit.

2 g = 2000 mg (moving decimal three places to right)

Problem 2

Convert 250 mL to liters.

Solution

Change a smaller unit to a larger unit.

250 mL = 0.25 L (moving decimal three places to left)

2. Apothecary measures such as grain, dram, minim, and ounce are not commonly used in the clinical setting.
3. Commonly used household measures include drop, teaspoon, tablespoon, ounce, pint, and cup.

C. Additional common drug measures
  1. **Milliequivalent**
     a. **Milliequivalent** is abbreviated mEq.
     b. The **milliequivalent** is an expression of the number of grams of a medication contained in 1 mL of a solution.
     c. For example, the measure of serum potassium is given in **milliequivalents**.
  2. **Unit**
     a. **Unit** measures a medication in terms of its action, not its physical weight.
     b. For example, penicillin, heparin sodium, and insulin are measured in units.

Calculating medication doses and intravenous flow rates

Identifying the adverse effects of and contraindications to medication or IV therapy

Monitoring for alterations in body systems

Monitoring laboratory values

I. MEDICATION ADMINISTRATION (Box 17-1)

II. DRUG MEASUREMENT SYSTEMS

A. Metric system (Box 17-2)
  1. The basic units of metric measures are meter, liter, and gram.
  2. Meter measures length; liter measures volume; gram measures mass.

B. Apothecary and household systems (Box 17-3)
  1. The apothecary and household systems are the oldest of the medication measurement systems.

III. CONVERSIONS

A. **Conversion** between metric units (Box 17-4)
  1. The metric system is a decimal system; therefore **conversions** between the units in this system

Box 17-5 Ratio and Proportion

Ratio: The relationship between two numbers, separated by a colon; for example, 1:2 (1 to 2).
Proportion: The relationship between two ratios, separated by a double colon (::) or an equal sign (=).

Formula:

H (on hand):V (vehicle) :: (=) (desired dose):X (unknown)

   To solve a ratio and proportion problem: The middle numbers (means) are multiplied and the end numbers (extremes) are multiplied.

Sample Problem

H = 1
V = 2
Desired dose = 3
X = unknown
Set up the formula:
1:2::3:X
Solve: Multiply means and extremes.
1X = 6
X = 6

Box 17-6 Calculating Equivalents Between Two Systems

Calculating equivalents between two systems may be done by using the method of ratio and proportion.

Problem
The physician prescribes nitroglycerin, grain (gr) $\frac{1}{150}$. The medication label reads 0.4 milligrams (mg) per tablet. The nurse prepares to administer how many tablets to the client?

Ratio and Proportion Formula
H (on hand):V (vehicle) :: (=) (desired dose):X
1 gr:60 mg :: $\frac{1}{150}$ gr:X mg
$60 \times \frac{1}{150} = X$
X = 0.4 mg (1 tablet)

Box 17-7 Celsius and Fahrenheit Temperature

Fahrenheit to Celsius
To convert Fahrenheit to Celsius, subtract 32 and divide the result by 1.8.

Formula:

$$C = \frac{(F - 32)}{1.8}$$

Celsius to Fahrenheit
To convert Celsius to Fahrenheit, multiply by 1.8 and add 32.

Formula:

$$F = (1.8 \times C) + 32$$

can be done by dividing or multiplying by 1000 or by moving the decimal point three places to the right or three places to the left.
   2. In the metric system, to convert larger to smaller, multiply by 1000 or move the decimal point three places to the right.
   3. In the metric system, to convert smaller to larger, divide by 1000 or move the decimal point three places to the left.

B. **Conversion** between household and metric systems
   1. Household and metric measures are equivalent and not equal measures.
   2. **Conversion** to equivalent measures between systems is necessary when a medication prescription is written in one system but the medication label is stated in another.
   3. Medications are not always prescribed and prepared in the same system of measurement; therefore **conversion** of units from one system to another is necessary.
   4. Calculating equivalents between two systems may be done by using the method of ratio and proportion (Boxes 17-5 and 17-6).

⚠ Conversion is the first step in the calculation of dosages.

IV. CELSIUS AND FAHRENHEIT TEMPERATURE (Box 17-7)

A. To convert Fahrenheit to Celsius, subtract 32 and divide the result by 1.8.
B. To convert Celsius to Fahrenheit, multiply by 1.8 and add 32.

Box 17-8 Medication Prescriptions

Name of client
Date and time when prescription is written
Name of medication to be given
Dosage of medication
Medication route
Time and frequency of administration
Signature of person writing the prescription

V. MEDICATION LABELS

A. A medication label contains the **generic name** and the **trade name** of the medication.
B. Always check expiration dates on medication labels. ◀

VI. MEDICATION PRESCRIPTIONS (Box 17-8)

A. In a medication prescription, the name of the medication is written first, followed by the dosage, route, and frequency (depending on the frequency of the prescription, times of administration are usually established by the health care agency and written in an agency policy).

B. Medication prescriptions need to be written using accepted abbreviations, acronyms, and symbols approved by The Joint Commission; also follow agency guidelines.

⚠ If the nurse has any questions about or sees inconsistencies in the written prescription, the nurse must contact the person who wrote the prescription immediately and must verify the prescription.

VII. ORAL MEDICATIONS

A. Scored tablets contain an indented mark to be used for possible breakage into partial doses; when necessary, scored tablets (those marked for division) can be divided into halves or quarters.

B. Enteric-coated tablets and sustained-released capsules delay absorption until the medication reaches the small intestine; these medications should not be crushed.

C. Capsules contain a powdered or oily medication in a gelatin cover.

D. Orally administered liquids are supplied in solution form and contain a specific amount of medication in a given amount of solution, as stated on the label.

E. The medicine cup

  1. The medicine cup has a capacity of 30 mL or 1 oz and is used for orally administered liquids.

  2. The medicine cup is calibrated to measure teaspoons, tablespoons, and ounces.

  3. To pour accurately, place the medication cup on a level surface at eye level and then pour the liquid while reading the measuring markings.

F. Volumes of less than 5 mL are measured by using a syringe with the needle removed.

⚠ A calibrated dropper is used for giving medicine to children or for adding small amounts of liquid to water or juice; calibrations are in milliliters or drops.

VIII. PARENTERAL MEDICATIONS

A. **Parenteral** always means an injection route and **parenteral** medications are administered by intravenous, intramuscular, subcutaneous, or intradermal injection (see Fig. 17-1 for angles of injection).

B. **Parenteral** medications are packaged in single-use ampules, in single- and multiple-use rubber-stoppered vials, and in premeasured syringes and cartridges.

C. The nurse should not administer more than 3 mL per intramuscular or 1 mL per subcutaneous injection site; larger volumes are difficult for an injection site to absorb and, if prescribed, need to be verified.

D. The standard 3-mL syringe is used to measure most injectable medications and is calibrated in tenths (0.1) of a milliliter.

E. The calibrations on a syringe are read from the top black ring on the syringe, not the middle section and not the bottom ring (Fig. 17-2).

⚠ Always question and verify excessively large or small volumes of medication.

F. Prefilled medication cartridge

  1. The medication cartridge slips into the cartridge holder, which provides a plunger for injection of the medication.

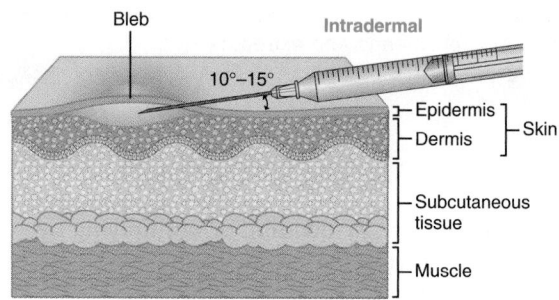

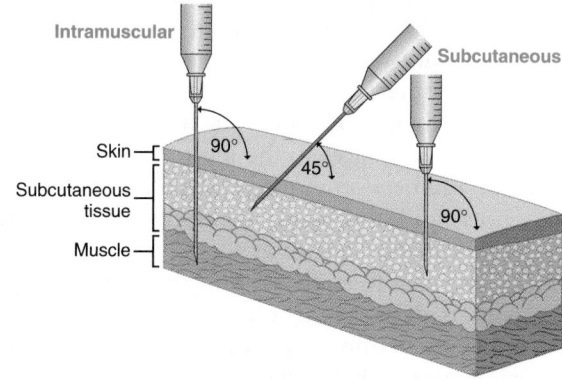

▲ **FIGURE 17-1** Angles of injection. (From Kee, J., & Marshall, S. [2009]. *Clinical calculations: With applications to general and specialty areas* [6th ed.]. St. Louis: Saunders.)

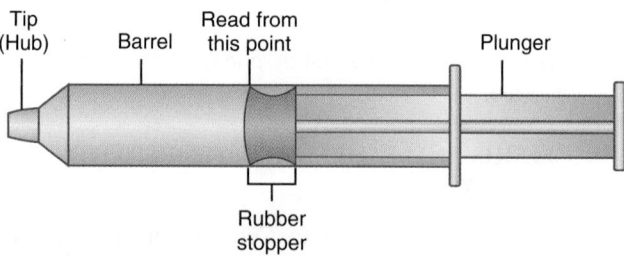

▲ **FIGURE 17-2** Parts of a syringe. (From Kee, J., & Marshall, S. [2009]. *Clinical calculations: With applications to general and specialty areas* [6th ed.]. St. Louis: Saunders.)

2. The cartridge is designed to provide sufficient capacity to allow for the addition of a second medication when combined dosages are prescribed.
3. The prefilled medication cartridge is to be used once and discarded; if a nurse is to give less than the full single dose provided, the nurse needs to discard the extra amount before giving the client the injection, following agency policies and procedures.

G. Generally, standard medication doses for adults are to be rounded to the nearest tenth (0.1 mL) of a milliliter and measured on the milliliter scale; for example, 1.25 mL is rounded to 1.3 mL (follow agency policy for rounding medication doses).

H. When volumes larger than 3 mL are required, the nurse may use a 5-mL syringe; these syringes are calibrated in fifths (0.2 mL) (Fig. 17-3).

I. Other syringes sizes may be available (10, 20, and 50 mL) and may be used for medication administration requiring dilution.

J. Tuberculin syringe (Fig. 17-4)
1. The tuberculin syringe holds 1 mL and is used to measure small or critical amounts of medication, such as allergen extract, vaccine, or a child's medication.
2. The syringe is calibrated in hundredths (0.01) of a milliliter, with each one tenth (0.1) marked on the metric scale.

K. Insulin syringe (Fig. 17-5)

1. The standard 100-**unit** insulin syringe is calibrated for 100 units of insulin (100 units = 1 mL); low-dose insulin syringes (½- and 1-mL sizes) may also be used when administering smaller insulin doses.
2. Insulin should not be measured in any other type of syringe.

⚠ If the insulin prescription states to administer regular and NPH insulin, combine both types of insulin in the same syringe. Use the mnemonic RN: Draw *Regular* insulin into the insulin syringe first, and then draw the *NPH* insulin.

L. Safety needles contain shielding devices that are attached to the needle and slipped over the needle to reduce the incidence of needle stick injuries

IX. INJECTABLE MEDICATIONS IN POWDER FORM

A. Some medications become unstable when stored in solution form and are therefore packaged in powder form.

B. Powders must be dissolved with a sterile diluent before use; usually, sterile water or normal saline is used. The dissolving procedure is called **reconstitution** (Box 17-9).

X. CALCULATING THE CORRECT DOSAGE (See Box 17-10 for the standard formula)

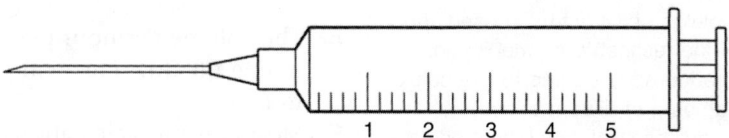

▲ **FIGURE 17-3** Five-milliliter syringe. (From Kee, J., & Marshall, S. [2009]. *Clinical calculations: With applications to general and specialty areas* [6th ed.]. St. Louis: Saunders.)

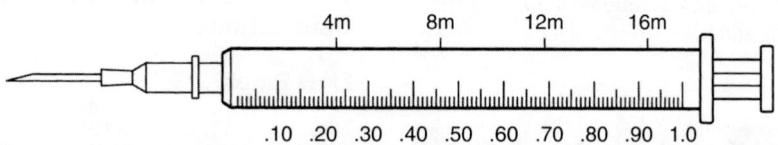

▲ **FIGURE 17-4** Tuberculin syringe. (From Kee, J., & Marshall, S. [2009]. *Clinical calculations: With applications to general and specialty areas* [6th ed.]. St. Louis: Saunders.)

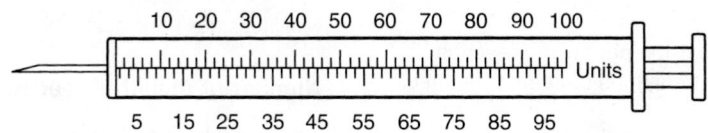

▲ **Figure 17-5** A 100-unit insulin syringe. (From Kee, J., & Marshall, S. [2009]. *Clinical calculations: With applications to general and specialty areas* [6th ed.]. St. Louis: Saunders.)

A. When calculating dosages of oral medications, check the calculation and question the prescription if the calculation calls for more than three tablets.

B. When calculating dosages of **parenteral** medications, check the calculation and question the prescription if the amount to be given is too large a dose.

C. Be sure that all measures are in the same system, and that all units are in the same size, converting when necessary; carefully consider what the reasonable amount of the medication that should be administered is.

D. Round standard injection doses to tenths and measure in a 3-mL syringe (follow agency policy).

E. Round small, critical amounts or children's doses to hundredths and measure in the 1-mL tuberculin syringe (follow agency policy).

F. In additional to using the standard formula (see Box 17-10), calculations can be done through the use of dimensional analysis; the required elements of a dimensional analysis equation include the desired answer units, **conversion** formula that includes the desired answer units and the units that need to be converted, and the original factors to convert including quantity and units.

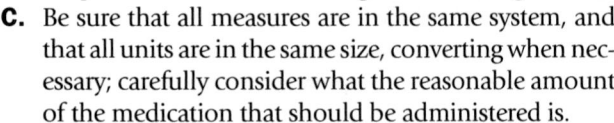 Regardless of the source or cause of a medication error, if a nurse gives an incorrect dose, the nurse is legally responsible for the action.

Box 17-9 Reconstitution

In reconstituting the medication, locate the instructions on the label or in the vial package insert, and read and follow the directions carefully.

Instructions will state the volume of diluent to be used and the resulting volume of the reconstituted medication.

Often, the powdered medication adds volume to the solution in addition to the amount of diluent added.

When reconstituting a multiple-dose vial, label the medication vial with the date and time of preparation, your initials, and the date of expiration.

Indicating the strength per volume on the medication label also is important.

The total volume of the prepared solution will exceed the volume of the diluent added.

Box 17-10 Standard Formula for Calculating a Medication Dosage

$$\frac{D}{A} \times Q = X$$

D (desired) is the dosage that the physician prescribed.
A (available) is the dosage strength as stated on the medication label.
Q (quantity) is the volume or form in which the dosage strength is available, such as tablets, capsules, or milliliters.

XI. PERCENTAGE AND RATIO SOLUTIONS

A. Percentage solutions
   1. Express the number of grams of the medication per 100 mL of solution.
   2. For example, calcium gluconate 10% is 10 g of pure medication per 100 mL of solution.

B. Ratio solutions
   1. Express the number of grams of the medication per total milliliters of solution.
   2. For example, epinephrine 1:1000 is 1 g of pure medication per 1000 mL solution.

XII. INTRAVENOUS FLOW RATES (Box 17-11)

A. Monitor IV flow rate frequently even if the IV solution is being administered through an electronic infusion device (follow agency policy regarding frequency).

B. If an IV is running behind schedule, collaborate with the physician to determine the client's ability to tolerate an increased flow rate, particularly for clients with cardiac, pulmonary, renal, or neurological conditions.

The nurse should never increase the rate (speed up) of an IV infusion to catch up if the infusion is running behind schedule.

C. Whenever a prescribed IV rate is increased, the nurse should assess the client for increased heart rate, increased respirations, and increased lung congestion, which could indicate fluid overload.

D. Intravenously administered fluids are prescribed most frequently based on milliliters per hour to be administered.

E. The volume per hour prescribed is administered by setting the flow rate, which is counted in drops per minute.

F. Most flow rate calculations involve changing milliliters per hour into drops per minute.

G. Intravenous tubing

Box 17-11 Formulas for Intravenous Calculations

Flow Rates

$$\frac{\text{Total volume} \times \text{drop factor}}{\text{Time in minutes}} = \text{Drops per minute}$$

Infusion Time

$$\frac{\text{Total volume to infuse}}{\text{Milliliters per hour being infused}} = \text{Infusion time}$$

Number of Milliliters per Hour

$$\frac{\text{Total volume in milliliters}}{\text{Number of hours}} = \text{Number of milliliters per hour}$$

1. Intravenous tubing sets are calibrated in drops per milliliter; this calibration is needed for calculating flow rates.
2. A standard or macrodrip set is used for routine adult IV administrations; depending on the manufacturer and type of tubing, the set will require 10, 15, or 20 gtt to equal 1 mL.
3. A minidrip or microdrip set is used when more exact measurements are needed, such as in intensive care units and pediatric units.
4. In a minidrip or microdrip set, 60 gtt is usually equal to 1 mL.
5. The calibration, in drops per milliliter, is written on the IV tubing package.

XIII. CALCULATION OF INFUSIONS ORDERED BY UNIT DOSAGE PER HOUR

A. The most common medications that will be ordered by **unit** dosage per hour and run by continuous infusion are heparin sodium and regular insulin.
B. Calculation of these infusions can be done by a two-step process (Box 17-12).
  1. Determine the amount of medication per 1 mL.
  2. Determine the infusion rate or milliliters per hour.

 MORE QUESTIONS ON THE CD!

Practice Questions: Alternate Item Format (Fill-In-The-Blank)

141. A physician's prescription reads 1000 mL of normal saline (NS) to infuse over 12 hours. The drop factor is 15 drops (gtt)/1 mL. A nurse prepares to set the flow rate at how many drops per minute? (Round answer to the nearest whole number.)
Answer: _____ drops per minute

142. A physician's prescription reads to administer an intravenous (IV) dose of 400,000 units of penicillin G benzathine (Bicillin). The label on the 10-mL ampule sent from the pharmacy reads penicillin G benzathine (Bicillin), 300,000 units/mL. A nurse prepares how much medication to administer the correct dose? (Round answer to the nearest tenth position.)
Answer: _____ mL

143. A physician's prescription reads potassium chloride 30 mEq to be added to 1000 mL normal saline (NS) and to be administered over a

---

Box 17-12 Infusions Ordered by Unit Dosage per Hour

Calculation of these problems can be done by a two-step process:
1. Determine the amount of medication per 1 mL.
2. Determine the infusion rate or milliliters per hour.

Problem 1
Order: Continuous heparin sodium by IV at 1000 units per hour
Available: IV bag of 500 mL D$_5$W with 20,000 units of heparin sodium
How many milliliters per hour are required to administer the correct dose?

Solution
Step 1: Calculate the amount of medication (units) per milliliter (mL).

$$\frac{\text{Known amount of medication in solution}}{\text{Total volume of diluent}} = \text{Amount of medication per milliliter}$$

$$\frac{20,000 \text{ units}}{500 \text{ mL}} = 40 \text{ units}/1 \text{ mL}$$

Step 2: Calculate milliliters per hour.

$$\frac{\text{Dose per hour desired}}{\text{Concentration per milliliter}} = \text{Infusion rate, or mL/hr}$$

$$\frac{1000 \text{ units}}{40 \text{ units}} = 25 \text{ mL/hr}$$

Problem 2
Order: Continuous regular insulin by IV at 10 units per hour
Available: IV bag of 100 mL NS with 50 units regular insulin
How many milliliters per hour are required to administer the correct dose?

Solution
Step 1: Calculate the amount of medication (units) per milliliter.

$$\frac{\text{Known amount of medication in solution}}{\text{Total volume of diluent}} = \text{Amount of medication per milliliter}$$

$$\frac{50 \text{ units}}{100 \text{ mL}} = 0.5 \text{ units}/1 \text{ mL}$$

Step 2: Calculate milliliters per hour.

$$\frac{\text{Dose per hour desired}}{\text{Concentration per milliliter}} = \text{Infusion rate, or mL/hr}$$

$$\frac{10 \text{ units}}{0.5 \text{ units/mL}} = 20 \text{ mL/hr}$$

10-hour period. The label on the medication bottle reads 40 mEq/20 mL. A nurse prepares how many milliliters of potassium chloride to administer the correct dose of medication?

Answer: _____ mL

144. A physician's prescription reads clindamycin phosphate (Cleocin Phosphate) 0.3 g in 50 mL normal saline (NS) to be administered intravenously over 30 minutes. The medication label reads clindamycin phosphate (Cleocin Phosphate) 900 mg in 6 mL. A nurse prepares how many milliliters of the medication to administer the correct dose?

Answer: _____ mL

145. A physician's prescription reads phenytoin (Dilantin) 0.2 g orally twice daily. The medication label states 100-mg capsules. A nurse prepares how many capsule(s) to administer one dose?

Answer: _____ capsule(s)

146. A physician prescribes 1000 mL of ½ normal saline (NS) to infuse over 8 hours. The drop factor is 15 drops (gtt)/1 mL. The nurse sets the flow rate at how many drops per minute? (Round answer to the nearest whole number.)

Answer: _____ drops per minute

147. A physician prescribes heparin sodium, 1300 units/hr by continuous intravenous (IV) infusion. The pharmacy prepares the medication and delivers an IV bag labeled heparin sodium 20,000 units/250 mL D_5W. An infusion pump must be used to administer the medication. The nurse sets the infusion pump at how many milliliters per hour to deliver 1300 units/hr? (Round answer to the nearest whole number.)

Answer: _____ mL per hour

148. A physician prescribes 3000 mL of D_5W to be administered over a 24-hour period. A nurse determines that how many milliliters per hour will be administered to the client?

Answer: _____ mL per hour

149. Gentamicin sulfate, 80 mg in 100 mL normal saline (NS), is to be administered over 30 minutes.

The drop factor is 10 drops (gtt)/mL. A nurse sets the flow rate at how many drops per minute? (Round answer to the nearest whole number.)

Answer: _____ drops per minute

150. A physician's prescription reads levothyroxine (Synthroid), 150 mcg orally daily. The medication label reads Synthroid, 0.1 mg/tablet. A nurse administers how many tablet(s) to the client?

Answer: _____ tablet(s)

151. Cefuroxime sodium, 1 g in 50 mL normal saline (NS), is to be administered over 30 minutes. The drop factor is 15 drops (gtt)/mL. A nurse sets the flow rate at how many drops per minute?

Answer: _____ drops per minute

152. A physician prescribes 1000 mL D_5W to infuse at a rate of 125 mL/hr. A nurse determines that it will take how many hours for 1 L to infuse?

Answer: _____ hour(s)

153. A physician prescribes 1 unit of packed red blood cells to infuse over 4 hours. The unit of blood contains 250 mL. The drop factor is 10 drops (gtt)/1 mL. A nurse prepares to set the flow rate at how many drops per minute? (Round answer to the nearest whole number.)

Answer: _____ drops per minute

154. A physician's prescription reads morphine sulfate, 8 mg stat. The medication ampule reads morphine sulfate, 10 mg/mL. A nurse prepares how many milliliters to administer the correct dose?

Answer: _____ mL

155. A physician prescribes regular insulin, 8 units/hr by continuous intravenous (IV) infusion. The pharmacy prepares the medication and then delivers an IV bag labeled 100 units of regular insulin in 100 mL normal saline (NS). An infusion pump must be used to administer the medication. The nurse sets the infusion pump at how many milliliters per hour to deliver 8 units/hr?

Answer: _____ mL

ANSWERS: ALTERNATE ITEM FORMAT (FILL-IN-THE-BLANK)

141. 21

Rationale: Use the intravenous (IV) flow rate formula.

Formula:

$$\frac{\text{Total volume} \times \text{Drop factor}}{\text{Time in minutes}} = \text{Drops per minute}$$

$$\frac{1000 \text{ mL} \times 15 \text{ gtt}}{720 \text{ minutes}} = \frac{15,000}{720} = 20.8, \text{ or } 21 \text{ gtt/min}$$

Test-Taking Strategy: Use the formula for calculating IV flow rates when answering the question. Once you have performed the calculation, verify your answer using a calculator and make sure that the answer makes sense. Remember to round the answer to the nearest whole number. Review the formula

to calculate IV infusion rates if you had difficulty with this question.
Level of Cognitive Ability: Applying
Client Needs: Physiological Integrity
Integrated Process: Nursing Process—Implementation
Content Area: Fundamental Skills—Medications/Blood & IV Therapy
Reference: Potter, P., & Perry, A. (2009). *Fundamentals of nursing* (7th ed., p. 1007). St Louis: Mosby.

142. 1.3

Rationale: Use the medication dose formula.
Formula:

$$\frac{\text{Desired} \times \text{mL}}{\text{Available}} = \text{Milliliters per dose}$$

$$\frac{400{,}000 \text{ units} \times 1 \text{ mL}}{300{,}000 \text{ units}} = \text{Milliliters per dose}$$

$$\frac{400{,}000}{300{,}000} = 1.33 = 1.3 \text{ mL}$$

Test-Taking Strategy: Follow the formula for the calculation of the correct medication dose. Once you have performed the calculation, verify your answer using a calculator and make sure that the answer makes sense. Remember to round the answer to the nearest tenth position. If you had difficulty with this question, review the formula for calculating medication doses.
Level of Cognitive Ability: Applying
Client Needs: Physiological Integrity
Integrated Process: Nursing Process—Implementation
Content Area: Fundamental Skills—Medications/Blood & IV Therapy
Reference: Kee, J. & Marshall, S. (2009). *Clinical calculations: With applications to general and specialty areas* (6th ed., p. 86). St. Louis: Saunders.

143. 15

Rationale: Use the medication calculation formula.
Formula:

$$\frac{\text{Desired} \times \text{mL}}{\text{Available}} = \text{Milliliters per dose}$$

$$\frac{30 \text{ mEq} \times 20 \text{ mL}}{40 \text{ mEq}} = 15 \text{ mL}$$

Test-Taking Strategy: Follow the formula for the calculation of the correct medication dose. Once you have performed the calculation, verify your answer using a calculator and make sure that the answer makes sense. If you had difficulty with this question, review the formula for calculating medication doses.
Level of Cognitive Ability: Applying
Client Needs: Physiological Integrity
Integrated Process: Nursing Process—Implementation
Content Area: Fundamental Skills—Medications/Blood & IV Therapy
Reference: Kee, J. & Marshall, S. (2009). *Clinical calculations: With applications to general and specialty areas* (6th ed., p. 86). St. Louis: Saunders.

144. 2

Rationale: You must convert 0.3 g to milligrams. In the metric system, to convert larger to smaller, multiply by 1000 or move the decimal three places to the right. Therefore

0.3 g = 300 mg. Following conversion from grams to milligrams, use the formula to calculate the correct dose.
Formula:

$$\frac{\text{Desired} \times \text{mL}}{\text{Available}} = \text{Milliliters per dose}$$

$$\frac{300 \text{ mg} \times 6 \text{ mL}}{900 \text{ mg}} = \frac{1800}{900} = 2 \text{ mL}$$

Test-Taking Strategy: In this medication calculation problem, first you must convert grams to milligrams. Once you have performed the calculation, verify your answer using a calculator and make sure that the answer makes sense. If you had difficulty with this question, review the formula for calculating medication doses.
Level of Cognitive Ability: Applying
Client Needs: Physiological Integrity
Integrated Process: Nursing Process—Implementation
Content Area: Fundamental Skills—Medications/Blood & IV Therapy
Reference: Kee, J. & Marshall, S. (2009). *Clinical calculations: With applications to general and specialty areas* (6th ed., p. 86). St. Louis: Saunders.

145. 2

Rationale: You must convert 0.2 g to milligrams. In the metric system, to convert larger to smaller, multiply by 1000 or move the decimal three places to the right. Therefore 0.2 g equals 200 mg. After conversion from grams to milligrams, use the formula to calculate the correct dose.
Formula:

$$\frac{\text{Desired} \times \text{Capsule(s)}}{\text{Available}} = \text{Capsule(s) per dose}$$

$$\frac{200 \text{ mg} \times 1 \text{ capsule}}{100 \text{ mg}} = 2 \text{ capsules}$$

Test-Taking Strategy: In this medication calculation problem, first you must convert grams to milligrams. Once you have done the conversion and reread the medication calculation problem, you will know that two capsules is the correct answer. Recheck your work using a calculator and make sure that the answer makes sense. If you had difficulty with this question, review the formula for calculating medication doses.
Level of Cognitive Ability: Applying
Client Needs: Physiological Integrity
Integrated Process: Nursing Process—Implementation
Content Area: Fundamental Skills—Medications/Blood & IV Therapy
Reference: Kee, J. & Marshall, S. (2009). *Clinical calculations: With applications to general and specialty areas* (6th ed., p. 86). St. Louis: Saunders.

146. 31

Rationale: Use the intravenous (IV) flow rate formula.
Formula:

$$\frac{\text{Total volume} \times \text{Drop factor}}{\text{Time in minutes}} = \text{Drops per minute}$$

$$\frac{1000 \text{ mL} \times 15 \text{ gtt}}{480 \text{ minutes}} = \frac{15{,}000}{480} = 31.2, \text{ or } 31 \text{ gtt/min}$$

Test-Taking Strategy: Use the formula for calculating IV flow rates when answering the question. Once you have performed

the calculation, verify your answer using a calculator and make sure that the answer makes sense. Remember to round the answer to the nearest whole number. Review the formula for calculating IV infusion rates if you had difficulty with this question.
Level of Cognitive Ability: Applying
Client Needs: Physiological Integrity
Integrated Process: Nursing Process—Implementation
Content Area: Fundamental Skills—Medications/Blood & IV Therapy
Reference: Potter, P., & Perry, A. (2009). *Fundamentals of nursing* (7th ed., p. 1007). St Louis: Mosby.

147. 16

Rationale: Calculation of this problem can be done using a two-step process. First, you need to determine the amount of heparin sodium in 1 mL. The next step is to determine the infusion rate, or milliliters per hour.

Step 1:

$$\frac{\text{Known amount of medication in solution}}{\text{Total volume of diluent}}$$
$$= \text{Amount of medication per milliliter}$$

$$\frac{20,000 \text{ units}}{250 \text{ mL}} = 80 \text{ units/mL}$$

Step 2:

$$\frac{\text{Dose per hour desired}}{\text{Concentration per milliliter}} = \text{Infusion rate, or mL/hr}$$

$$\frac{1300 \text{ units}}{80 \text{ units/mL}} = 16.25, \text{ or } 16 \text{ mL/hr}$$

Test-Taking Strategy: Read the question carefully, noting that two steps can be used to solve this medication problem. Follow the formula, verify your answer using a calculator, and make sure that the answer makes sense. Remember to round the answer to the nearest whole number. If you had difficulty with this question, learn these steps. These steps can be used for similar medication problems related to the administration of heparin sodium or regular insulin by IV infusion.
Level of Cognitive Ability: Applying
Client Needs: Physiological Integrity
Integrated Process: Nursing Process—Implementation
Content Area: Fundamental Skills—Medications/Blood & IV Therapy
Reference: Kee, J., & Marshall, S. (2009). *Clinical calculations: With applications to general and specialty areas* (4th ed., p. 236). St. Louis: Saunders.

148. 125

Rationale: Use the intravenous (IV) formula to determine milliliters per hour.
Formula:

$$\frac{\text{Total volume in milliliters}}{\text{Number of hours}} = \text{Milliliters per hour}$$

$$\frac{3000 \text{ mL}}{24 \text{ hours}} = 125 \text{ mL/hr}$$

Test-Taking Strategy: Read the question carefully, noting that the question is asking about milliliters per hour to be administered to the client. Use the formula for calculating milliliters per hour. Once you have performed the calculation,

verify your answer using a calculator and make sure that the answer makes sense. Review the IV formula for calculating milliliters per hour if you had difficulty with this question.
Level of Cognitive Ability: Understanding
Client Needs: Physiological Integrity
Integrated Process: Nursing Process—Planning
Content Area: Fundamental Skills—Medications/Blood & IV Therapy
Reference: Potter, P., & Perry, A. (2009). *Fundamentals of nursing* (7th ed., p. 1007). St Louis: Mosby.

149. 33

Rationale: Use the intravenous (IV) flow rate formula.
Formula:

$$\frac{\text{Total volume} \times \text{Drop factor}}{\text{Time in minutes}} = \text{Drops per minute}$$

$$\frac{100 \text{ mL} \times 10 \text{ gtt}}{30 \text{ minutes}} = \frac{1000}{30} = 33.3, \text{ or } 33 \text{ gtt/min}$$

Test-Taking Strategy: Use the formula for calculating IV flow rates when answering the question. Once you have performed the calculation, verify your answer using a calculator and make sure that the answer makes sense. Remember to round the answer to the nearest whole number. Review the formula for calculating IV infusion rates if you had difficulty with this question.
Level of Cognitive Ability: Applying
Client Needs: Physiological Integrity
Integrated Process: Nursing Process—Implementation
Content Area: Fundamental Skills—Medications/Blood & IV Therapy
Reference: Potter, P., & Perry, A. (2009). *Fundamentals of nursing* (7th ed., p. 1007). St Louis: Mosby.

150. 1.5

Rationale: You must convert 150 mcg to milligrams. In the metric system, to convert smaller to larger, divide by 1000 or move the decimal three places to the left. Therefore 150 mcg equals 0.15 mg. Next, use the formula to calculate the correct dose.
Formula:

$$\frac{\text{Desired}}{\text{Available}} \times \text{Tablet} = \text{Tablets per dose}$$

$$\frac{0.15 \text{ mg}}{0.1 \text{ mg}} \times 1 \text{ tablet} = 1.5 \text{ tablets}$$

Test-Taking Strategy: In this medication calculation problem, first you must convert micrograms to milligrams. Next, follow the formula for the calculation of the correct dose, verify your answer using a calculator, and make sure that the answer makes sense. If you had difficulty with this question, review the formula for calculating medication doses.
Level of Cognitive Ability: Applying
Client Needs: Physiological Integrity
Integrated Process: Nursing Process—Implementation
Content Area: Fundamental Skills—Medications/Blood & IV Therapy
Reference: Kee, J. & Marshall, S. (2009). *Clinical calculations: With applications to general and specialty areas* (6th ed., p. 86). St. Louis: Saunders.

151. 25

Rationale: Use the intravenous (IV) flow rate formula.

Formula:

$$\frac{\text{Total volume} \times \text{Drop factor}}{\text{Time in minutes}} = \text{Drops per minute}$$

$$\frac{50 \text{ mL} \times 15 \text{ gtt}}{30 \text{ minutes}} = \frac{750}{30} = 25 \text{ gtt/min}$$

Test-Taking Strategy: Use the formula for calculating IV flow rates when answering the question. Once you have performed the calculation, verify your answer using a calculator and make sure that the answer makes sense. Review the formula for calculating IV infusion rates if you had difficulty with this question.
Level of Cognitive Ability: Applying
Client Needs: Physiological Integrity
Integrated Process: Nursing Process—Implementation
Content Area: Fundamental Skills—Medications/Blood & IV Therapy
Reference: Potter, P., & Perry, A. (2009). *Fundamentals of nursing* (7th ed., p. 1007). St Louis: Mosby.

152. 8
Rationale: You must determine that 1 L equals 1000 mL. Next, use the formula for determining infusion time in hours.
Formula:

$$\frac{\text{Total volume to infuse}}{\text{Milliliters per hour being infused}} = \text{Infusion time}$$

$$\frac{1000 \text{ mL}}{125 \text{ mL}} = 8 \text{ hours}$$

Test-Taking Strategy: Read the question carefully, noting that the question is asking about infusion time in hours. First, convert 1 L to milliliters. Next, use the formula for determining infusion time in hours. Verify your answer using a calculator and make sure that the answer makes sense. Review the IV formula for calculating infusion time if you had difficulty with this question.
Level of Cognitive Ability: Understanding
Client Needs: Physiological Integrity
Integrated Process: Nursing Process—Planning
Content Area: Fundamental Skills—Medications/Blood & IV Therapy
Reference: Potter, P., & Perry, A. (2009). *Fundamentals of nursing* (7th ed., p. 1007). St Louis: Mosby.

153. 10
Rationale: Use the IV flow rate formula.
Formula:

$$\frac{\text{Total volume} \times \text{Drop factor}}{\text{Time in minutes}} = \text{Drops per minute}$$

$$\frac{250 \text{ mL} \times 10 \text{ gtt}}{240 \text{ minutes}} = \frac{2500}{240} = 10.4, \text{ or } 10 \text{ gtt/min}$$

Test-Taking Strategy: Use the formula for calculating IV flow rates when answering the question. Once you have performed the calculation, verify your answer using a calculator and make sure that the answer makes sense. Remember to round the answer to the nearest whole number. Review the formula for calculating IV infusion rates if you had difficulty with this question.
Level of Cognitive Ability: Applying
Client Needs: Physiological Integrity
Integrated Process: Nursing Process—Planning
Content Area: Fundamental Skills—Medications/Blood & IV Therapy

Reference: Potter, P., & Perry, A. (2009). *Fundamentals of nursing* (7th ed., p. 1007). St Louis: Mosby.

154. 0.8
Rationale: Use the formula to calculate the correct dose.
Formula:

$$\frac{\text{Desired} \times \text{mL}}{\text{Available}} = \text{Milliliters per dose}$$

$$\frac{8 \text{ mg} \times 1 \text{ mL}}{10 \text{ mg}} = 0.8 \text{ mL}$$

Test-Taking Strategy: Follow the formula for the calculation of the correct dose. Once you have performed the calculation, verify your answer using a calculator and make sure that the answer makes sense. If you had difficulty with this question, review the formula for calculating medication doses.
Level of Cognitive Ability: Applying
Client Needs: Physiological Integrity
Integrated Process: Nursing Process—Implementation
Content Area: Fundamental Skills—Medications/Blood & IV Therapy
Reference: Kee, J. & Marshall, S. (2009). *Clinical calculations: With applications to general and specialty areas* (6th ed., p. 86). St. Louis: Saunders.

155. 8
Rationale: Calculation of this problem can be done using a two-step process. First, you need to determine the amount of regular insulin in 1 mL. The next step is to determine the infusion rate, or milliliters per hour.
Formula:
Step 1:

$$\frac{\text{Known amount of medication in solution}}{\text{Total volume of diluent}} = \text{Amount of medication per milliliter}$$

$$\frac{100 \text{ units}}{100 \text{ mL}} = 1 \text{ unit/mL}$$

Step 2:

$$\frac{\text{Dose per hour desired}}{\text{Concentration per milliliter}} = \text{Infusion rate, or milliliters per hour}$$

$$\frac{8 \text{ units}}{1 \text{ unit/mL}} = 8 \text{ mL/hr}$$

Test-Taking Strategy: Read the question carefully, noting that two steps can be used to solve this medication problem. Once you have performed the calculation, verify your answer using a calculator and make sure that the answer makes sense. These steps can be used for similar medication problems related to the administration of heparin sodium or regular insulin by IV infusion. Learn these steps if you had difficulty with this question.
Level of Cognitive Ability: Applying
Client Need: Physiological Integrity
Integrated Process: Nursing Process—Implementation
Content Area: Fundamental Skills—Medications/Blood & IV Therapy
Reference: Kee, J., & Marshall, S. (2009). *Clinical calculations: With applications to general and specialty areas* (6th ed., p. 236). St. Louis: Saunders.

18

Cardiopulmonary Resuscitation Guidelines for Health Care Providers

PYRAMID TERMS

abdominal thrust maneuver Method to relieve a foreign body airway obstruction.

automated external defibrillator Machine that converts ventricular fibrillation into a perfusing rhythm and allows for early defibrillation by first responders.

basic life support Provision of oxygen to the brain, heart, and other vital organs until help arrives.

cardiopulmonary resuscitation An interchangeable term for basic life support.

head tilt–chin lift Preferred method to open a victim's airway.

jaw thrust maneuver Method used to open a victim's airway if a neck injury is suspected.

 THE PYRAMID TO SUCCESS

The Pyramid to Success focuses on emergency care guidelines and procedures performed by the health care provider (HCP). These include cardiopulmonary resuscitation (CPR), the abdominal thrust maneuver, and use of the automated external defibrillator (AED). In addition to CPR guidelines for the HCP, the American Heart Association has also developed CPR guidelines for the lay rescuer and guidelines for performing Hands-Only CPR. For information on lay rescuer CPR guidelines and Hands-Only CPR, access the American Heart Association Web site at www.americanheart.org.

 CLIENT NEEDS

Safe and Effective Care Environment

Acting as an advocate regarding the client's wishes
Considering ethical and legal responsibilities
Establishing priorities
Following advance directives regarding the client's documented requests
Implementing standard and transmission-based precautions and surgical asepsis techniques
Upholding client's rights

Health Promotion and Maintenance

Performing the techniques of physical assessment
Teaching significant others to perform Lay Rescuer CPR and the abdominal thrust maneuver

Psychosocial Integrity

Considering the client's cultural, religious, and spiritual preferences
Discussing end-of-life and grief and loss issues
Providing emotional support to significant others

Physiological Integrity

Administering emergency medications and intravenous solutions
Documenting the client's response to basic life support (BLS) measures
Handling medical emergencies
Identifying alterations in the cardiopulmonary system
Performing CPR or the abdominal thrust maneuver
Using special equipment

I. CARDIOPULMONARY RESUSCITATION (Box 18-1)

A. CPR is providing oxygen to the brain, heart, and other vital organs until help arrives.

B. CPR is also known as BLS.

II. ADULT CPR GUIDELINES FOR THE HEALTH CARE PROVIDER (Box 18-2 and Table 18-1; see Priority Nursing Actions on p. 204)

A. Description: An adult is defined as a person who is an adolescent or older (for lay rescuers, adults are defined as those 8 years of age or older).

🔺 Remember CAB for CPR—circulation, airway, breathing.

B. Airway
   1. For the HCP, assessment is the first step of the nursing process; assessing a victim of sudden illness or accident for unconsciousness is the initial action (assess for 5 to 10 seconds)

Box 18-1 The CAB for Cardiopulmonary Resuscitation for the Health Care Provider

C: Circulation
A: Airway
B: Breathing

Each step of CAB for cardiopulmonary resuscitation begins with assessment.

Box 18-2 Pyramid Points: CPR

Current CPR guidelines indicate that the health care provider follow the CAB procedure – circulation, airway, and breathing.

Immediate recognition of sudden cardiac arrest is based on assessing unresponsiveness and absence of normal breathing.

Ensure that the scene is safe before approaching the victim.

"Look, listen, and feel" is no longer a part of CPR procedures.

CPR should be continued until the return of the spontaneous circulation or resuscitative efforts are terminated.

Rapid defibrillation is done if indicated.

Refer to the American Heart Association at http://www.heart.org/HEARTORG/ and http://circ.ahajournals.org for updates to Table 18-1 and other information in the chapter.

TABLE 18-1 Summary of Cardiopulmonary Resuscitation ABCD Guidelines for Infants, Children, and Adults

Maneuver*	Adult[†]	Child[†]	Infant[‡]
Activate (call) emergency response number (one rescuer)	Call when victim is found unresponsive HCP: If asphyxial arrest is likely, call after five cycles (2 min) of cardio-pulmonary resuscitation (CPR)	Call after performing five cycles of CPR For sudden unwitnessed collapse, call after verifying that victim is unresponsive	Call after performing five cycles of CPR For sudden unwitnessed collapse, call after verifying that victim is unresponsive
Airway breaths	Head tilt–chin lift (HCP: If trauma is suspected, use jaw thrust) Two effective breaths at 1 sec per breath	Head tilt–chin lift (HCP: If trauma is suspected, use jaw thrust) Two effective breaths at 1 sec per breath	Head tilt–chin lift (HCP: If trauma is suspected, use jaw thrust) Two effective breaths at 1 sec per breath
HCP: Rescue breathing without chest compressions	10-12 breaths/min (one breath every 5-6 sec)	12-20 breaths/min (one breath every 3-5 sec)	12-20 breaths/min (one breath every 3-5 sec)
HCP: Rescue breathing for CPR with advanced airway	8-10 breaths/min (one breath every 6-8 sec)	8-10 breaths/min (one breath every 6-8 sec)	8-10 breaths/min (one breath every 6-8 sec)
Foreign body airway obstruction	Abdominal thrusts	Back slaps and chest thrusts	Back slaps and chest thrusts
CIRCULATION HCP: Pulse check (10 sec or less)	Carotid artery	HCP can use femoral artery in child	Brachial or femoral artery
Compression landmarks	Center of chest, between nipples	Center of chest, between nipples	Just below nipple line
Compression method: Push hard and fast Allow complete recoil	Two hands: Heel of one hand, other hand on top	Two hands: Heel of one hand with second on top *or* One hand: Heel of one hand only	One rescuer: two fingers HCP, two rescuers: Two-thumb–encircling hands technique
Compression depth	1½-2 inches	Approximately ⅓ to ½ the depth of the chest	Approximately ⅓ to ½ the depth of the chest
Compression rate	Approximately 100 per minute	Approximately 100 per minute	Approximately 100 per minute
Compression-to-ventilation ratio	30:2 (one or two rescuers)	30:2 (single rescuer) HCP: 15:2 (two rescuers)	30:2 (single rescuer) HCP: 15:2 (two rescuers)
DEFIBRILLATION Automatic external defibrillator (AED)	Use adult pads Do not use child pads or a child system HCP: For out-of-hospital response, you may provide five cycles (2 min) of CPR before shock if response time is longer than 4-5 min and arrest was not witnessed	HCP: Use AED as soon as possible for sudden and in-hospital collapse All: After five cycles of CPR (out of hospital) Use child pads and system for child 1-8 yr old if available If child pads and system are not available, use adult AED and pads	No recommendation for infants younger than 1 yr old

*Maneuver performed only by health care provider indicated by HCP.

[†]For lay rescuers, adults are defined as those 8 years of age or older; for HCPs, adolescent or older. For lay rescuers, children are those 1 to 8 years of age; for HCPs, 1 year to adolescent.

[‡]For all rescuers, infants are defined as those younger than 1 year of age.

Reprinted with permission. 2005 American Heart Association Guidelilnes for Cardiopulmonary Resuscitation and Emergency Cardiovascular Care, Part 3: Overview of CPR. *Circulation.* 2005;112:IV-12–IV-18. ©2005 American Heart Association, Inc.

2. Gently shake the victim's shoulders and ask, "Are you OK?"; be alert to the potential for a head or neck injury.

3. Call the emergency response number when the victim is found unconscious; for the HCP, if asphyxial arrest is likely, call after five cycles (2 minutes) of CPR.

4. Place the victim in a supine position on a firm, flat surface (logroll the victim, using spine precautions).

   a. One-person rescue: The rescuer is positioned on his or her knees, perpendicular to the victim's sternum and facing the victim.

   b. Two-person rescue: One rescuer faces the victim, kneeling perpendicular to the victim's head, maintains an open airway, monitors the carotid pulse, and performs the rescue breathing; the second rescuer moves to the opposite side and faces the victim, kneeling perpendicular to the victim's sternum, and performs the chest compressions.

   c. When two rescuers are present during CPR, the rescuers should rotate the compressor role every 2 minutes.

   d. The rescuers apply gloves and face shields, if available.

▲ For the HCP, determining unresponsiveness of the victim is the first action.

5. Open the airway.

6. The **head tilt–chin lift** is the preferred method for opening the airway; for the HCP, if the victim has a neck injury, the **jaw thrust maneuver** is used to open the airway (Figs. 18-1 and 18-2).

7. Look for foreign material, liquids, or solids in the victim's mouth; wipe out any foreign material.

▲ If a neck injury is suspected, the jaw thrust maneuver is used to open the victim's airway.

C. Breathing

1. Assess breathing and maintain an open airway.

2. The rescuer places his or her ear over the victim's nose and mouth and looks for the chest to rise and fall, listens for air moving in and out of the lungs, and feels for the flow of air (Fig. 18-3).

3. For the breathing victim, do the following:

   a. Place the victim on his or her side if no cervical trauma is suspected; logroll the victim onto the side as a unit (without twisting) to help maintain an open airway and decrease the risk of aspiration.

   b. If trauma or injury is suspected, do not move the victim.

4. For the nonbreathing victim, do the following:

   a. Maintain the **head tilt–chin lift**, pinch the nostrils closed, and give two, effective breaths

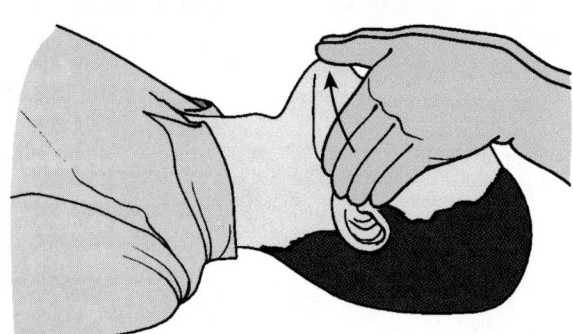

▲ **FIGURE 18-2** Opening the airway using the jaw thrust maneuver. (From Harkreader, H., Hogan, M., & Thobaben, M. [2007]. *Fundamentals of nursing: Caring and clinical judgment* [3rd ed.]. St. Louis: Saunders. Used with permission of the American Heart Association. [1992]. Guidelines for cardiopulmonary resuscitation and emergency cardiac care: An international consensus on science and circulation, *Circulation*, 102[Suppl], 217-222.)

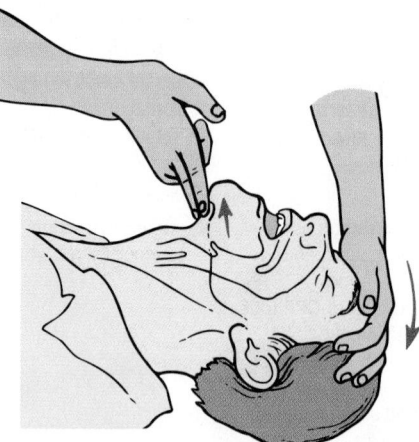

▲ **FIGURE 18-1** Opening the airway using the head tilt–chin lift maneuver. (From Lewis, S., Heitkemper, M., Dirksen, S., O'Brien, P., & Bucher, L. [2007]. *Medical-surgical nursing: Assessment and management of clinical problems* [7th ed.]. St. Louis: Mosby.)

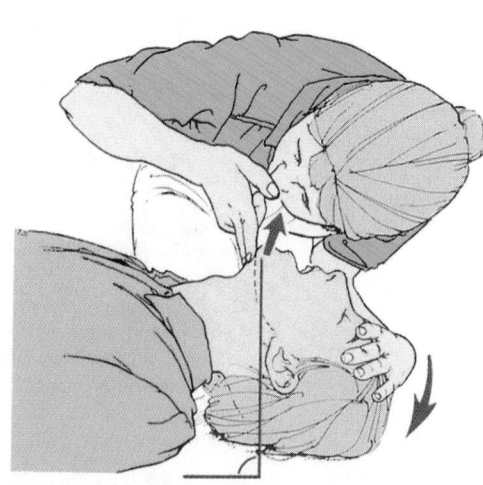

▲ **FIGURE 18-3** Listening and feeling for exhalation. (From Christensen, B., and Kockrow, E. [2011]. *Foundations and adult health nursing* [6th ed.]. St. Louis: Mosby.)

at 1 second per breath; thereafter, if rescue breathing is delivered without chest compressions, give 10 to 12 breaths per minute (one breath every 5 to 6 seconds) (Fig. 18-4).

b. Avoid delivering breaths that are too large or too forceful.

c. Try to use a resuscitation bag or face shield, if available, ensuring an adequate air seal; allow the victim to exhale fully between breaths.

d. If unsuccessful at giving the breath, reposition the victim's head and try again (improper chin and head position is a common cause of difficulty in ventilating the victim).

e. If still unsuccessful, check the victim's mouth for a foreign body or for loose dentures (remove dentures only if they interfere with the mouth seal), clear the airway, and try to ventilate again.

f. Be alert to gastric distention when giving ventilations.

⚠ When performing CPR, if you are unsuccessful at giving a breath, reposition the victim's head and try again.

5. Mouth to nose: This method is recommended when ventilating through the victim's mouth is impossible, the mouth cannot be opened, the mouth is seriously injured, or a tight mouth-to-mouth seal is difficult to achieve.

6. Mouth to stoma (advanced airway)

a. This method is used for the victim who has had a laryngectomy or has an advanced airway such as tracheostomy; to be effective, an adequate seal over the victim's mouth and nose is necessary.

b. With an advanced airway (endotracheal tube, laryngeal airway, tracheostomy, esophagotracheal Combitube), 8 to 10 breaths per minute (one breath every 6 to 8 seconds) is delivered

D. Circulation

1. Palpate the carotid artery to assess circulation; always check for the absence of a pulse before beginning chest compressions (Fig. 18-5).

2. Maintain an open airway and palpate for a carotid pulse for 10 seconds or less.

3. If there is a pulse, continue to give 10 to 12 breaths per minute.

4. If there is no pulse, chest compressions should begin.

E. Chest compression landmarks: center of the chest, between the nipples

⚠ To produce as much blood flow as possible, allow the chest to recoil (return to normal position) completely after delivery of each breath and each compression.

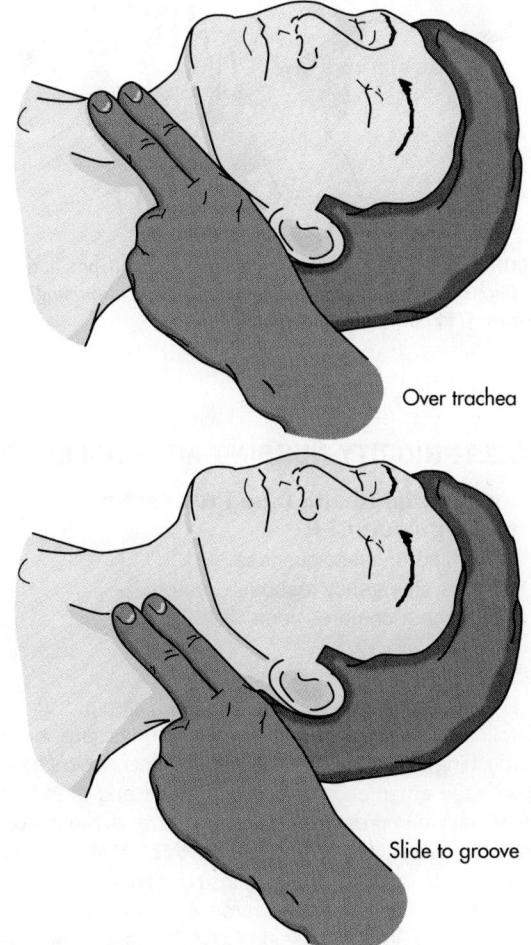

Over trachea

Slide to groove

▲ **FIGURE 18-5** Locating carotid artery. (From Monahan, F., Sands, J., Neighbors, M., Marek, J., & Green, C. [2007]. *Phipps' medical-surgical nursing: Health and illness perspectives* [8th ed.]. St. Louis: Mosby.)

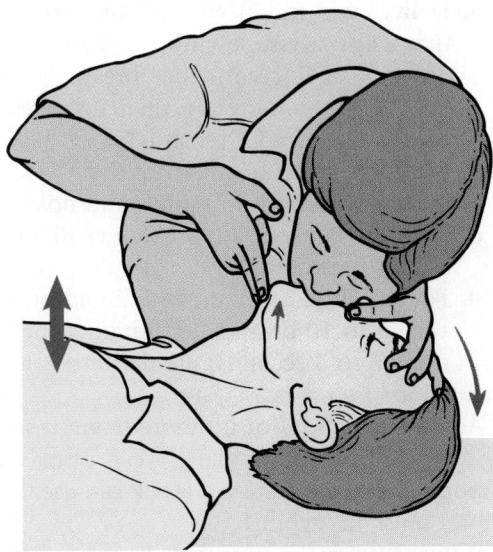

▲ **FIGURE 18-4** The chin is lifted and brought forward; the nostrils are then closed and two effective breaths are given at 1 second per breath (From Lewis, S., Heitkemper, M., Dirksen, S., O'Brien, P., & Bucher, L. [2007]. *Medical-surgical nursing: Assessment and management of clinical problems* [7th ed.]. St. Louis: Mosby.)

F. Chest compression method (Fig. 18-6)

1. The rescuer uses two hands; the heel of one hand is placed on the landmark and the other hand is placed on top.

2. The rescuer should push hard and fast and avoid interrupted compressions (every time that chest compressions are stopped, blood flow stops as well).

3. The rescuer should allow for complete recoil between compressions.

4. Compression depth should be 1½ to 2 inches.

5. Compression rate is approximately 100 times per minute.

6. The compression-to-ventilation ratio is 30:2 (for either one or two rescuers).

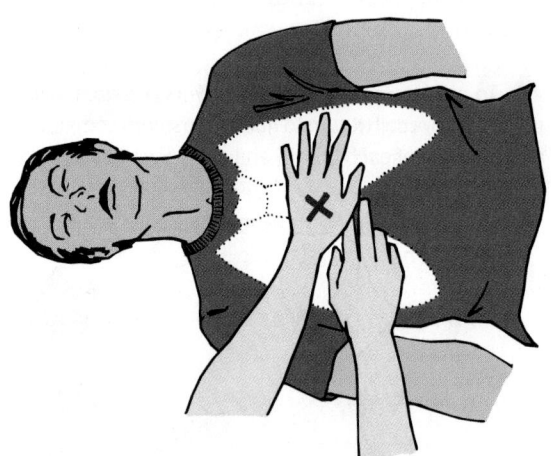

▲ **FIGURE 18-6** Chest compression—proper hand position for an adult. (From Perry, A., & Potter, P. [2010]. *Clinical nursing skills & techniques* [7th ed.]. St. Louis: Mosby.)

PRIORITY NURSING ACTIONS!

Actions for the Health Care Provider for Performing Adult CPR

1. Determine unconsciousness.
2. Activate emergency response system.
3. Begin chest compressions.
4. Open the airway.
5. Deliver rescue breaths.

The sequence for basic CPR for health care providers is as follows. Determine that the scene is safe before approaching a victim. After determining unconsciousness, activate the emergency response system, and then begin CPR. Chest compressions are initiated and the rescuer needs to push hard and fast at a depth of 2 inches for an adult at a rate of 100 compressions per minute. The airway is opened and breaths are delivered. A compression to ventilation ratio of 30 compressions to 2 ventilations is done.

Reference: Berg, R. et al. (2010). 2010 American Heart Association guidelines for cardiopulmonary resuscitation and emergency cardiovascular care. *Circulation.* 2010;122(suppl 3):S685–S705 @ http://circ.ahajournals.org

---

G. Complications of chest compressions

1. Laceration of internal organs
2. Punctured lungs
3. Fractured ribs or sternum

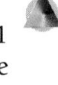 When performing chest compressions, push hard and fast, and avoid interrupted compressions.

III. PEDIATRIC CPR GUIDELINES FOR THE HEALTH CARE PROVIDER

A. Description

1. For HCPs, a child is defined as a person from 1 year to adolescent; for lay rescuers, children are 1 to 8 years of age.

2. For both HCPs and lay rescuers, an infant is defined as a person younger than 1 year of age.

3. For an unresponsive infant or child, the lone (one rescuer) HCP should perform five cycles (about 2 minutes of CPR) and then call the emergency response number; the HCP must assess the most likely cause of the arrest.

4. If the infant or child has a sudden witnessed collapse, the collapse is likely to be cardiac in origin (hypoxic cardiac arrest); in this situation, the emergency response number should be called after verifying that the victim is unresponsive.

B. Airway

1. Assess unresponsiveness.

2. Use the **head tilt–chin lift** to open the airway (the HCP would use the **jaw thrust maneuver** if neck trauma is suspected).

C. Breathing

1. Breathing victim: Keep the airway open.

2. Nonbreathing victim

   a. Deliver two initial effective breaths (breaths that cause a visible chest rise) to the infant or child at 1 second per breath; 12 to 20 breaths per minute are then delivered (one breath every 3 to 5 seconds)

   b. With the infant or small child, provide ventilations by mouth to mouth and nose.

   c. With the larger child, provide ventilations by mouth to mouth.

   d. For the child or infant with an advanced airway, 8 to 10 breaths per minute (one breath every 6 to 8 seconds) are delivered.

D. Circulation

1. Assess circulation for no more than 10 seconds.

2. If the victim is older than 1 year, assess circulation via the carotid artery (HCP can use the femoral pulse in a child).

3. If the victim is younger than 1 year, assess circulation via the brachial artery (HCP can use the femoral pulse in a child).

4. If there is a pulse, continue to give 12 to 20 breaths per minute (one breath every 3 to 5 seconds).

5. If there is no pulse, begin chest compressions.

⚠ The chest compression landmark for a child is in the center of the chest between the nipples. For the infant, the landmark is just below the nipple line.

6. Chest compression method
   a. Child: Use of two hands with the heel of one hand on the chest and the second hand on top; or use one hand with the heel of one hand only on the chest.
   b. Infant: One rescuer uses two fingers; for HCPs with two rescuers present, use two-thumb–encircling hands technique.
   c. Compression depth: ⅓ to ½ the depth of the chest
   d. Compression rate: Approximately 100 per minute
   e. Compression-to-ventilation ratio: 30:2 for a single rescuer; for the HCP, 15:2 for two rescuers

IV. **AUTOMATED EXTERNAL DEFIBRILLATOR BY THE HEALTH CARE PROVIDER**

A. Description
   1. The automated external defribulator (AED) is used to convert ventricular fibrillation into a perfusing rhythm.
   2. The AED differentiates nonventricular from ventricular fibrillation rhythms and allows for early defibrillation by first responders.
   3. The use of AEDs is recommended for children in cardiac arrest 1 year of age and older (not recommended for infants younger than 1 year).
   4. For sudden witnessed arrest in the child or adult in the out-of-hospital setting, the HCP should phone the emergency response number, retrieve the AED, and return to the victim to perform CPR and use the AED.

B. Adult
   1. Adult pads need to be used (child pads or a child system cannot be used on an adult).
   2. Out-of-hospital response: Provide five cycles (2 minutes) of CPR before defibrillating if response time was longer than 4 to 5 minutes and the arrest was not witnessed.

C. Child
   1. Child pads and child system are used for the child 1 to 8 years of age, if available (if child pads and system are not available, adult AED and pads are used).
   2. Out-of-hospital response: Provide five cycles of CPR before defibrillating (for sudden and in-hospital collapse, use AED as soon as possible).

⚠ When using the AED on an adult, do not use the child pads; these pads will not provide an effective shock.

D. Interventions
   1. Attach AED pads to the victim.
   2. Turn on the AED and push the button to activate the analyzer.

3. Follow instructions given for the AED, usually "assess," "stand back," "shock," and "reassess."
4. CPR guidelines to treat cardiac arrest associated with ventricular fibrillation or pulseless ventricular tachycardia recommend the delivery of single shocks followed immediately by a period of CPR; interruptions of chest compressions to check circulation should not be done until about five cycles or approximately 2 minutes of CPR have been provided after the shock.

V. **FOREIGN BODY AIRWAY OBSTRUCTION (FBAO)**

A. General guidelines
   1. The HCP needs to distinguish choking victims who require treatment (abdominal thrusts or back slaps and chest thrusts) from those who do not (mild versus severe airway obstruction).
   2. Signs of severe airway obstruction include poor air exchange and increased breathing difficulty, a silent cough, cyanosis, or inability to speak or breathe.
   3. Every time the airway is opened (with a **head tilt–chin lift**) to deliver rescue breaths, the rescuer should look in the mouth and remove an object only if one is seen.
   4. Abdominal thrusts are used for the adult; back slaps and chest thrusts are used for the child and infant.

⚠ Blind finger sweeps in the mouth of a victim with a foreign body airway obstruction (FBAO) should not be performed because of the risk of pushing the object further into the airway.

B. Conscious adult
   1. Ask the victim, "Are you choking?" (the victim will not be able to speak or cough if he or she is choking); if the victim nods "yes," help is needed.
   2. Relieve the obstruction by the **abdominal thrust maneuver** (Box 18-3 and Fig. 18-7).
   3. Continue abdominal thrusts until the object is dislodged or the victim becomes unconscious.

C. Unconscious adult
   1. Assess unconsciousness.
   2. Call for help.

Box 18-3 Abdominal Thrust Maneuver

Stand behind the victim.
Place arms around the victim's waist.
Make a fist.
Place the thumb side of the fist just above the umbilicus (belly button) and well below the xiphoid process.
Perform five quick in and up abdominal thrusts (between the umbilicus and the xiphoid process).
Use chest thrusts for the obese or the advanced pregnancy victim.

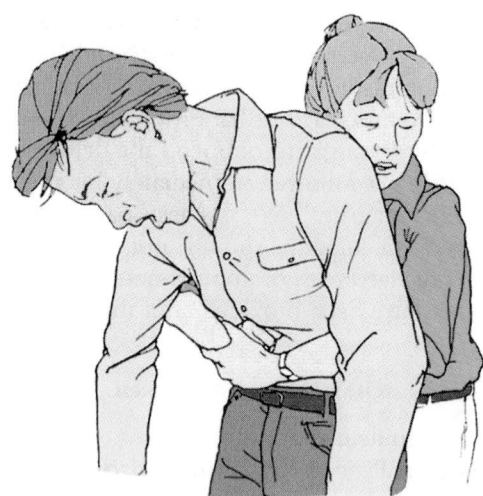

▲ **FIGURE 18-7** Abdominal thrust maneuver. (From Christensen, B., & Kockrow, E. [2006]. *Foundations of nursing* [5th ed.]. St. Louis: Mosby.)

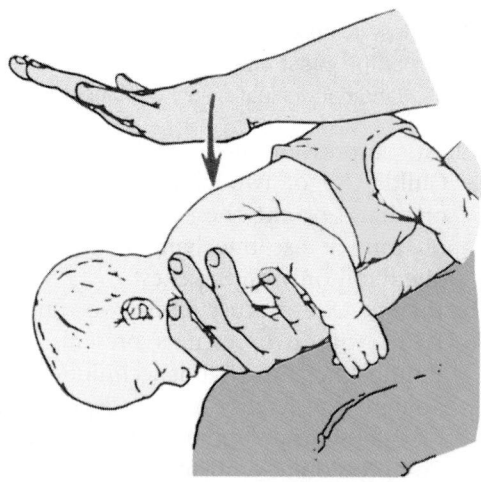

▲ **FIGURE 18-8** Clearing airway obstruction in an infant. (From Christensen, B., & Kockrow, E. [2006]. *Foundations of nursing* [5th ed.]. St. Louis: Mosby.)

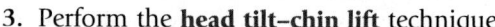

3. Perform the **head tilt–chin lift** technique.
4. Open the airway and look in the mouth; remove an object only if one is seen.
5. Attempt ventilation.
6. Reposition the head if unsuccessful; reattempt ventilation.
7. Relieve the obstruction by the **abdominal thrust maneuver** with five abdominal thrusts.
8. Reattempt ventilation.
9. Repeat the sequence of **head tilt–chin lift**, breaths, and **abdominal thrust maneuver** until successful.
10. Be sure to assess for the victim's carotid pulse and for the presence of spontaneous respirations.
11. Perform rescue breathing or CPR, if required.

⚠ To perform the abdominal thrust maneuver on an adult, straddle the victim's thighs, place the heel of one hand on top of the other, between the umbilicus and xiphoid process, and give five abdominal thrusts in and up with the heel of the bottom hand.

D. Choking child or infant
1. FBAO requiring intervention is when signs of severe airway obstruction exist.
2. For the conscious child:
    a. Assess for obstruction by asking the child, "Are you choking?" If the victim nods "yes," help is needed.
    b. Relieve the obstruction by the **abdominal thrust maneuver** until the obstruction is dislodged or the child becomes unconscious.
3. For the unconscious child, do the following:
    a. Assess unconsciousness.
    b. Open the airway by the **head tilt–chin lift** technique.

c. Check for breathing and look for a foreign object (remove only if seen).
d. Attempt ventilation.
e. If unsuccessful, reposition the head; reattempt ventilation.
f. Relieve the obstruction by using the **abdominal thrust maneuver**.
g. Look in the mouth and remove a foreign object only if one is seen.
h. Reattempt ventilation.
i. Repeat the sequence.
4. For the conscious infant, do the following:
    a. Assess for obstruction and note if mild or severe airway obstruction exists.
    b. Relieve the obstruction by five back slaps and five chest thrusts (Fig. 18-8).
    c. Straddle the infant over the arm, place the infant's head lower than the trunk, and support the head firmly, holding the jaw.
    d. Give five back slaps with the heel of the hand between the shoulder blades.
    e. Turn the infant; place the head lower than the trunk.
    f. Give five chest thrusts at the same location as for chest compressions.
    g. Check for the object and remove, if visible.
    h. Continue until the object is removed or the infant becomes unconscious.
5. For the unconscious infant, do the following:
    a. Assess unconsciousness by gentle taps.
    b. Open the airway by the **head tilt–chin lift** technique and check for breathing.
    c. Look in the mouth and remove any visualized foreign object every time the airway is opened
    d. Attempt ventilation.
    e. Reposition the head if unsuccessful; reattempt ventilation.

f. Relieve the obstruction by five back slaps and five chest thrusts.

g. Reattempt ventilation and repeat the sequence.

 In an infant, deliver five back slaps and then five chest thrusts to remove the foreign body from the airway.

VI. PREGNANT OR OBESE VICTIM

A. **Abdominal thrust maneuver** and relieving a FBAO

1. Place the arms under the woman's axillae and across the chest.
2. Place the thumb side of a clenched fist against the middle of the sternum, and place the other hand over the fist.
3. Perform backward chest thrusts until the foreign body is expelled or until the woman becomes unconscious.
4. If she becomes unconscious, place her on her back.

 If the victim of FBAO is pregnant, remember to place a wedge, such as a pillow or rolled blanket, under the right abdominal flank and hip to displace the uterus to the left side of the abdomen. This prevents supine hypotension.

5. If unable to ventilate, position the hands as for chest compressions and deliver chest thrusts firmly to remove the obstruction.

B. Defibrillation in the pregnant client: If defibrillation is needed, place the paddles one rib interspace higher than usual because the heart is displaced slightly by the enlarged uterus.

🔘 MORE QUESTIONS ON THE CD!

Practice Questions

156. A nurse on the day shift walks into a client's room and finds the client unresponsive. The client is not breathing and does not have a pulse, and the nurse immediately calls out for help. The next nursing action is which of the following?
1. Open the airway.
2. Give the client oxygen.
3. Start chest compressions.
4. Ventilate with a mouth-to-mask device.

157. A nurse witnesses a neighbor's husband sustain a fall from the roof of his house. The nurse rushes to the victim and determines the need to open the airway. The nurse opens the airway in this victim by using which method?
1. Flexed position
2. Head tilt–chin lift
3. Jaw thrust maneuver
4. Modified head tilt–chin lift

158. A nurse understands that which of the following is a correct guideline for adult cardiopulmonary resuscitation (CPR) for a health care provider?
1. One breath should be given for every five compressions.
2. Two breaths should be given for every 15 compressions.
3. Initially, two quick breaths should be given as rapidly as possible.
4. Each rescue breath should be given over 1 second and should produce a visible chest rise.

159. A nurse attempts to relieve an airway obstruction on a 3-year-old conscious child. The nurse performs this maneuver correctly by standing behind the child, placing her arms under the child's axillae and around the child, and positioning her hands to deliver the thrusts between the:
1. Groin and the abdomen
2. Umbilicus and the groin
3. Lower abdomen and the chest
4. Umbilicus and the xiphoid process

160. A nurse is performing cardiopulmonary resuscitation (CPR) on a 7-year-old child. The nurse delivers how many breaths per minute to the child?
1. 6
2. 8
3. 10
4. 20

161. A nurse is performing cardiopulmonary resuscitation (CPR) on an infant. When performing chest compressions, the nurse compresses at least:
1. 60 times per minute
2. 80 times per minute
3. 100 times per minute
4. 160 times per minute

162. A nurse is teaching cardiopulmonary resuscitation (CPR) to a group of nursing students. The nurse asks a student to describe the reason why blind finger sweeps are avoided in infants. The nurse determines that the student understands this reason if the student makes which statement?
1. "The object may have been swallowed."
2. "The infant may bite down on the finger."
3. "The mouth is too small to see the object."
4. "The object may be forced back farther into the throat."

163. A nurse is performing cardiopulmonary resuscitation (CPR) on an adult client. When performing chest compressions, the nurse should depress the sternum:
    1. ¾ inch
    2. 1 inch
    3. 2 inches
    4. 3 inches

164. A nursing instructor asks a nursing student to describe the procedure for performing abdominal thrusts on an unconscious pregnant woman at 8 months' gestation. The student describes a component of the procedure the procedure correctly if the student states that he will:
    1. Place his hands in the pelvis to perform the thrusts.
    2. Perform abdominal thrusts until the object is dislodged.
    3. Perform left lateral abdominal thrusts until the object is dislodged.
    4. Place a rolled blanket under the right abdominal flank and hip area.

Alternate Item Format: Prioritizing (Ordered Response)

165. A nursing student is asked to describe the correct steps for performing abdominal thrusts on an unconscious adult. Number in order of priority the steps for performing this procedure. (Number 1 is the first step and number 5 is the last step.)
    _____ Open the airway
    _____ Attempt ventilation
    _____ Assess unconsciousness
    _____ Perform abdominal thrusts
    _____ Look in the mouth and remove the object blocking the airway if seen

ANSWERS

156. 3

Rationale: The next nursing action would be to start chest compressions. The airway is then opened and breaths are delivered. Oxygen may be helpful at some point but giving oxygen is not the next action.

Test-Taking Strategy: Visualize the steps of cardiopulmonary resuscitation (CPR) to answer the question. Recalling CAB—circulation, airway, and breathing,—will assist in directing you to option 3. Review the steps of CPR if you had difficulty with this question.

Level of Cognitive Ability: Applying
Client Needs: Physiological Integrity
Integrated Process: Nursing Process—implementation
Content Area: Critical Care
Reference: Berg, R. et al. (2010). 2010 American Heart Association guidelines for cardiopulmonary resuscitation and emergency cardiovascular care. *Circulation.* 2010:122(suppl 3): S685-S705 @ http://circ.ahajournals.org

157. 3

Rationale: If a neck injury is suspected, the jaw thrust maneuver is used to open the airway. The head tilt–chin lift maneuver produces hyperextension of the neck and could cause complications if a neck injury is present. A flexed position is an inappropriate position for opening the airway.

Test-Taking Strategy: Use the process of elimination. Eliminate options 2 and 4 first because they are comparable or alike. Next, eliminate option 1 because this position would not open the airway. If you had difficulty with this question, review the appropriate methods to open an airway.

Level of Cognitive Ability: Applying
Client Needs: Physiological Integrity
Integrated Process: Nursing Process—Implementation
Content Area: Critical Care
Reference: Ignatavicius, D., & Workman, M. (2010). *Medical-surgical nursing: Patient-centered collaborative care* (6th ed., p. 136). St. Louis: Saunders.

158. 4

Rationale: In adult CPR, each rescue breath should be given over 1 second and should produce a visible chest rise. Excessive ventilation (too many breaths per minute or breaths that are too large or forceful) may be harmful and should not be performed. Health care providers should employ a 30:2 compression-to-ventilation ratio for the adult victim. Options 1, 2, and 3 are incorrect.

Test-Taking Strategy: Read each option carefully. Noting the words *visible chest rise* in option 4 will direct you to this option. Review CPR guidelines for the adult if you had difficulty with this question.

Level of Cognitive Ability: Understanding
Client Needs: Physiological Integrity
Integrated Process: Nursing Process—Implementation
Content Area: Critical Care
Reference: Perry, A., & Potter, P. (2010). *Clinical nursing skills & techniques* (7th ed., pp. 731, 734). St. Louis: Mosby.

159. 4

Rationale: To perform abdominal thrusts on a child, the rescuer stands behind the victim and places the arms directly under the victim's axillae and around the victim. The rescuer places the thumb side of one fist against the victim's abdomen in the midline, slightly above the umbilicus and well below the tip of the xiphoid process. The rescuer grasps the fist with the other hand and delivers up to five thrusts. One must take care not to touch the xiphoid process or the lower margins of the rib cage because force applied to these structures may damage internal organs. Options 1, 2, and 3 are incorrect hand placements.

Test-Taking Strategy: Use the process of elimination, noting the age of the child. Eliminate options 1 and 2 first because they are comparable or alike locations. From the remaining options, considering the anatomical location and the effect of the maneuver in dislodging an obstruction will direct you to option 4. If you had difficulty with this question, review the correct hand placement for performing abdominal thrusts.

Level of Cognitive Ability: Applying
Client Needs: Physiological Integrity
Integrated Process: Nursing Process—Implementation
Content Area: Critical Care
Reference: Hockenberry, M., & Wilson, D. (2009). *Wong's essentials of pediatric nursing* (8th ed., pp. 809–810). St. Louis: Mosby.

160. 4
Rationale: In a child between the ages of 1 and 8 years, 12 to 20 breaths per minute are delivered. Options 1, 2, and 3 are incorrect.
Test-Taking Strategy: Use the process of elimination and note the age of the child. Recalling the normal respiratory rate in a child at this age will assist in directing you to option 4. If you had difficulty with this question, review CPR guidelines for a child.
Level of Cognitive Ability: Applying
Client Needs: Physiological Integrity
Integrated Process: Nursing Process—Implementation
Content Area: Critical Care
Reference: McKinney, E., James, S., Murray, S., & Ashwill, J. (2009). *Maternal-child nursing* (3rd ed., p. 858). St. Louis: Saunders.

161. 3
Rationale: In an infant, the rate of chest compressions is at least 100 times per minute. Options 1 and 2 identify rates that are too low, and option 4 identifies a rate that is too high.
Test-Taking Strategy: Use the process of elimination, considering the normal heart rate of an infant. Eliminate options 1 and 2 because of the low rates identified in the options. Eliminate option 4 because this rate would be much too rapid for an infant. If you had difficulty with this question, review CPR for an infant.
Level of Cognitive Ability: Applying
Client Needs: Physiological Integrity
Integrated Process: Nursing Process—Implementation
Content Area: Critical Care
Reference: Lowdermilk, D., & Perry, S. (2007). *Maternity & women's health care* (9th ed., p. 753). St. Louis: Mosby.

162. 4
Rationale: Blind finger sweeps are not recommended for infants and children because of the risk of forcing the object farther down into the airway. Options 1, 2, and 3 are not related directly to the subject of the question, a blocked airway.
Test-Taking Strategy: Use the ABCDs—airway, breathing, circulation, and defibrillation or definitive treatment—to answer this question. Also focus on the subject of the question, a blocked airway. Option 4 addresses the concern of airway patency. If you had difficulty with this question, review obstructed airway management for an infant or a child.
Level of Cognitive Ability: Understanding
Client Needs: Physiological Integrity
Integrated Process: Teaching and Learning
Content Area: Critical Care
Reference: McKinney, E., James, S., Murray, S., & Ashwill, J. (2009). *Maternal-child nursing* (3rd ed., p. 859). St. Louis: Saunders.

163. 3
Rationale: When performing CPR on an adult client, the sternum is depressed 1½ to 2 inches. Options 1 and 2 identify

compression depths that would be ineffective in an adult. Option 4 identifies a depth that could cause injury to the client.
Test-Taking Strategy: Note the strategic word *adult* in the question. Consider the normal body structure of an adult to assist in directing you to option 3. If you had difficulty with this question, review the procedure for performing adult CPR.
Level of Cognitive Ability: Applying
Client Needs: Physiological Integrity
Integrated Process: Nursing Process—Implementation
Content Area: Critical Care
Reference: Perry, A., & Potter, P. (2010). *Clinical nursing skills & techniques* (7th ed., p. 731). St. Louis: Mosby.

164. 4
Rationale: To perform abdominal thrusts on an unconscious woman in an advanced gestational stage of pregnancy, the woman is placed on her back. A wedge, such as a pillow or rolled blanket, is placed under the right abdominal flank and hip to displace the uterus to the left side of the abdomen. This prevents supine hypotension that can occur if the gravid uterus rests on the aorta. Options 1, 2, and 3 are incorrect and can harm the woman and the fetus.
Test-Taking Strategy: Note that the victim is an unconscious pregnant woman at 8 months' gestation. Recall the causes associated with supine hypotension and vena caval syndrome to assist in directing you to option 4. Review the principles associated with performing abdominal thrusts on a pregnant woman if you had difficulty with this question.
Level of Cognitive Ability: Understanding
Client Needs: Physiological Integrity
Integrated Process: Teaching and Learning
Content Area: Critical Care
Reference: Lowdermilk, D., & Perry, A. (2007). *Maternity & women's health care* (9th ed., p. 861). St. Louis: Mosby.

ALTERNATE ITEM FORMAT: PRIORITIZING (ORDERED RESPONSE)
165. 2, 4, 1, 5, 3
Rationale: For health care providers, the sequence for removing a foreign body airway obstruction in an adult is as follows. After determining unconsciousness, the airway is opened and the rescuer looks into the mouth of the victim and removes the object blocking the airway if it is seen. Next, the health care provider attempts to ventilate the victim. If unsuccessful, the victim's head is repositioned and ventilation is reattempted. Five abdominal thrusts are then delivered. The sequence is repeated until successful.
Test-Taking Strategy: Visualize the procedure; the ABCs can be used as a guide in performing this procedure. Remember that determining unconsciousness is the first action. Next, open the airway; otherwise, you would not be able to look into the victim's mouth. Breathe: Attempt ventilation. Finally, perform the abdominal thrusts. Review the procedure for performing abdominal thrusts if you had difficulty with this question.
Level of Cognitive Ability: Applying
Client Needs: Physiological Integrity
Integrated Process: Teaching and Learning
Content Area: Critical Care
Reference: Ignatavicius, D., & Workman, M. (2010). *Medical-surgical nursing: Patient-centered collaborative care* (6th ed., p. 597). St. Louis: Saunders.

19

Perioperative Nursing Care

PYRAMID TERMS

atelectasis A collapsed or airless state of the lung that may be the result of airway obstruction caused by accumulated secretions or failure of the client to deep breathe or ambulate about after surgery; a postoperative complication that usually occurs 1 to 2 days after surgery.

extended postoperative stage The period of at least 1 to 4 days after surgery.

immediate postoperative stage The period of 1 to 4 hours after surgery.

intermediate postoperative stage The period of 4 to 24 hours after surgery.

perioperative nursing Nursing care given before (preoperative), during (intraoperative), and after surgery (postoperative).

wound dehiscence Separation of the wound edges.

wound evisceration Protrusion of internal organs through an incision.

 THE PYRAMID TO SUCCESS

Pyramid Points focus on teaching the client and family or significant other in the preoperative stage, preparing the client for the operative procedure, ensuring that prescribed preoperative tests and procedures such as x-ray films or laboratory studies have been performed, and ensuring that the results of the tests and procedures are within expected ranges and are documented. In the postoperative stage, Pyramid Points focus on monitoring for surgical complications and on the implementation of initial nursing measures if a complication arises. Because many surgical procedures are performed through ambulatory care units (1-day stay units), Pyramid Points also focus on preparing the client for discharge, teaching related to the prescribed treatments and medications, follow-up care, and the mobilization of home care support services.

 CLIENT NEEDS

Safe and Effective Care Environment

Acting as an advocate and upholding client's rights
Collaboration with the interdisciplinary team

Ensuring that advance directives documents are in the client's medical record
Establishing priorities
Informing the client of the surgical process
Maintaining continuity of care and initiating referrals to home care and other support services
Maintaining confidentiality
Maintaining standard and transmission based precautions and surgical asepsis
Obtaining informed consent for the surgical procedure
Preventing a surgical infection
Providing safety to the medicated client

Health Promotion and Maintenance

Discussing expected body image changes
Identifying lifestyle choices
Performing techniques of physical assessment
Providing client and family teaching related to the prescribed discharge plan
Providing health and wellness teaching to prevent complications

Psychosocial Integrity

Assessing psychosocial concerns
Assisting the client to develop coping methods
Communicating therapeutically
Considering cultural practices when planning care
Identifying support systems
Identifying unexpected body image changes
Promoting an environment that will allow the client to express concerns

Physiological Integrity

Administering intravenous (IV) fluids and blood products safely
Administering preoperative and postoperative medications safely
Initiating nursing interventions when surgical complications arise
Monitoring for unexpected responses to treatments and procedures

Monitoring for surgical complications
Monitoring for wound infection
Providing basic care and comfort
Providing respiratory therapy and other prescribed therapies

I. PREOPERATIVE CARE

⚠ A client may return home shortly after having a surgical procedure because many surgical procedures are done through ambulatory care or 1-day stay surgical units. Perioperative care procedures apply even when the client returns home the same day of the surgical procedure.

A. Obtaining informed consent
   1. The surgeon is responsible for obtaining the consent for surgery.
   2. Minors (clients younger than 18 years old) may need a parent or legal guardian to sign the consent form.
   3. Older clients may need a legal guardian to sign the consent form.
   4. No sedation should be administered to the client before the client signs the consent.
   5. The nurse may witness the client's signing of the consent form, but the nurse must be sure that the client has understood the surgeon's explanation of the surgery.
   6. The nurse needs to document the witnessing of the signing of the consent form after the client acknowledges understanding the procedure.

B. Nutrition
   1. Review the physician's prescriptions regarding the NPO status before surgery.
   2. Withhold solid foods and liquids as prescribed to avoid aspiration; usually for 6 to 8 hours before general anesthesia and for approximately 3 hours before surgery with local anesthesia.
   3. Insert an IV line and administer IV fluids, if prescribed; IV catheter size should be large enough to administer blood products if they are required.
   4. Administer parenteral nutrition (PN) as prescribed; usually PN is prescribed for clients who are malnourished, have protein or metabolic deficiencies from underlying disease, or cannot ingest foods.

C. Elimination
   1. If the client is to have intestinal or abdominal surgery, then an enema, laxative, or both may be prescribed the day or night before surgery.
   2. The client should void immediately before surgery.
   3. Insert a Foley catheter, if prescribed; Foley catheters should be emptied immediately before surgery, and the nurse should document the amount and characteristics of the urine.

D. Surgical site
   1. Clean the surgical site with a mild antiseptic or antibacterial soap the night before surgery, as prescribed.
   2. Shave the operative site, as prescribed; shaving may be done in the operative area.

⚠ Hair on the head or face (including the eyebrows) should be shaved only if prescribed.

E. Preoperative client teaching
   1. Inform the client about what to expect postoperatively.
   2. Inform the client to notify the nurse if the client experiences any pain postoperatively and that pain medication will be prescribed and given as the client requests.
   3. Demonstrate the use of a patient-controlled analgesia pump if prescribed.
   4. Inform the client that requesting an opioid after surgery will not make the client a drug addict.
   5. Instruct the client to use noninvasive pain relief techniques such as relaxation, distraction techniques, and guided imagery before the pain occurs and as soon as the pain is noticed.
   6. The nurse should instruct the client not to smoke (for at least 24 hours before surgery); discuss smoking cessation treatments and programs.
   7. Instruct the client in deep-breathing and coughing techniques, use of incentive spirometry, and the importance of performing the techniques postoperatively to prevent the development of pneumonia and **atelectasis** (Box 19-1).
   8. Instruct the client in leg and foot exercises to prevent venous stasis of blood and to facilitate venous blood return (Fig. 19-1; see Box 19-1).
   9. Instruct the client in how to splint an incision, turn, and reposition (Fig. 19-2; see Box 19-1).
   10. Inform the client of any invasive devices that may be needed after surgery, such as a nasogastric tube, drain, Foley catheter, epidural catheter, or IV or subclavian lines.
   11. Instruct the client not to pull on any of the invasive devices; they will be removed as soon as possible.

F. Psychosocial preparation
   1. Be alert to the client's level of anxiety.
   2. Answer any questions or concerns that the client may have regarding surgery.
   3. Allow time for privacy for the client to prepare for surgery psychologically.
   4. Provide support and assistance as needed.
   5. Take cultural aspects into consideration when providing care (Box 19-2)

Box 19-1 Client Teaching

Deep-Breathing and Coughing Exercises

Instruct the client that a sitting position gives the best lung expansion for coughing and deep-breathing exercises.

Instruct the client to breathe deeply three times, inhaling through the nostrils and exhaling slowly through pursed lips.

Instruct the client that the third breath should be held for 3 seconds; then the client should cough deeply three times.

The client should perform this exercise every 1 to 2 hours.

Incentive Spirometry

Instruct the client to assume a sitting or upright position.

Instruct the client to place the mouth tightly around the mouthpiece.

Instruct the client to inhale slowly to raise and maintain the flow rate indicator, usually between the 600 and 900 marks on the device.

Instruct the client to hold the breath for 5 seconds and then to exhale through pursed lips.

Instruct the client to repeat this process 10 times every hour.

Leg and Foot Exercises

Gastrocnemius (calf) pumping: Instruct the client to move both ankles by pointing the toes up and then down.

Quadriceps (thigh) setting: Instruct the client to press the back of the knees against the bed and then to relax the knees; this contracts and relaxes the thigh and calf muscles to prevent thrombus formation.

Foot circles: Instruct the client to rotate each foot in a circle.

Hip and knee movements: Instruct the client to flex the knee and thigh and to straighten the leg, holding the position for 5 seconds before lowering (not performed if the client is having abdominal surgery or if the client has a back problem).

Splinting the Incision

If the surgical incision is abdominal or thoracic, instruct the client to place a pillow, or one hand with the other hand on top, over the incisional area.

During deep breathing and coughing, the client presses gently against the incisional area to splint or support it.

Essential
Gastrocnemius (calf) pumping

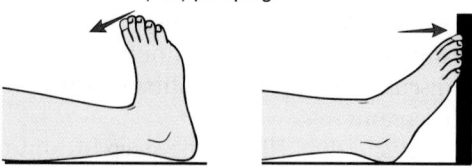

Quadriceps (thigh) setting

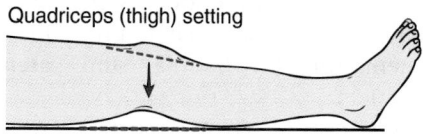

Desirable
Foot circles

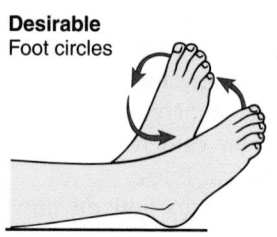

Hip and knee movements

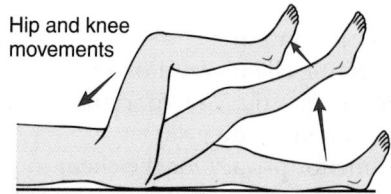

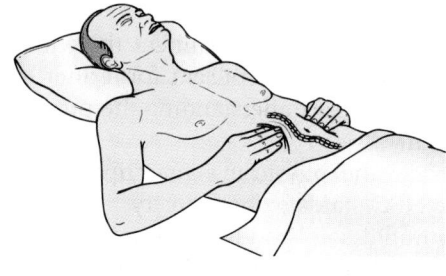

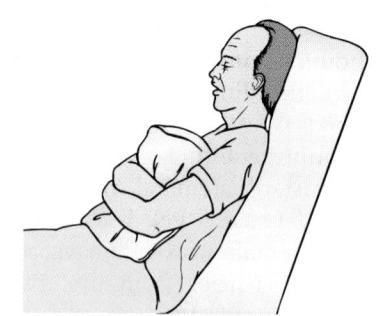

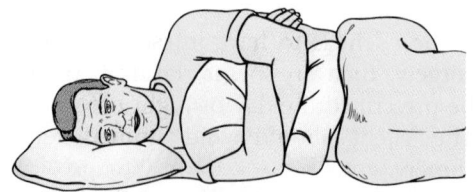

▲ **FIGURE 19-1** Postoperative leg exercises. (From Lewis, S., Heitkemper, M., & Dirksen, S. [2007]. *Medical-surgical nursing: Assessment and management of clinical problems* [7th ed.]. St. Louis: Mosby.)

▲ **FIGURE 19-2** Techniques for splinting a wound when coughing. (From Lewis, S., Heitkemper, M., & Dirksen, S. [2007]. *Medical-surgical nursing: Assessment and management of clinical problems* [7th ed.]. St. Louis: Mosby.)

Box 19-2 Cultural Aspects of Perioperative Nursing Care

Cultural assessment includes questions related to:
- Primary language spoken
- Feelings related to surgery and pain
- Pain management
- Expectations
- Support systems
- Feelings toward self
- Cultural practices and beliefs

Allow a family member to be present when and if appropriate.

Secure the help of a professional interpreter to communicate with non–English-speaking clients.

Use pictures or phrase cards to communicate and assess the non–English-speaking client's perception of pain or other feelings.

Provide preoperative and postoperative educational materials in the appropriate language.

Modified from Potter, P., & Perry, A. (2009). *Fundamentals of nursing* (7th ed., p. 1375). St. Louis: Mosby.

Box 19-3 Medical Conditions That Increase Risk During Surgery

Bleeding disorders such as thrombocytopenia, hemophilia
Diabetes mellitus
Chronic pain
Heart disease, such as a recent myocardial infarction, dysrhythmia, heart failure, or peripheral vascular disease
Obstructive sleep apnea
Upper respiratory infection
Liver disease
Fever
Chronic respiratory disease, such as emphysema, bronchitis, or asthma
Immunological disorders, such as leukemia, infection with human immunodeficiency virus, acquired immunodeficiency syndrome, bone marrow depression, or use of chemotherapy or immunosuppressive agents
Abuse of street drugs

Modified from Potter, P., & Perry, A. (2009). *Fundamentals of nursing* (7th ed., p. 1370). St. Louis: Mosby.

G. Preoperative checklist
  1. Ensure that the client is wearing an identification bracelet.
  2. Assess for allergies, including an allergy to latex (see Chapter 70 for information on latex allergy).
  3. Review the preoperative checklist to be sure that each item is addressed before the client is transported to surgery.
  4. Follow agency policies regarding preoperative procedures including informed consents, preoperative checklists, prescribed laboratory or radiological tests, or any other preoperative procedure.
  5. Ensure that informed consent forms have been signed for the operative procedure, any blood transfusions, disposal of a limb, or surgical sterilization procedures.
  6. Ensure that a history and physical examination have been completed and documented in the client's record (Box 19-3).
  7. Ensure that consultation requests have been completed and documented in the client's record.
  8. Ensure that prescribed laboratory results are documented in the client's record.
  9. Ensure that the electrocardiogram and chest radiography reports are documented in the client's record.
  10. Ensure that a blood type, screen, and crossmatch are performed and documented in the client's record.
  11. Remove jewelry, makeup, dentures, hairpins, nail polish (depending on agency procedures), glasses, and prostheses.
  12. Document that valuables have been given to the client's family members or locked in the hospital safe.
  13. Document the last time that the client ate or drank.
  14. Document that the client voided before surgery.
  15. Document that the prescribed preoperative medications were given (Box 19-4).
  16. Monitor and document the client's vital signs.

H. Preoperative medications
  1. Prepare to administer preoperative medications as prescribed before surgery.
  2. Instruct the client about the desired effects of the preoperative medication.

⚠ After administering the preoperative medications, keep the client in bed with the side rails up. Place the call bell next to the client; instruct the client not to get out of bed and to call for assistance if needed.

I. Arrival in the operating room
  1. Guidelines to eliminate wrong site and wrong procedure surgery
     a. The surgeon meets with the client in the preoperative area and uses indelible ink to mark the operative site.
     b. In the operating room, the nurse and surgeon ensure and reconfirm that the operative site has been appropriately marked.
     c. Just before starting the surgical procedure, a time out is conducted with all members of

Box 19-4 Substances That Can Affect the Client in Surgery

Antibiotics
Antibiotics potentiate the action of anesthetic agents.

Anticholinergics
Medications with anticholinergic effects increase the potential for confusion.

Anticoagulants
Anticoagulants alter normal clotting factors and increase the risk of hemorrhaging.
Aspirin (acetylsalicylic acid) and nonsteroidal anti-inflammatory drugs are commonly used medications that can alter clotting mechanisms.
These medications should be discontinued at least 48 hours before surgery or as specified by the surgeon.

Anticonvulsants
Long-term use of certain anticonvulsants can alter the metabolism of anesthetic agents.

Antidepressants
Antidepressants may lower the blood pressure during anesthesia.

Antidysrhythmics
Antidysrhythmic medications reduce cardiac contractility and impair cardiac conduction during anesthesia.

Antihypertensives
Antihypertensive medications can interact with anesthetic agents and cause bradycardia, hypotension, and impaired circulation.

Corticosteroids
Corticosteroids cause adrenal atrophy and reduce the ability of the body to withstand stress.
Before and during surgery, dosages may be increased temporarily.

Diuretics
Diuretics potentiate electrolyte imbalances after surgery.

Herbal Substances
Herbal substances can interact with anesthesia and cause a variety of adverse effects. These substances may need to be stopped at a specific time before surgery. During the preoperative period, the client needs to be asked if he or she is taking an herbal substance.

Insulin
The need for insulin after surgery in a diabetic may be reduced because the client's nutritional intake is decreased, or the need for insulin may be increased because of the stress response and intravenous administration of glucose solutions.

Modified from Potter, P., & Perry, A. (2009). *Fundamentals of nursing* (7th ed., p. 1373). St. Louis: Mosby.

the operative team present to identify the appropriate surgical site again.

2. When the client arrives in the operating room, the operating room nurse will verify the identification bracelet with the client's verbal response and will review the client's chart.
3. The client's chart will be checked for completeness and reviewed for informed consent forms, history and physical examination, and allergic reaction information.
4. Physicians' prescriptions will be verified and implemented.
5. The IV line may be initiated at this time (or in the preoperative area), if prescribed.
6. The anesthesia team will administer the prescribed anesthesia.

⚠ Verification of the client and the surgical operative site is critical.

II. POSTOPERATIVE CARE

A. Description
1. **Immediate postoperative stage**: The period of 1 to 4 hours after surgery
2. **Intermediate postoperative stage**: The period of 4 to 24 hours after surgery
3. **Extended postoperative stage**: The period of at least 1 to 4 days after surgery

B. Respiratory system

⚠ Assess breath sounds—stridor, wheezing, or a crowing sound can indicate partial obstruction, bronchospasm, or laryngospasm; crackles or rhonchi may indicate pulmonary edema.

1. Monitor vital signs.
2. Monitor airway patency and ensure adequate ventilation (prolonged mechanical ventilation during anesthesia may affect postoperative lung function).
3. Remember that extubated clients who are lethargic may not be able to maintain an airway.
4. Monitor for secretions; if the client is unable to clear the airway by coughing, suction the secretions from the client's airway.
5. Observe chest movement for symmetry and the use of accessory muscles.
6. Monitor oxygen administration if prescribed.
7. Monitor pulse oximetry.
8. Encourage deep breathing and coughing exercises as soon as possible after surgery.
9. Note the rate, depth, and quality of respirations; the respiratory rate should be greater than 10 and less than 30 breaths/min.
10. Monitor for signs of respiratory distress, **atelectasis**, or other respiratory complications.

C. Cardiovascular system
1. Monitor circulatory status, such as skin color, peripheral pulses, capillary refill, and for the absence of edema, numbness, and tingling.
2. Monitor for bleeding.
3. Assess the pulse for rate and rhythm (a bounding pulse may indicate hypertension, fluid overload, or client anxiety).
4. Monitor for signs of hypertension and hypotension.
5. Monitor for cardiac dysrhythmias.
6. Monitor for signs of thrombophlebitis, particularly in clients who were in the lithotomy position during surgery.
7. Encourage the use of antiembolism stockings, if prescribed, to promote venous return, strengthen muscle tone, and prevent pooling of blood in the extremities.

D. Musculoskeletal system
1. Assess the client for movement of the extremities.
2. Review physician's prescriptions regarding client positioning or restrictions.
3. Encourage ambulation if prescribed; before ambulation, instruct the client to sit at the edge of the bed with his or her feet supported to assume balance.
4. Unless contraindicated, place the client in a low Fowler's position after surgery to increase the size of the thorax for lung expansion.
5. Avoid positioning the postoperative client in a supine position until pharyngeal reflexes have returned; if the client is comatose or semicomatose, position on the side (additionally, an oral airway may be needed).
6. If the client is unable to get out of bed, turn the client every 1 to 2 hours.

E. Neurological system
1. Assess level of consciousness.
2. Make frequent periodic attempts to awaken the client until the client awakens.
3. Orient the client to the environment.
4. Speak in a soft tone; filter out extraneous noises in the environment.
5. Maintain the client's body temperature and prevent heat loss by providing the client with warm blankets and raising the room temperature as necessary.

F. Temperature control
1. Monitor temperature.
2. Monitor for signs of hypothermia that may result from anesthesia, a cool operating room, or exposure of the skin and internal organs during surgery.
3. Apply warm blankets and continue oxygen as prescribed if the client experiences shivering.

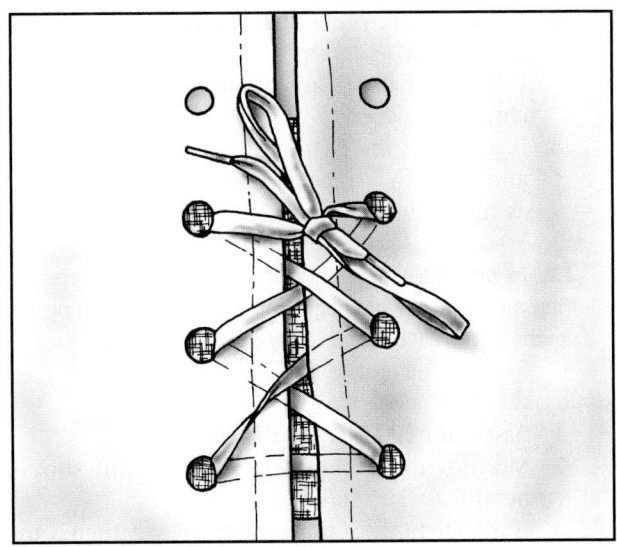

▲ **FIGURE 19-3** Montgomery straps may be used when frequent dressing changes are anticipated to help prevent skin irritation from frequent tape removal. (From Ignatavicius, D., & Workman, M. [2010]. *Medical-surgical nursing: Patient-centered collaborative care.* [6th ed.]. St. Louis: Saunders.)

G. Integumentary system
1. Assess surgical site, drains, and wound dressings (serous drainage may occur from an incision, but if excessive bleeding occurs from the site, notify the physician).
2. Assess the skin for redness, abrasions, or breakdown that may have resulted from surgical positioning.
3. Monitor body temperature and wound for signs of infection.
4. Maintain a dry, intact dressing.
5. Change dressings as prescribed, noting the amount of bleeding or drainage, odor, and intactness of sutures or staples (Fig. 19-3).
6. Wound drains should be patent; prepare to assist with the removal of drains (as prescribed by the physician) when the drainage amount becomes insignificant.
7. An abdominal binder may be prescribed for obese and debilitated individuals to prevent dehiscence of the incision

H. Fluid and electrolyte balance
1. Monitor IV fluid administration as prescribed.
2. Record intake and output.
3. Monitor for signs of fluid or electrolyte imbalances.

I. Gastrointestinal system
1. Monitor intake and output and for nausea and vomiting.
2. Maintain patency of the nasogastric tube if present.
3. Monitor for abdominal distention.
4. Monitor for passage of flatus and return of bowel sounds.
5. Administer frequent oral care, at least every 2 hours.

6. Maintain the NPO status until the gag reflex and peristalsis return.
7. When oral fluids are permitted, start with ice chips and water.
8. Ensure that the client advances to clear liquids and then to a regular diet, as prescribed and as the client can tolerate.

⚠ To prevent aspiration, turn the client to a side-lying position if vomiting occurs; have suctioning equipment available and ready to use.

J. Renal system
1. Assess the bladder for distention.
2. Monitor urine output (urinary output should be at least 30 mL/hr).
3. If the client does not have a Foley catheter, the client is expected to void within 6 to 8 hours postoperatively depending on the type of anesthesia administered; ensure that the amount is at least 200 mL.

K. Pain management
1. Assess the type of anesthetic used and preoperative medication that the client received, and note whether the client received any pain medications in the postanesthesia period.
2. Assess for pain and inquire about the type and location of pain; ask the client to rate the degree of pain on a scale of 1 to 10, with 10 being the most severe.
3. If the client is unable to rate the pain with a numerical pain scale, then use a descriptor scale that lists words that describe different levels of pain intensity, such as *no pain, mild pain, moderate pain,* and *severe pain.*
4. Monitor for objective data related to pain, such as facial expressions, body gestures, increased pulse rate, increased blood pressure, and increased respirations.
5. Inquire about the effectiveness of the last pain medication.
6. Administer pain medication as prescribed.
7. Ensure that the client with a patient-controlled analgesia pump understands how to use it.
8. If an opioid has been prescribed, after the initial administration, assess the client every 30 minutes for respiratory rate and pain relief.
9. Use noninvasive measures to relieve postoperative pain, including provision of distraction, comfort measures, positioning, backrubs, and a quiet and restful environment.
10. Document effectiveness of the pain medication and noninvasive pain relief measures.

⚠ Consider cultural practices and beliefs when planning pain management.

III. PNEUMONIA AND ATELECTASIS

A. Description (Box 19-5; Fig. 19-4)
1. Pneumonia: An inflammation of the alveoli caused by an infectious process that may develop 3 to 5 days postoperatively as a result of infection, aspiration, or immobility
2. **Atelectasis**: A collapsed or airless state of the lung that may be the result of airway obstruction caused by accumulated secretions or failure of the client to deep breathe or ambulate about after surgery; a postoperative complication that usually occurs 1 to 2 days after surgery

B. Assessment
1. Assess for factors that may increase the risk of pneumonia and **atelectasis**.
2. Assess for dyspnea and increased respiratory rate.
3. Assess for crackles over involved lung area.

Box 19-5 Postoperative Complications

Pneumonia and atelectasis
Hypoxemia
Pulmonary embolism
Hemorrhage
Shock
Thrombophlebitis
Urinary retention
Constipation
Paralytic ileus
Wound infection
Wound dehiscence
Wound evisceration

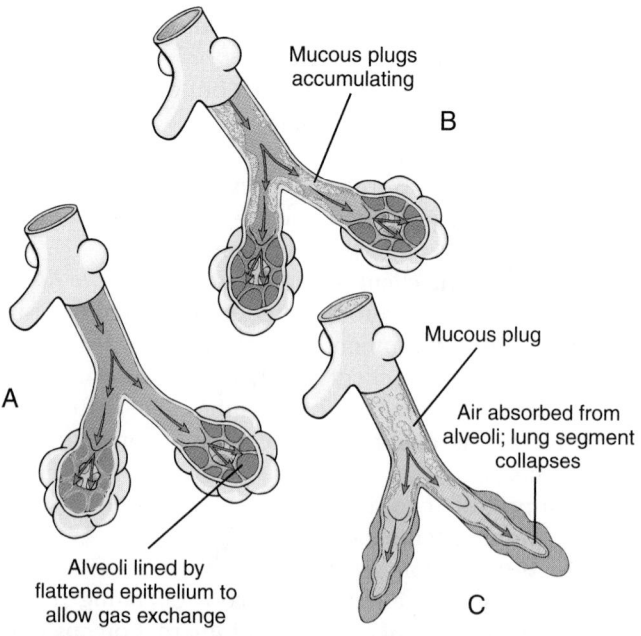

▲ **FIGURE 19-4** Postoperative atelectasis. **A,** Normal bronchiole and alveoli. **B,** Mucous plug in bronchiole. **C,** Collapse of alveoli caused by atelectasis following absorption of air. (From Lewis, S., Heitkemper, M., & Dirksen, S. [2004]. *Medical-surgical nursing: Assessment and management of clinical problems* [6th ed.]. St. Louis: Mosby.)

4. Assess for elevated temperature.
5. Assess for productive cough and chest pain.

C. Interventions
1. Assess lung and breath sounds.
2. Reposition the client every 1 to 2 hours.
3. Encourage the client to deep breathe, cough, and use the incentive spirometer.
4. Provide chest physiotherapy and postural drainage, as prescribed.
5. Encourage fluid intake and early ambulation.
6. Use suction to clear secretions if the client is unable to cough.

IV. HYPOXEMIA

A. Description: An inadequate concentration of oxygen in arterial blood; in the postoperative client, hypoxemia can be due to shallow breathing from the effects of anesthesia or medications.

B. Assessment
1. Restlessness
2. Dyspnea
3. Diaphoresis
4. Tachycardia
5. Hypertension
6. Cyanosis

C. Interventions
1. Monitor for signs of hypoxemia.
2. Notify the physician.
3. Monitor lung sounds and pulse oximetry.
4. Administer oxygen as prescribed.
5. Encourage deep breathing and coughing and use of the incentive spirometer.
6. Turn and reposition the client frequently; encourage ambulation.

V. PULMONARY EMBOLISM

A. Description: An embolus blocking the pulmonary artery and disrupting blood flow to one or more lobes of the lung.

B. Assessment
1. Sudden dyspnea
2. Sudden sharp chest or upper abdominal pain
3. Cyanosis
4. Tachycardia
5. A drop in blood pressure

C. Interventions
1. Notify the physician immediately because pulmonary embolism may be life-threatening and requires emergency action.
2. Monitor vital signs.
3. Administer oxygen and medications as prescribed.

VI. HEMORRHAGE

A. Description: The loss of a large amount of blood externally or internally in a short time period.

B. Assessment
1. Restlessness
2. Weak and rapid pulse
3. Hypotension
4. Tachypnea
5. Cool, clammy skin
6. Reduced urine output

C. Interventions
1. Provide pressure to the site of bleeding.
2. Notify the physician.
3. Administer oxygen, as prescribed.
4. Administer IV fluids and blood, as prescribed.
5. Prepare the client for a surgical procedure, if necessary.

VII. SHOCK

A. Description: Loss of circulatory fluid volume, which usually is caused by hemorrhage.

B. Assessment: Similar to assessment findings in hemorrhage

C. Interventions
1. If shock develops, elevate the legs.
2. Notify the physician.
3. Determine and treat the cause of shock.
4. Administer oxygen, as prescribed.
5. Monitor level of consciousness.
6. Monitor vital signs for increased pulse or decreased blood pressure.
7. Monitor intake and output.
8. Assess color, temperature, turgor, and moisture of the skin and mucous membranes.
9. Administer IV fluids, blood, and colloid solutions, as prescribed.

⚠ If the client had spinal anesthesia, do not elevate the legs any higher than placing them on the pillow; otherwise, the diaphragm muscles needed for effective breathing could be impaired.

VIII. THROMBOPHLEBITIS

A. Description
1. Thrombophlebitis is an inflammation of a vein, often accompanied by clot formation.
2. Veins in the legs are affected most commonly.

B. Assessment
1. Vein inflammation
2. Aching or cramping pain
3. Vein feels hard and cord-like and is tender to touch
4. Elevated temperature

C. Interventions
1. Monitor legs for swelling, inflammation, pain, tenderness, venous distention, and cyanosis; notify the physician if any of these signs are present.
2. Elevate the extremity 30 degrees without allowing any pressure on the popliteal area.

3. Encourage the use of antiembolism stockings as prescribed; remove stockings twice a day to wash and inspect the legs.
4. Use an intermittent pulsatile compression device as prescribed (Fig. 19-5).
5. Perform passive range-of-motion exercises every 2 hours if the client is confined to bedrest.
6. Encourage early ambulation, as prescribed.
7. Do not allow the client to dangle the legs.
8. Instruct the client not to sit in one position for an extended period of time.
9. Administer anticoagulants such as heparin sodium or warfarin (Coumadin), as prescribed.

IX. URINARY RETENTION

A. Description
1. Urinary retention is an involuntary accumulation of urine in the bladder as a result of loss of muscle tone.
2. It is caused by the effects of anesthetics or opioid analgesics and appears 6 to 8 hours after surgery.

B. Assessment
1. Inability to void
2. Restlessness and diaphoresis
3. Lower abdominal pain
4. Distended bladder
5. Hypertension
6. On percussion, bladder sounds like a drum

C. Interventions
1. Monitor for voiding.
2. Assess for a distended bladder.
3. Encourage ambulation when prescribed.
4. Encourage fluid intake unless contraindicated.
5. Assist the client to void by helping to stand.
6. Provide privacy.
7. Pour warm water over the perineum or allow the client to hear running water to promote voiding.
8. Contact the physician and catheterize the client as prescribed after all noninvasive techniques have been attempted.

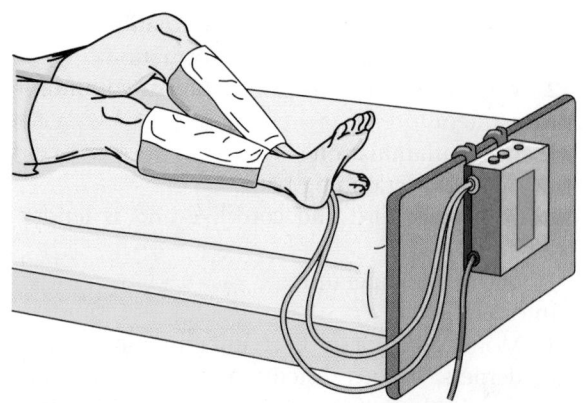

▲ **FIGURE 19-5** Intermittent pulsatile compression device. (From Monahan, F., Sands, J., Neighbors, M., Marek, J., & Green, C. [2007]. *Phipps' medical-surgical nursing: Health and illness perspectives* [8th ed.]. St. Louis: Mosby.)

X. CONSTIPATION

A. Description
1. Constipation is an abnormal infrequent passage of stool.
2. When the client resumes a solid diet postoperatively, failure to pass stool within 48 hours may indicate constipation.

B. Assessment
1. Absence of bowel movements
2. Abdominal distention
3. Anorexia, headache, and nausea

C. Interventions
1. Assess bowel sounds.
2. Encourage fluid intake up to 3000 mL/day unless contraindicated.
3. Encourage early ambulation.
4. Encourage consumption of fiber foods unless contraindicated.
5. Provide privacy and adequate time for bowel elimination.
6. Administer stool softeners and laxatives, as prescribed.

XI. PARALYTIC ILEUS

A. Description
1. Paralytic ileus is failure of appropriate forward movement of bowel contents.
2. The condition may occur as a result of anesthetic medications or of manipulation of the bowel during the surgical procedure.

B. Assessment
1. Vomiting postoperatively
2. Abdominal distention
3. Absence of bowel sounds, bowel movement, or flatus

C. Interventions
1. Monitor intake and output.
2. Maintain NPO status until bowel sounds return.
3. Maintain patency of a nasogastric tube if in place.
4. Encourage ambulation.
5. Administer IV fluids or PN, as prescribed.
6. Administer medications as prescribed to increase gastrointestinal motility and secretions.
7. If ileus occurs, it is treated first nonsurgically with bowel decompression by insertion of a nasogastric tube attached to intermittent or constant suction.

⚠ Vomiting postoperatively, abdominal distention, and absence of bowel sounds may be signs of paralytic ileus.

XII. WOUND INFECTION

A. Description
1. Wound infection may be caused by poor aseptic technique or a contaminated wound before

surgical exploration; existing client conditions such as diabetes mellitus or immunocompromise may place the client at risk.
2. Infection usually occurs 3 to 6 days after surgery.
3. Purulent material may exit from the drains or separated wound edges.

B. Assessment
1. Fever and chills
2. Warm, tender, painful, and inflamed incision site
3. Edematous skin at the incision and tight skin sutures
4. Elevated white blood cell count

C. Interventions
1. Monitor temperature.
2. Monitor incision site for approximation of suture line, edema, or bleeding, and signs of infection (*REEDA*: *r*edness, *e*rythema, *e*cchymosis, *d*rainage, *a*pproximation of the wound edges); notify the physician if signs of wound infection are present.
3. Maintain patency of drains, and assess drainage amount, color, and consistency.
4. Maintain asepsis and change the dressing, as prescribed.
5. Administer antibiotics, as prescribed.

XIII. WOUND DEHISCENCE AND EVISCERATION (Fig. 19-6)

A. Description
1. **Wound dehiscence** is separation of the wound edges at the suture line; it usually occurs 6 to 8 days after surgery.
2. **Wound evisceration** is protrusion of the internal organs through an incision; it usually occurs 6 to 8 days after surgery.
3. Evisceration is most common among obese clients, clients who have had abdominal surgery, or those who have poor wound-healing ability.

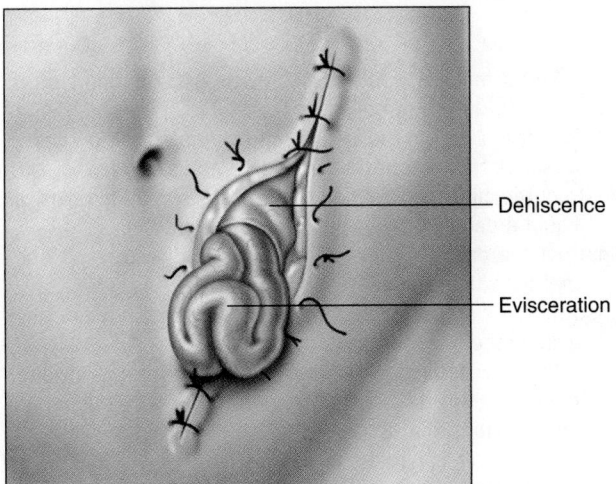

▲ **FIGURE 19-6** Complications of wound healing. (From Ignatavicius, D., & Workman, M. [2010]. *Medical-surgical nursing: Patient-centered collaborative care.* [6th ed.]. St. Louis: Saunders.)

4. **Wound evisceration** is an emergency.
B. Assessment: Dehiscence
1. Increased drainage
2. Opened wound edges
3. Appearance of underlying tissues through the wound
C. Assessment: Evisceration
1. Discharge of serosanguineous fluid from a previously dry wound
2. The appearance of loops of bowel or other abdominal contents through the wound
3. Client reports feeling a popping sensation after coughing or turning
D. Interventions (see Priority Nursing Actions)
1. Place the client in a low Fowler's position with the knees bent to prevent abdominal tension on an abdominal suture line.
2. Cover the wound with a sterile normal saline dressing.
3. Notify the physician.
4. Prevent wound infection through strict asepsis.

◼◼◼◼ **PRIORITY NURSING ACTIONS!** ◼◼◼◼

Actions to Take if Evisceration Occurs
1. Call for help; ask that the physician be notified and that needed supplies be brought to the client's room.
2. Stay with the client.
3. While waiting for supplies to arrive, place the client in a low Fowler's position with the knees bent.
4. Cover the wound with a sterile normal saline dressing and keep the dressing moist.
5. Take vital signs and monitor the client closely for signs of shock.
6. Prepare the client for surgery as necessary.
7. Document the occurrence, actions taken, and the client's response.

Wound evisceration is protrusion of the internal organs through an incision; it usually occurs 6 to 8 days after surgery. Evisceration is most common among obese clients, clients who have had abdominal surgery, or those who have poor wound-healing ability. Wound evisceration is an emergency. The nurse immediately calls for help and asks that the physician be notified and that needed supplies (vital sign measurement devices, sterile normal saline, and dressings) be brought to the client's room. The nurse stays with the client and while waiting for supplies to arrive, places the client in a low Fowler's position with the knees bent to prevent abdominal tension on an abdominal suture line. The nurse covers the wound with a sterile normal saline dressing as soon as supplies are available and keeps the dressing moist. Vital signs are monitored closely, and the client is monitored for signs of shock. The client is prepared for surgery if necessary. The nurse also documents the occurrence, actions taken, and client's response.

Reference: Ignatavicius, D., & Workman, M. (2010). *Medical-surgical nursing: Patient-centered collaborative care.* (7th ed., p. 296). St. Louis: Saunders.

5. Administer antiemetics as prescribed to prevent vomiting and further strain on the abdominal incision.
6. Instruct the client to splint the abdominal incision when coughing; this action assists in preventing or worsening these complications.
7. Prepare the client for surgery as necessary.

XIV. AMBULATORY SURGERY

A. General criteria for client discharge
1. Client is alert and oriented.
2. Client has voided.
3. Client has no respiratory distress.
4. Client is able to ambulate, swallow, and cough.
5. Client has minimal pain.
6. Client is not vomiting.
7. Client has minimal, if any, bleeding from the incision site.
8. Client has a responsible adult available to drive the client home.
9. The surgeon has signed a release form.

B. Discharge teaching (Box 19-6)
1. Discharge teaching should be performed before the date of the scheduled procedure.
2. Provide written instructions to the client and family regarding the specifics of care.
3. Instruct the client and family about postoperative complications that can occur.
4. Provide appropriate resources for home care support.
5. Instruct the client not to drive, make important decisions, or sign any legal documents for 24 hours after receiving general anesthesia.
6. Instruct the client to call the surgeon, ambulatory center, or emergency department if postoperative problems occur.
7. Instruct the client to keep follow-up appointments with the surgeon.

MORE QUESTIONS ON THE CD!

Practice Questions

166. A nurse has just reassessed the condition of a postoperative client who was admitted 1 hour ago to the surgical unit. The nurse plans to monitor which of the following parameters most carefully during the next hour?
    1. Urinary output of 20 mL/hr
    2. Temperature of 37.6° C (99.6° F)
    3. Blood pressure of 100/70 mm Hg
    4. Serous drainage on the surgical dressing

167. A postoperative client asks a nurse why it is so important to deep breathe and cough after surgery. When formulating a response, the nurse incorporates the understanding that retained pulmonary secretions in a postoperative client can lead to:
    1. Pneumonia
    2. Fluid imbalance
    3. Pulmonary embolism
    4. Carbon dioxide retention

168. A nurse is developing a plan of care for a client scheduled for surgery. The nurse should include which activity in the nursing care plan for the client on the day of surgery?
    1. Have the client void immediately before going into surgery.
    2. Avoid oral hygiene and rinsing with mouthwash.
    3. Verify that the client has not eaten for the last 24 hours.
    4. Report immediately any slight increase in blood pressure or pulse.

Box 19-6 Postoperative Discharge Teaching

Assess the client's readiness to learn, educational level, and desire to change or modify lifestyle.

Assess the need for resources needed for home care.

Demonstrate care of the incision and how to change the dressing.

Instruct the client to cover the incision with plastic if showering is allowed.

Be sure the client is provided with a 48-hour supply of dressings for home use.

Instruct the client on the importance of returning to the physician's office for follow-up.

Instruct the client that sutures usually are removed in the physician's office 7 to 10 days after surgery.

Inform the client that staples are removed 7 to 14 days after surgery and that the skin may become slightly reddened when they are ready to be removed.

Steri-Strips may be applied to provide extra support after the sutures are removed.

Instruct the client on the use of medications, their purpose, dosages, administration, and side effects.

Instruct the client on diet and to drink six to eight glasses of liquid a day.

Instruct the client about activity levels and to resume normal activities gradually.

Instruct the client to avoid lifting for 6 weeks if a major surgical procedure was performed.

Instruct the client with an abdominal incision not to lift anything weighing 10 pounds or more and not to engage in any activities that involve pushing or pulling.

The client usually can return to work in 6 to 8 weeks depending on the procedure and as prescribed by the physician.

Instruct the client about the signs and symptoms of complications and when to call a physician.

169. A client with a perforated gastric ulcer is scheduled for surgery. The client cannot sign the operative consent form because of sedation from opioid analgesics that have been administered. The nurse should take which appropriate action in the care of this client?
1. Obtain a court order for the surgery.
2. Send the client to surgery without the consent form being signed.
3. Have the hospital chaplain sign the informed consent immediately.
4. Obtain a telephone consent from a family member, following agency policy.

170. A preoperative client expresses anxiety to a nurse about upcoming surgery. Which response by the nurse is most likely to stimulate further discussion between the client and the nurse?
1. "If it's any help, everyone is nervous before surgery."
2. "I will be happy to explain the entire surgical procedure to you."
3. "Can you share with me what you've been told about your surgery?"
4. "Let me tell you about the care you'll receive after surgery and the amount of pain you can anticipate."

171. A nurse is conducting preoperative teaching with a client about the use of an incentive spirometer. The nurse should include which piece of information in discussions with the client?
1. Inhale as rapidly as possible.
2. Keep a loose seal between the lips and the mouthpiece.
3. After maximum inspiration, hold the breath for 15 seconds and exhale.
4. The best results are achieved when sitting up or with the head of the bed elevated 45 to 90 degrees.

172. A nurse has conducted preoperative teaching for a client scheduled for surgery in 1 week. The client has a history of arthritis and has been taking acetylsalicylic acid (aspirin). The nurse determines that the client needs additional teaching if the client states:
1. "Aspirin can cause bleeding after surgery."
2. "Aspirin can cause my ability to clot blood to be abnormal."
3. "I need to continue to take the aspirin until the day of surgery."
4. "I need to check with my physician about the need to stop the aspirin before the scheduled surgery."

173. A nurse assesses a client's surgical incision for signs of infection. Which finding by the nurse would be interpreted as a normal finding at the surgical site?
1. Red, hard skin
2. Serous drainage
3. Purulent drainage
4. Warm, tender skin

174. A nurse is monitoring the status of a postoperative client. The nurse would become most concerned with which of the following signs that could indicate an evolving complication?
1. Increasing restlessness
2. A pulse of 86 beats/min
3. Blood pressure of 110/70 mm Hg
4. Hypoactive bowel sounds in all four quadrants

175. A nurse is reviewing a physician's prescription sheet for a preoperative client that states that the client must be NPO after midnight. The nurse would telephone the physician to clarify that which of the following medications should be given to the client and not withheld?
1. Prednisone
2. Ferrous sulfate
3. Cyclobenzaprine (Flexeril)
4. Conjugated estrogen (Premarin)

176. A client who has undergone preadmission testing has had blood drawn for serum laboratory studies, including a complete blood count, coagulation studies, and electrolytes and creatinine levels. Which of the following laboratory results should be reported to the surgeon's office by the nurse, knowing that it could cause surgery to be postponed?
1. Sodium, 141 mEq/L
2. Hemoglobin, 8.0 g/dL
3. Platelets, 210,000/mm^3
4. Serum creatinine, 0.8 mg/dL

177. A nurse receives a telephone call from the postanesthesia care unit stating that a client is being transferred to the surgical unit. The nurse plans to do which of the following first on arrival of the client?
1. Assess the patency of the airway.
2. Check tubes or drains for patency.
3. Check the dressing to assess for bleeding.
4. Assess the vital signs to compare with preoperative measurements.

Alternate Item Format: Multiple Response

178. A client who has had abdominal surgery complains of feeling as though "something gave way" in the incisional site. The nurse removes the dressing and notes the presence of a loop of bowel protruding through the incision. Which nursing interventions should the nurse take? Select all that apply.

☐ 1. Contact the surgeon.
☐ 2. Instruct the client to remain quiet.
☐ 3. Prepare the client for wound closure.
☐ 4. Document the findings and actions taken
☐ 5. Place a sterile saline dressing and ice packs over the wound.
☐ 6. Place the client in a supine position without a pillow under the head.

ANSWERS

166. 1

Rationale: Urine output should be maintained at a minimum of 30 mL/hr for an adult. An output of less than 30 mL for each of 2 consecutive hours should be reported to the physician. A temperature higher than 37.7° C (100° F) or lower than 36.1° C (97° F) and a falling systolic blood pressure, lower than 90 mm Hg, are usually considered reportable immediately. The client's preoperative or baseline blood pressure is used to make informed postoperative comparisons. Moderate or light serous drainage from the surgical site is considered normal.

Test-Taking Strategy: To answer this question correctly, you must know the normal ranges for temperature, blood pressure, urinary output, and wound drainage. Through the process of elimination, you then can determine that the urinary output is the only observation that is not within the normal range. Review expected postoperative assessment findings if you had difficulty with this question.

Level of Cognitive Ability: Analyzing
Client Needs: Physiological Integrity
Integrated Process: Nursing Process—Planning
Content Area: Fundamental Skills—Perioperative Care
Reference: Ignatavicius, D., & Workman, M. (2010). *Medical-surgical nursing: Patient-centered collaborative care* (6th ed., p. 290). St. Louis: Saunders.

167. 1

Rationale: Postoperative respiratory problems are atelectasis, pneumonia, and pulmonary emboli. Pneumonia is the inflammation of lung tissue that causes productive cough, dyspnea, and lung crackles. Fluid imbalance can be a deficit or excess related to fluid loss or overload. Pulmonary embolus occurs as a result of a blockage of the pulmonary artery that disrupts blood flow to one or more lobes of the lung; this is usually due to clot formation. Carbon dioxide retention results from an inability to exhale carbon dioxide in conditions such as chronic obstructive pulmonary disease.

Test-Taking Strategy: Use the process of elimination. Focus on the relationship between the words *deep breathe* and *cough* in the question and pneumonia in the correct option. Review the postoperative complications if you had difficulty with this question.

Level of Cognitive Ability: Understanding
Client Needs: Physiological Integrity
Integrated Process: Teaching and Learning
Content Area: Fundamental Skills—Perioperative Care
Reference: Swearingen, P. (2008). *All-in-one care planning resource: Medical-surgical, pediatric, maternity, & psychiatric nursing care plans* (2nd ed., p. 58). St. Louis: Mosby.

168. 1

Rationale: The nurse would assist the client to void immediately before surgery so that the bladder will be empty. A slight increase in blood pressure and pulse is common during the preoperative period and is usually the result of anxiety. The client usually has a restriction of food and fluids for 6 to 8 hours before surgery instead of 24 hours. Oral hygiene is allowed, but the client should not swallow any water.

Test-Taking Strategy: Use the process of elimination and read each option carefully. Eliminate option 4 because of the words *immediately* and *slight*. Eliminate option 3, knowing that the client should be NPO for 6 to 8 hours before surgery. There is no useful reason for option 2; in fact, oral hygiene may make the client feel more comfortable. Review general preoperative care measures if you had difficulty with this question.

Level of Cognitive Ability: Applying
Client Needs: Physiological Integrity
Integrated Process: Nursing Process—Planning
Content Area: Fundamental Skills—Perioperative Care
Reference: Black, J., & Hawks, J. (2009). *Medical-surgical nursing: Clinical management for positive outcomes* (8th ed., p. 199). St. Louis: Saunders.

169. 4

Rationale: Every effort should be made to obtain permission from a responsible family member to perform surgery if the client is unable to sign the consent form. A telephone consent must be witnessed by two persons who hear the family member's oral consent. The two witnesses then sign the consent with the name of the family member, noting that an oral consent was obtained. Consent is not informed if it is obtained from a client who is confused, unconscious, mentally incompetent, or under the influence of sedatives. In an emergency, a client may be unable to sign and family members may not be available. In this situation, a physician is permitted legally to perform surgery without consent. Options 1 and 3 are not appropriate in this situation. Also, agency policies regarding informed consent should always be followed.

Test-Taking Strategy: Focus on the data in the question. Eliminate options 1 and 3 first. Option 1 will delay necessary surgery and option 3 is inappropriate. Select option 4 over option 2 because it is the most appropriate of the options presented and it is legally acceptable to obtain a telephone permission from a family member if it is witnessed by two persons. Review the procedures for obtaining informed consent if you had difficulty with this question.

Level of Cognitive Ability: Applying
Client Needs: Safe and Effective Care Environment
Integrated Process: Nursing Process—Implementation
Content Area: Fundamental Skills—Perioperative Care

Reference: Ignatavicius, D., & Workman, M. (2010). *Medical-surgical nursing: Patient-centered collaborative care* (6th ed., p. 254). St. Louis: Saunders.

170. 3

Rationale: Explanations should begin with the information that the client knows. By providing the client with individualized explanations of care and procedures, the nurse can assist the client in handling anxiety and fear for a smooth preoperative experience. Clients who are calm and emotionally prepared for surgery withstand anesthesia better and experience fewer postoperative complications. Options 1, 2, and 4 will produce anxiety in the client.

Test-Taking Strategy: Use the process of elimination. Note that the question contains the strategic words *most likely* and *stimulate further discussion.* Use the steps of the nursing process and therapeutic communication techniques. Option 3 addresses assessment and is the only therapeutic response. If this question was difficult, review the principles of therapeutic communication and the measures to relieve anxiety.

Level of Cognitive Ability: Applying
Client Needs: Psychosocial Integrity
Integrated Process: Communication and Documentation
Content Area: Fundamental Skills—Perioperative Care
References: Black, J., & Hawks, J. (2009). *Medical-surgical nursing: Clinical management for positive outcomes* (8th ed., p. 193). St. Louis: Saunders.
  Potter, P., & Perry, A. (2009). *Fundamentals of nursing* (7th ed., pp. 352–356). St. Louis: Mosby.

171. 4

Rationale: For optimal lung expansion with the incentive spirometer, the client should assume the semi-Fowler's or high Fowler's position. The mouthpiece should be covered completely and tightly while the client inhales slowly, with a constant flow through the unit. The breath should be held for 5 seconds before exhaling slowly.

Test-Taking Strategy: Use the process of elimination and visualize the procedure for using the incentive spirometer. Options 1, 2, and 3 are incorrect steps regarding incentive spirometer use. If you had difficulty with this question, review the correct procedure related to the use of an incentive spirometer.

Level of Cognitive Ability: Applying
Client Needs: Physiological Integrity
Integrated Process: Teaching and Learning
Content Area: Fundamental Skills—Perioperative Care
Reference: Potter, P., & Perry, A. (2009). *Fundamentals of nursing* (7th ed., p. 1382). St. Louis: Mosby.

172. 3

Rationale: Anticoagulants alter normal clotting factors and increase the risk of bleeding after surgery. Aspirin has properties that can alter the clotting mechanism and should be discontinued at least 48 hours before surgery. However, the client should always check with his or her physician regarding when to stop taking the aspirin when a surgical procedure is scheduled. Options 1, 2, and 4 are accurate client statements.

Test-Taking Strategy: Note the strategic words *the client needs additional teaching.* These words indicate a negative event query and that you need to select the incorrect client statement. Eliminate options 1 and 2 first because they are comparable or alike. From the remaining options, recalling that

aspirin has properties that can alter the clotting mechanism will direct you to option 3. If you had difficulty with this question, review the medications that affect the client preparing for surgery.

Level of Cognitive Ability: Evaluation
Client Needs: Physiological Integrity
Integrated Process: Teaching and Learning
Content Area: Fundamental Skills—Perioperative Care
Reference: Ignatavicius, D., & Workman, M. (2010). *Medical-surgical nursing: Patient-centered collaborative care* (6th ed., p. 254). St. Louis: Saunders.

173. 2

Rationale: Serous drainage is an expected finding at a surgical site. The other options indicate signs of wound infection. Signs and symptoms of infection include warm, red, and tender skin around the incision. Purulent material may exit from drains or from separated wound edges. Infection may be caused by poor aseptic technique or a contaminated wound before surgical exploration; existing client conditions such as diabetes mellitus or immunocompromise may place the client at risk. Wound infection usually appears 3 to 6 days after surgery. The client also may have a fever and chills.

Test-Taking Strategy: Use the process of elimination, noting the strategic words *normal finding.* Recalling the signs of a wound infection and noting these strategic words will direct you to option 2. Review the signs of a wound infection if you had difficulty with this question.

Level of Cognitive Ability: Understanding
Client Needs: Physiological Integrity
Integrated Process: Nursing Process—Assessment
Content Area: Fundamental Skills—Perioperative Care
Reference: Ignatavicius, D., & Workman, M. (2010). *Medical-surgical nursing: Patient-centered collaborative care* (6th ed., p. 291). St. Louis: Saunders.

174. 1

Rationale: Increasing restlessness is a sign that requires continuous and close monitoring because it could indicate a potential complication, such as hemorrhage, shock, or pulmonary embolism. Hypoactive bowel sounds heard in all four quadrants are a normal occurrence. A blood pressure of 110/70 mm Hg with a pulse of 86 beats/min is within normal limits.

Test-Taking Strategy: Use the process of elimination, noting the strategic words *indicate an evolving complication.* Eliminate each of the incorrect options because they are normal expected findings. If you had difficulty with this question, review the normal expected postoperative findings and the signs and symptoms of postoperative complications.

Level of Cognitive Ability: Analyzing
Client Needs: Physiological Integrity
Integrated Process: Nursing Process—Analysis
Content Area: Fundamental Skills—Perioperative Care
Reference: Ignatavicius, D., & Workman, M. (2010). *Medical-surgical nursing: Patient-centered collaborative care* (6th ed., p. 293). St. Louis: Saunders.

175. 1

Rationale: Prednisone is a corticosteroid. With prolonged use, corticosteroids cause adrenal atrophy, which reduces the ability of the body to withstand stress. When stress is severe, corticosteroids are essential to life. Before and during surgery, dosages may be increased temporarily. Ferrous sulfate is an oral iron preparation used to treat iron deficiency anemia. Cyclobenzaprine (Flexeril) is a skeletal muscle relaxant. Conjugated estrogen (Premarin) is an estrogen used for hormone replacement therapy in postmenopausal women. These last three medications may be withheld before surgery without undue effects on the client.

Test-Taking Strategy: Use the process of elimination and knowledge about medications that may have special implications for the surgical client. Remember that when stress is severe, corticosteroids are essential to life. Review the effects of corticosteroids on the surgical client if you had difficulty with this question.

Level of Cognitive Ability: Analyzing
Client Needs: Physiological Integrity
Integrated Process: Nursing Process—Analysis
Content Area: Fundamental Skills—Perioperative Care
Reference: Ignatavicius, D., & Workman, M. (2010). *Medical-surgical nursing: Patient-centered collaborative care* (6th ed., p. 254). St. Louis: Saunders.

176. 2

Rationale: Routine screening tests include a complete blood count, serum electrolyte analysis, coagulation studies, and a serum creatinine test. The complete blood count includes the hemoglobin analysis. All these values are within normal range except the hemoglobin. If a client has a low hemoglobin level, the surgery likely could be postponed by the surgeon.

Test-Taking Strategy: Use the process of elimination and knowledge of the normal laboratory values. The only option that identifies an abnormal laboratory value is option 2. Review these laboratory values if you had difficulty answering this question.

Level of Cognitive Ability: Understanding
Client Needs: Physiological Integrity
Integrated Process: Nursing Process—Implementation
Content Area: Fundamental Skills—Perioperative Care
Reference: Ignatavicius, D., & Workman, M. (2010). *Medical-surgical nursing: Patient-centered collaborative care* (6th ed., p. 251). St. Louis: Saunders.

177. 1

Rationale: The first action of the nurse is to assess the patency of the airway and respiratory function. If the airway is not patent, the nurse must take immediate measures for the survival of the client. The nurse then takes vital signs followed by checking the dressing and the tubes or drains. Options 2, 3, and 4 are all nursing actions that should be performed after a patent airway has been established.

Test-Taking Strategy: Use the principles of prioritization when answering this question. Remember the ABCs—airway, breathing, and circulation. Ensuring airway patency is the first action to be taken; therefore option 1 is correct. Review the initial care of the postoperative client if you had difficulty with this question.

Level of Cognitive Ability: Applying
Client Needs: Physiological Integrity
Integrated Process: Nursing Process—Planning
Content Area: Fundamental Skills—Perioperative Care
Reference: Ignatavicius, D., & Workman, M. (2010). *Medical-surgical nursing: Patient-centered collaborative care* (6th ed., p. 289). St. Louis: Saunders.

ALTERNATE ITEM FORMAT: MULTIPLE RESPONSE

178. 1, 2, 3, 4

Rationale: Wound dehiscence is the separation of the wound edges. Wound evisceration is protrusion of the internal organs through an incision. If wound dehiscence or evisceration occurs, the nurse should call for help, stay with the client, and ask another nurse to contact the surgeon and obtain needed supplies to care for the client. The nurse places the client in a low Fowler's position, and the client is kept quiet, and instructed not to cough. Protruding organs are covered with a sterile saline dressing. Ice is not applied because of its vasoconstrictive effect. The treatment for evisceration is usually immediate wound closure under local or general anesthesia. The nurse also documents the findings and actions taken.

Test-Taking Strategy: Focus on the information in the question to determine that the client is experiencing wound evisceration. Visualizing this occurrence will assist you in determining that the client would not be placed supine and that ice packs would not be placed on the incision. Review the interventions for the client with wound evisceration if you had difficulty with this question.

Level of Cognitive Ability: Applying
Client Needs: Physiological Integrity
Integrated Process: Nursing Process—Implementation
Content Area: Fundamental Skills—Perioperative Care
Reference: Ignatavicius, D., & Workman, M. (2010). *Medical-surgical nursing: Patient-centered collaborative care* (6th ed., pp. 291–292). St. Louis: Saunders.

20

Positioning Clients

PYRAMID TERMS

body mechanics The coordinated efforts of the musculoskeletal and nervous systems to maintain balance, posture, and body alignment during lifting, bending, and moving to perform activities safely.

ergonomic principles The anatomical, physiological, psychological, and mechanical principles affecting the efficient and safe use of an individual's energy.

Fowler's position The client is supine and the head of the bed is elevated to 45 to 60 degrees.

high Fowler's position The client is supine and the head of the bed is elevated to 90 degrees.

lateral (side-lying) position The client is lying on the side and the head and shoulders are aligned with the hips and the spine and are parallel to the edge of the mattress. The head, neck, and upper arm are supported by a pillow. The lower shoulder is pulled forward slightly and, along with the elbow, flexed at 90 degrees. The legs are flexed or extended. A pillow is placed to support the back.

lithotomy position The client is lying on the back with the hips and knees flexed at right angles and the feet in stirrups.

prone position The client is lying on the abdomen with head turned to the side.

reverse Trendelenburg's position The bed is tilted so that the client's foot of the bed is down.

semi-Fowler's position (low Fowler's) The client is supine and the head of the bed is elevated about 30 degrees.

Sims' position The client is lying on the side with the body turned prone at 45 degrees. The lower leg is extended, with the upper leg flexed at the hip and knee to a 45- to 90-degree angle.

supine position The client is lying on the back. The head and shoulders usually are elevated slightly (depending on the client's condition) with a small pillow. The arms and legs are extended, and the legs are slightly abducted.

Trendelenburg's position The bed is tilted so that the client's head of the bed is down. This position is contraindicated in clients with head injuries, increased intracranial pressure, spinal cord injuries, and certain respiratory and cardiac disorders.

THE PYRAMID TO SUCCESS

Nursing responsibility includes positioning clients safely and appropriately to provide safety and comfort. Knowledge regarding the client position required for a certain procedure or condition is expected. The nurse has the responsibility to reduce the likelihood and prevent the development of complications related to an existing condition, prescribed treatment, or medical or surgical procedure. The nurse must review the physician's prescriptions after treatments or procedures and take note of instructions regarding positioning and mobility (Figs. 20-1 and 20-2). The nurse must also be aware of various body pressure points when clients are positioned in the lying or sitting position (Fig. 20-3).

CLIENT NEEDS

Safe and Effective Care Environment

Establishing priorities
Ensuring environmental and personal safety
Ensuring home safety
Positioning the client appropriately and safely
Preventing accidents and injuries
Providing protective measures
Using equipment safely
Using ergonomic principles and body mechanics when moving a client

Health Promotion and Maintenance

Information regarding the need for prescribed therapies
Performing the techniques of physical assessment

Psychosocial Integrity

Assisting the client to use coping mechanisms
Keeping the family informed of client progress
Providing support to the client

Physiological Integrity

Assessing the mobility and immobility level of the client
Preventing the complications of immobility
Providing comfort measures for rest and sleep
Providing nutrition and oral intake
Providing personal hygiene as needed
Using assistive devices

Trendelenburg's
Fowler's
Reverse Trendelenburg's
Semi-Fowler's
Flat

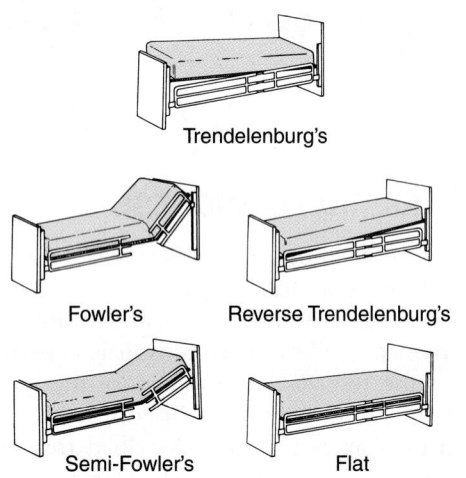

▲ **FIGURE 20-1** Common bed positions. (Potter, P., & Perry, A. [2009]. *Fundamentals of nursing* [7th ed.]. St. Louis: Mosby.)

I. GUIDELINES FOR POSITIONING

A. Client safety and comfort
1. Position client in a safe and appropriate manner to provide safety and comfort.
2. Select a position that will prevent the development of complications related to an existing condition, prescribed treatment, or medical or surgical procedure.

B. **Ergonomic principles** related to **body mechanics** (Box 20-1)

▲ Always review the physician's prescription, especially after treatments or procedures, and take note of instructions regarding positioning and mobility.

II. POSITIONS TO ENSURE SAFETY AND COMFORT

A. Integumentary system
1. Autograft: After surgery, the site is immobilized usually for 3 to 7 days to provide the time needed for the graft to adhere and attach to the wound bed.

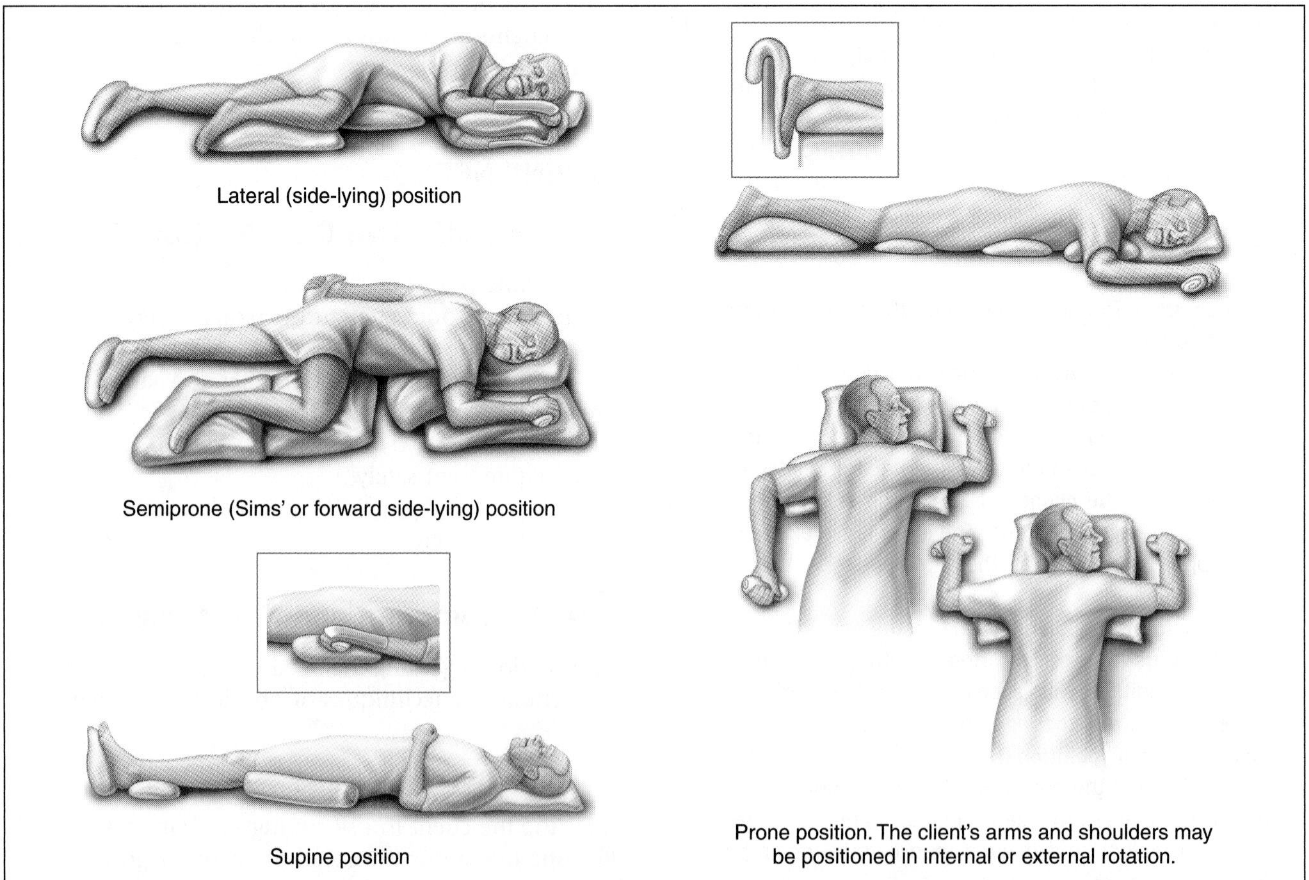

Lateral (side-lying) position
Semiprone (Sims' or forward side-lying) position
Supine position
Prone position. The client's arms and shoulders may be positioned in internal or external rotation.

▲ **FIGURE 20-2** Common client positions. (From Harkreader, H., Hogan, M., & Thobaben, M. [2007]. *Fundamentals of nursing: Caring and clinical judgment* [3rd ed.]. St. Louis: Saunders.)

2. Burns of the face and head: Elevate the head of the bed to prevent or reduce facial, head, and tracheal edema.

3. Circumferential burns of the extremities: Elevate the extremities above the level of the heart to prevent or reduce dependent edema.

4. Skin graft: Elevate and immobilize the graft site to prevent movement and shearing of the graft and disruption of tissue; avoid weight-bearing.

B. Reproductive system

1. Mastectomy

a. Position the client with the head of the bed elevated at least 30 degrees (**semi-Fowler's position**), with the affected arm elevated on a pillow to promote lymphatic fluid return after the removal of axillary lymph nodes.

b. Turn the client only to the back and unaffected side.

2. Perineal and vaginal procedures: Place the client in the **lithotomy position** (Fig. 20-4).

C. Endocrine system

1. Hypophysectomy: Elevate the head of the bed to prevent increased intracranial pressure.

Box 20-1 Body Mechanics (Ergonomic Principles) for Health Care Workers

When planning to move a client, arrange for adequate help. Use mechanical aids if help is unavailable.

Encourage the client to assist as much as possible.

Keep the back, neck and pelvis, and feet aligned. Avoid twisting.

Flex knees, and keep feet wide apart.

Position self close to the client (or object being lifted).

Use arms and legs (not back).

Slide client toward yourself using a pull sheet. When transferring a client onto a stretcher, a slide board is more appropriate.

Set (tighten) abdominal and gluteal muscles in preparation for the move.

Person with the heaviest load coordinates efforts of team involved by counting to three.

Modified from Potter, P., & Perry, A. (2009). *Fundamentals of nursing* (7th ed.). St. Louis: Mosby.

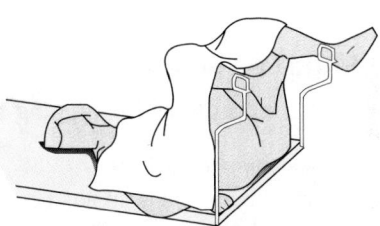

▲ **FIGURE 20-4** Lithotomy position for examination. (From Potter, P., & Perry, A. [2009]. *Fundamentals of nursing* [7th ed.]. St. Louis: Mosby.)

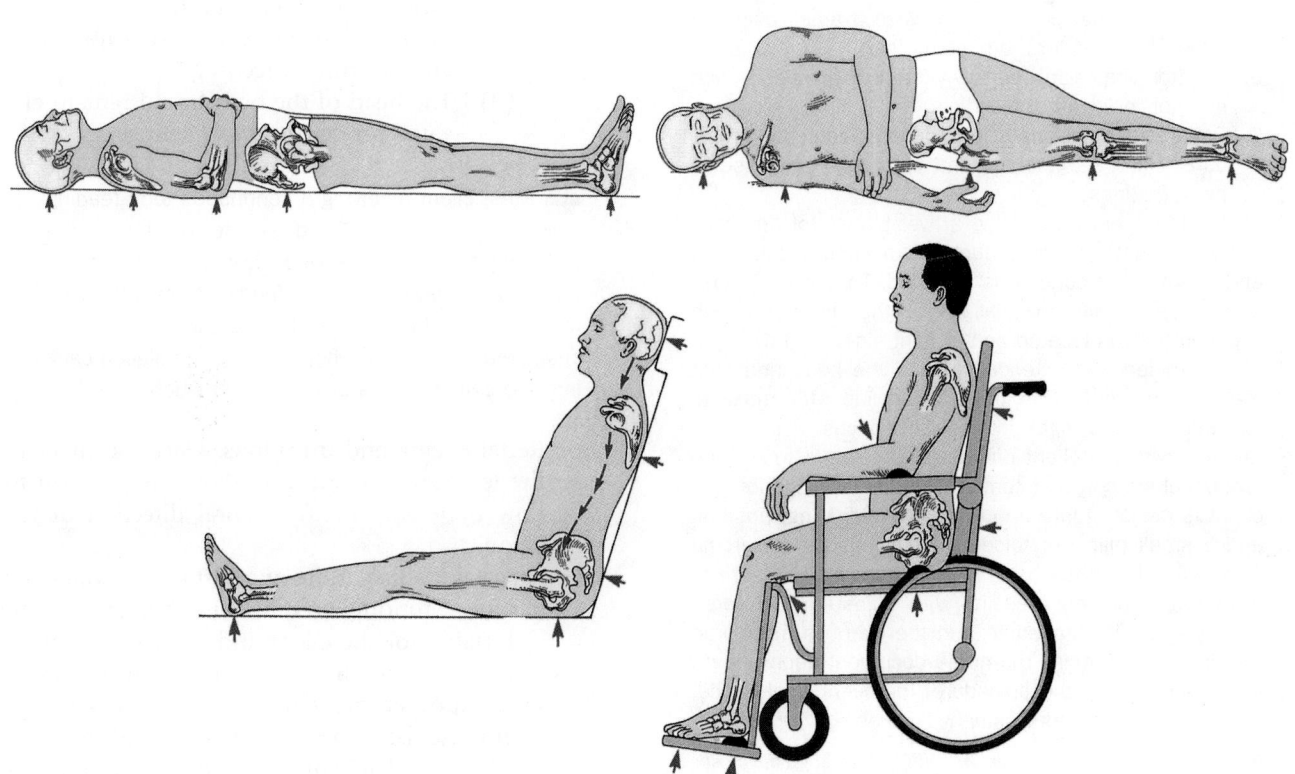

▲ **FIGURE 20-3** Pressure points in lying and sitting position. (From Elkin, M., Perry, A., & Potter, P. [2007] *Nursing interventions and clinical skills* [4th ed.]. St. Louis: Mosby.)

2. Thyroidectomy
   a. Place the client in the **semi-Fowler's** to **Fowler's position** to reduce swelling and edema in the neck area.
   b. Sandbags or pillows may be used to support the client's head or neck.
D. Gastrointestinal system
   1. Hemorrhoidectomy: Assist the client to a **lateral (side-lying) position** to prevent pain and bleeding.
   2. Gastroesophageal reflux disease: **Reverse Trendelenburg's position** may be prescribed to promote gastric emptying and prevent esophageal reflux.

   3. Liver biopsy (see Priority Nursing Actions)

▰▰▰▰▰ PRIORITY NURSING ACTIONS! ▰▰▰▰▰

Actions to Take for a Client Undergoing a Liver Biopsy

1. Explain the procedure to the client.
2. Ensure that an informed consent has been obtained.
3. Position the client supine, with the right side of the upper abdomen exposed; the client's right arm is raised and extended behind the head and over the left shoulder.
4. Remain with the client during the procedure.
5. After the procedure, assist the client into a right lateral (side-lying) position and place a small pillow or folded towel under the puncture site.
6. Monitor vital signs closely after the procedure and monitor for signs of bleeding.
7. Document appropriate information about the procedure, client's tolerance, and postprocedure assessment findings.

For the client undergoing a liver biopsy (or any invasive procedure), the procedure is explained to the client and an informed consent is obtained. The client is positioned supine, with the right side of the upper abdomen exposed (liver is located on the right side), and the right arm is raised and extended behind the head and over the left shoulder. This position provides for maximal exposure of the right intercostal spaces. The nurse remains with the client during the procedure to provide emotional support and comfort. After the procedure, the client is assisted into a right lateral (side-lying) position and a small pillow or folded towel is placed under the puncture site for at least 3 hours to provide pressure to the site and prevent bleeding. Vital signs are monitored closely after the procedure and the client is monitored for signs of bleeding. The nurse documents appropriate information about the procedure, the client's tolerance, and postprocedure assessment findings.

Reference: Pagana, K., & Pagana, T. (2009). *Mosby's diagnostic and laboratory test reference* (9th ed. pp. 604–605). St. Louis: Mosby.

---

a. During the procedure, do the following:
   (1) Position the client supine, with the right side of the upper abdomen exposed.
   (2) The client's right arm is raised and extended behind the head and over the left shoulder.
   (3) The liver is located on the right side; this position provides for maximal exposure of the right intercostal spaces.
b. After the procedure, do the following:
   (1) Assist the client into a right **lateral (side-lying) position**.
   (2) Place a small pillow or folded towel under the puncture site for at least 3 hours to provide pressure to the site and prevent bleeding.

4. Paracentesis: Client is usually positioned in a **semi-Fowler's position** in bed, or sitting upright on the side of the bed or in a chair with the feet supported; client is assisted to a position of comfort following the procedure.
5. Nasogastric tube
   a. Insertion
      (1) Position the client in a **high Fowler's position** with the head tilted forward.
      (2) This position will assist to close the trachea and open the esophagus.
   b. Irrigations and tube feedings
      (1) Elevate the head of the bed 30 to 45 degrees (**semi-Fowler's** to **Fowler's position**) to prevent aspiration.
      (2) Maintain head elevation for 1 hour after an intermittent feeding.
      (3) The head of the bed should remain elevated for continuous feedings.

⚠ If the client receiving a continuous tube feeding needs to be placed in a supine position when providing care, such as when giving a bed bath or changing linens, shut off the feeding to prevent aspiration. Remember to turn the feeding back on and check the rate of flow when the client is placed back into the semi-Fowler's or Fowler's position.

6. Rectal enema and irrigations: Place the client in the left **Sims' position** to allow the solution to flow by gravity in the natural direction of the colon.
7. Sengstaken-Blakemore and Minnesota tubes
   a. Not commonly used because they are uncomfortable for the client and can cause complications, but their use may be necessary when other interventions are not feasible.
   b. If prescribed, maintain elevation of the head of the bed to enhance lung expansion and reduce portal blood flow, permitting effective esophagogastric balloon tamponade.

E. Respiratory system
1. Chronic obstructive pulmonary disease: In advanced disease, place the client in a sitting position, leaning forward, with the client's arms over several pillows or an overbed table; this position will assist the client to breathe easier.
2. Laryngectomy (radical neck dissection): Place the client in a **semi-Fowler's** or **Fowler's position** to maintain a patent airway and minimize edema.
3. Bronchoscopy postprocedure: Place the client in a **semi-Fowler's position** to prevent choking or aspiration resulting from an impaired ability to swallow.
4. Postural drainage: The lung segment to be drained should be in the uppermost position; **Trendelenburg's position** may be used.
5. Thoracentesis
   a. During the procedure, to facilitate removal of fluid from the pleural space, position the client sitting on the edge of the bed and leaning over the bedside table with the feet supported on a stool, or lying in bed on the unaffected side with the head of the bed elevated about 45 degrees (**Fowler's position**).
   b. After the procedure, assist the client to a position of comfort.

⚠ Always check the physician's prescription regarding positioning for the client who had a thoracotomy, lung wedge resection, lobectomy of the lung, or pneumonectomy.

F. Cardiovascular system
1. Abdominal aneurysm resection
   a. After surgery, limit elevation of the head of the bed to 45 degrees (**Fowler's position**) to avoid flexion of the graft.
   b. The client may be turned from side to side.
2. Amputation of the lower extremity
   a. During the first 24 hours after amputation, elevate the foot of the bed (the stump is supported with pillows but not elevated because of the risk of flexion contractures) to reduce edema.
   b. Consult with the physician and, if prescribed, position the client in a **prone position** twice a day for a 20- to 30-minute period to stretch muscles and prevent flexion contractures of the hip.
3. Arterial vascular grafting of an extremity
   a. To promote graft patency after the procedure, bedrest usually is maintained for approximately 24 hours and the affected extremity is kept straight.
   b. Limit movement and avoid flexion of the hip and knee.

4. Cardiac catheterization
   a. If the femoral artery was accessed for the procedure, the client is maintained on bedrest for 4 to 6 hours (time for bedrest may vary depending on physician preference and if a vascular closure device was used); the client may turn from side to side.
   b. The affected extremity is kept straight and the head is elevated no more than 30 degrees (some physicians prefer the flat position) until hemostasis is adequately achieved.
5. Congestive heart failure and pulmonary edema: Position the client upright, preferably with the legs dangling over the side of the bed, to decrease venous return and lung congestion.

⚠ Most often, clients with respiratory and cardiac disorders should be positioned with the head of the bed elevated.

6. Peripheral arterial disease
   a. Obtain the physician's prescription for positioning.
   b. Because swelling can prevent arterial blood flow, clients may be advised to elevate their feet at rest, but they should not raise their legs above the level of the heart because extreme elevation slows arterial blood flow; some clients may be advised to maintain a slightly dependent position to promote perfusion.
7. Deep vein thrombosis
   a. If the extremity is red, edematous, and painful, and if traditional heparin sodium therapy may be initiated, bedrest with leg elevation may be prescribed for the client.
   b. Clients receiving low-molecular-weight heparin usually can be out of bed after 24 hours if pain level permits.
8. Varicose veins: Leg elevation above heart level usually is prescribed; the client also is advised to minimize prolonged sitting or standing during daily activities.
9. Venous insufficiency and leg ulcers: Leg elevation usually is prescribed.

G. Sensory system
1. Cataract surgery: Postoperatively, elevate the head of the bed (**semi-Fowler's** to **Fowler's position**) and position the client on the back or the nonoperative side to prevent the development of edema at the operative site.
2. Retinal detachment
   a. If the detachment is large, bedrest and bilateral eye patching may be prescribed to minimize eye movement and prevent extension of the detachment.
   b. Restrictions in activity and positioning following repair of the detachment depends on

the physician's preference and the surgical procedure performed.

H. Neurological system

1. Autonomic dysreflexia: Elevate the head of the bed to a **high Fowler's position** to assist with adequate ventilation and assist in the prevention of hypertensive stroke.

⚠ If autonomic dysreflexia occurs, immediately place the client in a high Fowler's position.

2. Cerebral aneurysm: Bedrest is maintained with the head of the bed elevated 30 to 45 degrees (**semi-Fowler's** to **Fowler's position**) to prevent pressure on the aneurysm site.

3. Cerebral angiography
   a. Maintain bedrest for the length of time as prescribed.
   b. The extremity into which the contrast medium was injected is kept straight and immobilized for about 6 to 8 hours.

4. Brain attack (stroke)
   a. In clients with hemorrhagic strokes, the head of the bed is usually elevated to 30 degrees to reduce intracranial pressure and to facilitate venous drainage.
   b. For clients with ischemic strokes, the head of the bed is usually kept flat.
   c. Maintain the head in a midline, neutral position to facilitate venous drainage from the head.
   d. Avoid extreme hip and neck flexion; extreme hip flexion may increase intrathoracic pressure, whereas extreme neck flexion prohibits venous drainage from the brain.

5. Craniotomy
   a. The client should not be positioned on the site that was operated on, especially if the bone flap has been removed, because the brain has no bony covering on the affected site.
   b. Elevate the head of the bed 30 to 45 degrees (**semi-Fowler's** to **Fowler's position**) and maintain the head in a midline, neutral position to facilitate venous drainage from the head.
   c. Avoid extreme hip and neck flexion.

6. Laminectomy
   a. Logroll the client.
   b. When the client is out of bed, the client's back is kept straight (the client is placed in a straight-backed chair) with the feet resting comfortably on the floor.

7. Increased intracranial pressure
   a. Elevate the head of the bed 30 to 45 degrees (**semi-Fowler's** to **Fowler's position**) and maintain the head in a midline, neutral position to facilitate venous drainage from the head.

   b. Avoid extreme hip and neck flexion.

⚠ Do not place a client with a head injury in a flat or Trendelenburg's position because of the risk of increased intracranial pressure.

8. Lumbar puncture
   a. During the procedure, assist the client to the **lateral (side-lying) position**, with the back bowed at the edge of the examining table, the knees flexed up to the abdomen, and the neck flexed so that the chin is resting on the chest.
   b. After the procedure, place the client in the **supine position** for 4 to 12 hours, as prescribed.

9. Myelogram postprocedure
   a. The head position varies according to the dye used.
   b. The head is usually elevated if an oil-based or water-soluble contrast agent is used and the head is usually positioned lower than the trunk if air contrast is used.

10. Spinal cord injury
    a. Immobilize the client on a spinal backboard, with the head in a neutral position, to prevent incomplete injury from becoming complete.
    b. Prevent head flexion, rotation, or extension; the head is immobilized with a firm, padded cervical collar.
    c. Logroll the client; no part of the body should be twisted or turned, nor should the client be allowed to assume a sitting position.

I. Musculoskeletal system

1. Total hip replacement
   a. Positioning depends on the surgical techniques used, the method of implantation, and the prosthesis.
   b. Avoid extreme internal and external rotation.
   c. Avoid adduction; side-lying on the operative side is not allowed (unless specifically prescribed by the physician).
   d. Maintain abduction when the client is in a **supine position** or positioned on the nonoperative side.
   e. Place a pillow between the client's legs to maintain abduction; instruct the client not to cross the legs (Box 20-2).
   f. Check the physician's prescriptions regarding elevation of the head of the bed; flexion usually is limited to 60 degrees during the first postoperative week (usually 90 degrees for 2 to 3 months thereafter).

2. Devices used to promote proper positioning (see Box 20-2)

Box 20-2 Devices Used for Proper Positioning

Bed Boards

These plywood boards are placed under the entire surface area of the mattress and are useful for increasing back support and body alignment.

Foot Boots

Foot boots are made of rigid plastic or heavy foam and keep the foot flexed at the proper angle. They should be removed two or three times a day to assess skin integrity and joint mobility.

Hand Rolls

Hand rolls maintain the fingers in a slightly flexed and functional position and keep the thumb slightly adducted in opposition to the fingers.

Hand-Wrist Splints

These splints are individually molded for the client to maintain proper alignment of the thumb in slight adduction and the wrist in slight dorsiflexion.

Pillows

Pillows provide support, elevate body parts, splint incisional areas, and reduce postoperative pain during activity, coughing, or deep breathing. They should be of the appropriate size for the body part to be positioned.

Sandbags

Sandbags are soft devices filled with a substance that can be shaped to body contours to provide support. They immobilize extremities and maintain specific body alignment.

Side Rails

These bars, positioned along the sides of the length of the bed, ensure client safety and are useful for increasing mobility. They also provide assistance in rolling from side to side or sitting up in bed.

Trapeze Bar

This bar descends from a securely fastened overhead bar attached to the bed frame. It allows the client to use the upper extremities to raise the trunk off the bed, assists in transfer from the bed to a wheelchair, and helps the client perform upper arm strengthening exercises.

Trochanter Rolls

These rolls prevent external rotation of the legs when the client is in the supine position. To form a roll, use a cotton bath blanket or a sheet folded lengthwise to a width extending from the greater trochanter of the femur to the lower border of the popliteal space.

Wedge Pillow

This triangular pillow is made of heavy foam and is used to maintain the legs in abduction following total hip replacement surgery.

Modified from Potter, P., & Perry, A. (2009). *Fundamentals of nursing* (7th ed.). St. Louis: Mosby.

 MORE QUESTIONS ON THE CD!

Practice Questions

179. A client is being prepared for a thoracentesis. A nurse assists the client to which position for the procedure?
1. Lying in bed on the affected side
2. Lying in bed on the unaffected side
3. Sims' position with the head of the bed flat
4. Prone with the head turned to the side and supported by a pillow

180. A nurse is preparing to insert a nasogastric tube into a client. The nurse places the client in which position for insertion?
1. Right side
2. Low Fowler's
3. High Fowler's
4. Supine with the head flat

181. A nurse develops a plan of care for a client with deep vein thrombosis. Which client position or activity in the plan will be included?
1. Out-of-bed activities as desired
2. Bedrest with the affected extremity kept flat
3. Bedrest with elevation of the affected extremity
4. Bedrest with the affected extremity in a dependent position

182. The nurse is caring for a client who is 1 day postoperative for a total hip replacement. Which is the best position in which the nurse should place the client?
1. Side-lying on the operative side
2. On the nonoperative side with the legs abducted
3. Side-lying with the affected leg internally rotated
4. Side-lying with the affected leg externally rotated

183. A nurse is providing instructions to a client and the family regarding home care after right eye cataract removal. Which statement by the client would indicate an understanding of the instructions?
1. "I should not sleep on my left side."
2. "I should not sleep on my right side."
3. "I should not sleep with my head elevated."
4. "I should not wear my glasses at any time."

184. A nurse is administering a cleansing enema to a client with a fecal impaction. Before administering the enema, the nurse places the client in which position?
1. Left Sims' position
2. Right Sims' position
3. On the left side of the body, with the head of the bed elevated 45 degrees
4. On the right side of the body, with the head of the bed elevated 45 degrees

185. A client has just returned to a nursing unit after an above-knee amputation of the right leg. A nurse places the client in which position?
1. Prone
2. Reverse Trendelenburg's
3. Supine, with the amputated limb flat on the bed
4. Supine, with the amputated limb supported with pillows

186. A nurse is caring for a client with a severe burn who is scheduled for an autograft to be placed on the lower extremity. The nurse develops a postoperative plan of care for the client and includes which of the following in the plan?
1. Maintain the client in a prone position.
2. Elevate and immobilize the grafted extremity.
3. Maintain the surgical extremity in a flat position.

4. Keep the surgical extremity covered with a blanket.

187. A nurse is preparing to care for a client who has returned to the nursing unit following cardiac catheterization performed through the femoral artery. The nurse checks the physician's prescription and plans to allow which client position or activity following the procedure?
1. Bedrest in high Fowler's position
2. Bedrest with bathroom privileges only
3. Bedrest with head elevation at 60 degrees
4. Bedrest with head elevation no greater than 30 degrees

Alternate Item Format:
Multiple Response

188. The nurse is caring for a client following a supratentorial craniotomy in which a large tumor was removed from the left side. Select the positions in which the nurse can safely place the client. Select all that apply.
❑ 1. On the left side
❑ 2. With the neck flexed
❑ 3. Supine on the left side
❑ 4. With extreme hip flexion
❑ 5. In a semi-Fowler's position
❑ 6. With the head in a midline position

ANSWERS
179. 2
Rationale: To facilitate removal of fluid from the chest, the client is positioned sitting at the edge of the bed leaning over the bedside table, with the feet supported on a stool or lying in bed on the unaffected side with the head of the bed elevated 30 to 45 degrees. The prone and Sims' positions are inappropriate positions for this procedure.
Test-Taking Strategy: Use the process of elimination. Eliminate option 1 first because, if the client was lying on the affected side, it would be difficult to perform the procedure. Option 3 can be eliminated next because the Sims' position is used primarily for rectal enemas or irrigations. Next, visualize the prone position. In the prone position, the client is lying on the abdomen, which is not an appropriate position for this procedure. Review the procedure for a thoracentesis if you had difficulty with this question.
Level of Cognitive Ability: Applying
Client Needs: Physiological Integrity
Integrated Process: Nursing Process—Implementation
Content Area: Fundamental Skills—Safety/Infection Control
Reference: Chernecky, C., & Berger, B. (2008). *Laboratory tests and diagnostic procedures* (5th ed., p. 1063). St. Louis: Saunders.

180. 3
Rationale: During insertion of a nasogastric tube, the client is placed in a sitting or high Fowler's position to reduce the risk of pulmonary aspiration if the client should vomit. Options 1, 2, and 4 will not facilitate insertion of the tube or prevent aspiration.
Test-Taking Strategy: Use the process of elimination. Recalling that a concern with insertion of a nasogastric tube is pulmonary aspiration will direct you to option 3. Review the procedure for inserting a nasogastric tube if you had difficulty with this question.
Level of Cognitive Ability: Applying
Client Needs: Physiological Integrity
Integrated Process: Nursing Process—Implementation
Content Area: Fundamental Skills—Safety/Infection Control
Reference: Potter, P., & Perry, A. (2009). *Fundamentals of nursing* (7th ed., p. 1204). St. Louis: Mosby.

181. 3
Rationale: For the client with deep vein thrombosis, elevation of the affected leg facilitates blood flow by the force of gravity and also decreases venous pressure, which in turn relieves edema and pain. Bedrest is indicated to prevent emboli and to prevent pressure fluctuations in the venous system that occur with walking.

Test-Taking Strategy: Use the process of elimination. Focus on the client's diagnosis and think about the principles related to gravity flow and edema to answer the question. If you had difficulty with this question review nursing care for a client with a venous disorder.
Level of Cognitive Ability: Applying
Client Needs: Physiological Integrity
Integrated Process: Nursing Process—Planning
Content Area: Fundamental Skills—Safety/Infection Control
Reference: Ignatavicius, D., & Workman, M. (2010). *Medical-surgical nursing: Patient-centered collaborative care* (6th ed., p. 818). St. Louis: Saunders.

182. 2
Rationale: Positioning following a total hip replacement depends on the surgical techniques used, the method of implantation, the prosthesis, and physician's preference. Abduction is maintained when the client is in a supine position or positioned on the nonoperative side. Internal and external rotation, adduction, or side-lying on the operative side (unless specifically prescribed by the physician) is avoided. Options 1, 3, and 4 are incorrect positions for this client.
Test-Taking Strategy: Use the process of elimination and knowledge regarding care of clients following total hip replacement to answer this question. Options 3 and 4 can be eliminated first because of the words *internally rotated* and *externally rotated*. From the remaining options, eliminate option 1 because lying on the operative side can disrupt the replacement. Review positioning after total hip replacement if you had difficulty with this question.
Level of Cognitive Ability: Applying
Client Needs: Physiological Integrity
Integrated Process: Implementation
Content Area: Fundamental Skills—Safety/Infection Control
Reference: Black, J., & Hawks, J. (2009). *Medical-surgical nursing: Clinical management for positive outcomes* (8th ed., pp. 480–481). St. Louis: Saunders.

183. 2
Rationale: After cataract surgery, the client should not sleep on the side of the body that was operated on to prevent edema formation and intraocular pressure. The client also should be placed in a semi-Fowler's position to assist in minimizing edema and intraocular pressure. During the day, the client may wear glasses or a protective shield; at night, the protective shield alone is sufficient.
Test-Taking Strategy: Use the process of elimination. Remember to instruct the client to remain off the operative side and to rest with the head elevated to minimize edema formation. This will assist you when answering questions related to cataract surgery. Review postoperative instructions for the client following cataract surgery if you had difficulty with this question.
Level of Cognitive Ability: Evaluating
Client Needs: Physiological Integrity
Integrated Process: Nursing Process—Evaluation
Content Area: Fundamental Skills—Safety/Infection Control
Reference: Black, J., & Hawks, J. (2009). *Medical-surgical nursing: Clinical management for positive outcomes* (8th ed., p. 1706). St. Louis: Saunders.

184. 1
Rationale: For administering an enema, the client is placed in a left Sims' position so that the enema solution can flow by gravity in the natural direction of the colon. The head of the bed is not elevated in the Sims' position.
Test-Taking Strategy: Use the process of elimination and knowledge regarding the anatomy of the bowel to answer the question. This will assist in eliminating options 2 and 4. Visualize the procedure for administering an enema and eliminate option 3 because the head of the bed should be flat during enema administration. Review the procedure for administering an enema if you had difficulty with this question.
Level of Cognitive Ability: Applying
Client Needs: Physiological Integrity
Integrated Process: Nursing Process—Implementation
Content Area: Fundamental Skills—Safety/Infection Control
Reference: Potter, P., & Perry, A. (2009). *Fundamentals of nursing* (7th ed., p. 1200). St. Louis: Mosby.

185. 4
Rationale: The amputated limb is usually supported on pillows for the first 24 hours following surgery to promote venous return and decrease edema. After the first 24 hours, the amputated limb usually is placed flat on the bed to reduce hip contracture. Edema also is controlled by limb-wrapping techniques. Additionally, it is important to check physician prescriptions regarding positioning following amputation. Options 1, 2, and 3 are inappropriate positions for the client immediately after surgery.
Test-Taking Strategy: Use the process of elimination. The subject of this question is that the client has just returned from surgery. Using basic principles related to immediate postoperative care will assist in directing you to option 4. If you had difficulty with this question, review postoperative positioning following amputation.
Level of Cognitive Ability: Applying
Client Needs: Physiological Integrity
Integrated Process: Nursing Process—Implementation
Content Area: Fundamental Skills—Safety/Infection Control
References: Black, J., & Hawks, J. (2009). *Medical-surgical nursing: Clinical management for positive outcomes* (8th ed., p. 1321). St. Louis: Saunders.

   Ignatavicius, D., & Workman, M. (2010). *Medical-surgical nursing: Patient-centered collaborative care* (6th ed., p. 1202). St. Louis: Saunders.

186. 2
Rationale: Autografts placed over joints or on lower extremities are elevated and immobilized following surgery for 3 to 7 days, depending on the surgeon's preference. This period of immobilization allows the autograft time to adhere and attach to the wound bed, and the elevation minimizes edema. Keeping the client in a prone position and covering the extremity with a blanket can disrupt the graft site.
Test-Taking Strategy: Use the process of elimination. Options 1 and 4 can be eliminated first because a prone position and a blanket can disrupt a graft easily. From the remaining options, recall the principles related to gravity and edema to assist in directing you to option 2. Review care for the client following an autograft if you had difficulty with this question.

Level of Cognitive Ability: Applying
Client Needs: Physiological Integrity
Integrated Process: Nursing Process—Planning
Content Area: Fundamental Skills—Safety/Infection Control
Reference: Black, J., & Hawks, J. (2009). *Medical-surgical nursing: Clinical management for positive outcomes* (8th ed., p. 1265). St. Louis: Saunders.

187. 4

Rationale: After cardiac catheterization, the extremity into which the catheter was inserted is kept straight for 4 to 6 hours. The client is maintained on bedrest for 4 to 6 hours (time for bedrest may vary depending on physician preference and if a vascular closure device was used) and the client may turn from side to side. The head is elevated no more than 30 degrees (although some physicians prefer the flat position) until hemostasis is adequately achieved.
Test-Taking Strategy: Use the process of elimination. Knowing that the head of the bed should not be elevated more than 30 degrees will assist in eliminating options 1 and 3. Remembering that bathroom privileges are not allowed in the immediate postcatheterization period will assist in eliminating option 2. If you had difficulty with this question, review care after cardiac catheterization.
Level of Cognitive Ability: Applying
Client Needs: Physiological Integrity
Integrated Process: Nursing Process—Planning
Content Area: Fundamental Skills—Safety/Infection Control
Reference: Ignatavicius, D., & Workman, M. (2010). *Medical-surgical nursing: Patient-centered collaborative care* (6th ed., p. 7240). St. Louis: Saunders.

ALTERNATE ITEM FORMAT: MULTIPLE RESPONSE

188. 5, 6

Rationale: Clients who have undergone supratentorial surgery should have the head of the bed elevated 30 degrees to promote venous drainage from the head. The client is positioned to avoid extreme hip or neck flexion and the head is maintained in a midline neutral position. If a large tumor has been removed, the client should be placed on the nonoperative side to prevent displacement of the cranial contents.
Test-Taking Strategy: Focus on the data in the question. Remember that a primary concern is the risk for increased intracranial pressure. Therefore use concepts related to preventing increased intracranial pressure to answer this question. Also remember that with *supra*tentorial surgery, the head is usually kept "up" and that the client is placed on the nonoperative side. Review positioning for a client after craniotomy if you had difficulty with this question.
Level of Cognitive Ability: Applying
Client Needs: Physiological Integrity
Integrated Process: Nursing Process—Implementation
Content Area: Fundamental Skills—Safety/Infection Control
Reference: Black, J., & Hawks, J. (2009). *Medical-surgical nursing: Clinical management for positive outcomes* (8th ed., p. 1932). St. Louis: Saunders.

Care of a Client With a Tube

PYRAMID TERMS

chest tube Tube that returns negative pressure to the intra-pleural space; used to remove abnormal accumulations of air and fluid from the pleural space.

endotracheal tube Tube used to maintain a patent airway; indicated when a client needs mechanical ventilation.

tracheostomy An opening made surgically directly into the trachea to establish an airway. A tracheostomy tube is inserted into the opening and the tube attaches to the mechanical ventilator or another type of oxygen delivery device.

THE PYRAMID TO SUCCESS

The Pyramid to Success focuses on the common types of tubes used in the medical-surgical and acute care clinical settings. The NCLEX-RN examination is likely to address content areas related to the appropriate care of certain tubes and the immediate interventions required if a complication arises. Focus on the specific assessment points related to the specific type of tube. Review procedures for inserting a particular tube, verifying correct placement, and administering medications or feedings, if appropriate. Remember that for certain types of tubes such as endotracheal, tracheostomy, urinary and renal, and chest tubes, implementing and maintaining surgical asepsis is critical. Pyramid Points also focus on interventions associated with complications or emergencies.

CLIENT NEEDS

Safe and Effective Care Environment

Acting as a client advocate
Collaborating with members of the health care team
Ensuring that advance directives are in the client's medical record
Ensuring client's rights
Establishing priorities
Handling of hazardous and infectious materials
Maintaining standard and transmission-based precautions as well as surgical asepsis

Obtaining informed consent for invasive procedures
Providing continuity of care
Using equipment safely

Health Promotion and Maintenance

Assisting the client to accept lifestyle changes
Preventing disease
Providing the client and family education regarding care at home
Performing techniques of physical assessment

Psychosocial Integrity

Discussing situational role changes
Identifying cultural, religious, and spiritual influences on health
Identifying support systems
Monitoring for sensory and perceptual alterations
Providing home care services

Physiological Integrity

Administering medications
Initiating emergency interventions for complications
Implementing measures to ensure basic care and comfort
Monitoring for potential complications associated with the tube
Monitoring laboratory values
Preparing for diagnostic tests to confirm accurate placement of a tube
Providing nutrition and oral hydration
Providing respiratory care

I. NASOGASTRIC TUBES

A. Description
1. These are tubes used to intubate the stomach.
2. The tube is inserted from the nose to the stomach.

B. Purpose
1. To decompress the stomach by removing fluids or gas to promote abdominal comfort

235

2. To allow surgical anastomoses to heal without distention
3. To decrease the risk of aspiration
4. To administer medications to clients who are unable to swallow
5. To provide nutrition by acting as a temporary feeding tube
6. To irrigate the stomach and remove toxic substances, such as in poisoning

C. Types of tubes
1. Levin tube (Fig. 21-1)
   a. Single-lumen nasogastric tube
   b. Used to remove gastric contents via intermittent suction or to provide tube feedings
2. Salem sump tube: A Salem sump is a double-lumen nasogastric tube with an air vent (pigtail) used for decompression with intermittent continuous suction (see Fig. 21-1).

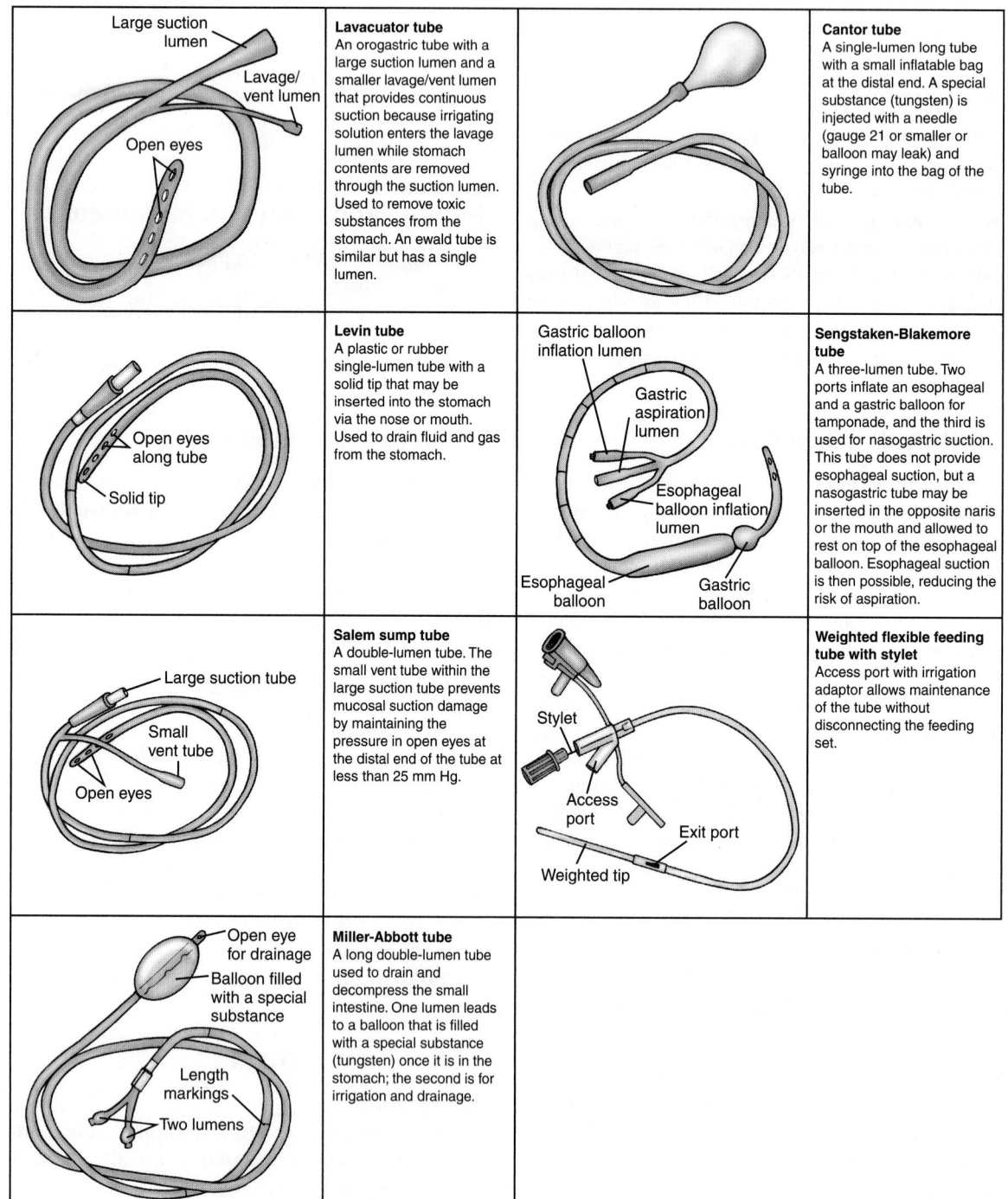

Lavacuator tube
An orogastric tube with a large suction lumen and a smaller lavage/vent lumen that provides continuous suction because irrigating solution enters the lavage lumen while stomach contents are removed through the suction lumen. Used to remove toxic substances from the stomach. An ewald tube is similar but has a single lumen.

Cantor tube
A single-lumen long tube with a small inflatable bag at the distal end. A special substance (tungsten) is injected with a needle (gauge 21 or smaller or balloon may leak) and syringe into the bag of the tube.

Levin tube
A plastic or rubber single-lumen tube with a solid tip that may be inserted into the stomach via the nose or mouth. Used to drain fluid and gas from the stomach.

Sengstaken-Blakemore tube
A three-lumen tube. Two ports inflate an esophageal and a gastric balloon for tamponade, and the third is used for nasogastric suction. This tube does not provide esophageal suction, but a nasogastric tube may be inserted in the opposite naris or the mouth and allowed to rest on top of the esophageal balloon. Esophageal suction is then possible, reducing the risk of aspiration.

Salem sump tube
A double-lumen tube. The small vent tube within the large suction tube prevents mucosal suction damage by maintaining the pressure in open eyes at the distal end of the tube at less than 25 mm Hg.

Weighted flexible feeding tube with stylet
Access port with irrigation adaptor allows maintenance of the tube without disconnecting the feeding set.

Miller-Abbott tube
A long double-lumen tube used to drain and decompress the small intestine. One lumen leads to a balloon that is filled with a special substance (tungsten) once it is in the stomach; the second is for irrigation and drainage.

▲ **FIGURE 21-1** Comparison of design and function of selected gastrointestinal tubes. (Modified from Monahan, F., & Neighbors, M. [1998]. *Medical-surgical nursing* [2nd ed.]. St. Louis: Saunders.)

⚠ The air vent on a Salem sump tube is not to be clamped and is to be kept above the level of the stomach. If leakage occurs through the air vent, instill 30 mL of air into the air vent and irrigate the main lumen with normal saline (NS).

D. Intubation procedures (Box 21-1)
E. Irrigation
1. Assess placement before irrigating (see Box 21-1).
2. Perform irrigation every 4 hours to assess and maintain the patency of the tube.
3. Gently instill 30 to 50 mL of water or NS (depending on agency policy) with an irrigation syringe.
4. Pull back on the syringe plunger to withdraw the fluid to check patency; repeat if the tube flow is sluggish.
F. Removal of a nasogastric tube: Ask the client to take a deep breath and hold; remove the tube slowly and evenly over the course of 3 to 6 seconds (coil the tube around the hand while removing it).

II. GASTROINTESTINAL TUBE FEEDINGS

A. Types of tubes and anatomical placement
1. Nasogastric: Nose to stomach
2. Nasoduodenal-nasojejunal: Nose to duodenum or jejunum
3. Gastrostomy: Stomach
4. Jejunostomy: Jejunum
B. Types of administration
1. Bolus
   a. A bolus resembles normal meal feeding patterns.
   b. Formula is administrated over a 30- to 60-minute period every 3 to 6 hours; the amount of formula is prescribed by the physician.
2. Continuous
   a. Feeding is administered continually for 24 hours.
   b. An infusion feeding pump regulates the flow.
3. Cyclical
   a. Feeding is administered in the daytime or nighttime for approximately 8 to 16 hours.
   b. An infusion feeding pump regulates the flow.

Box 21-1 Nasogastric Tubes: Intubation Procedures

1. Follow agency procedures.
2. Explain the procedure and its potential discomfort to the client.
3. Position the client with pillows behind the shoulders.
4. Determine which nostril is more patent.
5. Measure the length of the tube from the bridge of the nose to the earlobe to the xiphoid process and indicate this length with a piece of tape on the tube.
6. If the client is conscious and alert, have him or her swallow or drink water (follow agency procedure).
7. Lubricate the tip of the tube with water-soluble lubricant.
8. Gently insert the tube into the nasopharynx and advance the tube.
9. When the tube nears the back of the throat (first black measurement on the tube) instruct the client to swallow or drink sips of water (unless contraindicated). If resistance is met, then slowly rotate and aim the tube downward and toward the closer ear; in the intubated or semiconscious client, flex the head toward the chest while passing the tube.
10. Immediately withdraw the tube if any change is noted in the client's respiratory status.
11. Following insertion, obtain an abdominal x-ray study to confirm placement of the tube.
12. Connect the tube to suction, to either the intermittent or continuous suction setting, as prescribed.
13. Secure the tube to the client's nose with adhesive tape and to the client's gown (follow agency procedure and check for client allergy to tape).
14. Observe the client for nausea, vomiting, abdominal fullness, or distention and monitor output.
15. Check residual volumes every 4 hours, before each feeding, and before giving medications. Aspirate all stomach contents (residual) and measure the amount. Reinstill residual contents to prevent excessive fluid and electrolyte losses, unless the residual contents appear abnormal and the volume is large (follow agency procedure). Withhold the feeding if the amount is more than 100 mL or according to agency or nutritional consult recommendations.
16. Before the instillation of any substance through the tube (i.e., irrigation solution, feeding, medications) aspirate stomach contents and test the pH (a pH of 3.5 or lower indicates that the tip of the tube is in a gastric location).
17. If irrigation is indicated, use normal saline solution (check agency procedure).
18. Observe the client for fluid and electrolyte balance.
19. Instruct the client about movement to prevent nasal irritation and dislodgment of the tube.
20. On a daily basis, remove the adhesive tape that is securing the tube to the nose and clean and dry the skin; then reapply the tape.

Note: Gastrostomy or jejunostomy tubes are surgically inserted. A dressing is placed at the site of insertion. The dressing needs to be removed, the skin needs to be cleansed (with a solution determined by the physician or agency procedure), and a new sterile dressing needs to be applied every 8 hours (or as specified by agency policy). The skin at the insertion site is checked for signs of infection or other abnormalities, such as leakage of the feeding solution.

Modified from Ignatavicius, D., & Workman, M. (2010). *Medical-surgical nursing: Patient-centered collaborative care* (6th ed.). St. Louis: Saunders.

c. Feedings at night allow for more freedom during the day.

C. Administration of feedings

1. Check the physician's prescription and agency policy regarding residual amounts; usually, if the residual is less than 100 mL, feeding is administered; large-volume aspirates indicate delayed gastric emptying and place the client at risk for aspiration.

2. Assess bowel sounds; hold the feeding and notify the physician if bowel sounds are absent.

3. Position the client in a high Fowler's position; if comatose, place in high-Fowler's and on the right side.

4. Assess tube placement by aspirating gastric contents and measuring the pH (should be 3.5 or lower).

5. Aspirate all stomach contents (residual), measure the amount, and return the contents to the stomach to prevent electrolyte imbalances.

6. Warm the feeding to room temperature to prevent diarrhea and cramps.

7. Use an infusion feeding pump for continuous or cyclic feedings.

8. For bolus feeding, maintain the client in a high Fowler's position for 30 minutes after the feeding.

9. For a continuous feeding, keep the client in a semi-Fowler's position at all times.

D. Precautions

⚠ Always assess the placement of a gastrointestinal tube before instilling feeding solutions, medications, or any other solution. If the tube is incorrectly placed the client is at risk for aspiration.

1. Change the feeding container and tubing every 24 hours.

2. Do not hang more solution than required for a 4-hour period; this prevents bacterial growth.

3. Check the expiration date on the formula before administering.

4. Shake the formula well before pouring it into the container (feeding bag).

5. Always assess bowel sounds; do not administer any feedings if bowel sounds are absent.

6. Administer the feeding at the prescribed rate or via gravity flow (intermittent bolus feedings) with a 50- to 60-mL syringe with the plunger removed.

7. Gently flush with 30 to 50 mL of water or normal saline (depending on agency policy) with the irrigation syringe after the feeding.

E. Prevention of complications

1. Diarrhea
   a. Assess the client for lactose intolerance.
   b. Use fiber-containing feedings.
   c. Administer feeding slowly and at room temperature.

2. Aspiration
   a. Verify tube placement.
   b. Do not administer the feeding if residual is more than 100 mL (check physician's prescription and agency policy).
   c. Keep the head of the bed elevated.
   d. If aspiration occurs, suction as needed, assess respiratory rate, auscultate lung sounds, monitor temperature for aspiration pneumonia, and prepare to obtain chest radiograph.

3. Clogged tube
   a. Use liquid forms of medication, if possible.
   b. Flush the tube with 30 to 50 mL of water or NS (depending on agency policy) before and after medication administration and before and after bolus feeding.
   c. Flush with water every 4 hours for continuous feeding.

4. Vomiting
   a. Administer feedings slowly and, for bolus feedings, make feeding last for at least 30 minutes.
   b. Measure abdominal girth.
   c. Do not allow the feeding bag to empty.
   d. Do not allow air to enter the tubing.
   e. Administer the feeding at room temperature.
   f. Elevate the head of the bed.
   g. Administer antiemetics as prescribed.

⚠ If the client vomits, stop the tube feeding and place the client in a side-lying position; suction the client as needed.

F. Administration of medications (see Priority Nursing Actions)

▰▰▰▰ PRIORITY NURSING ACTIONS! ▰▰▰▰

Actions for Administering Medications via a Nasogastric or Gastrostomy Tube

1. Check the physician's prescription.
2. Prepare the medication for administration.
3. Ensure that the medication prescribed can be crushed or if it is a capsule that it can be opened; use elixir forms of medications if available.
4. Dissolve crushed medication or capsule contents in 15 to 30 mL of water.
5. Verify the client's identity and explain the procedure to the client.
6. Check tube placement and residual contents before instilling the medication; check for bowel sounds.
7. Draw up the medication into a catheter-tip syringe, clear excess air from the syringe, and insert the medication into the tube.
8. Flush with 30 to 50 mL of water or normal saline (NS), depending on agency policy.
9. Clamp the tube for 30 to 60 minutes, depending on medication and agency policy.
10. Document the administration of the medication and any other appropriate information.

The nurse always checks the physician's prescription before administering any medication to a client. Once the prescription is verified, the medication is prepared for administration. The nurse determines the reason for administration, checks for any contraindications to administering the medication, and for any potential interactions. When preparing medications for administration through a nasogastric or gastrostomy tube, the nurse needs to ensure that the medication prescribed can be crushed or if it is a capsule that it can be opened. Whole tablets or capsules cannot be administered through a tube because they can cause a tube blockage. Elixir forms of medications can also be used if available. The nurse then dissolves the crushed medication or capsule contents in 15 to 30 mL of water. Client identity is always verified before medication administration and the procedure is explained to the client. The nurse checks tube placement and residual contents before instilling the medication and checks for bowel sounds. The nurse also performs any additional assessments, such as checking the apical heart rate for cardiac medications or checking the blood pressure for antihypertensives. The medication is drawn up into a catheter-tip syringe, excess air is removed from the syringe, and the medication is inserted into the tube. The tube is flushed with 30 to 50 mL of water or NS (depending on agency policy) to ensure that all medication has been instilled. The tube is then clamped for 30 to 60 minutes (depending on the medication and agency policy) to ensure it is absorbed (if the tube is not clamped and is reattached to suction then the medication will be aspirated out with the suction). The nurse then documents the administration of the medication and any other appropriate information.

Reference: Potter, P., & Perry, A. (2009). *Fundamentals of nursing* (7th ed., p. 719). St. Louis: Mosby.

III. INTESTINAL TUBES

A. Description
1. The intestinal tube is passed nasally into the small intestine.
2. The tube may be used to decompress the bowel or to remove accumulated intestinal secretions when other interventions to decompress the bowel are not effective.
3. The tube enters the small intestine through the pyloric sphincter because of the weight of a small bag containing tungsten at the end.

B. Types of tubes include the Cantor tube (single lumen) or the Miller-Abbott tube (double lumen) (see Fig. 21-1)

C. Interventions
1. Assess the physician's prescriptions and agency policy for advancement and removal of the tube.
2. Position the client on the right side to facilitate passage of the weighted bag in the tube through the pylorus of the stomach and into the small intestine.
3. Do not secure the tube to the face with tape until it has reached final placement (may take several hours) in the intestines.
4. Radiography is performed to verify desired placement.
5. Monitor drainage from the tube.
6. If the tube becomes blocked, notify the physician. A small amount of air injected into the lumen may be prescribed to clear the tube; do not irrigate the tube with air or fluid without a prescription from the physician.
7. Assess the abdomen and measure abdominal girth.
8. To remove the tube, the tungsten is removed from the balloon portion of the tube with a syringe; the tube is removed gradually (6 inches every hour) as prescribed by the physician.
9. Dispose of the tube and tungsten in the appropriate manner as per agency policy.

IV. ESOPHAGEAL AND GASTRIC TUBES

A. Description
1. May be used to apply pressure against bleeding esophageal veins to control the bleeding when other interventions are not effective or they are contraindicated.
2. Not used if the client has ulceration or necrosis of the esophagus or has had previous esophageal surgery because of the risk of rupture

B. Sengstaken-Blakemore tube and Minnesota tube (see Fig. 21-1)
1. The Sengstaken-Blakemore tube is a triple-lumen gastric tube with an inflatable esophageal balloon, an inflatable gastric balloon, and a gastric aspiration lumen.
2. The gastric balloon applies pressure at the cardi-oesophageal junction to compress gastric varices directly and to decrease blood flow to esophageal varices; traction is applied to maintain the gastric balloon in place.
3. The esophageal balloon directly compresses esophageal varices.
4. If bleeding is not stopped with inflation of the gastric balloon, the esophageal balloon is inflated to 25 to 45 mm Hg as prescribed.
5. A radiograph of the upper abdomen and chest confirms placement.
6. Gastric contents are aspirated by gastric lavage or intermittent suction via the gastric aspiration port.
7. With the Sengstaken-Blakemore tube, a nasogastric tube also is inserted in the opposite naris to collect secretions that accumulate above the esophageal balloon.
8. The Minnesota tube is a modified Sengstaken-Blakemore tube with an additional lumen (a four-lumen gastric tube) for aspirating esophagopharyngeal secretions.

C. Interventions

1. Check patency and integrity of all balloons before insertion.
2. Label each lumen.
3. Place the client in the upright or Fowler's position for insertion.
4. Immediately after insertion, prepare for radiography to verify placement.
5. Maintain head elevation once the tube is in place.
6. Double-clamp the balloon ports to prevent air leaks.
7. Keep scissors at the bedside at all times; monitor for respiratory distress, and if it occurs, cut the tubes to deflate balloons.
8. To prevent ulceration or necrosis of the esophagus, release esophageal pressure at intervals as prescribed and per agency policy.
9. Monitor for increased bloody drainage, which may indicate persistent bleeding.
10. Monitor for signs of esophageal rupture, which includes a drop in blood pressure, increased heart rate, and back and upper abdominal pain. (Esophageal rupture is an emergency, and signs of esophageal rupture must be reported to the physician immediately.)

V. LAVAGE TUBES

A. Description: Used to remove toxic substances from the stomach

B. Types of tubes
1. Lavacuator (see Fig. 21-1)
   a. The Lavacuator is an orogastric tube with a large suction lumen and a smaller lavage–vent lumen that provides continuous suction.
   b. Irrigation solution enters the lavage lumen while stomach contents are removed through the suction lumen.
2. Ewald tube: A single-lumen large tube used for rapid one-time irrigation and evacuation

VI. URINARY AND RENAL TUBES

A. Types of urinary catheters
1. Single lumen: Usually used for straight catheterization to empty the client's bladder or to check the residual amount of urine after the client voids.
2. Double lumen: Used when an indwelling catheter is needed for continuous bladder drainage; one lumen is for drainage and the other is for balloon inflation.
3. Triple lumen: Used when bladder irrigation and drainage is necessary; one lumen is for instilling the bladder irrigant solution, one lumen is for continuous bladder drainage, and one lumen is for balloon inflation.

4. Strict aseptic technique is necessary for insertion and care of the catheter.

B. Routine urinary catheter care
1. Use gloves and wash the perineal area with warm soapy water.
2. With the nondominant hand, pull back the labia or foreskin to expose the meatus (in the adult male, return the foreskin to its normal position).
3. Cleanse along the catheter with soap and water.
4. Anchor the catheter to the thigh.
5. Maintain the catheter bag below the level of the bladder.

C. Ureteral and nephrostomy tubes
1. Never clamp the tube.
2. Maintain patency.
3. Irrigate only if prescribed by a physician, using strict aseptic technique; a maximum of 5 mL of sterile normal saline is instilled slowly and gently.
4. If patency cannot be established with the prescribed irrigation, immediately notify the physician.

⚠ If the client has a ureteral or nephrostomy tube, monitor output closely; urine output of less than 30 mL/hr or lack of output for more than 15 minutes should be reported to the physician immediately.

VII. RESPIRATORY SYSTEM TUBES

A. **Endotracheal tubes** (Fig. 21-2)
1. Description
   a. The **endotracheal tube** is used to maintain a patent airway.
   b. **Endotracheal tubes** are indicated when the client needs mechanical ventilation.
   c. If the client requires an artificial airway for longer than 10 to 14 days, a **tracheostomy** may be created to avoid mucosal and vocal cord damage that can be caused by the **endotracheal tube**.
   d. The cuff (located at the distal end of the tube), when inflated, produces a seal between the trachea and the cuff to prevent aspiration and ensure delivery of a set tidal volume when mechanical ventilation is used; an inflated cuff also prevents air from passing to the vocal cords, nose, or mouth.
   e. The pilot balloon permits air to be inserted into the cuff, prevents air from escaping, and is used as a guideline for determining the presence or absence of air in the cuff.
   f. The universal adapter enables attachment of the tube to mechanical ventilation tubing or other types of oxygen delivery systems.
   g. Types of tubes: Orotracheal and nasotracheal
2. Orotracheal tubes
   a. Inserted through the mouth and allows use of a larger diameter tube and reduces the work of breathing.

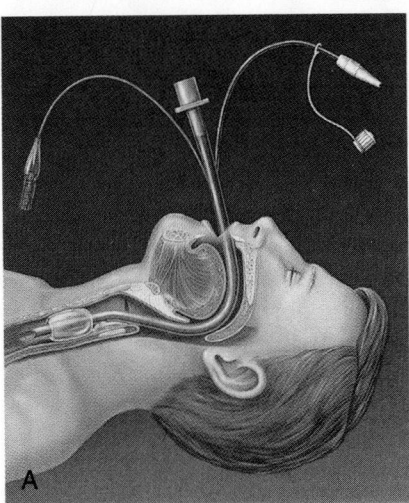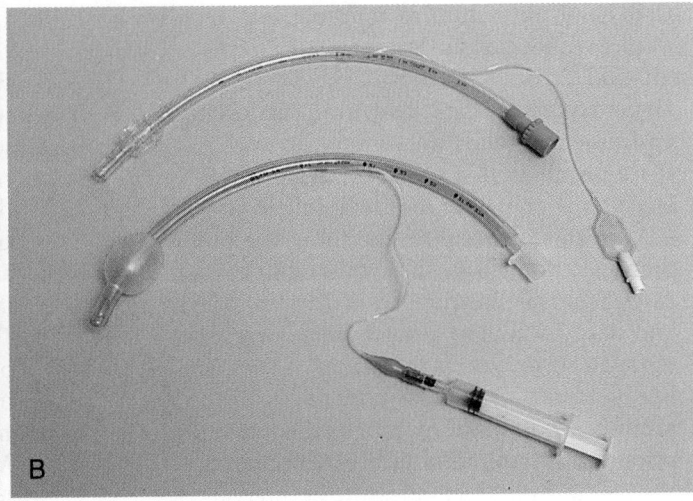

▲ **FIGURE 21-2 A,** Endotracheal (ET) tube with inflated cuff. **B,** ET tubes with uninflated and inflated cuffs and syringe for inflation (From Perry, A., & Potter, P. [2010]. *Clinical nursing skills & techniques* [7th ed.]. St. Louis: Mosby.)

   b. Indicated when the client has a nasal obstruction or a predisposition to epistaxis.
   c. Uncomfortable and can be manipulated by the tongue, causing airway obstruction; an oral airway may be needed to keep the client from biting on the tube.
  3. Nasotracheal tubes
   a. Inserted through a nostril; this smaller tube increases resistance and the client's work of breathing.
   b. Its use is avoided in clients with bleeding disorders.
   c. It is more comfortable for the client, and the client is unable to manipulate the tube with the tongue.
  4. Interventions
   a. Placement is confirmed by chest x-ray film (correct placement is 1 to 2 cm above the carina).
   b. Assess placement by auscultating both sides of the chest while manually ventilating with a resuscitation (Ambu) bag (if breath sounds and chest wall movement are absent in the left side, the tube may be in the right main stem bronchus).
   c. Perform auscultation over the stomach to rule out esophageal intubation.
   d. If the tube is in the stomach, louder breath sounds will be heard over the stomach than over the chest, and abdominal distention will be present.
   e. Secure the tube with adhesive tape immediately after intubation.
   f. Monitor the position of the tube at the lip or nose.
   g. Monitor skin and mucous membranes.
   h. Suction the tube only when needed.
   i. The oral tube needs to be moved to the opposite side of the mouth daily to prevent pressure and necrosis of the lip and mouth area, prevent nerve damage, and facilitate inspection and cleaning of the mouth; moving the tube to the opposite side of the mouth should be done by two health care providers.
   j. Prevent dislodgment and pulling or tugging on the tube; suction, coughing, and speaking attempts by the client place extra stress on the tube and can cause dislodgment.
   k. Assess the pilot balloon to ensure that the cuff is inflated; maintain cuff inflation, which creates a seal and allows complete mechanical control of respiration.
   l. Monitor cuff pressures at least every 8 hours per agency procedure to ensure that they do not exceed 20 mm Hg (an aneroid pressure manometer is used to measure cuff pressures); minimal leak and occlusive techniques are used for cuff inflation to check cuff pressures.

⚠ A resuscitation (Ambu) bag needs to be kept at the bedside of a client with an endotracheal tube or a tracheostomy tube at all times.

  5. Minimal leak technique
   a. This is used for cuff inflation and checking cuff pressures for cuffs without pressure relief valves.
   b. Inflate the cuff until a seal is established; no harsh sound should be heard through a stethoscope placed over the trachea when the client breathes in, but a slight air leak on peak inspiration is present and can be heard.
   c. The client cannot make verbal sounds, and no air is felt coming out of the client's mouth.
  6. Occlusive technique
   a. This is used for cuff inflation and checking cuff pressures for cuffs with pressure relief valves.
   b. Provides an adequate seal in the trachea at the lowest possible cuff pressure.

c. Uses same procedure as minimal leak technique, without an air leak.

7. Extubation
   a. Hyperoxygenate the client and suction the **endotracheal tube** and the oral cavity.
   b. Place the client in a semi-Fowler's position.
   c. Deflate the cuff; have the client inhale and, at peak inspiration, remove the tube, suctioning the airway through the tube while pulling it out.
   d. After removal, instruct the client to cough and deep breathe to assist in removing accumulated secretions in the throat.
   e. Apply oxygen therapy, as prescribed.
   f. Monitor for respiratory difficulty; contact the physician if respiratory difficulty occurs.

g. Inform the client that hoarseness or a sore throat is normal and that the client should limit talking if it occurs.

B. Tracheostomy (Fig. 21-3)
1. Description
   a. A **tracheostomy** is an opening made surgically directly into the trachea to establish an airway; **tracheostomy** tube is inserted into the opening and the tube attaches to the mechanical ventilator or another type of oxygen delivery device.
   b. The **tracheostomy** can be temporary or permanent. (See Box 21-2 for types of tracheostomies.)
2. Interventions
   a. Assess respirations and for bilateral breath sounds.
   b. Monitor arterial blood gases and pulse oximetry.
   c. Encourage coughing and deep breathing.
   d. Maintain a semi-Fowler's to high Fowler's position.
   e. Monitor for bleeding, difficulty with breathing, absence of breath sounds, and crepitus (subcutaneous emphysema), which are indications of hemorrhage or pneumothorax.
   f. Provide respiratory treatments as prescribed.
   g. Suction fluids as needed; hyperoxygenate the client before suctioning.
   h. If the client is allowed to eat, sit the client up for meals and ensure that the cuff is inflated (if the tube is not capped) for meals and for 1 hour after meals to prevent aspiration.
   i. Monitor cuff pressures as prescribed.
   j. Assess the stoma and secretions for blood or purulent drainage.

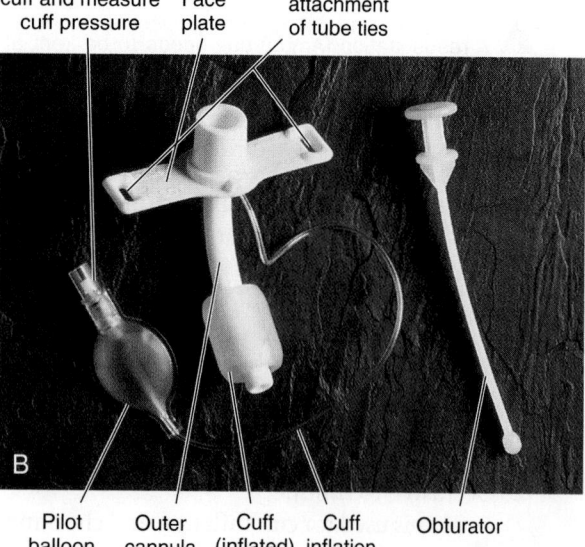

Valve used for cuff inflation, deflation, and pressure measurement | Face plate | Slots for tube ties

A

Pilot balloon | Outer cannula | Cuff (inflated) | Disposable inner cannula | Obturator

Valve used to inflate and deflate cuff and measure cuff pressure | Face plate | Slots for attachment of tube ties

B

Pilot balloon | Outer cannula | Cuff (inflated) | Cuff inflation tube | Obturator

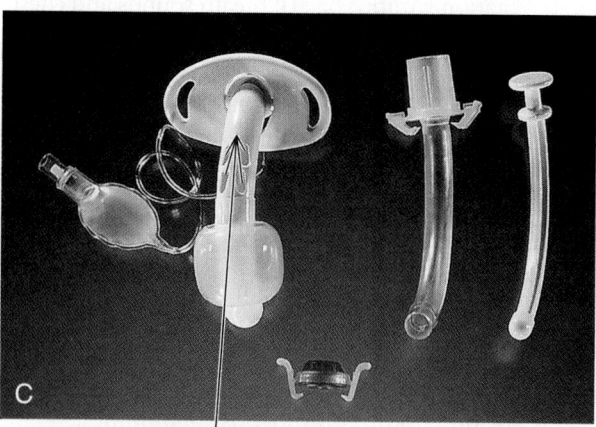

C

Fenestrations

▲ **FIGURE 21-3** Tracheostomy tubes. **A,** Double-lumen cuffed tracheostomy tube with disposable inner cannula. **B,** Single-lumen cannula cuffed tracheostomy tube. **C,** Double-lumen cuffed fenestrated tracheostomy tube with plug (red cap). (From Ignatavicius, D., & Workman, M. [2010]. *Medical-surgical nursing: Patient-centered collaborative care* [6th ed.]. St. Louis: Saunders.)

k. Follow the physician's prescriptions and agency policy for cleaning the **tracheostomy** site and inner cannula (many inner cannulas are disposable); usually, half-strength hydrogen peroxide is used.

l. Administer humidified oxygen as prescribed, because the normal humidification process is bypassed in a client with a **tracheostomy**.

m. Obtain assistance in changing **tracheostomy** ties; after placing the new ties, cut and remove the old ties holding the **tracheostomy** in place (some securing devices are soft and made with Velcro to hold the tube in place).

n. Keep a resuscitation (Ambu) bag, obturator, clamps, and a spare tracheostomy tube of the same size at the bedside.

3. Complications of a **tracheostomy** (Box 21-3; Table 21-1)

Box 21-2 Some Types of Tracheostomy Tubes

Double-Lumen Tube
The double-lumen tube has the following parts:

Outer cannula—fits into the stoma and keeps the airway open. The face plate indicates the size and type of tube and has small holes on both sides for securing the tube with tracheostomy ties or another device.

Inner cannula—fits snugly into the outer cannula and locks into place. It provides the universal adaptor for use with the ventilator and other respiratory therapy equipment. Some may be removed, cleaned, and reused; others are disposable.

Obturator—a stylet with a smooth end used to facilitate the direction of the tube when inserting or changing a tracheostomy tube. The obturator is removed immediately after tube placement and is always kept with the client and at the bedside in case of accidental decannulation.

Cuff—when inflated, seals the airway. The cuffed tube is used for mechanical ventilation, preventing aspiration of oral or gastric secretions, or for the client receiving a tube feeding to prevent aspiration. A pilot balloon attached to the outside of the tube indicates the presence or absence of air in the cuff.

Single-Lumen Tube
The single-lumen tube is similar to the double-lumen tube except that there is no inner cannula. More intensive nursing care is required with this tube because there is no inner cannula to ensure a patent lumen.

Fenestrated Tube
The fenestrated tube has a precut opening (fenestration) in the upper posterior wall of the outer cannula. The tube is used to wean the client from a tracheostomy by ensuring that the client can tolerate breathing through his or her natural airway before the entire tube is removed. This tube allows the client to speak.

Cuffed Fenestrated Tube
The cuffed fenestrated tube facilitates mechanical ventilation and speech and often is used for clients with spinal cord paralysis or neuromuscular disease who do not require ventilation at all times. When not on the ventilator, the client can have the cuff deflated and the tube capped (see Fig. 21-3 for fenestrated cuffed tube with red cap) for speech. A cuffed fenestrated tube is never used in weaning from a tracheostomy because the cuff, even fully deflated, may partially obstruct the airway.

Box 21-3 Complications of a Tracheostomy

Tube Obstruction
Assessment
Difficulty in breathing
Noisy respirations
Difficulty in inserting the suction catheter
Thick, dry secretions
Unexplained peak pressures if client is on a mechanical ventilator

Prevention and Interventions
Assist the client to cough and deep breathe.
Provide humidification and suctioning.
Clean the inner cannula regularly.
The physician repositions or replaces the tube if obstruction occurs as a result of cuff prolapse over the end of the tube.

Tube Dislodgment
Prevention and Interventions
Secure the tube in place. Minimize manipulation and traction on the tube. Ensure that the client does not pull on the tube. Ensure that a tracheostomy tube of the same type and size is at the client's bedside.

Be familiar with institutional policy regarding replacement of a tracheostomy tube as a nursing procedure.

During the first 72 hours following surgical placement of the tracheostomy, the nurse manually ventilates the client by using a manual resuscitation (Ambu) bag while another nurse calls the Rapid Response team for help.

After 72 hours following surgical placement of the tracheostomy:

■ Extend the client's neck and open the tissues of the stoma to secure the airway.

■ Grasp the retention sutures (if they are present) to spread the opening.

■ Use a tracheal dilator (curved clamp) to hold the stoma open.

■ Prepare to insert a tracheostomy tube; place the obturator into the tracheostomy tube, replace the tube, and remove the obturator.

■ Maintain ventilation by resuscitation (Ambu) bag.

■ Assess airflow and bilateral breath sounds.

■ If unable to secure an airway, call the Rapid Response team and the anesthesiologist.

TABLE 21-1 Complications of a Tracheostomy

Complications and Description	Manifestations	Management	Prevention
Tracheomalacia: Constant pressure exerted by the cuff causes tracheal dilation and erosion of cartilage.	An increased amount of air is required in the cuff to maintain the seal. A larger tracheostomy tube is required to prevent an air leak at the stoma. Food particles are seen in tracheal secretions. The client does not receive the set tidal volume on the ventilator.	No special management is needed unless bleeding occurs.	Use an uncuffed tube as soon as possible. Monitor cuff pressure and air volume closely to detect changes.
Tracheal stenosis: Narrowed tracheal lumen is the result of scar formation from irritation of tracheal mucosa by the cuff.	Stenosis is usually seen after the cuff is deflated or the tracheostomy tube is removed. The client has increased coughing, inability to expectorate secretions, or difficulty in breathing and talking.	Tracheal dilation or surgical intervention is used.	Prevent pulling of and traction on the tracheostomy tube. Properly secure the tube in the midline position. Maintain cuff pressure. Minimize oronasal intubation time.
Tracheoesophageal fistula (TEF): Excessive cuff pressure causes erosion of the posterior wall of the trachea. A hole is created between the trachea and the anterior esophagus. The client at highest risk also has a nasogastric tube present.	Similar to tracheomalacia: 1. Food particles are seen in tracheal secretions. 2. Increased air in cuff is needed to achieve a seal. 3. The client has increased coughing and choking while eating. 4. The client does not receive the set tidal volume on the ventilator.	Manually administer oxygen by mask to prevent hypoxemia. Use a small soft feeding tube instead of a nasogastric tube for tube feedings. A gastrostomy or jejunostomy may be performed. Monitor the client with a nasogastric tube closely; assess for TEF and aspiration.	Maintain cuff pressure. Monitor the amount of air needed for inflation to detect changes. Progress to a deflated or cuffless tube as soon as possible.
Trachea-innominate artery fistula: A malpositioned tube causes its distal tip to push against the lateral wall of the trachea. Continued pressure causes necrosis and erosion of the innominate artery. *This is a medical emergency.*	The tracheostomy tube pulsates in synchrony with the heartbeat. There is heavy bleeding from the stoma. *This is a life-threatening complication.*	Remove the tracheostomy tube immediately. Apply direct pressure to the innominate artery at the stoma site. Prepare the client for immediate repair surgery.	Use the correct tube size, length, and maintain the take in midline position. Prevent pulling or tugging of the tracheostomy tube. Immediately notify the physician of a pulsating tube.

From Ignatavicius, D., & Workman, M. (2010). *Medical-surgical nursing: Patient-centered collaborative care* (6th ed.). St. Louis: Saunders.

 Never insert a decannulation plug into a tracheostomy tube until the cuff is deflated and the inner cannula is removed; prior insertion prevents airflow to the client.

VIII. CHEST TUBE DRAINAGE SYSTEM

A. Description
1. The **chest tube** drainage system returns negative pressure to the intrapleural space.
2. The system is used to remove abnormal accumulations of air and fluids from the pleural space (Fig. 21-4).

B. Drainage collection chamber (Fig. 21-5)
1. The drainage collection chamber is located where the **chest tube** from the client connects to the system.
2. Drainage from the tube drains into and collects in a series of calibrated columns in this chamber.
C. Water seal chamber (see Fig. 21-5)
1. The tip of the tube is underwater, allowing fluid and air to drain from the pleural space and preventing air from entering the pleural space.
2. Water oscillates (moves up as the client inhales and moves down as the client exhales).

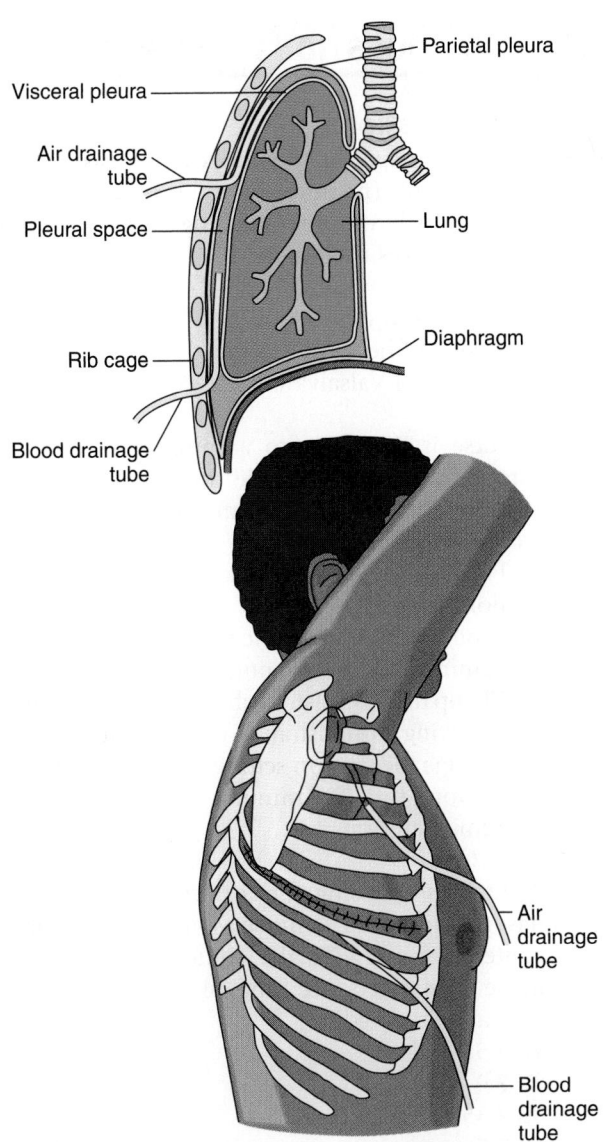

▲ **FIGURE 21-4** Chest tube placement. (From Ignatavicius, D., & Workman, M. [2010]. *Medical-surgical nursing: Patient-centered collaborative care.* [6th ed.]. St. Louis: Saunders.)

3. Excessive bubbling indicates an air leak in the **chest tube** system.

D. Suction control chamber (see Fig. 21-5)
　1. The suction control chamber provides the suction, which can be controlled to provide negative pressure to the chest.
　2. This chamber is filled with various levels of water to achieve the desired level of suction; without this control, lung tissue could be sucked into the **chest tube**.
　3. Gentle bubbling in this chamber indicates that there is suction and does not indicate that air is escaping from the pleural space.

E. Dry suction system
　1. This is another type of a chest drainage system and because this is a dry suction system, absence of bubbling is noted in the suction control chamber.

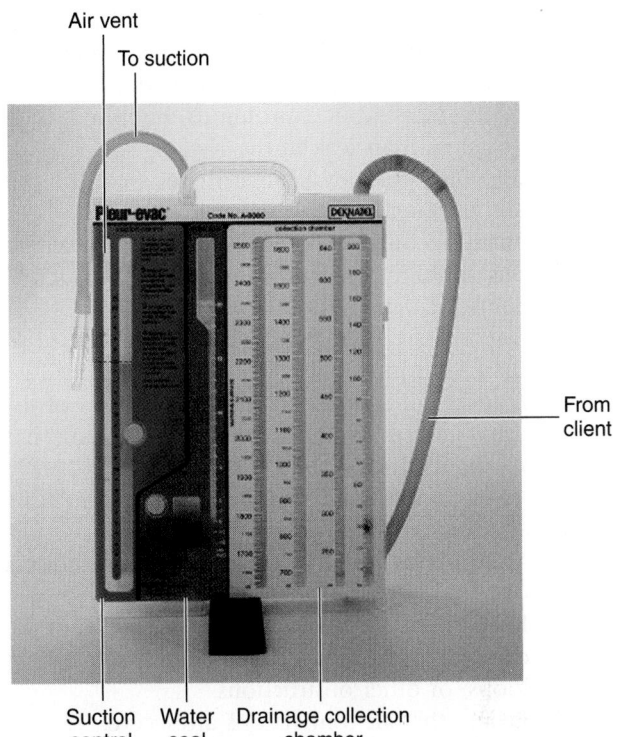

Suction control　Water seal　Drainage collection chamber

▲ **FIGURE 21-5** The Pleur-Evac drainage system, a commercial three-bottle chest drainage device. (From Ignatavicius, D., & Workman, M. [2010]. *Medical-surgical nursing: Patient centered collaborative care* [6th ed.]. St. Louis: Saunders.)

　2. A knob on the collection device is used to set the prescribed amount of suction; then the wall suction source dial is turned until a small orange floater valve appears in the window on the device (when the orange floater valve is in the window, the correct amount of suction is applied).

F. Portable chest drainage system: Small and portable chest drainage systems are also available and are dry systems that use a control flutter valve to prevent the backflow of air into the client's lung; principles of gravity and pressure, and the nursing care involved are the same for all types of systems and these systems allow greater ambulation and allow the client to go home with the **chest tubes** in place.

G. Interventions
　1. Collection chamber
　　a. Monitor drainage; notify the physician if drainage is more than 70 to 100 mL/hr or if drainage becomes bright red or increases suddenly.
　　b. Mark the **chest tube** drainage in the collection chamber at 1- to 4-hour intervals, using a piece of tape.
　2. Water seal chamber
　　a. Monitor for fluctuation of the fluid level in the water seal chamber.
　　b. Fluctuation in the water seal chamber stops if the tube is obstructed, if a dependent loop exists, if the suction is not working properly, or if the lung has reexpanded.

c. If the client has a known pneumothorax, intermittent bubbling in the water seal chamber is expected as air is drained from the chest, but continuous bubbling indicates an air leak in the system.

d. Notify the physician if there is continuous bubbling in the water seal chamber.

3. Suction control chamber: Gentle (not vigorous) bubbling should be noted in the suction control chamber.

4. An occlusive sterile dressing is maintained at the insertion site.

5. A chest radiograph assesses the position of the tube and determines whether the lung has reexpanded.

6. Assess respiratory status and auscultate lung sounds.

7. Monitor for signs of extended pneumothorax or hemothorax.

8. Keep the drainage system below the level of the chest and the tubes free of kinks, dependent loops, or other obstructions.

9. Ensure that all connections are secure.

10. Encourage coughing and deep breathing.

11. Change the client's position frequently to promote drainage and ventilation.

12. Do not strip or milk a **chest tube** unless specifically directed to do so by a physician and if agency policy allows it.

13. Keep a clamp (may be needed if the system needs to be changed) and a sterile occlusive dressing at the bedside at all times.

14. Never clamp a **chest tube** without a written prescription from the physician; also, determine agency policy for clamping a **chest tube**.

15. If the drainage system cracks or breaks, insert the **chest tube** into a bottle of sterile water, remove the cracked or broken system, and replace it with a new system.

16. When the **chest tube** is removed, the client is asked to take a deep breath and hold it, and the tube is removed; a dry sterile dressing, petroleum gauze dressing, or Telfa dressing (depending on the physician's preference) is taped in place after removal of the **chest tube**.

17. Depending on the physician's preference, when the **chest tube** is removed, the client may be asked to take a deep breath, exhale, and bear down (Valsalva maneuver).

⚠ If the chest tube is pulled out of the chest accidentally, pinch the skin opening together, apply an occlusive sterile dressing, cover the dressing with overlapping pieces of 2-inch tape, and call the physician immediately.

 MORE QUESTIONS ON THE CD!

Practice Questions

189. A nurse is preparing to remove a nasogastric tube from a client. The nurse should instruct the client to do which of the following just before the nurse removes the tube?
1. Exhale.
2. Inhale and exhale quickly.
3. Take and hold a deep breath.
4. Perform a Valsalva maneuver.

190. A nurse is preparing to administer medication through a nasogastric tube that is connected to suction. To administer the medication, the nurse would:
1. Position the client supine to assist in medication absorption.
2. Aspirate the nasogastric tube after medication administration to maintain patency.
3. Clamp the nasogastric tube for 30 to 60 minutes following administration of the medication.
4. Change the suction setting to low intermittent suction for 30 minutes after medication administration.

191. A nurse is assessing for correct placement of a nasogastric tube. The nurse aspirates the stomach contents and checks the contents for pH. The nurse verifies correct tube placement if which pH value is noted?
1. 3.5
2. 7.0
3. 7.35
4. 7.5

192. A nurse caring for a client with a chest tube turns the client to the side and the chest tube accidentally disconnects. The initial nursing action is to:
1. Call the physician.
2. Place the tube in a bottle of sterile water.
3. Immediately replace the chest tube system.
4. Place a sterile dressing over the disconnection site.

193. A registered nurse is preparing to insert a nasogastric tube in an adult client. To determine the accurate measurement of the length of the tube to be inserted, the nurse should:
1. Mark the tube at 10 inches.
2. Mark the tube at 32 inches.
3. Place the tube at the tip of the nose and measure by extending the tube to the earlobe and then down to the xiphoid process.

4. Place the tube at the tip of the nose and measure by extending the tube to the earlobe and then down to the top of the sternum.

194. A nurse is inserting a nasogastric tube in an adult client. During the procedure, the client begins to cough and has difficulty breathing. Which of the following is the appropriate nursing action?
1. Quickly insert the tube.
2. Notify the physician immediately.
3. Remove the tube and reinsert when the respiratory distress subsides.
4. Pull back on the tube and wait until the respiratory distress subsides.

195. A nurse is assisting a physician with the removal of a chest tube. The nurse should instruct the client to:
1. Exhale slowly.
2. Stay very still.
3. Inhale and exhale quickly.
4. Perform the Valsalva maneuver.

196. While changing the tapes on a tracheostomy tube, the client coughs and the tube is dislodged. The initial nursing action is to:
1. Call the physician to reinsert the tube.
2. Grasp the retention sutures to spread the opening.
3. Call the respiratory therapy department to reinsert the tracheotomy.
4. Cover the tracheostomy site with a sterile dressing to prevent infection.

197. A nurse is caring for a client immediately after removal of the endotracheal tube. The nurse reports which of the following signs immediately if experienced by the client?
1. Stridor
2. Occasional pink-tinged sputum
3. Respiratory rate of 24 breaths/min
4. A few basilar lung crackles on the right

198. The nurse checks for residual before administering a bolus tube feeding to a client with a nasogastric tube and obtains a residual amount of 150 mL. What is the appropriate action for the nurse to take?
1. Hold the feeding.
2. Reinstill the amount and continue with administering the feeding.
3. Elevate the client's head at least 45 degrees and administer the feeding.
4. Discard the residual amount and proceed with administering the feeding.

199. A nurse caring for a client with a pneumothorax and who has had a chest tube inserted notes continuous gentle bubbling in the suction control chamber. What action is appropriate?
1. Do nothing, because this is an expected finding.
2. Immediately clamp the chest tube and notify the physician.
3. Check for an air leak because the bubbling should be intermittent.
4. Increase the suction pressure so that the bubbling becomes vigorous.

Alternate Item Format: Multiple Response

200. A nurse is assessing the functioning of a chest tube drainage system in a client who has just returned from the recovery room following a thoracotomy with wedge resection. Select the expected assessment findings. **Select all that apply**.
- ❑ 1. Excessive bubbling in the water seal chamber
- ❑ 2. Vigorous bubbling in the suction control chamber
- ❑ 3. 50 mL of drainage in the drainage collection chamber
- ❑ 4. Drainage system maintained below the client's chest
- ❑ 5. Occlusive dressing in place over the chest tube insertion site
- ❑ 6. Fluctuation of water in the tube in the water seal chamber during inhalation and exhalation

ANSWERS

189. 3
Rationale: When the nurse removes a nasogastric tube, the client is instructed to take and hold a deep breath. This will close the epiglottis. This allows for easy withdrawal through the esophagus into the nose. The nurse removes the tube with one smooth, continuous pull. Therefore, options 1, 2, and 4 are incorrect.
Test-Taking Strategy: Use the process of elimination and focus on the subject, removing a nasogastric tube. Visualize the procedure as a guide, considering what each action identified in the options would produce. Review the procedure for removing a nasogastric tube if you had difficulty with this question.
Level of Cognitive Ability: Applying
Client Needs: Physiological Integrity
Integrated Process: Nursing Process—Implementation
Content Area: Fundamental Skills—Safety/Infection Control
Reference: Potter, P., & Perry, A. (2009). *Fundamentals of nursing* (7th ed., p. 1209). St. Louis: Mosby.

190. 3

Rationale: If a client has a nasogastric tube connected to suction, the nurse should wait 30 to 60 minutes before reconnecting the tube to the suction apparatus to allow adequate time for medication absorption. Aspirating the nasogastric tube will remove the medication just administered. Low intermittent suction also will remove the medication just administered. The client should not be placed in the supine position because of the risk for aspiration.

Test-Taking Strategy: Use the process of elimination. Eliminate options 2 and 4 first because these actions are comparable or alike and will produce the same effect. Recalling that the client should not be placed in a supine position will assist in eliminating option 1. If you had difficulty with this question, review the procedure for administering medications through a nasogastric tube.

Level of Cognitive Ability: Applying
Client Needs: Physiological Integrity
Integrated Process: Nursing Process—Implementation
Content Area: Fundamental Skills—Safety/Infection Control
Reference: Potter, P., & Perry, A. (2009). *Fundamentals of nursing* (7th ed., pp. 718, 1208). St. Louis: Mosby.

191. 1

Rationale: If the nasogastric tube is in the stomach, the pH of the contents will be acidic. Gastric aspirates have acidic pH values and should be 3.5 or lower. Option 2 indicates a slightly acidic pH. Option 3 indicates a neutral pH. Option 4 indicates an alkaline pH.

Test-Taking Strategy: Use the process of elimination and note the strategic word *verifies*. Recalling that gastric contents are acidic will direct you to option 1. If you had difficulty with this question, review the procedure for assessing nasogastric tube placement.

Level of Cognitive Ability: Understanding
Client Needs: Physiological Integrity
Integrated Process: Nursing Process—Assessment
Content Area: Fundamental Skills—Safety/Infection Control
Reference: Potter, P., & Perry, A. (2009). *Fundamentals of nursing* (7th ed., p. 1206). St. Louis: Mosby.

192. 2

Rationale: If the chest drainage system is disconnected, the end of the tube is placed in a bottle of sterile water held below the level of the chest. The system is replaced if it breaks or cracks or if the collection chamber is full. Placing a sterile dressing over the disconnection site will not prevent complications resulting from the disconnection. The physician may need to be notified, but this is not the initial action.

Test-Taking Strategy: Use the process of elimination and note the strategic word *initial* in the question. This indicates that a nursing action is required that will prevent a serious complication as a result of the disconnection. Eliminate options 1 and 3 because these actions delay required and immediate intervention. From the remaining options, recalling the complications that can occur from a disconnection will direct you to option 2. Review interventions related to the complications of a chest tube if you had difficulty with this question.

Level of Cognitive Ability: Applying

Client Needs: Physiological Integrity
Integrated Process: Nursing Process—Implementation
Content Area: Critical Care
References: Ignatavicius, D., & Workman, M. (2010). *Medical-surgical nursing: Patient-centered collaborative care* (6th ed., p. 648). St. Louis: Saunders.
Potter, P., & Perry, A. (2009). *Fundamentals of nursing* (7th ed., p. 955). St. Louis: Mosby.

193. 3

Rationale: Measuring the length of a nasogastric tube needed is done by placing the tube at the tip of the client's nose and extending the tube to the earlobe and then down to the xiphoid process. The average length for an adult is about 22 to 26 inches. Therefore options 1, 2, and 4 are incorrect.

Test-Taking Strategy: Use the process of elimination and visualize this procedure. Eliminate options 1 and 2 first because 10 inches is short and 32 inches is too long. Remember the abbreviation NEX, which stands for nose, earlobe, and xiphoid process, to assist in answering questions similar to this one. Review the procedure for measuring the length of a nasogastric tube for insertion if you had difficulty with this question.

Level of Cognitive Ability: Applying
Client Needs: Physiological Integrity
Integrated Process: Nursing Process—Assessment
Content Area: Fundamental Skills—Safety/Infection Control
Reference: Potter, P., & Perry, A. (2009). *Fundamentals of nursing* (7th ed., p. 1205). St. Louis: Mosby.

194. 4

Rationale: During the insertion of a nasogastric tube, if the client experiences difficulty breathing or any respiratory distress, withdraw the tube slightly, stop the tube advancement, and wait until the distress subsides. Options 2 and 3 are unnecessary. Quickly inserting the tube is not an appropriate action because, in this situation, it may be likely that the tube has entered the bronchus.

Test-Taking Strategy: Use the process of elimination. Eliminate option 1 first because of the word *quickly*. Visualizing the procedure and anticipating potential complications will assist in eliminating options 2 and 3 as unnecessary actions. Review the procedure and cautions related to inserting a nasogastric tube if you had difficulty with this question.

Level of Cognitive Ability: Applying
Client Needs: Physiological Integrity
Integrated Process: Nursing Process—Implementation
Content Area: Fundamental Skills—Safety/Infection Control
Reference: Potter, P., & Perry, A. (2009). *Fundamentals of nursing* (7th ed., p. 1206). St. Louis: Mosby.

195. 4

Rationale: When the chest tube is removed, the client is asked to perform the Valsalva maneuver (take a deep breath, exhale, and bear down). The tube is quickly withdrawn, and an airtight dressing is taped in place. An alternative instruction is to ask the client to take a deep breath and hold the breath while the tube is removed. Options 1, 2, and 3 are incorrect client instructions.

Test-Taking Strategy: Use the process of elimination and focus on the subject. Visualize the procedure, client

instructions, and the effect of each of the actions in the options to answer correctly. If you had difficulty with this question, review the procedure for removal of a chest tube.
Level of Cognitive Ability: Applying
Client Needs: Physiological Integrity
Integrated Process: Nursing Process—Implementation
Content Area: Fundamental Skills—Safety/Infection Control
Reference: Black, J., & Hawks, J. (2009). *Medical-surgical nursing: Clinical management for positive outcomes* (8th ed., p. 1624). St. Louis: Saunders.

196. 2
Rationale: If the tube is dislodged accidentally, the initial nursing action is to grasp the retention sutures and spread the opening. If agency policy permits, the nurse then attempts immediately to replace the tube. Covering the tracheostomy site will block the airway. Options 1 and 3 will delay treatment in this emergency situation.
Test-Taking Strategy: Use the process of elimination. Eliminate options 1 and 3 first because they are comparable or alike and will delay the immediate intervention needed. Eliminate option 4 because this action will block the airway. If you had difficulty with this question, review the intervention required if a tracheostomy tube dislodges.
Level of Cognitive Ability: Applying
Client Needs: Physiological Integrity
Integrated Process: Nursing Process—Implementation
Content Area: Critical Care
References: Black, J., & Hawks, J. (2009). *Medical-surgical nursing: Clinical management for positive outcomes* (8th ed., p. 1546). St. Louis: Saunders.
 Ignatavicius, D., & Workman, M. (2010). *Medical-surgical nursing: Patient-centered collaborative care* (6th ed., p. 580). St. Louis: Saunders.

197. 1
Rationale: Following removal of the endotracheal tube the nurse monitors the client for respiratory distress. The nurse reports stridor to the physician immediately. This is a high-pitched, coarse sound that is heard with the stethoscope over the trachea. Stridor indicates airway edema and places the client at risk for airway obstruction. Options 2, 3, and 4 are not signs that require immediate notification of the physician.
Test-Taking Strategy: Use the process of elimination. Recall that the prime danger after removal of an artificial airway is the client's inability to maintain a patent airway and breathe independently. In comparing each of the options with this risk in mind, eliminate options 2, 3, and 4. Because stridor indicates laryngeal edema and possible airway obstruction, it is the symptom that must be reported immediately. Review care to the client following removal of an endotracheal tube if you had difficulty with this question.
Level of Cognitive Ability: Analyzing
Client Needs: Physiological Integrity
Integrated Process: Nursing Process—Implementation
Content Area: Critical Care
Reference: Ignatavicius, D., & Workman, M. (2010). *Medical-surgical nursing: Patient-centered collaborative care* (6th ed., p. 697). St. Louis: Saunders.

198. 1
Rationale: Unless specifically indicated, residual amounts more than 100 mL require holding the feeding. Therefore options 2, 3, and 4 are incorrect. Additionally, the feeding is not discarded unless its contents are abnormal in color or characteristics.
Test-Taking Strategy: Use the process of elimination and note that the residual amount is 150 mL. Also note that options 2, 3, and 4 are comparable or alike and indicate administering the feeding. If you had difficulty with this question, review nursing interventions for clients with nasogastric tubes.
Level of Cognitive Ability: Applying
Client Needs: Physiological Integrity
Integrated Process: Nursing Process—Implementation
Content Area: Fundamental Skills—Safety/Infection Control
Reference: Ignatavicius, D., & Workman, M. (2010). *Medical-surgical nursing: Patient-centered collaborative care* (6th ed., p. 1399). St. Louis: Saunders.

199. 1
Rationale: Continuous gentle bubbling should be noted in the suction control chamber. Option 2 is incorrect. Chest tubes should only be clamped to check for an air leak or when changing drainage devices (according to agency policy). Option 3 is incorrect. Bubbling should be continuous in the suction control chamber and not intermittent. Option 4 is incorrect because bubbling should be gentle. Increasing the suction pressure only increases the rate of evaporation of water in the drainage system.
Test-Taking Strategy: Use the process of elimination and think about the physiology associated with each chamber of the chest tube drainage system. Remember that continuous gentle bubbling in the suction control chamber is expected. If you had difficulty with this question, review nursing interventions and expected findings for clients with chest tubes.
Level of Cognitive Ability: Applying
Client Needs: Physiological Integrity
Integrated Process: Nursing Process—Implementation
Content Area: Fundamental Skills—Safety/Infection Control
References: Black, J., & Hawks, J. (2009). *Medical-surgical nursing: Clinical management for positive outcomes* (8th ed., pp. 1622–1623). St. Louis: Saunders.
 Ignatavicius, D., & Workman, M. (2010). *Medical-surgical nursing: Patient-centered collaborative care* (6th ed., p. 1399). St. Louis: Saunders.

ALTERNATE ITEM FORMAT: MULTIPLE RESPONSE
200. 3, 4, 5, 6
Rationale: The bubbling of water in the water seal chamber indicates air drainage from the client and usually is seen when intrathoracic pressure is higher than atmospheric pressure, and may occur during exhalation, coughing, or sneezing. Excessive bubbling in the water seal chamber may indicate an air leak, an unexpected finding. Fluctuation of water in the tube in the water seal chamber during inhalation and exhalation is expected. An absence of fluctuation may indicate that the chest tube is obstructed or that the lung has reexpanded and that no more air is leaking into

the pleural space. Gentle (not vigorous) bubbling should be noted in the suction control chamber. A total of 50 mL of drainage is not excessive in a client returning to the nursing unit from the recovery room. Drainage that is more that 70 to 100 mL/hr is considered excessive and requires physician notification. The chest tube insertion site is covered with an occlusive (airtight) dressing to prevent air from entering the pleural space. Positioning the drainage system below the client's chest allows gravity to drain the pleural space.

Test-Taking Strategy: Thinking about the physiology associated with the functioning of a chest tube drainage system will assist in answering this question. The words *excessive bubbling* and *vigorous bubbling* will assist in eliminating these assessment findings. Review care for the client with a chest tube drainage system if you had difficulty with this question.

Level of Cognitive Ability: Analyzing

Client Needs: Physiological Integrity

Integrated Process: Nursing Process—Assessment

Content Area Fundamental Skills—Safety/Infection Control

Reference: Ignatavicius, D., & Workman, M. (2010). *Medical-surgical nursing: Patient-centered collaborative care* (6th ed., p. 648). St. Louis: Saunders.

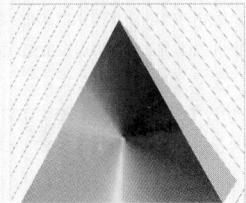

Maternity Nursing

PYRAMID TERMS

amniotic fluid Pale, straw-colored fluid in which the fetus floats. It serves as a cushion against injury from sudden blows or movements and helps maintain a constant body temperature for the fetus. The fetus modifies the amniotic fluid through the processes of swallowing, urinating, and movement through the respiratory tract.

ballottement Rebounding of the fetus against the examiner's finger on palpation. When the examiner taps the cervix, the fetus floats upward in the amniotic fluid. The examiner feels a rebound when the fetus falls back.

Chadwick's sign Violet coloration of the mucous membranes of the cervix, vagina, and vulva that occurs at about 4 weeks of pregnancy caused by increased vascularity. This is considered a probable sign of pregnancy.

delivery Actual event of birth; the expulsion or extraction of the neonate.

embryo Stage of fetal development that lasts from day 15 until approximately 8 weeks after conception or until the embryo measures 3 cm from crown to rump.

fertilization Uniting of the sperm and ovum, which occurs within 12 hours of ovulation and within 2 to 3 days of insemination, the average duration of viability for the ovum and sperm.

Goodell's sign Softening of the cervix that occurs at the beginning of the second month of gestation. This is considered a probable sign of pregnancy.

gravida A pregnant woman; called gravida I (primigravida) during the first pregnancy, gravida II during the second pregnancy, and so on.

Hegar's sign Compressibility and softening of the lower uterine segment that occurs at about week 6 of gestation. This is considered a probable sign of pregnancy.

implantation Embedding of the fertilized ovum in the uterine mucosa 6 to 10 days after conception.

infant A human born alive; also, a human from 28 days of age until the first birthday.

labor Coordinated sequence of rhythmic involuntary uterine contractions resulting in effacement and dilation of the cervix, followed by expulsion of the products of conception.

lecithin-to-sphingomyelin (L/S) ratio Ratio of two components of amniotic fluid, used for predicting fetal lung maturity; normal L/S ratio in amniotic fluid is 2:1 or greater when the fetal lungs are mature.

lochia Discharge from the uterus that consists of blood from the vessels of the placental site and debris from the decidua; lasts for 2 to 6 weeks after delivery.

Nägele's rule Determines the estimated date of birth based on the premise that the woman has a 28-day menstrual cycle. Add 7 days to the first day of the last menstrual period; subtract 3 months and add 1 year. Alternatively, add 7 days to the last menstrual period and count forward 9 months.

newborn A human from the time of birth to the twenty-eighth day of life; also called neonate.

parity Number of pregnancies that have reached viability regardless of whether the fetus was born alive or stillborn.

placenta Organ that provides for the exchange of nutrients and waste products between the fetus and the mother and produces hormones to maintain pregnancy. The placenta develops by the third month of gestation and is also called afterbirth.

quickening Maternal perception of fetal movement for the first time, occurring usually in the sixteenth to twentieth week of pregnancy.

surfactant Phospholipid that is necessary to keep the fetal lung alveoli from collapsing; amount is usually sufficient after 32 weeks' gestation.

uterus Organ located behind the symphysis pubis, between the bladder and the rectum. It has four parts— fundus (upper part), corpus (body), isthmus (lower segment), and cervix.

vagina Tubular structure located behind the bladder and in front of the rectum; it extends from the cervix to the vaginal opening in the perineum. It functions as the outflow tract for menstrual fluid and for vaginal and cervical secretions, the birth canal, and the organ for coitus.

viability Capability of the fetus to survive outside the uterus; about 22 to 24 weeks of gestation or fetal weight more than 500 g.

▲ PYRAMID TO SUCCESS

The Pyramid to Success focuses on the physiological and psychosocial aspects related to the experience of pregnancy, delivery, and the postpartum period. Pyramid Points begin with the assessment and knowledge of expected findings of the pregnant client and fetus during the antepartum period. Instructing the pregnant client in measures that promote a healthy environment for the mother and the fetus is included. The focus is on the importance of antepartum follow-up, nutrition, and interventions for common discomforts that occur during pregnancy. Knowledge of the purpose of the commonly prescribed diagnostic tests and procedures in the antepartum period is also part of the Pyramid to Success. The focus is on disorders that can occur during pregnancy, particularly gestational hypertension and diabetes mellitus. The labor and delivery process and the immediate interventions for conditions in which the maternal or fetal status is compromised, such as prolapsed cord or altered fetal heart rate, is part of the Pyramid to Success. Review of the fetus of a mother with human immunodeficiency virus or acquired immunodeficiency syndrome or a substance-abusing mother is recommended. The Pyramid to Success also includes a focus on the normal expectations of the postpartum period and the complications that can occur during this time. The next Pyramid Point focuses on the normal physical assessment findings and early identification of disorders in the neonate. The last Pyramid Point in this unit focuses on maternity and newborn medications.

CLIENT NEEDS

Safe and Effective Care Environment

Consulting with other health care team members
Delegating client care activities
Establishing priorities of care
Handling hazardous and infectious materials safely
Maintaining confidentiality
Managing the health care environment
Obtaining informed consent for diagnostic tests and procedures

Providing continuity of client care
Upholding client's rights
Using surgical asepsis when providing care
Using standard and transmission-based precautions when providing care

Health Promotion and Maintenance

Assessing for growth and development
Discussing expected body image changes with the client
Discussing family planning and birthing and parenting issues
Identifying at-risk clients during pregnancy
Identifying health and wellness concepts and providing health care screening
Identifying high-risk behaviors
Identifying lifestyle choices
Performing techniques of physical assessment
Providing antepartum, intrapartum, postpartum, and newborn care
Teaching regarding antepartum, intrapartum, and postpartum care
Teaching regarding care to the newborn

Psychosocial Integrity

Considering cultural, religious, and spiritual influences regarding birth and motherhood
Discussing situational role changes in the family
Ensuring therapeutic interactions within the family
Identifying available support systems
Identifying coping mechanisms

Physiological Integrity

Providing nonpharmacological comfort interventions and pharmacological pain management during labor
Identifying the action and contraindications for prescribed pharmacological agents
Monitoring for side effects and adverse effects related to prescribed pharmacological and parenteral therapies
Calculating medication dosages and administering medications safely
Monitoring for expected outcomes and effects related to pharmacological and parenteral therapies
Instructing the client about prescribed diagnostic tests and procedures
Providing interventions for unexpected events during pregnancy
Monitoring the client during the labor and delivery process
Monitoring for normal expectations during pregnancy
Teaching the client about nutrition during pregnancy and in the postpartum period
Teaching the client about the physiological changes that occur during pregnancy

Female Reproductive System

I. REPRODUCTIVE STRUCTURES (Fig. 22-1)

A. Ovaries
   1. Form and expel ova
   2. Secrete estrogen and progesterone
B. Fallopian tubes
   1. Muscular tubes (oviducts) approximate to the ovaries and connected to the **uterus**
   2. Tubes that propel the ova from the ovaries to the **uterus**
C. Uterus
   1. Muscular, pear-shaped cavity in which the fetus develops
   2. Cavity from which menstruation occurs
D. Cervix
   1. The internal os of the cervix opens into the body of the uterine cavity.
   2. The cervical canal is located between the internal os and the external os.
   3. The external cervical os opens into the **vagina**.
E. Vagina
   1. Muscular tube that extends from the cervix to the vaginal opening in the perineum
   2. Known as the birth canal
   3. Passage between the cervical os and the external environment
      a. Passageway for menstrual blood flow
      b. Passageway for fetus
      c. Passageway for penis for intercourse

II. MENSTRUAL CYCLE (Box 22-1)

A. Ovarian hormones
   1. Ovarian hormones include follicle-stimulating hormone (FSH) and luteinizing hormone (LH).
   2. The hormones are released by the anterior pituitary gland.
   3. The hormones produce changes in the ovaries.
   4. Secretion of ovarian hormones leads to changes in the endometrium.
   5. The menstrual cycle, the regularly recurring physiological changes in the endometrium that culminate in its shedding, may vary in length, with the average length being about 28 days.
B. Ovarian and uterine phases (see Box 22-1)

III. FEMALE PELVIS AND MEASUREMENTS

A. True pelvis
   1. Lies below the pelvic brim
   2. Consists of the pelvic inlet, midpelvis, and pelvic outlet
B. False pelvis
   1. Is the shallow portion above the pelvic brim
   2. Supports the abdominal viscera
C. Types of pelvis
   1. Gynecoid
      a. Normal female pelvis
      b. Transversely rounded or blunt

⚠ The gynecoid pelvis is most favorable for successful labor and birth.

   2. Anthropoid
      a. Oval shape
      b. Adequate outlet, with a narrow pubic arch
   3. Android
      a. Heart-shaped or angulated
      b. Resembles a male pelvis
      c. Not favorable for **labor** and birth
      d. Narrow pelvic planes can cause slow descent and midpelvic arrest.
   4. Platypelloid
      a. Flat with an oval inlet
      b. Wide transverse diameter, but short anteroposterior diameter, making **labor** and birth difficult
D. Pelvic inlet diameters
   1. Anteroposterior diameters
      a. Diagonal conjugate: Distance from the lower margin of the symphysis pubis to the sacral promontory
      b. True conjugate or conjugate vera: Distance from the upper margin of the symphysis pubis to the sacral promontory
      c. Obstetric conjugate: The smallest front-to-back distance through which the fetal head must pass in moving through the pelvic inlet
   2. Transverse diameter: The largest of the pelvic inlet diameters; located at right angles to the true conjugate

253

3. Oblique (diagonal) diameter: Not clinically measurable
4. Posterior sagittal diameter: Distance from the point where the anteroposterior and transverse diameters cross each other to the middle of the sacral promontory

E. Pelvic midplane diameters
1. Transverse diameter (interspinous diameter)
2. Midplane normally is the largest plane and has the longest diameter.

F. Pelvic outlet diameters
1. Transverse (intertuberous diameter)
2. Outlet presents the smallest plane of the pelvic canal.

IV. FERTILIZATION AND IMPLANTATION

A. Fertilization
1. **Fertilization** occurs in the ampulla of the fallopian (uterine) tube.
2. **Fertilization** occurs when sperm and ovum unite.
3. When fertilized, the membrane of the ovum undergoes changes that prevent entry of other sperm.
4. Each reproductive cell carries 23 chromosomes.
5. Sperm carry an X or a Y chromosome—XY, male; XX, female.

B. Implantation
1. The zygote is propelled toward the **uterus**.
2. The zygote implants 6 to 8 days after ovulation.

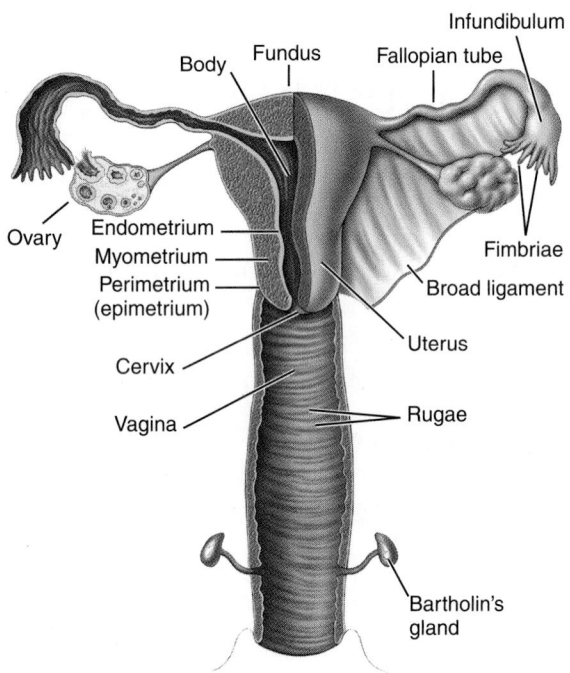

▲ **FIGURE 22-1** Female reproductive organs. (From Herlihy, B., & Maebius, N. [2007]. *The human body in health and illness* [3rd ed.] St. Louis: Saunders.)

Box 22-1 Menstrual Cycle

Ovarian Changes

Preovulatory Phase

Hypothalamus releases gonadotropin-releasing hormone through the portal system to the anterior pituitary system.

Secretion of follicle-stimulating hormone (FSH) by the anterior lobe of the pituitary gland stimulates growth of follicles.

Most follicles die, leaving one to mature into a large graafian follicle.

Estrogen produced by the follicle stimulates increased secretions of luteinizing hormone (LH) by the anterior lobe of the pituitary gland.

The follicle ruptures and releases an ovum into the peritoneal cavity.

Luteal Phase

Luteal phase begins with ovulation.

Body temperature decreases and then increases by 0.5° F to 1° F around the time of ovulation.

Corpus luteum is formed from follicle cells that remain in the ovary after ovulation.

Corpus luteum secretes estrogen and progesterone during the remaining 14 days of the cycle.

Corpus luteum degenerates if the ovum is not fertilized, and secretion of estrogen and progesterone declines.

Decline of estrogen and progesterone stimulates the anterior pituitary to secrete more FSH and LH, initiating a new reproductive cycle.

Uterine Changes

Menstrual Phase

Menstrual phase consists of 4 to 6 days of bleeding as the endometrium breaks down because of the decreased levels of estrogen and progesterone.

The level of FSH increases, enabling the beginning of a new cycle.

Proliferative Phase

Proliferative phase lasts about 9 days.

Estrogen stimulates proliferation and growth of the endometrium.

As estrogen increases, it suppresses secretion of FSH and increases secretion of LH.

Secretion of LH stimulates ovulation and the development of the corpus luteum.

Ovulation occurs between days 12 and 16.

Estrogen level is high, and progesterone level is low.

Secretory Phase

Secretory phase lasts about 12 days and follows ovulation.

This phase is initiated in response to the increase in LH level.

The graafian follicle is replaced by the corpus luteum.

The corpus luteum secretes progesterone and estrogen.

Progesterone prepares the endometrium for pregnancy if a fertilized ovum is implanted.

3. The blastocyst secretes chorionic gonadotropin to ensure that the corpus luteum remains viable and secretes estrogen and progesterone for the first 2 to 3 months of gestation.

V. FETAL DEVELOPMENT (Box 22-2)

A. Pre-embryonic period: First 2 weeks after conception

B. Embryonic period: Beginning at day 15 through approximately the eighth week after conception

C. Fetal period: Beginning at the ninth week after conception and ending with birth

VI. FETAL ENVIRONMENT

A. Amnion
1. Encloses the amniotic cavity

Box 22-2 Fetal Development

Pre-embryonic Period
First 2 weeks after conception

Embryonic Period
Beginning day 15 through approximately week 8 after conception

Fetal Period
Week 9 after conception to birth

Week 1
Blastocyst is free-floating.

Weeks 2 to 3
Embryo is 1.5 to 2 mm in length.
Lung buds appear
Blood circulation begins.
Heart is tubular and begins to beat.
Neural plate becomes brain and spinal cord.

Week 5
Embryo is 0.4 to 0.5 cm in length.
Embryo is 0.4 g.
Double heart chambers are visible.
Heart is beating.
Limb buds form.

Week 8
Embryo is 3 cm in length.
Embryo is 2 g.
Eyelids begin to fuse.
Circulatory system through umbilical cord is well established.
Every organ system is present.

Week 12
Fetus is 6 to 9 cm in length.
Fetus is 19 g.
Face is well formed
Limbs are long and slender.
Kidneys begin to form urine.
Spontaneous movements occur.
Heartbeat is detected by Doppler transducer between 10 and 12 weeks.
Sex is visually recognizable.

Week 16
Fetus is 11.5 to 13.5 cm in length.
Fetus is 100 g.
Active movements are present.
Fetal skin is transparent.
Lanugo hair begins to develop.
Skeletal ossification occurs.

Week 20
Fetus is 16 to 18.5 cm in length.

Fetus is 300 g.
Lanugo covers the entire body.
Fetus has nails.
Muscles are developed.
Enamel and dentin are depositing.
Heartbeat is detected by regular (nonelectronic) fetoscope.

Week 24
Fetus is 23 cm in length.
Fetus is 600 g.
Hair on head is well formed.
Skin is reddish and wrinkled.
Reflex hand grasp functions.
Vernix caseosa covers entire body.
Fetus has ability to hear.

Week 28
Fetus is 27 cm in length.
Fetus is 1100 g.
Limbs are well flexed.
Brain is developing rapidly.
Eyelids open and close.
Lungs are developed sufficiently to provide gas exchange (lecithin forming).
If born, neonate can breathe at this time.

Week 32
Fetus is 31 cm in length.
Fetus is 1800 to 2100 g.
Bones are fully developed.
Subcutaneous fat has collected.
Lecithin-to-sphingomyelin (L/S) ratio is 1.2:1.

Week 36
Fetus is 35 cm in length.
Fetus is 2200 to 2900 g.
Skin is pink and body is rounded.
Skin is less wrinkled.
Lanugo is disappearing.
L/S ratio is greater than 2:1.

Week 40
Fetus is 40 cm in length.
Fetus is more than 3200 g.
Skin is pinkish and smooth.
Lanugo is present on upper arms and shoulders.
Vernix caseosa decreases.
Fingernails extend beyond fingertips.
Sole (plantar) creases run down to the heel.
Testes are in the scrotum.
Labia majora are well developed.

2. Is the inner membrane that forms about the second week of embryonic development
3. Forms a fluid-filled sac that surrounds the **embryo** and later the fetus

B. Chorion
1. Is the outer membrane
2. Becomes vascularized and forms the fetal part of the **placenta**

C. Amniotic fluid
1. Consists of 800 to 1200 mL by the end of pregnancy
2. Surrounds, cushions, and protects the fetus and allows for fetal movement
3. Maintains the body temperature of the fetus
4. Contains fetal urine and is a measure of fetal kidney function
5. The fetus modifies the **amniotic fluid** through the processes of swallowing, urinating, and movement through the respiratory tract.

D. Placenta
1. The **placenta** provides for exchange of nutrients and waste products between the fetus and mother
2. The **placenta** begins to form at **implantation**; the structure is complete by week 12.
3. It produces hormones to maintain pregnancy and assumes full responsibility for the production of these hormones by the twelfth week of gestation.
4. In the third trimester, transfer of maternal immunoglobulin provides the fetus with passive immunity to certain diseases for the first few months after birth.
5. By week 10 to 12, genetic testing can be done via chorionic villus sampling (CVS).

⚠ Large particles such as bacteria cannot pass through the placenta, but nutrients, drugs, antibodies, and viruses can pass through the placenta.

VII. FETAL CIRCULATION

A. Umbilical cord
1. It contains two arteries and one vein.
2. The arteries carry deoxygenated blood and waste products from the fetus.
3. The vein carries oxygenated blood and provides oxygen and nutrients to the fetus.

B. Fetal heart rate (FHR)
1. FHR depends on gestational age; FHR is 160 to 170 beats/min in the first trimester, but slows with fetal growth to 120 to 160 beats/min near or at term.
2. FHR is about twice the maternal heart rate.

C. Fetal circulation bypass (Fig. 22-2)
1. Fetal circulation bypass is present because of nonfunctioning lungs.

2. Bypasses must close after birth to allow blood to flow through the lungs and the liver.
3. The ductus arteriosus connects the pulmonary artery to the aorta, bypassing the lungs.
4. The ductus venosus connects the umbilical vein and the inferior vena cava, bypassing the liver.
5. The foramen ovale is the opening between the right and left atria of the heart, bypassing the lungs.

⚠ The fetal heart rate is 160 to 170 beats/min in the first trimester, but slows with fetal growth to 120 to 160 beats/min near or at term. The physician must be notified if the fetal heart rate is outside these parameters.

VIII. FAMILY PLANNING

A. Description
1. Involves choosing when to have children
2. Includes contraception, prevention of pregnancy, and methods to achieve pregnancy

B. Birth control
1. The focus of counseling on contraception must meet the needs and feelings of the woman and her partner.
2. Several factors should be considered when choosing a method of birth control, including effectiveness, safety, and personal preference.
3. The woman's preferences are most important, and cultural practices and beliefs and religious or other personal beliefs may affect the choice of contraceptives.
4. Other factors that bear on selection of a contraceptive method include family-planning goals, age, frequency of intercourse, and the individual's capacity for compliance.
5. If planning goals have already been met, sterilization of either the male or female partner may be desirable (it is important for the couple to understand that tubal reconstruction may be unsuccessful).
6. For women who frequently engage in coitus, oral contraceptives or a long-term method such as implants or an intrauterine device (IUD) may be considered.
7. When sexual activity is limited, use of spermicide, condoms, or a diaphragm may be most appropriate.
8. Because some methods have adverse effects, an informed consent form may be needed.
9. For additional information on the use of contraceptives, see Chapter 55.

C. Infertility
1. Infertility is the involuntary inability to conceive when desired.

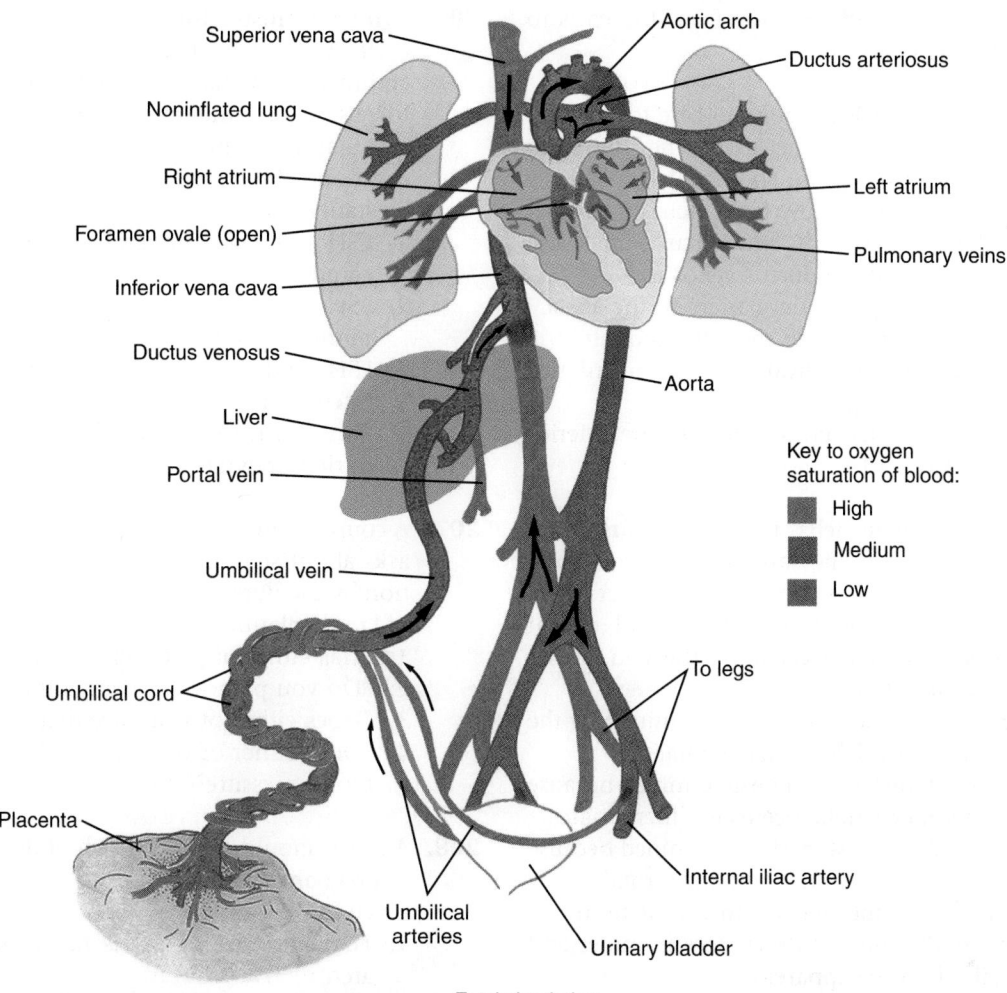

▲ **FIGURE 22-2** Fetal circulation. Three shunts (ductus venosus, ductus arteriosus, and foramen ovale) allow most blood from the placenta to bypass the fetal lungs and liver. (From McKinney, E., James, S., Murray, S., & Ashwill, J. [2009]. *Maternal-child nursing* [3rd ed.]. St. Louis: Saunders.)

2. Some factors contributing to infertility in men include abnormalities of the sperm, abnormal erections or ejaculations, or abnormalities of the seminal fluid.

3. Some factors that contribute to infertility in women include disorders of ovulation or abnormalities of the fallopian tubes or cervix.

4. Several diagnostic tests are available to determine the probable cause of infertility and the therapy recommended may depend on the cause of the infertility.

5. Infertility options
   a. Options include medication, surgical procedures, or therapeutic insemination.
   b. Other therapies are available, such as in vitro **fertilization**, surrogate mothers, or embryo hosts.
   c. Adoption may also be an option.

6. The nurse needs to provide support to the couple in their decision-making process and during therapy.

MORE QUESTIONS ON THE CD!

Practice Questions

201. A nursing student is preparing a prenatal class on the process of fetal circulation. The nursing instructor asks the student specifically to describe the process through the umbilical cord. Which of the following statements from the student is correct?
    1. "The one artery carries freshly oxygenated blood and nutrient-rich blood back from the placenta to the fetus."
    2. "The two arteries carry freshly oxygenated blood and nutrient-rich blood back from the placenta to the fetus."
    3. "The two arteries in the umbilical cord carry deoxygenated blood and waste products away from the fetus to the placenta."
    4. "The two veins in the umbilical cord carry blood that is high in carbon dioxide and

other waste products away from the fetus to the placenta."

202. A nursing student is assigned to care for a client in labor. A nursing instructor asks the student to describe fetal circulation, specifically the ductus venosus. The nursing instructor determines that the student understands fetal circulation if the student states that the ductus venosus:
1. Connects the pulmonary artery to the aorta
2. Is an opening between the right and left atria
3. Connects the umbilical vein to the inferior vena cava
4. Connects the umbilical artery to the inferior vena cava

203. A pregnant client tells the clinic nurse that she wants to know the sex of her baby as soon as it can be determined. The nurse understands that the client should be able to find out at 12 weeks' gestation because by the end of the twelfth week:
1. The sex of the fetus can be determined by the appearance of the external genitalia.
2. The sex of the fetus can be determined because the external genitalia begins to differentiate.
3. The sex of the fetus can be determined because the testes are descended into the scrotal sac.
4. The sex of the fetus can be determined because the internal differences in males and females become apparent.

204. A nurse is performing an assessment on a client who is at 38 weeks' gestation and notes that the fetal heart rate is 174 beats/min. On the basis of this finding, the appropriate nursing action is to:
1. Notify the physician.
2. Document the finding.
3. Check the mother's heart rate.
4. Tell the client that the fetal heart rate is normal.

205. A nurse is conducting a prenatal class on the female reproductive system. When a client in the class asks why the fertilized ovum stays in the fallopian tube for 3 days, the nurse responds that the reason for this is that it:
1. Promotes the fertilized ovum's chances of survival
2. Promotes the fertilized ovum's exposure to estrogen and progesterone
3. Promotes the fertilized ovum's normal implantation in the top portion of the uterus
4. Promotes the fertilized ovum's exposure to luteinizing hormone and follicle-stimulating hormone

206. A nursing instructor is reviewing the menstrual cycle with a nursing student who will be conducting a prenatal teaching session. The instructor asks the student to describe the follicle-stimulating hormone (FSH) and the luteinizing hormone (LH). The student accurately responds by stating that:
1. FSH and LH are secreted by the adrenal glands.
2. FSH and LH are released from the anterior pituitary gland.
3. FSH and LH are secreted by the corpus luteum of the ovary.
4. FSH and LH stimulate the formation of milk during pregnancy.

207. A couple comes to the family planning clinic and asks about sterilization procedures. Which question by the nurse would determine if this method of family planning would be appropriate?
1. "Has either of you ever had surgery?"
2. "Do you plan to have any other children?"
3. "Does either of you have diabetes mellitus?"
4. "Does either of you have problems with high blood pressure?"

208. A nurse should explain which of the following to a pregnant client found to have a gynecoid pelvis?
1. That her type of pelvis has a narrow pubic arch
2. That her type of pelvis is the most favorable for labor and birth
3. That her type of pelvis is a wide pelvis, but has a short diameter
4. That she will need a cesarean section because this type of pelvis is not favorable for a normal labor and vaginal delivery

209. A nurse explains some of the purposes of the placenta to a client during a prenatal visit. The nurse determines that the client understands some of these purposes when the client states that the placenta:
1. Cushions and protects the baby.
2. Maintains the temperature of the baby.
3. Is the way the baby gets food and oxygen.
4. Prevents all antibodies and viruses from passing to the baby.

Alternate Item Format: Multiple Response

210. A nursing instructor asks a nursing student to list the functions of the amniotic fluid. The student responds correctly by stating that which of the

following are functions of amniotic fluid? **Select all that apply**.
- ❑ 1. Allows for fetal movement
- ❑ 2. Is a measure of kidney function
- ❑ 3. Surrounds, cushions, and protects the fetus
- ❑ 4. Maintains the body temperature of the fetus
- ❑ 5. Prevents large particles such as bacteria from passing to the fetus
- ❑ 6. Provides an exchange of nutrients and waste products between the mother and the fetus

ANSWERS

201. 3

Rationale: Blood pumped by the embryo's heart leaves the embryo through two umbilical arteries. When oxygenated, the blood is returned by one umbilical vein. Arteries carry deoxygenated blood and waste products from the fetus, and veins carry oxygenated blood and provide oxygen and nutrients to the fetus.

Test-Taking Strategy: Recall that three umbilical vessels are within the umbilical cord (two arteries and one vein) and that the veins carry oxygenated blood and the arteries carry deoxygenated blood. If you had difficulty with this question, review fetal circulation.

Level of Cognitive Ability: Understanding
Client Needs: Physiological Integrity
Integrated Process: Teaching and Learning
Content Area: Maternity—Antepartum
Reference: McKinney, E., James, S., Murray, S., & Ashwill, J. (2009). *Maternal-child nursing* (3rd ed., pp. 245–246). St. Louis: Saunders.

202. 3

Rationale: The ductus venosus connects the umbilical vein to the inferior vena cava. Options 1, 2, and 4 are incorrect. The foramen ovale is a temporary opening between the right and left atria. The ductus arteriosus joins the aorta and the pulmonary artery.

Test-Taking Strategy: Focus on the subject, the description of the ductus venosus. Note the relationship of the word *venosus* in the question and *vein* in the correct option. Remember that the ductus venosus connects the umbilical vein to the inferior vena cava. Review fetal circulation if you had difficulty with this question.

Level of Cognitive Ability: Understanding
Client Needs: Physiological Integrity
Integrated Process: Teaching and Learning
Content Area: Maternity—Intrapartum
Reference: Perry, S., Hockenberry, M., Lowdermilk, D., & Wilson, D. (2010). *Maternal child nursing care* (4th ed., p. 180). St. Louis: Mosby.

203. 1

Rationale: By the end of the twelfth week, the external genitalia of the fetus have developed to such a degree that the sex of the fetus can be determined visually. Option 2 (differentiation of the external genitalia) occurs at the end of the ninth week. Option 3 occurs at the end of the thirty-eighth week (testes descend into the scrotal sac). Option 4 occurs at the end of the seventh week (internal differences in the male and female).

Test-Taking Strategy: Use knowledge regarding fetal development to answer this question. Remember that the sex of the fetus can be recognizable visually by the appearance of the external genitalia by gestational week 12. If you had difficulty with this question, review fetal development.

Level of Cognitive Ability: Understanding
Client Needs: Health Promotion and Maintenance
Integrated Process: Teaching and Learning
Content Area: Maternity—Antepartum
Reference: McKinney, E., James, S., Murray, S., & Ashwill, J. (2009). *Maternal-child nursing* (3rd ed., p. 237). St. Louis: Saunders.

204. 1

Rationale: The fetal heart rate (FHR) depends on gestational age and ranges from 160 to 170 beats/min in the first trimester, but slows with fetal growth to 120 to 160 beats/min near or at term. At or near term, if FHR is less than 120 beats/min or more than 160 beats/min with the uterus at rest, the fetus may be in distress. Because the FHR is increased from the reference range, the nurse should notify the physician. Options 3 and 4 are inappropriate actions based on the information in the question. Although the nurse documents the findings, based on the information in the question, the physician needs to be notified.

Test-Taking Strategy: Use the process of elimination and note the FHR and that the client is at 38 weeks of gestation. Remember that normal FHR at or near term is 120 to 160 beats/min. Review FHR if you had difficulty with this question.

Level of Cognitive Ability: Applying
Client Needs: Physiological Integrity
Integrated Process: Nursing Process—Implementation
Content Area: Maternity—Antepartum
Reference: McKinney, E., James, S., Murray, S., & Ashwill, J. (2009). *Maternal-child nursing* (3rd ed., p. 261). St. Louis: Saunders.

205. 3

Rationale: The tubal isthmus remains contracted until 3 days after conception to allow the fertilized ovum to develop within the tube. This initial growth of the fertilized ovum promotes its normal implantation in the fundal portion of the uterine corpus. Estrogen is a hormone produced by the ovarian follicles, corpus luteum, adrenal cortex, and placenta during pregnancy. Progesterone is a hormone secreted by the corpus luteum of the ovary, adrenal glands, and placenta during pregnancy. Luteinizing hormone and follicle-stimulating hormone are excreted by the anterior pituitary gland. The survival of the fertilized ovum does not depend on it staying in the fallopian tube for 3 days.

Test-Taking Strategy: Use knowledge of the anatomy and physiology of the female reproductive system. Remember that fertilization occurs in the fallopian tube and the fertilized ovum remains in the fallopian tube for about 3 days. This promotes its normal implantation. If you had difficulty with this question, review anatomy and physiology of the reproductive system.

Level of Cognitive Ability: Understanding
Client Needs: Physiological Integrity
Integrated Process: Teaching and Learning
Content Area: Maternity—Antepartum
Reference: McKinney, E., James, S., Murray, S., & Ashwill, J. (2009). *Maternal-child nursing* (3rd ed., p. 233). St. Louis: Saunders.

206. 2
Rationale: Follicle-stimulating hormone and luteinizing hormone, when stimulated by gonadotropin-releasing hormone from the hypothalamus, are released from the anterior pituitary gland to stimulate follicular growth and development, growth of the graafian follicle, and production of progesterone. Options 1, 3, and 4 are incorrect.
Test-Taking Strategy: Use your knowledge of anatomy and physiology concepts, recalling that follicle-stimulating hormone and luteinizing hormone are released from the anterior pituitary gland. If you had difficulty with this question, review the menstrual cycle.
Level of Cognitive Ability: Understanding
Client Needs: Physiological Integrity
Integrated Process: Teaching and Learning
Content Area: Maternity—Antepartum
Reference: McKinney, E., James, S., Murray, S., & Ashwill, J. (2009). *Maternal-child nursing* (3rd ed., p. 219). St. Louis: Saunders.

207. 2
Rationale: Sterilization is a method of contraception for couples who have completed their families. It should be considered a permanent end to fertility because reversal surgery is not always successful. The nurse would ask the couple about their plans for having children in the future. Options 1, 3, and 4 are unrelated to this procedure.
Test-Taking Strategy: Focus on the subject, sterilization procedure. Noting the relationship between the word *sterilization* and option 2 will direct you to this option. Review the effects of sterilization if you had difficulty with this question.
Level of Cognitive Ability: Applying
Client Needs: Health Promotion and Maintenance
Integrated Process: Nursing Process—Assessment
Content Area: Maternity—Antepartum
Reference: Perry, S., Hockenberry, M., Lowdermilk, D., & Wilson, D. (2010). *Maternal child nursing care* (4th ed., p. 154). St. Louis: Mosby.

208. 2
Rationale: A gynecoid pelvis is a normal female pelvis and is the most favorable for successful labor and birth. An android pelvis (resembling a male pelvis) would be unfavorable for labor because of the narrow pelvic planes. An anthropoid pelvis has an outlet that is adequate, with a normal or moderately narrow pubic arch. A platypelloid pelvis (flat pelvis) has a wide transverse diameter, but the anteroposterior diameter is short, making the outlet inadequate.

Test-Taking Strategy: Use knowledge of the anatomy of the female pelvis to answer the question. Recalling that the gynecoid pelvis is the normal female pelvis will direct you to the correct option. Review female pelvic types if you had difficulty with this question.
Level of Cognitive Ability: Understanding
Client Needs: Health Promotion and Maintenance
Integrated Process: Teaching and Learning
Content Area: Maternity—Antepartum
Reference: Perry, S., Hockenberry, M., Lowdermilk, D., & Wilson, D. (2010). *Maternal child nursing care* (4th ed., p. 381). St. Louis: Mosby.

209. 3
Rationale: The placenta provides an exchange of oxygen, nutrients, and waste products between the mother and the fetus. The amniotic fluid surrounds, cushions, and protects the fetus and maintains the body temperature of the fetus. Nutrients, drugs, antibodies, and viruses can pass through the placenta.
Test-Taking Strategy: Focus on the subject, the purpose of the placenta. Remember that the placenta provides oxygen and nutrients. If you had difficulty with this question, review the structure and function of the placenta and amniotic fluid.
Level of Cognitive Ability: Understanding
Client Needs: Health Promotion and Maintenance
Integrated Process: Teaching and Learning
Content Area: Maternity—Antepartum
Reference: Perry, S., Hockenberry, M., Lowdermilk, D., & Wilson, D. (2010). *Maternal child nursing care* (4th ed., pp. 177–179). St. Louis: Mosby.

ALTERNATE ITEM FORMAT: MULTIPLE RESPONSE
210. 1, 2, 3, 4
Rationale: The amniotic fluid surrounds, cushions, and protects the fetus. It allows the fetus to move freely, maintains the body temperature of the fetus, and helps assess kidney function because it contains urine from the fetus. The placenta prevents large particles such as bacteria from passing to the fetus and provides an exchange of nutrients and waste products between the mother and the fetus.
Test-Taking Strategy: Focus on the subject of the question: the functions of amniotic fluid. Visualizing the location of the amniotic fluid will assist in answering this question. If you had difficulty with this question, review the function of the amniotic fluid.
Level of Cognitive Ability: Understanding
Client Needs: Physiological Integrity
Integrated Process: Teaching and Learning
Content Area: Maternity—antepartum
Reference: Perry, S., Hockenberry, M., Lowdermilk, D., & Wilson, D. (2010). *Maternal child nursing care* (4th ed., p. 175). St. Louis: Mosby.

Obstetrical Assessment

I. GESTATION

A. Time from **fertilization** of the ovum until the estimated date of confinement or estimated date of **delivery**

B. About 280 days

C. **Nägele's rule** for estimating the date of confinement (**delivery**) (Box 23-1)

1. Use of **Nägele's rule** requires that the woman have a regular 28-day menstrual cycle.

2. Add 7 days to the first day of the last menstrual period, subtract 3 months, and then add 1 year to that date; alternatively, add 7 days to the date of the last menstrual period and count forward 9 months.

II. GRAVIDITY AND PARITY

A. Gravidity

1. **Gravida** refers to a pregnant woman.

2. Gravidity refers to the number of pregnancies.

3. Nulligravida is a woman who has never been pregnant.

4. Primigravida is a woman who is pregnant for the first time.

5. Multigravida is a woman in at least her second pregnancy.

B. **Parity**

1. **Parity** is the number of births (not the number of fetuses, e.g., twins) carried past 20 weeks' gestation, whether or not the fetus was born alive.

2. Nullipara is a woman who has not had a birth at more than 20 weeks of gestation.

3. Primipara is a woman who has had one birth that occurred after the twentieth week of gestation.

4. Multipara is a woman who has had two or more pregnancies to the stage of fetal viability.

C. Use of GTPAL: Pregnancy outcomes can be described with the acronym *GTPAL* (Box 23-2).

1. *G* is gravidity, the number of pregnancies, including the present one.

2. *T* is term births, the number born at term (longer than 37 weeks' gestation).

Box 23-1 Nägele's Rule for Estimating the Date of Confinement (Delivery)

First day of last menstrual period	September 12, 2011
Add 7 days	September 19, 2011
Subtract 3 months	June 19, 2011
Add 1 year	June 19, 2012
Estimated date of confinement (delivery)	June 19, 2012

Box 23-2 Describing Pregnancy Outcome with GTPAL

G Gravidity
T Term births
P Preterm births
A Abortions or miscarriages
L Current living children

Example: A woman is pregnant for the fourth time. She had one elective abortion in the first trimester, a daughter who was born at 40 weeks' gestation, and a son who was born at 36 weeks' gestation. She is gravida (G) 4, parity (number of births carried past 20 weeks) 2, and term (T) 1 (the daughter born at 40 weeks); preterm (P), 1 (the son born at 36 weeks); abortion (A), 1 (the abortion is counted in the gravidity, but is not included in the parity because it occurred before 20 weeks); living children (L), 2.
   GTPAL = 4, 1, 1, 1, 2

---

3. *P* is preterm births, the number born before 37 weeks' gestation.

4. *A* is abortions or miscarriages, the number of abortions or miscarriages (included in **gravida** if before 20 weeks' gestation; included in **parity** if past 20 weeks' gestation). A termination of the pregnancy after 20 weeks is referred to as a "therapeutic termination."

5. *L* is the number of current living children.

III. PREGNANCY SIGNS

A. Presumptive signs
1. Amenorrhea
2. Nausea and vomiting
3. Increased size and increased feeling of fullness in breasts
4. Pronounced nipples
5. Urinary frequency
6. **Quickening**: The first perception of fetal movement by the mother may occur the sixteenth to twentieth week of gestation.
7. Fatigue
8. Discoloration of the vaginal mucosa

B. Probable signs
1. Uterine enlargement
2. **Hegar's sign**: Compressibility and softening of the lower uterine segment that occurs at about week 6
3. **Goodell's sign**: Softening of the cervix that occurs at the beginning of the second month
4. **Chadwick's sign**: Violet coloration of the mucous membranes of the cervix, **vagina**, and vulva that occurs at about week 4
5. **Ballottement**: Rebounding of the fetus against the examiner's fingers on palpation
6. Braxton Hicks contractions (irregular painless contractions that may occur intermittently throughout pregnancy)
7. Positive pregnancy test for determination of the presence of human chorionic gonadotropin

C. Positive signs (diagnostic)
1. Fetal heart rate detected by electronic device (Doppler transducer) at 10 to 12 weeks and by nonelectronic device (fetoscope) at 20 weeks of gestation
2. Active fetal movements palpable by examiner
3. Outline of fetus via radiography or ultra-sonography

IV. FUNDAL HEIGHT (Box 23-3)

A. Fundal height is measured to evaluate the gestational age of the fetus.
B. During the second and third trimesters (weeks 18 to 30), fundal height in centimeters approximately equals fetal age in weeks ± 2 cm (Fig. 23-1).
C. At 16 weeks, the fundus can be found approximately halfway between the symphysis pubis and the umbilicus.
D. At 20 to 22 weeks, the fundus is approximately at the location of the umbilicus.

Box 23-3 Measuring Fundal Height

1. Place the client in the supine position.
2. Place the end of the tape measure at the level of the symphysis pubis.
3. Stretch the tape to the top of the uterine fundus.
4. Note and record the measurement.

E. At 36 weeks, the fundus is at the xiphoid process.

⚠ When assessing fundal height, monitor the client closely for supine hypotension when placed in the supine position.

V. MATERNAL RISK FACTORS

A. Maternal age: Women younger than 20 years and older than 35 years are at risk for adverse perinatal outcomes.
B. Adolescent pregnancy
1. Factors that result in adolescent pregnancy include the early onset of menarche, changing sexual behaviors in this age group, problems with family relationships, poverty, and lack of knowledge of reproduction and birth control.
2. Major concerns related to adolescent pregnancy include poor nutritional status; emotional and behavioral difficulties; lack of support systems; increased risk of stillbirth; low-birth-weight **infants**; fetal mortality; cephalopelvic disproportion; and increased risk of maternal complications, such as hypertension, anemia, prolonged **labor**, and infections.
3. The role of the nurse in reducing risks and consequences of adolescent pregnancy is twofold—first, to encourage early and continued prenatal care, and second, to refer the adolescent, if necessary, for appropriate assistance, which can help counter the effects of a negative socioeconomic environment.

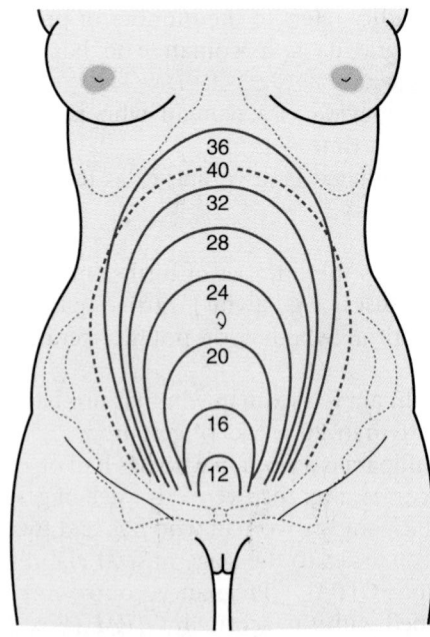

▲ **FIGURE 23-1** Height of fundus by weeks of normal gestation with a single fetus. *Dashed line*, Height after lightening (descent of the fetus toward the pelvic inlet before labor). (From Perry, S., Hockenberry, M., Lowdermilk, D., & Wilson, D. [2010]. *Maternal child nursing care* [4th ed.] St. Louis: Mosby.)

C. Nutrition: Adequate nutrition is necessary for normal fetal growth and development.

⚠ Women of childbearing age should take folic acid supplements to prevent neural tube defects and oro-facial clefts in the fetus.

D. Genetic considerations: Genetic abnormalities such as defective genes or transmissible inherited disorders can result in congenital anomalies; the nurse should perform a genetic risk assessment to determine an inheritable risk.

E. Health care: Failure to seek and obtain prenatal care, including dental care, increases the risk for preterm birth and low birth weight.

F. Abuse and violence: Physical abuse and violence can increase the risk for abruptio placentae, preterm birth, and infections from unwanted and forced sex.

G. Medical conditions: Concurrent medical conditions, such as but not limited to diabetes mellitus, hypertensive disorder, or cardiac disease, increase the risk of pregnancy.

H. German measles (rubella): Maternal infection during the first 8 weeks of gestation carries the highest rate of fetal infection.

I. Sexually transmitted infections
1. Syphilis
   a. Organism may cross the **placenta**.
   b. Infection usually leads to spontaneous abortions and increases the incidence of mental subnormality and physical deformities.
2. Condyloma acuminatum (human papillomavirus)
   a. Transmission may occur during vaginal birth.
   b. Infection is associated with the development of epithelial tumors of the mucous membranes of the larynx in children.
3. Gonorrhea
   a. Fetus is contaminated at the time of **delivery**.
   b. Maternal infection may result in postpartum infection of the **neonate**.
   c. Risks to the **neonate** include ophthalmia neonatorum, pneumonia, and sepsis.
4. Chlamydial infection
   a. Transmission may occur during vaginal birth and can result in neonatal conjunctivitis or pneumonitis.
   b. Infection can cause premature rupture of the membranes, premature labor, and postpartum endometritis.
5. Trichomoniasis: Associated with premature rupture of the membranes and postpartum endometritis
J. Human immunodeficiency virus (HIV)
1. HIV is transmitted through blood; blood products; and other bodily fluids, such as urine, semen, and vaginal secretions; the virus is also transmitted through exposure to infected secretions during birth and through breast milk.

2. Repeated exposure to the virus during pregnancy through unsafe sex practices or intravenous drug use can increase the risk of transmission to the fetus.
3. Perinatal administration of zidovudine may be recommended to decrease the risk of transmission of HIV from mother to fetus.
K. Substance abuse
1. Substance abuse threatens normal fetal growth and successful term completion of the pregnancy.
2. Substance abuse places the pregnancy at risk for fetal growth restriction, abruptio placentae, and fetal bradycardia.
3. Many substances cross the **placenta** and can be teratogenic; no drugs, including tobacco and over-the-counter medications, should be taken unless prescribed by a health care provider.
4. Smoking (tobacco) can result in low birth weight, a higher incidence of birth defects, and stillbirths.
5. Physical signs of drug abuse may include dilated or contracted pupils, fatigue, track (needle) marks, skin abscesses, inflamed nasal mucosa, and inappropriate behavior by the mother.
6. Consumption of alcohol during pregnancy may lead to fetal alcohol syndrome and can cause jitteriness, physical abnormalities, congenital anomalies, and growth deficits in the **newborn**.
L. Viral hepatitis (see Chapter 25 for information regarding hepatitis B infection)

 MORE QUESTIONS ON THE CD!

Practice Questions

211. A nurse is performing an assessment of a pregnant client who is at 28 weeks of gestation. The nurse measures the fundal height in centimeters and expects the finding to be which of the following?
1. 22 cm
2. 30 cm
3. 36 cm
4. 40 cm

212. A nurse is collecting data during an admission assessment of a client who is pregnant with twins. The client has a healthy 5-year-old child who was delivered at 38 weeks and tells the nurse that she does not have a history of any type of abortion or fetal demise. The nurse would document the GTPAL for this client as
1. G = 3, T = 2, P = 0, A = 0, L = 1
2. G = 2, T = 1, P = 0, A = 0, L = 1
3. G = 1, T = 1, P = 1, A = 0, L = 1
4. G = 2, T = 0, P = 0, A = 0, L = 1

213. A pregnant client is seen in a health care clinic for a regular prenatal visit. The client tells the nurse that she is experiencing irregular contractions, and the nurse determines that she is experiencing Braxton Hicks contractions. Based on this finding, which nursing action is appropriate?
1. Contact the physician.
2. Instruct the client to maintain bedrest for the remainder of the pregnancy.
3. Inform the client that these contractions are common and may occur throughout the pregnancy.
4. Call the maternity unit and inform them that the client will be admitted in a prelabor condition.

214. A nurse is providing instructions to a pregnant client with genital herpes about the measures that are needed to protect the fetus. The nurse tells the client that:
1. Total abstinence from sexual intercourse is necessary during the entire pregnancy.
2. Sitz baths need to be taken every 4 hours while awake if vaginal lesions are present.
3. Daily administration of acyclovir (Zovirax) is necessary during the entire pregnancy.
4. A cesarean section will be necessary if vaginal lesions are present at the time of labor.

215. A nurse is reviewing the record of a client who has just been told that a pregnancy test is positive. The physician has documented the presence of Goodell's sign. The nurse determines that this sign indicates:
1. A softening of the cervix
2. The presence of fetal movement
3. The presence of human chorionic gonadotropin in the urine
4. A soft blowing sound that corresponds to the maternal pulse during auscultation of the uterus

216. A client arrives at the clinic for the first prenatal assessment. The client tells a nurse that the first day of her last menstrual period was October 19, 2012. Using Nägele's rule, the nurse determines the estimated date of confinement is:
1. July 12, 2012
2. July 26, 2013

3. August 12, 2013
4. August 26, 2013

217. A nurse-midwife is assessing a pregnant client for the presence of ballottement. To make this determination, the nurse-midwife does which of the following?
1. Auscultates for fetal heart sounds
2. Assesses the cervix for compressibility
3. Palpates the abdomen for fetal movement
4. Initiates a gentle upward tap on the cervix

218. A pregnant client asks a nurse in the clinic when she will be able to begin to feel the fetus move. The nurse responds by telling the mother that fetal movements will be noted between which of the following weeks of gestation?
1. 6 and 8
2. 8 and 10
3. 10 and 12
4. 16 and 20

219. A nurse is performing an assessment of a primigravida who is being evaluated in a clinic during her second trimester of pregnancy. Which of the following indicates an abnormal physical finding that necessitates further testing?
1. Quickening
2. Braxton Hicks contractions
3. Fetal heart rate of 180 beats/min
4. Consistent increase in fundal height

Alternate Item Format: Multiple Response

220. A nurse is assisting in performing an assessment on a client who suspects that she is pregnant and is checking the client for probable signs of pregnancy. Which of the following are probable signs of pregnancy? **Select all that apply**.
❏ 1. Ballottement
❏ 2. Chadwick's sign
❏ 3. Uterine enlargement
❏ 4. Braxton Hicks contractions
❏ 5. Fetal heart rate detected by a nonelectronic device
❏ 6. Outline of fetus via radiography or ultrasonography

ANSWERS

211. 2
Rationale: During the second and third trimesters (weeks 18 to 30), fundal height in centimeters approximately equals the fetus' age in weeks ± 2 cm. At 16 weeks, the fundus can be located halfway between the symphysis pubis and the umbilicus. At 20 to 22 weeks, the fundus is at the umbilicus. At 36 weeks, the fundus is at the xiphoid process.

Test-Taking Strategy: Focus on the subject: the location of fundal height. Remember that during the second and third trimesters (weeks 18 to 30), fundal height in centimeters approximately equals the fetus' age in weeks ± 2 cm. If you

are unfamiliar with this assessment technique and expected findings related to fundal height, review this content area.
Level of Cognitive Ability: Understanding
Client Needs: Health Promotion and Maintenance
Integrated Process: Nursing Process—Assessment
Content Area: Maternity—Antepartum
Reference: Perry, S., Hockenberry, M., Lowdermilk, D., & Wilson, D. (2010). *Maternal child nursing care* (4th ed., p. 243). St. Louis: Mosby.

212. 2
Rationale: Pregnancy outcomes can be described with the acronym *GTPAL*. G is gravidity, the number of pregnancies; T is term births, the number born at term (longer than 37 weeks); P is preterm births, the number born before 37 weeks' gestation; A is abortions or miscarriages, the number of abortions or miscarriages (included in gravida if before 20 weeks' gestation; included in parity [number of births] if past 20 weeks' gestation); and L is the number of current living children. A woman who is pregnant with twins and has a child has a gravida of 2. Because the child was delivered at 38 weeks, the number of term births is 1, and the number of preterm births is 0. The number of abortions is 0, and the number of living children is 1.
Test-Taking Strategy: Focus on the data in the question. Recalling the meaning of the acronym *GTPAL* will direct you to option 2. If you had difficulty answering this question, review the *GTPAL* method of describing pregnancy outcomes.
Level of Cognitive Ability: Applying
Client Needs: Health Promotion and Maintenance
Integrated Process: Nursing Process—Assessment
Content Area: Maternity—Antepartum
Reference: McKinney, E., James, S., Murray, S., & Ashwill, J. (2009). *Maternal-child nursing* (3rd ed., p. 262). St. Louis: Saunders.

213. 3
Rationale: Braxton Hicks contractions are irregular, painless contractions that may occur intermittently throughout pregnancy. Because Braxton Hicks contractions may occur and are normal in some pregnant women during pregnancy, options 1, 2, and 4 are unnecessary and inappropriate actions.
Test-Taking Strategy: Use the process of elimination. Options 1 and 4 are comparable or alike and can be eliminated first. From the remaining options, knowing that Braxton Hicks contractions are common and normal and can occur throughout pregnancy will assist in directing you to option 3. Review the physiology associated with Braxton Hicks contractions if you had difficulty with this question.
Level of Cognitive Ability: Applying
Client Needs: Health Promotion and Maintenance
Integrated Process: Nursing Process—Implementation
Content Area: Maternity—Antepartum
Reference: McKinney, E., James, S., Murray, S., & Ashwill, J. (2009). *Maternal-child nursing* (3rd ed., pp. 261, 348). St. Louis: Saunders.

214. 4
Rationale: For women with active lesions, either recurrent or primary at the time of labor, delivery should be by cesarean section to prevent the fetus from being in contact with the genital herpes. The safety of acyclovir has not been established during pregnancy, and it should be used only when a life-threatening infection is present. Clients should be advised to abstain from sexual contact while the lesions are present. If this is an initial infection, clients should continue to abstain until they become culture-negative because prolonged viral shedding may occur in such cases. Keeping the genital area clean and dry promotes healing.
Test-Taking Strategy: Use the process of elimination. Eliminate options 1 and 3 first because of the close-ended word *entire* in these options. From the remaining options, recalling that the lesions should be kept clean and dry to promote healing will assist in eliminating option 2. If you had difficulty with this question, review the content related to genital herpes as a maternal risk factor.
Level of Cognitive Ability: Applying
Client Needs: Physiological Integrity
Integrated Process: Nursing Process—Implementation
Content Area: Maternity—Antepartum
Reference: From Perry, S., Hockenberry, M., Lowdermilk, D., & Wilson, D. (2010). *Maternal child nursing care* (4th ed., p. 106). St. Louis: Mosby.

215. 1
Rationale: At the beginning of the second month of gestation, the cervix becomes softer as a result of increased vascularity and hyperplasia, which cause Goodell's sign. Cervical softening is noted by the examiner during pelvic examination. Goodell's sign does not indicate the presence of fetal movement. Human chorionic gonadotropin noted in maternal urine is a probable sign of pregnancy. A soft blowing sound that corresponds to the maternal pulse may be auscultated over the uterus and is caused by blood circulating through the placenta.
Test-Taking Strategy: Think about the physiological findings in Goodell's sign to answer this question. Remember that Goodell's sign refers to a softening of the cervix. If you had difficulty with this question, review the changes in the cervix that occur during pregnancy.
Level of Cognitive Ability: Understanding
Client Needs: Health Promotion and Maintenance
Integrated Process: Nursing Process—Assessment
Content Area: Maternity—Antepartum
Reference: Perry, S., Hockenberry, M., Lowdermilk, D., & Wilson, D. (2010). *Maternal child nursing care* (4th ed., p. 214). St. Louis: Mosby.

216. 2
Rationale: Accurate use of Nägele's rule requires that the woman have a regular 28-day menstrual cycle. Add 7 days to the first day of the last menstrual period, subtract 3 months, and then add 1 year to that date: first day of the last menstrual period, October 19, 2012; add 7 days, October 26, 2012; subtract 3 months, July 26, 2012; add 1 year, July 26, 2013.
Test-Taking Strategy: Use knowledge regarding Nägele's rule to answer this question. This rule requires addition and subtraction, so read all the options carefully, noting the dates and years in the options, before selecting an answer. Review Nägele's rule if you had difficulty with this question.

Level of Cognitive Ability: Understanding
Client Needs: Health Promotion and Maintenance
Integrated Process: Nursing Process—Assessment
Content Area: Maternity—Antepartum
Reference: Perry, S., Hockenberry, M., Lowdermilk, D., & Wilson, D. (2010). *Maternal child nursing care* (4th ed., p. 230). St. Louis: Mosby.

217. 4

Rationale: Ballottement is a technique of palpating a floating structure by bouncing it gently and feeling it rebound. In the technique used to palpate the fetus, the examiner places a finger in the vagina and taps gently upward, causing the fetus to rise. The fetus then sinks, and the examiner feels a gentle tap on the finger. Options 1, 2, and 3 are not assessment techniques to check for ballottement. Option 2 is related to Hegar's sign. Options 1 and 3 are a part of fetal assessment.
Test-Taking Strategy: Focus on the subject: ballottement. Recalling the definition of ballottement—that it is a technique of palpating a floating structure by bouncing it gently and feeling it rebound—will direct you to option 4. Review this assessment technique if you had difficulty with this question.
Level of Cognitive Ability: Applying
Client Needs: Health Promotion and Maintenance
Integrated Process: Nursing Process—Assessment
Content Area: Maternity—Antepartum
Reference: Perry, S., Hockenberry, M., Lowdermilk, D., & Wilson, D. (2010). *Maternal child nursing care* (4th ed., p. 215). St. Louis: Mosby.

218. 4

Rationale: Quickening is fetal movement and may occur by the 16 to 20 week's gestation. The expectant mother first notices subtle fetal movements during this time, which gradually increase in intensity. Options 1, 2, and 3 are incorrect time frames because quickening does not occur this early during pregnancy.
Test-Taking Strategy: Use knowledge regarding the occurrence of quickening. In this situation, selecting the option that indicates the greatest length of gestational time is best. Review the process of quickening and its occurrence if you had difficulty with this question.
Level of Cognitive Ability: Applying
Client Needs: Health Promotion and Maintenance
Integrated Process: Nursing Process—Implementation
Content Area: Maternity—Antepartum
Reference: McKinney, E., James, S., Murray, S., & Ashwill, J. (2009). *Maternal-child nursing* (3rd ed., p. 237). St. Louis: Saunders.

219. 3

Rationale: The normal range of the fetal heart rate depends on gestational age. The heart rate is usually 160 to 170 beats/min in the first trimester and slows with fetal growth. Near and at term, the fetal heart rate ranges from 120 to 160 beats/min. Options 1, 2, and 4 are normal expected findings.
Test-Taking Strategy: Note the strategic words *indicates an abnormal physical finding*, and note that the client is in the second trimester of pregnancy. Recalling the normal fetal heart rate will direct you to option 3. Review normal assessment findings in pregnancy if you had difficulty with this question.
Level of Cognitive Ability: Understanding
Client Needs: Physiological Integrity
Integrated Process: Nursing Process—Assessment
Content Area: Maternity—Antepartum
Reference: McKinney, E., James, S., Murray, S., & Ashwill, J. (2009). *Maternal-child nursing* (3rd ed., p. 261). St. Louis: Saunders.

ALTERNATE ITEM FORMAT: MULTIPLE RESPONSE

220. 1, 2, 3, 4

Rationale: The probable signs of pregnancy include uterine enlargement, Hegar's sign (compressibility and softening of the lower uterine segment that occurs at about week 6), Goodell's sign (softening of the cervix that occurs at the beginning of the second month), Chadwick's sign (violet coloration of the mucous membranes of the cervix, vagina, and vulva that occurs at about week 4), ballottement (rebounding of the fetus against the examiner's fingers on palpation), Braxton Hicks contractions, and a positive pregnancy test for the presence of human chorionic gonadotropin. Positive signs of pregnancy include fetal heart rate detected by electronic device (Doppler transducer) at 10 to 12 weeks and by nonelectronic device (fetoscope) at 20 weeks of gestation, active fetal movements palpable by the examiner, and an outline of the fetus by radiography or ultrasonography.
Test-Taking Strategy: Focusing on the subject, probable signs of pregnancy, will assist in answering this question. Remember that detection of the fetal heart rate and an outline of the fetus via radiography or ultrasonography are positive signs of pregnancy. Review the probable signs of pregnancy if you had difficulty with this question.
Level of Cognitive Ability: Analyzing
Client Needs: Health Promotion and Maintenance
Integrated Process: Nursing Process—Assessment
Content Area: Maternity—Antepartum
Reference: McKinney, E., James, S., Murray, S., & Ashwill, J. (2009). *Maternal-child nursing* (3rd ed., p. 260). St. Louis: Saunders.

Prenatal Period

I. PHYSIOLOGICAL MATERNAL CHANGES

A. Cardiovascular system
1. Circulating blood volume increases, plasma increases, and total red blood cell volume increases (total volume increases by approximately 40% to 50%).
2. Physiological anemia occurs as the plasma increase exceeds the increase in production of red blood cells.
3. Iron requirements are increased.
4. Heart size increases, and the heart is elevated slightly upward and to the left because of displacement of the diaphragm as the **uterus** enlarges (Fig. 24-1).
5. Retention of sodium and water may occur.

B. Respiratory system
1. Oxygen consumption increases by approximately 15% to 20%.
2. Diaphragm is elevated because of the enlarged **uterus** (see Fig. 24-1).
3. Shortness of breath may be experienced.

⚠ During pregnancy, a woman's pulse rate may increase about 10 to 15 beats/min, the blood pressure slightly decreases in the second trimester, and the respiratory rate remains unchanged or slightly increases.

C. Gastrointestinal system
1. Nausea and vomiting may occur as a result of the secretion of human chorionic gonadotropin; it subsides by the third month.
2. Poor appetite may occur because of decreased gastric motility.
3. Alterations in taste and smell may occur.
4. Constipation may occur because of an increase in progesterone production or pressure of the **uterus** resulting in decreased gastrointestinal motility.
5. Flatulence and heartburn may occur because of decreased gastrointestinal motility and slowed emptying of the stomach caused by an increase in progesterone production.

6. Hemorrhoids may occur because of increased venous pressure.
7. Gum tissue may become swollen and easily bleed because of increasing levels of estrogen.
8. Ptyalism (excessive secretion of saliva) may occur because of increasing levels of estrogen.

D. Renal system
1. Frequency of urination increases in the first and third trimesters because of increased bladder sensitivity and pressure of the enlarging **uterus** on the bladder.
2. Decreased bladder tone may occur and is caused by an increase in progesterone and estrogen levels; bladder capacity increases in response to increasing levels of progesterone.
3. Renal threshold for glucose may be reduced.

E. Endocrine system
1. Basal metabolic rate increases and metabolic function increases.
2. The anterior lobe of the pituitary gland enlarges.
3. The thyroid enlarges slightly, and thyroid activity increases.
4. The parathyroid increases in size.
5. Aldosterone levels gradually increase.
6. Body weight increases.
7. Water retention is increased, which can contribute to weight gain.

F. Reproductive system
1. **Uterus**
   a. **Uterus** enlarges, increasing in mass from approximately 60 to 1000 g as a result of hyperplasia (influence of estrogen) and hypertrophy.
   b. Size and number of blood vessels and lymphatics increase.
   c. Irregular contractions occur.
2. Cervix
   a. Cervix becomes shorter, more elastic, and larger in diameter.
   b. Endocervical glands secrete a thick mucous plug, which is expelled from the canal when dilation begins.
   c. Increased vascularization and an increase in estrogen cause softening and a violet

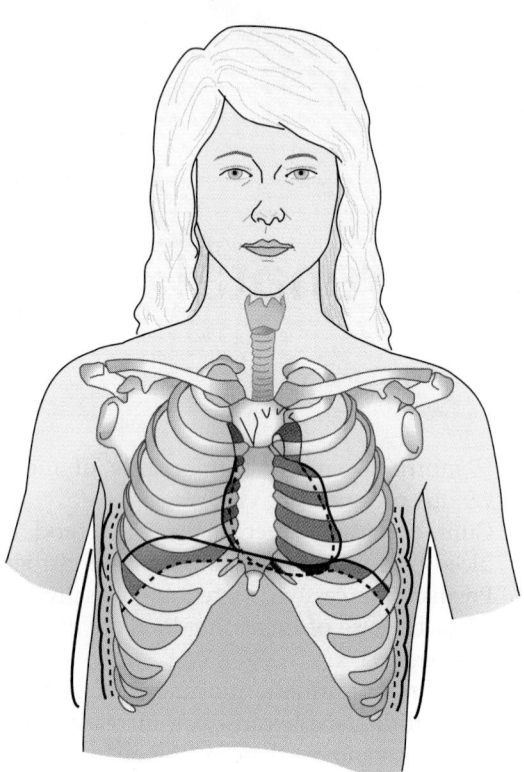

▲ **FIGURE 24-1** Changes in position of heart, lungs, and thoracic cage in pregnancy. *Broken line*, nonpregnant state; *solid line*, change that occurs in pregnancy. (From Perry, S., Hockenberry, M., Lowdermilk, D., & Wilson, D. [2010]. *Maternal child nursing care* [4th ed.]. St. Louis: Mosby.)

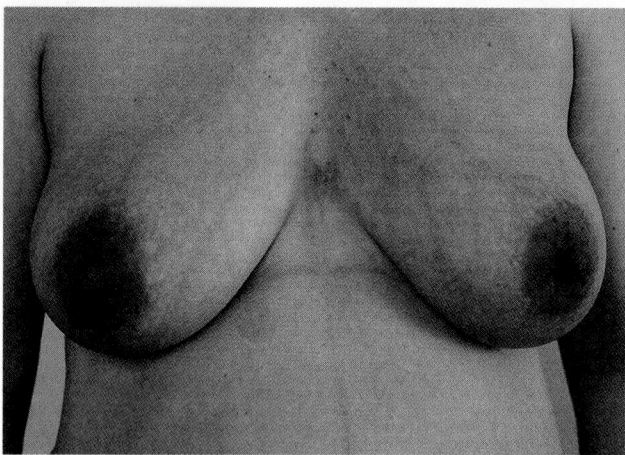

▲ **FIGURE 24-2** Enlarged breasts in pregnancy with venous network and darkened areolae and nipples. (From Perry, S., Hockenberry, M., Lowdermilk, D., & Wilson, D. [2010]. *Maternal child nursing care* [4th ed.]. St. Louis: Mosby.)

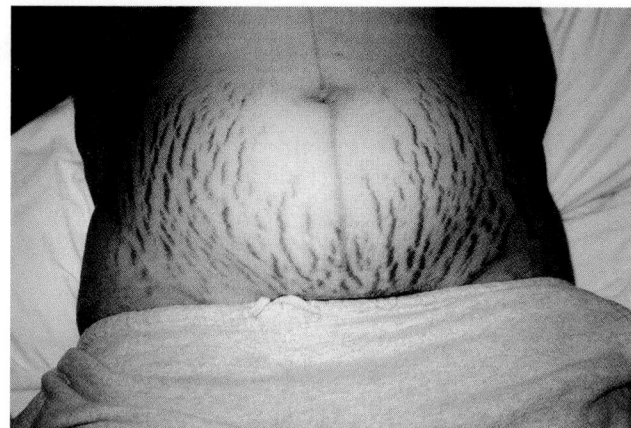

▲ **FIGURE 24-3** Striae gravidarum and linea nigra in a dark-skinned woman. (From Perry, S., Hockenberry, M., Lowdermilk, D., & Wilson, D. [2010]. *Maternal child nursing care* [4th ed.]. St. Louis: Mosby. Courtesy Shannon Perry, Phoenix, AZ.)

discoloration known as Chadwick's sign, which occurs at about 4 weeks of gestation.

   3. Ovaries

     a. A major function of the ovaries is to secrete progesterone for the first 6 to 7 weeks of pregnancy.

     b. The maturation of new follicles is blocked.

     c. The ovaries cease ovum production.

   4. Vagina

     a. Hypertrophy and thickening of the muscle occur.

     b. An increase in vaginal secretions is experienced; secretions are usually thick, white, and acidic.

   5. Breasts: Breast changes occur because of the increasing effects of estrogen and progesterone (Fig. 24-2).

     a. Breast size increases, and breasts may be tender.

     b. Nipples become more pronounced.

     c. The areolae become darker in color.

     d. Superficial veins become prominent.

     e. Hypertrophy of Montgomery's follicles occurs.

     f. Colostrum may leak from the breast.

G. Skin

   1. Some changes occur because the levels of melanocyte-stimulating hormone increase as a result of an increase in estrogen and progesterone levels; these changes include the following:

     a. Increased pigmentation

     b. Dark streak down the midline of the abdomen (linea nigra) (Fig. 24-3)

     c. Chloasma (mask of pregnancy)—a blotchy brownish hyperpigmentation, over the forehead, cheeks, and nose

     d. Reddish purple stretch marks (striae) on the abdomen, breasts, thighs, and upper arms (see Fig. 24-3)

   2. Vascular spider nevi may occur on the neck, chest, face, arms, and legs.

   3. Rate of hair growth may increase.

H. Skeletal system: Changes in the center of gravity begin in the second trimester and are caused by the hormones relaxin and progesterone.

⚠ During pregnancy, postural changes occur as the increased weight of the uterus causes a forward pull of the bony pelvis. It is important for the nurse to encourage the client to implement measures that maintain correct posture to prevent a backache.

II. PSYCHOLOGICAL MATERNAL CHANGES

A. Ambivalence
1. Ambivalence occurs early in pregnancy, even when the pregnancy is planned.
2. The mother may experience a dependence-independence conflict and ambivalence related to role changes.
3. The father may experience ambivalence related to the new role that he is assuming, increased financial responsibilities, and sharing the wife's attention with the child.

B. Acceptance: Factors that may be related to acceptance of the pregnancy are the woman's readiness for the experience and her identification with the motherhood role.

C. Emotional lability
1. Emotional lability may be manifested by frequent changes of emotional states or extremes in emotional states.
2. These emotional changes are common, but the mother may think that these changes are abnormal.

D. Body image changes
1. The changes in a woman's perception of her image during pregnancy occur gradually and may be positive or negative.
2. The physical changes and symptoms that the woman experiences during pregnancy contribute to her body image.

E. Relationship with the fetus
1. The woman may daydream to prepare for motherhood and think about the maternal qualities that she would like to possess.
2. The woman first accepts the biological fact that she is pregnant.
3. The woman next accepts the growing fetus as distinct from herself and a person to nurture.
4. Finally, the woman prepares realistically for the birth and parenting of the child.

III. DISCOMFORTS OF PREGNANCY

A. Nausea and vomiting
1. Occurs in the first trimester and subsides by the third month
2. Caused by elevated levels of human chorionic gonadotropin and changes in carbohydrate metabolism
3. Interventions
   a. Eating dry crackers before arising
   b. Avoiding brushing teeth immediately after arising
   c. Eating small, frequent, low-fat meals during the day
   d. Drinking liquids between meals rather than at meals
   e. Avoiding fried foods and spicy foods
   f. Asking the physician or nurse-midwife about acupressure (some types may require a prescription)
   g. Asking the physician or nurse-midwife about the use of herbal remedies

B. Syncope
1. Usually occurs in the first trimester; supine hypotension occurs particularly in the second and third trimesters
2. May be triggered hormonally or caused by the increased blood volume, anemia, fatigue, sudden position changes, or lying supine
3. Interventions
   a. Sitting with the feet elevated
   b. Changing positions slowly

⚠ The nurse needs to instruct the pregnant woman to avoid lying in the supine position, particularly in the second and third trimesters. The supine position places the woman at risk for supine hypotension, which occurs as a result of pressure of the uterus on the inferior vena cava.

C. Urinary urgency and frequency
1. Usually occurs in the first and third trimesters
2. Caused by pressure of the **uterus** on the bladder
3. Interventions
   a. Drinking adequate amounts of fluid during the day
   b. Limiting fluid intake in the evening
   c. Voiding at regular intervals
   d. Sleeping side-lying at night
   e. Wearing perineal pads, if necessary
   f. Performing Kegel exercises

D. Breast tenderness
1. Can occur in the first through the third trimesters
2. Caused by increased levels of estrogen and progesterone
3. Interventions
   a. Wearing a supportive bra
   b. Avoiding the use of soap on the nipples and areolar area to prevent drying of skin

E. Increased vaginal discharge
1. Can occur in the first through the third trimesters
2. Caused by hypertrophy and thickening of the vaginal mucosa and increased mucus production
3. Interventions
   a. Using proper cleansing and hygiene techniques
   b. Wearing cotton underwear
   c. Avoiding douching
   d. Consulting the physician or nurse-midwife if infection is suspected

F. Nasal stuffiness
1. Occurs in the first through third trimesters
2. Results from increased estrogen, which causes swelling of the nasal tissues and dryness
3. Interventions
   a. Encouraging the use of a humidifier
   b. Avoiding the use of nasal sprays or antihistamines (the physician or nurse-midwife should be consulted about their use)

G. Fatigue
  1. Occurs usually in the first and third trimesters
  2. Usually results from hormonal changes
  3. Interventions
     a. Arranging frequent rest periods throughout the day
     b. Using correct posture and body mechanics
     c. Obtaining regular exercise
     d. Performing muscle relaxation and strengthening exercises for the legs and hip joints
     e. Avoiding eating and drinking foods containing stimulants throughout the pregnancy

H. Heartburn
  1. Occurs in the second and the third trimesters
  2. Results from increased progesterone levels, decreased gastrointestinal motility, esophageal reflux, and displacement of the stomach by the enlarging **uterus**
  3. Interventions
     a. Eating small, frequent meals
     b. Sitting upright for 30 minutes after a meal
     c. Drinking milk between meals
     d. Avoiding fatty and spicy foods
     e. Performing tailor-sitting exercises
     f. Consulting with the physician or nurse-midwife about the use of antacids

I. Ankle edema
  1. Usually occurs in the second and the third trimesters
  2. Results from vasodilation, venous stasis, and increased venous pressure below the **uterus**
  3. Interventions
     a. Elevating the legs at least twice a day and when resting
     b. Sleeping in a side-lying position
     c. Wearing supportive stockings or support hose
     d. Avoiding sitting or standing in one position for long periods

J. Varicose veins
  1. Usually occur in the second and the third trimesters
  2. Result from weakening walls of the veins or valves and venous congestion
  3. Interventions
     a. Wearing supportive stockings or support hose
     b. Elevating the feet when sitting
     c. Lying with the feet and hips elevated
     d. Avoiding long periods of standing or sitting
     e. Moving about while standing to improve circulation
     f. Avoiding leg crossing
     g. Avoiding constricting articles of clothing such as knee-high stockings

K. Headaches
  1. Usually occur in the second and the third trimesters
  2. Result from changes in blood volume and vascular tone

  3. Interventions
     a. Changing position slowly
     b. Applying a cool cloth to the forehead
     c. Eating a small snack
     d. Using acetaminophen (Tylenol) only if prescribed by the physician or nurse-midwife

L. Hemorrhoids
  1. Usually occur in the second and the third trimesters
  2. Result from increased venous pressure and constipation
  3. Interventions
     a. Soaking in a warm sitz bath
     b. Sitting on a soft pillow
     c. Eating high-fiber foods and drinking sufficient fluids to avoid constipation
     d. Increasing exercise, such as walking
     e. Applying ointments, suppositories, or compresses as prescribed by the physician or nurse-midwife

M. Constipation
  1. Usually occurs in the second and the third trimesters
  2. Results from an increase in progesterone production, decreased intestinal motility, displacement of the intestines, pressure of the **uterus**, and taking iron supplements
  3. Interventions
     a. Eating high-fiber foods
     b. Drinking sufficient fluids
     c. Exercising regularly
     d. Consulting with the physician or nurse-midwife about interventions such as the use of stool softeners, laxatives, or enemas

N. Backache
  1. Usually occurs in the second and the third trimesters
  2. Caused by an exaggerated lumbosacral curve resulting from an enlarged **uterus**
  3. Interventions
     a. Obtaining rest
     b. Using correct posture and body mechanics
     c. Wearing low-heeled, comfortable, and supportive shoes
     d. Performing pelvic tilt (rock) exercises and conscious relaxation exercises
     e. Sleeping on a firm mattress

O. Leg cramps
  1. Usually occur in the second and the third trimesters
  2. Result from an altered calcium-phosphorus balance and pressure of the **uterus** on nerves or from fatigue
  3. Interventions
     a. Getting regular exercise, especially walking
     b. Dorsiflexing the foot of the affected leg
     c. Increasing calcium intake

P. Shortness of breath
1. Can occur in the second and the third trimesters
2. Results from pressure on the diaphragm from the enlarged **uterus**
3. Interventions
   a. Taking frequent rest periods
   b. Sitting and sleeping with the head elevated or on the side
   c. Avoiding overexertion

IV. ANTEPARTUM DIAGNOSTIC TESTING

The usual schedule for antepartum health care visits is every 4 weeks for the first 28 to 32 weeks, every 2 weeks from 32 to 36 weeks, and every week from 36 to 40 weeks.

A. Blood type and Rh factor
1. ABO typing is performed to determine the woman's blood type in the ABO antigen system.
2. Rh typing is done to determine the woman's blood type in the rhesus antigen system. (Rh positive indicates the presence of the antigen; Rh negative indicates the absence of the antigen.)
3. If the client is Rh negative and has a negative antibody screen, she will need repeat antibody screens and should receive $Rh_o(D)$ immune globulin (RhoGAM) at 28 weeks' gestation.

B. Rubella titer
1. If the client has a negative titer (less than 1:8), indicating susceptibility to the rubella virus, she should receive the appropriate immunization postpartum.
2. The client must be using effective birth control at the time of the immunization and must be counseled not to become pregnant for 1 to 3 months after immunization (as specified by health care provider) and to avoid contact with anyone who is immunocompromised.
3. If the rubella vaccine is administered at the same time as $Rh_o(D)$ immune globulin, it may not be effective.

Rubella vaccine is not given during pregnancy because the live attenuated virus may cross the placenta and present a risk to the developing fetus.

C. Hemoglobin and hematocrit levels
1. Hemoglobin and hematocrit levels decline during gestation as a result of increased plasma volume.
2. A decrease in the hemoglobin level to less than 10 g/dL or in the hematocrit level to less than 30% indicates anemia.

D. Papanicolaou's smear is done during the initial prenatal examination to screen for cervical neoplasia.

E. Sexually transmitted infections (Table 24-1)

F. Sickle cell screening
1. Screening is indicated for clients at risk for sickle cell disease.

TABLE 24-1 Monitoring for Sexually Transmitted Infections

Disease	Laboratory Test
Gonorrhea	Vaginal culture is done during initial prenatal examination to screen for gonorrhea. Culture may be repeated during third trimester in high-risk clients
Syphilis	Culture is done of lesions (if present) during initial prenatal examination to screen for syphilis. Diagnosis depends on microscopic examination of primary and secondary lesion tissue and serology (Venereal Disease Research Laboratory [VDRL] or rapid plasma reagin [RPR] test) during latency and late infection. Culture may be repeated during third trimester in high-risk clients
Condyloma acuminatum (human papillomavirus)	Culture is indicated for clients with positive history or with active lesions. Test is performed to determine route of delivery. Weekly cultures may be done at week 35 or 36 of pregnancy until delivery
Chlamydia	Vaginal culture is indicated for all pregnant clients if client is in a high-risk group or if infants from previous pregnancies have developed neonatal conjunctivitis or pneumonia
Trichomoniasis	Normal saline wet smear of vaginal secretions is checked for presence of protozoa. Associated with premature rupture of membranes and postpartum endometritis

2. A positive test may indicate a need for further screening.

G. Tuberculin skin test
1. The health care provider may prefer to perform this skin test after **delivery**.
2. A positive skin test indicates the need for a chest radiograph (using an abdominal lead shield) to rule out active disease; in a pregnant client, chest radiography would not be performed until after 20 weeks of gestation (after the fetal organs are formed).
3. Converters to positive may be referred for treatment with medication after **delivery**.

H. Hepatitis B surface antigens
1. Testing for hepatitis antigens is recommended for all women because of the prevalence of the disease in the general population.
2. Vaccination for hepatitis B antigen may be specifically indicated for the following:

a. Health care workers

b. Intravenous drug users

c. Clients born in Asia, Africa, Haiti, or the Pacific islands

d. Clients with previously undiagnosed jaundice or chronic liver disease

e. Clients with tattoos

f. Clients with histories of blood transfusions

g. Clients with histories of multiple episodes of sexually transmitted infections

h. Clients who have been rejected previously as blood donors

i. Clients with histories of dialysis or renal transplantation

j. Clients from households having members infected with hepatitis B or hemodialysis clients

3. Hepatitis B vaccine is not contraindicated during pregnancy and may be recommended by the health care provider

4. See Chapter 56 for additional information about hepatitis.

I. Urinalysis and urine culture

1. A urine specimen for glucose and protein determinations should be obtained at every antepartum visit.

2. Glycosuria is a common result of decreased renal threshold that occurs during pregnancy.

3. If glycosuria persists, it may indicate diabetes.

4. White blood cells in the urine may indicate infection.

5. Ketonuria may result from insufficient food intake or vomiting.

6. Levels of 2+ to 4+ protein in the urine may indicate infection or preeclampsia.

J. Ultrasonography

1. Outlines and identifies fetal and maternal structures

2. Assists in confirming gestational age and estimated date of **delivery** and evaluating **amniotic fluid** volume (**amniotic fluid** index), which is done via special measurements

3. May be done abdominally or transvaginally during pregnancy

4. Interventions

a. If an abdominal ultrasound is being performed, the woman may need to drink water to fill the bladder before the procedure to obtain a better image of the fetus.

b. If a transvaginal ultrasound is being performed, a lubricated probe is inserted into the **vagina**.

c. The client should be informed that the test presents no known risks to the client or the fetus.

K. Biophysical profile

1. Noninvasive assessment of the fetus that includes fetal breathing movements, fetal movements, fetal tone, **amniotic fluid** index, and fetal heart rate patterns via a nonstress test

2. Normal fetal biophysical activities indicate that the central nervous system is functional and that the fetus is not hypoxemic

L. Doppler blood flow analysis: Noninvasive (ultrasonography) method of studying the blood flow in the fetus and **placenta**

M. Percutaneous umbilical blood sampling

1. Percutaneous umbilical blood sampling is performed if fetal blood sampling is necessary; it involves insertion of a needle directly into the fetal umbilical vessel under ultrasound guidance.

2. Fetal heart rate monitoring is necessary for 1 hour after the procedure, and a follow-up ultrasound to check for bleeding or hematoma formation is done 1 hour after the procedure.

N. Alpha-fetoprotein screening

1. Assesses the quantity of fetal serum proteins; elevated levels of protein are associated with open neural tube and abdominal wall defects

2. Can detect spina bifida and Down syndrome

3. Interventions

a. Alpha-fetoprotein level is determined by a maternal blood sample drawn between 16 and 18 weeks' gestation.

b. If the level is elevated and the gestation is less than 18 weeks, a second sample is drawn and screened.

c. An ultrasound is performed for elevated levels to rule out fetal abnormalities or multiple gestation.

O. Chorionic villus sampling

1. The physician aspirates a small sample of chorionic villus tissue at 10 to 13 weeks' gestation.

2. The test is performed for the purpose of detecting genetic abnormalities.

3. Interventions

a. Obtain informed consent.

b. The client may need to drink water to fill the bladder before the procedure to aid in the visualization of the **uterus** for catheter insertion.

c. Obtain baseline vital signs and fetal heart rate; monitor frequently after the procedure.

d. Rh-negative women may be given $Rh_o(D)$ immune globulin because chorionic villus sampling increases the risk of Rh sensitization.

P. Amniocentesis

1. Aspiration of **amniotic fluid**; best performed between 15 and 20 weeks of pregnancy because **amniotic fluid** volume is adequate and many viable fetal cells are present in the fluid by this time

2. Performed to determine genetic disorders, metabolic defects, and fetal lung maturity

3. Risks

a. Maternal hemorrhage

b. Infection

c. Rh isoimmunization
d. Abruptio placentae
e. **Amniotic fluid** emboli
f. Premature rupture of the membranes
4. Interventions
   a. Obtain informed consent.
   b. If less than 20 weeks' gestation, the client should have a full bladder to support the **uterus**; if performed after 20 weeks' gestation, the client should have an empty bladder to minimize chance of puncture.
   c. Prepare the client for ultrasonography, which is performed to locate the **placenta** and avoid puncture.
   d. Obtain baseline vital signs and fetal heart rate; monitor every 15 minutes.
   e. Position the client supine during the examination and on the left side after the procedure.

⚠ After chorionic villus sampling and amniocentesis, instruct the client that if chills, fever, bleeding, leakage of fluid at the needle insertion site, decreased fetal movement, uterine contractions, or cramping occurs, she must notify the physician or nurse-midwife.

Q. Kick counts (fetal movement counting)
1. The client sits quietly or lies down on her side and counts fetal kicks for a period of time, as instructed.
2. Instruct the client to notify the physician or nurse-midwife if there are fewer than 10 kicks in a 12-hour period or as instructed by the physician or nurse-midwife.
R. Fern test
1. The fern test is a microscopic slide test to determine the presence of **amniotic fluid** leakage.

2. Using sterile technique, a specimen is obtained from the external os of the cervix and vaginal pool and is examined on a slide under a microscope.
3. A fern-like pattern produced by the effects of salts of the **amniotic fluid** indicates the presence of **amniotic fluid**.
4. Interventions
   a. Position the client in the dorsal lithotomy position.
   b. Instruct the client to cough, which causes the **amniotic fluid** to leak from the **uterus** if the membranes are ruptured.
S. Nitrazine test
1. A nitrazine test strip is used to detect the presence of **amniotic fluid** in vaginal secretions.
2. Vaginal secretions have a pH of 4.5 to 5.5 and do not affect the nitrazine strip or swab.
3. **Amniotic fluid** has a pH of 7.0 to 7.5 and turns the nitrazine strip or swab blue.
4. Interventions
   a. Position the client in the dorsal lithotomy position.
   b. Touch the test tape to the fluid.
   c. Assess the test tape for a blue-green, blue-gray, or deep blue color, which indicates that the membranes are ruptured causing leakage of **amniotic fluid**.
T. Nonstress test (Box 24-1)
U. Contraction stress test (Box 24-2)

V. NUTRITION

A. General guidelines
1. A MyPyramid Web site designed specifically for pregnant and breast-feeding mothers provides unique, individualized nutrition guidance to

---

Box 24-1 Nonstress Test

Description
Test is performed to assess placental function and oxygenation.
Test determines fetal well-being.
Test evaluates fetal heart rate (FHR) response to fetal movement.

Interventions
An external ultrasound transducer and tocodynamometer are applied to the client, and a tracing of at least 20 minutes' duration is obtained so that FHR and uterine activity can be observed.
Baseline blood pressure is obtained, and blood pressure is monitored frequently.
The client is placed in the lateral (side-lying) position to avoid vena cava compression.
The client may be asked to press a button every time she feels fetal movement; the monitor records a mark at

each point of fetal movement, which is used as a reference point to assess FHR response.

Results
Reactive Nonstress Test (Normal, Negative)
"Reactive" indicates a healthy fetus.
The result requires two or more FHR accelerations of at least 15 beats/min, lasting at least 15 seconds from the beginning of the acceleration to the end, in association with fetal movement, during a 20-minute period.

Nonreactive Nonstress Test (Abnormal)
No accelerations or accelerations of less than 15 beats/min or lasting less than 15 seconds in duration occur during a 40-minute observation.

Unsatisfactory
The result cannot be interpreted because of the poor quality of the FHR tracing.

Box 24-2 Contraction Stress Test

Description
- Test assesses placental oxygenation and function.
- Test determines fetal ability to tolerate labor and determines fetal well-being.
- Fetus is exposed to the stress of contractions to assess the adequacy of placental perfusion under simulated labor conditions.
- Test is performed if nonstress test is abnormal.

Interventions
External fetal monitor is applied to the client, and a 20- to 30-minute baseline strip is recorded.

The uterus is stimulated to contract by the administration of a dilute dose of oxytocin (Pitocin) or by having the client use nipple stimulation until three palpable contractions with a duration of 40 seconds or more in a 10-minute period have been achieved.

Frequent maternal blood pressure readings are done, and the mother is monitored closely while increasing doses of oxytocin are given.

Results
Negative Contraction Stress Test (Normal)
A negative result is represented by no late decelerations of fetal heart rate (FHR).

Positive Contraction Stress Test (Abnormal)
A positive result is represented by late decelerations of FHR, with 50% or more of the contractions in the absence of hyperstimulation of the uterus.

Equivocal
An equivocal result contains decelerations, but with less than 50% of the contractions, or uterine activity shows a hyperstimulated uterus.

Unsatisfactory
An unsatisfactory result means that adequate uterine contractions cannot be achieved, or FHR tracing is of insufficient quality for adequate interpretation.

---

meet the needs of the pregnant woman. The woman should be assisted with accessing this site and preparing a nutritional plan (http://www.mypyramid.gov).

2. The average expected weight gain during pregnancy is 25 to 35 lb for women with a normal prepregnancy weight.
3. An increase of about 300 cal/day is needed during pregnancy.
4. Calorie needs are greater in the last two trimesters than in the first.
5. An increase of about 500 cal/day is needed during lactation.
6. A diet high in folic acid and folic acid supplements are recommended.
7. A diet high in folic acid is necessary for all women of childbearing age to prevent neural tube defects and orofacial clefts in the fetus.
8. At least 8 to 10 (8-oz) glasses of fluid are needed each day, of which 4 to 6 glasses should be water.
9. Sodium is not restricted unless specifically prescribed by the physician or nurse-midwife.

B. Vegetarianism (see Box 12-9)
  1. Ensure that the client eats a sufficient amount of varied foods to meet normal nutrient and energy needs.
  2. Clients should be educated about consuming complementary proteins over the course of each day to ensure that all essential amino acids are provided.
  3. Potential deficiencies in vegetarian diets include energy, protein, vitamin B_{12}, zinc, iron, calcium,

omega-3 fatty acids, and vitamin D (if limited exposure to sunlight).
  4. Protein consumption can be increased by consumption of a variety of vegetable protein sources based on whole grains, legumes, seeds, nuts, and vegetables combined to provide all essential amino acids.
  5. To enhance absorption of iron, vegetarians should include a good source of iron and vitamin C with each meal.
  6. Foods commonly eaten include tofu, tempeh, soy milk and soy products, meat analogues, legumes, nuts and seeds, sprouts, and a variety of fruits and vegetables.

C. Lactose intolerance
  1. Lactose consumed by an individual with lactose intolerance can cause abdominal distention, discomfort, nausea, vomiting, cramps, and loose stools.
  2. Clients with lactose intolerance need to incorporate sources of calcium other than dairy products into their dietary patterns regularly.
  3. Milk may be tolerated in cooked form, such as in custards or fermented dairy products.
  4. Cheese and yogurt sometimes are tolerated.
  5. Lactase, an enzyme, may be prescribed and is taken before ingesting milk or milk products.
  6. Lactase-treated milk or lactose-free products are also available commercially.

D. Pica
  1. Pica refers to eating nonfood substances, such as dirt, clay, starch, and freezer frost.

2. The cause is unknown; cultural values, such as beliefs regarding the effect of a material on the mother or fetus, may make pica a common practice.

3. Iron deficiency anemia may occur as a result of pica.

E. Cultural considerations: See Chapter 6 for information on cultural considerations in nutrition.

MORE QUESTIONS ON THE CD!

Practice Questions

221. A nurse is providing instructions to a pregnant client who is scheduled for an amniocentesis. The nurse tells the client that:
1. Strict bed rest is required after the procedure.
2. An informed consent needs to be signed before the procedure.
3. Hospitalization is necessary for 24 hours after the procedure.
4. A fever is expected after the procedure because of the trauma to the abdomen.

222. A pregnant client in the first trimester calls a nurse at a health care clinic and reports that she has noticed a thin, colorless vaginal drainage. The nurse should make which statement to the client?
1. "Come to the clinic immediately."
2. "Report to the emergency department at the maternity center immediately."
3. "The vaginal discharge may be bothersome, but is a normal occurrence."
4. "Use tampons if the discharge is bothersome, but to be sure to change the tampons every 2 hours."

223. A nurse has performed a nonstress test on a pregnant client and is reviewing the fetal monitor strip. The nurse interprets the test as reactive and understands that this indicates:
1. Normal findings
2. Abnormal findings
3. The need for further evaluation
4. That the findings on the monitor were difficult to interpret

224. A nonstress test is performed on a client who is pregnant, and the results of the test indicate nonreactive findings. The physician prescribes a contraction stress test, and the results are documented as negative. A nurse interprets the finding of the contraction stress test as indicating:

1. A normal test result
2. An abnormal test result
3. A high risk for fetal demise
4. The need for a cesarean delivery

225. A pregnant client tells a nurse that she has been craving "unusual foods." The nurse gathers additional assessment data from the client and discovers that the client has been ingesting daily amounts of white clay dirt from her backyard. Laboratory studies are performed on the client. The nurse reviews the results and determines that which of the following indicates a physiological consequence of the client's practice?
1. Hematocrit 38%
2. Glucose 86 mg/dL
3. Hemoglobin 9.1 g/dL
4. White blood cell count 12,400/mm^3

226. A pregnant client asks a nurse about the types of exercises that are allowable during pregnancy. The nurse should instruct the client that the safest exercise to engage in is which of the following?
1. Swimming
2. Scuba diving
3. Low-impact gymnastics
4. Bicycling with the legs in the air

227. A physician has prescribed transvaginal ultrasonography for a client in the first trimester of pregnancy and the client asks a nurse about the procedure. The nurse tells the client that:
1. The procedure takes about 2 hours.
2. It will be necessary to drink 1 to 2 quarts of water before the examination.
3. Gel is spread over the abdomen, and a round disk transducer will be moved over the abdomen to obtain the picture.
4. The probe that will be inserted into the vagina will be covered with a disposable cover and coated with a gel.

228. A clinic nurse has instructed a pregnant client in measures to prevent varicose veins during pregnancy. Which statement by the client indicates a need for further instructions?
1. "I should wear panty hose."
2. "I should wear support hose."
3. "I should wear flat nonslip shoes that have good support."
4. "I should wear knee-high hose, but I should not leave them on longer than 8 hours."

229. A pregnant client calls a clinic and tells a nurse that she is experiencing leg cramps that awaken

her at night. To provide relief from the leg cramps, the nurse tells the client the following:
1. "Bend your foot toward your body while flexing the knee when the cramps occur."
2. "Bend your foot toward your body while extending the knee when the cramps occur."
3. "Point your foot away from your body while flexing the knee when the cramps occur."
4. "Point your foot away from your body while extending the knee when the cramps occur."

230. A clinic nurse is providing instructions to a pregnant client regarding measures that assist in alleviating heartburn. Which statement by the client indicates an understanding of the instructions?
1. "I should avoid between-meal snacks."
2. "I should lie down for an hour after eating."
3. "I should use spices for cooking rather than using salt."
4. "I should avoid eating foods that produce gas, such as beans and some vegetables, and fatty foods such as deep-fried chicken."

231. A nurse in a health care clinic is instructing a pregnant client how to perform "kick counts." Which statement by the client indicates a need for further instructions?
1. "I will record the number of movements or kicks."
2. "I need to lie flat on my back to perform the procedure."
3. "If I count fewer than 10 kicks in a 12-hour period, I need to contact the physician."
4. "I should place my hands on the largest part of my abdomen and concentrate on the fetal movements to count the kicks."

232. A nurse is providing instructions regarding treatment of hemorrhoids to a client who is in the second trimester of pregnancy. Which statement by the client indicates a need for further instruction?
1. "I should avoid straining during bowel movements."
2. "I can gently replace the hemorrhoids into the rectum."
3. "I can apply ice packs to the hemorrhoids to reduce the swelling."

4. "I should apply heat packs to the hemorrhoids to help the hemorrhoids shrink."

233. A nurse is providing instructions to a client in the first trimester of pregnancy regarding measures to assist in reducing breast tenderness. The nurse tells the client to:
1. Avoid wearing a bra.
2. Wash the breasts with warm water and keep them dry.
3. Wear tight-fitting blouses or dresses to provide support.
4. Wash the nipples and areolar area daily with soap, and massage the breasts with lotion.

234. A nurse is describing cardiovascular system changes that occur during pregnancy to a client and understands that which finding would be normal for a client in the second trimester?
1. Increase in pulse rate
2. Increase in blood pressure
3. Frequent bowel elimination
4. Decrease in red blood cell production

Alternate Item Format: Multiple Response

235. A rubella titer result of a 1-day postpartum client is less than 1:8, and a rubella virus vaccine is prescribed to be administered before discharge. The nurse provides which information to the client about the vaccine? **Select all that apply**.
❑ 1. Breast-feeding needs to be stopped for 3 months.
❑ 2. Pregnancy needs to be avoided for 1 to 3 months.
❑ 3. The vaccine is administered by the subcutaneous route.
❑ 4. A hypersensitivity reaction can occur if the client has an allergy to eggs.
❑ 5. Exposure to immunosuppressed individuals needs to be avoided.
❑ 6. The area of the injection needs to be covered with a sterile gauze for 1 week.

ANSWERS

221. 2

Rationale: Because amniocentesis is an invasive procedure, informed consent needs to be obtained before the procedure. After the procedure, the client is instructed to rest, but may resume light activity after the cramping subsides. The client is instructed to keep the puncture site clean and to report any complications, such as chills, fever, bleeding, leakage of fluid at the needle insertion site, decreased fetal movement, uterine contractions, or cramping. Amniocentesis is an outpatient procedure and may be done in a physician's private office or in a special prenatal testing unit. Hospitalization is not necessary after the procedure.

Test-Taking Strategy: Use the process of elimination. Recalling that this procedure is invasive will direct you to option 2. If you had difficulty with this question, review amniocentesis.
Level of Cognitive Ability: Applying
Client Needs: Physiological Integrity
Integrated Process: Teaching and Learning
Content Area: Maternity—Antepartum
References: Chernecky, C., & Berger, B. (2008). *Laboratory tests and diagnostic procedures* (5th ed., p. 131). St. Louis: Saunders.

McKinney, E., James, S., Murray, S., & Ashwill, J. (2009). *Maternal-child nursing* (3rd ed., pp. 17–18, 327–328). St. Louis: Saunders.

222. 3
Rationale: Leukorrhea begins during the first trimester. Many clients notice a thin, colorless or yellow vaginal discharge throughout pregnancy. Some clients become distressed about this condition, but it does not require that the client report to the health care clinic or emergency department immediately. If vaginal discharge is profuse, the client may use panty liners, but she should not wear tampons because of the risk of infection. If the client uses panty liners, she should change them frequently.
Test-Taking Strategy: Use the process of elimination. Eliminate options 1 and 2 first because they are comparable or alike indicating that the client requires medical attention. From the remaining options, recalling that this manifestation is a normal physiological occurrence or that tampons should be avoided will assist in directing you to the correct option. Review the normal occurrences related to vaginal discharge in a pregnant client if you had difficulty with this question.
Level of Cognitive Ability: Applying
Client Needs: Health Promotion and Maintenance
Integrated Process: Nursing Process—Implementation
Content Area: Maternity—Antepartum
Reference: Perry, S., Hockenberry, M., Lowdermilk, D., & Wilson, D. (2010). *Maternal child nursing care* (4th ed., p. 216). St. Louis: Mosby.

223. 1
Rationale: A reactive nonstress test is a normal result. To be considered reactive, the baseline fetal heart rate must be within normal range (120 to 160 beats/min) with good long-term variability. In addition, two or more fetal heart rate accelerations of at least 15 beats/min must occur, each with a duration of at least 15 seconds, in a 20-minute interval.
Test-Taking Strategy: Use the process of elimination. Eliminate options 2, 3, and 4 because they are comparable or alike indicating that an alteration from normal is present. If you had difficulty with this question and are unfamiliar with the interpretation of the results of a nonstress test, review this content.
Level of Cognitive Ability: Analyzing
Client Needs: Physiological Integrity
Integrated Process: Nursing Process—Analysis
Content Area: Maternity—Antepartum
Reference: McKinney, E., James, S., Murray, S., & Ashwill, J. (2009). *Maternal-child nursing* (3rd ed., p. 329). St. Louis: Saunders.

224. 1
Rationale: Contraction stress test results may be interpreted as negative (normal), positive (abnormal), or equivocal. A negative test result indicates that no late decelerations occurred in the fetal heart rate, although the fetus was stressed by three contractions of at least 40 seconds' duration in a 10-minute period. Options 2, 3, and 4 are incorrect interpretations.
Test-Taking Strategy: Use the process of elimination, noting that options 2, 3, and 4 are comparable or alike in that they indicate an abnormal test result finding. If you had difficulty with this question and are unfamiliar with the interpretation of the results of a contraction stress test, review this content.
Level of Cognitive Ability: Analyzing
Client Needs: Physiological Integrity
Integrated Process: Nursing Process—Analysis
Content Area: Maternity—Antepartum
Reference: McKinney, E., James, S., Murray, S., & Ashwill, J. (2009). *Maternal-child nursing* (3rd ed., pp. 330–331). St. Louis: Saunders.

225. 3
Rationale: Pica cravings often lead to iron deficiency anemia, resulting in a decreased hemoglobin level. The laboratory values in options 1, 2, and 4 are normal for the pregnant client.
Test-Taking Strategy: Use the process of elimination, recalling that pica results in anemia. This will assist in eliminating options 2 and 4. From the remaining options, recall the normal laboratory values in a pregnant client to assist in directing you to option 3. Review the physiological effects of pica and the normal laboratory values in a pregnant client if you had difficulty with this question.
Level of Cognitive Ability: Analyzing
Client Needs: Physiological Integrity
Integrated Process: Nursing Process—Analysis
Content Area: Maternity—Antepartum
Reference: Perry, S., Hockenberry, M., Lowdermilk, D., & Wilson, D. (2010). *Maternal child nursing care* (4th ed., p. 285). St. Louis: Mosby.

226. 1
Rationale: Non–weight-bearing exercises are preferable to weight-bearing exercises during pregnancy. Exercises to avoid are shoulder standing and bicycling with the legs in the air because the knee-chest position should be avoided. Competitive or high-risk sports such as scuba diving, water skiing, downhill skiing, horseback riding, basketball, volleyball, and gymnastics should be avoided. Non–weight-bearing exercises such as swimming are allowable.
Test-Taking Strategy: Focus on the subject, safe exercise to engage in during pregnancy. Identify the activities or exercises that could cause an injury to the fetus. This should direct you to option 1. If you had difficulty with this question, review the teaching points related to exercising for a client who is pregnant.
Level of Cognitive Ability: Applying
Client Needs: Health Promotion and Maintenance
Integrated Process: Teaching and Learning
Content Area: Maternity—Antepartum
Reference: McKinney, E., James, S., Murray, S., & Ashwill, J. (2009). *Maternal-child nursing* (3rd ed., p. 274). St. Louis: Saunders.

227. 4

Rationale: Transvaginal ultrasonography allows clear visibility of the uterus, gestational sac, embryo, and deep pelvic structures, such as the ovaries and fallopian tubes. The client is placed in a lithotomy position and a transvaginal probe, encased in a disposable cover and coated with a gel that provides lubrication and promotes conductivity, is inserted into the vagina. The client may feel more comfortable if she is allowed to insert the probe. The procedure takes about 10 to 15 minutes. Options 2 and 3 identify components of abdominal ultrasound.

Test-Taking Strategy: Use the process of elimination. Note the strategic words *transvaginal ultrasonography*. Also, note the relationship of the name of the test and the description in the correct option. If you had difficulty with this question, review the procedure for transvaginal ultrasonography.

Level of Cognitive Ability: Applying
Client Needs: Physiological Integrity
Integrated Process: Teaching and Learning
Content Area: Maternity—Antepartum
Reference: Perry, S., Hockenberry, M., Lowdermilk, D., & Wilson, D. (2010). *Maternal child nursing care* (4th ed., p. 194). St. Louis: Mosby.

228. 4

Rationale: Varicose veins often develop in the lower extremities during pregnancy. Any constrictive clothing, such as knee-high hose, impedes venous return from the lower legs and places the client at risk for developing varicosities. The client should be encouraged to wear support hose or panty hose. Flat nonslip shoes with proper support are important to assist the pregnant woman to maintain proper posture and balance and to minimize falls.

Test-Taking Strategy: Use the process of elimination and note the strategic words *a need for further instructions*. These words indicate a negative event query and ask you to select an option that is an incorrect statement. Focus on the subject of the question as it relates to preventing varicose veins. Recall that anything that constricts the lower vessels and impedes venous return from the lower legs would place the client at risk for varicosities. If you had difficulty with this question, review measures to prevent varicose veins.

Level of Cognitive Ability: Analyzing
Client Needs: Health Promotion and Maintenance
Integrated Process: Teaching and Learning
Content Area: Maternity—Antepartum
Reference: McKinney, E., James, S., Murray, S., & Ashwill, J. (2009). *Maternal-child nursing* (3rd ed., p. 271). St. Louis: Saunders.

229. 2

Rationale: Leg cramps occur when the pregnant client stretches her leg and plantar flexes her foot. Dorsiflexion of the foot while extending the knee stretches the affected muscle, prevents the muscle from contracting, and stops the cramping. Options 1, 3, and 4 are not measures that provide relief from leg cramps.

Test-Taking Strategy: Use the process of elimination and focus on the subject of the question, to provide relief from the leg cramps. Visualize each of the descriptions in the options to assist in directing you to option 2. If you had

difficulty with this question, review measures that assist in alleviating muscle cramps.

Level of Cognitive Ability: Applying
Client Needs: Health Promotion and Maintenance
Integrated Process: Teaching and Learning
Content Area: Maternity—Antepartum
Reference: McKinney, E., James, S., Murray, S., & Ashwill, J. (2009). *Maternal-child nursing* (3rd ed., p. 270). St. Louis: Saunders.

230. 4

Rationale: Lying down is likely to lead to reflux of stomach contents, especially immediately after a meal. The client should be instructed to avoid spices, along with salt, because spices trigger heartburn. Salt produces edema. The client should be encouraged to eat between-meal snacks and should be instructed that to control heartburn, eating smaller, more frequent portions is preferred over eating three large meals. The client also should limit or avoid gas-producing and fatty foods.

Test-Taking Strategy: Use the process of elimination and note the strategic words *indicates an understanding of the instructions*. Recalling that the client needs to limit or avoid gas-producing and fatty foods will assist in directing you to option 4. If you had difficulty with this question, review the measures that alleviate heartburn in the pregnant client.

Level of Cognitive Ability: Evaluating
Client Needs: Health Promotion and Maintenance
Integrated Process: Nursing Process—Evaluation
Content Area: Maternity—Antepartum
References: McKinney, E., James, S., Murray, S., & Ashwill, J. (2009). *Maternal-child nursing* (3rd ed., p. 270). St. Louis: Saunders.

Nix, S. (2009). *Williams' basic nutrition and diet therapy* (13th ed., pp. 175–176). St. Louis: Mosby.

231. 2

Rationale: The client should sit or lie quietly on her side to perform kick counts. Lying flat on the back is not necessary to perform this procedure, can cause discomfort, and presents a risk of vena caval (supine hypotensive) syndrome. The client is instructed to place her hands on the largest part of the abdomen and concentrate on the fetal movements. The client records the number of movements felt during a specified time period. The client needs to notify the physician or nurse-midwife if there are fewer than 10 kicks in a 12-hour period or as instructed by the physician or nurse-midwife.

Test-Taking Strategy: Use the process of elimination, noting the strategic words *a need for further instructions*. These words indicate a negative event query and ask you to select an option that is an incorrect statement. If you are unfamiliar with this procedure, recalling that the risk of vena caval (supine hypotensive) syndrome exists when the client lies on her back will direct you to option 2. Review the procedure for kick counts if you had difficulty with this question.

Level of Cognitive Ability: Evaluating
Client Needs: Health Promotion and Maintenance
Integrated Process: Teaching and Learning
Content Area: Maternity—Antepartum
Reference: McKinney, E., James, S., Murray, S., & Ashwill, J. (2009). *Maternal-child nursing* (3rd ed., p. 333). St. Louis: Saunders.

232. 4

Rationale: Measures that provide relief from hemorrhoids include avoiding constipation and straining during bowel movements; applying ice packs to reduce the hemorrhoidal swelling; gently replacing the hemorrhoids into the rectum; using stool softeners, ointments, or sprays as prescribed; and assuming certain positions to relieve pressure on the hemorrhoids. Heat packs increase the blood flow to the area and worsen the discomfort from hemorrhoids.

Test-Taking Strategy: Use the process of elimination, noting the strategic words *need for further instruction*. These words indicate a negative event query and ask you to select an option that is an incorrect statement. Recalling the principles regarding heat and cold will assist in directing you to option 4. If you had difficulty with this question, review the measures for the treatment of hemorrhoids.

Level of Cognitive Ability: Evaluating
Client Needs: Physiological Integrity
Integrated Process: Teaching and Learning
Content Area: Maternity—Antepartum
Reference: McKinney, E., James, S., Murray, S., & Ashwill, J. (2009). *Maternal-child nursing* (3rd ed., p. 271). St. Louis: Saunders.

233. 2

Rationale: The pregnant client should be instructed to wash the breasts with warm water and keep them dry. The client should be instructed to avoid using soap on the nipples and areolar area to prevent the drying of tissues. Wearing a supportive bra with wide adjustable straps can decrease breast tenderness. Tight-fitting blouses or dresses cause discomfort. The client is instructed to wear soft-textured clothing to decrease nipple tenderness and to use breast pads inside the bra to prevent leakage through the clothing if colostrum is a problem.

Test-Taking Strategy: Focusing on the subject of the question—reducing breast tenderness—and visualizing each of the measures identified in the options will direct you to option 2. Also, noting the word *warm* and the word *dry* in option 2 will direct you to this option. If you had difficulty with this question, review treatment measures for the client with breast tenderness.

Level of Cognitive Ability: Applying
Client Needs: Health Promotion and Maintenance
Integrated Process: Teaching and Learning
Content Area: Maternity—Antepartum
References: McKinney, E., James, S., Murray, S., & Ashwill, J. (2009). *Maternal-child nursing* (3rd ed., p. 274). St. Louis: Saunders.
　　Perry, S., Hockenberry, M., Lowdermilk, D., & Wilson, D. (2010). *Maternal child nursing care* (4th ed., p. 217). St. Louis: Mosby.

234. 1

Rationale: Between 14 and 20 weeks' gestation, the pulse rate increases about 10 to 15 beats/min, which then persists to term. Options 2, 3, and 4 are incorrect. During pregnancy, the blood pressure usually is the same as the prepregnancy level, but then gradually decreases up to about 20 weeks of gestation. During the second trimester, systolic and diastolic pressures decrease by about 5 to 10 mm Hg. Constipation

may occur as a result of decreased gastrointestinal motility or pressure of the uterus. During pregnancy, there is an accelerated production of red blood cells.

Test-Taking Strategy: Focus on the subject of the question, the findings that would be considered normal for a client in her second trimester. Think about the physiological occurrences during pregnancy and remember that between 14 and 20 weeks' gestation, the pulse increases about 10 to 15 beats/min. If you had difficulty with this question, review normal physiological changes during the second trimester of pregnancy.

Level of Cognitive Ability: Understanding
Client Needs: Physiological Integrity
Integrated Process: Teaching and Learning
Content Area: Maternity—Antepartum
References: McKinney, E., James, S., Murray, S., & Ashwill, J. (2009). *Maternal-child nursing* (3rd ed., p. 266). St. Louis: Saunders.
　　Perry, S., Hockenberry, M., Lowdermilk, D., & Wilson, D. (2010). *Maternal child nursing care* (4th ed., p. 221). St. Louis: Mosby.

ALTERNATE ITEM FORMAT: MULTIPLE RESPONSE

235. 2, 3, 4, 5

Rationale: Rubella vaccine is administered to women who have not had rubella or women who are not serologically immune. The vaccine may be administered in the immediate postpartum period to prevent the possibility of contracting rubella in future pregnancies. The live attenuated rubella virus is not communicable in breast milk; breast-feeding does not need to be stopped. The client is counseled not to become pregnant for 1 to 3 months after immunization as specified by the health care provider because of a possible risk to a fetus from the live virus vaccine; the client must be using effective birth control at the time of the immunization. The client should avoid contact with immunosuppressed individuals because of their low immunity toward live viruses and because the virus is shed in the urine and other body fluids. The vaccine is administered by the subcutaneous route. A hypersensitivity reaction can occur if the client has an allergy to eggs because the vaccine is made from duck eggs. There is no useful or necessary reason for covering the area of the injection with a sterile gauze.

Test-Taking Strategy: Focus on the subject: client instructions regarding the rubella vaccine. Recalling that the rubella vaccine is a live virus vaccine will assist in selecting options 2 and 5. Next, recalling the route of administration and the contraindications associated with its use will assist in selecting options 3 and 4. Review client instructions related to the rubella vaccine if you had difficulty with this question.

Level of Cognitive Ability: Applying
Client Needs: Health Promotion and Maintenance
Integrated Process: Teaching and Learning
Content Area: Maternity—Postpartum
References: McKinney, E., James, S., Murray, S., & Ashwill, J. (2009). *Maternal-child nursing* (3rd ed., p. 462). St. Louis: Saunders.
　　Perry, S., Hockenberry, M., Lowdermilk, D., & Wilson, D. (2010). *Maternal child nursing care* (4th ed., p. 546). St. Louis: Mosby.

Risk Conditions Related to Pregnancy

I. ABORTION

A. Description: A pregnancy that ends before 20 weeks' gestation, spontaneously or electively
B. Types (Box 25-1)
C. Assessment
   1. Spontaneous vaginal bleeding occurs.
   2. Low uterine cramping or contractions occur.
   3. Blood clots or tissue through the vagina.
   4. Hemorrhage and shock can result if bleeding is excessive.
D. Interventions
   1. Maintain bed rest as prescribed.
   2. Monitor vital signs.
   3. Monitor for cramping and bleeding.
   4. Count perineal pads to evaluate blood loss, and save expelled tissues and clots.
   5. Maintain intravenous fluids as prescribed; monitor for signs of hemorrhage or shock.
   6. Prepare the client for dilation and curettage as prescribed for incomplete abortion.
   7. Rh$_o$(D) immune globulin (RhoGAM) is prescribed for an Rh-negative woman.

II. ANEMIA

A. Description
   1. Iron deficiency anemia is a condition that develops as a result of an inadequate amount of serum iron.
   2. Anemia predisposes the client to postpartum infection.
B. Assessment
   1. Fatigue
   2. Headache
   3. Pallor
   4. Tachycardia
   5. Hemoglobin value is usually less than 10 g/dL; hematocrit value is usually less than 30%.
C. Interventions
   1. Monitor hemoglobin and hematocrit levels every 2 weeks.
   2. Administer and instruct the client about iron and folic acid supplements.

Box 25-1 Types of Abortions	
Spontaneous	Pregnancy ends because of natural causes
Induced	Therapeutic or elective reasons exist for terminating pregnancy
Threatened	Spotting and cramping without cervical change occur
Inevitable	Spotting and cramping occur and cervix begins to dilate and efface
Incomplete	Loss of some of the products of conception occurs, with part of the products retained (most often placenta is retained)
Complete	Loss of all products of conception occurs
Missed	Products of conception are retained in utero after fetal death
Habitual	Spontaneous abortions occur in three or more successive pregnancies

   3. Instruct the client to take iron with a source of vitamin C to increase its absorption and to avoid taking iron with tea.
   4. Instruct the client to eat foods high in iron, folic acid, and protein.
   5. Teach the client to monitor for signs and symptoms of infection.
   6. Prepare to administer parenteral iron; this may be prescribed for severe anemia.
   7. Prepare to administer blood transfusions for severe anemia, if prescribed.
   8. Prepare for the administration of oxytocic medications in the postpartum period if excessive bleeding is a concern.

III. CARDIAC DISEASE

A. Description: A pregnant client with cardiac disease may be unable physiologically to cope with the added plasma volume and increased cardiac output that occur during pregnancy; blood volume is at a maximum during the last weeks of the second trimester.
B. Maternal cardiac disease risk groups (Box 25-2)
C. Functional classification of heart disease (Box 25-3)

Box 25-2 Maternal Cardiac Disease Risk Groups

Group I (Mortality Rate 1%)
Corrected tetralogy of Fallot
Pulmonic or tricuspid disease
Mitral stenosis (classes I and II)
Patent ductus arteriosus
Ventricular septal defect
Atrial septal defect
Porcine valve

Group II (Mortality Rate 5%-15%)
Mitral stenosis with atrial fibrillation
Artificial heart valves
Mitral stenosis (classes III and IV)
Uncorrected tetralogy
Aortic coarctation (uncomplicated)
Aortic stenosis

Group III (Mortality Rate 25%-50%)
Aortic coarctation (complicated)
Myocardial infarction
Marfan syndrome
True cardiomyopathy
Pulmonary hypertension

Modified from Perry, S., Hockenberry, M., Lowdermilk, D., & Wilson, D. (2010). *Maternal child nursing care* (4th ed., p. 311). St. Louis: Mosby.

Box 25-3 New York Heart Association Functional Classification of Heart Disease*

Class I	Uncompromised; no limitation of physical activity; asymptomatic with ordinary activity
Class II	Slightly compromised, requiring slight limitation of physical activity; client is comfortable at rest, but ordinary physical activity causes symptoms such as fatigue, dyspnea, palpitations, or anginal pain
Class III	Markedly compromised; marked limitation of physical activity; client is comfortable at rest, but less than ordinary activity causes excessive fatigue, palpitations, dyspnea, or anginal pain
Class IV	Inability to perform any physical activity without discomfort; symptoms of cardiac insufficiency are present even at rest

*Generally, maternal and fetal risks for classes I and II disease are small, but risks are greatly increased with classes III and IV.
Modified from Perry, S., Hockenberry, M., Lowdermilk, D., & Wilson, D. (2010). *Maternal child nursing care* (4th ed., p. 311). St. Louis: Mosby; and McKinney, E., James, S., Murray, S., & Ashwill, J. (2009). *Maternal-child nursing* (3rd ed., p. 646). St. Louis: Saunders.

D. Assessment
1. Signs and symptoms of cardiac decompensation
   a. Cough and respiratory congestion
   b. Dyspnea and fatigue
   c. Palpitations and tachycardia
   d. Peripheral edema
   e. Chest pain
2. Signs of respiratory infection
3. Signs of heart failure and pulmonary edema
E. Interventions
1. Monitor vital signs, fetal heart rate, and condition of the fetus.
2. Limit physical activities, and stress the need for sufficient rest.
3. Monitor for signs of cardiac stress and decompensation, such as cough, fatigue, dyspnea, chest pain, and tachycardia.
4. Encourage adequate nutrition to prevent anemia, which would worsen the cardiac status; additionally, a low-sodium diet may be prescribed to prevent fluid retention and heart failure.
5. Avoid excessive weight gain.
6. Monitor for signs of heart failure, pulmonary edema, and cardiac decompensation.
7. During **labor**, prepare to do the following:
   a. Monitor vital signs frequently.
   b. Place the client on a cardiac monitor and on an external fetal monitor.
   c. Maintain bed rest, with the client lying on her side with her head and shoulders elevated.
   d. Administer oxygen as prescribed.

⚠ Excessive weight gain places stress on the heart. Additionally, obesity places the client at increased risk for complications during pregnancy.

IV. CHORIOAMNIONITIS

A. Description
1. Bacterial infection of the amniotic cavity; can result from premature rupture of the membranes, vaginitis, amniocentesis, or intrauterine procedures
2. May result in the development of postpartum endometritis
B. Assessment
1. Uterine tenderness and contractions
2. Elevated temperature
3. Maternal or fetal tachycardia
4. Foul odor to **amniotic fluid**
5. Leukocytosis
C. Interventions
1. Monitor maternal vital signs and fetal heart rate.
2. Monitor for uterine tenderness, contractions, and fetal activity.
3. Monitor results of blood cultures.
4. Prepare for amniocentesis to obtain **amniotic fluid** for Gram stain and leukocyte count.
5. Administer antibiotics as prescribed after cultures are obtained.
6. Administer oxytocic medications as prescribed to increase uterine tone.
7. Prepare to obtain neonatal cultures after **delivery**.

V. DIABETES MELLITUS

A. Description
  1. Pregnancy places demands on carbohydrate metabolism and causes insulin requirements to change.
  2. Maternal glucose crosses the **placenta**, but insulin does not.
  3. During the first trimester, maternal insulin needs decrease.
  4. During the second and third trimesters, increases in placental hormones cause an insulin-resistant state, requiring an increase in the client's insulin dose.
  5. After placental **delivery**, placental hormone levels abruptly decrease and insulin requirements decrease.
  6. The fetus produces its own insulin and pulls glucose from the mother, which predisposes the mother to hypoglycemic reactions.
  7. The **newborn** of a diabetic mother may be large in size, but has functions related to gestational age rather than size.
  8. The **newborn** of a diabetic mother is at risk for hypoglycemia, hyperbilirubinemia, respiratory distress syndrome, hypocalcemia, and congenital anomalies.

B. Gestational diabetes mellitus
  1. Gestational diabetes occurs in pregnancy (during the second or third trimester) in clients not previously diagnosed as diabetic and occurs when the pancreas cannot respond to the demand for more insulin.
  2. Pregnant women should be screened for gestational diabetes between 24 and 28 weeks of pregnancy.
  3. A 3-hour oral glucose tolerance test is performed to confirm gestational diabetes mellitus.
  4. Gestational diabetes frequently can be treated by diet alone; however, some clients may need insulin.
  5. Most women with gestational diabetes return to a euglycemic state after **delivery**; however, these individuals have an increased risk of developing diabetes mellitus in their lifetimes.

⚠ Oral hypoglycemic agents are never prescribed for use during pregnancy.

C. Predisposing conditions to gestational diabetes
  1. Older than 35 years
  2. Obesity
  3. Multiple gestation
  4. Family history of diabetes mellitus

D. Assessment
  1. Excessive thirst
  2. Hunger
  3. Weight loss
  4. Frequent urination
  5. Blurred vision
  6. Recurrent urinary tract infections and vaginal yeast infections
  7. Glycosuria and ketonuria
  8. Signs of gestational hypertension
  9. Polyhydramnios
  10. Large fetus for gestational age

E. Interventions
  1. Employ diet, insulin (if diet cannot control blood glucose levels), exercise, and blood glucose determinations to maintain blood glucose levels between 65 mg/dL and 130 mg/dL.
  2. Observe for signs of hyperglycemia, glycosuria and ketonuria, and hypoglycemia.
  3. Monitor weight.
  4. Increase calorie intake as prescribed, with adequate insulin therapy so that glucose moves into the cells.
  5. Assess for signs of maternal complications such as preeclampsia (hypertension, proteinuria, and edema).
  6. Monitor for signs of infection.
  7. Instruct the client to report burning and pain on urination, vaginal discharge or itching, or any other signs of infection to the health care provider.
  8. Assess fetal status and monitor for signs of fetal compromise.

F. Interventions during **labor**
  1. Monitor fetal status continuously for signs of distress and, if noted, prepare the client for immediate cesarean section.
  2. Carefully regulate insulin and provide glucose intravenously as prescribed because **labor** depletes glycogen.

G. Interventions during the postpartum period
  1. Observe the mother closely for a hypoglycemic reaction because a precipitous decline in insulin requirements normally occurs (the mother may not require insulin for the first 24 hours).
  2. Reregulate insulin needs as prescribed after the first day, according to blood glucose testing.
  3. Assess dietary needs based on blood glucose testing and insulin requirements.
  4. Monitor for signs of infection or postpartum hemorrhage.

VI. DISSEMINATED INTRAVASCULAR COAGULATION (DIC)

A. Description: DIC is a maternal condition in which the clotting cascade is activated, resulting in the formation of clots in the microcirculation (Fig. 25-1).

⚠ The rapid and extensive formation of clots that occurs in DIC causes the platelets and clotting factors to be depleted; this results in bleeding and the potential vascular occlusion of organs from thromboembolus formation.

B. Predisposing conditions (Box 25-4)

C. Assessment
1. Uncontrolled bleeding
2. Bruising, purpura, petechiae, and ecchymosis
3. Presence of occult blood in excretions such as stool
4. Hematuria, hematemesis, or vaginal bleeding
5. Signs of shock
6. Decreased fibrinogen level, platelet count, and hematocrit level
7. Increased prothrombin time and partial thromboplastin time, clotting time, and fibrin degradation products

D. Interventions
1. Remove underlying cause.
2. Monitor vital signs; assess for bleeding and signs of shock.
3. Prepare for oxygen therapy, volume replacement, blood component therapy, and possibly heparin therapy.

4. Monitor for complications associated with fluid and blood replacement and heparin therapy.
5. Monitor urine output and maintain at 30 mL/hr (renal failure is a complication of DIC).

VII. ECTOPIC PREGNANCY

A. Description
1. **Implantation** of the fertilized ovum outside of the uterine cavity
2. Most common location is the ampulla of the fallopian tube (Fig. 25-2)

B. Assessment
1. Missed menstrual period
2. Abdominal pain
3. Vaginal spotting to bleeding that is dark red or brown
4. Rupture: Increased pain, referred shoulder pain, signs of shock

C. Interventions
1. Obtain assessment data and vital signs.
2. Monitor bleeding and initiate measures to prevent rupture and shock.
3. Methotrexate (Trexall), a folic acid antagonist, may be prescribed to inhibit cell division in the developing **embryo**.
4. Prepare the client for laparotomy and removal of the pregnancy and tube, if necessary, or repair of the tube.
5. Administer antibiotics; $Rh_o(D)$ immune globulin is prescribed for Rh-negative women.

VIII. ENDOMETRITIS

A. Description
1. Endometritis is an infection of the lining of the **uterus** occurring in the postpartum period and caused by bacteria that invade the **uterus** at the placental site.

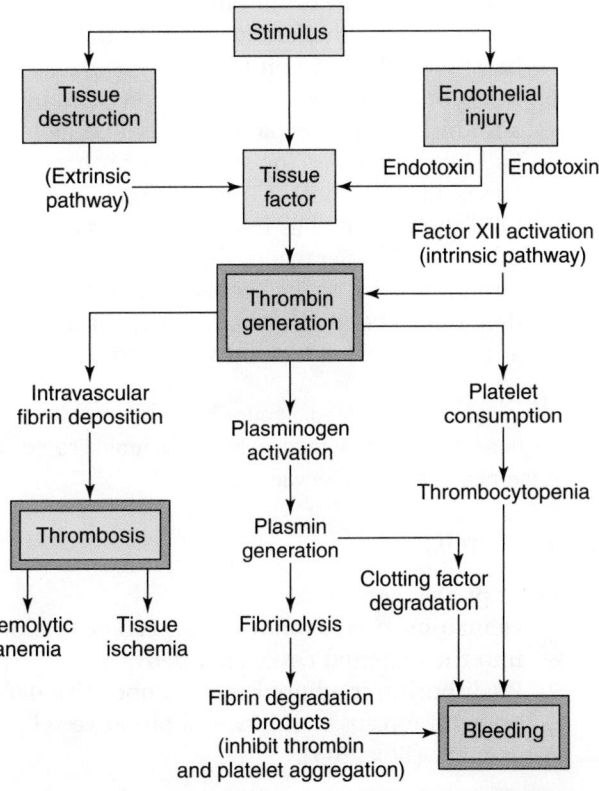

▲ **FIGURE 25-1** Pathophysiology of disseminated intravascular coagulation. (From Monahan, F., Sands, J., Neighbors, M., Marek, J., & Green, C. [2007]. *Phipps' medical-surgical nursing: Health and illness perspectives* [8th ed.]. St. Louis: Mosby.)

Box 25-4 Predisposing Conditions for Disseminated Intravascular Coagulation

Abruptio placentae	Intrauterine fetal death
Amniotic fluid embolism	Liver disease
Gestational hypertension	Sepsis

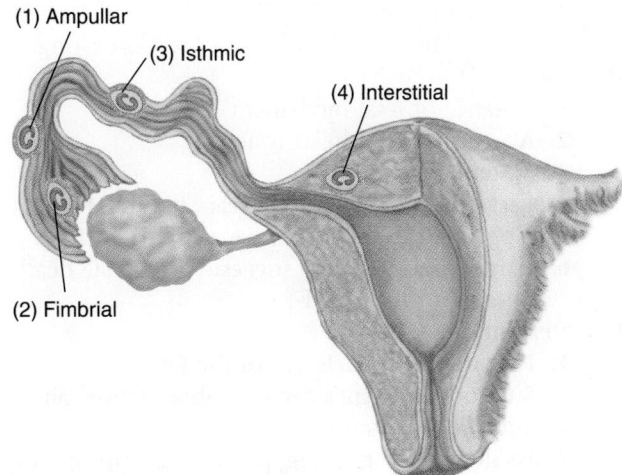

▲ **FIGURE 25-2** Sites of tubal ectopic pregnancy. Numbers indicate order of prevalence. (From McKinney, E., James, S., Murray, S., & Ashwill, J. [2009]. *Maternal-child nursing* [3rd ed.]. St. Louis: Saunders.)

2. The infection may spread and involve the entire endometrium and cause peritonitis or pelvic thrombophlebitis.
B. Assessment
1. Chills and fever
2. Increased pulse
3. Decreased appetite
4. Headache
5. Backache
6. Prolonged, severe afterpains
7. Tender, large **uterus**
8. Foul odor to **lochia** or reddish brown **lochia**
9. Ileus
10. Elevated white blood cell count, with left shift of immature cells
C. Interventions
1. Monitor vital signs.
2. Position the client in Fowler's position to facilitate drainage of **lochia**.
3. Provide a private room for the mother; inform the mother that isolation of the **newborn** from the mother is unnecessary.
4. Instruct the mother in proper handwashing techniques.
5. Initiate contact precautions as necessary.
6. Monitor intake and output and encourage fluid intake.
7. Administer antibiotics as prescribed.
8. Administer comfort measures such as back rubs and position changes and pain medications as prescribed.
9. Administer oxytocic medications as prescribed to improve uterine tone.

IX. FETAL DEATH IN UTERO

A. Description
1. Fetal death in utero refers to the death of a fetus after the twentieth week of gestation and before birth.
2. The client can develop DIC if the dead fetus is retained in the **uterus** for 3 to 4 weeks or longer.
B. Assessment
1. Absence of fetal movement
2. Absence of fetal heart tones
3. Maternal weight loss
4. Lack of fetal growth or decrease in fundal height
5. No evidence of fetal cardiac activity
6. Other characteristics suggestive of fetal death noted on ultrasound
C. Interventions
1. Prepare for the **delivery** of the fetus.
2. Support the client's decision about **labor**, birth, and the postpartum period.
3. Facilitate the grieving process as appropriate considering cultural practices and beliefs.
4. Accept behaviors such as anger and hostility from the parents.
5. Refer the parents to an appropriate support group.

Cultural and religious practices and beliefs are important to consider when caring for the parents of a fetus who has died. Be aware of the cultural and religious practices and beliefs of the client.

X. HEPATITIS B

A. Description
1. The risks of prematurity, low birth weight, and neonatal death increase if the mother has hepatitis B infection.
2. Hepatitis is transmitted through blood, saliva, vaginal secretions, semen, and breast milk and across the placental barrier.
B. Interventions
1. Minimize the risk for intrapartum ascending infections (limit the number of vaginal examinations).
2. Remove maternal blood from the neonate immediately after birth.
3. Suction the fluids from the neonate immediately after birth.
4. Bathe the neonate before any invasive procedures.
5. Clean and dry the face and eyes of the neonate before instilling eye prophylaxis.
6. Infection of the neonate can be prevented by the administration of hepatitis B immune globulin and hepatitis B vaccine soon after birth.
7. Discourage the mother from kissing the neonate until the neonate has received the vaccine.
8. Inform the mother that the hepatitis B vaccine will be administered to the neonate and that a second dose should be administered at 1 month after birth and a third dose at 6 months after birth.

Support breast-feeding after neonatal treatment for hepatitis B; breast-feeding is not contraindicated if the neonate has been vaccinated.

XI. HEMATOMA

A. Description
1. Hematoma occurs following the escape of blood into the maternal tissue after **delivery**.
2. Predisposing conditions include operative **delivery** with forceps or injury to a blood vessel.
B. Assessment (Box 25-5)

Box 25-5 Hematoma: Assessment Findings

Abnormal, severe pain
Pressure in perineal area (client states that she feels like she has to have a bowel movement)
Palpable, sensitive swelling in the perineal area, with discolored skin
Inability to void
Decreased hemoglobin and hematocrit levels
Signs of shock, such as pallor, tachycardia, and hypotension, if significant blood loss has occurred

C. Interventions
1. Monitor vital signs.
2. Monitor client for abnormal pain, especially when forceps **delivery** has been performed.
3. Apply ice to the hematoma site.
4. Administer analgesics as prescribed.
5. Monitor intake and output.
6. Encourage fluids and voiding; prepare for urinary catheterization if the client is unable to void.
7. Administer blood replacements as prescribed.
8. Monitor for signs of infection, such as increased temperature, pulse rate, and white blood cell count.
9. Administer antibiotics as prescribed because infection is common after hematoma formation.
10. Prepare for incision and evacuation of the hematoma if necessary.

XII. HUMAN IMMUNODEFICIENCY VIRUS (HIV) AND ACQUIRED IMMUNODEFICIENCY SYNDROME (AIDS)

A. Description
1. HIV is the causative agent of AIDS.
2. Women infected with HIV may first show symptoms at the time of pregnancy or possibly develop life-threatening infections because normal pregnancy involves some suppression of the maternal immune system.
3. Zidovudine (Retrovir) is recommended for the prevention of maternal-to-fetal HIV transmission and is administered orally beginning after 14 weeks' gestation, intravenously during **labor**, and in the form of syrup to the **newborn** for 6 weeks after birth.

B. Transmission
1. Sexual exposure to genital secretions of an infected person
2. Parenteral exposure to infected blood and tissue
3. Perinatal exposure of an **infant** to infected maternal secretions through birth or breast-feeding

C. Risks to the mother: A mother with HIV is managed as high risk because she is vulnerable to infections.

D. Diagnosis
1. Tests used to determine the presence of antibodies to HIV include enzyme-linked immunosorbent assay (ELISA), Western blot, and immunofluorescence assay (IFA).
2. A single reactive ELISA test by itself cannot be used to diagnose HIV, and the test should be repeated with the same blood sample; if the result is again reactive, follow-up tests using Western blot or IFA should be done.
3. A positive Western blot or IFA is considered confirmatory for HIV.
4. A positive ELISA that fails to be confirmed by Western blot or IFA should not be considered

negative, and repeat testing should be done in 3 to 6 months.
5. See Chapter 11 for additional laboratory tests.

E. Assessment (Box 25-6)

F. Interventions
1. Prenatal period
   a. Prevent opportunistic infections.
   b. Avoid procedures that increase the risk of perinatal transmission, such as amniocentesis and fetal scalp sampling.
2. Intrapartum period
   a. If the fetus has not been exposed to HIV in utero, the highest risk exists during **delivery** through the birth canal.
   b. Avoid the use of internal scalp electrodes for monitoring of the fetus.
   c. Avoid episiotomy to decrease the amount of maternal blood in and around the birth canal.
   d. Avoid the administration of oxytocin (Pitocin) because contractions induced by oxytocin can be strong, causing vaginal tears or necessitating an episiotomy.
   e. Place heavy absorbent pads under the mother's hips to absorb **amniotic fluid** and maternal blood.
   f. Minimize the neonate's exposure to maternal blood and body fluids; promptly remove the neonate from the mother's blood after **delivery**.
   g. Suction fluids from the neonate promptly.
   h. Prepare to administer zidovudine as prescribed to the mother during **labor** and **delivery**.

Box 25-6 Stages of Acquired Immunodeficiency Syndrome (AIDS)

Stage 1
Fever
Headache
Lymphadenopathy
Myalgia

Stage 2
Infection is active but asymptomatic and may remain so for years
Client may experience outbreak of herpes zoster (shingles)
Client may experience transient thrombocytopenia

Stage 3
Client is symptomatic
Immune dysfunction is evident
All body systems can show signs of immune dysfunction
Integumentary and gynecological problems are common

Stage 4
Advanced infection
Client vulnerable to common bacterial infections
Development of opportunistic infections
Serious immune compromise

3. Postpartum period
   a. Monitor for signs of infection.
   b. Place the mother in protective isolation if she is immunosuppressed.
   c. Restrict breast-feeding.
   d. Instruct the mother to monitor for signs of infection and report any signs if they occur.
G. The **newborn** and HIV
   1. Description
      a. Neonates born to HIV-positive clients may test positive because antibodies received from the mother may persist for 18 months after birth; all neonates acquire maternal antibody to HIV infection, but not all acquire infection.
      b. The use of antiviral medication, reduced exposure of the neonate to maternal blood and body fluids, and early identification of HIV in pregnancy reduce the risk of transmission to the neonate.
   2. Interventions
      a. Bathe the neonate carefully before any invasive procedure, such as the administration of vitamin K, heel sticks, or venipunctures; clean the umbilical cord stump meticulously every day until healed.
      b. The **newborn** can room with the mother.
      c. Administer zidovudine to the **newborn** as prescribed for the first 6 weeks of life.
      d. All HIV-exposed **newborns** should be treated with medication to prevent infection by *Pneumocystis jiroveci*.
      e. HIV culture is recommended at 1 and 4 months after birth; **infants** at risk for HIV infection should be seen by the physician at birth and 1 week, 2 weeks, 1 month, 2 months, and 4 months of age.
      f. The child may be asymptomatic for the first several years of life and should be monitored for early signs of immunodeficiency

⚠ Infants at risk for HIV infection need to receive all recommended immunizations at the regular schedule; however, no live vaccines should be administered.

XIII. HYDATIDIFORM MOLE

A. Description
   1. Hydatidiform mole is a form of gestational trophoblastic disease that occurs when the trophoblasts, which are the peripheral cells that attach the fertilized ovum to the uterine wall, develop abnormally.
   2. The mole manifests as an edematous grape-like cluster that may be nonmalignant or may develop into choriocarcinoma.
B. Assessment
   1. Fetal heart rate not detectable

2. Vaginal bleeding, which may occur by the fourth week or not until the second trimester; may be bright red or dark brown in color and may be slight, profuse, or intermittent
3. Symptoms of gestational hypertension, such as elevated blood pressure, edema, and proteinuria, before the twentieth week of gestation
4. Fundal height greater than expected for gestational date
5. Elevated human chorionic gonadotropin levels
6. Characteristic snowstorm pattern shown on ultrasound
C. Interventions
   1. Prepare the client for uterine evacuation (before evacuation, diagnostic tests are done to detect metastatic disease).
   2. Evacuation of the mole is done by vacuum aspiration; oxytocin is administered after evacuation to contract the **uterus**.
   3. Monitor for postprocedure hemorrhage and infection.
   4. Tissue is sent to the laboratory for evaluation, and follow-up is important to detect changes suggestive of malignancy.
   5. Human chorionic gonadotropin levels are monitored every 1 to 2 weeks until normal prepregnancy levels are attained; levels are checked every 1 to 2 months for 1 year.
   6. Instruct the client and her partner about birth control measures so that pregnancy can be prevented during the 1-year follow-up.

XIV. HYPEREMESIS GRAVIDARUM

A. Description: Intractable nausea and vomiting during the first trimester that causes disturbances in nutrition and fluid and electrolyte balance
B. Assessment
   1. Nausea most pronounced on arising; may occur at other times during the day
   2. Persistent vomiting
   3. Weight loss
   4. Signs of dehydration
   5. Fluid and electrolyte imbalances
C. Interventions
   1. Initiate measures to alleviate nausea, including medication therapy; if unsuccessful, and weight loss and fluid and electrolyte imbalances occur, intravenously administered fluid and electrolyte replacement or parenteral nutrition may be necessary.
   2. Monitor vital signs, intake and output, weight, and calorie count.
   3. Monitor laboratory data and for signs of dehydration and electrolyte imbalances.
   4. Monitor urine for ketones.
   5. Monitor fetal heart rate, activity, and growth.

6. Encourage intake of small portions of food (low-fat, easily digestible carbohydrates, such as cereals, rice, and pasta).
7. Liquids should be taken between meals to avoid distending the stomach and triggering vomiting.
8. Encourage the client to sit upright after meals.

XV. GESTATIONAL HYPERTENSION

A. Description and types: Hypertension can be mild or severe, leading to preeclampsia and then eclampsia (seizures) (Table 25-1).

⚠ Signs of preeclampsia are hypertension, generalized edema, and proteinuria.

B. Assessment (Table 25-2)
C. Predisposing conditions
   1. Primigravida
   2. Women younger than 19 years or older than 40 years
   3. Chronic renal disease
   4. Chronic hypertension
   5. Diabetes mellitus
   6. Rh incompatibility

7. History of or family history of gestational hypertension
D. Complications of gestational hypertension
   1. Abruptio placentae
   2. Disseminated intravascular coagulation
   3. Thrombocytopenia

TABLE 25-1 Classification of Hypertensive Stages of Pregnancy

Type	Description
Gestational Hypertensive Disorders	
Gestational hypertension	Blood pressure elevation detected first time after mid-pregnancy without proteinuria
Transient hypertension	Gestational hypertension with no signs of preeclampsia present at time of birth and hypertension resolves by 12 weeks after birth
Preeclampsia	Pregnancy-specific syndrome that usually occurs after 20 weeks of gestation and is determined by gestational hypertension plus proteinuria
Eclampsia	Occurrence of seizures in a preeclamptic woman
Chronic Hypertensive Disorders	
Chronic hypertension	Hypertension that is present and observable before pregnancy or that is diagnosed before week 20 of gestation
Preeclampsia superimposed on chronic hypertension	Chronic hypertension with new proteinuria or exacerbation of hypertension (previously well controlled) or proteinuria, thrombocytopenia, or increases in hepatocellular enzymes

Modified from Perry, S., Hockenberry, M., Lowdermilk, D., & Wilson, D. (2010). *Maternal child nursing care* (4th ed., p. 335). St. Louis: Mosby.

TABLE 25-2 Mild Versus Severe Preeclampsia

Parameter Evaluated	Mild	Severe
Systolic blood pressure	≥140 but <160 mm Hg	≥160 mm Hg (two readings, 6 hr apart, while on bed rest)
Diastolic blood pressure	≥90 but <110 mm Hg	≥110 mm Hg
Proteinuria (24-hr specimen is preferred to eliminate hour-to-hour variations)	≥0.3 but <2 g in 24-hr specimen (1+ on random dipstick)	≥5 g in 24-hr specimen (≥3+ on random dipstick sample)
Creatinine, serum (renal function)	Normal	Elevated (>1.2 mg/dL)
Platelets	Normal	Decreased (<100,000 cells/mm^3)
Liver enzymes (alanine aminotransferase or aspartate aminotransferase)	Normal or minimal increase in levels	Elevated levels
Urine output	Normal	Oliguria common, often <500 mL/day
Severe, unrelenting headache not attributable to other cause; mental confusion (cerebral edema)	Absent	Often present
Persistent right upper quadrant or epigastric pain or pain penetrating to back (distention of liver capsule); nausea and vomiting	Absent	May be present and often precedes seizure
Visual disturbances (spots or "sparkles"; temporary blindness; photophobia)	Absent to minimal	Common
Pulmonary edema; heart failure; cyanosis	Absent	May be present
Fetal growth restriction	Normal growth	Growth restriction; reduced amniotic fluid volume

From McKinney, E., James, S., Murray, S., & Ashwill, J. (2009). *Maternal-child nursing* (3rd ed., p. 625). St. Louis: Saunders.

4. Placental insufficiency
5. Intrauterine growth restriction
6. Intrauterine fetal death

E. Interventions for mild hypertension
1. Monitor blood pressure.
2. Monitor fetal activity and fetal growth.
3. Encourage frequent rest periods, instructing the client to lie in the lateral position.
4. Administer antihypertensive medications as prescribed; teach client about the importance of the medications.
5. Monitor intake and output.
6. Evaluate renal function through prescribed studies such as blood urea nitrogen, serum creatinine, and 24-hour urine levels for creatinine clearance and protein.

F. Interventions for mild preeclampsia
1. Provide bedrest and place the client in the lateral position.
2. Monitor blood pressure and weight.
3. Monitor neurological status because changes can indicate cerebral hypoxia or impending seizure.
4. Monitor deep tendon reflexes and for the presence of clonus because hyperreflexia indicates increased central nervous system irritability (Box 25-7).
5. Provide adequate fluids.
6. Monitor intake and output; a urinary output of 30 mL/hr indicates adequate renal perfusion.
7. Increase dietary protein and carbohydrates with no added salt.
8. Administer medications as prescribed to reduce blood pressure; blood pressure should not be reduced drastically because placental perfusion can be compromised.
9. Monitor for HELLP syndrome, a laboratory diagnosis for severe preeclampsia characterized by *h*emolysis, *e*levated *l*iver enzyme levels, and *l*ow *p*latelet count.

G. Interventions for severe preeclampsia
1. Maintain bed rest.
2. Administer magnesium sulfate (use a controlled infusion device) as prescribed to prevent seizures; magnesium sulfate may be continued for 24 to 48 hours postpartum.
3. Monitor for signs of magnesium toxicity, including flushing, sweating, hypotension, depressed deep tendon reflexes, and central nervous system depression including respiratory depression; keep antidote (calcium gluconate) at the client's bedside.
4. Administer antihypertensives as prescribed.
5. Prepare for the induction of **labor**.

H. Eclampsia
1. Assessment: Characterized by generalized seizures (Box 25-8)
2. Interventions (see Priority Nursing Actions)

Box 25-7 Assessment of Reflexes

Biceps
Position thumb over client's biceps tendon, supporting client's elbow with the palm of the hand
Strike a downward blow over the thumb with percussion hammer
Normal response: Flexion of the arm at the elbow

Patellar
Position client with her legs dangling over the edge of the examining table or lying on her back with her legs slightly flexed
Strike patellar tendon just below kneecap with percussion hammer
Normal response: Extension or kicking out of the leg

Clonus
Position client with her legs dangling over the edge of examining table
Support the leg with one hand and sharply dorsiflex client's foot with the other hand
Maintain the dorsiflexed position for a few seconds and then release foot
Normal response (negative clonus response)
- Foot remains steady in dorsiflexed position
- No rhythmic oscillations or jerking of foot is felt
- When released, foot drops to plantar-flexed position with no oscillations
Abnormal response (positive clonus response)
- Rhythmic oscillations occur when foot is dorsiflexed
- Similar oscillations are noted when foot drops to plantar-flexed position

Grading Response
0   Reflex absent
1+ Reflex present but hypoactive
2+ Normal reflex
3+ Hyperactive reflex
4+ Hyperactive reflex with clonus present

Box 25-8 Eclampsia

Seizure typically begins with twitching around the mouth
Body then becomes rigid in a state of tonic muscular contractions that last 15 to 20 seconds
Facial muscles and then all body muscles alternately contract and relax in rapid succession (clonic phase may last about 1 minute)
Respiration ceases during seizure because diaphragm tends to remain fixed (breathing resumes shortly after the seizure)
Postictal sleep occurs

XVI. INCOMPETENT CERVIX

A. Description
1. Incompetent cervix refers to premature dilation of the cervix, which occurs most often in the fourth or fifth month of pregnancy and is associated with structural or functional defects of the cervix.

■■■ **PRIORITY NURSING ACTIONS!** ■■■

Actions to Take in the Event of Eclampsia

1. Remain with the client and call for help.
2. Ensure an open airway, turn the client on her side, and administer oxygen by face mask at 8 to 10 L/min.
3. Monitor fetal heart rate patterns.
4. Administer medications to control the seizures as prescribed.
5. After the seizure, insert an oral airway and suction the client's mouth as needed.
6. Prepare for delivery of the fetus after stabilization of the client, if warranted.
7. Document occurrence, client's response, and outcome.

Eclampsia refers to the occurrence of a seizure. It is a potentially preventable extension of severe pre-eclampsia; early identification of preeclampsia in a pregnant client allows intervention before the condition reaches the seizure state. If eclampsia occurs, the nurse remains with the client and calls for help. The nurse ensures an open airway. If the client is not on her side already, the nurse attempts to turn the client on her side. The side-lying position permits greater circulation through the placenta and may help prevent aspiration. The nurse administers oxygen by face mask at 8 to 10 L/min to ensure adequate placental oxygenation. The nurse also notes the time the seizure began and the duration of the seizure and protects the client from injury during the event. The nurse monitors fetal heart rate patterns closely and administers medications as prescribed (magnesium sulfate may be prescribed). After the seizure, the nurse inserts an oral airway to maintain airway patency and suctions the client's mouth as needed. If warranted, the nurse prepares for the delivery of the fetus after stabilization of the client. The nurse documents the occurrence, the client's response, and the outcome.

References: McKinney, E., James, S., Murray, S., & Ashwill, J. (2009). *Maternal-child nursing.* (3rd ed., p. 629). St. Louis: Saunders.
Perry, S., Hockenberry, M., Lowdermilk, D., & Wilson, D. (2010). *Maternal child nursing care* (4th ed., p. 347). St. Louis: Mosby.

2. Treatment involves surgical placement of a cervical cerclage.
   B. Assessment
   1. Vaginal bleeding
   2. Fetal membranes visible through the cervix
   C. Interventions
   1. Provide bed rest, hydration, and tocolysis, as prescribed, to inhibit uterine contractions.
   2. Prepare for cervical cerclage (at 10 to 14 weeks' gestation) in which a band of fascia or nonabsorbable ribbon is placed around the cervix beneath the mucosa to constrict the internal os.
   3. After cervical cerclage, the client is told to refrain from intercourse and to avoid prolonged standing and heavy lifting.

4. The cervical cerclage is removed at 37 weeks' gestation or left in place and a cesarean birth is performed; if removed, cerclage must be repeated with each successive pregnancy.
5. After placement of the cervical cerclage, monitor for contractions, rupture of the membranes, and signs of infection.
6. Instruct the client to report to the health care provider immediately any postprocedure vaginal bleeding or increased uterine contractions.

XVII. INFECTIONS

A. Toxoplasmosis
   1. Caused by infection with the intracellular protozoan parasite *Toxoplasma gondii*
   2. Produces a rash and symptoms of acute, flu-like infection in the mother
   3. Transmitted to the mother through raw meat or handling of cat litter of infected cats
   4. Organism transmitted to the fetus across the **placenta**
   5. Can cause spontaneous abortion in the first trimester
B. Rubella (German measles)
   1. Teratogenic in the first trimester
   2. Organism transmitted to the fetus across the **placenta**
   3. Causes congenital defects of the eyes, heart, ears, and brain
   4. If not immune (titer less than 1:8), the client should be vaccinated in the postpartum period; the client must wait 1 to 3 months (as specified by health care provider) before becoming pregnant.
C. Cytomegalovirus
   1. Organism is transmitted through close personal contact; it is transmitted across the **placenta** to the fetus, or the fetus may be infected through the birth canal.
   2. The mother may be asymptomatic; most **infants** are asymptomatic at birth.
   3. Cytomegalovirus causes low birth weight, intrauterine growth restriction, enlarged liver and spleen, jaundice, blindness, hearing loss, and seizures.
   4. Antiviral medications may be prescribed for severe infections in the mother, but these medications are toxic and may only temporarily suppress shedding of the virus.
D. Herpes simplex virus
   1. Herpes simplex virus affects the external genitalia, **vagina**, and cervix and causes draining, painful vesicles.
   2. Virus usually is transmitted to the fetus during birth through the infected **vagina** or via an ascending infection after rupture of the membranes.

3. No vaginal examinations are done in the presence of active vaginal herpetic lesions.
4. Herpes can cause death or severe neurological impairment in the **newborn**.
5. **Delivery** of the fetus is usually by cesarean section if active lesions are present in the **vagina**; **delivery** may be performed vaginally if the lesions are in the anal, perineal, or inner thigh area (strict precautions are necessary to protect the fetus during **delivery**).
6. Maintain contact precautions.

E. Group B streptococcus (GBS)
1. GBS is a leading cause of life-threatening perinatal infections.
2. The gram-positive bacterium colonizes the rectum, **vagina**, cervix, and urethra of pregnant and nonpregnant women.
3. Meningitis, fasciitis, and intra-abdominal abscess can occur in the pregnant client if she is infected at the time of birth.
4. Transmission occurs during vaginal **delivery**.
5. Early-onset **newborn** GBS occurs within the first week after birth, usually within 48 hours, and can include infections such as sepsis, pneumonia, or meningitis; permanent neurological disability can result.
6. Diagnosis of the mother is done via vaginal and rectal cultures at 35 to 37 weeks' gestation.
7. Antibiotics such as penicillin may be prescribed for the mother during **labor** and birth; intravenous antibiotics may be prescribed for infected **infants**.

XVIII. MULTIPLE GESTATION

A. Description
1. Multiple gestation results from **fertilization** of two ova (fraternal or dizygotic) or a splitting of one fertilized ovum (identical or monozygotic).
2. Complications include spontaneous abortion, anemia, congenital anomalies, hyperemesis gravidarum, intrauterine growth restriction, gestational hypertension, polyhydramnios, postpartum hemorrhage, premature rupture of membranes, and preterm **labor** and **delivery**.

B. Assessment
1. Excessive fetal activity
2. **Uterus** large for gestational age
3. Palpation of three or four large parts in the **uterus**
4. Auscultation of more than one fetal heart rate
5. Excessive weight gain

C. Interventions
1. Monitor vital signs.
2. Monitor fetal heart rates, activity, and growth.
3. Monitor for cervical changes.
4. Prepare the client for ultrasound as prescribed.

5. Monitor for anemia; administer supplemental vitamins as prescribed.
6. Monitor for preterm **labor**, and treat preterm **labor** promptly.
7. Prepare for cesarean **delivery** for abnormal presentations.
8. Prepare to administer oxytocic medications after **delivery** to prevent postpartum hemorrhage from uterine overdistention.

XIX. PYELONEPHRITIS

A. Description
1. Results from bacterial infections that extend upward from the bladder through the blood vessels and lymphatics
2. Frequently follows untreated urinary tract infections and is associated with increased incidence of anemia, low birth weight, gestational hypertension, premature **labor** and **delivery**, and premature rupture of the membranes

B. Assessment
1. Flank pain
2. Burning or painful urination
3. Increased frequency of urination
4. Chills, malaise, nausea, and vomiting
5. Increased temperature, pulse rate, and fetal heart rate
6. Uterine contractions
7. Elevated white blood cell count

C. Interventions
1. Monitor vital signs.
2. Monitor fetal heart rate.
3. Monitor for uterine contractions.
4. Encourage fluids; monitor intake and output.
5. Monitor renal function.
6. Administer antibiotics as prescribed.
7. Administer antipyretics such as acetaminophen (Tylenol) as prescribed.
8. Obtain urine cultures every 2 to 4 weeks after resolution of infection.

XX. SEXUALLY TRANSMITTED INFECTIONS

A. *Chlamydia*
1. Description
   a. Sexually transmitted pathogen associated with an increased risk for premature birth, stillbirth, neonatal conjunctivitis, and **newborn** chlamydial pneumonia
   b. Can cause salpingitis, pelvic abscesses, ectopic pregnancy, chronic pelvic pain, and infertility
   c. Diagnostic test is culture for *Chlamydia trachomatis*
2. Assessment
   a. Usually asymptomatic
   b. Bleeding between periods or after coitus
   c. Mucoid or purulent cervical discharge
   d. Dysuria and pelvic pain

3. Interventions
   a. Screen the client to determine whether she is high risk; a vaginal culture is indicated for all pregnant clients if the client is in a high-risk group or if **infants** from previous pregnancies have developed neonatal conjunctivitis or pneumonia.
   b. Instruct the client in the importance of re-screening because reinfection can occur as the client nears term.
   c. Ensure that the sexual partner is treated.

B. Syphilis
   1. Description
      a. Syphilis is a chronic infectious disease caused by the organism *Treponema pallidum.*
      b. Transmission is by physical contact with syphilitic lesions, which usually are found on the skin, mucous membranes of the mouth, or genitals.
      c. The infection may cause abortion or premature **labor** and is passed to the fetus after the fourth month of pregnancy as congenital syphilis.
   2. Assessment (Box 25-9)
   3. Interventions
      a. Obtain a serum test (Venereal Disease Research Laboratory or rapid plasma reagin) for syphilis on the first prenatal visit; prepare to repeat the test at 36 weeks' gestation because the disease may be acquired after the initial visit.
      b. If the test result is positive, treatment with an antibiotic such as penicillin may be necessary.
      c. Instruct the client that treatment of her partner is necessary if infection is present.

Box 25-9 Stages of Syphilis

Primary Stage
Most infectious stage
Appearance of ulcerative, painless lesions produced by spirochetes at point of entry into the body

Secondary Stage
Highly infectious stage
Appearance of lesions about 6 weeks to 6 months after primary stage located anywhere on skin and mucous membranes
Generalized lymphadenopathy

Tertiary Stage
Entrance of spirochetes into internal organs, causing permanent damage; symptoms occur 10 to 30 years after untreated primary lesion
Invasion of central nervous system, causing meningitis, ataxia, general paresis, and progressive mental deterioration
Deleterious effects on aortic valve and aorta

C. Gonorrhea
   1. Description
      a. Gonorrhea is an infection caused by *Neisseria gonorrhoeae* that causes inflammation of the mucous membranes of the genital and urinary tracts.
      b. Transmission of the organism is by sexual intercourse.
      c. Infection may be transmitted to the **newborn's** eyes during **delivery**, causing blindness (ophthalmia neonatorum).
   2. Assessment: Usually asymptomatic; vaginal discharge, urinary frequency, and lower abdominal pain possible
   3. Interventions
      a. Obtain a vaginal culture during the initial prenatal examination to screen for gonorrhea; the culture may be repeated during the third trimester in high-risk clients.
      b. Instruct the client that treatment of her partner is necessary if infection is present.

D. Condyloma acuminatum (human papillomavirus)
   1. Description
      a. Condyloma acuminatum is caused by human papillomavirus.
      b. Infection affects the cervix, urethra, anus, penis, and scrotum.
      c. A culture is indicated for clients with a positive history or with active lesions, and weekly cultures may be done at week 35 or 36 of pregnancy until **delivery**; the test is performed to determine the route of **delivery**.
      d. Human papillomavirus is transmitted through sexual contact.
   2. Assessment
      a. Infection produces small to large wart-like growths on the genitals.
      b. Cervical cell changes may be noted because human papillomavirus is associated with cervical malignancies.
   3. Interventions
      a. Lesions are removed by the use of cytotoxic agents, cryotherapy, electrocautery, and laser.
      b. Encourage annual Papanicolaou smear.
      c. Sexual contact should be avoided until lesions are healed (condoms reduce transmission).

E. Trichomoniasis
   1. Description
      a. Trichomoniasis is caused by *Trichomonas vaginalis* and is transmitted via sexual contact.
      b. A normal saline wet smear of vaginal secretions indicates the presence of protozoa.
      c. Infection is associated with premature rupture of the membranes and postpartum endometritis.

2. Assessment
   a. Yellowish to greenish, frothy, mucopurulent, copious, malodorous vaginal discharge
   b. Inflammation of vulva, **vagina**, or both may occur
3. Interventions
   a. Metronidazole (Flagyl) may be prescribed.
   b. Sexual partner may need to be treated.

F. Bacterial vaginosis
1. Description
   a. Caused by *Haemophilus vaginalis* (*Gardnerella vaginalis*) and transmitted via sexual contact
   b. Associated with premature **labor** and birth
2. Assessment
   a. Client complains of "fishy odor" to vaginal secretions and increased odor after intercourse.
   b. Microscopic examination of vaginal secretions identifies the infection.
3. Interventions
   a. Oral metronidazole (Flagyl) may be prescribed.
   b. Sexual partner may need to be treated.

G. Vaginal candidiasis
1. Description
   a. *Candida albicans* is the most common causative organism.
   b. Predisposing factors include use of antibiotics, diabetes mellitus, and obesity.
   c. Vaginal candidiasis is diagnosed by identifying spores of *Candida albicans*.
2. Assessment
   a. Vulvar and vaginal pruritus
   b. White, lumpy, cottage cheese–like discharge from **vagina**
3. Interventions
   a. An antifungal vaginal preparation such as miconazole (Monistat) may be prescribed.
   b. For extensive irritation and swelling, sitz baths may be prescribed.
   c. Sexual partner may need to be treated.

XXI. TUBERCULOSIS

A. Description
1. Highly communicable disease caused by *Mycobacterium tuberculosis*
2. Transmitted by the airborne route
3. Multidrug-resistant strains of tuberculosis can result from improper compliance, noncompliance with treatment programs, or development of mutations in tubercle bacillus.

B. Transmission
1. Transplacental transmission is rare.
2. Transmission can occur during birth through aspiration of infected **amniotic fluid**.
3. The **newborn** can become infected from contact with infected individuals.

C. Risk to mother: Active disease during pregnancy has been associated with an increase in hypertensive disorders of pregnancy.

D. Diagnosis: If a chest radiograph is required for the mother, it is done only after 20 weeks of gestation, and a lead shield for the abdomen is required.

⚠ Tuberculin skin testing is safe during pregnancy; however the health care provider may want to delay testing until after delivery.

E. Assessment
1. Mother
   a. Possibly asymptomatic
   b. Fever and chills
   c. Night sweats
   d. Weight loss
   e. Fatigue
   f. Cough with hemoptysis or green or yellow sputum
   g. Dyspnea
   h. Pleural pain
2. Neonate
   a. Fever
   b. Lethargy
   c. Poor feeding
   d. Failure to thrive
   e. Respiratory distress
   f. Hepatosplenomegaly
   g. Meningitis
   h. Disease may spread to all major organs

F. Interventions
1. Pregnant client
   a. Administration of isoniazid (INH), pyrazinamide, and rifampin (Rifadin) daily for 9 months (as prescribed); ethambutol (Myambutol) is added if medication resistance is likely.
   b. Pyridoxine (vitamin B_6) should be administered with INH to the pregnant client to prevent fetal neurotoxicity caused by the INH.
   c. Promote breast-feeding only if the client is noninfectious.
2. **Newborn**
   a. Management focuses on preventing disease and treating early infection.
   b. Skin testing is performed on the **infant** at birth, and the infant may be placed on INH therapy; the skin test is repeated in 3 to 4 months, and INH may be stopped if the skin test results remain negative.
   c. If the skin test result is positive, the **infant** should receive INH for at least 6 months (as prescribed).
   d. If the mother's sputum is free of organisms, the **infant** does not need to be isolated from the mother while in the hospital.

XXII. URINARY TRACT INFECTION

A. Description: A urinary tract infection can occur during pregnancy (pregnancy is a predisposing factor); if untreated, the client can develop pyelonephritis.

B. Predisposing conditions
1. History of urinary tract infections
2. Sickle cell trait
3. Poor hygiene
4. Anemia
5. Diabetes mellitus

C. Assessment
1. Possibly asymptomatic during pregnancy
2. Burning and pain on urination
3. Increased frequency of urination
4. Lower abdominal pain and costovertebral angle tenderness
5. Fever
6. Proteinuria, hematuria, bacteriuria, and white blood cells in urine

D. Interventions
1. Monitor vital signs.
2. Monitor fetal heart rate.
3. Increase fluid intake and monitor intake and output.
4. Monitor urine for consistency and odor.
5. Monitor for signs and symptoms of pyelonephritis (dipstick test of urine for increase in protein, glucose, and ketone levels with each prenatal visit).
6. Obtain urine sample for culture and sensitivity.
7. Provide heat to lower abdomen or back.
8. Administer antibiotics as prescribed.
9. Instruct the client to complete the course of antibiotics if prescribed.
10. Instruct the client regarding the need to repeat the culture after treatment is completed.

● MORE QUESTIONS ON THE CD!

Practice Questions

236. A nurse is providing instructions to a pregnant client with human immunodeficiency virus (HIV) infection regarding care to the newborn infant after delivery. The client asks the nurse about the feeding options that are available. The best response by the nurse is:
1. "You will need to bottle-feed the newborn infant."
2. "You will need to feed the newborn infant by nasogastric tube feeding."
3. "You will be able to breast-feed for 6 months and then will need to switch to bottle-feeding."
4. "You will be able to breast-feed for 9 months and then will need to switch to bottle-feeding."

237. A home care nurse visits a pregnant client who has a diagnosis of mild preeclampsia. Which assessment finding indicates a worsening of the preeclampsia and the need to notify the physician?
1. Urinary output has increased.
2. Dependent edema has resolved.
3. Blood pressure reading is at the prenatal baseline.
4. The client complains of a headache and blurred vision.

238. A stillborn infant was delivered in the birthing suite a few hours ago. After the delivery, the family remained together, holding and touching the infant. Which statement by the nurse would further assist the family in their initial period of grief?
1. "What can I do for you?"
2. "Now you have an angel in heaven."
3. "Don't worry, there is nothing you could have done to prevent this from happening."
4. "We will see to it that you have an early discharge so that you don't have to be reminded of this experience."

239. A nurse implements a teaching plan for a pregnant client who is newly diagnosed with gestational diabetes mellitus. Which statement made by the client indicates a need for further teaching?
1. "I should stay on the diabetic diet."
2. "I should perform glucose monitoring at home."
3. "I should avoid exercise because of the negative effects on insulin production."
4. "I should be aware of any infections and report signs of infection immediately to my health care provider."

240. A pregnant client in the last trimester has been admitted to the hospital with a diagnosis of severe preeclampsia. A nurse monitors for complications associated with the diagnosis and assesses the client for:
1. Enlargement of the breasts
2. Complaints of feeling hot when the room is cool
3. Periods of fetal movement followed by quiet periods
4. Evidence of bleeding, such as in the gums, petechiae, and purpura

241. A nurse in a maternity unit is reviewing the records of the clients on the unit. Which client would the nurse identify as being at the greatest risk for developing disseminated intravascular coagulation?
1. A primigravida with mild preeclampsia
2. A primigravida who delivered a 10-lb infant 3 hours ago
3. A gravida II who has just been diagnosed with dead fetus syndrome
4. A gravida IV who delivered 8 hours ago and has lost 500 mL of blood

242. A client in the first trimester of pregnancy arrives at a health care clinic and reports that she has been experiencing vaginal bleeding. A threatened abortion is suspected, and the nurse instructs the client regarding management of care. Which statement made by the client indicates a need for further instructions?
1. "I will watch for the evidence of the passage of tissue."
2. "I will maintain strict bedrest throughout the remainder of the pregnancy."
3. "I will count the number of perineal pads used on a daily basis and note the amount and color of blood on the pad."
4. "I will avoid sexual intercourse until the bleeding has stopped, and for 2 weeks following the last evidence of bleeding."

243. The nurse is assessing a pregnant client with type 1 diabetes mellitus about her understanding regarding changing insulin needs during pregnancy. The nurse determines that teaching is needed if the client makes which statement?
1. "I will need to increase my insulin dosage during the first 3 months of pregnancy."
2. "My insulin dose will likely need to be increased during the second and third trimesters."
3. "Episodes of hypoglycemia are more likely to occur during the first 3 months of pregnancy."
4. "My insulin needs should return to normal within 7 to 10 days after birth if I am bottle-feeding."

244. A pregnant client reports to a health care clinic, complaining of loss of appetite, weight loss, and fatigue. After assessment of the client, tuberculosis is suspected. A sputum culture is obtained and identifies *Mycobacterium tuberculosis*. The nurse provides instructions to the client regarding therapeutic management of the tuberculosis and the nurse tells the client that:
1. Therapeutic abortion is required.
2. She will have to stay at home until treatment is completed.
3. Medication will not be started until after delivery of the fetus.
4. Isoniazid (INH) plus rifampin (Rifadin) will be required for 9 months.

245. A nurse is providing instructions to a maternity client with a history of cardiac disease regarding appropriate dietary measures. Which statement, if made by the client, indicates an

understanding of the information provided by the nurse?
1. "I should increase my sodium intake during pregnancy."
2. "I should lower my blood volume by limiting my fluids."
3. "I should maintain a low-calorie diet to prevent any weight gain."
4. "I should drink adequate fluids and increase my intake of high-fiber foods."

246. A clinic nurse is performing a psychosocial assessment of a client who has been told that she is pregnant. Which assessment finding indicates to the nurse that the client is at high risk for contracting human immunodeficiency virus (HIV)?
1. A client who has a history of intravenous drug use
2. A client who has a significant other who is heterosexual
3. A client who has a history of sexually transmitted diseases
4. A client who has had one sexual partner for the past 10 years

247. A nurse in a maternity unit is providing emotional support to a client and her husband who are preparing to be discharged from the hospital after the birth of a dead fetus. Which statement made by the client indicates a component of the normal grieving process?
1. "We want to attend a support group."
2. "We never want to try to have a baby again."
3. "We are going to try to adopt a child immediately."
4. "We are okay, and we are going to try to have another baby immediately."

248. A nurse evaluates the ability of a hepatitis B–positive mother to provide safe bottle-feeding to her infant during postpartum hospitalization. Which maternal action best exemplifies the mother's knowledge of potential disease transmission to the infant?
1. The mother requests that the window be closed before feeding.
2. The mother holds the infant properly during feeding and burping.
3. The mother tests the temperature of the formula before initiating feeding.
4. The mother washes and dries her hands before and after self-care of the perineum and asks for a pair of gloves before feeding.

Alternate Item Format: Multiple Response

249. A home care nurse is monitoring a pregnant client with gestational hypertension who is at risk for preeclampsia. At each home care visit, the nurse assesses the client for which classic signs of preeclampsia? **Select all that apply**.

❑ 1. Proteinuria
❑ 2. Hypertension
❑ 3. Low-grade fever
❑ 4. Generalized edema
❑ 5. Increased pulse rate
❑ 6. Increased respiratory rate

ANSWERS

236. 1

Rationale: Perinatal transmission of human immunodeficiency virus (HIV) can occur during the antepartal period, during labor and birth, or in the postpartum period if the mother is breast-feeding. Clients who have HIV are advised not to breast-feed. There is no physiological reason why the newborn needs to be fed by nasogastric tube.

Test-Taking Strategy: Use the process of elimination and knowledge regarding the transmission of HIV. Eliminate options 3 and 4 first because these options are comparable or alike in that they both address breast-feeding. From the remaining options, select option 1, knowing that it is unnecessary to feed the infant by nasogastric tube. Review feeding options for newborns of HIV-positive clients if you had difficulty with this question.

Level of Cognitive Ability: Applying
Client Needs: Safe and Effective Care Environment
Integrated Process: Teaching and Learning
Content Area: Maternity—Postpartum
Reference: McKinney, E., James, S., Murray, S., & Ashwill, J. (2009). *Maternal-child nursing* (3rd ed., pp. 751, 754). St. Louis: Saunders.

237. 4

Rationale: If the client complains of a headache and blurred vision, the physician should be notified because these are signs of worsening preeclampsia. Options 1, 2, and 3 are normal signs.

Test-Taking Strategy: Use the process of elimination, noting the strategic word *worsening* in the question. Eliminate options 1, 2, and 3 because these options indicate normal findings. Review the signs that indicate a worsening of preeclampsia if you had difficulty with this question.

Level of Cognitive Ability: Analyzing
Client Needs: Physiological Integrity
Integrated Process: Nursing Process—Assessment
Content Area: Maternity—Antepartum
Reference: Perry, S., Hockenberry, M., Lowdermilk, D., & Wilson, D. (2010). *Maternal-child nursing care* (4th ed., pp. 336, 342). St. Louis: Mosby.

238. 1

Rationale: When a loss or death occurs, the nurse should ensure that parents have been honestly told about the situation by their physician or others on the health care team. It is important for the nurse to be with the parents at this time and to use therapeutic communication techniques. The nurse must also consider cultural and religious practices and beliefs.

Option 1 provides a supportive, giving, and caring response. Options 2, 3, and 4 are blocks to communication and devalue the parents' feelings.

Test-Taking Strategy: Use the process of elimination and knowledge of therapeutic communication techniques to answer the question. Option 1 is the only option that reflects use of therapeutic communication techniques. Review these techniques and the nursing strategies for caring for parents who experience perinatal death if you had difficulty with this question.

Level of Cognitive Ability: Applying
Client Needs: Psychosocial Integrity
Integrated Process: Caring
Content Area: Maternity—Postpartum
Reference: Perry, S., Hockenberry, M., Lowdermilk, D., & Wilson, D. (2010). *Maternal child nursing care* (4th ed., pp. 601–602). St. Louis: Mosby.

239. 3

Rationale: Exercise is safe for a client with gestational diabetes mellitus and is helpful in lowering the blood glucose level. Dietary modifications are the mainstay of treatment, and the client is placed on a standard diabetic diet. Many clients are taught to perform blood glucose monitoring. If the client is not performing the blood glucose monitoring at home, it is performed at the clinic or health care provider's office. Signs of infection need to be reported to the health care provider.

Test-Taking Strategy: Use the process of elimination, noting the strategic words *need for further teaching*. These words indicate a negative event query and the need to select an incorrect client statement. Noting these strategic words and the close-ended word *avoid* in option 3 will assist in answering the question. If you had difficulty with this question, review the teaching points for a client with gestational diabetes mellitus.

Level of Cognitive Ability: Evaluating
Client Needs: Physiological Integrity
Integrated Process: Teaching and Learning
Content Area: Maternity—Antepartum
Reference: McKinney, E., James, S., Murray, S., & Ashwill, J. (2009). *Maternal-child nursing* (3rd ed., p. 641). St. Louis: Saunders.

240. 4

Rationale: Severe preeclampsia can trigger disseminated intravascular coagulation (DIC) because of the widespread damage to vascular integrity. Bleeding is an early sign of

DIC and should be reported to the health care provider if noted on assessment. Options 1, 2, and 3 are normal occurrences in the last trimester of pregnancy.

Test-Taking Strategy: Focus on the subject, a complication of severe preeclampsia. Eliminate options 1, 2, and 3 because they are normal occurrences in the last trimester of pregnancy. Review the assessment findings in DIC if you had difficulty with this question.

Level of Cognitive Ability: Analyzing
Client Needs: Physiological Integrity
Integrated Process: Nursing Process—Assessment
Content Area: Maternity—Antepartum
Reference: Perry, S., Hockenberry, M., Lowdermilk, D., & Wilson, D. (2010). *Maternal child nursing care* (4th ed., p. 367). St. Louis: Mosby.

241. 3
Rationale: In a pregnant client, disseminated intravascular coagulation (DIC) is a condition in which the clotting cascade is activated, resulting in the formation of clots in the microcirculation. Dead fetus syndrome is considered a risk factor for DIC. Severe preeclampsia is considered a risk factor for DIC; a mild case is not. Delivering a large infant is not considered a risk factor for DIC. Hemorrhage is a risk factor for DIC; however, a loss of 500 mL is not considered hemorrhage.

Test-Taking Strategy: Focus on the subject, the client at greatest risk for DIC. Think about the pathophysiology associated with DIC and recall that dead fetus syndrome is a risk factor. This will direct you to option 3. If you had difficulty answering this question, review the risk factors for DIC.

Level of Cognitive Ability: Analyzing
Client Needs: Physiological Integrity
Integrated Process: Nursing Process—Analysis
Content Area: Maternity—Intrapartum
Reference: Perry, S., Hockenberry, M., Lowdermilk, D., & Wilson, D. (2010). *Maternal-child nursing care* (4th ed., p. 367). St. Louis: Mosby.

242. 2
Rationale: Strict bedrest throughout the remainder of the pregnancy is not required for a threatened abortion. The client is advised to curtail sexual activities until bleeding has ceased and for 2 weeks after the last evidence of bleeding or as recommended by the physician or other health care provider. The client is instructed to count the number of perineal pads used daily and to note the quantity and color of blood on the pad. The client also should watch for the evidence of the passage of tissue.

Test-Taking Strategy: Use the process of elimination. Note the strategic words *need for further instructions* in the question. These words indicate a negative event query and the need to select an incorrect client statement. Noting the word *strict* in option 2 will assist in directing you to this option. Review therapeutic management for a threatened abortion if you had difficulty with this question.

Level of Cognitive Ability: Evaluating
Client Needs: Physiological Integrity
Integrated Process: Teaching and Learning
Content Area: Maternity—Antepartum

Reference: McKinney, E., James, S., Murray, S., & Ashwill, J. (2009). *Maternal-child nursing* (3rd ed., p. 608). St. Louis: Saunders.

243. 1
Rationale: Insulin needs decrease in the first trimester of pregnancy because of increased insulin production by the pancreas and increased peripheral sensitivity to insulin. The statements in options 2, 3, and 4 are accurate and signify that the client understands control of her diabetes during pregnancy.

Test-Taking Strategy: Note the strategic words *teaching is needed*. These words indicate a negative event query and the need to select an incorrect client statement. Eliminate options 2, 3, and 4 because they are accurate statements. Remember that insulin needs decrease in the first trimester of pregnancy. Review the insulin needs of the pregnant client with diabetes mellitus if you had difficulty with this question.

Level of Cognitive Ability: Evaluating
Client Needs: Physiological Integrity
Integrated Process: Teaching and Learning
Content Area: Maternity—Antepartum
Reference: Perry, S., Hockenberry, M., Lowdermilk, D., & Wilson, D. (2010). *Maternal child nursing care* (4th ed., pp. 297–298). St. Louis: Mosby.

244. 4
Rationale: More than one medication may be used to prevent the growth of resistant organisms in a pregnant client with tuberculosis. Treatment must continue for a prolonged period. The preferred treatment for the pregnant client is isoniazid (INH) plus rifampin daily for 9 months. Ethambutol is added initially if medication resistance is suspected. Pyridoxine (vitamin B$_6$) often is administered with INH to prevent fetal neurotoxicity. The client does not need to stay at home during treatment, and therapeutic abortion is not required.

Test-Taking Strategy: Focus on the subject, the therapeutic management for a client with tuberculosis. Recalling the pathophysiology associated with tuberculosis and its treatment will assist in eliminating options 1, 2, and 3. If you had difficulty with this question, review the treatment measures for the client with tuberculosis.

Level of Cognitive Ability: Applying
Client Needs: Physiological Integrity
Integrated Process: Teaching and Learning
Content Area: Maternity—Antepartum
Reference: McKinney, E., James, S., Murray, S., & Ashwill, J. (2009). *Maternal-child nursing* (3rd ed., p. 658). St. Louis: Saunders.

245. 4
Rationale: Valsalva maneuver should be avoided in clients with cardiac disease because it can cause blood to rush to the heart and overload the cardiac system. Constipation can cause the client to use Valsalva maneuver. High-fiber foods are important. A low-calorie diet is not recommended during pregnancy and could be harmful to the fetus. Diets low in fluid can cause a decrease in blood volume, which could deprive the fetus of nutrients, so adequate fluid intake and high-fiber foods are important. Sodium should be restricted as prescribed by the physician because excess

sodium would cause an overload to the circulating blood volume and contribute to cardiac complications.

Test-Taking Strategy: Use the process of elimination. Think about the physiology of the cardiac system, maternal and fetal needs, and the factors that increase the workload on the heart. This will direct you to option 4. If you had difficulty with this question, review nursing measures for a pregnant client with cardiac disease.

Level of Cognitive Ability: Evaluating
Client Needs: Physiological Integrity
Integrated Process: Nursing Process—Evaluation
Content Area: Maternity—Antepartum
Reference: Perry, S., Hockenberry, M., Lowdermilk, D., & Wilson, D. (2010). *Maternal child nursing care* (4th ed., p. 314). St. Louis: Mosby.

246. 1
Rationale: Human immunodeficiency virus (HIV) is transmitted by intimate sexual contact and the exchange of body fluids, exposure to infected blood, and passage from an infected woman to her fetus. Clients who fall into the high-risk category for HIV infection include individuals with persistent and recurrent sexually transmitted infections, individuals who have a history of multiple sexual partners, and individuals who have used intravenous drugs. A client with a heterosexual partner, particularly a client who has had only one sexual partner in 10 years, does not have a high risk for contracting HIV.

Test-Taking Strategy: Use the process of elimination. Recalling that exchange of blood and body fluids places the client at high risk for HIV infection will direct you to option 1. If you had difficulty with this question, review the risk factors for HIV.

Level of Cognitive Ability: Analyzing
Client Needs: Safe and Effective Care Environment
Integrated Process: Nursing Process—Assessment
Content Area: Maternity—Antepartum
Reference: Perry, S., Hockenberry, M., Lowdermilk, D., & Wilson, D. (2010). *Maternal child nursing care* (4th ed., p. 97). St. Louis: Mosby.

247. 1
Rationale: A support group can help the parents work through their pain by nonjudgmental sharing of feelings. Option 1 identifies a statement that would indicate positive, normal grieving. Although the other options may indicate reactions of the client and significant other, they are not specifically a part of the normal grieving process.

Test-Taking Strategy: Read all the options carefully before selecting an answer and focus on the subject of the question, the normal grieving process. Note that options 2, 3, and 4 are comparable or alike in that they relate to childbearing. If you had difficulty with this question, review the components of the normal grieving process.

Level of Cognitive Ability: Analyzing
Client Needs: Psychosocial Integrity
Integrated Process: Caring
Content Area: Maternity—Postpartum
Reference: Perry, S., Hockenberry, M., Lowdermilk, D., & Wilson, D. (2010). *Maternal child nursing care* (4th ed., p. 606). St. Louis: Mosby.

248. 4
Rationale: Hepatitis B virus is highly contagious and is transmitted by direct contact with blood and body fluids of infected persons. The rationale for identifying childbearing clients with this disease is to provide adequate protection of the fetus and the newborn, to minimize transmission to other individuals, and to reduce maternal complications. Option 4 provides the best evaluation of maternal understanding of disease transmission. Option 1 will not affect disease transmission. Options 2 and 3 are appropriate feeding techniques for bottle-feeding, but do not minimize disease transmission for hepatitis B.

Test-Taking Strategy: Focus on the subject of the question, disease transmission to the infant. This focus and the process of elimination will direct you to option 4. Review measures to prevent transmission of hepatitis if you had difficulty with this question.

Level of Cognitive Ability: Evaluating
Client Needs: Safe and Effective Care Environment
Integrated Process: Nursing Process—Evaluation
Content Area: Maternity—Postpartum
Reference: Perry, S., Hockenberry, M., Lowdermilk, D., & Wilson, D. (2010). *Maternal child nursing care* (4th ed., pp. 750–751). St. Louis: Mosby.

ALTERNATE ITEM FORMAT: MULTIPLE RESPONSE
249. 1, 2, 4
Rationale: The three classic signs of preeclampsia are hypertension, generalized edema, and proteinuria. A low-grade fever, increased pulse rate, or increased respiratory rate is not associated with preeclampsia.

Test-Taking Strategy: Focus on the subject, the classic signs of preeclampsia. Thinking about the pathophysiology associated with preeclampsia will direct you to the correct options. Remember that the three classic signs of preeclampsia are hypertension, generalized edema, and proteinuria. Review the signs of preeclampsia if you had difficulty with this question.

Level of Cognitive Ability: Analyzing
Client Needs: Physiological Integrity
Integrated Process: Nursing Process—Assessment
Content Area: Maternity—Antepartum
Reference: Perry, S., Hockenberry, M., Lowdermilk, D., & Wilson, D. (2010). *Maternal child nursing care* (4th ed., p. 337). St. Louis: Mosby.

Labor and Delivery

I. PROCESS OF LABOR—FOUR *P*'s

A. Description
 1. **Labor**: Coordinated sequence of involuntary, intermittent uterine contractions
 2. **Delivery**: Actual event of birth
B. Four major factors (four *P*'s) interact during normal childbirth; the four *P*'s are interrelated and depend on each other for a safe **delivery** (Box 26-1).
C. Powers: Uterine contractions
 1. Forces acting to expel the fetus
 2. Effacement: Shortening and thinning of the cervix during the first stage of **labor**
 3. Dilation: Enlargement of cervical os and cervical canal during the first stage of **labor**
 4. Pushing efforts of mother during the second stage
D. Passageway: The mother's rigid bony pelvis and the soft tissues of the cervix, pelvic floor, **vagina**, and introitus (external opening to the **vagina**)
E. Passenger: The fetus, membranes, and **placenta**
F. Psyche: A woman's emotional structure that can determine her entire response to **labor** and influence physiological and psychological functioning; the mother may experience anxiety or fear.
G. Attitude
 1. Attitude is the relationship of the fetal body parts to one another.
 2. Normal intrauterine attitude is flexion, in which the fetal back is rounded, the head is forward on the chest, and the arms and legs are folded in against the body. The other attitude, extension, tends to present larger fetal diameters.
H. Lie
 1. Relationship of the spine of the fetus to the spine of the mother
 2. Longitudinal or vertical (Fig. 26-1)
  a. Fetal spine is parallel to the mother's spine.
  b. Fetus is in cephalic or breech presentation.
 3. Transverse or horizontal (see Fig. 26-1)
  a. Fetal spine is at a right angle, or perpendicular, to the mother's spine.
  b. Presenting part is the shoulder.
  c. **Delivery** by cesarean section is necessary.

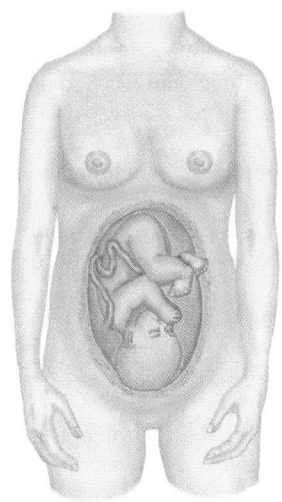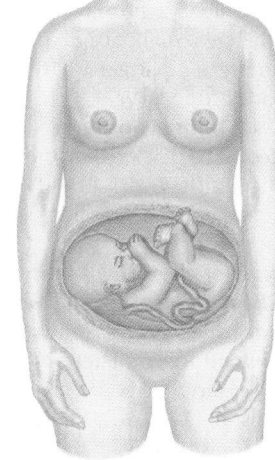

A   Longitudinal lie   B   Transverse lie

▲ **FIGURE 26-1** Fetal lie. **A,** In a longitudinal lie, the long axis of the fetus is parallel to the long axis of the mother. **B,** In a transverse lie, the long axis of the fetus is at a right angle to the long axis of the mother. The mother's abdomen has a wide, short appearance. (From McKinney, E., James, S., Murray, S., & Ashwill, J. [2009]. *Maternal-child nursing* [3rd ed.]. St. Louis: Saunders.)

I. Presentation
 1. Portion of the fetus that enters the pelvic inlet first
 2. Cephalic: Head first
  a. Cephalic is the most common presentation.
  b. Cephalic presentation has four variations—vertex, military, brow, and face.
 3. Breech: Buttocks present first.
  a. **Delivery** by cesarean section may be required, although vaginal birth is often possible.
  b. Breech presentation has three variations—frank, full (complete), and footling

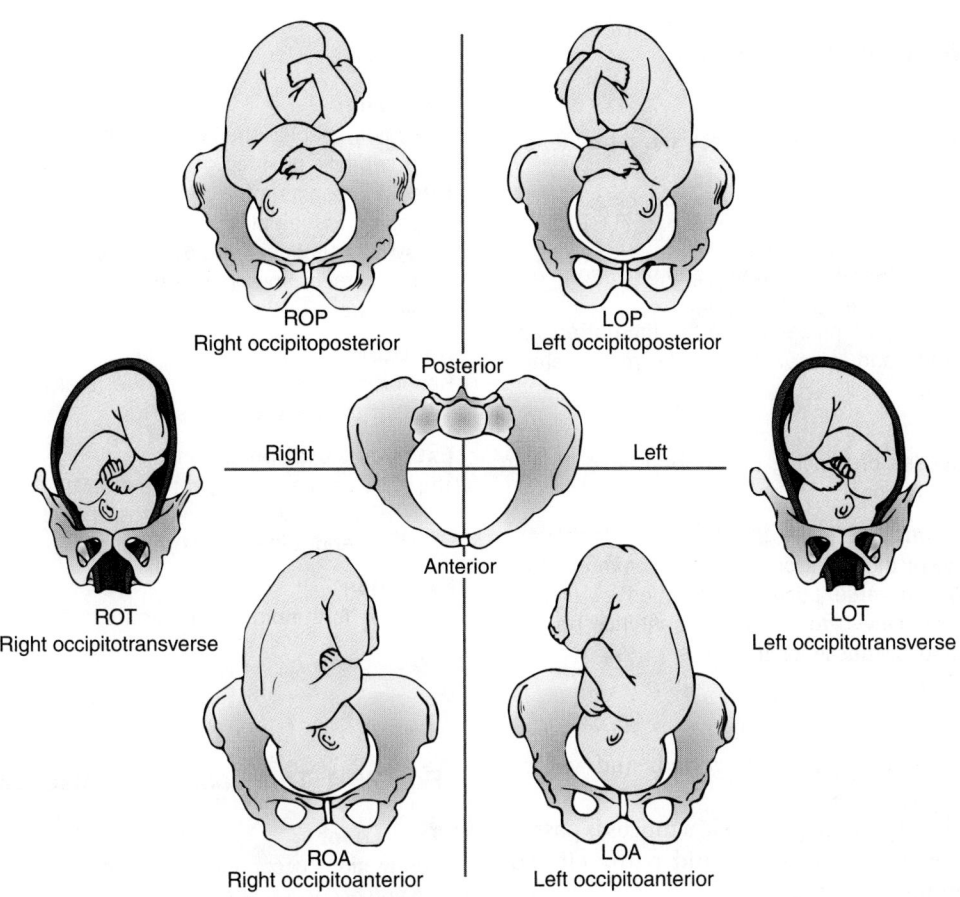

Right occipitoposterior — ROP

Left occipitoposterior — LOP

Posterior

Right

Left

Anterior

ROT
Right occipitotransverse

LOT
Left occipitotransverse

ROA
Right occipitoanterior

LOA
Left occipitoanterior

Lie: Longitudinal or vertical
Presentation: Vertex
Reference point: Occiput
Attitude: Complete flexion

▲ FIGURE 26-2 Fetal vertex (occiput) presentations in relation to the front, back, or side of the maternal pelvis. (From Perry, S., Hockenberry, M., Lowdermilk, D., & Wilson, D. [2010]. *Maternal child nursing care* [4th ed.]. St. Louis: Mosby.)

4. Shoulder
   a. Fetus is in a transverse lie, or the arm, back, abdomen, or side could present.
   b. If the fetus does not spontaneously rotate, or if it is impossible to turn the fetus manually, a cesarean section may need to be performed.
J. **Presenting part:** The specific fetal structure lying nearest to the cervix
K. **Position:** Relationship of assigned area of the presenting part or landmark to the maternal pelvis (Fig. 26-2, Box 26-2)
L. Station
   1. The measurement of the progress of descent in centimeters above or below the midplane from the presenting part to the ischial spine
   2. Station 0: At ischial spine
   3. Minus station: Above ischial spine
   4. Plus station: Below ischial spine
   5. Engagement: When the widest diameter of the presenting part has passed the inlet; usually corresponds to a 0 station

Box 26-2 Fetal Positions

ROA	Right occipitoanterior
LOA	Left occipitoanterior
ROP	Right occipitoposterior
LOP	Left occipitoposterior
ROT	Right occipitotransverse
LOT	Left occipitotransverse
RMA	Right mentum anterior
LMA	Left mentoanterior
RMP	Right mentoposterior
LSA	Left sacroanterior
LSP	Left sacroposterior

II. MECHANISMS OF LABOR (Box 26-3)

A. Assessment
   1. Lightening or dropping: Is also known as engagement and occurs when the fetus descends into the pelvis about 2 weeks before **delivery**; lightening or dropping is most noticeable in first pregnancies
   2. Braxton Hicks contractions increase.

Box 26-3 Mechanisms of Labor

Engagement
Engagement is the mechanism whereby the fetus nestles into the pelvis.
Engagement also is termed *lightening* or *dropping*.

Descent
Descent is the process that the fetal head undergoes as it begins its journey through the pelvis.
Descent is a continuous process from the time of engagement until birth and is assessed by the measurement called station.

Flexion
Flexion is a process of nodding of the fetal head forward toward the fetal chest.

Internal Rotation
Internal rotation of the fetus occurs most commonly from the occipitotransverse position, assumed at engagement into the pelvis, to the occipitoanterior position while continuously descending.

Extension
Extension enables the head to emerge when the fetus is in a cephalic position.
Extension begins after the head crowns.
Extension is complete when the head passes under the symphysis pubis and occiput, and the anterior fontanel, brow, face, and chin pass over the sacrum and coccyx and are over the perineum.

Restitution
Restitution is realignment of the fetal head with the body after the head emerges.

External Rotation
The shoulders externally rotate after the head emerges and restitution occurs, so that the shoulders are in the anteroposterior diameter of the pelvis.

Expulsion
Expulsion is the birth of the entire body.

---

3. The vaginal mucosa is congested, and vaginal discharge increases.
4. Brownish or blood-tinged cervical mucus is passed.
5. Cervix ripens, becomes soft and partly effaced, and may begin to dilate.
6. The mother has a sudden burst of energy, also known as "nesting," often 24 to 48 hours before onset of **labor**.
7. Weight loss of 1 to 3 lb results from fluid shifts produced by the changes in progesterone and estrogen levels 24 to 48 hours before the onset of **labor**.
8. Spontaneous rupture of membranes occurs.
B. True **labor**: Contractions may manifest as back pain in some women; contractions often resemble menstrual cramps during early **labor** (Box 26-4).
C. False **labor**: Also known as prodromal **labor**, contractions are felt in the abdomen and groin and may be more annoying than painful (see Box 26-4).

⚠️ In true labor, contractions increase in duration and intensity. In false labor, contractions are irregular and do not produce dilation, effacement, or descent.

III. LEOPOLD'S MANEUVERS

A. Description: Methods of palpation to determine presentation and position of the fetus and aid in location of fetal heart sounds
B. If the head is in the fundus, a hard, round, movable object is felt. The buttocks feel soft and have an irregular shape and are more difficult to move.
C. The fetus' back, which is a smooth, hard surface, should be felt on one side of the abdomen.

Box 26-4 True Labor and False Labor

True Labor
Contractions occur regularly, become stronger, last longer, and occur closer together.
Cervical dilation and effacement are progressive.
The fetus usually becomes engaged in the pelvis and begins to descend.

False Labor
False labor does not produce dilation, effacement, or descent.
Contractions are irregular, without progression.
Activity, such as walking, often relieves false labor.
Example: If a woman has been sleeping and wakes up with contractions, gets up, and moves around, and her contractions become stronger and closer together, this is true labor. If the contractions go away, this is false labor.

D. Irregular knobs and lumps, which may be the hands, feet, elbows, and knees, are felt on the opposite side of the abdomen.

IV. BREATHING TECHNIQUES (Box 26-5)

A. Provide a focus during contractions, interfering with pain sensory transmission
B. Promote relaxation and oxygenation
C. Begin with simple breathing patterns and progress to more complex ones as needed.

V. FETAL MONITORING

A. Description
1. The fetal monitor displays the fetal heart rate (FHR).

Box 26-5 Breathing Techniques

First-Stage Breathing

Cleansing Breath
Each contraction begins and ends with a deep inspiration and expiration.

Slow-Paced Breathing
Slow-paced breathing promotes relaxation.
Slow-paced breathing is used as long as possible during labor.

Modified-Paced Breathing
Modified-paced breathing is used when slow-paced breathing is no longer effective.
Breathing is shallow and fast.

Pattern-Paced Breathing
Pattern-paced breathing sometimes is referred to as pant-blow.
After a certain number of breaths (modified-paced breathing), the woman exhales with a slight blow, and then begins modified-paced breathing again.

Breathing to Prevent Pushing
The woman blows repeatedly using short puffs when the urge to push is strong.

Second-Stage Breathing
Several variations of breathing can be used in the pushing stage of labor, and the woman may grunt, groan, sigh, or moan as she pushes. Prolonged breath holding while pushing with a closed glottis may result in a decrease in cardiac output. If breath holding while pushing is used, the open glottis method or limiting breath holding to less than 6 to 8 seconds should be done.

2. The device monitors uterine activity.
3. The monitor assesses frequency, duration, and intensity of contractions.
4. The monitor assesses FHR in relation to maternal contractions.
5. Baseline FHR is measured between contractions; the normal FHR at term is 120 to 160 beats/min.

B. External fetal monitoring
1. External fetal monitoring is noninvasive and is performed using a tocotransducer or Doppler ultrasonic transducer.
2. Leopold's maneuvers are performed to determine on which side the fetal back is located, and the ultrasound transducer is placed over this area (fasten with a belt).
3. The tocotransducer is placed over the fundus of the uterus where contractions feel the strongest (fasten with a belt).
4. The client is allowed to assume a comfortable position, avoiding vena cava compression (maternal supine hypotensive syndrome).
5. The preferred position is to have the client lie on her side to increase perfusion.

Box 26-6 Variability in Fetal Heart Rate

Absent variability: Undetected variability
Minimal variability: Greater than undetected but not more than 5 beats/min
Moderate variability: Fetal heart rate fluctuations are 6 to 25 beats/min
Marked variability: Fetal heart rate fluctuations are greater than 25 beats/min

C. Internal fetal monitoring
1. Internal fetal monitoring is invasive and requires rupturing of the membranes and attaching an electrode to the presenting part of the fetus.
2. The client must be dilated 2 to 3 cm to perform internal monitoring.

D. Periodic patterns in FHR
1. Fetal bradycardia and tachycardia
   a. Bradycardia: FHR is less than 120 beats/min for 10 minutes or longer.
   b. Tachycardia: FHR is more than 160 beats/min for 10 minutes or longer.

⚠ If fetal bradycardia or tachycardia occurs, change the position of the mother, administer oxygen, and assess the mother's vital signs. Notify the health care provider as soon as possible.

2. Variability (Box 26-6)
   a. Fluctuations in baseline FHR
   b. Absent or undetected variability is considered nonreassuring.
   c. Decreased variability can result from fetal hypoxemia, acidosis, or certain medications.
   d. A temporary decrease in variability can occur when the fetus is in a sleep state (sleep states do not usually last longer than 30 minutes).
3. Accelerations
   a. Brief, temporary increases in FHR of at least 15 beats more than baseline and lasting at least 15 seconds
   b. Usually are a reassuring sign, reflecting a responsive, nonacidotic fetus
   c. Usually occur with fetal movement
   d. May be nonperiodic (having no relation to contractions) or periodic
   e. May occur with uterine contractions, vaginal examinations, or mild cord compression, or when the fetus is in a breech presentation.
4. Early decelerations (Fig. 26-3)
   a. Early decelerations are decreases in FHR below baseline; the rate at the lowest point of the deceleration usually remains greater than 100 beats/min.
   b. Early decelerations occur during contractions as the fetal head is pressed against the

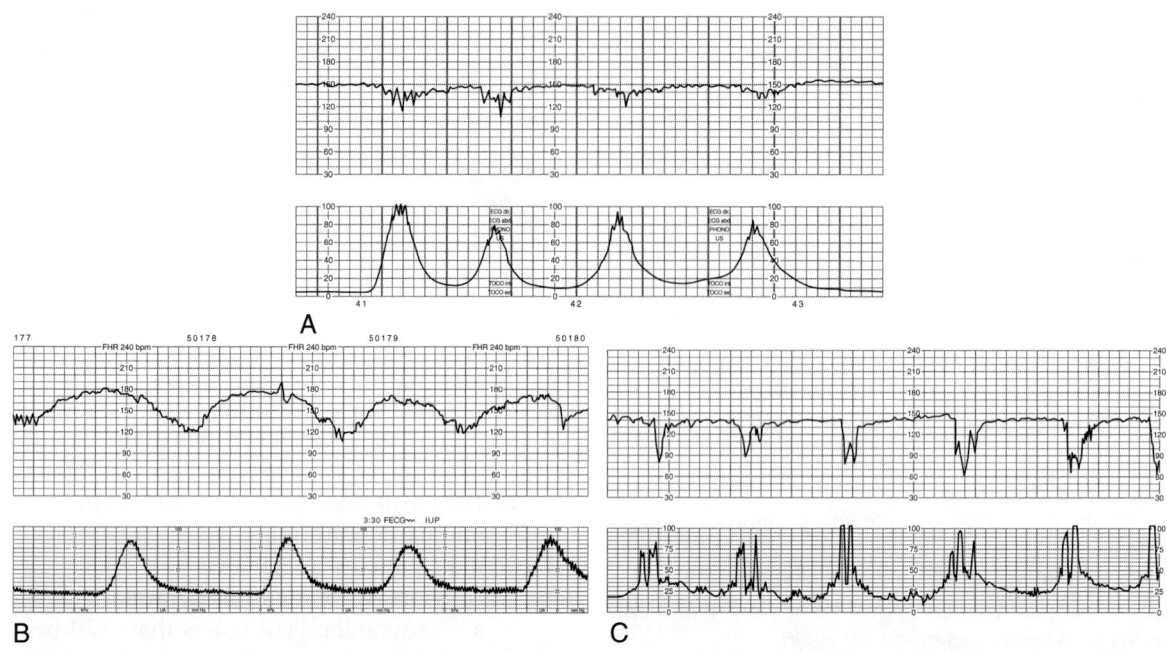

▲ **FIGURE 26-3** Deceleration patterns. **A,** Early decelerations caused by head compression. **B,** Late decelerations caused by uteroplacental insufficiency. **C,** Variable decelerations caused by cord compression. (From Perry, S., Hockenberry, M., Lowdermilk, D., & Wilson, D. [2010]. *Maternal child nursing care* [4th ed.]. St. Louis: Mosby.)

mother's pelvis or soft tissues, such as the cervix, and return to baseline FHR by the end of the contraction.

   c. Tracing shows a uniform shape and mirror image of uterine contractions.

   d. Early decelerations are not associated with fetal compromise and require no intervention.

5. Late decelerations (see Fig. 26-3)

   a. Late decelerations are nonreassuring patterns that reflect impaired placental exchange or uteroplacental insufficiency.

   b. The patterns look similar to early decelerations, but begin well after the contraction begins and return to baseline after the contraction ends.

   c. The degree of decline in FHR from baseline is not related to the amount of uteroplacental insufficiency.

⚠ Interventions for late decelerations include improving placental blood flow and fetal oxygenation.

6. Variable decelerations (see Fig. 26-3)

   a. Variable decelerations are caused by conditions that restrict flow through the umbilical cord.

   b. Variable decelerations do not have the uniform appearance of early and late decelerations.

   c. The shape, duration, and degree of decline below baseline FHR are variable; these fall and rise abruptly with the onset and relief of cord compression.

   d. Variable decelerations also may be nonperiodic, occurring at times unrelated to contractions.

   e. Baseline rate and variability are considered when evaluating variable decelerations.

Box 26-7 Nonreassuring FHR Patterns

Bradycardia
Tachycardia
Late decelerations
Prolonged decelerations
Hypertonic uterine activity
Decreased or absent variability
Variable decelerations falling to less than 70 beats/min for longer than 60 seconds

   f. Variable decelerations are significant when FHR repeatedly declines to less than 70 beats/min and persists at that level for at least 60 seconds before returning to baseline.

7. Hypertonic uterine activity

   a. Assessment of uterine activity includes frequency, duration, intensity of contractions, and uterine resting tone.

   b. The **uterus** should relax between contractions for 60 seconds or longer.

   c. Uterine contraction intensity is about 50 to 75 mm Hg (with intrauterine catheter) during **labor** and may reach 110 mm Hg with pushing during the second stage.

   d. The average resting tone is 5 to 15 mm Hg.

   e. In hypertonic uterine activity, the uterine resting tone between contractions is high, reducing uterine blood flow and decreasing fetal oxygen supply.

8. Nonreassuring FHR patterns (Box 26-7)

9. Interventions for nonreassuring patterns (see Priority Nursing Actions)

■■■■ **PRIORITY NURSING ACTIONS!** ■■■■

Actions to Take for a Nonreassuring Fetal Heart Rate Pattern

1. Identify the cause.
2. Discontinue oxytocin (Pitocin) infusion.
3. Change the mother's position.
4. Administer oxygen by face mask at 8 to 10 L/min and infuse intravenous fluids as prescribed.
5. Prepare to initiate continuous electronic fetal monitoring with internal devices if not contraindicated.
6. Prepare for cesarean delivery if necessary.
7. Document the event, actions taken, and the mother's response.

Nonreassuring fetal heart rate patterns include bradycardia, tachycardia, late decelerations, prolonged decelerations, hypertonic uterine activity, decreased or absent variability, or variable decelerations falling to less than 70 beats/min for longer than 60 seconds. If a nonreassuring fetal heart rate pattern is noted, the physician or nurse-midwife is notified as soon as possible (the nurse stays with the client and asks another nurse to contact the health care provider). The nurse needs to identify the cause of the pattern immediately. This includes checking for a prolapsed umbilical cord and checking maternal vital signs to identify hypotension, hypertension, or fever that can contribute to the fetal response associated with the nonreassuring pattern. If the mother is receiving an oxytocin (Pitocin) infusion, it is stopped because oxytocin causes uterine stimulation, which can worsen the nonreassuring pattern. A tocolytic may be prescribed. The mother is repositioned because this may improve placental perfusion (avoid the supine position). Oxygen is administered by face mask at 8 to 10 L/min to increase maternal blood oxygen saturation making more oxygen available to the fetus, and intravenous fluids are infused to expand the mother's blood volume and improve placental perfusion. If not contraindicated, the nurse prepares to initiate continuous electronic fetal monitoring with internal devices. Cesarean delivery may be necessary, and the nurse should prepare for this procedure. Birth preparation should also include neonatal resuscitation. The nurse documents the event, actions taken, the mother's response, and any other pertinent data.

Reference: McKinney, E., James, S., Murray, S., & Ashwill, J. (2009). *Maternal-child nursing* (3rd ed., p. 397). St. Louis: Saunders.

VI. FOUR STAGES OF LABOR (Table 26-1)

A. Stage 1: Latent phase
1. Description: Stage 1 is the longest. A **labor** curve, often called a Friedman curve, may be used to identify whether a woman's cervical dilation is progressing at the expected rate (Fig. 26-4).
2. Assessment
   a. Cervical dilation is 1 to 4 cm.
   b. Uterine contractions occur every 15 to 30 minutes, are 15 to 30 seconds in duration, and are of mild intensity.

TABLE 26-1 Four Stages of Labor

First Stage	Second Stage	Third Stage	Fourth Stage
Effacement and dilation of cervix	Expulsion of fetus	Separation of placenta	Physical recovery
Three stages— latent, active, and transition	Pushing stage	Expulsion of placenta	1–4 hr after expulsion of placenta
Mother is talkative and eager in latent phase, becoming tired, restless, and anxious as labor intensifies and contractions become stronger	Mother has intense concentration on pushing with contractions; may fall asleep between contractions	Mother is relieved after birth of infant; mother is usually very tired	Mother is tired, but is eager to become acquainted with her newborn

3. Interventions
   a. Encourage mother and partner to participate in care.
   b. Assist with comfort measures, changes of position, and ambulation.
   c. Keep mother and partner informed of progress.
   d. Offer fluids and ice chips.
   e. Encourage voiding every 1 to 2 hours.
B. Stage 1: Active phase
1. Assessment
   a. Cervical dilation is 4 to 7 cm.
   b. Uterine contractions occur every 3 to 5 minutes, are 30 to 60 seconds in duration, and are of moderate intensity.
2. Interventions
   a. Encourage maintenance of effective breathing patterns.
   b. Provide a quiet environment.
   c. Keep mother and partner informed of progress.
   d. Promote comfort with back rubs, sacral pressure, pillow support, and position changes.
   e. Instruct partner in effleurage (light stroking of abdomen).
   f. Offer fluids and ice chips and ointment for dry lips.
   g. Encourage voiding every 1 to 2 hours.
C. Stage 1: Transition phase
1. Assessment
   a. Cervical dilation is 8 to 10 cm.
   b. Uterine contractions occur every 2 to 3 minutes, are 45 to 90 seconds in duration, and are of strong intensity.
2. Interventions
   a. Encourage rest between contractions.
   b. Wake mother at beginning of contraction so she can begin breathing pattern.

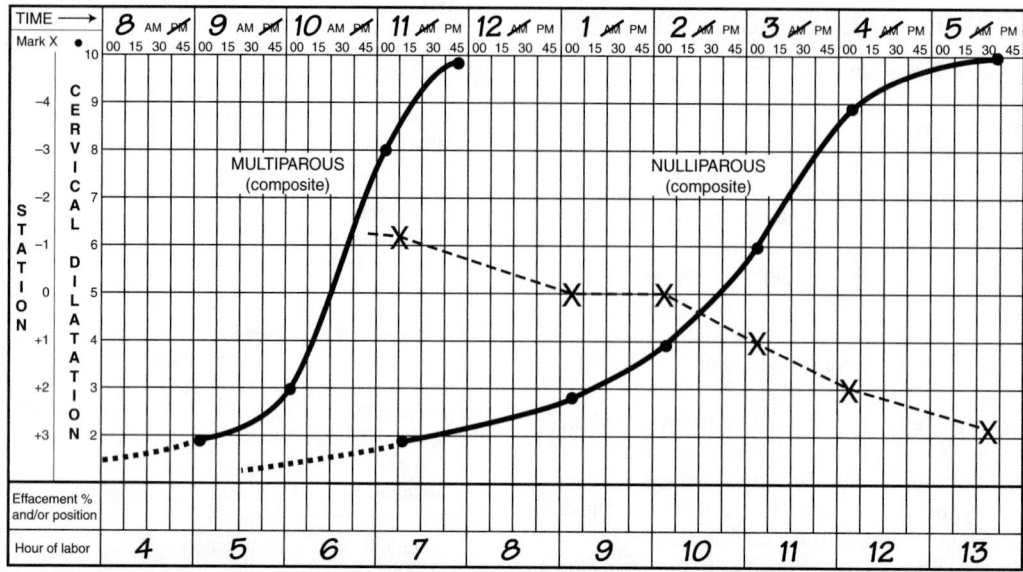

▲ **FIGURE 26-4** A labor curve, often called a Friedman curve, may be used to identify whether a woman's cervical dilation is progressing at the expected rate. The symbol for station (X) may be added to the labor curve. Typical labor curves for a multiparous woman and a nulliparous woman are illustrated for comparison of patterns. (From McKinney, E., James, S., Murray, S., & Ashwill, J. [2009]. *Maternal-child nursing* [3rd ed.]. St. Louis: Saunders.)

c. Keep mother and partner informed of progress.
d. Provide privacy.
e. Offer fluids and ice chips and ointment for dry lips.
f. Encourage voiding every 1 to 2 hours.

D. Interventions throughout stage 1
1. Monitor maternal vital signs.
2. Monitor FHR via ultrasound Doppler, fetoscope, or electronic fetal monitor.
3. Assess FHR before, during, and after a contraction, noting that the normal FHR is 120 to 160 beats/min.
4. Monitor uterine contractions by palpation or tocodynamometer, determining frequency, duration, and intensity.
5. Assess status of cervical dilation and effacement.
6. Assess fetal station presentation and position by Leopold's maneuvers.
7. Assist with pelvic examination and prepare for a fern test.

⚠ Assess the color of the amniotic fluid if the membranes have ruptured because meconium-stained fluid can indicate fetal distress.

E. Stage 2
1. Assessment
   a. Cervical dilation is complete.
   b. Progress of **labor** is measured by descent of fetal head through the birth canal (change in fetal station).

c. Uterine contractions occur every 2 to 3 minutes, lasting 60 to 75 seconds, and are of strong intensity.
d. Increase in bloody show occurs.
e. Mother feels urge to bear down; assist mother in pushing efforts.

2. Interventions
   a. Perform assessments every 5 minutes.
   b. Monitor maternal vital signs.
   c. Monitor FHR via ultrasound Doppler, fetoscope, or electronic fetal monitor.
   d. Assess FHR before, during, and after a contraction, noting that normal FHR is 120 to 160 beats/min.
   e. Monitor uterine contractions by palpation or tocodynamometer, determining frequency, duration, and intensity.
   f. Provide mother with encouragement and praise and provide for rest between contractions.
   g. Keep mother and partner informed of progress.
   h. Maintain privacy.
   i. Provide ice chips and ointment for dry lips.
   j. Assist mother into a position that promotes comfort and facilitates pushing efforts, such as lithotomy, semisitting, kneeling, side-lying, or squatting.
   k. Monitor for signs of approaching birth, such as perineal bulging or visualization of the fetal head.
   l. Prepare for birth (expulsion of the fetus).

F. Stage 3
1. Assessment
   a. Contractions occur until the **placenta** is expelled.
   b. Placental separation and expulsion occur.
   c. Expulsion of the **placenta** occurs 5 to 30 minutes after the birth of the infant.
   d. Schultze mechanism: Center portion of the **placenta** separates first, and its shiny fetal surface emerges from the **vagina**.
   e. Duncan mechanism: Margin of the **placenta** separates, and the dull, red, rough maternal surface emerges from the **vagina** first.
2. Interventions
   a. Assess maternal vital signs.
   b. Assess uterine status.
   c. Provide parents with an explanation regarding expulsion of the **placenta**.
   d. After expulsion of the **placenta**, uterine fundus remains firm and is located 2 fingerbreadths below the umbilicus.
   e. Examine **placenta** for cotyledons and membranes to verify that it is intact.
   f. Assess mother for shivering and provide warmth.
   g. Promote parental-neonatal attachment.
G. Stage 4
1. Description: Period 1 to 4 hours after **delivery**
2. Assessment
   a. Blood pressure returns to prelabor level.
   b. Pulse is slightly lower than during **labor**.
   c. Fundus remains contracted, in the midline, 1 or 2 fingerbreadths below the umbilicus.

⚠ Monitor lochia discharge. Lochia may be moderate in amount and red in color in stage 4.

3. Interventions
   a. Perform maternal assessments every 15 minutes for 1 hour, every 30 minutes for 1 hour, and hourly for 2 hours (or as per agency policy).
   b. Provide warm blankets.
   c. Apply ice packs to the perineum.
   d. Massage the **uterus** if needed, and teach the mother to massage the **uterus**.
   e. Provide breast-feeding support as needed.
   f. See Chapter 30 for information on caring for the **newborn**.

VII. ANESTHESIA

A. Local anesthesia
1. Local anesthesia is used for blocking pain during episiotomy.
2. Local anesthesia is administered just before the birth of the infant.
3. The anesthetic has no effect on the fetus.

B. Pudendal block
1. A pudendal block is administered just before the birth of the infant.
2. Injection site is at the pudendal nerve through a transvaginal route.
3. Anesthetic blocks the perineal area for episiotomy.
4. Its effect lasts about 30 minutes.
5. Anesthetic has no effect on contractions or the fetus.
C. Lumbar epidural block
1. Injection site is in epidural space at L3 to L4.
2. The block is administered after **labor** is established or just before a scheduled cesarean birth.
3. The anesthetic relieves pain from contractions and numbs the **vagina** and perineum.
4. The block may cause hypotension, bladder distention, and a prolonged second stage.
5. The anesthetic does not cause a headache because the dura mater is not penetrated.
6. Assess maternal blood pressure and assess bladder frequently.
7. Maintain the mother in a side-lying position or place a rolled blanket beneath the right hip to displace the **uterus** from the vena cava.
8. Administer intravenous fluids as prescribed.
9. Increase fluids as prescribed if hypotension occurs.
10. Observe for any adverse effects from opioid epidurals, such as nausea and vomiting, pruritus, or respiratory depression.
D. Intrathecal opioid analgesics
1. The medication is injected into the subarachnoid space and has a rapid onset of action.
2. It may be used in combination with a lumbar epidural block.
E. Subarachnoid (spinal) block
1. Injection site is in the spinal subarachnoid space at L3 to L5.
2. The block is administered just before birth.
3. The anesthetic relieves uterine and perineal pain and numbs the **vagina**, perineum, and lower extremities.
4. The anesthetic may cause maternal hypotension.
5. The anesthetic may cause postpartum headache.
6. The mother must lie flat for 8 to 12 hours after spinal injection.
7. Administer intravenous fluids as prescribed.
F. General anesthesia
1. General anesthesia may be used for some surgical interventions.
2. The mother is not awake.

⚠ General anesthesia presents a danger of respiratory depression, vomiting, and aspiration.

TABLE 26-2 Factors of the Bishop Score

	Score			
	0	1	2	3
Dilation of cervix (cm)	0	1-2	3-4	>5
Effacement of cervix (%)	0-30	40-50	60-70	>80
Consistency of cervix	Firm	Medium	Soft	—
Position of cervix	Posterior	Midposition	Anterior	—
Station of presenting part	−3	−2	−1	+1, +2

VIII. OBSTETRICAL PROCEDURES

A. Bishop score (Table 26-2)
   1. The Bishop score is used to determine maternal readiness for **labor** and evaluates cervical status and fetal position.
   2. The Bishop score is indicated before the induction of **labor**.
   3. The five factors are assigned a score of 0 to 3, and the total score is calculated.
   4. A score of 6 or more indicates a readiness for **labor** induction.

B. Induction
   1. Induction is a deliberate initiation of uterine contractions that stimulates **labor**.
   2. Elective induction may be accomplished by oxytocin (Pitocin) infusion.
   3. Obtain baseline tracing of uterine contractions and FHR.
   4. Increase the intravenous dosage of oxytocin as prescribed only after assessing contractions, FHR, and maternal blood pressure and pulse.
   5. Do not increase the rate of oxytocin when the desired contraction pattern is obtained (contraction frequency of 2 to 3 minutes and lasting 60 seconds).

⚠ An oxytocin (Pitocin) infusion is discontinued if uterine contraction frequency is less than 2 minutes or duration is longer than 90 seconds, or if fetal distress is noted.

C. Amniotomy
   1. Artificial rupture of the membranes is performed by the physician or nurse-midwife to stimulate **labor**.
   2. Amniotomy is performed if the fetus is at 0 or a plus station.
   3. Amniotomy increases the risk of prolapsed cord and infection.

   4. Monitor FHR before and after amniotomy.
   5. Record time of amniotomy, FHR, and characteristics of the fluid.
   6. Meconium-stained **amniotic fluid** may be associated with fetal distress.
   7. Bloody **amniotic fluid** may indicate abruptio placentae or fetal trauma.
   8. An unpleasant odor to **amniotic fluid** is associated with infection.
   9. Polyhydramnios is associated with maternal diabetes and certain congenital disorders.
   10. Oligohydramnios is associated with intrauterine growth restriction and congenital disorders.
   11. Expect more variable decelerations after rupture of the membranes as a result of possible cord compression during contractions.
   12. Limit client activity if prescribed.

D. External version
   1. External version is the manipulation of the fetus from an abnormal position into a normal presentation.
   2. External version is indicated for an abnormal presentation that exists after the thirty-fourth week.
   3. Monitor vital signs.
   4. If the mother is Rh-negative, ensure that $Rh_o(D)$ immune globulin (RhoGAM) was given at 28 weeks' gestation.
   5. Prepare for a nonstress test to evaluate fetal well-being.
   6. Intravenous fluids and tocolytic therapy may be administered to relax the **uterus** and permit easier manipulation of the fetus.
   7. Ultrasound is used during the procedure to evaluate fetal position and placental placement and guide direction of the fetus.
   8. The abdominal wall is manipulated to direct the fetus into a cephalic presentation if possible.
   9. Monitor blood pressure to identify vena cava compression.
   10. Monitor for unusual pain.
   11. After the procedure, do the following:
       a. Perform a nonstress test to evaluate fetal well-being.
       b. Monitor for uterine activity, bleeding, ruptured membranes, and decreased fetal activity.
       c. With Rh-negative clients, perform Kleihauer-Betke test as prescribed to detect the presence and amount of fetal blood in the maternal circulation and to identify clients who need additional $Rh_o(D)$ immune globulin.

E. Episiotomy
   1. An episiotomy is an incision made into the perineum to enlarge the vaginal outlet and facilitate **delivery**.
   2. Check the episiotomy site.

3. Institute measures to relieve pain.
4. Provide ice packs during the first 24 hours.
5. Instruct the client in the use of sitz baths.
6. Apply analgesic spray or ointment as prescribed.
7. Provide perineal care, using clean technique.
8. Instruct the client in the proper care of the incision.
9. Instruct the client to dry the perineal area from front to back and to blot the area rather than wipe it.
10. Instruct the client to shower rather than bathe in a tub.
11. Apply a perineal pad without touching the inside surface of the pad.
12. Report any bleeding or discharge from the episiotomy site to the physician.

F. Forceps delivery
1. Two double-crossed, spoon-like articulated blades are used to assist in the **delivery** of the fetal head.
2. Reassure the mother and explain the need for forceps.
3. Monitor the mother and fetus during **delivery**.
4. Check neonate and mother after **delivery** for any possible injury.
5. Assist with repair of any lacerations.

G. Vacuum extraction
1. A cap-like suction device is applied to the fetal head to facilitate extraction.
2. Suction is used to assist in **delivery** of the fetal head.
3. Traction is applied during uterine contractions until descent of the fetal head is achieved.
4. The suction device should not be kept in place any longer than 25 minutes.
5. Monitor FHR every 5 minutes if external fetal monitoring is not used.
6. Assess **infant** at birth and throughout the postpartum period for signs of cerebral trauma.
7. Monitor for developing cephalhematoma.
8. Caput succedaneum is normal and resolves in 24 hours.

H. Cesarean delivery
1. Cesarean section is **delivery** of the fetus usually through a transabdominal, low-segment incision of the **uterus**.
2. Preoperative
   a. If planned, prepare the mother and partner.
   b. If an emergency, quickly explain the need and procedure to the mother and partner.
   c. Obtain informed consent.
   d. Ensure that the preoperative diagnostic tests are done, including Rh factor determination.
   e. Prepare to insert an intravenous line and a Foley catheter.
   f. Prepare the abdomen as prescribed.
   g. Monitor the mother and fetus continuously.
   h. Provide emotional support.

   i. Administer preoperative medications as prescribed.
3. Postoperative
   a. Monitor vital signs.
   b. Provide pain relief.
   c. Encourage turning, coughing, and deep breathing.
   d. Encourage ambulation.
   e. Monitor for signs of infection and bleeding.
   f. Burning and pain on urination may indicate a bladder infection.
   g. A tender **uterus** and foul-smelling **lochia** may indicate endometritis.
   h. A productive cough or chills may indicate pneumonia.
   i. Pain, redness, or edema of an extremity may indicate thrombophlebitis.

MORE QUESTIONS ON THE CD!

Practice Questions

250. A nurse is caring for a client in labor. The nurse determines that the client is beginning the second stage of labor when which of the following assessments is noted?
1. The contractions are regular.
2. The membranes have ruptured.
3. The cervix is dilated completely.
4. The client begins to expel clear vaginal fluid.

251. A nurse in the labor room is caring for a client in the active stage of labor. The nurse is assessing the fetal patterns and notes a late deceleration on the monitor strip. The appropriate nursing action is to:
1. Administer oxygen via face mask.
2. Place the mother in a supine position.
3. Increase the rate of the oxytocin (Pitocin) intravenous infusion.
4. Document the findings and continue to monitor the fetal patterns.

252. A nurse is performing an assessment of a client who is scheduled for a cesarean delivery. Which assessment finding would indicate a need to contact the physician?
1. Hemoglobin of 11 g/dL
2. Fetal heart rate of 180 beats/min
3. Maternal pulse rate of 85 beats/min
4. White blood cell count of 12,000/mm^3

253. A nurse is reviewing the record of a client in the labor room and notes that the nurse-midwife has documented that the fetus is at −1 station. The nurse determines that the fetal presenting part is:

1. 1 inch below the coccyx
2. 1 inch below the iliac crest
3. 1 cm above the ischial spine
4. 1 fingerbreadth below the symphysis pubis

254. A client arrives at a birthing center in active labor. Her membranes are still intact, and the nurse-midwife prepares to perform an amniotomy. A nurse who is assisting the nurse-midwife explains to the client that after this procedure, she will most likely have:
1. Less pressure on her cervix
2. Decreased number of contractions
3. Increased efficiency of contractions
4. The need for increased maternal blood pressure monitoring

255. A nurse is monitoring a client in labor. The nurse suspects umbilical cord compression if which of the following is noted on the external monitor tracing during a contraction?
1. Variability
2. Accelerations
3. Early decelerations
4. Variable decelerations

256. A client in labor is transported to the delivery room and prepared for a cesarean delivery. After the client is transferred to the delivery room table, a nurse places her in:
1. Supine position with a wedge under the right hip
2. Trendelenburg's position with the legs in stirrups
3. Prone position with the legs separated and elevated
4. Semi-Fowler's position with a pillow under the knees

257. A nurse has provided discharge instructions to a client who delivered a healthy infant by cesarean delivery. Which statement made by the client indicates a need for further instructions?
1. "I will begin abdominal exercises immediately."
2. "I will notify the physician if I develop a fever."
3. "I will turn on my side and push up with my arms to get out of bed."
4. "I will lift nothing heavier than the newborn infant for at least 2 weeks."

258. A nurse is monitoring a client in active labor and notes that the client is having contractions every 3 minutes that last 45 seconds. The nurse notes that the fetal heart rate between contractions is 100 beats/min. Which of the following nursing actions is appropriate?
1. Notify the physician or nurse-midwife.
2. Continue monitoring the fetal heart rate.

3. Encourage the client to continue pushing with each contraction.
4. Instruct the client's coach to continue to encourage breathing techniques.

259. A nurse is caring for a client in labor and is monitoring the fetal heart rate patterns. The nurse notes the presence of episodic accelerations on the electronic fetal monitor tracing. Which of the following actions is appropriate?
1. Notify the physician or nurse-midwife of the findings.
2. Reposition the mother and check the monitor for changes in the fetal tracing.
3. Take the mother's vital signs and tell the mother that bedrest is required to conserve oxygen.
4. Document the findings and tell the mother that the pattern on the monitor indicates fetal well-being.

260. A nurse is admitting a pregnant client to the labor room and attaches an external electronic fetal monitor to the client's abdomen. After attachment of the electronic fetal monitor, the initial nursing assessment is which of the following?
1. Identify the types of accelerations.
2. Assess the baseline fetal heart rate.
3. Determine the intensity of the contractions.
4. Determine the frequency of the contractions.

261. A nurse is reviewing true and false labor signs with a multiparous client. The nurse determines that the client understands the signs of true labor if she makes which statement?
1. "I won't be in labor until my baby drops."
2. "My contractions will be felt in my abdominal area."
3. "My contractions will not be as painful if I walk around."
4. "My contractions will increase in duration and intensity."

262. After an amniotomy has been performed, a nurse should first assess:
1. For cervical dilation
2. For bladder distention
3. The maternal blood pressure
4. The fetal heart rate pattern

263. A client in labor has been pushing effectively for 1 hour. A nurse determines that the client's primary physiological need at this time is to:
1. Ambulate
2. Rest between contractions
3. Change positions frequently
4. Consume oral food and fluids

Alternate Item Format: Prioritizing (Ordered Response)

264. A nurse is monitoring a client in labor who is receiving oxytocin (Pitocin) and notes that the client is experiencing hypertonic uterine contractions. List in order of priority the actions that the nurse takes. (Number 1 is the first action, and number 6 is the last action.)

____ Reposition the client.
____ Stop the oxytocin infusion.
____ Perform a vaginal examination.
____ Check the client's blood pressure.
____ Administer oxygen by face mask at 8 to 10 L/min.
____ Administer medication as prescribed to reduce uterine activity

ANSWERS

250. 3
Rationale: The second stage of labor begins when the cervix is dilated completely and ends with birth of the neonate. Options 1, 2, and 4 are not specific assessment findings of the second stage of labor and occur in stage 1.
Test-Taking Strategy: Use the process of elimination. Eliminate options 2 and 4 first because they are comparable or alike. From the remaining options, recalling that regular contractions occur before the second stage of labor will direct you to option 3. Review the stages of labor if you had difficulty with this question.
Level of Cognitive Ability: Analyzing
Client Needs: Health Promotion and Maintenance
Integrated Process: Nursing Process—Assessment
Content Area: Maternity—Intrapartum
Reference: Perry, S., Hockenberry, M., Lowdermilk, D., & Wilson, D. (2010). *Maternal child nursing care* (4th ed., p. 466). St. Louis: Mosby.

251. 1
Rationale: Late decelerations are due to uteroplacental insufficiency and occur because of decreased blood flow and oxygen to the fetus during the uterine contractions. Hypoxemia results; oxygen at 8 to 10 L/min via face mask is necessary. The supine position is avoided because it decreases uterine blood flow to the fetus. The client should be turned onto her side to displace pressure of the gravid uterus on the inferior vena cava. An intravenous oxytocin infusion is discontinued when a late deceleration is noted. The oxytocin would cause further hypoxemia because of increased uteroplacental insufficiency resulting from stimulation of contractions by this medication. Although the nurse would document the occurrence, option 4 would delay necessary treatment.
Test-Taking Strategy: Use the ABCs—airway, breathing, and circulation—and knowledge related to the significance of a late deceleration to answer this question. Review the nursing actions to take if late decelerations occur if you had difficulty with this question.
Level of Cognitive Ability: Applying
Client Needs: Physiological Integrity
Integrated Process: Nursing Process—Implementation
Content Area: Maternity—Intrapartum
Reference: Perry, S., Hockenberry, M., Lowdermilk, D., & Wilson, D. (2010). *Maternal child nursing care* (4th ed., p. 467). St. Louis: Mosby.

252. 2
Rationale: Normal fetal heart rate is 120 to 160 beats/min. Fetal heart rate of 180 beats/min could indicate fetal distress

and would warrant immediate notification of the physician. White blood cell counts in a normal pregnancy begin to increase in the second trimester and peak in the third trimester, with a normal range of 11,000 to 15,000/mm³ (up to 18,000/mm³). During the immediate postpartum period, white blood cell count may be 25,000 to 30,000/mm³ because of increased leukocytosis that occurs during delivery. By full term, a normal maternal hemoglobin range is 11 to 13 g/dL because of the hemodilution caused by an increase in plasma volume during pregnancy. The maternal pulse rate during pregnancy increases 10 to 15 beats/min over prepregnancy readings to facilitate increased cardiac output, oxygen transport, and kidney filtration.
Test-Taking Strategy: Use the process of elimination, noting the strategic words *indicate a need to contact the physician.* Knowledge regarding the normal and abnormal findings in a pregnant client and fetus will direct you to option 2. If you are unfamiliar with these normal and abnormal findings and the normal fetal heart rate, review this content.
Level of Cognitive Ability: Analyzing
Client Needs: Physiological Integrity
Integrated Process: Nursing Process—Analysis
Content Area: Maternity—Intrapartum
Reference: McKinney, E., James, S., Murray, S., & Ashwill, J. (2009). *Maternal-child nursing* (3rd ed., pp. 261, 388). St. Louis: Saunders.

253. 3
Rationale: Station is the relationship of the presenting part to an imaginary line drawn between the ischial spines, measured in centimeters, and noted as a negative number above the line and a positive number below the line. At negative 1 (−1) station, the fetal presenting part is 1 cm above the ischial spines.
Test-Taking Strategy: Recalling that station is measured in centimeters and uses the ischial spines as a reference point will assist in answering this question. Options 1, 2, and 4 are comparable or alike in the use of the word *below,* which would be represented by a positive measurement in determining station. Review stations of the presenting part if you had difficulty with this question.
Level of Cognitive Ability: Understanding
Client Needs: Health Promotion and Maintenance
Integrated Process: Nursing Process—Assessment
Content Area: Maternity—Intrapartum
Reference: McKinney, E., James, S., Murray, S., & Ashwill, J. (2009). *Maternal-child nursing* (3rd ed., pp. 337, 350). St. Louis: Saunders.

254. 3
Rationale: Amniotomy (artificial rupture of the membranes) can be used to induce labor when the condition of the cervix

is favorable (ripe) or to augment labor if the progress begins to slow. Rupturing of the membranes allows the fetal head to contact the cervix more directly and may increase the efficiency of contractions. Increased monitoring of maternal blood pressure is unnecessary following this procedure. The fetal heart rate needs to be monitored frequently, however.

Test-Taking Strategy: Focus on the subject, an amniotomy. Recalling that amniotomy is performed to augment labor if the progress begins to slow will direct you to option 3. Review the purpose of amniotomy if you had difficulty with this question.

Level of Cognitive Ability: Applying
Client Needs: Physiological Integrity
Integrated Process: Nursing Process—Implementation
Content Area: Maternity—Intrapartum
Reference: Perry, S., Hockenberry, M., Lowdermilk, D., & Wilson, D. (2010). *Maternal child nursing care* (4th ed., pp. 505–506). St. Louis: Mosby.

255. 4
Rationale: Variable decelerations occur if the umbilical cord becomes compressed, reducing blood flow between the placenta and the fetus. Variability refers to fluctuations in the baseline fetal heart rate. Accelerations are a reassuring sign and usually occur with fetal movement. Early decelerations result from pressure on the fetal head during a contraction.

Test-Taking Strategy: Use the process of elimination, focusing on the subject, umbilical cord compression. Recalling that variable decelerations occur if the umbilical cord becomes compressed will direct you to option 4. Review the findings that occur in umbilical cord compression if you had difficulty with this question.

Level of Cognitive Ability: Analyzing
Client Needs: Physiological Integrity
Integrated Process: Nursing Process—Assessment
Content Area: Maternity—Intrapartum
Reference: McKinney, E., James, S., Murray, S., & Ashwill, J. (2009). *Maternal-child nursing* (3rd ed., p. 403). St. Louis: Saunders.

256. 1
Rationale: Vena cava and descending aorta compression by the pregnant uterus impedes blood return from the lower trunk and extremities. This leads to decreasing cardiac return, cardiac output, and blood flow to the uterus and subsequently the fetus. The best position to prevent this would be side-lying, with the uterus displaced off the abdominal vessels. Positioning for abdominal surgery necessitates a supine position; however, a wedge placed under the right hip provides displacement of the uterus. Trendelenburg's position places pressure from the pregnant uterus on the diaphragm and lungs, decreasing respiratory capacity and oxygenation. A semi-Fowler's position or prone position is not practical for this type of abdominal surgery.

Test-Taking Strategy: Focus on the subject, positioning the pregnant woman. Use the process of elimination, visualizing each of the positions identified in the options and considering the effect that the position may have on the mother and the fetus. If you had difficulty with this question, review care for the mother requiring cesarean delivery.

Level of Cognitive Ability: Applying
Client Needs: Physiological Integrity
Integrated Process: Nursing Process—Implementation

Content Area: Maternity—Intrapartum
Reference: McKinney, E., James, S., Murray, S., & Ashwill, J. (2009). *Maternal-child nursing* (3rd ed., p. 452). St. Louis: Saunders.

257. 1
Rationale: A cesarean delivery requires an incision made through the abdominal wall and into the uterus. Abdominal exercises should not start immediately after abdominal surgery; the client should wait at least 3 to 4 weeks postoperatively to allow for healing of the incision. Options 2, 3, and 4 are appropriate instructions for the client after a cesarean delivery.

Test-Taking Strategy: Note the strategic words *indicates a need for further instructions*. These words indicate a negative event query and ask you to select an option that is an incorrect statement. Keeping in mind that the client had a cesarean delivery and noting the word *immediately* in option 1 will assist in directing you to this option. Review home care instructions for a client after cesarean delivery if you had difficulty with this question.

Level of Cognitive Ability: Evaluating
Client Needs: Health Promotion and Maintenance
Integrated Process: Teaching and Learning
Content Area: Maternity—Postpartum
Reference: McKinney, E., James, S., Murray, S., & Ashwill, J. (2009). *Maternal-child nursing* (3rd ed., p. 475). St. Louis: Saunders.

258. 1
Rationale: A normal fetal heart rate is 120 to 160 beats/min, and the fetal heart rate should be within this range between contractions. Fetal bradycardia between contractions may indicate the need for immediate medical management, and the physician or nurse-midwife needs to be notified. Options 2, 3, and 4 are inappropriate nursing actions in this situation and delay necessary intervention.

Test-Taking Strategy: Focus on the data in the question. Knowledge that the normal fetal heart rate is 120 to 160 beats/min will assist you to recognize that fetal bradycardia is present. If you had difficulty with this question, review the expected and unexpected findings during the labor process.

Level of Cognitive Ability: Applying
Client Needs: Physiological Integrity
Integrated Process: Nursing Process—Implementation
Content Area: Maternity—Intrapartum
Reference: McKinney, E., James, S., Murray, S., & Ashwill, J. (2009). *Maternal-child nursing* (3rd ed., pp. 363, 366). St. Louis: Saunders.

259. 4
Rationale: Accelerations are transient increases in the fetal heart rate that often accompany contractions or are caused by fetal movement. Episodic accelerations are thought to be a sign of fetal well-being and adequate oxygen reserve. Options 1, 2, and 3 are inaccurate nursing actions and are unnecessary.

Test-Taking Strategy: Use the process of elimination. Options 1, 2, and 3 are comparable or alike in that they indicate the need for further intervention. Also, knowing that accelerations indicate fetal well-being will direct you to option 4. Review the significance of episodic accelerations if you had difficulty with this question.

Level of Cognitive Ability: Applying
Client Needs: Physiological Integrity
Integrated Process: Nursing Process—Implementation
Content Area: Maternity—Intrapartum
Reference: Perry, S., Hockenberry, M., Lowdermilk, D., & Wilson, D. (2010). *Maternal child nursing care* (4th ed., pp. 429–430). St. Louis: Mosby.

260. 2

Rationale: Assessing the baseline fetal heart rate is important so that abnormal variations of the baseline rate can be identified if they occur. The intensity of contractions is assessed by an internal fetal monitor, not an external fetal monitor. Options 1 and 4 are important to assess, but not as the first priority. Fetal heart rate is evaluated by assessing baseline and periodic changes. Periodic changes occur in response to the intermittent stress of uterine contractions and the baseline beat-to-beat variability of the fetal heart rate.

Test-Taking Strategy: Note the strategic word *initial* in the question. Use the ABCs—airway, breathing, and circulation. Fetal heart rate reflects the ABCs. Review the concepts related to external fetal monitoring if you had difficulty with this question.

Level of Cognitive Ability: Applying
Client Needs: Physiological Integrity
Integrated Process: Nursing Process—Assessment
Content Area: Maternity—Intrapartum
Reference: McKinney, E., James, S., Murray, S., & Ashwill, J. (2009). *Maternal-child nursing* (3rd ed., pp. 392–393). St. Louis: Saunders.

261. 4

Rationale: True labor is present when contractions increase in duration and intensity. Lightening or dropping is also known as engagement and occurs when the fetus descends into the pelvis about 2 weeks before delivery. Contractions felt in the abdominal area and contractions that ease with walking are signs of false labor.

Test-Taking Strategy: Focus on the subject, the signs of true labor. Noting the word *true* in the question and its relationship to the words *increase in duration and intensity* in option 4 will direct you to this option. Review the signs of true and false labor if you had difficulty with this question.

Level of Cognitive Ability: Evaluating
Client Needs: Health Promotion and Maintenance
Integrated Process: Nursing Process—Evaluation
Content Area: Maternity—Intrapartum
Reference: McKinney, E., James, S., Murray, S., & Ashwill, J. (2009). *Maternal-child nursing* (3rd ed., pp. 348, 352). St. Louis: Saunders.

262. 4

Rationale: Fetal heart rate is assessed immediately after amniotomy to detect any changes that may indicate cord compression or prolapse. Bladder distention or maternal blood pressure would not be the first things to check after an amniotomy. When the membranes are ruptured, minimal vaginal examinations would be done because of the risk of infection.

Test-Taking Strategy: Note the strategic word *first.* Because of the risk of a prolapsed cord after an amniotomy, the first action is to check the fetal heart rate for signs of nonreassuring fetal heart rate patterns. Review care after an amniotomy if you had difficulty with this question.

Level of Cognitive Ability: Applying
Client Needs: Physiological Integrity
Integrated Process: Nursing Process—Assessment
Content Area: Maternity—Intrapartum
Reference: Perry, S., Hockenberry, M., Lowdermilk, D., & Wilson, D. (2010). *Maternal-child nursing care* (4th ed., pp. 506–507). St. Louis: Mosby.

263. 2

Rationale: The birth process expends a great deal of energy, particularly during the transition stage. Encouraging rest between contractions conserves maternal energy, facilitating voluntary pushing efforts with contractions. Uteroplacental perfusion also is enhanced, which promotes fetal tolerance of the stress of labor. Changing positions frequently is not the primary physiological need. Ambulation is encouraged during early labor. Ice chips should be provided. Food and fluids likely are to be withheld at this time.

Test-Taking Strategy: Use the process of elimination. Focusing on the strategic words *pushing effectively* will assist in directing you to option 2. Review care for the client in the transition stage of labor if you had difficulty with this question.

Level of Cognitive Ability: Analyzing
Client Needs: Physiological Integrity
Integrated Process: Nursing Process—Analysis
Content Area: Maternity—Intrapartum
References: McKinney, E., James, S., Murray, S., & Ashwill, J. (2009). *Maternal-child nursing* (3rd ed., p. 369). St. Louis: Saunders.

Perry, S., Hockenberry, M., Lowdermilk, D., & Wilson, D. (2010). *Maternal child nursing care* (4th ed., p. 458). St. Louis: Mosby.

ALTERNATE ITEM FORMAT: PRIORITIZING (ORDERED RESPONSE)

264. 2, 1, 4, 5, 3, 6

Rationale: If uterine hypertonicity occurs, the nurse would immediately intervene to reduce uterine activity and increase fetal oxygenation. The nurse would stop the oxytocin infusion and increase the rate of the nonadditive solution, position the client in a side-lying position, and administer oxygen by face mask at 8 to 10 L/min. The nurse then would attempt to determine the cause of the uterine hypertonicity and perform a vaginal examination to check for a prolapsed cord. The nurse would check maternal blood pressure for the presence of hypertension or hypotension. The nurse stays with the client and contacts the physician as soon as possible (or asks another nurse to contact the physician) and then implements prescribed physician prescriptions, including the administration of medications to reduce uterine activity.

Test-Taking Strategy: Noting that the client is experiencing uterine hypertonicity will assist in determining that the first action would be to stop the oxytocin infusion. The mother's position would then be changed because this would immediately provide oxygen to the fetus. Because fetal oxygenation is a concern, oxygen would be administered next. The nurse then would determine the cause of the uterine hypertonicity by performing a vaginal examination to check for a prolapsed cord and checking the client's blood pressure. Medications cannot be administered without a physician's prescription; medication administration would be the last action in this situation. Review care for the client experiencing hypertonic uterine contractions if you had difficulty with this question.

Level of Cognitive Ability: Applying
Client Needs: Physiological Integrity
Integrated Process: Nursing Process—Implementation
Content Area: Maternity—Intrapartum
Reference: Perry, S., Hockenberry, M., Lowdermilk, D., & Wilson, D. (2010). *Maternal child nursing care* (4th ed., pp. 508–510). St. Louis: Mosby.

Problems With Labor and Delivery

I. SUPINE HYPOTENSION (VENA CAVA SYNDROME)

A. Description
1. Supine hypotension (also known as vena cava syndrome) occurs when the venous return to the heart is impaired by the weight of the **uterus** on the vena cava.
2. The syndrome results in partial occlusion of the vena cava and aorta and in reduced cardiac return, cardiac output, and blood pressure.

B. Assessment
1. Pallor
2. Faintness, dizziness, breathlessness
3. Tachycardia, hypotension
4. Sweating, cool and damp skin
5. Fetal distress

C. Interventions
1. Position the client on her side to shift the weight of the fetus off the vena cava until her signs and symptoms subside and vital signs stabilize.
2. Monitor vital signs and fetal heart rate.

⚠ Place a pillow or wedge under the client's hip to displace the gravid uterus off the vena cava. Avoid the supine position.

II. PREMATURE RUPTURE OF THE MEMBRANES

A. Description
1. Premature rupture of the membranes refers to spontaneous rupture of the amniotic membrane before the onset of **labor**.
2. Gestational age usually determines the plan and intervention.
3. When the rupture of membranes is before term and **delivery** will be delayed, infection becomes a risk.

B. Assessment
1. There is evidence of fluid pooling in vaginal vault; nitrazine test is positive.
2. Amount, color, consistency, and odor of fluid needs to be assessed.
3. Vital signs are monitored; an elevated temperature may indicate the presence of infection.
4. Fetal monitoring is necessary; tachycardia may indicate infection.

C. Interventions
1. Assist with tests to assess gestational age.
2. Avoid vaginal examinations because of the risk of infection.
3. Monitor maternal and fetal status for signs of compromise or infection.
4. Administer antibiotics as prescribed.

III. PROLAPSED UMBILICAL CORD

A. Description: The umbilical cord is displaced between the presenting part and the amnion or protruding through the cervix, causing compression of the cord and compromising fetal circulation (Fig. 27-1).

B. Assessment
1. The client has a feeling that something is coming through the **vagina**.
2. Umbilical cord is visible or palpable.
3. Fetal heart rate is irregular and slow.
4. Fetal heart monitor shows variable decelerations or bradycardia after rupture of the membranes.
5. If fetal hypoxia is severe, violent fetal activity may occur and then cease.

C. Interventions (see Priority Nursing Actions)

IV. PLACENTA PREVIA

A. Description
1. **Placenta** previa is an improperly implanted **placenta** in the lower uterine segment near or over the internal cervical os (Fig. 27-2).
2. Total: The internal cervical os is covered entirely by the **placenta** when the cervix is dilated fully.
3. Partial: The lower border of the **placenta** is within 3 cm of the internal cervical os, but does not fully cover it.
4. Marginal: The **placenta** is implanted in the lower **uterus**, but its lower border is greater than 3 cm from the internal cervical os.
5. Management depends on the classification of the previa and gestational age of the fetus.

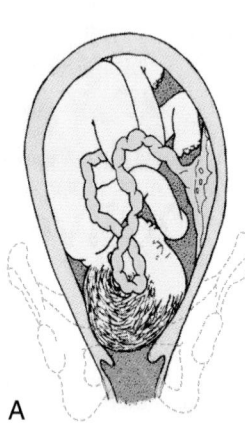 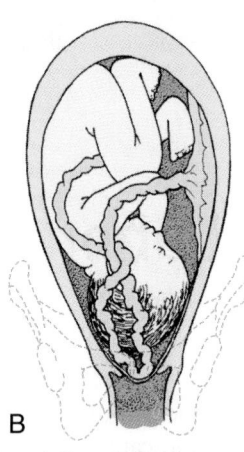 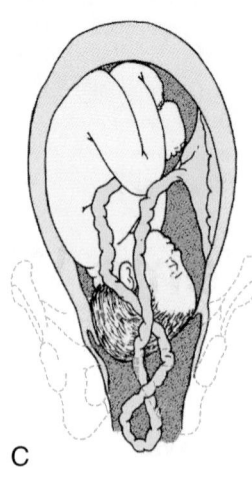 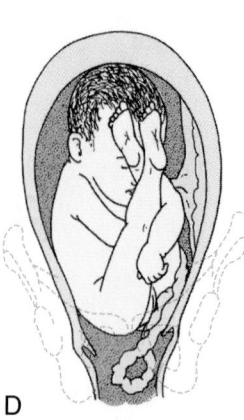

A   B   C   D

▲ **FIGURE 27-1** Prolapse of umbilical cord. Note the pressure of the presenting part on the umbilical cord, which endangers fetal circulation. **A,** Occult (hidden) prolapse of cord. **B,** Complete prolapse of cord. Membranes are intact. **C,** Cord presenting in front of the fetal head may be seen in the vagina. **D,** Frank breech presentation with prolapsed cord. (From Perry, S., Hockenberry, M., Lowdermilk, D., & Wilson, D. [2010]. *Maternal child nursing care* [4th ed., p. 521]. St. Louis: Mosby.)

■■■■■ ■PRIORITY NURSING ACTIONS! ■■■■■

Steps to Take if Umbilical Cord Prolapse Is Suspected

1. Elevate the fetal presenting part that is lying on the cord by applying finger pressure with a gloved hand.
2. Place the client into extreme Trendelenburg's or modified Sims' position or a knee-chest position.
3. Administer oxygen, 8 to 10 L/min, by face mask to the client.
4. Monitor fetal heart rate and assess the fetus for hypoxia.
5. Prepare to start intravenous fluids or increase the rate of an existing solution.
6. Prepare for immediate birth.
7. Document the event, actions taken, and the client's response.

If umbilical cord prolapse occurs, the cord is lying alongside or below the presenting part of the fetus and can be seen or felt in or protruding from the vagina. The nurse stays with the client and asks another nurse to call the health care provider immediately. The nurse must relieve cord pressure immediately so that the fetus receives adequate oxygenation. The nurse can relieve cord pressure by elevating the fetal presenting part that is lying on the cord; the nurse does this by quickly gloving the hand and inserting two fingers into the vagina to the cervix and exerting upward pressure on the presenting part. The nurse also relieves cord pressure by placing the client into extreme Trendelenburg's or modified Sims' position or a knee-chest position (a rolled towel is placed under the client's hip). The nurse administers oxygen, 8 to 10 L/min, by face mask to the client, monitors fetal heart rate and fetal heart rate patterns, and assesses the fetus for hypoxia. The client is prepared for immediate birth (vaginal or cesarean). The nurse documents the event, actions taken, the client's response, and any additional pertinent information. The nurse never attempts to push the cord into the uterus. If the umbilical cord is protruding from the vagina, the cord is wrapped loosely in a sterile towel saturated with warm sterile normal saline.

Reference: Perry, S., Hockenberry, M., Lowdermilk, D., & Wilson, D. (2010). *Maternal child nursing care* (4th ed., p. 467). St. Louis: Mosby.

Marginal   Partial

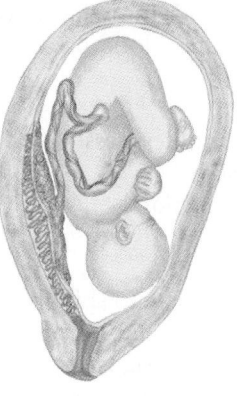 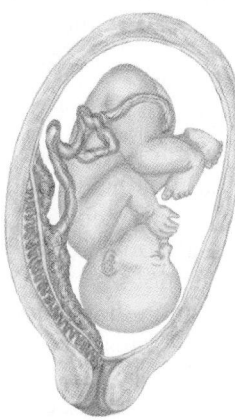

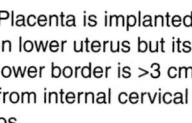

Placenta is implanted in lower uterus but its lower border is >3 cm from internal cervical os.

Lower border of placenta is within 3 cm of internal cervical os but does not fully cover it.

Total

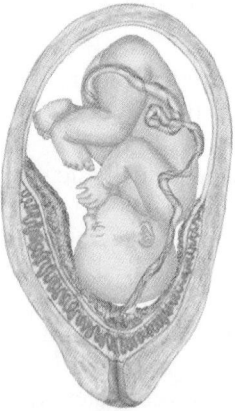

Placenta completely covers internal cervical os.

▲ **FIGURE 27-2** Three classifications of placenta previa. (From McKinney, E., James, S., Murray, S., & Ashwill, J. [2009]. *Maternal-child nursing* [3rd ed., p. 614]. St. Louis: Saunders.)

B. Assessment
1. Sudden onset of painless, bright red vaginal bleeding occurs in the last half of pregnancy.
2. **Uterus** is soft, relaxed, and nontender.
3. Fundal height may be more than expected for gestational age.

C. Interventions
1. Monitor maternal vital signs, fetal heart rate, and fetal activity.
2. Prepare for ultrasound to confirm the diagnosis.
3. Vaginal examinations or any other actions that would stimulate uterine activity are avoided.
4. Maintain bedrest in a side-lying position as prescribed.
5. Monitor amount of bleeding (treat signs of shock).
6. Administer intravenous fluids, blood products, or tocolytic medications as prescribed.
7. If bleeding is heavy, a cesarean **delivery** may be performed.

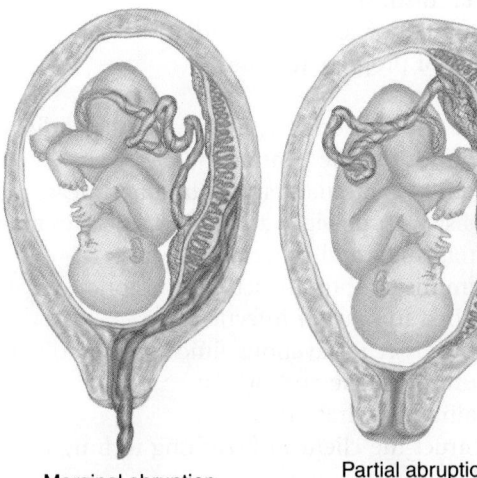

Marginal abruption with external bleeding

Partial abruption with concealed bleeding

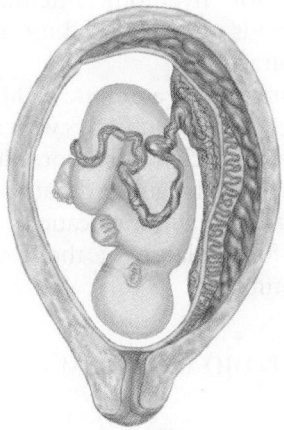

Complete abruption with concealed bleeding

▲ **FIGURE 27-3** Types of abruptio placentae. (From McKinney, E., James, S., Murray, S., & Ashwill, J. [2009]. *Maternal-child nursing* [3rd ed., p. 616]. St. Louis: Saunders.)

V. ABRUPTIO PLACENTAE

A. Description: Premature separation of the **placenta** from the uterine wall after the twentieth week of gestation and before the fetus is delivered (Fig. 27-3)

B. Assessment
1. Dark red vaginal bleeding. If the bleeding is high in the **uterus** or is minimal, there can be an absence of visible blood.
2. Uterine pain or tenderness or both
3. Uterine rigidity
4. Severe abdominal pain
5. Signs of fetal distress
6. Signs of maternal shock if bleeding is excessive

C. Interventions
1. Monitor maternal vital signs and fetal heart rate.
2. Assess for excessive vaginal bleeding, abdominal pain, and an increase in fundal height.
3. Maintain bedrest; administer oxygen, intravenous fluids, and blood products as prescribed.
4. Place the client in Trendelenburg's position if indicated to decrease the pressure of the fetus on the **placenta**, or place in the lateral position with the head of the bed flat if hypovolemic shock occurs.
5. Monitor and report any uterine activity.
6. Prepare for **delivery** of the fetus as quickly as possible, with vaginal **delivery** preferable if the fetus is healthy and stable and the presenting part is in the pelvis; emergency cesarean **delivery** is performed if the fetus is alive but shows signs of distress.
7. Monitor for signs of disseminated intravascular coagulation in the postpartum period.

⚠ Know the differences between placenta previa and abruptio placentae. In placenta previa, there is painless, bright red vaginal bleeding, and the uterus is soft, relaxed, and nontender. In abruptio placentae, there is dark red vaginal bleeding, uterine pain or tenderness or both, and uterine rigidity.

VI. PLACENTAL ABNORMALITIES

A. Description: **Placenta** accreta is an abnormally adherent **placenta**; **placenta** increta occurs when the **placenta** penetrates the uterine muscle itself; **placenta** percreta occurs when the **placenta** goes all the way through the **uterus**.

B. Assessment: May cause hemorrhage immediately after birth because the **placenta** does not separate cleanly

C. Intervention
1. Monitor for hemorrhage and shock.
2. Prepare the client for a hysterectomy if a large portion of the **placenta** is abnormally adherent.

VII. PRETERM LABOR

A. Description
1. Preterm **labor** occurs after the twentieth week but before the thirty-seventh week of gestation.

2. Risk factors include a history of medical conditions; present and past obstetric problems; infection; and social and environmental factors, including substance abuse.
3. Additional risk factors include a multifetal pregnancy, which contributes to overdistention of the **uterus**; anemia, which decreases oxygen supply to the **uterus**; and age younger than 18 years or first pregnancy and age older than 40 years.

B. Assessment
1. Uterine contractions (painful or painless)
2. Abdominal cramping (may be accompanied by diarrhea)
3. Low back pain
4. Pelvic pressure or heaviness
5. Change in character and amount of usual discharge—may be thicker or thinner, bloody, brown or colorless, odorous
6. Rupture of amniotic membranes

C. Interventions
1. Focus on stopping the **labor**: identify and treat infection, restrict activity, and ensure hydration.
2. Maintain bedrest and a lateral position.
3. Monitor fetal status.
4. Administer fluids.
5. Administer medications as prescribed and monitor for side effects of tocolytics (see Table 31-1 for a description of medications used to treat preterm **labor**).

VIII. PRECIPITOUS LABOR AND DELIVERY

A. Description: **Labor** lasting less than 3 hours
B. Interventions
1. Have a precipitous **delivery** tray available (hemostats, scissors, and cord clamp).
2. Stay with the client at all times.
3. Provide emotional support and keep the client calm.
4. Encourage the client to pant between contractions.
5. Prepare for rupturing membranes when the head crowns, if they are not already ruptured.
6. Do not try to keep the fetus from being delivered.
7. If **delivery** is necessary before the arrival of the health care provider, do the following:
   a. Apply gentle pressure to the fetal head upward toward the **vagina** to prevent damage to the fetal head and vaginal lacerations.
   b. Support the **infant's** body during **delivery**.
   c. Deliver the **infant** between contractions, checking for the cord around the neck.
   d. Use restitution to deliver the posterior shoulder.
   e. Use gentle downward pressure to move the anterior shoulder under the pubic symphysis.
   f. Clear the **infant's** mouth.
   g. Dry and cover the **infant** to keep the body warm.
   h. Allow the **placenta** to separate naturally.
   i. Place the **infant** on the mother's abdomen or breast to induce uterine contractions.

IX. DYSTOCIA

A. Description
1. Dystocia is difficult **labor** that is prolonged or more painful.
2. Dystocia occurs because of problems caused by uterine contractions, the fetus, or the bones and tissues of the maternal pelvis.
3. The fetus may be excessively large, malpositioned, or in an abnormal presentation.
4. Contractions may be hypotonic or hypertonic.
5. Hypotonic contractions are short, irregular, and weak; amniotomy and oxytocin (Pitocin) infusion may be treatment measures.
6. Hypertonic contractions are painful, occur frequently, and are uncoordinated; treatment depends on the cause and includes pain relief measures and rest.
7. Dystocia can result in maternal dehydration, infection, fetal injury, or death.

B. Assessment
1. Excessive abdominal pain
2. Abnormal contraction pattern
3. Fetal distress
4. Maternal or fetal tachycardia
5. Lack of progress in **labor**

C. Interventions
1. Assess fetal heart rate; monitor for fetal distress.
2. Monitor uterine contractions.
3. Monitor maternal temperature and heart rate.
4. Assist with pelvic examination, measurements, ultrasound, and other procedures.
5. Administer prophylactic antibiotics as prescribed to prevent infection.
6. Administer intravenous fluids as prescribed.
7. Monitor intake and output.
8. Maintain hydration.
9. Instruct the client in breathing techniques and relaxation exercises.
10. Perform fetal monitoring if oxytocin is prescribed for hypotonic uterine contractions (oxytocin is not prescribed for hypertonic uterine contractions).
11. Monitor color of **amniotic fluid**.
12. Provide rest and comfort as with a normal **delivery**, such as back rubs and position changes.
13. Assess client's fatigue and pain, and administer sedatives and pain medications as prescribed.
14. Assess for prolapse of the cord after membranes rupture.

X. AMNIOTIC FLUID EMBOLISM

A. Description
1. **Amniotic fluid** embolism is the escape of **amniotic fluid** into the maternal circulation.
2. The debris-containing **amniotic fluid** deposits in the pulmonary arterioles and is usually fatal to the mother.

B. Assessment
1. Abrupt onset of respiratory distress and chest pain
2. Cyanosis
3. Seizures
4. Heart failure and pulmonary edema
5. Fetal bradycardia and distress if **delivery** has not occurred at the time of the embolism

C. Intervention
1. Institute emergency measures to maintain life.
2. Administer oxygen, 8 to 10 L/min, by face mask or resuscitation bag delivering 100% oxygen.
3. Prepare for intubation and mechanical ventilation.
4. Position the client on her side.
5. Administer intravenous fluids, blood products, and medications to correct coagulation failure.
6. Monitor fetal status.
7. Prepare for emergency **delivery** when the client is stabilized.
8. Provide emotional support to the client, partner, and family.

XI. FETAL DISTRESS

A. Assessment
1. Fetal heart rate less than 120 beats/min or greater than 160 beats/min
2. Meconium-stained **amniotic fluid**
3. Fetal hyperactivity
4. Progressive decrease in baseline variability
5. Severe variable decelerations
6. Late decelerations

B. Interventions
1. Place the client in a lateral position.
2. Administer oxygen, 8 to 10 L/min, via face mask.
3. Discontinue oxytocin if infusing.
4. Monitor maternal and fetal status.

⚠ In the event of fetal distress, prepare the client for emergency cesarean delivery.

XII. INTRAUTERINE FETAL DEMISE

A. Assessment
1. Loss of fetal movement
2. Absence of fetal heart tones
3. Disseminated intravascular coagulation (DIC) screen (monitor for coagulation abnormalities because DIC is a complication related to intrauterine fetal demise)
4. Low hemoglobin and hematocrit; low platelet count; prolonged bleeding and clotting time
5. Bleeding from puncture sites (could indicate DIC)

B. Interventions
1. Encourage the client and her family to verbalize feelings; provide emotional support.
2. Incorporate religious and cultural health care beliefs and practices in the plan of care.
3. Allow the client choices relating to **labor** and **delivery**.

4. Administer intravenous fluids, medications, and blood and blood products as prescribed if DIC occurs.

XIII. RUPTURE OF THE UTERUS

A. Description
1. Complete or incomplete separation of the uterine tissue as a result of a tear in the wall of the **uterus** from the stress of **labor**
2. Complete: Direct communication between the uterine and peritoneal cavities
3. Incomplete: Rupture into the peritoneum covering the **uterus**, but not into the peritoneal cavity
4. Manifestations vary with the degree of rupture.

B. Assessment
1. Abdominal pain or tenderness
2. Chest pain
3. Contractions may stop or fail to progress
4. Rigid abdomen
5. Absent fetal heart rate
6. Signs of maternal shock
7. Fetus palpated outside the **uterus** (complete rupture)

C. Interventions
1. Monitor for and treat signs of shock (administer oxygen, intravenous fluids, and blood products).
2. Prepare client for cesarean **delivery** (possible hysterectomy may be necessary).
3. Provide emotional support for the client and partner.

XIV. UTERINE INVERSION

A. Description
1. **Uterus** completely or partly turns inside out.
2. This can occur during **delivery** or after **delivery** of the **placenta**.

B. Assessment
1. A depression in the fundal area of the **uterus** is noted.
2. The interior of the **uterus** may be seen through the cervix or protruding through the **vagina**.
3. The client has severe pain.
4. Hemorrhage is evident.
5. The client shows signs of shock.

C. Intervention
1. Monitor for hemorrhage and signs of shock and treat shock.
2. Prepare the client for a return of the **uterus** to the correct position via the **vagina**; if unsuccessful, laparotomy with replacement to the correct position is done.

🔘 MORE QUESTIONS ON THE CD!

Practice Questions

265. A nurse is assessing a pregnant client in the second trimester of pregnancy who was admitted

to the maternity unit with a suspected diagnosis of abruptio placentae. Which of the following assessment findings would the nurse expect to note if this condition is present?
1. Soft abdomen
2. Uterine tenderness
3. Absence of abdominal pain
4. Painless, bright red vaginal bleeding

266. A maternity nurse is preparing for the admission of a client in the third trimester of pregnancy who is experiencing vaginal bleeding and has a suspected diagnosis of placenta previa. The nurse reviews the physician's prescriptions and would question which prescription?
1. Prepare the client for an ultrasound.
2. Obtain equipment for a manual pelvic examination.
3. Prepare to draw a hemoglobin and hematocrit blood sample.
4. Obtain equipment for external electronic fetal heart rate monitoring.

267. An ultrasound is performed on a client at term gestation who is experiencing moderate vaginal bleeding. The results of the ultrasound indicate that abruptio placentae is present. Based on these findings, the nurse would prepare the client for:
1. Delivery of the fetus
2. Strict monitoring of intake and output
3. Complete bedrest for the remainder of the pregnancy
4. The need for weekly monitoring of coagulation studies until the time of delivery

268. A nurse is performing an initial assessment on a client who has just been told that a pregnancy test is positive. Which assessment finding would indicate that the client is at risk for preterm labor?
1. The client is a 35-year-old primigravida.
2. The client has a history of cardiac disease.
3. The client's hemoglobin level is 13.5 g/dL.
4. The client is a 20-year-old primigravida of average weight and height.

269. A nurse is monitoring a client who is in the active stage of labor. The client has been experiencing contractions that are short, irregular, and weak. The nurse documents that the client is experiencing which type of labor dystocia?
1. Hypotonic
2. Precipitous
3. Hypertonic
4. Preterm labor

270. After a precipitous delivery, a nurse notes that the new mother is passive and only touches her newborn infant briefly with her fingertips. The nurse

should do which of the following to help the woman process what has happened?
1. Encourage the mother to breast-feed soon after birth.
2. Support the mother in her reaction to the newborn infant.
3. Tell the mother that it is important to hold the newborn infant.
4. Document a complete account of the mother's reaction on the birth record.

271. A nurse in a labor room is monitoring a client with dysfunctional labor for signs of fetal or maternal compromise. Which of the following assessment findings would alert the nurse to a compromise?
1. Maternal fatigue
2. Coordinated uterine contractions
3. Progressive changes in the cervix
4. Persistent nonreassuring fetal heart rate

272. A nurse in a labor room is preparing to care for a client with hypertonic uterine contractions. The nurse is told that the client is experiencing uncoordinated contractions that are erratic in their frequency, duration, and intensity. The priority nursing intervention in caring for the client is to:
1. Provide pain relief measures.
2. Prepare the client for an amniotomy.
3. Promote ambulation every 30 minutes.
4. Monitor the oxytocin (Pitocin) infusion closely.

273. A nurse is reviewing the physician's prescriptions for a client admitted for premature rupture of the membranes. Gestational age of the fetus is determined to be 37 weeks. Which physician's prescription should the nurse question?
1. Perform a vaginal examination every shift.
2. Monitor maternal vital signs frequently.
3. Monitor fetal heart rate continuously.
4. Administer ampicillin 1 g as an intravenous piggyback every 6 hours.

274. A nurse has developed a plan of care for a client experiencing dystocia and includes several nursing interventions in the plan of care. The nurse prioritizes the plan of care and selects which intervention as the highest priority?
1. Providing comfort measures
2. Monitoring the fetal heart rate
3. Changing the client's position frequently
4. Keeping the significant other informed of the progress of the labor

275. Fetal distress is occurring with a laboring client. As the nurse prepares the client for a cesarean birth, what other intervention should be performed?

1. Slow the intravenous flow rate.
2. Place the client in a high Fowler's position.
3. Continue the oxytocin (Pitocin) drip if infusing.
4. Administer oxygen, 8 to 10 L/min, via face mask.

276. A nurse in the postpartum unit is caring for a client who has just delivered a newborn infant following a pregnancy with a placenta previa. The nurse reviews the plan of care and prepares to monitor the client for which risk associated with placenta previa?
1. Infection
2. Hemorrhage
3. Chronic hypertension
4. Disseminated intravascular coagulation

277. A nurse in a labor room is performing a vaginal assessment on a pregnant client in labor. The nurse notes the presence of the umbilical cord protruding from the vagina. Which of the following is an initial nursing action?

1. Gently push the cord into the vagina.
2. Place the client in Trendelenburg's position.
3. Find the closest telephone and page the physician stat.
4. Call the delivery room to notify the staff that the client will be transported immediately.

Alternate Item Format: Multiple Response
278. A nurse is performing an assessment on a client diagnosed with placenta previa. Which of these assessment findings would the nurse expect to note? **Select all that apply.**
❏ 1. Uterine rigidity
❏ 2. Uterine tenderness
❏ 3. Severe abdominal pain
❏ 4. Bright red vaginal bleeding
❏ 5. Soft, relaxed, nontender uterus
❏ 6. Fundal height may be greater than expected for gestational age

ANSWERS
265. 2
Rationale: Abruptio placentae is the premature separation of the placenta from the uterine wall after the twentieth week of gestation and before the fetus is delivered. Painless, bright red vaginal bleeding in the second or third trimester of pregnancy is a sign of placenta previa. In abruptio placentae, acute abdominal pain is present. Uterine tenderness accompanies placental abruption, especially with a central abruption and trapped blood behind the placenta. The abdomen feels hard and board-like on palpation as the blood penetrates the myometrium and causes uterine irritability.
Test-Taking Strategy: Focus on the subject, abruption placentae. Remember that the difference between placenta previa and abruptio placentae involves the presence of uterine pain and tenderness with abruptio placentae, as opposed to painless bleeding with placenta previa. Review the signs of abruptio placentae if you had difficulty with this question.
Level of Cognitive Ability: Analyzing
Client Needs: Physiological Integrity
Integrated Process: Nursing Process—Assessment
Content Area: Maternity—Intrapartum
Reference: McKinney, E., James, S., Murray, S., & Ashwill, J. (2009). *Maternal-child nursing* (3rd ed., p. 616). St. Louis: Saunders.

266. 2
Rationale: Placenta previa is an improperly implanted placenta in the lower uterine segment near or over the internal cervical os. Manual pelvic examinations are contraindicated when vaginal bleeding is apparent until a diagnosis is made and placenta previa is ruled out. Digital examination of the cervix can lead to hemorrhage. A diagnosis of placenta previa is made by ultrasound. The hemoglobin and hematocrit

levels are monitored, and external electronic fetal heart rate monitoring is initiated. Electronic fetal monitoring (external) is crucial in evaluating the status of the fetus, who is at risk for severe hypoxia.
Test-Taking Strategy: Use knowledge of the pathophysiology associated with placenta previa. Note the strategic words *would question which prescription* in the event query. Also, note that option 2 is the only procedure that is invasive to the pregnancy and endangers the physiological safety of the client and the fetus. Review care for the client with placenta previa if you had difficulty with this question.
Level of Cognitive Ability: Applying
Client Needs: Physiological Integrity
Integrated Process: Nursing Process—Implementation
Content Area: Maternity—Intrapartum
Reference: McKinney, E., James, S., Murray, S., & Ashwill, J. (2009). *Maternal-child nursing* (3rd ed., p. 615). St. Louis: Saunders.

267. 1
Rationale: Abruptio placentae is the premature separation of the placenta from the uterine wall after the twentieth week of gestation and before the fetus is delivered. The goal of management in abruptio placentae is to control the hemorrhage and deliver the fetus as soon as possible. Delivery is the treatment of choice if the fetus is at term gestation or if the bleeding is moderate to severe and the client or fetus is in jeopardy. Because delivery of the fetus is necessary, options 2, 3, and 4 are incorrect regarding management of a client with abruptio placentae.
Test-Taking Strategy: Use the process of elimination and knowledge regarding the management of abruptio placentae to answer the question. Note the strategic words *term gestation* and *moderate vaginal bleeding*. Knowing that the goal is to deliver the fetus will direct you easily to option 1. If you had difficulty with this question or are unfamiliar with the management of abruptio placentae, review this content.

Level of Cognitive Ability: Applying
Client Needs: Physiological Integrity
Integrated Process: Nursing Process—Planning
Content Area: Maternity—Intrapartum
Reference: McKinney, E., James, S., Murray, S., & Ashwill, J. (2009). *Maternal-child nursing* (3rd ed., p. 616). St. Louis: Saunders.

268. 2
Rationale: Preterm labor occurs after the twentieth week but before the thirty-seventh week of gestation. Several factors are associated with preterm labor, including a history of medical conditions, present and past obstetric problems, social and environmental factors, and substance abuse. Other risk factors include a multifetal pregnancy, which contributes to overdistention of the uterus; anemia, which decreases oxygen supply to the uterus; and age younger than 18 years or first pregnancy at age older than 40 years.
Test-Taking Strategy: Use the process of elimination and note that option 2 is the only option that identifies an abnormal condition. Options 1, 3, and 4 are average and normal findings. Review the risk factors for preterm labor if you had difficulty with this question.
Level of Cognitive Ability: Analyzing
Client Needs: Physiological Integrity
Integrated Process: Nursing Process—Assessment
Content Area: Maternity—Antepartum
References: McKinney, E., James, S., Murray, S., & Ashwill, J. (2009). *Maternal-child nursing* (3rd ed., pp. 674-675). St. Louis: Saunders.
    Perry, S., Hockenberry, M., Lowdermilk, D., & Wilson, D. (2010). *Maternal child nursing care* (4th ed., pp. 192, 487). St. Louis: Mosby.

269. 1
Rationale: Hypotonic labor contractions are short, irregular, and weak and usually occur during the active phase of labor. Hypertonic dystocia usually occurs during the latent phase of labor, and contractions are painful, frequent, and usually uncoordinated. Precipitous labor is labor that lasts in its entirety for 3 hours or less. Preterm labor is the onset of labor after 20 weeks of gestation and before the thirty-seventh week of gestation.
Test-Taking Strategy: Use the process of elimination. Note the relationship between the words *short, irregular, and weak* in the question and *hypotonic* in the correct option. If you are unfamiliar with dysfunctional labor (dystocia), review this content.
Level of Cognitive Ability: Understanding
Client Needs: Physiological Integrity
Integrated Process: Communication and Documentation
Content Area: Maternity—Intrapartum
Reference: Perry, S., Hockenberry, M., Lowdermilk, D., & Wilson, D. (2010). *Maternal child nursing care* (4th ed., p. 498). St. Louis: Mosby.

270. 2
Rationale: Precipitous labor is labor that lasts less than 3 hours. Women who have experienced precipitous labor often describe feelings of disbelief that their labor progressed so rapidly. To assist the client to process what has happened, the best option is to support the client in her reaction to the newborn infant. Options 1, 3, and 4 do not acknowledge the client's feelings.

Test-Taking Strategy: Use therapeutic communication techniques. Option 2 is the only option that acknowledges the client's feelings. If you had difficulty with this question, review these techniques and care to the mother after a precipitous labor.
Level of Cognitive Ability: Applying
Client Needs: Psychosocial Integrity
Integrated Process: Caring
Content Area: Maternity—Postpartum
Reference: McKinney, E., James, S., Murray, S., & Ashwill, J. (2009). *Maternal-child nursing* (3rd ed., pp. 664, 667). St. Louis: Saunders.

271. 4
Rationale: Signs of fetal or maternal compromise include a persistent, nonreassuring fetal heart rate, fetal acidosis, and the passage of meconium. Maternal fatigue and infection can occur if the labor is prolonged, but do not indicate fetal or maternal compromise. Progressive changes in the cervix and coordinated uterine contractions are a reassuring pattern in labor.
Test-Taking Strategy: Focus on the subject of the question, signs of fetal or maternal compromise. Use the process of elimination, noting that options 1, 2, and 3 are normal expectations during labor. Review the assessment findings that indicate fetal or maternal compromise if you had difficulty with this question.
Level of Cognitive Ability: Analyzing
Client Needs: Physiological Integrity
Integrated Process: Nursing Process—Assessment
Content Area: Maternity—Intrapartum
Reference: McKinney, E., James, S., Murray, S., & Ashwill, J. (2009). *Maternal-child nursing* (3rd ed., p. 366). St. Louis: Saunders.

272. 1
Rationale: Hypertonic uterine contractions are painful, occur frequently, and are uncoordinated. Management of hypertonic labor depends on the cause. Relief of pain is the primary intervention to promote a normal labor pattern. An amniotomy and oxytocin infusion are not treatment measures for hypertonic contractions; however, these treatments may be used in clients with hypotonic dysfunction. A client with hypertonic uterine contractions would not be encouraged to ambulate every 30 minutes, but would be encouraged to rest.
Test-Taking Strategy: Focus on the strategic word *hypertonic*. This strategic word and knowledge of the therapeutic management for this condition will assist in directing you to option 1. Options 2, 3, and 4 are therapeutic measures for hypotonic dysfunction. If you had difficulty with this question, review the therapeutic management for hypertonic uterine contractions.
Level of Cognitive Ability: Applying
Client Needs: Physiological Integrity
Integrated Process: Nursing Process—Implementation
Content Area: Maternity—Intrapartum
Reference: Perry, S., Hockenberry, M., Lowdermilk, D., & Wilson, D. (2010). *Maternal child nursing care* (4th ed., p. 498). St. Louis: Mosby.

273. 1
Rationale: Vaginal examinations should not be done routinely on a client with premature rupture of the membranes because of the risk of infection. The nurse would expect to administer an antibiotic, monitor maternal vital signs, and monitor fetal heart rate.
Test-Taking Strategy: Note the strategic word *question*. This word indicates the activity that the nurse should not implement without clarification. Options 2, 3, and 4 are expected activities for the nurse to perform for a client with premature rupture of the membranes. Performing a vaginal examination every shift should not be done on a client with premature rupture of the membranes because of the risk of infection, so the nurse would question this prescription. Review care for the client with premature rupture of the membranes if you had difficulty with this question.
Level of Cognitive Ability: Analyzing
Client Needs: Physiological Integrity
Integrated Process: Nursing Process—Implementation
Content Area: Maternity—Intrapartum
Reference: McKinney, E., James, S., Murray, S., & Ashwill, J. (2009). *Maternal-child nursing* (3rd ed., pp. 673–674). St. Louis: Saunders.

274. 2
Rationale: Dystocia is difficult labor that is prolonged or more painful than expected. The priority is to monitor the fetal heart rate. Although providing comfort measures, changing the client's position frequently, and keeping the significant other informed of the progress of the labor are components of the plan of care, the fetal status would be the priority.
Test-Taking Strategy: Note the strategic words *highest priority*. Use Maslow's Hierarchy of Needs theory and the ABCs—airway, breathing, and circulation—to assist in answering the question. Review priority nursing interventions for the client with dystocia if you had difficulty with this question.
Level of Cognitive Ability: Applying
Client Needs: Physiological Integrity
Integrated Process: Nursing Process—Planning
Content Area: Maternity—Intrapartum
Reference: Perry, S., Hockenberry, M., Lowdermilk, D., & Wilson, D. (2010). *Maternal child nursing care* (4th ed., p. 504). St. Louis: Mosby.

275. 4
Rationale: Oxygen is administered, 8 to 10 L/min, via face mask to optimize oxygenation of the circulating blood. Option 1 is incorrect because the intravenous infusion should be increased to increase the maternal blood volume. Option 2 is incorrect because the client is placed in the lateral position with her legs raised to increase maternal blood volume and improve fetal perfusion. Option 3 is incorrect because oxytocin stimulation of the uterus is discontinued if fetal heart rate patterns change for any reason.
Test-Taking Strategy: Use the ABCs—airway, breathing, and circulation. Oxygen is the only option that would improve cardiac output and improve perfusion to the fetus. The other options would not improve perfusion to the fetus. Review

care for the laboring client experiencing fetal distress if you had difficulty with this question.
Level of Cognitive Ability: Applying
Client Needs: Physiological Integrity
Integrated Process: Nursing Process—Implementation
Content Area: Maternity—Intrapartum
Reference: McKinney, E., James, S., Murray, S., & Ashwill, J. (2009). *Maternal-child nursing* (3rd ed., p. 400). St. Louis: Saunders.

276. 2
Rationale: In placenta previa, the placenta is implanted in the lower uterine segment. The lower uterine segment does not contain the same intertwining musculature as the fundus of the uterus, and this site is more prone to bleeding. Options 1, 3, and 4 are not risks that are related specifically to placenta previa.
Test-Taking Strategy: Use the process of elimination, focusing on the subject of the question, placenta previa. Recalling that bleeding is a primary concern in this client will direct you easily to option 2. Review the complications associated with placenta previa if you had difficulty with this question.
Level of Cognitive Ability: Analyzing
Client Needs: Physiological Integrity
Integrated Process: Nursing Process—Assessment
Content Area: Maternity—Postpartum
Reference: Perry, S., Hockenberry, M., Lowdermilk, D., & Wilson, D. (2010). *Maternal child nursing care* (4th ed., p. 364). St. Louis: Mosby.

277. 2
Rationale: When cord prolapse occurs, prompt actions are taken to relieve cord compression and increase fetal oxygenation. The client should be positioned with the hips higher than the head to shift the fetal presenting part toward the diaphragm. The nurse should push the call light to summon help, and other staff members should call the physician and notify the delivery room. If the cord is protruding from the vagina, no attempt should be made to replace it because to do so could traumatize it and reduce blood flow further. The examiner may place a gloved hand into the vagina, however, and hold the presenting part off the umbilical cord. Oxygen, 8 to 10 L/min, by face mask is administered to the client to increase fetal oxygenation.
Test-Taking Strategy: Note the strategic words *umbilical cord protruding from the vagina*. Options 3 and 4 can be eliminated first because these actions delay necessary and immediate treatment. Recalling that the goal is to relieve cord compression and to increase fetal oxygenation will direct you to option 2. Also remember that the cord should not be pushed back into the vagina. Review priority nursing measures for prolapsed cord if you had difficulty with this question.
Level of Cognitive Ability: Applying
Client Needs: Physiological Integrity
Integrated Process: Nursing Process—Implementation
Content Area: Maternity—Intrapartum
Reference: McKinney, E., James, S., Murray, S., & Ashwill, J. (2009). *Maternal-child nursing* (3rd ed., pp. 688–689). St. Louis: Saunders.

ALTERNATE ITEM FORMAT: MULTIPLE RESPONSE

278. 4, 5, 6

Rationale: Placenta previa is an improperly implanted placenta in the lower uterine segment near or over the internal cervical os. Painless, bright red vaginal bleeding in the second or third trimester of pregnancy is a sign of placenta previa. The client has a soft, relaxed, nontender uterus, and fundal height may be more than expected for gestational age. In abruptio placentae, severe abdominal pain is present. Uterine tenderness accompanies placental abruption. Additionally, in abruptio placentae, the abdomen feels hard and board-like on palpation as the blood penetrates the myometrium and causes uterine irritability.

Test-Taking Strategy: First eliminate options 1 and 2 because they are comparable or alike. Next, remember that the difference between placenta previa and abruptio placentae involves the presence of uterine pain and tenderness with abruptio placentae, as opposed to painless bleeding with placenta previa. Review the signs of placenta previa and abruptio placentae if you had difficulty with this question.

Level of Cognitive Ability: Analyzing
Client Needs: Physiological Integrity
Integrated Process: Nursing Process—Assessment
Content Area: Maternity—Intrapartum
Reference: Perry, S., Hockenberry, M., Lowdermilk, D., & Wilson, D. (2010). *Maternal child nursing care* (4th ed., pp. 361–362). St. Louis: Mosby.

Postpartum Period

I. POSTPARTUM

A. Description: Period when the reproductive tract returns to the normal, nonpregnant state

B. The postpartum period starts immediately after **delivery** and is usually completed by week 6 following **delivery**.

II. PHYSIOLOGICAL MATERNAL CHANGES

A. Involution
1. Description
   a. Involution is the rapid decrease in the size of the **uterus** as it returns to the nonpregnant state.
   b. Clients who breast-feed may experience a more rapid involution because of the release of oxytocin during breast-feeding.

2. Assessment
   a. The weight of the **uterus** decreases from approximately 2 lb to 2 oz in 6 weeks.
   b. The endometrium regenerates.
   c. The fundus steadily descends into the pelvis.
   d. Fundal height decreases about 1 fingerbreadth (1 cm) per day (Fig. 28-1).
   e. By 10 days postpartum, the **uterus** cannot be palpated abdominally.
   f. A flaccid fundus indicates uterine atony and should be massaged until firm; a tender fundus indicates an infection (Fig. 28-2).
   g. Afterpains decrease in frequency after the first few days.

B. Lochia
1. Description: Discharge from the **uterus** that consists of blood from the vessels of the placental site and debris from the decidua

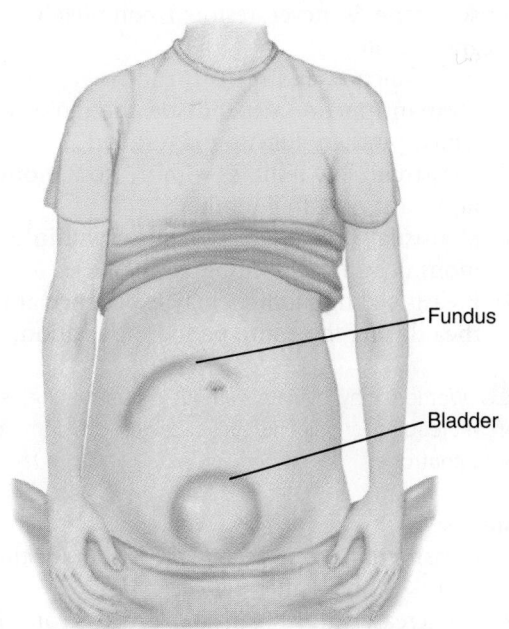

▲ **FIGURE 28-1** Involution of the uterus. The height of the uterine fundus decreases by approximately 1 cm/day. (From McKinney, E., James, S., Murray, S., & Ashwill, J. [2009]. *Maternal-child nursing* [3rd ed., p. 457]. St. Louis: Saunders.)

▲ **FIGURE 28-2** A full bladder displaces and prevents contraction of the uterus. (From McKinney, E., James, S., Murray, S., & Ashwill, J. [2009]. *Maternal-child nursing* [3rd ed., p. 460]. St. Louis: Saunders.)

Box 28-1 Amount of Lochia

Scant: Less than 2.5 cm (<1 inch) on menstrual pad in 1 hour
Light: Less than 10 cm (<4 inches) on menstrual pad in 1 hour
Moderate: Less than 15 cm (<6 inches) on menstrual pad in 1 hour
Heavy: Saturated menstrual pad in 1 hour
Excessive: Menstrual pad saturated in 15 minutes

From McKinney, E., James, S., Murray, S., & Ashwill, J. (2009). *Maternal-child nursing* (3rd ed., p. 457). St. Louis: Saunders.

Box 28-2 Breast Care for Non–Breast-Feeding Mothers

Avoid nipple stimulation.
Apply a breast binder, wear a snug-fitting bra, apply ice packs, or take a mild analgesic.
Engorgement usually resolves within 24 to 36 hours after it begins.

TABLE 28-1 Normal Postpartum Vital Signs

Vital Sign	Description
Temperature	May increase to 100.4° F because of dehydrating effects of labor. Any higher elevation may be caused by infection and must be reported
Pulse	May decrease to 50 beats/min (normal puerperal bradycardia). Pulse >100 beats/min may indicate excessive blood loss or infection
Blood pressure	Should be normal; suspect hypovolemia if it decreases
Respirations	Rarely change; if respirations increase significantly, suspect pulmonary embolism, uterine atony, or hemorrhage

2. Assessment (Box 28-1)
   a. Rubra is bright red discharge that occurs from **delivery** day to day 3.
   b. Serosa is brownish pink discharge that occurs from days 4 to 10.
   c. Alba is white discharge that occurs from days 11 to 14.
   d. The discharge should smell like normal menstrual flow.
   e. Discharge decreases daily in amount.
   f. Discharge may increase with ambulation.

   ⚠ To determine most accurately the amount of lochial flow, weigh the perineal pad before and after use and identify the amount of time between pad changes.

C. Cervix: Cervical involution occurs, and the muscle begins to regenerate after 1 week.
D. **Vagina**: Vaginal distention decreases, although muscle tone is never restored completely to the pregravid state.
E. Ovarian function and menstruation
   1. Ovarian function depends on the rapidity with which pituitary function is restored.
   2. Menstrual flow resumes within 1 to 2 months in non–breast-feeding mothers.
   3. Menstrual flow usually resumes within 3 to 6 months in breast-feeding mothers.
   4. Breast-feeding mothers may experience amenorrhea during the entire period of lactation.

   ⚠ Women may ovulate without menstruating, so breast-feeding should not be considered a form of birth control.

F. Breasts
   1. Breasts continue to secrete colostrum for the first 48 to 72 hours after **delivery**.
   2. A decrease in estrogen and progesterone levels after **delivery** stimulates increased prolactin levels, which promote breast milk production.
   3. Breasts become distended with milk on the third day.
   4. Engorgement occurs on approximately day 4 in non–breast-feeding mothers. Box 28-2 summarizes care of breasts for non–breast-feeding mothers.
   5. Breast-feeding relieves engorgement.
G. Urinary tract
   1. The client may have urinary retention as a result of loss of elasticity and tone and loss of sensation in the bladder from trauma, medications, anesthesia, and lack of privacy.
   2. Diuresis usually begins within the first 12 hours after **delivery**.
H. Gastrointestinal tract
   1. Clients are usually hungry after **delivery**.
   2. Constipation can occur, with bowel movement (soft, formed stool) by the second or third postpartum day.
   3. Hemorrhoids are common.
I. Vital signs (Table 28-1)
   1. Temperature may be elevated during the first 24 hours because of dehydration.
   2. Bradycardia is common during the first week (range of 50 to 70 beats/min).
   3. Blood pressure remains unchanged.

III. POSTPARTUM INTERVENTIONS

A. Assessment
1. Monitor vital signs.
2. Assess pain level.
3. Assess height, consistency, and location of the fundus (have client empty the bladder before fundal assessment) (see Fig. 28-2).
4. Monitor color, amount, and odor of **lochia**.
5. Assess breasts for engorgement.
6. Monitor perineum for swelling or discoloration.
7. Monitor episiotomy for healing.
8. Assess incisions or dressings of client who had a cesarean birth.
9. Monitor bowel status.
10. Monitor intake and output.
11. Encourage frequent voiding.
12. Encourage ambulation.
13. Assess extremities for thrombophlebitis (redness, tenderness, or warmth of the leg).
14. Administer Rh$_o$(D) immune globulin (Rho-GAM) as prescribed within 72 hours postpartum to Rh-negative client who has given birth to Rh-positive **infant**.
15. Assess bonding with the **newborn infant**.
16. Assess emotional status.

B. Client teaching
1. Demonstrate **newborn** care skills as necessary.
2. Provide the opportunity for the client to bathe the **newborn infant**.
3. Instruct in feeding technique.
4. Instruct the client to avoid heavy lifting for at least 3 weeks.
5. Instruct the client to plan at least one rest period per day.
6. Instruct the client that contraception should begin after **delivery** or with the initiation of intercourse (intercourse should be postponed at least until **lochia** ceases).
7. Instruct the client in the importance of follow-up, which should be scheduled at 4 to 6 weeks.
8. Instruct the client to report any signs of chills, fever, increased **lochia**, or depressed feelings to the physician immediately.

IV. POSTPARTUM DISCOMFORTS

A. Afterbirth pains
1. Afterbirth pains occur as a result of contractions of the **uterus**.
2. Afterbirth pains are more common in multiparas, breast-feeding mothers, clients treated with oxytocin (Pitocin), and clients who had an overdistended **uterus** during pregnancy, such as with carrying twins.

B. Perineal discomfort
1. Apply ice packs to the perineum during the first 24 hours to reduce swelling.

Box 28-3 Signs and Symptoms of Postpartum Depression

Anxiety	Irritability and agitation
Appetite changes	Lack of energy
Crying, sadness	Less responsive to the infant
Difficulty concentrating or making decisions	Loss of pleasure in normal activities
Fatigue, unable to sleep	Suicide thoughts
Feelings of guilt	

Modified from McKinney, E., James, S., Murray, S., & Ashwill, J. (2009). *Maternal-child nursing* (3rd ed., p. 712). St. Louis: Saunders.

---

2. After the first 24 hours, apply warmth by sitz baths.

C. Episiotomy
1. Instruct the client to administer perineal care after each voiding.
2. Encourage the use of an analgesic spray as prescribed.
3. Administer analgesics as prescribed if comfort measures are unsuccessful.

D. Perineal lacerations
1. Care as for an episiotomy; administer perineal care and use analgesic spray and analgesics for comfort.
2. Rectal suppositories and enemas may be contraindicated (to avoid injury to sutures).

E. Breast discomfort from engorgement
1. Encourage the client to wear a support bra at all times, even while she is sleeping.
2. Encourage the use of ice packs between feedings if the client is breast-feeding.
3. Encourage the use of warm soaks or a warm shower before feeding for the breast-feeding mother.
4. Administer analgesics as prescribed if comfort measures are unsuccessful.

F. Constipation
1. Encourage adequate intake of fluids (2000 mL/day).
2. Encourage diet high in fiber.
3. Encourage ambulation.
4. Administer stool softener, laxative, enema, or suppository if needed and prescribed.

G. Postpartum depression (Box 28-3).
1. Acknowledge the client's feelings and demonstrate a caring attitude.
2. Determine availability of family support and other support systems and resources as needed.
3. Encourage and assist the client to verbalize her feelings.
4. Monitor **newborn** for appropriate growth and development expectations.
5. Assist the significant other and other appropriate family members to discuss feelings and identify ways to assist the client.

⚠ All clients should be assessed for depression during pregnancy and in the postpartum period.

V. NUTRITIONAL COUNSELING

A. Discuss caloric intake with breast-feeding and non–breast-feeding mothers.

B. Nutritional needs depend on prepregnancy weight, ideal weight for height, and whether the client is breast-feeding.

C. If the client is breast-feeding, calorie needs increase by 200 to 500 cal/day, and the client may require increased fluids and the continuance of prenatal vitamins and minerals.

VI. BREAST-FEEDING

A. Interventions

1. Put the **infant** to the mother's breast as soon as the mother's and **infant**'s conditions are stable (on **delivery** table, if possible).

2. Stay with the client each time she nurses until she feels secure and confident with the **infant** and her feelings.

3. Assess *LATCH* (*l*atch achieved by **infant**; *a*udible swallowing; *t*ype of nipple; *c*omfort of mother; *h*elp given to mother with nursing).

4. Uterine cramping may occur the first day after **delivery** while the client is nursing, when oxytocin stimulation causes the **uterus** to contract.

5. Instruct the client to use general hygiene and wash the breasts once daily.

6. If engorgement occurs, breast-feed frequently, apply warm packs before feeding, apply ice packs between feedings, and massage the breasts.

7. The client should not use soap on the breasts because it tends to remove natural oils, which increases the chance of cracked nipples.

8. If cracked nipples develop, the client should expose the nipples to air for 10 to 20 minutes after feeding, rotate the position of the **infant** for each feeding, and ensure that the **infant** is latched on to the areola, not just the nipple.

9. The bra should be well-fitted and supporting.

10. Breasts may leak between feedings or during coitus; place breast pad in bra.

11. Calories should be increased by 200 to 500 cal/day, and the diet should include additional fluids; prenatal vitamins should be taken as prescribed.

12. **Infant**'s stools are usually light yellow, seedy, watery, and frequent.

13. Medications, including over-the-counter medications, need to be avoided unless prescribed because they may be unsafe when breast-feeding.

14. Gas-producing foods and caffeine should be avoided.

15. Hormonal contraceptives may cause a decrease in the milk supply and are best avoided during the first 6 weeks after birth.

Box 28-4 Breast-Feeding Procedure for the Mother

Wash hands and assume a comfortable position.
Start with the breast with which the last feeding ended.
Brush the newborn infant's lower lip with nipple.
Tickle the lips to have the infant open the mouth wide.
Guide the nipple and surrounding areola into the infant's mouth.
Encourage the infant to nurse on each breast for 15 to 20 minutes
After the infant has nursed, release suction by depressing the infant's chin or inserting a clean finger into the infant's mouth.
Burp the infant after the first breast.
Repeat the procedure on the second breast until the infant stops nursing.
Burp the infant again.
Listen for audible sucking and swallowing.

16. Oral contraceptives containing estrogen are not recommended for breast-feeding mothers; progestin-only birth control pills are less likely to interfere with the milk supply.

17. The **infant** will develop his or her own feeding schedule.

B. Breast-feeding procedure for client (Box 28-4)

 MORE QUESTIONS ON THE CD!

Practice Questions

279. A postpartum nurse is taking the vital signs of a client who delivered a healthy infant 4 hours ago. The nurse notes that the client's temperature is 100.2° F. Which of the following actions would be appropriate?
    1. Notify the physician.
    2. Document the findings.
    3. Retake the temperature in 15 minutes.
    4. Increase hydration by encouraging oral fluids.

280. A nurse is assessing a client who is 6 hours postpartum after delivering a full-term healthy infant. The client complains to the nurse of feelings of faintness and dizziness. Which nursing action would be most appropriate?
    1. Elevate the client's legs.
    2. Determine hemoglobin and hematocrit levels.
    3. Instruct the client to request help when getting out of bed.
    4. Inform the nursery room nurse to avoid bringing the newborn infant to the client until the feelings of faintness and dizziness have subsided.

281. A postpartum nurse is providing instructions to a client after delivery of a healthy infant. The nurse instructs the client that she should expect normal bowel elimination to return:
    1. 3 days postpartum
    2. 7 days postpartum
    3. On the day of delivery
    4. Within 2 weeks postpartum

282. A nurse is planning care for a postpartum client who had a vaginal delivery 2 hours ago. The client had a midline episiotomy and has several hemorrhoids. What is the priority nursing diagnosis for this client?
    1. *Acute pain*
    2. *Disturbed body image*
    3. *Impaired urinary elimination*
    4. *Risk for imbalanced fluid volume*

283. A nurse is monitoring the amount of lochia drainage in a client who is 2 hours postpartum and notes that the client has saturated a perineal pad in 1 hour. The nurse reports the amount of lochial flow as:
    1. Scant
    2. Light
    3. Heavy
    4. Excessive

284. A nurse is teaching a postpartum client about breast-feeding. Which of the following instructions should the nurse include?
    1. The diet should include additional fluids.
    2. Prenatal vitamins should be discontinued.
    3. Soap should be used to cleanse the breasts.
    4. Birth control measures are unnecessary while breast-feeding.

285. A nurse is preparing to perform a fundal assessment on a postpartum client. The initial nursing action in performing this assessment is which of the following?
    1. Ask the client to turn on her side.
    2. Ask the client to urinate and empty her bladder.

    3. Massage the fundus gently before determining the level of the fundus.
    4. Ask the client to lie flat on her back with the knees and legs flat and straight.

286. A nurse is caring for four 1-day postpartum clients. Which client has an abnormal finding that would require further intervention?
    1. The client with mild afterpains
    2. The client with a pulse rate of 60 beats/min
    3. The client with colostrum discharge from both breasts
    4. The client with lochia that is red and has a foul-smelling odor

287. When performing a postpartum assessment on a client, a nurse notes the presence of clots in the lochia. The nurse examines the clots and notes that they are larger than 1 cm. Which nursing action is appropriate?
    1. Notify the physician.
    2. Document the findings.
    3. Reassess the client in 2 hours.
    4. Encourage increased oral intake of fluids.

Alternate Item Format: Multiple Response

288. A nurse is providing postpartum instructions to a client who will be breast-feeding her newborn. The nurse determines that the client has understood the instructions if she makes which of the following statements? **Select all that apply**.
    ❏ 1. "I should wear a bra that provides support."
    ❏ 2. "Drinking alcohol can affect my milk supply."
    ❏ 3. "The use of caffeine can decrease my milk supply."
    ❏ 4. "I will start my estrogen birth control pills again as soon as I get home."
    ❏ 5. "I know if my breasts get engorged I will limit my breast-feeding and supplement the baby."
    ❏ 6. "I plan on having bottled water available in the refrigerator so I can get additional fluids easily."

ANSWERS
279. 4
Rationale: The client's temperature should be taken every 4 hours while she is awake. Temperatures up to 100.4° F (38° C) in the first 24 hours after birth often are related to the dehydrating effects of labor. The appropriate action is to increase hydration by encouraging oral fluids, which should bring the temperature to a normal reading. Although the nurse also would document the findings, the appropriate action would be to increase hydration. Contacting the physician is not necessary. Taking the temperature in another 15 minutes is an unnecessary action.

Test-Taking Strategy: Use the process of elimination and knowledge regarding the physiological findings in the immediate postpartum period to assist in answering this question. Recalling that a temperature elevation often is related to the dehydrating effects of labor will direct you to the correct option. Also, increasing hydration relates to a physiological client need. Review normal postpartum assessment findings if you had difficulty with this question.
Level of Cognitive Ability: Applying
Client Needs: Physiological Integrity
Integrated Process: Nursing Process—Implementation
Content Area: Maternity—Postpartum

References: McKinney, E., James, S., Murray, S., & Ashwill, J. (2009). *Maternal-child nursing* (3rd ed., p. 466). St. Louis: Saunders.

Swearingen, P. (2008). *All-in-one care planning resource: Medical-surgical, pediatric, maternity, & psychiatric nursing care plans* (2nd ed., p. 705). St. Louis: Mosby.

280. 3

Rationale: Orthostatic hypotension may be evident during the first 8 hours after birth. Feelings of faintness or dizziness are signs that caution the nurse to focus interventions on the client's safety. The nurse should advise the client to get help the first few times she gets out of bed. Option 1 is not the most appropriate or helpful action in this situation. Option 2 requires a physician's prescription. Option 4 is unnecessary.

Test-Taking Strategy: Focus on the subject of the question, client safety. Option 4 is inappropriate and should be eliminated first. Elevating the client's legs is not an appropriate or helpful nursing intervention. From the remaining options, recall that safety is a primary issue. This should assist in directing you to the correct option. If you had difficulty with this question, review postpartum nursing interventions.

Level of Cognitive Ability: Applying
Client Needs: Safe and Effective Care Environment
Integrated Process: Nursing Process—Implementation
Content Area: Maternity—Postpartum
Reference: McKinney, E., James, S., Murray, S., & Ashwill, J. (2009). *Maternal-child nursing* (3rd ed., p. 466). St. Louis: Saunders.

281. 1

Rationale: After birth, the nurse should auscultate the client's abdomen in all four quadrants to determine the return of bowel sounds. Normal bowel elimination usually returns 2 to 3 days postpartum. Surgery, anesthesia, and the use of opioids and pain control agents also contribute to the longer period of altered bowel functions. Options 2, 3, and 4 are incorrect.

Test-Taking Strategy: Use the process of elimination and general principles related to postpartum care to assist in answering this question. Eliminate options 2 and 4 first because of the length of time stated in these options. From the remaining options, eliminate option 3 because it would seem unreasonable that bowel function would return that quickly in the postpartum woman. Review normal gastrointestinal functions in the postpartum client if you had difficulty with this question.

Level of Cognitive Ability: Applying
Client Needs: Physiological Integrity
Integrated Process: Teaching and Learning
Content Area: Maternity—Postpartum
Reference: McKinney, E., James, S., Murray, S., & Ashwill, J. (2009). *Maternal-child nursing* (3rd ed., p. 459). St. Louis: Saunders.

282. 1

Rationale: The priority nursing diagnosis for a client who delivered 2 hours ago and who has a midline episiotomy and hemorrhoids is *Acute pain*. Most clients have some degree of discomfort during the immediate postpartum period. There are no data in the question that indicate the presence of *Disturbed body image, Impaired urinary elimination,* or *Risk for imbalanced fluid volume.*

Test-Taking Strategy: Note the strategic word *priority.* Use Maslow's Hierarchy of Needs theory to eliminate option 2 because this is a psychosocial, not a physiological, need. From the remaining options, focus on the data in the question to direct you to option 1. Review the discomforts that can occur in the postpartum client if you had difficulty with this question.

Level of Cognitive Ability: Analyzing
Client Needs: Physiological Integrity
Integrated Process: Nursing Process—Analysis
Content Area: Maternity—Postpartum
Reference: Perry, S., Hockenberry, M., Lowdermilk, D., & Wilson, D. (2010). *Maternal child nursing care* (4th ed., p. 539). St. Louis: Mosby.

283. 3

Rationale: Lochia is the discharge from the uterus in the postpartum period that consists of blood from the vessels of the placental site and debris from the decidua. The following can be used as a guide to determine the amount of flow: scant = less than 2.5 cm (<1 inch) on menstrual pad in 1 hour; light = less than 10 cm (<4 inches) on menstrual pad in 1 hour; moderate = less than 15 cm (<6 inches) on menstrual pad in 1 hour; heavy = saturated menstrual pad in 1 hour; and excessive = menstrual pad saturated in 15 minutes.

Test-Taking Strategy: Focus on the data in the question. The data and the use of guidelines to determine the amount of lochial flow will direct you to the correct option. If you had difficulty with this question, review postpartum assessment of the amount of lochial flow.

Level of Cognitive Ability: Understanding
Client Needs: Health Promotion and Maintenance
Integrated Process: Nursing Process—Assessment
Content Area: Maternity—Postpartum
References: McKinney, E., James, S., Murray, S., & Ashwill, J. (2009). *Maternal-child nursing* (3rd ed., pp. 457, 700). St. Louis: Saunders.

Perry, S., Hockenberry, M., Lowdermilk, D., & Wilson, D. (2010). *Maternal child nursing care* (4th ed., pp. 526–527). St. Louis: Mosby.

284. 1

Rationale: The diet for a breast-feeding client should include additional fluids. Prenatal vitamins should be taken as prescribed, and soap should not be used on the breast because it tends to remove natural oils, which increases the chance of cracked nipples. Breast-feeding is not a method of contraception, so birth control measures should be resumed.

Test-Taking Strategy: Use the process of elimination, noting the subject of the question, teaching for the breast-feeding client. Remember that fluids and calories should be increased when the client is breast-feeding. If you had difficulty with this question, review breast-feeding interventions.

Level of Cognitive Ability: Applying
Client Needs: Physiological Integrity
Integrated Process: Teaching and Learning
Content Area: Maternity—Postpartum

Reference: Swearingen, P. (2008). *All-in-one care planning resource: Medical-surgical, pediatric, maternity, & psychiatric nursing care plans* (2nd ed., p. 727). St. Louis: Mosby.

285. 2
Rationale: Before starting the fundal assessment, the nurse should ask the client to empty her bladder so that an accurate assessment can be done. When the nurse is performing fundal assessment, the nurse asks the client to lie flat on her back with the knees flexed. Massaging the fundus is inappropriate unless the fundus is boggy or soft, and then it should be massaged gently until firm.
Test-Taking Strategy: Note the strategic words *initial nursing action* in the query. Visualize the procedure when answering the question. This should direct you to option 2. Remember that a full bladder displaces the uterus. If you had difficulty with this question, review the procedure for performing fundal assessment in the postpartum period.
Level of Cognitive Ability: Applying
Client Needs: Health Promotion and Maintenance
Integrated Process: Nursing Process—Implementation
Content Area: Maternity—Postpartum
Reference: Perry, S., Hockenberry, M., Lowdermilk, D., & Wilson, D. (2010). *Maternal child nursing care* (4th ed., p. 483). St. Louis: Mosby.

286. 4
Rationale: Lochia, the discharge present after birth, is red for the first 1 to 3 days and gradually decreases in amount. Normal lochia has a fleshy odor or an odor similar to menstrual flow. Foul-smelling or purulent lochia usually indicates infection, and these findings are not normal. The other options are normal findings for a 1-day postpartum client.
Test-Taking Strategy: Note the strategic words *abnormal finding*. Noting the word *foul* in option 4 will direct you to this option. If you had difficulty with this question, review normal assessment findings in the postpartum client.
Level of Cognitive Ability: Analyzing
Client Needs: Physiological Integrity
Integrated Process: Nursing Process—Analysis
Content Area: Maternity—Postpartum
Reference: McKinney, E., James, S., Murray, S., & Ashwill, J. (2009). *Maternal-child nursing* (3rd ed., p. 469). St. Louis: Saunders.

287. 1
Rationale: Normally, a few small clots may be noted in the lochia in the first 1 to 2 days after birth from pooling of the blood in the vagina. Clots larger than 1 cm are considered abnormal. The cause of these clots, such as uterine atony or retained placental fragments, needs to be determined and treated to prevent further blood loss. Although the findings would be documented, the appropriate action is to notify the physician. Reassessing the client in 2 hours would delay necessary treatment. Increasing oral intake of fluids would not be a helpful action in this situation.
Test-Taking Strategy: Focus on the strategic words *larger than 1 cm*. Knowledge regarding the presence of clots in the postpartum period and their significance will direct you to option 1. If you had difficulty with this question, review normal findings in the postpartum client.
Level of Cognitive Ability: Applying
Client Needs: Physiological Integrity
Integrated Process: Nursing Process—Implementation
Content Area: Maternity—Postpartum
References: McKinney, E., James, S., Murray, S., & Ashwill, J. (2009). *Maternal-child nursing* (3rd ed., p. 700). St. Louis: Saunders.
Perry, S., Hockenberry, M., Lowdermilk, D., & Wilson, D. (2010). *Maternal child nursing care* (4th ed., pp. 539–540). St. Louis: Mosby.
Swearingen, P. (2008). *All-in-one care planning resource: Medical-surgical, pediatric, maternity, & psychiatric nursing care plans* (2nd ed., p. 708). St. Louis: Mosby.

ALTERNATE ITEM FORMAT: MULTIPLE RESPONSE
288. 1, 2, 3, 6
Rationale: The postpartum client should wear a bra that is well-fitted and supportive. Breasts may leak between feedings or during coitus, and the client is taught to place a breast pad in the bra. Breast-feeding clients should increase their daily fluid intake; having bottled water available indicates that the postpartum client understands the importance of increasing fluids. If engorgement occurs, the client should not limit breast-feeding, but should breast-feed frequently. Oral contraceptives containing estrogen are not recommended for breast-feeding mothers. Common causes of decreased milk supply include formula use; inadequate rest or diet; smoking by the mother or others in the home; and use of caffeine, alcohol, or other medications.
Test-Taking Strategy: Note the strategic words *understood the instructions*. Think about the physiology associated with milk production and the complications of breast-feeding. This will direct you to the correct options. Review postpartum instructions for a breast-feeding client if you had difficulty with this question.
Level of Cognitive Ability: Evaluating
Client Needs: Health Promotion and Maintenance
Integrated Process: Nursing Process—Evaluation
References: McKinney, E., James, S., Murray, S., & Ashwill, J. (2009). *Maternal-child nursing* (3rd ed., p. 568). St. Louis: Saunders.
Perry, S., Hockenberry, M., Lowdermilk, D., & Wilson, D. (2010). *Maternal child nursing care* (4th ed., pp. 694–695). St. Louis: Mosby.

Postpartum Complications

I. CYSTITIS

A. Description: Infection of the bladder

B. Assessment
   1. Burning and pain on urination
   2. Lower abdominal pain
   3. Increased frequency of urination
   4. Costovertebral angle tenderness
   5. Fever
   6. Proteinuria, hematuria, bacteriuria, white blood cells in the urine

C. Interventions
   1. Palpate bladder for distention.
   2. Palpate fundus.
   3. Obtain urine specimen for culture and sensitivity if prescribed.
   4. Institute measures to assist the client to void.
   5. Encourage frequent and complete emptying of the bladder.
   6. Encourage fluids to 3000 mL/day.
   7. Administer antibiotics as prescribed.
   8. Instruct the client in the methods of prevention and treatment of cystitis.

⚠ Obtain urine specimen for culture and sensitivity before initiating antibiotic therapy.

II. HEMATOMA

A. Description
   1. Hematoma is a localized collection of blood into the tissues of the reproductive sac after **delivery**; vulvar hematomas are the most common (Fig. 29-1).
   2. Predisposing conditions include operative **delivery** with forceps and injury to a blood vessel.
   3. Hematoma can be a life-threatening condition.

B. Assessment
   1. Abnormal severe pain
   2. Pressure in the perineal area
   3. Sensitive, bulging mass in the perineal area with discolored skin
   4. Inability to void
   5. Decreased hemoglobin and hematocrit levels

   6. Signs of shock, such as pallor, tachycardia, and hypotension, if significant blood loss has occurred

C. Interventions
   1. Monitor vital signs.
   2. Monitor client for abnormal pain or perineal pressure, especially when forceps **delivery** has occurred.
   3. Place ice at the hematoma site.
   4. Administer analgesics as prescribed.
   5. Monitor intake and output.
   6. Encourage fluids and voiding.
   7. Prepare for urinary catheterization if the client is unable to void.
   8. Administer blood products as prescribed.
   9. Monitor for signs of infection, such as increased temperature, pulse rate, and white blood cell count.
   10. Administer antibiotics as prescribed because infection is common after hematoma formation.
   11. Prepare for incision and evacuation of hematoma if necessary.

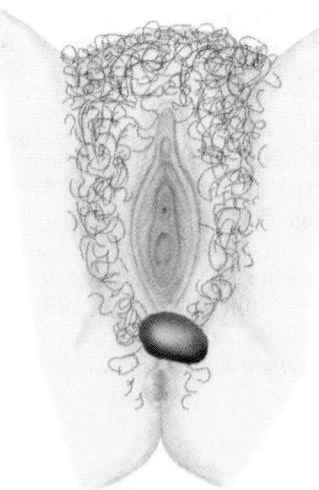

▲ **FIGURE 29-1** A vulvar hematoma is caused by rapid bleeding into soft tissue. It causes severe pain and feelings of pressure. (From Murray, S., & McKinney, E. [2010]. *Foundations of maternal-newborn and women's health nursing* [5th ed.]. St. Louis: Saunders.)

III. HEMORRHAGE

A. Description
1. Bleeding of 500 mL or more after **delivery**
2. Primary cause of maternal mortality that demands prompt recognition and intervention

B. Assessment (Box 29-1)
1. Early: Hemorrhage occurs during the first 24 hours after **delivery**.
2. Late: Hemorrhage occurs after the first 24 hours following **delivery**.

Box 29-1 Postpartum Hemorrhage

Causes
Uterine atony
Laceration of the vagina
Hematoma development in the cervix, perineum, or labia
Retained placental fragments

Predisposing Factors
Previous history of postpartum hemorrhage
Placenta previa
Abruptio placentae
Overdistention of the uterus—polyhydramnios, multiple gestation, large neonate
Infection
Multiparity
Dystocia or labor that is prolonged
Operative delivery—cesarean or forceps delivery, intrauterine manipulation

---

C. Interventions for signs of bleeding or shock
1. Massage fundus for uterine atony, with care not to overmassage (Fig. 29-2).
2. Remain with the client.
3. Ask another nurse to notify the physician or midwife.
4. Monitor vital signs and fundus every 5 to 15 minutes; monitor for early signs of hemorrhaging, including restlessness and increased pulse rate (a decrease in blood pressure is a later sign of hemorrhage).
5. Assess and estimate blood loss by pad count.
6. Turn the client to assess for pooled blood underneath her.
7. Assess level of consciousness.
8. Administer fluids and monitor intake and output.
9. Monitor hemoglobin and hematocrit levels.
10. Maintain asepsis because hemorrhage predisposes to infection.
11. Prepare for the administration of oxytocin (Pitocin) if prescribed.
12. Prepare for the administration of intravenous fluids and blood transfusions if prescribed.

IV. INFECTION

A. Description: Any infection of the reproductive organs that occurs within 28 days of **delivery** or abortion
B. Assessment
1. Fever

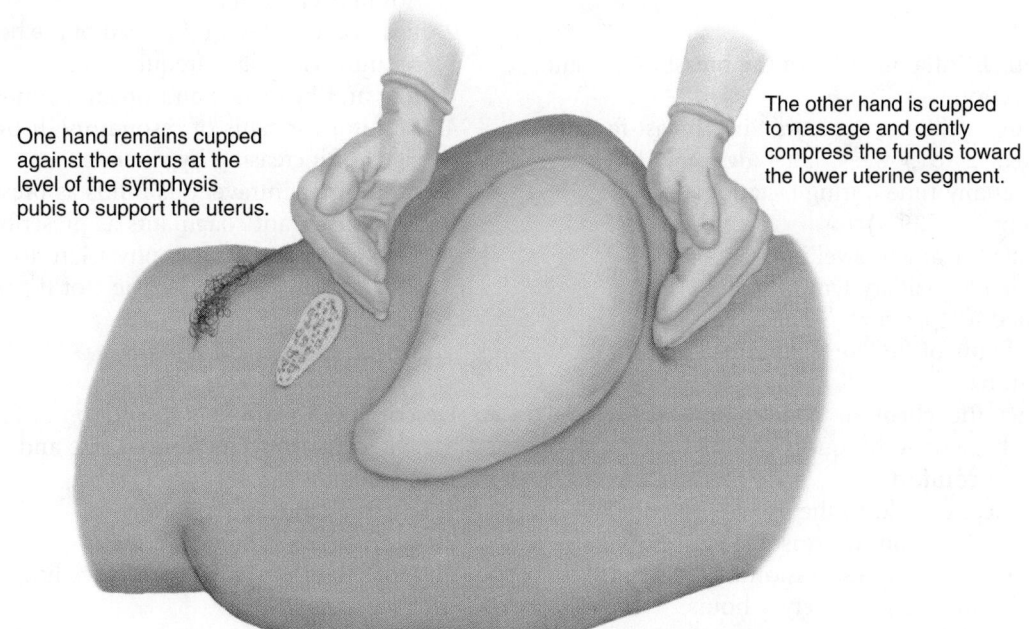

▲ **FIGURE 29-2** Technique for fundal massage. One hand remains cupped against the uterus at the level of the symphysis pubis to support the uterus. The other hand is cupped to massage and compress the fundus gently toward the lower uterine segment. (From McKinney, E., James, S., Murray, S., & Ashwill, J. [2009]. *Maternal-child nursing* [3rd ed., p. 697]. St. Louis: Saunders.)

One hand remains cupped against the uterus at the level of the symphysis pubis to support the uterus.

The other hand is cupped to massage and gently compress the fundus toward the lower uterine segment.

2. Chills
3. Anorexia
4. Pelvic discomfort or pain
5. Vaginal discharge that is malodorous; normal vaginal discharge has a fleshy odor or an odor similar to a menstrual period.
6. Elevated white blood cell count

⚠ A temperature of 100.4° F is normal during the first 24 hours postpartum because of dehydration; a temperature of 100.4° F or greater after 24 hours postpartum indicates infection.

C. Interventions
1. Monitor vital signs and temperature every 2 to 4 hours.
2. Make the client as comfortable as possible; position the client to promote drainage.
3. Keep the client warm if chilled.
4. Isolate the infant from the client only if the client can infect the infant.
5. Provide nutritious, high-calorie, high-protein diet.
6. Encourage fluids to 3000 to 4000 mL/day, if not contraindicated.
7. Encourage frequent voiding and monitor intake and output.
8. Monitor culture results if cultures were prescribed.
9. Administer antibiotics according to identified organism, as prescribed.

V. MASTITIS

A. Description
1. Mastitis is inflammation of the breast as a result of infection.
2. Mastitis primarily occurs in breast-feeding mothers 2 to 3 weeks after **delivery**, but may occur at any time during lactation.
B. Assessment (Fig. 29-3)
1. Localized heat and swelling
2. Pain; tender axillary lymph nodes
3. Elevated temperature
4. Complaints of flu-like symptoms
C. Interventions
1. Instruct the client in good handwashing and breast hygiene techniques.
2. Promote comfort.
3. Apply heat or cold to the site as prescribed.
4. Maintain lactation in breast-feeding mothers.
5. Encourage manual expression of breast milk or use of a breast pump every 4 hours.
6. Encourage the client to support the breasts by wearing a supportive bra.
7. Administer analgesics as prescribed.
8. Administer antibiotics as prescribed.

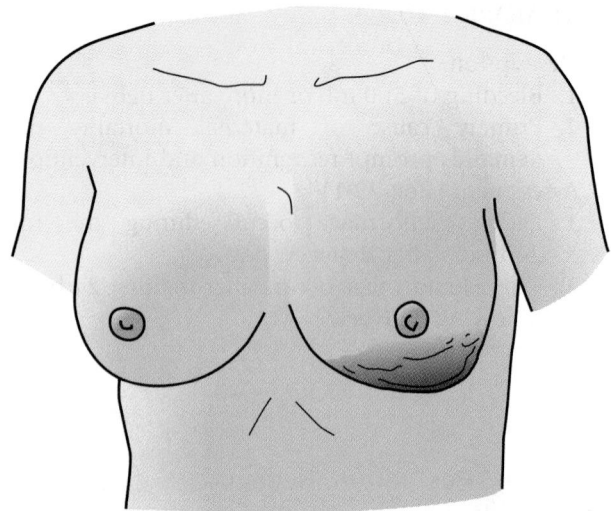

▲ **FIGURE 29-3** Mastitis. (From Perry, S., Hockenberry, M., Lowdermilk, D., & Wilson, D. [2010]. *Maternal child nursing care* [4th ed., p. 586]. St. Louis: Mosby.)

VI. PULMONARY EMBOLISM

A. Description: Passage of a thrombus, often originating in a uterine or other pelvic vein, into the lungs, where it disrupts the circulation of the blood
B. Assessment
1. Sudden dyspnea and chest pain
2. Tachypnea and tachycardia
3. Cough and lung crackles
4. Hemoptysis
5. Feeling of impending doom
C. Interventions
1. Administer oxygen.
2. Position client with the head of the bed elevated.
3. Monitor vital signs frequently, especially respiratory and heart rate and breath sounds.
4. Monitor for signs of respiratory distress and for signs of increasing hypoxemia.
5. Administer intravenous fluids as prescribed.
6. Administer anticoagulants as prescribed.
7. Prepare to assist the physician to administer medications to dissolve the clot if prescribed.

VII. SUBINVOLUTION

A. Description: Incomplete involution or failure of the **uterus** to return to its normal size and condition
B. Assessment
1. Uterine pain on palpation
2. **Uterus** larger than expected
3. More than normal vaginal bleeding
C. Interventions
1. Assess vital signs.
2. Assess **uterus** and fundus.
3. Monitor for uterine pain and vaginal bleeding.
4. Elevate legs to promote venous return.

Box 29-2 Assessment of Types of Thrombophlebitis

Superficial
Palpable thrombus that feels bumpy and hard
Tenderness and pain in affected lower extremity
Warm and pinkish red color over the thrombus area

Femoral
Malaise
Chills and fever
Possible positive Homans' sign (not always present)
Diminished peripheral pulses
Shiny white skin over affected area
Pain, stiffness, and swelling of affected leg

Pelvic
Severe chills
Dramatic body temperature changes
Pulmonary embolism may be the first sign

5. Encourage frequent voiding.
6. Monitor hemoglobin and hematocrit.
7. Prepare to administer methylergonovine maleate (Methergine), which provides sustained contraction of the uterus, as prescribed.

VIII. THROMBOPHLEBITIS

A. Description
1. A clot forms in a vessel wall as a result of the inflammation of the vessel wall.
2. A partial obstruction of the vessel can occur.
3. Increased blood-clotting factors in the postpartum period place the client at risk.
4. Early ambulation in the postoperative period after cesarean section is a preventive measure.
B. Types
1. Superficial thrombophlebitis
2. Femoral thrombophlebitis
3. Pelvic thrombophlebitis
C. Assessment (Box 29-2)
D. Interventions
1. Specific therapies may depend on the location of thrombophlebitis.
2. Assess the lower extremities for edema, tenderness, varices, and increased skin temperature.
3. Maintain bedrest.
4. Elevate affected leg.
5. Apply a bed cradle and keep bedclothes off affected leg.
6. Never massage the leg.
7. Monitor for manifestations of pulmonary embolism.
8. Apply hot packs or moist heat to the affected site as prescribed to alleviate discomfort.
9. Apply elastic stockings (support hose) if prescribed.
10. Administer analgesics as prescribed.

Box 29-3 Client Education for Thrombophlebitis

Never massage the leg.
Avoid crossing the legs.
Avoid prolonged sitting.
Avoid constrictive clothing.
Avoid pressure behind the knees.
Know how to apply elastic stockings (support hose) if prescribed.
Understand the importance of anticoagulant therapy if prescribed.
Understand the importance of follow-up with the health care provider.

11. Administer antibiotics if prescribed.
12. Heparin sodium intravenously may be prescribed for femoral or pelvic thrombophlebitis to prevent further thrombus formation.
E. Client education (Box 29-3)

IX. PERINATAL LOSS

A. Description
1. Perinatal loss is associated with miscarriage, neonatal death, stillbirth, and therapeutic abortion.
2. Loss and grief may also occur with the birth of a preterm **infant**, an **infant** with complications of birth, or an **infant** with congenital anomalies; it may also occur in a client who is giving up a child for adoption.
B. Interventions

Not all interventions are appropriate for every woman and her significant family. It is crucial to consider religious and cultural health care practices and beliefs when planning care for a woman and family who have experienced perinatal loss.

1. Communicate therapeutically and actively listen, providing parents time to grieve.
2. Notify the hospital chaplain or other religious person.
3. Discuss with the parents options such as seeing, holding, bathing, or dressing the deceased **infant**; visitation by other family members or friends; religious or cultural rituals; and funeral arrangements.
4. Prepare a special memories box with keepsakes such as footprints, handprints, locks of hair, and pictures, if appropriate.
5. Admit the mother to a private room; if possible, mark the door to the room with a special card (per agency procedure and maintaining confidentiality) that denotes to hospital staff that this family has experienced a loss.
6. See Chapter 27 for additional information on intrauterine fetal demise.

MORE QUESTIONS ON THE CD!

Practice Questions

289. A nurse is monitoring a client in the immediate postpartum period for signs of hemorrhage. Which of the following signs, if noted, would be an early sign of excessive blood loss?
1. A temperature of 100.4° F
2. A blood pressure change from 130/88 to 124/80 mm Hg
3. An increase in the pulse rate from 88 to 102 beats/min
4. An increase in the respiratory rate from 18 to 22 breaths/min

290. A nurse is preparing to assess the uterine fundus of a client in the immediate postpartum period. When the nurse locates the fundus, she notes that the uterus feels soft and boggy. Which nursing intervention would be appropriate initially?
1. Elevate the client's legs.
2. Encourage the client to void.
3. Massage the fundus until it is firm.
4. Push on the uterus to assist in expressing clots.

291. A nurse is providing instructions about measures to prevent postpartum mastitis to a client who is breast-feeding her newborn. Which of the following, if stated by the client, would indicate a need for further instructions?
1. "I should breast-feed every 2 to 3 hours."
2. "I should change the breast pads frequently."
3. "I should wash my hands well before breast-feeding."
4. "I should wash my nipples daily with soap and water."

292. A postpartum nurse is assessing a client who delivered a healthy infant by cesarean section for signs and symptoms of superficial venous thrombosis. Which of the following signs or symptoms would the nurse note if superficial venous thrombosis were present?
1. Paleness of the calf area
2. Coolness of the calf area
3. Enlarged, hardened veins
4. Palpable dorsalis pedis pulses

293. A client in a postpartum unit complains of sudden sharp chest pain and dyspnea. The nurse notes that the client is tachycardic and the respiratory rate is elevated. The nurse suspects a pulmonary embolism. Which of the following would be the initial nursing action?
1. Initiate an intravenous line.
2. Assess the client's blood pressure.
3. Prepare to administer morphine sulfate.
4. Administer oxygen, 8 to 10 L/min, by face mask.

294. A nurse is assessing a client in the fourth stage of labor and notes that the fundus is firm, but that bleeding is excessive. Which of the following would be the initial nursing action?
1. Record the findings.
2. Notify the physician.
3. Massage the fundus.
4. Place the client in Trendelenburg's position.

295. A nurse is preparing to care for four assigned clients. Which client is at highest risk for hemorrhage?
1. A primiparous client who delivered 4 hours ago
2. A multiparous client who delivered 6 hours ago
3. A primiparous client who delivered 6 hours ago and had epidural anesthesia
4. A multiparous client who delivered a large fetus after oxytocin (Pitocin) induction

296. A postpartum client is diagnosed with cystitis. The nurse plans for which priority nursing intervention in the care of the client?
1. Providing sitz baths
2. Encouraging fluid intake
3. Placing ice on the perineum
4. Monitoring hemoglobin and hematocrit levels

297. A nurse is monitoring a postpartum client who received epidural anesthesia for delivery for the presence of a vulvar hematoma. Which of the following assessment findings would best indicate the presence of a hematoma?
1. Changes in vital signs
2. Signs of heavy bruising
3. Complaints of intense pain
4. Complaints of a tearing sensation

298. A nurse is developing a plan of care for a postpartum client with a small vulvar hematoma. The nurse includes which specific intervention in the plan during the first 12 hours after delivery?
1. Assess vital signs every 4 hours.
2. Measure fundal height every 4 hours.
3. Prepare an ice pack for application to the area.
4. Inform the health care provider of assessment findings.

Alternate Item Format: Multiple Response

299. A nurse is preparing a list of self-care instructions for a postpartum client who was diagnosed with mastitis. Which of the following instructions would be included on the list? **Select all that apply.**
❑ 1. Wear a supportive bra.
❑ 2. Rest during the acute phase.
❑ 3. Maintain a fluid intake of at least 3000 mL.
❑ 4. Continue to breast-feed if the breasts are not too sore.
❑ 5. Take the prescribed antibiotics until the soreness subsides.
❑ 6. Avoid decompression of the breasts by breast-feeding or breast pump.

ANSWERS

289. 3

Rationale: During the fourth stage of labor, the maternal blood pressure, pulse, and respiration should be checked every 15 minutes during the first hour. An increasing pulse is an early sign of excessive blood loss because the heart pumps faster to compensate for reduced blood volume. The blood pressure decreases as the blood volume diminishes, but a decreased blood pressure would not be the earliest sign of hemorrhage. A slight increase in temperature is normal. The respiratory rate is slightly increased from normal.

Test-Taking Strategy: Use the process of elimination, noting the strategic word *early* in the question. Think about the physiological occurrences of shock and the expected findings in the postpartum period. This should assist in directing you to option 3. Review signs of early hemorrhage if you had difficulty with this question.

Level of Cognitive Ability: Analyzing
Client Needs: Physiological Integrity
Integrated Process: Nursing Process—Analysis
Content Area: Maternity—Postpartum
Reference: McKinney, E., James, S., Murray, S., & Ashwill, J. (2009). *Maternal-child nursing* (3rd ed., pp. 364, 381). St. Louis: Saunders.

290. 3

Rationale: If the uterus is not contracted firmly, the initial intervention is to massage the fundus until it is firm and to express clots that may have accumulated in the uterus. Pushing on an uncontracted uterus can invert the uterus and cause massive hemorrhage. Elevating the client's legs and encouraging the client to void would not assist in managing uterine atony. If the uterus does not remain contracted as a result of the uterine massage, the problem may be a distended bladder, and the nurse should assist the mother to urinate, but this would not be the initial action if the uterus is soft and boggy.

Test-Taking Strategy: Note the strategic word *initially* in the question. Focus on the subject of the question, that the uterus is soft and boggy. Recalling the therapeutic management for uterine atony will assist in directing you to the correct option. If you had difficulty with this question, review therapeutic management for the client with uterine atony.

Level of Cognitive Ability: Applying
Client Needs: Physiological Integrity
Integrated Process: Nursing Process—Implementation
Content Area: Maternity—Postpartum
Reference: McKinney, E., James, S., Murray, S., & Ashwill, J. (2009). *Maternal-child nursing* (3rd ed., p. 381). St. Louis: Saunders.

291. 4

Rationale: Mastitis is inflammation of the breast as a result of infection. It generally is caused by an organism that enters through an injured area of the nipples, such as a crack or blister. Measures to prevent the development of mastitis include changing nursing pads when they are wet and avoiding continuous pressure on the breasts. Soap is drying and could lead to cracking of the nipples, and the client should be instructed to avoid using soap on the nipples. The mother is taught about the importance of handwashing and that she should breast-feed every 2 to 3 hours.

Test-Taking Strategy: Note the strategic words *a need for further instructions.* These words indicate a negative event query and the need to select the option that identifies the incorrect client statement. Recalling that the use of soap is drying to the skin and could cause cracking and provide an entry point for organisms will direct you easily to option 4. Review these measures if you had difficulty with this question.

Level of Cognitive Ability: Evaluating
Client Needs: Health Promotion and Maintenance
Integrated Process: Teaching and Learning
Content Area: Maternity—Postpartum
Reference: McKinney, E., James, S., Murray, S., & Ashwill, J. (2009). *Maternal-child nursing* (3rd ed., p. 571). St. Louis: Saunders.

292. 3

Rationale: Thrombosis of superficial veins usually is accompanied by signs and symptoms of inflammation, including swelling, redness, tenderness, and warmth of the involved extremity. It also may be possible to palpate the enlarged, hard vein. Clients sometimes experience pain when they walk. Palpable dorsalis pedis pulses is a normal finding.

Test-Taking Strategy: Use the process of elimination, eliminating option 4 first because this is a normal and expected finding. Next eliminate options 1 and 2 because they are comparable or alike. If you had difficulty with this question, review the clinical manifestations associated with superficial venous thrombosis.

Level of Cognitive Ability: Analyzing
Client Needs: Physiological Integrity
Integrated Process: Nursing Process—Assessment
Content Area: Maternity—Postpartum
Reference: McKinney, E., James, S., Murray, S., & Ashwill, J. (2009). *Maternal-child nursing* (3rd ed., pp. 702–703). St. Louis: Saunders.

293. 4

Rationale: If pulmonary embolism is suspected, oxygen should be administered, 8 to 10 L/min, by face mask. Oxygen

is used to decrease hypoxia. The client also is kept on bedrest with the head of the bed slightly elevated to reduce dyspnea. Morphine sulfate may be prescribed for the client, but this would not be the initial nursing action. An intravenous line also will be required, and vital signs need to be monitored, but these actions would follow the administration of oxygen.
Test-Taking Strategy: Use the process of elimination, noting the strategic word *initial* in the query. Use the ABCs—airway, breathing, and circulation—to assist in directing you to option 4. If you had difficulty with this question, review the initial nursing interventions and therapeutic management of a client with pulmonary embolism.
Level of Cognitive Ability: Applying
Client Needs: Physiological Integrity
Integrated Process: Nursing Process—Implementation
Content Area: Maternity—Postpartum
Reference: McKinney, E., James, S., Murray, S., & Ashwill, J. (2009). *Maternal-child nursing* (3rd ed., pp. 704–705). St. Louis: Saunders.

294. 2

Rationale: If bleeding is excessive, the cause may be laceration of the cervix or birth canal. Massaging the fundus if it is firm would not assist in controlling the bleeding. Trendelenburg's position should be avoided because it may interfere with cardiac and respiratory function. Although the nurse would record the findings, the initial nursing action would be to notify the physician.
Test-Taking Strategy: Read the question carefully, noting the subject of the question and the clinical manifestations identified in the question. Eliminate option 3 first because, if the uterus is firm, it would not be necessary to perform fundal massage. Knowing that Trendelenburg's position is not advised will assist in eliminating this option. From the remaining options, noting the strategic words *bleeding is excessive* will assist in directing you to option 2. Review the interventions related to a client who is hemorrhaging if you had difficulty with this question.
Level of Cognitive Ability: Applying
Client Needs: Physiological Integrity
Integrated Process: Nursing Process—Implementation
Content Area: Maternity—Postpartum
Reference: McKinney, E., James, S., Murray, S., & Ashwill, J. (2009). *Maternal-child nursing* (3rd ed., p. 700). St. Louis: Saunders.

295. 4

Rationale: The causes of postpartum hemorrhage include uterine atony; laceration of the vagina; hematoma development in the cervix, perineum, or labia; and retained placental fragments. Predisposing factors for hemorrhage include a previous history of postpartum hemorrhage, placenta previa, abruptio placentae, overdistention of the uterus from polyhydramnios, multiple gestation, a large neonate, infection, multiparity, dystocia or labor that is prolonged, operative delivery such as a cesarean or forceps delivery, and intrauterine manipulation. The multiparous client who delivered a large fetus after oxytocin induction has more risk factors associated with postpartum hemorrhage than the other clients. Additionally, there are no specific data in the client descriptions in options 1, 2, or 3 that present the risk for hemorrhage.

Test-Taking Strategy: Focus on the subject, the client at highest risk for hemorrhage. Read the client description in each option. Noting the words *large* and *oxytocin* in option 4 will direct you to this option. Review delegating and assignment-making guidelines if you had difficulty with this question.
Level of Cognitive Ability: Analyzing
Client Needs: Health Promotion and Maintenance
Integrated Process: Nursing Process—Planning
Content Area: Leadership and Management—Delegating/Prioritizing
Reference: Perry, S., Hockenberry, M., Lowdermilk, D., & Wilson, D. (2010). *Maternal child nursing care* (4th ed., pp. 479, 579). St. Louis: Mosby.

296. 2

Rationale: Cystitis is an infection of the bladder. The client should consume 3000 mL of fluids per day if not contraindicated. Sitz baths and ice would be appropriate interventions for perineal discomfort. Hemoglobin and hematocrit levels would be monitored with hemorrhage.
Test-Taking Strategy: Focus on the subject, priority intervention for the client with cystitis. Remember that increased fluids are a priority intervention. Review these interventions for a client with cystitis if you had difficulty with this question.
Level of Cognitive Ability: Applying
Client Needs: Physiological Integrity
Integrated Process: Nursing Process—Implementation
Content Area: Maternity—Postpartum
Reference: McKinney, E., James, S., Murray, S., & Ashwill, J. (2009). *Maternal-child nursing* (3rd ed., p. 782). St. Louis: Saunders.

297. 1

Rationale: Because the client has had epidural anesthesia and is anesthetized, she cannot feel pain, pressure, or a tearing sensation. Changes in vital signs indicate hypovolemia in an anesthetized postpartum client with vulvar hematoma. Option 2 (heavy bruising) may be seen, but vital sign changes indicate hematoma caused by blood collection in the perineal tissues.
Test-Taking Strategy: Use the process of elimination, noting the strategic words *epidural anesthesia*. With this in mind, eliminate options 3 and 4. From the remaining options, use the ABCs—airway, breathing, and circulation—to direct you to option 1. Review the signs of a vulvar hematoma in a client who had epidural anesthesia if you had difficulty with this question.
Level of Cognitive Ability: Analyzing
Client Needs: Physiological Integrity
Integrated Process: Nursing Process—Assessment
Content Area: Maternity—Postpartum
Reference: McKinney, E., James, S., Murray, S., & Ashwill, J. (2009). *Maternal-child nursing* (3rd ed., p. 698). St. Louis: Saunders.

298. 3

Rationale: A hematoma is a localized collection of blood into the tissues of the reproductive sac after delivery. Vulvar hematoma is the most common. Application of ice reduces swelling caused by hematoma formation in the vulvar area. Options 1, 2, and 4 are not interventions that are specific to the plan of care for a client with a small vulvar hematoma.

Test-Taking Strategy: Use the process of elimination, noting the strategic words *small* and *specific intervention* in the question. This focus will assist in directing you to option 3. Review nursing care of the client with a hematoma if you had difficulty with this question.
Level of Cognitive Ability: Applying
Client Needs: Physiological Integrity
Integrated Process: Nursing Process—Planning
Content Area: Maternity—Postpartum
Reference: McKinney, E., James, S., Murray, S., & Ashwill, J. (2009). *Maternal-child nursing* (3rd ed., pp. 382, 446). St. Louis: Saunders.

ALTERNATE ITEM FORMAT: MULTIPLE RESPONSE
299. 1, 2, 3, 4
Rationale: Mastitis is an infection of the lactating breast. Client instructions include resting during the acute phase, maintaining a fluid intake of at least 3000 mL/day (if not contraindicated), and taking analgesics to relieve discomfort.

Antibiotics may be prescribed and are taken until the complete prescribed course is finished. They are not stopped when the soreness subsides. Additional supportive measures include the use of moist heat or ice packs and wearing a supportive bra. Continued decompression of the breast by breast-feeding or breast pump is important to empty the breast and prevent the formation of an abscess.
Test-Taking Strategy: Think about the pathophysiology associated with mastitis. Recalling that supportive measures include rest, moist heat or ice packs, antibiotics, analgesics, increased fluid intake, breast support, and decompression of the breasts will assist in answering the question. Review the measures to treat mastitis if you had difficulty with this question.
Level of Cognitive Ability: Applying
Client Needs: Physiological Integrity
Integrated Process: Teaching and Learning
Content Area: Maternity—Postpartum
Reference: McKinney, E., James, S., Murray, S., & Ashwill, J. (2009). *Maternal-child nursing* (3rd ed., p. 708). St. Louis: Saunders.

Care of the Newborn

I. INITIAL CARE OF THE NEWBORN

A. Assessment
1. Observe or assist with initiation of respirations.
2. Assess Apgar score.
3. Note characteristics of cry.
4. Monitor for nasal flaring, grunting, retractions, and abnormal respirations, such as a seesaw respiratory pattern (rise and fall of the chest and abdomen do not occur together).
5. Assess for cyanosis.
6. Obtain vital signs.
7. Observe the **newborn** for signs of hypothermia or hyperthermia.
8. Assess for gross anomalies.

B. Interventions
1. Suction the mouth first and then the nares with a bulb syringe.
2. Dry the **newborn** and stimulate crying by rubbing.
3. Maintain temperature stability; wrap the **newborn** in warm blankets and place a stockinette cap on the **newborn's** head.
4. Keep the **newborn** with the mother to facilitate bonding.
5. Place the **newborn** at mother's breast if breastfeeding is planned, or place the **newborn** on the mother's abdomen.
6. Place the **newborn** in radiant warmer (incubator).
7. Position the **newborn** on the side with a rolled blanket at the back to facilitate drainage of mucus.
8. Ensure the **newborn's** proper identification.
9. Footprint the **newborn** and fingerprint the mother on the identification sheet per agency policies and procedures.
10. Place matching identification bracelets on the mother and the **newborn**.

C. Apgar scoring system
1. Assess each of five items to be scored and add the points to determine the **newborn's** total score.
2. Five vital indicators (Table 30-1)
3. Interventions: Apgar score (Table 30-2)

⚠ The newborn's Apgar score is assessed and recorded at 1 minute and at 5 minutes after birth.

TABLE 30-1 Five Vital Indicators of Apgar Scoring

Indicator	0 Points	1 Point	2 Points
Heart rate	Absent	<100 beats/min	>100 beats/min
Respiratory rate	Absent	Slow, irregular, weak cry	Good, vigorous cry
Muscle tone	Flaccid, limp	Minimal flexion of extremities	Good flexion, active motion
Reflex irritability	No response	Minimal response (grimace) to suction or to gentle slap on soles	Responds promptly with a cry or active movement
Skin color	Pallor or cyanosis	Body skin normal, extremities blue	Body and extremity skin color normal

II. INITIAL PHYSICAL EXAMINATION

A. General guidelines
1. Keep the **newborn** warm during the examination.
2. Begin with general observations, and then perform assessments that are least disturbing to the **newborn** first.
3. Initiate nursing interventions for abnormal findings and document findings.

B. Vital signs
1. Heart rate (resting): 100 to 160 beats/min (apical); auscultate at the fourth intercostal space for 1 full minute to detect abnormalities
2. Respirations: 30 to 60 breaths/min; assess for 1 full minute
3. Assess heart rate and respiratory rate first while the **newborn** is resting or sleeping.
4. Axillary temperature: 96.8° F to 99° F
5. Blood pressure: 73/55 mm Hg

C. Body measurements (approximate)
1. Length: 45 to 55 cm (18 to 22 inches)
2. Weight: 2500 to 4300 g (5.5 to 9.5 lb)
3. Head circumference: 33 to 35 cm (13.2 to 14 inches)

TABLE 30-2 Apgar Score Interventions

Score	Intervention
8-10	No intervention required except to support newborn's spontaneous efforts
4-7	Gently stimulate; rub newborn's back; administer oxygen to newborn
0-3	Newborn requires resuscitation

TABLE 30-3 Fontanels

Fontanel	Characteristics	Closure
Anterior	Soft, flat, diamond-shaped; 3-4 cm wide × 2-3 cm long	Between 12 and 18 mo of age
Posterior	Triangular; 0.5-1 cm wide Located between occipital and parietal bones	Between birth and 2-3 mo of age

D. Head
  1. Head should be one-fourth of the body length (cephalocaudal development).
  2. Bones of the skull are not fused.
  3. Sutures (connective tissue between the skull bones) are palpable and may be overlapping because of head molding, but should not be widened.
  4. Fontanels are unossified membranous tissue at the junction of the sutures (Table 30-3).
  5. Molding is asymmetry of the head resulting from pressure in the birth canal; molding disappears in about 72 hours (Fig. 30-1).
  6. Masses from birth trauma
     a. Caput succedaneum is edema of the soft tissue over bone (crosses over suture line); it subsides within a few days.
     b. Cephalhematoma is swelling caused by bleeding into an area between the bone and its periosteum (does not cross over suture line); it usually is absorbed within 6 weeks with no treatment.
  7. Head lag
     a. Common when pulling the **newborn** to a sitting position
     b. When prone, the **newborn** should be able to lift the head slightly and turn the head from side to side.

E. Eyes
  1. Slate gray (light skin), dark blue, or brown-gray (dark skin)
  2. Symmetrical and clear
  3. Pupils equal, round, react to light and by accommodation
  4. Blink reflex present

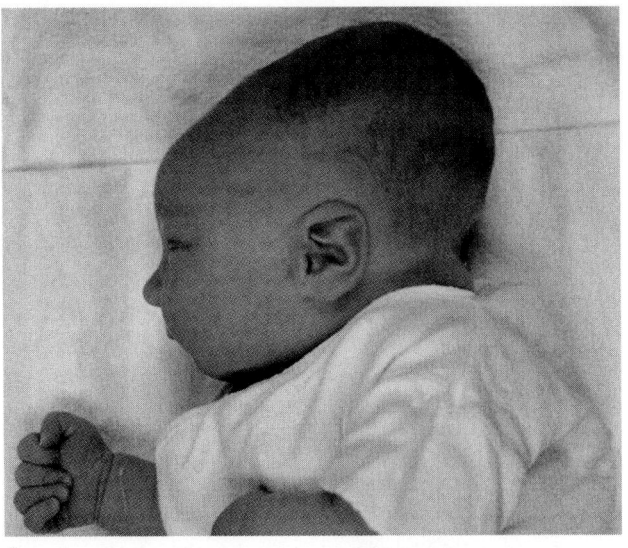

A

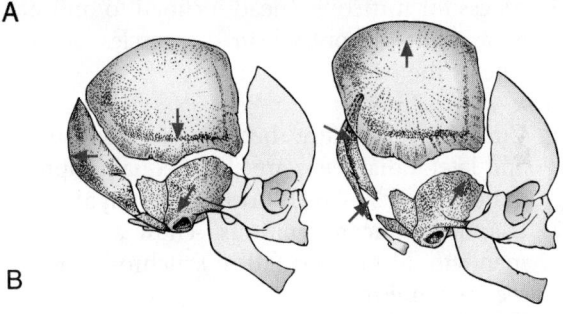

B

▲ **FIGURE 30-1** Molding. **A,** Significant molding after vaginal birth. **B,** Schematic of bones of skull when molding is present. (From Perry, S., Hockenberry, M., Lowdermilk, D., & Wilson, D. [2010]. *Maternal child nursing care* [4th ed.]. St. Louis: Mosby. Courtesy of Kim Molloy, Knoxville, IA.)

  5. Eyes cross because of weak extraocular muscles
  6. Ability to track and fixate momentarily
  7. Red reflex present
  8. Eyelids often edematous as a result of pressure during the birth process and the effects of eye medication

F. Ears
  1. Symmetrical
  2. Firm cartilage with recoil
  3. Top of pinna on or above line drawn from outer canthus of eye
  4. Low-set ears associated with Down syndrome

G. Nose
  1. Flat, broad, in center of face
  2. Obligatory nose breathing
  3. Occasional sneezing to remove obstructions
  4. Nares are patent and should not flare (flaring is an indication of respiratory distress).

H. Mouth
  1. Pink, moist gums
  2. Soft and hard palates intact
  3. Epstein's pearls (small, white cysts) may be present on hard palate.
  4. Uvula in midline

5. Freely moving tongue, symmetrical, has short frenulum
6. Sucking and crying movements symmetrical
7. Able to swallow
8. Root and gag reflexes present

⚠ When assessing the newborn's mouth, look for the presence of thrush (*Candida albicans*), which are white patchy areas on the tongue or gums that cannot be removed with a washcloth; these may be painful.

I. Neck
1. Short and thick
2. Head held in midline
3. Trachea on midline
4. Good range of motion and ability to flex and extend
5. Assess for torticollis (head inclined to one side as a result of contraction of muscles on that side of the neck)

J. Chest
1. Circular appearance because anteroposterior and lateral diameters are about equal (approximately 30 to 33 cm [12 to 13.2 inches] at birth)
2. Diaphragmatic respirations—chest and abdomen should rise and fall in synchrony, not in seesaw pattern
3. Bronchial sounds heard on auscultation
4. Nipples prominent and often edematous; milky secretion (witch's milk) common
5. Breast tissue present
6. Clavicles need to be palpated to assess for fractures.

K. Skin
1. Pinkish red (light-skinned **newborn**) to pinkish brown or pinkish yellow (dark-skinned **newborn**)
2. Vernix caseosa, a cheesy white substance, can be found on entire body, but is more prominent between folds.
3. Lanugo, fine hair, might be seen, especially on the back.
4. Milia, small white sebaceous glands, appear on the forehead, nose, and chin.
5. Dry, peeling skin
6. Dark red color common in premature **newborns**
7. Cyanosis may be noted with hypothermia, infection, and hypoglycemia and with cardiac, respiratory, or neurological abnormalities.
8. Acrocyanosis (peripheral cyanosis) is normal in the first few hours after birth and may be noted intermittently for the next 7 to 10 days (Fig. 30-2).
9. Assessment for ecchymosis and petechiae resulting from trauma of birth
10. Assessment of skin turgor over the abdomen to determine hydration status

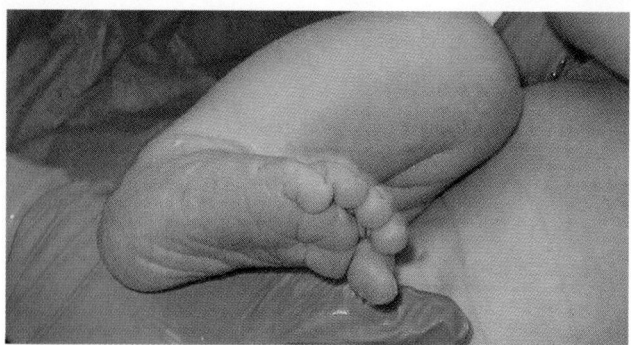

▲ **FIGURE 30-2** Acrocyanosis. (From McKinney, E., James, S., Murray, S., & Ashwill, J. [2009]. *Maternal-child nursing* [3rd ed.]. St. Louis: Saunders. Courtesy of Todd Shiros, Santa Fe Springs, CA.)

11. Observation for forceps marks
12. Harlequin sign
    a. Deep pink or red color develops over one side of **newborn's** body while the other side remains pale or of normal color.
    b. Harlequin sign may indicate shunting of blood that occurs with a cardiac problem or may indicate sepsis.
13. Birthmarks (Table 30-4)

L. Abdomen
1. Umbilical cord
   a. Umbilical cord should have three vessels—two arteries and one vein; if fewer than three vessels are noted, notify the physician.
   b. Small, thin cord may be associated with poor fetal growth.
   c. Assess for intact cord, and ensure that the cord clamp is secured.
   d. Cord should be clamped for at least the first 24 hours after birth; clamp can be removed when the cord is dried and occluded and is no longer bleeding.
   e. Note any bleeding or drainage from the cord.
   f. Hospital protocol and physician's preference determine the technique and skin preparation used for cord care; protocols include the use of antibiotic ointment, triple dye, alcohol, soap and water, sterile water, povidone-iodine, or another treatment.
   g. If symptoms of infection, such as moistness, oozing, discharge, and a reddened base, occur, antibiotic treatment is prescribed.
2. Gastrointestinal
   a. Monitor cord for meconium staining.
   b. Assess for umbilical hernia.
   c. Assess for abdominal depression associated with diaphragmatic hernia.
   d. Assess for abdominal distention associated with obstruction, mass, or sepsis.
   e. Monitor bowel sounds, which should occur within 1 to 2 hours after birth.

TABLE 30-4 Birthmarks

Birthmark	Characteristics
Telangiectatic nevi (stork bites)	Pale pink or red, flat, dilated capillaries On eyelids, nose, lower occipital bone, and nape of neck Blanch easily More noticeable during crying periods Disappear by age 2 yr
Nevus flammeus (port-wine stain)	Capillary angioma directly below epidermis Nonelevated, sharply demarcated, red to purple, dense areas of capillaries Commonly appear on face No fading with time May require future surgery
Nevus vasculosus (strawberry mark)	Capillary hemangioma Raised, clearly delineated, dark red, with rough surface Common in head region Disappears by age 7-9 yr
Mongolian spots	Bluish black pigmentation On lumbar dorsal area and buttocks Gradually fade during first and second years of life Common in Asian and dark-skinned individuals

3. Anus
   a. Ensure that the anal opening is patent.
   b. First stool meconium should pass within first 24 hours.
M. Genitals
   1. Female
      a. Labia are edematous; clitoris is enlarged.
      b. Smegma may be present (thick, white mucous discharge).
      c. Pseudomenstruation, caused from the withdrawal of the maternal hormone estrogen, is possible (blood-tinged mucus).
      d. Hymen tag may be visible.
      e. First voiding should occur within 24 hours.
   2. Male
      a. Prepuce (foreskin) covers glans penis.
      b. Scrotum is edematous.
      c. Verify meatus at tip of penis.
      d. Testes are descended, but may retract with cold.
      e. Assess for hernia or hydrocele.
      f. First voiding should occur within 24 hours.
N. Spine
   1. Straight
   2. Posture flexed
   3. Supportive of head momentarily when prone
   4. Arms and legs flexed
   5. Chin flexed on upper chest
   6. Well-coordinated, sporadic movements
   7. A degree of hypotonicity or hypertonicity may indicate central nervous system damage.

8. Assess for hair tufts and dimples along the spinal column (may be indicative of a possible opening).
O. Extremities
   1. Flexed
   2. Full range of motion; symmetrical movements
   3. Fists clenched
   4. Ten fingers and 10 toes, all separate
   5. Legs bowed
   6. Major gluteal folds even
   7. Creases on soles of feet
   8. Assessment for fractures (especially clavicle) or dislocations (hip)
   9. Assessment for developmental dysplasia of the hip; when thighs are rotated outward, no clicks should be heard (Ortolani's sign and Barlow's sign are the two assessment tools for developmental dysplasia of the hip)
   10. Pulses palpable (radial, brachial, femoral)

⚠ Slight tremors noted in the newborn may be a common finding, but could also be a sign of hypoglycemia or drug withdrawal.

III. **BODY SYSTEMS ASSESSMENT AND INTERVENTIONS**

A. Cardiovascular system
   1. Keep the **newborn** warm.
   2. Measure the apical heart rate for 1 full minute.
   3. Listen for murmurs; assess oxygen saturation via pulse oximetry if a murmur is heard.
   4. Palpate pulses.
   5. Assess for cyanosis; blanch the skin on the trunk and extremities to assess circulation.
   6. Observe for cardiac distress when the **newborn** is feeding.
B. Respiratory system
   1. Suction the airway as necessary: use a bulb syringe for upper airway suctioning (compress bulb before insertion) and a French catheter for deeper suctioning.
   2. Observe for respiratory distress and hypoxemia.
      a. Nasal flaring
      b. Increasingly severe retractions
      c. Grunting
      d. Cyanosis
      e. Bradycardia and periods of apnea lasting longer than 15 seconds
   3. Administer oxygen via hood if necessary and as prescribed.
C. Hepatic system
   1. Normal or physiological jaundice appears after the first 24 hours in full-term **newborns** and after the first 48 hours in premature **newborns**; jaundice occurring before this time (pathological jaundice) may indicate early hemolysis of

red blood cells and must be reported to the physician.

2. Physiological jaundice peaks about the fifth day of life (indirect bilirubin levels 6 to 7 mg/dL).

3. Monitor serum bilirubin levels.

4. Feed early to stimulate intestinal activity and to keep the bilirubin level low.

5. Prevent chilling because hypothermia can cause acidosis that interferes with bilirubin conjugation and excretion.

6. Liver stores the iron passed from the mother for 5 to 6 months.

7. Glycogen storage occurs in the liver.

8. The **newborn** is at risk for hemorrhagic disorders; coagulation factors synthesized in the liver depend on vitamin K, which is not synthesized until intestinal bacteria are present.

9. Handle the **newborn** carefully and monitor for any bruising or bleeding episodes.

10. Watch for meconium stool and subsequent stools.

11. Administer intramuscular dose of vitamin K to the **newborn** as prescribed to prevent hemorrhagic disorders (usually 0.5 to 1 mg is prescribed); administer in lateral aspect of the middle third of the vastus lateralis muscle.

12. Assess the **newborn's** hemoglobin and blood glucose levels.

D. Renal system

1. The immature kidneys are unable to concentrate urine.

2. A weight loss of 5% to 15% during the first week of life occurs as a result of voiding and limited intake; birth weight should be regained by 10 to 14 days after birth.

3. Weigh the **newborn** daily.

4. Monitor intake and output; weigh diapers if necessary (1 g of diaper weight equals 1 mL of urine).

5. If the diaper requires weighing, record the weight before putting it on the **newborn**; after the **newborn** voids, reweigh the diaper and subtract the prevoided weight.

6. Measure specific gravity of urine if necessary.

7. Assess for signs of dehydration (dry mucous membranes, sunken eyeballs, poor skin turgor, sunken fontanels).

E. Immune system

1. **Newborn** receives passive immunity via the **placenta** (immunoglobulin G).

2. **Newborn** receives passive immunity from colostrum (immunoglobulin A).

3. Elevations in immunoglobulin M indicate infection in utero.

4. Use aseptic technique when caring for the **newborn**.

5. Observe standard precautions when handling the **newborn**.

6. Ensure meticulous handwashing.

7. Ensure that an infection-free staff cares for the **newborn**.

8. Monitor the **newborn's** temperature.

9. Observe for any cracks or openings in the skin.

10. Administer eye medication within 1 hour after birth to prevent ophthalmia neonatorum.

a. Agent used varies depending on agency protocols, but usually ophthalmic forms of erythromycin (0.5%) or tetracycline (1%) are prescribed because they are bacteriostatic and bactericidal and provide prophylaxis against *Neisseria gonorrhoeae* and *Chlamydia trachomatis*.

b. Silver nitrate (1%) solution may be prescribed, but its use is minimal because it does not protect against chlamydial infection and it can cause chemical conjunctivitis.

11. Provide cord care.

a. Umbilical clamp can be removed after 24 hours if cord is dried and occluded and is not bleeding.

b. Teach the client how to perform cord care.

c. Keep the cord clean and dry; soap and water may be prescribed for cleaning the cord.

d. Keep the diaper from covering the cord; fold the diaper below the cord.

e. Assess cord for odor, swelling, or discharge.

f. The **newborn** is washed via a sponge bath until the cord falls off (within 2 weeks).

12. Provide circumcision care.

a. Apply petroleum jelly gauze to the penis except when a PlastiBell is used.

b. Remove petroleum jelly gauze, if applied, after the first voiding following circumcision.

c. Observe for swelling, infection, or bleeding from the circumcision site.

d. Teach the client how to care for circumcision site.

e. Clean the penis after each voiding by squeezing warm water over the penis.

f. A milky covering over the glans penis is normal and should not be disrupted.

g. Monitor for urinary retention.

F. Metabolic system and gastrointestinal system

1. **Newborns** are able to digest simple carbohydrates, but are unable to digest fats because of the lack of lipase.

2. Proteins may be broken down only partially, so they may serve as antigens and provoke an allergic reaction.

3. The **newborn** has a small stomach capacity (about 90 mL), with rapid intestinal peristalsis (bowel emptying time is 2.5 to 3 hours).

4. Breast-feeding usually can begin immediately after birth; based on physician preference and agency protocols, bottle-fed **newborns** may be

offered a few milliliters of sterile water or 5% dextrose 1 to 4 hours after birth before a feeding with formula.

5. Observe feeding reflexes, such as rooting, sucking, and swallowing.
6. Assist the client with breast-feeding or formula feeding; breast-feeding should be done every 2 to 3 hours, and formula feeding (minimum of 30 mL, or 1 oz) should be done every 3 to 4 hours (or per physician preference or agency protocols).
7. Burp the **newborn** during and after feeding.
8. Assess for regurgitation or vomiting.
9. Position the **newborn** on the right side after feeding; however, the side-lying position is not recommended for sleep because this position makes it easy for the **newborn** to roll to the prone position (prone position is contraindicated because the prone position increases the risk of sudden **infant** death syndrome).
10. Observe for normal stool and the passage of meconium.
    a. Meconium stool, which is greenish black with a thick, sticky, tar-like consistency, usually is passed within the first 24 hours of life.
    b. Transitional stool, the second type of stool excreted by the **newborn**, is greenish brown and of looser consistency than meconium.
    c. Seedy, yellow stools are usually noted in breast-fed **newborns**; pale yellow to light brown stools are usually seen in formula-fed **newborns**.
11. Perform a **newborn** screening test (including the test for phenylketonuria) as prescribed before discharge after sufficient protein intake occurs; the **newborn** should be on formula or breast milk for 24 hours before screening.

G. Neurological system
1. **Newborn** head size is proportionally larger than that of an adult because of cephalocaudal development.
2. Myelinization of nerve fibers is incomplete, so primitive reflexes are present.
3. Fontanels are open to allow for brain growth.
4. Assess for an abnormal head size and a bulging or depressed anterior fontanel.
5. Measure and graph the head circumference in relation to chest circumference and length.
6. Assess the **newborn's** movements, noting symmetry, posture, and abnormal movements.
7. Observe for jitteriness, marked tremors, and seizures.
8. Test the **newborn's** reflexes.
9. Assess for lethargy.
10. Assess pitch of cry.

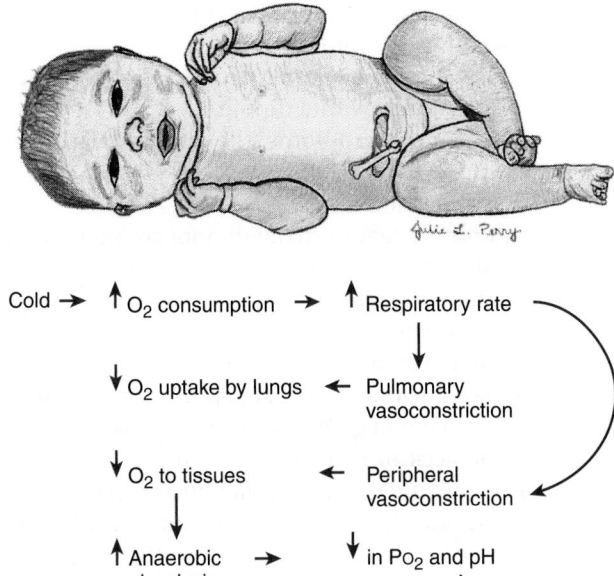

Cold → ↑O_2 consumption → ↑ Respiratory rate

↓ O_2 uptake by lungs ← Pulmonary vasoconstriction

↓ O_2 to tissues ← Peripheral vasoconstriction

↑ Anaerobic glycolysis → ↓ in Po_2 and pH

Metabolic acidosis

▲ **FIGURE 30-3** Effects of cold stress. When a newborn is stressed by cold, oxygen consumption increases, and pulmonary and peripheral vasoconstriction occur, decreasing oxygen uptake by the lungs and oxygen to the tissues; anaerobic glycolysis increases; and there is a decrease in Po_2 and pH, leading to metabolic acidosis. (From Perry, S., Hockenberry, M., Lowdermilk, D., & Wilson, D. [2010]. *Maternal child nursing care* [4th ed.]. St. Louis: Mosby).

H. Thermal regulatory system
1. Prevent cold stress (Fig. 30-3).
2. **Newborns** do not shiver to produce heat.
3. **Newborns** have brown fat deposits, which produce heat.
4. Prevent heat loss resulting from evaporation by keeping the **newborn** dry and well wrapped with a blanket.
5. Prevent heat loss resulting from radiation by keeping the **newborn** away from cold objects and outside walls.
6. Prevent heat loss resulting from convection by shielding the **newborn** from drafts.
7. Prevent heat loss resulting from conduction by performing all treatments on a warm, padded surface.
8. Keep the temperature in room warm.
9. Take the **newborn's** axillary temperature every hour for the first 4 hours of life, every 4 hours for the remainder of the first 24 hours, and then every shift (as per agency protocol).

⚠ Cold stress causes oxygen consumption and energy to be diverted from maintaining normal brain cell function and cardiac function resulting in serious metabolic and physiological conditions.

I. Reflexes
1. Sucking and rooting
   a. Touch the **newborn's** lip, cheek, or corner of the mouth with a nipple.
   b. The **newborn** turns the head toward the nipple, opens the mouth, takes hold of the nipple, and sucks.
   c. Rooting reflex usually disappears after 3 to 4 months, but may persist for 1 year.
2. Swallowing reflex
   a. Swallowing reflex occurs spontaneously after sucking and obtaining fluids.
   b. **Newborn** swallows in coordination with sucking without gagging, coughing, or vomiting.
3. Tonic neck or fencing
   a. While the **newborn** is falling asleep or sleeping, gently and quickly turn the head to one side.
   b. As the **newborn** faces the left side, the left arm and leg extend outward while the right arm and leg flex.
   c. When the head is turned to the right side, the right arm and leg extend outward while the left arm and leg flex.
   d. Response usually disappears within 3 to 4 months.
4. Palmar-plantar grasp
   a. Place a finger in the palm of the **newborn's** hand and then place a finger at the base of the toes.
   b. The **newborn's** fingers curl around the examiner's fingers, and the **newborn's** toes curl downward.
   c. Palmar response lessens within 3 to 4 months.
   d. Plantar response lessens within 8 months.
5. Moro reflex
   a. Hold the **newborn** in a semi-sitting position and then allow the head and trunk to fall backward to at least a 30-degree angle.
   b. The **newborn** assumes sharp extension and abduction of the arms with the thumbs and forefingers in a "C" position; this is followed by flexion and adduction to an "embrace" position (legs follow a similar pattern).
   c. The Moro reflex is present at birth and is absent by 6 months of age if neurological maturation is not delayed.
   d. A body jerk motion may be the response between 8 and 18 weeks.
   e. A persistent response lasting more than 6 months may indicate a neurological abnormality.
6. Startle reflex
   a. The response is best elicited if the **newborn** is a least 24 hours old.
   b. The examiner makes a loud noise or claps hands to elicit the response.

   c. The **newborn's** arms adduct while the elbows flex.
   d. The hands stay clenched.
   e. The reflex should disappear within 4 months.
7. Pull-to-sit response
   a. Pull the **newborn** up by the wrist while the **newborn** is in the supine position.
   b. The head lags until the **newborn** is in an upright position, and then the head is level with the chest and shoulders momentarily before falling forward.
   c. The head then lifts for a few minutes.
   d. The response depends on the **newborn's** general muscle tone and condition and on maturity level.
8. Babinski sign: Plantar reflex
   a. Beginning at the heel of the foot, use a finger to stroke gently upward along the lateral aspect of the sole, and then move the finger along the ball of the foot.
   b. The **newborn's** toes hyperextend while the big toe dorsiflexes.
   c. The reflex disappears after the **newborn** is 1 year old.
   d. Absence of this reflex indicates the need for a neurological examination.
9. Stepping or walking
   a. Hold the **newborn** in a vertical position, allowing one foot to touch a table surface.
   b. The **newborn** simulates walking, alternately flexing and extending the feet.
   c. The reflex is usually present for 3 to 4 months.
10. Crawling
   a. Place the **newborn** on the abdomen
   b. The **newborn** begins making crawling movements with the arms and legs.
   c. The reflex usually disappears after about 6 weeks.

IV. NEWBORN SAFETY

A. **Newborn** identification
1. Information bracelets are applied to the mother and **newborn** immediately after birth and before the mother and **newborn** are separated; additionally, identification pictures of the **newborn** and footprints from the **newborn** may be obtained before the **newborn** leaves the mother's side in the delivery room.
2. The bracelets include name, sex, date, time of birth, and identification numbers.
3. Some agencies use identification bracelets that have radiofrequency transmitters that set off alarms if the **newborn** is removed from a certain area.

Box 30-1 Precautions to Prevent Infant Abduction

All personnel must wear identification that is easily visible at all times.

Teach parents to allow only hospital staff with proper identification to take their infants from them.

Question anyone with a newborn near an exit or in an unusual part of the facility.

Never leave a newborn unattended.

Teach the parents that the newborn must be observed at all times.

When the newborn is in the mother's room, position the crib away from the doorway.

Teach the parents home safety precautions; suggest that the parents not place announcements in the paper or signs in their yard that might alert an abductor that a new infant is in the home.

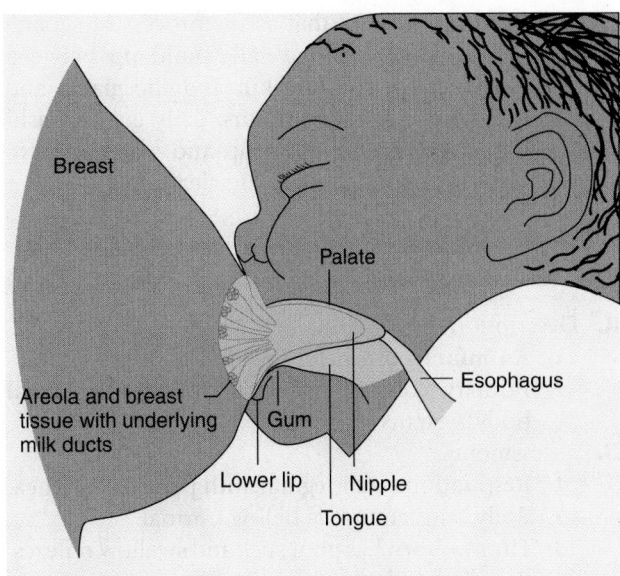

▲ **FIGURE 30-4** Correct attachment (latch-on) of a newborn at breast. (From Perry, S., Hockenberry, M., Lowdermilk, D., & Wilson, D. [2010]. *Maternal child nursing care* [4th ed.]. St. Louis: Mosby.)

4. Agencies also conduct unit and hospital-wide drills to prevent **newborn** abductions.

B. Newborn abduction

1. The client is taught to check the identification of any person who comes to remove the **infant** from her room and is taught other precautions to prevent **newborn** abduction (nurses must be wearing photo identification or some other security badge) (Box 30-1).

2. Closed-circuit televisions, code-alert bands, computer monitoring systems, or other monitoring systems may be used in some agencies.

3. The **newborn** is wheeled in a bassinette, not carried in a staff member's arms.

▲ **V. PARENT TEACHING**

A. Formula feeding

1. Teach sterilization techniques if the water supply is located in areas where the purification process of the water is questionable.

2. Remind the client not to heat the bottle of formula in a microwave oven.

3. Inform the client that formula is a sufficient diet for the first 4 to 6 months.

4. Assess the client's ability to burp the **newborn**.

B. Breast-feeding

1. Assess the **newborn's** ability to attach to the mother's breast and suck (Fig. 30-4).

2. Teach the client about engorgement.

3. Teach the client how to pump her breasts and how to store breast milk properly.

4. Inform the client that breast milk is a sufficient diet for the first 4 to 6 months.

5. Give the client the phone numbers of local organizations that offer support to breast-feeding mothers.

C. Bathing

1. Bathe the **newborn** in a warm room before feeding.

2. Have all equipment for bathing available.

3. Use a mild soap (not on the face).

4. Proceed from the cleanest area to the dirtiest.

5. Clean eyes from the inner canthus outward.

6. Special care should be taken to clean under the folds of the neck, underarms, groin, and genitals.

7. Make bath time enjoyable for the **newborn** and the mother.

D. Clothing

1. Assess diaper and clothing needs for the **newborn** with the client.

2. Instruct the client that the **newborn's** head should be covered in cold weather to prevent heat loss.

3. Instruct the client to layer the **newborn's** clothing in cooler weather.

4. To be comfortable, the **newborn** should be dressed in one more layer of clothing than what the parents are wearing.

E. Cord care: See earlier for cord care, "Body Systems Assessment and Interventions."

F. Circumcision: See earlier for circumcision care, "Body Systems Assessment and Interventions."

G. Uncircumcised **newborn**

1. Inform the client that the foreskin and glans are two similar layers of cells that separate from each other and that the separation process normally is complete by 3 years of age, although the layers can remain adhered until puberty.

2. Instruct the client not to pull back the foreskin, but to allow for the natural separation to occur.

3. Inform the client that as the process of separation occurs, sloughed cells build up between the layers of the foreskin and the glans, and that when retraction occurs, daily gentle washing of the glans with soap and water is sufficient to maintain adequate cleanliness.

VI. PRETERM NEWBORN

A. Description
  1. An **infant** born before 37 weeks of gestation
  2. Primary concern relates to immaturity of all body systems
B. Assessment
  1. Respirations are irregular with periods of apnea.
  2. Body temperature is below normal.
  3. The **newborn** has poor suck and swallow reflexes.
  4. Bowel sounds are diminished.
  5. Urinary output is increased or decreased.
  6. Extremities are thin, with minimal creasing on soles and palms.
  7. The **newborn** extends extremities and does not maintain flexion.
  8. Lanugo, on skin and in the hair on the **newborn's** head, is present in woolly patches.
  9. Skin is thin, with visible blood vessels and minimal subcutaneous fat pads.
  10. Skin may appear jaundiced.
  11. Testes are undescended in boys.
  12. Labia are narrow in girls.
C. Interventions
  1. Monitor vital signs every 2 to 4 hours.
  2. Maintain airway and cardiopulmonary functions.
  3. Administer oxygen and humidification as prescribed.
  4. Monitor intake and output and electrolyte balance.
  5. Monitor daily weight.
  6. Maintain the **newborn** in a warming device.
  7. Reposition the **newborn** every 1 to 2 hours, and handle the **newborn** carefully.
  8. Avoid exposure to infections.
  9. Provide the **newborn** with appropriate stimulation, such as touch and cuddling.

VII. POST-TERM NEWBORN

A. Description: **Infant** born after 42 weeks of gestation
B. Assessment
  1. Hypoglycemia
  2. Parchment-like skin (dry and cracked) without lanugo
  3. Long fingernails, extended over ends of fingers
  4. Profuse scalp hair
  5. Long and thin body
  6. Wasting of fat and muscle in extremities
  7. Meconium staining possibly present on nails and umbilical cord

C. Interventions
  1. Provide normal **newborn** care.
  2. Monitor for hypoglycemia.
  3. Maintain **newborn's** temperature.
  4. Monitor for meconium aspiration.

VIII. SMALL FOR GESTATIONAL AGE

A. Description: **Newborn** who is plotted at or below the 10th percentile on the intrauterine growth curve
B. Assessment
  1. Fetal distress
  2. Gestational age and physical maturity
  3. Decreased or elevated body temperature
  4. Physical abnormalities
  5. Hypoglycemia
  6. Signs of polycythemia
    a. Ruddy appearance
    b. Cyanosis
    c. Jaundice
  7. Signs of infection
  8. Signs of aspiration of meconium
C. Interventions
  1. Maintain airway and cardiopulmonary function.
  2. Maintain body temperature.
  3. Observe for signs of respiratory distress.
  4. Monitor for infection and initiate measures to prevent sepsis.
  5. Monitor blood glucose levels and for signs of hypoglycemia.
  6. Initiate early feedings and monitor for signs of aspiration.
  7. Provide stimulation (e.g., touch and cuddling).

IX. LARGE FOR GESTATIONAL AGE

A. Description: **Newborn** who is plotted at or above the 90th percentile on the intrauterine growth curve
B. Assessment
  1. Gestational age
  2. Birth trauma or injury
  3. Respiratory distress
  4. Hypoglycemia
C. Interventions
  1. Monitor vital signs.
  2. Monitor blood glucose levels and for signs of hypoglycemia.
  3. Initiate early feedings.
  4. Monitor for infection and initiate measures to prevent sepsis.
  5. Provide stimulation, such as touch and cuddling.

X. RESPIRATORY DISTRESS SYNDROME

A. Description: Serious lung disorder caused by immaturity and inability to produce **surfactant**, resulting in hypoxia and acidosis

B. Assessment
1. Tachypnea
2. Flaring nares
3. Expiratory grunting
4. Retractions
5. Seesaw respirations
6. Decreased breath sounds
7. Apnea
8. Pallor and cyanosis
9. Hypothermia
10. Poor muscle tone

C. Interventions
1. Monitor color, respiratory rate, and degree of effort in breathing.
2. Maintain airway and cardiopulmonary function and support respirations as prescribed.
3. Monitor arterial blood gases and oxygen saturation levels as prescribed (arterial blood gases from umbilical artery).
4. Monitor arterial blood gases so that oxygen administered to the **newborn** is at the lowest possible concentration necessary to maintain adequate arterial oxygenation.
5. Any premature **newborn** who required oxygen support should be scheduled for an eye examination before discharge to assess for retinal damage.
6. Suction every 2 hours or more often as necessary.
7. Position the **newborn** on the side or back, with the neck slightly extended.
8. Administer respiratory therapy (percussion and vibration) as prescribed; use padded small plastic cup or small oxygen mask for percussion; use padded electric toothbrush for vibration.
9. Provide nutrition.
10. Support bonding.
11. Prepare parents for short-term to long-term period of oxygen dependency if necessary.
12. Encourage the mother to pump the breasts for future breast-feeding if she so desires.
13. Encourage as much parental participation in the **newborn's** care as the condition allows.

⚠ Prepare to administer surfactant replacement therapy (instilled into the endotracheal tube) to a newborn with respiratory distress syndrome.

XI. MECONIUM ASPIRATION SYNDROME

A. Description
1. Occurs in term or post-term **newborns**
2. Fetal distress increases intestinal peristalsis, relaxing the anal sphincter and releasing meconium into the **amniotic fluid**.
3. Aspiration can occur in utero or with the first breath.

B. Assessment
1. Respiratory distress is present at birth; tachypnea, cyanosis, retractions, nasal flaring, grunting, crackles, and rhonchi may be present.

2. The **newborn's** nails, skin, and umbilical cord may be stained a yellow-green color.

C. Interventions
1. Suctioning must be done immediately after the head is delivered and before the first breath is taken; vocal cords should be viewed to see if the airway is clear before stimulation and crying.
2. **Newborns** with severe meconium aspiration syndrome may benefit from extracorporeal membrane oxygenation; this therapy uses a modified heart-lung machine and provides oxygen to the circulation allowing the lungs to rest and decreasing pulmonary hypertension and hypoxemia in some conditions, such as meconium aspiration.

XII. BRONCHOPULMONARY DYSPLASIA

A. Description
1. This chronic pulmonary condition affects **newborns** who have experienced respiratory failure or have been oxygen-dependent for more than 28 days.
2. X-ray findings are abnormal, indicating areas of overinflation and atelectasis.

B. Assessment
1. Tachypnea
2. Tachycardia
3. Retractions
4. Nasal flaring
5. Labored breathing
6. Crackles and decreased air movement
7. Occasional expiratory wheezing

C. Interventions
1. Monitor airway and cardiopulmonary function; provide oxygen therapy.
2. Fluid restriction may be prescribed.
3. Medications include **surfactant**, diuretics, corticosteroids, and bronchodilators.

XIII. TRANSIENT TACHYPNEA OF THE NEWBORN

A. Description
1. Respiratory condition that results from incomplete evacuation of fetal lung fluid in full-term **newborns**
2. Usually disappears within 24 to 48 hours

B. Assessment
1. Tachypnea
2. Expiratory grunting
3. Retractions
4. Nasal flaring
5. Wet lung sounds per auscultation
6. Cyanosis

C. Interventions
1. Supportive care
2. Oxygen administration

XIV. INTRAVENTRICULAR HEMORRHAGE

A. Description
 1. Bleeding within the ventricles of the brain
 2. Risk factors include prematurity, respiratory distress syndrome, trauma, and asphyxia.

B. Assessment: Diminished or absent Moro reflex, lethargy, apnea, poor feeding, high-pitched shrill cry, seizure activity

C. Interventions: Supportive treatment

XV. RETINOPATHY OF PREMATURITY

A. Description
 1. Vascular disorder involving gradual replacement of retina by fibrous tissue and blood vessels
 2. Primarily caused by prematurity and use of supplemental oxygen (>30 days)

B. Assessment: Leukorrhea (white tissue on the retrolental space), vitreous hemorrhage, myopia, strabismus, cataracts (check for red reflex)

C. Interventions: Laser photocoagulation surgery

XVI. NECROTIZING ENTEROCOLITIS

A. Description
 1. Acute inflammatory disease of the gastrointestinal tract
 2. Usually occurs 4 to 10 days after birth in a term **newborn**

B. Assessment: Increased abdominal girth, decreased or absent bowel sounds, bowel loop distention, vomiting, bile-stained emesis, abdominal tenderness, occult blood in stool

C. Interventions
 1. Hold oral feedings.
 2. Insert oral gastric tube to decompress the abdomen.
 3. Intravenous antibiotics
 4. Intravenous fluids to correct fluid, electrolyte, and acid-base imbalances
 5. Surgery if indicated

XVII. HYPERBILIRUBINEMIA

A. Description
 1. Elevated serum bilirubin level
 2. Evaluation is indicated when serum levels are greater than 12 mg/dL in a term **newborn**.
 3. Therapy is aimed at preventing kernicterus, which results in permanent neurological damage resulting from the deposition of bilirubin in the brain cells.

B. Assessment
 1. Jaundice
 2. Elevated serum bilirubin levels
 3. Enlarged liver
 4. Poor muscle tone
 5. Lethargy
 6. Poor sucking reflex

C. Interventions
 1. Monitor for the presence of jaundice; assess skin and sclera for jaundice.
  a. Examine the **newborn's** skin color in natural light.
  b. Press a finger over a bony prominence or tip of the **newborn's** nose to press out capillary blood from the tissues.
  c. Note that jaundice starts at the head first and spreads to the chest, abdomen, arms and legs, and hands and feet, which are the last to be jaundiced.
 2. Keep the **newborn** well hydrated to maintain blood volume.
 3. Facilitate early, frequent feeding to hasten passage of meconium and encourage excretion of bilirubin.
 4. Report to the physician any signs of jaundice in the first 24 hours of life and any abnormal signs and symptoms.
 5. Prepare for phototherapy, and monitor the **newborn** closely during the treatment.

⚠ At any serum bilirubin level, the appearance of jaundice during the first day of life indicates a pathological process.

D. Phototherapy
 1. Description
  a. Phototherapy is use of intense fluorescent lights to reduce serum bilirubin levels in the **newborn**.
  b. Adverse effects from treatment, such as eye damage, dehydration, or sensory deprivation, can occur.
 2. Interventions
  a. Expose as much of the **newborn's** skin as possible.
  b. Cover the genital area, and monitor the genital area for skin irritation or breakdown.
  c. Cover the **newborn's** eyes with eye shields or patches; ensure that the eyelids are closed when shields or patches are applied.
  d. Remove the shields or patches at least once per shift (during a feeding time) to inspect the eyes for infection or irritation and to allow for eye contact and bonding with the parents.
  e. Measure the lamp energy output to ensure efficacy of the treatment (done with a special device known as a photometer).
  f. Monitor skin temperature closely.
  g. Increase fluids to compensate for water loss.
  h. Expect loose green stools and green urine.
  i. Monitor the **newborn's** skin color with the fluorescent light turned off, every 4 to 8 hours.
  j. Monitor the skin for bronze baby syndrome, a grayish brown discoloration of the skin.
  k. Reposition the **newborn** every 2 hours.

l. Provide stimulation.

m. After treatment, continue monitoring for signs of hyperbilirubinemia because rebound elevations are normal after therapy is discontinued.

n. Turn off the phototherapy lights before drawing a blood specimen for serum bilirubin levels, and do not leave the blood specimen uncovered under fluorescent lights (to prevent the breakdown of bilirubin in the blood specimen).

XVIII. ERYTHROBLASTOSIS FETALIS

A. Description
1. Erythroblastosis fetalis is the destruction of red blood cells that results from an antigen-antibody reaction.
2. The disorder is characterized by hemolytic anemia or hyperbilirubinemia.
3. Exchange of fetal and maternal blood occurs primarily when the **placenta** separates at birth (Fig. 30-5).
4. Antibodies are harmless to the mother, but attach to the erythrocytes in the fetus and cause hemolysis.
5. Sensitization is rare with the first pregnancy.
6. ABO incompatibility is usually less severe.

B. Assessment
1. Anemia
2. Jaundice that develops rapidly after birth and before 24 hours
3. Edema

C. Interventions
1. Administer $Rh_o(D)$ immune globulin (Rho-GAM) to the mother during the first 72 hours after **delivery** if the Rh-negative mother delivers an Rh-positive fetus but remains unsensitized.

2. Assist with exchange transfusion after birth or intrauterine transfusion as prescribed.
3. The **newborn's** blood is replaced with Rh-negative blood to stop the destruction of the **newborn's** red blood cells; the Rh-negative blood is replaced with the **newborn's** own blood gradually.
4. Reassure the mother that the **newborn** will experience no untoward effects from the condition.

XIX. SEPSIS

A. Description: Generalized infection resulting from the presence of bacteria in the blood

B. Assessment
1. Pallor
2. Tachypnea, tachycardia
3. Poor feeding
4. Abdominal distention
5. Temperature instability

C. Interventions
1. Assess for periods of apnea or irregular respirations.
2. If apnea is present, stimulate by gently rubbing the chest or foot.
3. Administer oxygen as prescribed.
4. Monitor vital signs; assess for fever.
5. Maintain warmth in a radiant warmer.
6. Provide isolation as necessary.
7. Monitor intake and output, and obtain daily weight.
8. Monitor for diarrhea.
9. Assess feeding and sucking reflex, which may be poor.
10. Assess for jaundice.
11. Assess for irritability and lethargy.
12. Administer antibiotics as prescribed, and observe carefully for toxicity because a **newborn's** liver and kidneys are immature.

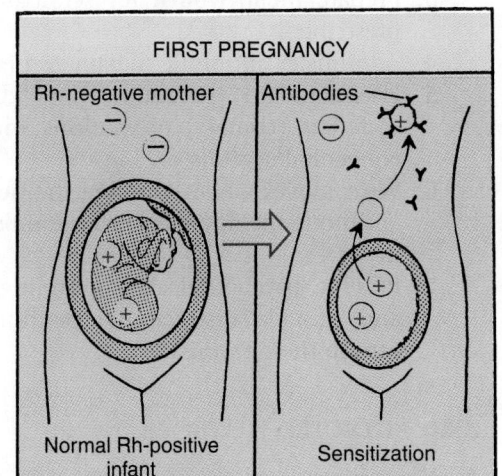
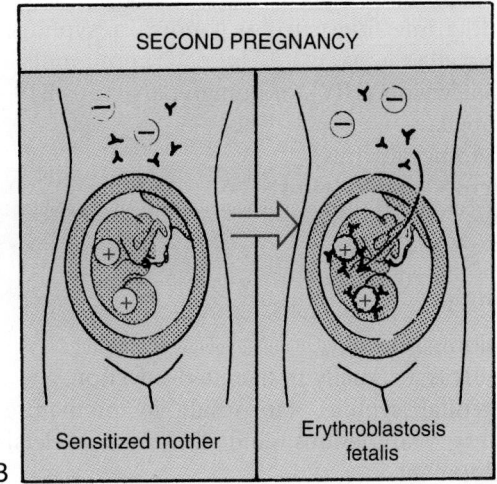

▲ **FIGURE 30-5** Development of maternal sensitization to Rh antigens. **A,** Fetal Rh-positive erythrocytes enter maternal system. Maternal anti-Rh antibodies are formed. **B,** Anti-Rh antibodies cross placenta and attack fetal erythrocytes. (From Hockenberry, M., & Wilson, D. [2009]. *Wong's essentials of pediatric nursing* [8th ed.]. St. Louis: Mosby.)

TABLE 30-5 Infections Included in TORCH Syndrome

Infection	Characteristics and Description
Toxoplasmosis	Caused by protozoan infection Produces no serious effects in mother Organism can be transmitted to fetus Infection can result in severe physical, developmental abnormalities Common carriers include cat feces, raw beef
Other infections	Can include syphilis, gonorrhea, varicella, hepatitis B, HIV, human parvovirus B19
Rubella	Systemic viral infection Rubella causes congenital rubella syndrome—includes congenital heart disease, cataracts, growth retardation, and pneumonia if mother becomes infected within first trimester Deafness and some learning disabilities can occur if mother becomes infected during first trimester
Cytomegalovirus	Viral infection that persists in the body indefinitely; has periods of reactivation without symptoms Can infect fetus or newborn during delivery or after birth through breast milk, blood transfusions, or contact with infected secretions May cause microcephaly, blindness, deafness, mental and motor retardation
Herpes simplex virus	Sexually transmitted infection Has periods of reactivation Newborn commonly infected during delivery by direct contact with lesions in genital tract Can cause neurological impairment or death

HIV, human immunodeficiency virus.

XX. TORCH INFECTIONS

A. Description
   1. TORCH infections are infections that occur in the fetus or **newborn**.
   2. Infection is caused by one of the following:
      a. *T*oxoplasmosis
      b. *O*ther infections such as gonorrhea, syphilis, varicella, hepatitis B, human immunodeficiency virus (HIV), or human parvovirus B19
      c. *R*ubella
      d. *C*ytomegalovirus
      e. *H*erpes simplex virus
B. Infections (Table 30-5)

XXI. SYPHILIS

A. Description
   1. Syphilis is a sexually transmitted infection.
   2. Congenital syphilis can result in premature **delivery**, skin lesions, and abnormal skeletal development.
   3. The causative organism, *Treponema pallidum*, a spirochete, is able to cross the **placenta**

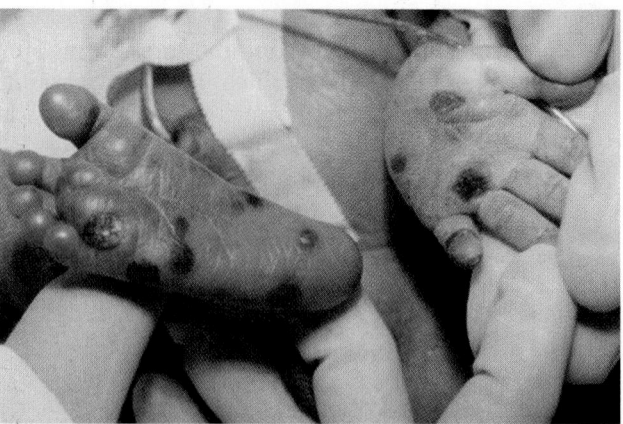

▲ **FIGURE 30-6** Neonatal syphilitic lesions on hands and feet. (From Lowdermilk, D., & Perry, S. [2007]. *Maternity & women's health care* [9th ed.]. St. Louis: Mosby. Courtesy of Mahesh Kotwal, MD, Phoenix, AZ.)

throughout pregnancy and infect the fetus, usually after 18 weeks' gestation.
   4. Risks include preterm birth, stillbirth, and low birth weight.
   5. Congenital effects are irreversible and may include central nervous system damage and hearing loss.
B. Assessment
   1. Hepatosplenomegaly
   2. Joint swelling
   3. Palmar rash and lesions (Fig. 30-6)
   4. Anemia
   5. Jaundice
   6. Snuffles
   7. Ascites
   8. Pneumonitis
   9. Cerebrospinal fluid changes
C. Interventions
   1. Monitor the **newborn** for signs of syphilis.
   2. Monitor for palmar rash and snuffles.
   3. Prepare the **newborn** for serological testing if prescribed.
   4. Administer antibiotic therapy as prescribed.
   5. Use standard precautions and drainage and secretion (contact) precautions with suspected congenital syphilis.
   6. Wear gloves when handling the **newborn** until antibiotic therapy has been administered for 24 hours.
   7. Provide psychological support to the mother, and provide instructions regarding follow-up care to the **newborn**.

XXII. ADDICTED NEWBORN

A. Description
   1. A **newborn** can become passively addicted to drugs that have passed through the **placenta**.

2. Assessment findings and withdrawal times may vary depending on the specific addicting drug.
3. See also fetal alcohol syndrome.

B. Assessment
   1. Irritability
   2. Tremors
   3. Hyperactivity and hypertonicity
   4. Respiratory distress
   5. Vomiting
   6. High-pitched cry
   7. Sneezing
   8. Fever
   9. Diarrhea
   10. Excessive sweating
   11. Poor feeding
   12. Extreme sucking of fists
   13. Seizures

C. Interventions
   1. Monitor respiratory and cardiac status frequently.
   2. Monitor temperature and vital signs.
   3. Hold **newborn** firmly and close to the body during feeding and when giving care.
   4. Initiate seizure precautions (pad sides of the crib).
   5. Provide small frequent feedings and allow a longer period for feeding.
   6. Monitor intake and output.
   7. Administer intravenous hydration if prescribed.
   8. Protect the **newborn's** skin from injury that can be caused by the constant rubbing from hyperactive jitters.
   9. Swaddle the **newborn**.
   10. Place the **newborn** in a quiet room and reduce stimulation.
   11. Allow the mother to express feelings such as anxiety and guilt.
   12. Refer the mother for treatment of the substance abuse problem.

XXIII. FETAL ALCOHOL SYNDROME

A. Description
   1. Fetal alcohol syndrome is caused by maternal alcohol use during pregnancy.
   2. The syndrome is a result of teratogenesis.
   3. The syndrome causes mental and physical retardation.

B. Assessment
   1. Facial changes (Fig. 30-7)
      a. Short palpebral fissures
      b. Hypoplastic philtrum
      c. Short, upturned nose
      d. Flat midface
      e. Thin upper lip
      f. Low nasal bridge

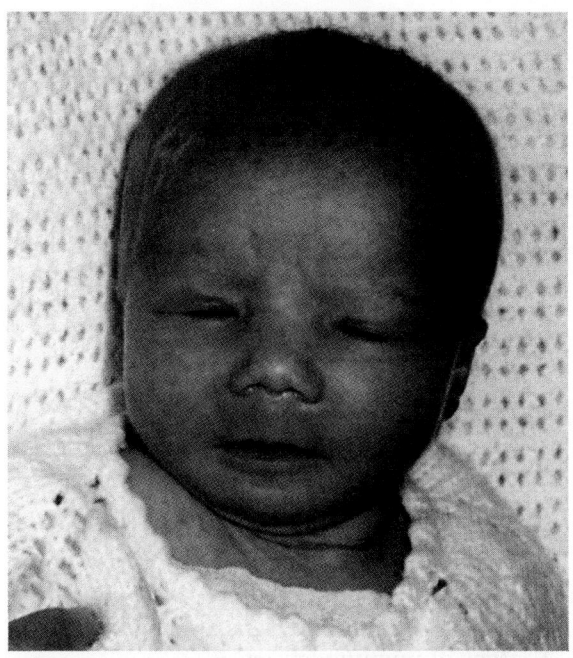

▲ **FIGURE 30-7** Infant with fetal alcohol syndrome. (From Perry, S., Hockenberry, M., Lowdermilk, D., & Wilson, D. [2010]. *Maternal child nursing care* [4th ed.]. St. Louis: Mosby.)

   2. Abnormal palmar creases
   3. Respiratory distress (apnea, cyanosis)
   4. Congenital heart disorders
   5. Irritability and hypersensitivity to stimuli
   6. Tremors
   7. Poor feeding
   8. Seizures

C. Interventions
   1. Monitor for respiratory distress.
   2. Position the **newborn** on the side to facilitate drainage of secretions.
   3. Keep resuscitation equipment at the bedside.
   4. Monitor for hypoglycemia.
   5. Assess suck and swallow reflex.
   6. Administer small feedings and burp well.
   7. Suction as necessary.
   8. Monitor intake and output.
   9. Monitor weight and head circumference.
   10. Decrease environmental stimuli.

XXIV. NEWBORN OF A MOTHER WITH HUMAN IMMUNODEFICIENCY VIRUS (HIV)

A. Description
   1. The fetus of a client who is positive for HIV antibody should be monitored closely throughout the pregnancy.
   2. Serial ultrasound screenings should be done during pregnancy to identify intrauterine growth restriction.
   3. Weekly nonstress testing after 32 weeks of gestation and biophysical profiles may be necessary during pregnancy.

4. **Newborns** born to HIV-positive clients may test positive because the mother's antibodies may persist in the **newborn** for 18 months after birth.

5. The use of antiviral medication, the reduction of **newborn** exposure to maternal blood and body fluids, and the early identification of HIV in pregnancy reduce the risk of transmission to the **newborn**.

6. All **newborns** born to HIV-positive mothers acquire maternal antibody to HIV infection, but not all acquire the infection.

7. The **newborn** may be asymptomatic for the first several months to years of life.

B. Transmission
1. Across placental barrier
2. During **labor** and **delivery**
3. Breast milk

C. Assessment
1. Possibly no outward signs at birth
2. Signs of immunodeficiency
3. Hepatomegaly
4. Splenomegaly
5. Lymphadenopathy
6. Impairment in growth and development

D. Interventions
1. Clean the **newborn's** skin carefully before any invasive procedure, such as the administration of vitamin K, heel sticks, or venipunctures.
2. Circumcisions are not done on **newborns** with HIV-positive mothers until the **newborn's** status is determined.
3. **Newborn** can room with mother.
4. All HIV-exposed **newborns** should be treated with medication to prevent infection by *Pneumocystis jiroveci*.
5. Antiretroviral medications may be administered as prescribed for the first 6 weeks of life.
6. Monitor for early signs of immunodeficiency, such as enlarged spleen or liver, lymphadenopathy, and impairment in growth and development.
7. **Newborns** at risk for HIV infection should be seen by the physician at birth and at 1 week, 2 weeks, 1 month, and 2 months of age.
8. Inform the client that HIV culture is recommended at 1 month and after 4 months of age.

E. Immunizations
1. Immunizations with live vaccines, such as measles-mumps-rubella and varicella, should not be done until the **newborn's**, **infant's**, or child's status is confirmed.
2. If infected, live vaccine will not be given.

⚠ Newborns at risk for HIV infection need to receive all recommended immunizations at the regular schedule.

XXV. NEWBORN OF A DIABETIC MOTHER

A. Description
1. **Infant** born to mother with insulin-dependent diabetes or gestational diabetes
2. Hypoglycemia, hyperbilirubinemia, respiratory distress syndrome, hypocalcemia, birth trauma, and congenital anomalies may be present.

B. Assessment
1. Excessive size and weight as a result of excess fat and glycogen in the tissues
2. Edema or puffiness in the face and cheeks
3. Signs of hypoglycemia, such as twitching, apnea, difficulty in feeding, lethargy, seizures, and cyanosis
4. Hyperbilirubinemia
5. Signs of respiratory distress, such as tachypnea, cyanosis, retractions, grunting, and nasal flaring

C. Interventions
1. Monitor for signs of respiratory distress, birth trauma, and congenital anomalies.
2. Monitor bilirubin and blood glucose levels.
3. Monitor weight.
4. Feed the **newborn** soon after birth with glucose in water, breast milk, or formula as prescribed.
5. Administer glucose intravenously to treat hypoglycemia if necessary and as prescribed.
6. Monitor for edema.
7. Monitor for respiratory distress, tremors, or seizures.

XXVI. HYPOGLYCEMIA

A. Description
1. Hypoglycemia is an abnormally low level of glucose in the blood (<40 mg/dL in the first 72 hours of life or <45 mg/dL after the first 3 days of life).
2. Normal blood glucose level is 40 to 60 mg/dL in a 1-day-old **newborn** and 50 to 90 mg/dL in a **newborn** older than 1 day.

B. Assessment
1. Increased respiratory rate
2. Twitching, nervousness, or tremors
3. Unstable temperature
4. Lethargy, apnea, seizures, cyanosis

C. Interventions
1. Prevent low blood glucose level through early feedings.
2. Administer glucose orally or intravenously as prescribed.
3. Monitor blood glucose levels as prescribed.
4. Monitor for feeding problems.
5. Monitor for apneic periods.
6. Assess for shrill or intermittent cries.
7. Evaluate lethargy and poor muscle tone.

MORE QUESTIONS ON THE CD!

Practice Questions

300. A nurse in a delivery room is assisting with the delivery of a newborn. After delivery, the nurse prepares to prevent heat loss in the newborn resulting from evaporation by:
1. Warming the crib pad
2. Closing the doors to the room
3. Drying the infant with a warm blanket
4. Turning on the overhead radiant warmer

301. The mother of a newborn calls a clinic and reports to a nurse that when cleaning the umbilical cord, the mother noticed that the cord was moist and that discharge was present. The appropriate nursing instruction to the mother is which of the following?
1. Bring the infant to the clinic.
2. This is a normal occurrence.
3. Increase the number of times that the cord is cleaned per day.
4. Monitor the cord for another 24 to 48 hours and call the clinic if the discharge continues.

302. A nurse in a newborn nursery receives a telephone call to prepare for the admission of a 43-week gestation newborn with Apgar scores of 1 and 4. In planning for admission of this newborn, the nurse's highest priority should be to:
1. Turn on the apnea and cardiorespiratory monitors.
2. Connect the resuscitation bag to the oxygen outlet.
3. Set up the intravenous line with 5% dextrose in water.
4. Set the radiant warmer control temperature at 36.5° C (97.6° F).

303. A nurse is assessing a newborn infant after circumcision and notes that the circumcised area is red with a small amount of bloody drainage. Which of the following nursing actions is appropriate?
1. Contact the physician.
2. Apply gentle pressure.
3. Reinforce the dressing.
4. Document the findings.

304. A nurse in a newborn nursery is monitoring a preterm newborn for respiratory distress syndrome. Which assessment signs noted in the newborn would alert the nurse to the possibility of this syndrome?
1. Tachypnea and retractions
2. Acrocyanosis and grunting
3. Hypotension and bradycardia
4. Presence of a barrel chest with acrocyanosis

305. A postpartum nurse is providing instructions to the mother of a newborn with hyperbilirubinemia who is being breast-fed. The nurse provides which appropriate instruction to the mother?
1. Feed the newborn less frequently.
2. Continue to breast-feed every 2 to 4 hours.
3. Switch to bottle-feeding the infant for 2 weeks.
4. Stop breast-feeding and switch to bottle-feeding permanently.

306. A nurse is assessing a newborn who was born to a mother who is addicted to drugs. Which assessment finding would the nurse expect to note during the assessment of this newborn?
1. Lethargy
2. Sleepiness
3. Incessant crying
4. Cuddles when being held

307. A nurse notes hypotonia, irritability, and a poor sucking reflex in a full-term newborn on admission to the nursery. The nurse suspects fetal alcohol syndrome and is aware that which additional sign would be consistent with fetal alcohol syndrome?
1. Length of 19 inches
2. Abnormal palmar creases
3. Birth weight of 6 lb, 14 oz
4. Head circumference appropriate for gestational age

308. A nurse is preparing a plan of care for a newborn with fetal alcohol syndrome. The nurse should include which priority intervention in the plan of care?
1. Allow the newborn to establish own sleep-rest pattern.
2. Maintain the newborn in a brightly lighted area of the nursery.
3. Encourage frequent handling of the newborn by staff and parents.
4. Monitor the newborn's response to feedings and weight gain pattern.

309. A nurse administers erythromycin ointment (0.5%) to the eyes of a newborn and the mother asks the nurse why this is performed. The nurse explains to the mother that this is routinely done to:
1. Protect the newborns eyes from possible infections acquired while hospitalized.
2. Prevent cataracts in the newborn born to a woman who is susceptible to rubella.
3. Minimize the spread of microorganisms to the newborn from invasive procedures during labor.
4. Prevent ophthalmia neonatorum from occurring after delivery in a newborn born to a woman with an untreated gonococcal infection.

310. A nurse prepares to administer a vitamin K injection to a newborn, and the mother asks the nurse why her infant needs the injection. The best response by the nurse would be:
  1. "Your newborn needs vitamin K to develop immunity."
  2. "The vitamin K will protect your newborn from being jaundiced."
  3. "Newborns have sterile bowels, and vitamin K promotes the growth of bacteria in the bowel."
  4. "Newborns are deficient in vitamin K, and this injection prevents your newborn from bleeding."

311. A nurse develops a plan of care for a woman with human immunodeficiency virus infection and her newborn. The nurse includes which intervention in the plan of care?
  1. Monitoring the newborn's vital signs routinely
  2. Maintaining standard precautions at all times while caring for the newborn
  3. Initiating referral to evaluate for blindness, deafness, learning problems, or behavioral problems
  4. Instructing the breast-feeding mother regarding the treatment of the nipples with nystatin ointment

312. A nurse is planning care for a newborn of a diabetic mother. A priority nursing diagnosis for this infant is:

  1. *Hyperthermia* related to excess fat and glycogen
  2. *Risk for injury* related to low blood glucose levels
  3. *Risk for delayed development* related to excessive size
  4. *Risk for aspiration* related to impaired suck and swallow reflexes

313. The nurse determines that a new mother understands the teaching about prevention of newborn abduction if she states:
  1. "I will place my baby's crib close to the door."
  2. "Some health care personnel won't have name badges."
  3. "It's OK to allow the nurse assistant to carry my newborn to the nursery."
  4. "I will ask the nurse to attend to my infant if I am napping and my husband is not here."

Alternate Item Format: Multiple Response

314. The nurse is preparing to care for a newborn receiving phototherapy. Which interventions are appropriate? **Select all that apply.**
  ☐ 1. Avoid stimulation.
  ☐ 2. Decrease fluid intake.
  ☐ 3. Expose all of the newborn's skin.
  ☐ 4. Monitor skin temperature closely.
  ☐ 5. Reposition the newborn every 2 hours.
  ☐ 6. Cover the newborn's eyes with eye shields or patches.

ANSWERS
300. 3
Rationale: Evaporation of moisture from a wet body dissipates heat along with the moisture. Keeping the newborn dry by drying the wet newborn at birth prevents hypothermia via evaporation. Hypothermia caused by conduction occurs when the newborn is on a cold surface, such as a cold pad or mattress, and heat from the newborn's body is transferred to the colder object (direct contact). Warming the crib pad assists in preventing hypothermia by conduction. Convection occurs as air moves across the newborn's skin from an open door and heat is transferred to the air. Radiation occurs when heat from the newborn radiates to a colder surface (indirect contact).
Test-Taking Strategy: Note the strategic word *evaporation* in the question to assist in selecting the correct option. Recalling that evaporation of moisture from a wet body dissipates heat along with the moisture will assist in directing you to option 3. Review the methods of heat loss in a newborn if you had difficulty with this question.
Level of Cognitive Ability: Applying
Client Needs: Physiological Integrity

Integrated Process: Nursing Process—Planning
Content Area: Maternity—Postpartum
Reference: McKinney, E., James, S., Murray, S., & Ashwill, J. (2009). *Maternal-child nursing* (3rd ed., pp. 495–496). St. Louis: Saunders.

301. 1
Rationale: Symptoms of umbilical cord infection are moistness, oozing, discharge, and a reddened base around the cord. If symptoms of infection occur, the client should be instructed to notify a health care provider. If these symptoms occur, antibiotics may be necessary. Options 2, 3, and 4 are inappropriate nursing interventions for the description given in the question.
Test-Taking Strategy: Focus on the clinical manifestations provided in the question to assist in directing you to the correct option. Noting the strategic word *discharge* in the question will assist in directing you to the option that indicates that the newborn needs to be seen by the health care provider. Review interventions related to cord care and the signs of infection if you had difficulty with this question.

Level of Cognitive Ability: Applying
Client Needs: Physiological Integrity
Integrated Process: Nursing Process—Implementation
Content Area: Maternity—Postpartum
Reference: McKinney, E., James, S., Murray, S., & Ashwill, J. (2009). *Maternal-child nursing* (3rd ed., p. 555). St. Louis: Saunders.

302. 2
Rationale: The highest priority on admission to the nursery for a newborn with a low Apgar score is the airway, which would involve preparing respiratory resuscitation equipment and oxygen. The remaining options are also important, although they are of lower priority. The newborn would be placed on an apnea and cardiorespiratory monitor. Setting up an intravenous line with 5% dextrose in water would provide circulatory support. The radiant warmer would provide an external heat source, which is necessary to prevent further respiratory distress.
Test-Taking Strategy: Note the strategic words *highest priority*. This question asks you to prioritize care on the basis of information about a newborn's condition. Use the ABCs—airway, breathing, and circulation. A method of planning for airway support is to have the resuscitation bag connected to an oxygen source. Review care for a newborn with low Apgar scores if you had difficulty with this question.
Level of Cognitive Ability: Analyzing
Client Needs: Physiological Integrity
Integrated Process: Nursing Process—Planning
Content Area: Critical Care
Reference: McKinney, E., James, S., Murray, S., & Ashwill, J. (2009). *Maternal-child nursing* (3rd ed., pp. 374–375, 377). St. Louis: Saunders.

303. 4
Rationale: The penis is normally red during the healing process after circumcision. A yellow exudate may be noted in 24 hours, and this is part of normal healing. The nurse would expect that the area would be red with a small amount of bloody drainage. Only if the bleeding were excessive would the nurse apply gentle pressure with a sterile gauze. If bleeding cannot be controlled, the blood vessel may need to be ligated, and the nurse would notify the physician. Because the findings identified in the question are normal, the nurse would document the assessment findings.
Test-Taking Strategy: Use the process of elimination. Note the strategic words *small amount of bloody drainage*. This should assist in directing you to option 4 because this is a normal occurrence after circumcision. If you had difficulty with this question, review the expected findings after circumcision.
Level of Cognitive Ability: Applying
Client Needs: Physiological Integrity
Integrated Process: Nursing Process—Implementation
Content Area: Maternity—Postpartum
Reference: Perry, S., Hockenberry, M., Lowdermilk, D., & Wilson, D. (2010). *Maternal child nursing care* (4th ed., p. 669). St. Louis: Mosby.

304. 1
Rationale: A newborn infant with respiratory distress syndrome may present with clinical signs of cyanosis, tachypnea or apnea, nasal flaring, chest wall retractions, or audible grunts. Acrocyanosis is bluish discoloration of the hands and feet, is associated with immature peripheral circulation, and is common in the first few hours of life. Options 2, 3, and 4 do not indicate clinical signs of respiratory distress syndrome.
Test-Taking Strategy: Use the process of elimination. Recalling that acrocyanosis may be a normal sign in a newborn infant will assist in eliminating options 2 and 4. From the remaining options, you must be familiar with the signs of respiratory distress syndrome. Also, note the relationship between the diagnosis and the signs noted in option 1. If you had difficulty with this question, review the signs of respiratory distress syndrome.
Level of Cognitive Ability: Analyzing
Client Needs: Physiological Integrity
Integrated Process: Nursing Process—Assessment
Content Area: Maternity—Postpartum
References: Hockenberry, M., & Wilson, D. (2009). *Wong's essentials of pediatric nursing* (8th ed., p. 286). St. Louis: Mosby.
   McKinney, E., James, S., Murray, S., & Ashwill, J. (2009). *Maternal-child nursing* (3rd ed., p. 505). St. Louis: Saunders.

305. 2
Rationale: Hyperbilirubinemia is an elevated serum bilirubin level. At any serum bilirubin level, the appearance of jaundice during the first day of life indicates a pathological process. Early and frequent feeding hastens the excretion of bilirubin. Breast-feeding should be initiated within 2 hours after birth and every 2 to 4 hours thereafter. The infant should not be fed less frequently. Switching to bottle-feeding for 2 weeks or stopping breast-feeding permanently is unnecessary.
Test-Taking Strategy: Options 3 and 4 are comparable or alike. These options discourage the continuation of breast-feeding and should be eliminated. From the remaining options, recalling the pathophysiology associated with hyperbilirubinemia will assist you in eliminating option 1. Review client instructions related to hyperbilirubinemia in the newborn if you had difficulty with this question.
Level of Cognitive Ability: Applying
Client Needs: Physiological Integrity
Integrated Process: Teaching and Learning
Content Area: Maternity—Postpartum
Reference: McKinney, E., James, S., Murray, S., & Ashwill, J. (2009). *Maternal-child nursing* (3rd ed., p. 573). St. Louis: Saunders.

306. 3
Rationale: A newborn of a woman using drugs is irritable. The infant is overloaded easily by sensory stimulation. The infant may cry incessantly and be difficult to console. The infant would hyperextend and posture rather than cuddle when being held.
Test-Taking Strategy: Options 1 and 2 are comparable or alike in that they indicate hypoactivity of the newborn and can be eliminated. From the remaining options, recalling the pathophysiology associated with an infant born to a drug-addicted mother and that the newborn is irritable will assist you in eliminating option 4. Review assessment findings for the newborn of a drug-addicted mother if you had difficulty with this question.

Level of Cognitive Ability: Analyzing
Client Needs: Physiological Integrity
Integrated Process: Nursing Process—Assessment
Content Area: Maternity—Postpartum
Reference: McKinney, E., James, S., Murray, S., & Ashwill, J. (2009). *Maternal-child nursing* (3rd ed., p. 757). St. Louis: Saunders.

307. 2
Rationale: Fetal alcohol syndrome is caused by maternal alcohol use during pregnancy. Features of newborns diagnosed with fetal alcohol syndrome include craniofacial abnormalities, intrauterine growth restriction, cardiac abnormalities, abnormal palmar creases, and respiratory distress. Options 1, 3, and 4 are normal assessment findings in the full-term newborn infant.
Test-Taking Strategy: Use knowledge regarding normal assessment findings in the full-term newborn infant to answer this question. Options 1, 3, and 4 are comparable or alike and represent normal assessment findings in a full-term newborn. If you had difficulty with this question, review the content related to normal newborn assessment findings and fetal alcohol syndrome.
Level of Cognitive Ability: Analyzing
Client Needs: Physiological Integrity
Integrated Process: Nursing Process—Assessment
Content Area: Maternity—Postpartum
References: Hockenberry, M., & Wilson, D. (2009). *Wong's essentials of pediatric nursing* (8th ed., p. 311). St. Louis: Mosby.
   McKinney, E., James, S., Murray, S., & Ashwill, J. (2009). *Maternal-child nursing* (3rd ed., p. 1547). St. Louis: Saunders.

308. 4
Rationale: Fetal alcohol syndrome is caused by maternal alcohol use during pregnancy. A primary nursing goal for the newborn diagnosed with fetal alcohol syndrome is to establish nutritional balance after delivery. These newborns may exhibit hyperirritability, vomiting, diarrhea, or an uncoordinated sucking and swallowing ability. A quiet environment with minimal stimuli and handling would help establish appropriate sleep-rest cycles in the newborn as well. Options 1, 2, and 3 are inappropriate interventions.
Test-Taking Strategy: Use the process of elimination and think about the pathophysiology that occurs in a newborn with this condition. Recalling that these newborns may exhibit hyperirritability, vomiting, diarrhea, or an uncoordinated sucking and swallowing ability will direct you easily to option 4. Review care of a newborn with fetal alcohol syndrome if you had difficulty with this question.
Level of Cognitive Ability: Applying
Client Needs: Physiological Integrity
Integrated Process: Nursing Process—Planning
Content Area: Maternity—Postpartum
Reference: McKinney, E., James, S., Murray, S., & Ashwill, J. (2009). *Maternal-child nursing* (3rd ed., p. 1548). St. Louis: Saunders.

309. 4
Rationale: Erythromycin ophthalmic ointment 0.5% is used as a prophylactic treatment for ophthalmia neonatorum,

which is caused by the bacterium *Neisseria gonorrhoeae*. Preventive treatment of gonorrhea is required by law. Options 1, 2, and 3 are not the purposes for administering this medication to a newborn infant.
Test-Taking Strategy: Use knowledge of the purpose of administering erythromycin ophthalmic ointment to a newborn infant. Remember that this is done to prevent ophthalmia neonatorum. If you had difficulty with this question, review initial eye care for the newborn infant.
Level of Cognitive Ability: Applying
Client Needs: Health Promotion and Maintenance
Integrated Process: Teaching and Learning
Content Area: Maternity—Postpartum
Reference: McKinney, E., James, S., Murray, S., & Ashwill, J. (2009). *Maternal-child nursing* (3rd ed., p. 539). St. Louis: Saunders.

310. 4
Rationale: Vitamin K is necessary for the body to synthesize coagulation factors. Vitamin K is administered to the newborn to prevent bleeding disorders. Vitamin K promotes liver formation of the clotting factors II, VII, IX, and X. Newborns are vitamin K–deficient because the bowel does not have the bacteria necessary for synthesizing fat-soluble vitamin K. The normal flora in the intestinal tract produces vitamin K. The newborn's bowel does not support the normal production of vitamin K until bacteria adequately colonize it. The bowel becomes colonized by bacteria as food is ingested. Vitamin K does not promote the development of immunity or prevent the infant from becoming jaundiced.
Test-Taking Strategy: Note the strategic word *best*. Because immunity and jaundice are not related to the action of vitamin K, eliminate options 1 and 2. From the remaining options, recall the action of vitamin K to direct you to option 4. Remember that vitamin K does not promote the growth of bacteria, but is administered to prevent bleeding. If you had difficulty with this question, review the purpose of administering a vitamin K injection to a newborn.
Level of Cognitive Ability: Applying
Client Needs: Physiological Integrity
Integrated Process: Teaching and Learning
Content Area: Maternity—Postpartum
Reference: Hockenberry, M., & Wilson, D. (2009). *Wong's essentials of pediatric nursing* (8th ed., p. 222). St. Louis: Mosby.

311. 2
Rationale: An infant born to a mother infected with human immunodeficiency virus (HIV) must be cared for with strict attention to standard precautions. This prevents the transmission of HIV from the newborn, if infected, to others and prevents transmission of other infectious agents to the possibly immunocompromised newborn. Mothers infected with HIV should not breast-feed. Options 1 and 3 are not associated specifically with the care of a potentially HIV-infected newborn.
Test-Taking Strategy: Use knowledge regarding care of an infant born to an HIV-infected mother. Eliminate options 1 and 3 first because they are not associated specifically with the care of a potentially HIV-infected newborn.

Recalling that HIV-infected mothers should not breast-feed will direct you to option 2. Review care of an infant born to an HIV-infected mother if you had difficulty with this question.
Level of Cognitive Ability: Applying
Client Needs: Safe and Effective Care Environment
Integrated Process: Nursing Process—Planning
Content Area: Maternity—Postpartum
Reference: McKinney, E., James, S., Murray, S., & Ashwill, J. (2009). *Maternal-child nursing* (3rd ed., p. 1054). St. Louis: Saunders.

312. 2
Rationale: The newborn of a diabetic mother is at risk for hypoglycemia, so *Risk for injury* related to low blood glucose levels would be a priority nursing diagnosis. The newborn would also be at risk for hyperbilirubinemia, respiratory distress, hypocalcemia, and congenital anomalies. Hyperthermia, risk for delayed development, and risk for aspiration are not expected problems.
Test-Taking Strategy: Note the strategic word *priority*. Read each option thoroughly and eliminate options 1, 3, and 4 because newborns of diabetic mothers are not at risk for these problems. Also, note the relationship of the word *diabetic* in the question and the word *glucose* in option 2. Review nursing interventions for newborns of diabetic mothers if you had difficulty with this question.
Level of Cognitive Ability: Analyzing
Client Needs: Physiological Integrity
Integrated Process: Nursing Process—Planning
Content Area: Maternity-Postportum
Reference: McKinney, E., James, S., Murray, S., & Ashwill, J. (2009). *Maternal-child nursing* (3rd ed., p. 755). St. Louis: Saunders.

313. 4
Rationale: Precautions to prevent infant abduction include placing a newborn's crib away from the door, transporting a newborn only in the crib and never carrying the newborn, expecting health care personnel to wear identification that is easily visible at all times, and asking a nurse to attend to the newborn if the mother is napping and no family member is available to watch the newborn (the newborn is never left unattended). If the mother states that she will ask the nurse to watch the newborn while she is sleeping, she has understood the teaching. Options 1, 2, and 3 are incorrect and would indicate that the mother needs further teaching.
Test-Taking Strategy: Focus on the subject, that the client understands precautions to prevent infant abduction. Read each option carefully and select the option that provides protection to the infant. This will direct you to option 4. Review

precautions to prevent newborn abduction if you had difficulty with this question.
Level of Cognitive Ability: Evaluating
Client Needs: Safe and Effective Care Environment
Integrated Process: Nursing Process—Evaluation
Content Area: Maternity—Postpartum
Reference: McKinney, E., James, S., Murray, S., & Ashwill, J. (2009). *Maternal-child nursing* (3rd ed., p. 547). St. Louis: Saunders.

ALTERNATE ITEM FORMAT: MULTIPLE RESPONSE
314. 4, 5, 6
Rationale: Phototherapy is the use of intense fluorescent lights to reduce serum bilirubin levels in the newborn. Adverse effects from treatment, such as eye damage, dehydration, or sensory deprivation, can occur. Interventions include exposing as much of the newborn's skin as possible; however, the genital area is covered. The newborn's eyes are also covered with eye shields or patches, ensuring that the eyelids are closed when shields or patches are applied. The shields or patches are removed at least once per shift to inspect the eyes for infection or irritation and to allow eye contact. The nurse measures the lamp energy output to ensure efficacy of the treatment (done with a special device known as a photometer), monitors skin temperature closely, and increases fluids to compensate for water loss. The newborn will have loose green stools and green-colored urine. The newborn's skin color is monitored with the fluorescent light turned off every 4 to 8 hours and is monitored for bronze baby syndrome, a grayish brown discoloration of the skin. The newborn is repositioned every 2 hours, and stimulation is provided. After treatment, the newborn is monitored for signs of hyperbilirubinemia because rebound elevations can occur after therapy is discontinued.
Test-Taking Strategy: Focus on the subject, phototherapy. Recalling that adverse effects from treatment, such as eye damage, dehydration, or sensory deprivation, can occur will assist in determining the correct interventions. Review the interventions for a newborn receiving phototherapy if you had difficulty with this question.
Level of Cognitive Ability: Applying
Client Needs: Safe and Effective Care Environment
Integrated Process: Nursing Process—Implementation
Content Area: Maternity—Postpartum
References: Hockenberry, M., & Wilson, D. (2009). *Wong's essentials of pediatric nursing* (8th ed., pp. 279–280). St. Louis: Mosby.
  McKinney, E., James, S., Murray, S., & Ashwill, J. (2009). *Maternal-child nursing* (3rd ed., p. 750). St. Louis: Saunders.

31

Maternity and Newborn Medications

I. Rh$_o$(D) IMMUNE GLOBULIN (RhoGAM)

A. Description
1. Prevention of anti-Rh$_o$(D) antibody formation is most successful if the medication is administered twice, at 28 weeks of gestation and again within 72 hours after **delivery**.
2. Rh$_o$(D) immune globulin also should be administered within 72 hours after potential or actual exposure to Rh-positive blood and must be given with each subsequent exposure or potential exposure to Rh-positive blood.

B. Use: To prevent isoimmunization in Rh-negative clients who are exposed or potentially exposed to Rh-positive red blood cells by transfusion, termination of pregnancy, amniocentesis, chorionic villus sampling, abdominal trauma, or bleeding during pregnancy or the birth process

C. Adverse reactions and contraindications
1. Elevated temperature
2. Tenderness at the injection site
3. Contraindicated for Rh-positive clients
4. Contraindicated in clients with a history of systemic allergic reactions to preparations containing human immunoglobulins
5. Not administered to a **newborn**

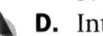

D. Interventions
1. Administer to the client by the intramuscular injection at 28 weeks' gestation and within 72 hours after **delivery**.
2. Never administer by intravenous route.
3. Monitor for temperature elevation.
4. Monitor injection site for tenderness.

⚠ Rh$_o$(D) immune globulin (RhoGAM) is of no benefit when the client has developed a positive antibody titer to the Rh antigen.

II. TOCOLYTICS

A. Description: Tocolytics are medications that produce uterine relaxation and suppress uterine activity in an attempt to halt uterine contractions and prevent preterm birth (Box 31-1 and Table 31-1).

B. Uses: To halt uterine contractions and prevent preterm birth

C. Adverse reactions and contraindications
1. See Table 31-1 for a description of adverse reactions.
2. Maternal contraindications include severe preeclampsia and eclampsia, active vaginal bleeding, intrauterine infection, cardiac disease, and medical or obstetric condition that contraindicates continuation of pregnancy.
3. Fetal contraindications include estimated gestational age greater than 37 weeks, cervical dilation greater than 4 cm, fetal demise, lethal fetal anomaly, chorioamnionitis, acute fetal distress, and chronic intrauterine growth restriction.

D. Interventions for the client receiving tocolytic therapy
1. Position the client on her side to enhance **placental** perfusion and reduce pressure on the cervix.
2. Monitor maternal vital signs, fetal status, and **labor** status frequently according to agency protocol.
3. Monitor for signs of adverse reactions to the medication.
4. Monitor daily weight and input and output status, and provide fluid intake as prescribed.
5. Offer comfort measures and provide psychosocial support to the client and family.
6. See Table 31-1 for interventions specific to each tocolytic medication.

III. MAGNESIUM SULFATE

A. Description (see Table 31-1)
1. Magnesium sulfate is a central nervous system depressant and anticonvulsant.
2. The medication causes smooth muscle relaxation.
3. The antidote is calcium gluconate.

Box 31-1 Tocolytics

Prostaglandin inhibitor: Indomethacin (Indocin)
Magnesium sulfate
Calcium channel blocker: Nifedipine (Procardia, Adalat, Nifedical)
β$_2$-selective adrenergic agonist: Terbutaline (Brethine)

B. Uses
  1. Stopping preterm **labor** to prevent preterm birth
  2. Preventing and controlling seizures in preeclamptic and eclamptic clients
C. Adverse reactions and contraindications
  1. Magnesium sulfate can cause respiratory depression, depressed reflexes, flushing, hypotension, extreme muscle weakness, decreased urine output, pulmonary edema, and elevated serum magnesium levels.
  2. Continuous intravenous infusion increases the risk of magnesium toxicity in the **newborn**.
  3. Intravenous administration should not be used for 2 hours preceding **delivery**.

TABLE 31-1 Tocolytics

Medication, Classification, and Actions	Adverse Reactions	Nursing Interventions
Indomethacin (Indocin)—prostaglandin inhibitor; relaxes uterine smooth muscle	*Maternal*—nausea and vomiting, dyspepsia, dizziness	Used when other methods fail only if gestational age is <32 wk
	Fetal—premature closure of ductus arteriosus	Not used in clients with bleeding potential, peptic ulcer disease, or oligohydramnios
	Newborn—bronchopulmonary dysplasia, respiratory distress syndrome, intracranial pressure, necrotizing enterocolitis, hyperbilirubinemia	Follow agency protocol for administration
		Prepare to determine amniotic fluid volume and function of ductus arteriosus before therapy and within 48 hr of discontinuing therapy
Magnesium sulfate—central nervous system depressant; relaxes smooth muscle, including the uterus; used to halt preterm labor contractions; used for preeclamptic clients to prevent seizures	*Maternal*—depressed respirations, depressed DTRs, hypotension, extreme muscle weakness, flushing, decreased urine output, pulmonary edema, serum magnesium levels >9 mg/dL	Use intravenous controller pump for administration
	Newborn—hypotonia and sleepiness	Follow agency protocol for administration
		Discontinue infusion and notify physician if adverse reactions occur
		Monitor for respirations <12/min, urine output <100 mL/4 hr (25-30 mL/hr)
		Monitor DTRs
		Monitor magnesium levels and report values outside therapeutic range (4-7.5 mEq/L [5-8 mg/dL])
		Keep calcium gluconate at bedside (antidote)
Nifedipine (Procardia, Adalat, Nifedical)—calcium channel blocker; relaxes smooth muscles, including the uterus, by blocking calcium entry	*Maternal*—tachycardia, hypotension, dizziness, headache, nervousness, facial flushing, fatigue, nausea	Follow agency protocol for administration
	Newborn—hypotension	Avoid use or use cautiously with magnesium sulfate because severe hypotension can occur
		Monitor for adverse reactions
Terbutaline (Brethine)—β-adrenergic agonist; relaxes smooth muscles, inhibiting uterine activity and causing bronchodilation	*Maternal*—tachycardia, palpitations, pulmonary edema, chest pain, myocardial ischemia, hypotension, tremors, hypokalemia, hyperglycemia	Monitor for adverse reactions and notify physician if they occur
	Newborn—tachycardia, hypotension, ileus, hypocalcemia, hyperbilirubinemia, hyperinsulinemia with hypoglycemia	Teach client and family to monitor for adverse reactions and when to notify physician

DTRs, deep tendon reflexes.

4. Magnesium sulfate may be prescribed for the first 12 to 24 hours postpartum if it is used for preeclampsia.
5. High doses can cause loss of deep tendon reflexes, heart block, respiratory paralysis, and cardiac arrest.
6. The medication is contraindicated in clients with heart block, myocardial damage, or renal failure.
7. The medication is used with caution in clients with severe renal impairment.

D. Interventions
1. Monitor maternal vital signs, especially respirations, every 30 to 60 minutes.
2. Assess renal function and electrocardiogram for cardiac function.
3. Monitor magnesium levels—the target range is 4 to 7.5 mEq/L (5 to 8 mg/dL); if the magnesium level increases, notify the health care provider.
4. Always administer by intravenous infusion via an infusion monitoring device such as a controller pump; carefully monitor the dose being administered, and follow agency protocol for administration.
5. Keep calcium gluconate on hand in case of a magnesium sulfate overdose because calcium gluconate antagonizes the effect of magnesium sulfate.
6. Monitor deep tendon reflexes hourly for signs of developing toxicity.
7. Test the patellar reflex or knee jerk reflex before administering a repeat parenteral dose (used as an indicator of central nervous system depression; suppressed reflex may be a sign of impending respiratory arrest) (Fig. 31-1 and Table 31-2).
8. Patellar reflex must be present and respiratory rate must be greater than 16 breaths/min (or as designated by agency protocol) before each parenteral dose.
9. Monitor intake and output hourly; output should be maintained at 25 to 30 mL/hr because the medication is eliminated through the kidneys.

⚠ Monitor a client receiving magnesium sulfate intravenously closely for signs of toxicity. Call the health care provider if respirations are less than 12 breaths/min, which indicate respiratory depression, or if any other adverse reactions occur.

IV. BETAMETHASONE AND DEXAMETHASONE

A. Description: Corticosteroids that increase the production of **surfactant** to accelerate fetal lung maturity and reduce the incidence or severity of respiratory distress syndrome
B. Use: For a client in preterm **labor** between 28 and 32 weeks' gestation whose **labor** can be inhibited for 48 hours without jeopardizing the mother or fetus
C. Adverse reactions and contraindications
1. May decrease the mother's resistance to infection
2. Pulmonary edema secondary to sodium and fluid retention can occur.

3. Elevated blood glucose levels can occur in a client with diabetes mellitus.
D. Interventions
1. Monitor maternal vital signs, lung sounds, and for edema.
2. Monitor mother for signs of infection.
3. Monitor white blood cell count.
4. Monitor blood glucose levels.

V. OPIOID ANALGESICS

A. Description
1. Used to relieve moderate to severe pain associated with **labor**
2. Administered by intramuscular or intravenous route
3. Regular use of opioids during pregnancy may produce withdrawal symptoms in the **newborn** (irritability, excessive crying, tremors, hyperactive reflexes, fever, vomiting, diarrhea, yawning, sneezing, and seizures).
4. Antidotes for opioids
   a. Naloxone (Narcan) is usually the treatment of choice because it rapidly reverses opioid toxicity; the dose may need to be repeated every few hours until opioid concentrations have decreased to nontoxic levels.

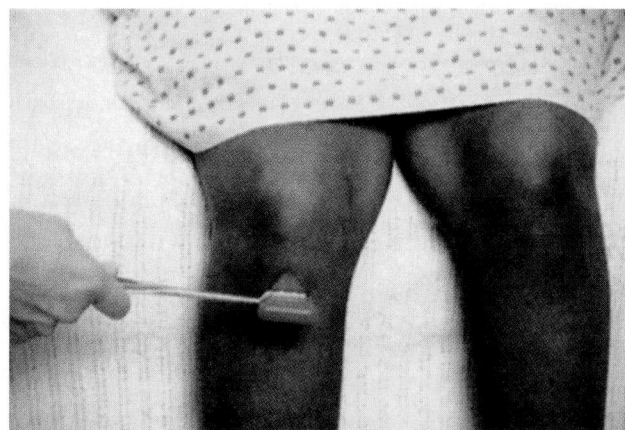

▲ **FIGURE 31-1** Patellar reflex, with client's legs hanging freely over end of examining table. (From Perry, S., Hockenberry, M., Lowdermilk, D., & Wilson, D. [2010]. *Maternal child nursing care* [4th ed.]. St. Louis: Mosby. Courtesy Shannon Perry, Phoenix, AZ.)

TABLE 31-2 Assessing Deep Tendon Reflexes

Grade	Deep Tendon Reflex Response
0	No response
1	Sluggish or diminished
2	Active or expected response
3	More brisk than expected, slightly hyperactive
4	Brisk, hyperactive, with intermittent or transient clonus

From Seidel, H., Ball, J., Dains, J., & Benedict, G. (2006). *Mosby's guide to physical examination* (5th ed.). St. Louis: Mosby.

b. Nalmefene (Revex) is a long-acting opioid antagonist that does not require repeat doses.

c. These medications can cause withdrawal in opioid-dependent clients.

B. Meperidine hydrochloride (Demerol) and hydromorphone hydrochloride (Dilaudid)

1. Can cause dizziness, nausea, vomiting, sedation, decreased blood pressure, decreased respirations, diaphoresis, flushed face, urinary retention

2. May be prescribed to be administered with an antiemetic such as promethazine (Phenergan) to prevent nausea

3. High dosages may result in respiratory depression, skeletal muscle flaccidity, cold clammy skin, cyanosis, and extreme somnolence progressing to seizures, stupor, and coma.

4. Used cautiously in clients delivering preterm infants

5. Not administered in early **labor** because it may slow the **labor** process

6. Not administered in advanced **labor** (within 1 hour of expected **delivery**); if the medication is not adequately removed from the fetal circulation, respiratory depression can occur.

C. Fentanyl (Sublimaze) and sufentanil (Sufenta): Can cause respiratory depression, dizziness, drowsiness, hypotension, urinary retention, fetal narcosis and distress

D. Butorphanol tartrate (Stadol) and nalbuphine (Nubain)

1. Can cause confusion, sedation, sweating, nausea, vomiting, hypotension, sinusoidal-like fetal heart rhythm

2. Use with caution in a client with preexisting opioid dependency because these medications can precipitate withdrawal symptoms in the client and the **newborn.**

E. Interventions

1. Monitor vital signs, particularly respiratory status; if respirations are 12 breaths/min or less, withhold the medication and contact the health care provider.

2. Monitor the fetal heart rate and characteristics of uterine contractions.

3. Monitor for blood pressure changes (hypotension); maintain the client in a recumbent position (elevate the hip with a wedge pillow or other device).

4. Record the client's response and level of pain relief.

5. Monitor the bladder for distention and retention.

6. Have the antidote naloxone (Narcan) available, especially if **delivery** is expected to occur during peak drug absorption time.

⚠ Obtain a drug history before the administration of an opioid analgesic. Some medications may be contraindicated if the client has a history of opioid dependency because these medications can precipitate withdrawal symptoms in the client and newborn.

VI. PROSTAGLANDINS (Box 31-2)

A. Description

1. Ripen the cervix, making it softer and causing it to begin to dilate and efface

2. Stimulate uterine contractions

3. Administered vaginally

B. Uses

1. Preinduction cervical ripening (ripening of the cervix before the induction of **labor** when the Bishop score is ≤4)

2. Induction of **labor**

3. Induction of abortion (abortifacient agent)

C. Adverse reactions and contraindications

1. Gastrointestinal effects, including diarrhea, nausea, vomiting, and stomach cramps

2. Fever, chills, flushing, headache, hypotension

3. Tachysystole (≥12 uterine contractions in 20 minutes without an alteration in the fetal heart rate pattern)

4. Hyperstimulation of the **uterus**

5. Fetal passage of meconium

6. Contraindications (Box 31-3)

D. Interventions

1. Monitor maternal vital signs, fetal heart rate pattern, and status of pregnancy including indications for cervical ripening or the induction of **labor**, signs of **labor** or impending **labor**, and the Bishop score (see Table 26-2 for information about the Bishop score).

2. Monitor for adverse reactions to the medication.

3. Have the client void before administration of medication and then have her maintain a supine with lateral tilt or side-lying position for 30 to 60 minutes (gel) up to 2 hours (insert) after administration, depending on the medication administered.

Box 31-2 Prostaglandins

Prostaglandin E$_2$: Dinoprostone (Cervidil vaginal insert, Prepidil gel)

Box 31-3 Contraindications to the Use of Prostaglandins

Active cardiac, hepatic, pulmonary, or renal disease
Acute pelvic inflammatory disease
Clients in whom vaginal delivery is not indicated
Fetal malpresentation
History of cesarean section or major uterine surgery
History of difficult labor or traumatic labor
Hypersensitivity to prostaglandins
Maternal fever or infection
Nonreassuring fetal heart rate pattern
Placenta previa or unexplained vaginal bleeding
Regular progressive uterine contractions
Significant cephalopelvic disproportion

4. Treatment is discontinued when the Bishop score is 8 or more (cervix ripens) or an effective contraction pattern is established (three or more contractions in a 10-minute period); additionally, signs of adverse reactions indicate that the treatment needs to be discontinued.
5. Follow agency protocol for the induction of **labor** if cervical ripening has occurred and **labor** has not begun; oxytocin (Pitocin) can be initiated if needed 6 to 12 hours after discontinuation of prostaglandin therapy.

VII. UTERINE STIMULANTS (OXYTOCICS): OXYTOCIN (PITOCIN)

A. Description
1. Oxytocin stimulates the smooth muscle of the **uterus** and increases the force, frequency, and duration of uterine contractions.
2. Oxytocin also promotes milk letdown.
3. For induction of **labor**, oxytocin is administered by the intravenous route (other routes of administration include intranasal and intramuscular).
4. Minimal cervical change usually is noted until the active phase of **labor** is achieved.

B. Uses
1. Induces or augments **labor**
2. Controls postpartum bleeding
3. Promotes milk letdown and facilitates breastfeeding (intranasal route)
4. Manages an incomplete abortion

C. Adverse reactions and contraindications
1. Adverse reactions include allergies, dysrhythmias, changes in blood pressure, uterine rupture, and water intoxication; intranasal administration may cause nasal vasoconstriction.
2. Oxytocin may produce uterine hypertonicity, resulting in fetal or maternal adverse effects.
3. High doses may cause hypotension, with rebound hypertension.
4. Postpartum hemorrhage can occur and should be monitored for because the **uterus** may become atonic when the medication wears off.
5. Oxytocin should not be used in a client who cannot deliver vaginally or in a client with hypertonic uterine contractions; it is also contraindicated in a client with active genital herpes.

D. Interventions
1. Monitor maternal vital signs (every 15 minutes), especially the blood pressure and heart rate; weight; intake and output; level of consciousness; and lung sounds.
2. Monitor frequency, duration, and force of contractions and resting uterine tone every 15 minutes.
3. Monitor fetal heart rate every 15 minutes, and notify the health care provider if significant changes occur; use of an internal fetal scalp electrode may be prescribed.

4. Administered by intravenous infusion via an infusion monitoring device; prescribed additive solution is piggybacked at the port nearest the point of venous insertion (prescribed additive solution may be normal saline, lactated Ringer's, or 5% dextrose in water)
5. Carefully monitor the dose being administered; do not leave the client unattended while the oxytocin is infusing.
6. Administer oxygen if prescribed.
7. Monitor for hypertonic contractions or a nonreassuring fetal heart rate and notify the health care provider if these occur (See Priority Nursing Actions).

■■■■■ PRIORITY NURSING ACTIONS! ■■■■■

Steps to Take if Hypertonic Contractions or a Nonreassuring Fetal Heart Rate Occurs During Oxytocin (Pitocin) Infusion

1. Stop the oxytocin (Pitocin) infusion.
2. Turn the client on her side, stay with the client, and ask another nurse to contact the health care provider.
3. Increase the flow rate of the intravenous additive solution.
4. Administer oxygen, 8 to 10 L/min, by snug face mask.
5. Assess maternal vital signs; fetal heart rate and patterns; and frequency, duration, and force of contractions.
6. Document the event, actions taken, and the response.

Oxytocin (Pitocin) is a uterine stimulant and stimulates the smooth muscle of the uterus and increases the force, frequency, and duration of uterine contractions. It is administered to induce or augment labor. The presence of hypertonic contractions or a nonreassuring fetal heart rate indicates the need to institute emergency measures to reduce uterine stimulation and increase fetal oxygenation. The nurse would always follow the agency's protocol regarding the procedure to follow in this event. Keeping the emergency goals of care in mind (to reduce uterine stimulation and increase fetal oxygenation) guides the nurse's actions. The oxytocin infusion needs to be stopped to reduce uterine contractions. The nurse turns the client on her side to increase placental oxygenation. The nurse never leaves a client if an emergency situation is present; the nurse asks another nurse to contact the health care provider. The flow rate of the intravenous additive solution is increased, and oxygen is administered. These actions also facilitate the goals of care. When these emergency actions are taken, the nurse assesses and continuously monitors maternal vital signs; fetal heart rate and patterns; and frequency, duration, and force of contractions. The nurse also implements any additional prescriptions and documents the event, actions taken, and the response.

References: McKinney, E., James, S., Murray, S., & Ashwill, J. (2009). *Maternal-child nursing* (3rd ed., p. 440). St. Louis: Saunders.
Perry, S., Hockenberry, M., Lowdermilk, D., & Wilson, D. (2010). *Maternal child nursing care* (4th ed., pp. 508-509). St. Louis: Mosby.

8. Stop the medication if uterine hyperstimulation or a nonreassuring fetal heart rate occurs; turn the client on her side, increase the intravenous rate of the normal saline, and administer oxygen via face mask.
9. Monitor for signs of water intoxication.
10. Have emergency equipment available.
11. Document the dose of the medication and the time the medication was started, increased, maintained, and discontinued; document the client's response.
12. Keep the client and family informed of the client's progress.

VIII. MEDICATIONS USED TO MANAGE POSTPARTUM HEMORRHAGE (Box 31-4)

A. Ergot alkaloids
1. Description
   a. Ergonovine maleate or ergometrine (Ergotrate Maleate) and methylergonovine maleate (Methergine) are ergot alkaloids.
   b. Directly stimulate uterine muscle, increase the force and frequency of contractions, and produce a firm tetanic contraction of the **uterus**
   c. Can produce arterial vasoconstriction and vasospasm of the coronary arteries
   d. Ergot alkaloids are not administered before the **delivery** of the **placenta.**
2. Uses
   a. Postpartum hemorrhage
   b. Postabortal hemorrhage resulting from atony or involution
3. Adverse reactions and contraindications
   a. Can cause nausea, uterine cramping, bradycardia, dysrhythmias, myocardial infarction, and severe hypertension
   b. High doses are associated with peripheral vasospasm or vasoconstriction, angina, miosis, confusion, respiratory depression, seizures, or unconsciousness; uterine tetany can occur.
   c. Contraindicated during pregnancy and in clients with significant cardiovascular disease, peripheral vascular disease, or hypertension
4. Interventions
   a. Monitor maternal vital signs, weight, intake and output, level of consciousness, and lung sounds.
   b. Monitor the blood pressure closely; the medication produces vasoconstriction, and if an increase in blood pressure is noted, withhold

Box 31-4 Medications Used to Manage Postpartum Bleeding

Ergonovine maleate, ergometrine (Ergotrate Maleate)
Methylergonovine (Methergine)
Oxytocin (Pitocin)
Prostaglandin $F_{2\alpha}$: Carboprost tromethamine (Hemabate)

the medication and notify the health care provider.
   c. Monitor uterine contractions (frequency, strength, and duration).
   d. Assess for chest pain, headache, shortness of breath, itching, pale or cold hands or feet, nausea, diarrhea, or dizziness.
   e. Assess the extremities for color, warmth, movement, and pain.
   f. Assess vaginal bleeding.
   g. Notify the health care provider if chest pain or other adverse reactions occur.
   h. Administer analgesics as prescribed; they may be required because the medication produces painful uterine contractions.

⚠ Check the client's blood pressure before administering an ergot alkaloid. These medications can cause severe hypertension and are contraindicated in a client with hypertension.

B. Prostaglandin $F_{2\alpha}$ (carboprost tromethamine [Hemabate])
1. Description: Contracts the **uterus**
2. Uses: Postpartum hemorrhage
3. Adverse reactions and contraindications
   a. Can cause headache, nausea, vomiting, diarrhea, fever, tachycardia, hypertension
   b. Contraindicated if client has asthma
4. Interventions
   a. Monitor vital signs.
   b. Monitor vaginal bleeding and uterine tone.

C. Oxytocin (Pitocin): see section on uterine stimulants

IX. RUBELLA VACCINE

A. Given subcutaneously before hospital discharge to a nonimmune postpartum client
B. Administered if the rubella titer is less than 1:8
C. Adverse reactions: Transient rash, hypersensitivity
D. Contraindicated in a client with an allergy to duck eggs
E. Interventions
1. Assess for allergy to duck eggs and notify the health care provider before administration if an allergy exists
2. Do not administer if the client or other family members are immunocompromised.

⚠ The client should avoid pregnancy for 1 to 3 months (or as prescribed) after immunization with rubella vaccine. Inform the client about the need for using a contraception method during this time.

X. LUNG SURFACTANTS (Box 31-5)

A. Description
1. Lung **surfactants** replenish **surfactant** and restore surface activity to the lungs to prevent and treat respiratory distress syndrome.

2. Lung **surfactants** are administered by the intra-tracheal route.
B. Use: To prevent or treat respiratory distress syndrome in premature infants
C. Adverse reactions and contraindications
  1. Adverse effects include transient bradycardia and oxygen desaturation; pulmonary hemorrhage, mucus plugging, and endotracheal tube reflux can also occur.
  2. **Surfactants** are administered with caution in infants at risk for circulatory overload.
D. Interventions
  1. Instill **surfactant** through the catheter inserted into the **newborn's** endotracheal tube; avoid suctioning for at least 2 hours after administration.
  2. Monitor for bradycardia and decreased oxygen saturation during administration.
  3. Monitor respiratory status and lung sounds and for signs of adverse reactions.

XI. EYE PROPHYLAXIS FOR THE NEWBORN

A. Description
  1. Preventive eye treatment against ophthalmia neonatorum in the **newborn** is required by law in the United States.
  2. Agent used varies depending on agency protocols, but usually ophthalmic forms of erythromycin (0.5%) or tetracycline (1%) are prescribed because they are bacteriostatic and bactericidal and provide prophylaxis against *Neisseria gonorrhoeae* and *Chlamydia trachomatis*.
  3. Silver nitrate (1%) solution may be prescribed, but its use is minimal because it does not protect against chlamydial infection and can cause chemical conjunctivitis.
B. Use: As a prophylactic measure to protect against *N. gonorrhoeae* and *C. trachomatis*
C. Adverse reaction: Silver nitrate (1%) solution can cause chemical conjunctivitis.
D. Interventions
  1. Clean the **newborn's** eyes before instilling the medication.
  2. Do not flush the eyes after instillation.

⚠ Instillation of eye medication can be delayed for 1 hour after birth to facilitate eye contact and parent-newborn attachment and bonding.

Box 31-5 Lung Surfactant Replacement Therapy

Beractant (Survanta)
Calfactant (Infasurf)
Poractant alfa (Curosurf)

XII. VITAMIN K

A. Description
  1. The **newborn** is at risk for hemorrhagic disorders; coagulation factors synthesized in the liver depend on vitamin K, which is not synthesized until intestinal bacteria are present.
  2. **Newborns** are deficient in vitamin K for the first 5 to 8 days of life because of the lack of intestinal bacteria.
B. Use: Prophylaxis and treatment of hemorrhagic disease of the **newborn**
C. Adverse reaction: Vitamin K can cause hyperbilirubinemia in the **newborn**.
D. Interventions
  1. Protect the medication from light.
  2. Administer during the early **newborn** period.
  3. Administer in the lateral aspect of the middle third of the vastus lateralis muscle of the thigh.
  4. Monitor for bruising at the injection site and for bleeding from the cord.
  5. Monitor for jaundice and monitor the bilirubin level because the medication can cause hyperbilirubinemia in the **newborn**.

XIII. HEPATITIS B VIRUS (HBV) VACCINE

A. Description: Given intramuscularly to the **newborn** before discharge home
B. Use: Recommended for all **newborns** to prevent hepatitis B
C. Adverse reaction: Rash, fever, erythema, and pain at injection site
D. Interventions
  1. Parental consent must be obtained.
  2. Administer intramuscularly in the lateral aspect of the middle third of the vastus lateralis muscle.
  3. If the **infant** was born to a mother positive for hepatitis B surface antigen, hepatitis B immune globulin should be given within 12 hours of birth in addition to HBV vaccine. Then follow the regularly scheduled HBV vaccination schedule.
  4. Document immunization administration on a vaccination card for the parents to have a record that it was administered.

💿 **MORE QUESTIONS ON THE CD!**

Practice Questions

315. A nurse is caring for a client who is receiving oxytocin (Pitocin) to induce labor. The nurse discontinues the oxytocin infusion if which of the following is noted on assessment of the client?
  1. Fatigue
  2. Drowsiness
  3. Uterine hyperstimulation
  4. Early decelerations of the fetal heart rate

316. A pregnant client is receiving magnesium sulfate for the management of preeclampsia. A nurse determines that the client is experiencing toxicity from the medication if which of the following is noted on assessment?
1. Proteinuria of 3+
2. Respirations of 10 breaths/min
3. Presence of deep tendon reflexes
4. Serum magnesium level of 6 mEq/L

317. Methylergonovine (Methergine) is prescribed for a client with postpartum hemorrhage. Before administering the medication, a nurse contacts the health care provider who prescribed the medication if which condition is documented in the client's medical history?
1. Hypotension
2. Hypothyroidism
3. Diabetes mellitus
4. Peripheral vascular disease

318. A nursing instructor asks a nursing student to describe the procedure for administering erythromycin ointment to the eyes of a newborn. The instructor determines that the student needs to research this procedure further if the student states that:
1. "I will flush the eyes after instilling the ointment."
2. "I will clean the newborn's eyes before instilling ointment."
3. "I need to administer the eye ointment within 1 hour after delivery."
4. "I will instill the eye ointment into each of the newborn's conjunctival sacs."

319. A client in preterm labor (31 weeks) who is dilated to 4 cm has been started on magnesium sulfate and contractions have stopped. If the client's labor can be inhibited for the next 48 hours, what medication does the nurse anticipate will be prescribed?
1. Betamethasone
2. Nalbuphine (Nubain)
3. Rh$_o$(D) immune globulin (RhoGAM)
4. Dinoprostone (Cervidil vaginal insert)

320. Methylergonovine (Methergine) is prescribed for a woman to treat postpartum hemorrhage. Before administration of methylergonovine, the priority nursing assessment is to check the:

1. Uterine tone
2. Blood pressure
3. Amount of lochia
4. Deep tendon reflexes

321. A nurse is preparing to administer beractant (Survanta) to a premature infant who has respiratory distress syndrome. The nurse plans to administer the medication by which of the following routes?
1. Intradermal
2. Intratracheal
3. Subcutaneous
4. Intramuscular

322. An opioid analgesic is administered to a client in labor. The nurse assigned to care for the client ensures that which medication is readily available if respiratory depression occurs?
1. Betamethasone
2. Morphine sulfate
3. Naloxone (Narcan)
4. Meperidine hydrochloride (Demerol)

323. Rh$_o$(D) immune globulin (RhoGAM) is prescribed for a client after delivery and the nurse provides information to the client about the purpose of the medication. The nurse determines that the woman understands the purpose of the medication if the woman states that it will protect her next baby from which of the following?
1. Having Rh-positive blood
2. Developing a rubella infection
3. Developing physiological jaundice
4. Being affected by Rh incompatibility

Alternate Item Format: Multiple Response

324. A nurse is monitoring a client in preterm labor who is receiving intravenous magnesium sulfate. The nurse monitors for which adverse reactions of this medication? **Select all that apply.**
❑ 1. Flushing
❑ 2. Hypertension
❑ 3. Increased urine output
❑ 4. Depressed respirations
❑ 5. Extreme muscle weakness
❑ 6. Hyperactive deep tendon reflexes

ANSWERS
315. 3
Rationale: Oxytocin stimulates uterine contractions and is a common pharmacological method to induce labor. Adverse reactions associated with administration of the medication are hyperstimulation of uterine contractions and nonreassuring fetal heart rate patterns. Oxytocin infusion must be stopped when any signs of uterine hyperstimulation are present. Drowsiness and fatigue may be caused by the labor experience. Early decelerations of the fetal heart rate are a reassuring sign and do not indicate fetal distress.

Test-Taking Strategy: Use the process of elimination, focusing on the subject, an adverse reaction to oxytocin. Options 1 and 2 are comparable or alike and can be eliminated first. From the remaining options, recalling that early decelerations of the fetal heart rate are a reassuring sign will direct you to option 3. Review the nursing responsibilities associated with the administration of oxytocin if you had difficulty with this question.
Level of Cognitive Ability: Applying
Client Needs: Physiological Integrity
Integrated Process: Nursing Process—Implementation
Content Area: Maternity—Intrapartum
References: Hodgson, B., & Kizior, R. (2009). *Saunders nursing drug handbook 2009* (pp. 883–884). St. Louis: Saunders.
McKinney, E., James, S., Murray, S., & Ashwill, J. (2009). *Maternal-child nursing* (3rd ed., p. 331). St. Louis: Saunders.

316. 2
Rationale: Magnesium toxicity can occur from magnesium sulfate therapy. Signs of magnesium sulfate toxicity relate to the central nervous system depressant effects of the medication and include respiratory depression, loss of deep tendon reflexes, and a sudden decline in fetal heart rate and maternal heart rate and blood pressure. Therapeutic serum levels of magnesium are 4 to 7.5 mEq/L. Proteinuria of 3+ is an expected finding in a client with preeclampsia.
Test-Taking Strategy: Use the process of elimination and eliminate option 3 first because it is a normal finding. Next, eliminate option 4, knowing that the therapeutic serum level of magnesium is 4 to 7.5 mEq/L. From the remaining options, recalling that proteinuria of 3+ would be noted in a client with preeclampsia will direct you to the correct option. Review the adverse effects of magnesium sulfate if you had difficulty with this question.
Level of Cognitive Ability: Analyzing
Client Needs: Physiological Integrity
Integrated Process: Nursing Process—Assessment
Content Area: Maternity—Intrapartum
References: Hodgson, B., & Kizior, R. (2009). *Saunders nursing drug handbook 2009* (p. 711). St. Louis: Saunders.
McKinney, E., James, S., Murray, S., & Ashwill, J. (2009). *Maternal-child nursing* (3rd ed., p. 625). St. Louis: Saunders.

317. 4
Rationale: Methylergonovine is an ergot alkaloid used to treat postpartum hemorrhage. Ergot alkaloids are contraindicated in clients with significant cardiovascular disease, peripheral vascular disease, hypertension, preeclampsia, or eclampsia. These conditions are worsened by the vasoconstrictive effects of the ergot alkaloids. Options 1, 2, and 3 are not contraindications related to the use of ergot alkaloids.
Test-Taking Strategy: Focus on the purpose and action of methylergonovine. Recalling that ergot alkaloids produce vasoconstriction will direct you to option 4. Review the effects of this medication and the associated contraindications if you had difficulty with this question.
Level of Cognitive Ability: Analyzing
Client Needs: Physiological Integrity
Integrated Process: Nursing Process—Implementation
Content Area: Maternity—Postpartum
References: Hodgson, B., & Kizior, R. (2009). *Saunders nursing drug handbook 2009* (p. 744). St. Louis: Saunders.

McKinney, E., James, S., Murray, S., & Ashwill, J. (2009). *Maternal-child nursing* (3rd ed., pp. 697–698). St. Louis: Saunders.

318. 1
Rationale: Eye prophylaxis protects the newborn against *Neisseria gonorrhoeae* and *Chlamydia trachomatis*. The eyes are not flushed after instillation of the medication because the flush would wash away the administered medication. Options 2, 3, and 4 are correct statements regarding the procedure for administering eye medication to the newborn.
Test-Taking Strategy: Note the strategic words *needs to research*. These words indicate a negative event query and ask you to select an option that is an incorrect statement. Eliminate options 3 and 4 first because they are comparable or alike and relate to instilling the eye medication. From the remaining options, visualize the effect of each. This will direct you to option 1. Review the procedure for administering eye medication to the newborn if you had difficulty with this question.
Level of Cognitive Ability: Evaluating
Client Needs: Health Promotion and Maintenance
Integrated Process: Teaching and Learning
Content Area: Maternity—Postpartum
Reference: McKinney, E., James, S., Murray, S., & Ashwill, J. (2009). *Maternal-child nursing* (3rd ed., p. 539). St. Louis: Saunders.

319. 1
Rationale: Betamethasone, a glucocorticoid, is given to increase the production of surfactant to stimulate fetal lung maturation. It is administered to clients in preterm labor at 28 to 32 weeks of gestation if the labor can be inhibited for 48 hours. Nalbuphine (Nubain) is an opioid analgesic. Rh$_o$(D) immune globulin (RhoGAM) is given to Rh-negative clients to prevent sensitization. Dinoprostone (Cervidil vaginal insert) is a prostaglandin given to ripen and soften the cervix and to stimulate uterine contractions.
Test-Taking Strategy: Note the strategic words *client in preterm labor (31 weeks)* and recall that the preterm infant is at risk for respiratory distress syndrome because of immaturity and the inability to produce surfactant. Next, recalling the actions of the medications in the options and that betamethasone is used to increase the production of surfactant will direct you to option 1. Review the purpose and actions of the medications listed in the options if you had difficulty with this question.
Level of Cognitive Ability: Analyzing
Client Needs: Physiological Integrity
Integrated Process: Nursing Process—Analysis
Content Area: Maternity—Intrapartum
Reference: McKinney, E., James, S., Murray, S., & Ashwill, J. (2009). *Maternal-child nursing* (3rd ed., p. 683). St. Louis: Saunders.

320. 2
Rationale: Methylergonovine, an ergot alkaloid, is used to prevent or control postpartum hemorrhage by contracting the uterus. Methylergonovine causes continuous uterine contractions and may elevate the blood pressure. A priority assessment before the administration of the medication is to

check the blood pressure. The physician should be notified if hypertension is present. Although options 1, 3, and 4 may be components of the postpartum assessment, option 2, blood pressure, is related specifically to the administration of this medication.

Test-Taking Strategy: Eliminate options 1 and 3 first because they are comparable or alike and related to one another. To choose from the remaining options, use the ABCs—airway, breathing, and circulation. Blood pressure is a method of assessing circulation. Review the adverse effects of methylergonovine if you had difficulty with this question.

Level of Cognitive Ability: Applying
Client Needs: Physiological Integrity
Integrated Process: Nursing Process—Assessment
Content Area: Maternity—Postpartum
References: Hodgson, B., & Kizior, R. (2009). *Saunders nursing drug handbook 2009* (p. 744). St. Louis: Saunders.

McKinney, E., James, S., Murray, S., & Ashwill, J. (2009). *Maternal-child nursing* (3rd ed., pp. 697–698). St. Louis: Saunders.

321. 2

Rationale: Respiratory distress syndrome is a serious lung disorder caused by immaturity and the inability to produce surfactant, resulting in hypoxia and acidosis. It is common in premature infants and may be due to lung immaturity as a result of surfactant deficiency. The mainstay of treatment is the administration of exogenous surfactant, which is administered by the intratracheal route. Options 1, 3, and 4 are not routes of administration for this medication.

Test-Taking Strategy: Use the process of elimination. Note the relationship between the diagnosis *respiratory distress syndrome* and the correct option, *intratracheal*. Review the route of administration of beractant (Survanta) if you had difficulty with this question.

Level of Cognitive Ability: Understanding
Client Needs: Physiological Integrity
Integrated Process: Nursing Process—Planning
Content Area: Maternity—Postpartum
References: Hockenberry, M., & Wilson, D. (2009). *Wong's essentials of pediatric nursing* (8th ed., p. 287). St. Louis: Mosby.

Hodgson, B., & Kizior, R. (2009). *Saunders nursing drug handbook 2009* (pp. 126–127). St. Louis: Saunders.

322. 3

Rationale: Opioid analgesics may be prescribed to relieve moderate to severe pain associated with labor. Opioid toxicity can occur and cause respiratory depression. Naloxone (Narcan) is a opioid antagonist, which reverses the effects of opioids and is given for respiratory depression. Morphine sulfate and meperidine hydrochloride are opioid analgesics. Betamethasone is a corticosteroid administered to enhance fetal lung maturity.

Test-Taking Strategy: Use the process of elimination, focusing on the subject of the question, the antidote for respiratory depression. Eliminate options 2 and 4 first because they are comparable or alike and are opioid analgesics. Next, eliminate option 1, knowing that this medication is a corticosteroid. Review the purpose and actions of the medications identified in the options and the antidote for opioid toxicity if you had difficulty with this question.

Level of Cognitive Ability: Applying
Client Needs: Physiological Integrity
Integrated Process: Nursing Process—Planning
Content Area: Maternity—Postpartum
Reference: McKinney, E., James, S., Murray, S., & Ashwill, J. (2009). *Maternal-child nursing* (3rd ed., p. 421). St. Louis: Saunders.

323. 4

Rationale: Rh incompatibility can occur when an Rh-negative mother becomes sensitized to the Rh antigen. Sensitization may develop when an Rh-negative woman becomes pregnant with a fetus who is Rh positive. During pregnancy and at delivery, some of the fetus' Rh-positive blood can enter the maternal circulation, causing the mother's immune system to form antibodies against Rh-positive blood. Administration of $Rh_o(D)$ immune globulin (RhoGAM) prevents the mother from developing antibodies against Rh-positive blood by providing passive antibody protection against the Rh antigen.

Test-Taking Strategy: Use the process of elimination and note the subject of the question, the purpose of $Rh_o(D)$ immune globulin. Noting the relationship between the name of the medication, $Rh_o(D)$ immune globulin, and the word *incompatibility* in option 4 will direct you to this option. Review the purpose of $Rh_o(D)$ immune globulin if you had difficulty with this question.

Level of Cognitive Ability: Evaluating
Client Needs: Physiological Integrity
Integrated Process: Nursing Process—Evaluation
Content Area: Maternity—Postpartum
Reference: Edmunds, M. (2010). *Introduction to clinical pharmacology* (6th ed., p. 371). St. Louis: Mosby.

ALTERNATE ITEM FORMAT: MULTIPLE RESPONSE
324. 1, 4, 5

Rationale: Magnesium sulfate is a central nervous system depressant and relaxes smooth muscle, including the uterus. It is used to halt preterm labor contractions and is used for preeclamptic clients to prevent seizures. Adverse effects include flushing, depressed respirations, depressed deep tendon reflexes, hypotension, extreme muscle weakness, decreased urine output, pulmonary edema, and elevated serum magnesium levels.

Test-Taking Strategy: Focus on the subject, adverse effects of magnesium sulfate. Recalling that this medication is a central nervous system depressant and relaxes smooth muscle will assist you in choosing the correct answer. Review the adverse effects of this medication if you had difficulty with this question.

Level of Cognitive Ability: Analyzing
Client Needs: Physiological Integrity
Integrated Process: Nursing Process—Assessment
Content Area: Maternity—Intrapartum
References: Gahart, B., & Nazareno, A. (2009). *Intravenous medications* (25th ed., p. 831). St. Louis: Mosby.

McKinney, E., James, S., Murray, S., & Ashwill, J. (2009). *Maternal-child nursing* (3rd ed., p. 625). St. Louis: Saunders.

UNIT VI

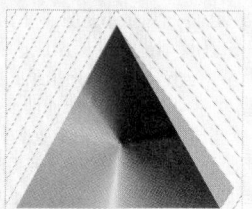

Growth and Development Across the Life Span

PYRAMID TERMS

abuse The willful infliction of pain, injury, mental anguish, or unreasonable confinement. Abuse can include verbal assaults, the demand to perform demeaning tasks, theft, or mismanagement of personal belongings (exploitation). Abuse inflicted can be physical, emotional, or sexual.

auscultation The physical assessment technique that involves listening to sounds within the body. Special equipment such as a stethoscope may be needed to perform this technique.

dementia An organic syndrome identified by gradual and progressive deterioration in intellectual functioning. Long- and short-term memory losses occur with impairment in judgment, abstract thinking, problem-solving ability, and behavior, resulting in a self-care deficit. A common type of dementia is Alzheimer's disease.

depression A mood disorder that can be identified by feelings of sadness, hopelessness, and worthlessness, and a decreased interest in activities.

ego One's "sense of self"; provides functions such as problem solving, mobilization of defense mechanisms, reality testing, and the capability of functioning independently; the mediator between the id and the superego.

id Source of all primitive drives and instincts; considered to be the reservoir of all psychic energy.

inspection The first physical assessment technique that begins the moment that the examiner meets the client. It involves a visual assessment of the client during the health history and making observations during the physical examination of specific body systems.

neglect The lack of providing services necessary for physical or mental health; includes failure to prevent injury.

objective data Information about the client that is obtained by the examiner through the physical examination and reviewing the results of laboratory, radiological, or other diagnostic studies.

palpation A physical assessment technique that involves using the hands to feel certain parts of the client's body, including some organs. The examiner uses this technique to assess texture, size, and consistency of the body part being examined.

percussion A physical assessment technique that involves tapping the body to assess the size, borders, and consistency of some organs and to assess for the presence of fluid within body cavities. Direct percussion is performed by striking the fingers directly on the body surface. Indirect percussion is performed by striking a finger of one hand on a finger of the other hand as it is placed on the body surface, such as over an organ.

polypharmacy Taking multiple prescription and/or over-the-counter medications together.

play An activity that is spontaneous or organized and provides entertainment or diversion. It is a part of childhood that is necessary for the development of a normal personality and social, physical and intellectual skills.

safety Instituting measures that ensure protection and the prevention of an accident or injury.

self-neglect The choice to avoid medical care or other services that could improve optimal function. Unless declared legally incompetent, an individual has the right to refuse care.

subjective data Information obtained from the client during history-taking. It is what the client says about himself or herself.

superego The moral component of personality, including internalization of the values, ideals, and moral standards of society.

THE PYRAMID TO SUCCESS

Normal growth and development proceed in an orderly, systematic, and predictable pattern, which provides a basis for identifying and assessing an individual's abilities. Understanding the normal path of growth and development across the life span assists the nurse in identifying appropriate and expected human behavior. The Pyramid to Success focuses on Sigmund Freud's theory of psychosexual development, Jean Piaget's theory of cognitive development, Erik Erikson's psychosocial theory, and Lawrence Kohlberg's theory of moral development. Growth and development concepts also focus on the health and physical assessment of the adult client; on the aging process; and on physical characteristics, nutritional behaviors, skills, play, and specific safety measures relevant to a particular age group that will ensure a safe and hazard-free environment. When a question is presented on the NCLEX-RN examination, if an age is identified in the question, note the age and think about the associated growth and developmental concepts to answer the question correctly.

CLIENT NEEDS

Safe and Effective Care Environment

Acting as a client advocate
Consulting with members of the health care team
Ensuring home safety and security plans
Establishing priorities
Maintaining confidentiality
Preventing accidents
Providing care following ethical and legal standards
Respecting client and family needs based on their preferences
Upholding client's rights

Health Promotion and Maintenance

Discussing high-risk behaviors and lifestyle choices

Identifying changes that occur as a result of the aging process
Identifying developmental stages and transitions
Maintaining health and wellness and self-care measures
Monitoring growth and development
Performing the techniques associated with the health and physical assessment of the client
Providing client and family education
Respecting health care beliefs and preferences

Psychosocial Integrity

Assessing for abuse and neglect
Considering grief and loss issues and end-of life care
Identifying coping mechanisms
Identifying loss of quantity and quality of relationships with the older client
Identifying cultural practices and beliefs of the client and appropriate support systems
Monitoring for adjustment to potential deterioration in physical and mental health and well-being in the older client
Monitoring for changes and adjustment in role function in the older client (threat to independent functioning)
Monitoring for sensory and perceptual alterations
Providing resources for the client and family

Physiological Integrity

Administering medication safely and teaching the client about prescribed medications
Identifying practices or restrictions related to procedures and treatments
Monitoring for alterations in body systems and the related risks associated with the client's age
Providing basic care and comfort needs
Providing care using a nonjudgmental approach
Providing interventions compatible with the client's age, cultural, religious, and health care beliefs, education level, and language.

Theories of Growth and Development

I. PSYCHOSOCIAL DEVELOPMENT AND ERIK ERIKSON

A. The theory
1. Erikson's theory of psychosocial development describes the human life cycle as a series of eight **ego** developmental stages from birth to death.
2. Each stage presents a psychosocial crisis, the goal of which is to integrate physical, maturation, and societal demands.
3. The result of one stage may not be permanent, but can be changed by experience(s) later in life.
4. The theory focuses on psychosocial tasks that are accomplished throughout the life cycle.

B. Psychosocial development: Occurs through a lifelong series of crises affected by social and cultural factors

⚠ According to Erikson's theory of psychosocial development, each psychosocial crisis must be resolved for the child or adult to progress emotionally. Unsuccessful resolution leaves the person emotionally disabled.

C. Stages of psychosocial development (Table 32-1)

II. COGNITIVE DEVELOPMENT AND JEAN PIAGET

A. The theory
1. Piaget's theory of cognitive development defines cognitive acts as ways in which the mind organizes and adapts to its environment (i.e., "mental mapping").
2. Schema refers to an individual's cognitive structure or framework of thought.
3. Schemata
   a. Schemata are categories that an individual forms in his or her mind to organize and understand the world.
   b. A young child has only a few schemata with which to understand the world, and gradually these are increased.
   c. Adults use a wide variety of schemata to understand the world.
4. Assimilation
   a. Assimilation is the ability to incorporate new ideas, objects, and experiences into the framework of one's thoughts.
   b. The growing child will perceive and give meaning to new information according to what is already known and understood.
5. Accommodation
   a. Accommodation is the ability to change a schema to introduce new ideas, objects, or experiences.
   b. Accommodation changes the mental structure so that new experiences can be added.

B. Stages of cognitive development
1. Sensorimotor stage
   a. Birth to 2 years
   b. Development proceeds from reflex activity to imagining and solving problems through the senses and movement.
   c. The infant or toddler learns about reality and how it works.
   d. The infant or toddler does not recognize that objects continue to be in existence, even if out of the visual field.
2. Preoperational stage
   a. 2 to 7 years
   b. The child learns to think in terms of past, present, and future.
   c. The child moves from knowing the world through sensation and movement to prelogical thinking and finding solutions to problems.
   d. The child is egocentric.
   e. The child is unable to conceptualize and requires concrete examples.
3. Concrete operational
   a. 7 to 11 years
   b. The child is able to classify, order, and sort facts.
   c. The child moves from prelogical thought to solving concrete problems through logic.
   d. The child begins to develop abstract thinking.
4. Formal operations
   a. 11 years to adulthood
   b. The person is able to think abstractly and logically.

TABLE 32-1 Erik Erikson's Stages of Psychosocial Development

Age	Psychosocial Crisis	Task	Resolution of Crisis	
			Successful	**Unsuccessful**
Infancy (birth to 18 months)	Trust versus mistrust	Attachment to the mother	Trust in persons; faith and hope about the environment and future	General difficulties relating to persons effectively; suspicion; trust-fear conflict, fear of the future
Early childhood (18 months to 3 years)	Autonomy versus shame and doubt	Gaining some basic control over self and environment	Sense of self-control and adequacy; will power	Independence-fear conflict; severe feelings of self-doubt
Late childhood (3-6 years)	Initiative versus guilt	Becoming purposeful and directive	Ability to initiate one's own activities; sense of purpose	Aggression-fear conflict; sense of inadequacy or guilt
School age (6-12 years)	Industry versus inferiority	Developing social, physical, and learning skills	Competence; ability to learn and work	Sense of inferiority; difficulty learning and working
Adolescence (12-20 years)	Identity versus role confusion	Developing sense of id-entity	Sense of personal identity	Confusion about who one is; identity submerged in relationships or group memberships
Early adulthood (20-35 years)	Intimacy versus isolation	Establishing intimate bonds of love and friendship	Ability to love deeply and commit oneself	Emotional isolation, egocentricity
Middle adulthood (35-65 years)	Generativity versus stagnation	Fulfilling life goals that involve family, career, and society	Ability to give and care for others	Self-absorption; inability to grow as a person
Later adulthood (65 years to death)	Integrity versus despair	Looking back over one's life and accepting its meaning	Sense of integrity and fulfillment	Dissatisfaction with life

Modified from Varcarolis, E. (2010). *Foundations of psychiatric mental health nursing* (6th ed.). St. Louis: Saunders.

   c. Logical thinking is expanded to include solving abstract and concrete problems.

III. MORAL DEVELOPMENT AND LAWRENCE KOHLBERG

A. Moral development
  1. Moral development is a complicated process involving the acceptance of the values and rules of society in a way that shapes behavior.
  2. Moral development is classified in a series of levels and behaviors.
  3. Moral development is sequential but people do not automatically go from one stage or level to the next as they mature.
  4. Stages or levels of moral development cannot be skipped.
B. Levels of moral development (Box 32-1)

IV. PSYCHOSEXUAL DEVELOPMENT AND SIGMUND FREUD

A. Components of the theory (Box 32-2)
B. Levels of awareness

  1. Conscious level of awareness
   a. The conscious mind is logical and is regulated by the Reality Principle.
   b. Consciousness includes all experiences that are within an individual's awareness and that the individual is able to control and includes all information that is remembered easily and is immediately available to an individual.
  2. Preconscious level of awareness
   a. The preconscious is called the *subconscious*.
   b. The preconscious includes experiences, thoughts, feelings, or desires that might not be in immediate awareness but can be recalled to consciousness.
   c. The subconscious can help repress unpleasant thoughts or feelings and can examine and censor certain wishes and thinking.
  3. Unconscious level of awareness
   a. The unconscious is not logical and is governed by the Pleasure Principle, which refers to seeking immediate tension reduction.
   b. Memories, feelings, thoughts, or wishes are repressed and are not available to the conscious mind.

Box 32-1 Moral Development and Lawrence Kohlberg

Level One: Preconventional Morality
Stage 0 (Birth to 2 years): Egocentric Judgment
The infant has no awareness of right or wrong.

Stage 1 (2 to 3 years): Punishment-Obedience Orientation
At this stage, children cannot reason as mature members of society.
Children view the world in a selfish way, with no real understanding of right or wrong.
The child obeys rules and demonstrates acceptable behavior to avoid punishment and to avoid displeasing those who are in power, and because the child fears punishment from a superior force, such as a parent.
A toddler typically is at the first substage of the preconventional stage, involving punishment and obedience orientation, in which the toddler makes judgments based on avoiding punishment or obtaining a reward.
Physical punishment and withholding privileges tend to give the toddler a negative view of morals.
Withdrawing love and affection as punishment leads to feelings of guilt in the toddler.
Appropriate discipline includes providing simple explanations why certain behaviors are unacceptable, praising appropriate behavior, and using distractions when the toddler is headed for an unsafe action.

Stage 2 (4 to 7 years): Instrumental Relativist Orientation
The child conforms to rules to obtain rewards or have favors returned.
The child's moral standards are those of others, and the child observes them either to avoid punishment or obtain rewards.
A preschooler is in the preconventional stage of moral development.
In this stage, conscience emerges and the emphasis is on external control.

Level Two: Conventional Morality
The child conforms to rules to please others.
The child has increased awareness of others' feelings.
A concern for social order begins to emerge.
A child views good behavior as that which those in authority will approve.
If the behavior is not acceptable, the child feels guilty.

Stage 3 (7 to 10 years): Good Boy—Nice Girl Orientation
Conformity occurs to avoid disapproval or dislike by others.

This stage involves living up to what is expected by individuals close to the child or what individuals generally expect of others in their roles such as daughter, son, brother, sister, and friend.
Being good is important and is interpreted as having good motives and showing concern about others.
Being good also means maintaining mutual relationships, such as trust, loyalty, respect, and gratitude.

Stage 4 (10 to 12 years): Law and Order Orientation
The child has more concern with society as a whole.
Emphasis is on obeying laws to maintain social order.
Moral reasoning develops as the child shifts the focus of living to society.
The school-age child is at the conventional level of the conformity stage and has an increased desire to please others.
The child observes and to some extent internalizes the standards of others.
The child wants to be considered "good" by those individuals whose opinions matter to her or him.

Level Three: Postconventional Morality
The individual focuses on individual rights and principles of conscience.
The focus is on concerns regarding what is best for all.

Stage 5: Social Contract and Legalistic Orientation
The person is aware that others hold a variety of values and opinions and that most values and rules are relative to the group.
The adolescent in this stage gives and takes and does not expect to get something without paying for it.

Stage 6: Universal Ethical Principles Orientation
Conformity is based on universal principles of justice and occurs to avoid self-condemnation.
This stage involves following self-chosen ethical principles.
The development of the postconventional level of morality occurs in the adolescent at about age 13 years, marked by the development of an individual conscience and a defined set of moral values.
The adolescent can now acknowledge a conflict between two socially accepted standards and try to decide between them.
Control of conduct is now internal in standards observed and in reasoning about right and wrong.

c. These repressed memories, thoughts, or feelings, if made prematurely conscious, can cause anxiety.

C. Agencies of the mind: **Id**, **ego**, and **superego**

Box 32-2 Psychosexual Development and Sigmund Freud: Components of the Theory

Levels of awareness
Agencies of the mind (id, ego, superego)
Concept of anxiety and defense mechanisms
Psychosexual stages of development

⚠ The id, ego, and superego are the three systems of personality. These psychological processes follow different operating principles. In a mature and well-adjusted personality, they work together as a team under the leadership of the ego.

1. The **id**
   a. Source of all drives
   b. Present at birth
   c. Includes genetic inheritance, reflexes, capacities to respond, instincts, basic drives, needs, and wishes that motivate an individual
   d. Operates according to the Pleasure Principle
   e. Does not tolerate uncomfortable states and seeks to discharge the tension and return to a more comfortable, constant level of energy
   f. Acts immediately in an impulsive, irrational way and pays no attention to the consequences of its actions; therefore often behaves in ways harmful to self and others
   g. The primary process is a psychological activity in which the **id** attempts to reduce tension.
   h. The primary process can include hallucinating or forming an image of the object that will satisfy its needs and remove the tension.
   i. The primary process by itself is not capable of reducing tension; therefore a secondary psychological process must develop if the individual is to survive. When this occurs, the structure of the second system of the personality, the **ego**, begins to take form.

2. The **ego**
   a. Functions include reality testing and problem solving
   b. Begins its development during the fourth or fifth month of life
   c. Emerges out of the **id** and acts as an intermediary between the **id** and the external world
   d. Emerges because the needs, wishes, and demands of the **id** require appropriate exchanges with the outside world of reality
   e. The **ego** distinguishes between things in the mind and things in the external world.
   f. Reality testing is a function of the **ego**, and the **ego** uses realistic thinking.
   g. The **ego** follows the Reality Principle and operates by means of the secondary process—that is, realistic thinking.
   h. The aim of the Reality Principle is to satisfy the **id's** impulses in the external world with an object that is suitable; the Reality Principle determines whether an experience is true or false and whether it has external existence.
   i. The **ego** devises a plan and tests the plan by some type of action to see whether it will work.

3. The **superego**
   a. Necessary part of socialization that develops during the phallic stage at 3 to 6 years of age
   b. Develops from interactions with the child's parents during the extended period of childhood dependency
   c. Includes internalization of the values, ideals, and moral standards of society

   d. Child internalizes moral standards of the parents and society
   e. **Superego** consists of the conscience and the **ego** ideal
   f. Conscience refers to capacity for self-evaluation and criticism; when moral codes are violated, the conscience punishes the individual by instilling guilt.
   g. What parents approve of and what they reward the child for doing become incorporated as the **ego** ideal by the mechanism of introjection.
   h. The **superego** strives for perfection rather than pleasure and represents the ideal rather than the real.
   i. Living up to one's **ego** ideal results in the individual feeling proud and increases self-esteem.

D. Anxiety and defense mechanisms
   1. The **ego** develops defenses or defense mechanisms to fight off anxiety.
   2. Defense mechanisms operate on an unconscious level, except for suppression, so the individual is not aware of their operation.
   3. Defense mechanisms deny, falsify, or distort reality to make it less threatening.
   4. An individual cannot survive without defense mechanisms; however, if the individual becomes too extreme in distorting reality, then interference with healthy adjustment and personal growth may occur.

E. Psychosexual stages of development (Box 32-3 on next page)
   1. Human development proceeds through a series of stages from infancy to adulthood.
   2. Each stage is characterized by the inborn tendency of all individuals to reduce tension and seek pleasure.
   3. Each stage is associated with a particular conflict that must be resolved before the child can move successfully to the next stage.
   4. Experiences during the early stages determine an individual's adjustment patterns and the personality traits that the individual has as an adult.

⦿ MORE QUESTIONS ON THE CD!

Practice Questions

325. A clinic nurse is preparing to discuss the concepts of moral development with a mother. The nurse understands that according to Kohlberg's theory of moral development, in the preconventional level, moral development is thought to be motivated by which of the following?
   1. Peer pressure
   2. Social pressures

Box 32-3 Freud's Psychosexual Stages of Development

Oral Stage (Birth to 1 Year)

During this stage, the infant is concerned with self-gratification.

The infant is all id, operating on the Pleasure Principle and striving for immediate gratification of needs.

When the infant experiences gratification of basic needs, a sense of trust and security begins.

The ego begins to emerge as the infant begins to see self as separate from the mother; this marks the beginning of the development of a sense of self.

Anal Stage (1 to 3 Years)

Toilet training occurs during this period, and the child gains pleasure from the elimination of the feces and from their retention.

The conflict of this stage is between those demands from society and the parents and the sensations of pleasure associated with the anus.

The child begins to gain a sense of control over instinctive drives and learns to delay immediate gratification to gain a future goal.

Phallic Stage (3 to 6 Years)

The child experiences pleasurable and conflicting feelings associated with the genital organs.

The pleasures of masturbation and the fantasy life of children set the stage for the Oedipus complex.

The child's unconscious sexual attraction to and wish to possess the parent of the opposite gender, the hostility and desire to remove the parent of the same gender, and the subsequent guilt about these wishes is the conflict the child faces.

The conflict is resolved when the child identifies with the parent of the same gender.

The emergence of the superego is the solution to and the result of these intense impulses.

Latency Stage (6 to 12 Years)

The latency stage is a tapering off of conscious biological and sexual urges.

The sexual impulses are channeled and elevated into a more culturally accepted level of activity.

Growth of ego functions and the ability to care about and relate to others outside the home is the task of this stage of development.

Genital Stage (12 Years and Beyond)

The genital stage emerges at adolescence with the onset of puberty, when the genital organs mature.

The individual gains gratification from his or her own body.

During this stage, the individual develops satisfying sexual and emotional relationships with members of the opposite gender.

The individual plans life goals and gains a strong sense of personal identity.

---

3. Parents' behavior
4. Punishment and reward

326. A maternity nurse is providing instructions to a new mother regarding the psychosocial development of the newborn infant. Using Erikson's psychosocial development theory, the nurse instructs the mother to:
1. Allow the newborn infant to signal a need.
2. Anticipate all the needs of the newborn infant.
3. Attend to the newborn infant immediately when crying.
4. Avoid the newborn infant during the first 10 minutes of crying.

327. A mother of a 3-year-old tells a clinic nurse that the child is rebelling constantly and having temper tantrums. Using Erikson's psychosocial development theory, the nurse tells the mother to:
1. Set limits on the child's behavior.
2. Ignore the child when this behavior occurs.
3. Allow the behavior, because this is normal at this age period.
4. Punish the child every time the child says "no" to change the behavior.

328. The mother of an 8-year-old child tells the clinic nurse that she is concerned about the child because the child seems to be more attentive to friends than anything else. Using Erikson's psychosocial development theory, the appropriate nursing response is which of the following?
1. "You need to be concerned."
2. "You need to monitor the child's behavior closely."
3. "At this age, the child is developing his own personality."
4. "You need to provide more praise to the child to stop this behavior."

329. The mother of a 4-year-old child calls the clinic nurse and expresses concern because the child has been masturbating. Using Freud's psychosexual stages of development, the appropriate response by the nurse is which of the following?
1. "This is a normal behavior at this age."
2. "Children usually begin this behavior at age 8 years."
3. "This is not normal behavior, and the child should be seen by the physician."
4. "The child is very young to begin this behavior and should be brought to the clinic."

330. A nursing instructor asks a nursing student to present a clinical conference to peers regarding Freud's psychosexual stages of development,

specifically the anal stage. The student plans the conference, knowing that which of the following most appropriately relates to this stage of development?
1. This stage is associated with toilet training.
2. This stage is characterized by the gratification of self.
3. This stage is characterized by a tapering off of conscious biological and sexual urges.
4. This stage is associated with pleasurable and conflicting feelings about the genital organs.

331. A nursing instructor asks a nursing student to describe the formal operations stage of Piaget's cognitive developmental theory. The appropriate response by the nursing student is:
1. "The child has the ability to think abstractly."
2. "The child begins to understand the environment."
3. "The child is able to classify, order, and sort facts."
4. "The child learns to think in terms of past, present, and future."

Alternate Item Format: Multiple Response

332. A nurse educator is preparing to conduct a session to the nursing staff regarding the theories of growth and development and plans to discuss Kohlberg's theory of moral development. Which of the following should the nurse include in the session? **Select all that apply.**
❑ 1. Individuals move through all six stages in a sequential fashion.
❑ 2. Moral development progresses in relationship to cognitive development.
❑ 3. A person's ability to make moral judgments develops over a period of time.
❑ 4. The theory provides a framework for understanding how individuals determine a moral code to guide their behavior.
❑ 5. In stage 1 (punishment-obedience orientation), children are expected to reason as mature members of society.
❑ 6. In stage 2 (instrumental relativist orientation), the child conforms to rules to obtain rewards or have favors returned.

ANSWERS

325. 4
Rationale: In the preconventional stage, morals are thought to be motivated by punishment and reward. If the child is obedient and is not punished, then the child is being moral. The child sees actions as good or bad. If the child's actions are good, the child is praised. If the child's actions are bad, the child is punished. Options 1, 2, and 3 are incorrect for this stage of moral development.
Test-Taking Strategy: Eliminate options 1 and 2 because they are comparable or alike because peer pressure is the same as social pressures. To select from the remaining options, recalling that the preconventional stage occurs between birth and 7 years will assist in directing you to option 4 from the remaining options. If you had difficulty with this question, review the preconventional stage of Kohlberg's theory of moral development.
Level of Cognitive Ability: Understanding
Client Needs: Health Promotion and Maintenance
Integrated Process: Teaching and Learning
Content Area: Fundamental Skills—Developmental Stages
Reference: Hockenberry, M., & Wilson, D. (2009). *Wong's essentials of pediatric nursing* (8th ed., p. 439). St. Louis: Mosby.

326. 1
Rationale: According to Erikson, the caregiver should not try to anticipate the newborn infant's needs at all times but must allow the newborn infant to signal needs. If a newborn infant is not allowed to signal a need, the newborn will not learn how to control the environment. Erikson believed that a delayed or prolonged response to a newborn infant's signal would inhibit the development of trust and lead to mistrust of others.

Test-Taking Strategy: Use the process of elimination. Eliminate options 2, 3, and 4 because of the close-ended words *all, immediately,* and *avoid* in these options. Review Erikson's stage of psychosocial development for infancy if you had difficulty with this question.
Level of Cognitive Ability: Applying
Client Needs: Health Promotion and Maintenance
Integrated Process: Teaching and Learning
Content Area: Fundamental Skills—Developmental Stages
Reference: Hockenberry, M., & Wilson, D. (2009). *Wong's essentials of pediatric nursing* (8th ed., p. 327). St. Louis: Mosby.

327. 1
Rationale: According to Erikson, the child focuses on gaining some basic control over self and the environment and independence between ages 1 and 3 years. Gaining independence often means that the child has to rebel against the parents' wishes. Saying things like "no" or "mine" and having temper tantrums are common during this period of development. Being consistent and setting limits on the child's behavior are necessary elements. Options 2 and 3 do not address the child's behavior. Option 4 is likely to produce a negative response during this normal developmental pattern.
Test-Taking Strategy: Use the process of elimination. Options 2 and 3 can be eliminated first because they are comparable or alike indicating that the mother should not address the child's behavior. Next, eliminate option 4 because this action is likely to produce a negative response during this normal developmental pattern. Review psychosocial development of the toddler according the Erikson if you had difficulty with this question.
Level of Cognitive Ability: Applying

Client Needs: Health Promotion and Maintenance
Integrated Process: Teaching and Learning
Content Area: Fundamental Skills—Developmental Stages
Reference: McKinney, E., James, S., Murray, S., & Ashwill, J. (2009). *Maternal-child nursing* (3rd ed., p. 56). St. Louis: Saunders.

328. 3
Rationale: According to Erikson, during school-age years (6 to 12 years of age), the child begins to move toward peers and friends and away from the parents for support. The child also begins to develop special interests that reflect his or her own developing personality instead of the parents. Therefore options 1, 2, and 4 are incorrect responses.
Test-Taking Strategy: Use knowledge of Erikson's psychosocial development theory related to middle childhood. Options 1 and 2 can be eliminated first because they are comparable or alike and indicate that the mother should be concerned about the child. Eliminate option 4 next because, although praising the child for accomplishments is important at this age, the behavior that the child is exhibiting is normal. Review psychosocial development of the school-age child according to Erikson if you had difficulty with this question.
Level of Cognitive Ability: Applying
Client Needs: Health Promotion and Maintenance
Integrated Process: Nursing Process—Implementation
Content Area: Fundamental Skills—Developmental Stages
Reference: Hockenberry, M., & Wilson, D. (2009). *Wong's essentials of pediatric nursing* (8th ed., p. 80). St. Louis: Mosby.

329. 1
Rationale: According to Freud's psychosexual stages of development, between the ages of 3 and 6 the child is in the phallic stage. At this time, the child devotes much energy to examining his or her genitalia, masturbating, and expressing interest in sexual concerns. Therefore options 2, 3, and 4 are incorrect.
Test-Taking Strategy: Use the process of elimination. Eliminate options 3 and 4 first because they are comparable or alike indicating that the child's behavior is abnormal. Next, focus on the subject of the question and note the words *age 8 years* in option 2 to assist in eliminating this option. If you had difficulty with this question, review Freud's psychosexual stages of development.
Level of Cognitive Ability: Applying
Client Needs: Health Promotion and Maintenance
Integrated Process: Nursing Process—Implementation
Content Area: Fundamental Skills—Developmental Stages
Reference: McKinney, E., James, S., Murray, S., & Ashwill, J. (2009). *Maternal-child nursing* (3rd ed., p. 56). St. Louis: Saunders.

330. 1
Rationale: Generally, toilet training occurs during the anal stage. According to Freud, the child gains pleasure from the elimination of feces and from their retention. Option 2 relates to the oral stage. Option 3 relates to the latency period. Option 4 relates to the phallic stage.
Test-Taking Strategy: Use the process of elimination. Note the relationship between the words *anal* in the question and *toilet*

training in the correct option. If you had difficulty with this question, review Freud's psychosexual stages of development.
Level of Cognitive Ability: Understanding
Client Needs: Health Promotion and Maintenance
Integrated Process: Teaching and Learning
Content Area: Fundamental Skills—Developmental Stages
Reference: McKinney, E., James, S., Murray, S., & Ashwill, J. (2009). *Maternal-child nursing* (3rd ed., p. 56). St. Louis: Saunders.

331. 1
Rationale: In the formal operations stage, the child has the ability to think abstractly and logically. Option 2 identifies the sensorimotor stage. Option 3 identifies the concrete operational stage. Option 4 identifies the preoperational stage.
Test-Taking Strategy: Focus on the subject, the formal operations stage of Piaget's cognitive developmental theory, and note the relationship between the subject and the description in option 1. Remember that in the formal operations stage, the child has the ability to think abstractly and logically. If you had difficulty with this question, review these concepts.
Level of Cognitive Ability: Understanding
Client Needs: Health Promotion and Maintenance
Integrated Process: Teaching and Learning
Content Area: Fundamental Skills—Developmental Stages
Reference: Hockenberry, M., & Wilson, D. (2009). *Wong's essentials of pediatric nursing* (8th ed., p. 80). St. Louis: Mosby.

ALTERNATE ITEM FORMAT: MULTIPLE RESPONSE
332. 2, 3, 4, 6
Rationale: Kohlberg's theory states that individuals move through the six stages of development in a sequential fashion but that not everyone reaches stages 5 and 6 in his or her development of personal morality. The theory provides a framework for understanding how individuals determine a moral code to guide their behavior. It states that moral development progresses in relationship to cognitive development and that a person's ability to make moral judgments develops over a period of time. In stage 1, ages 2 to 3 years (punishment-obedience orientation), children cannot reason as mature members of society. In stage 2, ages 4 to 7 years, (instrumental relativist orientation), the child conforms to rules to obtain rewards or have favors returned.
Test-Taking Strategy: Read each option carefully. Recalling that the theory provides a framework for understanding how individuals determine a moral code to guide their behavior and recalling the ages associated with each stage will assist in answering the question. Also noting the word *all* in option 1 and the word *mature* in option 5 will assist in eliminating these options. If you had difficulty with this question, review Kohlberg's theory of moral development.
Level of Cognitive Ability: Applying
Client Needs: Health Promotion and Maintenance
Integrated Process: Teaching and Learning
Content Area: Fundamental Skills—Developmental Stages
Reference: McKinney, E., James, S., Murray, S., & Ashwill, J. (2009). *Maternal-child nursing* (3rd ed., pp. 56–57). St. Louis: Saunders.

Developmental Stages

I. THE HOSPITALIZED INFANT AND TODDLER

A. Separation anxiety
1. Protest
   a. Crying, screaming, searching for a parent; avoidance and rejection of contact with strangers
   b. Verbal attacks on others
   c. Physical fighting: kicking, biting, hitting, pinching
2. Despair
   a. Withdrawn, depressed, uninterested in the environment
   b. Loss of newly learned skills
3. Detachment
   a. Detachment is uncommon and occurs only after lengthy separations from the parent.
   b. Superficially, the toddler appears to have adjusted to the loss.
   c. During the detachment phase, the toddler again becomes more interested in the environment, plays with others, and seems to form new relationships; this behavior is a form of resignation and is not a sign of contentment.
   d. The toddler detaches from the parents in an effort to escape the emotional pain of desiring the parent's presence.
   e. During the detachment phase, the toddler copes by forming shallow relationships with others, becoming increasingly self-centered, and attaching primary importance to material objects.
   f. Detachment is the most serious phase because reversal of the potential adverse effects is less likely to occur once detachment is established. In most situations, the temporary separation imposed by hospitalization does not cause such prolonged parental absence that the toddler enters into detachment.

B. Fear of injury and pain: Affected by previous experiences, separation from parents, and preparation for the experience

C. Loss of control
1. Hospitalization, with its own set of rituals and routines, can severely disrupt the life of a toddler.
2. The lack of control often is exhibited in behaviors related to feeding, toileting, playing, and bedtime.
3. The toddler may demonstrate regression.

D. Interventions
1. Provide cuddling and touch and talk softly to the infant.
2. Provide opportunities for sucking and oral stimulation for the infant using a pacifier if the infant is NPO (not to receive anything by mouth).
3. Provide stimulation, if appropriate, for the infant, using objects of contrasting colors and textures.
4. Provide choices as much as possible to the toddler to enable him or her to have some control.
5. Approach the toddler with a positive attitude.
6. Allow the toddler to express feelings of protest.
7. Encourage the toddler to talk about parents or others in their lives.
8. Accept regressive behavior without ridiculing the toddler.
9. Provide the toddler with favorite and comforting objects.
10. Allow the toddler as much mobility as possible.
11. Anticipate temper tantrums from the toddler, and maintain a safe environment for physical acting out.
12. Employ pain reduction techniques, as appropriate.

⚠ For the hospitalized toddler, provide routines and rituals as close as possible to what he or she is used to at home.

II. THE HOSPITALIZED PRESCHOOLER

A. Separation anxiety
1. Separation anxiety is generally less obvious and less serious than in the toddler.
2. As stress increases, the preschooler's ability to separate from the parents decreases.
3. Protest

      a. Protest is less direct and aggressive than in the toddler.

      b. The preschooler may displace feelings onto others.

    4. Despair

      a. The preschooler reacts in a manner similar to that of the toddler.

      b. The preschooler is quietly withdrawn, depressed, and uninterested in the environment.

      c. The child exhibits loss of newly learned skills.

      d. The preschooler becomes generally uncooperative, refusing to eat or take medication.

      e. The preschooler repeatedly asks when the parents will be visiting.

    5. Detachment: Similar to the toddler

B. Fear of injury and pain

    1. The preschooler has a general lack of understanding of body integrity.

    2. The child fears invasive procedures and mutilation.

    3. The child imagines things to be much worse than they are.

    4. Preschoolers believe that they are ill because of something they did or thought.

C. Loss of control

    1. The preschooler likes familiar routines and rituals and may show regression if not allowed to maintain some control.

    2. The child has attained a good deal of independence and self-care at home and may expect that to continue in the hospital.

D. Interventions

    1. Provide a safe and secure environment.

    2. Take time for communication.

    3. Allow the preschooler to express anger.

    4. Acknowledge fears and anxieties.

    5. Accept regressive behavior; assist the preschooler in moving from regressive to appropriate behaviors according to age.

    6. Encourage rooming-in or leaving a favorite toy.

    7. Allow mobility and provide **play** and diversional activities.

    8. Place the preschooler with other children of the same age if possible.

    9. Encourage the preschooler to be independent.

    10. Explain procedures simply, on the preschooler's level.

    11. Avoid intrusive procedures when possible.

    12. Allow wearing of underpants.

III. THE HOSPITALIZED SCHOOL-AGE CHILD

A. Separation anxiety

    1. The school-age child is accustomed to periods of separation from the parents, but as stressors are added, the separation becomes more difficult.

    2. The child is more concerned with missing school and the fear that friends will forget her or him.

    3. Usually, the stages of behavior of protest, despair, and detachment do not occur with school-age children.

B. Fear of injury and pain

    1. The school-age child fears bodily injury and pain.

    2. The child fears illness itself, disability, death, and intrusive procedures in genital areas.

    3. The child is uncomfortable with any type of sexual examination.

    4. The child groans or whines, holds rigidly still, and communicates about pain.

C. Loss of control

    1. The child is usually highly social, independent, and involved with activities.

    2. The child seeks information and asks relevant questions about tests and procedures and the illness.

    3. The child associates his or her actions with the cause of the illness.

    4. The child may feel helpless and dependent if physical limitations occur.

D. Interventions

    1. Encourage rooming-in.

    2. Focus on the school-age child's abilities and needs.

    3. Encourage the school-age child to become involved with his or her own care.

    4. Accept regression but encourage independence.

    5. Provide choices to the school-age child.

    6. Allow expression of feelings verbally and nonverbally.

    7. Acknowledge fears and concerns and allow for discussion.

    8. Explain all procedures, using body diagrams or outlines.

    9. Provide privacy.

    10. Avoid intrusive procedures if possible.

    11. Allow the school-age child to wear underpants.

    12. Involve the school-age child in activities appropriate to developmental level and illness.

    13. Encourage the school-age child to contact friends.

    14. Provide for educational needs.

    15. Use appropriate interventions to relieve pain.

IV. THE HOSPITALIZED ADOLESCENT

A. Separation anxiety

    1. Adolescents are not sure whether they want their parents with them when they are hospitalized.

    2. Adolescents become upset if friends go on with their lives, excluding them.

⚠ For the hospitalized adolescent, separation from friends is a source of anxiety.

B. Fear of injury and pain
   1. Adolescents fear being different from others and their peers.
   2. Adolescents may give the impression that they are not afraid, even though they are terrified.
   3. Adolescents become guarded when any areas related to sexual development are examined.

C. Loss of control
   1. Behaviors exhibited include anger, withdrawal, and uncooperativeness.
   2. Adolescents seek help and then reject it.

D. Interventions
   1. Encourage questions about appearance and effects of the illness on the future.
   2. Explore feelings about the hospital and the significance that the illness might have for relationships.
   3. Encourage adolescents to wear their own clothes and carry out normal grooming activities.
   4. Allow favorite foods to be brought in to the hospital if possible.
   5. Provide privacy.
   6. Use body diagrams to prepare for procedures.
   7. Introduce them to other adolescents in the nursing unit.
   8. Encourage maintaining contact with peer groups.
   9. Provide for educational needs.
   10. Identify formation of future plans.
   11. Help develop positive coping mechanisms.

V. COMMUNICATION APPROACHES

A. General guidelines (Box 33-1)

B. Infant
   1. Infants respond to nonverbal communication behaviors of adults, such as holding, rocking, patting, cuddling, and touching.
   2. Use a slow approach and allow the infant to get to know the nurse.
   3. Use a calm, soft, soothing voice.
   4. Be responsive to cries.
   5. Talk and read to infants.
   6. Allow security objects such as blankets and pacifiers if the infant has them.

C. Toddler
   1. Approach the toddler cautiously.
   2. Remember that toddlers accept verbal communications of others literally.
   3. Learn the toddler's words for common items and use them in conversations.
   4. Use short, concrete terms.
   5. Prepare the toddler for procedures immediately before the event.
   6. Repeat explanations and descriptions.
   7. Use **play** for demonstrations.
   8. Use visual aids such as picture books, puppets, and dolls.

Box 33-1 General Guidelines for Communication

Allow the child to feel comfortable with the nurse.
Communicate through the use of objects.
Allow the child to express fears and concerns.
Speak clearly and in a quiet, unhurried voice.
Offer choices when possible.
Be honest with the child.
Set limits with the child as appropriate.

   9. Allow the toddler to handle the equipment or instruments; explain what the equipment or instrument does and how it feels.
   10. Encourage the use of comfort objects.

D. Preschooler
   1. Seek opportunities to offer choices.
   2. Speak in simple sentences.
   3. Be concise and limit the length of explanations.
   4. Allow asking questions.
   5. Describe procedures as they are about to be performed.
   6. Use **play** to explain procedures and activities.
   7. Allow handling the equipment or instruments, which will ease fear and help answer questions.

E. School-age child
   1. Establish limits.
   2. Provide reassurance to help in alleviating fears and anxieties.
   3. Engage in conversations that encourage thinking.
   4. Use medical **play** techniques.
   5. Use photographs, books, dolls, and videos to explain procedures.
   6. Explain in clear terms.
   7. Allow time for composure and privacy.

F. Adolescent
   1. Remember that the adolescent may be preoccupied with body image.
   2. Encourage and support independence.
   3. Provide privacy.
   4. Use photographs, books, and videos to explain procedures.
   5. Engage in conversations about adolescent's interests.
   6. Avoid becoming too abstract, too detailed, and too technical.
   7. Avoid responding by prying, confrontation, or judgmental attitudes.

VI. DEVELOPMENTAL CHARACTERISTICS

A. Infant
   1. Physical
      a. Height increases by ¾ inch per month.
      b. Weight is doubled at 5 to 6 months and tripled at 12 months.

Box 33-2 Vital Signs: Newborn and 1-Year-Old Infant

Newborn
Temperature: Axillary, 97.9° to 98° F
Apical heart rate: 120 to 140 beats/min
Respirations: 30 to 60 (average 40) breaths/min
Blood pressure: 73/55 mm Hg

1-Year-Old Infant
Temperature: Axillary, 97° to 99° F
Apical heart rate: 90 to 130 beats/min
Respirations: 20 to 40 breaths/min
Blood pressure: 90/56 mm Hg

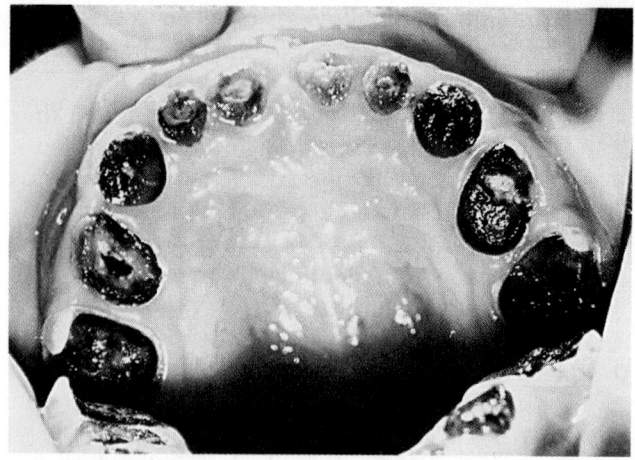

▲ **FIGURE 33-1** Nursing caries. (From Hockenberry, M., & Wilson, D. [2009]. *Wong's essentials of pediatric nursing* [8th ed., p. 426]. St. Louis: Mosby. Courtesy Bruce Carter, DDS, Texas Children's Hospital, Houston.)

c. At birth, head circumference is 33 to 35 cm (13.2 to 14 inches), approximately 2 to 3 cm more than chest circumference.

d. By 1 to 2 years of age, head circumference and chest circumference are equal.

e. Anterior fontanel (soft and flat in a normal infant) closes by 12 to 18 months of age.

f. Posterior fontanel (soft and flat in a normal infant) closes by the end of the second month.

g. Infant has 10 upper and 10 lower deciduous teeth by 2½ years of age.

h. Lower central incisors are present by 6 to 8 months.

i. Sleep patterns vary among infants; generally, by 3 to 4 months of age, most infants have developed a nocturnal pattern of sleep that lasts 9 to 11 hours.

2. Vital signs (Box 33-2)

3. Nutrition

a. The infant may breast-feed or bottle-feed (with iron-fortified formula), depending on the mother's choice; however, human milk is the preferred form of nutrition for all infants, especially during the first 6 months.

b. All infants should receive daily vitamin D supplementation (200 IU) starting in the first 2 months of life to prevent rickets and vitamin D deficiency.

c. Iron stores from birth are depleted by 4 months of age; if the infant is being only breast-fed, iron supplementation usually with iron-fortified cereal is needed.

d. Whole milk, low-fat milk, skim milk, other animal milk, or imitation milk should not be given to infants as a primary source of nutrition because these food sources lack the necessary components needed for growth and have limited digestibility.

e. Fluoride supplementation may be needed at about 6 months of age, depending on the infant's intake of fluoridated tap water.

f. Solid foods (strained, pureed, or finely mashed) are introduced at about 5 to 6 months of age; introduce solid foods one at a time, usually at intervals of 4 to 5 days, to identify food allergens.

g. Sequence of the introduction of solid foods varies depending on physician's preference and usually is as follows: iron-fortified rice cereal, fruits, vegetables, then meats.

h. At 12 months of age, eggs can be given (introduce egg whites in small quantities to detect an allergy); cheese may be used as a substitute for meat.

i. Avoid solid foods that place the infant at risk for choking, such as nuts, foods with seeds, raisins, popcorn, grapes, and hot dog pieces.

j. Avoid microwaving baby bottles and baby food.

k. Never mix food or medications with formula.

l. Avoid adding honey to formula, water, or other fluid to prevent botulism.

m. Offer fruit juice from a cup (12 to 13 months or at a prescribed age) rather than a bottle to prevent nursing (bottle-mouth) caries; fruit juice is limited because of its high sugar content (Fig. 33-1).

4. Skills (Box 33-3)

5. **Play**

a. Solitary

b. Birth to 3 months: Verbal, visual, and tactile stimuli

c. 4 to 6 months: Initiation of actions and recognition of new experiences

d. 6 to 12 months: Awareness of self, imitation, repetition of pleasurable actions

e. Enjoyment of soft stuffed animals, crib mobiles with contrasting colors, squeeze

Box 33-3 Infant Skills

2 to 3 Months
Smiles
Turns head side to side
Cries
Follows objects
Holds head in midline

4 to 5 Months
Grasps objects
Switches objects from hands
Rolls over for the first time
Enjoys social interaction
Begins to show memory
Aware of unfamiliar surroundings

6 to 7 Months
Creeps
Sits with support
Imitates
Exhibits fear of strangers
Holds arms out
Frequent mood swings
Waves "bye-bye"

8 to 9 Months
Sits steadily unsupported
Crawls
May stand while holding on
Begins to stand without help

10 to 11 Months
Can change from prone to sitting position
Walks while holding on to furniture
Stands securely
Entertains self for periods of time

12 to 13 Months
Walks with one hand held
Can take a few steps without falling
Can drink from a cup

14 to 15 Months
Walks alone
Can crawl up stairs
Shows emotions such as anger and affection
Will explore away from mother in familiar surroundings

g. Avoid offering food that is round and similar to the size of the airway to prevent choking.
h. Be sure toys have no small pieces.
i. Toys or mobiles hanging over the crib should be well out of reach to prevent strangulation.
j. Avoid placing large toys in the crib because an older infant may use them as steps to climb.
k. Cribs should be positioned away from curtains and blind cords.
l. Cover electrical outlets.
m. Remove hazardous objects from low, reachable places.
n. Remove chemicals such as cleaning or other household products, medications, poisons, and plants from the infant's reach.
o. Keep the Poison Control Center number available.

⚠ Never shake an infant because of the risk of causing a closed head injury known as shaken baby syndrome.

B. Toddler
1. Physical
a. Height and weight increase in phases, reflecting growth spurts and lags.
b. Head circumference increases about 1 inch between ages 1 and 2; thereafter head circumference increases about ½ inch per year until age 5.
c. Anterior fontanel closes between ages 12 and 18 months.
d. Weight gain is slower than in infancy; by age 2, the average weight is 22 to 27 pounds.
e. Normal height changes include a growth of about 3 inches per year; the average height of the toddler is 34 inches at age 2 years.
f. Lordosis (pot belly) is noted.
g. The toddler should see a dentist soon after the first teeth erupt, usually around 1 year of age and oral hygiene measures should be instituted; regular dental care is essential, and the toddler will require assistance with brushing and flossing of teeth (fluoride supplements may be necessary if the water is not fluoridated).
h. A toddler should never be allowed to fall asleep with a bottle containing milk, juice, soda pop, sweetened water, or any other sweet liquid because of the risk of nursing (bottle-mouth) caries (see Fig. 33-1).
i. Typically, the toddler sleeps through the night and has one daytime nap; the daytime nap is normally discontinued at about age 3.
j. A consistent bedtime ritual helps prepare the toddler for sleep.
k. Security objects at bedtime may assist in sleep.
2. Vital signs (Box 33-4)

toys, rattles, musical toys, water toys during the bath, large picture books, and push toys after he or she begins to walk
6. Safety
a. Parents must baby-proof the home.
b. Guard the infant when on a bed or changing table.
c. Use gates to protect the infant from stairs.
d. Be sure that bath water is not hot; do not leave the infant unattended in the bath.
e. Do not hold the infant while drinking or working near hot liquids or items such as a stove.
f. Cool vaporizers should be used if needed, instead of steam, to prevent burn injuries.

Box 33-4 The Toddler's Vital Signs

Temperature: Axillary, 97.5° to 98.6° F
Apical heart rate: 80 to 120 beats/min
Respirations: 20 to 30 breaths/min
Blood pressure: Average, 92/55 mm Hg

Box 33-5 Signs of Readiness for Toilet Training

Child is able to stay dry for 2 hours.
Child is waking up dry from a nap.
Child is able to sit, squat, and walk.
Child is able to remove clothing.
Child recognizes the urge to defecate or urinate.
Child expresses willingness to please a parent.
Child is able to sit on the toilet for 5 to 10 minutes without fussing or getting off.

Modified from Hockenberry, M., & Wilson, D. (2009). *Wong's essentials of pediatric nursing* (8th ed., p. 417). St. Louis: Mosby.

3. Nutrition
   a. The MyPyramid for Kids food guide provides dietary guidelines and applies to children as young as 2 years of age (see www.mypyramid.gov).
   b. The toddler should average an intake of two to three servings of milk daily (24 to 30 oz) to ensure an adequate amount of calcium and phosphorus (low-fat milk may be given after 2 years of age).
   c. Trans-fatty acids and saturated fats need to be restricted; otherwise fat restriction is not appropriate for a toddler (mothers should be taught about the types of food that contain fat that should be selected).
   d. Iron-fortified cereal and a high-iron diet, adequate amounts of calcium and vitamin D, and vitamin C (4 to 6 oz of juice daily) are essential components for the toddler's diet.
   e. Most toddlers prefer to feed themselves.
   f. The toddler generally does best by eating several small nutritious meals each day rather than three large meals.
   g. Offer a limited number of foods at any one time.
   h. Offer finger foods and avoid concentrated sweets and empty calories.
   i. The toddler is at risk for aspiration of small foods that are not chewed easily, such as nuts, foods with seeds, raisins, popcorn, grapes, and hot dog pieces.
   j. Physiological anorexia may occur and is normal because of the alternating stages of fast and slow growth.
   k. Sit the toddler in a high chair at the family table for meals.
   l. Allow sufficient time to eat, but remove food when the toddler begins to **play** with it.
   m. The toddler drinks well from a cup held with both hands.
   n. Avoid using food as a reward or punishment.
4. Skills
   a. The toddler begins to walk with one hand held by age 12 to 13 months.
   b. The toddler runs by age 2 years and walks backward and hops on one foot by age 3 years.
   c. The toddler usually cannot alternate feet when climbing stairs.
   d. The toddler begins to master fine motor skills for building, undressing, and drawing lines.
   e. The young toddler often uses "no" even when he or she means "yes" to assert independence.
   f. The toddler begins to use short sentences and has a vocabulary of about 300 words by age 2.
5. Bowel and bladder control
   a. Certain signs indicate that a toddler is ready for toilet training (Box 33-5).
   b. Bowel control develops before bladder control.
   c. By age 3, the toddler achieves fairly good bowel and bladder control.
   d. The toddler may stay dry during the day but may need a diaper at night until about age 4.
6. **Play**
   a. The major socializing mechanism is parallel **play**, and therapeutic **play** can begin at this age.
   b. The toddler has a short attention span, causing the toddler to change toys often.
   c. The toddler explores body parts of self and others.
   d. Typical toys include push-pull toys, blocks, sand, finger paints and bubbles, large balls, crayons, trucks and dolls, containers, Play-Doh, toy telephones, cloth books, and wooden puzzles.
7. Safety

   ⚠ Toddlers are eager to explore the world around them they need to be supervised at play to ensure safety.

   a. Use back burners on the stove to prepare a meal; turn pot handles inward and toward the middle of the stove.
   b. Keep dangling cords from small appliances away from the toddler.
   c. Place inaccessible locks on windows and doors, and keep furniture away from windows.
   d. Secure screens on all windows.

Box 33-6 The Preschooler's Vital Signs

Temperature: Axillary, 97.5° to 98.6° F
Apical heart rate: 70 to 110 beats/min
Respirations: 16 to 22 breaths/min
Blood pressure: Average, 95/57 mm Hg

   e. Place safety gates at stairways.
   f. Do not allow the toddler to sleep or **play** in an upper bunk bed.
   g. Never leave the toddler alone near a bathtub, pail of water, swimming pool, or any other body of water.
   h. Keep toilet lids closed.
   i. Keep all medicines, poisons, household plants, and toxic products in high areas and locked out of reach.
   j. Keep the Poison Control Center number available.
C. Preschooler
   1. Physical
      a. The preschooler grows 2½ to 3 inches per year.
      b. Average height is 37 inches at age 3, 40½ inches at age 4, and 43 inches at age 5.
      c. The preschooler gains approximately 5 pounds per year; average weight is 35 to 40 pounds at age 5.
      d. The preschooler requires about 12 hours of sleep each day.
      e. A security object and a nightlight help with sleeping.
      f. At the beginning of the preschool period, the eruption of the deciduous (primary) teeth is complete.
      g. Regular dental care is essential, and the preschooler may require assistance with brushing and flossing of teeth; fluoride supplements may be necessary if the water is not fluoridated.
   2. Vital signs (Box 33-6)
   3. Nutrition
      a. Nutritional needs are similar to those required for the toddler although the daily amounts of minerals, vitamins, and protein may increase with age.
      b. The MyPyramid for Kids food guide is appropriate for preschoolers (see www.mypyramid.gov).
      c. The preschooler exhibits food fads and certain taste preferences and may exhibit finicky eating.
      d. By 5 years old, the child tends to focus on social aspects of eating, table conversations, manners, and willingness to try new foods.
   4. Skills
      a. The preschooler has good posture.
      b. The child develops fine motor coordination.
      c. The child can hop, skip, and run more smoothly.
      d. Athletic abilities begin to develop.
      e. The preschooler demonstrates increased skills in balancing.
      f. The child alternates feet when climbing stairs.
      g. The child can tie shoelaces by age 6.
      h. The child may talk continuously and ask many "why" questions.
      i. Vocabulary increases to about 900 words by age 3 and to 2100 words by age 5.
      j. By age 3, the preschooler usually talks in three- or four-word sentences and speaks in short phrases.
      k. By age 4, the preschooler speaks five- or six-word sentences and, by age 5, speaks in longer sentences that contain all parts of speech.
      l. The child can be understood readily by others and can understand clearly what others are saying.
   5. Bowel and bladder control
      a. By age 4, the preschooler has daytime control of bowel and bladder but may experience bed-wetting accidents at night.
      b. By age 5, the preschooler achieves bowel and bladder control, although accidents may occur in stressful situations.
   6. **Play**
      a. The preschooler is cooperative.
      b. The preschooler has imaginary playmates.
      c. The child likes to build and create things, and **play** is simple and imaginative.
      d. The child understands sharing and is able to interact with peers.
      e. The child requires regular socialization with mates of similar age.
      f. **Play** activities include a large space for running and jumping.
      g. The preschooler likes dress-up clothes, paints, paper, and crayons for creative expression.
      h. Swimming and sports aid in growth development.
      i. Puzzles and toys aid with fine motor development.
   7. Safety
      a. Preschoolers are active and inquisitive.
      b. Because of their magical thinking, they may believe that daring feats seen in cartoons are possible and may attempt them.
      c. The preschooler can learn simple safety practices because they can follow simple verbal directions and their attention span is longer.
      d. Teach the preschooler basic safety rules to ensure safety when playing in a playground such as near swings and ladders.

e. Teach the preschooler never to **play** with matches or lighters.

f. The preschooler should be taught what to do in the event of a fire or if clothes catch fire; fire drills should be practiced with the preschooler.

g. Guns should be stored unloaded and secured under lock and key (ammunition should be locked in a separate place).

h. Teach the preschooler his or her full name, address, parents' names, and telephone number.

i. Teach the preschooler how to dial 911 in an emergency situation.

j. Keep the Poison Control Center number available.

⚠ Teach a preschooler and school-age child to leave an area immediately if a gun is visible and to tell an adult. The preschooler should also be taught never to point a toy gun at another person.

D. School-age child
1. Physical
   a. Girls usually grow faster than boys.
   b. Growth is about 2 inches per year between ages 6 and 12.
   c. Height ranges from 45 inches at age 6 to 59 inches at age 12.
   d. School-age children gain weight at a rate of about 4½ to 6½ pounds per year.
   e. Average weight is 46 pounds at age 6 and 88 pounds at age 12.
   f. The first permanent (secondary) teeth erupt around age 6, and deciduous teeth are lost gradually.
   g. Regular dentist visits are necessary, and the school-age child needs to be supervised with brushing and flossing teeth; fluoride supplements may be necessary if the water is not fluoridated.
   h. For school-age children with primary and permanent dentition, the best toothbrush is one with soft nylon bristles and an overall length of about 6 inches.
   i. Sleep requirements range from 10 to 12 hours a night.
2. Vital signs (Box 33-7)
3. Nutrition
   a. School-age children will have increased growth needs as they approach adolescence.
   b. Children require a balanced diet from foods in the MyPyramid Food Guide; healthy snacks should continue to be emphasized to prevent childhood obesity.
   c. Children still may be picky eaters but are usually willing to try new foods.

Box 33-7 The School-Age Child's Vital Signs

Temperature: Oral, 97.5° to 98.6° F
Apical heart rate: 60 to 100 beats/min
Respirations: 18 to 20 breaths/min
Blood pressure: Average, 107/64 mm Hg

4. Skills
   a. School-age children exhibit refinement of fine motor skills.
   b. Development of gross motor skills continues.
   c. Strength and endurance increase.
5. **Play**
   a. **Play** is more competitive.
   b. Rules and rituals are important aspects of **play** and games.
   c. The school-age child enjoys drawing, collecting items, dolls, pets, guessing games, board games, listening to the radio, TV, reading, watching videos or DVDs, and computer games.
   d. The child participates in team sports.
   e. The child may participate in secret clubs, group peer activities, and scout organizations.
6. Safety
   a. The school-age child experiences less fear in **play** activities and frequently imitates real life by using tools and household items.
   b. Major causes of injuries include bicycles, skateboards, and team sports as the child increases in motor abilities and independence.
   c. Children should always wear a helmet when riding a bike or using in-line skates or skateboards.
   d. Teach the child water safety rules.
   e. Instruct the child to avoid teasing or playing roughly with animals.
   f. Teach the child never to **play** with matches or lighters.
   g. The child should be taught what to do in the event of a fire or if clothes catch fire; fire drills should be practiced with the child.
   h. Guns should be stored unloaded and secured under lock and key (ammunition should be locked in a separate place).
   i. Teach the child traffic safety rules.
   j. Teach the child how to dial 911 in an emergency situation.
   k. Keep the Poison Control Center number available.

⚠ Teach the preschooler and school-age child that if another person touches his or her body in an inappropriate way, an adult should be told. Also teach the child to avoid speaking to strangers and never to accept a ride, toys, or gifts from a stranger.

E. Adolescent
  1. Physical
     a. Puberty is the maturational, hormonal, and growth process that occurs when the reproductive organs begin to function and the secondary sex characteristics develop.
     b. Body mass increases to adult size.
     c. Sebaceous and sweat glands become active and fully functional.
     d. Body hair distribution occurs.
     e. Increases in height, weight, breast development, and pelvic girth occur in girls.
     f. Menstrual periods occur about 2½ years after the onset of puberty.
     g. In boys, increases in height, weight, muscle mass, and penis and testicle size occur.
     h. The voice deepens in boys.
     i. Normal weight gain during puberty: Girls gain 15 to 55 pounds; boys gain 15 to 65 pounds.
     j. Careful brushing and care of the teeth are important, and many adolescents need to wear braces.
     k. Sleep patterns include a tendency to stay up late; therefore, in an attempt to catch up on missed sleep, adolescents sleep late whenever possible; an overall average of 8 hours per night is recommended.
  2. Vital signs (Box 33-8)
  3. Nutrition
     a. Teaching about the MyPyramid Food Guide is important.
     b. Adolescents typically eat whenever they have a break in activities.
     c. Calcium, zinc, iron, folic acid, and protein are especially important nutritional needs.
     d. Adolescents tend to snack on empty calories and the importance of adequate and healthy nutrition needs to be stressed.
     e. Body image is important.
  4. Skills
     a. Gross and fine motor skills are well developed.
     b. Strength and endurance increase.
  5. **Play**
     a. Games and athletic activities are the most common forms of **play**.
     b. Competition and strict rules are important.
     c. Adolescents enjoy activities such as sports, videos, movies, reading, parties, dancing, hobbies, computer games, music, communicating via the Internet, and experimenting, such as with makeup and hairstyles.
     d. Friends are important, and adolescents like to gather in small groups.
  6. Safety
     a. Adolescents are risk takers.
     b. Adolescents have a natural urge to experiment and to be independent.

Box 33-8 The Adolescent's Vital Signs

Temperature: Oral, 97.5° to 98.6° F
Apical heart rate: 55 to 90 beats/min
Respirations: 12 to 20 breaths/min
Blood pressure: Average, 121/70 mm Hg

     c. Reinforce instructions about the dangers related to cigarette smoking, caffeine ingestion, alcohol, and drugs.
     d. Help adolescents recognize that they have choices when difficult or potentially dangerous situations arise.
     e. Ensure that the adolescent uses a seat belt.
     f. Instruct adolescents in the consequences of injuries that motor vehicle accidents can cause.
     g. Instruct adolescents in water safety and emphasize that they should enter the water feet first as opposed to diving, especially when the depth of the water is unknown.
     h. Instruct adolescents about the dangers associated with guns, violence, and gangs.
     i. Instruct adolescents about the complications associated with body piercing, tattooing, and sun tanning.

Discuss issues such as date rape, sexual relationships, and transmission of sexually transmitted infections with the adolescent. Also discuss the dangers of the Internet related to communicating and setting up meetings (dates) with unknown persons.

F. Early adulthood
  1. Description: Period between the late teens and mid to late 30s
  2. Physical changes
     a. Person has completed physical growth by the age of 20.
     b. Person is active.
     c. Severe illnesses are less common than in older age groups.
     d. Person tends to ignore physical symptoms and postpone seeking health care.
     e. Lifestyle habits such as smoking, stress, lack of exercise, poor personal hygiene, and family history of disease increase the risk of future illness.
  3. Cognitive changes
     a. Person has rational thinking habits.
     b. Conceptual, problem-solving, and motor skills increase.
     c. Person identifies preferred occupational areas.
  4. Psychosocial changes
     a. Person separates from family of origin.

b. Person gives much attention to occupational and social pursuits to improve socioeconomic status.

c. Person makes decisions regarding career, marriage, and parenthood.

d. Person needs to adapt to new situations.

5. Sexuality
   a. Person has the emotional maturity to develop mature sexual relationships.
   b. Person is at risk for sexually transmitted infections.

G. Middle adulthood
   1. Description: Period between the mid to late 30s and mid 60s
   2. Physical changes
      a. Physical changes occur between 40 and 65 years of age.
      b. Individual becomes aware that changes in reproductive and physical abilities signify the beginning of another stage in life.
      c. Menopause occurs in women and climacteric occurs in men.
      d. Physiological changes often have an impact on self-concept and body image.
      e. Physiological concerns include stress, level of wellness, and the formation of positive health habits.
   3. Cognitive changes
      a. Person may be interested in learning new skills.
      b. Person may become involved in educational or vocational programs for entering the job market or for changing careers.
   4. Psychosocial changes
      a. Changes may include expected events, such as children moving away from home (postparental family stage), or unexpected events, such as the death of a close friend.
      b. Time and financial demands decrease as children move away from home, and couples face redefining their relationship.
      c. Adults may become grandparents.
      d. Adults are achieving generativity.
   5. Sexuality
      a. Many couples renew their relationships and find increased marital and sexual satisfaction.
      b. The onset of menopause and climacteric may affect sexual health.
      c. Stress, health, and medications can affect sexuality.

H. Later adulthood (period between 65 years to death): refer to Chapter 35.

VII. CAR SAFETY SEATS AND GUIDELINES

A. The safest place for all children to ride, regardless of age, is in the back seat of the car.

B. There are different types of car safety seats and the manufacturer's guidelines need to be followed.

C. LATCH (Lower Anchors and Tethers for Children): An attachment or anchor system that is in the vehicle and on the car safety seat that improves safety because it eliminates the need to use seat belts to secure the car safety seat; if the vehicle or car safety seat does not have this anchor system, the seat belts need to be used to install the car safety system.

D. A rear-facing car safety seat is never placed in the front seat of a vehicle because if the air bag inflates it will hit the back of the car safety seat (where the child's head is) and cause serious injury.

E. Make sure that the safety seat is installed tightly and that the seat is at the correct angle so that the infant's head does not fall forward.

F. Lock the car doors; four-door cars should be equipped with child safety locks on the back doors.

G. The harness placed around the infant or child should be snug.

H. Infants should ride in a car in a semireclined, rear-facing position in an infant-only seat or a convertible seat until they weigh at least 20 pounds and have reached at least 1 year of age. (Convertible seats can be used rear-facing for infants and then converted to a forward-facing position once the child is old enough and big enough to do so safely.)

I. The toddler can be placed in an upright forward-facing position in a car safety seat (convertible restraint with a full harness); the transition point for switching to a forward-facing position is defined by the manufacturer of the car seat but is generally at a body weight of at least 20 pounds (9 kg) and 1 year of age (Fig. 33-2).

J. Booster seats are used for children shorter than 4 feet, 9 inches tall and weigh more than 40 pounds (typically between 4 and 8 years of age); a booster seat is used until the child can sit against the back of the seat with feet hanging down and legs bent at the knees and adult belts fit correctly (usually when the child is between 8 and 12 years of age and reaches 4 feet, 9 inches tall) (Fig. 33-3).

K. Once the child has outgrown the booster seat, the child should ride in a lap and shoulder belt in the back seat until 13 years of age (shoulder strap should be away from neck and face).

🔘 MORE QUESTIONS ON THE CD!

Practice Questions

333. A 4-year old child diagnosed with leukemia is hospitalized for chemotherapy. The child is fearful of the hospitalization. Which nursing intervention would be most appropriate to alleviate the child's fears?

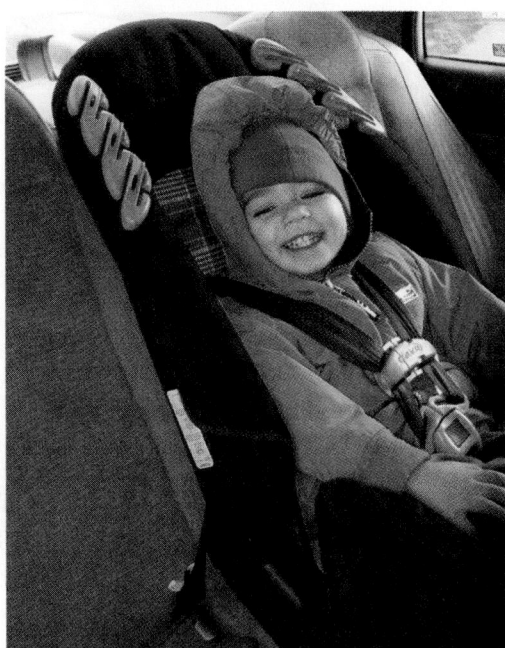

▲ **FIGURE 33-2** When the child reaches 1 year of age and 20 pounds, the car safety seat can be adjusted to a forward-facing, upright position. The seat is appropriate for the toddler until the child weighs about 40 pounds. The safety straps should be adjusted to provide a snug fit, and the seat should be placed in the back seat of the car, ideally in the middle. (From McKinney, E., James, S., Murray, S., & Ashwill, J. [2009]. *Maternal-child nursing* [3rd ed.]. St. Louis: Saunders.)

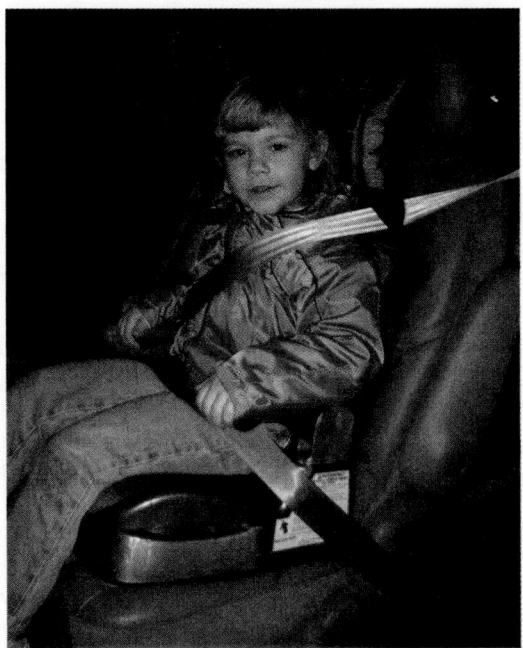

▲ **FIGURE 33-3** A high-backed booster seat designed to hold car lap and shoulder belts properly is strongly recommended for children who have outgrown a child safety seat. Booster seats raise the young child high enough to allow the car seat belt to be positioned correctly over the child's chest and pelvis. (From McKinney, E., James, S., Murray, S., & Ashwill, J. [2009]. *Maternal-child nursing* [3rd ed.]. St. Louis: Saunders. Photo courtesy of Michele M. Hayden.)

1. Encourage the child's parents to stay with the child.
2. Encourage play with other children of the same age.
3. Advise the family to visit only during the scheduled visiting hours.
4. Provide a private room, allowing the child to bring the favorite toys from home.

334. A 16-year-old is admitted to the hospital for acute appendicitis and an appendectomy is performed. Which nursing intervention is appropriate to facilitate normal growth and development postoperatively?
1. Encourage the child to rest and read.
2. Encourage the parents to room in with the child.
3. Allow the child to interact with others in his or her same age group.
4. Allow the family to bring in the child's favorite computer games.

335. A nurse prepares to administer digoxin (Lanoxin) to a 3-year-old child with a diagnosis of congestive heart failure and notes that the apical heart rate is 110 beats/min. Based on this finding which nursing action is appropriate?
1. Hold the medication.
2. Notify the physician.

3. Administer the digoxin.
4. Recheck the apical rate in 15 minutes.

336. Which of the following car safety devices should be used for a child who is 8 years old and is 4 feet tall?
1. Seat belt
2. Booster seat
3. Rear-facing convertible seat
4. Front-facing convertible seat

337. A nurse assesses the vital signs of a 12-month-old infant with a respiratory infection and notes that the respiratory rate is 35 breaths/min. Based on this finding, which action is appropriate?
1. Administer oxygen.
2. Notify the physician.
3. Document the findings.
4. Reassess the respiratory rate in 15 minutes.

338. A nurse is monitoring a 3-month-old infant for signs of increased intracranial pressure. On palpation of the fontanels, the nurse notes that the anterior fontanel is soft and flat. Based on this finding, which nursing action is appropriate?
1. Increase oral fluids.
2. Notify the physician.
3. Document the finding.
4. Elevate the head of the bed to 90 degrees.

339. A nurse is evaluating the developmental level of a 2-year-old. Which of the following does the nurse expect to observe in this child?
1. Uses a fork to eat
2. Uses a cup to drink
3. Pours own milk into a cup
4. Uses a knife for cutting food

340. A 2-year-old child is treated in the emergency room for a burn to the chest and abdomen. The child sustained the burn by grabbing a cup of hot coffee that was left on the kitchen counter. The nurse reviews safety principles with the parents before discharge. Which statement by the parents indicates an understanding of measures to provide safety in the home?
1. "We will be sure not to leave hot liquids unattended."
2. "I guess my children need to understand what the word *hot* means."
3. "We will be sure that the children stay in their rooms when we work in the kitchen."
4. "We will install a safety gate as soon as we get home so the children cannot get into the kitchen."

341. A mother arrives at a clinic with her toddler and tells a nurse that she has a difficult time getting the child to go to bed at night. Which of the following is appropriate for the nurse to suggest to the mother?
1. Avoid a nap during the day.
2. Allow the child to set bedtime limits.
3. Allow the child to have temper tantrums.
4. Inform the child of bedtime a few minutes before it is time for bed.

342. A mother of a 3-year-old asks a clinic nurse about appropriate and safe toys for the child. The nurse tells the mother that the most appropriate toy for a 3-year-old is which of the following?

1. A wagon
2. A golf set
3. A farm set
4. A jack set with marbles

343. The mother of a 3-year-old is concerned because her child still is insisting on a bottle at nap time and at bedtime. Which of the following is the appropriate suggestion to the mother?
1. Allow the bottle if it contains juice.
2. Allow the bottle if it contains water.
3. Do not allow the child to have the bottle.
4. Allow the bottle during naps but not at bedtime.

344. A nurse is preparing to care for a 5-year-old who has been placed in traction following a fracture of the femur. The nurse plans care, knowing that which of the following is the most appropriate activity for this child?
1. A radio
2. A sports video
3. Large picture books
4. Crayons and a coloring book

Alternate Item Format: Multiple Response
345. Which interventions are appropriate for the care of an infant? **Select all that apply.**
- 1. Provide swaddling.
- 2. Talk in a loud voice.
- 3. Provide the infant with a bottle of juice at nap time.
- 4. Hang mobiles with black and white contrast designs.
- 5. Caress the infant while bathing or during diaper changes.
- 6. Allow the infant to cry for at least 10 minutes before responding.

ANSWERS
333. 1
Rationale: Although the preschooler already may be spending some time away from parents at a day care center or preschool, illness adds a stressor that makes separation more difficult. The child may ask repeatedly when parents will be coming for a visit or may constantly want to call the parents. Options 3 and 4 increase stress related to separation anxiety. Option 2 is unrelated to the subject of the question and, in addition, may not be appropriate for a child who may be immunocompromised and at risk for infection.
Test-Taking Strategy: Note that the subject relates to the child's fear and use the process of elimination. Options 3 and 4 will increase anxiety and fear further and should be eliminated. Bearing the subject of the question in mind and

considering the child's diagnosis will assist you in eliminating option 2. Review interventions to prevent or minimize separation anxiety in the preschooler if you had difficulty with this question.
Level of Cognitive Ability: Applying
Client Needs: Health Promotion and Maintenance
Integrated Process: Caring
Content Area: Fundamental Skills—Developmental Stages
Reference: McKinney, E., James, S., Murray, S., & Ashwill, J. (2009). *Maternal-child nursing* (3rd ed., p. 886). St. Louis: Saunders.

334. 3
Rationale: Adolescents often are not sure whether they want their parents with them when they are hospitalized. Because of the importance of their peer group, separation from friends

is a source of anxiety. Ideally, the members of the peer group will support their ill friend. Options 1, 2, and 4 isolate the child from the peer group.
Test-Taking Strategy: Consider the psychosocial needs of the adolescent when answering the question and remember that the peer group is very important. Options 1, 2, and 4 are comparable or alike in that they isolate the child from his or her own peer group. If you had difficulty with this question, review the psychosocial needs of the adolescent.
Level of Cognitive Ability: Applying
Client Needs: Health Promotion and Maintenance
Integrated Process: Caring
Content Area: Fundamental Skills—Developmental Stages
Reference: McKinney, E., James, S., Murray, S., & Ashwill, J. (2009). *Maternal-child nursing* (3rd ed., p. 891). St. Louis: Saunders.

335. 3
Rationale: The normal apical heart rate for a 3-year-old is 80 to 120 beats/min. Because the apical rate is within the normal range, options 1, 2, and 4 are inappropriate and unnecessary.
Test-Taking Strategy: Use the process of elimination and knowledge of the normal apical heart rate for a 3-year-old to answer the question. Recalling that a heart rate of 110 beats/min is within the normal range will direct you to option 3. Review the normal vital signs for a 3-year-old if you had difficulty with this question.
Level of Cognitive Ability: Applying
Client Needs: Physiological Integrity
Integrated Process: Nursing Process—Implementation
Content Area: Fundamental Skills—Developmental Stages
Reference: McKinney, E., James, S., Murray, S., & Ashwill, J. (2009). *Maternal-child nursing* (3rd ed., pp. 817, 1272). St. Louis: Saunders.

336. 2
Rationale: Children should remain in a booster seat until they are 8 to 12 years old and at least 4 feet, 9 inches tall. Infants should ride in a car in a semireclined, rear-facing position in an infant-only seat or a convertible seat until they weigh at least 20 pounds and are at least 1 year of age. The transition point for switching to the forward-facing position is defined by the manufacturer of the convertible car safety seat but is generally at a body weight of 9 kg (20 pounds) and 1 year of age.
Test-Taking Strategy: Note the age and height of the child to identify the appropriate safety device. Remember that children should remain in a booster seat until they are 8 to 12 years old and at least 4 feet, 9 inches tall. If you had difficulty with this question, review the physical development requirements for car safety devices.
Level of Cognitive Ability: Understanding
Client Needs: Safe and Effective Care Environment
Integrated Process: Nursing Process—Planning
Content Area: Fundamental Skills—Developmental Stages
Reference: McKinney, E., James, S., Murray, S., & Ashwill, J. (2009). *Maternal-child nursing* (3rd ed., p. 119). St. Louis: Saunders.

337. 3
Rationale: The normal respiratory rate in a 12-month-old infant is 20 to 40 breaths/min. The normal apical heart

rate is 90 to 130 beats/min, and the average blood pressure is 90/56 mm Hg. The nurse would document the findings.
Test-Taking Strategy: Focus on the data in the question. Recalling the normal vital signs of an infant and noting that the respiratory rate identified in the question is within the normal range will direct you to the correct option. If you had difficulty with this question, review the normal vital signs for an infant.
Level of Cognitive Ability: Applying
Client Needs: Physiological Integrity
Integrated Process: Nursing Process—Implementation
Content Area: Fundamental Skills—Developmental Stages
References: Hockenberry, M., & Wilson, D. (2009). *Wong's essentials of pediatric nursing* (8th ed., p. 129). St. Louis: Mosby.
   McKinney, E., James, S., Murray, S., & Ashwill, J. (2009). *Maternal-child nursing* (3rd ed., p. 817). St. Louis: Saunders.

338. 3
Rationale: The anterior fontanel is diamond-shaped and located on the top of the head. The fontanel should be soft and flat in a normal infant, and it normally closes by 12 to 18 months of age. The nurse would document the finding because it is normal. There is no useful reason to increase oral fluids, notify the physician, or elevate the head of the bed to 90 degrees.
Test-Taking Strategy: Use the process of elimination and note the strategic words *soft* and *flat*. This should provide you with the clue that this is a normal finding. A bulging or tense fontanel may result from crying or increased intracranial pressure. If you had difficulty with this question, review normal assessment findings in an infant related to the fontanels.
Level of Cognitive Ability: Applying
Client Needs: Health Promotion and Maintenance
Integrated Process: Nursing Process—Implementation
Content Area: Fundamental Skills—Developmental Stages
Reference: McKinney, E., James, S., Murray, S., & Ashwill, J. (2009). *Maternal-child nursing* (3rd ed., p. 1468). St. Louis: Saunders.

339. 2
Rationale: By age 2 years, the child can use a cup and spoon correctly but with some spilling. By age 3 to 4, the child begins to use a fork. By the end of the preschool period, the child should be able to pour milk into a cup and begin to use a knife for cutting.
Test-Taking Strategy: Note the age of the child and use the process of elimination. Option 4 can be eliminated first because of the word *knife*. Next, think about the fine motor skills that need to be developed in selecting the correct option. With this in mind, eliminate options 1 and 3. If you had difficulty with this question, review the developmental skills of a 2-year-old.
Level of Cognitive Ability: Understanding
Client Needs: Health Promotion and Maintenance
Integrated Process: Nursing Process—Assessment
Content Area: Fundamental Skills—Developmental Stages
Reference: McKinney, E., James, S., Murray, S., & Ashwill, J. (2009). *Maternal-child nursing* (3rd ed., p. 110). St. Louis: Saunders.

340. 1

Rationale: Toddlers, with their increased mobility and development of motor skills, can reach hot water or hot objects placed on counters and stoves and can reach open fires or stove burners above their eye level. The nurse should encourage parents to remain in the kitchen when preparing a meal, use the back burners on the stove, and turn pot handles inward and toward the middle of the stove. Hot liquids should never be left unattended or within the child's reach, and the toddler should always be supervised. The statements in options 2, 3, and 4 do not indicate an understanding of the principles of safety.
Test-Taking Strategy: Use the process of elimination, noting the strategic words *indicates an understanding*. Option 2 can be eliminated because it is mandating that the toddler understand what is and what is not safe. The toddler is not developmentally able to understand danger. Options 3 and 4 are comparable or alike in that they isolate the child from the environment. Option 1 is the only option that reflects an understanding of safety principles by the parents. Review the home safety principles for the toddler if you had difficulty with this question.
Level of Cognitive Ability: Evaluating
Client Needs: Safe and Effective Care Environment
Integrated Process: Nursing Process—Evaluation
Content Area: Fundamental Skills—Developmental Stages
Reference: McKinney, E., James, S., Murray, S., & Ashwill, J. (2009). *Maternal-child nursing* (3rd ed., p. 120). St. Louis: Saunders.

341. 4

Rationale: Toddlers often resist going to bed. Bedtime protests may be reduced by establishing a consistent before-bedtime routine and enforcing consistent limits regarding the child's bedtime behavior. Informing the child of bedtime a few minutes before it is time for bed is the most appropriate option. Most toddlers take an afternoon nap and, until their second birthday, also may require a morning nap. Firm, consistent limits are needed for temper tantrums or when toddlers try stalling tactics.
Test-Taking Strategy: Use the process of elimination. Eliminate options 1, 2, and 3 by using concepts related to growth and development. Remember that preparing the toddler for an event will minimize resistive behavior. Review concepts related to sleep patterns and the toddler if you had difficulty with this question.
Level of Cognitive Ability: Applying
Client Needs: Health Promotion and Maintenance
Integrated Process: Teaching and Learning
Content Area: Fundamental Skills—Developmental Stages
Reference: Hockenberry, M., & Wilson, D. (2009). *Wong's essentials of pediatric nursing* (8th ed., p. 424). St. Louis: Mosby.

342. 1

Rationale: Toys for the toddler must be strong, safe, and too large to swallow or place in the ear or nose. Toddlers need supervision at all times. Push-pull toys, large balls, large crayons, large trucks, and dolls are some of the appropriate toys. A farm set, a golf set, and jacks with marbles may contain items that the child could swallow.

Test-Taking Strategy: Use the process of elimination and focus on the subject, the appropriate toy for a 3-year-old. Options 2, 3, and 4 can be eliminated because they are comparable or alike and could contain items that the child could swallow. Remember that large and strong toys are safest for the toddler. Review the safety principles related to play activities and the toddler if you had difficulty with this question.
Level of Cognitive Ability: Applying
Client Needs: Safe and Effective Care Environment
Integrated Process: Teaching and Learning
Content Area: Fundamental Skills—Developmental Stages
Reference: Hockenberry, M., & Wilson, D. (2009). *Wong's essentials of pediatric nursing* (8th ed., p. 416). St. Louis: Mosby.

343. 2

Rationale: A toddler should never be allowed to fall asleep with a bottle containing milk, juice, soda pop, sweetened water, or any other sweet liquid because of the risk of nursing (bottle-mouth) caries. If a bottle is allowed at nap time or bedtime, it should contain only water.
Test-Taking Strategy: Use the process of elimination. Eliminate options 3 and 4 first because they are comparable or alike statements. From the remaining options, recalling that nursing (bottle-mouth) caries is a concern in a child will assist in directing you to option 2. Review dental health principles related to children if you had difficulty with this question.
Level of Cognitive Ability: Applying
Client Needs: Health Promotion and Maintenance
Integrated Process: Teaching and Learning
Content Area: Fundamental Skills—Developmental Stages
Reference: Hockenberry, M., & Wilson, D. (2009). *Wong's essentials of pediatric nursing* (8th ed., p. 426). St. Louis: Mosby.

344. 4

Rationale: In the preschooler, play is simple and imaginative, and includes activities such as crayons and coloring books, puppets, felt and magnetic boards, and Play-Doh. A radio or sports video are most appropriate for the adolescent. Large picture books are most appropriate for the infant.
Test-Taking Strategy: Note the age of the child, and think about the age-related activity that would be most appropriate. Eliminate options 1 and 2, knowing that they are most appropriate for the adolescent. From the remaining options, the word *large* in option 3 should provide you with the clue that this activity would be more appropriate for a child younger than age 5. If you had difficulty with this question, review the appropriate play activities for a preschooler.
Level of Cognitive Ability: Applying
Client Needs: Health Promotion and Maintenance
Integrated Process: Nursing Process—Planning
Content Area: Fundamental Skills—Developmental Stages
Reference: Hockenberry, M., & Wilson, D. (2009). *Wong's essentials of pediatric nursing* (8th ed., pp. 673–674). St. Louis: Mosby.

ALTERNATE ITEM FORMAT: MULTIPLE RESPONSE

345. 1, 4, 5

Rationale: Holding, caressing, and swaddling provide warmth and tactile stimulation for the infant. To provide auditory stimulation, the nurse should talk to the infant in a soft voice and should instruct the mother to do so also. Additional interventions include playing a music box, radio, or television, or having a ticking clock or metronome nearby. Hanging a bright shiny object in midline within 20 to 25 cm of the infant's face and hanging mobiles with contrasting colors, such as black and white, provide visual stimulation. Crying is an infant's way of communicating; therefore the nurse would respond to the infant's crying. The mother is taught to do so also. An infant or child should never be allowed to fall asleep with a bottle containing milk, juice, soda pop, sweetened water, or another sweet liquid because of the risk of nursing (bottle-mouth) caries.

Test-Taking Strategy: Focus on the subject, care of the infant. Noting the word *loud* and the words *at least 10 minutes before responding* will assist in eliminating these interventions. Also, recalling the concerns related to dental caries will assist in eliminating option 3. Review the guidelines related to the care of an infant if you had difficulty with this question.

Level of Cognitive Ability: Applying
Client Needs: Health Promotion and Maintenance
Integrated Process: Nursing Process—Implementation
Content Area: Fundamental Skills—Developmental Stages
References: Hockenberry, M., & Wilson, D. (2009). *Wong's essentials of pediatric nursing* (8th ed., p. 103). St. Louis: Mosby.

McKinney, E., James, S., Murray, S., & Ashwill, J. (2009). *Maternal-child nursing* (3rd ed., pp. 486–488). St. Louis: Saunders.

Health and Physical Assessment of the Adult Client

I. ENVIRONMENT/SETTING

A. Establish a relationship and explain the procedure to the client.

B. Ensure privacy and make the client feel comfortable (comfortable room temperature, sufficient lighting, remove distractions such as noise or objects, avoid interruptions).

C. Sit down for the interview (avoid barriers such as a desk), maintain an appropriate social distance, and maintain eye level.

D. Use therapeutic communication techniques and open-ended questions to obtain information about the client's symptoms and concerns; allow time for the client to ask questions.

E. Consider religious and cultural characteristics such as language (the need for an interpreter), values and beliefs, health practices, eye contact, and touch.

F. Keep note-taking to a minimum so the client is the focus of attention.

G. Types of health and physical assessments (Box 34-1)

II. HEALTH HISTORY

A. General state of health: Body features and physical characteristics, body movements, body posture, level of consciousness, nutritional status, speech

B. Chief complaint and history of present illness (direct client quotes) that directs the client to seek care

C. Family history: The health status of direct blood relatives as well as the client's spouse

D. Social history
  1. Data about the client's lifestyle with a focus on factors that may impact health.
  2. Information about alcohol, drug, and tobacco use; sexual practices; tattoos; body piercing; travel history; and work setting to identify occupational hazards

E. Domestic violence screening
  1. Done to determine if the client is experiencing any form of domestic violence.
  2. Conducted during a one-to-one interview with client while obtaining the health history.

III. MENTAL STATUS EXAM

A. The mental status can be assessed while obtaining **subjective data** from the client during the health history interview.

B. Appearance
  1. Note appearance, including posture, body movements, dress, and hygiene and grooming.
  2. An inappropriate appearance and poor hygiene may be indicative of **depression**, manic disorder, **dementia**, organic brain disease, or another disorder.

C. Behavior
  1. Level of consciousness: Assess alertness and awareness and the client's ability to interact appropriately with the environment.
  2. Facial expression and body language: Check for appropriate eye contact and determine whether facial expression and body language are appropriate to the situation; this assessment also provides information regarding the client's mood and affect.
  3. Speech: Assess speech pattern for articulation and appropriateness of conversation.

D. Cognitive level of functioning (Box 34-2)

IV. PHYSICAL EXAM

A. Overview
  1. Gather equipment needed for the examination.
  2. Use the senses of sight, smell, touch, and hearing to collect data.
  3. Assessment includes **inspection, palpation, percussion**, and **auscultation**; these skills are performed one at a time, in this order (except the abdominal assessment).

B. Assessment techniques
  1. **Inspection**
     a. The first assessment technique, which uses vision and smell senses while observing the client
     b. Requires good lighting, adequate exposure, and possibly the use of certain instruments such as an otoscope or ophthalmoscope
  2. **Palpation**
     a. Uses the sense of touch; warm the hands before touching the client.

Box 34-1 Types of Health and Physical Assessments

Complete assessment: Includes a complete health history and physical examination and forms a baseline database.

Focused assessment: Focuses on a limited or short-term problem, such as the client's complaint.

Episodic/follow-up assessment: Focuses on evaluating a client's progress.

Emergency assessment: Involves the rapid collection of data, often during the provision of lifesaving measures.

Box 34-2 The Mental-Status Examination: Cognitive Level of Functioning

Orientation: Assess client's orientation to person, place, and time.

Attention span: Assess client's ability to concentrate.

Recent memory: Assessed by asking the client to recall a recent occurrence (e.g., the means of transportation used to get to the health care agency for the physical assessment).

Remote memory: Assessed by asking the client about a verifiable past event (e.g., a vacation).

New learning: Used to assess the client's ability to recall unrelated words identified by the nurse; nurse selects four words and asks the client to recall the words 5, 10, and 30 minutes later.

Judgment: Determine whether the client's actions or decisions regarding discussions during the interview are realistic.

Thought processes and perceptions: The way the client thinks and what the client says should be logical, coherent, and relevant; the client should be consistently aware of reality.

Box 34-3 Characteristics of Skin Color

Cyanosis: Mottled bluish coloration
Erythema: Redness
Pallor: Pale, whitish coloration
Jaundice: Yellow coloration

Box 34-4 Assessing Capillary Filling Time

Depress the nail bed to produce blanching.
Release and observe for the return of color.
Color will return within 3 seconds if arterial capillary perfusion is normal.

C. Vital signs
   1. Includes temperature, radial pulse (apical pulse may be measured during the cardiovascular assessment), respirations, blood pressure, pulse oximetry, and presence of pain
   2. Height and weight and nutritional status are also assessed.

V. BODY SYSTEMS ASSESSMENT

A. Integumentary system: Involves **inspection** and **palpation** of skin, hair, and nails.
   1. **Subjective data:** Self-care behaviors, history of skin disease, medications being taken, environmental or occupational hazards and exposure to toxic substances, changes in skin color or pigmentation, change in a mole or a sore that does not heal
   2. **Objective data:** Color, temperature (hypothermia or hyperthermia); excessive dryness or moisture; skin turgor; texture (smoothness, firmness); excessive bruising, itching, rash; hair loss (alopecia) or nail abnormalities such as pitting; lesions (may be inspected with a magnifier and light or with the use of a Wood's light [ultraviolet light used in a darkened room]; scars or birthmarks; edema; capillary filling time (Boxes 34-3 and 34-4; Table 34-1)

⚠ To test skin turgor, pinch a large fold of skin and assess the ability of the skin to return to its place when released. Poor turgor occurs in severe dehydration or extreme weight loss.

   3. Client teaching
      a. Provide information about factors that can be harmful to the skin, such as sun exposure.
      b. Encourage performing self-examination of the skin monthly.

B. Head, neck, and lymph nodes: Involves **inspection** and **palpation** of the head, neck, and lymph nodes
   1. Ask the client about headaches, episodes of dizziness (lightheadedness) or vertigo (spinning

   b. Identify tender areas and palpate them last.
   c. Start with light palpation to detect surface characteristics, then perform deeper palpation.
   d. Assess texture, temperature, and moisture of the skin, as well as organ location and size.
   e. Assess for swelling, vibration or pulsation, rigidity or spasticity, and crepitation.
   f. Assess for the presence of lumps or masses, as well as the presence of tenderness or pain.

   3. **Percussion**
      a. Involves tapping the client's skin to assess underlying structures and to determine vibrations and sounds related to intensity, duration, pitch, quality, and location.
      b. Provides information related to the presence of air, fluid, or solid masses as well as organ size, shape and position.
   4. **Auscultation:** Involves listening to sounds produced by the body, such as heart, lung, or bowel sounds

TABLE 34-1 Pitting Edema Scale

Scale	Description	"Measurement"*
1 +	A barely perceptible pit	2 mm (³⁄₃₂ in)
2 +	A deeper pit, rebounds in a few seconds	4 mm (⁶⁄₃₂ in)
3 +	A deep pit, rebounds in 10-20 seconds	6 mm (¼ in)
4 +	A deeper pit, rebounds in >30 seconds	8 mm (⁵⁄₁₆ in)

+1 — 2 mm   +2 — 4 mm   +3 — 6 mm   +4 — 8 mm   G.J.Wassilchenko

*"Measurement" is in quotation marks because depth of edema is rarely actually measured but is included as a frame of reference.
From Wilson, A., & Giddens, J., (2009). *Health assessment for nursing practice* (4th ed., p. 255). St. Louis: Mosby. Descriptions column data from Kirton, C. Assessing edema, *Nursing 96* 26(7):54, 1996. Illustrations from Canobblo, M. (1990). *Cardiovascular disorders*. St. Louis: Mosby.

sensation), history of head injury, loss of consciousness, seizures, episodes of neck pain, limitations of range of motion, numbness or tingling in the shoulders, arms, or hands, lumps or swelling in the neck, difficulty swallowing, medications being taken, and history of surgery in the head and neck region.

2. Head
   a. Inspect and palpate: Size, shape, masses or tenderness, and symmetry of the skull
   b. Palpate temporal arteries, located above the cheekbone between the eye and the top of the ear.
   c. Temporomandibular joint: Ask the client to open his or her mouth; note any crepitation, tenderness, or limited range of motion.
   d. Face: Inspect facial structures for shape, symmetry, involuntary movements, or swelling, such as periorbital edema (swelling around the eyes).
3. Neck
   a. Inspect for symmetry of accessory neck muscles.
   b. Assess range of motion.
   c. Test cranial nerve XI (spinal accessory nerve) to assess muscle strength: Ask the client to rotate the head forcibly against resistance applied to the side of the chin; also ask the client to shrug the shoulders against resistance.
   d. Palpate the trachea: It should be midline, without any deviations.
   e. Thyroid gland: Inspect the neck as the client takes a sip of water and swallows (thyroid tissue moves up with a swallow); palpate using an anterior-posterior approach (usually the normal adult thyroid cannot be palpated); if it is enlarged, auscultate for a bruit.
4. Lymph nodes
   a. Palpate using a gentle pressure and a circular motion of the finger pads.

   b. Begin with the preauricular lymph nodes (in front of the ear); move to the posterior auricular lymph nodes and then downward toward the supraclavicular lymph nodes.
   c. Palpate with both hands, comparing the two sides for symmetry.
   d. If nodes are palpated, note their size, shape, location, mobility, consistency, and tenderness.
5. Client teaching: Instruct the client to notify the health care provider if persistent headache, dizziness, or neck pain occurs, if swelling or lumps are noted in the head and neck region, or if a neck or head injury occurs.

⚠ Neck movements are never performed if the client has sustained a neck injury or a neck injury is suspected.

C. Eyes: Includes **inspection, palpation,** vision-testing procedures, and the use of an ophthalmoscope
   1. **Subjective data:** Difficulty with vision (e.g., decreased acuity, double vision, blurring, blind spots); pain, redness, swelling, watery or other discharge from the eye; use of glasses or contact lenses; medications being taken; history of eye problems
   2. **Objective data**
      a. Inspect the external eye structures, including eyebrows, for symmetry; eyelashes for even distribution; eyelids for ptosis (drooping); eyeballs for exophthalmos (protrusion) or enophthalmos (sunken).
      b. Inspect the conjunctiva (should be clear), sclera (should be white), and lacrimal apparatus (check for excessive tearing, redness, tenderness, or swelling); cornea and lens (should be smooth and clear); iris (should

be flat, with a round regular shape and even coloration); eyelids, and pupils (Box 34-5)

3. Snellen eye chart
   a. Position the client in a well-lit spot 20 feet from the chart, with the chart at eye level, and ask the client to read the smallest line that he or she can discern.
   b. Instruct the client to leave on glasses or leave in contact lenses; if the glasses are for reading only, they are removed because they blur distant vision.
   c. Test one eye at a time
   d. Record result using the fraction at the end of the last line successfully read on the chart.
   e. Normal visual acuity is 20/20 (distance in feet at which the client is standing from the chart/distance in feet at which a normal eye could have read that particular line).

4. Near vision
   a. Use a hand-held vision screener (held about 14 inches from the eye) that contains various sizes of print or ask the client to read from a magazine.
   b. Test each eye separately with the client's glasses on or contact lenses in.
   c. Normal result is 14/14 (distance in inches at which the subject holds the card from the eye/distance in inches at which a normal eye could have read that particular line).

5. Confrontation test
   a. Used to measure peripheral vision and compare the client's peripheral vision with the nurse's (assuming that the nurse's peripheral vision is normal)
   b. The client covers one eye and looks straight ahead; the nurse, positioned 2 feet away, covers his or her eye opposite the client's covered eye.
   c. The nurse advances a finger or other small object in from the periphery from several directions; the client should see the object at the same time the nurse does.

6. Corneal light reflex
   a. Used to assess for parallel alignment of the axes of the eyes
   b. Client is asked to gaze straight ahead as the nurse holds a light about 12 inches from the client
   c. The nurse looks for reflection of the light on the corneas in exactly the same spot in each eye

7. Cover test
   a. Used to check for slight degrees of deviated alignment
   b. Each eye is tested separately.
   c. The nurse asks the client to gaze straight ahead and cover one eye.
   d. The nurse examines the uncovered eye, expecting to note a steady, fixed gaze

8. Six cardinal positions of gaze
   a. Used to check for muscle weakness in the eyes
   b. The client is asked to hold the head steady, then follow movement of an object through the positions of gaze.
   c. The client should follow the object in a parallel manner with the two eyes.
   d. Assess for nystagmus, an oscillating movement of the eye, best noted around the iris.

9. Color vision
   a. Ishihara chart is a tool used to assess color vision; it determines the client's ability to distinguish a pattern of color (a number) in a series of color plates.
   b. The nurse tests each eye separately and asks the client to identify the number that he or she sees on the chart.
   c. The ability to read the number correctly depends on the normal functioning of color vision.

10. Examination of the internal structures
    a. An ophthalmoscope is used to inspect the fundus, including the retina, choroids, optic nerve disc, macula, fovea centralis, and retinal vessels.
    b. The nurse inspects the size, color, and clarity of the disc, the integrity of the vessels, and the appearance of the macula, and fovea and looks for retinal lesions
    c. Performed in a darkened room

d. The client's eyeglasses are removed (contact lenses are left in place)

e. The nurse and the client face each other with the eyes at the same height, the ophthalmoscope light is switched on, and the lens is rotated to 0.

f. As the client gazes straight ahead with both eyes open, the nurse (standing about 10 inches from the client and about 25 degrees lateral to the client's central line of vision) shines the light on the pupil.

g. A bright-orange glow (red reflex) can be seen by the nurse; the nurse slowly moves toward the pupil, focusing on the red reflex.

h. Rotating the lens on the ophthalmoscope, the nurse brings the internal structures into focus.

11. Client teaching

a. Instruct the client to notify the health care provider if alterations in vision occur or any redness, swelling, or drainage from the eye is noted.

b. Inform the client of the importance of regular eye examinations.

D. Ears: Includes **inspection**, **palpation**, hearing tests, and the use of an otoscope

1. **Subjective data**: Difficulty hearing, earaches, drainage from the ears, dizziness, ringing in the ears, exposure to environment noise, use of a hearing aid, medications being taken, history of ear problems or infections

2. **Objective data**

a. Inspect and palpate the external ear, noting size, shape, symmetry, skin color, and the presence of pain.

b. Inspect the external auditory meatus for size, swelling, redness, discharge, and foreign bodies; some cerumen (ear wax) may be present.

3. Conductive and sensorineural hearing loss

a. A conductive hearing loss occurs as a result of a physical obstruction to the transmission of sound waves.

b. A sensorineural hearing loss occurs as a result of a pathological process in the inner ear or of the sensory fibers that lead to the cerebral cortex.

4. Voice test

a. Used to determine whether hearing loss has occurred

b. One ear is tested at a time (the ear not being tested is occluded by the client)

c. The nurse stands 1 to 2 feet from the client, covers his or her mouth so that the client cannot read the lips, exhales fully, and softly whispers two-syllable words in the direction of the unoccluded ear; the client points a finger up during the test when the

nurse's voice is heard (a ticking watch may also be used to test hearing acuity).

5. Pure-tone audiometry testing: Provides a precise quantitative measure of hearing by assessing the client's ability to hear sounds of varying frequencies (done by a person skilled in performing audiometry testing)

6. Tuning fork tests

a. Used to measure hearing on the basis of air conduction or bone conduction; includes the Weber and Rinne tests

b. To activate the tuning fork, the nurse holds the base and lightly taps the tines against the other hand, setting the fork in vibration.

7. Weber test

a. Stem of the vibrating tuning fork is placed in the midline of the client's skull and the client is asked if the tone sounds the same in both ears or better in one ear.

b. The client hears the tone by bone conduction and the sound should be heard equally in both ears.

8. Rinne test

a. Stem of the vibrating tuning fork is placed on the client's mastoid process.

b. When the client no longer hears the sound, the tuning fork is quickly inverted and placed near the ear canal; the client should still hear a sound.

c. Normally the sound is heard twice as long by way of air conduction (near the ear canal) than by way of bone conduction (at the mastoid process).

9. Otoscopic exam

a. An otoscope is used; for best visualization, the largest speculum that fits comfortably into the client's ear canal should be used.

b. The nurse asks the client to tilt the head slightly away, to the opposite shoulder; next the nurse pulls the pinna up and back (on an adult or older child), holds the otoscope upside down, and inserts the speculum slightly down and forward, approximately half an inch, into the ear canal.

c. The normal tympanic membrane is translucent, shiny, and pearly gray.

⚠ Before performing an otoscopic exam and inserting the speculum, check the auditory canal for foreign bodies. Instruct the client not to move the head during the examination to avoid damage to the canal and tympanic membrane.

10. Client teaching

a. Instruct the client to notify the health care provider if an alteration in hearing or ear pain or ringing in the ears occurs, or redness, swelling, or drainage from the ear is noted.

b. Instruct the client in the proper method of cleaning the ear canal.

c. The client should cleanse the ear canal with the corner of a moistened washcloth and should never insert sharp objects or cotton-tipped applicators into the ear canal.

E. Nose, mouth, and throat: Includes **inspection** and **palpation**

1. **Subjective data**

a. Nose: Ask about discharge or nosebleed (epistaxis); facial or sinus pain; history of frequent colds; altered sense of smell; allergies; medications being taken; history of nose trauma or surgery.

b. Mouth and throat: Ask about the presence of sores or lesions; bleeding from the gums or elsewhere; altered sense of taste; toothaches; use of dentures or other appliances; tooth- and mouth-care hygiene habits; at-risk behaviors (e.g., smoking, alcohol consumption); history of infection, trauma, or surgery.

2. **Objective data**

a. External nose should be midline and in proportion to other facial features.

b. Patency of the nostrils can be tested by pushing each nasal cavity closed and asking the client to sniff inward through the other nostril.

c. Use of a nasal speculum and penlight or a short, wide-tipped speculum attached to an otoscope head is used to inspect for redness, swelling, discharge, bleeding, or foreign bodies; the nasal septum is assessed for deviation.

d. The nurse presses the frontal sinuses (located below the eyebrows) and over the maxillary sinuses (located below the cheekbones); the client should feel firm pressure but no pain.

e. The external and inner surfaces of the lips are assessed for color, moisture, cracking, or lesions.

f. The teeth are inspected for condition and number (should be white, spaced evenly, straight, and clean, free of debris and decay).

g. The alignment of the upper and lower jaw is assessed by having the client bite down.

h. The gums are inspected for swelling, bleeding, discoloration, and retraction of gingival margins (gums normally appear pink).

i. The tongue is inspected for color, surface characteristics, moisture, white patches, nodules, and ulcerations (dorsal surface is normally rough; ventral surface is smooth and glistening, with visible veins).

j. The nurse retracts the cheek with a tongue depressor to check for the buccal mucosa for color and the presence of nodules or lesions; normal mucosa is glistening, pink, soft, moist, and smooth.

k. Using a penlight and tongue depressor, the nurse inspects the hard and soft palates for color, shape, texture, and defects; the hard palate (roof of the mouth), which is located anteriorly, should be white and dome-shaped, and the soft palate, which extends posteriorly, should be light pink and smooth.

l. The uvula is inspected for midline location; the nurse asks the client to say "ahhh" and watches for the soft palate and uvula to rise in the midline (this tests one function of cranial nerve X, the vagus nerve).

m. Using a penlight and tongue depressor, the nurse inspects the throat for color, presence of tonsils, and the presence of exudate or lesions; cranial nerve XII is tested (the hypoglossal nerve) by asking the client to stick out the tongue (should protrude in the midline).

3. Client teaching

a. Emphasize the importance of hygiene and tooth care, as well as regular dental examinations and the use of fluoridated water or fluoride supplements.

b. Encourage the client to avoid at-risk behaviors (e.g., smoking, alcohol consumption).

c. Stress the importance of reporting pain or abnormal occurrence (e.g., nodules, lesions, signs of infection).

F. Lungs

1. **Subjective data**: Cough; expectoration of sputum; shortness of breath or dyspnea; chest pain on breathing; smoking history; environmental exposure to pollution or chemicals; medications being taken; history of respiratory disease or infection; last tuberculosis test, chest radiograph, pneumonia, and any influenza immunizations including the H1N1 vaccine (H and N refer to *hemagglutanin* and *neuraminadase*, respectively, which are surface antigens, and the number 1 refers to the specific subtype of those antigens).

2. **Objective data**: Includes **inspection**, **palpation**, **percussion**, and **auscultation**

3. **Inspection** of the anterior and posterior chest: Note skin color and condition and the rate and quality of respirations, look for lumps or lesions, note the shape and configuration of the chest wall, note the position the client takes to breathe.

4. **Palpation**: Palpate the entire chest wall, noting skin temperature and moisture and looking for areas of tenderness and lumps, lesions, or masses; assess chest excursion and tactile or vocal fremitus (Box 34-6).

5. **Percussion**

a. Starting at the apices, percuss across the top of the shoulders, moving to the interspaces, making a side-to-side comparison all the way down the lung area (Fig. 34-1).

Box 34-6 Palpation of the Chest

Chest Excursion

Posterior: The nurse places the thumbs along the spinal processes at the 10th rib, with the palms in light contact with the posterolateral surfaces.

The nurse's thumbs should be about 2 inches apart, pointing toward the spine, with the fingers pointing laterally

Anterior: The nurse places the hands on the anterolateral wall with the thumbs along the costal margins, pointing toward the xiphoid process.

The nurse instructs the client to take a deep breath after exhaling.

Normal Findings

The nurse notes movement of the thumbs.

Chest excursion should be symmetrical, separating the thumbs approximately 2 inches.

Tactile or Vocal Fremitus

The nurse places the ball or lower palm of the hand over the chest.

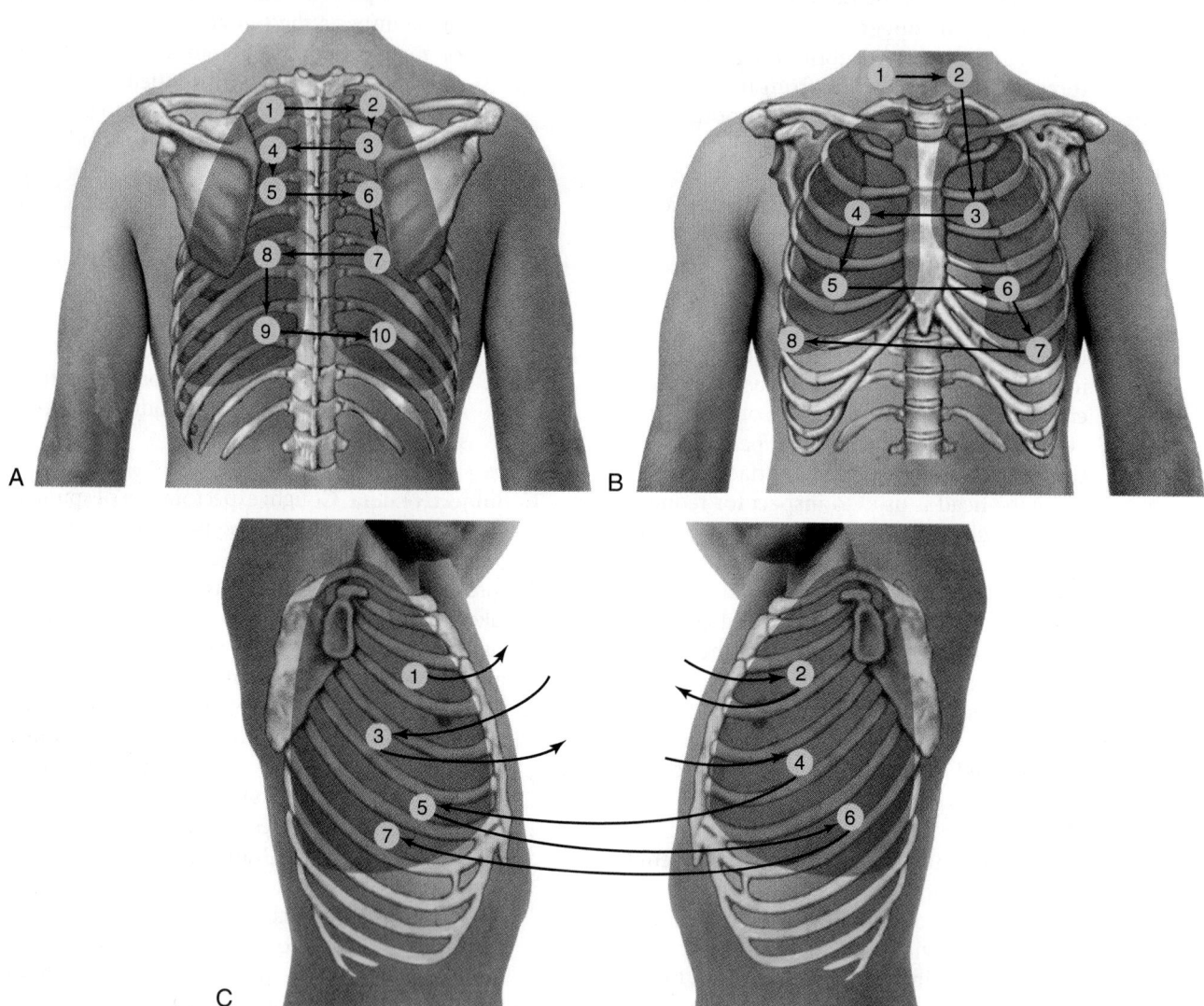

▲ FIGURE 34-1 Landmarks for chest auscultation and percussion. **A,** Posterior view. **B,** Anterior view. **C,** Lateral view. (From Wilson, A. F., & Giddens, J. F. [2009]. *Health assessment for nursing practice* (4th ed., p. 218). St. Louis: Mosby).

    b. Determine the predominant note; resonance is noted in healthy lung tissue.

    c. Hyperresonance is noted when excessive air is present and a dull note indicates lung density.

  6. **Auscultation**

    a. Use the flat diaphragm end piece of the stethoscope, hold it firmly against the chest

wall, and listen to at least one full respiration in each location (anterior, posterior, and lateral).

    b. Posterior: Start at the apices and move side to side for comparison (see Fig. 34-1)

    c. Anterior: Auscultate the lung fields from the apices in the supraclavicular area down

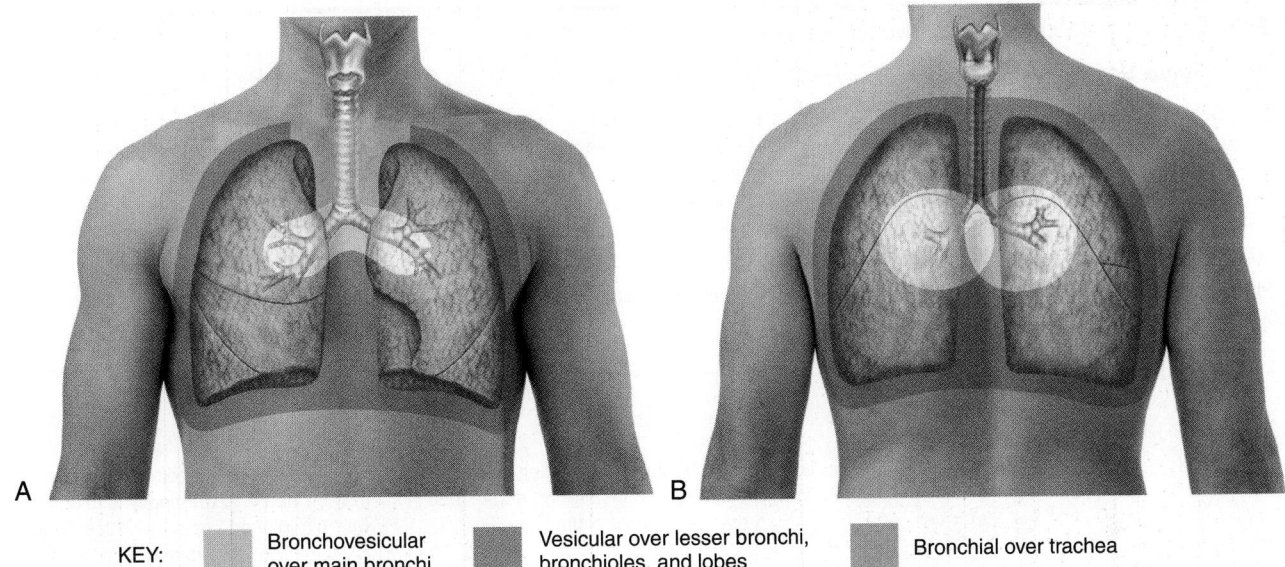

KEY: | Bronchovesicular over main bronchi | Vesicular over lesser bronchi, bronchioles, and lobes | Bronchial over trachea

▲ **FIGURE 34-2** Auscultatory sounds. **A,** Anterior thorax. **B,** Posterior thorax. (From Wilson, A. F., & Giddens, J. F. [2009]. *Health assessment for nursing practice* [4th ed., p. 219]. St. Louis: Mosby).

to the sixth rib; avoid **percussion** and **auscultation** over female breast tissue (displace this tissue) because a dull sound will be produced (see Fig. 34-1).

   d. Compare findings on each side.

7. Normal breath sounds: Three types of breath sounds are considered normal in certain parts of the thorax, including vesicular, bronchovesicular, and bronchial; breath sounds should be clear to **auscultation** (Fig. 34-2).

8. Abnormal breath sounds: Also known as adventitious sounds (Table 34-2)

9. Voice sounds (Box 34-7)
   a. Performed when a pathological lung condition is suspected
   b. Auscultate over the chest wall; the client is asked to vocalize words or a phrase while the nurse listens to the chest.
   c. Normal voice transmission is soft and muffled; the nurse can hear the sound but is unable to distinguish exactly what is being said.

⚠ When auscultating breath sounds, instruct the client to breathe through the mouth and monitor the client for dizziness.

10. Client teaching
   a. Encourage the client to avoid exposure to environmental hazards, including smoking (discuss smoking cessation programs as appropriate).
   b. Client should undergo periodic examinations as prescribed (e.g., chest x-ray study, tuberculosis skin testing).

   c. Encourage the client to obtain pneumonia and influenza immunizations.
   d. Health care provider should be notified if client experiences persistent cough, shortness of breath, or other respiratory symptoms.

G. Heart and peripheral vascular system
1. **Subjective data**: Chest pain, dyspnea, cough, fatigue, edema, nocturia, leg pain or cramps (claudication), changes in skin color, obesity, medications being taken, cardiovascular risk factors, family history of cardiac or vascular problems, personal history of cardiac or vascular problems

2. **Objective data**: May include **inspection, palpation, percussion**, and **auscultation**

3. **Inspection**: Inspect the anterior chest for pulsations (apical impulse) created as the left ventricle rotates against the chest wall during systole; not always visible.

4. **Palpation**
   a. Palpate the apical impulse at the fourth or fifth interspace, or medial to the midclavicular line (not palpable in obese clients or clients with thick chest walls).
   b. Palpate the apex, left sternal border, and base for pulsations; normally none are present.

5. **Percussion**: May be performed to outline the heart's borders and to check for cardiac enlargement (denoted by resonance over the lung and dull notes over the heart).

6. **Auscultation**
   a. Areas of the heart (Fig. 34-3)
   b. Auscultate heart rate and rhythm; check for a pulse deficit (auscultate the apical heartbeat while palpating an artery) if an irregularity is noted.

TABLE 34-2 Characteristics of Adventitious Sounds

Adventitious Sounds	Characteristics	Clinical Examples
Crackles (previously called *rales*) fine crackles	Fine. high-pitched crackling and popping noises (discontinuous sounds) heard during the end of inspiration. Not cleared by cough.	May be heard in pneumonia, heart failure, asthma, and restrictive pulmonary diseases.
Medium crackles	Medium-pitched, moist sound heard about halfway through inspiration. Not cleared by cough.	Same as above, but condition is worse.
Coarse crackles	Low-pitched, bubbling or gurgling sounds that start early in inspiration and extend into the first part of expiration.	Same as above, but condition is worse or may be heard in terminally ill clients with diminished gag reflex. Also heard in pulmonary edema and pulmonary fibrosis.
Wheeze (also called *sibilant* wheeze)	High-pitched, musical sound similar to a squeak. Heard more commonly during expiration, but may also be heard during inspiration. Occurs in small airways.	Heard in narrowed airway diseases such as asthma.
Rhonchi (also called *sonorous* wheeze)	Low-pitched, coarse, loud, low snoring or moaning tone. Actually sounds like snoring. Heard primarily during expiration, but may also be heard during inspiration. Coughing may clear.	Heard in disorders causing obstruction of the trachea or bronchus, such as chronic bronchitis.
Pleural friction rub	A superficial, low-pitched, coarse rubbing or grating sound. Sounds like two surfaces rubbing together. Heard throughout inspiration and expiration. Loudest over the lower anterolateral surface. Not cleared by cough.	Heard in individuals with pleurisy (inflammation of the pleural surfaces).

From Wilson, A. F., & Giddens, J. F. (2009). *Health assessment for nursing practice* (4th ed., p. 221). St. Louis: Mosby.

Box 34-7 Voice Sounds

Bronchophony
Ask the client to repeat the words "ninety-nine."
Normal voice transmission is soft, muffled, and indistinct.

Egophony
Ask the client to repeat a long "ee-ee-ee" sound.
Normally the nurse would hear the "ee-ee-ee" sound.

Whispered Pectoriloquy
Ask the client to whisper the word "ninety-nine."
Normal voice transmission is faint, muffled, and almost inaudible.

c. Assess S1 ("lub") and S2 ("dub") sounds, and listen for extra heart sounds, as well as the presence of murmurs (gentle, blowing or swooshing noise).

7. Peripheral vascular system
   a. Assess adequacy of blood flow to the extremities by palpating arterial pulses for equality and symmetry and checking the condition of the skin and nails.
   b. Check for pretibial edema and measure calf circumference (see Table 34-1).
   c. Measure blood pressure.
   d. Palpate superficial inguinal nodes (using firm but gentle pressure), beginning in the inguinal area and moving down toward the inner thigh.
   e. An ultrasonic stethoscope may be needed to amplify the sounds of a pulse wave if the pulse cannot be palpated.
   f. Carotid artery: Located in the groove between the trachea and sternocleidomastoid muscle, medial to and alongside the muscle

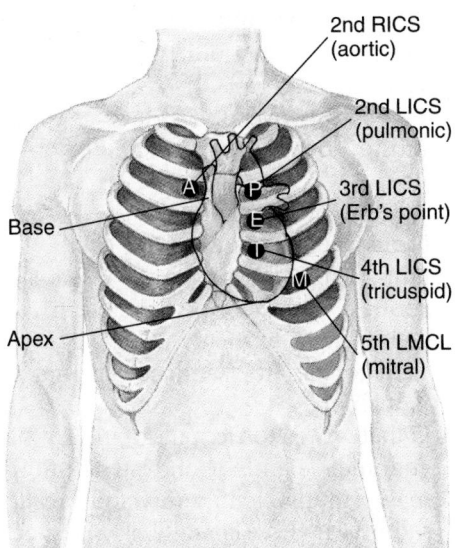

▲ **FIGURE 34-3** Auscultation areas of the heart. (From Wilson, A., & Giddens, J. [2009]. *Health assessment for nursing practice* [4th ed., p. 262]. St. Louis: Mosby).

2nd RICS (aortic)
2nd LICS (pulmonic)
3rd LICS (Erb's point)
4th LICS (tricuspid)
5th LMCL (mitral)
Base
Apex

Box 34-8 Arterial Pulse Points and Grading the Force of Pulses

Arteries in the Arms and Hands

Radial pulse: Located at the radial side of the forearm at the wrist

Ulnar pulse: Located on the opposite side of the location of the radial pulse at the wrist

Brachial pulse: Located above the elbow at the antecubital fossa, between the biceps and triceps muscles

Arteries in the Legs

Femoral pulse: Located below the inguinal ligament, midway between the symphysis pubis and the anterosuperior iliac spine

Popliteal pulse: Located behind the knee

Dorsalis pedis pulse: Located at the top of the foot, in line with the groove between the extensor tendons of the great and first toes

Posterior tibial pulse: Located inside of the ankle, behind and below the medial malleolus (ankle bone)

Grading the Force

4+ = strong and bounding
3+ = full pulse, increased
2+ = normal, easily palpable
1+ = weak, barely palpable

g. Palpate one carotid artery at a time to avoid compromising blood flow to the brain.

h. Auscultate each carotid artery for the presence of a bruit (a blowing, swishing sound), which indicates blood flow turbulence); normally a bruit is not present.

i. Palpate the arteries in the extremities (Box 34-8).

8. Client teaching
   a. Advise client to modify lifestyle for risk factors associated with heart and vascular disease.
   b. Encourage the client to seek regular physical examinations.
   c. Client should seek medical assistance for signs of heart or vascular disease.

H. Breasts
   1. **Subjective data**: Pain or tenderness, lumps or thickening, swollen axillary lymph nodes, nipple discharge, rash or swelling, medications being taken, personal or family history of breast disease, trauma or injury to the breasts, previous surgery on the breasts, breast self-examination compliance, mammograms as prescribed
   2. **Objective data: Inspection** and **palpation**
   3. **Inspection**
      a. Performed with the client's arms raised above the head, the hands pressed against the hips, and the arms extended straight ahead while the client sits and leans forward
      b. Assess size and symmetry (one breast is often larger than the other); masses, flattening, retraction, or dimpling; color and venous pattern; size, color, shape, and discharge in the nipple and areola; and the direction in which nipples point.
   4. **Palpation**
      a. Client lies supine, with the arm on the side being examined behind the head and a small pillow under the shoulder.
      b. The nurse uses the pads of the first three fingers to compress the breast tissue gently against the chest wall, noting tissue consistency.
      c. **Palpation** is performed systematically ensuring that the entire breast and tail are palpated.
      d. The nurse notes the consistency of the breast tissue, which normally feels dense, firm, and elastic.
      e. The nurse gently palpates the nipple and areola and compresses the nipple, noting any discharge.
   5. Axillary lymph nodes
      a. The nurse faces the client and stands on the side being examined, supporting the client's arm in a slightly flexed position, and abducts the arm away from the chest wall.
      b. The nurse places the free hand against the client's chest wall and high in the axillary hollow, then, with the fingertips, gently presses down, rolling soft tissue over the surface of the ribs and muscles.
      c. Lymph nodes are normally not palpable.
   6. Client teaching
      a. Encourage and teach the client to perform breast self-examination (BSE) (refer to Chapter 52 for information on performing the BSE).

b. BSE should be performed 7 to 10 days after the menses; postmenopausal clients or clients who have had a hysterectomy should select a specific day of the month and perform BSE monthly on that day.

c. Regular physical examinations and mammograms should be obtained as prescribed.

d. Client should report lumps or masses to the healthcare provider immediately.

I. Abdomen

1. **Subjective data**: Changes in appetite or weight, difficulty swallowing, dietary intake, intolerance to certain foods, nausea or vomiting, pain, bowel habits, medications currently being taken, history of abdominal problems or abdominal surgery

2. **Objective data**
   a. Ask the client to empty the bladder.
   b. Be sure to warm the hands and the end piece of the stethoscope.
   c. Examine painful areas last.

▲ When performing an abdominal assessment, the specific order for assessment techniques is inspection, auscultation, percussion, and palpation.

3. **Inspection**
   a. Contour: Look down at the abdomen and then across the abdomen from the rib margin to the public bone; describe as flat, rounded, concave or protuberant.
   b. Symmetry: Note any bulging or masses.
   c. Umbilicus: Should be midline and inverted
   d. Skin surface: Should be smooth and even
   e. Pulsations from the aorta may be noted in the epigastric area, and peristaltic waves may be noted across the abdomen.

4. **Auscultation**
   a. Performed before **percussion** and **palpation**, which can increase peristalsis.
   b. Hold the stethoscope lightly against the skin and listen for bowel sounds in all four quadrants; begin in the right lower quadrant (bowel sounds are normally heard here).
   c. Note the character and frequency of normal bowel sounds: high-pitched gurgling sounds occurring irregularly from 5 to 30 times a minute.
   d. Identify as normal, hypoactive, or hyperactive (borborygmus).
   e. Absent sounds: Auscultate for 5 minutes before determining that sounds are absent.
   f. Auscultate over the aorta, renal arteries, iliac arteries, and femoral arteries for vascular sounds or bruits.

5. **Percussion**
   a. All four quadrants are percussed lightly.
   b. Borders of the liver and spleen are percussed.

c. Tympany should predominate over the abdomen with dullness over the liver and spleen.
   d. **Percussion** over the kidney at the 12th rib (costovertebral angle) should produce no pain.

6. **Palpation**
   a. Begin with light **palpation** of all four quadrants, using the fingers to depress the skin about 1 cm; next perform deep **palpation**, depressing 5 to 8 cm.
   b. Palpate the liver and spleen (may not be palpable).
   c. Palpate the aortic pulsation in the upper abdomen slightly to the left of midline; normally it pulsates in a forward direction (pulsation expands laterally if an aneurysm is present).

7. Client teaching
   a. Encourage the client to consume a balanced diet.
   b. Substances that can cause gastric irritation should be avoided.
   c. The regular use of laxatives is discouraged.
   d. Lifestyle behaviors that can cause gastric irritation (e.g., smoking, spicy foods) should be modified.
   e. Regular physical examinations are important.
   f. The client should report gastrointestinal problems to the health care provider.

J. Musculoskeletal system

1. **Subjective data**: Joint pain or stiffness; redness, swelling, or warm joints; limited motion of joints; muscle pain, cramps, or weakness; bone pain; limitations in activities of daily living; exercise patterns; exposure to occupational hazards (e.g., heavy lifting, prolonged standing or sitting); medications being taken; history of joint, muscle, or bone injuries; history of surgery of the joints, muscles, or bones

2. **Objective data**: **inspection** and **palpation**

3. **Inspection**: Inspect gait and posture, and for cervical, thoracic, and lumbar curves (Box 34-9).

4. **Palpation**: Palpate all bones, joints, and surrounding muscles.

5. Range of motion
   a. Perform active and passive range-of-motion exercises of each major joint.

Box 34-9 Common Postural Abnormalities

Lordosis (swayback): increased lumbar curvature
Kyphosis (hunchback): Exaggeration of the posterior curvature of the thoracic spine
Scoliosis: lateral spinal curvature

b. Check for pain, limited mobility, spastic movement, joint instability, stiffness, and contractures.

c. Normally joints are nontender, without swelling, and move freely.

6. Muscle tone and strength
   a. Assess during measurement of range of motion.
   b. Ask client to flex the muscle to be examined and then to resist while applying opposing force against the flexion.
   c. Assess for increased tone (hypertonicity) or little tone (hypotonicity).

7. Grading muscle strength (Table 34-3)

8. Client teaching
   a. The client should consume a balanced diet, including foods high in calcium and vitamin D.
   b. Activities that cause muscle strain or stress to the joints should be avoided.
   c. Encourage the client to maintain a normal weight.
   d. Participation in a regular exercise program is beneficial.
   e. The client should contact the health care provider if joint or muscle pain or problems occur or if limitations in range of motion or muscle strength develop.

K. Neurological system (refer to Chapter 66)
1. **Subjective data**: Headaches, dizziness or vertigo, tremors, weakness, incoordination, numbness or tingling in any area of the body, difficulty speaking or swallowing, medications being taken, history of seizures, history of head injury or surgery, exposure to environmental or occupational hazards (e.g., chemicals, alcohol, drugs)
2. **Objective data**: Assessment of cranial nerves, level of consciousness, pupils, motor function, cerebellar function, coordination, sensory function, and reflexes
3. Note mental and emotional status, behavior and appearance, language ability, and intellectual functioning, including memory, knowledge, abstract thinking, association, and judgment.
4. Vital signs: Check temperature, pulse, respirations, and blood pressure; monitor for blood pressure or pulse changes, which may indicate increased intracranial pressure (see Chapter 66 for abnormal respiratory patterns).
5. Cranial nerves (Table 34-4)
6. Level of consciousness
   a. Assess the client's behavior to determine level of consciousness (e.g., alertness, confusion, delirium, unconsciousness, stupor, coma); assessment becomes increasingly invasive as the client is less responsive.
   b. Speak to client.
   c. Assess appropriateness of behavior and conversation.
   d. Lightly touch the client (as culturally appropriate).
7. Pupils
   a. Assess size, equality, and reaction to light (brisk, slow, or fixed) and note any unusual eye movements (check direct light and consensual light reflex).
   b. This component of the neurological examination may be performed during assessment of the eye.
8. Motor function
   a. Assess muscle tone, including strength and equality.
   b. Assess for voluntary and involuntary movements and purposeful and nonpurposeful movements.
   c. This component of the neurological examination may be performed during assessment of the musculoskeletal system.
9. Cerebellar function
   a. Monitor gait as the client walks in a straight line, heel to toe (tandem walking).
   b. Romberg test: Client is asked to stand with the feet together and the arms at the sides and to close the eyes and hold the position;

TABLE 34-3 Criteria for Grading and Recording Muscle Strength

Functional Level	Lovett Scale	Grade	Percent of Normal
No evidence of contractility	Zero (0)	0	0
Evidence of slight contractility	Trace (T)	1	10
Complete range of motion with gravity eliminated	Poor (P)	2	25
Complete range of motion with gravity	Fair (F)	3	50
Complete range of motion against gravity with some resistance	Good (G)	4	75
Complete range of motion against gravity with full resistance	Normal (N)	5	100

From Wilson, A., & Giddens, J. (2009). *Health assessment for nursing practice* (4th ed., p. 330). St. Louis: Mosby.

TABLE 34-4 Assessment of the Cranial Nerves

Cranial Nerve	Test
Cranial nerve I: Olfactory Sensory Controls the sense of smell	Have the client close the eyes and occlude one nostril with a finger. Ask the client to identify nonirritating and familiar odors (e.g., coffee, tea, cloves, soap, chewing gum, peppermint). Repeat the test on the other nostril.
Cranial nerve II: Optic Sensory Controls vision	Assess visual acuity with a Snellen chart and perform an ophthalmoscopic exam. Check peripheral vision by confrontation. Check color vision.
Cranial nerve III: Oculomotor Motor Controls pupillary constriction, upper-eyelid elevation, and most eye movement. Cranial nerve IV: Trochlear Motor Controls downward and inward eye movement. Cranial nerve VI: Abducens Motor Controls lateral eye movement	The motor functions of these nerves overlap; therefore they should be tested together. Inspect the eyelids for ptosis (drooping), then assess ocular movements and note any eye deviation. Test accommodation and direct and consensual light reflexes.
Cranial Nerve V: Trigeminal Sensory and motor Controls sensation in the cornea, nasal and oral mucosa, and facial skin, as well as mastication	To test motor function, ask the client to clench the teeth and assess the muscles of mastication; then try to open the client's jaws after asking the client to keep them tightly closed. Test the corneal reflex by lightly touching the client's cornea with a cotton wisp (this test may be omitted if the client is alert and blinking normally). Check sensory function by asking the client to close the eyes; lightly touch forehead, cheeks, and chin, noting whether the touch is felt equally on the two sides.
Cranial nerve VII: Facial Sensory and motor Controls movement of the face and taste sensation	Test taste perception on the anterior two thirds of the tongue; the client should be able to taste salty and sweet tastes. Have the client smile, frown, and show the teeth. Ask the client to puff out the cheeks. Attempt to close the client's eyes against resistance.
Cranial nerve VIII: Acoustic Sensory Controls hearing and vestibular function	Assessing the client's ability to hear tests the cochlear portion. Assessing the client's sense of equilibrium tests the vestibular portion. Check the client's hearing using acuity tests. Observe the client's balance and watch for swaying when he or she is walking or standing. Assessment of sensorineural hearing loss may be done with the Weber or Rinne test.
Cranial nerve IX: Glossopharyngeal Sensory and motor Controls swallowing ability, sensation in the pharyngeal soft palate and tonsillar mucosa, taste perception on the posterior third of the tongue, and salivation Usually cranial nerves IX and X are tested together	Test taste perception on the posterior one third of the tongue or pharynx; the client should be able to taste bitter and sour tastes. Inspect the soft palate and watch for symmetrical elevation when the client says "aaah." Touch the posterior pharyngeal wall with a tongue depressor to elicit the gag reflex.
Cranial nerve X: Vagus Sensory and motor Controls swallowing and phonation, sensation in the exterior ear's posterior wall, and sensation behind the ear Controls sensation in the thoracic and abdominal viscera Usually cranial nerves IX and X are tested together	Refer to cranial nerve IX.
Cranial nerve XI: Spinal accessory Motor Controls strength of neck and shoulder muscles	The nurse palpates and inspects the sternocleidomastoid muscle as the client pushes the chin against the nurse's hand. The nurse palpates and inspects the trapezius muscle as the client shrugs the shoulders against the nurse's resistance.
Cranial nerve XII: Hypoglossal Motor Controls tongue movements involved in swallowing and speech	Observe the tongue for asymmetry, atrophy, deviation to one side, and fasciculations (uncontrollable twitching). Ask the client to push the tongue against a tongue depressor, then have the client move the tongue rapidly in and out and from side to side.

normally the client can maintain posture and balance.

c. If appropriate, ask the client to perform a shallow knee bend or to hop in place on one leg and then the other.

10. Coordination
   a. Assess by asking the client to perform rapid alternating movements of the hands (e.g., turning the hands over and patting the knees continuously).
   b. The nurse asks the client to touch the nurse's finger, then his or her own nose; the client keeps the eyes open and the nurse moves the finger to different spots to ensure that the client's movements are smooth and accurate.
   c. Heel-to-shin test: Assist the client into a supine position, then ask the client to place the heel on the opposite knee and run it down the shin; normally the client moves the heel down the shin in a straight line.

11. Sensory function
   a. Pain: Assess by applying an object with a sharp point and one with a dull point to the client's body in random order; ask the client to identify the sharp and dull feelings.
   b. Light touch: Brush a piece of cotton over the client's skin at various locations in a random order and ask the client to say when the touch is felt.
   c. Vibration: Use a tuning fork to test the client's ability to feel vibrations over bony prominences; ask the client to announce when the vibration starts and stops.
   d. Position sense (kinesthesia): Move the client's finger or toe up or down and ask the client which way it has been moved; this tests the client's ability to perceive passive movement.
   e. Stereognosis: Tests the client's ability to recognize objects placed in his or her hand
   f. Graphesthesia: Tests the client's ability to identify a number traced on the client's hand
   g. Two-point discrimination: Tests the client's ability to discriminate two simultaneous pinpricks on the skin

12. Deep tendon reflexes
   a. Includes testing the following reflexes: Biceps, triceps, brachioradialis, patella, achilles
   b. Limb should be relaxed.
   c. The tendon is tapped quickly with a reflex hammer, which should cause contraction of muscle.
   d. Scoring deep tendon reflex activity (Box 34-10).

13. Plantar reflex
   a. A cutaneous (superficial) reflex is tested with a pointed but not sharp object.

Box 34-10 Scoring Deep Tendon Reflex Activity

0 = No response
1+ = Sluggish or diminished
2+ = Active or expected response
3+ = Slightly hyperactive, more brisk than normal; not necessarily pathologic
4+ = Brisk, hyperactive with intermittent clonus associated with disease

Modified from Wilson, A. F., & Giddens, J. F. (2009). *Health assessment for nursing practice* (4th ed., p. 387). St. Louis: Mosby.

   b. The sole of the client's foot is stroked from the heel, up the lateral side, and then across the ball of the foot to the medial side.
   c. The normal response is plantar flexion of all toes.

⚠ Dorsiflexion of the great toe and fanning of the other toes (Babinski's sign) is abnormal in anyone older than 2 years and indicates the presence of central nervous system disease.

14. Client teaching
   a. Client should avoid exposure to environmental hazards (e.g., insecticides, lead).
   b. High-risk behaviors that can result in head and spinal cord injuries should be avoided.
   c. Protective devices (e.g., a helmet, body pads) should be worn when participating in high-risk behaviors.

L. Female genitalia and reproductive tract
   1. **Subjective data**: Urinary difficulties or symptoms such as frequency, urgency, or burning, vaginal discharge, pain, menstrual and obstetrical histories, onset of menopause, medications being taken, sexual activity and the use of contraceptives, history of sexually transmitted infections
   2. **Objective data**
      a. Use a calm and relaxing approach; the examination is embarrassing for many women and may be a difficult experience for an adolescent.
      b. Consider the client's cultural background and her beliefs with regard to examination of the genitalia.
      c. A complete examination will include the external genitalia and a vaginal examination.
      d. The nurse's role is to prepare the client for the examination and to assist the physician, nurse practitioner, or nurse midwife.
      e. The client is asked to empty her bladder before the examination.
      f. The client is placed in the lithotomy position, and a drape is placed across the client

3. External genitalia
   a. Quantity and distribution of hair
   b. Characteristics of labia majora and minora (make note of any inflammation, edema, lesions, or lacerations)
   c. Urethral orifice is observed for color and position.
   d. Vaginal orifice (introitus) is inspected for inflammation, edema, discoloration, discharge, and lesions.
   e. The examiner may check Skene's and Bartholin's glands for tenderness or discharge (if discharge is present, color, odor, and consistency are noted and a culture of the discharge is obtained).
   f. The client is assessed for the presence of a cystocele (a portion of the vaginal wall and bladder prolapse or fall into the orifice anteriorly) or a rectocele (bulging of the posterior wall of the vagina caused by prolapse of the rectum).
4. Speculum examination of the internal genitalia
   a. Performed by the physician, nurse practitioner, or nurse midwife
   b. Permits visualization of the cervix and vagina
   c. Papanicolaou smear: A painless screening test for cervical cancer is done; the specimen is obtained during the speculum examination, and the nurse helps prepare the specimen for laboratory analysis.
5. Client teaching
   a. Stress the importance of personal hygiene.
   b. Explain the purpose and recommended frequency of Papanicolaou (Pap) tests.
   c. Explain the signs of sexually transmitted infections.
   d. Educate the client on the measures to prevent a sexually transmitted infection.
   e. Inform the client with a sexually transmitted infection that she must inform her sexual partner of the need for an examination.

M. Male genitalia
1. **Subjective data**: Urinary difficulty (e.g., frequency, urgency, hesitancy or straining, dysuria, nocturia), pain, lesions, or discharge on or from the penis, pain or lesions in the scrotum, medications being taken, sexual activity and the use of contraceptives, history of sexually transmitted infections
2. **Objective data**
   a. Includes assessment (**inspection** and **palpation**) of the external genitalia and inguinal ring and canal
   b. Client may stand or lie down for this examination.
   c. Genitalia are manipulated gently to avoid causing erection or discomfort.
   d. Sexual maturity is assessed by noting the size and shape of the penis and testes, the color

and texture of the scrotal skin, and the character and distribution of pubic hair.
   e. The penis is checked for the presence of lesions or discharge; a culture is obtained if a discharge is present.
   f. The scrotum is inspected for size, shape, and symmetry (normally the left testicle hangs lower than the right) and is palpated for the presence of lumps.
   g. Inguinal ring and canal; **inspection** (asking the client to bear down) and **palpation** are performed to assess for the presence of a hernia.
3. Client teaching
   a. Stress the importance of personal hygiene.
   b. Teach the client how to perform testicular self-examination (TSE); a day of the month is selected and the exam is performed on the same day each month after a shower or bath when the hands are warm and soapy and the scrotum is warm. (Refer to Chapter 52 for information on performing the TSE.)
   c. Explain the signs of sexually transmitted infections.
   d. Educate the client on measures to prevent sexually transmitted infections.
   e. Inform the client with a sexually transmitted infection that he must inform his sexual partner of the need for an examination.

N. Rectum and anus
1. **Subjective data**: Usual bowel pattern; any change in bowel habits; rectal pain, bleeding from the rectum, or black or tarry stools; dietary habits; problems with urination; previous screening for colorectal cancer; medications being taken; history of rectal or colon problems; family history of rectal or colon problems
2. **Objective data**
   a. Examination can detect colorectal cancer in its early stages; in men, the rectal examination can also detect prostate tumors.
   b. Women may be examined in the lithotomy position after examination of the genitalia.
   c. A man is best examined by having the client bend forward with his hips flexed and upper body resting over the examination table.
   d. A nonambulatory client may be examined in the left lateral (Sims') position.
   e. The external anus is inspected for lumps or lesions, rashes, inflammation or excoriation, scars, or hemorrhoids.
   f. Digital examination will most likely be performed by the physician or nurse practitioner.
   g. Digital examination is performed to assess sphincter tone; to check for tenderness, irregularities, polyps, masses, or nodules in the rectal wall; and to assess the prostate gland

h. The prostate gland is normally firm, without bogginess, tenderness, or nodules (hardness or nodules may indicate the presence of a cancerous lesion).
  3. Client teaching
   a. Diet should include high-fiber and low fat foods and plenty of liquids.
   b. The client should obtain regular digital examinations.
   c. Identify the symptoms of colorectal cancer or prostatic cancer (men).
   d. The client should follow the American Cancer Society's guidelines for screening for colorectal cancer.

VI. DOCUMENTING HEALTH AND PHYSICAL ASSESSMENT FINDINGS

A. Documentation of findings may be either written or recorded electronically (depending on agency protocol).
B. Whether written or electronic, the documentation is a legal document and a permanent record of the client's health status.
C. Principles of documentation need to be followed and data need to be recorded accurately, concisely, completely, legibly, and objectively without bias or opinions; always follow agency protocol for documentation.
D. Documentation findings serve as a source of client information for other health care providers.
E. Record findings about the client's health history and physical examination as soon as possible after completion of the health assessment.
F. Refer to Chapter 7 for additional information about documentation guidelines.

🔘 MORE QUESTIONS ON THE CD!

Practice Questions

346. A Spanish-speaking client arrives at the triage desk in the emergency department and states to the nurse, "No speak English, need interpreter." What is the best action for the nurse to take?
  1. Have one of the client's family members interpret.
  2. Have the Spanish speaking triage receptionist interpret.
  3. Page an interpreter from the hospital's interpreter services.
  4. Obtain a Spanish-English dictionary and attempt to triage the client.

347. A client with a diagnosis of asthma is admitted to the hospital with respiratory distress. What type of adventitious lung sounds would the nurse expect to hear when performing a respiratory assessment on this client?
  1. Stridor
  2. Crackles
  3. Wheezes
  4. Diminished

348. The nurse is performing a neurological assessment on a client and elicits a positive Romberg's sign. The nurse makes this determination based on which observation?
  1. An involuntary rhythmic, rapid, twitching of the eyeballs.
  2. A dorsiflexion of the ankle and great toe with fanning of the other toes.
  3. A significant sway when the client stands erect with feet together, arms at the side, and the eyes closed.
  4. A lack of normal sense of position when the client is unable to return extended fingers to a point of reference.

349. The nurse notes documentation that a client is exhibiting Cheyne-Stokes respirations. On assessment of the client, the nurse expects to note which of the following?
  1. Rhythmic respirations with periods of apnea
  2. Regular rapid and deep, sustained respirations
  3. Totally irregular respiration in rhythm and depth
  4. Irregular respirations with pauses at the end of inspiration and expiration

350. The nurse notes documentation that a client has conductive hearing loss. The nurse understands that this type of hearing loss is caused by which of the following?
  1. A defect in the cochlea.
  2. A defect in the 8th cranial nerve.
  3. A physical obstruction to the transmission of sound waves.
  4. A defect in the sensory fibers that lead to the cerebral cortex.

351. While performing a cardiac assessment on a client with an incompetent heart valve, the nurse auscultates a murmur. Which of the following best describes the sound of a heart murmur?
  1. Lub-dub sounds
  2. Scratchy, leathery heart noise
  3. Gentle, blowing or swooshing noise
  4. Abrupt, high-pitched snapping noise

352. The nurse is testing the extraocular movements in a client to assess for muscle weakness in the eyes. The nurse implements which physical

assessment technique to assess for muscle weakness in the eye?
1. Tests the corneal reflexes
2. Tests the six cardinal positions of gaze.
3. Tests visual acuity using a Snellen eye chart
4. Tests sensory function by asking the client to close eyes and then lightly touching the forehead, cheeks, and chin.

353. The nurse is instructing a client how to perform a testicular self-examination (TSE). The nurse explains that the best time to perform this exam is:
1. After a shower or bath
2. While standing to void
3. After having a bowel movement
4. While lying in bed before arising

354. The nurse is assessing a client for meningeal irritation and elicits a positive Brudzinski's sign. Which finding did the nurse observe?
1. The client rigidly extends the arms with pronated forearms and plantar flexion of the feet.
2. The client flexes a leg at the hip and knee and reports pain in the vertebral column when the leg is extended.

3. The client passively flexes the hip and knee in response to neck flexion and reports pain in the vertebral column.
4. The client's upper arms are flexed and held tightly to the sides of the body and the legs are extended and internally rotated.

Alternate Item Format: Multiple Response

355. The clinic nurse prepares to perform a focused assessment on a client who is complaining of symptoms of a cold, a cough, and lung congestion. Which of the following would the nurse include for this type of assessment? **Select all that apply**.
☐ 1. Auscultating lung sounds
☐ 2. Obtaining the client's temperature
☐ 3. Assessing the strength of peripheral pulses
☐ 4. Obtaining information about the client's respirations
☐ 5. Performing a musculoskeletal and neurological examination
☐ 6. Asking the client about a family history of any illness or disease

ANSWERS
346. 3
Rationale: The best action is to have a professional hospital-based interpreter translate for the client. English-speaking family members may not appropriately understand what is asked of them and may paraphrase what the client is actually saying. Also, client confidentiality as well as accurate information may be compromised when a family member or a non–health care provider acts as interpreter.
Test-Taking Strategy: Note the strategic word *best*. Initially focus on what the client needs. In this case the client needs and asks for an interpreter. Next keep in mind the issue of confidentiality and making sure that information is obtained in the most efficient and accurate way. This will assist in eliminating options 1, 2, and 4. Review the best nursing actions to take to obtain data from a non–English-speaking client if you had difficulty with this question.
Level of Cognitive Ability: Applying
Client Needs: Psychosocial Integrity
Integrated Process: Communication and Documentation
Content Area: Adult Health—Health Assessment/Physical Exam
Reference: Jarvis, C. (2008). *Physical examination and health assessment* (5th ed., p. 37). St. Louis: Saunders.

347. 3
Rationale: Asthma is a respiratory disorder characterized by recurring episodes of dyspnea, constriction of the bronchi, and wheezing. Wheezes are described as high-pitched musical sounds heard when air passes through an obstructed or narrowed lumen of a respiratory passageway. Stridor is a harsh

sound noted with an upper airway obstruction and often signals a life-threatening emergency. Crackles are produced by air passing over retained airway secretions or fluid, or the sudden opening of collapsed airways. Diminished lung sounds are heard over lung tissue where poor oxygen exchange is occurring.
Test-Taking Strategy: Note the client's diagnosis and think about the pathophysiology that occurs in this disorder. Recalling that bronchial constriction occurs will assist in directing you to option 3. Also, thinking about the definition of each adventitious lung sound identified in the options will direct you to option 3. Review the characteristics of adventitious lung sounds if you had difficulty with this question.
Level of Cognitive Ability: Analyzing
Client Needs: Physiological Integrity
Integrated Process: Nursing Process—Assessment
Content Area: Adult Health—Health Assessment/Physical Exam
Reference: Wilson, S., & Giddens, J. (2009). *Health assessment for nursing practice* (4th ed., p. 221). St. Louis: Mosby.

348. 3
Rationale: In Romberg's test, the client is asked to stand with the feet together and the arms at the sides, and to close the eyes and hold the position; normally the client can maintain posture and balance. A positive Romberg's sign is a vestibular neurological sign that is found when a client exhibits a loss of balance when closing the eyes. This may occur with cerebellar ataxia, loss of proprioception, and loss of vestibular function. A lack of normal sense of position coupled with an inability to return extended fingers to a point of reference is a finding that indicates a problem with coordination. A positive gaze

nystagmus evaluation results in an involuntary rhythmic, rapid, twitching of the eyeballs. A positive Babinski's test results in dorsiflexion of the ankle and great toe with fanning of the other toes; if this occurs in anyone older than 2 years it indicates the presence of central nervous system disease.
Test-Taking Strategy: Specific knowledge regarding the technique for performing the Romberg test is needed to answer this question. You can easily answer this question if you can recall that the client's balance is tested in this test. Review the procedure for performing Romberg's test and the purpose of the test if you had difficulty with this question.
Level of Cognitive Ability: Analyzing
Client Needs: Physiological Integrity
Integrated Process: Nursing Process—Assessment
Content Area: Adult Health—Health Assessment/Physical Exam
Reference: Wilson, S., & Giddens, J. (2009). *Health assessment for nursing practice* (4th ed., p. 383). St. Louis: Mosby.

349. 1
Rationale: Cheyne-Stokes respirations are rhythmic respirations with periods of apnea and can indicate a metabolic dysfunction in the cerebral hemisphere or basal ganglia. Neurogenic hyperventilation is a regular, rapid and deep, sustained respiration that can indicate a dysfunction in the low midbrain and middle pons. Ataxic respirations are totally irregular in rhythm and depth and indicate a dysfunction in the medulla. Apneustic respirations are irregular respirations with pauses at the end of inspiration and expiration and can indicate a dysfunction in the middle or caudal pons.
Test-Taking Strategy: Focus on the subject, the characteristics of Cheyne-Stokes respirations. Recalling that periods of apnea occur with this type of respiration will help direct you to correctly answer this question. Review the characteristics of Cheyne-Stokes respirations if you had difficulty with this question.
Level of Cognitive Ability: Understanding
Client Needs: Physiological Integrity
Integrated Process: Nursing Process—Assessment
Content Area: Adult Health—Health Assessment/Physical Exam
Reference: Jarvis, C. (2008). *Physical examination and health assessment* (5th ed., p. 469). St. Louis: Saunders.

350. 3
Rationale: A conductive hearing loss occurs as a result of a physical obstruction to the transmission of sound waves. A sensorineural hearing loss occurs as a result of a pathological process in the inner ear, a defect in the 8th cranial nerve, or a defect of the sensory fibers that lead to the cerebral cortex.
Test-Taking Strategy: Focus on the subject, a conductive hearing loss. Noting the relationship of the word *conductive* in the question and *transmission* in option 3 will direct you to this option. Review the causes of a conductive and a sensorineural hearing loss if you had difficulty with this question.
Level of Cognitive Ability: Understanding
Client Needs: Physiological Integrity
Integrated Process: Nursing Process—Assessment
Content Area: Adult Health—Health Assessment/Physical Exam

Reference: Jarvis, C. (2008). *Physical examination and health assessment* (5th ed., pp. 370–372). St. Louis: Saunders.

351. 3
Rationale: A heart murmur is an abnormal heart sound and is described as a gentle, blowing, swooshing sound. Lub-dub sounds are normal and represent the S1 (first heart sound) and S2 (second heart sound), respectively. A pericardial friction rub is described as a scratchy, leathery heart sound. A click is described as an abrupt, high-pitched snapping sound.
Test-Taking Strategy: Focus on the subject, characteristics of a murmur. Eliminate option 1 because it describes normal heart sounds. Next use the process of elimination recalling that a murmur occurs as a result of the manner in which the blood is flowing through the cardiac chambers and valves. This will direct you to option 3. Review the characteristics of a murmur if you had difficulty with this question.
Level of Cognitive Ability: Analyzing
Client Needs: Physiological Integrity
Integrated Process: Nursing Process—Assessment
Content Area: Adult Health—Health Assessment/Physical Exam
References: Jarvis, C. (2008). *Physical examination and health assessment* (5th ed., p. 488). St. Louis: Saunders.
Wilson, S., & Giddens, J. (2009). *Health assessment for nursing practice* (4th ed., p. 264). St. Louis: Mosby.

352. 2
Rationale: Testing the six cardinal positions of gaze is done to assess for muscle weakness in the eyes. The client is asked to hold the head steady, then to follow movement of an object through the positions of gaze. The client should follow the object in a parallel manner with the two eyes. A Snellen eye chart assesses visual acuity and cranial nerve II (optic). Testing sensory function by having the client close his or her eyes and then lightly touching areas of the face and testing the corneal reflexes assess cranial nerve V (trigeminal).
Test-Taking Strategy: Focus on the subject, assessing for muscle weakness in the eyes. Note the relationship between the words *extraocular movements* in the question and *positions of gaze* in the correct option. Review the physical assessment technique for assessing for muscle weakness in the eyes if you had difficulty with this question.
Level of Cognitive Ability: Applying
Client Needs: Physiological Integrity
Integrated Process: Nursing Process—Assessment
Content Area: Adult Health—Health Assessment/Physical Exam
Reference: Ignatavicius, D., & Workman, M. (2010). *Medical-surgical nursing: Patient-centered collaborative care* (6th ed., p. 1078). St. Louis: Saunders.

353. 1
Rationale: The nurse needs to teach the client how to perform a testicular self-examination (TSE). The nurse should instruct the client to perform the exam on the same day each month. The nurse should also instruct the client that the best time to perform a TSE is after a shower or bath when the hands are warm and soapy and the scrotum is warm. Palpation is easier and the client will be better able to identify any abnormalities. The client would stand to perform the

exam, but it would be difficult to perform the exam while voiding. Having a bowel movement is unrelated to performing the TSE.

Test-Taking Strategy: Think about the purpose of the TSE and visualize this assessment technique. Review the instructions for performing the TSE if you had difficulty with this question. Eliminate option 3 because having a bowel movement is unrelated to performing the TSE. Next eliminate options 2 and 4 because it would be difficult to perform this self-exam while lying down or during voiding.

Level of Cognitive Ability: Applying
Client Needs: Health Promotion and Maintenance
Integrated Process: Teaching and Learning
Content Area: Adult Health—Health Assessment/Physical Exam
Reference: Jarvis, C. (2008). *Physical examination and health assessment* (5th ed., p. 727). St. Louis: Saunders.

354. 3

Rationale: Brudzinski's sign is tested with the client in the supine position. The nurse flexes the client's head (gently moves the head to the chest) and there should be no reports of pain or resistance to the neck flexion. A positive Brudzinski's sign is observed if the client passively flexes the hip and knee in response to neck flexion and reports pain in the vertebral column. Kernig's sign also tests for meningeal irritation and is positive when the client flexes the legs at the hip and knee and complains of pain along the vertebral column when the leg is extended. Decorticate posturing is abnormal flexion and is noted when the client's upper arms are flexed and held tightly to the sides of the body and the legs are extended and internally rotated. Decerebrate posturing is abnormal extension and occurs when the arms are fully extended, forearms pronated, wrists and fingers flexed, jaws clenched, neck extended, and feet plantar-flexed.

Test-Taking Strategy: Focus on the subject: a positive Brudzinski's sign. Recalling that a positive sign is elicited if the client reports pain will assist in eliminating options 1 and 4. Next it is necessary to know that a positive Brudzinski's sign is observed if the client passively flexes the hip and knee in response to neck flexion and reports pain in the vertebral column. Review the findings in a positive Brudzinski's sign if you had difficulty with this question.

Level of Cognitive Ability: Analyzing
Client Needs: Physiological Integrity
Integrated Process: Nursing Process—Assessment
Content Area: Adult Health—Health Assessment/Physical Exam
Reference: Wilson, S., & Giddens, J. (2009). *Health assessment for nursing practice* (4th ed., p. 392). St. Louis: Mosby.

ALTERNATE ITEM FORMAT: MULTIPLE RESPONSE
355. 1, 2, 4
Rationale: A focused assessment focuses on a limited or short-term problem, such as the client's complaint. Because the client is complaining of symptoms of a cold, a cough, and lung congestion, the nurse would focus on the respiratory system and the presence of an infection. A complete assessment includes a complete health history and physical examination and forms a baseline database. Assessing the strength of peripheral pulses relates to a vascular assessment, which is not related to this client's complaints. A musculoskeletal and neurological examination also is not related to this client's complaints. However strength of peripheral pulses and a musculoskeletal and neurological examination would be included in a complete assessment. Likewise, asking the client about a family history of any illness or disease would be included in a complete assessment.

Test-Taking Strategy: Note the strategic words *focused assessment*. Noting that the client's symptoms relate to the respiratory system and the presence of an infection will direct you to options 1, 2, and 4. Review the types of health and physical assessments and the components of a focused assessment if you had difficulty with this question.

Level of Cognitive Ability: Applying
Client Needs: Health Promotion and Maintenance
Integrated Process: Nursing Process—Assessment
Content Area: Adult Health—Health Assessment/Physical Exam
Reference: Wilson, S., & Giddens, J. (2009). *Health assessment for nursing practice* (4th ed., p. 3). St. Louis: Mosby.

Care of the Older Client

I. AGING AND GERONTOLOGY

A. Aging is the biopsychosocial process of change that occurs in a person between birth and death.

B. Gerontology is the study of the aging process.

II. PHYSIOLOGICAL CHANGES

A. Integumentary system
1. Loss of pigment in hair and skin
2. Wrinkling of the skin
3. Thinning of the epidermis and easy bruising and tearing of the skin (Fig. 35-1)
4. Decreased skin turgor, elasticity, and subcutaneous fat
5. Increased nail thickness and decreased nail growth
6. Decreased perspiration
7. Dry, itchy, scaly skin
8. Seborrheic dermatitis and keratosis formation (overgrowth and thickening of the skin)

B. Neurological system
1. Slowed reflexes
2. Slight tremors and difficulty with fine motor movement
3. Loss of balance
4. Increased incidence of awakening after sleep onset
5. Increased susceptibility to hypothermia and hyperthermia
6. Short-term memory decline possible
7. Long-term memory usually maintained

C. Musculoskeletal system
1. Decreased muscle mass and strength and atrophy of muscles
2. Decreased mobility, range of motion, flexibility, coordination, and stability
3. Change of gait, with shortened step and wider base
4. Posture and stature changes causing a decrease in height (Fig. 35-2)
5. Increased brittleness of the bones
6. Deterioration of joint capsule components
7. Kyphosis of the dorsal spine (increased convexity in the curvature of the spine)

The older client is at risk for falls because of the changes that occur in the neurological and musculoskeletal systems.

D. Cardiovascular system
1. Diminished energy and endurance, with lowered tolerance to exercise
2. Decreased compliance of the heart muscle, with heart valves becoming thicker and more rigid
3. Decreased cardiac output and decreased efficiency of blood return to the heart
4. Decreased compensatory response, so less able to respond to increased demands on the cardiovascular system
5. Decreased resting heart rate
6. Weak peripheral pulses
7. Increased blood pressure but susceptibility to postural hypotension

E. Respiratory system
1. Decreased stretch and compliance of the chest wall
2. Decreased strength and function of respiratory muscles
3. Decreased size and number of alveoli
4. The respiratory rate usually remains unchanged
5. Decreased depth of respirations and oxygen intake
6. Decreased ability to cough and expectorate sputum

F. Hematological system
1. Hemoglobin and hematocrit average levels toward the low end of normal
2. Prone to increased blood clotting
3. Decreased protein available for protein-bound medications

G. Immune system
1. Tendency for lymphocyte counts to be low with altered immunoglobulin production
2. Decreased resistance to infection and disease

H. Gastrointestinal system
1. Decreased need for calories because of lowered basal metabolic rate
2. Decreased appetite, thirst, and oral intake
3. Decreased lean body weight
4. Decreased stomach emptying time
5. Increased tendency toward constipation

411

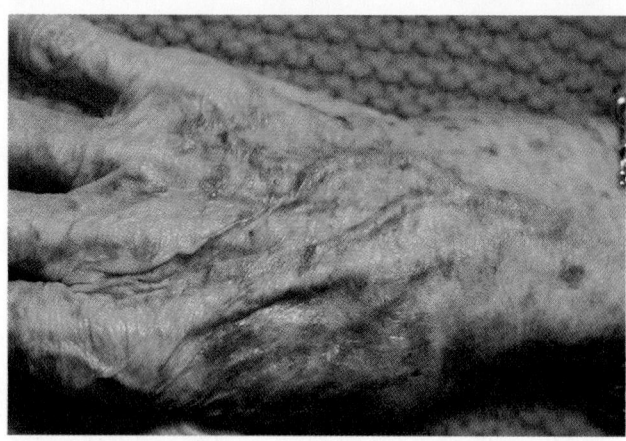

▲ **FIGURE 35-1** Paper-thin, transparent skin. (From Ignatavicius, D., & Workman, M. [2010]. *Medical-surgical nursing: Patient-centered collaborative care.* [6th ed., p. 465]. St. Louis: Saunders.)

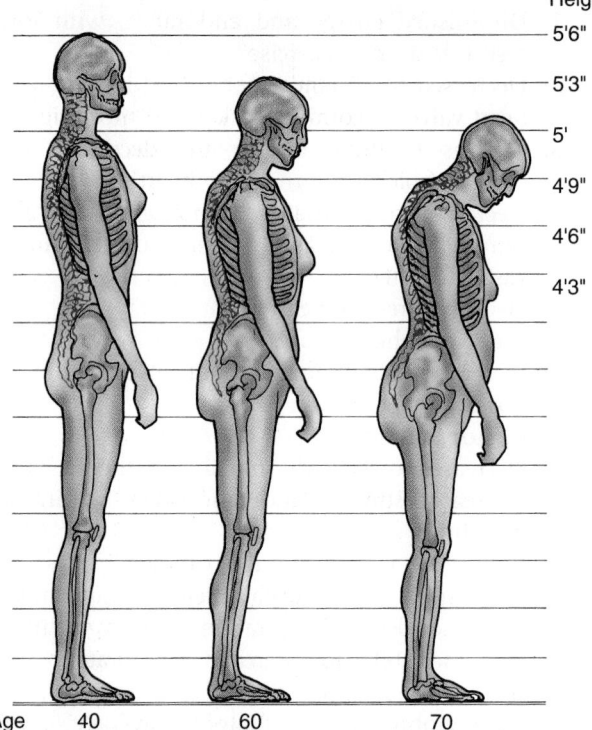

▲ **FIGURE 35-2** A normal spine at age 40 years of age and osteoporotic changes at 60 and 70 years of age. These changes can cause a loss of as much as 6 inches in height and can result in the so-called dowager's hump (far right) in the upper thoracic vertebrae. (From Ignatavicius, D., & Workman, M. [2010]. *Medical-surgical nursing: Patient-centered collaborative care.* [6th ed., p. 1156]. St. Louis: Saunders.)

6. Increased susceptibility for dehydration
7. Tooth loss
8. Difficulty in chewing and swallowing food

I. Endocrine system
   1. Decreased secretion of hormones, with specific changes related to each hormone's function
   2. Decreased metabolic rate
   3. Decreased glucose tolerance, with resistance to insulin in peripheral tissues

J. Renal system
   1. Decreased kidney size, function, and ability to concentrate urine
   2. Decreased glomerular filtration rate
   3. Decreased capacity of the bladder
   4. Increased residual urine and increased incidence of infection and possibly incontinence
   5. Impaired medication excretion

K. Reproductive system
   1. Decreased testosterone production and decreased size of the testes
   2. Changes in the prostate gland, leading to urinary problems
   3. Decreased secretion of hormones with the cessation of menses
   4. Vaginal changes, including decreased muscle tone and lubrication
   5. Impotence or sexual dysfunction for both genders; sexual function varies and depends on general physical condition, mental health status, and medications

L. Special senses
   1. Decreased visual acuity
   2. Decreased accommodation in eyes, requiring increased adjustment time to changes in light
   3. Decreased peripheral vision and increased sensitivity to glare
   4. Presbyopia and cataract formation
   5. Possible loss of hearing ability; low-pitched tones are heard more easily
   6. Inability to discern taste of food
   7. Decreased sense of smell
   8. Changes in touch sensation
   9. Decreased pain awareness

III. PSYCHOSOCIAL CONCERNS

A. Adjustment to deterioration in physical and mental health and well-being
B. Threat to independent functioning and fear of becoming a burden to loved ones
C. Adjustment to retirement and loss of income
D. Loss of skills and competencies developed early in life
E. Coping with changes in role function and social life
F. Diminished quantity and quality of relationships and coping with loss
G. Dependence on governmental and social systems
H. Access to social support systems
I. Costs of health care and medications

IV. MENTAL HEALTH CONCERNS (Box 35-1)

A. Depression: The increased dependency that older adults may experience can lead to hopelessness, helplessness, lowered sense of self-control, and decreased self-esteem and self-worth; these changes can interfere with daily functioning and lead to **depression**.

Box 35-1 Mental Health Concerns

Depression
Grief
Isolation
Suicide

Box 35-2 Nonspecific Symptoms That Possibly Indicate Illness or Infection

Apathy	Fatigue
Anorexia	Incontinence
Changes in functional status	Self-neglect
Confusion	Shortness of breath
Dyspnea	Tachypnea
Falling	Vital sign changes

B. Grief: Client reacts to the perception of loss, including physical, psychological, social, and spiritual aspects.

C. Isolation: Client is alone and desires contact with others but is unable to make that contact.

D. Suicide: **Depression** can lead to thoughts of self-harm.

⚠ Any suicide threat from an older client should be taken seriously.

V. PAIN

A. Description
1. Pain can occur from numerous causes and most often occurs from degenerative changes in the musculoskeletal system.
2. The failure to alleviate pain in the older client can lead to functional limitations affecting his or her ability to function independently.

B. Assessment
1. Restlessness
2. Verbal reporting of pain
3. Agitation
4. Moaning
5. Crying

C. Interventions
1. Monitor the client for signs of pain.
2. Identify the pattern of pain.
3. Identify the precipitating factor(s) for the pain.
4. Monitor the impact of the pain on activities of daily living.
5. Provide pain relief through measures such as distraction, relaxation, massage, and biofeedback.
6. Administer pain medication as prescribed, and instruct the client in its use.
7. Evaluate the effects of pain-reducing measures.

VI. INFECTION (Box 35-2)

A. Confusion is a common sign of infection in the older adult, especially infection of the urinary tract.

B. Carefully monitor the older adult with infection because of the diminished and altered immune response.

C. Nonspecific symptoms may indicate illness or infection (see Box 35-2).

VII. MEDICATIONS

A. Major problems with prescriptive medications include adverse effects, medication interactions, medication errors, noncompliance, and cost.

B. Determine the use of over-the-counter medications. ⚠

C. **Polypharmacy**
1. Routinely monitor the number of prescription and nonprescription medications used and determine whether any can be eliminated or combined.
2. Keep the use of medications to a minimum.
3. Overprescribing medications leads to increased problems with more side effects, increased interaction between medications, replication of medication treatment, diminished quality of life, and increased costs.

D. Medication dosages normally are prescribed at one third to one half of normal adult dosages.

E. Closely monitor the client for adverse effects and response to therapy because of the increased risk for medication toxicity. ⚠

F. Assess for medication interactions in the client taking multiple medications.

G. Advise the client to use one pharmacy and notify the consulting physician(s) of the medications taken. ⚠

⚠ A common sign of an adverse reaction to a medication in the older client is an acute change in mental status.

H. Administration of medications ⚠
1. The client should be in a sitting position when taking medication.
2. The mouth is checked for dryness because medication may stick and dissolve in the mouth.
3. Liquid preparations can be used if the client has difficulty swallowing tablets.
4. Tablets can be crushed if necessary and given with textured food (nectar, applesauce) if not contraindicated.
5. Enteric-coated tablets are not crushed and capsules are not opened.
6. If administering a suppository, avoid inserting the suppository immediately after removing it from the refrigerator; a suppository may take

a while to dissolve because of decreased body core temperature.

7. When administering parenteral solution or medication, monitor the site, because it may ooze or bleed because of decreased tissue elasticity; an immobile limb is not used for administering parenteral medication.

8. Monitor client compliance with taking prescribed medications.

9. Monitor the client for **safety** in correctly taking medications, including an assessment of their ability to read the instructions and discriminate among the pills and their color and shape.

10. Use a medication cassette to facilitate proper administration of medication.

VIII. ABUSE OF THE OLDER ADULT

A. **Abuse** involves physical, emotional, or sexual **abuse** and also can involve **neglect** or economic exploitation.

B. Categories of mistreatment to the older client.
1. Domestic mistreatment takes place in the home of the older adult and is usually carried out by a family member or significant other; this can include physical maltreatment, **neglect**, or abandonment.
2. Institutional mistreatment takes place when an older adult experiences **abuse** when hospitalized or living somewhere other than home (e.g., long-term care facility).
3. **Self-neglect** is the choice by a mentally competent individual to avoid medical care or other services that could improve optimal function, lack caring for oneself, and engage in actions that negatively affect his or her personal **safety**; unless declared legally incompetent, an individual has the right to refuse care.

⚠️ Individuals at most risk for abuse include those who are dependent because of their immobility or altered mental status.

C. Factors that contribute to **abuse** and **neglect** include long-standing family violence, caregiver stress, and the individual's increasing dependence on others.

D. Abusers tend to be male, engage in substance **abuse**, and have a mental illness or **dementia**; in addition, they tend to depend on the older client for financial assistance or other resources.

E. Victims may attempt to dismiss injuries as accidental, and abusers may prevent victims from receiving proper medical care to avoid discovery.

F. Victims often are isolated socially by their abusers.

G. For additional information on **abuse** of the older client, see Chapter 76.

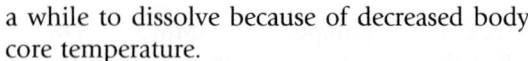 **MORE QUESTIONS ON THE CD!**

Practice Questions

356. The nurse is providing medication instructions to an older client who is taking digoxin (Lanoxin) daily. The nurse notes that which age-related body changes could place the client at risk for digoxin toxicity?
1. Decreased muscle strength and loss of bone density
2. Decreased cough efficiency and decreased vital capacity
3. Decreased salivation and decreased gastrointestinal motility
4. Decreased lean body mass and decreased glomerular filtration rate

357. The nurse employed in a long-term care facility is caring for an older male client. Which nursing action contributes to encouraging autonomy in the client?
1. Planning his meals
2. Decorating his room
3. Scheduling his barber appointments
4. Allowing him to choose social activities

358. The home care nurse is visiting an older female client whose husband died 6 months ago. Which behavior by the client indicates ineffective coping?
1. Neglecting her personal grooming
2. Looking at old snapshots of her family
3. Participating in a senior citizens' program
4. Visiting her husband's grave once a month

359. The nurse is providing instructions to a nursing assistant regarding care of an older client with hearing loss. The nurse tells the assistant that clients with a hearing loss:
1. Are often distracted
2. Have middle ear changes
3. Respond to low-pitched tones
4. Develop moist cerumen production

360. The nurse is providing an educational session to new employees, and the topic is abuse of the older client. The nurse helps the employees identify that which client is most typical of a victim of abuse?
1. A 75-year-old man who has moderate hypertension
2. A 68-year-old man who has newly diagnosed cataracts
3. A 90-year-old woman who has advanced Parkinson's disease
4. A 70-year-old woman who has early diagnosed Lyme disease

361. The nurse is performing an assessment on an older client who is having difficulty sleeping at night. Which statement, if made by the client, indicates that teaching about improving sleep is necessary?
1. "I swim three times a week."
2. "I have stopped smoking cigars."
3. "I drink hot chocolate before bedtime."
4. "I read for 40 minutes before bedtime."

362. The visiting nurse observes that the older male client is confined by his daughter-in-law to his room. When the nurse suggests that he walk to the den and join the family, he says, "I'm in everyone's way; my daughter-in-law needs me to stay here." The most important action for the nurse to take is to:
1. Say nothing, because it is best for the nurse to remain neutral and wait to be asked for help.
2. Suggest to the client and daughter-in-law that they consider a nursing home for the client.
3. Say to the daughter-in-law, "Confining your father-in-law to his room is inhuman."
4. Suggest appropriate resources to the client and daughter-in-law, such as respite care and a senior citizens' center.

363. The nurse is performing an assessment on an older adult client. Which assessment data would indicate a potential complication associated with the skin of this client?

1. Crusting
2. Wrinkling
3. Deepening of expression lines
4. Thinning and loss of elasticity in the skin

364. The home health nurse is visiting a client for the first time. While assessing the client's medication, it is noted that there are at least 19 prescription and several over-the-counter medications that the client has been taking. Which intervention should the nurse take first?
1. Check for drug-drug interactions.
2. Determine whether there are any adverse side effects.
3. Determine whether there are medication duplications.
4. Call the prescribing physician and report any polypharmacy.

Alternate Item Format: Multiple Response
365. Which of the following are normal age-related physiological changes? **Select all that apply**.
❑ 1. Increased heart rate
❑ 2. Decline in visual acuity
❑ 3. Decreased respiratory rate
❑ 4. Decline in long-term memory
❑ 5. Increased susceptibility to urinary tract infections
❑ 6. Increased incidence of awakening after sleep onset

ANSWERS
356. 4
Rationale: The older client is at risk for medication toxicity because of decreased lean body mass and an age-associated decreased glomerular filtration rate. Although options 1, 2, and 3 identify age-related changes that occur in the older client, they are not associated specifically with this risk.
Test-Taking Strategy: Use the process of elimination and focus on the subject age-related body changes that could place the client at risk for medication toxicity. Note that option 4 is the only option that addresses renal excretion. If you had difficulty with this question, review the physiological changes associated with aging and those that place the older client at risk for medication toxicity.
Level of Cognitive Ability: Understanding
Client Needs: Physiological Integrity
Integrated Process: Teaching and Learning
Content Area: Fundamental Skills—Developmental Stages
References: Ebersole, P., Hess, P., Touhy, T., Jett, K., & Luggen, A. (2008). *Toward healthy aging* (7th ed., p. 309). St. Louis: Mosby.

Ignatavicius, D., & Workman, M. (2010). *Medical-surgical nursing: Patient-centered collaborative care* (6th ed., p. 19). St. Louis: Saunders.
Perry, A., & Potter, P. (2010). *Clinical nursing skills & techniques* (7th ed., pp. 510–511). St. Louis: Mosby.

357. 4
Rationale: Autonomy is the personal freedom to direct one's own life as long as it does not impinge on the rights of others. An autonomous person is capable of rational thought. This individual can identify problems, search for alternatives, and select solutions that allow continued personal freedom as long as others and their rights and property are not harmed. Loss of autonomy, and therefore independence, is a real fear of older clients. Option 4 is the only option that allows the client to be a decision maker.
Test-Taking Strategy: Use the process of elimination, focusing on the subject encouraging autonomy. Recalling the definition of autonomy will direct you to the correct option. Remember that giving the client choices is essential to promote independence. Review the concept of autonomy as it relates to the older client if you had difficulty with this question.

Level of Cognitive Ability: Applying
Client Needs: Safe and Effective Care Environment
Integrated Process: Caring
Content Area: Fundamental Skills—Developmental Stages
Reference: Potter, P., & Perry, A. (2009). *Fundamentals of nursing* (7th ed., pp. 9–10, 314, 348). St. Louis: Mosby.

358. 1

Rationale: Coping mechanisms are behaviors used to decrease stress and anxiety. In response to a death, ineffective coping is manifested by an extreme behavior that in some cases may be harmful to the individual physically or psychologically. Option 1 is indicative of a behavior that identifies an ineffective coping behavior in the grieving process.
Test-Taking Strategy: Note the subject, an ineffective coping behavior. Eliminate options 2, 3, and 4 because they are comparable or alike and are positive activities in which the individual is engaging to get on with her life. Review coping mechanisms in response to grief and loss if you had difficulty with this question.
Level of Cognitive Ability: Analyzing
Client Needs: Psychosocial Integrity
Integrated Process: Nursing Process—Assessment
Content Area: Mental Health
References: Ebersole, P., Hess, P., Touhy, T., Jett, K., & Luggen, A. (2008). *Toward healthy aging* (7th ed., p. 643). St. Louis: Mosby.
Touhy, T., & Jett, K. (2010). *Ebersole and Hess' gerontological nursing & healthy aging* (3rd ed., pp. 382–383). St. Louis: Mosby.

359. 3

Rationale: Presbycusis refers to the age-related irreversible degenerative changes of the inner ear that lead to decreased hearing ability. As a result of these changes, the older client has a decreased response to high-frequency sounds. Low-pitched voice tones are heard more easily and can be interpreted by the older client. Options 1, 2, and 4 are not accurate characteristics related to aging.
Test-Taking Strategy: Think about the age-related changes that occur in the older client. Recalling that the client with a hearing loss responds to low-pitched tones will direct you to option 3. If you had difficulty with this question, review the characteristics associated with presbycusis and hearing loss.
Level of Cognitive Ability: Applying
Client Needs: Physiological Integrity
Integrated Process: Teaching and Learning
Content Area: Fundamental Skills—Developmental Stages
Reference: Ebersole, P., Hess, P., Touhy, T., Jett, K., & Luggen, A. (2008). *Toward healthy aging* (7th ed., pp. 351–352). St. Louis: Mosby.

360. 3

Rationale: Elder abuse includes physical, sexual, or psychological abuse, misuse of property, and violation of rights. The typical abuse victim is a woman of advanced age with few social contacts and at least one physical or mental impairment that limits her ability to perform activities of daily living. In addition, the client usually lives alone or with the abuser and depends on the abuser for care.
Test-Taking Strategy: Read each option carefully and identify the client who is most defenseless as the result of the disease

process. This will direct you to option 3. If you had difficulty with this question review the characteristics associated with elder abuse.
Level of Cognitive Ability: Applying
Client Needs: Psychosocial Integrity
Integrated Process: Teaching and Learning
Content Area: Mental Health
Reference: Ebersole, P., Hess, P., Touhy, T., Jett, K., & Luggen, A. (2008). *Toward healthy aging* (7th ed., p. 453). St. Louis: Mosby.

361. 3

Rationale: Many nonpharmacological sleep aids can be used to influence sleep. However, the client should avoid caffeinated beverages and stimulants such as tea, cola, and chocolate. The client should exercise regularly, because exercise promotes sleep by burning off tension that accumulates during the day. A 20- to 30-minute walk, swim, or bicycle ride three times a week is helpful. The client should sleep on a bed with a firm mattress. Smoking and alcohol should be avoided. The client should avoid large meals; peanuts, beans, fruit, raw vegetables, and other foods that produce gas; and snacks that are high in fat because they are difficult to digest.
Test-Taking Strategy: Note the strategic words *that teaching about improving sleep is necessary.* These words indicate a negative event query and ask you to select an option that is an incorrect statement. Options 1, 2, and 4 are positive statements indicating that the client understands the methods of improving sleep. Review the factors that can interfere with sleep in the older client if you had difficulty with this question.
Level of Cognitive Ability: Analyzing
Client Needs: Physiological Integrity
Integrated Process: Teaching and Learning
Content Area: Fundamental Skills—Developmental Stages
Reference: Touhy, T., & Jett, K. (2010). *Ebersole and Hess' gerontological nursing & healthy aging* (3rd ed., p. 155). St. Louis: Mosby.

362. 4

Rationale: Assisting clients and families to become aware of available community support systems is a role and responsibility of the nurse. Observing that the client has begun to be confined to his room makes it necessary for the nurse to intervene legally and ethically, so option 1 is not appropriate and is passive in terms of advocacy. Option 2 suggests committing the client to a nursing home and is a premature action on the nurse's part. Although the data provided tell the nurse that this client requires nursing care, the nurse does not know the extent of the nursing care required. Option 3 is incorrect and judgmental.
Test-Taking Strategy: Note the strategic words *most important action.* Using principles related to the ethical and legal responsibility of the nurse and knowledge of the nurse's role will direct you to option 4. Option 1 avoids the situation, option 2 is a premature action, and option 3 is a nontherapeutic statement. Review the roles and responsibilities of the nurse in caring for the older client if you had difficulty with this question.
Level of Cognitive Ability: Applying
Client Needs: Safe and Effective Care Environment

Integrated Process: Nursing Process—Implementation
Content Area: Fundamental Skills—Developmental Stages
Reference: Touhy, T., & Jett, K. (2010). *Ebersole and Hess' gerontological nursing & healthy aging* (3rd ed., pp. 452–454). St. Louis: Mosby.

363. 1
Rationale: The normal physiological changes that occur in the skin of older adults include thinning of the skin, loss of elasticity, deepening of expression lines, and wrinkling. Crusting noted on the skin would indicate a potential complication.
Test-Taking Strategy: Note the strategic words *potential complication.* Think about the normal physiological changes that occur in the aging process to direct you to option 1. Review these age-related skin changes if you had difficulty with this question.
Level of Cognitive Ability: Analyzing
Client Needs: Health Promotion and Maintenance
Integrated Process: Nursing Process—Assessment
Content Area: Fundamental Skills—Developmental Stages
References: Copstead-Kirkhorn, L., & Banasik, J. (2010). *Pathophysiology* (4th ed., p. 1227). St. Louis: Mosby.

Perry, A., & Potter, P. (2010). *Clinical nursing skills & techniques* (7th ed., p. 120). St. Louis: Mosby.

364. 3
Rationale: Polypharmacy is a concern in the older client. Duplication of medications needs to be identified before drug-drug interactions or adverse side effects can be determined because the nurse needs to know what the client is taking. The phone call to the health care provider is the intervention after all other information has been collected.
Test-Taking Strategy: Note the strategic word *first.* Also note that the nurse is visiting the client for the first time. Note that options 1, 2, and 3 relate to obtaining data. Therefore, think about the order of action with these options; option 3 is the first action. Options 1, 2, and 4 should be done after possible medication duplication has been identified. Review the interventions related to polypharmacy in the older client if you had difficulty with this question.

Level of Cognitive Ability: Applying
Client Needs: Physiological Integrity
Integrated Process: Nursing Process—Implementation
Content Area: Pharmacology
References: Ebersole, P., Hess, P., Touhy, T., Jett, K., & Luggen, A. (2008). *Toward healthy aging* (7th ed., pp. 301–302). St. Louis: Mosby.

Touhy, T., & Jett, K. (2010). *Ebersole and Hess' gerontological nursing & healthy aging* (3rd ed., p. 226). St. Louis: Mosby.

ALTERNATE ITEM FORMAT: MULTIPLE RESPONSE
365. 2, 5, 6
Rationale: Anatomical changes to the eye affect the individual's visual ability, leading to potential problems with activities of daily living. Light adaptation and visual fields are reduced. Although lung function may decrease, the respiratory rate usually remains unchanged. Heart rate decreases and heart valves thicken. Age-related changes that affect the urinary tract increase an older client's susceptibility to urinary tract infections. Short-term memory may decline with age, but long-term memory usually is maintained. Change in sleep patterns is a consistent, age-related change. Older persons experience an increased incidence of awakening after sleep onset.
Test-Taking Strategy: Specific knowledge regarding normal age-related changes is needed to answer this question. Read each characteristic carefully and think about the physiological changes that occur with aging to select the correct items. Review the normal age-related changes if you had difficulty with this question.
Level of Cognitive Ability: Understanding
Client Needs: Health Promotion and Maintenance
Integrated Process: Nursing Process—Assessment
Content Area: Fundamental Skills—Developmental Stages
Reference: Potter, P., & Perry, A. (2009). *Fundamentals of nursing* (7th ed., p. 198). St. Louis: Mosby.

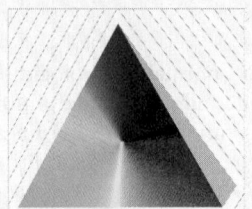

Pediatric Nursing

PYRAMID TERMS

abuse Nonaccidental physical injury or the nonaccidental act of omission of care by a parent or person responsible for a child; includes neglect, physical, sexual, or emotional maltreatment.

active immunity A form of long-term acquired antibody protection that develops naturally after an initial infection or exposure to antigens, or artificially after a vaccination.

atresia Congenital absence or closure of a body orifice.

attenuated vaccines Vaccines derived from microorganisms or viruses; their virulence has been weakened as a result of passage through another host.

crackles Audible high-pitched crackling or popping sounds heard during lung auscultation; result from fluid in the airways, and are not cleared by coughing (formerly referred to as "rales").

chronological age Age in years.

cyanosis The bluish color that results in tissues, nail beds, and mucous membranes when tissues are deprived of adequate amounts of oxygen.

developmental age Age based on a child's maturational progress. It is determined by standardized resources such as body size, physical and psychological functioning, motor skills, and aptitude tests.

functional age The age equivalent at which a child actually is able to perform specific self-care or related tasks.

growth Measurable physical and physiological body changes that occur over time.

grunting The sound made by forced expiration, which is the body's attempt to improve oxygenation when hypoxemia is present.

hereditary Refers to the transmission of genetic characteristics from parent to offspring.

inactivated vaccines Vaccines that contain killed microorganisms.

nasal flaring A widening of the nares to enable an infant or child to take in more oxygen; a serious indicator of air hunger.

passive immunity A form of acquired immunity that occurs artificially through injection or is acquired naturally as the result of antibody transfer through the placenta to a fetus or through colostrum to an infant; is not permanent and does not last as long as active immunity.

prodromal Pertaining to early symptoms that mark the onset of a disease.

puberty The period of time during which the adolescent experiences a growth spurt, develops secondary sex characteristics, and achieves reproductive maturity.

regurgitation An abnormal backward flow of body fluid.

retraction An abnormal movement of the chest wall during inspiration in which the skin appears to be drawn in between the ribs, and above and/or below the clavicle, and scapula; indicates respiratory difficulty.

shunt Movement of blood or body fluid through an abnormal anatomical or surgically created opening.

stenosis The narrowing or constriction of an opening.

stridor A shrill harsh sound heard during inspiration, expiration, or both, produced by the flow of air through a narrowed segment of the respiratory tract.

vaccine A suspension of attenuated or killed microorganisms administered to induce active immunity to infectious disease.

wheezing High-pitched musical whistle sounds heard with or without a stethoscope as air is compressed through narrowed or obstructed airways because of swelling, secretions, or tumors.

PYRAMID TO SUCCESS

Pyramid Points focus on growth and development, safety, and age-appropriate measures to ensure a safe and hazard-free environment for the child, protection of the child and the prevention of accidents, and on acute disorders that can occur in children. The focus is on nutrition, specific feeding techniques, positioning techniques, and interventions that will provide and maintain adequate airway, breathing, and circulation patterns in the child. Additionally, neglect and abuse of a child is a focus. On the NCLEX-RN examination, be alert to the age of the child if the age is presented in a question. If an age is presented in the question, think about the specific growth and development characteristics of the age group to answer the question correctly.

CLIENT NEEDS

Safe and Effective Care Environment

Considering issues related to informed consent regarding minors

Ensuring environmental safety, including home safety and personal safety, related to the developmental age of the child

Establishing priorities

Instituting measures related to the spread and control of infectious agents, particularly regarding communicable diseases

Maintaining confidentiality

Preventing accidents

Providing continuity of care

Providing protective measures

Protecting the child and other contacts to prevent illness

Upholding parent and child rights

Health Promotion and Maintenance

Ensuring that immunization schedules are up to date

Focusing on developmental stages when planning care

Performing physical assessment techniques specific to the pediatric client

Preventing disease in the pediatric population

Providing health promotion programs for the pediatric client

Providing instructions to the child and parents regarding care at home

Psychosocial Integrity

Assessment for child neglect and abuse

Communicating with the pediatric client

Considering concepts of family dynamics when planning care

Considering cultural, religious, and spiritual beliefs when planning care

Considering end-of-life issues and grief and loss in the pediatric population

Identifying family and support systems for the child

Providing play therapies

Physiological Integrity

Following medication administration procedures

Following nutritional guidelines for the pediatric population

Identifying comfort measures appropriate for the child

Maintaining sensitivity for intrusive procedures needed for the pediatric client

Managing childhood illnesses

Monitoring elimination patterns

Monitoring for age-appropriate normal body structure and function

Monitoring for infectious diseases of the pediatric client

Monitoring for potential alterations in body systems from disease

Monitoring for responses to treatments

Providing for consistent rest and sleep patterns

Responding to medical emergencies

36

Neurological, Cognitive, and Psychosocial Disorders

I. ATTENTION-DEFICIT/HYPERACTIVITY DISORDER

A. Description
   1. Behavior disorder characterized by developmentally inappropriate degrees of inattention, overactivity, and impulsivity
   2. Childhood problems include lowered intellectual development, some minor physical abnormalities, sleeping disturbances, behavioral or emotional disorders, and difficulty in social relationships.
   3. Early diagnosis is important to prevent impaired emotional and psychological development.
   4. Diagnosis is established based on self-reports, parent and teacher reports, and use of assessment tools.

B. Assessment
   1. Fidgets with hands or feet or squirms in the seat
   2. Easily distracted with external or internal stimuli
   3. Difficulty with following through on instructions
   4. Poor attention span
   5. Shifts from one uncompleted activity to another
   6. Talks excessively
   7. Interrupts or intrudes on others
   8. Engages in physically dangerous activities without considering the possible consequences

C. Interventions
   1. Provide parents with information about the disorder and treatment plan; encourage support groups for parents.
   2. Treatment includes behavioral therapy, medication, maintaining a consistent environment, and appropriate classroom placement.
   3. Behavioral therapy focuses on preventing undesirable behavior.
   4. Maintain a consistent home and classroom environment, and provide environmental and physical safety measures.
   5. Promote self-esteem.
   6. Stimulant medications may be prescribed; possible side effects include appetite suppression and weight loss, nervousness, tics, insomnia, and increased blood pressure.

   7. Instruct the child and parents about medication administration and the need for regular follow-up.

II. AUTISM

A. Description
   1. A severe form of an autism spectrum disorder (pervasive developmental disorder)
   2. Symptoms are usually noticed by the parents by 3 years of age.
   3. The cause of the disorder is not specifically known; however, it has been linked to a wide range of antepartum, intrapartum, and postpartum conditions and exposure to hazardous chemicals; genetic predisposition is also linked to the disorder.
   4. The disorder is accompanied by intellectual and social behavioral deficits, and the child exhibits peculiar and bizarre characteristics with social interactions, communication, and behaviors.
   5. Diagnosis is established based on symptoms and the use of several screening tools.

B. Assessment
   1. Social
      a. Abnormal or lack of comfort-seeking behaviors
      b. Abnormal or lack of social play
      c. Impairment in peer relationships
      d. Lack of awareness of the existence or feelings of others
      e. Abnormal or lack of imitation of others
   2. Communication
      a. Lack of, impaired, or abnormal speech such as producing a monotone voice or echolalia
      b. Abnormal nonverbal communication (does not use gestures to communicate)
      c. Lack of imaginative play
   3. Behavior
      a. Persistent preoccupation or attachment to objects; range of interests restricted
      b. Self-injurious behaviors
      c. Must maintain routine; any environmental change produces marked distress
      d. Produces repetitive body movements such as rocking or head banging

C. Interventions
1. Determine the child's routines, habits, and preferences and maintain consistency as much as possible.
2. Determine the specific ways in which the child communicates and use these methods.
3. Avoid placing demands on the child.
4. Evaluate the child for safety.
5. Implement safety precautions as necessary for self-injurious behaviors such as head banging.
6. Initiate referrals to special programs as required.
7. Provide support to parents.

⚠ Ensuring a safe environment for a child with autism is a priority.

III. CEREBRAL PALSY

A. Description
1. Disorder characterized by impaired movement and posture resulting from an abnormality in the extrapyramidal or pyramidal motor system
2. The most common clinical type is spastic cerebral palsy, which represents an upper motor neuron type of muscle weakness.
3. Less common types of cerebral palsy are athetoid, ataxic, and mixed.

B. Assessment
1. Extreme irritability and crying
2. Feeding difficulties
3. Abnormal motor performance
4. Alterations of muscle tone; stiff and rigid arms or legs
5. Delayed developmental milestones
6. Persistence of primitive infantile reflexes (Moro, tonic neck) after 6 months (most primitive reflexes disappear by 3 to 4 months of age)
7. Abnormal posturing, such as opisthotonos (exaggerated arching of the back) (Fig. 36-1)
8. Seizures may occur

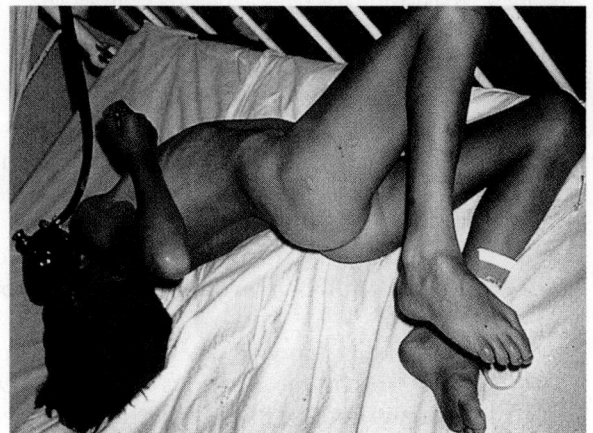

▲ **FIGURE 36-1** Abnormal posturing: opisthotonos. (From *Mosby's dictionary of medicine, nursing & health professions* [8th ed., p. 1328]. [2009]. St. Louis: Mosby. *Farrar* 1992.)

C. Interventions
1. The goal of management is early recognition and interventions to maximize the child's abilities.
2. A multidisciplinary team approach is implemented to meet the many needs of the child.
3. Therapeutic management includes physical therapy, occupational therapy, speech therapy, education, and recreation.
4. Assess the child's developmental level and intelligence.
5. Encourage early intervention and participation in school programs.
6. Prepare for using mobilizing devices to help prevent or reduce deformities.
7. Encourage communication and interaction with the child on his or her developmental level, rather than **chronological age** level.
8. Provide a safe environment by removing sharp objects, using a protective helmet if the child falls frequently, and implementing seizure precautions if necessary.
9. Provide safe, appropriate toys for the child's age and developmental level.
10. Position the child upright after meals.
11. Medications may be prescribed to relieve muscle spasms, which cause intense pain; antiseizure medications may also be prescribed.
12. Provide the parents with information about the disorder and treatment plan; encourage support groups for parents.

IV. CHILD ABDUCTION

A. Description
1. Child abduction is the kidnapping of a child (or infant) by an older person.
2. Occurrences
   a. A stranger may kidnap a child for criminal or mischievous purposes.
   b. A stranger may kidnap a child (or infant) to bring up him or her as that person's own child.
   c. A parent removes or retains a child from the other parent's care (often in the course of or after divorce proceedings).
3. Because of the increased independence that occurs in the preschool-age child, parents are less able to provide the constant protection they once did when the child reaches this age; interventions (including teaching the child) that ensure protection are necessary.

B. Interventions
1. Instruct the parents to teach a child basic guidelines about personal safety that include the following:
   a. Do not go anywhere alone.
   b. Always tell an adult where he or she is going and when he or she will return.
   c. Say *no* if he or she feels uncomfortable with a situation.

Box 36-1 Child Neglect and Abuse: Assessment Findings

Neglect
Inadequate weight gain
Poor hygiene
Consistent hunger
Inconsistent school attendance
Constant fatigue
Reports of lack of child supervision
Delinquency

Physical Abuse
Unexplained bruises, burns, or fractures
Bald spots on the scalp
Apprehensive child
Extreme aggressiveness or withdrawal
Fear of parents
Lack of crying (older infant, toddler, or young preschool child) when approached by a stranger

Emotional Abuse
Speech disorders

Habit disorders such as sucking, biting, and rocking
Psychoneurotic reactions
Learning disorders
Suicide attempts

Sexual Abuse
Difficulty walking or sitting
Torn, stained, or bloody underclothing
Pain, swelling, or itching of genitals
Bruises, bleeding, or lacerations in genital or anal area
Unwillingness to change clothes or unwillingness to participate in gym activities
Poor peer relations

Shaken Baby Syndrome
External signs of trauma are usually absent
Ophthalmoscopic examination reveals retinal hemorrhages
Full bulging fontanels and head circumference greater than expected

d. Do not talk with strangers or get into their cars.
e. Do not help anyone look for a lost dog or cat and do not accept candy from a stranger.
f. If lost in a store, do not wander around looking for the parent; go at once to a clerk or guard.
2. Children need to learn their full name, address, and parent's name.
3. Watch for posttraumatic stress disorder in any child who has experienced an abduction.

V. CHILD ABUSE

A. Description
1. **Abuse** is the nonaccidental physical injury or the nonaccidental act of omission of care by a parent or person responsible for a child; **abuse** comprises neglect and physical, sexual, and emotional maltreatment.
2. Neglect can be in the form of physical or emotional neglect and involves the deprivation of basic needs, supervision, medical care, or education and failure to meet a child's needs for attention and affection.
3. Sexual **abuse** can involve incest, molestation, exhibitionism, pornography, prostitution, or pedophilia; findings associated with sexual **abuse** may not be easily apparent in a child.
4. Shaken baby syndrome is caused by the violent shaking of an infant younger than 1 year and results in intracranial (usually subdural hemorrhage) trauma; this can lead to cerebral edema and death.

B. Assessment (Box 36-1)
C. Interventions
1. Support the child during a thorough physical assessment.
2. Assess injuries.

3. If shaken baby syndrome is suspected, monitor the infant for a decrease in level of consciousness, which can indicate increased intracranial pressure (ICP).
4. Report a case of suspected **abuse**; nurses are legally required to report all cases of suspected child **abuse** to the appropriate local or state agency.
5. Place the child in an environment that is safe, preventing further injury.
6. Document information related to the suspected **abuse** in an objective manner.
7. Assess parents' strengths and weaknesses, normal coping mechanisms, and presence or absence of support systems.
8. Assist the family in identifying stressors, support systems, and resources.
9. Refer the family to appropriate support groups.

⚠ Nurses are legally required to report all cases of suspected child abuse to the appropriate local or state agency.

VI. HEAD INJURY

A. Description
1. Head injury is the pathological result of any mechanical force to the skull, scalp, meninges, or brain (Fig. 36-2).
a. Open head injury occurs when there is a fracture of the skull or penetration of the skull by an object.
b. Closed head injury is the result of blunt trauma (this is more serious than an open head injury because of the chance of increased ICP in a "closed" vault); this type of injury can also be caused by shaken baby syndrome.

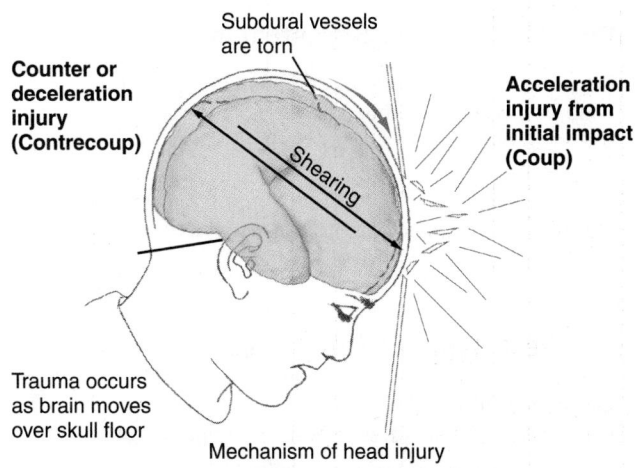

Mechanism of head injury

▲ **FIGURE 36-2** Mechanism of head injury. (From Marcoux, K. [2005]. Management of increased intravascular pressure in the critically ill child. *AACU Clinical Issues* 16[2], 212–213. Reprinted with permission.)

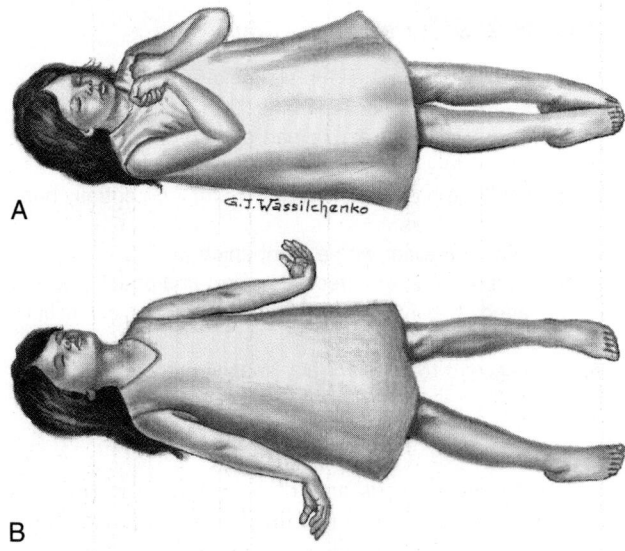

▲ **FIGURE 36-3 A,** Decorticate (flexion) posturing. **B,** Decerebrate (extension) posturing. (From Hockenberry, M., & Wilson, D. [2009]. *Wong's essentials of pediatric nursing* [8th ed., p. 979]. St. Louis: Mosby.)

2. Manifestations depend on the type of injury and the subsequent amount of increased ICP.

B. Assessment: Increased ICP

⚠️ The child's level of consciousness provides the earliest indication of an improvement or deterioration of the neurological condition.

1. Early signs
   a. Slight change in vital signs
   b. Slight change in level of consciousness
   c. Infant: Irritability, high-pitched cry, bulging fontanel, increased head circumference, dilated scalp veins, Macewen's sign (cracked-pot sound on percussion of the head), setting sun sign (sclera visible above the iris)
   d. Child: Headache, nausea, vomiting, visual disturbances (diplopia), seizures
2. Late signs
   a. Decrease in level of consciousness
   b. Bradycardia
   c. Decreased motor and sensory responses
   d. Alteration in pupil size and reactivity
   e. Decorticate (flexion) posturing: Adduction of the arms at the shoulders; arms are flexed on the chest with the wrists flexed and the hands fisted, and the lower extremities are extended and adducted; seen with severe dysfunction of cerebral cortex (Fig. 36-3)
   f. Decerebrate (extension) posturing: Rigid extension and pronation of the arms and the legs; sign of dysfunction at the level of the midbrain (see Fig. 36-3)
   g. Cheyne-Stokes respirations
   h. Coma

C. Interventions

⚠️ Immobilize the neck and spine after a head injury if a cervical or other spinal injury is suspected. When a spinal cord injury is ruled out, elevate the head of the bed 15 to 30 degrees, if not contraindicated and as prescribed, to facilitate venous drainage.

1. Monitor the airway; administer oxygen as prescribed.
2. Assess injuries. (See Chapter 66 for information on spinal cord injuries.)
3. Position the client so that the head is maintained midline to avoid jugular vein compression, which can increase ICP.
4. Monitor vital signs and neurological function (assess level of consciousness closely).
5. Keep stimuli to a minimum; attempt to minimize crying in an infant.
6. Withhold sedating medications during the acute phase of the injury so that changes in levels of consciousness can be assessed.
7. Initiate seizure precautions (Box 36-2).
8. Monitor for decreased responsiveness to pain (a significant sign of altered level of consciousness).
9. Maintain NPO status or provide clear liquids, if prescribed, until it is determined that vomiting will not occur.
10. Monitor prescribed intravenous fluids carefully to avoid aggravating any cerebral edema and to minimize the possibility of overhydration.
11. Monitor for a fluid or electrolyte alteration (could indicate injury to the hypothalamus or posterior pituitary)

Box 36-2 Seizure Precautions

Raise side rails when child is sleeping or resting.
Pad side rails and other hard objects.
Place waterproof mattress or pad on bed or crib.
Instruct child to wear or carry medical identification.
Instruct child in precautions to take during potentially hazardous activities.
Instruct child to swim with a companion.
Instruct child to use a protective helmet and padding when engaged in bicycle riding, skateboarding, and in-line skating.
Alert caregivers to need for any special precautions.

Box 36-3 Signs of Brainstem Involvement

Deep, rapid, or intermittent and gasping respirations
Wide fluctuations or noticeable slowing of pulse
Widening pulse pressure or extreme fluctuations in blood pressure
Sluggish, dilated, or unequal pupils
Notify physician immediately if these signs develop!

Box 36-4 Types of Hydrocephalus

Communicating
Hydrocephalus occurs as a result of impaired absorption within the subarachnoid space.
Interference of the cerebrospinal fluid in the ventricular system does not occur.

Noncommunicating
Obstruction of cerebrospinal fluid flow in the ventricular system does occur.

12. Assess wounds and dressings for the presence of drainage, and monitor for nose or ear drainage, which could indicate leakage of cerebrospinal fluid (CSF).
13. Administer tepid sponge baths or place the child on a hypothermia blanket as prescribed if hyperthermia occurs.
14. Avoid suctioning through the nares because of the possibility of the catheter entering the brain through a fracture, which places the child at high risk for a secondary infection.
15. As prescribed, administer acetaminophen (Tylenol) for headache, anticonvulsants for seizures, and antibiotics if a laceration is present; prepare to administer prophylactic tetanus toxoid.
16. A corticosteroid or osmotic diuretic may be prescribed to reduce cerebral edema.
17. Monitor for signs of brainstem involvement (Box 36-3).
18. Monitor for signs of epidural hematoma: Asymmetrical pupils (one dilated, nonreactive pupil) may indicate a neurosurgical emergency that requires evacuation of the hematoma.

⚠ Drainage from the nose or ear needs to be tested for the presence of glucose. Drainage that is positive for glucose (as tested with reagent strips) indicates leakage of CSF. The physician must be notified immediately if the drainage tests positive for glucose.

VII. HYDROCEPHALUS

A. Description
1. An imbalance of CSF absorption or production caused by malformations, tumors, hemorrhage, infections, or trauma
2. Results in head enlargement and increased ICP
B. Types (Box 36-4)
C. Assessment
1. Infant
a. Increased head circumference
b. Thin, widely separated bones of the head that produce a cracked-pot sound (Macewen's sign) on percussion
c. Anterior fontanel tense, bulging, and nonpulsating
d. Dilated scalp veins
e. Frontal bossing
f. Setting sun eyes
2. Child
a. Behavior changes, such as irritability and lethargy
b. Headache on awakening
c. Nausea and vomiting
d. Ataxia
e. Nystagmus
3. Late signs: High, shrill cry and seizures
D. Surgical interventions
1. The goal of surgical treatment is to prevent further CSF accumulation by bypassing the blockage and draining the fluid from the ventricles to a location where it may be reabsorbed.
2. In a ventriculoperitoneal **shunt**, the CSF drains into the peritoneal cavity from the lateral ventricle (Fig. 36-4).
3. In a ventriculoatrial **shunt**, CSF drains into the right atrium of the heart from the lateral ventricle, bypassing the obstruction (used in older children and in children with pathological conditions of the abdomen).
4. **Shunt** revision may be necessary as the child grows.
5. An alternative to **shunt** placement is endoscopic third ventriculostomy, in which a small opening in the floor of the third ventricle is made that allows CSF to bypass the fourth ventricle and return to the circulation to be absorbed; this treatment may not be appropriate for some types of hydrocephalus.

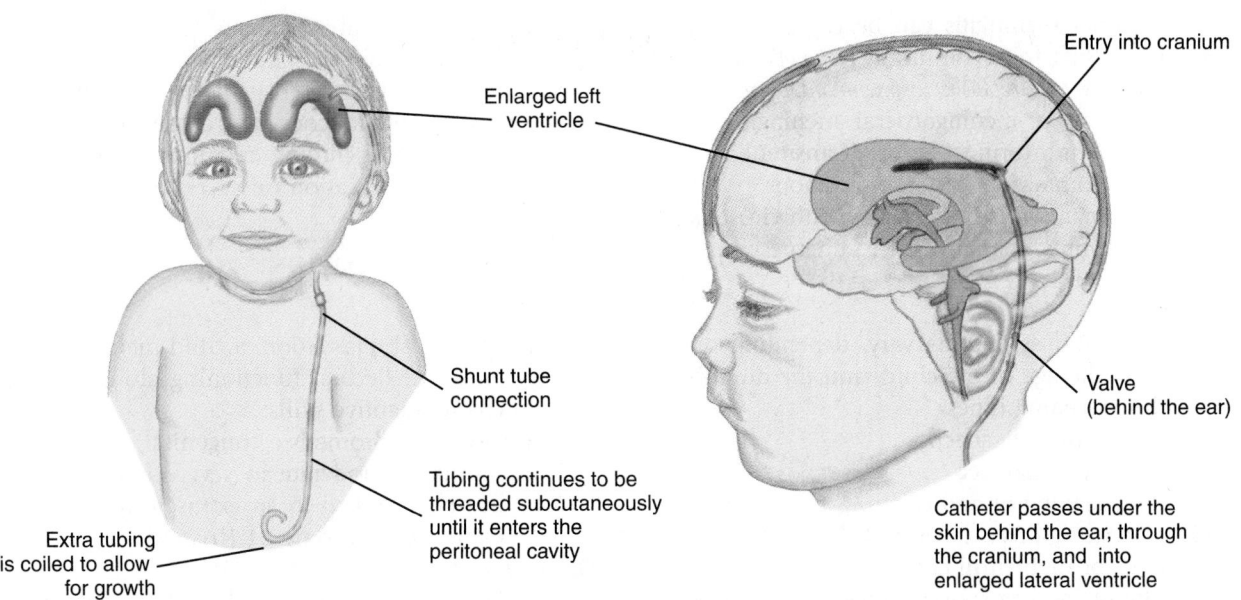

Enlarged left ventricle

Entry into cranium

Shunt tube connection

Valve (behind the ear)

Tubing continues to be threaded subcutaneously until it enters the peritoneal cavity

Extra tubing is coiled to allow for growth

Catheter passes under the skin behind the ear, through the cranium, and into enlarged lateral ventricle

▲ **FIGURE 36-4** Ventriculoperitoneal shunt. (From McKinney, E., James, S., Murray, S., & Ashwill, J. [2009]. *Maternal-child nursing* [3rd ed.]. St. Louis: Saunders.)

E. Preoperative interventions
1. Monitor intake and output; give small, frequent feedings as tolerated until preoperative NPO status is prescribed.
2. Reposition the head frequently and use special devices such as an egg crate mattress under the head to prevent pressure sores.
3. Prepare the child and family for diagnostic procedures and surgery.

F. Postoperative interventions
1. Monitor vital signs and neurological signs.
2. Position the child on the unoperated side to prevent pressure on the **shunt** valve.
3. Keep the child flat as prescribed to avoid rapid reduction of intracranial fluid.
4. Observe for increased ICP; if increased ICP occurs, elevate the head of the bed to 15 to 30 degrees to enhance gravity flow through the **shunt**.
5. Measure head circumference.
6. Monitor for signs of infection and assess dressings for drainage.
7. Monitor intake and output.
8. Provide comfort measures and administer medications as prescribed.
9. Instruct parents on how to recognize **shunt** infection or malfunction.
10. In an infant, irritability, a high shrill cry, lethargy, and feeding poorly may indicate **shunt** malfunction or infection.
11. In a toddler, headache and a lack of appetite are the earliest common signs of **shunt** malfunction.
12. In older children, an indicator of **shunt** malfunction is an alteration in the child's level of consciousness.

⚠ A high shrill cry in an infant can be a sign of increased ICP.

VIII. LATCHKEY CHILDREN

A. Description
1. Children who do not have adult supervision before or after school hours; they are left to care for themselves during these times
2. Occurs when children are members of a single-parent family or both parents work and need to leave the home before children are brought to school
3. This situation induces a stress-provoking environment for the children and places the children at risk for injury and delinquent behavior.

B. Interventions
1. Identify the latchkey child.
2. Encourage the parent to teach the child about self-care and self-help skills.
3. Inform the parent about available community resources such as after-school programs for children.

IX. MENINGITIS

A. Description
1. Meningitis is an infectious process of the central nervous system caused by bacteria or viruses that may be acquired as a primary disease or as a result of complications of neurosurgery, trauma, infection of the sinuses or ears, or systemic infections.
2. Diagnosis of bacterial meningitis is made by testing CSF obtained by lumbar puncture; the fluid is cloudy with increased pressure, increased white blood cell count, elevated protein, and decreased glucose levels.

3. Bacterial meningitis can be caused by various organisms, most commonly *Haemophilus influenzae* type b, *Streptococcus pneumoniae*, or *Neisseria meningitidis*; meningococcal meningitis occurs in epidemic form and can be transmitted by droplets from nasopharyngeal secretions.

4. Viral meningitis is associated with viruses such as mumps, paramyxovirus, herpesvirus, and enterovirus.

B. Assessment

1. Signs and symptoms vary, depending on the type, the age of the child, and the duration of the preceding illness.
2. Fever, chills, headache
3. Vomiting, diarrhea
4. Poor feeding or anorexia
5. Nuchal rigidity
6. Poor or high shrill cry
7. Altered level of consciousness, such as lethargy or irritability
8. Bulging anterior fontanel in an infant
9. Positive Kernig's sign (inability to extend the leg when the thigh is flexed anteriorly at the hip) and Brudzinski's sign (neck flexion causes adduction and flexion movements of the lower extremities) in children and adolescents
10. Muscle or joint pain (meningococcal infection and *H. influenzae* infection)
11. Petechial or purpuric rashes (meningococcal infection)
12. Ear that chronically drains (pneumococcal meningitis)

C. Interventions

1. Provide respiratory isolation precautions and maintain it for at least 24 hours after antibiotics are initiated.
2. 'Administer antibiotics and antipyretics as prescribed (administer antibiotics as soon as they are prescribed after lumbar puncture); antiseizure medications may also be prescribed.
3. Perform neurological assessment and monitor for seizures; assess for the complication of inappropriate antidiuretic hormone secretion, causing fluid retention (cerebral edema) and dilutional hyponatremia.
4. Assess for changes in level of consciousness and irritability.
5. Monitor for a purpuric or petechial rash and for signs of thromboemboli.
6. Assess nutritional status; monitor intake and output.
7. Monitor for hearing loss.
8. Determine close contacts of the child with meningitis because the contacts need prophylactic treatment.

9. Pneumococcal conjugate **vaccine** is recommended for all children beginning at age 2 months to protect against meningitis; streptococcal pneumococci can cause many bacterial infections including meningitis (see Chapter 48 for information on **vaccines**).

X. MENTAL RETARDATION

A. Description

1. In mental retardation, a child manifests subaverage intellectual functioning along with deficits in adaptive skills.
2. Down syndrome is a congenital condition that results in moderate to severe retardation and has been linked to an extra group G chromosome, chromosome 21 (trisomy 21).

B. Assessment

1. Deficits in cognitive skills and level of adaptive functioning
2. Delays in fine and gross motor skills
3. Speech delays
4. Decreased spontaneous activity
5. Nonresponsiveness
6. Irritability
7. Poor eye contact during feeding

C. Interventions

1. Medical strategies are focused on correcting structural deformities and treating associated behaviors.
2. Implement community and educational services using a multidisciplinary approach.
3. Promote care skills as much as possible.
4. Assist with communication and socialization skills.
5. Facilitate appropriate play time.
6. Initiate safety precautions as necessary.
7. Assist the family with decisions regarding care.
8. Provide information regarding support services and community agencies.

XI. NEAR-DROWNING

A. Description

1. Survival of at least 24 hours after submersion in a fluid medium
2. Hypoxia and asphyxiation is the primary problem because it results in extensive cell damage; cerebral cells sustain irreversible damage after 4 to 6 minutes of submersion.
3. Additional problems include aspiration and hypothermia.
4. Outcome is predicted based on the length of submersion in nonicy water; outcome may be good if submersion was for less than 5 minutes and the child exhibits neurological responsiveness, reactive pupils, and a normal cardiac rhythm.

5. A child who was submerged for more than 10 minutes and does not respond to cardiopulmonary life support measures within 25 minutes has an extremely poor prognosis (severe neurological impairment or death).
B. Interventions
1. Provide ventilatory and circulatory support; if the child has had a severe cerebral insult, endotracheal intubation and mechanical ventilation may be required.
2. Monitor respiratory status because respiratory compromise and cerebral edema may occur 24 hours after the incident.
3. Monitor for aspiration pneumonia.
4. Monitor neurological status closely; if spontaneous purposeful movement and normal brainstem function are not apparent 24 hours after the event, the child most likely has sustained severe neurological deficits.
5. Teach parents to provide adequate supervision of infants and small children around water to prevent accidents.

XII. REYE'S SYNDROME

A. Description
1. Reye's syndrome is an acute encephalopathy that follows a viral illness and is characterized pathologically by cerebral edema and fatty changes in the liver; a definitive diagnosis is made by liver biopsy.
2. The exact cause is unclear; it most commonly follows a viral illness such as influenza or varicella.
3. Administration of aspirin and aspirin-containing products is not recommended for children with a febrile illness or children with varicella or influenza because of its association with Reye's syndrome.
4. Acetaminophen (Tylenol) is considered the medication of choice for pediatric clients.
5. Early diagnosis and aggressive treatment are important; the goal of treatment is to maintain effective cerebral perfusion and control increasing ICP.
B. Assessment
1. History of systemic viral illness 4 to 7 days before the onset of symptoms
2. Fever
3. Nausea and vomiting
4. Signs of altered hepatic function such as lethargy
5. Progressive neurological deterioration
C. Interventions
1. Provide rest and decrease stimulation in the environment.
2. Assess neurological status.
3. Monitor for altered level of consciousness and signs of increased ICP.

4. Monitor for signs of altered hepatic function and results of liver function studies.
5. Monitor intake and output.
6. Monitor for signs of bleeding and signs of impaired coagulation, such as a prolonged bleeding time.

XIII. SEIZURE DISORDERS

A. Description (see Chapter 66 for additional information on seizures)
1. Excessive and unorganized neuronal discharges in the brain that activate associated motor and sensory organs
2. Classified as generalized, partial, or unclassified, depending on the area of the brain involved
3. Types of generalized seizures include tonic-clonic, absence, myoclonic, and atonic.
4. Partial seizures arise from a specific area in the brain and cause limited symptoms; types include simple partial and complex partial.
B. Assessment
1. Obtain information from the parents about the time of onset, precipitating events, and behavior before and after the seizure.
2. Determine the child's history related to seizures.
3. Ask the child about the presence of an aura (a warning sign of impending seizure).
4. Monitor for apnea and **cyanosis**.
5. Postseizure: The child is disoriented and sleepy.
C. Seizure precautions (see Box 36-2)
D. Interventions (Box 36-5)
E. Anticonvulsant medications (see Chapter 67 for information on medications)

Box 36-5 Interventions for Seizures

Ensure airway patency.
Have suction equipment and oxygen available.
Time the seizure episode.
If the child is standing or sitting, ease the child down to the floor and place the child in a side-lying position.
Place a pillow or folded blanket under the child's head; if no bedding is available, place your own hands under the child's head or place the child's head in your own lap.
Loosen restrictive clothing.
Remove eyeglasses from the child if present.
Clear the area of any hazards or hard objects.
Allow the seizure to proceed and end without interference.
If vomiting occurs, turn the child to one side as a unit.
Do not restrain the child, place anything in the child's mouth, or give any food or liquids to the child.
Prepare to administer medications as prescribed.
Remain with the child until the child fully recovers.
Observe for incontinence, which may have occurred during the seizure.
Document the occurrence.

⚠ Never place anything, including an airway device or a padded tongue blade, into the mouth of a child experiencing a seizure.

XIV. SPINA BIFIDA

A. Description
1. This central nervous system defect results from failure of the neural tube to close during embryonic development.
2. Associated deficits include sensorimotor disturbance, dislocated hips, talipes equinovarus (clubfoot), and hydrocephalus.
3. Defect closure is performed soon after birth.

B. Types
1. Spina bifida occulta
   a. Posterior vertebral arches fail to close in the lumbosacral area.
   b. Spinal cord remains intact and usually is not visible.
   c. Meninges are not exposed on the skin surface.
   d. Neurological deficits are not usually present.
2. Spina bifida cystica
   a. Protrusion of the spinal cord or its meninges or both occurs.
   b. Defect results in incomplete closure of the vertebral and neural tubes, resulting in a sac-like protrusion in the lumbar or sacral area, with varying degrees of nervous tissue involvement.
   c. Defect can include meningocele, myelomeningocele, lipomeningocele, and lipomeningomyelocele.
3. Meningocele
   a. Protrusion involves meninges and a sac-like cyst that contains CSF in the midline of the back, usually in the lumbosacral area.
   b. Spinal cord is not involved.
   c. Neurological deficits are usually not present.
4. Myelomeningocele
   a. Protrusion of the meninges, CSF, nerve roots, and a portion of the spinal cord occurs.
   b. The sac (defect) is covered by a thin membrane prone to leakage or rupture.
   c. Neurological deficits are evident.

C. Assessment
1. Depends on the spinal cord involvement
2. Visible spinal defect
3. Flaccid paralysis of the legs
4. Altered bladder and bowel function
5. Hip and joint deformities
6. Hydrocephalus

D. Interventions
1. Evaluate the sac and measure the lesion.
2. Perform neurological assessment.
3. Monitor for increased ICP, which might indicate developing hydrocephalus.

4. Measure head circumference; assess anterior fontanel for fullness.
5. Protect the sac; cover with a sterile, moist (normal saline), nonadherent dressing to maintain the moisture of the sac and contents.
6. Change the dressing covering the sac on a regular schedule or whenever it becomes soiled because of the risk of infection; diapering may be contraindicated until the defect has been repaired.
7. Use aseptic technique to prevent infection.
8. Assess the sac for redness, clear or purulent drainage, abrasions, irritation, and signs of infection.
9. Early signs of infection include elevated temperature (axillary), irritability, lethargy, and nuchal rigidity.
10. Place in a prone position to minimize tension on the sac and the risk of trauma; the head is turned to one side for feeding.
11. Assess for physical impairments such as hip and joint deformities.
12. Prepare the child and family for surgery.
13. Administer antibiotics preoperatively and postoperatively, as prescribed, to prevent infection.
14. Teach the parents and eventually the child about long-term home care.
    a. Positioning, feeding, skin care, and range-of-motion exercises
    b. Instituting a bladder elimination program and performing clean intermittent catheterization technique
    c. Administering antispasmodics (that act on the smooth muscle of the bladder) as prescribed to increase bladder capacity and improve continence
    d. Implement a bowel program including a high-fiber diet, increased fluids, and suppositories as needed.
    e. The child is at high risk for allergy to latex and rubber products because of the frequent exposure to latex during implementation of care measures.

🔘 MORE QUESTIONS ON THE CD!

Practice Questions

366. A nurse is caring for a child recently diagnosed with cerebral palsy, and the parents of the child ask the nurse about the disorder. The nurse bases her response on the understanding that cerebral palsy is:

1. An infectious disease of the central nervous system
2. An inflammation of the brain as a result of a viral illness
3. A congenital condition that results in moderate to severe retardation
4. A chronic disability characterized by impaired muscle movement and posture

367. A nurse performs an admission assessment on a child and suspects physical abuse. Based on this suspicion, the primary legal nursing responsibility is which of the following?
1. Refer the family to the appropriate support groups.
2. Assist the family in identifying resources and support systems.
3. Report the case in which the abuse is suspected to the local authorities.
4. Document the child's physical assessment findings accurately and thoroughly.

368. A mother arrives at an emergency department with her 5-year-old child and states that the child fell off a bunk bed. A head injury is suspected, and a nurse checks the child's airway status and assesses the child for signs of increased intracranial pressure (ICP). Which of the following is a late sign of increased ICP in this child?
1. Nausea
2. Bradycardia
3. Bulging fontanel
4. Dilated scalp veins

369. A nurse is assigned to care for an 8-year-old child with a diagnosis of a basilar skull fracture. The nurse reviews the physician's prescriptions and contacts the physician to question which prescriptions?
1. Suction as needed.
2. Obtain daily weight.
3. Provide clear liquid intake.
4. Maintain a patent intravenous line.

370. A nurse is caring for an infant with a diagnosis of hydrocephalus. Preoperatively, a priority nursing intervention is to:
1. Test the urine for protein.
2. Reposition the infant frequently.
3. Provide a stimulating environment.
4. Assess blood pressure every 15 minutes.

371. A nurse is reviewing the record of a child with increased intracranial pressure and notes that the child has exhibited signs of decerebrate posturing. On assessment of the child, the nurse expects to note which of the following if this type of posturing is present?

1. Flaccid paralysis of all extremities
2. Adduction of the arms at the shoulders
3. Rigid extension and pronation of the arms and legs
4. Abnormal flexion of the upper extremities and extension and adduction of the lower extremities

372. A child is diagnosed with Reye's syndrome. A nurse develops a nursing care plan for the child and includes which intervention in the plan?
1. Assessing hearing loss
2. Monitoring urine output
3. Changing body position every 2 hours
4. Providing a quiet atmosphere with dimmed lighting

373. A nurse develops a plan of care for a child at risk for tonic-clonic seizures. In the plan of care, the nurse identifies seizure precautions and documents that which item(s) need to be placed at the child's bedside?
1. Emergency cart
2. Tracheotomy set
3. Padded tongue blade
4. Suctioning equipment and oxygen

374. A lumbar puncture is performed on a child suspected to have bacterial meningitis, and cerebrospinal fluid (CSF) is obtained for analysis. A nurse reviews the results of the CSF analysis and determines that which of the following results would verify the diagnosis?
1. Clear CSF, decreased pressure, and elevated protein level
2. Clear CSF, elevated protein, and decreased glucose levels
3. Cloudy CSF, elevated protein, and decreased glucose levels
4. Cloudy CSF, decreased protein, and decreased glucose levels

375. A nurse is planning care for a child with acute bacterial meningitis. Based on the mode of transmission of this infection, which of the following should be included in the plan of care?
1. Maintain enteric precautions.
2. Maintain neutropenic precautions.
3. No precautions are required as long as antibiotics have been started.
4. Maintain respiratory isolation precautions for at least 24 hours after the initiation of antibiotics.

Alternate Item Format: Multiple Response

376. A nurse is developing a plan of care for a child who is at risk for seizures. Which interventions apply if the child has a seizure? **Select all that apply.**
❑ 1. Time the seizure.
❑ 2. Restrain the child.
❑ 3. Stay with the child.
❑ 4. Place the child in a prone position.
❑ 5. Move furniture away from the child.
❑ 6. Insert a padded tongue blade in the child's mouth.

ANSWERS

366. 4
Rationale: Cerebral palsy is a chronic disability characterized by impaired movement and posture resulting from an abnormality in the extrapyramidal or pyramidal motor system. Meningitis is an infectious process of the central nervous system. Encephalitis is an inflammation of the brain that occurs as a result of viral illness or central nervous system infection. Down syndrome is an example of a congenital condition that results in moderate to severe retardation.
Test-Taking Strategy: Use the process of elimination. Eliminate options 1 and 2 first, noting that they are comparable or alike. Next, note the relationship between the words *palsy* in the question and *impaired muscle movement* in option 4. If you had difficulty with this question, review the characteristics associated with cerebral palsy.
Level of Cognitive Ability: Understanding
Client Needs: Physiological Integrity
Integrated Process: Teaching and Learning
Content Area: Child Health—Neurological/Musculoskeletal
References: McKinney, E., James, S., Murray, S., & Ashwill, J. (2009). *Maternal-child nursing* (3rd ed., p. 1480). St. Louis: Saunders.
Swearingen, P. (2008). *All-in-one care planning resource: Medical-surgical, pediatric, maternity, & psychiatric nursing care plans* (2nd ed., p. 609). St. Louis: Mosby.

367. 3
Rationale: Abuse is the nonaccidental physical injury or the nonaccidental act of omission of care by a parent or person responsible for a child. It includes neglect and physical, sexual, and emotional maltreatment. The primary legal nursing responsibility when child abuse is suspected is to report the case. All states and provinces in North America have laws for mandatory reporting of child maltreatment. Suspected child abuse should be reported to the local authorities. Although documentation of assessment findings, assisting the family, and referring the family to appropriate resources and support groups are important, the primary legal responsibility is to report the suspected case.
Test-Taking Strategy: Use the process of elimination, noting the strategic words *primary* and *legal*. In addition to the many implications associated with child abuse, abuse is a crime. With this in mind, option 3, reporting the case of abuse, is the primary responsibility. If you had difficulty with this question, review the responsibilities of the nurse when child abuse is suspected.
Level of Cognitive Ability: Applying
Client Needs: Psychosocial Integrity
Integrated Process: Nursing Process—Implementation
Content Area: Child Health—Neurological/Musculoskeletal
Reference: Hockenberry, M., & Wilson, D. (2009). *Wong's essentials of pediatric nursing* (8th ed., p. 486). St. Louis: Mosby.

368. 2
Rationale: Head injury is the pathological result of any mechanical force to the skull, scalp, meninges, or brain. A head injury can cause bleeding in the brain and result in increased intracranial pressure (ICP). Late signs of increased ICP include a significant decrease in level of consciousness, bradycardia, decreased motor and sensory responses, alterations in pupil size and reactivity, posturing, Cheyne-Stokes respirations, and coma. A bulging fontanel and dilated scalp veins are early signs of increased ICP and would be noted in an infant, not a 5-year-old child. Nausea is an early sign of increased ICP.
Test-Taking Strategy: Use the process of elimination, and note the age of the child and the strategic word *late*. Options 3 and 4 can be eliminated first because these signs would be noted in an infant, not a 5-year-old child. Focusing on the strategic word *late* will direct you to option 2 from the remaining options. If you had difficulty with this question, review the early and late signs of increased ICP in an infant and in a child.
Level of Cognitive Ability: Analyzing
Client Needs: Physiological Integrity
Integrated Process: Nursing Process—Assessment
Content Area: Child Health—Neurological/Musculoskeletal
Reference: Hockenberry, M., & Wilson, D. (2009). *Wong's essentials of pediatric nursing* (8th ed., p. 976). St. Louis: Mosby.

369. 1
Rationale: A basilar skull fracture is a type of head injury. Nasotracheal suctioning is contraindicated in a child with a basilar skull fracture. Because of the nature of the injury, there is a high risk of secondary infection and the probability of the catheter entering the brain through the fracture. Fluid balance is monitored closely by daily weight, intake and output measurement, and serum osmolality determination to detect early signs of water retention, excessive dehydration, and states of hypertonicity or hypotonicity. The child is maintained on NPO status or restricted to clear liquids until it is determined that vomiting will not occur. An intravenous line is maintained to administer fluids or medications if necessary.
Test-Taking Strategy: Note the strategic words *question which prescription*. Eliminate options 2, 3, and 4 because they are comparable or alike in that they address the subject of fluids. Remember that nasotracheal suctioning is contraindicated in a child with a skull fracture because of the risk of infection. If you had difficulty with this question, review the care of a child with a skull fracture.
Level of Cognitive Ability: Analyzing
Client Needs: Physiological Integrity
Integrated Process: Nursing Process—Implementation

Content Area: Child Health—Neurological/Musculoskeletal
Reference: Hockenberry, M., & Wilson, D. (2009). *Wong's essentials of pediatric nursing* (8th ed., p. 992). St. Louis: Mosby.

370. 2

Rationale: Hydrocephalus occurs as a result of an imbalance of cerebrospinal fluid absorption or production that is caused by malformations, tumors, hemorrhage, infections, or trauma. It results in head enlargement and increased intracranial pressure. In infants with hydrocephalus, the head grows at an abnormal rate, and if the infant is not repositioned frequently, pressure ulcers can occur on the back and side of the head. An egg crate mattress under the head is also a nursing intervention that can help prevent skin breakdown. Proteinuria is not specific to hydrocephalus. Stimulus should be kept at a minimum because of the increase in intracranial pressure. It is not necessary to check the blood pressure every 15 minutes.
Test-Taking Strategy: Focus on the child's diagnosis. Eliminate option 4 because of the words *15 minutes*. From the remaining options, recall that because of the severe head enlargement, the nursing intervention that has priority is to reposition the infant frequently to prevent development of pressure areas. Review the complications associated with hydrocephalus if you had difficulty with this question.
Level of Cognitive Ability: Applying
Client Needs: Physiological Integrity
Integrated Process: Nursing Process—Implementation
Content Area: Child Health—Neurological/Musculoskeletal
Reference: McKinney, E., James, S., Murray, S., & Ashwill, J. (2009). *Maternal-child nursing* (3rd ed., p. 1478). St. Louis: Saunders.

371. 3

Rationale: Decerebrate (extension) posturing is characterized by the rigid extension and pronation of the arms and legs. Option 1 is incorrect. Options 2 and 4 describe decorticate (flexion) posturing.
Test-Taking Strategy: Focus on the data in the question. Recalling the clinical manifestations associated with decerebrate posturing will direct you to the correct option. Remember that decerebrate posturing is characterized by the rigid extension and pronation of the arms and legs. Review the characteristics of decorticate and decerebrate posturing if you had difficulty with this question.
Level of Cognitive Ability: Analyzing
Client Needs: Physiological Integrity
Integrated Process: Nursing Process—Assessment
Content Area: Child Health—Neurological/Musculoskeletal
Reference: Hockenberry, M., & Wilson, D. (2009). *Wong's essentials of pediatric nursing* (8th ed., p. 979). St. Louis: Mosby.

372. 4

Rationale: Reye's syndrome is an acute encephalopathy that follows a viral illness and is characterized pathologically by cerebral edema and fatty changes in the liver. A definitive diagnosis is made by liver biopsy. In Reye's syndrome, supportive care is directed toward monitoring and managing cerebral edema. Decreasing stimuli in the environment by providing a quiet environment with dimmed lighting would decrease the stress on the cerebral tissue and neuron responses. Hearing loss and urine output are not affected. Changing the body position every 2 hours would not affect the cerebral edema directly. The child should be positioned with the head elevated to decrease the progression of the cerebral edema and promote drainage of cerebrospinal fluid.
Test-Taking Strategy: Think about the pathophysiology associated with Reye's syndrome. Recalling that cerebral edema is a concern for a child with Reye's syndrome will direct you to option 4. If you had difficulty with this question, review the appropriate plan of nursing care for a child with Reye's syndrome.
Level of Cognitive Ability: Applying
Client Needs: Physiological Integrity
Integrated Process: Nursing Process—Planning
Content Area: Child Health—Neurological/Musculoskeletal
References: Hockenberry, M., & Wilson, D. (2009). *Wong's essentials of pediatric nursing* (8th ed., p. 1004). St. Louis: Mosby.
McKinney, E., James, S., Murray, S., & Ashwill, J. (2009). *Maternal-child nursing* (3rd ed., p. 1499). St. Louis: Saunders.

373. 4

Rationale: A seizure results from the excessive and unorganized neuronal discharges in the brain that activate associated motor and sensory organs. A type of generalized seizure is a tonic-clonic seizure. This type of seizure causes rigidity of all body muscles, followed by intense jerking movements. Because increased oral secretions and apnea can occur during and after the seizure, oxygen and suctioning equipment are placed at the bedside. A tracheotomy is not performed during a seizure. No object, including a padded tongue blade, is placed into the child's mouth during a seizure. An emergency cart would not be left at the bedside, but would be available in the treatment room or nearby on the nursing unit.
Test-Taking Strategy: Use the process of elimination and note the strategic words *need to be placed at the child's bedside*. Eliminate option 2 knowing that a tracheotomy is not performed. Next, recalling that no object is placed into the mouth of a child experiencing a seizure assists in eliminating option 3. From the remaining options, focus on the primary concern during seizure activity. This will direct you to option 4. If you had difficulty with this question, review the plan of care associated with seizure precautions.
Level of Cognitive Ability: Applying
Client Needs: Physiological Integrity
Integrated Process: Nursing Process—Planning
Content Area: Child Health—Neurological/Musculoskeletal
Reference: Hockenberry, M., & Wilson, D. (2009). *Wong's essentials of pediatric nursing* (8th ed., p. 1015). St. Louis: Mosby.

374. 3

Rationale: Meningitis is an infectious process of the central nervous system caused by bacteria and viruses; it may be acquired as a primary disease or as a result of complications of neurosurgery, trauma, infection of the sinus or ears, or systemic infections. Meningitis is diagnosed by testing cerebrospinal fluid obtained by lumbar puncture. In the case of bacterial meningitis, findings usually include an elevated pressure; turbid or cloudy cerebrospinal fluid; and elevated leukocyte, elevated protein, and decreased glucose levels.

Test-Taking Strategy: Use the process of elimination and knowledge regarding the diagnostic findings in meningitis. Eliminate options 1 and 2 first because clear cerebrospinal fluid is not likely to be found in an infectious process such as meningitis. From this point, recall that an elevated protein level indicates a possible diagnosis of meningitis to direct you to the correct option. If you had difficulty with this question, review the diagnostic findings associated with a diagnosis of meningitis.

Level of Cognitive Ability: Analyzing
Client Needs: Physiological Integrity
Integrated Process: Nursing Process—Analysis
Content Area: Child Health—Neurological/Musculoskeletal
References: McKinney, E., James, S., Murray, S., & Ashwill, J. (2009). *Maternal-child nursing* (3rd ed., p. 1494). St. Louis: Saunders.

Swearingen, P. (2008). *All-in-one care planning resource: Medical-surgical, pediatric, maternity, & psychiatric nursing care plans* (2nd ed., pp. 281–282). St. Louis: Mosby.

375. 4

Rationale: Meningitis is an infectious process of the central nervous system caused by bacteria and viruses; it may be acquired as a primary disease or as a result of complications of neurosurgery, trauma, infection of the sinus or ears, or systemic infections. A major priority of nursing care for a child suspected to have meningitis is to administer the prescribed antibiotic as soon as it is ordered. The child also is placed on respiratory isolation precautions for at least 24 hours while culture results are obtained and the antibiotic is having an effect. Enteric precautions and neutropenic precautions are not associated with the mode of transmission of meningitis. Enteric precautions are instituted when the mode of transmission is through the gastrointestinal tract. Neutropenic precautions are instituted when a child has a low neutrophil count.

Test-Taking Strategy: Use the process of elimination and knowledge regarding the mode of transmission of meningitis. Eliminate options 1 and 2 first because enteric and neutropenic precautions are unrelated to the mode of transmission. Recalling that it takes about 24 hours for antibiotics to reach a therapeutic blood level will assist in directing you to option 4. If you had difficulty with this question, review the mode of transmission of meningitis.

Level of Cognitive Ability: Applying
Client Needs: Safe and Effective Care Environment
Integrated Process: Nursing Process—Planning
Content Area: Child Health—Neurological/Musculoskeletal
Reference: Hockenberry, M., & Wilson, D. (2009). *Wong's essentials of pediatric nursing* (8th ed., p. 1001). St. Louis: Mosby.

ALTERNATE ITEM FORMAT: MULTIPLE RESPONSE
376. 1, 3, 5

Rationale: A seizure is a disorder that occurs as a result of excessive and unorganized neuronal discharges in the brain that activate associated motor and sensory organs. During a seizure, the child is placed on his or her side in a lateral position. Positioning on the side prevents aspiration because saliva drains out the corner of the child's mouth. The child is not restrained because this could cause injury to the child. The nurse would loosen clothing around the child's neck and ensure a patent airway. Nothing is placed into the child's mouth during a seizure because this action may cause injury to the child's mouth, gums, or teeth. The nurse would stay with the child to reduce the risk of injury and allow for observation and timing of the seizure.

Test-Taking Strategy: Visualize this clinical situation. Recalling that airway patency and safety is the priority will assist in determining the appropriate interventions. Review care of the child experiencing a seizure if you had difficulty with this question.

Level of Cognitive Ability: Applying
Client Needs: Physiological Integrity
Integrated Process: Nursing Process—Implementation
Content Area: Child Health—Neurological/Musculoskeletal
Reference: Hockenberry, M., & Wilson, D. (2009). *Wong's essentials of pediatric nursing* (8th ed., p. 1014). St. Louis: Mosby.

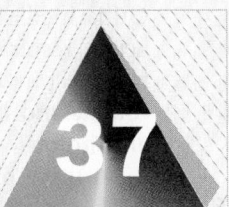

Eye, Ear, and Throat Disorders

I. STRABISMUS

A. Description
1. Called "squint" or "lazy eye"
2. Condition in which the eyes are not aligned because of lack of coordination of the extraocular muscles
3. Most often results from muscle imbalance or paralysis of extraocular muscles, but also may result from a congenital defect
4. Amblyopia (reduced visual acuity) may occur if not treated early because the brain receives two messages as a result of the unparallel visual axes.
5. Permanent loss of vision can occur if not treated early.
6. This condition may be normally found in a young infant, but should not be present after about age 4 months.
7. Treatment of the condition depends on the cause.

B. Assessment
1. Crossed eyes
2. Squinting; tilts the head or closes one eye to see
3. Loss of binocular vision
4. Impairment of depth perception
5. Frequent headaches
6. Diplopia; photophobia

C. Interventions
1. Corrective lenses may be indicated.
2. Instruct the parents regarding patching (occlusion therapy) of the "good" eye to strengthen the weak eye.
3. Prepare for surgery to realign the weak muscles as prescribed if nonsurgical interventions are unsuccessful; this is usually performed before age 2 years.
4. Instruct the parents about the need for follow-up visits.

II. CONJUNCTIVITIS

A. Description
1. Also known as "pinkeye"; an inflammation of the conjunctiva
2. Conjunctivitis usually is caused by allergy, infection, or trauma.

3. Bacterial or viral conjunctivitis is extremely contagious.

B. Assessment
1. Itching, burning, or scratchy eyelids
2. Redness
3. Edema
4. Discharge

⚠ Chlamydial conjunctivitis is rare in older children; if diagnosed in a child who is not sexually active, the child should be assessed for possible sexual abuse.

C. Interventions
1. Instruct in infection control measures such as good handwashing and not sharing towels and washcloths.
2. Administer antibiotic or antiviral eye drops or ointment as prescribed if infection is present (severe infection may require therapy with systemic antibiotics).
3. Instruct the child and parents about the administration of the prescribed medications.
4. Instruct the parents that the child should be kept home from school or day care until antibiotics have been administered for 24 hours.
5. Instruct about the use of cool compresses to lessen irritation and wearing dark glasses if photophobia occurs.
6. Instruct the child to avoid rubbing the eye to prevent injury.
7. Instruct a child who is wearing contact lenses to discontinue wearing them and to obtain new lenses to eliminate the chance of reinfection that can occur from the use of the old lenses.
8. Instruct an adolescent that eye makeup should be discarded and replaced.

III. OTITIS MEDIA

A. Description
1. An inflammatory disorder usually caused by an infection of the middle ear occurring as a result of a blocked eustachian tube, which prevents normal drainage; can be acute or chronic.

2. Otitis media is a common complication of an acute respiratory infection (most commonly from respiratory syncytial virus or influenza).
3. Infants and children have eustachian tubes that are shorter, wider, and straighter, which makes them more prone to otitis media.

B. Prevention
1. Feed infants in upright position, to prevent reflux.
2. Maintain routine immunizations.
3. Encourage breast-feeding for at least the first 6 months of life.
4. Avoid exposure to tobacco smoke and allergens.

C. Assessment
1. Fever
2. Acute onset of ear pain
3. Crying, irritability, lethargy
4. Loss of appetite
5. Rolling of head from side to side
6. Pulling on or rubbing the ear
7. Purulent ear drainage may be present
8. Red, opaque, bulging, immobile tympanic membrane on otoscopic examination
9. Signs of hearing loss (indicative of chronic otitis media)

D. Interventions
1. Encourage fluid intake (may be difficult if the child is in pain).
2. Instruct the child to avoid chewing as much as possible during the acute period because chewing increases pain.
3. Provide local heat or cold as prescribed to relieve discomfort, and have the child lie with the affected ear down.
4. Instruct the parents in the appropriate procedure to clean drainage from the external ear canal with sterile swabs or gauze; frequent cleansing and the application of moisture barriers may be prescribed to prevent ear excoriation from the drainage.
5. Instruct the parents in the administration of analgesics or antipyretics such as acetaminophen (Tylenol) or ibuprofen (Motrin) to decrease fever and pain.
6. Instruct the parents in the administration of antibiotics if prescribed, emphasizing that the prescribed period of administration is necessary to eliminate infective organisms.
7. Instruct the parents that screening for hearing loss may be necessary.
8. Instruct the parents about the procedure for administering ear medications such as topical pain relief drops if prescribed.

⚠ To administer ear medications in a child younger than age 3, pull the ear lobe down and back. In a child older than 3 years, pull the pinna up and back.

E. Myringotomy
1. Description
    a. A surgical incision into the tympanic membrane to provide drainage of the purulent middle ear fluid; may be done by a laser-assisted procedure
    b. Tympanoplasty tubes may be inserted into the middle ear to allow continued drainage and to equalize pressure and allow ventilation of the middle ear.
2. Postoperative interventions
    a. Instruct the parents and child to keep the ears dry.
    b. The client should wear earplugs while bathing, shampooing, and swimming (diving and submerging under water are not allowed).
    c. Parents can administer an analgesic such as acetaminophen (Tylenol) or ibuprofen (Motrin) to relieve discomfort after insertion of tympanoplasty tubes.
    d. Parents should be taught that the child should not blow his or her nose for 7 to 10 days after surgery.
    e. Instruct the parents that if the tubes fall out, it is not an emergency, but the physician should be notified; inform the parents of the appearance of the tubes (tiny, white, spool-shaped tubes).

IV. TONSILLITIS AND ADENOIDITIS

A. Description
1. Tonsillitis refers to inflammation and infection of the tonsils, which is lymphoid tissue located in the pharynx (Fig. 37-1).
2. Adenoiditis refers to inflammation and infection of the adenoids (pharyngeal tonsils), located on the posterior wall of the nasopharynx.

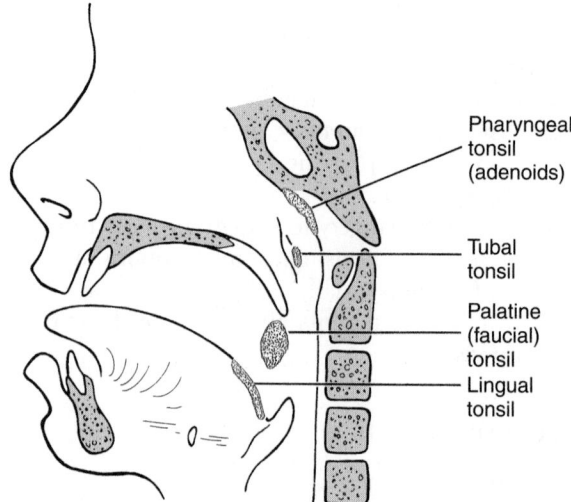

▲ **FIGURE 37-1** Location of various tonsillar masses. (From Perry, S., Hockenberry, M., Lowdermilk, D., & Wilson, D. [2010]. *Maternal child nursing care* [4th ed., p. 1312]. St. Louis: Mosby.)

3. Tonsillectomy (surgical removal of the tonsils) and adenoidectomy (surgical removal of the adenoids) may be necessary.

B. Assessment
   1. Persistent or recurrent sore throat
   2. Enlarged, bright red tonsils that may be covered with white exudate
   3. Difficulty in swallowing
   4. Mouth breathing and an unpleasant mouth odor
   5. Fever
   6. Cough
   7. Enlarged adenoids may cause nasal quality of speech, mouth breathing, hearing difficulty, snoring, or obstructive sleep apnea.

C. Preoperative interventions
   1. Assess for signs of active infection.
   2. Assess bleeding and clotting studies because the throat is vascular.
   3. Prepare the child for a sore throat postoperatively, and inform the child that he or she will need to drink liquids.
   4. Assess for any loose teeth to decrease the risk of aspiration during surgery.

D. Interventions postoperatively
   1. Position the child prone or side-lying to facilitate drainage.
   2. Have suction equipment available, but do not suction unless there is an airway obstruction.
   3. Monitor for signs of bleeding (frequent swallowing may indicate bleeding); if bleeding occurs, turn the child to the side and notify the physician.
   4. Discourage coughing, clearing the throat, or nose blowing to prevent bleeding.
   5. Provide an ice collar or analgesics (rectally or intravenously) for discomfort.
   6. Administer antiemetics to prevent vomiting if prescribed.
   7. Provide clear, cool, noncitrus and noncarbonated fluids (crushed ice, ice pops).
   8. Avoid red, purple, or brown liquids, which simulate the appearance of blood if the child vomits.
   9. Avoid milk products such as milk, ice cream, and pudding initially because they coat the throat causing the child to cough to clear the throat.
   10. Soft foods may be prescribed 1 to 2 days postoperatively.
   11. Do not give the child any straws, forks, or sharp objects that can be put into the mouth.
   12. Mouth odor, slight ear pain, and a low-grade fever may occur for a few days postoperatively, but the parents should be instructed to notify the physician if bleeding, persistent earache, or fever occurs.
   13. Instruct the parents to keep the child away from crowds until healing has occurred; usually the child is able to resume normal activities after 1 to 2 weeks postoperatively.

V. EPISTAXIS (NOSEBLEEDS)

A. Description
   1. The nose, especially the septum, is a highly vascular structure, and bleeding usually results from direct trauma, foreign bodies, and nose picking or from mucosal inflammation.
   2. Recurrent epistaxis and severe bleeding may indicate an underlying disease.

B. Interventions
   1. See Priority Nursing Actions.
   2. If bleeding cannot be controlled, packing or cauterization of the bleeding vessel may be prescribed.

◾◾◾◾ PRIORITY NURSING ACTIONS! ◾◾◾◾

Actions to Take if a Child Has a Nosebleed
1. Remain calm and keep the child calm and quiet.
2. Have the child sit up and lean forward (not lying down).
3. Apply continuous pressure to the nose with the thumb and forefinger for at least 10 minutes.
4. Insert cotton or wadded tissue into each nostril, and apply ice or a cold cloth to the bridge of the nose if bleeding persists.

If a nosebleed occurs in a child, it is important for the nurse to remain calm; otherwise, the child becomes agitated and it is difficult to get the child to cooperate with the necessary interventions. The child should be assisted to a sitting up and leaning forward position to prevent aspiration of blood. The child should not be placed in a lying down position. Nosebleeds usually originate in the anterior part of the nasal septum and can be controlled by applying pressure to the soft lower portion of the nose with the thumb and forefinger for at least 10 minutes. If bleeding persists, cotton or wadded tissue should be placed into each nostril, and ice or a cold cloth should be applied to the bridge of the nose. If bleeding does persist, the physician needs to be notified, and the nose may require packing by the physician. After the nosebleed has been stopped, petroleum or a water-soluble jelly may be inserted into each nostril to prevent crusting of old blood and to lessen the likelihood of the child picking at the crusted lesions and restarting the bleeding. Repeated bleeding episodes that last longer than 30 minutes may be an indication of the need for evaluation of a bleeding disorder.

Reference: Perry, S., Hockenberry, M., Lowdermilk, D., & Wilson, D. (2010). *Maternal child nursing care* (4th ed., p. 1507). St. Louis: Mosby.

MORE QUESTIONS ON THE CD!

Practice Questions

377. After a tonsillectomy, a child begins to vomit bright red blood. The initial nursing action is to:
1. Notify the physician.
2. Maintain NPO status.
3. Turn the child to the side.
4. Administer the prescribed antiemetic.

378. A day care nurse is observing a 2-year-old child and suspects that the child may have strabismus. Which observation made by the nurse might indicate this condition?
1. The child has difficulty hearing.
2. The child consistently tilts the head to see.
3. The child consistently turns the head to see.
4. The child does not respond when spoken to.

379. The mother of a 6-year-old child arrives at a clinic because the child has been experiencing scratchy, red, and swollen eyes. The nurse notes a discharge from the eyes and sends a culture to the laboratory for analysis. Chlamydial conjunctivitis is diagnosed. Based on this diagnosis, the nurse determines that which of the following requires further investigation?
1. Possible trauma
2. Possible sexual abuse
3. Presence of an allergy
4. Presence of a respiratory infection

380. A nurse prepares a teaching plan for a mother of a child diagnosed with bacterial conjunctivitis. Which of the following, if stated by the mother, indicates a need for further teaching?
1. "I need to wash my hands frequently."
2. "I need to clean the eye as prescribed."
3. "It is okay to share towels and washcloths."
4. "I need to give the eye drops as prescribed."

381. A nurse is reviewing the laboratory results for a child scheduled for tonsillectomy. The nurse determines that which laboratory value is most significant to review?
1. Creatinine level
2. Prothrombin time
3. Sedimentation rate
4. Blood urea nitrogen level

382. A nurse is preparing to care for a child after a tonsillectomy. The nurse documents on the plan of care to place the child in which appropriate position?

1. Supine
2. Side-lying
3. High Fowler's
4. Trendelenburg's

383. After a tonsillectomy, a nurse reviews the physician's postoperative prescriptions. Which of the following physician's prescriptions does the nurse question?
1. Monitor for bleeding.
2. Suction every 2 hours.
3. Give no milk or milk products.
4. Give clear, cool liquids when awake and alert.

384. A nurse is caring for a child after a tonsillectomy. The nurse monitors the child, knowing that which of the following indicates that the child is bleeding?
1. Frequent swallowing
2. A decreased pulse rate
3. Complaints of discomfort
4. An elevation in blood pressure

385. Antibiotics are prescribed for a child with otitis media who underwent a myringotomy with insertion of tympanostomy tubes. The nurse provides discharge instructions to the parents regarding the administration of the antibiotics. Which statement, if made by the parents, indicates that they understood the instructions?
1. "Administer the antibiotics until they are gone."
2. "Administer the antibiotics if the child has a fever."
3. "Administer the antibiotics until the child feels better."
4. "Begin to taper the antibiotics after 3 days of a full course."

Alternate Item Format: Multiple Response

386. A child has been diagnosed with acute otitis media of the right ear. Which interventions should the nurse include in the plan of care? **Select all that apply.**
☐ 1. Provide a soft diet.
☐ 2. Position the child on the left side.
☐ 3. Administer an antihistamine twice daily.
☐ 4. Irrigate the right ear with normal saline every 8 hours.
☐ 5. Administer acetaminophen (Tylenol) for fever every 4 hours as prescribed and as needed.
☐ 6. Instruct the parents about the need to administer the antibiotics for the full course of prescribed therapy.

ANSWERS

377. 3

Rationale: After tonsillectomy, if bleeding occurs, the nurse immediately turns the child to the side to prevent aspiration and then notifies the physician. NPO status would be maintained, and an antiemetic may be prescribed; however, the initial nursing action would be to turn the child to the side.

Test-Taking Strategy: Note the strategic word *initial* in the event query. Although all the options may be appropriate to maintain physiological integrity, the initial action is to turn the child to the side to prevent aspiration. Review the initial action to take if a postoperative child vomits if you had difficulty with this question.

Level of Cognitive Ability: Applying
Client Needs: Physiological Integrity
Integrated Process: Nursing Process—Implementation
Content Area: Leadership and Management—Delegating/Prioritizing
References: Hockenberry, M., & Wilson, D. (2009). *Wong's essentials of pediatric nursing* (8th ed., p. 764). St. Louis: Mosby.
   McKinney, E., James, S., Murray, S., & Ashwill, J. (2009). *Maternal-child nursing* (3rd ed., p. 1184). St. Louis: Saunders.

378. 2

Rationale: Strabismus is a condition in which the eyes are not aligned because of lack of coordination of the extraocular muscles. The nurse may suspect strabismus in a child when the child complains of frequent headaches, squints, or tilts the head to see. Other manifestations include crossed eyes, closing one eye to see, diplopia, photophobia, loss of binocular vision, or impairment of depth perception. Options 1, 3, and 4 are not indicative of this condition.

Test-Taking Strategy: Use the process of elimination. Eliminate options 1 and 4 first because they are comparable or alike. To select from the remaining options, recall that this is a condition in which the eyes are not aligned because of lack of coordination of the extraocular muscles. Review the signs of strabismus if you had difficulty with this question.

Level of Cognitive Ability: Analyzing
Client Needs: Physiological Integrity
Integrated Process: Nursing Process—Assessment
Content Area: Child Health—Eye/Ear/Throat/Respiratory/Cardiovascular
Reference: McKinney, E., James, S., Murray, S., & Ashwill, J. (2009). *Maternal-child nursing* (3rd ed., p. 1561). St. Louis: Saunders.

379. 2

Rationale: Conjunctivitis is an inflammation of the conjunctiva. A diagnosis of chlamydial conjunctivitis in a child who is not sexually active should signal the health care provider to assess the child for possible sexual abuse. Allergy, infection, and trauma can cause conjunctivitis, but the causative organism is not likely to be chlamydia.

Test-Taking Strategy: Note the age of the child and the organism that is identified in the question. This will assist in directing you to option 2. Options 1, 3, and 4 can be recognized as the common causes of conjunctivitis. These options are comparable or alike in that they relate to a physiological problem. Review the causes of chlamydial conjunctivitis if you had difficulty with this question.

Level of Cognitive Ability: Analyzing
Client Needs: Psychosocial Integrity
Integrated Process: Nursing Process—Assessment
Content Area: Child Health—Integumentary/AIDS/Infectious Diseases
Reference: McKinney, E., James, S., Murray, S., & Ashwill, J. (2009). *Maternal-child nursing* (3rd ed., p. 1563). St. Louis: Saunders.

380. 3

Rationale: Conjunctivitis is an inflammation of the conjunctiva. Bacterial conjunctivitis is highly contagious, and the nurse should teach infection control measures. These include good handwashing and not sharing towels and washcloths. Options 1, 2, and 4 are correct treatment measures.

Test-Taking Strategy: Note the strategic words *need for further teaching*. These words indicate a negative event query and ask you to select an option that is an incorrect statement. Options 1, 2, and 4 can be eliminated by recalling that bacterial conjunctivitis is highly contagious. If you had difficulty with this question, review infection control measures for bacterial conjunctivitis.

Level of Cognitive Ability: Evaluating
Client Needs: Safe and Effective Care Environment
Integrated Process: Teaching and Learning
Content Area: Child Health—Integumentary/AIDS/Infectious Diseases
Reference: McKinney, E., James, S., Murray, S., & Ashwill, J. (2009). *Maternal-child nursing* (3rd ed., p. 1563). St. Louis: Saunders.

381. 2

Rationale: A tonsillectomy is the surgical removal of the tonsils. Because the tonsillar area is so vascular, postoperative bleeding is a concern. Prothrombin time, partial thromboplastin time, platelet count, hemoglobin and hematocrit, white blood cell count, and urinalysis are performed preoperatively. The prothrombin time results would identify a potential for bleeding. Creatinine level, sedimentation rate, and blood urea nitrogen would not determine the potential for bleeding.

Test-Taking Strategy: Focus on the surgical procedure and the subject of the question. The subject of the question relates to the potential for bleeding. Options 1 and 4 can be eliminated because they relate to kidney function. Similarly, option 3 can be eliminated because it is unrelated to the subject of the question. Review preoperative care of the child scheduled for tonsillectomy if you had difficulty with this question.

Level of Cognitive Ability: Analyzing
Client Needs: Physiological Integrity
Integrated Process: Nursing Process—Assessment
Content Area: Child Health—Eye/Ear/Throat/Respiratory/Cardiovascular
Reference: McKinney, E., James, S., Murray, S., & Ashwill, J. (2009). *Maternal-child nursing* (3rd ed., p. 1183). St. Louis: Saunders.

382. 2

Rationale: A tonsillectomy is the surgical removal of the tonsils. The child should be placed in a prone or side-lying position after the surgical procedure to facilitate drainage. Options 1, 3, and 4 would not achieve this goal.

Test-Taking Strategy: Focus on the surgical procedure and visualize each of the positions described in the options. Keeping in mind that the goal is to facilitate drainage will direct you to option 2. Review positioning procedures after tonsillectomy if you had difficulty with this question.
Level of Cognitive Ability: Applying
Client Needs: Physiological Integrity
Integrated Process: Nursing Process—Planning
Content Area: Child Health—Eye/Ear/Throat/Respiratory/Cardiovascular
References: Hockenberry, M., & Wilson, D. (2009). *Wong's essentials of pediatric nursing* (8th ed., p. 764). St. Louis: Mosby.
    McKinney, E., James, S., Murray, S., & Ashwill, J. (2009). *Maternal-child nursing* (3rd ed., p. 1184). St. Louis: Saunders.

383. 2

Rationale: A tonsillectomy is the surgical removal of the tonsils. After tonsillectomy, suction equipment should be available, but suctioning is not performed unless there is an airway obstruction because of the risk of trauma to the surgical site. Monitoring for bleeding is an important nursing intervention after any type of surgery. Milk and milk products are avoided initially because they coat the throat, cause the child to clear the throat, and increase the risk of bleeding. Clear, cool liquids are encouraged.
Test-Taking Strategy: Focus on the subject, the prescription that the nurse questions. Option 1 can be eliminated first because this is a nursing action, not a medical prescription. From the remaining options, consider the anatomical location of the surgery. This should direct you to option 2. Review postoperative care after tonsillectomy if you had difficulty with this question.
Level of Cognitive Ability: Analyzing
Client Needs: Physiological Integrity
Integrated Process: Nursing Process—Implementation
Content Area: Child Health—Eye/Ear/Throat/Respiratory/Cardiovascular
References: Hockenberry, M., & Wilson, D. (2009). *Wong's essentials of pediatric nursing* (8th ed., p. 764). St. Louis: Mosby.
    McKinney, E., James, S., Murray, S., & Ashwill, J. (2009). *Maternal-child nursing* (3rd ed., p. 1184). St. Louis: Saunders.

384. 1

Rationale: A tonsillectomy is the surgical removal of the tonsils. Frequent swallowing, restlessness, a fast and thready pulse, and vomiting bright red blood are signs of bleeding. An elevated blood pressure and complaints of discomfort are not indications of bleeding.
Test-Taking Strategy: Use the concepts related to the signs of shock to assist in answering this question. These concepts should assist in eliminating options 2 and 4. From the remaining options, recalling that discomfort is expected and does not indicate bleeding will direct you to option 1. Review the signs of bleeding after tonsillectomy if you had difficulty with this question.
Level of Cognitive Ability: Analyzing
Client Needs: Physiological Integrity
Integrated Process: Nursing Process—Assessment
Content Area: Child Health—Eye/Ear/Throat/Respiratory/Cardiovascular
References: Hockenberry, M., & Wilson, D. (2009). *Wong's essentials of pediatric nursing* (8th ed., p. 764). St. Louis: Mosby.
    McKinney, E., James, S., Murray, S., & Ashwill, J. (2009). *Maternal-child nursing* (3rd ed., p. 1183). St. Louis: Saunders.

385. 1

Rationale: A myringotomy is the insertion of tympanoplasty tubes into the middle ear to promote drainage of purulent middle ear fluid and to equalize pressure and keep the ear aerated. The nurse must instruct parents regarding the administration of antibiotics. Antibiotics need to be taken as prescribed, and the full course needs to be completed. Options 2, 3, and 4 are incorrect. Antibiotics are not tapered, but are administered for the full course of therapy.
Test-Taking Strategy: Note the strategic words *understood the instructions.* Use the process of elimination and recall that antibiotics must be taken for the full course, regardless of whether the child is feeling better. This will assist in directing you to option 1. Review concepts related to the administration of antibiotics if you had difficulty with this question.
Level of Cognitive Ability: Evaluating
Client Needs: Physiological Integrity
Integrated Process: Nursing Process—Evaluation
Content Area: Child Health—Eye/Ear/Throat/Respiratory/Cardiovascular
References: Hockenberry, M., & Wilson, D. (2009). *Wong's essentials of pediatric nursing* (8th ed., p. 767). St. Louis: Mosby.
    McKinney, E., James, S., Murray, S., & Ashwill, J. (2009). *Maternal-child nursing* (3rd ed., p. 1181). St. Louis: Saunders.

ALTERNATE ITEM FORMAT: MULTIPLE RESPONSE

386. 1, 5, 6

Rationale: Acute otitis media is an inflammatory disorder caused by an infection of the middle ear. The child often has fever, pain, loss of appetite, and possible ear drainage. The child also is irritable and lethargic and may roll the head or pull on or rub the affected ear. Otoscopic examination may reveal a red, opaque, bulging, and immobile tympanic membrane. Hearing loss may be noted particularly in chronic otitis media. The child's fever should be treated with acetaminophen (Tylenol) or ibuprofen (Motrin). The child is positioned on his or her affected side to facilitate drainage. A soft diet is recommended during the acute stage to avoid pain that can occur with chewing. Antibiotics are prescribed to treat the bacterial infection and should be administered for the full prescribed course. The ear should not be irrigated with normal saline because it can exacerbate the inflammation further. Antihistamines are not usually recommended as a part of therapy.
Test-Taking Strategy: Focus on the child's diagnosis and note the strategic words, *acute* and *right ear.* Think about the pathophysiology associated with the disorder and the associated manifestations to select the correct options. Review the interventions and the treatment for acute otitis media if you had difficulty with this question.
Level of Cognitive Ability: Applying
Client Needs: Physiological Integrity
Integrated Process: Nursing Process—Planning
Content Area: Child Health—Eye/Ear/Throat/Respiratory/Cardiovascular
References: Hockenberry, M., & Wilson, D. (2009). *Wong's essentials of pediatric nursing* (8th ed., pp. 766–767). St. Louis: Mosby.
    McKinney, E., James, S., Murray, S., & Ashwill, J. (2009). *Maternal-child nursing* (3rd ed., p. 1181). St. Louis: Saunders.

Respiratory Disorders

I. EPIGLOTTITIS

A. Description
1. Bacterial form of croup
2. Inflammation of the epiglottis occurs, which may be caused by *Haemophilus influenzae* type b or *Streptococcus pneumoniae*; children immunized with *H. influenzae* type b (Hib **vaccine**) are at less risk for epiglottitis.
3. Occurs most frequently in children 2 to 8 years old, but can occur from infancy to adulthood
4. Onset is abrupt, and the condition occurs most often in the winter.
5. Considered an emergency situation because it can progress rapidly to severe respiratory distress

B. Assessment
1. High fever
2. Sore, red, and inflamed throat (large, cherry red, edematous epiglottis) and pain on swallowing (Fig. 38-1)
3. Absence of spontaneous cough
4. Drooling
5. Agitation
6. Muffled voice
7. **Retractions** and child struggles to breathe
8. Inspiratory **stridor** aggravated by the supine position
9. Tachycardia
10. Tachypnea progressing to more severe respiratory distress (hypoxia, hypercapnia, respiratory acidosis, decreased level of consciousness)
11. Tripod positioning: While supporting the body with the hands, the child leans forward, thrusts the chin forward and opens the mouth in an attempt to widen the airway

C. Interventions
1. Maintain a patent airway.
2. Assess respiratory status and breath sounds, noting **nasal flaring**, the use of accessory muscles, **retractions**, and the presence of **stridor**.
3. Assess temperature by the axillary route, not the oral route.
4. Monitor pulse oximetry.
5. Prepare the child for lateral neck films to confirm the diagnosis (accompany the child to the radiology department).
6. Maintain NPO status.
7. Do not leave the child unattended.
8. Avoid placing the child in a supine position because this position would affect the respiratory status further.
9. Do not restrain the child or take any other measure that may agitate the child.
10. Administer intravenous fluids as prescribed; insertion of an intravenous line may need to be delayed until an adequate airway is established because this procedure may agitate the child.
11. Administer intravenous antibiotics as prescribed; these are usually followed by oral antibiotics.
12. Administer analgesics and antipyretics (acetaminophen [Tylenol] or ibuprofen [Motrin]) to reduce fever and throat pain as prescribed.
13. Administer corticosteroids to decrease inflammation and reduce throat edema as prescribed.
14. Nebulized epinephrine (racemic epinephrine) may be prescribed for severe cases (causes mucosal vasoconstriction and reduces edema); heliox (mixture of helium and oxygen) may also be prescribed to reduce mucosal edema.
15. Provide cool mist oxygen therapy as prescribed; high humidification cools the airway and decreases swelling.
16. Have resuscitation equipment available, and prepare for endotracheal intubation or tracheotomy for severe respiratory distress.
17. Ensure that the child is up to date with immunizations, including Hib conjugate **vaccine** (see Chapter 48).

⚠ If epiglottitis is suspected, no attempts should be made to visualize the posterior pharynx, obtain a throat culture, or take an oral temperature. Otherwise, spasm of the epiglottis can occur leading to complete airway occlusion.

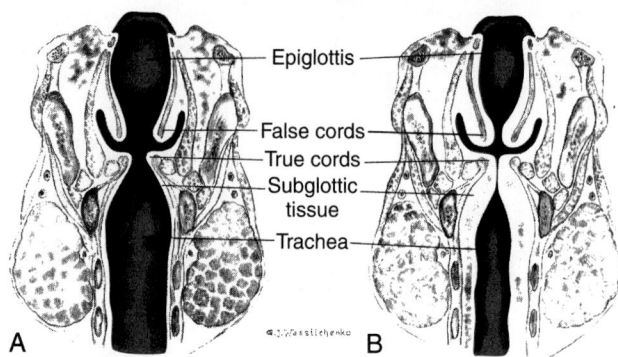

▲ **FIGURE 38-1 A,** Normal larynx. **B,** Obstruction and narrowing resulting from edema of croup. (From Hockenberry, M., & Wilson, D. [2007]. *Wong's nursing care of infants and children* [8th ed.]. St. Louis: Mosby.)

II. LARYNGOTRACHEOBRONCHITIS

A. Description
  1. Inflammation of the larynx, trachea, and bronchi
  2. Most common type of croup; may be viral or bacterial and most frequently occurs in children younger than 5 years
  3. Common causative organisms include parainfluenzae virus types 1 and 2, respiratory syncytial virus (RSV), *Mycoplasma pneumoniae*, and influenza.
  4. Characterized by gradual onset that may be preceded by an upper respiratory infection

B. Assessment (Box 38-1)

C. Interventions
  1. Maintain a patent airway.
  2. Assess respiratory status and monitor pulse oximetry; monitor for **nasal flaring**, sternal **retraction**, and inspiratory **stridor** (Fig. 38-2).
  3. Monitor for adequate respiratory exchange; monitor for pallor or **cyanosis**.
  4. Elevate the head of the bed and provide rest.
  5. Provide humidified oxygen via a cool air or mist tent as prescribed for a hospitalized child (Table 38-1).
  6. Instruct the parents to use a cool air vaporizer at home; other measures include having the child breathe in the cool night air or the air from an open freezer or taking the child to a cool basement or garage.
  7. Provide and encourage fluid intake; intravenous fluids may be prescribed to maintain hydration status if the child is unable to take fluids orally.
  8. Administer analgesics as prescribed to reduce fever.
  9. Teach the parents to avoid administering cough syrups or cold medicines, which may dry and thicken secretions.
  10. Administer corticosteroids if prescribed to reduce inflammation and edema.

Box 38-1 Progression of Symptoms in Laryngotracheobronchitis

Stage I
Low-grade fever
Hoarseness
Seal bark and brassy cough (croup cough)
Inspiratory stridor
Fear
Irritability and restlessness

Stage II
Continuous respiratory stridor
Retractions
Use of accessory muscles
Crackles and wheezing
Labored respirations

Stage III
Continued restlessness
Anxiety
Pallor
Diaphoresis
Tachypnea
Signs of anoxia and hypercapnia

Stage IV
Intermittent cyanosis progressing to permanent cyanosis
Apneic episodes progressing to cessation of breathing

Modified from Perry, S., Hockenberry, M., Lowdermilk, D., & Wilson, D. (2010). *Maternal child nursing care.* (4th ed., p. 1320). St. Louis: Mosby.

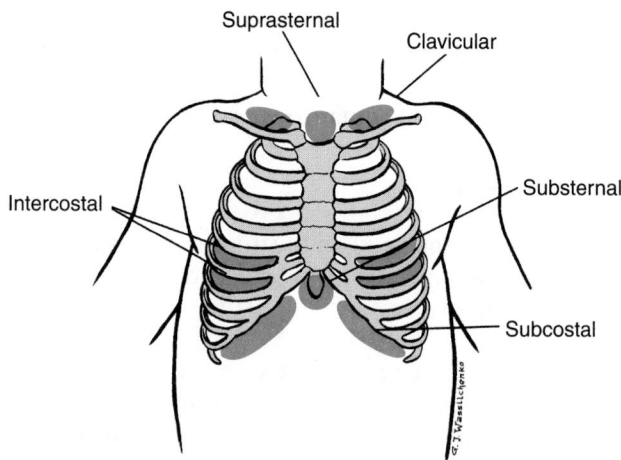

▲ **FIGURE 38-2** Location of retractions. (From Hockenberry, M., & Wilson, D. [2007]. *Wong's nursing care of infants and children* [8th ed.]. St. Louis: Mosby.)

  11. Administer nebulized epinephrine (racemic epinephrine) as prescribed; this may be prescribed for children with severe disease experiencing **stridor** at rest, **retractions**, or difficulty breathing.
  12. Administer antibiotics as prescribed, noting that they are not indicated unless a bacterial infection is present.

TABLE 38-1 Advantages and Disadvantages of Oxygen Delivery Systems

Systems	Advantages	Disadvantages
Oxygen mask	Various sizes available; delivers higher O_2 concentration than cannula Able to provide a predictable concentration of oxygen (with Venturi mask) whether child breathes through nose or mouth	Skin irritation Fear of suffocation Accumulation of moisture on face Possibility of aspiration of vomitus Difficulty in controlling O_2 concentrations (except with Venturi mask)
Nasal cannula	Provides low-moderate O_2 concentration (22%-40%) Child able to eat and talk while getting O_2 Possibility of more complete observation of child because nose and mouth remain unobstructed	Must have patent nasal passages May cause abdominal distention and discomfort or vomiting Difficulty controlling O_2 concentrations if child breathes through mouth Inability to provide mist if desired
Oxygen tent	Provides lower O_2 concentrations (F_{IO_2} up to 0.3-0.5) Child able to receive desired inspired O_2 concentrations, even while eating	Necessity for tight fit around bed to prevent leakage of oxygen Cool and wet tent environment Poor access to child; inspired O_2 levels fall when tent is entered
Oxygen hood, face tent	Provides high O_2 concentrations (F_{IO_2} up to 1.00) Free access to child's chest for assessment	High-humidity environment Need to remove child for feeding and care

From Hockenberry, M., & Wilson, D. (2007). *Wong's nursing care of infants and children* (8th ed.). St. Louis: Mosby.

13. Heliox (mixture of helium and oxygen) may be prescribed; this medication reduces the work of breathing, reduces airway turbulence, and helps to relieve airway obstruction.
14. Have resuscitation equipment available.
15. Provide appropriate reassurance and education to the parents or caregivers.

Isolation precautions should be implemented for a hospitalized child with an upper respiratory infection until the cause of the infection is known.

III. BRONCHITIS

A. Description
1. Inflammation of the trachea and bronchi; may be referred to as tracheobronchitis
2. Usually occurs in association with an upper respiratory infection
3. Is usually a mild disorder; causative agent is most often viral

B. Assessment
1. Fever
2. Dry, hacking, and nonproductive cough that is worse at night and becomes productive in 2 to 3 days

C. Interventions
1. Treat symptoms as necessary.
2. Monitor for respiratory distress.
3. Provide cool, humidified air to the child.
4. Encourage increased fluid intake; child may drink beverages that he or she likes as long as the respiratory status is stable.
5. Administer antipyretics for fever as prescribed.

6. Cough suppressants may be prescribed to promote rest.

IV. BRONCHIOLITIS AND RESPIRATORY SYNCYTIAL VIRUS (RSV)

A. Description
1. Bronchiolitis is an inflammation of the bronchioles that causes production of thick mucus that occludes bronchiole tubes and small bronchi.
2. RSV causes an acute viral infection and is a common cause of bronchiolitis (other organisms that cause bronchiolitis include adenoviruses, parainfluenza viruses, and human metapneumovirus).
3. RSV, although not airborne, is highly communicable and is usually transferred by direct contact with respiratory secretions.
4. RSV occurs primarily in the winter and spring.
5. RSV is rarer in children older than 2 years, with a peak incidence at approximately 6 months of age.
6. At-risk children include children older than 1 year of age who have a chronic or disabling condition.
7. Identification of the virus is done via testing of nasal or nasopharyngeal secretions.
8. Prevention measures include encouraging breast-feeding; avoiding tobacco smoke exposure; using good handwashing techniques; and administering palivizumab (Synagis), a monoclonal antibody, to high-risk infants. Palivizumab is administered via intramuscular injection monthly for a 5-month period (usually from November to March).

B. Assessment (Box 38-2)

Box 38-2 Assessment: Respiratory Syncytial Virus

Initial Manifestations
Rhinorrhea
Eye or ear drainage
Pharyngitis
Coughing
Sneezing
Wheezing
Intermittent fever

Manifestations as Disease Progresses
Increased coughing and wheezing
Signs of air hunger
Tachypnea and retractions
Periods of cyanosis

Manifestations in Severe Illness
Tachypnea more than 70 breaths/min
Decreased breath sounds and poor air exchange
Listlessness
Apneic episodes

Modified from Perry, S., Hockenberry, M., Lowdermilk, D., & Wilson, D. (2010). *Maternal child nursing care* (4th ed., p. 1322). St. Louis: Mosby.

C. Interventions
  1. For a child with bronchiolitis, interventions are aimed at treating symptoms and include airway maintenance, cool humidified air and oxygen, adequate fluid intake, and medications.
  2. For a hospitalized child with RSV, isolate the child in a single room or place in a room with another child with RSV.
  3. Ensure that nurses caring for a child with RSV do not care for other high-risk children.
  4. Use contact and standard precautions during care; using good handwashing techniques and wearing gloves and gowns are necessary.
  5. Monitor airway status and maintain a patent airway.
  6. For most effective airway maintenance, position the child at a 30- to 40-degree angle with the neck slightly extended to maintain an open airway and decrease pressure on the diaphragm.
  7. Provide cool, humidified oxygen as prescribed.
  8. Monitor pulse oximetry levels.
  9. Encourage fluids; fluids administered intravenously may be necessary until the acute stage has passed.
  10. Periodic suctioning may be necessary if nasal secretions are copious; use of a bulb syringe for suctioning may be effective. Suctioning should be done before feeding to promote comfort and adequate intake.
  11. Administer ribavirin (Virazole), an antiviral medication, if prescribed (administered via the inhalation route).

⚠ Cough suppressants are administered with caution because they can interfere with the clearance of respiratory secretions.

V. PNEUMONIA

A. Description
  1. Inflammation of the pulmonary parenchyma or alveoli or both caused by a virus, mycoplasmal agents, bacteria, or aspiration of foreign substances.
  2. The causative agent usually is introduced into the lungs through inhalation or from the bloodstream.
  3. Viral pneumonia occurs more frequently than bacterial pneumonia, is seen in children of all ages, and often is associated with a viral upper respiratory infection.
  4. Primary atypical pneumonia, usually caused by *Mycoplasma pneumoniae* or *Chlamydia pneumoniae*, occurs most often in the fall and winter months and is more common in crowded living conditions; it is most often seen in children 5 to 12 years old.
  5. Bacterial pneumonia is often a serious infection requiring hospitalization when pleural effusion or empyema accompanies the disease; hospitalization is also necessary for children with staphylococcal pneumonia (*Streptococcus pneumoniae* is a common cause).
  6. Aspiration pneumonia occurs when food, secretions, liquids, or other materials enter the lung and cause inflammation and a chemical pneumonitis. Classic symptoms include an increasing cough or fever with foul-smelling sputum, deteriorating results on chest x-rays, and other signs of airway involvement.
  7. Prevention of viral and bacterial pneumonia includes immunization of infants and children with pneumococcal **vaccine** (see Chapter 48).

B. Viral pneumonia
  1. Assessment
     a. Acute or insidious onset
     b. Symptoms range from mild fever, slight cough, and malaise to high fever, severe cough, and diaphoresis.
     c. Nonproductive or productive cough of small amounts of whitish sputum
     d. Wheezes or fine **crackles**
  2. Interventions
     a. Treatment is symptomatic.
     b. Administer oxygen with cool humidified air as prescribed.
     c. Increase fluid intake.
     d. Administer antipyretics for fever as prescribed.
     e. Administer chest physiotherapy and postural drainage as prescribed.

C. Primary atypical pneumonia
1. Assessment
   a. Acute or insidious onset
   b. Fever (lasting several days to 2 weeks), chills, anorexia, headache, malaise, and myalgia (muscle pain)
   c. Rhinitis; sore throat; and dry, hacking cough
   d. Nonproductive cough initially progressing to production of seromucoid sputum that becomes mucopurulent or blood-streaked
2. Interventions
   a. Treatment is symptomatic.
   b. Recovery generally occurs in 7 to 10 days.

D. Bacterial pneumonia
1. Assessment
   a. Acute onset
   b. Infant: Irritability, lethargy, poor feeding; abrupt fever (may be accompanied by seizures); respiratory distress (air hunger, tachypnea, and circumoral **cyanosis)**
   c. Older child: Headache, chills, abdominal pain, chest pain, meningeal symptoms (meningism)
   d. Hacking, nonproductive cough
   e. Diminished breath sounds or scattered **crackles**
   f. With consolidation, decreased breath sounds are more pronounced.
   g. As the infection resolves, the cough becomes productive, and the child expectorates purulent sputum; coarse **crackles** and **wheezing** are noted.
2. Interventions
   a. Antibiotic therapy is initiated as soon as the diagnosis is suspected; in a hospitalized infant or child, intravenous antibiotics are usually prescribed.
   b. Administer oxygen for respiratory distress as prescribed, and monitor oxygen saturation via pulse oximetry.
   c. Place the child in a cool mist tent as prescribed; cool humidification moistens the airways and assists in temperature reduction.
   d. Suction mucus from the infant using a bulb syringe to maintain a patent airway if the infant is unable to handle secretions.
   e. Administer chest physiotherapy and postural drainage every 4 hours as prescribed.
   f. Promote bed rest to conserve energy.
   g. Encourage the child to lie on the affected side (if pneumonia is unilateral) to splint the chest and reduce the discomfort caused by pleural rubbing.
   h. Encourage fluid intake (administer cautiously to prevent aspiration); intravenously administered fluids may be necessary.
   i. Administer antipyretics for fever and bronchodilators as prescribed.
   j. Monitor temperature frequently because of the risk for febrile seizures.
   k. Institute isolation precautions with pneumococcal or staphylococcal pneumonia (according to agency policy).
   l. Administer cough suppressant as prescribed before rest times and meals if the cough is disturbing.
   m. Continuous closed chest drainage may be instituted if purulent fluid is present (usually noted in *Staphylococcus* infections).
   n. Fluid accumulation in the pleural cavity may be removed by thoracentesis; thoracentesis also provides a means for obtaining fluid for culture and for instilling antibiotics directly into the pleural cavity.

⚠ Children with a respiratory disorder should be monitored for weight loss and for signs of dehydration. Signs of dehydration include a sunken fontanel, nonelastic skin turgor, decreased and concentrated urinary output, dry mucous membranes, and decreased tear production.

VI. ASTHMA

A. Description
1. Asthma is a chronic inflammatory disease of the airways (see Chapter 58).
2. Asthma is classified based on disease severity; management includes medications, environmental control of allergens, and child and family education.
3. The allergic reaction in the airways caused by the precipitant can result in an immediate reaction with obstruction occurring, and it can result in a late bronchial obstructive reaction several hours after the initial exposure to the precipitant.
4. Mast cell release of histamine leads to a bronchoconstrictive process, bronchospasm, and obstruction.
5. Diagnosis is made based on the child's symptoms, history and physical examination, chest radiograph, and laboratory tests (Box 38-3).
6. Precipitants may trigger an asthma attack (Box 38-4).
7. Status asthmaticus is an acute asthma attack, and the child displays respiratory distress despite vigorous treatment measures; this is a medical emergency that can result in respiratory failure and death if not treated.

B. Assessment
1. Child has episodes of dyspnea, **wheezing,** breathlessness, chest tightness, and cough, particularly at night or in the early morning or both.

Box 38-3 Laboratory Tests to Assist in Diagnosing Asthma

Pulmonary function tests: Spirometry testing assesses presence and degree of disease and can determine response to treatment.

Peak expiratory flow rate measurement: Measures maximum flow of air that can be forcefully exhaled in 1 second; child uses a peak expiratory flowmeter to determine a "personal best value" that can be used for comparison at other times, such as during and after an asthma attack.

Bronchoprovocation testing: Testing that is done to identify inhaled allergens; mucous membranes are directly exposed to suspected allergen in increasing amounts.

Skin testing: Done to identify specific allergens.

Exercise challenges: Exercise is used to identify the occurrence of exercise-induced bronchospasm.

Radioallergosorbent test: Blood test used to identify a specific allergen.

Chest radiograph: May show hyperexpansion of the airways.

Note: Some tests place the child at risk for an asthma attack; testing should be done under close supervision.

Box 38-4 Precipitants Triggering an Asthma Attack

Allergens
　Outdoor: trees, shrubs, weeds, grasses, molds, pollen, air pollution, spores
　Indoor: dust, dust mites, mold, cockroach antigen
Irritants: tobacco smoke, wood smoke, odors, sprays
Exposure to occupational irritants
Exercise
Cold air
Changes in weather or temperature
Environmental change: moving to a new home, starting a new school
Colds and infections
Animals: cats, dogs, rodents, horses
Medications: aspirin, nonsteroidal anti-inflammatory drugs, antibiotics, β-blockers
Strong emotions: fear, anger, laughing, crying
Conditions: gastroesophageal reflux disease, tracheoesophageal fistula
Food additives: sulfite preservatives
Foods: nuts, milk and other dairy products
Endocrine factors: menses, pregnancy, thyroid disease

From Perry, S., Hockenberry, M., Lowdermilk, D., & Wilson, D. (2010). *Maternal child nursing care* (4th ed., p. 1335). St. Louis: Mosby.

2. Acute asthma attacks
　a. Episodes include progressively worsening shortness of breath, cough, **wheezing**, chest tightness, decreases in expiratory airflow secondary to bronchospasm, mucosal edema, and mucus plugging; air is trapped behind occluded or narrow airways, and hypoxemia can occur.
　b. The attack begins with irritability, restlessness, headache, feeling tired, or chest tightness; just before the attack, the child may present with itching localized at the front of the neck or over the upper part of the back.
　c. Respiratory symptoms include a hacking, irritable, nonproductive cough caused by bronchial edema.
　d. Accumulated secretions stimulate the cough; the cough becomes rattling, and there is production of frothy, clear, gelatinous sputum.
　e. The child experiences **retractions**.
　f. Hyperresonance on percussion of the chest is noted.
　g. Breath sounds are coarse and loud, with **crackles**, coarse rhonchi, and inspiratory and expiratory **wheezing**; expiration is prolonged.
　h. Child may be pale or flushed, and the lips may have a deep, dark red color that may progress to **cyanosis** (also observed in the nail beds and skin, especially around the mouth).
　i. Restlessness, apprehension, and diaphoresis occur.
　j. Child speaks in short, broken phrases.
　k. Younger children assume the tripod sitting position; older children sit upright, with the shoulders in a hunched-over position, the hands on the bed or a chair, and the arms braced to facilitate the use of the accessory muscles of breathing (child refuses to lie down).
　l. Exercise-induced attack: Cough, shortness of breath, chest pain or tightness, **wheezing**, and endurance problems occur during exercise.
　m. Severe spasm or obstruction: Breath sounds and **wheezing** cannot be heard (silent chest), and cough is ineffective (represents a lack of air movement).
　n. Ventilatory failure and asphyxia: Shortness of breath, with air movement in the chest restricted to the point of absent breath sounds, is noted; this is accompanied by a sudden increase in the respiratory rate.
C. Interventions: Acute episode (see Priority Nursing Actions)

■■■ PRIORITY NURSING ACTIONS! ■■■

Actions to Take in the Event of an Acute Asthma Attack

1. Assess airway patency and respiratory status.
2. Administer humidified oxygen by nasal cannula or face mask.
3. Administer quick-relief (rescue) medications.
4. Initiate an intravenous (IV) line.
5. Prepare the child for a chest radiograph if prescribed.
6. Prepare to obtain a blood sample for determining arterial blood gas levels if prescribed.

In the event of an acute asthma attack, several interventions are necessary. First, the nurse assesses airway status to ensure airway patency. If the airway is not patent, emergency interventions such as endotracheal intubation may be necessary. The nurse also quickly assesses the child's respiratory status. If the airway is patent, the nurse administers oxygen by nasal cannula or mask as prescribed. Quick-relief (rescue) medications are administered as prescribed to treat the symptoms. An IV line is initiated so that IV medications can be administered if prescribed.

The nurse prepares the child for a chest x-ray to assess airway status and to assist in ruling out a respiratory infection. Blood samples are obtained, and an arterial blood gas may be obtained. When the laboratory results are obtained, the nurse administers medications as prescribed to correct dehydration, acidosis, or electrolyte imbalances. During the episode and during treatment, the nurse continuously monitors respiratory status, pulse oximetry, and color. The nurse also needs to be alert to decreased wheezing or a silent chest, which may signal the inability to move air.

References: Hockenberry, M., & Wilson, D. (2007). *Wong's essentials of pediatric nursing* (8th ed., p. 790). St. Louis: Mosby. McKinney, E., James, S., Murray, S., & Ashwill, J. (2009). *Maternal-child nursing* (3rd ed., p. 1204). St. Louis: Saunders.

D. Medications
 1. Quick-relief medications (rescue medications): Used to treat symptoms and exacerbations (Box 38-5)
 2. Long-term control medications (preventer medications): Used to achieve and maintain control of inflammation (Box 38-6)
 3. Nebulizer, metered-dose inhaler (MDI): May be used to administer medications; if the child has difficulty using the MDI, medication can be administered by nebulization (medication is mixed with saline and then nebulized with compressed air by a machine).
 4. If the MDI is used to administer a corticosteroid, a spacer should be used to prevent yeast infections in the child's mouth.
 5. The child's **growth** patterns need to be monitored when corticosteroids are prescribed.

Box 38-5 Quick-Relief Medications (Rescue Medications)

Short-acting β₂ agonists (for bronchodilation)
Anticholinergics (for relief of acute bronchospasm)
Systemic corticosteroids (for anti-inflammatory action to treat reversible airflow obstruction)

Box 38-6 Long-Term Control (Preventer Medications)

Corticosteroids (for anti-inflammatory action)
Antiallergic medications (to prevent an adverse response on exposure to an allergen)
Nonsteroidal anti-inflammatory drugs (for anti-inflammatory action)
Long-acting β₂ agonists (for long-acting bronchodilation)
Leukotriene modifiers (to prevent bronchospasm and inflammatory cell infiltration)
Monoclonal antibody (blocks binding of IgE to mast cells to inhibit inflammation)

E. Chest physiotherapy
 1. Includes breathing exercises, clapping and vibration procedures with postural drainage, and suctioning when necessary
 2. Chest physiotherapy strengthens the respiratory musculature and produces more efficient breathing patterns.
 3. Chest physiotherapy is not recommended during an acute exacerbation.
F. Allergen control
 1. Testing may be done to identify allergens.
 2. Teach the child and parents about measures to prevent and reduce exposure to allergens (see Box 38-4)
G. Home care measures
 1. Instruct the family in measures to eliminate environmental allergens.
 2. Avoid extremes of environmental temperature; in cold temperatures, instruct the child to breathe through the nose, not the mouth, and to cover the nose and mouth with a scarf.
 3. Avoid exposure to individuals with a respiratory infection.
 4. Instruct the child and family in how to recognize early symptoms of an asthma attack.
 5. Teach the child and family how to administer medications as prescribed.
 6. Teach the child and family how to use a nebulizer, MDI, or peak expiratory flowmeter.
 7. Instruct the child and family about the importance of home monitoring of the peak expiratory flow rate; a decrease in the expiratory flow rate may indicate impending infection or exacerbation.

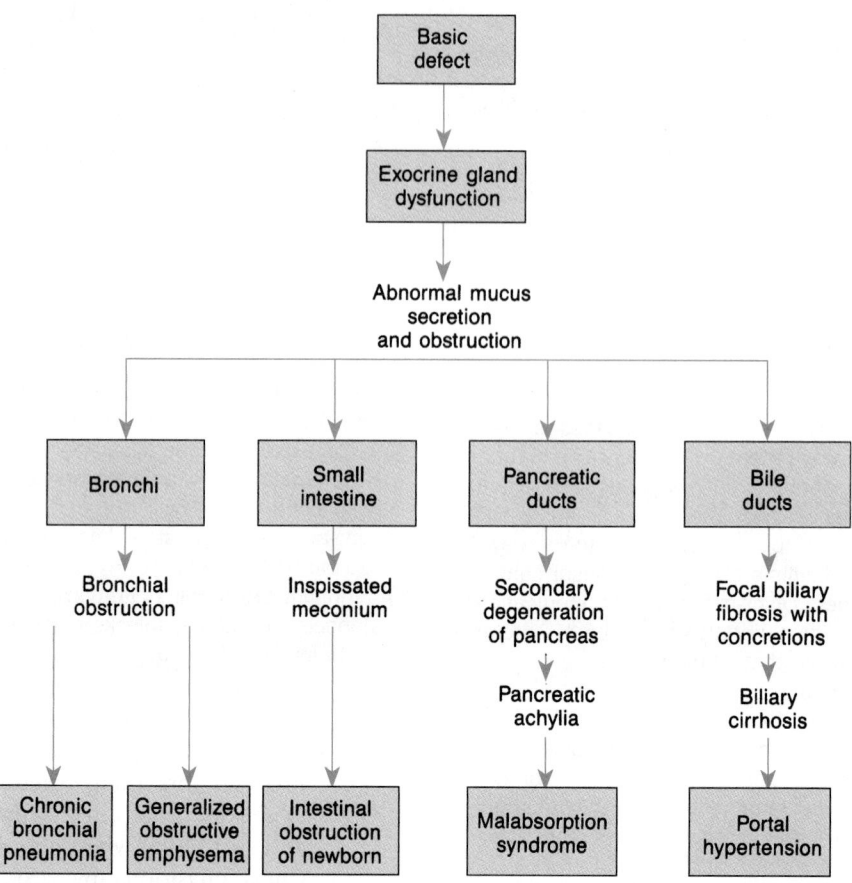

▲ **FIGURE 38-3** Various effects of exocrine gland dysfunction in cystic fibrosis. (From Hockenberry, M., & Wilson, D. [2007]. *Wong's nursing care of infants and children* [8th ed.]. St. Louis: Mosby.)

8. Instruct the child in the cleaning of devices used for inhaled medications (yeast infections can occur with the use of aerosolized corticosteroids).
9. Encourage adequate rest, sleep, and a well-balanced diet.
10. Instruct the child in the importance of adequate fluid intake to liquefy secretions.
11. Assist in developing an exercise program.
12. Instruct the child in the procedure for respiratory treatments and exercises as prescribed.
13. Encourage the child to cough effectively.
14. Encourage the parents to keep immunizations up to date; annual influenza vaccinations are recommended for children 6 months of age and older.
15. Inform other health care providers and school personnel of the asthma condition.
16. Allow the child to take control of self-care measures based on age appropriateness.

VII. CYSTIC FIBROSIS

A. Description (Fig. 38-3)
1. A chronic multisystem disorder (autosomal recessive trait disorder) characterized by exocrine gland dysfunction

2. The mucus produced by the exocrine glands is abnormally thick, tenacious, and copious, causing obstruction of the small passageways of the affected organs, particularly in the respiratory, gastrointestinal, and reproductive systems.
3. Common symptoms are associated with pancreatic enzyme deficiency and pancreatic fibrosis caused by duct blockage, progressive chronic lung disease as a result of infection, and sweat gland dysfunction resulting in increased sodium and chloride sweat concentrations.
4. An increase in sodium and chloride in sweat and saliva forms the basis for one diagnostic test, the sweat chloride test (Box 38-7).
5. Cystic fibrosis is a progressive and incurable disorder, and respiratory failure is a common cause of death; organ transplantations may be an option to increase survival rates.

B. Respiratory system
1. Symptoms are produced by the stagnation of mucus in the airway, leading to bacterial colonization and destruction of lung tissue.
2. Emphysema and atelectasis occur as the airways become increasingly obstructed.

Box 38-7 Quantitative Sweat Chloride Test

Production of sweat is stimulated (pilocarpine iontophoresis), sweat is collected, and sweat electrolytes are measured (more than 75 mg of sweat is needed).

Normally, sweat chloride concentration is less than 40 mEq/L.

Chloride concentration greater than 60 mEq/L is a positive test result (higher than 40 mEq/L is diagnostic in infants younger than 3 months of age).

Chloride concentrations of 40 to 60 mEq/L are highly suggestive of cystic fibrosis and require a repeat test.

3. Chronic hypoxemia causes contraction and hypertrophy of the muscle fibers in pulmonary arteries and arterioles, leading to pulmonary hypertension and eventual cor pulmonale.
4. Pneumothorax from ruptured bullae and hemoptysis from erosion of the bronchial wall occur as the disease progresses.
5. Other respiratory symptoms
   a. **Wheezing** and cough
   b. Dyspnea
   c. **Cyanosis**
   d. Clubbing of the fingers and toes
   e. Barrel chest
   f. Repeated episodes of bronchitis and pneumonia
C. Gastrointestinal system
   1. Meconium ileus in the newborn is the earliest manifestation.
   2. Intestinal obstruction (distal intestinal obstructive syndrome) caused by thick intestinal secretions can occur; signs include pain, abdominal distention, nausea, and vomiting.
   3. Stools are frothy and foul-smelling.
   4. Deficiency of the fat-soluble vitamins A, D, E, and K, which can result in easy bruising, bleeding, and anemia, occurs.
   5. Malnutrition and failure to thrive is a concern.
   6. Demonstration of hypoalbuminemia can occur from diminished absorption of protein, resulting in generalized edema.
   7. Rectal prolapse can result from the large, bulky stools and increased intra-abdominal pressure.
   8. Pancreatic fibrosis can occur and places the child at risk for diabetes mellitus.
D. Integumentary system
   1. Abnormally high concentrations of sodium and chloride in sweat is noted.
   2. Parents report that the infant tastes "salty" when kissed.
   3. Dehydration and electrolyte imbalances can occur, especially during hyperthermic conditions.
E. Reproductive system
   1. Cystic fibrosis can delay **puberty** in girls.

2. Fertility can be inhibited by the highly viscous cervical secretions, which act as a plug and block sperm entry.
3. Males are usually sterile, caused by the blockage of the vas deferens by abnormal secretions or by failure of normal development of duct structures.
F. Diagnostic tests
   1. Quantitative sweat chloride test is positive (see Box 38-7).
   2. Newborn screening may be done in some states and may consist of immunoreactive trypsinogen analysis and direct DNA analysis for mutant genes.
   3. Chest x-ray reveals atelectasis and obstructive emphysema.
   4. Pulmonary function tests provide evidence of abnormal small airway function.
   5. Stool, fat, enzyme analysis: A 72-hour stool sample is collected to check the fat or enzyme (trypsin) content, or both (food intake is recorded during the collection).
G. Interventions: Respiratory system
   1. Goals of treatment include preventing and treating pulmonary infection by improving aeration, removing secretions, and administering antibiotic medications.
   2. Monitor respiratory status including lung sounds and the presence and characteristics of a cough.
   3. Chest physiotherapy (percussion and postural drainage) on awakening and in the evening (more frequently during pulmonary infection) needs to be done every day to maintain pulmonary hygiene; chest physiotherapy should not be performed before or immediately after a meal.
   4. A Flutter Mucus Clearance Device (a small, hand-held plastic pipe with a stainless steel ball on the inside) facilitates the removal of mucus and may be prescribed; store away from small children because if the device separates, the steel ball poses a choking hazard.
   5. Hand-held percussors or a special vest device that provides high-frequency chest wall oscillation may be prescribed to help loosen secretions.
   6. A positive expiratory pressure mask may be prescribed; use of this mask forces secretion to the upper airway for expectoration.
   7. The child should be taught the forced expiratory technique (huffing) to mobilize secretions for expectoration.
   8. Bronchodilator medication by aerosol may be prescribed; the medication opens the bronchi for easier expectoration (administered before chest physiotherapy when the child has

reactive airway disease or is **wheezing**). Medications that decrease the viscosity of mucus may also be prescribed.

9. A physical exercise program with the aim of stimulating mucus expectoration and establishing an effective breathing pattern should be instituted.

10. Aerosolized or intravenous antibiotics may be prescribed and administered at home through a central venous access device.

11. Oxygen may be prescribed during acute episodes; monitor closely for oxygen narcosis (signs include nausea and vomiting, malaise, fatigue, numbness and tingling of extremities, substernal distress) because a child with cystic fibrosis may have chronic carbon dioxide retention.

12. Monitor for hemoptysis; more than 250 mL in 24 hours for an older child (less for a younger child) needs to be reported to the health care provider and treated immediately.

13. Hemoptysis may be controlled with measures such as bedrest, antibiotics if an infection is present, blood replacement therapy, and vitamin K; if hemoptysis persists, the site of bleeding may need to be cauterized.

H. Interventions: Gastrointestinal system

1. A child with cystic fibrosis requires a high-calorie, high-protein, and well-balanced diet to meet energy and **growth** needs; multivitamins and vitamins A, D, E, and K are also administered.

2. Monitor weight and for failure to thrive.

3. Monitor stool patterns and for signs of intestinal obstruction.

4. The goal of treatment for pancreatic insufficiency is to replace pancreatic enzymes; pancreatic enzymes are administered within 30 minutes of eating and administered with all meals and all snacks (enzymes should not be given if the child is NPO).

5. The amount of pancreatic enzymes administered depends on the physician's preference and usually is adjusted to achieve normal **growth** and a decrease in the number of stools to two or three daily (additional enzymes are needed if the child is consuming high-fat foods).

6. Enteric-coated pancreatic enzymes should not be crushed or chewed; capsules can be taken apart and the contents can be sprinkled on a small amount of food for administration.

7. Monitor for constipation, intestinal obstruction, and rectal prolapse.

8. Monitor for signs of gastroesophageal reflux; place the infant in an upright position after eating, and teach the child to sit upright after eating.

I. Additional interventions

1. Monitor blood glucose levels and for signs of diabetes mellitus.

2. Ensure adequate salt intake and fluids that provide an adequate supply of electrolytes during extremely hot weather and when the child has a fever.

3. Monitor bone **growth** in the child.

4. Monitor for signs of retinopathy or nephropathy.

5. Provide emotional support to the parents, particularly when the child is diagnosed; parents will be fearful and uncertain about the disorder and the care involved.

6. Provide support to the child as he or she transitions through the stages of **growth**.

7. Teach the child and parents about the care involved and encourage independence in the child for self-care as age-appropriate.

J. Home care

1. Home care involves educating the parents and the child about all of the aspects of care for the disorder.

2. Informing the parents and child about the signs of complications and actions to take and that the importance of follow-up care is crucial.

3. Instruct the parents to ensure that the child receives the recommended immunizations on schedule; additionally, annual influenza vaccinations are recommended for children 6 months of age and older.

4. Inform the child and parents about the Cystic Fibrosis Foundation.

⚠ An alteration in respiratory status can be a frightening experience for the child and parents. A calm and reassuring nursing approach assists in reducing fear.

VIII. SUDDEN INFANT DEATH SYNDROME (SIDS)

A. Description

1. SIDS refers to unexpected death of an apparently healthy infant younger than 1 year for whom an investigation of the death and a thorough autopsy fails to show an adequate cause of death.

2. Several theories are proposed regarding the cause of SIDS, but the exact cause is unknown.

3. SIDS most frequently occurs during winter months.

4. Death usually occurs during sleep periods, but not necessarily at night.

5. SIDS most frequently affects infants 2 to 3 months of age.

6. Incidence is higher in boys.

7. Incidence is higher in Native Americans, African Americans, and Hispanics and in lower socioeconomic groups.

8. Incidence has been found to be lower in breastfed infants and infants sleeping with a pacifier
9. High-risk conditions for SIDS
   a. Prone position
   b. Use of soft bedding, sleeping in a noninfant bed such as a sofa
   c. Overheating (thermal stress)
   d. Cosleeping
   e. Mother who smoked cigarettes or abused substances during pregnancy
   f. Exposure to tobacco smoke after birth
B. Assessment
1. Infant is apneic, blue, and lifeless.
2. Frothy blood-tinged fluid is in the nose and mouth.
3. Infant may be found in any position, but typically is found in a disheveled bed, with blankets over the head, and huddled in a corner.
4. Infants may appear to have been clutching bedding.
5. Diaper may be wet and full of stool.
C. Prevention and interventions
1. Infants should be placed in the supine position for sleep.
2. Mother needs to be taught about the risk factors: cigarette smoking and substance **abuse** during pregnancy; use of soft bedding, sleeping in a noninfant bed such as a sofa, overheating (thermal stress), cosleeping, exposure to tobacco smoke after birth; stuffed animals or other toys should be removed from the crib while the infant is sleeping.
3. Teach the parents to monitor for positional plagiocephaly caused by the supine sleeping position; signs include flattened posterior occiput and development of a bald spot in the posterior occiput area.
4. To assist in preventing positional plagiocephaly, teach the parents to alter head position during sleep, avoid excessive time in infant seats and bouncers, and place the infant in a prone position while awake (monitor the infant when in the prone position).
5. If SIDS occurs, the parents need a great deal of support as they grieve and mourn, especially because the event was sudden, unexpected, and unexplained.

IX. FOREIGN BODY ASPIRATION

A. Description (Fig. 38-4)
1. Swallowing and aspiration of a foreign body into the air passages
2. Most inhaled foreign bodies lodge in the main stem or lobar bronchus.
3. Most common offending foods are round in shape and include items such as hot dogs, candy, peanuts, popcorn, or grapes.
B. Assessment
1. Initially, choking, gagging, coughing, and **retractions** are general findings.
2. If the condition worsens, **cyanosis** may occur.
3. Laryngotracheal obstruction leads to dyspnea, **stridor**, cough, and hoarseness.
4. Bronchial obstruction produces paroxysmal cough, **wheezing**, asymmetrical breath sounds, and dyspnea.

FIRST-DEGREE OBSTRUCTION

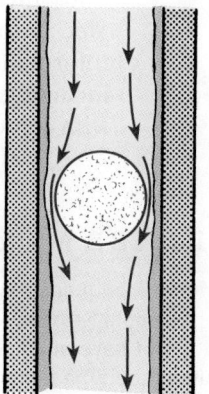

Obstruction allows passage of air in both directions

SECOND-DEGREE OBSTRUCTION

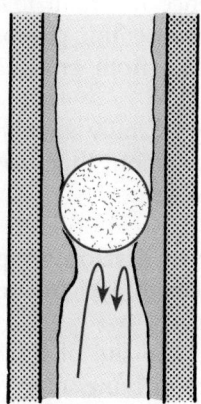

Inhalation
Air able to move past the obstruction in one direction only. Air passages enlarge during inspiration and diminish during expiration.

Expiration

COMPLETE OBSTRUCTION

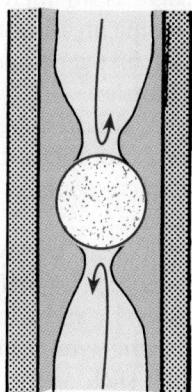

Air unable to move in either direction. FB and edematous mucosa obliterate passage.

▲ **FIGURE 38-4** Mechanisms of airway obstruction by a foreign body (FB). (From Hockenberry, M., & Wilson, D. [2007]. *Wong's nursing care of infants and children* [8th ed.]. St. Louis: Mosby.)

5. If any obstruction progresses, unconsciousness and asphyxiation may occur.
6. Partial obstructions may occur without symptoms.
7. Distressed child cannot speak, becomes cyanotic, and collapses.

C. Interventions
1. Emergency care (see Chapter 18)
2. Nonemergency management entails removal by endoscopy.
   a. After endoscopy, the child receives high-humidity air.
   b. Observe for signs and symptoms of airway edema.
3. Prevention
   a. Keep small objects including rubber balloons out of reach of small children.
   b. Avoid giving small children small, round food items.
4. Parent, day care provider, babysitter education
   a. Teach about the hazards of aspiration.
   b. Discuss potential situations in which small items may be aspirated.
   c. Teach about the symptoms of aspiration.
   d. Teach how to perform emergency care measures.

X. TUBERCULOSIS

A. Description
1. Tuberculosis is a contagious disease caused by *Mycobacterium tuberculosis*, an acid-fast bacillus (see Chapter 58).
2. Multidrug-resistant strains of *M. tuberculosis* occur because of child or family noncompliance with therapeutic regimens.
3. The route of transmission of *M. tuberculosis* is through inhalation of droplets from an individual with active tuberculosis.
4. There is an increased incidence in urban low-income areas, nonwhite racial or ethnic groups, and first-generation immigrants from endemic countries.
5. Most children are infected by a family member or by another individual with whom they have frequent contact, such as a babysitter.

B. Assessment
1. Child may be asymptomatic or develop symptoms such as malaise, fever, cough, weight loss, anorexia, and lymphadenopathy.
2. Specific symptoms related to the site of infection, such as the lungs, brain, or bone, may be present.
3. With increased time, asymmetrical expansion of the lungs, decreased breath sounds, **crackles**, and dullness to percussion develop.

C. Mantoux test (Box 38-8)
1. The test produces a positive reaction 2 to 10 weeks after the initial infection.

2. The test determines whether a child has been infected and has developed a sensitivity to the protein of the tubercle bacillus; a positive reaction does not confirm the presence of active disease (exposure versus presence).
3. After a child reacts positively, the child will always react positively; a positive reaction in a previously negative child indicates that the child has been infected since the last test.
4. Tuberculosis testing should not be done at the same time as measles immunization (viral interference from the measles **vaccine** may cause a false-negative result).

D. Sputum culture
1. A definitive diagnosis is made by showing the presence of mycobacteria in a culture.
2. Chest x-rays are supplemental to sputum cultures and are not definitive alone.
3. Because an infant or young child often swallows sputum rather than expectorates it, gastric washings (aspiration of lavaged contents from the fasting stomach) may be done to obtain a specimen; the specimen is obtained in the early morning before breakfast.

E. Interventions
1. Medications
   a. A 9-month course of isoniazid (INH) may be prescribed to prevent a latent infection from progressing to clinically active tuberculosis and to prevent initial infection in children in high-risk situations; a 12-month course may be prescribed for a child infected with human immunodeficiency virus (HIV).
   b. Recommendation for a child with clinically active tuberculosis may include combination administration of isoniazid, rifampin (Rifadin), and pyrazinamide daily for 2 months, and then isoniazid and rifampin twice weekly for 4 months.
   c. Inform the parents and child that bodily fluids including urine may turn an orange-red color with some tuberculosis medications.

Box 38-8 Mantoux Test Interpretation

Induration measuring 15 mm or more is considered to be a positive reaction in children 4 years or older who do not have any risk factors.

Induration measuring 10 mm or more is considered to be a positive reaction in children younger than 4 years and in children with chronic illness or at high risk for exposure to tuberculosis.

Induration measuring 5 mm or more is considered to be positive for the highest risk groups, such as children with immunosuppressive conditions or human immunodeficiency virus infection.

d. Directly observed therapy may be necessary for some children.

2. Place children with active disease who are contagious on respiratory isolation until medications have been initiated, sputum cultures show a diminished number of organisms, and cough is improving; this includes use of a personally fitted air-purifying N95 or N100 respirator (mask) by the nurse caring for the child.

3. Stress the importance of adequate rest and adequate diet.

4. Instruct the child and family about measures to prevent the transmission of tuberculosis.

5. Case finding and follow-up with known contacts is crucial to decrease the number of cases of individuals with active tuberculosis.

 MORE QUESTIONS ON THE CD!

Practice Questions

387. A 10-year-old child with asthma is treated for acute exacerbation in the emergency department. A nurse caring for the child monitors for which of the following, knowing that it indicates a worsening of the condition?
1. Warm, dry skin
2. Decreased wheezing
3. Pulse rate of 90 beats/min
4. Respirations of 18 breaths/min

388. The mother of an 8-year-old child being treated for right lower lobe pneumonia at home calls the clinic nurse. The mother tells the nurse that the child complains of discomfort on the right side and that the ibuprofen (Motrin) is not effective. The nurse should tell the mother to:
1. Increase the dose of the ibuprofen.
2. Increase the frequency of the ibuprofen.
3. Encourage the child to lie on the left side.
4. Encourage the child to lie on the right side.

389. A new mother expresses concern to a nurse regarding sudden infant death syndrome (SIDS). She asks the nurse how to position her new infant for sleep. The nurse appropriately tells the mother that the infant should be placed on the:
1. Side or prone
2. Back or prone
3. Stomach with the face turned
4. Back rather than on the stomach

390. A clinic nurse is providing instructions to a mother of a child with cystic fibrosis regarding the immunization schedule for the child. Which statement would the nurse make to the mother?

1. "The immunization schedule will need to be altered."
2. "The child should not receive any hepatitis vaccines."
3. "The child will receive all the immunizations except for the polio series."
4. "The child will receive the recommended basic series of immunizations along with a yearly influenza vaccination."

391. An emergency department nurse is caring for a child diagnosed with epiglottitis. Assessing the child, the nurse monitors for which indication that the child may be experiencing airway obstruction?
1. The child exhibits nasal flaring and bradycardia.
2. The child is leaning forward, with the chin thrust out.
3. The child has a low-grade fever and complains of a sore throat.
4. The child is leaning backward, supporting himself or herself with the hands and arms.

392. A child with laryngotracheobronchitis (croup) is placed in a cool mist tent. The mother becomes concerned because the child is frightened, consistently crying and trying to climb out of the tent. The appropriate nursing action is to:
1. Tell the mother that the child must stay in the tent.
2. Call the physician and obtain a prescription for a mild sedative.
3. Place a toy in the tent to make the child feel more comfortable.
4. Let the mother hold the child and direct the cool mist over the child's face.

393. A nurse is caring for an infant with bronchiolitis, and diagnostic tests have confirmed respiratory syncytial virus (RSV). Based on this finding, which of the following is the appropriate nursing action?
1. Initiate strict enteric precautions.
2. Move the infant to a room with another child with RSV.
3. Leave the infant in the present room because RSV is not contagious.
4. Inform the staff that they must wear a mask, gloves, and a gown when caring for the child.

394. A clinic nurse reads the results of a Mantoux test on a 3-year-old child. The results indicate an area of induration measuring 10 mm. The nurse would interpret these results as:
1. Positive
2. Negative

3. Inconclusive

4. Definitive and requiring a repeat test

395. The mother of a hospitalized 2-year-old child with viral laryngotracheobronchitis (croup) asks a nurse why the physician did not prescribe antibiotics. The appropriate response is:

1. "The child may be allergic to antibiotics."

2. "The child is too young to receive antibiotics."

3. "Antibiotics are not indicated unless a bacterial infection is present."

4. "The child still has the maternal antibodies from birth and does not need antibiotics."

Alternate Item Format: Multiple Response

396. A nurse is preparing for the admission of an infant with a diagnosis of bronchiolitis caused by respiratory syncytial virus (RSV). Which interventions would the nurse include in the plan of care? **Select all that apply.**

❏ 1. Place the infant in a private room.

❏ 2. Ensure that the infant's head is in a flexed position.

❏ 3. Wear a mask at all times when in contact with the infant.

❏ 4. Place the infant in a tent that delivers warm humidified air.

❏ 5. Position the infant side-lying, with the head lower than the chest.

❏ 6. Ensure that nurses caring for the infant with RSV do not care for other high-risk children.

ANSWERS

387. 2

Rationale: Asthma is a chronic inflammatory disease of the airways. Decreased wheezing in a child with asthma may be interpreted incorrectly as a positive sign when it may actually signal an inability to move air. A "silent chest" is an ominous sign during an asthma episode. With treatment, increased wheezing actually may signal that the child's condition is improving. Warm, dry skin indicates an improvement in the child's condition because the child is normally diaphoretic during exacerbation. The normal pulse rate in a 10-year-old is 70 to 110 beats/min. The normal respiratory rate in a 10-year-old is 16 to 20 breaths/min.

Test-Taking Strategy: Use the process of elimination and note the strategic word *worsening* in the question. Options 3 and 4 can be eliminated because they are normal vital signs. From the remaining options, recall that a "silent chest" is an ominous sign during an asthma episode and indicates severe bronchial spasm or obstruction. Review the clinical manifestations of severe bronchial spasm or obstruction in a child with asthma if you had difficulty with this question.

Level of Cognitive Ability: Analyzing

Client Needs: Physiological Integrity

Integrated Process: Nursing Process—Analysis

Content Area: Critical Care

Reference: Swearingen, P. (2008). *All-in-one care planning resource: Medical-surgical, pediatric, maternity, & psychiatric nursing care plans* (2nd ed., p. 577). St. Louis: Mosby.

388. 4

Rationale: Pneumonia is an inflammation of the pulmonary parenchyma or alveoli or both caused by a virus, mycoplasmal agents, bacteria, or aspiration of foreign substances. Splinting of the affected side by lying on that side may decrease discomfort. It would be inappropriate to advise the mother to increase the dose or frequency of the ibuprofen. Lying on the left side would not be helpful in alleviating discomfort.

Test-Taking Strategy: Use the process of elimination. Options 1 and 2 can be eliminated because the nurse does not adjust the dose or frequency of medications. Recalling the principles related to splinting an incision in the postoperative client will assist in directing you to option 4 because these principles can be applied in this situation. Review care of a child with pneumonia if you had difficulty with this question.

Level of Cognitive Ability: Applying

Client Needs: Physiological Integrity

Integrated Process: Nursing Process—Implementation

Content Area: Child Health—Eye/Ear/Throat/Respiratory/Cardiovascular

Reference: McKinney, E., James, S., Murray, S., & Ashwill, J. (2009). *Maternal-child nursing* (3rd ed., p. 1196). St. Louis: Saunders.

389. 4

Rationale: Sudden infant death syndrome (SIDS) is the unexpected death of an apparently healthy infant younger than 1 year for whom an investigation of the death and a thorough autopsy fails to show an adequate cause of death. Several theories are proposed regarding the cause, but the exact cause is unknown. Nurses should encourage parents to place the infant on the back (supine) for sleep. Infants in the prone position (on the stomach) may be unable to move their heads to the side, increasing the risk of suffocation. The infant may have the ability to turn to a prone position from the side-lying position.

Test-Taking Strategy: Use the process of elimination. Eliminate options 1, 2, and 3 because they are comparable or alike. Remember that the infant needs to be placed on his or her back. Review positioning of the healthy infant for sleep and the preventive measures for SIDS if you had difficulty with this question.

Level of Cognitive Ability: Applying

Client Needs: Safe and Effective Care Environment

Integrated Process: Teaching and Learning

Content Area: Child Health—Eye/Ear/Throat/Respiratory/ Cardiovascular
Reference: Perry, S., Hockenberry, M., Lowdermilk, D., & Wilson, D. (2010). *Maternal child nursing care* (4th ed., p. 1008). St. Louis: Mosby.

390. 4
Rationale: Cystic fibrosis is a chronic multisystem disorder (autosomal recessive trait disorder) characterized by exocrine gland dysfunction. The mucus produced by the exocrine glands is abnormally thick, tenacious, and copious, causing obstruction of the small passageways of the affected organs, particularly in the respiratory, gastrointestinal, and reproductive systems. Adequately protecting children with cystic fibrosis from communicable diseases by immunization is essential. In addition to the basic series of immunizations, a yearly influenza immunization is recommended for children with cystic fibrosis. Options 1, 2, and 3 are incorrect.
Test-Taking Strategy: Use the process of elimination. Eliminate options 1, 2, and 3 because they are comparable or alike indicating that the immunization schedule will be adjusted in some way. Recalling the importance of protection from communicable diseases, particularly in children with a disorder such as cystic fibrosis, will assist in directing you to option 4. Review the immunization schedule for a child with cystic fibrosis if you had difficulty with this question.
Level of Cognitive Ability: Applying
Client Needs: Health Promotion and Maintenance
Integrated Process: Teaching and Learning
Content Area: Child Health—Eye/Ear/Throat/Respiratory/ Cardiovascular
Reference: Perry, S., Hockenberry, M., Lowdermilk, D., & Wilson, D. (2010). *Maternal child nursing care* (4th ed., p. 1352). St. Louis: Mosby.

391. 2
Rationale: Epiglottitis is a bacterial form of croup. A primary concern is that it can progress to acute respiratory distress. Clinical manifestations suggestive of airway obstruction include tripod positioning (leaning forward while supported by arms, chin thrust out, mouth open), nasal flaring, the use of accessory muscles for breathing, and the presence of stridor. Option 4 is an incorrect position. Options 1 and 3 are incorrect because epiglottitis causes a high fever and tachycardia.
Test-Taking Strategy: Use the process of elimination. Eliminate option 1 first because tachycardia rather than bradycardia would occur in a child experiencing respiratory distress. Eliminate option 3 next, knowing that a high fever occurs with epiglottitis. From the remaining options, visualize the descriptions in each and determine which position would best assist a child experiencing respiratory distress. Review the manifestations of epiglottitis and airway obstruction if you had difficulty with this question.
Level of Cognitive Ability: Analyzing
Client Needs: Physiological Integrity
Integrated Process: Nursing Process—Assessment
Content Area: Critical Care
References: Hockenberry, M., & Wilson, D. (2009). *Wong's essentials of pediatric nursing* (8th ed., p. 771). St. Louis: Mosby.
McKinney, E., James, S., Murray, S., & Ashwill, J. (2009). *Maternal-child nursing* (3rd ed., p. 1190). St. Louis: Saunders.

392. 4
Rationale: Laryngotracheobronchitis (croup) is the inflammation of the larynx, trachea, and bronchi and is the most common type of croup. Cool mist therapy may be prescribed to liquefy secretions and to assist in breathing. If the use of a tent or hood is causing distress, treatment may be more effective if the child is held by the parent and a cool mist is directed toward the child's face. A mild sedative would not be administered to the child. Crying would increase hypoxia and aggravate laryngospasm, which may cause airway obstruction. Options 1 and 3 would not alleviate the child's fear.
Test-Taking Strategy: Focus on the subject of the question, the child's fear. Options 1, 2, and 3 are comparable or alike in that they do not address the fear. Option 4 is the option that addresses the subject of the question. Review care of a child in a mist tent if you had difficulty with this question.
Level of Cognitive Ability: Applying
Client Needs: Psychosocial Integrity
Integrated Process: Caring
Content Area: Child Health—Eye/Ear/Throat/Respiratory/ Cardiovascular
Reference: McKinney, E., James, S., Murray, S., & Ashwill, J. (2009). *Maternal-child nursing* (3rd ed., p. 1188). St. Louis: Saunders.

393. 2
Rationale: Respiratory syncytial virus (RSV) is a highly communicable disorder and is not transmitted via the airborne route. The virus usually is transferred by the hands. Use of contact and standard precautions during care is necessary. Using good handwashing techniques and wearing gloves and gowns are also necessary. Masks are not required. An infant with RSV is isolated in a single room or placed in a room with another child with RSV. Enteric precautions are unnecessary.
Test-Taking Strategy: Use the process of elimination, recalling the method of viral transmission. Remember that the virus is not transmitted via the airborne route and is usually transferred by the hands. An infant with RSV is isolated in a single room or placed in a room with another child with RSV. Review the nursing care required for an infant with RSV if you had difficulty with this question.
Level of Cognitive Ability: Applying
Client Needs: Safe and Effective Care Environment
Integrated Process: Nursing Process—Implementation
Content Area: Child Health—Eye/Ear/Throat/Respiratory/ Cardiovascular
Reference: Perry, S., Hockenberry, M., Lowdermilk, D., & Wilson, D. (2010). *Maternal child nursing care* (4th ed., p. 1323). St. Louis: Mosby.

394. 1
Rationale: Induration measuring 10 mm or more is considered to be a positive result in children younger than 4 years of age and in children with chronic illness or at high risk for exposure to tuberculosis. A reaction of 5 mm or more is considered to be a positive result for the highest risk groups, such as a child with an immunosuppressive condition or a child with human immunodeficiency virus (HIV) infection. A reaction of 15 mm or more is positive in children 4 years or older without any risk factors.

Test-Taking Strategy: Use the process of elimination. Options 3 and 4 are comparable or alike and can be eliminated first. From the remaining options, focus on the data in the question and note the child's age to assist in directing you to option 1. If you had difficulty with this question, review the analysis of the Mantoux test in children.
Level of Cognitive Ability: Analyzing
Client Needs: Physiological Integrity
Integrated Process: Nursing Process—Analysis
Content Area: Child Health—Eye/Ear/Throat/Respiratory/Cardiovascular
Reference: Perry, S., Hockenberry, M., Lowdermilk, D., & Wilson, D. (2010). *Maternal child nursing care* (4th ed., p. 1329). St. Louis: Mosby.

395. 3

Rationale: Laryngotracheobronchitis (croup) is the inflammation of the larynx, trachea, and bronchi and is the most common type of croup. It can be viral or bacterial. Antibiotics are not indicated in the treatment of croup unless a bacterial infection is present. Options 1, 2, and 4 are incorrect. In addition, no supporting data in the question indicate that the child may be allergic to antibiotics.
Test-Taking Strategy: Use the process of elimination. Eliminate option 1 because no supporting data are in the question regarding the potential for allergies. Noting the strategic word *viral* in the question and noting the age of the child will assist in eliminating options 2 and 4. Review the indications for the use of antibiotics in a child with croup if you had difficulty with this question.
Level of Cognitive Ability: Applying
Client Needs: Physiological Integrity
Integrated Process: Teaching and Learning
Content Area: Child Health—Eye/Ear/Throat/Respiratory/Cardiovascular
Reference: McKinney, E., James, S., Murray, S., & Ashwill, J. (2009). *Maternal-child nursing* (3rd ed., p. 1187). St. Louis: Saunders.

ALTERNATE ITEM FORMAT: MULTIPLE RESPONSE
396. 1, 6

Rationale: Respiratory syncytial virus (RSV) is a highly communicable disorder and is not transmitted via the airborne route. The virus usually is transferred by the hands. Use of contact and standard precautions during care (wearing gloves and a gown) reduce nosocomial transmission of RSV. A mask is unnecessary. Additionally, it is important to ensure that nurses caring for a child with RSV do not care for other high-risk children to prevent the transmission of the infection. An infant with RSV should be isolated in a private room or in a room with another infant with RSV infection. The infant should be positioned with the head and chest at a 30- to 40-degree angle and the neck slightly extended to maintain an open airway and decrease pressure on the diaphragm. Cool humidified oxygen is delivered to relieve dyspnea, hypoxemia, and insensible water loss from tachypnea.
Test-Taking Strategy: Recalling the mode of transmission of RSV will assist in determining that the infant needs to be placed in a private room or in a room with another infant with RSV infection and that contact precautions need to be maintained. Recalling the need to maintain a patent airway (edema and the accumulation of mucus obstruct the bronchioles) will assist in determining that the infant needs to be observed closely, the infant's head should be elevated, and the infant should receive cool humidified oxygen. Review care of a child with bronchiolitis and RSV if you had difficulty with this question.
Level of Cognitive Ability: Applying
Client Needs: Physiological Integrity
Integrated Process: Nursing Process—Planning
Content Area: Child Health—Eye/Ear/Throat/Respiratory/Cardiovascular
Reference: McKinney, E., James, S., Murray, S., & Ashwill, J. (2009). *Maternal-child nursing* (3rd ed., pp. 1187, 1193). St. Louis: Saunders.

Cardiovascular Disorders

I. CONGESTIVE HEART FAILURE (CHF)

A. Description
1. CHF (Box 39-1) is the inability of the heart to pump a sufficient amount of oxygen to meet the metabolic needs of the body.
2. In infants and children, inadequate cardiac output most commonly is caused by congenital heart defects (**shunt**, obstruction, or a combination of both) that produce an excessive volume or pressure load on the myocardium.
3. In infants and children, a combination of left-sided and right-sided heart failure is usually present.
4. The goals of treatment are to improve cardiac function, remove accumulated fluid and sodium, decrease cardiac demands, improve tissue oxygenation, and decrease oxygen consumption.

B. Assessment of early signs
1. Tachycardia, especially during rest and slight exertion
2. Tachypnea
3. Profuse scalp diaphoresis, especially in infants
4. Fatigue and irritability
5. Sudden weight gain
6. Respiratory distress

C. Interventions
1. Monitor for early signs of CHF.
2. Monitor for respiratory distress (count respirations for 1 minute).
3. Monitor apical pulse (count apical pulse for 1 minute), and monitor for dysrhythmias.
4. Monitor temperature for hyperthermia and for other signs of infection, particularly respiratory infection.
5. Monitor strict intake and output; weigh diapers as appropriate for most accurate output.
6. Monitor daily weight to assess for fluid retention; a weight gain of 0.5 kg (1 lb) in 1 day is caused by the accumulation of fluid.
7. Monitor for facial or peripheral dependent edema, auscultate lung sounds, and report abnormal findings indicating excessive fluid in the body.
8. Elevate the head of the bed in a semi-Fowler's position.
9. Maintain a neutral thermal environment to prevent cold stress in infants.
10. Provide rest and decrease environmental stimuli.
11. Administer cool humidified oxygen as prescribed, using an oxygen hood for young infants and a nasal cannula or face mask for older infants and children.
12. Organize nursing activities to allow for uninterrupted sleep.
13. Maintain adequate nutritional status.
14. Feed when hungry and soon after awakening, conserving energy and oxygen supply.
15. Provide small, frequent feedings, conserving energy and oxygen supply.
16. Administer sedation as prescribed during the acute stage to promote rest.
17. Administer digoxin (Lanoxin) as prescribed.
    a. Assess apical heart rate for 1 minute before administration.
    b. Hold digoxin if the apical pulse is less than 90 to 110 beats/min in infants and young children and less than 70 beats/min in older children, as prescribed.
    c. Be aware that infants rarely receive more than 1 mL (50 mcg or 0.05 mg) of digoxin in one dose.
18. Monitor digoxin levels and for signs of digoxin toxicity, including anorexia, poor feeding, nausea, vomiting, bradycardia, and dysrhythmias.
    a. Normal digoxin level is 0.5 to 2 ng/mL.
    b. Digoxin toxicity is present when level is greater than 2 ng/mL.
19. Administer angiotensin-converting enzyme inhibitors as prescribed.
    a. Monitor for hypotension, renal dysfunction, and cough when angiotensin-converting enzyme inhibitors are administered.
    b. Assess blood pressure; serum protein, albumin, blood urea nitrogen, and creatinine levels; white blood cell count; urine output; urinary specific gravity; and urinary protein level.

Box 39-1 Signs and Symptoms of Congestive Heart Failure

Left-Sided Failure	Right-Sided Failure
Crackles and wheezes	Ascites
Cough	Hepatosplenomegaly
Dyspnea	Jugular vein distention
Grunting (infants)	Oliguria
Head bobbing (infants)	Peripheral edema, especially
Nasal flaring	dependent edema, and
Orthopnea	periorbital edema
Periods of cyanosis	Weight gain
Retractions	
Tachypnea	

Box 39-2 Home Care Instructions for Administering Digoxin (Lanoxin)

Administer as prescribed.
Administer 1 hour before or 2 hours after feedings.
Use a calendar to mark off the dose administered.
Do not mix medication with foods or fluid.
If a dose is missed and more than 4 hours has elapsed, withhold the dose and give the next dose at the scheduled time; if less than 4 hours has elapsed, administer the missed dose.
If the child vomits, do not administer a second dose.
If more than two consecutive doses have been missed, notify the physician; do not increase or double the dose for missed doses.
If the child has teeth, give water after the medication; if possible, brush the teeth to prevent tooth decay from the sweetened liquid.
Monitor for signs of toxicity, such as poor feeding or vomiting.
If the child becomes ill, notify the physician.
Keep the medication in a locked cabinet.
Call the poison control center immediately if accidental overdose occurs.

20. Administer diuretics such as furosemide (Lasix) as prescribed.
    a. Monitor for signs and symptoms of hypokalemia (serum potassium level <3.5 mEq/L), including muscle weakness and cramping, confusion, irritability, restlessness, and inverted T waves or prominent U waves on the electrocardiogram.
    b. If signs and symptoms of hypokalemia are present and the child is also being administered digoxin, monitor closely for digoxin toxicity because hypokalemia potentiates digoxin toxicity.
21. Administer potassium supplements and provide dietary sources of potassium as prescribed.
    a. Supplemental potassium should be given only if indicated by serum potassium levels and if adequate renal function is evident and is usually necessary when administering a non–potassium-sparing diuretic such as furosemide (Lasix).
    b. Encourage foods that the child will eat that are high in potassium, as appropriate, such as bananas, baked potato skins, and peanut butter.
22. Monitor serum electrolyte levels, particularly the potassium level (normal level is 3.5 to 5.1 mEq/L).
23. Limit fluid intake as prescribed in the acute stage.
24. Monitor for signs and symptoms of dehydration, including sunken fontanel, nonelastic skin turgor, dry mucous membranes, decreased tear production, decreased urine output, and concentrated urine.
25. Monitor sodium levels as prescribed.
    a. Normal level is 135 to 145 mEq/L.
    b. Many infant formulas have slightly more sodium than breast milk.
26. Instruct the parents regarding the description of the diagnosis and administration of medications (Box 39-2).
27. Instruct the parents in cardiopulmonary resuscitation (CPR) (see Chapter 18).

⚠ The parents should be provided with a medication guide for any medication prescribed for the infant or child. Additionally, the nurse needs to review the instructions in the guide and provide an opportunity for the parents to demonstrate medication administration procedures.

II. DEFECTS WITH INCREASED PULMONARY BLOOD FLOW (Box 39-3)

A. Description
1. Intracardiac communication along the septum or an abnormal connection between the great arteries allows blood to flow from the high-pressure left side of the heart to the low-pressure right side of the heart.
2. The infant typically shows signs and symptoms of CHF.
B. Atrial septal defect (ASD)
1. ASD is an abnormal opening between the atria that causes an increased flow of oxygenated blood into the right side of the heart.
2. Right atrial and ventricular enlargement occurs.
3. Infant may be asymptomatic or may develop CHF.
4. Signs and symptoms of decreased cardiac output may be present (Box 39-4).
5. Types
    a. ASD 1 (ostium primum): Opening is at the lower end of the septum.
    b. ASD 2 (ostium secundum): Opening is near the center of the septum.

Box 39-3 Defects with Increased Pulmonary Blood Flow

Atrial septal defect
Atrioventricular canal defect
Patent ductus arteriosus
Ventricular septal defect

Box 39-4 Signs and Symptoms of Decreased Cardiac Output

Decreased peripheral pulses
Exercise intolerance
Feeding difficulties
Hypotension
Irritability, restlessness, lethargy
Oliguria
Pale, cool extremities
Tachycardia

c. ASD 3 (sinus venosus defect): Opening is near the junction of the superior vena cava and the right atrium.
6. Management
   a. Defect may be closed during a cardiac catheterization.
   b. Open repair with cardiopulmonary bypass may be performed and usually is performed before school age.
C. Atrioventricular canal defect
   1. The defect results from incomplete fusion of the endocardial cushions.
   2. The defect is the most common cardiac defect in Down syndrome.
   3. A characteristic murmur is present.
   4. The infant usually has mild to moderate CHF, with **cyanosis** increasing with crying.
   5. Signs and symptoms of decreased cardiac output may be present.
   6. Management can include pulmonary artery banding for infants with severe symptoms (palliative) or complete repair via cardiopulmonary bypass.
D. Patent ductus arteriosus
   1. Patent ductus arteriosus is failure of the fetal ductus arteriosus (artery connecting the aorta and the pulmonary artery) to close within the first weeks of life.
   2. A characteristic machinery-like murmur is present.
   3. An infant may be asymptomatic or may show signs of CHF.
   4. A widened pulse pressure and bounding pulses are present.
   5. Signs and symptoms of decreased cardiac output may be present.

Box 39-5 Obstructive Defects

Aortic stenosis
Coarctation of the aorta
Pulmonary stenosis

6. Management
   a. Indomethacin (Indocin), a prostaglandin inhibitor, may be administered to close a patent ductus in premature infants and some newborns.
   b. The defect may be closed during cardiac catheterization, or the defect may require surgical management.
E. Ventricular septal defect (VSD)
   1. VSD is an abnormal opening between the right and left ventricles.
   2. Many VSDs close spontaneously during the first year of life in children having small or moderate defects.
   3. A characteristic murmur is present.
   4. Signs and symptoms of CHF are commonly present.
   5. Signs and symptoms of decreased cardiac output may be present.
   6. Management
      a. Closure during cardiac catheterization may be possible.
      b. Open repair may be done with cardiopulmonary bypass.

III. OBSTRUCTIVE DEFECTS (Box 39-5)

A. Description
   1. Blood exiting a portion of the heart meets an area of anatomical narrowing (**stenosis**), causing obstruction to blood flow.
   2. The location of narrowing is usually near the valve of the obstructive defect.
   3. Infants and children exhibit signs of CHF.
   4. Children with mild obstruction may be asymptomatic.
B. Aortic **stenosis**
   1. Aortic **stenosis** is a narrowing or stricture of the aortic valve, causing resistance to blood flow from the left ventricle into the aorta, resulting in decreased cardiac output, left ventricular hypertrophy, and pulmonary vascular congestion.
   2. Valvular **stenosis** is the most common type and usually is caused by malformed cusps, resulting in a bicuspid rather than a tricuspid valve, or fusion of the cusps.
   3. A characteristic murmur is present.
   4. Infants with severe defects show signs of decreased cardiac output.
   5. Children show signs of exercise intolerance, chest pain, and dizziness when standing for long periods.

6. Management
   a. Dilation of the narrowed valve may be done during cardiac catheterization.
   b. Surgical aortic valvotomy (palliative) may be done; a valve replacement may be required at a second procedure.

C. Coarctation of the aorta
   1. Coarctation of the aorta is localized narrowing near the insertion of the ductus arteriosus.
   2. Blood pressure is higher in the upper extremities than the lower extremities; bounding pulses in the arms, weak or absent femoral pulses, and cool lower extremities may be present.
   3. Signs of CHF may occur in infants.
   4. Signs and symptoms of decreased cardiac output may be present.
   5. Children may experience headaches, dizziness, fainting, and epistaxis resulting from hypertension.
   6. Management of the defect may be done via balloon angioplasty in children; restenosis can occur.
   7. Surgical management
      a. Mechanical ventilation and medications to improve cardiac output are often necessary before surgery.
      b. Resection of the coarcted portion with end-to-end anastomosis of the aorta or enlargement of the constricted section using a graft may be required.
      c. Because the defect is outside the heart, cardiopulmonary bypass is not required, and a thoracotomy incision is used.

⚠ With coarctation of the aorta, the blood pressure is higher in the upper extremities than the lower extremities. Additionally, bounding pulses in the arms, weak or absent femoral pulses, and cool lower extremities may be present.

D. Pulmonary **stenosis**
   1. Pulmonary **stenosis** is narrowing at the entrance to the pulmonary artery.
   2. Resistance to blood flow causes right ventricular hypertrophy and decreased pulmonary blood flow; the right ventricle may be hypoplastic.
   3. Pulmonary **atresia** is the extreme form of pulmonary **stenosis** in that there is total fusion of the commissures and no blood flows to the lungs.
   4. A characteristic murmur is present.
   5. Infants or children may be asymptomatic.
   6. Newborns with severe narrowing are cyanotic.
   7. If pulmonary **stenosis** is severe, CHF occurs.
   8. Signs and symptoms of decreased cardiac output may occur.
   9. Management: Dilation of the narrowed valve may be done during cardiac catheterization.

Box 39-6 Defects with Decreased Pulmonary Blood Flow

Tetralogy of Fallot
Tricuspid atresia

---

10. Surgical management
    a. In infants: Transventricular (closed) valvotomy procedure
    b. In children: Pulmonary valvotomy with cardiopulmonary bypass

IV. DEFECTS WITH DECREASED PULMONARY BLOOD FLOW (Box 39-6)

A. Description
   1. Obstructed pulmonary blood flow and an anatomical defect (ASD or VSD) between the right and left sides of the heart are present.
   2. Pressure on the right side of the heart increases, exceeding pressure on the left side, which allows desaturated blood to **shunt** right to left, causing desaturation in the left side of the heart and in the systemic circulation.
   3. Typically hypoxemia and **cyanosis** appear.

B. Tetralogy of Fallot
   1. Tetralogy of Fallot includes four defects—VSD, pulmonary **stenosis**, overriding aorta, and right ventricular hypertrophy.
   2. If pulmonary vascular resistance is higher than systemic resistance, the **shunt** is from right to left; if systemic resistance is higher than pulmonary resistance, the **shunt** is left to right.
   3. Infants
      a. An infant may be acutely cyanotic at birth or may have mild **cyanosis** that progresses over the first year of life as the pulmonic **stenosis** worsens.
      b. A characteristic murmur is present.
      c. Acute episodes of **cyanosis** and hypoxia (hypercyanotic spells), called blue spells or tet spells, occur when the infant's oxygen requirements exceed the blood supply, such as during periods of crying, feeding, or defecating.
   4. Children: With increasing **cyanosis**, squatting, clubbing of the fingers, and poor **growth** may occur.
      a. Squatting is a compensatory mechanism to facilitate increased return of blood flow to the heart for oxygenation.
      b. Clubbing is an abnormal enlargement in the distal phalanges seen in the fingers.
   5. Surgical management: Palliative **shunt**
      a. The **shunt** increases pulmonary blood flow and increases oxygen saturation in infants who cannot undergo primary repair.

b. The **shunt** provides blood flow to the pulmonary arteries from the left or right subclavian artery.

6. Surgical management: Complete repair
   a. Complete repair usually is performed in the first year of life.
   b. The repair requires a median sternotomy and cardiopulmonary bypass.

C. Tricuspid **atresia**
1. Tricuspid **atresia** is failure of the tricuspid valve to develop.
2. No communication exists from the right atrium to the right ventricle.
3. Blood flows through an ASD or a patent foramen ovale to the left side of the heart and through a VSD to the right ventricle and out to the lungs.
4. The defect often is associated with pulmonic **stenosis** and transposition of the great arteries.
5. The defect results in complete mixing of unoxygenated and oxygenated blood in the left side of the heart, resulting in systemic desaturation, pulmonary obstruction, and decreased pulmonary blood flow.
6. **Cyanosis**, tachycardia, and dyspnea are seen in the newborn.
7. Older children exhibit signs of chronic hypoxemia and clubbing.
8. Management: If the ASD is small, the defect may be closed during cardiac catheterization; otherwise, surgery is needed.

⚠ Clubbing is symptomatic of chronic hypoxia. Peripheral circulation is diminished and oxygenation of vital organs and tissues is compromised.

V. **MIXED DEFECTS** (Box 39-7)

A. Description
1. Fully saturated systemic blood flow mixes with the desaturated blood flow, causing a desaturation of the systemic blood flow.
2. Pulmonary congestion occurs and cardiac output decreases.
3. Signs of CHF are present; symptoms vary with the degree of desaturation.

B. Hypoplastic left heart syndrome
1. Underdevelopment of the left side of the heart occurs, resulting in a hypoplastic left ventricle and aortic **atresia**.
2. Mild **cyanosis** and signs of CHF occur until the ductus arteriosus closes; then progressive deterioration with **cyanosis** and decreased cardiac output are seen, leading to cardiovascular collapse.
3. The defect is fatal in the first few months of life without intervention.
4. Surgical treatment
   a. Surgical treatment is necessary; transplantation in the newborn period may be considered.

   b. In the preoperative period, the newborn requires mechanical ventilation and a continuous infusion of prostaglandin E_1 to maintain ductal patency, ensuring adequate systemic blood flow.

C. Transposition of the great arteries or transposition of the great vessels
1. The pulmonary artery leaves the left ventricle, and the aorta exits from the right ventricle.
2. No communication exists between the systemic and pulmonary circulation.
3. Infants with minimal communication are severely cyanotic and depressed at birth.
4. Infants with large septal defects or a patent ductus arteriosus may be less severely cyanotic, but may have symptoms of CHF.
5. Cardiomegaly is evident a few weeks after birth.
6. Nonsurgical management
   a. Prostaglandin E_1 may be initiated to increase blood mixing temporarily if systemic and pulmonary mixing are inadequate.
   b. Balloon atrial septostomy during cardiac catheterization may be performed to increase mixing and to maintain cardiac output over a longer period.
7. Surgical management: The arterial switch procedure re-establishes normal circulation with the left ventricle acting as the systemic pump and creation of a new aorta.

D. Total anomalous pulmonary venous connection
1. The defect is a failure of the pulmonary veins to join the left atrium.
2. The defect results in mixed blood being returned to the right atrium and shunted from the right to the left through an ASD.
3. The right side of the heart hypertrophies, whereas the left side of the heart may remain small.
4. Signs and symptoms of CHF develop.
5. **Cyanosis** worsens with pulmonary vein obstruction; when obstruction occurs, the infant's condition deteriorates rapidly.
6. Surgical management
   a. Corrective repair is performed in early infancy.
   b. The pulmonary vein is anastomosed to the left atrium, the ASD is closed, and the anomalous pulmonary venous connection is ligated.

E. Truncus arteriosus
   1. Truncus arteriosus is failure of normal septation and division of the embryonic bulbar trunk into the pulmonary artery and the aorta, resulting in a single vessel that overrides both ventricles.
   2. Blood from both ventricles mixes in the common great artery, causing desaturation and hypoxemia.
   3. A characteristic murmur is present.
   4. The infant exhibits moderate to severe CHF and variable **cyanosis**, poor **growth**, and activity intolerance.
   5. Surgical management: Corrective surgical repair is performed in the first few months of life.

VI. **INTERVENTIONS: CARDIOVASCULAR DEFECTS**

   A. Monitor for signs of a defect in the infant or child (see descriptions of defects earlier).
   B. Monitor vital signs closely.
   C. Monitor respiratory status for the presence of **nasal flaring**, use of accessory muscles, and other signs of impending respiratory distress, and notify the physician if any changes occur.
   D. Auscultate breath sounds for **crackles**, rhonchi, or **wheezes**.
   E. If respiratory effort is increased, place the child in a reverse Trendelenburg position, elevating the head and upper body, to decrease the work of breathing.
   F. Administer humidified oxygen as prescribed.
   G. Provide endotracheal tube and ventilator care as prescribed.
   H. Monitor for hypercyanotic spells and intervene immediately if they occur (see Priority Nursing Actions).
   I. Assess for signs of CHF, such as periorbital edema or dependent edema in the hands and feet.
   J. Assess peripheral pulses.
   K. Maintain fluid restriction if prescribed.
   L. Monitor intake and output, and notify the physician if a decrease in urine output occurs.
   M. Obtain daily weight.
   N. Provide adequate nutrition (high calorie requirements) as prescribed.
   O. Administer medications as prescribed.
   P. Plan interventions to allow maximal rest for the child; keep the child as stress-free as possible.
   Q. Prepare the child and parents for cardiac catheterization, if appropriate.

VII. **CARDIAC CATHETERIZATION**

   A. Description
      1. Invasive diagnostic procedure to determine cardiac defects.
      2. Provides information about oxygen saturation of blood in great vessels and heart chambers.
      3. May be done for diagnostic, interventional, or electrophysiological reasons.
      4. May be carried out on an outpatient basis.

■■■ PRIORITY NURSING ACTIONS! ■■■

Actions to Take if a Hypercyanotic Spell Occurs in an Infant
1. Place the infant in a knee-chest position.
2. Administer 100% oxygen.
3. Administer morphine sulfate.
4. Administer fluids intravenously.
5. Document occurrence, actions taken, and the infant's response.

Hypercyanotic spells are also known as tet spells or blue spells and occur in infants or children with certain types of heart defects. The infant or child becomes acutely cyanotic and hyperpneic because of the sudden infundibular spasm. These spells may occur as a result of stressful procedures or from feeding, crying, or defecation. If a spell occurs, the nurse needs to provide a calm and comforting approach while immediately placing the infant in the knee-chest position; this assists breathing and increases oxygenation to body tissues. Oxygen is administered by face mask or blow by. Morphine sulfate is administered as prescribed subcutaneously or through an existing intravenous line (morphine sulfate helps reduce the infundibular spasm). Intravenous fluids are administered to replace fluids and to keep the infant well hydrated and to keep the hematocrit and blood viscosity within acceptable limits. Depending on the infant's response, a repeated dose of morphine sulfate may be prescribed. Finally, the nurse documents the occurrence, actions taken, and the infant's response.

Reference: Perry, S., Hockenberry, M., Lowdermilk, D., & Wilson, D. (2010). *Maternal child nursing care* (4th ed., pp. 1465-1466). St. Louis: Mosby.

---

      5. Risks include hemorrhage from the entry site, clot formation and subsequent blockage distally, and transient dysrhythmias.
      6. General anesthesia is usually unnecessary.
      7. See Chapter 60.
   B. Preprocedure nursing interventions
      1. Assess accurate height and weight because this helps with the selection of the correct catheter size.
      2. Obtain a history of the presence of allergic reactions to iodine.
      3. Assess for symptoms of infection, including a diaper rash.
      4. Assess and mark bilateral pulses, such as the dorsalis pedis and posterior tibial.
      5. Assess baseline oxygen saturation.
      6. Familiarize the parents and child with hospital procedures and equipment.
      7. Educate the child, if age appropriate, and the parents about the procedure.
      8. Allow the parents and child to verbalize feelings and concerns regarding the procedure and the disorder.

Box 39-8 Home Care After Cardiac Surgery

Omit play outside for several weeks.

Avoid activities in which the child could fall and be injured, such as bike riding, for 2 to 4 weeks.

Avoid crowds for 2 weeks after discharge.

Follow a no-added-salt diet if prescribed.

Do not add any new foods to the infant's diet (if an allergy exists to the new food, the manifestations may be interpreted as a postoperative complication).

Do not place creams, lotions, or powders on the incision until completely healed.

The child may return to school usually the third week after discharge, starting with half-days.

The child should not participate in physical education for 2 months.

Instruct the parents to discipline the child normally.

Instruct the parents about the importance of the 2-week follow-up.

Avoid immunizations, invasive procedures, and dental visits for 2 months; following this time period, the immunization schedule and dental visits need to be resumed.

Advise the parents regarding the importance of a dental visit every 6 months after age 3 years and to inform the dentist of the cardiac problem so that antibiotics can be prescribed if necessary.

Instruct the parents to call the physician if coughing, tachypnea, cyanosis, vomiting, diarrhea, anorexia, pain, or fever occur, or any swelling, redness, or drainage occurs at the site of the incision.

C. Postprocedure nursing interventions
  1. Monitor findings on the cardiac monitor and oxygen saturation for 4 hours after procedure.
  2. Assess pulses below the catheter site for equality and symmetry.
  3. Assess the temperature and color of the affected extremity and report coolness, which may indicate arterial obstruction.
  4. Monitor vital signs frequently, usually every 15 minutes four times, every half-hour four times, and then every hour four times.
  5. Assess the pressure dressing for intactness and signs of hemorrhage.
  6. Check the bed sheets under the extremity for blood, which may indicate bleeding from the entry site.
  7. If bleeding is present, apply continuous, direct pressure at the cardiac catheter entry site and report it immediately.
  8. Immobilize the affected extremity in a flat position for at least 4 to 6 hours for venous entry site and 6 to 8 hours for arterial entry site as prescribed.
  9. Hydrate the child via the oral or intravenous route or both routes as prescribed.
  10. Administer acetaminophen (Tylenol) or ibuprofen (Motrin) for pain or discomfort as prescribed.
  11. Prepare the parents and child, if appropriate, for surgery.

D. Discharge teaching for the child and parents
  1. Remove the dressing on the day after the procedure and cover it with a Band-Aid for 2 or 3 days as prescribed.
  2. Keep the site clean and dry.
  3. Avoid tub baths for 2 to 3 days.
  4. Observe for redness, edema, drainage, bleeding, and fever, and report any of these signs immediately.
  5. Avoid strenuous activity, if applicable.
  6. The child may return to school, if appropriate.
  7. Provide a diet as tolerated.

  8. Administer acetaminophen or ibuprofen for pain, discomfort, or fever.
  9. Keep follow-up appointment with primary care provider.

VIII. CARDIAC SURGERY

A. Postoperative interventions
  1. Monitor vital signs frequently, especially temperature, and notify the physician if fever occurs.
  2. Monitor for signs of sepsis, such as fever, chills, diaphoresis, lethargy, and altered levels of consciousness.
  3. Maintain strict aseptic technique.
  4. Monitor lines, tubes, or catheters that are in place, and monitor for signs and symptoms of infection.
  5. Assess for signs of discomfort, such as irritability, restlessness, changes in heart rate, respiratory rate, and blood pressure.
  6. Administer pain medications as prescribed.
  7. Administer antibiotics and antipyretics as prescribed.
  8. Promote rest and sleep periods.
  9. Facilitate parent-child contact as soon as possible.

B. Postoperative home care (Box 39-8)

IX. RHEUMATIC FEVER

A. Description
  1. Rheumatic fever is an inflammatory autoimmune disease that affects the connective tissues of the heart, joints, subcutaneous tissues, and blood vessels of the central nervous system.
  2. The most serious complication is rheumatic heart disease, which affects the cardiac valves, particularly the mitral valve.
  3. Rheumatic fever manifests 2 to 6 weeks after an untreated or partially treated group A beta-hemolytic streptococcal infection of the upper respiratory tract.

Box 39-9 Jones Criteria for Diagnosis of Rheumatic Fever

Major Criteria

Carditis
Arthralgia
Chorea
Erythema marginatum
Subcutaneous nodules

Minor Criteria

Fever
Arthralgia
Elevated erythrocyte sedimentation rate or positive C-reactive protein level
Prolonged P-R interval on electrocardiogram

Note: For making a diagnosis, two major or one major and two minor manifestations must be accompanied by supporting evidence of a preceding streptococcal infection (positive throat culture for group A streptococcus and an elevated or increasing antistreptolysin O titer).

4. Jones criteria are used to help determine the diagnosis (Box 39-9).

B. Assessment (Fig. 39-1)
   1. Fever: Low-grade fever that spikes in the late afternoon
   2. Elevated antistreptolysin O titer
   3. Elevated erythrocyte sedimentation rate
   4. Elevated C-reactive protein level
   5. Aschoff bodies (lesions): Found in the heart, blood vessels, brain, and serous surfaces of the joints and pleura

⚠ Assessment of a child with suspected rheumatic fever includes inquiring about a recent sore throat because rheumatic fever manifests 2 to 6 weeks after an untreated or partially treated group A beta-hemolytic streptococcal infection of the upper respiratory tract.

C. Interventions
   1. Assess vital signs.
   2. Control joint pain and inflammation with massage and alternating hot and cold applications as prescribed.
   3. Provide bed rest during the acute febrile phase.
   4. Limit physical exercise in a child with carditis.
   5. Administer antibiotics (penicillin) as prescribed.
   6. Administer salicylates and anti-inflammatory agents as prescribed; these medications should not be administered before the diagnosis is confirmed because the medications mask the polyarthritis.
   7. Initiate seizure precautions if the child is experiencing chorea.
   8. Instruct the parents about the importance of follow-up and the need for antibiotic prophylaxis for dental work, infection, and invasive procedures.

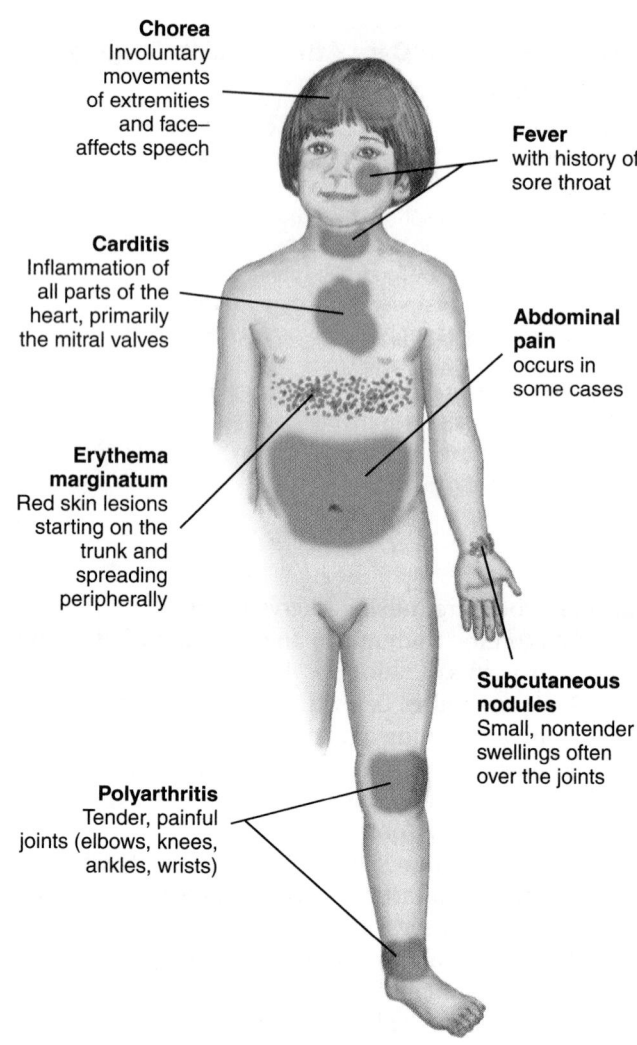

Chorea
Involuntary movements of extremities and face—affects speech

Fever
with history of sore throat

Carditis
Inflammation of all parts of the heart, primarily the mitral valves

Abdominal pain
occurs in some cases

Erythema marginatum
Red skin lesions starting on the trunk and spreading peripherally

Subcutaneous nodules
Small, nontender swellings often over the joints

Polyarthritis
Tender, painful joints (elbows, knees, ankles, wrists)

▲ **FIGURE 39-1** Clinical manifestations of rheumatic fever. (From McKinney, E., James, S., Murray, S., & Ashwill, J. [2009]. *Maternal-child nursing* [3rd ed.]. St. Louis: Saunders.)

   9. Advise the child to inform the parents if anyone in school develops a streptococcal throat infection.

X. KAWASAKI DISEASE

A. Description
   1. Kawasaki disease is also known as mucocutaneous lymph node syndrome and is an acute systemic inflammatory illness.
   2. The cause is unknown, but may be associated with an infection from an organism or toxin.
   3. Cardiac involvement is the most serious complication; aneurysms can develop.

B. Assessment
   1. Acute stage
      a. Fever
      b. Conjunctival hyperemia
      c. Red throat
      d. Swollen hands, rash, and enlargement of cervical lymph nodes

Box 39-10 Parent Education for Kawasaki Disease

Follow-up care is essential to recovery.

Signs and symptoms of Kawasaki disease include the following:

Irritability that may last for 2 months after the onset of symptoms.

Peeling of the hands and feet may occur.

Pain in the joints may persist for several weeks.

Stiffness in the morning, after naps, and in cold temperatures may occur.

Record the temperature (because fever is expected) until the child has been afebrile for several days.

Notify the physician if the temperature is 101° F or higher.

Salicylates such as acetylsalicylic acid (aspirin) may be prescribed.

Signs of aspirin toxicity include tinnitus, headache, vertigo, and bruising; do not administer aspirin or aspirin-containing products if the child has been exposed to chickenpox or the flu.

Signs and symptoms of bleeding include epistaxis (nosebleeds), hemoptysis (coughing up blood), hematemesis (vomiting up blood), hematuria (blood in urine), melena (blood in stool), and bruises on the body.

Signs and symptoms of cardiac complications include chest pain or tightness (older children), cool and pale extremities, abdominal pain, nausea and vomiting, irritability, restlessness, and uncontrollable crying.

The child should avoid contact sports, if age appropriate, if taking aspirin or anticoagulants.

Avoid administration of measles, mumps, and rubella (MMR) or varicella vaccine to the child for 11 months after intravenous immunoglobulin therapy, if appropriate.

10. Administer acetylsalicylic acid (aspirin) as prescribed for its antipyretic and antiplatelet effects (additional anticoagulation may be necessary if aneurysms are present).

11. Administer immunoglobulin intravenously as prescribed to reduce the duration of the fever and the incidence of coronary artery lesions and aneurysms; intravenous immunoglobulin is a blood product, so blood precautions when administering it are warranted.

12. Parent education (Box 39-10)

MORE QUESTIONS ON THE CD!

Practice Questions

397. A nurse caring for an infant with congenital heart disease is monitoring the infant closely for signs of congestive heart failure (CHF). The nurse assesses the infant for which early sign of CHF?
    1. Pallor
    2. Cough
    3. Tachycardia
    4. Slow and shallow breathing

398. A nurse is caring for a child with a suspected diagnosis of rheumatic fever. The nurse reviews the laboratory results, knowing that which laboratory study would assist in confirming the diagnosis?
    1. Immunoglobulin
    2. Red blood cell count
    3. White blood cell count
    4. Antistreptolysin O titer

399. A nurse is preparing for the admission of a child with a diagnosis of acute-stage Kawasaki disease. On assessment of the child, the nurse expects to note which clinical manifestation of the acute stage of the disease?
    1. Cracked lips
    2. Normal appearance
    3. Conjunctival hyperemia
    4. Desquamation of the skin

400. A nurse provides home care instructions to the parents of a child with congestive heart failure regarding the procedure for administration of digoxin (Lanoxin). Which statement made by the parent indicates the need for further instructions?
    1. "I will not mix the medication with food."
    2. "If more than one dose is missed, I will call the physician."
    3. "I will take the child's pulse before administering the medication."
    4. "If the child vomits after medication administration, I will repeat the dose."

2. Subacute stage
    a. Cracking lips and fissures
    b. Desquamation of the skin on the tips of the fingers and toes
    c. Joint pain
    d. Cardiac manifestations
    e. Thrombocytosis
3. Convalescent stage: Child appears normal, but signs of inflammation may be present.

C. Interventions
    1. Monitor temperature frequently.
    2. Assess heart sounds and heart rate and rhythm.
    3. Assess extremities for edema, redness, and desquamation.
    4. Examine eyes for conjunctivitis.
    5. Monitor mucous membranes for inflammation.
    6. Monitor strict intake and output.
    7. Administer soft foods and liquids that are neither too hot nor too cold.
    8. Weigh child daily.
    9. Provide passive range-of-motion exercises to facilitate joint movement.

401. A physician has prescribed oxygen as needed for an infant with congestive heart failure. In which situation should the nurse administer the oxygen to the infant?
1. During sleep
2. When changing the infant's diapers
3. When the mother is holding the infant
4. When drawing blood for electrolyte level testing

402. An infant with congestive heart failure is receiving diuretic therapy, and a nurse is closely monitoring the intake and output. The nurse uses which most appropriate method to assess the urine output?
1. Weighing the diapers
2. Inserting a Foley catheter
3. Comparing intake with output
4. Measuring the amount of water added to formula

403. A clinic nurse reviews the record of a child just seen by a physician and diagnosed with suspected aortic stenosis. The nurse expects to note documentation of which clinical manifestation specifically found in this disorder?
1. Pallor
2. Hyperactivity
3. Exercise intolerance
4. Gastrointestinal disturbances

404. A nurse has provided home care instructions to the mother of a child who is being discharged after cardiac surgery. Which statement made by the mother indicates a need for further instructions?
1. "A balance of rest and exercise is important."
2. "I can apply lotion or powder to the incision if it is itchy."
3. "Activities in which my child could fall need to be avoided for 2 to 4 weeks."
4. "Large crowds of people need to be avoided for at least 2 weeks after surgery."

405. A nurse receives a telephone call from the admitting office and is told that a child with rheumatic fever will be arriving in the nursing unit for admission. On admission, the nurse prepares to ask the mother which question to elicit assessment information specific to the development of rheumatic fever?
1. "Has the child complained of back pain?"
2. "Has the child complained of headaches?"
3. "Has the child had any nausea or vomiting?"
4. "Did the child have a sore throat or fever within the last 2 months?"

Alternate Item Format: Figure/Illustration

406. Assessment findings of an infant admitted to the hospital reveal a machinery-like murmur on auscultation of the heart and signs of congestive heart failure. The nurse reviews congenital cardiac anomalies and identifies the infant's condition as which of the following? Refer to the circled area in the figure to determine the condition.
1. Aortic stenosis
2. Atrial septal defect
3. Patent ductus arteriosus
4. Ventricular septal defect

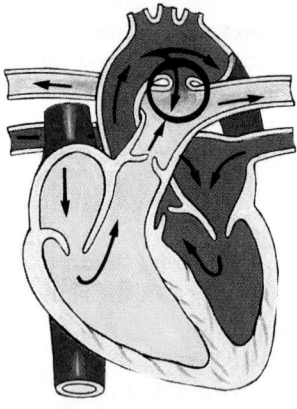

(From Hockenberry, M., & Wilson, D. [2007]. *Wong's nursing care of infants and children* [8th ed.]. St. Louis: Saunders.)

ANSWERS
397. 3

Rationale: Congestive heart failure (CHF) is the inability of the heart to pump a sufficient amount of oxygen to meet the metabolic needs of the body. The early signs of CHF include tachycardia, tachypnea, profuse scalp sweating, fatigue and irritability, sudden weight gain, and respiratory distress. A cough may occur in CHF as a result of mucosal swelling and irritation, but is not an early sign. Pallor may be noted in an infant with CHF, but is not an early sign.

Test-Taking Strategy: Note the strategic word *early*. Think about the physiology and the effects on the heart when fluid overload occurs. These concepts will assist in directing you to option 3. If you had difficulty with this question, review the early signs of CHF in an infant.
Level of Cognitive Ability: Analyzing
Client Needs: Physiological Integrity
Integrated Process: Nursing Process—Assessment
Content Area: Child Health—Eye/Ear/Throat/Respiratory/Cardiovascular

Reference: Hockenberry, M., & Wilson, D. (2009). *Wong's essentials of pediatric nursing* (8th ed., p. 878). St. Louis: Mosby.

398. 4
Rationale: Rheumatic fever is an inflammatory autoimmune disease that affects the connective tissues of the heart, joints, subcutaneous tissues, and blood vessels of the central nervous system. A diagnosis of rheumatic fever is confirmed by the presence of two major manifestations or one major and two minor manifestations from the Jones criteria. In addition, evidence of a recent streptococcal infection is confirmed by a positive antistreptolysin O titer, Streptozyme assay, or anti-DNase B assay. Options 1, 2, and 3 would not help to confirm the diagnosis of rheumatic fever.
Test-Taking Strategy: Use the process of elimination. Recalling that rheumatic fever characteristically is associated with streptococcal infection will direct you to option 4. If you had difficulty with this question, review the Jones criteria and diagnostic tests for rheumatic fever.
Level of Cognitive Ability: Analyzing
Client Needs: Physiological Integrity
Integrated Process: Nursing Process—Analysis
Content Area: Child Health—Eye/Ear/Throat/Respiratory/Cardiovascular
Reference: Hockenberry, M., & Wilson, D. (2009). *Wong's essentials of pediatric nursing* (8th ed., p. 893). St. Louis: Mosby.

399. 3
Rationale: Kawasaki disease is also known as mucocutaneous lymph node syndrome and is an acute systemic inflammatory illness. In the acute stage, the child has a fever, conjunctival hyperemia, red throat, swollen hands, rash, and enlargement of the cervical lymph nodes. In the subacute stage, cracking lips and fissures, desquamation of the skin on the tips of the fingers and toes, joint pain, cardiac manifestations, and thrombocytosis occur. In the convalescent stage, the child appears normal, but signs of inflammation may be present.
Test-Taking Strategy: Use the process of elimination. Option 2 can be eliminated first because a normal appearance is not likely in the acute stage. From the remaining options, focusing on the strategic words *acute stage* in the question will assist in directing you to option 3. Review the clinical manifestations associated with each stage of Kawasaki disease if you had difficulty with this question.
Level of Cognitive Ability: Analyzing
Client Needs: Physiological Integrity
Integrated Process: Nursing Process—Assessment
Content Area: Child Health—Eye/Ear/Throat/Respiratory/Cardiovascular
Reference: McKinney, E., James, S., Murray, S., & Ashwill, J. (2009). *Maternal-child nursing* (3rd ed., p. 1269). St. Louis: Saunders.

400. 4
Rationale: Digoxin is a cardiac glycoside. The parents need to be instructed that if the child vomits after digoxin is administered, they are not to repeat the dose. Options 1, 2, and 3 are accurate instructions regarding the administration of this medication. In addition, the parents should be instructed that

if a dose is missed and is not identified until 4 hours later, the dose should not be administered.
Test-Taking Strategy: Note the strategic words *need for further instructions*. These words indicate a negative event query and ask you to select an option that is an incorrect statement. General knowledge regarding digoxin administration will assist in eliminating option 3. Principles related to administering medications to children will assist in eliminating option 1. From the remaining options, select option 4 because if the child vomits, it would be difficult to determine whether the medication also was vomited or was absorbed by the body. Review home care instructions regarding the administration of digoxin if you had difficulty with this question.
Level of Cognitive Ability: Evaluating
Client Needs: Physiological Integrity
Integrated Process: Teaching and Learning
Content Area: Child Health—Eye/Ear/Throat/Respiratory/Cardiovascular
Reference: Perry, S., Hockenberry, M., Lowdermilk, D., & Wilson, D. (2010). *Maternal child nursing care* (4th ed., p. 1242). St. Louis: Mosby.

401. 4
Rationale: Congestive heart failure (CHF) is the inability of the heart to pump a sufficient amount of oxygen to meet the metabolic needs of the body. Crying exhausts the limited energy supply, increases the workload of the heart, and increases the oxygen demands. Oxygen administration may be prescribed for stressful periods, especially during bouts of crying or invasive procedures. Options 1, 2, and 3 are not likely to produce crying in the infant.
Test-Taking Strategy: Use the process of elimination. Recall the situations that would place stress and an increased workload on the heart; this should direct you to option 4. Drawing blood is an invasive procedure, which would likely cause the infant to cry. Review care of a child with CHF if you had difficulty with this question.
Level of Cognitive Ability: Analyzing
Client Needs: Physiological Integrity
Integrated Process: Nursing Process—Implementation
Content Area: Child Health—Eye/Ear/Throat/Respiratory/Cardiovascular
References: Hockenberry, M., & Wilson, D. (2009). *Wong's essentials of pediatric nursing* (8th ed., pp. 878–879, 883). St. Louis: Mosby.
    McKinney, E., James, S., Murray, S., & Ashwill, J. (2009). *Maternal-child nursing* (3rd ed., p. 1240). St. Louis: Saunders.

402. 1
Rationale: Congestive heart failure is the inability of the heart to pump a sufficient amount of oxygen to meet the metabolic needs of the body. The most appropriate method for assessing urine output in an infant receiving diuretic therapy is to weigh the diapers. Comparing intake with output would not provide an accurate measure of urine output. Measuring the amount of water added to formula is unrelated to the amount of output. Although Foley catheter drainage is most accurate in determining output, it is not the most appropriate method in an infant and places the infant at risk for infection.
Test-Taking Strategy: Use the process of elimination. Eliminate options 3 and 4 first because they will not provide an

indication of urine output. Note the words *most appropriate* in the question. These words will direct you to option 1 from the remaining options. Review care of an infant receiving diuretic therapy if you had difficulty with this question.
Level of Cognitive Ability: Applying
Client Needs: Physiological Integrity
Integrated Process: Nursing Process—Assessment
Content Area: Child Health—Eye/Ear/Throat/Respiratory/Cardiovascular
Reference: McKinney, E., James, S., Murray, S., & Ashwill, J. (2009). *Maternal-child nursing* (3rd ed., p. 1240). St. Louis: Saunders.

403. 3
Rationale: Aortic stenosis is a narrowing or stricture of the aortic valve, causing resistance to blood flow in the left ventricle, decreased cardiac output, left ventricular hypertrophy, and pulmonary vascular congestion. A child with aortic stenosis shows signs of exercise intolerance, chest pain, and dizziness when standing for long periods. Pallor may be noted, but is not specific to this type of disorder alone. Options 2 and 4 are not related to this disorder.
Test-Taking Strategy: Use the process of elimination, focusing on the disorder. Options 2 and 4 can be eliminated first because they are not associated with a cardiac disorder. From the remaining options, noting the word *specifically* in the question will direct you to option 3. Review the manifestations associated with aortic stenosis if you had difficulty with this question.
Level of Cognitive Ability: Analyzing
Client Needs: Physiological Integrity
Integrated Process: Communication and Documentation
Content Area: Child Health—Eye/Ear/Throat/Respiratory/Cardiovascular
Reference: McKinney, E., James, S., Murray, S., & Ashwill, J. (2009). *Maternal-child nursing* (3rd ed., p. 1250). St. Louis: Saunders.

404. 2
Rationale: The mother should be instructed that lotions and powders should not be applied to the incision site after cardiac surgery. Lotions and powders can irritate the surrounding skin, which could lead to skin breakdown and subsequent infection of the incision site. Options 1, 3, and 4 are accurate instructions regarding home care after cardiac surgery.
Test-Taking Strategy: Note the strategic words *indicates a need for further instructions*. These words indicate a negative event query and ask you to select an option that is an incorrect statement. Using general principles related to postoperative incisional site care will direct you to option 2. Review home care instructions after cardiac surgery if you had difficulty with this question.
Level of Cognitive Ability: Evaluating
Client Needs: Physiological Integrity

Integrated Process: Teaching and Learning
Content Area: Child Health—Eye/Ear/Throat/Respiratory/Cardiovascular
Reference: McKinney, E., James, S., Murray, S., & Ashwill, J. (2009). *Maternal-child nursing* (3rd ed., p. 1260). St. Louis: Saunders.

405. 4
Rationale: Rheumatic fever is an inflammatory autoimmune disease that affects the connective tissues of the heart, joints, subcutaneous tissues, and blood vessels of the central nervous system. Rheumatic fever characteristically manifests 2 to 6 weeks after an untreated or partially treated group A beta-hemolytic streptococcal infection of the upper respiratory tract. Initially, the nurse determines whether the child had a sore throat or an unexplained fever within the past 2 months. Options 1, 2, and 3 are unrelated to rheumatic fever.
Test-Taking Strategy: Use the process of elimination and note the similarity between the words rheumatic *fever* in the question and the word *fever* in the correct option. If you had difficulty with this question, review the etiology related to rheumatic fever.
Level of Cognitive Ability: Analyzing
Client Needs: Physiological Integrity
Integrated Process: Nursing Process—Assessment
Content Area: Child Health—Eye/Ear/Throat/Respiratory/Cardiovascular
Reference: Hockenberry, M., & Wilson, D. (2009). *Wong's essentials of pediatric nursing* (8th ed., p. 893). St. Louis: Mosby.

ALTERNATE ITEM FORMAT: FIGURE/ILLUSTRATION
406. 3
Rationale: A patent ductus arteriosus is failure of the fetal ductus arteriosus (artery connecting the aorta and the pulmonary artery) to close. A characteristic machinery-like murmur is present, and the infant may show signs of congestive heart failure. Aortic stenosis is a narrowing or stricture of the aortic valve. Atrial septal defect is an abnormal opening between the atria. Ventricular septal defect is an abnormal opening between the right and left ventricles.
Test-Taking Strategy: Focus on the figure and the location of the defect. Recalling the anatomical locations in the heart will direct you to option 3. Review congenital heart defects if you had difficulty with this question.
Level of Cognitive Ability: Analyzing
Client Needs: Physiological Integrity
Integrated Process: Nursing Process—Assessment
Content Area: Child Health—Eye/Ear/Throat/Respiratory/Cardiovascular
Reference: McKinney, E., James, S., Murray, S., & Ashwill, J. (2009). *Maternal-child nursing* (3rd ed., pp. 1245–1246). St. Louis: Saunders.

Gastrointestinal Disorders

I. VOMITING

A. Description
1. The major concerns when a child is vomiting are the risk of dehydration, the loss of fluid and electrolytes, and the development of metabolic alkalosis.
2. Additional concerns include aspiration and the development of atelectasis or pneumonia.
3. Causes of vomiting include acute infectious diseases, increased intracranial pressure, toxic ingestions, food intolerance, mechanical obstruction of the gastrointestinal tract, metabolic disorders, and psychogenic disorders.

B. Assessment
1. Character of vomitus
2. Signs of aspiration
3. Presence of pain and abdominal cramping
4. Signs of dehydration
5. Signs of fluid and electrolyte imbalances
6. Signs of metabolic alkalosis

C. Interventions
1. Maintain a patent airway.
2. Position the child on the side to prevent aspiration.
3. Monitor vital signs.
4. Monitor the character, amount, and frequency of vomiting.
5. Assess the force of the vomiting; projectile vomiting indicates pyloric **stenosis** or increased intracranial pressure.
6. Monitor strict intake and output.
7. Monitor for signs and symptoms of dehydration, such as a sunken fontanel (age-appropriate), nonelastic skin turgor, dry mucous membranes, decreased tear production, and oliguria.
8. Monitor electrolyte levels.
9. Provide oral rehydration therapy as tolerated and as prescribed; begin feeding slowly, with small amounts of fluid at frequent intervals.
10. Assess for abdominal pain or diarrhea.
11. Advise the parents to inform the physician if signs of dehydration, blood in vomitus, forceful vomiting, or abdominal pain are present.

II. DIARRHEA

A. Description
1. Acute diarrhea is a cause of dehydration, particularly in children younger than 5 years.
2. Causes of acute diarrhea include acute infectious disorders of the gastrointestinal tract, antibiotic therapy, and parasitic infestation.
3. Causes of chronic diarrhea include rotavirus, malabsorption syndromes, inflammatory bowel disease, immunodeficiencies, food intolerances, and nonspecific factors.
4. Rotavirus is a cause of serious gastroenteritis and is a nosocomial (hospital-acquired) pathogen that is most severe in children 3 to 24 months old; children younger than 3 months have some protection because of maternally acquired anti-bodies.

B. Assessment
1. Character of stools
2. Presence of pain and abdominal cramping
3. Signs of dehydration
4. Signs of fluid and electrolyte imbalances
5. Signs of metabolic acidosis

C. Interventions
1. Monitor vital signs.
2. Monitor character, amount, and frequency of diarrhea.
3. Provide enteric isolation as required; instruct the parents in effective handwashing technique (the child should be taught this technique also).
4. Monitor skin integrity.
5. Monitor strict intake and output.
6. Monitor electrolyte levels.
7. Monitor for signs and symptoms of dehydration.
8. For mild to moderate dehydration, provide oral rehydration therapy with Pedialyte or a similar rehydration solution as prescribed; avoid carbonated beverages because they are gas-producing and fluids that contain high amounts of sugar, such as apple juice.
9. For severe dehydration, maintain NPO status to place the bowel at rest and provide fluid and electrolyte replacement by the intravenous

(IV) route as prescribed; if potassium is prescribed for IV administration, ensure that the child has voided before administering and has adequate renal function.

10. Reintroduce a normal diet when rehydration is achieved.

⚠ The major concerns when a child is having diarrhea are the risk of dehydration, the loss of fluid and electrolytes, and the development of metabolic acidosis.

III. CLEFT LIP AND CLEFT PALATE

A. Description
1. Cleft lip and cleft palate are congenital anomalies that occur as a result of failure of soft tissue or bony structure to fuse during embryonic development.
2. The defects involve abnormal openings in the lip and palate that may occur unilaterally or bilaterally and are readily apparent at birth.
3. Causes include **hereditary**, and environmental factors—exposure to radiation or rubella virus, chromosome abnormalities, and teratogenic factors.
4. Closure of cleft lip defect precedes closure of the cleft palate and is usually performed by age 3 to 6 months.

5. Cleft palate repair is performed sometime between 6 and 24 months of age to allow for the palatal changes that occur with normal **growth**; a cleft palate is closed as early as possible to facilitate speech development.
6. A child with cleft palate is at risk for developing frequent otitis media; this can result in hearing loss.
7. A multidisciplinary team approach, including audiologists, orthodontists, plastic surgeons, and occupational and speech therapists, is taken to address the many needs of the child.

B. Assessment (Fig. 40-1)
1. Cleft lip can range from a slight notch to a complete separation from the floor of the nose.
2. Cleft palate can include nasal distortion, midline or bilateral cleft, and variable extension from the uvula and soft and hard palate.

C. Interventions
1. Assess the ability to suck, swallow, handle normal secretions, and breathe without distress.
2. Assess fluid and calorie intake daily.
3. Monitor daily weight.
4. Modify feeding techniques; plan to use specialized feeding techniques, obturators, and special nipples and feeders.

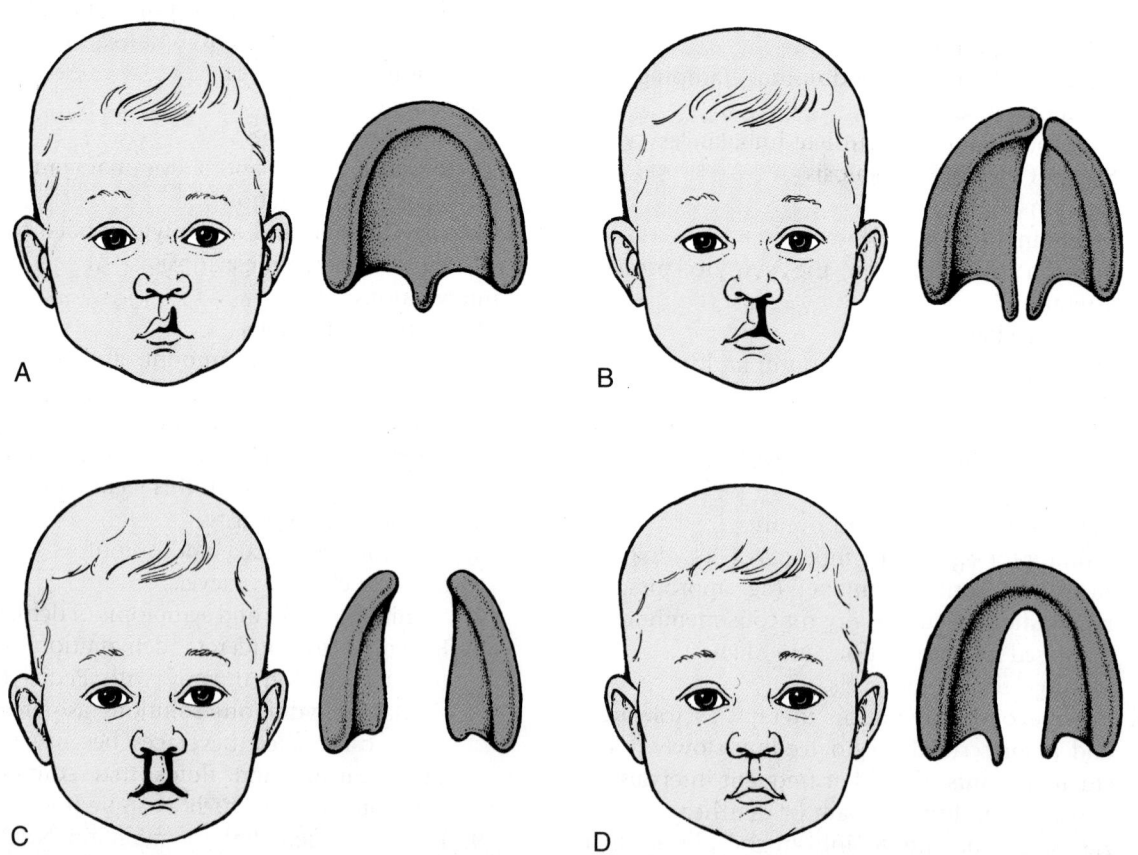

▲ **FIGURE 40-1** Variations in clefts of lip and palate at birth. **A,** Notch in vermilion border. **B,** Unilateral cleft lip and palate. **C,** Bilateral cleft lip and palate. **D,** Cleft palate. (From Hockenberry, M., & Wilson, D. [2009]. *Wong's essentials of pediatric nursing* [8th ed.]. St. Louis: Mosby.)

5. Hold the infant in an upright position and direct the formula to the side and back of the mouth to prevent aspiration.
6. Feed small amounts gradually and burp frequently.
7. Keep suction equipment and a bulb syringe at the bedside.
8. Teach the parents special feeding or suctioning techniques.
9. Teach the parents the *ESSR* method of feeding—*e*nlarge the nipple, *s*timulate the sucking reflex, *s*wallow, *r*est to allow the infant to finish swallowing what has been placed in the mouth.
10. Encourage parents to express their feelings about the disorder.
11. Encourage parental bonding with the infant, including holding the infant and calling the infant by name.

D. Postoperative interventions
1. Cleft lip repair
   a. Provide lip protection; a metal appliance or adhesive strips may be taped securely to the cheeks to prevent trauma to the suture line.
   b. Avoid positioning the infant on the side of the repair or in the prone position because these positions can cause rubbing of the surgical site on the mattress (position on the back upright and position to prevent airway obstruction by secretions, blood, or the tongue).
   c. Keep the surgical site clean and dry; after feeding, gently cleanse the suture line of formula or serosanguineous drainage with a solution such as normal saline or as designated by agency procedure.
   d. Apply antibiotic ointment to the site as prescribed.
   e. Elbow restraints should be used to prevent the infant from injuring or traumatizing the surgical site.

   f. Monitor for signs and symptoms of infection at the surgical site.
2. Cleft palate repair
   a. Feedings are resumed by bottle, breast, or cup per surgeon preference; some surgeons prescribe the use of an Asepto syringe for feeding or a soft cup such as a Sippy cup.
   b. Oral packing may be secured to the palate (usually removed in 2 to 3 days).
   c. Do not allow the child to brush his or her teeth.
   d. Instruct the parents to avoid offering hard food items to the child, such as toast or cookies.
3. Soft elbow or jacket restraints may be used (check agency policies and procedures) to keep the child from touching the repair site; remove restraints at least every 2 hours (or per agency procedure) to assess skin integrity and circulation and to allow for exercising the arms.
4. Avoid the use of oral suction or placing objects in the mouth such as a tongue depressor, thermometer, straws, spoons, forks, or pacifiers.
5. Provide analgesics for pain as prescribed.
6. Instruct the parents in feeding techniques and in the care of the surgical site.
7. Instruct the parents to monitor for signs of infection at the surgical site, such as redness, swelling, or drainage.
8. Encourage the parents to hold the child.
9. Initiate appropriate referrals such as a dental referral and speech therapy referral.

IV. ESOPHAGEAL ATRESIA AND TRACHEOESOPHAGEAL FISTULA (Fig. 40-2)

A. Description
1. The esophagus terminates before it reaches the stomach, ending in a blind pouch, or a fistula is present that forms an unnatural connection with the trachea.

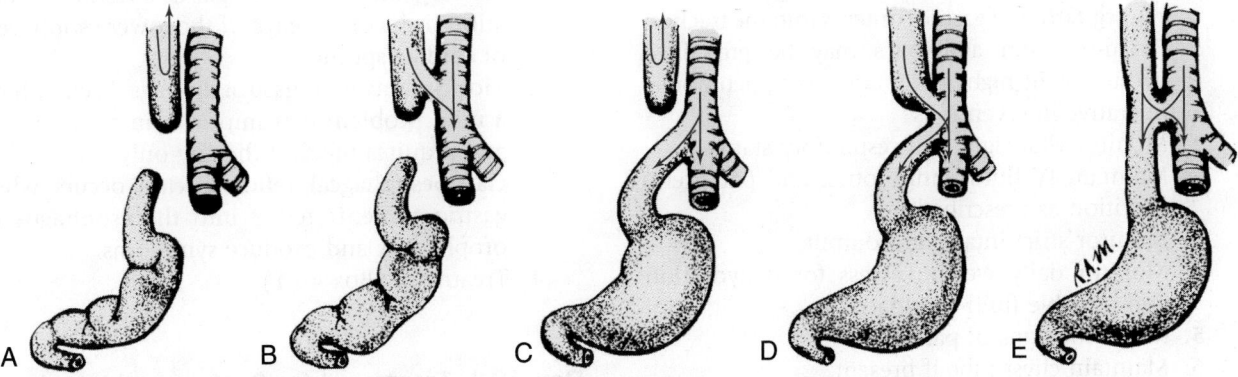

▲ **FIGURE 40-2** Congenital atresia of esophagus and tracheoesophageal fistula. **A,** Upper and lower segments of esophagus end in blind sac (occurring in 5% to 8% of such infants). **B,** Upper segment of esophagus ends in atresia and connects to trachea by fistulous tract (occurring rarely). **C,** Upper segment of esophagus ends in blind pouch; lower segment connects with trachea by small fistulous tract (occurring in 80% to 95% of such infants). **D,** Both segments of esophagus connect by fistulous tracts to trachea (occurring in <1% of such infants). Infant may aspirate with first feeding. **E,** Esophagus is continuous, but connects by fistulous tract to trachea—known as H-type. (From Hockenberry, M., & Wilson, D. [2007]. *Wong's nursing care of infants and children* [8th ed.]. St. Louis: Mosby.)

2. The condition causes oral intake to enter the lungs or a large amount of air to enter the stomach, presenting a risk of coughing and choking; severe abdominal distention can occur.

3. Aspiration pneumonia and severe respiratory distress may develop, and death is likely to occur without surgical intervention.

4. Treatment includes maintenance of a patent airway, prevention of aspiration pneumonia, gastric or blind pouch decompression, supportive therapy, and surgical repair.

B. Assessment
1. Frothy saliva in the mouth and nose and excessive drooling
2. The "3 C's"—*c*oughing and *c*hoking during feedings and unexplained **cyanosis**
3. **Regurgitation** and vomiting
4. Abdominal distention
5. Increased respiratory distress during and after feeding

C. Preoperative interventions
1. The infant may be placed in an incubator or radiant warmer in which humidified oxygen is administered (intubation and mechanical ventilation may be necessary if respiratory distress occurs).
2. Maintain NPO status.
3. Maintain IV fluids as prescribed.
4. Monitor respiratory status closely.
5. Suction accumulated secretions from the mouth and pharynx.
6. Maintain in a supine upright position (at least 30 degrees upright) to facilitate drainage and prevent aspiration of gastric secretions.
7. Keep the blind pouch empty of secretions by intermittent or continuous suction as prescribed; monitor its patency closely because clogging from mucus can easily occur.
8. If a gastrostomy tube is inserted, it may be left open so that air entering the stomach through the fistula can escape, minimizing the risk of **regurgitation** of gastric contents into the trachea.
9. Broad-spectrum antibiotics may be prescribed because of the high risk for aspiration pneumonia.

D. Postoperative interventions
1. Monitor vital signs and respiratory status.
2. Maintain IV fluids, antibiotics, and parenteral nutrition as prescribed.
3. Monitor strict intake and output.
4. Monitor daily weight; assess for dehydration and possible fluid overload.
5. Assess for signs of pain.
6. Maintain chest tube if present.
7. Inspect the surgical site for signs and symptoms of infection.
8. Monitor for anastomotic leaks as evidenced by purulent drainage from the chest tube, increased temperature, and increased white blood cell count.

9. If a gastrostomy tube is present, it is usually attached to gravity drainage until the infant can tolerate feedings and the anastomosis is healed (usually postoperative day 5 to 7); then feedings are prescribed.
10. Before oral feedings and removal of the chest tube, prepare for an esophagogram as prescribed to check the integrity of the esophageal anastomosis.
11. Before feeding, elevate the gastrostomy tube and secure it above the level of the stomach to allow gastric secretions to pass to the duodenum and swallowed air to escape through the open gastrostomy tube.
12. Administer oral feedings with sterile water, followed by frequent small feedings of formula as prescribed.
13. Assess the cervical esophagostomy site, if present, for redness, breakdown, or exudate; remove accumulated drainage frequently, and apply protective ointment, barrier dressing, or a collection device as prescribed.
14. Provide non-nutritive sucking using a pacifier for infants who remain NPO for extended periods (a pacifier should not be used if the infant is unable to handle secretions).
15. Instruct the parents in the techniques of suctioning, gastrostomy tube care and feedings, and skin site care as appropriate.
16. Instruct the parents to identify behaviors that indicate the need for suctioning, signs of respiratory distress, and signs of a constricted esophagus (e.g., poor feeding, dysphagia, drooling, coughing during feedings, regurgitated undigested food).

V. GASTROESOPHAGEAL REFLUX DISEASE

A. Description
1. Gastroesophageal reflux is backflow of gastric contents into the esophagus as a result of relaxation or incompetence of the lower esophageal or cardiac sphincter.
2. Most infants with gastroesophageal reflux have a mild problem that improves in about 1 year and requires medical therapy only.
3. Gastroesophageal reflux disease occurs when gastric contents reflux into the esophagus or oropharynx and produce symptoms.
4. Treatment (Box 40-1)

Box 40-1 Treatment for Gastroesophageal Reflux Disease

Diet
Positioning
Medications
Surgery: Performed when severe complications occur

B. Assessment
1. Passive **regurgitation** or emesis
2. Poor weight gain
3. Irritability
4. Hematemesis
5. Melena
6. Heartburn (in older children)
7. Anemia from blood loss

C. Interventions
1. Assess amount and characteristics of emesis.
2. Assess the relationship of vomiting to the times of feedings and infant activity.
3. Monitor breath sounds before and after feedings.
4. Assess for signs of aspiration, such as drooling, coughing, or dyspnea, after feeding.
5. Place suction equipment at the bedside.
6. Monitor intake and output.
7. Monitor for signs and symptoms of dehydration.
8. Maintain IV fluids as prescribed.

⚠ Complications of gastroesophageal reflux disease include esophagitis, esophageal strictures, aspiration of gastric contents, and aspiration pneumonia.

D. Positioning
1. The infant is placed in the supine position during sleep (to reduce the incidence of sudden infant death syndrome) unless the risk of death from aspiration or other serious complications of gastroesophageal reflux disease greatly outweighs the risks associated with the prone position (check physician's prescription); otherwise, the prone position is acceptable only while the infant is awake and can be monitored.
2. In children older than 1 year, position with the head of the bed elevated.

E. Diet
1. Provide small, frequent feedings with predigested formula to decrease the amount of **regurgitation**.
2. Nutrition via nasogastric tube feedings may be prescribed if severe **regurgitation** and poor **growth** are present.
3. For infants, formula may be thickened by adding rice cereal to the formula (follow agency procedure); cross-cut the nipple.
4. Breast-feeding may continue, and the mother may provide more frequent feeding times or express milk for thickening with rice cereal.
5. Burp the infant frequently when feeding and handle the infant minimally after feedings; monitor for coughing during feeding and other signs of aspiration.
6. For toddlers, feed solids first, followed by liquids.
7. Instruct the parents to avoid feeding the child fatty foods, chocolate, tomato products, carbonated liquids, fruit juices, citrus products, and spicy foods.

8. Instruct the parents that the child should avoid vigorous play after feeding and avoid feeding just before bedtime.

F. Medications
1. Antacids for symptom relief
2. Proton pump inhibitors and histamine 2 (H_2)-receptor antagonists to decrease gastric acid secretion
3. Prokinetics to accelerate gastric emptying

G. Surgery
1. Fundoplication, in which a wrap to the stomach fundus is made around the distal esophagus (restores the competence of the lower esophageal sphincter), is performed.
2. A gastrostomy may be performed at the same time as fundoplication for decompression of the stomach postoperatively.
3. Fundoplication may be combined with pyloroplasty in children with gastroesophageal reflux who also have delayed gastric emptying.
4. Postoperative care is similar to care after other types of abdominal surgery.
5. Instruct the parents about potential postoperative problems, such as bloating symptoms or discomfort after consuming large, solid meals.

VI. HYPERTROPHIC PYLORIC STENOSIS (Fig. 40-3)

A. Description
1. Hypertrophy of the circular muscles of the pylorus causes narrowing of the pyloric canal between the stomach and the duodenum.
2. The **stenosis** usually develops in the first few weeks of life, causing projectile vomiting, dehydration, metabolic alkalosis, and failure to thrive.

B. Assessment
1. Vomiting that progresses from mild **regurgitation** to forceful and projectile vomiting; it usually occurs after a feeding.
2. Vomitus contains gastric contents such as milk or formula, may contain mucus, may be blood-tinged, and does not usually contain bile.
3. The child exhibits hunger and irritability.
4. Peristaltic waves are visible from left to right across the epigastrium during or immediately after a feeding.
5. An olive-shaped mass is in the epigastrium just right of the umbilicus.
6. Dehydration and malnutrition can occur.
7. Electrolyte imbalances can occur.
8. Metabolic alkalosis can occur.

C. Interventions
1. Monitor vital signs.
2. Monitor strict intake and output.
3. Monitor vomiting episodes and stools.
4. Obtain daily weights.
5. Monitor for signs of dehydration and electrolyte imbalances.
6. Prepare the child and parents for pyloromyotomy if prescribed.

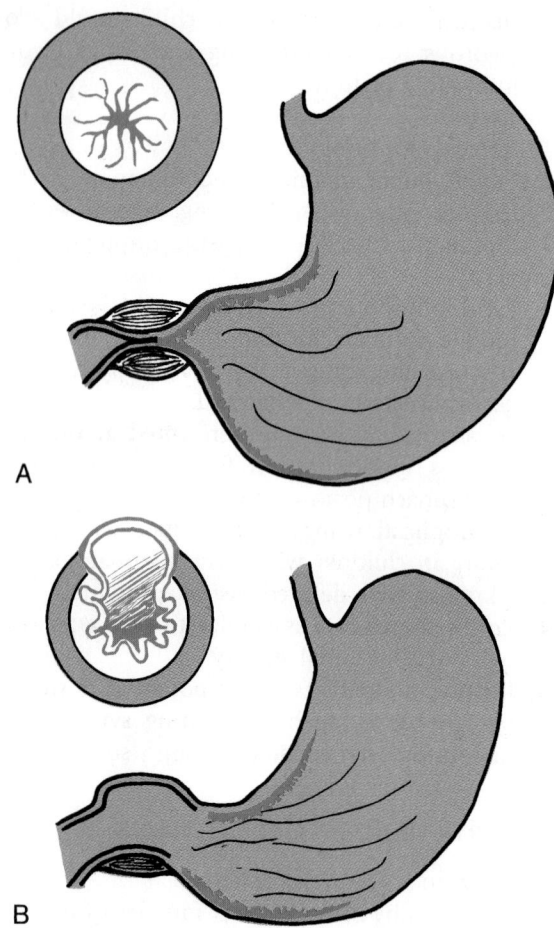

A

B

▲ **FIGURE 40-3** Hypertrophic pyloric stenosis. **A**, Enlarged muscular area nearly obliterates pyloric channel. **B**, Longitudinal surgical division of muscle down to submucosa establishes adequate passageway. (From Hockenberry, M., & Wilson, D. [2009]. *Wong's essentials of pediatric nursing* [8th ed.]. St. Louis: Mosby.)

D. Pyloromyotomy
1. Description: An incision through the muscle fibers of the pylorus; may be performed by laparoscopy
2. Preoperative interventions
   a. Monitor hydration status by daily weights, intake and output, and urine for specific gravity.
   b. Correct fluid and electrolyte imbalances; administer fluids intravenously as prescribed for rehydration.
   c. Maintain NPO status as prescribed.
   d. Monitor the number and character of stools.
   e. Maintain patency of the nasogastric tube placed for stomach decompression.
3. Postoperative interventions
   a. Monitor intake and output.
   b. Begin small, frequent feedings postoperatively as prescribed.
   c. Gradually increase amount and interval between feedings until a full feeding schedule has been reinstated.

d. Feed the infant slowly, burping frequently and handle the infant minimally after feedings.
e. Monitor for abdominal distention.
f. Monitor the surgical wound and for signs of infection.
g. Instruct the parents about wound care and feeding.

VII. LACTOSE INTOLERANCE

A. Description: Inability to tolerate lactose as a result of an absence or deficiency of lactase, an enzyme found in the secretions of the small intestine that is required for the digestion of lactose
B. Assessment
1. Symptoms occur after the ingestion of milk products.
2. Abdominal distention
3. Crampy, abdominal pain; colic
4. Diarrhea and excessive flatus
C. Interventions
1. Eliminate the offending dairy product, or administer an enzyme tablet replacement.
2. Provide information to the parents about enzyme tablets that predigest the lactose in milk or supplement the body's own lactase.
3. Substitute soy-based formulas for cow's milk formula or human milk.
4. Limit milk consumption to one glass at a time.
5. Instruct the child and family that the child should drink milk with other foods rather than by itself.
6. Encourage consumption of hard cheese, cottage cheese, and yogurt, which contain the inactive lactase enzyme.
7. Encourage consumption of small amounts of dairy foods daily to help colonic bacteria adapt to ingested lactose.
8. Instruct the parents about the foods that contain lactose, including hidden sources.

▲ A child with lactose intolerance can develop calcium and vitamin D deficiency. Instruct the parents about the importance of providing these supplements.

VIII. CELIAC DISEASE

A. Description
1. Celiac disease also is known as gluten enteropathy or celiac sprue.
2. Intolerance to gluten, the protein component of wheat, barley, rye, and oats, is characteristic.
3. Celiac disease results in the accumulation of the amino acid glutamine, which is toxic to intestinal mucosal cells.
4. Intestinal villous atrophy occurs, which affects absorption of ingested nutrients.
5. Symptoms of the disorder occur most often between the ages of 1 and 5 years.

Box 40-2 Basics of a Gluten-Free Diet

Foods Allowed

Meat such as beef, pork, poultry, and fish; eggs; milk and dairy products; vegetables, fruits, rice, corn, gluten-free flour, puffed rice, cornflakes, cornmeal, and precooked gluten-free cereals are allowed.

Foods Prohibited

Commercially prepared ice cream; malted milk; prepared puddings; and grains, including anything made from wheat, rye, oats, or barley, such as breads, rolls, cookies, cakes, crackers, cereal, spaghetti, macaroni noodles, beer, and ale, are prohibited.

6. There is usually an interval of 3 to 6 months between the introduction of gluten in the diet and the onset of symptoms.
7. Strict dietary avoidance of gluten minimizes the risk of developing malignant lymphoma of the small intestine and other gastrointestinal malignancies.

B. Assessment
1. Acute or insidious diarrhea
2. Steatorrhea
3. Anorexia
4. Abdominal pain and distention
5. Muscle wasting, particularly in the buttocks and extremities
6. Vomiting
7. Anemia
8. Irritability

C. Celiac crisis
1. Precipitated by infection, fasting, or ingestion of gluten
2. Causes profuse watery diarrhea and vomiting
3. Can lead to electrolyte imbalance, rapid dehydration, and severe acidosis

D. Interventions
1. Maintain a gluten-free diet, substituting corn, rice, and millet as grain sources.
2. Instruct the parents and child about lifelong elimination of gluten sources such as wheat, rye, oats, and barley.
3. Administer mineral and vitamin supplements, including iron, folic acid, and fat-soluble vitamins A, D, E, and K.
4. Teach the child and parents about a gluten-free diet and about reading food labels carefully for hidden sources of gluten (Box 40-2).
5. Instruct the parents in measures to prevent celiac crisis.
6. Inform the parents about the Celiac Sprue Association.

IX. APPENDICITIS

A. Description
1. Inflammation of the appendix

2. When the appendix becomes inflamed or infected, perforation may occur within a matter of hours, leading to peritonitis, sepsis, septic shock, and potentially death.
3. Treatment is surgical removal of the appendix before perforation occurs.

B. Assessment
1. Pain in periumbilical area that descends to the right lower quadrant
2. Abdominal pain that is most intense at McBurney's point
3. Referred pain indicating the presence of peritoneal irritation
4. Rebound tenderness and abdominal rigidity
5. Elevated white blood cell count
6. Side-lying position with abdominal guarding (legs flexed) to relieve pain
7. Difficulty walking and pain in the right hip
8. Low-grade fever
9. Anorexia, nausea, and vomiting after pain develops
10. Diarrhea

C. Peritonitis
1. Description: Results from a perforated appendix
2. Assessment
   a. Increased fever
   b. Progressive abdominal distention
   c. Tachycardia and tachypnea
   d. Pallor
   e. Chills
   f. Restlessness and irritability

⚠ An indication of a perforated appendix is the sudden relief of pain and then a subsequent increase in pain accompanied by right guarding of the abdomen.

D. Appendectomy
1. Description: Surgical removal of the appendix
2. Interventions preoperatively
   a. Maintain NPO status.
   b. Administer IV fluids and electrolytes as prescribed to prevent dehydration and correct electrolyte imbalances.
   c. Monitor for changes in the level of pain.
   d. Monitor for signs of a ruptured appendix and peritonitis.
   e. Avoid the use of pain medications so as not to mask pain changes associated with perforation.
   f. Administer antibiotics as prescribed.
   g. Monitor bowel sounds.
   h. Position in a right side-lying or low to semi-Fowler's position to promote comfort.
   i. Apply ice packs to the abdomen for 20 to 30 minutes every hour if prescribed.
   j. Avoid the application of heat to the abdomen.
   k. Avoid laxatives or enemas.

3. Postoperative interventions
   a. Monitor vital signs, particularly temperature.
   b. Maintain NPO status until bowel function has returned, advancing the diet gradually as tolerated and as prescribed when bowel sounds return.
   c. Assess the incision for signs of infection, such as redness, swelling, drainage, and pain.
   d. Monitor drainage in Penrose drain, which may be inserted if perforation occurred.
   e. Position the child in a right side-lying or low to semi-Fowler's position with the legs slightly flexed to facilitate drainage.
   f. Change the dressing as prescribed, and record the type and amount of drainage.
   g. Perform wound irrigations if prescribed.
   h. Maintain nasogastric tube suction and patency of the tube if present.
   i. Administer antibiotics and analgesics as prescribed.

X. HIRSCHSPRUNG'S DISEASE (Fig. 40-4)

A. Description
1. Hirschsprung's disease is a congenital anomaly also known as congenital aganglionosis or aganglionic megacolon.
2. The disease occurs as the result of an absence of ganglion cells in the rectum and other areas of the affected intestine.
3. Mechanical obstruction results because of inadequate motility in an intestinal segment.
4. The disease may be a familial congenital defect or may be associated with other anomalies, such as Down syndrome and genitourinary abnormalities.
5. A rectal biopsy specimen shows histological evidence of the absence of ganglionic cells.

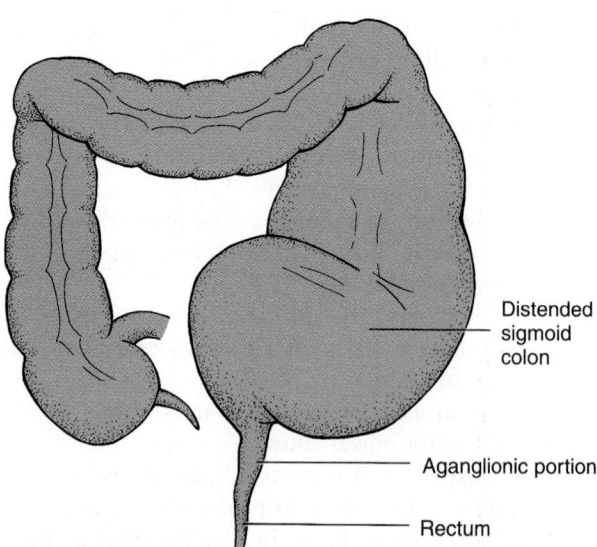

Distended sigmoid colon

Aganglionic portion

Rectum

▲ **FIGURE 40-4** Hirschsprung's disease. (From Perry, S., Hockenberry, M., Lowdermilk, D., & Wilson, D. [2010]. *Maternal child nursing care* [4th ed.]. St. Louis: Mosby.)

6. The most serious complication is enterocolitis; signs include fever, severe prostration, gastrointestinal bleeding, and explosive watery diarrhea.
7. Treatment for mild or moderate disease is based on relieving the chronic constipation with stool softeners and rectal irrigations; however, many children require surgery.
8. Treatment for moderate to severe disease involves a two-step surgical procedure.
   a. Initially, in the neonatal period, a temporary colostomy is created to relieve obstruction and allow the normally innervated, dilated bowel to return to its normal size.
   b. When the bowel returns to its normal size, a complete surgical repair is performed via a pull-through procedure to excise portions of the bowel; at this time, the colostomy is closed.

B. Assessment
1. Newborn infants
   a. Failure to pass meconium stool
   b. Refusal to suck
   c. Abdominal distention
   d. Bile-stained vomitus
2. Children
   a. Failure to gain weight and delayed **growth**
   b. Abdominal distention
   c. Vomiting
   d. Constipation alternating with diarrhea
   e. Ribbon-like and foul-smelling stools

C. Interventions: Medical management
1. Maintain a low-fiber, high-calorie, high-protein diet; parenteral nutrition may be necessary in extreme situations.
2. Administer stool softeners as prescribed.
3. Administer daily rectal irrigations with normal saline to promote adequate elimination and prevent obstruction as prescribed.

D. Surgical management: Preoperative interventions
1. Assess bowel function.
2. Administer bowel preparation as prescribed.
3. Maintain NPO status.
4. Monitor hydration and fluid and electrolyte status; provide fluids intravenously as prescribed for hydration.
5. Administer antibiotics or colonic irrigations with an antibiotic solution as prescribed to clear the bowel of bacteria.
6. Monitor strict intake and output.
7. Obtain daily weight.
8. Measure abdominal girth daily
9. Avoid taking the temperature rectally.
10. Monitor for respiratory distress associated with abdominal distention.

E. Surgical management: Postoperative interventions
1. Monitor vital signs, avoiding taking the temperature rectally.
2. Measure abdominal girth daily and PRN.

3. Assess the surgical site for redness, swelling, and drainage.
4. Assess the stoma if present for bleeding or skin breakdown (stoma should be red and moist).
5. Assess the anal area for the presence of stool, redness, or discharge.
6. Maintain NPO status as prescribed and until bowel sounds return or flatus is passed, usually within 48 to 72 hours.
7. Maintain nasogastric tube to allow intermittent suction until peristalsis returns.
8. Maintain IV fluids until the child tolerates appropriate oral intake, advancing the diet from clear liquids to regular as tolerated and as prescribed.
9. Assess for dehydration and fluid overload.
10. Monitor strict intake and output.
11. Obtain daily weight.
12. Assess for pain and provide comfort measures as required.
13. Provide the parents with instructions regarding colostomy care and skin care.
14. Teach the parents about the appropriate diet and the need for adequate fluid intake.

XI. INTUSSUSCEPTION (Fig. 40-5)

A. Description
1. Telescoping of one portion of the bowel into another portion
2. The condition results in obstruction to the passage of intestinal contents.

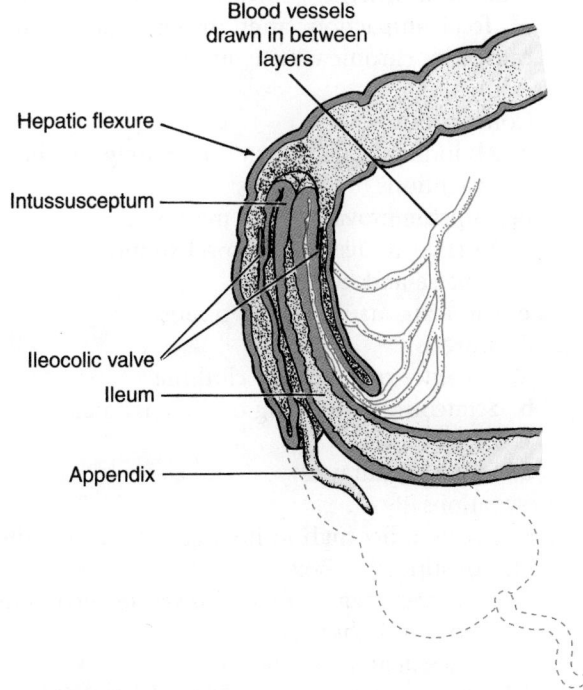

▲ **FIGURE 40-5** Ileocolic intussusception. (From Hockenberry, M., & Wilson, D. [2009]. *Wong's essentials of pediatric nursing* [8th ed.]. St. Louis: Mosby.)

B. Assessment
1. Colicky abdominal pain that causes the child to scream and draw the knees to the abdomen, similar to the fetal position
2. Vomiting of gastric contents
3. Bile-stained fecal emesis
4. Currant jelly–like stools containing blood and mucus
5. Hypoactive or hyperactive bowel sounds
6. Tender distended abdomen, possibly with a palpable sausage-shaped mass in the upper right quadrant

C. Interventions
1. Monitor for signs of perforation and shock as evidenced by fever, increased heart rate, changes in level of consciousness or blood pressure, and respiratory distress, and report immediately.
2. Antibiotics, IV fluids, and decompression via nasogastric tube may be prescribed.
3. Monitor for the passage of normal, brown stool, which indicates that the intussusception has reduced itself.
4. Prepare for hydrostatic reduction as prescribed, if no signs of perforation or shock occur (in hydrostatic reduction, air or fluid is used to exert pressure on area involved to lessen, diminish, or rid the intestine of prolapse).
5. Posthydrostatic reduction
   a. Monitor for the return of normal bowel sounds, for the passage of barium, and the characteristics of stool.
   b. Administer clear fluids, and advance the diet gradually as prescribed.
6. If surgery is required, postoperative care is similar to care after any abdominal surgery.

XII. ABDOMINAL WALL DEFECTS

A. Omphalocele
1. Omphalocele refers to herniation of the abdominal contents through the umbilical ring, usually with an intact peritoneal sac.
2. The protrusion is covered by a translucent sac that may contain bowel or other abdominal organs.
3. Rupture of the sac results in evisceration of the abdominal contents.
4. Immediately after birth, the sac is covered with sterile gauze soaked in normal saline to prevent drying of abdominal contents; a layer of plastic wrap is placed over the gauze to provide additional protection against moisture loss.
5. Monitor vital signs frequently (every 2 to 4 hours), particularly temperature, because the infant can lose heat through the sac.
6. Preoperatively: Maintain NPO status, administer IV fluids as prescribed to maintain hydration and electrolyte balance, monitor for signs of

infection, and handle the infant carefully to prevent rupture of the sac.

7. Postoperatively: Control pain, prevent infection, maintain fluid and electrolyte balance, and ensure adequate nutrition.

B. Gastroschisis

1. Gastroschisis occurs when the herniation of the intestine is lateral to the umbilical ring.
2. No membrane covers the exposed bowel.
3. The exposed bowel is covered loosely in saline-soaked pads, and the abdomen is loosely wrapped in a plastic drape; wrapping directly around the exposed bowel is contraindicated because if the exposed bowel expands, wrapping could cause pressure and necrosis.
4. Preoperatively: Care is similar to that for omphalocele; surgery is performed within several hours after birth because no membrane is covering the sac.
5. Postoperatively: Most infants develop prolonged ileus, require mechanical ventilation, and need parenteral nutrition; otherwise, care is similar to that for omphalocele.

XIII. UMBILICAL HERNIA

A. Description

1. A hernia is a protrusion of the bowel through an abnormal opening in the abdominal wall.
2. In children, hernias most commonly occur at the umbilicus and through the inguinal canal.
3. A hydrocele is the presence of abdominal fluid in the scrotal sac.

B. Assessment

1. Umbilical hernia: Soft swelling or protrusion around the umbilicus that is usually reducible with the finger
2. Inguinal hernia
   a. Inguinal hernia refers to painless inguinal swelling that is reducible.
   b. Swelling may disappear during periods of rest and is most noticeable when the infant cries or coughs.
3. Incarcerated hernia
   a. Incarcerated hernia occurs when the descended portion of the bowel becomes tightly caught in the hernial sac, compromising blood supply.
   b. This represents a medical emergency requiring surgical repair.
   c. Assessment findings include irritability, tenderness at site, anorexia, abdominal distention, and difficulty defecating.
   d. Complete intestinal obstruction and gangrene may occur.
4. Noncommunicating hydrocele
   a. Noncommunicating hydrocele occurs when residual peritoneal fluid is trapped with no communication to the peritoneal cavity.
   b. Hydrocele usually disappears by age 1 year.

5. Communicating hydrocele
   a. Communicating hydrocele is associated with a hernia that remains open from the scrotum to the abdominal cavity.
   b. Assessment includes a bulge in the inguinal area or the scrotum that increases with crying or straining and decreases when the infant is at rest.

C. Postoperative interventions (hernia)

1. Monitor vital signs.
2. Assess for wound infection.
3. Monitor for redness or drainage.
4. Monitor input and output and hydration status.
5. Advance the diet as tolerated.
6. Administer analgesics as prescribed.

D. Postoperative interventions (hydrocele)

1. Provide ice bags and a scrotal support to relieve pain and swelling.
2. Instruct the child and parents to avoid tub bathing until the incision heals.
3. Instruct the child and parents to avoid strenuous physical activities.

XIV. CONSTIPATION AND ENCOPRESIS

A. Description

1. Constipation is the infrequent and difficult passage of dry, hard stools.
2. Encopresis is constipation with fecal incontinence; children often complain that soiling is involuntary and occurs without warning.
3. If the child does not have a neurological or anatomical disorder, encopresis is usually the result of fecal impaction and an enlarged rectum caused by chronic constipation.

B. Assessment

1. Constipation
   a. Abdominal pain and cramping without distention
   b. Palpable movable fecal masses
   c. Normal or decreased bowel sounds
   d. Malaise and headache
   e. Anorexia, nausea, and vomiting
2. Encopresis
   a. Evidence of soiling of clothing
   b. Scratching or rubbing of the anal area
   c. Fecal odor
   d. Social withdrawal

C. Interventions

1. Maintain a diet high in fiber and fluids for simple constipation (Box 40-3).
2. Monitor treatment regimen for severe encopresis for 3 to 6 months.
3. Decrease sugar and milk intake.
4. Administer enemas as prescribed until impaction is cleared.
5. Monitor for hypernatremia or hyperphosphatemia when administering repeated enemas.

Box 40-3 High-Fiber Foods

Bread, grains
- Whole-grain bread or rolls
- Whole-grain cereals
- Bran
- Pancakes, waffles, and muffins with fruit or bran
- Unrefined (brown) rice

Vegetables
- Raw vegetables, especially broccoli, cabbage, carrots, cauliflower, celery, lettuce, and spinach
- Cooked vegetables including those listed above and asparagus, beans, Brussels sprouts, corn, potatoes, rhubarb, squash, string beans, and turnips

Fruits
- Prunes, raisins, or other dried fruits
- Raw fruits, especially those with skins or seeds, other than ripe banana or avocado

Miscellaneous
- Legumes (beans), popcorn, nuts, and seeds
- High-fiber snack bars

From Perry, S., Hockenberry, M., Lowdermilk, D., & Wilson, D. (2010). *Maternal child nursing care* (4th ed., p. 1391). St. Louis: Mosby.

a. Signs of hypernatremia include increased thirst; dry, sticky mucous membranes; flushed skin; increased temperature; nausea and vomiting; oliguria; and lethargy.
b. Signs of hyperphosphatemia include tetany, muscle weakness, dysrhythmias, and hypotension.
6. Administer stool softeners or laxatives as prescribed.
7. Encourage the child to sit on the toilet for 5 to 10 minutes approximately 20 to 30 minutes after breakfast and dinner to assist with defecation.

XV. IRRITABLE BOWEL SYNDROME

A. Description
1. Irritable bowel syndrome results from increased motility, which can lead to spasm and pain.
2. The diagnosis is based on the elimination of pathological conditions.
3. The syndrome is a self-limiting, intermittent problem with no definitive treatment.
4. Stress and emotional factors may contribute to its occurrence.

B. Assessment
1. Diffuse abdominal pain unrelated to meals or activity
2. Alternating constipation and diarrhea with the presence of undigested food and mucus in the stool

C. Interventions
1. Reassure the parents and child that the problem is self-limiting and intermittent and will resolve.
2. Anticholinergics may be prescribed (antidepressants may be needed in severe cases).

Box 40-4 Assessment Findings: Imperforate Anus

Failure to pass meconium stool
Absence or stenosis of the anal rectal canal
Presence of an anal membrane
External fistula to the perineum

3. Encourage the maintenance of a healthy, well-balanced, moderate-fiber, and low-fat diet.
4. Encourage health promotion activities such as exercise and school activities.
5. Inform the parents of psychosocial resources if required.

XVI. IMPERFORATE ANUS

A. Description: Incomplete development or absence of the anus in its normal position in the perineum
B. Types
1. A membrane is noted over the anal opening, with a normal anus just above the membrane.
2. There is complete absence of the anus (anal agenesis) with a rectal pouch ending some distance above.
3. Rectum ends blindly or has a fistula connection to the perineum, urethra, bladder, or vagina.
C. Assessment (Box 40-4)
D. Preoperative interventions
1. Determine patency of the anus.
2. Monitor for the presence of stool in the urine and vagina (indicates a fistula) and report immediately.
3. Administer IV fluids as prescribed.
4. Prepare the child and parents for the surgical procedures, including the potential for colostomy.
E. Postoperative interventions
1. Monitor the skin for signs of infection.
2. The preferred position is a side-lying prone position with the hips elevated or a supine position with the legs suspended at a 90-degree angle to the trunk to reduce edema and pressure on the surgical site.
3. Keep the anal surgical incision clean and dry, and monitor for redness, swelling, or drainage.
4. Maintain NPO status and nasogastric tube if in place.
5. Maintain IV fluids until gastrointestinal motility returns.
6. Provide care for colostomy, if present, as prescribed.
7. A new colostomy stoma is red and edematous, but this should decrease with time.
8. Instruct the parents to perform anal dilation if prescribed to achieve and maintain bowel patency.
9. Instruct the parents to use only dilators supplied by the physician and a water-soluble lubricant and to insert the dilator no more than 1 to 2 cm into the anus to prevent damage to the mucosa.

XVII. HEPATITIS

A. This section contains specific information regarding hepatitis as it relates to infants and children; see also Chapters 25 and 56.

B. Description: An acute or chronic inflammation of the liver that may be caused by a virus, a medication reaction, or another disease process

C. Hepatitis A (HAV)
1. Highest incidence of HAV infection occurs among preschool or school-age children younger than 15 years.
2. Many infected children are asymptomatic, but mild nausea, vomiting, and diarrhea may occur.
3. Infected children who are asymptomatic still can spread HAV to others.

D. Hepatitis B (HBV)
1. Most HBV infection in children is acquired perinatally.
2. Newborn infants are at risk if the mother is infected with HBV or was a carrier of HBV during pregnancy.
3. Possible routes of maternal-fetal (infant) transmission include leakage of the virus across the placenta late in pregnancy or during labor, ingestion of amniotic fluid or maternal blood, and breast-feeding, especially if the mother has cracked nipples.
4. The severity in the infant varies from no liver disease to fulminant (severe acute course) or chronic active disease.
5. In children and adolescents, HBV occurs in specific high-risk groups, including children with hemophilia or other disorders requiring multiple blood transfusions, children or adolescents involved in IV drug **abuse**, institutionalized children, preschool children in endemic areas, and children who have had heterosexual activity or sexual activity with homosexual men.
6. Infection with HBV can cause a carrier state and lead to eventual cirrhosis or hepatocellular carcinoma in adulthood.

E. Hepatitis C (HCV)
1. Transmission of HCV is primarily by the parenteral route.
2. Some children may be asymptomatic, but HCV often becomes a chronic condition and can cause cirrhosis and hepatocellular carcinoma.

F. Hepatitis D
1. Infection occurs in children already infected with HBV.
2. Acute and chronic forms tend to be more severe than HBV and can lead to cirrhosis.
3. Children with hemophilia are more likely to be infected, as are children who are IV drug users.

G. Hepatitis E
1. Infection is uncommon in children.

2. Infection is not a chronic condition, does not cause chronic liver disease, and has no carrier state.

H. Hepatitis G
1. Hepatitis G virus is blood-borne and is similar to HCV.
2. High-risk groups include transfusion recipients, IV drug users, and individuals infected with HCV.
3. Individuals are often asymptomatic, and most infections are chronic.

I. Assessment (Box 40-5)

J. Diagnostic evaluation: See Chapter 11.

K. Prevention
1. Immunoglobulin provides **passive immunity** and may be effective for pre-exposure prophylaxis to prevent HAV infection.
2. Hepatitis B immunoglobulin provides **passive immunity** and may be effective in preventing infection after a one-time exposure (should be given immediately after exposure), such as an accidental needle puncture or other contact of contaminated material with mucous membranes; immunoglobulin should also be given to newborns whose mothers are positive for hepatitis B surface antigen.
3. Hepatitis A **vaccine** and hepatitis B **vaccine**: See Chapter 48.

⚠ Proper handwashing and standard precautions can prevent the spread of viral hepatitis.

L. Interventions
1. Strict handwashing is required.
2. Hospitalization is required in the event of coagulopathy or fulminant hepatitis.
3. Standard precautions and enteric precautions are followed during hospitalization.
4. Provide enteric precautions for at least 1 week after the onset of jaundice with HAV.

Box 40-5 Assessment Findings: Hepatitis

Prodromal or Anicteric Phase
Lasts 5 to 7 days
Absence of jaundice
Anorexia, malaise, lethargy, easy fatigability
Fever (especially in adolescents)
Nausea and vomiting
Epigastric or right upper quadrant abdominal pain
Arthralgia and rashes (more likely with hepatitis B virus)
Hepatomegaly

Icteric Phase
Jaundice, which is best assessed in the sclera, nail beds, and mucous membranes
Dark urine and pale stools
Pruritus

5. The hospitalized child usually is not isolated in a separate room unless he or she is fecally incontinent and items are likely to become contaminated with feces.
6. Children are discouraged from sharing toys.
7. Instruct the child and parents in effective hand-washing techniques.
8. Instruct the parents to disinfect diaper-changing surfaces thoroughly with a solution of 1/4 cup bleach in 1 gallon of water.
9. Maintain comfort, and provide adequate rest and sleep.
10. Provide a low-fat, well-balanced diet.
11. Inform the parents that because HAV is not infectious 1 week after the onset of jaundice, the child may return to school at that time if he or she feels well enough.
12. Inform the parents that jaundice may appear worse before it resolves.
13. Caution the parents about administering any medications to the child; explain the role of the liver in detoxification and excretion of medications in understandable terms.
14. Instruct the parents about the signs of the child's condition worsening, such as changes in neurological status, bleeding, and fluid retention.

XVIII. INGESTION OF POISONS (see Priority Nursing Actions)

PRIORITY NURSING ACTIONS!

Actions to Take in the Emergency Department in the Event of a Poisoning
1. Assess the child.
2. Terminate exposure to the poison.
3. Identify the poison.
4. Take measures to prevent absorption of the poison.
5. Document the occurrence, assessment findings, poison ingested, treatment measures, and the child's response.

In the event of a poisoning, the nurse treats the child first, not the poison. The ABCs—airway, breathing, and circulation—and vital signs are assessed. Cardiopulmonary resuscitation is initiated immediately if necessary. Exposure to the poison is terminated next, such as emptying the mouth of pills or other materials or flushing the skin or other body area. The poison is identified next by questioning the parents or witnesses of the event to determine the appropriate treatment. The nurse administers the antidote or takes other measures as prescribed by the physician, such as administering activated charcoal. The nurse documents the occurrence, assessment findings, poison ingested, treatment measures, and the child's response.

Reference: Perry, S., Hockenberry, M., Lowdermilk, D., & Wilson, D. (2010). *Maternal child nursing care* (4th ed., pp. 1427-1430). St. Louis: Mosby.

A. Lead poisoning
1. Description: Excessive accumulation of lead in the blood
2. Causes
   a. The pathway for exposure may be food, air, or water.
   b. Dust and soil contaminated with lead may be a source of exposure.
   c. Lead enters the child's body through ingestion or inhalation or through placental transmission to an unborn child when the mother is exposed; the most common route is hand to mouth from contaminated objects, such as loose paint chips, pottery, or ceramic ware coupled with the inhalation of lead dust in the environment.
   d. When lead enters the body, it affects the erythrocytes, bones and teeth, and organs and tissues, including the brain and nervous system; the most serious consequences are the effects on the central nervous system.
3. Universal screening
   a. Screening is recommended for children 1 to 2 years old; children at high risk should be screened earlier.
   b. Any child between the ages of 3 and 6 years who has not been screened should be tested.
4. Targeted screening
   a. Targeted screening is acceptable in low-risk areas.
   b. A child at the age of 1 to 2 years (or a child between the ages of 3 and 6 years who has not been screened) may be targeted for screening if determined to be at risk.
5. Blood lead level test: Used for screening and diagnosis (Table 40-1)
6. Erythrocyte protoporphyrin test
   a. Indicator of anemia
   b. Normal value for a child: 35 mcg/100 mL of whole blood or lower
7. Chelation therapy
   a. Chelation therapy removes lead from the circulating blood and from some organs and tissues.
   b. Therapy does not counteract any effects of the lead.
   c. Medications include calcium disodium edetate ($CaNa_2EDTA$), and succimer (Chemet), an oral preparation; British anti-Lewisite (BAL, dimercaprol) is used in conjunction with EDTA.
   d. British anti-Lewisite is administered by the IV route or via deep intramuscular route and is contraindicated in children with an allergy to peanuts because the medication is prepared in a peanut oil solution; it is also contraindicated in children with glucose 6-phosphate dehydrogenase (G6PD) deficiency and should not be given with iron.

TABLE 40-1 Blood Lead Level Test Results and Intervention

Level (mcg/dL)	Intervention
<10	Reassess or rescreen in 1 yr or sooner if exposure status changes
10-14	Provide family lead education, follow-up testing, and social service referral for home assessment if necessary
15-19	Provide family lead education, follow-up testing, and social service referral if necessary; on follow-up testing, initiate actions for blood lead level of 20-44 mcg/dL
20-44	Provide coordination of care and clinical management, including treatment, environmental investigation, and lead-hazard control
45-69	Provide coordination of care and clinical management within 48 hr, including treatment, environmental investigation, and lead-hazard control (the child must not remain in a lead-hazardous environment if resolution is necessary)
≥70	Medical treatment is provided immediately, including coordination of care, clinical management, environmental investigation, and lead-hazard control

Modified from Perry, S., Hockenberry, M., Lowdermilk, D., & Wilson, D. (2010). *Maternal child nursing care* (4th ed., p. 1436). St. Louis: Mosby.

   e. The function of the renal, hepatic, and hematological systems must be monitored closely.
   f. Ensure adequate urinary output before administering the medication, and monitor the output and pH of the urine closely during and after therapy.
   g. Provide adequate hydration and monitor kidney function for nephrotoxicity when the medication is given because the medication is excreted via the kidneys.
   h. Follow-up of lead levels needs to be done to monitor progress.
   i. Provide instructions to parents about safety from lead hazards, medication administration, and the need for follow-up.
   j. Confirm that the child will be discharged to a home without lead hazards.
B. Acetaminophen (Tylenol)
   1. Description
      a. Seriousness of ingestion is determined by the amount ingested and the length of time before intervention
      b. Toxic dose is 150 mg/kg or higher in children.
   2. Assessment
      a. First 2 to 4 hours: Malaise, nausea, vomiting, sweating, pallor, weakness

   b. Latent period: 24 to 36 hours; child improves
   c. Hepatic involvement: May last 7 days and may be permanent; right upper quadrant pain, jaundice, confusion, stupor, elevated liver enzyme and bilirubin levels, prolonged prothrombin time
   3. Interventions
      a. Administer antidote: *N*-acetyl cysteine (Mucomyst)
      b. Dilute antidote in juice or soda because of its offensive odor.
      c. Loading dose is followed by maintenance doses.
      d. In an unconscious child, prepare to administer gastric lavage with activated charcoal to decrease the absorption of acetaminophen.
      e. If using activated charcoal with lavage, do not also use *N*-acetyl cysteine because activated charcoal inactivates the antidote.
C. Acetylsalicylic acid (aspirin)
   1. Description
      a. Overdose may be caused by acute ingestion or chronic ingestion.
      b. Acute: Severe toxicity with 300 to 500 mg/kg
      c. Chronic: Ingestion of more than 100 mg/kg per day for 2 days or more, which can be more serious than acute ingestion
   2. Assessment
      a. Gastrointestinal effects: Nausea, vomiting, and thirst from dehydration
      b. Central nervous system effects: Hyperpnea, confusion, tinnitus, convulsions, coma, respiratory failure, circulatory collapse
      c. Renal effects: Oliguria
      d. Hematopoietic effects: Bleeding tendencies
      e. Metabolic effects: Diaphoresis, fever, hyponatremia, hypokalemia, dehydration, hypoglycemia, metabolic acidosis
   3. Interventions
      a. Prepare to administer activated charcoal to decrease absorption of salicylate.
      b. Emesis or cathartic measures may be prescribed.
      c. Administer IV fluids; sodium bicarbonate may be prescribed to correct metabolic acidosis.
      d. Other interventions include external cooling, anticonvulsants, vitamin K (if bleeding), and oxygen.
      e. Prepare the child for dialysis as prescribed if the child is unresponsive to the therapy.
D. Corrosives
   1. Description
      a. Items that can cause poisoning include household cleaners, detergents, bleach, paint or paint thinners, or batteries.
      b. Liquid corrosives can cause more damage to the victim than other types of corrosives, such as granular.

2. Assessment
   a. Severe burning in the mouth, throat, or stomach
   b. Edema of the mucous membranes, lips, tongue, and pharynx
   c. Vomiting
   d. Drooling and inability to clear secretions
3. Interventions
   a. Dilute corrosive with water or milk as prescribed (usually no more than 4 oz)
   b. Inducing vomiting is contraindicated because vomiting redamages the mucous membranes.
   c. Neutralization of the ingested corrosive is not done because it can cause a reaction producing heat and burns.

⚠ Educate parents to call the poison control center immediately in the event of poisoning. The parents need to be instructed to post the poison control center telephone number near each phone in the house.

XIX. INTESTINAL PARASITES

A. Description: Common infections in children are giardiasis and pinworm infestation.
   1. Giardiasis is caused by protozoa and is prevalent among children in crowded environments, such as classrooms or day care centers.
   2. Pinworms (enterobiasis) are universally present in temperate climate zones and are easily transmitted in crowded environments.
B. Assessment
   1. Giardiasis
      a. Diarrhea and vomiting
      b. Anorexia
      c. Failure to thrive
      d. Abdominal cramps with intermittent loose stools and constipation
      e. Steatorrhea
      f. Resolves in 4 to 6 weeks spontaneously
      g. Stool specimens from three or more collections are used for diagnosis.
   2. Pinworms
      a. Intense perianal itching
      b. Irritability, restlessness
      c. Poor sleeping
      d. Bed wetting
C. Interventions
   1. Giardiasis
      a. Medications that may be prescribed include metronidazole (Flagyl), tinidazole (Tindamax), nitazoxanide (Alinia), or albendazole (Albenza).
      b. Caregivers should wash hands meticulously.
      c. Provide education to family and caregivers regarding sanitary practices.
   2. Pinworms

a. Perform a visual inspection of the anus with a flashlight 2 to 3 hours after sleep.
b. The tape test is the most common diagnostic test.
c. Educate the family and caregivers regarding the tape test. A loop of transparent tape is placed firmly against the child's perianal area; it is removed in the morning and placed in a glass jar or plastic bag and transported to the primary care provider for analysis.
d. Medications that may be prescribed include mebendazole (Vermox), pyrantel pamoate (Pin-Rid, Antiminth), and albendazole (Albenza); these medications are not used in children younger than 2 years.
e. The medication regimen may be repeated in 2 weeks to prevent reinfection.
f. All members of the family are treated for the infection.
g. Teach the family and caregivers about the importance of meticulous handwashing and about washing all clothes and bed linens in hot water.

MORE QUESTIONS ON THE CD!

Practice Questions

407. A nurse is preparing to care for a child with a diagnosis of intussusception. The nurse reviews the child's record and expects to note which symptom of this disorder documented?
    1. Watery diarrhea
    2. Ribbon-like stools
    3. Profuse projectile vomiting
    4. Bright red blood and mucus in the stools

408. A clinic nurse reviews the record of an infant and notes that the physician has documented a diagnosis of suspected Hirschsprung's disease. The nurse reviews the assessment findings documented in the record, knowing that which symptom most likely led the mother to seek health care for the infant?
    1. Diarrhea
    2. Projectile vomiting
    3. Regurgitation of feedings
    4. Foul-smelling ribbon-like stools

409. An infant has just returned to the nursing unit after a surgical repair of a cleft lip on the right side. The nurse places the infant in which best position at this time?
    1. Prone position
    2. On the stomach
    3. Left lateral position
    4. Right lateral position

410. A nurse reviews the record of a newborn infant and notes that a diagnosis of esophageal atresia with tracheoesophageal fistula is suspected. The nurse expects to note which most likely sign of this condition documented in the record?
1. Incessant crying
2. Coughing at nighttime
3. Choking with feedings
4. Severe projectile vomiting

411. A nurse provides feeding instructions to a mother of an infant diagnosed with gastroesophageal reflux disease. To assist in reducing the episodes of emesis, the nurse tells the mother to:
1. Provide less frequent, larger feedings.
2. Burp the infant less frequently during feedings.
3. Thin the feedings by adding water to the formula.
4. Thicken the feedings by adding rice cereal to the formula.

412. A child is hospitalized because of persistent vomiting. The nurse monitors the child closely for:
1. Diarrhea
2. Metabolic acidosis
3. Metabolic alkalosis
4. Hyperactive bowel sounds

413. A nurse is caring for a newborn infant with a suspected diagnosis of imperforate anus. The nurse monitors the infant, knowing that which of the following is a clinical manifestation associated with this disorder?
1. Bile-stained fecal emesis
2. The passage of currant jelly–like stools
3. Failure to pass meconium stool in the first 24 hours after birth
4. Sausage-shaped mass palpated in the upper right abdominal quadrant

414. A nurse admits a child to the hospital with a diagnosis of pyloric stenosis. On admission assessment, which data would the nurse expect to obtain when asking the mother about the child's symptoms?
1. Watery diarrhea
2. Projectile vomiting
3. Increased urine output
4. Vomiting large amounts of bile

415. A nurse provides home care instructions to the parents of a child with celiac disease. The nurse teaches the parents to include which food item in the child's diet?
1. Rice
2. Oatmeal
3. Rye toast
4. Wheat bread

Alternate Item Format: Multiple Response

416. Which interventions would a nurse include when preparing a care plan for a child with hepatitis? **Select all that apply**.
❑ 1. Providing a low-fat, well-balanced diet.
❑ 2. Notifying the physician if jaundice is present.
❑ 3. Teaching the child effective handwashing techniques.
❑ 4. Scheduling playtime in the playroom with other children.
❑ 5. Instructing the parents to avoid administering medications unless prescribed.
❑ 6. Arranging for indefinite home schooling because the child will not be able to return to school.

ANSWERS

407. 4
Rationale: Intussusception is a telescoping of one portion of the bowel into another. The condition results in an obstruction to the passage of intestinal contents. A child with intussusception typically has severe abdominal pain that is crampy and intermittent, causing the child to draw in the knees to the chest. Vomiting may be present, but is not projectile. Bright red blood and mucus are passed through the rectum and commonly are described as currant jelly–like stools. Watery diarrhea and ribbon-like stools are not manifestations of this disorder.
Test-Taking Strategy: Focus on the diagnosis and think about the pathophysiology that occurs. Recalling that a classic manifestation is currant jelly–like stools will assist in directing you to option 4. Review the manifestations of intussusception if you had difficulty with this question.
Level of Cognitive Ability: Analyzing
Client Needs: Physiological Integrity
Integrated Process: Nursing Process—Assessment
Content Area: Child Health—Gastrointestinal/Renal
Reference: Hockenberry, M., & Wilson, D. (2009). *Wong's essentials of pediatric nursing* (8th ed., pp. 852–853). St. Louis: Mosby.

408. 4
Rationale: Hirschsprung's disease is a congenital anomaly also known as congenital aganglionosis or aganglionic megacolon. It occurs as the result of an absence of ganglion cells in the rectum and other areas of the affected intestine. Chronic

constipation beginning in the first month of life and resulting in pellet-like or ribbon-like stools that are foul-smelling is a clinical manifestation of this disorder. Delayed passage or absence of meconium stool in the neonatal period is also a sign. Bowel obstruction especially in the neonatal period, abdominal pain and distention, and failure to thrive are also clinical manifestations. Options 1, 2, and 3 are not associated specifically with this disorder.
Test-Taking Strategy: Use the process of elimination and knowledge regarding the pathophysiology associated with Hirschsprung's disease to direct you to option 4. Remember that chronic constipation beginning in the first month of life and resulting in pellet-like or ribbon-like, foul-smelling stools is a clinical manifestation of this disorder. If you are unfamiliar with the manifestations of Hirschsprung's disease, review these assessment findings.
Level of Cognitive Ability: Analyzing
Client Needs: Physiological Integrity
Integrated Process: Nursing Process—Assessment
Content Area: Child Health—Gastrointestinal/Renal
Reference: Perry, S., Hockenberry, M., Lowdermilk, D., & Wilson, D. (2010). *Maternal child nursing care* (4th ed., p. 1392). St. Louis: Mosby.

409. 3
Rationale: A cleft lip is a congenital anomaly that occurs as a result of failure of soft tissue or bony structure to fuse during embryonic development. After cleft lip repair, a nurse avoids positioning an infant on the side of the repair or in the prone position because these positions can cause rubbing of the surgical site on the mattress. The nurse positions the infant on the side lateral to the repair or on the back upright and positions the infant to prevent airway obstruction by secretions, blood, or the tongue. From the options provided, placing the infant on the left side immediately after surgery is best to prevent the risk of aspiration if the infant vomits.
Test-Taking Strategy: Eliminate options 1 and 2 because they are comparable or alike positions. Consider the anatomical location of the surgical site and note the strategic words *right side* to direct you to the correct option from the remaining options. Review postoperative positioning techniques after cleft lip repair if you had difficulty with this question.
Level of Cognitive Ability: Applying
Client Needs: Physiological Integrity
Integrated Process: Nursing Process—Implementation
Content Area: Child Health—Gastrointestinal/Renal
Reference: McKinney, E., James, S., Murray, S., & Ashwill, J. (2009). *Maternal-child nursing* (3rd ed., p. 1095). St. Louis: Saunders.

410. 3
Rationale: In esophageal atresia and tracheoesophageal fistula, the esophagus terminates before it reaches the stomach, ending in a blind pouch, and a fistula is present that forms an unnatural connection with the trachea. Any child who exhibits the "3 C's"—coughing and choking with feedings and unexplained cyanosis—should be suspected to have tracheoesophageal fistula. Options 1, 2, and 4 are not specifically associated with tracheoesophageal fistula.
Test-Taking Strategy: Focus on the diagnosis and think about the pathophysiology of the disorder. Recalling the "3 C's" associated with this disorder will assist in directing

you to the correct option. Review the clinical manifestations associated with esophageal atresia and tracheoesophageal fistula if you had difficulty with this question.
Level of Cognitive Ability: Analyzing
Client Needs: Physiological Integrity
Integrated Process: Nursing Process—Assessment
Content Area: Child Health—Gastrointestinal/Renal
Reference: McKinney, E., James, S., Murray, S., & Ashwill, J. (2009). *Maternal-child nursing* (3rd ed., p. 1098). St. Louis: Saunders.

411. 4
Rationale: Gastroesophageal reflux is backflow of gastric contents into the esophagus as a result of relaxation or incompetence of the lower esophageal or cardiac sphincter. Small, more frequent feedings with frequent burping often are prescribed in the treatment of gastroesophageal reflux. Feedings thickened with rice cereal may reduce episodes of emesis. If thickened formula is used, cross-cutting of the nipple may be required.
Test-Taking Strategy: Use the process of elimination and basic principles related to feeding an infant to assist in eliminating options 1 and 2. Noting the strategic words *reducing the episodes of emesis* will assist in directing you to select option 4 over option 3. Review therapeutic interventions associated with gastroesophageal reflux disease if you had difficulty with this question.
Level of Cognitive Ability: Applying
Client Needs: Physiological Integrity
Integrated Process: Teaching and Learning
Content Area: Child Health—Gastrointestinal/Renal
Reference: McKinney, E., James, S., Murray, S., & Ashwill, J. (2009). *Maternal-child nursing* (3rd ed., p. 1105). St. Louis: Saunders.

412. 3
Rationale: Vomiting causes the loss of hydrochloric acid and subsequent metabolic alkalosis. Metabolic acidosis would occur in a child experiencing diarrhea because of the loss of bicarbonate. Diarrhea might or might not accompany vomiting. Hyperactive bowel sounds are not associated with vomiting.
Test-Taking Strategy: Use the process of elimination. Recalling that gastric fluids are acidic and that the loss of these fluids leads to alkalosis will assist you in answering the question. No data in the question support options 1 and 4. Review the manifestations associated with vomiting if you had difficulty with this question.
Level of Cognitive Ability: Analyzing
Client Needs: Physiological Integrity
Integrated Process: Nursing Process—Assessment
Content Area: Child Health—Gastrointestinal/Renal
Reference: McKinney, E., James, S., Murray, S., & Ashwill, J. (2009). *Maternal-child nursing* (3rd ed., p. 1082). St. Louis: Saunders.

413. 3
Rationale: Imperforate anus is the incomplete development or absence of the anus in its normal position in the perineum. During the newborn assessment, this defect should be identified easily on sight. A rectal thermometer or tube may be necessary, however, to determine patency if meconium is not passed in the

first 24 hours after birth. Other assessment findings include absence or stenosis of the anal rectal canal, presence of an anal membrane, and an external fistula to the perineum. Options 1, 2, and 4 are findings noted in intussusception.

Test-Taking Strategy: Focus on the newborn's diagnosis. Use the process of elimination and the definition of the word *imperforate* to assist in answering this question. This should direct you to option 3. Review the assessment findings associated with imperforate anus if you had difficulty with this question.

Level of Cognitive Ability: Analyzing
Client Needs: Physiological Integrity
Integrated Process: Nursing Process—Assessment
Content Area: Child Health—Gastrointestinal/Renal
References: Hockenberry, M., & Wilson, D. (2009). *Wong's essentials of pediatric nursing* (8th ed., p. 854). St. Louis: Mosby.

McKinney, E., James, S., Murray, S., & Ashwill, J. (2009). *Maternal-child nursing* (3rd ed., pp. 1101–1102). St. Louis: Saunders.

414. 2

Rationale: In pyloric stenosis, hypertrophy of the circular muscles of the pylorus causes narrowing of the pyloric canal between the stomach and the duodenum. Clinical manifestations of pyloric stenosis include projectile vomiting, irritability, hunger and crying, constipation, and signs of dehydration including a decrease in urine output.

Test-Taking Strategy: Considering the anatomical location of this disorder and its potential effects will assist in eliminating options 1 and 3. Thinking about the pathophysiology of the disorder and recalling that a major clinical manifestation is projectile vomiting will assist in directing you to option 2 from the remaining options. Review the clinical manifestations of pyloric stenosis if you had difficulty with this question.

Level of Cognitive Ability: Analyzing
Client Needs: Physiological Integrity
Integrated Process: Nursing Process—Assessment
Content Area: Child Health—Gastrointestinal/Renal
Reference: Hockenberry, M., & Wilson, D. (2009). *Wong's essentials of pediatric nursing* (8th ed., pp. 849–850). St. Louis: Mosby.

415. 1

Rationale: Celiac disease also is known as gluten enteropathy or celiac sprue and refers to an intolerance to gluten, the protein component of wheat, barley, rye, and oats. The important factor to remember is that all wheat, rye, barley, and oats should be eliminated from the diet and replaced with corn, rice, or millet. Vitamin supplements—especially the fat-soluble vitamins, iron, and folic acid—may be needed to correct deficiencies. Dietary restrictions are likely to be lifelong.

Test-Taking Strategy: Focus on the disorder. Recalling that corn, rice, and millet are substitute food replacements in this disease will direct you to option 1. Review the dietary management in celiac disease if you had difficulty with this question.

Level of Cognitive Ability: Applying
Client Needs: Health Promotion and Maintenance
Integrated Process: Teaching and Learning
Content Area: Child Health—Gastrointestinal/Renal
Reference: Perry, S., Hockenberry, M., Lowdermilk, D., & Wilson, D. (2010). *Maternal child nursing care* (4th ed., p. 1423). St. Louis: Saunders.

ALTERNATE ITEM FORMAT: MULTIPLE RESPONSE

416. 1, 3, 5

Rationale: Hepatitis is an acute or chronic inflammation of the liver that may be caused by a virus, a medication reaction, or another disease process. Because hepatitis can be viral, standard precautions should be instituted in the hospital. The child should be discouraged from sharing toys, so playtime in the playroom with other children is not part of the plan of care. The child will be allowed to return to school 1 week after the onset of jaundice, so indefinite home schooling would not need to be arranged. Jaundice is an expected finding with hepatitis and would not warrant notification of the physician. Provision of a low-fat, well-balanced diet is recommended. Parents are cautioned about administering any medication to the child because normal doses of many medications may become dangerous owing to the liver's inability to detoxify and excrete them. Handwashing is the most effective measure for control of hepatitis in any setting, and effective handwashing can prevent the immunocompromised child from contracting an opportunistic type of infection.

Test-Taking Strategy: Use the process of elimination. Eliminate any intervention that would be inappropriate for a child with hepatitis. Thinking about the pathophysiology associated with hepatitis and the method of transmission will assist you in answering the question. Playing with other children in the playroom, planning for an indefinite period of home schooling, and notifying the physician of jaundice would not be appropriate interventions. Review care for a child with hepatitis if you had difficulty with this question.

Level of Cognitive Ability: Applying
Client Needs: Safe and Effective Care Environment
Integrated Process: Nursing Process—Planning
Content Area: Child Health—Gastrointestinal/Renal
Reference: Hockenberry, M., & Wilson, D. (2009). *Wong's essentials of pediatric nursing* (8th ed., p. 841). St. Louis: Mosby.

Metabolic and Endocrine Disorders

I. FEVER

A. Description
1. Fever is an abnormal body temperature elevation.
2. A child's temperature can vary depending on activity, emotional stress, disease processes, medications, type of clothing the child is wearing, and temperature of the environment.
3. Assessment findings associated with the fever provide important indications of the seriousness of the fever.

B. Assessment
1. Temperature elevation: Normal temperature range for a child is 36.4° C to 37° C (97.5° F to 98.6° F); 38° C (100.4° F) is considered to be fever.
2. Flushed skin, warm to touch
3. Diaphoresis
4. Chills
5. Restlessness or lethargy

C. Interventions
1. Monitor vital signs; take the temperature via the tympanic or axillary route or per agency procedures.
2. Remove excess clothing and blankets, reduce the room temperature, and increase the air circulation; use other cooling measures such as the application of a cool compress to the forehead if appropriate.
3. Administer a sponge bath with tepid water for 20 to 30 minutes and gently squeeze water from a facecloth over the back and chest, and recheck the temperature 30 minutes after the bath; do not use alcohol because it can cause peripheral vasoconstriction.
4. Administer antipyretics such as acetaminophen (Tylenol) or ibuprofen (Motrin) as prescribed.
5. Aspirin (acetylsalicylic acid) should not be administered, unless specifically prescribed, because of the risk of Reye's syndrome.
6. Retake the temperature 30 to 60 minutes after the antipyretic is administered.
7. Provide adequate fluid intake as tolerated and as prescribed.
8. Monitor for signs and symptoms that indicate dehydration and electrolyte imbalances; monitor laboratory values.
9. Instruct the parents in how to take the temperature, how to medicate the child safely, and when it is necessary to call the physician.

II. DEHYDRATION (Box 41-1)

A. Description
1. Dehydration is a common fluid and electrolyte imbalance in infants and children.
2. In infants and children, the organs that conserve water are immature, placing them at risk for fluid volume deficit.
3. Causes can include decreased fluid intake, diaphoresis, vomiting, diarrhea, diabetic ketoacidosis, and extensive burns or other serious injuries.

⚠ Infants and children are more vulnerable to fluid volume deficit because more of their body water is in the extracellular fluid compartment.

B. Assessment (Table 41-1)
C. Interventions
1. Treat and eliminate the cause of the dehydration.
2. Monitor vital signs.
3. Monitor for signs of dehydration.
4. Monitor weight and monitor for changes, including fluid gains and losses.
5. Monitor intake and output and urine for specific gravity.
6. Monitor level of consciousness.
7. Monitor skin turgor and mucous membranes for dryness.
8. For mild to moderate dehydration, provide oral rehydration therapy with Pedialyte or a similar rehydration solution as prescribed; avoid carbonated beverages because they are gas-producing and fluids that contain high amounts of sugar, such as apple juice.
9. For severe dehydration, maintain NPO status to place the bowel at rest and provide fluid and electrolyte replacement by the intravenous

(IV) route as prescribed; if potassium is prescribed for IV administration, ensure that the child has voided before administering and has adequate renal function.

10. Reintroduce a normal diet when rehydration is achieved.

11. Provide instructions to the parents about the types and amounts of fluid to encourage, signs of dehydration, and indications of the need to notify the physician.

III. PHENYLKETONURIA

A. Description

1. Phenylketonuria is a genetic disorder (autosomal recessive disorder) that results in central nervous system damage from toxic levels of phenylalanine (an essential amino acid) in the blood.

Box 41-1 Types of Dehydration

Isotonic dehydration: Electrolyte and water deficits occur in approximately balanced proportions

Hypertonic dehydration: Water loss exceeds electrolyte loss

Hypotonic dehydration: Electrolyte loss exceeds water loss

---

2. It is characterized by blood phenylalanine levels greater than 20 mg/dL (normal level is 1.2 to 3.4 mg/dL in newborns and 0.8 to 1.8 mg/dL thereafter).

3. All 50 states require routine screening of all newborns for phenylketonuria.

B. Assessment

1. In all children
   a. Digestive problems and vomiting
   b. Seizures
   c. Musty odor of the urine
   d. Mental retardation
2. In older children
   a. Eczema
   b. Hypertonia
   c. Hypopigmentation of the hair, skin, and irises
   d. Hyperactive behavior

C. Interventions

1. Screening of newborn infants for phenylketonuria: The infant should have begun formula or breast milk feeding before specimen collection.
2. If initial screening is positive, a repeat test is performed, and further diagnostic evaluation is required to verify the diagnosis.
3. Rescreen infants by 14 days of age if the initial screening was done before 48 hours of age.
4. If phenylketonuria is diagnosed, prepare to implement the following:

TABLE 41-1 Evaluating the Extent of Dehydration

| | Level of Dehydration | | |
Clinical Signs	Mild	Moderate	Severe
Weight loss—infants	3%-5%	6%-9%	≥10%
Weight loss—children	3%-4%	6%-8%	10%
Pulse	Normal	Slightly increased	Very increased
Respiratory rate	Normal	Slight tachypnea (rapid)	Hyperpnea (deep and rapid)
Blood pressure	Normal	Normal to orthostatic (>10 mm Hg change)	Orthostatic to shock
Behavior	Normal	Irritable, more thirsty	Hyperirritable to lethargic
Thirst	Slight	Moderate	Intense
Mucous membranes*	Normal	Dry	Parched
Tears	Present	Decreased	Absent; sunken eyes
Anterior fontanel	Normal	Normal to sunken	Sunken
External jugular vein	Visible when supine	Not visible except with supraclavicular pressure	Not visible even with supraclavicular pressure
Skin*	Capillary refill >2 sec	Slowed capillary refill (2-4 sec [decreased turgor])	Very delayed capillary refill (>4 sec) and tenting; skin cool, acrocyanotic or mottled
Urine specific gravity	>1.020	>1.020; oliguria	Oliguria or anuria

*These signs are less prominent in the child who has hypernatremia.
Data from Jospe, N., Forbes, G. Fluids and electrolytes—Clinical aspects, *Pediatrics in Review* 17(11):395-403, 1996; and Steiner, M.J., DeWalt, D.A., Byerley, J.S. Is this child dehydrated? *Journal of the American Medical Association* 291(22):2746-2754, 2004. Table from Perry, S., Hockenberry, M., Lowdermilk, D., & Wilson, D. (2010). *Maternal child nursing care* (4th ed., p. 1382). St. Louis: Mosby.

a. Restrict phenylalanine intake; high-protein foods (meats and dairy products) and aspartame are avoided because they contain large amounts of phenylalanine.

b. Monitor physical, neurological, and intellectual development.

c. Stress the importance of follow-up treatment.

d. Encourage the parents to express their feelings about the diagnosis and discuss the risk of phenylketonuria in future children.

e. Educate the parents about use of special preparation formulas and about the foods that contain phenylalanine.

f. Consult with social care services to assist the parents with the financial burdens of purchasing special prepared formulas.

IV. DIABETES MELLITUS

A. Description (Fig. 41-1)

1. Type 1 diabetes mellitus is characterized by the destruction of the pancreatic beta cells, which produce insulin; this results in absolute insulin deficiency.

2. Type 2 diabetes mellitus usually arises because of insulin resistance, in which the body fails to use insulin properly, combined with relative (rather than absolute) insulin deficiency.

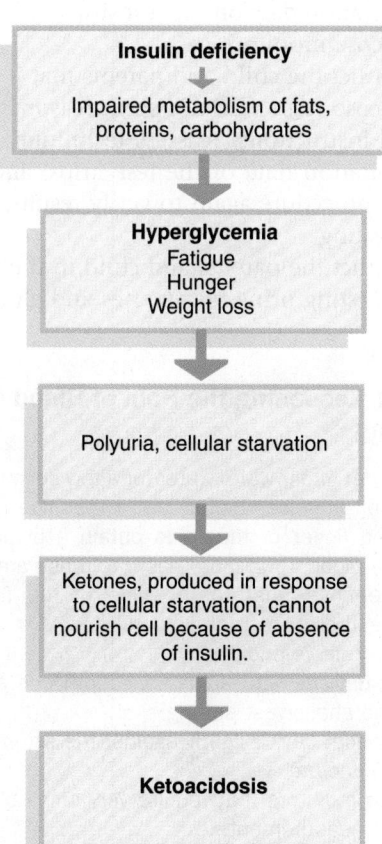

▲ **FIGURE 41-1** Insulin deficiency leading to ketoacidosis. (From McKinney, E., James, S., Murray, S., & Ashwill, J. [2009]. *Maternal-child nursing* [3rd ed.]. St. Louis: Saunders.)

3. Complete insulin deficiency requires the use of exogenous insulin to promote appropriate glucose use and to prevent complications related to elevated blood glucose levels, such as hyperglycemia, diabetic ketoacidosis, and death.

4. Diagnosis is based on the presence of classic symptoms and an elevated blood glucose level (normal blood glucose level is 70 to 110 mg/dL).

5. Children may need to be admitted directly to the pediatric intensive care unit because of the manifestations of diabetic ketoacidosis, which may be the initial occurrence leading to diagnosis of diabetes mellitus.

B. Assessment

1. Polyuria, polydipsia, polyphagia
2. Hyperglycemia
3. Weight loss
4. Unexplained fatigue or lethargy
5. Headaches
6. Stomachaches
7. Occasional enuresis in a previously toilet-trained child
8. Vaginitis in adolescent girls (caused by *Candida*, which thrives in hyperglycemic tissues)
9. Fruity odor to breath
10. Dehydration
11. Blurred vision
12. Slow wound healing
13. Changes in level of consciousness

C. Long-term effects

1. Failure to grow at a normal rate
2. Delayed maturation
3. Recurrent infections
4. Neuropathy
5. Cardiovascular disease
6. Retinal microvascular disease
7. Renal microvascular disease

D. Complications

1. Hypoglycemia
2. Hyperglycemia
3. Diabetic ketoacidosis
4. Coma
5. Hypokalemia
6. Hyperkalemia
7. Microvascular changes
8. Cardiovascular changes

⚠ For a child with diabetes mellitus, plan to initiate a consultation with the diabetic specialist to plan the child's care.

E. Diet

1. Normal healthy nutrition is encouraged, and the total number of calories is individualized based on the child's age and **growth** expectations.

2. As prescribed by the physician, the child may be instructed to follow the dietary guidelines

(MyPyramid) issued by the U.S. Departments of Agriculture and Health and Human Services or the food exchange diet from the American Diabetic Association.

3. Dietary intake should include three well-balanced meals per day, eaten at regular intervals, plus a midafternoon snack and a bedtime snack; a consistent intake of the prescribed protein, fats, and carbohydrates at each meal and snack is needed (concentrated sweets are discouraged).

4. Instruct the child and parents that the child should carry a source of glucose, such as glucose tablets, with him or her at all times to treat hypoglycemia if it occurs.

5. Incorporate the diet into the individual child's needs, likes and dislikes, lifestyle, and cultural and socioeconomic patterns.

6. Allow the child to participate in making food choices to provide a sense of control.

F. Exercise
1. Instruct the child in dietary adjustments when exercising.
2. Extra food needs to be consumed for increased activity, usually 10 to 15 g of carbohydrates for every 30 to 45 minutes of activity.
3. Instruct the child to monitor the blood glucose level before exercising.
4. Plan an appropriate exercise regimen with the child, taking the developmental stage into account.

G. Insulin
1. Diluted insulin may be required for some infants to provide small enough doses to avoid hypoglycemia; diluted insulin should be labeled clearly to avoid dosage errors.
2. Laboratory evaluation of glycosylated hemoglobin should be performed every 3 months.
3. Illness, infection, and stress increase the need for insulin, and insulin should not be withheld during illness, infection, or stress because hyperglycemia and ketoacidosis can result.
4. When the child is not receiving anything by mouth for a special procedure, verify with the physician the need to withhold the morning insulin, and when food, fluids, and insulin are to be resumed.
5. Instruct the child and parents in the administration of insulin.
6. Instruct the child and parents to recognize symptoms of hypoglycemia and hyperglycemia.
7. Instruct the parents in the administration of glucagon intramuscularly or subcutaneously if the child has a hypoglycemic reaction and is unable to consume anything orally (if semiconscious or unconscious).
8. Instruct the child and parents always to have a spare bottle of insulin available.

9. Advise the parents to obtain a Medic-Alert bracelet indicating the type and daily insulin dosage prescribed for the child.
10. See Chapter 55 for information on insulin types, administration sites, and administration procedure.

H. Blood glucose monitoring
1. Results provide information needed to maintain good glycemic control.
2. Blood glucose monitoring is more accurate than urine testing.
3. Monitoring requires that the child prick himself or herself several times a day as prescribed (Box 41-2).
4. Instruct the child and parents about the proper procedure for obtaining the blood glucose level.
5. Inform the child and parents that the procedure must be done precisely to obtain accurate results.
6. Stress the importance of handwashing before and after performing the procedure to prevent infection.
7. Stress the importance of following the manufacturer's instructions for the blood glucose monitoring device.
8. Instruct the child and parents to calibrate the monitor as instructed by the manufacturer.
9. Instruct the child and parents to check the expiration date on the test strips used for blood glucose monitoring.
10. Instruct the child and parents that if the blood glucose results do not seem reasonable, reread the instructions, reassess technique, check the expiration date of the test strips, and perform the procedure again to verify results.

I. Urine testing
1. Instruct the parents and child in the procedure for testing urine for ketones and glucose.

Box 41-2 Lessening the Pain of Blood Glucose Monitoring

Hold the finger under warm water for a few seconds before puncture (enhances blood flow to the finger).

Use the ring finger or thumb to obtain a blood sample because blood flows more easily to these areas; puncture the finger just to the side of the finger pad because there are more blood vessels in this area and fewer nerve endings.

Use lancet devices with adjustable-depth tips and begin using the shallowest setting.

Press the lancet device lightly against the skin to prevent a deep puncture.

Use glucose monitors that require very small blood samples for measurement.

Modified from Perry, S., Hockenberry, M., Lowdermilk, D., & Wilson, D. (2010). *Maternal child nursing care* (4th ed., p. 1627). St. Louis: Mosby.

2. Teach the child that the second voided urine specimen is most accurate.
3. The presence of ketones may indicate impending ketoacidosis.

⚠ Urine glucose testing is an unreliable method of monitoring the glucose level; however, the urine should be tested for ketones when the child is ill or when the blood glucose level is greater than 240 mg/dL.

J. Hypoglycemia
   1. Description
      a. Hypoglycemia is a blood glucose level less than 70 mg/dL.
      b. Hypoglycemia results from too much insulin, not enough food, or excessive activity.
   2. Signs include headache, nausea, sweating, tremors, lethargy, hunger, confusion, slurred speech, tingling around the mouth, and anxiety.
   3. Interventions (Boxes 41-3 and 41-4; see also Priority Nursing Actions)

■■■■ PRIORITY NURSING ACTIONS! ■■■■

Actions to Take When a Hospitalized Child With Diabetes Mellitus Experiences Hypoglycemia
1. Check the child's blood glucose level.
2. Give the child ½ cup of fruit juice or other acceptable item.
3. Take the child's vital signs.
4. Retest the blood glucose level.
5. Give the child a small snack of carbohydrate and protein.
6. Document the child's complaints, actions taken, and outcome.

If a child with diabetes mellitus experiences hypoglycemia, the nurse first would check the child's blood glucose level to verify that the child is experiencing hypoglycemia. When this is verified, the nurse gives the child 10 to 15 g of carbohydrates. The nurse retests the blood glucose level in 15 minutes. In the meantime, the nurse checks the child's vital signs. If the child's symptoms of hypoglycemia do not resolve, the nurse gives the child another 10- to 15-g carbohydrate food item. Otherwise, the nurse provides a small snack of carbohydrates and protein if the child's next scheduled meal is more than 1 hour away from the time of the occurrence. After treatment and resolution of the hypoglycemic event, the nurse documents the occurrence, actions taken, and outcome.

References: Ignatavicius, D., & Workman, M. (2010). *Medical-surgical nursing: Patient-centered collaborative care.* (6th ed., pp. 1507-1508). Philadelphia: Saunders.
Perry, S., Hockenberry, M., Lowdermilk, D., & Wilson, D. (2010). *Maternal child nursing care* (4th ed., pp. 1621, 1624). St. Louis: Mosby.

K. Hyperglycemia
   1. Description: Elevated blood glucose level (>250 mg/dL, or as specified by the physician)
   2. Signs include polydipsia, polyuria, polyphagia, blurred vision, weakness, weight loss, and syncope.
   3. Interventions (Box 41-5)
   4. Sick day rules (Box 41-6)
L. Diabetic ketoacidosis
   1. Description
      a. Diabetic ketoacidosis is a complication of diabetes mellitus that develops when a severe insulin deficiency occurs.

Box 41-3 Interventions for Hypoglycemia

If possible, confirm hypoglycemia with a blood glucose reading.
Administer glucose immediately; rapid-releasing glucose is followed by a complex carbohydrate and protein, such as a slice of bread or a peanut butter cracker.
Give an extra snack if the next meal is not planned for more than 30 minutes or if activity is planned.
If the child becomes unconscious, squeeze cake frosting or glucose paste onto the gums and retest the blood glucose level if the child does not improve within 15 to 20 minutes; if the reading remains low, administer additional glucose.
If the child remains unconscious, the administration of glucagon may be necessary.
In the hospital, prepare to administer dextrose intravenously if the child is unable to consume an oral glucose product.

Box 41-4 Food Items to Treat Hypoglycemia

½ cup orange juice or sugar-sweetened carbonated beverage
8 oz of milk
1 small box of raisins
3 to 4 hard candies
4 sugar cubes (1 tbsp of sugar)
3 to 4 LifeSavers candies
1 candy bar
1 tsp honey
2 or 3 glucose tablets

Box 41-5 Interventions for Hyperglycemia

Instruct the parents to notify the physician when the following occur:
■ Blood glucose results remain elevated (usually >240 mg/dL)
■ Moderate or high ketonuria is present
■ Child is unable to take food or fluids
■ Child vomits more than once
■ Illness persists

b. Diabetic ketoacidosis is a life-threatening condition.

c. Hyperglycemia that progresses to metabolic acidosis occurs.

d. Diabetic ketoacidosis develops over several hours to days.

e. The blood glucose level is greater than 300 mg/dL, and urine and serum ketone tests are positive.

⚠ Manifestations include signs of hyperglycemia, Kussmaul's respirations, acetone (fruity) breath odor, increasing lethargy, and decreasing level of consciousness.

2. Interventions
   a. Restore circulating blood volume, and protect against cerebral, coronary, or renal hypoperfusion.
   b. Correct dehydration with IV infusions of 0.9% or 0.45% saline as prescribed.
   c. Correct hyperglycemia with IV regular insulin administration as prescribed.
   d. Monitor vital signs, urine output, and mental status closely.
   e. Correct acidosis and electrolyte imbalances as prescribed.
   f. Administer oxygen as prescribed.
   g. Monitor blood glucose level frequently.
   h. Monitor potassium level closely because when the child receives insulin to reduce the blood glucose level, the serum potassium level changes; if the potassium level decreases, potassium replacement may be required.
   i. The child should be voiding adequately before administering potassium; if the child does not have an adequate output, hyperkalemia may result.

Box 41-6 Sick Day Rules for a Diabetic Child

Always give insulin, even if the child does not have an appetite, or contact the physician for specific instructions.
Test blood glucose levels at least every 4 hours.
Test for urinary ketones with each voiding.
Notify the physician if moderate or large amounts of urinary ketones are present.
Follow the child's usual meal plan.
Encourage calorie-free liquids to aid in clearing ketones.
Encourage rest, especially if urinary ketones are present.
Notify the physician if vomiting, fruity odor to the breath, deep rapid respirations, decreasing level of consciousness, or persistent hyperglycemia occurs.

Modified from McKinney, E., James, S., Murray, S., & Ashwill, J. (2009). *Maternal-child nursing* (3rd ed., p. 1451). St. Louis: Saunders.

---

j. Monitor the child closely for signs of fluid overload.

k. IV dextrose is added as prescribed when the blood glucose reaches an appropriate level.

l. Treat the cause of hyperglycemia.

💿 **MORE QUESTIONS ON THE CD!**

Practice Questions

417. A school-age child with type 1 diabetes mellitus has soccer practice three afternoons a week. The school nurse provides instructions regarding how to prevent hypoglycemia during practice. The school nurse tells the child to:
1. Eat twice the amount normally eaten at lunch time.
2. Take half the amount of prescribed insulin on practice days.
3. Take the prescribed insulin at noontime rather than in the morning.
4. Eat a small box of raisins or drink a cup of orange juice before soccer practice.

418. The mother of a 6-year-old child who has type 1 diabetes mellitus calls a clinic nurse and tells the nurse that the child has been sick. The mother reports that she checked the child's urine and it was positive for ketones. The nurse instructs the mother to:
1. Hold the next dose of insulin.
2. Come to the clinic immediately.
3. Administer an additional dose of regular insulin.
4. Encourage the child to drink calorie-free liquids.

419. A physician prescribes an IV solution of 5% dextrose and half-normal saline (0.45%) with 40 mEq of potassium chloride for a child with hypotonic dehydration. The nurse performs which priority assessment before administering this IV prescription?
1. Obtains a weight
2. Takes the temperature
3. Takes the blood pressure
4. Checks the amount of urine output

420. An adolescent client with type 1 diabetes mellitus is admitted to the emergency department for treatment of diabetic ketoacidosis. Which assessment findings should the nurse expect to note?
1. Sweating and tremors
2. Hunger and hypertension
3. Cold, clammy skin and irritability
4. Fruity breath odor and decreasing level of consciousness

421. A mother brings her 3-week-old infant to a clinic for a phenylketonuria rescreening blood test. The test indicates a serum phenylalanine level of 1 mg/dL. The nurse interprets this result as:
1. Positive
2. Negative
3. Inconclusive
4. Requiring rescreening at age 6 weeks

422. A child has fluid volume deficit. The nurse performs an assessment and determines that the child is improving and the deficit is resolving if:
1. The child has no tears.
2. Urine specific gravity is 1.030.
3. Urine output is less than 1 mL/kg/hr.
4. Capillary refill is less than 2 seconds.

423. A child with type 1 diabetes mellitus is brought to the emergency department by the mother, who states that the child has been complaining of abdominal pain and has a fruity odor of the breath. Diabetic ketoacidosis is diagnosed. Anticipating the plan of care, the nurse prepares to administer:
1. Potassium IV infusion.
2. NPH insulin IV infusion.
3. 5% dextrose IV infusion.
4. Normal saline IV infusion.

424. A nurse has just administered acetaminophen (Tylenol) to a child with a temperature of 38.8° C (102° F). The nurse should also take which action?
1. Withhold oral fluids for 8 hours.
2. Sponge the child with cold water.
3. Plan to administer salicylate (aspirin) in 4 hours.
4. Remove excess clothing and blankets from the child.

Alternate Item Format: Multiple Response
425. The nurse would implement which interventions for a child older than 2 years with type 1 diabetes mellitus who has a blood glucose level of 60 mg/dL? **Select all that apply.**
❑ 1. Administer regular insulin.
❑ 2. Encourage the child to ambulate.
❑ 3. Give the child a teaspoon of honey.
❑ 4. Provide electrolyte replacement therapy intravenously.
❑ 5. Wait 30 minutes and confirm the blood glucose reading.
❑ 6. Prepare to administer glucagon subcutaneously if unconsciousness occurs.

ANSWERS
417. 4
Rationale: Hypoglycemia is a blood glucose level less than 70 mg/dL and results from too much insulin, not enough food, or excessive activity. An extra snack of 15 to 30 g of carbohydrates eaten before activities such as soccer practice would prevent hypoglycemia. A small box of raisins or a cup of orange juice provides 15 to 30 g of carbohydrates. The child or parents should not be instructed to adjust the amount or time of insulin administration. Meal amounts should not be doubled.
Test-Taking Strategy: Use general medication guidelines to eliminate options 2 and 3 first because insulin doses and times should not be adjusted. From the remaining options, recalling the definition of hypoglycemia and the manifestations and treatment associated with hypoglycemia will direct you to option 4. Review treatment to prevent hypoglycemia if you had difficulty with this question.
Level of Cognitive Ability: Applying
Client Needs: Physiological Integrity
Integrated Process: Teaching and Learning
Content Area: Child Health—Metabolic/Endocrine
Reference: Hockenberry, M., & Wilson, D. (2009). *Wong's essentials of pediatric nursing* (8th ed., p. 1052). St. Louis: Mosby.

418. 4
Rationale: When the child is sick, the mother should test for urinary ketones with each voiding. If ketones are present, liquids are essential to aid in clearing the ketones. The child should be encouraged to drink calorie-free liquids. Bringing the child to the clinic immediately is unnecessary. Insulin doses should not be adjusted or changed.
Test-Taking Strategy: Use general medication guidelines. Eliminate options 1 and 3 first because insulin doses should not be adjusted or changed. From the remaining options, note the words *positive for ketones*. Recalling that liquids are essential to aid in clearing the ketones will direct you to the correct option. Review home care instructions for a sick diabetic child if you had difficulty with this question.
Level of Cognitive Ability: Applying
Client Needs: Physiological Integrity
Integrated Process: Nursing Process—Implementation
Content Area: Child Health—Metabolic/Endocrine
Reference: McKinney, E., James, S., Murray, S., & Ashwill, J. (2009). *Maternal-child nursing* (3rd ed., p. 1451). St. Louis: Saunders.

419. 4
Rationale: In hypotonic dehydration, electrolyte loss exceeds water loss. The priority assessment before administering potassium chloride intravenously would be to assess the status of the urine output. Potassium chloride should never be administered in the presence of oliguria or anuria. If the urine output is less than 1 to 2 mL/kg/hr, potassium chloride should not be administered. Although options 1, 2, and 3 are appropriate assessments for a child with dehydration, these assessments are not related specifically to the IV administration of potassium chloride.

Test-Taking Strategy: Focus on the IV prescription. Recalling that the kidneys play a key role in the excretion and reabsorption of potassium will direct you to option 4. Review the nursing considerations when administering potassium chloride if you had difficulty with this question.
Level of Cognitive Ability: Analyzing
Client Needs: Physiological Integrity
Integrated Process: Nursing Process—Assessment
Content Area: Child Health—Metabolic/Endocrine
Reference: McKinney, E., James, S., Murray, S., & Ashwill, J. (2009). *Maternal-child nursing* (3rd ed., p. 1076). St. Louis: Saunders.

420. 4
Rationale: Diabetic ketoacidosis is a complication of diabetes mellitus that develops when a severe insulin deficiency occurs. Hyperglycemia occurs with diabetic ketoacidosis. Signs of hyperglycemia include fruity breath odor and a decreasing level of consciousness. Hunger can be a sign of hypoglycemia or hyperglycemia, but hypertension is not a sign of diabetic ketoacidosis. Hypotension occurs because of a decrease in blood volume related to the dehydrated state that occurs during diabetic ketoacidosis. Cold clammy skin, irritability, sweating, and tremors all are signs of hypoglycemia.
Test-Taking Strategy: Focus on the subject, the signs of diabetic ketoacidosis, and recall that in this condition the blood glucose level is elevated. Eliminate options 1, 2, and 3 because these signs do not occur with hyperglycemia. Recall that fruity breath odor and a change in the level of consciousness can occur during diabetic ketoacidosis. Review the signs and symptoms of hypoglycemia and hyperglycemia and the signs of diabetic ketoacidosis if you had difficulty with this question.
Level of Cognitive Ability: Analyzing
Client Needs: Physiological Integrity
Integrated Process: Nursing Process—Assessment
Content Area: Child Health—Metabolic/Endocrine
Reference: Swearingen, P. (2008). *All-in-one care planning resource: Medical-surgical, pediatric, maternity, & psychiatric nursing care plans* (2nd ed., p. 387). St. Louis: Mosby.

421. 2
Rationale: Phenylketonuria is a genetic disorder (autosomal recessive disorder) that results in central nervous system damage from toxic levels of phenylalanine (an essential amino acid) in the blood. It is characterized by blood phenylalanine levels greater than 20 mg/dL (normal level is 1.2 to 3.4 mg/dL in newborns and 0.8 to 1.8 mg/dL thereafter). A result of 1 mg/dL is a negative test result.
Test-Taking Strategy: Use the process of elimination. Eliminate options 3 and 4 first because they are comparable or alike. Note that the level identified in the question is a low level; this should assist in directing you to option 2. Review the phenylketonuria screening test if you had difficulty with this question.
Level of Cognitive Ability: Understanding
Client Needs: Physiological Integrity
Integrated Process: Nursing Process—Assessment
Content Area: Child Health—Metabolic/Endocrine
Reference: McKinney, E., James, S., Murray, S., & Ashwill, J. (2009). *Maternal-child nursing* (3rd ed., p. 1425). St. Louis: Saunders.

422. 4
Rationale: Indicators that fluid volume deficit is resolving would be capillary refill less than 2 seconds, specific gravity of 1.002 to 1.025, urine output of at least 1 mL/kg/hr, and adequate tear production. A capillary refill time less than 2 seconds is the only indicator that the child is improving. Urine output of less than 1 mL/kg/hr, a specific gravity of 1.030, and no tears would indicate that the deficit is not resolving.
Test-Taking Strategy: Focus on the subject, that the fluid volume deficit is resolving. Recall the parameters that indicate adequate hydration status. The only option that indicates an improving fluid balance is option 4. The other options indicate fluid imbalance. Review the normal parameters for fluid balance if you had difficulty with this question.
Level of Cognitive Ability: Evaluating
Client Needs: Physiological Integrity
Integrated Process: Nursing Process—Evaluation
Content Area: Child Health—Metabolic/Endocrine
Reference: McKinney, E., James, S., Murray, S., & Ashwill, J. (2009). *Maternal-child nursing* (3rd ed., p. 1073). St. Louis: Saunders.

423. 4
Rationale: Diabetic ketoacidosis is a complication of diabetes mellitus that develops when a severe insulin deficiency occurs. Hyperglycemia occurs with diabetic ketoacidosis. Rehydration is the initial step in resolving diabetic ketoacidosis. Normal saline is the initial IV rehydration fluid. NPH insulin is never administered by the IV route. Dextrose solutions are added to the treatment when the blood glucose level decreases to an acceptable level. Intravenously administered potassium may be required, depending on the potassium level, but would not be part of the initial treatment.
Test-Taking Strategy: Use the process of elimination. Eliminate option 3, knowing that dextrose would not be administered in a hyperglycemic state. Eliminate option 2 next, knowing that NPH insulin is never administered by the IV route. Recalling that hydration is the initial treatment in diabetic ketoacidosis will direct you to option 4. Review the treatment for diabetic ketoacidosis if you had difficulty with this question.
Level of Cognitive Ability: Analyzing
Client Needs: Physiological Integrity
Integrated Process: Nursing Process—Planning
Content Area: Child Health—Metabolic/Endocrine
Reference: McKinney, E., James, S., Murray, S., & Ashwill, J. (2009). *Maternal-child nursing* (3rd ed., p. 1452). St. Louis: Saunders.

424. 4
Rationale: After administering acetaminophen, excess clothing and blankets should be removed. The child can be sponged with tepid water, but not cold water because the cold water can cause shivering, which increases metabolic requirements above those already caused by the fever. Aspirin is not administered to a child with fever because of the risk of Reye's syndrome. Fluids should be encouraged to prevent dehydration, so oral fluids should not be withheld.
Test-Taking Strategy: Use the process of elimination and remember that cooling measures such as removing excess clothing should be done when a child has a fever. Options

1, 2, and 3 would not be done if a child has a fever. Review interventions to reduce an elevated temperature if you had difficulty with this question.
Level of Cognitive Ability: Applying
Client Needs: Physiological Integrity
Integrated Process: Nursing Process—Implementation
Content Area: Child Health—Metabolic/Endocrine
References: Hockenberry, M., & Wilson, D. (2009). *Wong's essentials of pediatric nursing* (8th ed., p. 704). St. Louis: Mosby.

McKinney, E., James, S., Murray, S., & Ashwill, J. (2009). *Maternal-child nursing* (3rd ed., p. 941). St. Louis: Saunders.

ALTERNATE ITEM FORMAT: MULTIPLE RESPONSE
425. 3, 6
Rationale: Hypoglycemia is defined as a blood glucose level less than 70 mg/dL. Hypoglycemia occurs as a result of too much insulin, not enough food, or excessive activity. If possible, the nurse should confirm hypoglycemia with a blood glucose reading. Glucose is administered orally immediately; rapid-releasing glucose is followed by a complex carbohydrate and protein, such as a slice of bread or a peanut butter cracker. An extra snack is given if the next meal is not planned for more than 30 minutes or if activity is planned. If the child becomes unconscious, cake frosting or glucose paste is squeezed onto the gums, and the blood glucose level is retested if the child does not improve in 15 minutes; if the reading remains low, additional glucose is administered. If the child remains unconscious, administration of glucagon may be necessary, and the nurse should be prepared for this intervention. Encouraging the child to ambulate and administering regular insulin would result in a lowered blood glucose level. Providing electrolyte replacement therapy intravenously is an intervention to treat diabetic ketoacidosis. Waiting 30 minutes to confirm the blood glucose level delays necessary intervention.
Test-Taking Strategy: Focus on the information in the question. Think about the pathophysiology associated with hypoglycemia. Recalling that a blood glucose level of 60 mg/dL indicates hypoglycemia will assist in determining the correct interventions. Review the interventions for hypoglycemia if you had difficulty with this question.
Level of Cognitive Ability: Applying
Client Needs: Physiological Integrity
Integrated Process: Nursing Process—Implementation
Content Area: Child Health—Metabolic/Endocrine
References: Hockenberry, M., & Wilson, D. (2009). *Wong's essentials of pediatric nursing* (8th ed., pp. 1047–1048). St. Louis: Mosby.

McKinney, E., James, S., Murray, S., & Ashwill, J. (2009). *Maternal-child nursing* (3rd ed., pp. 1448–1449). St. Louis: Saunders.

Renal and Urinary Disorders

I. GLOMERULONEPHRITIS

A. Description
1. Glomerulonephritis refers to a group of kidney disorders characterized by inflammatory injury in the glomerulus, most of which are caused by an immunological reaction.
2. The disorder results in proliferative and inflammatory changes within the glomerular structure.
3. Destruction, inflammation, and sclerosis of the glomeruli of the kidneys occur.
4. Inflammation of the glomeruli results from an antigen-antibody reaction produced by an infection elsewhere in the body.
5. Loss of kidney function develops.

B. Causes
1. Immunological diseases
2. Autoimmune diseases
3. Antecedent group A beta-hemolytic streptococcal infection of the pharynx or skin
4. History of pharyngitis or tonsillitis 2 to 3 weeks before symptoms

C. Types (Box 42-1)

D. Complications
1. Renal failure
2. Hypertensive encephalopathy
3. Pulmonary edema
4. Heart failure

E. Assessment
1. Periorbital and facial edema that is more prominent in the morning
2. Anorexia
3. Decreased urinary output
4. Cloudy, smoky, brown-colored urine (hematuria)
5. Pallor, irritability, lethargy
6. In an older child: Headaches, abdominal or flank pain, dysuria
7. Hypertension
8. Proteinuria that produces a persistent and excessive foam in the urine
9. Azotemia
10. Increased blood urea nitrogen and creatinine levels

11. Increased antistreptolysin O titer (used to diagnose disorders caused by streptococcal infections)

F. Interventions
1. Monitor vital signs, weight, intake and output, and characteristics of urine.
2. Limit activity; provide safety measures.
3. Provide high-quality nutrient foods.
   a. Restrictions depend on the stage and severity of the disease, especially the extent of the edema.
   b. In uncomplicated cases, a regular diet is permitted, but sodium is restricted to a "no added salt to foods" diet.
   c. Moderate sodium and fluid restriction is prescribed for a child with hypertension or edema.
   d. Foods high in potassium are restricted during periods of oliguria.
   e. Protein is restricted if the child has severe azotemia resulting from prolonged oliguria.
4. Monitor for complications (e.g., renal failure, hypertensive encephalopathy, seizures, pulmonary edema, heart failure).
5. Administer diuretics (if significant edema and fluid overload are present), antihypertensives (for hypertension), and antibiotics (to a child with evidence of persistent streptococcal infections) as prescribed.
6. Initiate seizure precautions and administer anticonvulsants as prescribed for seizures associated with hypertensive encephalopathy.
7. Instruct parents to report signs of bloody urine, headache, or edema.
8. Instruct parents that the child needs to obtain appropriate adequate treatment for infections, specifically for sore throats, upper respiratory infections, and skin infections.

⚠ Measuring the daily weight and assessing for changes is the most useful and effective measure for determining fluid balance.

II. NEPHROTIC SYNDROME

A. Description

1. Nephrotic syndrome is a kidney disorder characterized by massive proteinuria, hypoalbuminemia (hypoproteinemia), and edema (Fig. 42-1).

2. The primary objectives of therapeutic management are to reduce the excretion of urinary protein, maintain protein-free urine, reduce edema, prevent infection, and minimize complications.

B. Assessment (Box 42-2)

⚠ The classic manifestations of nephrotic syndrome are massive proteinuria, hypoalbuminemia, and edema.

Box 42-1 Types of Glomerulonephritis

Acute	Occurs 2 to 3 weeks after a streptococcal infection
Chronic	Can occur after the acute phase or slowly over time

C. Interventions

1. Monitor vital signs, intake and output, and daily weights.

2. Monitor urine for specific gravity and protein.

3. Monitor for edema.

4. Nutrition: A regular diet without added salt may be prescribed if the child is in remission; sodium is restricted during periods of massive edema (fluids may also be restricted).

Box 42-2 Assessment Findings in Nephrotic Syndrome

Child gains weight
Periorbital and facial edema most prominent in the morning
Leg, ankle, labial, or scrotal edema
Urine output decreases; urine dark and frothy
Ascites (fluid in abdominal cavity)
Blood pressure normal or slightly decreased
Lethargy, anorexia, and pallor
Massive proteinuria
Decreased serum protein (hypoproteinemia) and elevated serum lipid levels

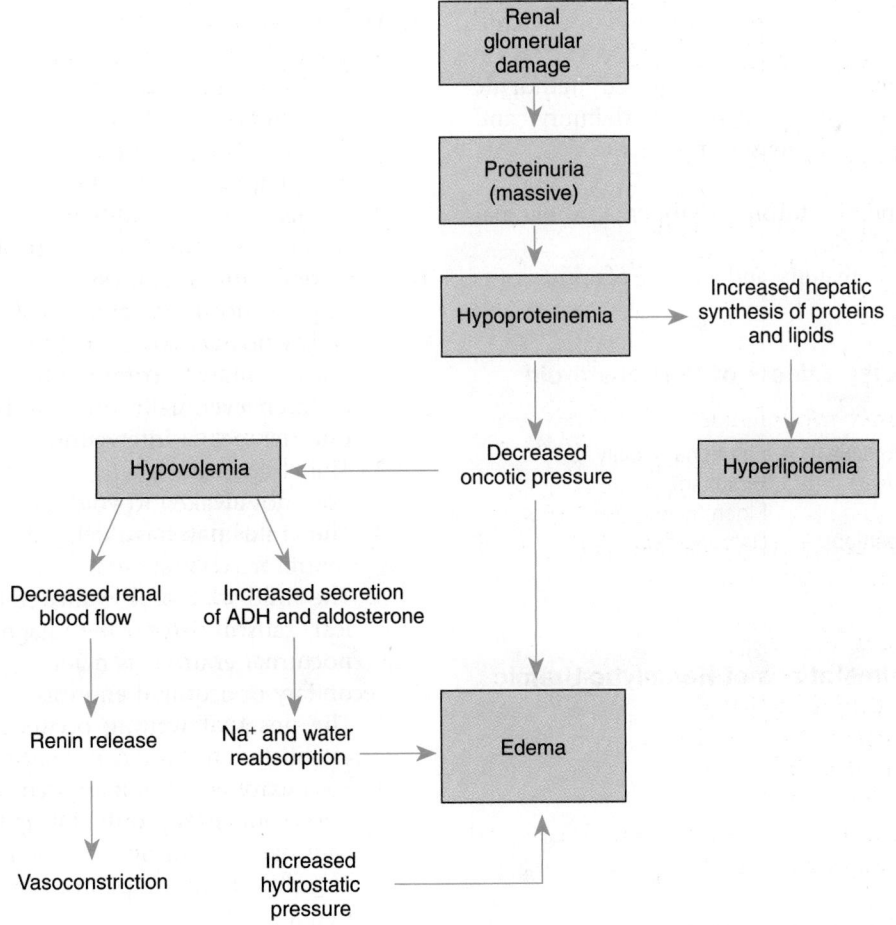

▲ **FIGURE 42-1** Sequence of events in nephrotic syndrome. (From Perry, S., Hockenberry, M., Lowdermilk, D., & Wilson, D. [2010]. *Maternal child nursing care* [4th ed.]. St. Louis: Mosby.)

5. Corticosteroid therapy is prescribed as soon as the diagnosis has been determined; monitor the child closely for signs of infection and other adverse effects (Box 42-3).
6. Immunosuppressant therapy may be prescribed to reduce the relapse rate and induce long-term remission, or, if the child is nonresponsive to corticosteroid therapy, therapy may be administered along with the corticosteroid.
7. Diuretics may be prescribed to reduce edema.
8. Plasma expanders such as salt-poor human albumin may be prescribed for a severely edematous child.
9. Instruct parents about testing the urine for protein, medication administration, side effects of medications, and general care of the child.
10. Instruct parents regarding the signs of infection and the need to avoid contact with other children who may be infectious.

III. HEMOLYTIC-UREMIC SYNDROME

A. Description
1. Hemolytic-uremic syndrome is thought to be associated with bacterial toxins, chemicals, and viruses that cause acute renal failure in children.
2. It occurs primarily in infants and small children 6 months to 5 years old.
3. Clinical features include acquired hemolytic anemia, thrombocytopenia, renal injury, and central nervous system symptoms.

B. Assessment
1. Triad of anemia, thrombocytopenia, and renal failure (Box 42-4)
2. Proteinuria, hematuria, and presence of urinary casts

Box 42-3 Adverse Effects of Corticosteroid Therapy

Impaired wound healing	Emotional lability
Hyperglycemia	Hirsutism
Skin fragility	Moon facies
Abnormal fat deposition	Osteoporosis

Box 42-4 Manifestations of Hemolytic-Uremic Syndrome

Vomiting
Irritability
Lethargy
Marked pallor
Hemorrhagic manifestations: Bruising, petechiae, jaundice, bloody diarrhea
Oliguria or anuria
Central nervous system involvement: Seizures, stupor, coma

3. Blood urea nitrogen and serum creatinine levels elevated; hemoglobin and hematocrit levels decreased.

C. Interventions
1. Hemodialysis or peritoneal dialysis may be prescribed if a child is anuric.
   a. Hemodialysis requires venous access (e.g., an arteriovenous fistula), and treatment is usually 3 to 8 hours in length (three times per week); peritoneal dialysis requires surgical placement of an abdominal catheter (correction of fluid and electrolyte imbalance is slower with peritoneal dialysis than hemodialysis).
   b. Dialysate solution is prescribed to meet the child's electrolyte needs.
2. Strict monitoring of fluid balance is necessary; fluid restrictions may be prescribed if the child is anuric.
3. Institute measures to prevent infection.
4. Provide adequate nutrition.
5. Other treatments include medications to treat manifestations and the administration of blood products to treat severe anemia (administered with caution to prevent fluid overload).

IV. ENURESIS

A. Description
1. Enuresis refers to a condition in which a child is unable to control bladder function, even though the child has reached an age at which control of voiding is expected or the child has successfully completed a bladder control program.
2. By age 5, most children are aware of bladder fullness and are able to control voiding.

B. Primary nocturnal enuresis
1. Primary nocturnal enuresis is bed-wetting in a child who has never been dry for extended periods.
2. The condition is common in children, and most children eventually outgrow bed-wetting without therapeutic intervention.
3. The child is unable to sense a full bladder and does not awaken to void.
4. The child may have delayed maturation of the central nervous system.
5. The child should be evaluated for any pathological causes before the diagnosis of primary nocturnal enuresis is made.

C. Secondary or acquired enuresis
1. The onset of wetting occurs after a period of established urinary continence.
2. Secondary enuresis may occur during nighttime sleep (nocturnal), only during the waking hours (diurnal), or during daytime and nighttime.
3. The child may complain of dysuria, urgency, or frequency.
4. The child should be assessed for urinary tract infections.

D. Assessment: History of bed-wetting with no extended period of dryness in a child older than age 5 years

E. Interventions

1. Perform urinalysis and urine culture as prescribed to rule out infection or an existing disorder.
2. Assist the family with identifying a treatment plan that best fits the needs of the child.
3. Limit fluid intake at night, and encourage the child to void just before going to bed.
4. Involve the child in caring for the wet sheets and changing the bed to assist the child to take ownership of the problem.
5. Provide reward systems as appropriate for the child.
6. Incorporate behavioral conditioning techniques.
7. Encourage follow-up to determine the effectiveness of the treatment.

V. CRYPTORCHIDISM

A. Description: Cryptorchidism is a condition in which one or both testes fail to descend through the inguinal canal into the scrotal sac.

B. Assessment: Testes are not palpable or easily guided into the scrotum.

C. Interventions

1. Monitor during the first 12 months of life to determine whether spontaneous descent occurs.
2. After age 1 year, medical or surgical treatment may be instituted.
3. Human chorionic gonadotropin, a pituitary hormone that stimulates the production of testosterone, may be prescribed for an older child.
4. Surgical correction, if needed, is done by orchiopexy before the child's second birthday (preferably between 1 and 2 years of age) if the testes do not descend spontaneously.
5. Monitor for bleeding and infection postoperatively.
6. Instruct parents in postoperative home care measures, including preventing infection, pain control, and activity restrictions.
7. Provide an opportunity for parental counseling if the parents are concerned about the future fertility of the child.

VI. EPISPADIAS AND HYPOSPADIAS (Fig. 42-2)

A. Description

1. Epispadias and hypospadias are congenital defects involving abnormal placement of the urethral orifice of the penis.
2. These anatomical defects can lead to the easy entry of bacteria into the urine.

B. Assessment

1. Epispadias: Urethral orifice is located on the dorsal surface of the penis; the condition often occurs with exstrophy of the bladder.

2. Hypospadias: Urethral orifice is located below the glans penis along the ventral surface.

C. Surgical interventions: Surgery is done before the age of toilet training, preferably between 16 and 18 months of age.

⚠ Circumcision is not performed on a newborn with epispadias or hypospadias because the foreskin may be used in surgical reconstruction of the defect.

D. Postoperative interventions

1. The child has a pressure dressing and may have some type of urinary diversion or a urinary stent (used to maintain patency of the urethral opening) while the meatus is healing.
2. Monitor vital signs.
3. Encourage fluid intake to maintain adequate urine output and maintain patency of the stent.
4. Monitor intake and output and the urine for cloudiness or a foul odor.
5. Notify the physician if there is no urinary output for 1 hour because this may indicate kinks

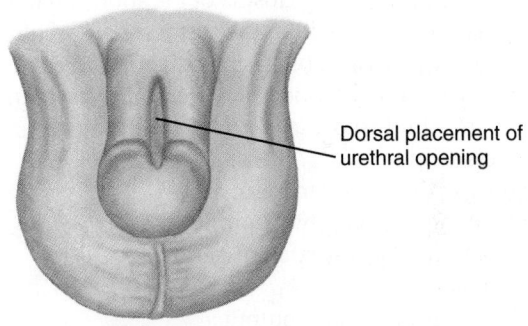

Epispadias

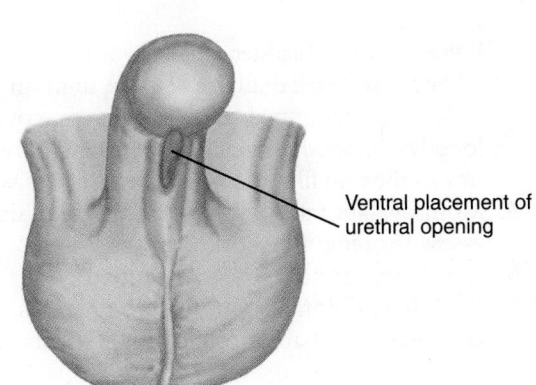

Hypospadias

▲ **FIGURE 42-2** Epispadias and hypospadias are genital anomalies in which the urethral opening is above or below its normal location on the glans of the penis. (From James, S., Ashwill, J., & Droske, S. [2007]. *Nursing care of children: Principles and practice* [3rd ed.]. St. Louis: Saunders.)

in the urinary diversion or stent or obstruction by sediment.

6. Provide pain medication or medication to relieve bladder spasms (anticholinergic) as prescribed.
7. Administer antibiotics as prescribed.
8. Instruct parents in the care of the child who has a urinary diversion or stent.
9. Instruct parents to avoid giving the child a tub bath until the stent, if present, is removed.
10. Instruct parents about fluid intake, medication administration, signs and symptoms of infection, and need for physician follow-up for dressing removal after surgery as prescribed.

VII. BLADDER EXSTROPHY

A. Description
1. Bladder exstrophy is a congenital anomaly characterized by extrusion of the urinary bladder to the outside of the body through a defect in the lower abdominal wall.
2. The cause is unknown.
3. Treatment requires surgical management and occurs in a series of staged reconstructions.
4. Initial surgery for closure of the abdominal defect should occur within the first few days of life.
5. The goal of subsequent surgeries is to reconstruct the bladder and genitalia and enable the child to achieve urinary continence.

B. Assessment
1. Exposed bladder mucosa
2. Widened symphysis pubis
3. Defects of the external genitalia

C. Interventions
1. Monitor urinary output.
2. Monitor for signs of urinary tract or wound infection.
3. Maintain the integrity of the exposed bladder mucosa.
4. Prevent the bladder tissue from drying, while allowing the drainage of urine, until surgical closure is performed; the bladder is covered loosely with sterile, nonadherent clear plastic wrap or a sterile thin film dressing without adhesive.
5. Monitor laboratory values and urinalysis to assess for renal function.
6. Administer antibiotics as prescribed.
7. Provide emotional support to the parents, and encourage verbalization of their fears and concerns.

 Applying petroleum jelly to the bladder mucosa is avoided because it tends to dry out, adhere to the bladder mucosa, and damage the delicate tissues when the dressing is removed.

 MORE QUESTIONS ON THE CD!

Practice Questions

426. A nurse is assigned to care for a child suspected to have glomerulonephritis. The nurse reviews the child's record and notes that which finding is associated with the diagnosis of glomerulonephritis?
1. Hypotension
2. Brown-colored urine
3. Low urinary specific gravity
4. Low blood urea nitrogen level

427. A nurse is performing an admission assessment on a 2-year-old child who has been diagnosed with nephrotic syndrome. The nurse understands that the most common characteristic associated with nephrotic syndrome is:
1. Hypertension
2. Generalized edema
3. Increased urinary output
4. Frank, bright red blood in the urine

428. A nurse is planning care for a child with hemolytic-uremic syndrome. The child has been anuric and will be receiving peritoneal dialysis treatment. The nurse plans to:
1. Restrict fluids as prescribed.
2. Encourage foods high in potassium.
3. Administer analgesics as prescribed.
4. Care for the arteriovenous fistula.

429. A 7-year-old child is seen in a clinic, and the primary health care provider documents a diagnosis of primary nocturnal enuresis. When the mother asks a nurse about the diagnosis, the nurse plans to respond knowing that:
1. Primary nocturnal enuresis does not respond to treatment.
2. Primary nocturnal enuresis is caused by a psychiatric problem.
3. Primary nocturnal enuresis requires surgical intervention to improve the problem.
4. Most children outgrow the bed-wetting problem without therapeutic intervention.

430. A nurse has provided discharge instructions to the mother of a 2-year-old child who had an orchiopexy to correct cryptorchidism. Which statement by the mother of the child indicates that further teaching is necessary?
1. "I'll check his temperature."
2. "I'll give him medication so he'll be comfortable."

3. "I'll check his voiding to be sure there's no problem."
4. "I'll let him decide when to return to his play activities."

431. A nurse collects a urine specimen preoperatively from a child with epispadias who is scheduled for surgical repair. When the nurse is analyzing the results of the urinalysis, which of the following would the nurse most likely expect to note?
1. Hematuria
2. Proteinuria
3. Bacteriuria
4. Glucosuria

432. A nurse is reviewing a treatment plan with the parents of a newborn infant with hypospadias. Which statement by the parents indicates their understanding of the plan?
1. "Caution should be used when straddling the infant on a hip."
2. "Vital signs should be taken daily to check for bladder infection."
3. "Catheterization will be necessary when the infant does not void."
4. "Circumcision has been delayed to save tissue for surgical repair."

433. A nurse is caring for an infant with a diagnosis of bladder exstrophy. To protect the exposed bladder tissue, the nurse plans to:
1. Cover the bladder with petroleum jelly gauze.
2. Cover the bladder with a nonadhering plastic wrap.
3. Apply sterile distilled water dressings over the bladder mucosa.
4. Keep the bladder tissue dry by covering it with dry sterile gauze.

434. A nurse interviews the parents of a child recently diagnosed with glomerulonephritis. The nurse understands that which information collected during the assessment most often is associated with the diagnosis of glomerulonephritis?
1. Child fell off a bike onto the handlebars
2. Nausea and vomiting for the last 24 hours
3. Urticaria and itching for 1 week before diagnosis
4. Streptococcal throat infection 2 weeks before diagnosis

Alternate Item Format: Multiple Response

435. A nurse is performing an assessment on a child admitted to the hospital with a probable diagnosis of nephrotic syndrome. What assessment findings would the nurse expect to observe? **Select all that apply.**
❑ 1. Pallor
❑ 2. Edema
❑ 3. Anorexia
❑ 4. Proteinuria
❑ 5. Weight loss
❑ 6. Decreased serum lipids

ANSWERS
426. 2
Rationale: Glomerulonephritis refers to a group of kidney disorders characterized by inflammatory injury in the glomerulus. Gross hematuria, resulting in dark, smoky, cola-colored or brown-colored urine, is a classic symptom of glomerulonephritis. Hypertension is also common. Blood urea nitrogen levels may be elevated. A moderately elevated to high urinary specific gravity is associated with glomerulonephritis.
Test-Taking Strategy: Use the process of elimination. Eliminate options 1 and 3 first because hypertension and a high specific gravity are most likely to occur in this kidney disorder. Recalling that this is a renal disorder and that blood urea nitrogen levels increase will assist in directing you to option 2. If you had difficulty with this question, review the clinical manifestations associated with glomerulonephritis.
Level of Cognitive Ability: Analyzing
Client Needs: Physiological Integrity
Integrated Process: Nursing Process—Assessment
Content Area: Child Health—Gastrointestinal/Renal
Reference: Hockenberry, M., & Wilson, D. (2009). *Wong's essentials of pediatric nursing* (8th ed., p. 961). St. Louis: Mosby.

427. 2
Rationale: Nephrotic syndrome is defined as massive proteinuria, hypoalbuminemia, hyperlipemia, and edema. Other manifestations include weight gain; periorbital and facial edema that is most prominent in the morning; leg, ankle, labial, or scrotal edema; decreased urine output and urine that is dark and frothy; abdominal swelling; and blood pressure that is normal or slightly decreased.
Test-Taking Strategy: Recall the pathophysiology associated with nephrotic syndrome. Associate edema with nephrotic syndrome. This will help you answer questions similar to this one. If you had difficulty with this question, review the manifestations of nephrotic syndrome.
Level of Cognitive Ability: Understanding
Client Needs: Physiological Integrity
Integrated Process: Nursing Process—Assessment
Content Area: Child Health—Gastrointestinal/Renal
Reference: Perry, S., Hockenberry, M., Lowdermilk, D., & Wilson, D. (2010). *Maternal child nursing care* (4th ed., p. 1537). St. Louis: Mosby.

428. 1
Rationale: Hemolytic-uremic syndrome is thought to be associated with bacterial toxins, chemicals, and viruses that cause

acute renal failure in children. Clinical manifestations of the disease include acquired hemolytic anemia, thrombocytopenia, renal injury, and central nervous system symptoms. A child with hemolytic-uremic syndrome undergoing peritoneal dialysis because of anuria would be on fluid restriction. Pain is not associated with hemolytic-uremic syndrome, and potassium would be restricted, not encouraged, if the child is anuric. Peritoneal dialysis does not require an arteriovenous fistula (only hemodialysis).

Test-Taking Strategy: Focus on the child's diagnosis and recall knowledge about the care of a client with acute renal failure. Also focus on the data in the question. Noting the word *peritoneal* will assist in eliminating option 4. From the remaining options, remember that because the child is anuric, fluids will be restricted. Review care of the child with hemolytic-uremic syndrome if this question was difficult.

Level of Cognitive Ability: Analyzing
Client Needs: Physiological Integrity
Integrated Process: Nursing Process—Planning
Content Area: Child Health—Gastrointestinal/Renal
Reference: McKinney, E., James, S., Murray, S., & Ashwill, J. (2009). *Maternal-child nursing* (3rd ed., p. 1163). St. Louis: Saunders.

429. 4

Rationale: Primary nocturnal enuresis occurs in a child who has never been dry at night for extended periods. The condition is common in children, and most children eventually outgrow bed-wetting without therapeutic intervention. The child is unable to sense a full bladder and does not awaken to void. The child may have delayed maturation of the central nervous system. The condition is not caused by a psychiatric problem.

Test-Taking Strategy: Use the process of elimination, noting the relationship between the words *enuresis* in the question and *bed-wetting* in the correct option. If you had difficulty with this question, review the characteristics associated with enuresis.

Level of Cognitive Ability: Understanding
Client Needs: Physiological Integrity
Integrated Process: Nursing Process—Planning
Content Area: Child Health—Gastrointestinal/Renal
Reference: Hockenberry, M., & Wilson, D. (2009). *Wong's essentials of pediatric nursing* (8th ed., p. 537). St. Louis: Mosby.

430. 4

Rationale: Cryptorchidism is a condition in which one or both testes fail to descend through the inguinal canal into the scrotal sac. Surgical correction may be necessary. All vigorous activities should be restricted for 2 weeks after surgery to promote healing and prevent injury. This prevents dislodging of the suture, which is internal. Normally, 2-year-olds want to be active; allowing the child to decide when to return to his play activities may prevent healing and cause injury. The parent should be taught to monitor the temperature, provide analgesics as needed, and monitor the urine output.

Test-Taking Strategy: Note the strategic words *further teaching is necessary*. These words indicate a negative event query and ask you to select an option that is an incorrect statement.

Option 1 is an important action to recognize signs of infection. Option 2 is appropriate to keep pain to a minimum. Option 3 monitors voiding pattern, which is also important after this type of surgery. If you had difficulty with this question, review the discharge instructions after surgical correction of cryptorchidism.

Level of Cognitive Ability: Evaluating
Client Needs: Physiological Integrity
Integrated Process: Teaching and Learning
Content Area: Child Health—Gastrointestinal/Renal
Reference: Hockenberry, M., & Wilson, D. (2009). *Wong's essentials of pediatric nursing* (8th ed., p. 958). St. Louis: Mosby.

431. 3

Rationale: Epispadias is a congenital defect involving abnormal placement of the urethral orifice of the penis. The urethral opening is located anywhere on the dorsum of the penis. This anatomical characteristic facilitates entry of bacteria into the urine. Options 1, 2, and 4 are not characteristically noted in this condition.

Test-Taking Strategy: Visualize the anatomical characteristics of epispadias and use the process of elimination to answer the question. Options 1, 2, and 4 do not relate to the potential for infection, which can be associated with epispadias. If you had difficulty with this question, review the diagnostic findings associated with epispadias.

Level of Cognitive Ability: Analyzing
Client Needs: Physiological Integrity
Integrated Process: Nursing Process—Assessment
Content Area: Child Health—Gastrointestinal/Renal
References: Hockenberry, M., & Wilson, D. (2009). *Wong's essentials of pediatric nursing* (8th ed., p. 953). St. Louis: Mosby.

McKinney, E., James, S., Murray, S., & Ashwill, J. (2009). *Maternal-child nursing* (3rd ed., pp. 1143, 1152–1153). St. Louis: Saunders.

432. 4

Rationale: Hypospadias is a congenital defect involving abnormal placement of the urethral orifice of the penis. In hypospadias, the urethral orifice is located below the glans penis along the ventral surface. The infant should not be circumcised because the dorsal foreskin tissue will be used for surgical repair of the hypospadias. Options 1, 2, and 3 are unrelated to this disorder.

Test-Taking Strategy: Note the strategic words *indicates their understanding*. Recalling that hypospadias is a congenital defect involving abnormal placement of the urethral orifice of the penis will direct you to option 4. Review the treatment plan related to the repair of the hypospadias if you had difficulty with this question.

Level of Cognitive Ability: Evaluating
Client Needs: Physiological Integrity
Integrated Process: Nursing Process—Evaluation
Content Area: Child Health—Gastrointestinal/Renal
References: Hockenberry, M., & Wilson, D. (2009). *Wong's essentials of pediatric nursing* (8th ed., p. 226). St. Louis: Mosby.

McKinney, E., James, S., Murray, S., & Ashwill, J. (2009). *Maternal-child nursing* (3rd ed., p. 549). St. Louis: Saunders.

433. 2

Rationale: In bladder exstrophy, the bladder is exposed and external to the body. In this disorder, one must take care to protect the exposed bladder tissue from drying, while allowing the drainage of urine. This is accomplished best by covering the bladder with a nonadhering plastic wrap. The use of petroleum jelly gauze should be avoided because this type of dressing can dry out, adhere to the mucosa, and damage the delicate tissue when removed. Dry sterile dressings and dressings soaked in solutions (that can dry out) also damage the mucosa when removed.

Test-Taking Strategy: Focus on the diagnosis and visualize this disorder. Noting the strategic word *nonadhering* in option 2 will direct you to this option. If you had difficulty with this question, review care of an infant with bladder exstrophy.

Level of Cognitive Ability: Applying
Client Needs: Physiological Integrity
Integrated Process: Nursing Process—Planning
Content Area: Child Health—Gastrointestinal/Renal
Reference: Hockenberry, M., & Wilson, D. (2009). *Wong's essentials of pediatric nursing* (8th ed., p. 958). St. Louis: Mosby.

434. 4

Rationale: Glomerulonephritis refers to a group of kidney disorders characterized by inflammatory injury in the glomerulus. Group A beta-hemolytic streptococcal infection is a cause of glomerulonephritis. Often, a child becomes ill with streptococcal infection of the upper respiratory tract and then develops symptoms of acute poststreptococcal glomerulonephritis after an interval of 1 to 2 weeks. The assessment data in options 1, 2, and 3 are unrelated to a diagnosis of glomerulonephritis.

Test-Taking Strategy: Use the process of elimination. Option 1 relates to a kidney injury, not an infectious process. From the remaining options, recalling a streptococcal infection 1 to 2 weeks before the development of glomerulonephritis is the classic assessment finding will assist in directing you to option 4. If you had difficulty with this question, review the causes of glomerulonephritis.

Level of Cognitive Ability: Understanding
Client Needs: Physiological Integrity
Integrated Process: Nursing Process—Assessment
Content Area: Child Health—Gastrointestinal/Renal
Reference: Perry, S., Hockenberry, M., Lowdermilk, D., & Wilson, D. (2010). *Maternal child nursing care* (4th ed., p. 1538). St. Louis: Mosby.

ALTERNATE ITEM FORMAT: MULTIPLE RESPONSE

435. 1, 2, 3, 4

Rationale: Nephrotic syndrome is a kidney disorder characterized by massive proteinuria, hypoalbuminemia, edema, elevated serum lipids, anorexia, and pallor. The child gains weight.

Test-Taking Strategy: Note the child's diagnosis. Thinking about the pathophysiology associated with this disorder and recalling the assessment findings for nephrotic syndrome will direct you to the correct options. Review the clinical manifestations associated with nephrotic syndrome if you had difficulty with this question.

Level of Cognitive Ability: Analyzing
Client Needs: Physiological Integrity
Integrated Process: Nursing Process—Assessment
Content Area: Child Health—Gastrointestinal/Renal
Reference: Perry, S., Hockenberry, M., Lowdermilk, D., & Wilson, D. (2010). *Maternal child nursing care* (4th ed., p. 1537). St. Louis: Mosby.

Integumentary Disorders

I. ECZEMA (ATOPIC DERMATITIS)

A. Description
1. Superficial inflammatory process involving primarily the epidermis
2. Associated with family history of the disorder, allergies, asthma, or allergic rhinitis
3. The major goals of management are to relieve pruritus, lubricate the skin, reduce inflammation, and prevent or control secondary infections.

B. Forms of eczema (Box 43-1)

C. Assessment
1. Redness
2. Scaliness
3. Itching
4. Minute papules (firm elevated circumscribed lesions <1 cm in diameter) and vesicles (similar to papules, but fluid-filled)
5. Weeping, oozing, and crusting of lesions
6. Adolescent and early adult forms: Commonly occur in antecubital and popliteal areas

D. Interventions
1. Avoid exposure to skin irritants such as soaps, detergents, fabric softeners, diaper wipes, and powder.
2. Avoid excessive bathing and washing of affected areas; bathing water should be tepid, and the skin should be lubricated immediately after the bath.
3. Intermittently apply cool, wet compresses for short periods to soothe the skin and alleviate itching; pat skin dry between cooling treatments.
4. Administer antihistamines and topical corticosteroids as prescribed; corticosteroids are applied in a thin layer and are rubbed into the area thoroughly.
5. Administer immunomodulator medications as prescribed.
6. Administer prescribed antibiotics if secondary infections occur.
7. Prevent or minimize scratching; keep nails short and clean, and place gloves or cotton socks over the hands.
8. Eliminate conditions that increase itching, such as wet diapers, excessive bathing, ambient heat, woolen clothes or blankets, and proximity to rough fabrics or furry stuffed animals; exposure to latex should also be avoided.
9. Instruct parents to wash clothing in a mild detergent and rinse thoroughly; putting the clothes through a second complete wash cycle without detergent minimizes the residue remaining on the fabric.
10. Instruct parents about measures to prevent skin infections.
11. Instruct parents to monitor lesions for signs of infection (honey-colored crusts with surrounding erythema) and to seek immediate medical intervention if such signs are noted.

⚠ A child with an integumentary disorder needs to be monitored for signs of either a skin infection or a systemic infection.

II. IMPETIGO

A. Description
1. Impetigo is a contagious bacterial infection of the skin caused by beta-hemolytic streptococci or staphylococci, or both; it occurs most commonly during hot, humid months.
2. Impetigo can occur because of poor hygiene; it can be a primary infection or occur secondarily at a site that has been injured or at a site that was originally a rash, such as caused by exposure to poison ivy or poison oak.
3. The most common sites of infection are on the face and around the mouth, and then on the hands, neck, and extremities.
4. The lesions begin as vesicles or pustules surrounded by edema and redness (a pustule is similar to a vesicle except its fluid content is purulent).
5. The lesions progress to an exudative and crusting stage; after the crusting of the lesions, the initially serous vesicular fluid becomes cloudy, and the vesicles rupture, leaving honey-colored crusts covering ulcerated bases.

B. Assessment (Fig. 43-1)
1. Lesions
2. Erythema

Box 43-1 Forms of Eczema

Infantile: Usually begins at 2 to 6 months of age and decreases in incidence with aging; spontaneous remission may occur by 3 years
Childhood: May follow the infantile form; occurs at 2 to 3 years of age
Preadolescent and adolescent: Begins at about 12 years of age and may continue into the early adult years or indefinitely

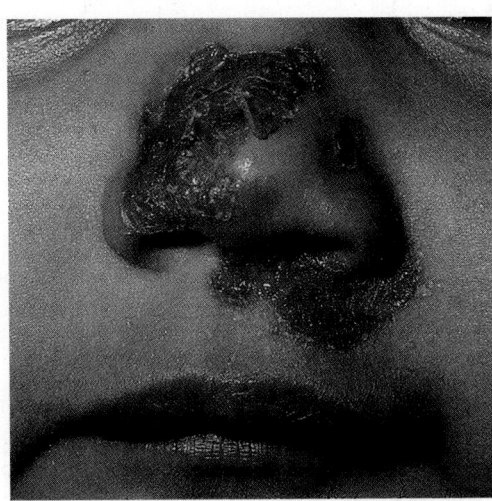

▲ **FIGURE 43-1** Impetigo contagiosa. (From Hockenberry, M., Wilson, D., Winkelstein, M., & Kline, N. [2007]. *Wong's nursing care of infants and children* [8th ed.]. St. Louis: Mosby.)

3. Pruritus
4. Burning
5. Secondary lymph node involvement

C. Interventions
1. Institute contact isolation; use standard precautions and implement agency-specific isolation procedures for the hospitalized child; strict hygiene practices are important because impetigo is a highly contagious condition.
2. Allow lesions to dry by air exposure.
3. Assist the child with daily bathing with antibacterial soap, as prescribed.
4. Apply warm saline or other prescribed compresses to the lesions two or three times daily, followed by a mild soap and water to remove crusts and allow for healing; Burow's solution may also be prescribed to soften the crusts.
5. Apply topical antibiotic ointments and instruct parents in their use; the infection is still communicable for 48 hours beyond initiation of antibiotic treatment.
6. Administer oral antibiotics, which may be prescribed if there is no response to topical

antibiotic treatment; it is extremely important to comply with the prescribed antibiotic regimen because secondary infections such as glomerulonephritis may result if the infectious agent is of a streptococcal type that can affect the nephrons.
7. To prevent skin cracking, apply emollients and instruct parents in the use of emollients.
8. Instruct parents in the methods to prevent the spread of the infection, especially careful handwashing.
9. Inform parents that the child needs to use separate towels, linens, and dishes.
10. Inform parents that all linens and clothing used by the child should be washed with detergent in hot water separately from linens and clothing of other household members.

III. PEDICULOSIS CAPITIS (LICE)

A. Description
1. Pediculosis capitis refers to an infestation of the hair and scalp with lice.
2. The most common sites of involvement are the occipital area, behind the ears at the nape of the neck, and occasionally the eyebrows and eyelashes.
3. The female louse lays her eggs (nits) on the hair shaft, close to the scalp; the incubation period is 7 to 10 days.
4. Lice can survive for 48 hours away from the host; nits shed in the environment can hatch in 7 to 10 days.
5. Head lice live and reproduce only on humans and are transmitted by direct and indirect contact, such as sharing of brushes, hats, towels, and bedding.
6. All contacts of the infested child, especially siblings, should be examined for lice infestation and referred for treatment as appropriate.

B. Assessment (Box 43-2 and Fig. 43-2)
C. Interventions
1. Use a pediculicide product (usually permethrin 1% cream rinse [Nix]) as prescribed; follow package instructions for timing the application and for contraindications for use in children.
2. Daily removal of nits with an extra-fine-tooth metal nit comb should be done as a control measure after use of the pediculicide product (gloves should be worn for removal of nits); hairbrushes or combs should be discarded or soaked in boiling water for 10 minutes or in a commercially available lice-killing product for 1 hour.
3. Instruct parents that siblings may also need treatment; grooming items should not be shared, and a single comb or brush should be used for each individual child.

4. Instruct parents that bedding and clothing used by the child should be changed daily, laundered in hot water with detergent, and dried in a hot dryer for 20 minutes; this process should continue for 1 week.
5. Instruct parents that nonessential bedding and clothing can be stored in a tightly sealed bag for 2 weeks and then washed.
6. Instruct parents to seal toys that cannot be washed or dry-cleaned in a plastic bag for 2 weeks.
7. Instruct parents that furniture and carpets need to be vacuumed frequently and that the dust bag from the vacuum should be discarded after vacuuming.
8. Teach the child not to share clothing, headwear, brushes, and combs.
9. Lice of the eyelashes or eyebrows may need to be removed manually.

 IV. SCABIES

A. Description
1. Scabies is a parasitic skin disorder caused by an infestation of *Sarcoptes scabiei* (itch mite) (see Chapter 50).

Box 43-2 Assessment Findings: Pediculosis Capitis

Child scratches scalp excessively.
Pruritus is caused by the crawling insect and insect saliva on the skin.
Nits (white eggs) are observable on the hair shaft (it is important to differentiate nits from lint or dandruff, which flakes away easily).
Adult lice are difficult to see and appear as small tan or grayish specks, which may crawl fast.

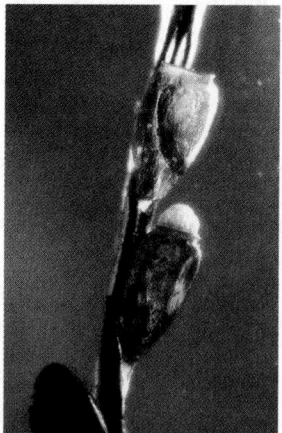

▲ **FIGURE 43-2** Viable nits. (From Morse, S., Ballard, R., Holmes, K., Moreland, A. [2003]. *Atlas of sexually transmitted diseases and AIDS* [3rd ed]. London: Mosby.)

2. Scabies is endemic among schoolchildren and institutionalized populations as a result of close personal contact.
3. Incubation period
   a. The female mite burrows into the epidermis, lays eggs, and dies in the burrow after 4 to 5 weeks.
   b. The eggs hatch in 3 to 5 days, and larvae mature and complete their life cycle.
4. Infectious period: During the entire course of the infestation
B. Assessment (Box 43-3 and Fig. 43-3)

⚠ Scabies is transmitted by close personal contact with an infected person. Household members and contacts of an infected child need to be treated simultaneously.

C. Interventions
1. Topical application of a scabicide such as permethrin (Elimite) kills the mites.
2. Lindane, an alternative product that may be prescribed, should not be used in children younger than 2 years because of the risk of neurotoxicity and seizures.
3. Instruct parents in the application of the scabicide.
4. When permethrin is used, it is applied to cool dry skin at least 30 minutes after bathing, the cream is massaged thoroughly and gently into all skin surfaces (not just the areas that have the rash) from the head to the soles of

---

Box 43-3 Assessment Findings: Scabies

Pruritic papular rash
Burrows on the skin (fine grayish red lines that may be difficult to see)

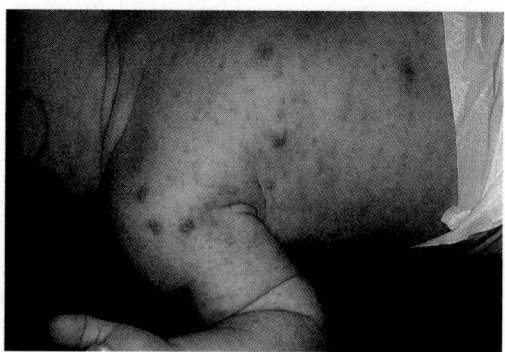

▲ **FIGURE 43-3** Scabies rash on an infant. (From *Mosby's dictionary of medicine, nursing, & health professions* [8th ed.]. [2009]. St. Louis: Mosby.)

the feet (avoid contact with the eyes), left on the skin for 8 to 14 hours, and then removed by bathing; a repeat treatment may be necessary.

5. Instruct the parents about the importance of frequent handwashing.

6. Instruct the parents that all clothing, bedding, and pillowcases used by the child need to be changed daily, washed in hot water with detergent, dried in a hot dryer, and ironed before reuse; this process should continue for 1 week.

7. Instruct parents that nonwashable toys and other items should be sealed in plastic bags for at least 4 days.

8. Anti-itch topical treatment may be necessary, and antibiotics may be prescribed if a secondary infection develops.

V. BURN INJURIES (see Priority Nursing Actions)

PRIORITY NURSING ACTIONS!

Actions to Take in the Event of a Major Burn Injury

1. Stop the burning process.
2. Assess the ABCs—assess for an adequate airway, breathing, and circulation.
3. Begin resuscitation if the child is not breathing.
4. Remove burned clothing and jewelry.
5. Cover the wound with a clean cloth.
6. Keep the child warm.
7. Transport the child to the emergency department.

The initial management of the burn injury begins at the scene of the injury. The first priority is to stop the burning process; this must be done before other interventions. To stop the burning process, flames should be smothered. The child should be placed in a horizontal position because a vertical position may cause the hair to ignite or the inhalation of flames, heat, or smoke. The child should be rolled in a blanket or other article taking care not to cover the face and head because of the danger of inhaling smoke and fumes. As soon as the flames are extinguished, the child is assessed for adequate airway, breathing, and circulation. Measures are taken immediately if resuscitation is necessary. Burned clothing and jewelry are removed to prevent further burning of the skin and disruption of skin integrity, and then the burn is covered with a clean cloth, which prevents contamination of the wound, reduces pain by eliminating air contact, and prevents hypothermia. The child is also kept warm to prevent hypothermia and is immediately transported to the nearest emergency facility.

Reference: Perry, S., Hockenberry, M., Lowdermilk, D., & Wilson, D. (2010). *Maternal child nursing care* (4th ed., pp. 1664-1665). St. Louis: Mosby.

A. Pediatric considerations

1. Very young children who have been burned severely have a higher mortality rate than older children and adults with comparable burns.

2. Lower burn temperatures and shorter exposure to heat can cause a more severe burn in a child than in an adult because a child's skin is thinner.

3. The degree of pain experienced by the child and the ability to communicate it are different than in an adult with the same exposure.

4. Severely burned children are at increased risk for fluid and heat loss, dehydration, and metabolic acidosis compared with adults.

5. The higher proportion of body fluid to mass in children increases the risk of cardiovascular problems.

6. Burns involving more than 10% of the total body surface area require some form of fluid resuscitation.

7. Infants and children are at increased risk for protein and calorie deficiency because they have smaller muscle mass and less body fat than adults.

8. Scarring is more severe in a child; disturbed body image is a distinct issue for a child or adolescent, especially as **growth** continues.

9. An immature immune system presents an increased risk of infection for infants and young children.

10. A delay in **growth** may occur after a burn.

B. Extent of burn injury

1. The rule of nines, used for adults with burn injuries, gives an inaccurate estimate in children because of the difference in body proportions between children and adults.

2. In a pediatric client, the extent of the burn is expressed as a percent of the total body surface area using age-related charts (Fig. 43-4).

C. Fluid replacement therapy

⚠ To determine adequacy of fluid resuscitation, vital signs (especially heart rate), urine output, adequacy of capillary filling, and sensorium status are assessed.

1. Fluid replacement is necessary during the initial 24-hour period after burn injury because of the fluid shifts that occur as a result of the injury.

2. Several formulas are available to calculate the child's fluid needs, and the formula used depends on the physician's preference.

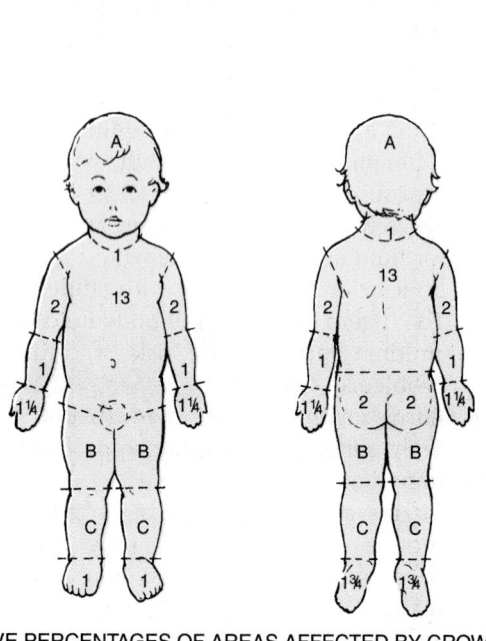

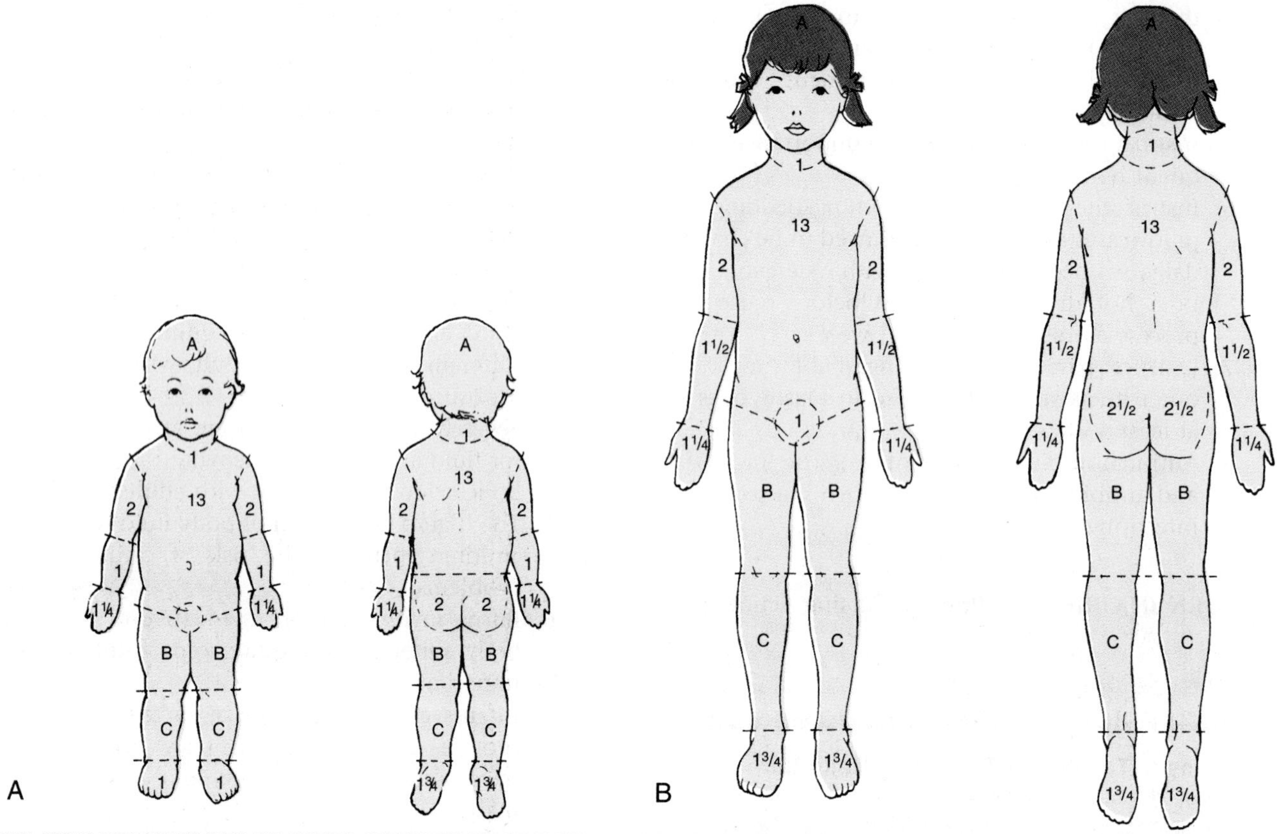

RELATIVE PERCENTAGES OF AREAS AFFECTED BY GROWTH

AREA	BIRTH	AGE 1 YR	AGE 5 YR
A = ½ of head	9½	8½	6½
B = ½ of one thigh	2¾	3¼	4
C = ½ of one leg	2½	2½	2¾

RELATIVE PERCENTAGES OF AREAS AFFECTED BY GROWTH

AREA	AGE 10 YR	AGE 15 YR	ADULT
A = ½ of head	5½	4½	3½
B = ½ of one thigh	4½	4½	4¾
C = ½ of one leg	3	3¼	3½

▲ **FIGURE 43-4** Estimation of distribution of burns in children. **A,** Children from birth to age 5 years. **B,** Older children. (From Perry, S., Hockenberry, M., Lowdermilk, D., & Wilson, D. [2010]. *Maternal child nursing care* [4th ed.]. St. Louis: Mosby.)

3. Crystalloid solutions are used during the initial phase of therapy; colloid solutions such as albumin, Plasma-Lyte (combined electrolyte solution), or fresh-frozen plasma are useful in maintaining plasma volume.
4. See also Chapter 50.

💿 MORE QUESTIONS ON THE CD!

Practice Questions

436. A nurse is monitoring a child with burns during treatment for burn shock. The nurse understands that which of the following assessments provides the most accurate guide to determining the adequacy of fluid resuscitation?
1. Skin turgor
2. Neurological assessment
3. Level of edema at burn site
4. Quality of peripheral pulses

437. A mother of a 3-year-old child arrives at a clinic and tells a nurse that the child has been scratching the skin continuously and has developed a rash. The nurse assesses the child and suspects the presence of scabies. The nurse bases this suspicion on which finding noted on assessment of the child's skin?
1. Fine grayish red lines
2. Purple-colored lesions
3. Thick, honey-colored crusts
4. Clusters of fluid-filled vesicles

438. Permethrin (Elimite) is prescribed for a 4-year-old child with a diagnosis of scabies. A clinic nurse instructs the mother regarding the use of this treatment and tells the mother:

1. Apply the lotion and leave it on for 6 hours.
2. Apply the lotion to areas of the rash only.
3. Avoid putting clothes on the child over the lotion.
4. Apply the lotion to cool, dry skin at least 30 minutes after bathing.

439. A school nurse has provided an instructional session about impetigo to parents of the children attending the school. Which statement, if made by a parent, indicates a need for further instructions?
1. "It is extremely contagious."
2. "It is most common in humid weather."
3. "Lesions most often are located on the arms and chest."
4. "It might show up in an area of broken skin, such as an insect bite."

440. A clinic nurse is reviewing the physician's prescription for a child who has been diagnosed with scabies. Lindane has been prescribed for the child. The nurse questions the prescription if which of the following is noted in the child's record?
1. The child is 18 months old.
2. The child is being bottle-fed.
3. A sibling is using lindane for the treatment of scabies.
4. The child has a history of frequent respiratory infections.

441. A school nurse is conducting pediculosis capitis (head lice) assessments. A child with a "positive" head check would have:
1. Maculopapular lesions behind the ears
2. Lesions in the scalp that extend to the hairline or neck
3. White flaky particles throughout the entire scalp region

4. White sacs attached to the hair shafts in the occipital area

442. A topical corticosteroid is prescribed by a physician for a child with atopic dermatitis (eczema). A nurse instructs the mother in how to apply the cream and tells the mother to:
1. Apply the cream over the entire body.
2. Apply a thick layer of cream to affected areas only.
3. Avoid cleansing the area before application of the cream.
4. Apply a thin layer of cream and rub it into the area thoroughly.

Alternate Item Format: Multiple Response

443. A nurse caring for a child who sustained a burn injury plans care based on which pediatric considerations associated with this injury? **Select all that apply.**
☐ 1. Scarring is less severe in a child than in an adult.
☐ 2. A delay in growth may occur after a burn injury.
☐ 3. Fluid resuscitation is unnecessary unless the burned area is more than 25% of the total body surface area.
☐ 4. An immature immune system presents an increased risk of infection for infants and young children.
☐ 5. The lower proportion of body fluid to mass in a child increases the risk of cardiovascular problems.
☐ 6. Infants and young children are at increased risk for protein and calorie deficiency because they have smaller muscle mass and less body fat than adults.

ANSWERS

436. 2
Rationale: Sensorium is an accurate guide to determine the adequacy of fluid resuscitation. The burn injury itself does not affect the sensorium, so the child should be alert and oriented. Any alteration in sensorium should be evaluated further. A neurological assessment would determine the level of sensorium in the child. Options 1, 3, and 4 would not provide an accurate assessment of the adequacy of fluid resuscitation.
Test-Taking Strategy: Note the strategic words *most accurate* in the event query. Although options 1, 3, and 4 may provide some information related to fluid volume, in a burn injury, neurological assessment, is most accurate from the options provided. Review assessments during fluid resuscitation and treatment for burn shock if you had difficulty with this question.

Level of Cognitive Ability: Evaluating
Client Needs: Physiological Integrity
Integrated Process: Nursing Process—Evaluation
Content Area: Child Health—Integumentary/AIDS/Infectious Diseases
References: McKinney, E., James, S., Murray, S., & Ashwill, J. (2009). *Maternal-child nursing* (3rd ed., pp. 1070, 1374). St. Louis: Saunders.
   Perry, S., Hockenberry, M., Lowdermilk, D., & Wilson, D. (2010). *Maternal child nursing care* (4th ed., p. 1537). St. Louis: Mosby.

437. 1
Rationale: Scabies is a parasitic skin disorder caused by an infestation of *Sarcoptes scabiei* (itch mite). Scabies appears as burrows or fine, grayish red, thread-like lines. They may be difficult to see if they are obscured by excoriation and inflammation. Purple-colored lesions may indicate various

disorders, including systemic conditions. Thick, honey-colored crusts are characteristic of impetigo or secondary infection in eczema. Clusters of fluid-filled vesicles are seen in herpesvirus infection.

Test-Taking Strategy: Think about the characteristic of this parasitic skin disorder. Recalling that scabies infestation produces burrows will assist in directing you to option 1. If you are unfamiliar with the clinical manifestations associated with scabies, review this content.

Level of Cognitive Ability: Analyzing
Client Needs: Physiological Integrity
Integrated Process: Nursing Process—Assessment
Content Area: Child Health—Integumentary/AIDS/Infectious Diseases
Reference: McKinney, E., James, S., Murray, S., & Ashwill, J. (2009). *Maternal-child nursing* (3rd ed., p. 1353). St. Louis: Saunders.

438. 4

Rationale: Permethrin is massaged thoroughly and gently into all skin surfaces (not just the areas that have the rash) from the head to the soles of the feet. Care should be taken to avoid contact with the eyes. The lotion should not be applied until at least 30 minutes after bathing and should be applied only to cool, dry skin. The lotion should be kept on for 8 to 14 hours, and then the child should be given a bath. The child should be clothed during the 8 to 14 hours of treatment contact time.

Test-Taking Strategy: Use the process of elimination. Option 3 can be eliminated because the child should be clothed. Eliminate option 2 next because of the close-ended word *only* in this option. From the remaining options, recalling the procedure for the application of this lotion will direct you to option 4. Review the treatment of scabies using permethrin if you had difficulty with this question.

Level of Cognitive Ability: Applying
Client Needs: Physiological Integrity
Integrated Process: Teaching and Learning
Content Area: Child Health—Integumentary/AIDS/Infectious Diseases
Reference: McKinney, E., James, S., Murray, S., & Ashwill, J. (2009). *Maternal-child nursing* (3rd ed., p. 1353). St. Louis: Saunders.

439. 3

Rationale: Impetigo is a contagious bacterial infection of the skin caused by beta-hemolytic streptococci or staphylococci, or both. Impetigo is most common during hot, humid summer months. Impetigo may begin in an area of broken skin, such as an insect bite or atopic dermatitis. Impetigo is extremely contagious. Lesions usually are located around the mouth and nose, but may be present on the hands and extremities.

Test-Taking Strategy: Use the process of elimination, noting the strategic words *need for further instructions*. These words indicate a negative event query and ask you to select an option that is an incorrect statement. Knowledge regarding the cause and manifestations of impetigo will direct you to option 3. If you are unfamiliar with the manifestations of impetigo, review this content.

Level of Cognitive Ability: Evaluating
Client Needs: Safe and Effective Care Environment

Integrated Process: Teaching and Learning
Content Area: Child Health—Integumentary/AIDS/Infectious Diseases
Reference: McKinney, E., James, S., Murray, S., & Ashwill, J. (2009). *Maternal-child nursing* (3rd ed., p. 1342). St. Louis: Saunders.

440. 1

Rationale: Lindane is a pediculicide product that may be prescribed to treat scabies. It is contraindicated for children younger than 2 years because they have more permeable skin, and high systemic absorption may occur, placing the children at risk for central nervous system toxicity and seizures. Lindane also is used with caution in children between the ages of 2 and 10 years. Siblings and other household members should be treated simultaneously. Options 2 and 4 are unrelated to the use of lindane. Lindane is not recommended for use by a breast-feeding woman because the medication is secreted into breast milk.

Test-Taking Strategy: Use the process of elimination and recall the concepts related to the body surface area of children and medication administration. These concepts will direct you to option 1. If you are unfamiliar with the use of lindane, review this medication and the contraindications associated with its use.

Level of Cognitive Ability: Analyzing
Client Needs: Physiological Integrity
Integrated Process: Nursing Process—Analysis
Content Area: Child Health—Integumentary/AIDS/Infectious Diseases
References: Hockenberry, M., & Wilson, D. (2009). *Wong's essentials of pediatric nursing* (8th ed., p. 1079). St. Louis: Mosby.

Skidmore-Roth, L. (2009). *Mosby's drug guide for nurses* (8th ed., p. 559). St. Louis: Mosby.

441. 4

Rationale: Pediculosis capitis is an infestation of the hair and scalp with lice. The nits are visible and attach firmly to the hair shaft near the scalp. The occiput is an area in which nits can be seen. White flaky particles are indicative of dandruff. Maculopapular lesions behind the ears or lesions that extend to the hairline or neck are indicative of an infectious process, not pediculosis.

Test-Taking Strategy: Focus on the subject, the characteristics of pediculosis capitis. Option 3 can be eliminated first because white flaky particles are indicative of dandruff. Recalling that in this infestation, nit sacs attach to the hair shaft will direct you to option 4. Review assessment findings with pediculosis capitis if you had difficulty with this question.

Level of Cognitive Ability: Understanding
Client Needs: Physiological Integrity
Integrated Process: Nursing Process—Assessment
Content Area: Child Health—Integumentary/AIDS/Infectious Diseases
Reference: Hockenberry, M., & Wilson, D. (2009). *Wong's essentials of pediatric nursing* (8th ed., pp. 1079–1080). St. Louis: Mosby.

442. 4

Rationale: Atopic dermatitis is a superficial inflammatory process involving primarily the epidermis. A topical corticosteroid may be prescribed and should be applied sparingly (thin layer) and rubbed into the area thoroughly. The affected area should be cleaned gently before application. A topical corticosteroid should not be applied over extensive areas. Systemic absorption is more likely to occur with extensive application.

Test-Taking Strategy: Use the process of elimination. Eliminate option 3 first because it does not make sense not to clean an affected area. Eliminate option 1 because medicated cream should be applied only to areas that are affected. Eliminate option 2 because of the word *thick*. Review the procedure for the application of a topical corticosteroid if you had difficulty with this question.

Level of Cognitive Ability: Applying
Client Needs: Physiological Integrity
Integrated Process: Teaching and Learning
Content Area: Child Health—Integumentary/AIDS/Infectious Diseases
References: Hockenberry, M., & Wilson, D. (2009). *Wong's essentials of pediatric nursing* (8th ed., pp. 1087–1088). St. Louis: Mosby.

McKinney, E., James, S., Murray, S., & Ashwill, J. (2009). *Maternal-child nursing* (3rd ed., p. 1355). St. Louis: Saunders.

ALTERNATE FORMAT ITEM: MULTIPLE RESPONSE

443. 2, 4, 6
Rationale: Pediatric considerations in the care of a burn victim include the following: Scarring is more severe in a child than in an adult. A delay in growth may occur after a burn injury. Burns involving more than 10% of total body surface area require some form of fluid resuscitation. An immature immune system presents an increased risk of infection for infants and young children. The higher proportion of body fluid to mass in a child increases the risk of cardiovascular problems. Infants and young children are at increased risk for protein and calorie deficiencies because they have smaller muscle mass and less body fat than adults.

Test-Taking Strategy: Focus on the subject, pediatric considerations in the care of a child who sustained a burn injury. To answer correctly, read each option carefully and think about the physiology of a child related to body size. Review the pediatric considerations related to a burn injury if you had difficulty with this question.

Level of Cognitive Ability: Applying
Client Needs: Physiological Integrity
Integrated Process: Nursing Process—Planning
Content Area: Child Health—Integumentary (AIDS) Infectious Diseases
References: McKinney, E., James, S., Murray, S., & Ashwill, J. (2009). *Maternal-child nursing* (3rd ed., p. 1365). St. Louis: Saunders.

Swearingen, P. (2008). *All-in-one care planning resource: Medical-surgical, pediatric, maternity, & psychiatric nursing care plans* (2nd ed., pp. 603, 605, 607). St. Louis: Mosby.

44

Musculoskeletal Disorders

I. DEVELOPMENTAL DYSPLASIA OF THE HIP

A. Description
1. Disorders related to abnormal development of the hip that may develop during fetal life, infancy, or childhood; in these disorders, the head of the femur is seated improperly in the acetabulum, or hip socket, of the pelvis
2. Degrees of developmental dysplasia of the hip (Box 44-1)

B. Assessment (Fig. 44-1)
1. Neonate: Laxity of the ligaments around the hip
2. Infant
   a. Shortening of the limb on the affected side (Galeazzi's sign, Allis' sign)
   b. Restricted abduction of the hip on the affected side when the infant is placed supine with knees and hips flexed
   c. Unequal gluteal folds when the infant is prone and legs are extended against the examining table
   d. Positive Ortolani's test: Ortolani's maneuver is a test to assess for hip instability. The examiner abducts the thigh and applies gentle pressure forward over the greater trochanter. A "clunking" sensation indicates a dislocated femoral head moving into the acetabulum.
   e. Positive Barlow's test: The examiner adducts the hips and applies gentle pressure down and back with the thumbs. In hip dysplasia, the examiner can feel the femoral head move out of the acetabulum.
3. Older infant and child
   a. Affected leg is shorter than the other.
   b. The head of the femur can be felt to move up and down in the buttock when the extended thigh is pushed first toward the child's head and then pulled distally.
   c. Positive Trendelenburg's sign: The child stands on one foot and then the other foot, holding onto a support and bearing weight on the affected hip; the pelvis tilts downward on the normal side instead of upward, as it would with normal stability.
   d. Greater trochanter is prominent.
   e. Marked lordosis or waddling gait is noted in bilateral dislocations.

C. Interventions
1. Birth to 6 months of age: Splinting of the hips with a Pavlik harness to maintain flexion and abduction and external rotation (worn continuously until hip is stable in about 3 to 6 months) (Fig. 44-2)
2. Age 6 to 18 months: Gradual reduction by traction followed by closed reduction or open reduction (if necessary) under general anesthesia; child is then placed in a hip spica cast for 2 to 4 months until the hip is stable, and then a flexion-abduction brace is applied for approximately 3 months
3. Older child: Operative reduction and reconstruction is usually required.
4. Parents are instructed regarding proper care of a Pavlik harness, spica cast, or abduction brace.

II. CONGENITAL CLUBFOOT

A. Description
1. Complex deformity of the ankle and foot that includes forefoot adduction, midfoot

---

Box 44-1 Degrees of Developmental Dysplasia of the Hip

Acetabular Dysplasia (Preluxation)
Mildest form
Neither subluxation nor dislocation
Delay in acetabular development occurs
Femoral head remains in acetabulum

Subluxation
Incomplete dislocation of the hip
Femoral head remains in acetabulum
Stretched capsule and ligamentum teres causes head of the femur to be partially displaced

Dislocation
Femoral head loses contact with acetabulum and is displaced posteriorly and superiorly over fibrocartilaginous rim
Ligamentum teres is elongated and taut

supination, hindfoot varus, and ankle equinus; defect may be unilateral or bilateral

2. The goal of treatment is to achieve a painless plantigrade (able to walk on the sole of the foot with the heel on the ground) and stable foot.

3. Long-term interval follow-up care is required until the child reaches skeletal maturity.

B. Assessment: Deformities are described based on the position of the ankle and foot.

1. Talipes varus: Inversion or bending inward
2. Talipes valgus: Eversion or bending outward
3. Talipes equinus: Plantar flexion in which the toes are lower than the heel
4. Talipes calcaneus: Dorsiflexion in which the toes are higher than the heel

C. Interventions

1. Treatment begins as soon after birth as possible.
2. Manipulation and casting are performed weekly for about 8 to 12 weeks because of the rapid growth of early infancy; a splint is then applied if casting and manipulation are successful.
3. Surgical intervention may be necessary if normal alignment is not achieved by about 6 to 12 weeks of age.
4. Monitor for pain, and monitor the neurovascular status of the toes.

⚠ Contact the physician immediately if signs of neurovascular impairment are noted in a child with a cast or brace.

III. IDIOPATHIC SCOLIOSIS

A. Description

1. Three-dimensional spinal deformity that usually involves lateral curvature, spinal rotation

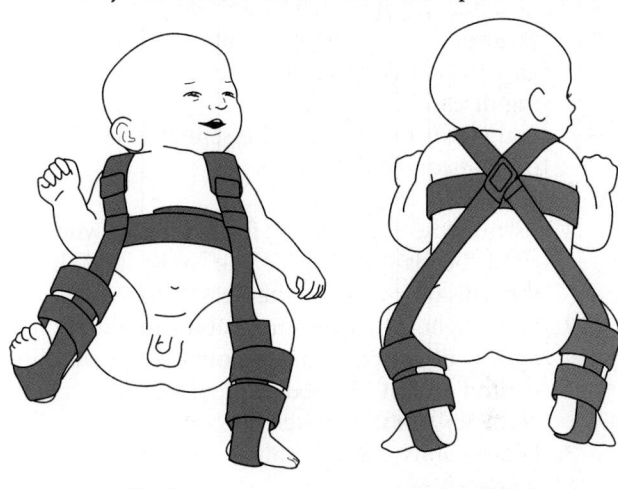

Front   Back

▲ **FIGURE 44-2** Child in Pavlik harness. (From Hockenberry, M., Wilson, S., Winkelstein, M. [2009]. *Wong's essentials of pediatric nursing* [8th ed.]. St. Louis: Mosby.)

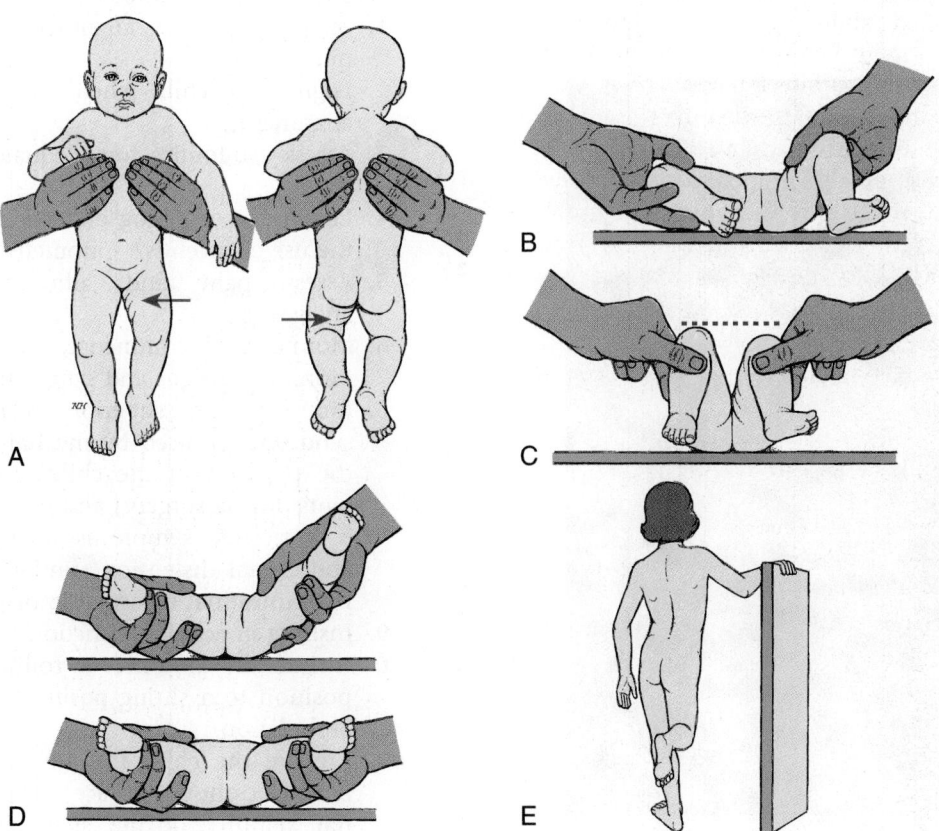

▲ **FIGURE 44-1** Signs of development dysplasia of the hip. **A,** Asymmetry of gluteal and thigh folds. **B,** Limited hip abduction, as seen in flexion. **C,** Apparent shortening of the femur, as indicated by the level of the knees in flexion. **D,** Ortolani click (if infant is younger than 4 weeks old). **E,** Positive Trendelenburg's sign or gait (if child is weight bearing). (From Hockenberry, M., Wilson, S., Winkelstein, M. [2009]. *Wong's essentials of pediatric nursing* [8th ed.]. St. Louis: Mosby.)

resulting in rib asymmetry, and hypokyphosis of the thorax (Fig. 44-3)

2. Idiopathic scoliosis usually is diagnosed during the preadolescent growth spurt; screenings are important when growth spurts occur.

3. Surgical (spinal fusion, placement of an instrumentation system) and nonsurgical (bracing) interventions are used; the type of treatment depends on the location and degree of the curvatures, the age of the child, the amount of growth that is yet anticipated, and any underlying disease processes.

4. Long-term monitoring is essential to detect any progression of the curve.

B. Assessment

1. Asymmetry of the ribs and flanks is noted when the child bends forward at the waist and hangs the arms down toward the feet (Adams' test).

2. Hip height, rib positioning, and shoulder height are asymmetrical (can be noted when standing behind an undressed child); leg-length discrepancy is also apparent.

3. Radiographs are obtained to confirm the diagnosis.

C. Interventions

1. Monitor progression of the curvatures.

2. Prepare the child and parents for the use of a brace if prescribed.

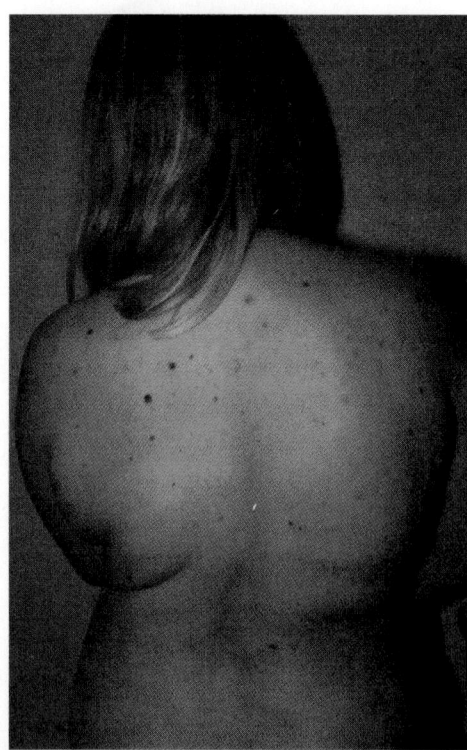

▲ **FIGURE 44-3** Scoliosis in a standing erect posture. (From Lewis, S., Heitkemper, M., & Dirksen, S. [2007]. *Medical-surgical nursing: Assessment and management of clinical problems* [7th ed.]. St. Louis: Mosby.)

3. Prepare the child and parents for surgery (spinal fusion, placement of internal instrumentation systems) if prescribed.

⚠ The potential for altered role performance, body image disturbance, fear, anger, and isolation exists for a child with a disabling condition and a condition that requires wearing a body brace.

D. Braces

1. Braces are not curative, but may slow the progression of the curvature to allow skeletal growth and maturity.

2. Braces usually are prescribed to be worn 16 to 23 hours a day.

3. Inspect the skin for signs of redness or breakdown.

4. Keep the skin clean and dry, and avoid lotions and powders because these cake and lead to skin breakdown.

5. Advise the child to wear soft nonirritating clothing under the brace.

6. Instruct in prescribed exercises (exercises help maintain and strengthen spinal and abdominal muscles during treatment).

7. Encourage verbalization about body image and other psychosocial issues.

E. Postoperative interventions

1. Maintain proper alignment; avoid twisting movements.

2. Logroll the child when turning to maintain alignment.

3. Assess extremities for adequate neurovascular status.

4. Encourage coughing and deep breathing and the use of incentive spirometry.

5. Assess pain and administer prescribed analgesics.

6. Monitor for incontinence.

7. Monitor for signs and symptoms of infection.

8. Monitor for superior mesenteric artery syndrome (caused by mechanical changes in the position of the child's abdominal contents during surgery) and notify the physician if it occurs; symptoms include emesis and abdominal distention similar to what occurs with intestinal obstruction or paralytic ileus.

9. Instruct in activity restrictions.

10. Instruct the child how to roll from a side-lying position to a sitting position, and assist with ambulation.

11. Prepare the child for the use of a molded plastic orthosis (brace) to provide external stability of the spine when resuming activities.

12. Address a body image disturbance when formulating a plan of nursing care.

IV. JUVENILE IDIOPATHIC ARTHRITIS

A. Description
1. Autoimmune inflammatory disease affecting the joints and other tissues, such as articular cartilage, that most often occurs in girls.
2. Treatment is supportive (there is no cure) and directed toward preserving joint function, controlling inflammation, minimizing deformity, and reducing the impact that the disease may have on the development of the child.
3. Treatment includes medications, physical and occupational therapies, and child and family education.
4. Surgical intervention may be implemented if the child has problems with joint contractures and unequal growth of extremities.

B. Assessment (Box 44-2)
1. There are no definitive tests to diagnose juvenile idiopathic arthritis.
2. Some laboratory tests, such as an elevated erythrocyte sedimentation rate or determination of the presence of leukocytosis, may support evidence of the disease.
3. Radiographs may show soft tissue swelling and joint space widening from increased synovial fluid in the joint.

C. Interventions
1. Facilitate social and emotional development.
2. Instruct parents and child in the administration of medications; medications may be given alone or in combination and are prescribed in a step-like manner depending on the disease response to each level (Box 44-3).
3. Assist the child with range-of-motion exercises and instruct in prescribed exercises.
4. Encourage normal performance of activities of daily living.
5. Instruct parents and child in the use of hot or cold packs, splinting, and positioning the affected joint in a neutral position during painful episodes.
6. Encourage and support prescribed physical and occupational therapy.
7. Instruct in the importance of preventive eye care and reporting visual disturbances.
8. Assess the child's and family's perceptions regarding the chronic illness; plan to discuss the nature of a chronic illness and the associated life alterations that result from the chronic progression of the disorder.

V. MARFAN SYNDROME

A. Description
1. Disorder of connective tissue that affects the skeletal system, cardiovascular system, eyes, and skin.
2. Marfan syndrome is caused by defects in the fibrillin-1 gene, which serves as a building block for elastic tissue in the body; also, the disorder may be inherited.
3. There is no cure for the disorder.

B. Assessment
1. Tall and thin body structure: slender fingers, long arms and legs, curvature of the spine
2. Presence of visual problems
3. Presence of cardiac problems

C. Interventions
1. Monitor for vision problems and obtain visual examinations on a regular schedule.
2. Monitor for curvature of the spine, especially during adolescence.
3. Cardiac medications may be prescribed to slow the heart rate, to decrease stress on the aorta.
4. Instruct parents that the child should avoid participating in competitive athletics and contact sports to avoid injuring the heart.

Box 44-3 Medications Used in Juvenile Idiopathic Arthritis

Nonsteroidal Anti-inflammatory Drugs (NSAIDs)
First medications used
May cause gastrointestinal irritation and easy bruising

Methotrexate
Used if NSAIDs are ineffective
Complete blood cell counts and liver function studies are monitored closely

Corticosteroids
Potent immunosuppressives used for life-threatening complications, incapacitating arthritis, and uveitis
Administered at lowest effective dose for the shortest time period; discontinued on a tapering schedule
Prolonged use can cause Cushing's syndrome, osteoporosis, increased infection risk, glucose intolerance, hypokalemia, cataracts, growth suppression

Tumor Necrosis Factor Receptor Inhibitors
Etanercept (Enbrel)
Infliximab (Remicade)
Adverse effects include allergic reaction at injection site, increased risk for infection, demyelinating disease, pancytopenia

Slower Acting Antirheumatic Drugs
Usually prescribed in combination with NSAIDs
Sulfasalazine (Azulfidine), hydroxychloroquine (Plaquenil), gold sodium thiomalate (Myochrysine), penicillamine

Box 44-2 Assessment Findings: Juvenile Idiopathic Arthritis

Stiffness, swelling, and limited motion occur in affected joints.
Affected joints are warm to touch, tender, and painful.
Joint stiffness is present on arising in the morning and after inactivity.
Uveitis (inflammation of structures in the uveal tract) can occur and cause blindness.

5. Instruct parents to inform the dentist of the condition; antibiotics should be taken before dental procedures to prevent endocarditis.
6. Surgical replacement of the aortic root and valve may be necessary.

VI. FRACTURES

A. Description (see also Chapter 68)
1. A break in the continuity of the bone as a result of trauma, twisting, or bone decalcification
2. Fractures in children usually occur as a result of increased mobility and inadequate or immature motor and cognitive skills; they may result from trauma or bone diseases such as congenital bone disease or bone tumors.

⚠ Fractures in infancy are generally rare and warrant further investigation to rule out the possibility of child abuse and to recognize bone structure defects.

B. Assessment
1. Pain or tenderness over the involved area
2. Obvious deformity
3. Edema
4. Ecchymosis
5. Muscle spasm
6. Loss of function
7. Crepitation

C. Initial care of a fracture (see Priority Nursing Actions)

PRIORITY NURSING ACTIONS!

Actions to Take if a Child Sustains an Extremity Fracture

1. Assess extent of injury and immobilize the affected extremity.
2. If a compound fracture exists, cover the wound with a sterile dressing (apply a clean dressing if a sterile dressing is unavailable).
3. Elevate the injured extremity.
4. Apply cold to injured area.
5. Continue to monitor neurovascular status.
6. Transport to the nearest emergency department.

If a child sustains a fracture, the extent of the injury is immediately assessed using the five "P's"—pain and point of tenderness, pulses distal to fracture site, pallor, paresthesia (sensation) distal to the fracture site, and paralysis (movement distal to fracture site). The extremity is immobilized to prevent movement and further injury to soft tissues. If an open wound is present, it is covered to reduce the risk of infection. The extremity is elevated to reduce swelling, and cold packs are applied to assist in reducing the swelling and to reduce the pain. The neurovascular status is monitored closely, and the child is transported to the nearest emergency facility.

Reference: Perry, S., Hockenberry, M., Lowdermilk, D., & Wilson, D. (2010). *Maternal child nursing care* (4th ed., p. 1684). St. Louis: Mosby.

D. Interventions
1. Reduction
   a. Restoring the bone to proper alignment
   b. Closed reduction: Accomplished by manual alignment of the fragments, followed by immobilization
   c. Open reduction: Surgical insertion of internal fixation devices, such as rods, wires, or pins, that help maintain alignment while healing occurs
2. Retention: Application of traction or a cast to maintain alignment until healing occurs

E. Traction (see Chapter 68)
1. Russell skin traction
   a. Used to stabilize a fractured femur before surgery
   b. Similar to Buck's traction, but provides a double pull using a knee sling that pulls at the knee and foot
2. Balanced suspension
   a. Used with skin or skeletal traction to approximate fractures of the femur, tibia, or fibula
   b. Balanced suspension is produced by a counterforce other than the child.
   c. Provide pin care if pins are used with the skeletal traction.
3. 90-degree–90-degree traction
   a. The lower leg is supported by a boot cast or a calf sling.
   b. A skeletal Steinmann pin or Kirschner wire is placed in the distal fragment of the femur, allowing 90-degree flexion at the hip and the knee.
4. Interventions
   a. Maintain correct amount of weight as prescribed.
   b. Ensure that weights hang freely.
   c. Check all ropes for fraying and all knots for tightness; be sure that the ropes are appropriately tracking in the grooves of the pulley wheels.
   d. Monitor neurovascular status of the involved extremity.
   e. Protect the skin from breakdown.
   f. Monitor for signs and symptoms of complications of immobilization, such as constipation, skin breakdown, lung congestion, renal complications, and disuse syndrome of unaffected extremities.
   g. Provide therapeutic and diversional play.

F. Casts (see Chapter 68)
1. Description
   a. Made of plaster or fiberglass to provide immobilization of bone and joints after a fracture or injury
   b. Fractures of the hip or knee may require a spica cast.

2. Interventions
   a. Examine the cast for pressure areas.
   b. Ensure that no rough casting material remains in contact with the skin; petal the cast edges as necessary (Fig. 44-4).
   c. If a hip spica cast is placed, the cast edges around the perineum and buttocks may need to be taped with waterproof tape.
   d. Monitor the extremity for circulatory impairment, such as pain greater than that expected for the type of injury, edema, rubor, pallor, numbness and tingling, coolness, decreased sensation or mobility, or diminished pulse.
   e. Notify the physician if circulatory impairment occurs.
   f. Prepare for bivalving or cutting the cast if circulatory impairment occurs; prepare for emergency fasciotomy if cast removal does not improve the neurocirculatory compromise.
   g. Instruct parents and child not to stick objects down the cast.
   h. Teach parents and child to keep the cast clean and dry.
   i. Instruct parents and child in isometric exercises to prevent muscle atrophy.

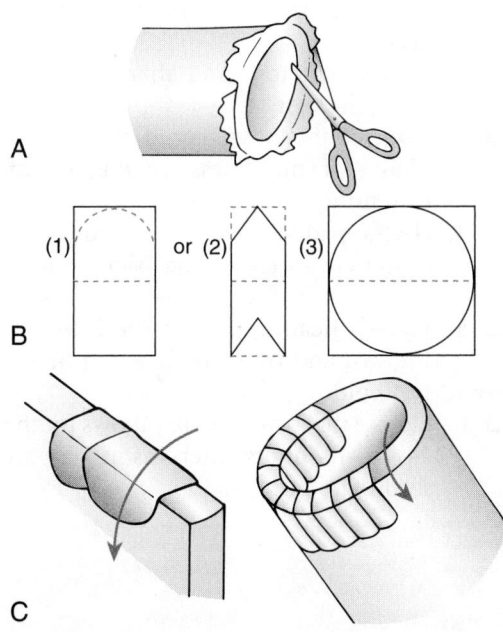

A

(1)   or (2)   (3)

B

C

▲ **FIGURE 44-4** Petaling edges of a cast with waterproof adhesive strips. **A,** Cast must be thoroughly dry. The nurse trims excess sheet wadding and stretches stockinette over cast edge (when possible). **B,** Several strips (petals) of waterproof adhesive tape (2-inch-wide strips for small areas, each 1 inch long) are made in advance. **C,** Uncut end of tape is placed beneath cast edge. Each succeeding petal overlaps the previous one by ½ inch, ensuring a smooth cast edge. (From Lewis, S., Heitkemper, M., & Dirksen, S. [2007]. *Medical-surgical nursing: Assessment and management of clinical problems* [7th ed.]. St. Louis: Mosby.)

MORE QUESTIONS ON THE CD!

Practice Questions

444. A child has a right femur fracture caused by a motor vehicle accident and is placed in skin traction temporarily until surgery can be performed. During assessment, the nurse notes that the dorsalis pedal pulse is absent on the right foot. What action should the nurse take?
1. Notify the physician.
2. Administer an analgesic.
3. Release the skin traction.
4. Apply ice to the extremity.

445. A child is placed in skeletal traction for treatment of a fractured femur. The nurse develops a plan of care for the child and includes which intervention in the plan?
1. Ensure that all ropes are outside the pulleys.
2. Ensure that the weights are resting lightly on the floor.
3. Restrict diversional and play activities until the child is out of traction.
4. Check the physician's prescriptions for the amount of weight to be applied.

446. A 4-year-old child sustains a fall at home and is brought to the emergency department by the mother. After an x-ray examination, the child is determined to have a fractured arm and a plaster cast is applied. The nurse provides instructions to the mother regarding care for the child's cast. Which statement by the mother indicates a need for further instructions?
1. "The cast may feel warm as the cast dries."
2. "I can use lotion or powder around the cast edges to relieve itching."
3. "A small amount of white shoe polish can touch up a soiled white cast."
4. "If the cast becomes wet, a blow drier set on the cool setting may be used to dry the cast."

447. A mother brings her 2-week-old infant to a clinic for treatment after a diagnosis of clubfoot made at birth. Which statement by the mother indicates a need for further teaching regarding this disorder?
1. "Treatment needs to be started as soon as possible."
2. "I realize my infant will require follow-up care until full grown."
3. "I need to bring my infant back to the clinic in 1 month for a new cast."
4. "I need to come to the clinic every week with my infant for the casting."

448. The mother of a child with juvenile idiopathic arthritis calls the clinic nurse because the child is experiencing a painful exacerbation of the disease. The mother asks the nurse if the child can perform range-of-motion exercises at this time. The appropriate nursing response is:
1. "Avoid all exercise during painful periods."
2. "Range-of-motion exercises must be performed every day."
3. "Have the child perform simple isometric exercises during this time."
4. "Administer additional pain medication before performing range-of-motion exercises."

449. A nurse is caring for a child after spinal fusion for scoliosis treatment. The child complains of abdominal discomfort and begins to have episodes of vomiting. On further assessment, the nurse notes abdominal distention. Based on these findings, the nurse should take which action?
1. Notify the physician.
2. Administer an antiemetic.
3. Increase the intravenous fluids.
4. Place the child in a Sims' position.

450. A nurse is providing instructions to the parents of a child with scoliosis regarding the use of a brace. Which statement by the parents indicates a need for further instructions?
1. "I will encourage my child to perform prescribed exercises."
2. "I will have my child wear soft fabric clothing under the brace."
3. "I should apply lotion under the brace to prevent skin breakdown."
4. "I should avoid the use of powder because it will cake under the brace."

451. A nurse is assisting a physician during the examination of an infant with developmental dysplasia of the hip. The physician performs an Ortolani maneuver. The nurse is aware that this maneuver is performed to:
1. Assess for hip instability.
2. Assess for movement of the hips.
3. Push the femoral head out of the acetabulum.
4. Ensure that hyperextension and full range of motion exists.

452. A 1-month-old infant is seen in a clinic and is diagnosed with developmental dysplasia of the hip. The nurse assesses the infant, knowing that which of the following findings would be noted in this condition?
1. Limited range of motion in the affected hip
2. An apparent lengthened femur on the affected side
3. Asymmetrical adduction of the affected hip when the infant is placed supine with the knees and hips flexed
4. Symmetry of the gluteal skinfolds when the infant is placed prone and the legs are extended against the examining table

Alternate Item Format: Multiple Response

453. A nurse prepares a list of home care instructions for the parents of a child who has a plaster cast applied to the left forearm. Which instructions would be included on the list? **Select all that apply**.
❏ 1. Use the fingertips to lift the cast while it is drying.
❏ 2. Keep small toys and sharp objects away from the cast.
❏ 3. Contact the physician if the child complains of numbness or tingling in the extremity.
❏ 4. Use a padded ruler or another padded object to scratch the skin under the cast if it itches.
❏ 5. Place a heating pad on the lower end of the cast and over the fingers if the fingers feel cold.
❏ 6. Elevate the extremity on pillows for the first 24 to 48 hours after casting to prevent swelling.

ANSWERS
444. 1
Rationale: An absent pulse to an extremity of the affected limb after a bone fracture could mean that the child is developing or experiencing compartment syndrome. This is an emergency situation, and the physician should be notified immediately. Applying ice to an extremity with absent perfusion is incorrect. Ice may be prescribed when perfusion is adequate to decrease swelling. Administering analgesics would not improve circulation. The skin traction should not be released without a physician's prescription.

Test-Taking Strategy: Use the ABCs—airway, breathing, and circulation—to assist in answering this question. Focusing on the data in the question indicates that circulation is impaired. This should direct you to option 1. Review care of the child in traction and the complications of a fracture if you had difficulty with this question.

Level of Cognitive Ability: Applying
Client Needs: Physiological Integrity
Integrated Process: Nursing Process—Implementation
Content Area: Child Health—Neurological/Musculoskeletal
Reference: Hockenberry, M., & Wilson, D. (2009). *Wong's essentials of pediatric nursing* (8th ed., p. 1120). St. Louis: Mosby.

445. 4

Rationale: When a child is in traction, the nurse would check the physician's prescription to verify the prescribed amount of traction weight. The nurse would maintain the correct amount of weight as prescribed, ensure that the weights hang freely, check the ropes for fraying and ensure that they are on the pulleys appropriately, monitor the neurovascular status of the involved extremity, and monitor for signs and symptoms of immobilization. The nurse would provide therapeutic and diversional play activities for the child.
Test-Taking Strategy: Use the process of elimination. Eliminate option 3 first because of the word *restrict*. Next recall the general principles related to traction, recalling that weights should hang freely and ropes should remain in the pulleys. Review care of the child in traction and the principles of traction care if you had difficulty with this question.
Level of Cognitive Ability: Applying
Client Needs: Physiological Integrity
Integrated Process: Nursing Process—Planning
Content Area: Child Health—Neurological/Musculoskeletal
References: Hockenberry, M., & Wilson, D. (2009). *Wong's essentials of pediatric nursing* (8th ed., p. 1120). St. Louis: Mosby.
   McKinney, E., James, S., Murray, S., & Ashwill, J. (2009). *Maternal-child nursing* (3rd ed., pp. 1384–1385). St. Louis: Saunders.

446. 2

Rationale: Teaching about cast care is essential to prevent complications from the cast. The mother needs to be instructed not to use lotion or powders on the skin around the cast edges or inside the cast. Lotions or powders can become sticky or caked and cause skin irritation. Options 1, 3, and 4 are appropriate statements.
Test-Taking Strategy: Note the strategic words *indicates a need for further instructions*. These words indicate a negative event query and ask you to select an option that is an incorrect statement. Remember that lotions or powders can become sticky or caked and cause skin irritation. Review home care instructions regarding cast care if you had difficulty with this question.
Level of Cognitive Ability: Evaluating
Client Needs: Physiological Integrity
Integrated Process: Teaching and Learning
Content Area: Child Health—Neurological/Musculoskeletal
Reference: McKinney, E., James, S., Murray, S., & Ashwill, J. (2009). *Maternal-child nursing* (3rd ed., p. 1387). St. Louis: Saunders.

447. 3

Rationale: Clubfoot is a complex deformity of the ankle and foot that includes forefoot adduction, midfoot supination, hindfoot varus, and ankle equinus; the defect may be unilateral or bilateral. Treatment for clubfoot is started as soon as possible after birth. Serial manipulation and casting are performed at least weekly. If sufficient correction is not achieved in 3 to 6 months, surgery usually is indicated. Because clubfoot can recur, all children with clubfoot require long-term interval follow-up until they reach skeletal maturity to ensure an optimal outcome.
Test-Taking Strategy: Use the process of elimination and note the strategic words *indicates a need for further teaching*. These words indicate a negative event query and ask you to select an option that is an incorrect statement. This will assist you in eliminating options 1 and 2. Recalling that serial manipulations and casting are required weekly will assist in directing you to option 3. Review these treatment procedures if you had difficulty with this question.
Level of Cognitive Ability: Evaluating
Client Needs: Physiological Integrity
Integrated Process: Teaching and Learning
Content Area: Child Health—Neurological/Musculoskeletal
Reference: Hockenberry, M., & Wilson, D. (2009). *Wong's essentials of pediatric nursing* (8th ed., p. 1126). St. Louis: Mosby.

448. 3

Rationale: Juvenile idiopathic arthritis is an autoimmune inflammatory disease affecting the joints and other tissues, such as articular cartilage. During painful episodes of juvenile idiopathic arthritis, hot or cold packs and splinting and positioning the affected joint in a neutral position help reduce the pain. Although resting the extremity is appropriate, beginning simple isometric or tensing exercises as soon as the child is able is important. These exercises do not involve joint movement.
Test-Taking Strategy: Use the process of elimination. Eliminate options 1, 2, and 4 because of the words *all, must,* and *additional* in these options. Review pain management and care during exacerbations of juvenile idiopathic arthritis if you had difficulty with this question.
Level of Cognitive Ability: Applying
Client Needs: Physiological Integrity
Integrated Process: Teaching and Learning
Content Area: Child Health—Neurological/Musculoskeletal
Reference: McKinney, E., James, S., Murray, S., & Ashwill, J. (2009). *Maternal-child nursing* (3rd ed., p. 1409). St. Louis: Saunders.

449. 1

Rationale: Scoliosis is a three-dimensional spinal deformity that usually involves lateral curvature, spinal rotation resulting in rib asymmetry, and hypokyphosis of the thorax. A complication after surgical treatment of scoliosis is superior mesenteric artery syndrome. This disorder is caused by mechanical changes in the position of the child's abdominal contents, resulting from lengthening of the child's body. The disorder results in a syndrome of emesis and abdominal distention similar to that which occurs with intestinal obstruction or paralytic ileus. Postoperative vomiting in children with body casts or children who have undergone spinal fusion warrants attention because of the possibility of superior mesenteric artery syndrome. Options 2, 3, and 4 are incorrect.
Test-Taking Strategy: Use the process of elimination. Eliminate option 3 first because it should not be implemented

unless prescribed by the physician. Eliminate option 4 next because this child requires logrolling, and Sims' position may cause injury after surgery. From the remaining options, note the assessment signs and symptoms in the question. These should alert you that notification of the physician is necessary. Review the manifestations of superior mesenteric artery syndrome if you had difficulty with this question.
Level of Cognitive Ability: Applying
Client Needs: Physiological Integrity
Integrated Process: Nursing Process—Implementation
Content Area: Child Health—Neurological/Musculoskeletal
Reference: McKinney, E., James, S., Murray, S., & Ashwill, J. (2009). *Maternal-child nursing* (3rd ed., p. 1418). St. Louis: Saunders.

450. 3

Rationale: A brace may be prescribed to treat scoliosis. Braces are not curative, but may slow the progression of the curvature to allow skeletal growth and maturity. The use of lotions or powders under a brace should be avoided because they can become sticky and cake under the brace, causing irritation. Options 1, 2, and 4 are appropriate interventions in the care of a child with a brace.
Test-Taking Strategy: Note the strategic words *need for further instructions* in the question. These words indicate a negative event query and ask you to select an option that is an incorrect statement. Careful reading of the options will assist in directing you to option 3. Also, applying the principles associated with cast care will direct you to the correct option. Review home care instructions regarding the care of a child in a brace if you had difficulty with this question.
Level of Cognitive Ability: Evaluating
Client Needs: Physiological Integrity
Integrated Process: Teaching and Learning
Content Area: Child Health—Neurological/Musculoskeletal
Reference: McKinney, E., James, S., Murray, S., & Ashwill, J. (2009). *Maternal-child nursing* (3rd ed., p. 1417). St. Louis: Saunders.

451. 1

Rationale: In developmental dysplasia of the hip, the head of the femur is seated improperly in the acetabulum or hip socket of the pelvis. Ortolani's maneuver is a test to assess for hip instability. The examiner abducts the thigh and applies gentle pressure forward over the greater trochanter. A "clunking" sensation indicates a dislocated femoral head moving into the acetabulum. This maneuver does not assess for hip movement or ensure that hyperextension and full range of motion exists. Pushing the femoral head out of the acetabulum is not a purpose of Ortolani's maneuver.
Test-Taking Strategy: Use the process of elimination. Options 2 and 4 can be eliminated first because they are comparable or alike. To select from the remaining options, remember that Ortolani's maneuver is an assessment technique. This will direct you to option 1. Review the purpose of Ortolani's maneuver if you had difficulty with this question.
Level of Cognitive Ability: Understanding

Client Needs: Physiological Integrity
Integrated Process: Nursing Process—Implementation
Content Area: Child Health—Neurological/Musculoskeletal
Reference: Hockenberry, M., & Wilson, D. (2009). *Wong's essentials of pediatric nursing* (8th ed., pp. 1122–1123). St. Louis: Mosby.

452. 1

Rationale: In developmental dysplasia of the hip, the head of the femur is seated improperly in the acetabulum or hip socket of the pelvis. Asymmetrical abduction of the affected hip, when the child is placed supine with the knees and hips flexed, would be an assessment finding in developmental dysplasia of the hip in infants beyond the newborn period. Other findings include an apparent short femur on the affected side, asymmetry of the gluteal skinfolds, and limited range of motion in the affected extremity.
Test-Taking Strategy: Note the age of the infant and focus on the infant's diagnosis. Visualizing each of the assessment findings described in the options will direct you to option 1. If you had difficulty with this question, review the assessment findings in developmental dysplasia of the hip.
Level of Cognitive Ability: Analyzing
Client Needs: Physiological Integrity
Integrated Process: Nursing Process—Assessment
Content Area: Child Health—Neurological/Musculoskeletal
Reference: McKinney, E., James, S., Murray, S., & Ashwill, J. (2009). *Maternal-child nursing* (3rd ed., p. 1390). St. Louis: Saunders.

ALTERNATE ITEM FORMAT: MULTIPLE RESPONSE

453. 2, 3, 6

Rationale: While the cast is drying, the palms of the hands are used to lift the cast. If the fingertips are used, indentations in the cast could occur and cause constant pressure on the underlying skin. Small toys and sharp objects are kept away from the cast, and no objects (including padded objects) are placed inside the cast because of the risk of altered skin integrity. The extremity is elevated to prevent swelling, and the physician is notified immediately if any signs of neurovascular impairment develop. A heating pad is not applied to the cast or fingers. Cold fingers could indicate neurovascular impairment, and the physician should be notified.
Test-Taking Strategy: Use of the ABCs—airway, breathing, and circulation—and safety principles related to care of a child with a cast will assist in answering this question. Review the general principles of cast care if you had difficulty with this question.
Level of Cognitive Ability: Applying
Client Needs: Physiological Integrity
Integrated Process: Teaching and Learning
Content Area: Child Health—Neurological/Musculoskeletal
Reference: McKinney, E., James, S., Murray, S., & Ashwill, J. (2009). *Maternal-child nursing* (3rd ed., p. 1388). St. Louis: Saunders.

45

Hematological Disorders

I. SICKLE CELL ANEMIA

A. Description

1. Sickle cell anemia constitutes a group of diseases termed *hemoglobinopathies,* in which hemoglobin A is partly or completely replaced by abnormal sickle hemoglobin S.

2. It is caused by the inheritance of a gene for a structurally abnormal portion of the hemoglobin chain.

3. Risk factors include having parents heterozygous for hemoglobin S or being of African-American descent.

4. Hemoglobin S is sensitive to changes in the oxygen content of the red blood cell.

5. Insufficient oxygen causes the cells to assume a sickle shape, and the cells become rigid and clumped together, obstructing capillary blood flow (Fig. 45-1)

6. The clinical manifestations primarily occur as a result of obstruction caused by sickled red blood cells and increased red blood cell destruction.

7. Situations that precipitate sickling include fever, dehydration, and emotional or physical stress; any condition that increases the need for oxygen or alters the transport of oxygen can result in sickle cell crisis (acute exacerbation).

8. Sickle cell crises are acute exacerbations of the disease, which vary considerably in severity and frequency; these include vaso-occlusive crisis, splenic sequestration, and aplastic crisis.

9. The sickling response is reversible under conditions of adequate oxygenation and hydration; after repeated sickling, the cell becomes permanently sickled.

10. A multidisciplinary approach to care is needed, and care focuses on the prevention (preventing exposure to infection and maintaining normal hydration) and treatment (oxygen, hydration, pain management, and bedrest) of the crisis.

B. Assessment of the crisis (Box 45-1)

Box 45-1 Sickle Cell Crisis

Vaso-Occlusive Crisis
Caused by stasis of blood with clumping of cells in the microcirculation, ischemia, and infarction
Manifestations: Fever; painful swelling of hands, feet, and joints; and abdominal pain

Splenic Sequestration
Caused by pooling and clumping of blood in the spleen (hypersplenism)
Manifestations: Profound anemia, hypovolemia, and shock

Aplastic Crisis
Caused by diminished production and increased destruction of red blood cells, triggered by viral infection or depletion of folic acid
Manifestations: Profound anemia and pallor

C. Interventions

1. Maintain adequate hydration and blood flow through oral and intravenously administered fluids; electrolyte replacement is also provided as needed.

2. Administer oxygen and blood transfusions as prescribed to increase tissue perfusion; exchange transfusions, which reduce the number of circulating sickle cells and the risk of complications, may also be prescribed.

3. Administer analgesics as prescribed (around the clock).

4. Assist the child to assume a comfortable position so that the child keeps the extremities extended to promote venous return; elevate the head of the bed no more than 30 degrees, avoid putting strain on painful joints, and do not raise the knee gatch of the bed.

5. Encourage consumption of a high-calorie, high-protein diet, with folic acid supplementation.

6. Administer antibiotics as prescribed to prevent infection.

7. Monitor for signs of complications, including increasing anemia, decreased perfusion, and shock (mental status changes, pallor, vital sign changes).

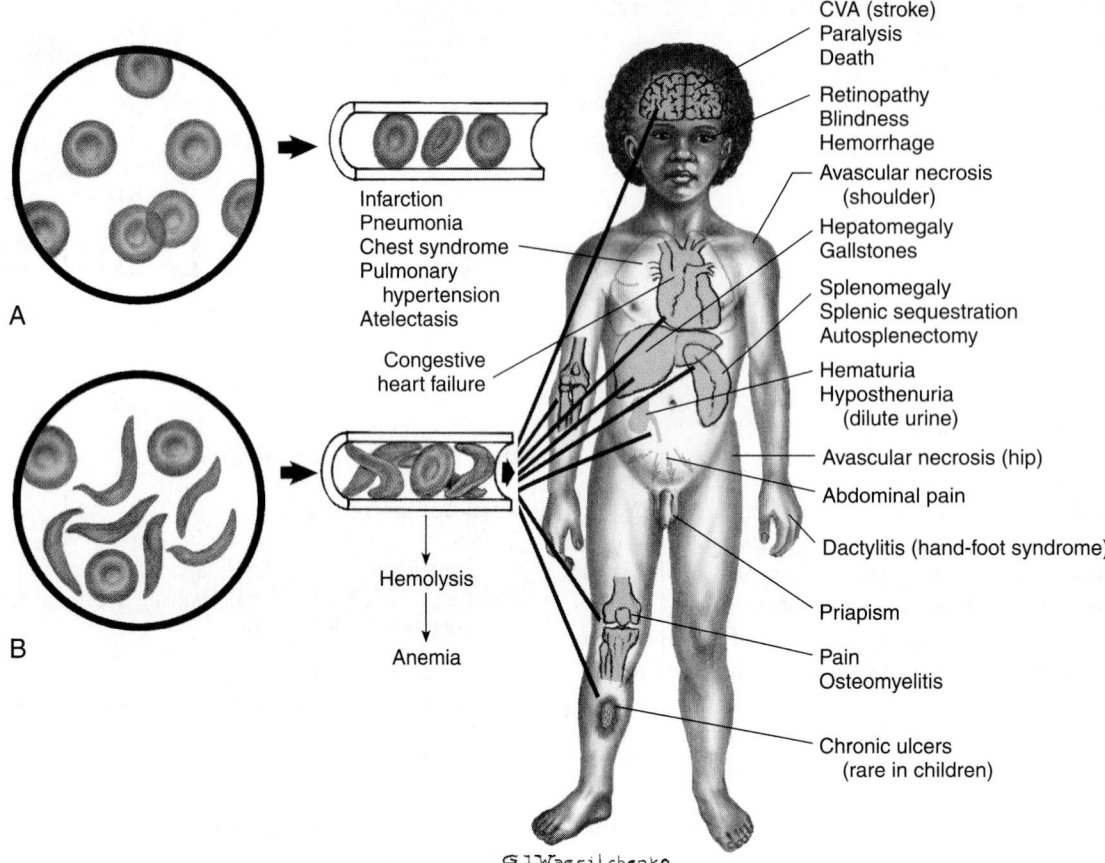

▲ **FIGURE 45-1** Differences between effects of (**A**) normal red blood cells and (**B**) sickled red blood cells on circulation, with related complications. (From Hockenberry, M., & Wilson, D. [2007]. *Nursing care of infants and children* [8th ed.]. St. Louis: Mosby.)

8. Instruct the child and parents about the early signs and symptoms of crisis and the measures to prevent crisis.

9. Ensure that the child receives pneumococcal and meningococcal **vaccines** and an annual influenza **vaccine** because of susceptibility to infection secondary to functional asplenia.

10. A splenectomy may be necessary for clients who experience recurrent splenic sequestration.

11. Inform parents of the **hereditary** aspects of the disorder.

⚠ Administration of meperidine (Demerol) for pain is avoided because of the risk of normeperidine-induced seizures.

II. IRON DEFICIENCY ANEMIA

A. Description

1. Iron stores are depleted, resulting in a decreased supply of iron for the manufacture of hemoglobin in red blood cells.

2. Iron deficiency anemia commonly results from blood loss, increased metabolic demands, syndromes of gastrointestinal malabsorption, and dietary inadequacy.

B. Assessment

1. Pallor

2. Weakness and fatigue

3. Irritability

4. Low hemoglobin and hematocrit levels

5. Red blood cells that are microcytic and hypochromic

C. Interventions

1. Increase oral intake of iron; iron-fortified formula is needed for an infant.

2. Instruct the child and parents in food choices that are high in iron (Box 45-2).

3. Administer iron supplements as prescribed.

4. Intramuscular injections of iron (using Z-track method) or intravenous administration of iron may be prescribed in severe cases of anemia.

5. Teach parents how to administer the iron supplements.

   a. Give iron supplements between meals for maximum absorption.

   b. Give iron supplements with a multivitamin or fruit juice because vitamin C increases absorption.

Box 45-2 Iron-Rich Foods

Breads and cereals	Molasses
Dark green, leafy vegetables	Nuts
Dried fruits	Potatoes
Egg yolks	Prune juice
Iron-enriched infant formula and cereal	Raisins
	Seeds
Kidney beans	Shellfish
Legumes	Tofu
Liver	Whole grains
Meats	

c. Do not give iron supplements with milk or antacids because these items decrease absorption.
6. Instruct the child and parents about the side effects of iron supplements (black stools, constipation, and foul aftertaste).

⚠ Liquid iron preparation stains the teeth. Teach the parents and child that liquid iron should be taken through a straw and that the teeth should be brushed after administration.

III. APLASTIC ANEMIA

A. Description
1. Aplastic anemia is a deficiency of circulating erythrocytes and all other formed elements of blood, resulting from the arrested development of cells within the bone marrow.
2. It can be primary (present at birth) or secondary (acquired).
3. Several possible causes exist, including chronic exposure to myelotoxic agents, viruses, infection, autoimmune disorders, and allergic states.
4. The definitive diagnosis is determined by bone marrow aspiration (shows conversion of red bone marrow to fatty bone marrow).
5. Therapeutic management focuses on restoring function to the bone marrow and involves immunosuppressive therapy and bone marrow transplantation (treatment of choice if a suitable donor exists).
6. If the cause is a myelotoxic medication that is being administered for another purpose, the medication may be discontinued to improve bone marrow function.

B. Assessment
1. Pancytopenia (deficiency of erythrocytes, leukocytes, and thrombocytes)
2. Petechiae, purpura, bleeding, pallor, weakness, tachycardia, and fatigue

C. Interventions
1. Prepare the child for bone marrow transplantation if planned.

Box 45-3 Hemophilia

Hemophilia A (classic hemophilia): Results from deficiency of factor VIII
Hemophilia B (Christmas disease): Results from deficiency of factor IX

2. Administer immunosuppressive medications as prescribed; antilymphocyte globulin or antithymocyte globulin may be prescribed to suppress the autoimmune response.
3. Colony-stimulating factors may be prescribed to enhance bone marrow production.
4. Corticosteroids and cyclosporine (sandimmune) may be prescribed.
5. Administer blood transfusions if prescribed and monitor for transfusion reactions.
6. Monitor for signs related to the disease and to complications of the treatments and medications administered.

IV. HEMOPHILIA

A. Description
1. Hemophilia refers to a group of bleeding disorders resulting from a deficiency of specific coagulation proteins.
2. Identifying the specific coagulation deficiency is important so that definitive treatment with the specific replacement agent can be implemented; aggressive replacement therapy is initiated to prevent the chronic crippling effects from joint bleeding.
3. The most common types are factor VIII deficiency (hemophilia A or classic hemophilia) and factor IX deficiency (hemophilia B or Christmas disease) (Box 45-3).
4. Hemophilia is transmitted as an X-linked recessive disorder (it may also occur as a result of a gene mutation).
5. Carrier females pass on the defect to affected males; female offspring are rarely born with the disorder, but may be if they inherit an affected gene from their mother and are offspring of a father with hemophilia.
6. The primary treatment is replacement of the missing clotting factor; additional medications, such as agents to relieve pain or corticosteroids, may be prescribed depending on the source of bleeding from the disorder.

B. Assessment
1. Abnormal bleeding in response to trauma or surgery (sometimes is detected after circumcision)
2. Epistaxis (nosebleeds)
3. Joint bleeding causing pain, tenderness, swelling, and limited range of motion
4. Tendency to bruise easily

5. Results of tests that measure platelet function are normal; results of tests that measure clotting factor function may be abnormal.

C. Interventions

1. Monitor for bleeding and maintain bleeding precautions.
2. Prepare to administer replacement factors as prescribed.
3. DDAVP (1-deamino-8-D-arginine vasopressin), a synthetic form of vasopressin, increases plasma factor VIII and may be prescribed to treat mild hemophilia.
4. Monitor for joint pain; immobilize the affected extremity if joint pain occurs.
5. Assess neurological status (child is at risk for intracranial hemorrhage).
6. Monitor urine for hematuria.
7. Control joint bleeding by immobilization, elevation, and application of ice; apply pressure (15 minutes) for superficial bleeding.
8. Instruct the child and parents about the signs of internal bleeding.
9. Instruct parents in how to control the bleeding.
10. Instruct parents regarding activities for the child, emphasizing the avoidance of contact sports and the need for protective devices while learning to walk; assist in developing an appropriate exercise plan.
11. Instruct the child to wear protective devices such as helmets and knee and elbow pads when participating in sports such as bicycling and skating.

V. VON WILLEBRAND'S DISEASE

A. Description
1. von Willebrand's disease is a **hereditary** bleeding disorder that occurs in males and females and is characterized by a deficiency of or a defect in a protein termed *von Willebrand factor*.
2. The disorder causes platelets to adhere to damaged endothelium; the von Willebrand factor protein also serves as a carrier protein for factor VIII.
3. It is characterized by an increased tendency to bleed from mucous membranes.

B. Assessment
1. Epistaxis
2. Gum bleeding
3. Easy bruising
4. Excessive menstrual bleeding

C. Interventions
1. Treatment and care are similar to measures implemented for hemophilia, including administration of clotting factors.
2. Provide emotional support to the child and parents, especially if the child is experiencing an episode of bleeding.

Box 45-4 Types of β-Thalassemia

Thalassemia minor: Asymptomatic silent carrier case
Thalassemia trait: Produces mild microcytic anemia
Thalassemia intermedia: Manifested as splenomegaly and moderate to severe anemia
Thalassemia major: Results in severe anemia requiring transfusion support to sustain life (also known as Cooley's anemia)

⚠ A child with a bleeding disorder needs to wear a Medic-Alert bracelet.

VI. β-THALASSEMIA MAJOR

A. Description (Box 45-4)
1. β-thalassemia major is an autosomal recessive disorder characterized by the reduced production of one of the globin chains in the synthesis of hemoglobin (both parents must be carriers to produce a child with β-thalassemia major).
2. The incidence is highest in individuals of Mediterranean descent, such as Italians, Greeks, Syrians, or their offspring.
3. Treatment is supportive; the goal of therapy is to maintain normal hemoglobin levels by the administration of blood transfusions.
4. Bone marrow transplantation may be offered as an alternative therapy.
5. A splenectomy may be performed in a child with severe splenomegaly who requires repeated transfusions (assists in relieving abdominal pressure and may increase the life span of supplemental red blood cells).

B. Assessment
1. Frontal bossing
2. Maxillary prominence
3. Wide-set eyes with a flattened nose
4. Greenish yellow skin tone
5. Hepatosplenomegaly
6. Severe anemia
7. Microcytic, hypochromic red blood cells

C. Interventions
1. Administer blood transfusions as prescribed; monitor for transfusion reactions.
2. Monitor for iron overload; chelation therapy with deferasirox (Exjade) or deferoxamine (Desferal) may be prescribed to treat iron overload and to prevent organ damage from the elevated levels of iron caused by the multiple transfusion therapy.
3. If the child has had a splenectomy, instruct parents to report any signs of infection because of the risk of sepsis.

4. Ensure that parents understand the importance of the child receiving pneumococcal and meningococcal **vaccines** in addition to an annual influenza vaccine and the regularly schedules **vaccines**.

5. Provide genetic counseling to parents.

 MORE QUESTIONS ON THE CD!

Practice Questions

454. A home care nurse is instructing the parents of a child with iron deficiency anemia regarding the administration of a liquid oral iron supplement. The nurse tells the mother to:
1. Administer the iron at mealtimes.
2. Administer the iron through a straw.
3. Mix the iron with cereal to administer.
4. Add the iron to formula for easy administration.

455. A nurse analyzes the laboratory results of a child with hemophilia. The nurse understands that which of the following would most likely be abnormal in this child?
1. Platelet count
2. Hematocrit level
3. Hemoglobin level
4. Partial thromboplastin time

456. A nurse is providing home care instructions to the mother of a 10-year-old child with hemophilia. Which of the following activities should the nurse suggest that the child could participate in safely with peers?
1. Soccer
2. Basketball
3. Swimming
4. Field hockey

457. A nursing student is presenting a clinical conference and discusses the cause of β-thalassemia. The nursing student informs the group that a child at greatest risk of developing this disorder is:
1. A child of Mexican descent
2. A child of Mediterranean descent
3. A child whose intake of iron is extremely poor
4. A breast-fed child of a mother with chronic anemia

458. A child with β-thalassemia is receiving long-term blood transfusion therapy for the treatment of this disorder. Chelation therapy is prescribed to prevent organ damage from the presence of too much iron in the body as a result of the transfusions. Which of the following medications would

the nurse anticipate to be prescribed in chelation therapy?
1. Meropenem (Merrem)
2. Metoprolol (Toprol-XL)
3. Deferoxamine (Desferal)
4. Dalteparin sodium (Fragmin)

459. A clinic nurse instructs the mother of a child with sickle cell anemia about the precipitating factors related to sickle cell crisis. Which of the following, if identified by the mother as a precipitating factor, indicates the need for further instructions?
1. Stress
2. Trauma
3. Infection
4. Fluid overload

460. A 10-year-old child with hemophilia A has slipped on the ice and bumped his knee. The nurse should prepare to administer an:
1. Injection of factor X
2. Intravenous infusion of iron
3. Intravenous infusion of factor VIII
4. Intramuscular injection of iron using the Z-track method

461. Laboratory studies are performed for a child suspected to have iron deficiency anemia. The nurse reviews the laboratory results, knowing that which of the following results would indicate this type of anemia?
1. Elevated hemoglobin level
2. Decreased reticulocyte count
3. Elevated red blood cell count
4. Red blood cells that are microcytic and hypochromic

Alternate Item Format: Multiple Response

462. A nurse is reviewing a physician's prescriptions for a child with sickle cell anemia who was admitted to the hospital for the treatment of vaso-occlusive crisis. Which prescriptions documented in the child's record should the nurse question? **Select all that apply.**
- ❑ 1. Restrict fluid intake.
- ❑ 2. Position for comfort.
- ❑ 3. Avoid strain on painful joints.
- ❑ 4. Apply nasal oxygen at 2 L/min.
- ❑ 5. Provide a high-calorie, high-protein diet.
- ❑ 6. Give meperidine (Demerol), 25 mg intravenously, every 4 hours for pain.

463. Which of the following are characteristics of von Willebrand's disease? **Select all that apply.**
- ❑ 1. Easy bruising occurs.

❏ 2. Gum bleeding occurs.
❏ 3. It is a hereditary bleeding disorder.
❏ 4. It is characterized by extremely high creatinine levels.

❏ 5. The disorder causes platelets to adhere to damaged endothelium.
❏ 6. Treatment and care are similar to that for hemophilia.

ANSWERS

454. 2

Rationale: In iron deficiency anemia, iron stores are depleted, resulting in a decreased supply of iron for the manufacture of hemoglobin in red blood cells. An oral iron supplement should be administered through a straw or medicine dropper placed at the back of the mouth because the iron stains the teeth. The parents should be instructed to brush or wipe the child's teeth or have the child brush the teeth after administration. Iron is administered between meals because absorption is decreased if there is food in the stomach. Iron requires an acid environment to facilitate its absorption in the duodenum. Iron is not added to formula or mixed with cereal or other food items.

Test-Taking Strategy: Use the process of elimination. Eliminate options 3 and 4 first because they are comparable or alike and because medication should not be added to formula and food. Note the strategic word *liquid* in the question. This should assist you in recalling that iron in liquid form stains teeth. Review the teaching points related to the administration of oral liquid iron if you had difficulty with this question.

Level of Cognitive Ability: Applying
Client Needs: Physiological Integrity
Integrated Process: Teaching and Learning
Content Area: Child Health—Hematological/Oncological
Reference: McKinney, E., James, S., Murray, S., & Ashwill, J. (2009). *Maternal-child nursing* (3rd ed., p. 1282). St. Louis: Saunders.

455. 4

Rationale: Hemophilia refers to a group of bleeding disorders resulting from a deficiency of specific coagulation proteins. Results of tests that measure platelet function are normal; results of tests that measure clotting factor function may be abnormal. Abnormal laboratory results in hemophilia indicate a prolonged partial thromboplastin time. The platelet count, hemoglobin level, and hematocrit level are normal in hemophilia.

Test-Taking Strategy: Use the process of elimination and knowledge regarding the laboratory tests used to monitor hemophilia. Recalling the pathophysiology associated with this disorder and recalling that it results from a deficiency of specific coagulation proteins will direct you to option 4. Review these laboratory tests if you had difficulty with this question.

Level of Cognitive Ability: Understanding
Client Needs: Physiological Integrity
Integrated Process: Nursing Process—Assessment
Content Area: Child Health—Hematological/Oncological
Reference: McKinney, E., James, S., Murray, S., & Ashwill, J. (2009). *Maternal-child nursing* (3rd ed., p. 1292). St. Louis: Saunders.

456. 3

Rationale: Hemophilia refers to a group of bleeding disorders resulting from a deficiency of specific coagulation proteins. Children with hemophilia need to avoid contact sports and to take precautions such as wearing elbow and knee pads and helmets with other sports. The safe activity for them is swimming.

Test-Taking Strategy: Use the process of elimination and note the strategic word *safely* in the question. Recalling that bleeding is a major concern in this condition will assist in directing you to option 3. Eliminate options 1, 2, and 4 because these activities present the potential for injury. Review home care and safety instructions for a child with hemophilia if you had difficulty with this question.

Level of Cognitive Ability: Applying
Client Needs: Safe and Effective Care Environment
Integrated Process: Teaching and Learning
Content Area: Child Health—Hematological/Oncological
Reference: McKinney, E., James, S., Murray, S., & Ashwill, J. (2009). *Maternal-child nursing* (3rd ed., p. 1295). St. Louis: Saunders.

457. 2

Rationale: β-thalassemia is an autosomal recessive disorder characterized by the reduced production of one of the globin chains in the synthesis of hemoglobin (both parents must be carriers to produce a child with β-thalassemia major). This disorder is found primarily in individuals of Mediterranean descent. Options 1, 3, and 4 are incorrect.

Test-Taking Strategy: Think about the pathophysiology of the disorder. Also, recall that this disorder occurs primarily in individuals of Mediterranean descent. If you are unfamiliar with β-thalassemia, review the information associated with its incidence and cause.

Level of Cognitive Ability: Applying
Client Needs: Physiological Integrity
Integrated Process: Teaching and Learning
Content Area: Child Health—Hematological/Oncological
Reference: McKinney, E., James, S., Murray, S., & Ashwill, J. (2009). *Maternal-child nursing* (3rd ed., p. 1289). St. Louis: Saunders.

458. 3

Rationale: β-thalassemia is an autosomal recessive disorder characterized by the reduced production of one of the globin chains in the synthesis of hemoglobin (both parents must be carriers to produce a child with β-thalassemia major). The major complication of long-term transfusion therapy is hemosiderosis. To prevent organ damage from too much iron, chelation therapy with either deferasirox (Exjade) or deferoxamine (Desferal) may be prescribed. Deferoxamine is classified as an antidote for acute iron toxicity. Dalteparin is

an anticoagulant used as prophylaxis for postoperative deep vein thrombosis. Meropenem is an antibiotic. Metoprolol is a β-blocker used to treat hypertension.
Test-Taking Strategy: Specific knowledge regarding the antidote for iron toxicity is needed to answer this question. One way to remember this is to look at the prefix in the generic name of the medication used to treat iron overdose. Remember to associate *defer-* and removal of iron. If you had difficulty with this question, review the medications used for chelation therapy.
Level of Cognitive Ability: Analyzing
Client Needs: Physiological Integrity
Integrated Process: Nursing Process—Analysis
Content Area: Child Health—Hematological/Oncological
References: Hockenberry, M., & Wilson, D. (2009). *Wong's essentials of pediatric nursing* (8th ed., p. 924). St. Louis: Mosby.
   McKinney, E., James, S., Murray, S., & Ashwill, J. (2009). *Maternal-child nursing* (3rd ed., p. 1290). St. Louis: Saunders.

459. 4
Rationale: Sickle cell crises are acute exacerbations of the disease, which vary considerably in severity and frequency; these include vaso-occlusive crisis, splenic sequestration, and aplastic crisis. Sickle cell crisis may be precipitated by infection, dehydration, hypoxia, trauma, or physical or emotional stress. The mother of a child with sickle cell disease should encourage fluid intake of 1½ to 2 times the daily requirement to prevent dehydration.
Test-Taking Strategy: Note the strategic words *the need for further instructions.* These words indicate a negative event query and ask you to select an option that is an incorrect statement. Recalling that fluids are a main component of treatment in sickle cell anemia to prevent crisis will direct you to option 4. Remember that fluids are required to prevent dehydration. Review the precipitating factors of sickle cell crisis if you had difficulty with this question.
Level of Cognitive Ability: Evaluating
Client Needs: Health Promotion and Maintenance
Integrated Process: Teaching and Learning
Content Area: Child Health—Hematological/Oncological
References: Perry, S., Hockenberry, M., Lowdermilk, D., & Wilson, D. (2010). *Maternal child nursing care* (4th ed., pp. 1495–1497). St. Louis: Mosby.
   McKinney, E., James, S., Murray, S., & Ashwill, J. (2009). *Maternal-child nursing* (3rd ed., p. 1287). St. Louis: Saunders.

460. 3
Rationale: Hemophilia refers to a group of bleeding disorders resulting from a deficiency of specific coagulation proteins. The primary treatment is replacement of the missing clotting factor; additional medications, such as agents to relieve pain, may be prescribed depending on the source of bleeding from the disorder. A child with hemophilia A is at risk for joint bleeding after a fall. Factor VIII would be prescribed intravenously to replace the missing clotting factor and minimize the bleeding. Factor X and iron are not used to treat children with hemophilia A.
Test-Taking Strategy: Focus on the child's diagnosis. Eliminate options 2 and 4 because they are comparable or alike. Recalling that a child with hemophilia A is missing clotting

factor VIII will direct you to the correct option from the remaining options. Review the treatment for bleeding episodes for children with hemophilia A if you had difficulty with this question.
Level of Cognitive Ability: Applying
Client Needs: Physiological Integrity
Integrated Process: Nursing Process—Planning
Content Area: Child Health—Hematological/Oncological
References: McKinney, E., James, S., Murray, S., & Ashwill, J. (2009). *Maternal-child nursing* (3rd ed., p. 1282). St. Louis: Saunders.
   Perry, S., Hockenberry, M., Lowdermilk, D., & Wilson, D. (2010). *Maternal child nursing care* (4th ed., p. 1503). St. Louis: Mosby.

461. 4
Rationale: In iron deficiency anemia, iron stores are depleted, resulting in a decreased supply of iron for the manufacture of hemoglobin in red blood cells. The results of a complete blood cell count in children with iron deficiency anemia show decreased hemoglobin levels and microcytic and hypochromic red blood cells. The red blood cell count is decreased. The reticulocyte count is usually normal or slightly elevated.
Test-Taking Strategy: Use the process of elimination. Eliminate options 1 and 3 first, knowing that the hemoglobin and red blood cell counts would be decreased. From the remaining options, select option 4 over option 2 because of the relationship between anemia and red blood cells. Review the laboratory findings in iron deficiency anemia if you had difficulty with this question.
Level of Cognitive Ability: Understanding
Client Needs: Physiological Integrity
Integrated Process: Nursing Process—Assessment
Content Area: Child Health—Hematological/Oncological
Reference: McKinney, E., James, S., Murray, S., & Ashwill, J. (2009). *Maternal-child nursing* (3rd ed., p. 1280). St. Louis: Saunders.

ALTERNATE ITEM FORMAT: MULTIPLE RESPONSE
462. 1, 6
Rationale: Sickle cell anemia is one of a group of diseases termed *hemoglobinopathies,* in which hemoglobin A is partly or completely replaced by abnormal sickle hemoglobin S. It is caused by the inheritance of a gene for a structurally abnormal portion of the hemoglobin chain. Hemoglobin S is sensitive to changes in the oxygen content of the red blood cell; insufficient oxygen causes the cells to assume a sickle shape, and the cells become rigid and clumped together, obstructing capillary blood flow. Oral and intravenous fluids are an important part of treatment. Meperidine (Demerol) is not recommended for a child with sickle cell disease because of the risk for normeperidine-induced seizures. Normeperidine, a metabolite of meperidine, is a central nervous system stimulant that produces anxiety, tremors, myoclonus, and generalized seizures when it accumulates with repetitive dosing. The nurse would question the prescription for restricted fluids and meperidine for pain control. Positioning for comfort, avoiding strain on painful joints, oxygen, and a high-calorie and high-protein diet are also important parts of the treatment plan.

Test-Taking Strategy: Focus on the pathophysiology that occurs in sickle cell disease to assist in identifying the prescriptions that need to be questioned. Recalling that fluids are an important component of the treatment plan will assist in identifying that a fluid restriction prescription would need to be questioned. Recalling the effects of meperidine will assist in identifying that this prescription needs to be questioned. Review care of a child with sickle cell anemia experiencing a crisis if you had difficulty with this question.

Level of Cognitive Ability: Analyzing
Client Needs: Physiological Integrity
Integrated Process: Nursing Process—Analysis
Content Area: Child Health—Hematological/Oncological
References: Hockenberry, M., & Wilson, D. (2009). *Wong's essentials of pediatric nursing* (8th ed., p. 921). St. Louis: Mosby.

McKinney, E., James, S., Murray, S., & Ashwill, J. (2009). *Maternal-child nursing* (3rd ed., p. 1285). St. Louis: Saunders.

463. 1, 2, 3, 5, 6

Rationale: von Willebrand's disease is a hereditary bleeding disorder characterized by a deficiency of or a defect in a protein termed *von Willebrand factor*. The disorder causes platelets to adhere to damaged endothelium. It is characterized by an increased tendency to bleed from mucous membranes. Assessment findings include epistaxis, gum bleeding, easy bruising, and excessive menstrual bleeding. An elevated creatinine level is not associated with this disorder.

Test-Taking Strategy: Focus on the child's diagnosis. Recalling that this disorder is characterized by an increased tendency to bleed from mucous membranes will direct you to select the correct options. Review the manifestations associated with von Willebrand's disease if you had difficulty with this question.

Level of Cognitive Ability: Analyzing
Client Needs: Physiological Integrity
Integrated Process: Nursing Process—Assessment
Content Area: Child Health—Hematological/Oncological
References: Hockenberry, M., & Wilson, D. (2009). *Wong's essentials of pediatric nursing* (8th ed., pp. 925–926). St. Louis: Mosby.

McKinney, E., James, S., Murray, S., & Ashwill, J. (2009). *Maternal-child nursing* (3rd ed., p. 1295). St. Louis: Saunders.

Oncological Disorders

I. LEUKEMIA

A. Description

1. Leukemia (Box 46-1) is a malignant increase in the number of leukocytes, usually at an immature stage, in the bone marrow.
2. Leukemia affects the bone marrow, causing anemia from decreased erythrocytes, infection from neutropenia, and bleeding from decreased platelet production (thrombocytopenia).
3. The cause is unknown; it seems to involve genetic damage of cells, leading to the transformation of cells from a normal state to a malignant state.
4. Risk factors include genetic, viral, immunological, and environmental factors and exposure to radiation, chemicals, and medications.
5. Acute lymphocytic leukemia is the most frequent type of cancer in children; peak onset is age 2 to 6 years.
6. Leukemia is more common in boys than girls after 1 year of age.
7. Prognosis depends on various factors such as age at diagnosis, initial white blood cell count, type of cell involved, and sex of the child.
8. Treatment involves chemotherapy and possibly radiation.
9. The phases of chemotherapy include induction, which achieves a complete remission or disappearance of leukemic cells; intensification or consolidation therapy, which decreases the tumor burden further; central nervous system prophylactic therapy, which prevents leukemic cells from invading the central nervous system;

Box 46-1 Classification of Leukemia

Acute Lymphocytic Leukemia
Mostly lymphoblasts present in bone marrow
Age of onset younger than 15 years

Acute Myelogenous Leukemia
Mostly myeloblasts present in bone marrow
Age of onset between 15 and 39 years

---

and maintenance, which serves to maintain the remission phase.
10. Hematopoietic stem cell transplantation also may be performed to treat some children with leukemia.

B. Assessment

1. Infiltration of the bone marrow by malignant cells causes fever, pallor, fatigue, anorexia, hemorrhage (usually petechiae), and bone and joint pain; pathological fractures can occur as a result of bone marrow invasion with leukemic cells.
2. Signs of infection occur as a result of neutropenia.
3. The child experiences hepatosplenomegaly and lymphadenopathy.
4. The child has a normal, elevated, or low white blood cell count, depending on the presence of infection or of immature versus mature white blood cells.
5. The child has decreased hemoglobin and hematocrit levels.
6. The child has a decreased platelet count.
7. A positive bone marrow biopsy specimen identifies leukemic blast (immature)-phase cells.
8. Signs of increased intracranial pressure, such as severe headache, vomiting, papilledema, irritability, lethargy, and eventually coma, occur as a result of central nervous system involvement.
9. The child shows signs of cranial nerve (cranial nerve VII, or the facial nerve, is most commonly affected) or spinal nerve involvement; clinical manifestations relate to the area involved.
10. Clinical manifestations indicate the invasion of leukemic cells to the kidneys, testes, prostate, ovaries, gastrointestinal tract, and lungs.

C. Infection (Box 46-2)

1. Infection can occur through self-contamination or cross-contamination.
2. The most common sites for infection are the skin (any break in the skin is a potential site of infection), respiratory tract, and gastrointestinal tract.

527

D. Bleeding (Box 46-3)
1. A child with a platelet count less than 20,000 cells/mm³ may need a platelet transfusion.
2. Packed red blood cells may be prescribed for a child with severe blood loss.

E. Fatigue and nutrition
1. Assist the parents and child in selecting a well-balanced diet.
2. Provide small meals that require little chewing and are not irritating to the oral mucosa.

3. If the child cannot take oral feedings, parenteral nutrition or enteral feedings may be prescribed.
4. Assist the child in self-care and mobility activities.
5. Allow adequate rest periods during care.
6. Do not perform nursing care activities unless they are essential.

F. Chemotherapy
1. Monitor for severe bone marrow suppression; during the period of greatest bone marrow

---

Box 46-2 Protecting the Child From Infection

Initiate protective isolation procedures.

Maintain frequent and thorough handwashing.

Maintain the child in a private room with high-efficiency particulate air filtration or laminar air flow system if possible.

Ensure that the child's room is cleaned daily.

Use strict aseptic technique for all nursing procedures.

Limit the number of caregivers entering the child's room, and ensure that anyone entering the child's room wears a mask.

Keep supplies for the child separate from supplies for other children.

Reduce exposure to environmental organisms by eliminating raw fruits and vegetables from the diet and not allowing fresh flowers in the child's room and by not leaving standing water in the child's room.

Assist the child with daily bathing, using antimicrobial soap.

Assist the child to perform oral hygiene frequently.

Assess for signs and symptoms of infection.

Monitor temperature, pulse, and blood pressure.

Change wound dressings daily, and inspect wounds for redness, swelling, or drainage.

Assess urine for color and cloudiness.

Assess the skin and oral mucous membranes for signs of infection.

Auscultate lung sounds.

Encourage the child to cough and deep-breathe.

Monitor white blood cell and neutrophil counts.

Notify the physician if signs of infection are present, and prepare to obtain specimens for culture of open lesions, urine, and sputum.

Initiate a bowel program to prevent constipation and rectal trauma.

Avoid invasive procedures such as injections, rectal temperatures, and urinary catheterization.

Administer antibiotic, antifungal, and antiviral medications as prescribed.

Administer granulocyte colony-stimulating factor as prescribed.

Instruct parents to keep the child away from crowds and individuals with infections.

Instruct parents that the child should not receive immunization with a live virus (measles, mumps, rubella, polio) because if the immune system is depressed, the attenuated virus can result in a life-threatening infection; also, the child should not receive the varicella vaccine.

The Salk (inactivated) vaccine for poliomyelitis may be administered.

Instruct parents to inform the teacher that they should be notified immediately if a case of a communicable disease occurs in another child at school.

Box 46-3 Protecting the Child From Bleeding

Examine the child for signs and symptoms of bleeding.

Handle the child gently.

Measure abdominal girth; an increase can indicate internal hemorrhage.

Instruct the child to use a soft toothbrush and avoid dental floss.

Provide soft foods that are cool to warm in temperature.

Avoid injections, if possible, to prevent trauma to the skin and bleeding.

Apply firm and gentle pressure to a needle stick site for at least 10 minutes.

Pad side rails and sharp corners of the bed and furniture.

Discourage the child from engaging in activities involving the use of objects that can be harmful.

Instruct the child to avoid constrictive or tight clothing.

Use caution when taking the blood pressure to prevent skin injury.

Instruct the child to avoid blowing his or her nose.

Avoid the use of rectal suppositories, enemas, and rectal thermometers.

Examine all body fluids and excrement for the presence of blood.

Count the number of pads or tampons used if the adolescent girl is menstruating.

Instruct the child about the signs and symptoms of bleeding.

Instruct parents to avoid administering nonsteroidal anti-inflammatory drugs and products that contain aspirin to the child.

suppression (the nadir), blood cell counts are extremely low.
2. Monitor for infection and bleeding.
3. Protect the child from life-threatening infections.
4. Monitor for nausea, vomiting, and diarrhea.
5. Administer stool softeners as prescribed.
6. Provide rectal hygiene gently as needed.
7. Administer antiemetics as prescribed.
8. Monitor for signs of dehydration.
9. Monitor for signs of hemorrhagic cystitis.
10. Monitor for signs of peripheral neuropathy.
11. Assess oral mucous membranes for mucositis; administer frequent mouth rinses per agency procedure and as prescribed; usually a mixture of normal saline with table salt or sodium bicarbonate is prescribed to promote healing or prevent infection (local oral anesthetics may also be prescribed).
12. Instruct the parents and child in the signs and symptoms to watch for after chemotherapy and when to notify the physician.
13. Inform the parents and child that hair loss may occur from chemotherapy (hair regrows in about 3 to 6 months and may be a slightly different color or texture).
14. Instruct the parents and child about the care of a central venous access device, as necessary (see Chapter 14).
15. Listen to the child and family, and encourage them to verbalize their feelings and express their concerns.
16. Introduce the family to other families of children with cancer.
17. Consult social services and chaplains as necessary.

⚠ Monitor a child receiving chemotherapy closely for signs of infection. Infection is a major cause of death in the immunosuppressed child.

II. HODGKIN'S DISEASE

A. Description
1. Hodgkin's disease (a type of lymphoma) is a malignancy of the lymph nodes that originates in a single lymph node or a single chain of nodes (Fig. 46-1).
2. The disease predictably metastasizes to non-nodal or extralymphatic sites, especially the spleen, liver, bone marrow, lungs, and mediastinum.
3. Hodgkin's disease is characterized by the presence of Reed-Sternberg cells noted in a lymph node biopsy specimen.
4. Peak incidence is in midadolescence.
5. Possible causes include viral infections and previous exposure to alkylating chemical agents.
6. The prognosis is excellent with long-term survival rates depending on the stage of the disease.

7. The primary treatment modalities are radiation and chemotherapy; each may be used alone or in combination, depending on the clinical stage of the disease.

B. Assessment
1. Painless enlargement of lymph nodes
2. Enlarged, firm, nontender, movable nodes in the supraclavicular area; in children, the "sentinel" node located near the left clavicle may be the first enlarged node
3. Nonproductive cough as a result of mediastinal lymphadenopathy
4. Abdominal pain as a result of enlarged retroperitoneal nodes
5. Advanced lymph node and extralymphatic involvement that may cause systemic symptoms, such as a low-grade or intermittent fever, anorexia, nausea, weight loss, night sweats, and pruritus
6. Positive biopsy specimen of a lymph node (presence of Reed-Sternberg cells) and positive bone marrow biopsy specimen
7. Computed tomography scan of the liver, spleen, and bone marrow may be done to detect metastasis.

C. Interventions
1. For early stages without mediastinal node involvement, the treatment of choice is extensive external radiation of the involved lymph node regions.
2. With more extensive disease, radiation and multidrug chemotherapy are used.
3. Monitor for drug-induced pancytopenia and an abnormal depression of all the cellular components

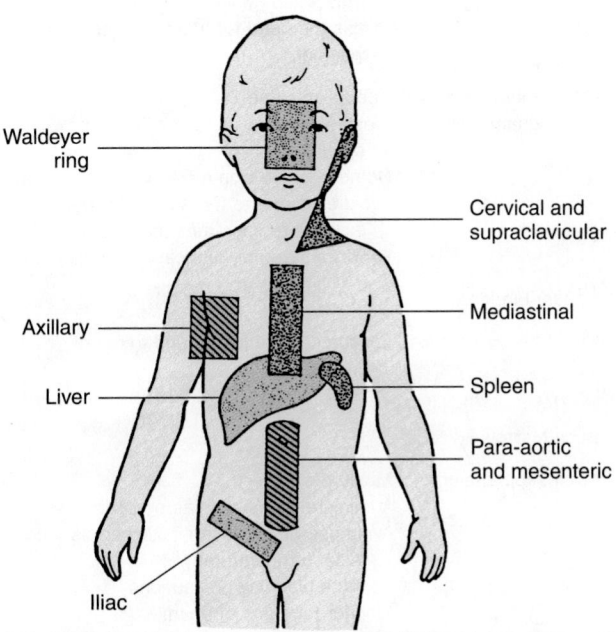

▲ **FIGURE 46-1** Main areas of lymphadenopathy and organ involvement in Hodgkin's disease. (From Hockenberry, M., Wilson, D., & Winkelstein, M. [2009]. *Wong's essentials of pediatric nursing* [8th ed.]. St. Louis: Mosby.)

of the blood, which increases the risk for infection, bleeding, and anemia.

4. Monitor for signs of infection and bleeding.
5. Protect the child from infection.
6. Provide a safe, hazard-free environment.
7. Monitor for side effects related to chemotherapy or radiation; the most common side effect of extensive irradiation is malaise, which can be difficult for older children and adolescents to tolerate physically and psychologically (Table 46-1).

TABLE 46-1 Side Effects of Radiation Therapy and Nursing Interventions

Body Area and Side Effects	Interventions
Gastrointestinal Tract	
Anorexia	Encourage fluids and foods as best tolerated Provide small, frequent meals Monitor for weight loss
Nausea, vomiting	Administer antiemetics around the clock Monitor for dehydration
Mucosal ulceration	Provide soothing oral hygiene and prescribed mouth rinses Topical anesthetic may be prescribed
Diarrhea	Administer antispasmodics and antidiarrheal preparations as prescribed Monitor for dehydration
Skin	
Alopecia (hair loss)	Introduce idea of a wig Provide scalp hygiene Stress the need for head covering in cold weather
Dry or moist desquamation	Keep skin clean Wash skin daily, using a mild soap sparingly Do not remove skin markings for radiation Avoid exposure to the sun and other extreme temperature changes For dryness, apply lubricant as prescribed
Urinary Bladder	
Cystitis	Encourage fluid intake and frequent voiding Monitor for hematuria
Bone Marrow	
Myelosuppression	Monitor for fever Administer antibiotics as prescribed Avoid use of suppositories, enemas, and rectal temperatures Institute bleeding precautions Monitor for signs of anemia

Modified from Hockenberry, M., & Wilson, D. (2007). Wong's nursing care of infants and children (8th ed.). St. Louis: Mosby; and McKinney, E., James, S., Murray, S., & Ashwill, J. (2009). Maternal-child nursing (3rd ed.). St. Louis: Saunders.

8. Monitor for nausea and vomiting, and administer antiemetics as prescribed.
9. Monitor for skin irritation and breakdown as a result of radiation therapy.

III. NEPHROBLASTOMA (WILMS' TUMOR)

A. Description
1. Wilms' tumor is the most common intra-abdominal and kidney tumor of childhood; it may manifest unilaterally and localized or bilaterally, sometimes with metastasis to other organs (Fig. 46-2).
2. The peak incidence is 3 years of age.
3. Occurrence is associated with a genetic inheritance and with several congenital anomalies.
4. Therapeutic management includes a combined treatment of surgery (partial to total nephrectomy) and chemotherapy with or without radiation, depending on the clinical stage and the histological pattern of the tumor.

B. Assessment
1. Swelling or mass within the abdomen (mass is characteristically firm, nontender, confined to one side, and deep within the flank)
2. Abdominal pain
3. Urinary retention or hematuria or both
4. Anemia (caused by hemorrhage within the tumor)
5. Pallor, anorexia, and lethargy (resulting from anemia)
6. Hypertension (caused by secretion of excess amounts of renin by the tumor)
7. Weight loss and fever
8. Symptoms of lung involvement, such as dyspnea, shortness of breath, and pain in the chest, if metastasis has occurred

C. Preoperative interventions
1. Monitor vital signs, particularly blood pressure.

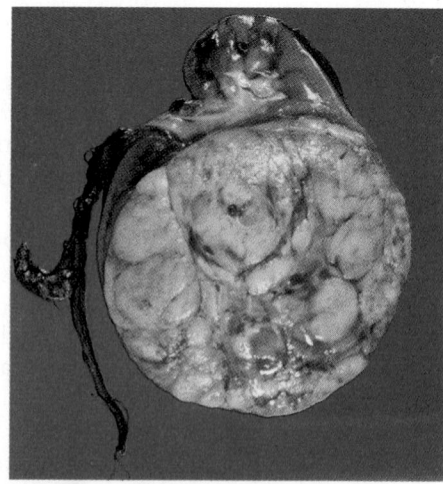

▲ **FIGURE 46-2** Wilms' tumor. (From *Mosby's dictionary of medicine, nursing and health professions* [8th ed.]. [2009]. St. Louis: Mosby.)

2. Avoid palpation of the abdomen; place a sign at bedside that reads, Do Not Palpate Abdomen.
3. Measure abdominal girth at least once daily.

D. Postoperative interventions
1. Monitor temperature and blood pressure closely.
2. Monitor for signs of hemorrhage and infection.
3. Monitor strict intake and urine output closely.
4. Monitor for abdominal distention; monitor bowel sounds and other signs of gastrointestinal activity because of the risk for intestinal obstruction.

⚠️ Avoid palpation of the abdomen in a child with Wilms' tumor and be cautious when bathing, moving, or handling the child. It is important to keep the encapsulated tumor intact. Rupture of the tumor can cause the cancer cells to spread throughout the abdomen, lymph system, and bloodstream.

IV. NEUROBLASTOMA

A. Description
1. Neuroblastoma is a tumor that originates from the embryonic neural crest cells that normally give rise to the adrenal medulla and the sympathetic ganglia.
2. Most tumors develop in the adrenal gland or the retroperitoneal sympathetic chain; other sites may be within the head, neck, chest, or pelvis.
3. Most children present with neuroblastoma before 10 years of age.
4. Most presenting signs are caused by the tumor compressing adjacent normal tissue and organs.
5. Diagnostic evaluation is aimed at locating the primary site of the tumor.
6. The prognosis is poor because of the frequency of invasiveness of the tumor and because, in most cases, a diagnosis is not made until after metastasis has occurred; the younger the child at diagnosis, the better the survival rate.
7. Therapeutic management
   a. Surgery is performed to remove as much of the tumor as possible and to obtain biopsy specimens; in the early stages, complete surgical removal of the tumor is the treatment of choice.
   b. Surgery usually is limited to biopsy in the later stages because of extensive metastasis.
   c. Radiation is used commonly with later stage disease and provides palliation for metastatic lesions in bones, lungs, liver, and brain.
   d. Chemotherapy is used for extensive local or disseminated disease.

B. Assessment
1. Firm, nontender, irregular mass in the abdomen that crosses the midline
2. Urinary frequency or retention from compression of the kidney, ureter, or bladder
3. Lymphadenopathy, especially in the cervical and supraclavicular areas

4. Bone pain if skeletal involvement
5. Supraorbital ecchymosis, periorbital edema, and exophthalmos as a result of invasion of retrobulbar soft tissue
6. Pallor, weakness, irritability, anorexia, weight loss
7. Signs of respiratory impairment (thoracic lesion)
8. Signs of neurological impairment (intracranial lesion)
9. Paralysis from compression of the spinal cord

C. Preoperative interventions
1. Monitor for signs and symptoms related to the location of the tumor.
2. Provide emotional support to the child and parents.

D. Postoperative interventions
1. Monitor for postoperative complications related to the location (organ) of the surgery.
2. Monitor for complications related to chemotherapy or radiation if prescribed.
3. Provide support to the parents and encourage them to express their feelings; many parents feel guilt for not having recognized signs in the child earlier.
4. Refer parents to appropriate community services.

V. OSTEOGENIC SARCOMA

A. Description
1. Osteogenic sarcoma is the most common bone cancer in children; it is also known as osteosarcoma (Fig. 46-3).
2. Cancer usually is found in the metaphysis of long bones, especially in the lower extremities, with most tumors occurring in the femur.
3. The peak age of incidence is between 10 and 25 years.

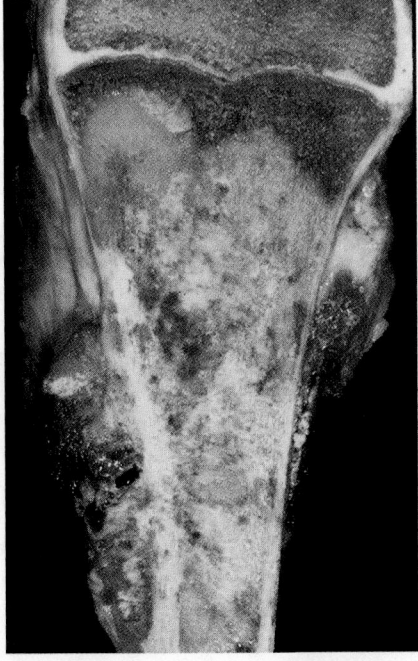

▲ **FIGURE 46-3** Osteosarcoma. (From *Mosby's dictionary of medicine, nursing and health professions* [8th ed.]. [2009]. St. Louis: Mosby.)

4. Symptoms in the earliest stage are almost always attributed to extremity injury or normal growing pains.
5. Treatment may include surgical resection (limb salvage procedure) to save a limb or remove affected tissue, or amputation.
6. Chemotherapy is used to treat the cancer and may be used before and after surgery.

B. Assessment
1. Localized pain at the affected site (may be severe or dull) that may be attributed to trauma or the vague complaint of "growing pains"; pain often is relieved by a flexed position.
2. Palpable mass
3. Limping if weight-bearing limb is affected
4. Progressive limited range of motion and the child's curtailing of physical activity
5. Child may be unable to hold heavy objects because of their weight and resultant pain in the affected extremity.
6. Pathological fractures occur at the tumor site.

C. Interventions
1. Prepare the child and family for prescribed treatment modalities, which may include surgical resection by limb salvage to remove affected tissue, amputation, and chemotherapy.
2. Communicate honestly with the child and family and provide support.
3. Prepare for prosthetic fitting as necessary.
4. Assist the child in dealing with problems of self-image.
5. Instruct the child and parents about the potential development of phantom limb pain that may occur after amputation, characterized by tingling, itching, and a painful sensation in the area where the limb was amputated.

VI. BRAIN TUMORS

A. Description
1. An infratentorial (below the tentorium cerebelli) tumor, the most common brain tumor, is located in the posterior third of the brain (primarily in the cerebellum or brainstem) and accounts for the frequency of symptoms resulting from increased intracranial pressure (ICP).
2. A supratentorial tumor is located within the anterior two thirds of the brain—mainly the cerebrum.
3. The signs and symptoms of a brain tumor depend on its anatomical location and size and, to some extent, the age of the child.
4. Therapeutic management includes surgery, radiation, and chemotherapy; the treatment of choice is total removal of the tumor without residual neurological damage.

B. Assessment
1. Headache that is worse on awakening and improves during the day

2. Vomiting that is unrelated to feeding or eating
3. Ataxia
4. Seizures
5. Behavioral changes
6. Clumsiness; awkward gait or difficulty walking
7. Diplopia
8. Facial weakness

⚠ Monitor for signs of increased ICP in a child with a brain tumor and after a craniotomy. If signs of increased ICP occur, notify the physician immediately.

C. Preoperative interventions
1. Perform a neurological assessment at least every 4 hours.
2. Institute seizure precautions and safety measures.
3. Assess weight loss and nutritional status.
4. Shave the child's head as prescribed (provide a favorite cap or hat for the child); shaving the head may also be done in the surgical suite.
5. Prepare the child as much as possible; tell the child that he or she will wake up with a large head dressing.

D. Postoperative interventions
1. Assess neurological and motor function and level of consciousness.
2. Monitor temperature closely, which may be elevated because of hypothalamus or brainstem involvement during surgery; maintain a cooling blanket by the bedside.
3. Monitor for signs of respiratory infection.
4. Monitor for signs of meningitis (opisthotonos, Kernig's and Brudzinski's signs).
5. Monitor for signs of increased ICP (Box 46-4; see also Chapter 36).
6. Monitor for hemorrhage, checking the back of the head dressing for posterior pooling of blood.
7. Assess pupillary response; sluggish, dilated, or unequal pupils are reported immediately because they may indicate increased ICP and potential brainstem herniation.
8. Monitor for colorless drainage on the dressing or from the ears or nose, which indicates cerebrospinal fluid and should be reported immediately; assess for the presence of glucose in the drainage (dipstick).
9. Assess the physician's prescription for positioning, including the degree of neck flexion (Box 46-5).
10. Monitor intravenous fluids closely.
11. Promote measures that prevent vomiting (vomiting increases intracranial pressure and the risk for incisional rupture).
12. Provide a quiet environment.
13. Administer analgesics as prescribed.
14. Provide emotional support to the child and parents, and promote optimal **growth** and development.

Box 46-4 Manifestations of Increased Intracranial Pressure in Infants and Children

Infants
Tense, bulging fontanel
Separated cranial sutures
Macewen's sign (cracked-pot sound on percussion)
Irritability
High-pitched cry
Increased head circumference
Distended scalp veins
Poor feeding
Crying when disturbed
Setting sun sign (eyes appear to look only downward, with the sclera prominent over the iris)

Children
Headache
Nausea
Forceful vomiting
Diplopia; blurred vision
Seizures

Personality and Behavior Signs
Irritability, restlessness
Indifference, drowsiness
Decline in school performance
Diminished physical activity and motor performance
Increased sleeping
Inability to follow simple commands
Lethargy

Late Signs
Bradycardia
Decreased motor response to command
Decreased sensory response to painful stimuli
Alterations in pupil size and reaction
Decerebrate (extension) or decorticate (flexion) posturing
Cheyne-Stokes respirations
Papilledema
Decreased consciousness
Coma

From Perry, S., Hockenberry, M., Lowdermilk, D., & Wilson, D. (2010). *Maternal child nursing care* (4th ed., p. 1552). St. Louis: Mosby.

Box 46-5 Positioning After Craniotomy

Assess the physician's prescription for positioning, including the degree of neck flexion.
If a large tumor has been removed, the child is not placed on the operative side because the brain may shift suddenly to that cavity.
In an infratentorial procedure, the child usually is positioned flat and on either side.
In a supratentorial procedure, the head usually is elevated above the heart level to facilitate cerebrospinal fluid drainage and to decrease excessive blood flow to the brain to prevent hemorrhage.
Never place the child in Trendelenburg's position because it increases intracranial pressure and the risk of hemorrhage.

MORE QUESTIONS ON THE CD!

Practice Questions

464. A nurse is monitoring a child for bleeding after surgery for removal of a brain tumor. The nurse checks the head dressing for the presence of blood and notes a colorless drainage on the back of the dressing. Which of the following is the appropriate nursing intervention?
    1. Notify the physician.
    2. Reinforce the dressing.
    3. Document the findings and continue to monitor.
    4. Circle the area of drainage and continue to monitor.

465. After surgical removal of a brain tumor, the physician writes a prescription to maintain the child in a flat position. During the postoperative period, a nurse is monitoring the child and notes that the child is restless, the pulse rate is elevated, and the blood pressure has decreased significantly from the baseline value. The nurse suspects that the child is in shock. Which of the following would be the appropriate nursing action?
    1. Notify the physician.
    2. Elevate the head of the bed.
    3. Increase intravenous fluids.
    4. Place the child in Trendelenburg's position.

466. The mother of a 4-year-old child brings the child to a clinic and tells a pediatric nurse specialist that the child's abdomen seems to be swollen. During further assessment of subjective data, the mother tells the nurse that the child is eating well and that the activity level of the child is unchanged. The nurse, suspecting the possibility of Wilms' tumor, would avoid which of the following during the physical assessment?
    1. Palpating the abdomen for a mass
    2. Assessing the urine for the presence of hematuria
    3. Monitoring the temperature for the presence of fever
    4. Monitoring the blood pressure for the presence of hypertension

467. A pediatric nurse specialist provides a teaching session to the nursing staff regarding osteogenic sarcoma. Which statement by a member of the

nursing staff indicates a need for clarification of the information presented?
1. "The femur is the most common site of this sarcoma."
2. "The child does not experience pain at the primary tumor site."
3. "Limping, if a weight-bearing limb is affected, is a clinical manifestation."
4. "The symptoms of the disease in the early stage are almost always attributed to normal growing pains."

468. The nurse analyzes the laboratory values of a child with leukemia who is receiving chemotherapy. The nurse notes that the platelet count is 19,500 cells/mm^3. Based on this laboratory result, which intervention would the nurse document in the plan of care?
1. Monitor closely for signs of infection.
2. Monitor the temperature every 4 hours.
3. Initiate protective isolation precautions.
4. Use a soft small toothbrush for mouth care.

469. A nurse is monitoring a 3-year-old child for signs and symptoms of increased intracranial pressure (ICP) after a craniotomy. The nurse plans to monitor for which early sign or symptom of increased ICP?
1. Excessive vomiting
2. Bulging anterior fontanel
3. Increasing head circumference
4. Complaints of a frontal headache

470. A 4-year-old child is admitted to the hospital for abdominal pain. The mother reports that the child has been pale and excessively tired and is bruising easily. On physical examination, lymphadenopathy and hepatosplenomegaly are noted. Diagnostic studies are being performed on the child because acute lymphocytic leukemia is suspected. The nurse understands that which diagnostic study would confirm this diagnosis?
1. Platelet count
2. Lumbar puncture
3. Bone marrow biopsy
4. White blood cell count

471. A 6-year-old child with leukemia is hospitalized and is receiving combination chemotherapy. Laboratory results indicate that the child is neutropenic, and protective isolation procedures are initiated. The

grandmother of the child visits and brings a fresh bouquet of flowers picked from her garden and asks the nurse for a vase for the flowers. The nurse responds to the grandmother by telling her:
1. "I have a vase in the utility room, and I will get it for you."
2. "I will get the vase and wash it well before you put the flowers in it."
3. "The flowers from your garden are beautiful, but should not be placed in the child's room at this time."
4. "When you bring the flowers into the room, place them on the bedside stand as far away from the child as possible."

472. A diagnosis of Hodgkin's disease is suspected in a 12-year-old child seen in a clinic. Several diagnostic studies are performed to determine the presence of this disease. Which diagnostic test results confirm the diagnosis of Hodgkin's disease?
1. Elevated vanillylmandelic acid urinary levels
2. The presence of blast cells in the bone marrow
3. The presence of Epstein-Barr virus in the blood
4. The presence of Reed-Sternberg cells in the lymph nodes

473. A nurse is performing an assessment on a 10-year-old child suspected to have Hodgkin's disease. The nurse understands that which of the following assessment findings is characteristic of this disease?
1. Fever and malaise
2. Anorexia and weight loss
3. Painful, enlarged inguinal lymph nodes
4. Painless, firm, and movable adenopathy in the cervical area

Alternate Item Format: Multiple Response

474. Which specific nursing interventions are implemented in the care of a child with leukemia who is at risk for infection? **Select all that apply.**
❏ 1. Maintain the child in a private room.
❏ 2. Reduce exposure to environmental organisms.
❏ 3. Use strict aseptic technique for all procedures.
❏ 4. Avoid the use of rectal suppositories and enemas.
❏ 5. Ensure that anyone entering the child's room wears a mask.
❏ 6. Apply firm pressure to a needle stick area for at least 10 minutes.

ANSWERS
464. 1
Rationale: Colorless drainage on the dressing in a child after craniotomy indicates the presence of cerebrospinal fluid and should be reported to the physician immediately. Options

2, 3, and 4 are inaccurate nursing interventions because they do not address the need for immediate intervention to prevent complications.
Test-Taking Strategy: Use the process of elimination. Eliminate options 2, 3, and 4 because they are comparable or alike and delay necessary intervention. Note the strategic words

colorless drainage. This should alert you quickly to the possibility of the presence of cerebrospinal fluid and direct you to option 1. If you had difficulty with this question, review the significance of the presence of colorless drainage on the surgical dressing after cranial surgery.
Level of Cognitive Ability: Applying
Client Needs: Physiological Integrity
Integrated Process: Nursing Process—Implementation
Content Area: Child Health—Hematological/Oncological
Reference: McKinney, E., James, S., Murray, S., & Ashwill, J. (2009). *Maternal-child nursing* (3rd ed., p. 1324). St. Louis: Saunders.

465. 1
Rationale: After craniotomy, a child is never placed in Trendelenburg's position because it increases intracranial pressure (ICP) and the risk of bleeding. In the event of shock, the physician is notified immediately before the nurse changes the child's position or increases intravenous fluids. Increasing intravenous fluids can cause an increase in ICP.
Test-Taking Strategy: Recall the complications associated with cranial surgery to answer this question. Eliminate option 2 because this intervention would not assist in alleviating shock. This action could cause harm to the child. Eliminate option 3 because this action could increase ICP. In addition, the nurse should not increase intravenous fluids without a physician's prescription. Eliminate option 4 because this position increases ICP. Review care of a child after surgical removal of a brain tumor if you had difficulty with this question.
Level of Cognitive Ability: Applying
Client Needs: Physiological Integrity
Integrated Process: Nursing Process—Implementation
Content Area: Child Health—Hematological/Oncological
Reference: McKinney, E., James, S., Murray, S., & Ashwill, J. (2009). *Maternal-child nursing* (3rd ed., p. 1324). St. Louis: Saunders.

466. 1
Rationale: Wilms' tumor is the most common intra-abdominal and kidney tumor of childhood. If Wilms' tumor is suspected, the tumor mass should not be palpated by the nurse. Excessive manipulation can cause seeding of the tumor and spread of the cancerous cells. Fever, hematuria, and hypertension are clinical manifestations associated with Wilms' tumor.
Test-Taking Strategy: Use the process of elimination and note the strategic word *avoid.* This word indicates a negative event query and asks you to select an option that is an incorrect action. Knowledge that this tumor is an intra-abdominal and kidney tumor will assist in eliminating options 2 and 4 because of the relationship of these options to renal function. Next, thinking about the effect of palpating the tumor will direct you to option 1 from the remaining options. Review the significant assessment procedures in a child with Wilms' tumor if you had difficulty with this question.
Level of Cognitive Ability: Applying
Client Needs: Physiological Integrity
Integrated Process: Nursing Process—Implementation
Content Area: Child Health—Hematological/Oncological
Reference: Perry, S., Hockenberry, M., Lowdermilk, D., & Wilson, D. (2010). *Maternal child nursing care* (4th ed., p. 1541). St. Louis: Mosby.

467. 2
Rationale: Osteogenic sarcoma is the most common bone cancer in children. Cancer usually is found in the metaphysis of long bones, especially in the lower extremities, with most tumors occurring in the femur. Osteogenic sarcoma is manifested clinically by progressive, insidious, and intermittent pain at the tumor site. By the time these children receive medical attention, they may be in considerable pain from the tumor. Options 1, 3, and 4 are accurate regarding osteogenic sarcoma.
Test-Taking Strategy: Use the process of elimination and note the strategic words *need for clarification of the information presented* in the question. These words indicate a negative event query and ask you to select an option that is an incorrect statement. Knowledge that osteogenic sarcoma is a malignant tumor of the bone will direct you to option 2. Review the clinical manifestations associated with osteogenic sarcoma if you had difficulty with this question.
Level of Cognitive Ability: Evaluating
Client Needs: Physiological Integrity
Integrated Process: Teaching and Learning
Content Area: Child Health—Hematological/Oncological
Reference: McKinney, E., James, S., Murray, S., & Ashwill, J. (2009). *Maternal-child nursing* (3rd ed., p. 1329). St. Louis: Saunders.

468. 4
Rationale: Leukemia is a malignant increase in the number of leukocytes, usually at an immature stage, in the bone marrow. It affects the bone marrow, causing anemia from decreased erythrocytes, infection from neutropenia, and bleeding from decreased platelet production (thrombocytopenia). If a child is severely thrombocytopenic and has a platelet count less than 20,000 cells/mm^3, bleeding precautions need to be initiated because of the increased risk of bleeding or hemorrhage. Precautions include limiting activity that could result in head injury, using soft toothbrushes, checking urine and stools for blood, and administering stool softeners to prevent straining with constipation. In addition, suppositories, enemas, and rectal temperatures are avoided. Options 1, 2, and 3 are related to the prevention of infection rather than bleeding.
Test-Taking Strategy: Use the process of elimination. Noting that the platelet count is low and that a low platelet count places the child at risk for bleeding will assist in directing you to option 4. In addition, note that options 1, 2, and 3 are comparable or alike because they relate to prevention of and monitoring for infection. Review interventions for a child who is at risk for bleeding if you had difficulty with this question.
Level of Cognitive Ability: Applying
Client Needs: Safe and Effective Care Environment
Integrated Process: Nursing Process—Planning
Content Area: Child Health—Hematological/Oncological
Reference: McKinney, E., James, S., Murray, S., & Ashwill, J. (2009). *Maternal-child nursing* (3rd ed., pp. 1314–1315). St. Louis: Saunders.

469. 1
Rationale: The brain, although well protected by the solid bony cranium, is highly susceptible to pressure that may accumulate within the enclosure. Volume and pressure must remain constant within the brain. A change in the size of

the brain, such as occurs with edema or increased volume of intracranial blood or cerebrospinal fluid without a compensatory change, leads to an increase in intracranial pressure (ICP), which may be life-threatening. Vomiting, an early sign of increased ICP, can become excessive as pressure builds up and stimulates the medulla in the brainstem, which houses the vomiting center. Children with open fontanels (posterior fontanel closes at 2 to 3 months; anterior fontanel closes at 12 to 18 months) compensate for ICP changes by skull expansion and subsequent bulging fontanels. When the fontanels have closed, nausea, excessive vomiting, diplopia, and headaches become pronounced, with headaches becoming more prevalent in older children.

Test-Taking Strategy: Note the strategic word *early*, focus on the age of the child, and use age as key to principles of growth and development. Knowing when the fontanels close and focusing on the child's age as 3 years eliminates options 2 and 3. The subjective symptom of headache in option 4 is unreliable in a 3-year-old, so eliminate this option. Review the pathophysiology of increased ICP if you had difficulty with this question.

Level of Cognitive Ability: Analyzing
Client Needs: Physiological Integrity
Integrated Process: Nursing Process—Assessment
Content Area: Child Health—Hematological/Oncological
Reference: McKinney, E., James, S., Murray, S., & Ashwill, J. (2009). *Maternal-child nursing* (3rd ed., p. 1468). St. Louis: Saunders.

470. 3

Rationale: Leukemia is a malignant increase in the number of leukocytes, usually at an immature stage, in the bone marrow. The confirmatory test for leukemia is microscopic examination of bone marrow obtained by bone marrow aspirate and biopsy. A lumbar puncture may be done to look for blast cells in the spinal fluid that indicate central nervous system disease. The white blood cell count may be normal, high, or low in leukemia. An altered platelet count occurs as a result of the disease, but also may occur as a result of chemotherapy and does not confirm the diagnosis.

Test-Taking Strategy: Use the process of elimination, and note the strategic word *confirm* in the question. This strategic word and knowledge that the bone marrow is affected in leukemia will direct you to option 3. If you had difficulty with this question, review the significance of the bone marrow biopsy in the diagnosis of leukemia.

Level of Cognitive Ability: Understanding
Client Needs: Physiological Integrity
Integrated Process: Nursing Process—Assessment
Content Area: Child Health—Hematological/Oncological
Reference: Hockenberry, M., & Wilson, D. (2009). *Wong's essentials of pediatric nursing* (8th ed., pp. 711, 931). St. Louis: Mosby.

471. 3

Rationale: Leukemia is a malignant increase in the number of leukocytes, usually at an immature stage, in the bone marrow. It affects the bone marrow, causing anemia from decreased erythrocytes, infection from neutropenia, and bleeding from decreased platelet production (thrombocytopenia). For a hospitalized neutropenic child, flowers or plants should not be kept in the room because standing water and damp soil harbor *Aspergillus* and *Pseudomonas aeruginosa*, to which the child is susceptible. In addition, fresh fruits and vegetables harbor molds and should be avoided until the white blood cell count increases.

Test-Taking Strategy: Use the process of elimination. Note that options 1 and 2 are comparable or alike and should be eliminated first. From the remaining options, select option 3 over option 4 because this nursing response maintains the protective isolation procedures required. Review protective isolation procedures for the neutropenic child if you had difficulty with this question.

Level of Cognitive Ability: Applying
Client Needs: Safe and Effective Care Environment
Integrated Process: Nursing Process—Implementation
Content Area: Child Health—Hematological/Oncological
Reference: McKinney, E., James, S., Murray, S., & Ashwill, J. (2009). *Maternal-child nursing* (3rd ed., p. 1315). St. Louis: Saunders.

472. 4

Rationale: Hodgkin's disease (a type of lymphoma) is a malignancy of the lymph nodes. The presence of giant, multinucleated cells (Reed-Sternberg cells) is the classic characteristic of this disease. The presence of blast cells in the bone marrow indicates leukemia. Epstein-Barr virus is associated with infectious mononucleosis. Elevated levels of vanillylmandelic acid in the urine may be found in children with neuroblastoma.

Test-Taking Strategy: Use the process of elimination and think about the pathophysiology associated with Hodgkin's disease. Remember that the Reed-Sternberg cell is characteristic of Hodgkin's disease. Review the clinical manifestations associated with Hodgkin's disease if you had difficulty with this question.

Level of Cognitive Ability: Understanding
Client Needs: Physiological Integrity
Integrated Process: Nursing Process—Assessment
Content Area: Child Health—Hematological/Oncological
Reference: Perry, S., Hockenberry, M., Lowdermilk, D., & Wilson, D. (2010). *Maternal child nursing care* (4th ed., p. 1514). St. Louis: Mosby.

473. 4

Rationale: Hodgkin's disease (a type of lymphoma) is a malignancy of the lymph nodes. Clinical manifestations specifically associated with Hodgkin's disease include painless, firm, and movable adenopathy in the cervical and supraclavicular areas. Hepatosplenomegaly also is noted. Although fever, malaise, anorexia, and weight loss are associated with Hodgkin's disease, these manifestations are seen in many disorders.

Test-Taking Strategy: Use the process of elimination, and note the strategic word *characteristic* in the question. Eliminate options 1 and 2 first because these symptoms are general and vague. Recalling that painless adenopathy is associated with Hodgkin's disease will direct you to option 4. Review the clinical manifestations related to Hodgkin's disease if you had difficulty with this question.

Level of Cognitive Ability: Analyzing
Client Needs: Physiological Integrity
Integrated Process: Nursing Process—Assessment
Content Area: Child Health—Hematological/Oncological
Reference: Perry, S., Hockenberry, M., Lowdermilk, D., & Wilson, D. (2010). *Maternal child nursing care* (4th ed., p. 1514). St. Louis: Mosby.

ALTERNATE ITEM FORMAT: MULTIPLE RESPONSE

474. 1, 2, 3, 4, 5

Rationale: Leukemia is a malignant increase in the number of leukocytes, usually at an immature stage, in the bone marrow. It affects the bone marrow, causing anemia from decreased erythrocytes, infection from neutropenia, and bleeding from decreased platelet production (thrombocytopenia). A common complication of treatment for leukemia is overwhelming infection secondary to neutropenia. Measures to prevent infection include the use of a private room, strict aseptic technique, restriction of visitors and health care personnel with active infection, strict handwashing, ensuring that anyone entering the child's room wears a mask, and reducing exposure to environmental organisms by eliminating raw fruits and vegetables from the diet and fresh flowers from the child's room and by not leaving standing water in the child's room. The other interventions listed are measures to prevent bleeding.

Test-Taking Strategy: Focus on the subject: preventing infection. Reading each intervention carefully and keeping this subject in mind will assist in answering the question. Applying firm pressure to a needle stick area for at least 10 minutes and avoiding the use of rectal suppositories and enemas are related to preventing bleeding. Review interventions for the child at risk for infection if you had difficulty with this question.

Level of Cognitive Ability: Applying
Client Needs: Physiological Integrity
Integrated Process: Nursing Process—Implementation
Content Area: Child Health—Hematological/Oncological
Reference: Hockenberry, M., & Wilson, D. (2009). *Wong's essentials of pediatric nursing* (8th ed., pp. 932–933, 935). St. Louis: Mosby.

47

Acquired Immunodeficiency Syndrome

I. ACQUIRED IMMUNODEFICIENCY SYNDROME (AIDS)

A. Description
1. AIDS is a disorder caused by human immunodeficiency virus (HIV) and characterized by generalized dysfunction of the immune system (Fig. 47-1).
2. HIV infects CD4+ T cells; a gradual decrease in CD4+ T cell count occurs and this results in a progressive immunodeficiency; the risk for opportunistic infections is present.
3. HIV is transmitted through blood, semen, vaginal secretions, and breast milk; the incubation period is months to years.
4. Horizontal transmission occurs through intimate sexual contact or parenteral exposure to blood or body fluids that contain the virus.
5. Vertical (perinatal) transmission occurs from an HIV-infected pregnant woman to her fetus (see Chapter 25).
6. The most common opportunistic infection that occurs in children infected with HIV is *Pneumocystis jiroveci* pneumonia (formerly known as *Pneumocystis carinii* pneumonia); *P. jiroveci* pneumonia most frequently occurs between the ages of 3 and 6 months, when HIV status may be indeterminate.

⚠ An infant or child infected with HIV is at risk for developing a life-threatening opportunistic infection. Monitor the infant or child closely for signs of infection and report these signs immediately if they occur.

B. Assessment (Boxes 47-1 and 47-2)
C. Diagnostic tests: Before testing, counseling should be provided to parents; issues that should be addressed include the causes of HIV, reasons for testing, implications of positive test results, confidentiality issues, and beneficial effects of early intervention (Table 47-1).

II. CARE OF THE CHILD WITH HIV INFECTION OR AIDS

A. A multidisciplinary health care approach is taken; primary goals are to decelerate the replication of the virus, prevent opportunistic infections, provide nutritional support, treat symptoms, and treat opportunistic infections.
B. Prophylaxis (*P. jiroveci* pneumonia and other opportunistic infections)
1. Provide prophylaxis as prescribed against *P. jiroveci* pneumonia and other opportunistic infections, particularly during the first year of life of an infant born to an HIV-infected mother.
2. After 1 year of age, the need for prophylaxis is determined based on the presence and severity of immunosuppression or a history of *P. jiroveci* pneumonia.
3. Continuing prophylaxis is based on the child's HIV status, history of opportunistic infections, and CD4+ counts.
C. Antiretroviral medications (Box 47-3)

⚠ Before administering an antiretroviral medication, ensure that the medication is safe for pediatric administration. Also check the contraindications for use and the adverse effects.

1. The goal of antiretroviral medications is to suppress viral replication to slow the decline in the number of CD4+ cells, preserve immune function, reduce the incidence and severity of opportunistic infections, and delay disease progression.
2. The medications affect different stages of the HIV life cycle to prevent reproduction of new virus particles.
3. Combination therapy may be prescribed and includes the use of more than one antiretroviral medication.
D. Immunizations

⚠ Immunization against childhood diseases is recommended for all children exposed to and infected with HIV.

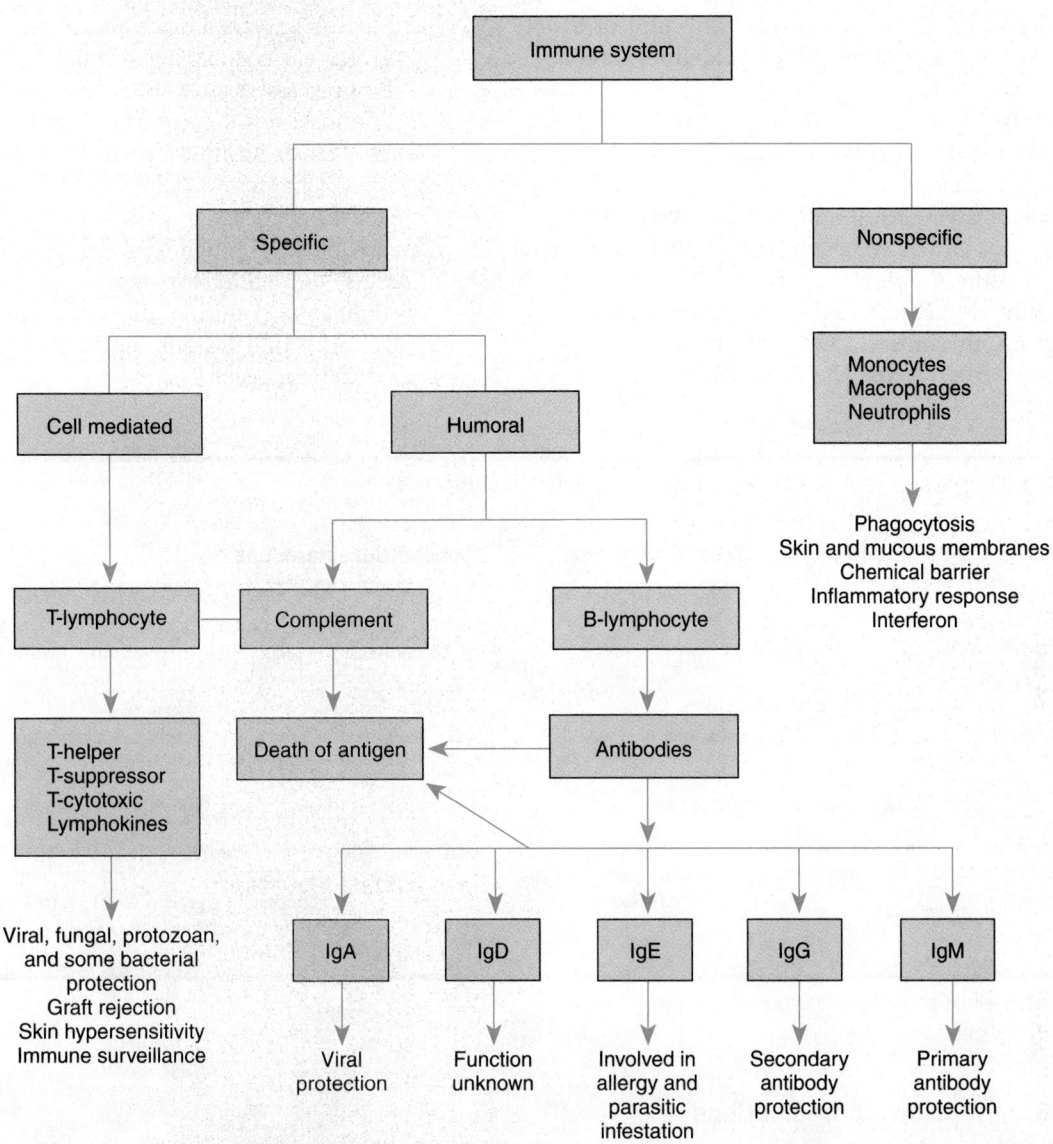

▲ **FIGURE 47-1** Components of the immune system. (From Hockenberry, M., & Wilson, D. [2007]. *Wong's nursing care of infants and children* [8th ed.]. St. Louis: Mosby.)

Box 47-1 Common Assessment Findings in Children With Human Immunodeficiency Virus Infection

Chronic cough
Chronic or recurrent diarrhea
Developmental delay or regression of developmental milestones
Failure to thrive
Hepatosplenomegaly
Lymphadenopathy
Malaise and fatigue
Night sweats
Oral candidiasis
Parotitis
Weight loss

Modified from Perry, S., Hockenberry, M., Lowdermilk, D., & Wilson, D. (2010). *Maternal child nursing care* (4th ed., p. 1517). St. Louis: Mosby.

Box 47-2 Common Acquired Immunodeficiency Syndrome (AIDS)–Defining Conditions in Children

Candidal esophagitis
Cryptosporidiosis
Cytomegalovirus disease
Herpes simplex disease
Human immunodeficiency virus encephalopathy
Lymphoid interstitial pneumonitis
Mycobacterium avium-intracellulare infection
Pneumocystis jiroveci pneumonia
Pulmonary candidiasis
Recurrent bacterial infections
Wasting syndrome

From Perry, S., Hockenberry, M., Lowdermilk, D., & Wilson, D. (2010). *Maternal child nursing care* (4th ed., p. 1517). St. Louis: Mosby.

1. If a child has symptomatic HIV infection or has severe immunosuppression, guidelines are as follows:
   a. Only the inactivated influenza **vaccine** that is given intramuscularly should be used (influenza vaccine should be given yearly).
   b. Measles **vaccine** should not be given; immunoglobulin may be prescribed after measles exposure.
   c. Only the inactivated polio **vaccine** that is given intramuscularly should be used.
   d. Rotavirus **vaccine** should not be given.
   e. Varicella-zoster virus **vaccine** should not be given; varicella-zoster immunoglobulin may be prescribed after chickenpox exposure.
   f. Tetanus immunoglobulin may be prescribed for tetanus-prone wounds.
2. See also Chapter 48.

E. Caretaker instructions
   1. Wash hands frequently.
   2. Assess the child for fever, malaise, fatigue, weight loss, vomiting, diarrhea, altered activity level, and oral lesions; notify the physician if any of these occur.

TABLE 47-1 Diagnostic Tests for Human Immunodeficiency Virus (HIV)

Test	Age-Appropriate Use	Test Determines	Special Considerations
Enzyme-linked immunosorbent assay	≥18 mo	Response of antibodies to HIV	If used and found to be positive in infants <18 mo, indicates only that mother is infected because maternal antibodies are transmitted transplacentally; use another diagnostic test
Western blot	≥18 mo	Presence of HIV antibodies	Same as above
Polymerase chain reaction	<18 mo	Presence of proviral DNA	Very accurate for diagnosing infants 1-4 mo of age
p24 antigen	<18 mo	HIV antigen specific	Very accurate for diagnosing infants 1-4 mo of age
CD4+ lymphocyte count, T-lymphocyte count	Infant–13 yr	Immune system status related specifically to suppression	Age adjustment is essential because normal counts are relatively high in infants and steadily decline until 6 yr of age Severe suppression in all age groups is <15% total lymphocytes (<750 cells/L in infant <12 mo, <500 cells/L in child 1-5 yr, <200 cells/L in child 6-12 yr)

Data from http://www.cdc.gov/hiv/topics/index.htm

Box 47-3 Antiretroviral Medications

Reverse Transcriptase Inhibitors
Action: Inhibit enzymes required for human immunodeficiency virus (HIV) replication

Nucleoside/Nucleotide Reverse Transcriptase Inhibitors
Abacavir (Ziagen)
Didanosine (Videx)
Emtricitabine (Emtriva)
Lamivudine (Epivir)
Stavudine (Zerit)
Tenofovir (Viread)
Zidovudine (Retrovir)

Non-nucleoside/Nucleotide Reverse Transcriptase Inhibitors
Delavirdine (Rescriptor)
Efavirenz (Sustiva)
Etravirine (Intelence)
Nevirapine (Viramune)

Integrase Inhibitor
Action: Inhibit enzymes required for HIV replication

Raltegravir (Isentress)

Protease Inhibitors
Action: Inhibit enzymes required for HIV replication
Amprenavir (Agenerase)
Atazanavir (Reyataz)
Darunavir (Prezista)
Fosamprenavir (Lexiva)
Indinavir (Crixivan)
Lopinavir/ritonavir (Kaletra)
Nelfinavir (Viracept)
Ritonavir (Norvir)
Saquinavir (Invirase)
Tipranavir (Aptivus)

Fusion Inhibitor
Action: Block viral entry into cells
Enfuvirtide (Fuzeon)

Chemokine Receptor 5 (CCR5) Antagonist
Action: Block viral entry into cells
Maraviroc (Selzentry)

Modified from Lehne, R. (2010) *Pharmacology for nursing care* (7th ed., p. 1092). St. Louis: Saunders.

3. Assess the child for signs and symptoms of opportunistic infections, such as pneumonia.
4. Administer antiretroviral medications and other medications to the child as prescribed.
5. The child needs to be restricted from having contact with persons who have infections or other contagious or potentially contagious illnesses.
6. Keep the child's immunizations up to date.
7. Keep the child home when sick.
8. Avoid direct unprotected contact with the child's body fluids.
9. Monitor the child's weight.
10. Provide a high-calorie and high-protein diet to the child.
11. Administer appetite stimulants to the child as prescribed and as needed.
12. Do not share eating utensils with the child.
13. Wash all eating utensils in the dishwasher.
14. Cover any of the child's unused food and formula and refrigerate (discard unused refrigerated formula and food after 24 hours).
15. Do not allow the child to eat fresh fruits or vegetables or raw meat or fish (neutropenic diet if immunosuppressed).
16. Wear gloves for caring for the child, especially when in contact with body fluids and changing diapers.
17. Change the child's diapers frequently, away from food areas.
18. Fold the child's soiled disposable diapers inward, close with the tabs, and dispose in a tightly covered plastic-lined container.
19. Dispose of trash daily.
20. Clean up any of the child's body fluid spills with a bleach solution (10:1 ratio of water to bleach).

F. Education for an adolescent infected with HIV
1. High-risk behaviors and the importance of avoiding high-risk behaviors
2. Methods of transmission of HIV
3. The importance of abstinence from sexual contact, such as intercourse
4. The importance of using safe condoms if intercourse is planned
5. Resources available for support and other issues

💿 MORE QUESTIONS ON THE CD!

Practice Questions

475. An infant of a mother infected with HIV is seen in the clinic each month and is being monitored for symptoms indicative of human immunodeficiency virus (HIV) infection. The nurse assesses the infant, knowing that the most common opportunistic infection of children infected with HIV is:
1. Meningitis
2. Gastroenteritis
3. Cytomegalovirus infection
4. *Pneumocystis jiroveci* pneumonia

476. The nurse provides home care instructions to the parent of a child with acquired immunodeficiency syndrome (AIDS). Which statement by the parent indicates the need for further teaching?
1. "I will wash my hands frequently."
2. "I will keep my child's immunizations up to date."
3. "I will avoid direct unprotected contact with my child's body fluids."
4. "I can send my child to day care if he has a fever, as long as it is a low-grade fever."

477. A clinic nurse is instructing the mother of a child with human immunodeficiency virus (HIV) infection regarding immunizations. The nurse tells the mother that:
1. The hepatitis B vaccine will not be given to the child.
2. The inactivated influenza vaccine will be given yearly.
3. The varicella vaccine will be given before 6 months of age.
4. A Western blot test needs to be performed and the results evaluated before immunizations.

478. A home care nurse provides instructions regarding basic infection control to the mother of an infant with human immunodeficiency virus (HIV) infection. Which statement, if made by the mother, indicates the need for further instructions?
1. "I will wash baby bottles, nipples, and pacifiers in the dishwasher."
2. "I will clean up any spills from the diaper with full-strength alcohol."
3. "I will be sure to prepare foods that are high in calories and high in protein."
4. "I will be sure to wash my hands carefully before and after caring for my infant."

479. A physician prescribes laboratory studies for an infant of a woman positive for human immunodeficiency virus (HIV) to determine the presence of HIV antigen in the infant. The nurse anticipates that which laboratory study will be prescribed for the infant?
1. Chest x-ray
2. Western blot
3. CD4+ cell count
4. p24 antigen assay

480. A mother with human immunodeficiency virus (HIV) infection brings her 10-month-old infant to the clinic for a routine checkup. The physician has documented that the infant is asymptomatic for HIV infection. After the checkup, the mother tells the nurse that she is so pleased that the infant will not get HIV. The appropriate nursing response to the mother is:
  1. "I am so pleased also that everything has turned out fine."
  2. "Because symptoms have not developed, it is unlikely that your infant will develop HIV infection."
  3. "Everything looks great, but be sure that you return with your infant next month for the scheduled visit."
  4. "Most children infected with HIV develop symptoms within the first 9 months of life, and some become symptomatic sometime before they are 3 years old."

481. A 6-year-old child with human immunodeficiency virus (HIV) has been admitted to the hospital for pain management. The child asks the nurse if the pain will ever go away. The nurse should make which best response to the child?
  1. "The pain will go away if you lie still and let the medicine work."
  2. "Try not to think about it. The more you think it hurts, the more it will hurt."
  3. "I know it must hurt, but if you tell me when it does, I will try and make it hurt a little less."
  4. "Every time it hurts, press on the call button and I will give you something to make the pain go all away."

482. A nurse is caring for a 4-year-old child with human immunodeficiency virus (HIV) infection. In planning care to address the child's psychosocial needs, the nurse expects that this child:
  1. Will express fear, withdrawal, and denial
  2. Begins to understand that something is wrong
  3. Is unable to grasp the concept of illness and death
  4. Begins to conceptualize the death process as involving physical harm

Alternate Item Format: Multiple Response

483. Which home care instructions would the nurse provide to the mother of a child with acquired immunodeficiency syndrome (AIDS)? **Select all that apply.**
  ❏ 1. Monitor the child's weight.
  ❏ 2. Frequent handwashing is important.
  ❏ 3. The child should avoid exposure to other illnesses.
  ❏ 4. The child's immunization schedule will need revision.
  ❏ 5. Clean up body fluid spills with bleach solution (10:1 ratio of water to bleach).
  ❏ 6. Fever, malaise, fatigue, weight loss, vomiting, and diarrhea are expected to occur and do not require special intervention.

ANSWERS
475. 4
Rationale: AIDS is a disorder caused by HIV and characterized by generalized dysfunction of the immune system. The most common opportunistic infection of children infected with HIV is *P. jiroveci* pneumonia, which occurs most frequently between the ages of 3 and 6 months, when HIV status may be indeterminate. Cytomegalovirus infection is also characteristic of HIV infection; however, it is not the most common opportunistic infection. Although gastrointestinal disturbances and neurological abnormalities may occur in a child with HIV infection, options 1 and 2 are not specific opportunistic infections noted in the HIV-infected child.
Test-Taking Strategy: Note the strategic words *most common opportunistic infection.* This focus will direct you to option 4. Remember the most common opportunistic infection of children infected with HIV is *P. jiroveci* pneumonia. Review the complications associated with HIV in an infant or child if you had difficulty with this question.
Level of Cognitive Ability: Understanding
Client Needs: Physiological Integrity
Integrated Process: Nursing Process—Assessment
Content Area: Child Health—Integumentary/AIDS/Infectious Diseases

Reference: Hockenberry, M., & Wilson, D. (2009). *Wong's essentials of pediatric nursing* (8th ed., p. 940). St. Louis: Mosby.

476. 4
Rationale: AIDS is a disorder caused by HIV and characterized by generalized dysfunction of the immune system. A child with AIDS who is sick or has a fever should be kept home and not brought to a day care center. Options 1, 2, and 3 are correct statements and would be actions a caretaker should take when the child has AIDS.
Test-Taking Strategy: Note the strategic words *indicates the need for further teaching.* These words indicate a negative event query and ask you to select an option that is an incorrect statement. Noting the word *fever* in option 4 will direct you to this option. Review teaching points and home care instructions related to the care of a child with AIDS if you had difficulty with this question.
Level of Cognitive Ability: Evaluating
Client Needs: Safe and Effective Care Environment
Integrated Process: Teaching and Learning
Content Area: Child Health—Integumentary/AIDS/Infectious Diseases

References: McKinney, E., James, S., Murray, S., & Ashwill, J. (2009). *Maternal-child nursing* (3rd ed., p. 1054). St. Louis: Saunders.

Perry, S., Hockenberry, M., Lowdermilk, D., & Wilson, D. (2010). *Maternal child nursing care* (4th ed., p. 1519). St. Louis: Mosby.

477. 2

Rationale: Immunizations against common childhood illnesses are recommended for all children exposed to or infected with HIV. The inactivated influenza vaccine that is given intramuscularly will be administered (influenza vaccine should be given yearly). The hepatitis B vaccine is administered according to the recommended immunization schedule. Varicella-zoster virus vaccine should not be given; varicella-zoster immunoglobulin may be prescribed after chickenpox exposure. Option 4 is unnecessary and is inaccurate.

Test-Taking Strategy: Use the process of elimination. Option 4 can be eliminated first because the Western blot is a diagnostic test, not an evaluative test. From the remaining options, recalling that the child infected with HIV is at risk for opportunistic infections and that live virus vaccines are not administered to an immunodeficient child will assist in directing you to option 2. Review immunizations in the immunodeficient child if you had difficulty with this question.

Level of Cognitive Ability: Applying
Client Needs: Health Promotion and Maintenance
Integrated Process: Teaching and Learning
Content Area: Child Health—Integumentary/AIDS/Infectious Diseases

References: Callen, N., & Schutze, G. (n.d.). *Immunizations for children with HIV/AIDS.* Available at: http://www.baylorcids.org/curriculum/files/20.pdf. Retrieved January 15, 2010.

McKinney, E., James, S., Murray, S., & Ashwill, J. (2009). *Maternal-child nursing* (3rd ed., p. 1054). St. Louis: Saunders.

478. 2

Rationale: HIV is transmitted through blood, semen, vaginal secretions, and breast milk. The mother of an infant with HIV should be instructed to use a bleach solution for disinfecting contaminated objects or cleaning up spills from the child's diaper. Alcohol would not be effective in destroying the virus. Options 1, 3, and 4 are accurate instructions related to basic infection control.

Test-Taking Strategy: Note the strategic words *need for further instructions.* These words indicate a negative event query and ask you to select an option that is an incorrect statement. Recalling basic infection control measures and the measures to prevent the spread of HIV will direct you to option 2. Review home care measures to prevent the transmission of HIV if you had difficulty with this question.

Level of Cognitive Ability: Evaluating
Client Needs: Safe and Effective Care Environment
Integrated Process: Teaching and Learning
Content Area: Child Health—Integumentary/AIDS/Infectious Diseases

Reference: McKinney, E., James, S., Murray, S., & Ashwill, J. (2009). *Maternal-child nursing* (3rd ed., p. 1054). St. Louis: Saunders.

479. 4

Rationale: The detection of HIV in infants is confirmed by a p24 antigen assay, virus culture of HIV, or polymerase chain reaction. A Western blot test confirms the presence of HIV antibodies. The CD4+ cell count indicates how well the immune system is working. A chest x-ray evaluates the presence of other manifestations of HIV infection, such as pneumonia.

Test-Taking Strategy: Note the strategic word *infant.* Recall the laboratory tests used to determine the presence of HIV infection to answer this question. If you are unfamiliar with the laboratory tests used to detect HIV in infants, review them. Specific laboratory tests to review include enzyme-linked immunosorbent assay, Western blot, CD4+ cell count, and p24 antigen assay.

Level of Cognitive Ability: Understanding
Client Needs: Physiological Integrity
Integrated Process: Nursing Process—Assessment
Content Area: Child Health—Integumentary/AIDS/Infectious Diseases

References: Pagana, K., & Pagana, T. (2009). *Mosby's diagnostic and laboratory test reference* (9th ed., pp. 524–527). St. Louis: Mosby.

Swearingen, P. (2008). *All-in-one care planning resource: Medical-surgical, pediatric, maternity, & psychiatric nursing care plans* (2nd ed., pp. 548–549). St. Louis: Mosby.

480. 4

Rationale: AIDS is caused by HIV and characterized by generalized dysfunction of the immune system. Most children infected with HIV develop symptoms within the first 9 months of life. The remaining infected children become symptomatic sometime before age 3 years. With their immature immune systems, children have a much shorter incubation period than adults. Options 1, 2, and 3 are incorrect.

Test-Taking Strategy: Use the process of elimination. Eliminate options 1, 2, and 3 because they are comparable or alike in content. Option 4 is the only option that provides specific and accurate data regarding HIV infection in an infant. Review assessment findings associated with HIV infection in an infant if you had difficulty with this question.

Level of Cognitive Ability: Applying
Client Needs: Psychosocial Integrity
Integrated Process: Nursing Process—Implementation
Content Area: Child Health—Integumentary/AIDS/Infectious Diseases

Reference: McKinney, E., James, S., Murray, S., & Ashwill, J. (2009). *Maternal-child nursing* (3rd ed., p. 1047). St. Louis: Saunders.

481. 3

Rationale: The multiple complications associated with HIV are accompanied by a high level of pain. Aggressive pain management is essential for the child to have an acceptable quality of life. A nurse must acknowledge the child's pain and let the child know that everything will be done to decrease the pain. Telling the child that movement or lack thereof would eliminate the pain is inaccurate. Allowing a child to think that he or she can control the pain simply by thinking or not thinking about it oversimplifies the pain cycle associated with HIV. Giving false hope by telling the child that the pain will be taken "all away" is neither truthful nor realistic.

Test-Taking Strategy: Recall the general concept of pain and growth and development concepts of a 6-year-old child. Giving the child information about the pain in words that he or she can understand, but without providing false hope or not telling the truth, should guide you to option 3. Options 1 and 2 provide inaccurate information about pain management. Option 4 provides false hope that the pain can be alleviated completely. Review the concepts associated with pain management in a child if you had difficulty with this question.
Level of Cognitive Ability: Applying
Client Needs: Physiological Integrity
Integrated Process: Nursing Process—Implementation
Content Area: Child Health—Integumentary/AIDS/Infectious Diseases
Reference: McKinney, E., James, S., Murray, S., & Ashwill, J. (2009). *Maternal-child nursing* (3rd ed., pp. 992, 994). St. Louis: Saunders.

482. 4
Rationale: A preschool child begins to conceptualize the death process as involving physical harm. A child from birth to 2 years of age is unable to grasp the concept of illness and death. A school-age child begins to understand that something is wrong. An adolescent expresses fear, withdrawal, and denial.
Test-Taking Strategy: Use concepts of growth and development and related psychosocial issues to answer the question. Noting the age of the child will assist in directing you to the correct option. Review growth and development concepts and psychosocial needs for the various age groups if you had difficulty with this question.
Level of Cognitive Ability: Analyzing
Client Needs: Psychosocial Integrity
Integrated Process: Nursing Process—Analysis
Content Area: Child Health—Integumentary/AIDS/Infectious Diseases
Reference: McKinney, E., James, S., Murray, S., & Ashwill, J. (2009). *Maternal-child nursing* (3rd ed., p. 1056). St. Louis: Saunders.

ALTERNATE ITEM FORMAT: MULTIPLE RESPONSE
483. 1, 2, 3, 5
Rationale: AIDS is a disorder caused by HIV and is characterized by a generalized dysfunction of the immune system. Home care instructions include the following: frequent handwashing; monitoring for fever, malaise, fatigue, weight loss, vomiting, and diarrhea and notifying the physician if these occur; monitoring for signs and symptoms of opportunistic infections; administering antiretroviral medications and other medications as prescribed; avoiding exposure to other illnesses; keeping immunizations up to date; monitoring weight and providing a high-calorie, high-protein diet; washing eating utensils in the dishwasher; and avoiding sharing eating utensils. Gloves are worn for care, especially when in contact with body fluids and changing diapers; diapers are changed frequently and away from food areas, and soiled disposable diapers are folded inward, closed with the tabs, and disposed of in a tightly covered plastic-lined container. Any body fluid spills are cleaned with a bleach solution (10:1 ratio of water to bleach).
Test-Taking Strategy: Focus on the subject, care of the child with AIDS. Recalling that AIDS is characterized by a generalized dysfunction of the immune system and recalling the modes of transmission of the virus will assist in selecting the correct home care instructions. Review the home care instructions that will prevent the transmission of AIDS and the measures that will protect the child if you had difficulty with this question.
Level of Cognitive Ability: Applying
Client Needs: Safe and Effective Care Environment
Integrated Process: Teaching and Learning
Content Area: Child Health—Integumentary/AIDS/Infectious Diseases
Reference: McKinney, E., James, S., Murray, S., & Ashwill, J. (2009). *Maternal-child nursing* (3rd ed., p. 1054). St. Louis: Saunders.

48

Infectious and Communicable Diseases

I. RUBEOLA (MEASLES)

A. Description

1. Agent: Paramyxovirus
2. Incubation period: 10 to 20 days
3. Communicable period: From 4 days before to 5 days after rash appears, mainly during **prodromal** stage (pertaining to early symptoms that may mark the onset of disease)
4. Source: Respiratory tract secretions, blood, or urine of infected person
5. Transmission: Airborne particles or direct contact with infectious droplets; transplacental

B. Assessment (Fig. 48-1)

1. Fever
2. Malaise
3. The three "C's"—coryza, cough, conjunctivitis
4. Rash appears as red, erythematous maculopapular eruption starting on the face and spreading downward to the feet; blanches easily with pressure and gradually turns a brownish color (lasts 6 to 7 days); may have desquamation
5. Koplik's spots: Small red spots with a bluish white center and a red base; located on the buccal mucosa and last 3 days

C. Interventions

1. Use airborne droplet precautions if the child is hospitalized.
2. Restrict child to quiet activities and bedrest.
3. Use a cool mist vaporizer for cough and coryza.
4. Dim lights if photophobia is present.
5. Administer antipyretics for fever.

II. ROSEOLA (EXANTHEMA SUBITUM)

A. Description

1. Agent: Human herpesvirus type 6
2. Incubation period: 5 to 15 days
3. Communicable period: Unknown, but thought to extend from the febrile stage to the time the rash first appears
4. Source: Unknown
5. Transmission: Unknown

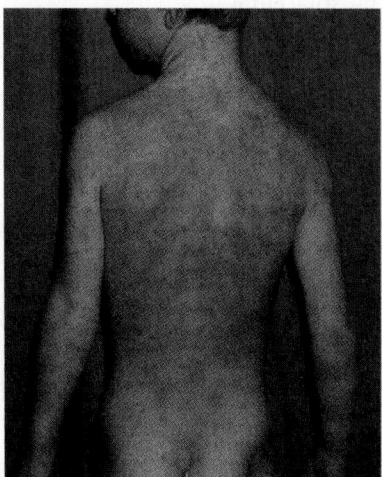

▲ **FIGURE 48-1** Rubeola (measles). (From Hockenberry, M., & Wilson, D. [2007]. *Wong's nursing care of infants and children* [8th ed.]. St. Louis: Mosby.)

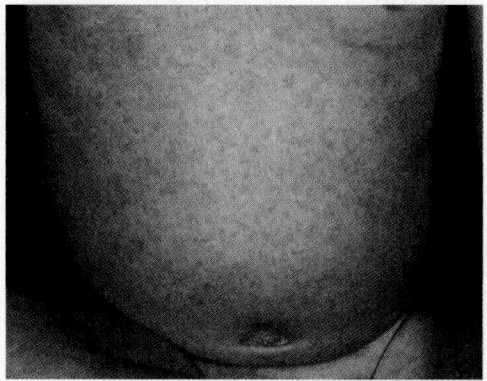

▲ **FIGURE 48-2** Roseola (exanthema subitum). (From Hockenberry, M., & Wilson, D. [2007]. *Wong's nursing care of infants and children* [8th ed.]. St. Louis: Mosby.)

B. Assessment (Fig. 48-2)

1. Sudden high (>38.8° C [>102° F]) fever of 3 to 5 days' duration in a child who appears well, followed by a rash (rose-pink macules that blanch with pressure)
2. Rash appears several hours to 2 days after the fever subsides and lasts 1 to 2 days.

C. Interventions: Supportive

III. RUBELLA (GERMAN MEASLES)

A. Description
1. Agent: Rubella virus
2. Incubation period: 14 to 21 days
3. Communicable period: From 7 days before to about 5 days after rash appears
4. Source: Nasopharyngeal secretions; virus is also present in blood, stool, and urine
5. Transmission
   a. Airborne or direct contact with infectious droplets
   b. Indirectly via articles freshly contaminated with nasopharyngeal secretions, feces, or urine
   c. Transplacental

B. Assessment (Fig. 48-3)
1. Low-grade fever
2. Malaise
3. Pinkish red maculopapular rash that begins on the face and spreads to the entire body within 1 to 3 days
4. Petechial red, pinpoint spots may occur on the soft palate.

C. Interventions
1. Use airborne droplet precautions if the child is hospitalized; provide supportive treatment.
2. Isolate the infected child from pregnant women.

IV. MUMPS

A. Description
1. Agent: Paramyxovirus
2. Incubation period: 14 to 21 days
3. Communicable period: Immediately before and after parotid gland swelling begins
4. Source: Saliva of infected person and possibly urine
5. Transmission: Direct contact or droplet spread from an infected person

B. Assessment
1. Fever
2. Headache and malaise
3. Anorexia
4. Jaw or ear pain aggravated by chewing, followed by parotid glandular swelling
5. Orchitis may occur

C. Interventions
1. Institute airborne droplet precautions.
2. Provide bedrest until the parotid gland swelling subsides.
3. Avoid foods that require chewing.
4. Apply hot or cold compresses as prescribed to the neck.
5. Apply warmth and local support with snug-fitting underpants to relieve orchitis.

V. CHICKENPOX (VARICELLA)

A. Description
1. Agent: Varicella-zoster virus
2. Incubation period: 13 to 17 days
3. Communicable period: From 1 to 2 days before the onset of the rash to 6 days after the first crop of vesicles, when crusts have formed
4. Source: Respiratory tract secretions of infected person; skin lesions
5. Transmission: Direct contact, droplet (airborne) spread, and contaminated objects

B. Assessment (Fig. 48-4)
1. Slight fever, malaise, and anorexia are followed by a macular rash that first appears on the trunk and scalp and moves to the face and extremities.
2. Lesions become pustules, begin to dry, and develop a crust.
3. Lesions may appear on the mucous membranes of the mouth, the genital area, and the rectal area.

C. Interventions
1. In the hospital, ensure strict isolation (contact and droplet precautions).
2. At home, isolate the infected child until the vesicles have dried.
3. Supportive care

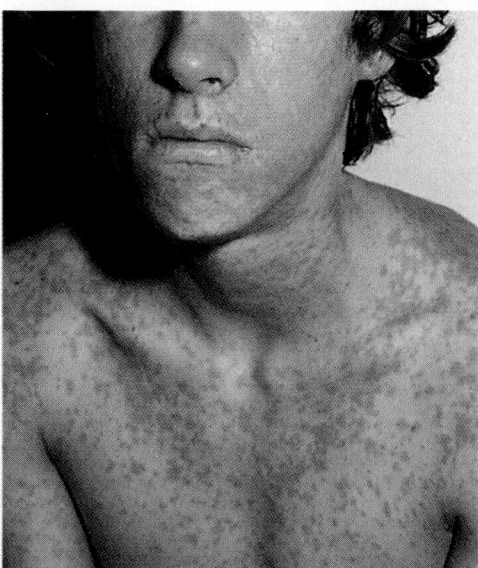

▲ **FIGURE 48-3** Rubella (German measles). (From Hockenberry, M., & Wilson, D. [2007]. *Wong's nursing care of infants and children* [8th ed.]. St. Louis: Mosby. Courtesy Dr Michael Sherlock.)

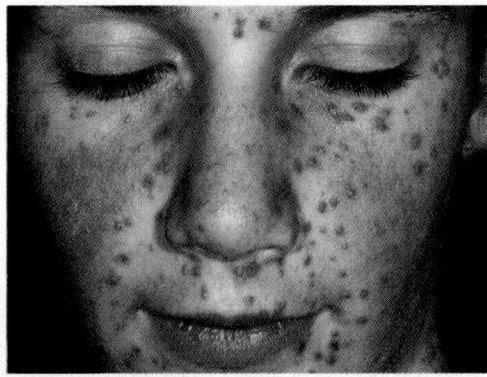

▲ **FIGURE 48-4** Chickenpox (varicella). (From Hockenberry, M., & Wilson, D. [2007]. *Wong's nursing care of infants and children* [8th ed.]. St. Louis: Mosby.)

⚠ Isolate high-risk children, such as children who have immunosuppressive disorders, from a child with a communicable disease.

VI. PERTUSSIS (WHOOPING COUGH)

A. Description
1. Agent: *Bordetella pertussis*
2. Incubation period: 5 to 21 days (usually 10 days)
3. Communicable period: Greatest during the catarrhal stage (when discharge from respiratory secretions occurs)
4. Source: Discharge from the respiratory tract of the infected person
5. Transmission: Direct contact or droplet spread from infected person; indirect contact with freshly contaminated articles

B. Assessment
1. Symptoms of respiratory infection followed by increased severity of cough, with a loud whooping inspiration
2. May experience **cyanosis**, respiratory distress, and tongue protrusion
3. Listlessness, irritability, anorexia

C. Interventions
1. Isolate child during the catarrhal stage; if the child is hospitalized, institute airborne droplet precautions.
2. Administer antimicrobial therapy as prescribed.
3. Reduce environmental factors that cause coughing spasms, such as dust, smoke, and sudden changes in temperature.
4. Ensure adequate hydration and nutrition.
5. Provide suction and humidified oxygen if needed.
6. Monitor cardiopulmonary status (via monitor as prescribed) and pulse oximetry.
7. Infants do not receive maternal immunity to pertussis.

VII. DIPHTHERIA

A. Description
1. Agent: *Corynebacterium diphtheriae*
2. Incubation period: 2 to 5 days
3. Communicable period: Variable, until virulent bacilli are no longer present (three negative cultures of discharge from the nose and nasopharynx, skin, and other lesions); usually 2 weeks, but can be 4 weeks
4. Source: Discharge from the mucous membrane of the nose and nasopharynx, skin, and other lesions of the infected person
5. Transmission: Direct contact with infected person, carrier, or contaminated articles

B. Assessment
1. Low-grade fever, malaise, sore throat
2. Foul-smelling, mucopurulent nasal discharge

3. Dense pseudomembrane formation of the throat that may interfere with eating, drinking, and breathing.
4. Lymphadenitis, neck edema, "bull neck"

C. Interventions
1. Ensure strict isolation for the hospitalized child.
2. Administer diphtheria antitoxin as prescribed (after a skin or conjunctival test to rule out sensitivity to horse serum).
3. Provide bedrest.
4. Administer antibiotics as prescribed.
5. Provide suction and humidified oxygen as needed.
6. Provide tracheostomy care if a tracheostomy is necessary.

VIII. POLIOMYELITIS

A. Description
1. Agent: Enteroviruses
2. Incubation period: 7 to 14 days
3. Communicable period: Unknown; the virus is present in the throat and feces shortly after infection and persists for about 1 week in the throat and 4 to 6 weeks in the feces
4. Source: Oropharyngeal secretions and feces of the infected person
5. Transmission: Direct contact with infected person; fecal-oral and oropharyngeal routes

B. Assessment
1. Fever, malaise, anorexia, nausea, headache, sore throat
2. Abdominal pain followed by soreness and stiffness of the trunk, neck, and limbs that may progress to central nervous system paralysis

C. Interventions
1. Enteric precautions
2. Supportive treatment
3. Bedrest
4. Monitoring for respiratory paralysis
5. Physical therapy

IX. SCARLET FEVER

A. Description
1. Agent: Group A beta-hemolytic streptococci
2. Incubation period: 1 to 7 days
3. Communicable period: About 10 days during the incubation period and clinical illness; during the first 2 weeks of the carrier stage, although may persist for months
4. Source: Nasopharyngeal secretions of infected person and carriers
5. Transmission: Direct contact with infected person or droplet spread; indirectly by contact with contaminated articles, ingestion of contaminated milk, or other foods

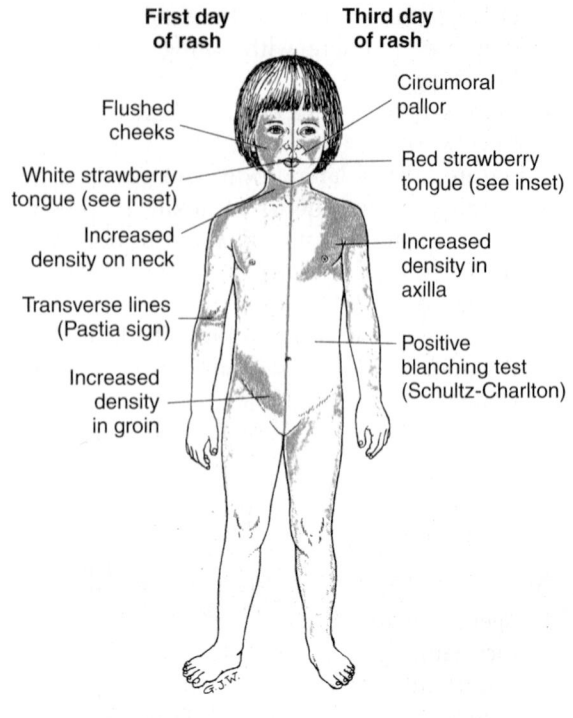

First day
of rash

Third day
of rash

Flushed
cheeks

Circumoral
pallor

White strawberry
tongue (see inset)

Red strawberry
tongue (see inset)

Increased
density on neck

Increased
density in
axilla

Transverse lines
(Pastia sign)

Positive
blanching test
(Schultz-Charlton)

Increased
density
in groin

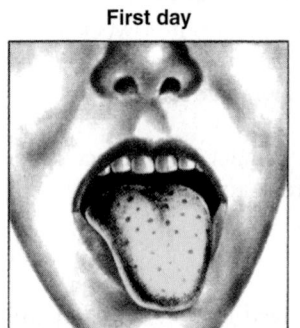

First day

White strawberry tongue

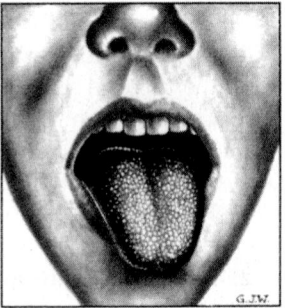

Third day

Red strawberry tongue

▲ **FIGURE 48-5** Scarlet fever. (From Hockenberry, M., & Wilson, D. [2007]. *Wong's nursing care of infants and children* [8th ed.]. St. Louis: Mosby.)

B. Assessment (Fig. 48-5)
1. Abrupt high fever, flushed cheeks, vomiting, headache, enlarged lymph nodes in the neck, malaise, abdominal pain
2. A red, fine sandpaper-like rash develops in the axilla, groin, and neck that spreads to cover the entire body except the face.
3. Rash blanches with pressure (Schultz-Charlton reaction) except in areas of deep creases and folds of the joints (Pastia's sign).
4. Desquamation, sheet-like sloughing of the skin on palms and soles, appears by weeks 1 to 3.
5. The tongue is initially coated with a white, furry covering with red projecting papillae (white strawberry tongue); by the third to fifth day, the white coat sloughs off, leaving a red swollen tongue (red strawberry tongue).

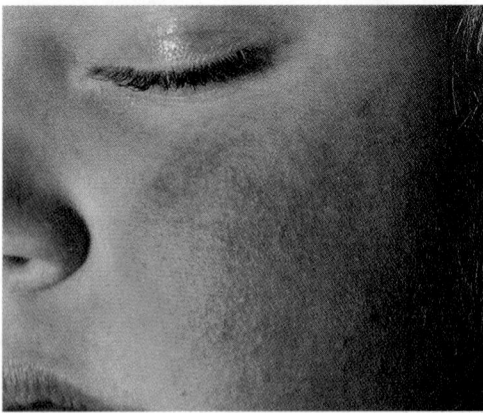

▲ **FIGURE 48-6** Erythema infectiosum (fifth disease): Slapped-face appearance. (From Hockenberry, M., & Wilson, D. [2007]. *Wong's nursing care of infants and children* [8th ed.]. St. Louis: Mosby.)

6. Tonsils are reddened, edematous, and covered with exudate.
7. Pharynx is edematous and beefy red.
C. Interventions
1. Institute respiratory precautions until 24 hours after initiation of antibiotic therapy.
2. Provide supportive therapy.
3. Provide bedrest.
4. Encourage fluid intake

X. ERYTHEMA INFECTIOSUM (FIFTH DISEASE)

A. Description
1. Agent: Human parvovirus B19
2. Incubation period: 4 to 14 days; may be 20 days
3. Communicable period: Uncertain, but before the onset of symptoms in most children
4. Source: Infected person
5. Transmission: Unknown; possibly respiratory secretions and blood
B. Assessment
1. Before rash: Asymptomatic or mild fever, malaise, headache, runny nose
2. Stages of rash
   a. Erythema of the face (slapped-cheek appearance) develops and disappears by 1 to 4 days (Fig. 48-6).
   b. About 1 day after the rash appears on the face, maculopapular red spots appear, symmetrically distributed on the extremities; the rash progresses from proximal to distal surfaces and may last a week or more.
   c. The rash subsides, but may reappear if the skin becomes irritated by the sun, heat, cold, exercise, or friction.
C. Interventions
1. Child is not usually hospitalized.
2. Pregnant women should avoid the infected individual.
3. Provide supportive care.

4. Administer antipyretics, analgesics, and anti-inflammatory medications as prescribed.

XI. INFECTIOUS MONONUCLEOSIS

A. Description
1. Agent: Epstein-Barr virus
2. Incubation period: 4 to 6 weeks
3. Communicable period: Unknown
4. Source: Oral secretions
5. Transmission: Direct intimate contact

B. Assessment
1. Fever, malaise, headache, fatigue, nausea, abdominal pain, sore throat, enlarged red tonsils
2. Lymphadenopathy and hepatosplenomegaly
3. Discrete macular rash most prominent over the trunk may occur.

C. Interventions
1. Provide supportive care.
2. Monitor for signs of splenic rupture

⚠️ Teach the parents of a child with mononucleosis to monitor for signs of splenic rupture, which include abdominal pain, left upper quadrant pain, and left shoulder pain.

XII. ROCKY MOUNTAIN SPOTTED FEVER

A. Description
1. Agent: *Rickettsia rickettsii*
2. Incubation period: 2 to 14 days
3. Source: Tick from a mammal, most often from wild rodents and dogs
4. Transmission: Bite of infected tick

B. Assessment
1. Fever, malaise, anorexia, vomiting, headache, myalgia
2. Maculopapular or petechial rash primarily on the extremities (ankles and wrists), but may spread to other areas, characteristically on the palms and soles

C. Interventions
1. Provide vigorous supportive care.
2. Administer antibiotics as prescribed.
3. Teach the child and parents about protection from tick bites (Box 48-1).

XIII. COMMUNITY-ASSOCIATED METHICILLIN-RESISTANT STAPHYLOCOCCUS AUREUS (MRSA)

A. Description
1. *Staphylococcus aureus* is a bacterium that is normally located on the skin or in the nose of healthy people; when present without symptoms, it is called colonization, and when symptoms are present, it is called an infection.
2. MRSA is a strain of *S. aureus* that is resistant to methicillin and most often occurs in people

---

Box 48-1 Measures to Protect the Child From Tick Bites

Wearing long-sleeved shirts, long pants tucked into long socks (socks should be pulled up over the pant legs), and a hat when walking in tick-infested areas

Wearing light-colored clothing to make ticks more visible if they get onto the child

Checking children for the presence of ticks after being in high-risk or tick-infested areas

Following paths rather than walking in tall grass and shrub areas because these are the places where most ticks are found

Applying insect repellents containing diethyltoluamide (DEET) and permethrin before possible exposure to areas where ticks are found (use with caution in infants and small children)

Keeping yards at home trimmed and free of accumulating leaves and other brush

Applying tick repellent to dogs

Saving the tick for later identification if it is removed from the child's body

---

who were hospitalized or treated at a health care facility (hospital-acquired MRSA).
3. Community-associated MRSA is a MRSA infection that occurs in a healthy person who has not been hospitalized or had a medical procedure done within the past year.
4. Persons at risk for community-associated MRSA include athletes, prisoners, day care attendees, military recruits, persons who **abuse** intravenous drugs, persons living in crowded settings, persons with poor hygiene practices, persons who use contaminated items, persons who get tattoos, and persons with a compromised immune system.
5. Community-associated MRSA is spread through person-to-person contact, through contact with contaminated items, or through infection of a preexisting cut or wound that is not protected by a dressing.
6. The bacteria can enter the bloodstream through the cut or wound and cause sepsis, cellulitis, endocarditis, osteomyelitis, septic arthritis, toxic shock syndrome, pneumonia, organ failure, and death.

B. Prevention measures
1. Handwashing and practicing good personal hygiene
2. Avoid sharing personal items
3. Regular cleaning of shared equipment such as athletic equipment, whirlpools, or saunas
4. Cleaning a cut or wound thoroughly

C. Assessment
1. Appearance of a skin infection: Red, swollen area, warmth around the area, drainage of pus, pain at the site, fever.

2. Symptoms of a more serious infection: Chest pain, cough, fatigue, chills, fever, malaise, headache, muscle aches, shortness of breath, rash

D. Interventions
1. Assess skin lesions.
2. Prepare to drain an infected skin site and culture the wound and wound drainage.
3. Prepare to obtain blood cultures, sputum cultures, and urine cultures.
4. Prepare to administer antibiotics as prescribed.
5. Educate the parent and family about the causes and modes of transmission, signs and symptoms, and importance of treatment measures prescribed.

XIV. H1N1 INFLUENZA

A. Description
1. H1N1 is also known as swine flu and is a strain of influenza.
2. It is a viral infection that affects the respiratory system and is highly contagious.
3. Children, pregnant women, persons with preexisting health conditions, and persons with a compromised immune system are at high risk for developing complications.
4. It is caused by contact with an infected person or by touching something such as a toy or tissue that the infected person has touched.

B. Prevention
1. H1N1 flu **vaccine**
   a. Children age 6 months and older need to be vaccinated.
   b. Children younger than 6 months are not old enough to receive the **vaccine**; family members and caregivers need to get vaccinated.
   c. Children 9 years and younger need two doses at least 3 weeks apart; children 10 years and older need one dose (it takes about 2 weeks after receiving the second dose or the first dose in children needing only one dose before immunity develops).
   d. The H1N1 **vaccine** and seasonal flu **vaccine** can be given at the same time.
   e. A nasal spray version of the H1N1 **vaccine** that contains a weakened live virus may be given to people 2 to 49 years old who do not have a chronic health condition.
2. Wash the child's hands frequently and teach handwashing techniques.
3. Avoid children who are ill.
4. Keep the child home from school or away from others until the child has been fever-free (without the use of antipyretics) for at least 24 hours.

⚠ The signs and symptoms of H1N1 infection are similar to those of seasonal flu and usually last a week. If they last longer, the presence of complications should be suspected.

C. Assessment
1. Fever that occurs suddenly and is high
2. Headache, body aches, fatigue, chills, cough, congestion, sore throat, loss of appetite, vomiting, diarrhea

D. Interventions
1. Antiviral medications if prescribed, fluids, rest, pain relievers such as acetaminophen (Tylenol) or ibuprofen (Motrin)
2. Family and child teaching about prevention measures

XV. IMMUNIZATIONS

A. Guidelines (see Priority Nursing Actions)
1. In the United States, the recommended age for beginning primary immunizations of infants is at birth.
2. Children who began primary immunizations at the recommended age but failed to receive all the required doses do not need to begin the series again; they need to receive only the missed doses.

▬▬▬ PRIORITY NURSING ACTIONS! ▬▬▬

Actions to Take When Administering a Parenteral Vaccine
1. Verify the prescription for the vaccine.
2. Obtain an immunization history from the parents and assess for allergies.
3. Provide information to the parents about the vaccine.
4. Obtain parental consent.
5. Check the lot number and expiration date and prepare the injection.
6. Select the appropriate site for administration.
7. Administer the vaccine.
8. Document the administration and site of administration and lot number and expiration date of the vaccine.
9. Provide a vaccination record to the parents.

The nurse should first verify the prescription and then obtain an immunization history from the parents to ensure that the immunizations are up to date. The nurse should also question the parents about the presence of any allergies in the child because some vaccines contain components to which the child may be allergic. The nurse next provides information to the parents about the vaccine and obtains consent. The expiration date and the lot number (located on the medication vial) of the vaccine should be checked before preparing the vaccine for administration. When the vaccine is prepared, the nurse prepares the child for the procedure, selects an appropriate site, and administers the vaccine. The nurse documents that the vaccination has been administered and provides an updated immunization record to the parents.

References: Hockenberry, M., & Wilson, D. (2009). *Wong's essentials of pediatric nursing* (8th ed., pp. 359, 363-364). St. Louis: Mosby.
McKinney, E., James, S., Murray, S., & Ashwill, J. (2009). *Maternal-child nursing* (3rd ed., pp. 68, 70). St. Louis: Saunders.

3. If there is suspicion that the parent will not bring the child to the pediatrician or health care clinic for follow-up immunizations according to the optimal immunization schedule, any of the recommended **vaccines** can be administered simultaneously.

B. General contraindications and precautions

1. A **vaccine** is contraindicated if the child experienced an anaphylactic reaction to a previously administered **vaccine** or a component in the **vaccine**.

2. Live virus **vaccines** generally are not administered to individuals with severely deficient immune systems, individuals with a severe sensitivity to gelatin, or pregnant women.

3. A **vaccine** is administered with caution to an individual with a moderate or severe acute illness, with or without fever.

4. See Section XVI, Recommended Childhood and Adolescent Immunizations, for specific information for each type of **vaccine**.

C. Guidelines for administration (Box 48-2)

⚠ Children born prematurely should receive the full dose of each vaccine at the appropriate chronological age.

XVI. RECOMMENDED CHILDHOOD AND ADOLESCENT IMMUNIZATIONS (Box 48-3)

A. Hepatitis B **vaccine** (HepB)

1. Protects against hepatitis B

2. Administered by the intramuscular route

3. First dose of hepatitis B **vaccine** (monovalent) should be administered soon after birth and before hospital discharge (the birth dose can be delayed in rare circumstances if the infant's mother tests negative for hepatitis B surface antigen [HBsAg]).

4. Monovalent HepB or a combination **vaccine** containing hepatitis B may be used to complete the series.

5. The second dose is administered at age 1 to 2 months.

6. The final dose should be given at 24 weeks or older (6 to 18 months of age).

7. Contraindications: Severe allergic reaction to previous dose or **vaccine** component (components include aluminum hydroxide, yeast protein)

8. Precautions: An infant weighing less than 2000 g or an infant with moderate or severe acute illness with or without fever.

9. HBsAg-positive mothers

   a. Infant should receive HepB **vaccine** and hepatitis B immunoglobulin (HBIG) within 12 hours of birth.

   b. Infant should be tested for HBsAg and antibody to HBsAg after completion of HepB series (9 to 18 months of age).

10. Mother whose HBsAg status is unknown

   a. Infant should receive the first dose of hepatitis **vaccine** series within 12 hours of birth.

   b. Maternal blood should be drawn as soon as possible to determine the mother's HBsAg status.

   c. If the mother's HBsAg test result is positive, the infant should receive HBIG as soon as possible (no later than 1 week of age).

B. Rotavirus **vaccine** (RV)

1. Rotavirus is a cause of serious gastroenteritis and is a nosocomial (hospital-acquired) pathogen that is most severe in children 3 to 24 months of age; children younger than 3 months have some protection because of maternally acquired antibodies.

Box 48-2 Guidelines for Administration of Vaccines

Follow manufacturer's recommendations for route of administration, storage, and reconstitution of the vaccine.

If refrigeration is necessary, store on a center shelf and not on the door; frequent temperature changes from opening the refrigerator door can alter the vaccine's potency.

A vaccine information statement needs to be given to the parents or individual, and informed consent for administration needs to be obtained.

Check the expiration date on the vaccine bottle.

Parenteral vaccines are given in separate syringes in different injection sites.

Vaccines administered intramuscularly are given in the vastus lateralis muscle (best site) or ventrogluteal muscle (the deltoid can be used for children 36 months and older); the dorsogluteal site (buttocks) is avoided.

Vaccines administered subcutaneously are given into the fatty areas in the lateral upper arms and anterior thighs.

Adequate needle length and gauge are as follows: intramuscular, 1 inch, 23-25 gauge; subcutaneous, ⅝ inch, 25 gauge (needle length may vary depending on the child's size).

Mild side effects include fever, soreness, swelling, or redness at injection site.

A topical anesthetic may be applied to injection site before the injection.

For painful or red injection sites, advise the parent to apply cool compresses for the first 24 hours, and then use warm or cold compresses as long as needed.

An age-appropriate dose of acetaminophen (Tylenol) or ibuprofen (Motrin) may be administered every 4 to 6 hours for vaccine-associated discomfort.

Maintain an immunization record—document day, month, year of administration; manufacturer and lot number of vaccine; name, address, title of person administering the vaccine; and site and route of administration.

A vaccine adverse event report needs to be filed and the health department needs to be notified if an adverse reaction to an immunization occurs.

Box 48-3 Recommended Childhood and Adolescent Immunizations

Birth: Hepatitis B vaccine (HepB)

1 month: HepB

2 months: Inactivated poliovirus vaccine (IPV); diphtheria, tetanus, acellular pertussis (DTaP) vaccine; *Haemophilus influenzae* type b conjugate vaccine (Hib); pneumococcal conjugate vaccine (PCV), rotavirus (RV)

4 months: DTaP, Hib, IPV, PCV, RV

6 months: DTaP, Hib, HepB, IPV, PCV, RV (dose may be needed depending on type of vaccine used for first and second doses)

12-15 months: Hib; measles, mumps, rubella (MMR) vaccine; PCV; hepatitis A, first dose (second dose is given 6 months after the first dose); varicella vaccine

15-18 months: DTaP

18-21 months: Hepatitis A, second dose (given 6 months after the first dose)

4-6 years: DTaP, IPV, MMR, varicella vaccine

11-12 years: MMR (if not administered at 4-6 years); diphtheria, tetanus, acellular pertussis adolescent preparation (Tdap); meningococcal vaccine (MCV4); human papillomavirus (HPV) (first dose to girls at age 11 to 12 years, second dose 2 months after first dose, and third dose 6 months after first dose).

Note: Influenza vaccine is recommended annually for children age 6 months through 18 years.

From Centers for Disease Control and Prevention (CDC). (2010). *Recommended immunization schedules for persons aged 0 through 18 years—United States, 2010.* Available at http://www.immunize.org/CDC/schedules/. Retrieved January 12, 2010.

2. Two **vaccines** are available (RotaTeq and Rotarix) and are administered by the oral route because the **vaccine** must replicate in the infant's gut.

3. **Vaccine** may be withheld if an infant is experiencing severe vomiting and diarrhea; it is administered as soon as the infant recovers.

4. RotaTeq: Three doses are needed; the first dose of the **vaccine** needs to be administered at age 6 to 14 weeks, the second is given 4 to 10 weeks after the first dose, and the third is given 4 to 10 weeks after the second dose (no later than 32 weeks of age).

5. Rotarix: Two doses are needed; the first dose of the **vaccine** needs to be administered at age 6 to 14 weeks, and the second is given 4 weeks after the first dose (series needs to be completed by 24 weeks of age).

C. Diphtheria, tetanus, acellular pertussis (DTaP); tetanus toxoid; reduced diphtheria toxoid and acellular pertussis **vaccine** (Tdap adolescent preparation)

1. Protect against diphtheria, tetanus, and pertussis

2. Administered by intramuscular route

3. DTaP is administered at 2, 4, and 6 months; between 15 and 18 months; and between 4 and 6 years of age.

4. The fourth dose of DTaP can be given at 12 months of age if 6 months have elapsed since the third dose and the child might not return for follow-up at 12 to 18 months of age.

5. The fifth (final) dose is administered at age 4 years or older.

6. The Tdap (adolescent preparation) is recommended at 11 to 12 years of age for children who have completed the recommended childhood DTaP series but have not received a tetanus and diphtheria toxoid (Td) booster dose; children 13 to 18 years old who have not received Tdap should receive a dose.

7. Td does not provide protection against pertussis; Td is used as a booster every 10 years after Tdap is administered at 11 to 18 years of age.

8. Encephalopathy is a complication.

9. Contraindications: Encephalopathy within 7 days of a previous dose or a severe allergic reaction to a previous dose or to a **vaccine** component.

D. *Haemophilus influenzae* type b conjugate **vaccine** (Hib)

1. Protects against numerous serious infections caused by *H. influenzae* type b, such as bacterial meningitis, epiglottitis, bacterial pneumonia, septic arthritis, and sepsis

2. Administered by intramuscular route

3. Hib is administered at 2, 4, and 6 months of age and between 12 and 15 months of age.

4. Depending on the brand of Hib **vaccine** used for the first and second doses, a dose at 6 months of age (third dose) may not be needed.

5. DTaP-Hib combination products should not be used for primary immunization in infants at 2, 4, or 6 months of age, but can be used as the final dose in children 12 months to 4 years of age.

6. Contraindications: Severe allergic reaction to a previous dose or **vaccine** component

E. Influenza **vaccine**

1. **Vaccine** is recommended annually for children 6 months to 18 years of age.

2. Refer to Section XIV for information on the H1N1 influenza virus and the H1N1 **vaccine**.

F. Inactivated poliovirus **vaccine** (IPV)

1. IPV protects against polio.

2. IPV is administered by the subcutaneous route (may also be given by the intramuscular route)

3. IPV is administered at 2, 4, and 6 to 18 months and 4 to 6 years of age.

4. The last dose of the IPV should be administered on or after age 4 years and at least 6 months after the previous dose; additionally, if four doses are administered before age 4 years, a fifth dose should be administered at age 4 to 6 years.

5. Contraindications: Severe allergic reaction to a previous dose or **vaccine** component; components may include formalin, neomycin, streptomycin, or polymyxin B

G. Measles, mumps, rubella (MMR) **vaccine**

1. MMR protects against measles, mumps, and rubella.

2. **Vaccine** is administered by the subcutaneous route.

3. The first dose of MMR is administered between 12 and 15 months of age; the second dose is recommended at 4 to 6 years of age (the second dose may be administered during any visit as long as at least 4 weeks have elapsed since the first dose).

4. Children who have not received the second dose previously should complete the schedule at the 11- to 12-year-old pediatric or health care clinic visit.

5. Contraindications: Severe allergic reaction to a previous dose or **vaccine** component (gelatin, neomycin, eggs), pregnancy, known immunodeficiency

6. If the child received immunoglobulin, the MMR **vaccine** should be postponed for at least 3 to 6 months (immunoglobulin can inhibit the immune response to the MMR **vaccine**).

H. Varicella **vaccine**

1. Varicella **vaccine** protects against chickenpox.

2. It is administered by the subcutaneous route.

3. Varicella **vaccine** is administered at 12 and 15 months of age and again at 4 to 6 years of age.

4. Children 13 years old and older (who have not had chickenpox or have not been previously vaccinated) need two doses given at least 28 days apart.

5. Children receiving the **vaccine** should avoid aspirin or aspirin-containing products because of the risk of Reye's syndrome.

6. Contraindications: Severe allergic reaction to a previous dose or **vaccine** component (gelatin, bovine albumin, neomycin), significant suppression of cellular immunity, pregnancy

I. Pneumococcal conjugate **vaccine** (PCV)

1. PCV prevents infection with *Streptococcus pneumoniae*, which may cause meningitis, pneumonia, septicemia, sinusitis, and otitis media.

2. It is administered by the intramuscular route.

3. **Vaccine** can be given concurrently with other childhood **vaccines** at 2, 4, 6, and 12 to 15 months of age (the final dose in the series is given at age 12 months or older).

4. Pneumococcal polysaccharide **vaccine** (PPSV) is recommended in addition to PCV for certain high-risk groups, such as children with chronic illness specifically associated with increased risk of pneumococcal disease or its complications; anatomical or functional asplenia; hemoglobinopathies; nephrotic syndrome; cerebrospinal fluid leaks; a cochlear implant; and conditions associated with immunosuppression (PPSV is given at least 8 weeks after the last dose of PCV).

5. Contraindications: Severe allergic reaction to a previous dose or **vaccine** component

J. Hepatitis A **vaccine** (HepA)

1. **Vaccine** protects against hepatitis A.

2. **Vaccine** is recommended for all children at age 1 year (12 to 23 months); two doses should be administered at least 6 months apart (vaccination of children older than 23 months is allowed for those at increased risk).

3. It is administered by the intramuscular route.

4. Contraindications: Severe allergic reaction to a previous dose or **vaccine** component

K. Meningococcal **vaccine** (MCV)

1. **Vaccine** protects against *Neisseria meningitidis*.

2. Meningococcal (MCV4) **vaccine** is the preferred type of **vaccine** and is given intramuscularly.

3. MCV4 should be administered to all children at age 11 to 12 years and to unvaccinated adolescents at high school entry (age 15 years); all college freshman living in dormitories should be vaccinated.

4. Revaccination is recommended for children who remain at increased risk after 3 years (if the first dose was administered at age 2 to 6 years) or after 5 years (if the first dose was administered at age 7 years or older).

5. It is contraindicated in children with a history of Guillain-Barré syndrome.

L. Human papillomavirus **vaccine** (HPV)

1. Depending on the type of **vaccine** used (HPV2 or HPV4), the HPV **vaccine** guards against diseases that are caused by HPV types 6, 11, 16, and 18, such as cervical cancer, cervical abnormalities that can lead to cervical cancer, and genital warts.

2. The **vaccine** is most effective for boys and girls if administered before exposure to HPV through sexual contact.

3. The **vaccine** is administered as three injections over 6 months—first dose to girls at age 11 to 12 years, second dose 2 months after the first dose, and third dose 6 months after the first dose.

4. A three-dose series may be administered to boys 9 to 18 years old to reduce their likelihood of acquiring genital warts.

5. The **vaccine** can cause pain, swelling, itching, and redness at the injection site; fever; nausea; and dizziness.

6. The **vaccine** is contraindicated in individuals with a reaction to a previous injection and in pregnant women.

XVII. REACTIONS TO A VACCINE

A. Local reactions

1. Tenderness, erythema, swelling at injection site

2. Low-grade fever

3. Behavioral changes such as drowsiness, unusual crying, decreased appetite

B. Minimizing local reactions

1. Select a needle of adequate length to deposit **vaccine** deep into the muscle or subcutaneous mass.

2. Inject into the appropriate recommended site.

C. Anaphylactic reactions
   1. Goals of treatment are to secure and protect the airway, restore adequate circulation, and prevent further exposure to the antigen.
   2. For a mild reaction with no evidence of respiratory distress or cardiovascular compromise, a subcutaneous injection of an antihistamine, such as diphenhydramine (Benadryl), and epinephrine (Adrenalin) may be administered.
   3. For moderate or severe distress, establish an airway; provide cardiopulmonary resuscitation if the child is not breathing; elevate the head; administer epinephrine, fluids, and vasopressors as prescribed; monitor vital signs; and monitor urine output.

 MORE QUESTIONS ON THE CD!

Practice Questions

484. A nurse provides home care instructions to the parents of a child hospitalized with pertussis. The child is in the convalescent stage and is being prepared for discharge. Which statement by a parent indicates a need for further instructions?
   1. "We need to encourage our child to drink fluids."
   2. "Coughing spells may be triggered by dust or smoke."
   3. "Vomiting may occur when our child has coughing episodes."
   4. "We need to maintain droplet precautions and a quiet environment for at least 2 weeks."

485. A 6-month-old infant receives a diphtheria, tetanus, and acellular pertussis (DTaP) immunization at a well-baby clinic. The mother returns home and calls the clinic to report that the infant has developed swelling and redness at the site of injection. A nurse tells the mother to:
   1. Monitor the infant for a fever.
   2. Bring the infant back to the clinic.
   3. Apply a hot pack to the injection site.
   4. Apply an ice pack to the injection site.

486. A child is scheduled to receive inactivated polio vaccine (IPV), and a nurse preparing to administer the vaccine reviews the child's record. The nurse questions the administration of IPV if which of the following is documented in the child's record?
   1. Recent recovery from a cold
   2. A history of frequent respiratory infections
   3. A history of an anaphylactic reaction to neomycin
   4. A local reaction at the site of injection of a previous IPV

487. A 12-year-old child is scheduled to receive a series of the hepatitis B vaccine. The child arrives at a clinic for the second dose. Before administering the vaccine, a nurse performs an assessment on the child and asks the child and parent about a history of a severe allergy to:
   1. Eggs
   2. Penicillin
   3. Sulfonamides
   4. A previous dose of hepatitis B vaccine or component

488. A child with rubeola (measles) is being admitted to the hospital. In preparing for the admission of the child, a nurse plans to place the child on which precautions?
   1. Neutropenic
   2. Enteric
   3. Airborne
   4. Protective

489. A home health nurse visits a child with infectious mononucleosis and provides home care instructions to the parents about the care of the child. The nurse tells the parents to:
   1. Maintain the child on bedrest for 2 weeks.
   2. Maintain respiratory precautions for 1 week.
   3. Notify the physician if the child develops a fever.
   4. Notify the physician if the child develops abdominal pain or left shoulder pain.

490. A mother brings her 4-month-old infant to a well-baby clinic for immunizations. The child is up to date with the immunization schedule. A nurse would prepare to administer which of the following immunizations to this infant?
   1. Diphtheria, tetanus, acellular pertussis (DTaP), *Haemophilus influenzae* type b (Hib), inactivated poliovirus vaccine (IPV), pneumococcal vaccine (PCV), rotavirus (RV)
   2. Varicella, HepB
   3. Measles, mumps, rubella (MMR), Hib, DTaP
   4. DTaP, MMR, IPV

491. A clinic nurse prepares to administer a measles, mumps, rubella (MMR) vaccine to a 5-year-old child. The nurse administers this vaccine by which best route and in which best site?
   1. Intramuscularly in the deltoid muscle
   2. Subcutaneously in the gluteal muscle
   3. Subcutaneously in the outer aspect of the upper arm
   4. Intramuscularly in the anterolateral aspect of the thigh

Alternate Item Format: Multiple Response

492. A clinic nurse is assessing a child who is scheduled to receive a live virus vaccine (immunization). Which of the following are general

contraindications associated with receiving a live virus vaccine? **Select all that apply**.
- ❑ 1. The child has symptoms of a cold.
- ❑ 2. The child had a previous anaphylactic reaction to the vaccine.
- ❑ 3. Mother reports that the child is having intermittent episodes of diarrhea.
- ❑ 4. Mother reports that the child has not had an appetite and has been fussy.
- ❑ 5. The child has a disorder that caused a severely deficient immune system.
- ❑ 6. Mother reports that the child has recently been exposed to an infectious disease.

ANSWERS

484. 4

Rationale: Pertussis is transmitted by direct contact or respiratory droplets from coughing. The communicable period occurs primarily during the catarrhal stage. Respiratory precautions are not required during the convalescent phase. Options 1, 2, and 3 are accurate components of home care instructions.

Test-Taking Strategy: Use the process of elimination and note the strategic word *convalescent* in the question. Also, note the words *need for further instructions*. These words indicate a negative event query and ask you to select an option that is an incorrect statement. Options 1 and 3 can be eliminated because they are generally associated with convalescence. Knowing that 2 weeks of respiratory precautions is not required during the convalescent period will direct you to option 4 from the remaining options. If you had difficulty with this question, review home care instructions for a child with pertussis.

Level of Cognitive Ability: Evaluating
Client Needs: Health Promotion and Maintenance
Integrated Process: Teaching and Learning
Content Area: Child Health—Integumentary/AIDS/Infectious Diseases
Reference: Hockenberry, M., & Wilson, D. (2009). *Wong's essentials of pediatric nursing* (8th ed., p. 460). St. Louis: Mosby.

485. 4

Rationale: Occasionally, tenderness, redness, or swelling may occur at the site of the DTaP injection. This can be relieved with cool packs for the first 24 hours, followed by warm or cold compresses if the inflammation persists. Bringing the infant back to the clinic is unnecessary. Option 1 may be an appropriate intervention, but is not specific to the subject of the question. Hot packs are not applied and can be harmful and cause burning of the skin.

Test-Taking Strategy: Use the process of elimination. Option 1 can be eliminated first because it does not relate specifically to the subject of the question. Eliminate option 2 next as an unnecessary intervention. From the remaining options, general principles related to the effects of heat and cold will direct you to option 4. Also noting the word *hot* in option 3 will assist in eliminating this option. Review interventions for redness and swelling at the site of a vaccine injection if you had difficulty with this question.

Level of Cognitive Ability: Applying
Client Needs: Physiological Integrity
Integrated Process: Nursing Process—Implementation

Content Area: Child Health—Integumentary/AIDS/Infectious Diseases
Reference: McKinney, E., James, S., Murray, S., & Ashwill, J. (2009). *Maternal-child nursing* (3rd ed., p. 70). St. Louis: Saunders.

486. 3

Rationale: Inactivated poliovirus vaccine (IPV) contains neomycin. A history of an anaphylactic reaction to neomycin is considered a contraindication to IPV. The presence of a minor illness such as the common cold is not a contraindication. In addition, a history of frequent respiratory infections is not a contraindication to receiving a vaccine. A local reaction to an immunization is not a contraindication to receiving a vaccine.

Test-Taking Strategy: Use the process of elimination. Recalling that a general contraindication to all immunizations is a severe illness (not a mild illness) will assist you in eliminating options 1 and 2. From the remaining options, note that option 4 identifies a local reaction. This will direct you to option 3, the systemic reaction and a potential life-threatening condition. Review the contraindications to receiving immunizations if you had difficulty with this question.

Level of Cognitive Ability: Analyzing
Client Needs: Physiological Integrity
Integrated Process: Nursing Process—Analysis
Content Area: Child Health—Integumentary/AIDS/Infectious Diseases
Reference: McKinney, E., James, S., Murray, S., & Ashwill, J. (2009). *Maternal-child nursing* (3rd ed., p. 68). St. Louis: Saunders.

487. 4

Rationale: A contraindication to receiving the hepatitis B vaccine is a previous anaphylactic reaction to a previous dose of hepatitis B vaccine or to a component (aluminum hydroxide or yeast protein) of the vaccine. An allergy to eggs, penicillin, and sulfonamides is unrelated to the contraindication to receiving this vaccine.

Test-Taking Strategy: Use the process of elimination and knowledge regarding the contraindications associated with the administration of vaccines. Note the relationship of the words *hepatitis B vaccine* in the question and option 4. Review receiving the hepatitis B vaccine if you had difficulty with this question.

Level of Cognitive Ability: Analyzing
Client Needs: Physiological Integrity
Integrated Process: Nursing Process—Assessment
Content Area: Child Health—Integumentary/AIDS/Infectious Diseases

Reference: Centers for Disease Control and Prevention (CDC). (n.d.). *Contraindications to vaccines chart.* Available at http://www.cdc.gov/vaccines/recs/vac-admin/contraindications-vacc.htm. Retrieved January 10, 2010.

488. 3

Rationale: Rubeola is transmitted via airborne particles or direct contact with infectious droplets. Airborne droplet precautions are required, and persons in contact with the child should wear masks. The child is placed in a private room if hospitalized, and the hospital room door remains closed. Gowns and gloves are unnecessary, but standard precautions are used. Articles that are contaminated should be bagged and labeled. Special enteric precautions and protective neutropenic isolation are not indicated in rubeola.
Test-Taking Strategy: Eliminate options 1 and 4 because they are comparable or alike. Remember that rubeola is transmitted via the airborne route. This will direct you to option 3. Review the route of transmission and therapeutic management of rubeola if you had difficulty with this question.
Level of Cognitive Ability: Applying
Client Needs: Safe and Effective Care Environment
Integrated Process: Nursing Process—Planning
Content Area: Child Health—Integumentary/AIDS/Infectious Diseases
Reference: McKinney, E., James, S., Murray, S., & Ashwill, J. (2009). *Maternal-child nursing* (3rd ed., p. 1016). St. Louis: Saunders.

489. 4

Rationale: Infectious mononucleosis is caused by Epstein-Barr virus. The parents need to be instructed to notify the physician if abdominal pain, especially in the left upper quadrant, or left shoulder pain occurs because this may indicate splenic rupture. Children with enlarged spleens also are instructed to avoid contact sports until splenomegaly resolves. Bedrest is unnecessary, and children usually self-limit their activity. Respiratory precautions are not required, although transmission can occur via direct intimate contact or contact with infected blood. Fever is treated with acetaminophen (Tylenol) or ibuprofen (Motrin).
Test-Taking Strategy: Use the process of elimination and knowledge regarding the organs affected in mononucleosis. Options 1 and 2 can be eliminated first because they are unnecessary interventions in this disease. From the remaining options, recalling that splenic rupture is a concern will direct you to option 4. Review the complications associated with infectious mononucleosis if you had difficulty with this question.
Level of Cognitive Ability: Applying
Client Needs: Physiological Integrity
Integrated Process: Teaching and Learning
Content Area: Child Health—Integumentary/AIDS/Infectious Diseases
References: Hockenberry, M., & Wilson, D. (2009). *Wong's essentials of pediatric nursing* (8th ed., p. 768). St. Louis: Mosby.
McKinney, E., James, S., Murray, S., & Ashwill, J. (2009). *Maternal-child nursing* (3rd ed., p. 1025). St. Louis: Saunders.

490. 1

Rationale: Diphtheria, tetanus, acellular pertussis vaccine (DTaP), *Haemophilus influenzae* type b conjugate vaccine (Hib), inactivated poliovirus vaccine (IPV), pneumococcal vaccine (PCV), and rotavirus vaccine (RV) are administered at 4 months of age. DTaP is administered at 2, 4, and 6 months of age; at 15 to 18 months of age; and at 4 to 6 years of age. Hib is administered at 2, 4, and 6 months of age and at 12 to 15 months of age. IPV is administered at 2, 4, and 6 months of age and at 4 to 6 years of age. PCV is administered at 2, 4, and 6 months of age and at 12 to 15 months of age. The first dose of measles, mumps, rubella (MMR) vaccine is administered at 12 to 15 months of age; the second dose is administered at 4 to 6 years of age (if the second dose was not given by 4 to 6 years of age, it should be given at the next visit). The first dose of hepatitis B vaccine is administered at birth, the second dose is administered at 1 month of age, and the third dose is administered at 6 months of age. Varicella-zoster vaccine is administered at 12 to 15 months of age and again at 4 to 6 years of age.
Test-Taking Strategy: Knowledge regarding the immunization schedule for infants and children is required to answer this question. Noting the age of the infant in the question will assist in directing you to option 1. If you are unfamiliar with the immunization schedule for children and adolescents, review this schedule.
Level of Cognitive Ability: Applying
Client Needs: Health Promotion and Maintenance
Integrated Process: Nursing Process—Implementation
Content Area: Child Health—Integumentary/AIDS/Infectious Diseases
References: Centers for Disease Control and Prevention (CDC). (2010). *Recommended immunization schedules for persons aged 0 through 18 years—United States, 2010.* Available at http://www.immunize.org/CDC/schedules/. Retrieved January 12, 2010.
McKinney, E., James, S., Murray, S., & Ashwill, J. (2009). *Maternal-child nursing* (3rd ed., p. 69). St. Louis: Saunders.

491. 3

Rationale: Measles, mumps, rubella (MMR) vaccine is administered subcutaneously in the outer aspect of the upper arm. The gluteal muscle is not recommended for injections. MMR vaccine is not administered by the intramuscular route.
Test-Taking Strategy: Use the process of elimination. Recalling that MMR vaccine is administered subcutaneously will assist you in eliminating options 1 and 4. From the remaining options, recalling that the gluteal muscle is not used for injections will assist in directing you to option 3. Review the procedures related to the administration of MMR vaccine if you had difficulty with this question.
Level of Cognitive Ability: Applying
Client Needs: Physiological Integrity
Integrated Process: Nursing Process—Implementation
Content Area: Child Health—Integumentary/AIDS/Infectious Diseases
References: Hockenberry, M., & Wilson, D. (2009). *Wong's essentials of pediatric nursing* (8th ed., p. 364). St. Louis: Mosby.
McKinney, E., James, S., Murray, S., & Ashwill, J. (2009). *Maternal-child nursing* (3rd ed., p. 70). St. Louis: Saunders.

ALTERNATE ITEM FORMAT: MULTIPLE RESPONSE

492. 2, 5

Rationale: The general contraindications for receiving live virus vaccines include a previous anaphylactic reaction to a vaccine or a component of a vaccine. Additionally, live virus vaccines generally are not administered to individuals with a severely deficient immune system, individuals with a severe sensitivity to gelatin, or pregnant women. A vaccine is administered with caution to an individual with a moderate or severe acute illness, with or without fever. Options 1, 3, 4, and 6 are not contraindications to receiving a vaccine.

Test-Taking Strategy: Note the strategic word *contraindications*. This word indicates that you need to select the situations in which a live virus vaccine cannot be given because doing so can cause harm to the child. Noting the word *anaphylactic* in option 2 and the words *severely deficient* in option 5 will direct you to these options. Review the contraindications to receiving a live virus vaccine if you had difficulty with this question.

Level of Cognitive Ability: Analyzing

Client Needs: Physiological Integrity

Integrated Process: Nursing Process—Assessment

Content Area: Child Health—Integumentary/AIDS/Infectious Diseases

References: Centers for Disease Control and Prevention (CDC). (n.d.). *Contraindications to vaccines chart.* Available at http://www.cdc.gov/vaccines/recs/vac-admin/contraindications-vacc.htm. Retrieved January 10, 2010.

McKinney, E., James, S., Murray, S., & Ashwill, J. (2009). *Maternal-child nursing* (3rd ed., pp. 68, 70). St. Louis: Saunders.

49

Pediatric Medication Administration and Calculations

I. ORAL MEDICATIONS

A. Most oral pediatric medications are in liquid or suspension form because children usually are unable to swallow a tablet.

B. Solutions may be measured by using an oral plastic syringe or other acceptable measurement or administration device; the device used depends on the developmental level of the child (Fig. 49-1).

C. Medications in suspension settle to the bottom of the bottle between uses, and thorough mixing is required before pouring the medication.

D. Suspensions must be administered immediately after measurement to prevent settling and resultant administration of an incomplete dose.

E. Administer oral medications with a child sitting in an upright position and with the head elevated to prevent aspiration if the child cries or resists.

F. Never pinch an infant or child's nostrils when administering medication.

G. If a medication is known to have an unpleasant taste, draw the required dose into a small syringe, and place the syringe into the side and toward the back of an infant's mouth; administer the medication slowly, allowing the infant to swallow.

H. Place a small child sideways on the lap; the child's closest arm should be placed under the adult's arm and behind the adult's back; cradle the child's head and hold the child's hand, and administer the medication slowly with a plastic spoon, small plastic cup, or syringe.

I. If a tablet or capsule has been administered, check the child's mouth to ensure that it has been swallowed; if swallowing is a problem, some tablets can be crushed and given in small amounts of puréed food or flavored syrup (enteric-coated tablets, timed-release tablets, and capsules should not be crushed).

J. Follow generally accepted medication administration guidelines for children (Box 49-1).

⚠ Newborns and infants have an immature liver and immature kidneys, so metabolism and elimination of medications is delayed.

II. PARENTERAL MEDICATIONS

A. Subcutaneously and intramuscularly administered medications
1. Medications most often given via the subcutaneous route are insulin and some immunizations.
2. Any site with sufficient subcutaneous tissue may be used for subcutaneous injections; common sites include the center third of the lateral aspect of the upper arm, the abdomen, and the center third of the anterior thigh.
3. The safe use of injection sites is based on normal muscle development and the size of the child; the preferred site for intramuscular injections in infants is the vastus lateralis, but agency policies and procedures need to be followed (Table 49-1 and Fig. 49-2).
4. The usual needle length and gauge for pediatric clients are ½ to 1 inch and 22 to 25 gauge; needle length also can be estimated by grasping the muscle between the thumb and forefinger—half the resulting distance would be the needle length.

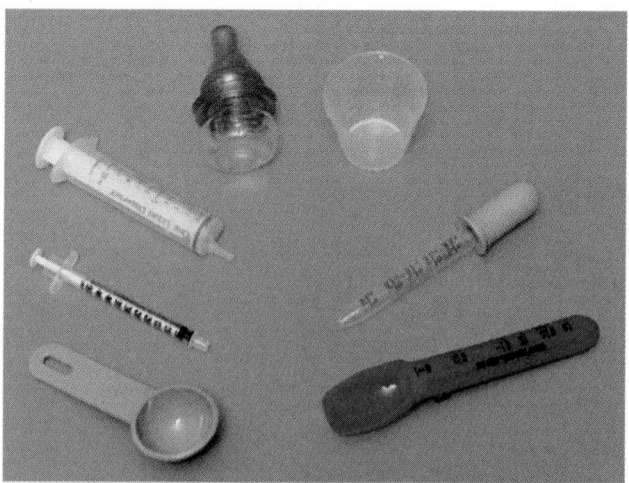

▲ FIGURE 49-1 Acceptable devices for measuring and administering oral medication to children (*clockwise from bottom left*): measuring spoon, plastic syringes, calibrated nipple, plastic medicine cup, calibrated dropper, hollow-handled medicine spoon. (From Hockenberry, M., Wilson, D., & Winkelstein, M. [2005]. *Wong's essentials of pediatric nursing* [7th ed.]. St. Louis: Mosby.)

5. Pediatric dosages for subcutaneous and intramuscular administration are calculated to the nearest hundredth and measured by using a tuberculin syringe; always follow agency guidelines.
6. Place an adhesive bandage or decorated Band-Aid over the puncture site to help the child view the experience in a pleasant way.

B. Intravenously administered medications
1. Intravenous (IV) medications are diluted for administration.

> ## Box 49-1 Medication Administration Guidelines for Children
>
> Two identifiers are required before medication administration—such as name, medical record number, birth date.
> Obtain information from parents about successful methods for administering medications to their children.
> Ask parents about any known allergies.
> To avoid aspiration, liquid forms of medication are safer to swallow than other forms.
> Straws often help older children swallow pills.
> Avoid putting medications in foods such as milk, cereal, or baby food because it may cause an unpleasant taste to the food, and the child may refuse to accept the same food in the future. Additionally, the child may not consume the entire serving and would not receive the required medication dosage.
> If the taste of the medication is unpleasant, have the child pinch the nose and drink the medication through a straw.
> Offer juice, a soft drink, or a frozen juice bar after the child swallows a medication.
> Always read the pharmacological indications for administration. Some items such as fruit syrups can be acidic and should not be used with medications that react negatively in an acid medium.
> Record the most successful method of administering medications and pertinent nursing prescriptions on the child's care plan for other nursing staff to follow; this notation also saves the child frustration, fear, and anxiety.

Modified from Potter, P., & Perry, A. (2009). *Fundamentals of nursing* (7th ed., p. 715). St. Louis: Mosby; and Perry, S., Hockenberry, M., Lowdermilk, D., & Wilson, D. (2010). *Maternal-child nursing care* (4th ed., p. 1274). St. Louis: Mosby.

2. When an infant or child is receiving an IV medication, the IV site needs to be assessed for signs of inflammation and infiltration or extravasation immediately before, during, and after completion of each medication.
3. IV medication may be administered continuously by adding the medication to an IV solution bag and infusing it through a primary infusion line.
4. IV medications may be administered intermittently; several doses may be administered in a 24-hour period.
5. Medications for IV administration are diluted according to the directions accompanying the medication and according to the physician's prescriptions and agency procedures.
6. Infusion time for IV medications is determined based on the directions accompanying the medication, the physician's prescription, and agency procedures.
7. Determine agency procedures related to the volume of flush for peripheral IV lines and for central lines.
8. The flush volume (3 to 20 mL) must be included in the child's intake; the flush is usually

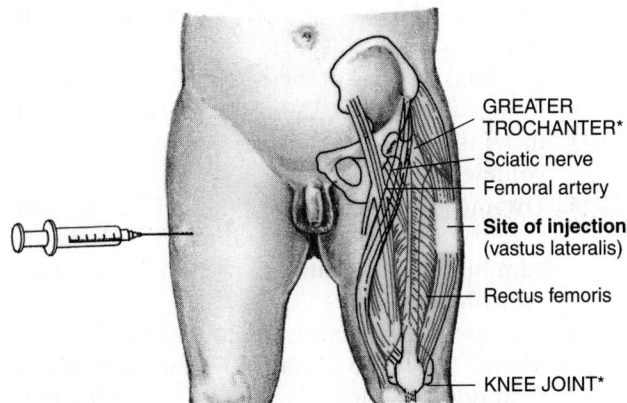

▲ **FIGURE 49-2** Intramuscular injection site—vastus lateralis. Landmarks are indicated by asterisks. (From Hockenberry, M., Wilson, D., & Winkelstein, M. [2009]. *Wong's essentials of pediatric nursing* [8th ed.]. St. Louis: Mosby.)

TABLE 49-1 Intramuscular Injections: Amount of Medication (mL) by Muscle Group

Muscle	Neonate	Infant (1-12 mo old)	Toddler (1-2 yr old)	Preschool to Child (3-12 yr old)	Adolescent (12-18 yr old)
Vastus lateralis	0.5	0.5-1	0.5-2	2	2
Rectus femoris	Not safe	Not safe	0.5-1	2	2
Ventrogluteal	Not safe	Not safe	Not safe	0.5-3	2-3
Dorsal gluteal	Not safe	Not safe	Not safe	0.5-2	2-3
Deltoid	Not safe	Not safe	0.5-1	0.5-1	1-1.5

Modified from Kee, J., & Marshall, S. (2009). *Clinical calculations: With applications to general and specialty areas* (6th ed., p. 261). St. Louis: Saunders.

administered before administering an IV medication and after the IV medication is completed and is infused at the same rate as the medication.

C. Intermittent IV medication administration
1. Children receiving IV medications intermittently may or may not have a primary IV solution infusing.
2. If a primary IV solution is infusing, the medication may be administered by IV piggyback via a secondary line.
3. If a primary IV solution does not exist, an indwelling infusion catheter is used for medication administration, and the medication may be administered by push, piggyback, or retrograde method; medication administration instructions must be checked for dilution and infusion time procedures.
4. All intermittent medication administrations are preceded and followed by a flush to ensure that the medication has cleared the IV tubing and that the total dose has been administered.
5. Electronic devices such as controllers or pumps are used to regulate and administer IV fluids and intermittent IV medications.

D. Special IV administration sets
1. Special IV administration sets, such as a burette, may be used for medication preparation and administration via piggyback.
2. These special sets are all microdrip sets calibrated to deliver 60 gtt/mL.
3. The total capacity of these special IV administration sets is 100 to 150 mL, calibrated in 1-mL increments so that exact measurements of small volumes are possible.
4. The medication is mixed with the appropriate amount of diluent, added to the special IV administration set, and allowed to infuse at the prescribed rate.
5. The special IV administration set needs to be labeled clearly to identify the medication and fluid dosage added.
6. During medication infusion time, a label is attached that indicates that the medication is infusing.
7. During the flush infusion time, a label is attached indicating that the flush is infusing.

E. Retrograde IV injection
1. In this method of administration, the medication is mixed with the appropriate amount of diluent in a syringe.
2. The IV tubing is clamped close to the child, the medication is injected through the port in the direction of the burette, the tubing is unclamped, the prescribed rate is set, and the medication is allowed to infuse over the prescribed time.

F. Syringe pump for IV medication administration
1. A syringe containing the medication is fitted into a pump that is connected to the IV tubing through a Y connector.

2. The medication is administered over the prescribed time.

⚠ The 24-hour fluid intake must be monitored closely, and all IV fluid amounts including the amount of flush volume need to be documented accurately to prevent overhydration. For children, the maximum amount of IV fluid administered in a 24-hour period varies and is usually based on body weight and other factors. Check the physician's prescription and agency guidelines for the procedures for the administration of IV fluids and medications.

III. CALCULATION OF MEDICATION DOSAGE BY BODY WEIGHT

A. Conversion of body weight (Box 49-2)
B. Calculation of daily dosages
1. Abbreviations (Box 49-3)
2. Dosages are expressed in terms of milligrams per kilogram per day, milligrams per pound per day, or milligrams per kilogram per dose.
3. The total daily dosage usually is administered in divided (more than one) doses per day.
4. Express the child's body weight in kilograms or pounds to correlate with the dosage specifications.
5. Calculate the total daily dosage.
6. Divide the total daily dosage by the number of doses to be administered in 1 day.

Box 49-2 Conversion of Body Weight

Measurements
1 lb = 16 oz
1 kg = 2.2 lb

Pounds to Kilograms
1 kg = 2.2 lb
When converting from pounds to kilograms, divide by 2.2. Kilograms are expressed to the nearest tenth.

Kilograms to Pounds
1 kg = 2.2 lb
When converting from kilograms to pounds, multiply by 2.2. Pounds are expressed to the nearest tenth.

Box 49-3 Abbreviations

BSA	body surface area
g	gram(s)
gr	grain(s)
kg	kilogram(s)
lb	pound(s)
m^2	square meters
mcg	microgram(s)
mg	milligram(s)
mL	milliliter(s)
SA	surface area

IV. CALCULATION OF BODY SURFACE AREA (BSA)

A. The BSA is determined by comparing body weight and height with averages or norms on a graph called a nomogram.

B. Not all children are the same size at the same age; the nomogram is used to determine the BSA of a child.

C. Look at the nomogram (Fig. 49-3), and note that the height is on the left-hand side of the chart and the weight is on the right-hand side of the chart.

D. Place a ruler across the chart.

E. Line up the left side of the ruler on the height and the right side of the ruler on the weight; read the BSA at the point where the straight edge of the ruler intersects the surface area (SA) column.

F. The estimated SA is given in square meters (m^2).

G. Box 49-4 gives a sample practice question using the nomogram.

V. CALCULATION BASED ON BSA

A. When dosage recommendations for children specify milligrams, micrograms, or units per square meter, calculating the dosage is simple multiplication (Box 49-5).

B. When dosage recommendations are specified only for adults, a formula is used to calculate a child's dosage from the adult dosage (Box 49-6).

Box 49-4 How to Use the Nomogram

Example: Use the nomogram (see Fig. 49-3) and calculate the body surface area (BSA) for a child whose height is 58 inches and weight is 12 kg.

Look at the nomogram chart and note that the height is on the left-hand side of the chart and the weight is on the right-hand side.

Place a ruler on the chart and line up the left side of the ruler on the height and the right side of the ruler on the weight; read the BSA at the point where the straight edge of the ruler intersects the surface area (SA) column.

The estimated SA is given in square meters.

Answer: 0.66 m^2

Box 49-5 Calculating Medication Dosage

When dosage recommendations for children specify milligrams, micrograms, or units per square meter, calculating the dosage is simple multiplication.

Example: The dosage recommendation is 4 mg/m^2. The child has a body surface area of 1.1 m^2. What is the dosage to be administered?

Answer: 1.1 × 4 mg = 4.4 mg

Box 49-6 Calculating a Child's Dosage From the Adult Dosage

When dosages are specified only for adults, a formula is used to calculate a child's dosage from the adult dosage. The adult dosage is based on a standardized body surface area (BSA) of 1.73 m^2.

Example: A physician has prescribed an antibiotic for a child. The average adult dose is 250 mg. The child has a BSA of 0.41 m^2. What is the dose for the child?

Answer: 59.24 mg

Formula:

$$\frac{\text{BSA of child (m}^2)}{1.73 \text{ m}^2} \times \text{Adult dose} = \text{Child's dose}$$

$$\frac{0.41}{1.73} \times 250 \text{ mg} = 59.24 \text{ mg}$$

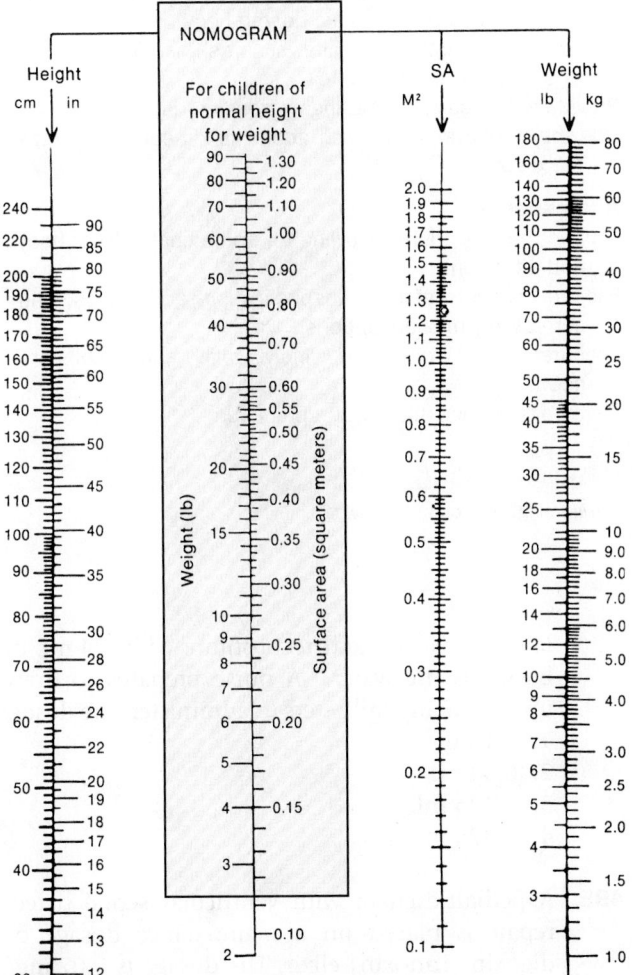

▲ FIGURE 49-3 West nomogram for estimation of surface areas in infants and children. First, find height; next, find weight; finally, draw a straight line connecting the height and weight. The body surface area (in square meters [m^2]) is indicated where a straight line connecting the height and weight intersects the surface area (SA) column or, if the child is approximately of normal proportion, from weight alone (*yellow area*). (From Hockenberry, M., Wilson, D., & Winkelstein, M. [2005]. *Wong's essentials of pediatric nursing* [7th ed.]. St. Louis: Mosby.)

VI. DEVELOPMENTAL CONSIDERATIONS FOR ADMINISTERING MEDICATIONS

A. When administering medications to children, **developmental age** must be taken into consideration to ensure safe and effective administration.

B. General interventions
   1. Always be prepared for the procedure with all necessary equipment and assistance.
   2. For a hospitalized child, ask the parent or child or both if the parent should or should not remain for the procedure.
   3. Determine appropriate preadministration and postadministration comfort measures.
   4. Try to make the event as pleasant as possible.

C. Box 49-7 lists developmental considerations when giving medications.

Box 49-7 Developmental Considerations for Administering Medications

Infants

Perform procedure quickly; then offer comfort measures, such as holding, rocking, and cuddling.

Allow self-comforting measures, such as the use of a pacifier.

Toddlers

Offer a brief, concrete explanation of the procedure and then perform it.

Accept aggressive behavior, within reasonable limits, as a healthy response, and provide outlets for the toddler.

Provide comfort measures immediately after the procedure, such as touch, holding, cuddling, and providing a favorite toy.

Preschoolers

Offer a brief, concrete explanation of the procedure and then perform it.

Accept aggressive behavior, within reasonable limits, as a healthy response, and provide outlets for the child.

Provide comfort measures after the procedure, such as touch, holding, or providing a favorite toy.

School-Age Children

Explain the procedure, allowing for some control over the body and situation.

Explore feelings and concepts through therapeutic play, drawings of own body and self in the hospital, and the use of books and realistic hospital equipment.

Set appropriate behavior limits, such as it is all right to cry or scream, but not to bite.

Provide activities for releasing aggression and anger.

Use the opportunity to teach about how medication helps the disorder.

Adolescents

Explain the procedure, allowing for some control over body and situation.

Explore concepts of self, hospitalization, and illness, and correct any misconceptions.

Encourage self-expression, individuality, and self-care needs.

Encourage participation in the procedure.

Modified from McKenry, L., and Salerno, E. (2003). *Mosby's pharmacology in nursing*. St. Louis: Mosby.

 MORE QUESTIONS ON THE CD!

Practice Questions

493. A nurse provides medication instructions to a mother. Which statement by the mother indicates a need for further instructions?
   1. "I should cuddle my child after giving the medication."
   2. "I can give my child a frozen juice bar after he swallows the medication."
   3. "I should mix the medication in the baby food and give it when I feed my child."
   4. "If my child does not like the taste of the medicine, I should encourage him to pinch his nose and drink the medication through a straw."

494. A physician's prescription reads "ampicillin sodium 125 mg IV every 6 hours." The medication label reads "1 g and reconstitute with 7.4 mL of bacteriostatic water." A nurse prepares to draw up how many milliliters to administer one dose?
   1. 1.1 mL
   2. 0.54 mL
   3. 7.425 mL
   4. 0.925 mL

495. A pediatric client with ventricular septal defect repair is placed on a maintenance dosage of digoxin (Lanoxin) elixir. The dosage is 0.07 mg/kg/day, and the client's weight is 7.2 kg. The physician orders the digoxin to be given twice daily. A nurse prepares how much digoxin to administer to the client at each dose?
   1. 0.5 mg
   2. 2.5 mg
   3. 0.25 mg
   4. 0.37 mg

496. Sulfisoxazole (Gantrisin), 1 g orally four times daily, is prescribed for an adolescent with a urinary tract infection. The medication label reads "500-mg tablets." A nurse has determined that the dosage prescribed is safe. The nurse administers how many tablets per dose to the adolescent?
1. ½ tablet
2. 1 tablet
3. 2 tablets
4. 3 tablets

497. A nurse prepares to administer an intramuscular injection to a 4-month-old infant. The nurse selects which site to administer the injection?
1. Ventrogluteal
2. Dorsal gluteal
3. Rectus femoris
4. Vastus lateralis

498. Penicillin G procaine (Wycillin), 1,000,000 units IM (intramuscularly), is prescribed for a child with an infection. The medication label reads "1,200,000 units per 2 mL." A nurse has determined that the dose prescribed is safe. The nurse administers how many milliliters per dose to the child?

1. 0.8 mL
2. 1.2 mL
3. 1.44 mL
4. 1.66 mL

Alternate Item Format: Figure and Fill-in-the-Blank

499. Atropine sulfate, 0.6 mg intramuscularly, is prescribed for a child preoperatively. A nurse has determined that the dose prescribed is safe and prepares to administer how many milliliters to the child? See figure.

_____ mL

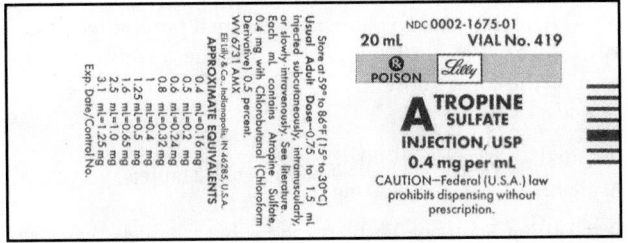

ANSWERS

493. 3

Rationale: The nurse would teach the mother to avoid putting medications in foods because it may cause an unpleasant taste to the food, and the child may refuse to accept the same food in the future. Additionally, the child may not consume the entire serving and would not receive the required medication dosage. If the taste of the medication is unpleasant, the child should pinch the nose and drink the medication through a straw. The mother should offer juice, a soft drink, or a frozen juice bar to the child after the child swallows the medication. The mother should provide comfort measures immediately after medication administration, such as touching, holding, cuddling, and providing a favorite toy.
Test-Taking Strategy: Note the strategic words *need for further instructions*. These words indicate a negative event query and the need to select the incorrect statement made by the mother. Read each statement carefully and think about the statement that may be unsafe and may not provide an accurate dose to the child. This will direct you to option 3. Review the procedures for administering medication to children if you had difficulty with this question.
Level of Cognitive Ability: Applying
Client Needs: Physiological Integrity
Integrated Process: Teaching and Learning
Content Area: Fundamental Skills—Medications/Blood & IV Therapy
Reference: Perry, S., Hockenberry, M., Lowdermilk, D., & Wilson, D. (2010). *Maternal child nursing care* (4th ed., p. 1274). St. Louis: Mosby.

494. 4

Rationale: Convert 1 g to milligrams. In the metric system, to convert larger to smaller, multiply by 1000 or move the decimal point three places to the right.
1 g = 1000 mg
Formula:

$$\frac{Desired}{Available} \times Volume = \frac{125\,mg}{1000\,mg} \times 7.4\,mL = 0.925\,mL\ per\ dose$$

Test-Taking Strategy: Focus on the subject, milliliters per dose. Convert grams to milligrams first. Next, use the formula to determine the correct dose, knowing that 1000 mg = 7.4 mL. Verify the answer using a calculator. Review the formula for calculating medication doses if you had difficulty with this question.
Level of Cognitive Ability: Applying
Client Needs: Physiological Integrity
Integrated Process: Nursing Process—Implementation
Content Area: Fundamental skills—Medications/Blood & IV Therapy
Reference: Kee, J., & Marshall, S. (2009). *Clinical calculations: With applications to general and specialty areas* (6th ed., p. 86). St. Louis: Saunders.

495. 3

Rationale: Calculate the dosage by weight first:
0.07 mg/day × 7.2 kg = 0.5 mg/day
The physician prescribes digoxin twice daily; two doses in 24 hours will be administered:

$$\frac{0.5\,mg/day}{2\,doses} = 0.25\,mg\ for\ each\ dose$$

Test-Taking Strategy: Read the question carefully, noting that the question states *twice daily* and *each dose*. Calculate the dosage per day by weight first, and then determine the milligrams per each dose. Verify the answer using a calculator. Review the formula for calculating dosage per kg of body weight if you had difficulty with this question.
Level of Cognitive Ability: Applying
Client Needs: Physiological Integrity
Integrated Process: Nursing Process—Implementation
Content Area: Fundamental Skills—Medications/Blood & IV Therapy
Reference: Kee, J., & Marshall, S. (2009). *Clinical calculations: With applications to general and specialty areas* (6th ed., p. 262). St. Louis: Saunders.

496. 3

Rationale: Change 1 g to milligrams, knowing that 1000 mg = 1 g. Also, when converting from grams to milligrams (larger to smaller), move the decimal point three places to the right: 1 g = 1000 mg. Next, use the formula for calculating the correct dose.
Formula:

$$\frac{\text{Desired}}{\text{Available}} \times \text{Tablet} = \frac{1000\,\text{mg}}{500\,\text{mg}} \times \text{Tablet} = 2\,\text{tablets}$$

Test-Taking Strategy: Focus on the subject, tablets per dose. Convert grams to milligrams first. Next, use the formula to determine the correct dose and verify the answer using a calculator. Review the formula for calculating medication doses if you had difficulty with this question.
Level of Cognitive Ability: Applying
Client Needs: Physiological Integrity
Integrated Process: Nursing Process—Implementation
Content Area: Fundamental Skills—Medications/Blood & IV Therapy
Reference: Kee, J., & Marshall, S. (2009). *Clinical calculations: With applications to general and specialty areas* (6th ed., p. 86). St. Louis: Saunders.

497. 4

Rationale: Intramuscular injection sites are selected based on the child's age and muscle development of the child. The vastus lateralis is the only safe muscle group to use for intramuscular injection in a 4-month-old infant. The sites identified in options 1, 2, and 3 are unsafe.
Test-Taking Strategy: Focus on the age of the child identified in the question and think about the physiological development of the muscle groups in an infant at 4 months of age. This will assist in directing you to option 4. Review the pediatric guidelines for administering intramuscular medications if you had difficulty with this question.

Level of Cognitive Ability: Applying
Client Needs: Physiological Integrity
Integrated Process: Nursing Process—Implementation
Content Area: Fundamental Skills—Medications/Blood & IV Therapy
Reference: Kee, J., & Marshall, S. (2009). *Clinical calculations: With applications to general and specialty areas* (6th ed., p. 261). St. Louis: Saunders.

498. 4

Rationale: Use the medication calculation formula.
Formula:

$$\frac{\text{Desired}}{\text{Available}} \times \text{Volume} = \frac{1,000,000}{1,200,000} \times 2\,\text{mL} = 1.66\,\text{mL per dose}$$

Test-Taking Strategy: Focus on the subject, milliliters per dose. Use the formula to determine the correct dose, and verify the answer using a calculator. Review the formula for calculating medication doses if you had difficulty with this question.
Level of Cognitive Ability: Applying
Client Needs: Physiological Integrity
Integrated Process: Nursing Process—Implementation
Content Area: Fundamental Skills—Medications/Blood & IV Therapy
Reference: Kee, J., & Marshall, S. (2009). *Clinical calculations: With applications to general and specialty areas* (6th ed., p. 86). St. Louis: Saunders.

ALTERNATE ITEM FORMAT: FIGURE AND FILL-IN-THE-BLANK

499. 1.5 mL

Rationale: Use the formula for calculating the medication dose.
Formula:

$$\frac{\text{Desired}}{\text{Available}} \times \text{Volume} = \frac{0.6\,\text{mg}}{0.4\,\text{mg}} \times 1\,\text{mL} = 1.5\,\text{mL}$$

Test-Taking Strategy: Focus on the subject, the milliliters to be administered. Note that the medication label indicates that there is 0.4 mg per mL. Use the formula to determine the correct dose, and verify the answer using a calculator. Review the formula for calculating medication doses if you had difficulty with this question.
Level of Cognitive Ability: Applying
Client Needs: Physiological Integrity
Integrated Process: Nursing Process—Implementation
Content Area: Fundamental Skills—Medications/Blood & IV Therapy
Reference: Kee, J., & Marshall, S. (2009). *Clinical calculations: With applications to general and specialty areas* (6th ed., p. 86, 271). St. Louis: Saunders.

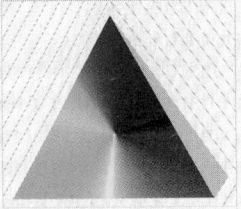

The Adult Client With an Integumentary Disorder

PYRAMID TERMS

burn Cell destruction of the layers of the skin resulting in local and systemic disruptions.

carbon monoxide poisoning Carbon monoxide is a colorless, odorless, and tasteless gas that has an affinity for hemoglobin 200 times greater than that of oxygen. Oxygen molecules are displaced, and carbon monoxide reversibly binds to hemoglobin to form carboxyhemoglobin. Tissue hypoxia occurs.

chemical burn Tissue injury caused by tissue contact with strong acids, alkalis, or organic compounds. Systemic toxicity from cutaneous absorption can occur.

deep full-thickness burn Involves injury to the muscle, bone, and tendons. Injured area appears black and eschar is hard and inelastic.

deep partial-thickness burn Injury extends into the skin dermis and the wound is red and dry, with white areas in deeper parts; can convert to a full-thickness burn if tissue damage increases with infection, hypoxia, or ischemia.

electrical burn Tissue injury caused by heat generated by electrical energy as it passes through the body; results in internal tissue damage.

full-thickness burn The injured area appears waxy white, deep red, yellow, brown, or black; injured surface appears dry. Edema is present under eschar.

herpes zoster (shingles) An acute viral infection of the nerve structure caused by varicella-zoster. Herpes zoster is contagious to individuals who never had chickenpox and have not been vaccinated against the disease.

pressure ulcer Area of tissue damage that occurs as a result of skin and underlying soft tissue compression from pressure between a surface and a bony prominence.

skin cancer A malignant lesion of the skin that may or may not metastasize. Overexposure to the sun is a primary cause. Diagnosis is confirmed by a skin biopsy that is positive for cancer cells.

smoke inhalation injury Respiratory injury that occurs when the victim is trapped in an enclosed, smoke-filled space.

superficial-thickness burn Involves injury to the epidermis. Mild to severe erythema is noted, and the skin blanches with pressure. The burn is painful.

superficial partial-thickness burn A mottled red base and broken epidermis and a wet shiny and weeping surface are present. Large blisters can be seen covering an extensive area. Skin is edematous and painful.

thermal burn Tissue injury caused by exposure to flames, hot liquids, steam, or hot objects.

PYRAMID TO SUCCESS

The Pyramid to Success focuses on the concept that the integumentary system provides the first line of defense against infections. Focus on the protective measures necessary to prevent infection, including methicillin-resistant *Staphlococcus aureus* (MRSA). Pyramid Points address the risk factors related to the development of integumentary disorders, and the preventive measures related to skin cancer. Focus on the emergency measures related to a client with a burn, fluid resuscitation, monitoring for complications, and skin grafting. Psychosocial issues relate to the body image disturbances that can occur as a result of the integumentary disorder.

CLIENT NEEDS

Safe and Effective Care Environment

Consulting with members of the health care team regarding treatments

Establishing priorities of care

Handling of hazardous and infectious materials

Instituting standard and other precautions

Maintaining confidentiality related to the disorder

Making referrals to appropriate health care providers

Obtaining informed consent for treatments and procedures

Practicing asepsis techniques and preventing infection

Health Promotion and Maintenance

Implementing disease prevention measures

Performing physical assessment techniques for the integumentary system

Promoting health screening and health promotion programs to prevent skin disorders

Providing instructions to the client regarding prevention measures and care of integumentary disorder

Psychosocial Integrity

Addressing end-of-life issues

Discussing unexpected body image changes

Identifying coping mechanisms

Identifying situational role changes

Using support systems

Physiological Integrity

Assessing for alterations in body systems

Providing adequate nutrition for healing

Providing basic care and comfort

Providing emergency care

Monitoring for expected effects of treatments

Monitoring for fluid and electrolyte imbalances and other complications

Monitoring laboratory values

50

Integumentary System

I. ANATOMY AND PHYSIOLOGY

A. The skin is the largest sensory organ of the body, with a surface area of 15 to 20 square feet and a weight of about 9 lb.

B. Functions
   1. Acts as the first line of defense against infections
   2. Protects underlying tissues and organs from injury
   3. Receives stimuli from the external environment; detects touch, pressure, pain, and temperature stimuli; relays information to the nervous system
   4. Maintains normal body temperature
   5. Excretes salts, water, and organic wastes
   6. Protects the body from excessive water loss
   7. Synthesizes vitamin D_3, which converts to calcitriol, for normal calcium metabolism
   8. Stores nutrients

C. Layers
   1. Epidermis
   2. Dermis
   3. Subcutaneous fat (adipose tissue)

D. Epidermal appendages
   1. Nails
   2. Hair
   3. Glands
      a. Sebaceous
      b. Sweat

E. Normal bacterial flora
   1. Types of normal bacterial flora include the following:
      a. Gram-positive and gram-negative staphylococci
      b. *Pseudomonas* sp.
      c. *Streptococcus* sp.
   2. Organisms are shed with normal exfoliation.
   3. A pH of 4.2 to 5.6 halts the growth of bacteria.

II. RISK FACTORS FOR INTEGUMENTARY DISORDERS

A. Exposure to chemical and environmental pollutants
B. Exposure to radiation
C. Race and age
D. Exposure to the sun or use of indoor tanning
E. Lack of personal hygiene habits
F. Use of harsh soaps or other harsh products

G. Some medications, such as long-term glucocorticoid use or herbal preparations
H. Nutritional deficiencies
I. Moderate to severe emotional stress
J. Infection, with injured areas as the potential entry points for infection
K. Repeated injury and irritation
L. Changes associated with developmental stages and aging
M. Inherited genetic mutations
N. Systemic illnesses

III. PSYCHOSOCIAL IMPACT

A. Change in body image, decreased general well-being, and decreased self-esteem
B. Social isolation and fear of rejection (because of embarrassment about changes in skin appearance)
C. Restrictions in physical activity
D. Pain
E. Disruption or loss of employment
F. Cost of medications, hospitalizations, and follow-up care including dressing supplies

IV. PHASES OF WOUND HEALING

A. Phases
   1. Inflammatory: Begins at the time of injury and lasts 3 to 5 days; manifestations include local edema, pain, redness, and warmth.
   2. Fibroblastic: Begins the 4th day after injury and lasts 2 to 4 weeks; scar tissue forms and granulation tissue forms in the tissue bed.
   3. Maturation: begins as early as 3 weeks after the injury and may last for 1 year; scar tissue becomes thinner and is firm and inelastic on palpation.

B. Healing by intention
   1. First intention: Wound edges are approximated and held in place (i.e., with sutures) until healing occurs; wound is easily closed and dead space is eliminated.
   2. Second intention: This type of healing occurs with injuries or wounds that have tissue loss and require gradual filling in of the dead space with connective tissue.

3. Third intention: This type of healing involves delayed primary closure and occurs with wounds that are intentionally left open for several days for irrigation or removal of debris and exudates; once debris has been removed and inflammation resolves, the wound is closed by first intention.

V. SKIN ASSESSMENT

A. Skin assessment techniques: Refer to Chapter 34 for assessment of the integumentary system and Chapter 35 for skin changes that occur with the aging process.

B. Dark-skinned client
   1. Cyanosis: Check lips and tongue for a gray color; nail beds, palms, and soles for a blue color; and conjunctiva for pallor.
   2. Jaundice: Check oral mucous membranes for a yellow color; check the sclera nearest to the iris for a yellow color.
   3. Bleeding: Look for skin swelling and darkening and compare the affected side with the unaffected side.
   4. Inflammation: check for warmth, a shiny or taut and pitting skin area, and compare with the unaffected side.

VI. DIAGNOSTIC TESTS

A. Skin biopsy
   1. Description
      a. Skin biopsy is the collection of a small piece of skin tissue for histopathological study.
      b. Methods include punch, excisional, and shave.
   2. Preprocedure interventions
      a. Obtain informed consent.
      b. Cleanse site as prescribed.
   3. Postprocedure interventions
      a. Place specimen when obtained by the physician in the appropriate container and send to pathology laboratory for analysis.
      b. Use surgically aseptic technique for biopsy site dressings.
      c. Assess the biopsy site for bleeding and infection.
      d. Instruct the client to keep dressing in place for at least 8 hours, and then clean daily and use antibiotic ointment as prescribed (sutures are usually removed in 7 to 10 days).
      e. Instruct the client to report signs of excessive drainage or redness or other signs of infection.

B. Skin cultures
   1. A small skin culture sample is obtained using a sterile applicator and the appropriate type of culture tube (e.g., bacterial or viral).
   2. Viral culture is placed immediately on ice.
   3. Sample is sent to laboratory to identify an existing organism.

⚠ Obtain skin culture samples or any other type of culture specimens before instituting antibiotic therapy.

C. Wood's light examination
   1. Description: Skin is viewed under ultraviolet light through a special glass (Wood's glass) to identify superficial infections of the skin.
   2. Preprocedure intervention: Darken the room before the examination.
   3. Postprocedure intervention: Assist the client during adjustment from the darkened room.

D. Diascopy
   1. Technique allows clearer inspection of lesions by eliminating the erythema caused by increased blood flow to the area.
   2. A glass slide is pressed over the lesion, causing blanching and revealing the lesion more clearly.

VII. *CANDIDA ALBICANS*

A. Description
   1. A superficial fungal infection of the skin and mucous membranes
   2. Also known as a yeast infection, or *thrush* when it occurs in the mouth
   3. Risk factors include immunosuppression, such as clients with acquired immunodeficiency syndrome; cancer clients receiving chemotherapy; clients on long-term antibiotic therapy; clients with diabetes mellitus; and obese clients.
   4. Common areas of occurrence include the mucous membranes of the mouth, perineum, vagina, axilla, and under the breasts.

B. Assessment
   1. Skin: Red and irritated appearance that itches and **burns**.
   2. Mucous membranes of the mouth: Red and whitish patches.

C. Interventions
   1. Teach the client to keep skin fold areas clean and dry.
   2. For the hospitalized client, inspect skin fold areas frequently, turn and reposition the client frequently, and keep the skin and bed linens clean and dry.
   3. Provide frequent mouth care as prescribed and avoid irritating products.
   4. Provide food and fluids that are tepid in temperature and nonirritating to mucous membranes.
   5. Antifungal medications may be prescribed.

VIII. HERPES ZOSTER (SHINGLES)

A. Description
   1. With a history of chickenpox, **shingles** is caused by the reactivation of the varicella-zoster virus; **shingles** can occur during any immunocompromised state in a client with a history of chickenpox.

2. The dormant virus is located in the dorsal nerve root ganglion of the sensory cranial and spinal nerves.
3. **Herpes zoster** eruptions occur in a segmental distribution on the skin area along the infected nerve and show up after several days of discomfort in the area.
4. Diagnosis is determined by visual examination, and by Tzanck smear and viral culture that identify the organism.
5. Postherpetic neuralgia (severe pain) can remain after the lesions resolve.
6. Herpes zoster is contagious to individuals who never had chickenpox and who have not been vaccinated against the disease.
7. Herpes simplex virus is another type of virus; type 1 infection causes a cold sore (usually on the lip) and type 2 causes genital herpes (both types are contagious).

B. Assessment: **Herpes zoster**
1. Unilaterally clustered skin vesicles along peripheral sensory nerves on the trunk, thorax, or face
2. Fever, malaise
3. Burning and pain
4. Pruritus
5. Paresthesia

C. Interventions
1. Isolate the client because exudate from the lesions contains the virus (maintain standard and other precautions as appropriate, such as contact precautions).
2. Assess for signs and symptoms of infection, including skin infections and eye infections; skin necrosis can also occur.
3. Assess neurovascular status and seventh cranial nerve function; Bell's palsy is a complication.
4. Use an air mattress and bed cradle on the client's bed if hospitalized, and keep the environment cool; warmth and touch aggravate the pain.
5. Prevent the client from scratching and rubbing the affected area.
6. Instruct the client to wear lightweight, loose cotton clothing and to avoid wool and synthetic clothing.
7. Teach the client about the prescribed therapies; astringent compresses may be prescribed to relieve irritation and pain and to promote crust formation and healing.
8. Teach the client about measures to keep the skin clean to prevent infection.
9. Teach the client about topical treatment or antiviral medications if prescribed.
10. Vaccination for **shingles** is recommended for adults 60 years of age and older to reduce the risk of occurrence and the associated long-term pain.
11. Antiviral medications may include acyclovir (Zovirax), valacyclovir (Valtrex), or famciclovir (Famvir); refer to Chapter 71 for information on antiviral medications.

IX. METHICILLIN-RESISTANT *STAPHYLOCOCCUS AUREUS* **(MRSA)**

A. Description
1. Skin or wound becomes infected with methicillin-resistant *Staphylococcus aureus* (MRSA).
2. Infection can range from mild to severe and can present as folliculitis or furuncles.
3. Folliculitis is a superficial infection of the follicle caused by *Staphylococcus* and presents as a raised red rash and pustules; furuncles are also caused by *Staphylococcus* and occur deep in the follicle, presenting as very painful large raised bumps that may or may not have a pustule.
4. If MRSA infects the blood, sepsis, organ damage, and death can occur.

MRSA is contagious and is spread to others by direct contact with infected skin or infected articles; for the client with MRSA, the infection can also be spread to other parts of the body.

B. Assessment: A culture and sensitivity test of the skin or wound confirms the presence of MRSA and leads to choice of appropriate antibiotic therapy.
C. Interventions
1. Maintain standard precautions and contact or isolation precautions as appropriate to prevent spread of infection to others.
2. Monitor the client closely for signs of further infection or worsening of the condition, which could indicate organ damage.
3. Administer antibiotic therapy as prescribed.
4. For additional information on MRSA, refer to Chapter 48.

X. ERYSIPELAS AND CELLULITIS

A. Description
1. Erysipelas is an acute, superficial, rapidly spreading inflammation of the dermis and lymphatics caused by *Streptococcus* group A, which enters the tissue via an abrasion, bite, trauma, or wound.
2. Cellulitis is a skin infection into the deeper dermis and subcutaneous fat; the causative organism is usually *Streptococcus pyogenes*.
B. Assessment
1. Pain
2. Itching
3. Swelling
4. Redness and warmth
C. Interventions
1. Promote rest of the affected area.
2. Apply warm compresses as prescribed to promote circulation and to decrease discomfort, erythema, and edema.
3. Clean the skin with an antibacterial type of soap as prescribed.

4. Administer antibiotics as prescribed for an infection; obtain a culture of the area before initiating the antibiotics.

XI. POISON IVY, POISON OAK, AND POISON SUMAC

A. Description: A dermatitis that develops from contact with urushiol from poison ivy, oak, or sumac plants

B. Assessment
1. Papulovesicular lesions
2. Severe itching

C. Interventions
1. Cleanse the skin of the plant oils immediately.
2. Apply cool, wet compresses to relieve the itching.
3. Apply topical products to relieve the itching and discomfort.
4. Topical or oral glucocorticoids may be prescribed for severe reactions.

XII. BITES AND STINGS

A. Spider bites
1. Almost all types of spider bites are venomous and most are not harmful, but bites or stings from brown recluse spiders, black widow spiders, tarantulas, scorpions, bees, and wasps can produce toxic reactions in humans.
2. Brown recluse spider
   a. Bite can cause a skin lesion, a necrotic wound, or systemic effects from the toxin (loxoscelism).
   b. Application of ice to decrease enzyme activity of the venom and limit tissue necrosis should be done immediately and intermittently for up to 4 days after the bite.
   c. Topical antiseptics and antibiotics may be necessary if the site becomes infected.
3. Black widow spider
   a. Bite causes a small red papule.
   b. Venom causes neurotoxicity.
   c. Ice is applied immediately to inhibit the action of the neurotoxin.
   d. Systemic toxicity can occur and the victim may require supportive therapy in the hospital.
4. Tarantulas
   a. Bite causes swelling, redness, numbness, lymph inflammation, and pain at the bite site.
   b. The tarantula launches its barbed hairs, which penetrate the skin and eyes of the victim, producing a severe inflammatory reaction.
   c. Tarantula hairs are removed as soon as possible using sticky tape to pull hairs from the skin, and the skin is thoroughly irrigated; saline irrigations are done for eye exposure.
   d. The involved extremity is elevated and immobilized to reduce pain and swelling.

e. Antihistamines and topical or systemic corticosteroids may be prescribed; tetanus prophylaxis is necessary.

B. Scorpion stings
1. Scorpions inject venom into the victim through a stinging apparatus on their tail.
2. Most stings cause local pain, inflammation, and mild systemic reactions that are treated with analgesics, wound care, and supportive treatment.
3. The bark scorpion can inflict a severe and fatal systemic response; the venom is neurotoxic; the victim is taken to the emergency department immediately (an antivenom is administered for bark scorpion bites).

C. Bees and wasps
1. Stings usually cause a wheal and flare reaction.
2. Emergency care involves quick removal of the stinger and application of an ice pack.
3. The stinger is removed by gently scraping or brushing it off with the edge of a needle or similar object; tweezers are not used because there is a risk of pinching the venom sac.
4. If the victim is allergic to the venom of a bee or wasp, a severe allergic response can occur (hives, pruritus, swelling of the lips and tongue) that can progress to life-threatening anaphylaxis; immediate emergency care is required.
5. Individuals who are allergic should carry an EpiPen for self-administration of intramuscular epinephrine if a bee or wasp sting occurs.

D. Snake bites
1. Some snakes are venomous and can cause a serious systemic reaction in the victim.
2. The victim should be immediately moved to a safe area away from the snake and should rest to decrease venom circulation; the extremity is immobilized and kept below the level of the heart.
3. Constricting clothing and jewelry are removed before swelling occurs.
4. The victim is kept warm and is not allowed to consume caffeinated or alcoholic beverages, which may speed absorption of the venom.
5. If transport to the emergency department is not done immediately, a constricting band may be applied proximal to the wound to slow the venom circulation; monitor the circulation frequently and loosen the band if edema occurs.
6. The wound is not incised or sucked to remove the venom; ice is not applied to the wound.
7. Emergency care in a hospital is required as soon as possible; an antivenom may be administered along with supportive care.

⚠ For spider bites, scorpion bites, or other stings or bites, the Poison Control Center should be contacted as soon as possible to determine the best initial management.

XIII. FROSTBITE

A. Description
1. Frostbite is damage to tissues and blood vessels as a result of prolonged exposure to cold.
2. Fingers, toes, face, nose, and ears often are affected.

B. Assessment
1. First-degree: Involves hyperemia and edema formation of the involved area
2. Second-degree: Large fluid-filled blisters with partial-thickness skin necrosis
3. Third-degree: Involves the formation of small blisters that contain dark fluid and an affected body part that is cool, numb, blue, or red and does not blanch; full-thickness and subcutaneous tissue necrosis require debridement.
4. Fourth-degree: No blisters or edema noted and the part is numb, cold, and bloodless; full-thickness necrosis extends into muscle and bone and gangrene develops, which may require amputation of the affected part.

C. Interventions
1. Rewarm the affected part rapidly and continuously with a warm water bath to thaw the frozen part (hot towels may be used if a warming tub is not available).
2. Handle the part gently and immobilize and elevate the part above heart level.
3. Avoid using dry heat, and never rub or massage the part, which may result in further tissue damage.
4. Rewarming process may be painful; analgesics may be necessary.
5. Avoid compression of the injured tissues and apply only loose and nonadherent sterile dressings.
6. Monitor for signs of compartment syndrome.
7. Tetanus prophylaxis is necessary, and topical and systemic antibiotics may be prescribed.
8. Debridement of necrotic tissue may be necessary; amputation may be necessary in those in whom gangrene develops.

XIV. ACTINIC KERATOSES

A. Actinic keratoses are caused by chronic exposure to the sun and appear as rough, scaly, red, or brown lesions that are usually found on the face, scalp, arms, and backs of the hands.
B. Lesions can progress to squamous cell carcinoma.
C. Treatment includes medications, excision, cryotherapy, curettage, and laser therapy.
D. Medications include fluorouracil (Carac, Efudex, Fluoroplex), diclofenac sodium (Solaraze), imiquimod 5% cream (Aldara), and aminolevulinic acid (Levulan Kerastick); see Chapter 51 for information on these medications.

XV. SKIN CANCER

A. Description
1. **Skin cancer** is a malignant lesion of the skin, which may or may not metastasize.
2. Overexposure to the sun is a primary cause; other causes and conditions that place the individual at risk include chronic skin damage from repeated injury and irritation, an inherited genetic mutation, ionizing radiation, light-skinned race, age older than 60 years, an outdoor occupation, and exposure to chemical carcinogens.
3. Diagnosis is confirmed by skin biopsy.

B. Types
1. Basal cell: Basal cell cancer arises from the basal cells contained in the epidermis; metastasis is rare but underlying tissue destruction can progress to organ tissue.
2. Squamous cell: Squamous cell cancer is a tumor of the epidermal keratinocytes and can infiltrate surrounding structures and metastasize to lymph nodes.
3. Melanoma: Melanoma may occur any place on the body, especially where birthmarks or new moles are apparent; it is highly metastatic to the brain, lungs, bone, and liver, with survival depending on early diagnosis and treatment.

C. Assessment (Box 50-1)
1. Change in color, size, or shape of preexisting lesion
2. Pruritus
3. Local soreness

The client needs to be informed about the risks associated with overexposure to the sun and taught about the importance of performing monthly self-skin assessments.

D. Interventions
1. Instruct the client regarding the risk factors and preventive measures.
2. Instruct the client to perform monthly self-skin assessments and to monitor for lesions that do not heal or that change characteristics.
3. Advise the client to have moles or lesions removed that are subject to chronic irritation.
4. Advise the client to avoid contact with chemical irritants.
5. Instruct the client to wear layered clothing and use sunscreen lotions with an appropriate skin protection factor when outdoors.
6. Instruct the client to avoid sun exposure between 10 AM and 4 PM.
7. Management may include surgical or nonsurgical interventions; if medication is prescribed provide instructions about its use.
8. Assist with surgical management, which may include cryosurgery, curettage and electrodessication, or surgical excision of the lesion.

Box 50-1 Appearance of Skin Cancer Lesions

Basal Cell Carcinoma

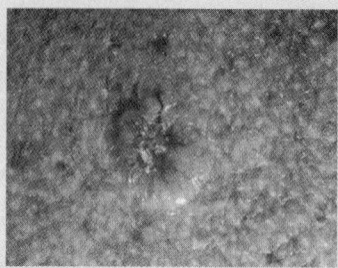

Waxy border
Papule, red, central crater
Metastasis is rare

Squamous Cell Carcinoma

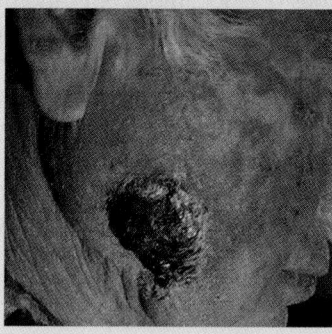

Oozing, bleeding, crusting lesion
Potentially metastatic
Larger tumors associated with a higher risk for metastasis

Melanoma

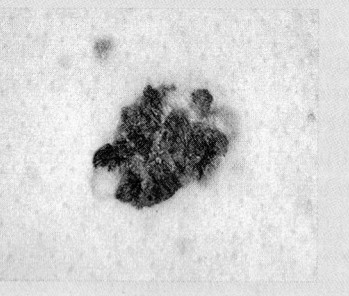

Irregular, circular, bordered lesion with hues of tan, black, or blue
Rapid infiltration into tissue, highly metastatic

Ignatavicius, D., & Workman, M. (2010). *Medical-surgical nursing: Patient-centered collaborative care* (6th ed.). St. Louis: Saunders.

XVI. PSORIASIS

A. Description
  1. Psoriasis is a chronic, noninfectious skin inflammation involving keratin synthesis that results in psoriatic patches.
  2. Various forms exist, with psoriasis vulgaris being the most common.
  3. Possible causes of the disorder include stress, trauma, infection, hormonal changes, obesity, an autoimmune reaction, and climate changes; a genetic predisposition may also be a cause.
  4. The disorder may be exacerbated by the use of certain medications.
  5. Koebner phenomenon is the development of psoriatic lesions at a site of injury, such as a scratched or sunburned area.
  6. In some individuals with psoriasis, arthritis develops that leads to joint changes similar to those seen in rheumatoid arthritis.
  7. The goal of therapy is to reduce cell proliferation and inflammation, and the type of therapy prescribed depends on the extent of the disease and the client's response to treatment.

B. Assessment
  1. Pruritus
  2. Shedding: Silvery, white scales on a raised, reddened, round plaque that usually affects the scalp, knees, elbows, extensor surfaces of arms and legs, and sacral regions
  3. Yellow discoloration, pitting, and thickening of the nails are noted if they are affected.
  4. Joint inflammation with psoriatic arthritis

C. Pharmacological therapy: Refer to Chapter 51 for medications used to treat psoriasis.

D. Interventions and client education
  1. Provide emotional support to the client with associated altered body image and decreased self-esteem.
  2. Instruct the client in the use of prescribed therapies and to avoid over-the-counter medications.
  3. Instruct the client not to scratch the affected areas and to keep the skin lubricated as prescribed to minimize itching.
  4. Monitor for and instruct the client to recognize the signs and symptoms of infection and to report these signs.
  5. Instruct the client to wear light cotton clothing over affected areas.
  6. Assist the client to identify ways to reduce stress if stress is a predisposing factor.

XVII. ACNE VULGARIS

A. Description
  1. Acne is a chronic skin disorder that usually begins in puberty and is more common in males; lesions develop on the face, neck, chest, shoulders, and back.
  2. Acne requires active treatment for control until it resolves.
  3. The types of lesions include comedones (open and closed), pustules, papules, and nodules.
  4. The exact cause is unknown but may include androgenic influence on sebaceous glands, increased sebum production, and proliferation

of *Propionibacterium acnes* (the enzymes reduce lipids to irritating fatty acids).

5. Exacerbations coincide with the menstrual cycle in female clients because of hormonal activity; oily skin and a genetic predisposition may be contributing factors.

B. Assessment
1. Closed comedones are whiteheads and noninflamed lesions that develop as follicles and enlarge, with the retention of horny cells.
2. Open comedones are blackheads that result from continuing accumulation of horny cells and sebum, which dilates the follicles.
3. Pustules and papules result as the inflammatory process progresses.
4. Nodules result from total disintegration of a comedone and subsequent collapse of the follicle.
5. Deep scarring can result from nodules.

C. Interventions
1. Instruct the client in prescribed skin-cleansing methods, with emphasis on not scrubbing the face and using only prescribed topical agents.
2. Instruct the client in the administration of topical or oral medications as prescribed.
3. Instruct the client not to squeeze, prick, or pick at lesions.
4. Instruct the client to use products labeled noncomedogenic and cosmetics that are water-based, and to avoid contact with products with an excessive oil base.
5. Instruct the client on the importance of follow-up treatment.
6. Refer to Chapter 51 for information on the medications used to treat acne.

XVIII. STEVENS-JOHNSON SYNDROME

A. A drug-induced skin reaction that occurs through an immunological response
B. Similar to toxic epidermal necrolysis, another drug-induced skin reaction that results in diffuse erythema and large blister formation
C. May be mild or severe, and may cause vesicles, erosions, and crusts on the skin; if severe, systemic reactions occur that involve the respiratory system, renal system, and eyes, resulting in blindness.
D. Most commonly occurs in clients with cancer who are receiving chemotherapy or immunotherapy
E. Treatment includes immediate discontinuation of the medication causing the syndrome; antibiotics, corticosteroids, and supportive therapy may be necessary.

XIX. PRESSURE ULCER

A. Description
1. A **pressure ulcer** causes impairment of skin integrity.

2. A **pressure ulcer** can occur anywhere on the body; tissue damage results when the skin and underlying tissue are compressed between a bony prominence and an external surface for an extended period of time.
3. The tissue compression restricts blood flow to the skin, which can result in tissue ischemia, inflammation, and necrosis; once a **pressure ulcer** forms, it is difficult to heal.
4. Prevention of skin breakdown in any part of the body is a major role of the nurse.

B. Risk factors
1. Skin pressure and skin shearing and friction
2. Immobility
3. Malnutrition
4. Excessive skin moisture such as that which occurs with incontinence
5. Decreased sensory perception

C. Assessment and staging (Box 50-2)
D. Interventions

⚠ Avoid direct massage to a reddened skin area because massage can damage the capillary beds and cause tissue necrosis.

1. Identify clients at risk for developing a **pressure ulcer**.
2. Institute measures to prevent **pressure ulcers** such as appropriate positioning, using pressure relief devices, ensuring adequate nutrition, and developing a plan for skin cleansing and care.
3. Perform frequent skin assessments and monitor for an alteration in skin integrity.
4. Keep the client's skin dry and the sheets wrinkle-free; if the client is incontinent, check the client frequently and change pads or any items placed under the client immediately after they are soiled.
5. Use creams and lotions to lubricate the skin and a barrier protection ointment for the incontinent client.
6. Turn and reposition the immobile client every 2 hours or more frequently if necessary; provide active and passive range of motion exercises at least every 8 hours.
7. If a **pressure ulcer** is present, record the location and size of the wound (length, width, depth), monitor and record the type and amount of exudates (a culture of the exudate may be prescribed), and assess for undermining and tunneling.
8. Serosanguineous exudate (blood-tinged amber fluid) is expected for the first 48 hours; purulent exudates indicate colonization of the wound with bacteria.
9. Use agency protocols for skin assessment and management of a wound.

Box 50-2 Stages of Pressure Ulcers

Stage I

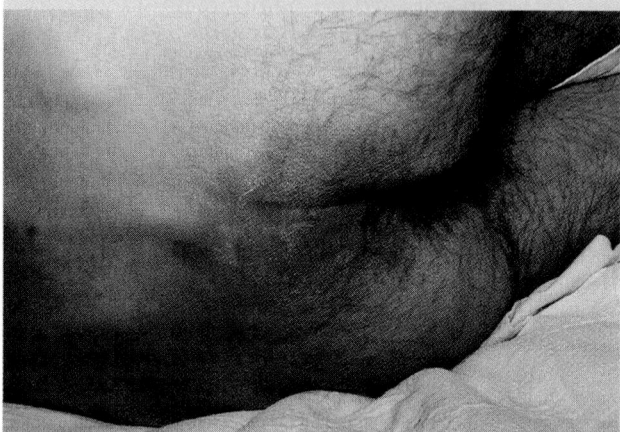

Skin is intact.
Area is red and does not blanch with external pressure.
Area may be painful, firm, soft, warmer or cooler compared with adjacent tissue.

Stage II

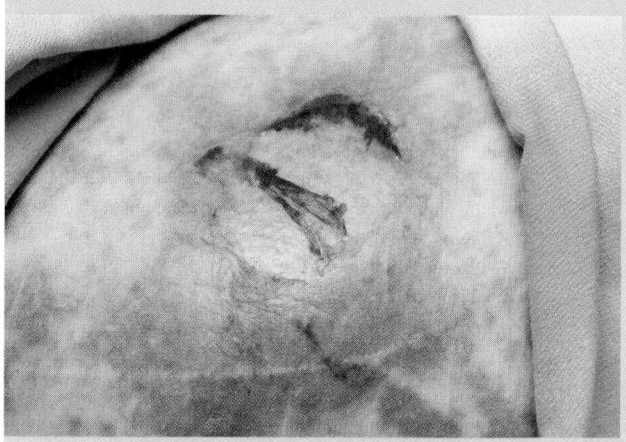

Skin is not intact.
Partial-thickness skin loss of the dermis occurs.
Presents as a shallow open ulcer with a red-pink wound bed or as intact or open/ruptured serum–filled blister.

Stage III

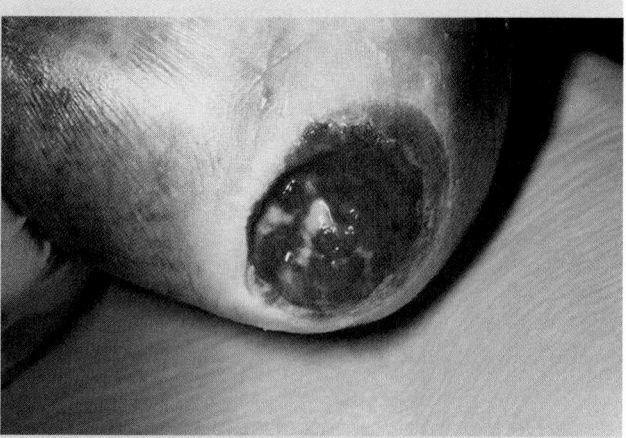

Full-thickness skin loss extends into the dermis and subcutaneous tissues, and slough may be present.
Subcutaneous tissue may be visible.
Undermining and tunneling may or may not be present.

Stage IV

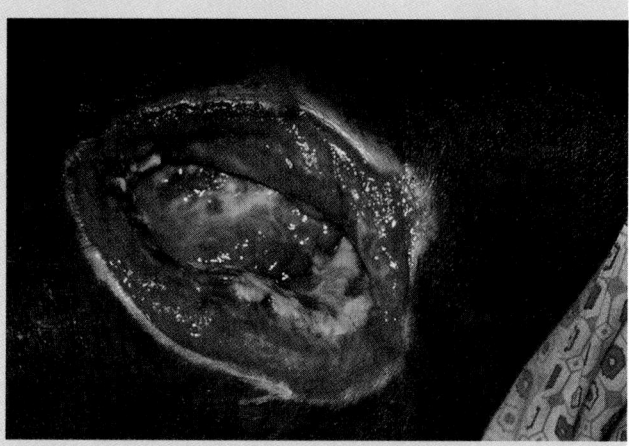

Full-thickness skin loss is present with exposed bone, tendon, or muscle.
Slough or eschar may be present.
Undermining and tunneling may develop.

Ignatavicius, D., & Workman, M. (2010). *Medical-surgical nursing: Patient-centered collaborative care* (6th ed.). St. Louis: Saunders.

10. Treatment may include wound dressings and debridement; skin grafting may be necessary (Tables 50-1 and 50-2).
11. Other treatments may include electrical stimulation to the wound area (increases blood vessel growth and stimulates granulation), vacuum-assisted wound closure (removes infectious material from the wound and promotes granulation), hyperbaric oxygen therapy (administration of oxygen under high pressure raises tissue oxygen concentration), and the use of topical growth factors (biologically active substances that stimulate cell growth).

XX. BURN INJURIES (see Priority Nursing Actions)

TABLE 50-1 Types of Dressings and Mechanism of Action

Dressing Type	Mechanism Of Action
Wet-to-damp saline-moistened gauze	Mechanically removes necrotic debris.
Continuous wet gauze	Wound is continually bathed with a prescribed solution; promotes dilution of exudates and softens dry eschar.
Topical enzyme preparations	Provides a proteolytic action on thick and adherent eschar; this causes breakdown of the denatured protein and more rapid separation of necrotic tissue.
Moisture-retentive dressing	Spontaneous separation of necrotic tissue is promoted by autolysis.

Modified from Ignatavicius, D., & Workman, M. (2010). *Medical-surgical nursing: Patient-centered collaborative care* (6th ed., p. 493). St. Louis: Saunders.

TABLE 50-2 Types of Dressing Materials

Type	Indications, Uses, Considerations	Frequency of Dressing Changes
Alginate	Provides hemostasis, debridement, absorption, and protection. Can be used as packing for deep wounds and for infected wounds. Requires a secondary dressing for securing.	When dressing is saturated (every 3 to 5 days) or more frequently
Biological	Provides protection, and debridement after eschar removal. May be used for dormant and nonhealing wounds that do not respond to other topical therapies. May be used for burns or before pigskin and cadaver skin grafts. Conforms to uneven wound surfaces; reduces pain. Requires a secondary dressing for securing.	Topical growth factors: changed daily. Skin substitutes: the need for dressing change varies.
Cotton gauze	Continuous dry dressing provides absorption and protection. Continuous wet dressing provides protection, a means for the delivery of topical treatment, and debridement. Wet to damp dressing provides atraumatic mechanical debridement. May be painful on removal.	Clean base: every 12 to 24 hours. Necrotic base: every 4 to 6 hours.
Foam	Provides absorption, protection, insulation, and debridement. Conforms to uneven wound surfaces. Requires a secondary dressing for securing.	When dressing is saturated or more frequently
Hydrocolloidal	Provides absorption, protection, and debridement. Is waterproof and is painless on removal.	Clean base: on leakage of exudates. Necrotic base: every 24 hours.
Hydrogel	Provides absorption, protection, and debridement. Conducive to use with topical agents. Conforms to uneven wound surfaces but allows only partial wound visualization. Requires a secondary dressing for securing. Can promote the growth of *Pseudomonas* and other microorganisms.	Clean base: every 24 hours. Necrotic base: every 6 to 8 hours.
Adhesive transparent film	Provides protection for partial-thickness lesions, debridement, and serves as a secondary (cover) dressing. Provides good wound visualization. Is waterproof and reduces pain. Use is limited to superficial lesions. Is nonabsorbent, adheres to normal and healing tissue. Dressing may be difficult to apply.	Clean base: on leakage of exudates. Necrotic base: every 24 hours.

Modified from Ignatavicius, D., & Workman, M. (2010). *Medical-surgical nursing: Patient-centered collaborative care* (6th ed., pp. 494-495). St. Louis: Saunders.

A. Description: Cell destruction of the layers of the skin that results in local and systemic disruptions

B. Burn size
   1. Small **burns**: The response of the body to injury is localized to the injured area
   2. Large or extensive **burns**
      a. Large **burns** consist of 25% or more of the total body surface area.
      b. The response of the body to the injury is systemic.
      c. The **burn** affects all major systems of the body.

PRIORITY NURSING ACTIONS!

Actions to Take in the Emergency Department for a Client With a Burn Injury

1. Assess for airway patency.
2. Administer oxygen as prescribed.
3. Obtain vital signs.
4. Initiate an intravenous (IV) line and begin fluid replacement as prescribed.
5. Elevate the extremities if no fractures are obvious.
6. Keep the client warm and place the client on an NPO status.

The primary goal for a burn injury is to maintain a patent airway, administer IV fluids to prevent hypovolemic shock, and preserve vital organ functioning. Therefore the priority action is to assess for airway patency and to maintain a patent airway. The nurse then prepares to administer oxygen. The type of oxygen delivery system is prescribed by the physician. Oxygen is necessary to perfuse tissues and organs. Vital signs should be assessed so that a baseline is obtained, which is needed for comparison of subsequent vital signs once fluid resuscitation is initiated. The nurse then initiates an IV line and begins fluid replacement as prescribed. The extremities are elevated (if no obvious fractures are present) to assist in preventing shock. The client is kept warm (using sterile linens) and is placed on NPO status because of the altered gastrointestinal function that occurs as a result of the burn injury. A Foley catheter may be inserted so that the response to the fluid resuscitation can be carefully monitored. Once these actions are taken the nurse performs a complete assessment, stays with the client, and monitors the client closely. Additionally, tetanus toxoid may be prescribed for prophylaxis.

Reference: Ignatavicius, D., & Workman, M. (2010). *Medical-surgical nursing: Patient-centered collaborative care* (6th ed., p. 528). St. Louis: Saunders.

Box 50-3 Method to Estimate Extent of Burn Injury

Rule of Nines (Adult)

Head:	9%
Anterior trunk:	18%
Posterior trunk:	18%
Arms (9% each):	18%
Legs (18% each):	36%
Perineum:	1%

The rule of nines provides a rapid method for calculating the size of the injury but overestimation of the total body surface area can occur with this method. Follow agency protocols for estimating the extent of the burn injury.

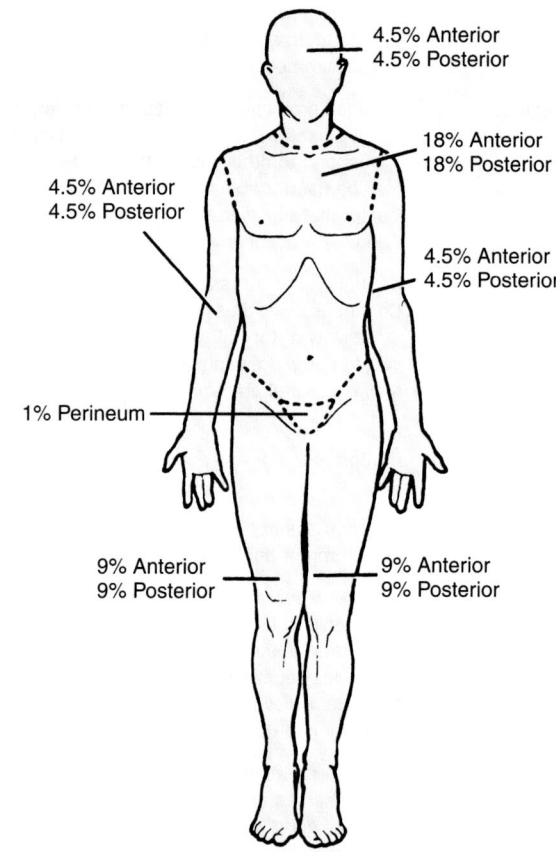

▲ **FIGURE 50-1** The rule of nines for estimating burn percentage. (Ignatavicius, D., & Workman, M. [2010]. *Medical-surgical nursing: Patient-centered collaborative care.* [6th ed.]. St. Louis: Saunders.)

C. Estimating the extent of injury (Box 50-3; Fig. 50-1)
D. **Burn** depth
   1. **Superficial-thickness burn** (Fig. 50-2)
      a. Involves injury to the epidermis; the blood supply to the dermis is still intact.
      b. Mild to severe erythema (pink to red) is present, but no blisters.
      c. Skin blanches with pressure.
      d. **Burn** is painful, with tingling sensation, and the pain is eased by cooling.
      e. Discomfort lasts about 48 hours; healing occurs in about 3 to 6 days.
      f. No scarring occurs and skin grafts are not required.
   2. **Superficial partial-thickness burn** (Fig. 50-3)
      a. Involves injury deeper into the dermis; the blood supply is reduced.
      b. Large blisters may cover an extensive area.
      c. Edema is present.
      d. Mottled pink to red base and broken epidermis, with a wet, shiny, and weeping surface is characteristic.
      e. **Burn** is painful and sensitive to cold air.
      f. Heals in 10 to 21 days with no scarring, but some minor pigment changes may occur.
      g. Grafts may be used if the healing process is prolonged.

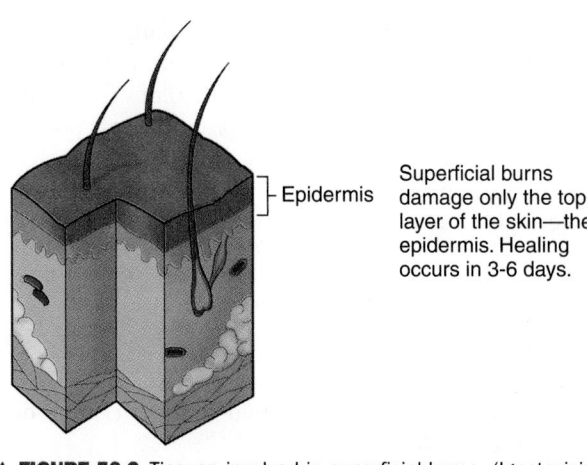

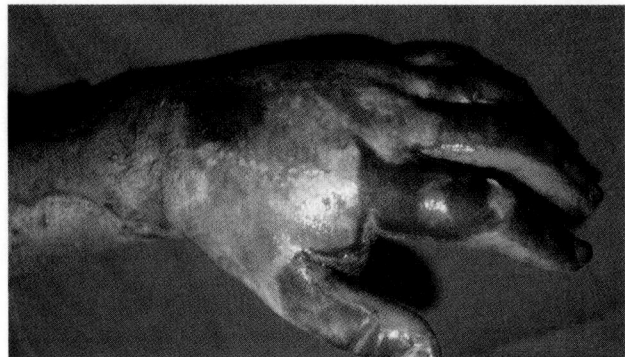

▲ **FIGURE 50-4** Typical appearance of deep partial-thickness burn injury. (Ignatavicius, D., & Workman, M. [2010]. *Medical-surgical nursing: Patient-centered collaborative care* [6th ed.]. St. Louis: Saunders.)

Superficial burns damage only the top layer of the skin—the epidermis. Healing occurs in 3-6 days.

Epidermis

▲ **FIGURE 50-2** Tissues involved in superficial burns. (Ignatavicius, D., & Workman, M. [2010]. *Medical-surgical nursing: Patient-centered collaborative care* [6th ed.]. St. Louis: Saunders.)

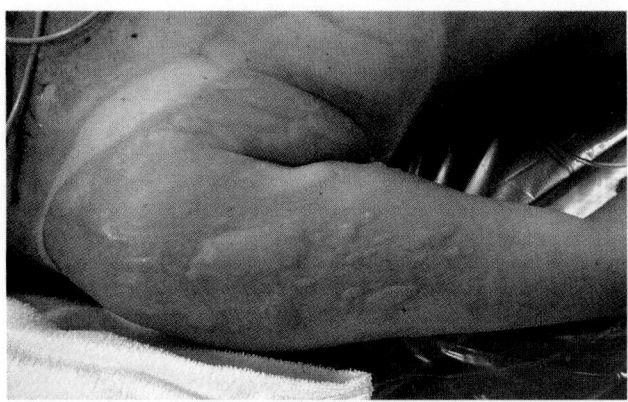

▲ **FIGURE 50-3** Typical appearance of superficial partial-thickness burn injury. (Ignatavicius, D., & Workman, M. [2010]. *Medical-surgical nursing: Patient-centered collaborative care* [6th ed.]. St. Louis: Saunders.)

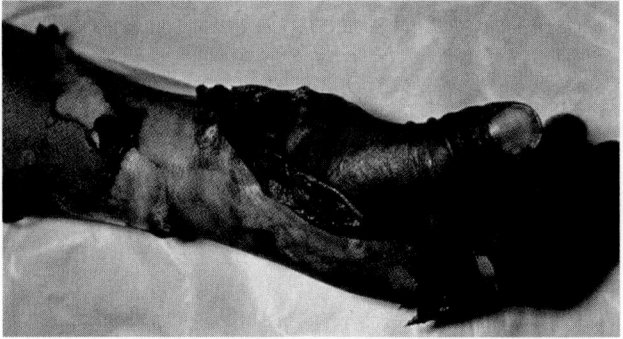

▲ **Figure 50-5** Typical appearance of full-thickness burn injury. (Ignatavicius, D., & Workman, M. [2010]. *Medical-surgical nursing: Patient-centered collaborative care* [6th ed.]. St. Louis: Saunders.)

3. **Deep partial-thickness burn** (Fig. 50-4)
   a. Extends deeper into the skin dermis
   b. Blister formation usually does not occur because the dead tissue layer is thick and sticks to underlying viable dermis.
   c. Wound surface is red and dry with white areas in deeper parts.
   d. May or may not blanch and edema is moderate
   e. Can convert to **full-thickness burn** if tissue damage increases with infection, hypoxia, or ischemia.
   f. Generally heals in 3 to 6 weeks, but scar formation results, and skin grafting may be necessary.
4. **Full-thickness burn** (Fig. 50-5)
   a. Involves injury and destruction of the epidermis and the dermis; the wound will not heal by re-epithelialization and grafting may be required.
   b. Appears as a dry, hard, leathery eschar (**burn** crust or dead tissue must slough off or be removed from the wound before healing can occur).

c. Appears waxy white, deep red, yellow, brown, or black.
   d. Injured surface appears dry.
   e. Edema is present under the eschar.
   f. Sensation is reduced or absent because of nerve ending destruction.
   g. Healing may take weeks to months and depends on establishing an adequate blood supply.
   h. **Burn** requires removal of eschar and split- or full-thickness skin grafting.
   i. If not prevented, scarring and wound contractures are likely to develop.
5. **Deep full-thickness burn** (Fig. 50-6)
   a. Injury extends beyond the skin into underlying fascia and tissues, and muscle, bone, and tendons are damaged.
   b. Injured area appears black and sensation is completely absent.
   c. Eschar is hard and inelastic.
   d. Healing time takes months and grafts are required.
E. Age and general health
   1. Mortality rates are higher for children younger than 4 years of age, particularly for children from birth to 1 year of age, and for clients older than 65 years.

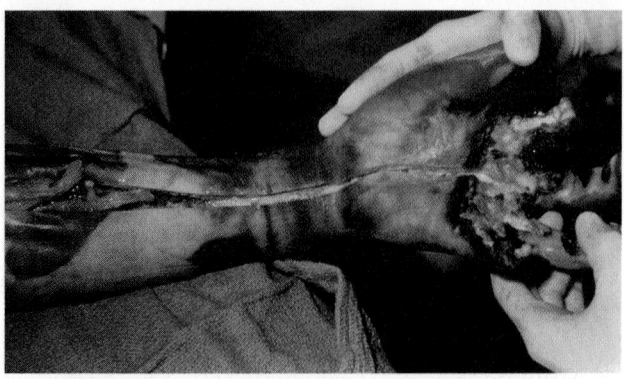

▲ **FIGURE 50-6** Typical appearance of deep full-thickness burn injury. (Ignatavicius, D., & Workman, M. [2010]. *Medical-surgical nursing: Patient-centered collaborative care* [6th ed.]. St. Louis: Saunders.)

2. Debilitating disorders, such as cardiac, respiratory, endocrine, and renal disorders, negatively influence the client's response to injury and treatment.
3. Mortality rate is higher when the client has a pre-existing disorder at the time of the **burn** injury.

F. Burn location
1. **Burns** of the head, neck, and chest are associated with pulmonary complications.
2. **Burns** of the face are associated with corneal abrasion.
3. **Burns** of the ear are associated with auricular chondritis.
4. Hands and joints require intensive therapy to prevent disability.
5. The perineal area is prone to autocontamination by urine and feces.
6. Circumferential **burns** of the extremities can produce a tourniquet-like effect and lead to vascular compromise (compartment syndrome).
7. Circumferential thorax **burns** lead to inadequate chest wall expansion and pulmonary insufficiency.

XXI. TYPES OF BURNS

A. Thermal burns are caused by exposure to flames, hot liquids, steam, or hot objects.
B. Chemical burns
1. **Burns** are caused by tissue contact with strong acids, alkalis, or organic compounds.
2. Systemic toxicity from cutaneous absorption can occur.
C. Electrical burns
1. **Burns** are caused by heat generated by electrical energy as it passes through the body.
2. **Electrical burns** result in internal tissue damage.
3. Cutaneous **burns** cause muscle and soft tissue damage that may be extensive, particularly in high-voltage electrical injuries.
4. The voltage, type of current, contact site, and duration of contact are important to identify.

5. Alternating current is more dangerous than direct current because it is associated with cardiopulmonary arrest, ventricular fibrillation, tetanic muscle contractions, and long bone or vertebral fractures.
D. Radiation **burns** are caused by exposure to ultraviolet light, x-rays, or radioactivity.

XXII. INHALATION INJURIES

A. Smoke inhalation injury
1. Description: Respiratory injury that occurs when the victim is trapped in an enclosed, hot, smoke-filled space

⚠ Airway is a priority concern in an inhalation injury.

2. Assessment
   a. Facial **burns**
   b. Erythema
   c. Swelling of oropharynx and nasopharynx
   d. Singed nasal hairs
   e. Flaring nostrils
   f. Stridor, wheezing, and dyspnea
   g. Hoarse voice
   h. Sooty (carbonaceous) sputum and cough
   i. Tachycardia
   j. Agitation and anxiety
B. Carbon monoxide poisoning
1. Description
   a. Carbon monoxide is a colorless, odorless, and tasteless gas that has an affinity for hemoglobin 200 times greater than that of oxygen.
   b. Oxygen molecules are displaced and carbon monoxide reversibly binds to hemoglobin to form carboxyhemoglobin.
   c. Tissue hypoxia occurs.
2. Assessment (Table 50-3)
C. Smoke poisoning
1. Description
   a. Smoke poisoning is caused by the inhalation of the byproducts of combustion.
   b. A localized inflammatory reaction occurs, causing a decrease in bronchial ciliary action and a decrease in surfactant.
2. Assessment
   a. Mucosal edema occurs in the airways.
   b. Wheezing is evident on auscultation.
   c. After several hours, sloughing of the tracheobronchial epithelium may occur, and hemorrhagic bronchitis may develop.
   d. Acute respiratory distress syndrome can result.
D. Direct thermal heat injury
1. Description
   a. Thermal heat injury can occur to the lower airways by the inhalation of steam or explosive gases or the aspiration of scalding liquids.

TABLE 50-3 Carbon Monoxide Poisoning

Blood Level (%)	Clinical Manifestations
1-10	Normal level
11-20 (mild poisoning)	Headache Flushing Decreased visual acuity Decreased cerebral functioning Slight breathlessness
21-40 (moderate poisoning)	Headache Nausea and vomiting Drowsiness Tinnitus and vertigo Confusion and stupor Pale to reddish-purple skin Decreased blood pressure Increased and irregular heart rate
41-60 (severe poisoning)	Coma Seizures
61-80 (fatal poisoning)	Death

Modified from Ignatavicius, D., & Workman, M. (2010). *Medical-surgical nursing: Patient-centered collaborative care* (6th ed., p. 530). St. Louis: Saunders.

   b. Injury can occur to the upper airways, which appear erythematous and edematous, with mucosal blisters and ulcerations.
   c. Mucosal edema can lead to upper airway obstruction, especially during the first 24 to 48 hours.
   d. All clients with head or neck **burns** should be monitored closely for the development of airway obstruction and are considered immediately for endotracheal intubation if obstruction occurs.
  2. Assessment
   a. Erythema and edema of the upper airways
   b. Mucosal blisters and ulcerations

XXIII. PATHOPHYSIOLOGY OF BURNS

A. Following the **burn**, vasoactive substances are released from the injured tissue, and these substances cause an increase in capillary permeability, allowing the plasma to seep into the surrounding tissues.

B. The direct injury to the vessels increases capillary permeability (capillary permeability decreases 18 to 26 hours after the **burn**, but does not normalize until 2 to 3 weeks following injury).

C. Extensive **burns** result in generalized body edema and a decrease in circulating intravascular blood volume.

D. The fluid losses result in a decrease in organ perfusion.

E. The heart rate increases, cardiac output decreases, and blood pressure drops.

F. Initially, hyponatremia and hyperkalemia occur.

G. The hematocrit level increases as a result of plasma loss; this initial increase falls to below normal at

the third to fourth day after the **burn** as a result of red blood cell damage and loss at the time of injury.

H. Initially, the body shunts blood from the kidneys, causing oliguria; then the body begins to reabsorb fluid, and diuresis of the excess fluid occurs over the next days to weeks.

I. Blood flow to the gastrointestinal tract is diminished, leading to intestinal ileus and gastrointestinal dysfunction.

J. Immune system function is depressed, resulting in immunosuppression and thus increasing the risk of infection and sepsis.

K. Pulmonary hypertension can develop, resulting in a decrease in the arterial oxygen tension level and a decrease in lung compliance.

L. Evaporative fluid losses through the **burn** wound are greater than normal, and the losses continue until complete wound closure occurs.

M. If the intravascular space is not replenished with intravenously administered fluids, hypovolemic shock and ultimately death occur.

XXIV. MANAGEMENT OF THE BURN INJURY

A. Resuscitation/emergent phase (Table 50-4)
  1. Prehospital care
   a. Prehospital care begins at the scene of the accident and ends when emergency care is obtained.
   b. Remove the victim from the source of the **burn**.
   c. Remove the source of heat.
   d. Assess the ABCs—airway, breathing, and circulation.
   e. Assess for associated trauma.
   f. Conserve body heat.
   g. Cover **burns** with sterile or clean cloths.
   h. Remove constricting jewelry and clothing.
   i. Assess the need for intravenous (IV) fluids.
   j. Transport to the emergency department.
  2. Emergency department care is a continuation of care administered at the scene of the injury.
  3. Major **burns**
   a. Evaluate the degree and extent of the **burn** and treat life-threatening conditions.
   b. Ensure a patent airway and administer 100% oxygen as prescribed if the **burn** occurred in an enclosed area.
   c. Monitor for respiratory distress and assess the need for intubation.
   d. Assess oropharynx for blisters and erythema.
   e. Monitor arterial blood gases and carboxyhemoglobin levels.
   f. For an inhalation injury, administer 100% oxygen via a tight-fitting non-rebreather face mask as prescribed until the carboxyhemoglobin level falls below 15%.

TABLE 50-4 Phases of Management of the Burn Injury

Phase	Goal
RESUSCITATION/EMERGENT PHASE Begins at the time of injury Ends with the restoration of normal capillary permeability Duration usually 48 to 72 hr Includes prehospital care and emergency department care	The primary goal is to maintain a patent airway, administer intravenous fluids to prevent hypovolemic shock, and preserve vital organ functioning.
RESUSCITATIVE PHASE Begins with the initiation of fluids Ends when capillary integrity returns to near-normal levels and large fluid shifts have decreased Amount of fluid administered based on client's weight and extent of injury (Most fluid replacement formulas are calculated from the time of injury and not from the time of arrival at the hospital.)	The goal is to prevent shock by maintaining adequate circulating blood volume and maintaining vital organ perfusion.
ACUTE PHASE Begins when the client is hemodynamically stable, capillary permeability is restored, and diuresis has begun Usually begins 48 to 72 hr after time of injury Focus on infection control, wound care, wound closure, nutritional support, pain management, physical therapy	The goal during this phase is placed on restorative therapy, and the phase continues until wound closure is achieved.
REHABILITATIVE PHASE Overlaps acute phase of care Extends beyond hospitalization	The goals of this phase are designed so that the client can gain independence and achieve maximal function.

TABLE 50-5 Common Fluid Resuscitation Formulas for First 24 Hours After a Burn Injury

Formula	Solution	Rate of Administration
MODIFIED BROOKE 0.5 mL to 15 mL/kg/% TBSA burn	Protenate or 5% albumin in isotonic saline Lactated Ringer's without dextrose	Half given in first 8 hr Half given in next 16 hr
PARKLAND (BAXTER) 4 mL/kg/% TBSA burn	Crystalloid only (lactated Ringer's)	Half given in first 8 hr, half given in next 16 hr
MODIFIED PARKLAND 4 mL/kg/% TBSA burn + 15 mL/m² of TBSA	Crystalloid only (lactated Ringer's)	Half given in first 8 hr, half given in next 16 hr

TBSA, *Total body surface area.*
Modified from Ignatavicius, D., & Workman, M. (2010). *Medical-surgical nursing: Patient-centered collaborative care* (6th ed., p. 533). St. Louis: Saunders.

g. Initiate peripheral IV access to nonburned skin proximal to any extremity **burn**, or prepare for the insertion of a central venous line as prescribed.
h. Assess for hypovolemia and prepare to administer fluids intravenously to maintain fluid balance.
i. Monitor vital signs closely.
j. Insert a Foley catheter as prescribed, and maintain urine output at 30 to 50 mL/hr.
k. Maintain an NPO status.
l. Insert a nasogastric tube as prescribed to remove gastric secretions and prevent aspiration.
m. Administer tetanus prophylaxis as prescribed.
n. Administer pain medication, as prescribed, by the IV route.
o. Prepare the client for an escharotomy or fasciotomy as prescribed.

4. Minor **burns**
   a. Administer pain medication as prescribed.
   b. Instruct the client in the use of oral analgesics as prescribed.
   c. Administer tetanus prophylaxis as prescribed.
   d. Administer wound care as prescribed, which may include cleansing, debriding loose tissue, and removing any damaging agents, followed by the application of topical antimicrobial cream and a sterile dressing.
   e. Instruct the client in follow-up care, including active range-of-motion exercises and wound care treatments.

B. Resuscitative phase (see Table 50-4)
   1. Fluid resuscitation (Table 50-5)
      a. The amount of fluid administered depends on how much IV fluid per hour is required to maintain a urinary output of 30 to 50 mL/hr.

b. Successful fluid resuscitation is evaluated by stable vital signs, an adequate urine output, palpable peripheral pulses, and a clear sensorium.

c. IV fluid replacement may be titrated (adjusted) based on urinary output plus serum electrolyte levels to meet the perfusion needs of the client with **burns**.

d. If the hemoglobin and hematocrit levels decrease or if the urinary output exceeds 50 mL/hr, the rate of IV fluid administration may be decreased.

⚠ Urinary output is the most reliable and most sensitive noninvasive assessment parameter for cardiac output and tissue perfusion.

2. Interventions

a. Monitor for tracheal or laryngeal edema and administer respiratory treatments as prescribed.

b. Monitor pulse oximetry and prepare for arterial blood gases and carboxyhemoglobin levels if inhalation injury is suspected.

c. Elevate the head of the bed to 30 degrees or more for **burns** of the face and head.

d. Initiate electrocardiographic monitoring.

e. Monitor temperature and assess for infection.

f. Initiate protective isolation techniques; maintain strict handwashing; use sterile sheets and linens when caring for the client; and use gloves, cap, masks, shoe covers, scrub clothes, and plastic aprons.

g. Shave or cut body hair around wound margins.

h. Monitor daily weights, expecting a weight gain of 15 to 20 pounds in the first 72 hours.

i. Monitor gastric output and pH levels and for gastric discomfort and bleeding, indicating a stress ulcer.

j. Administer antacids, H_2 receptor antagonists, and antiulcer medications as prescribed to prevent a stress ulcer.

k. Auscultate bowel sounds for ileus and monitor for abdominal distention and gastrointestinal dysfunction.

l. Monitor stools for occult blood.

m. Obtain urine specimen for myoglobin and hemoglobin levels.

n. Monitor IV fluids and hourly intake and output to determine the adequacy of fluid replacement therapy; notify the physician if urine output is less than 30 or greater than 50 mL/hr.

o. Elevate circumferential **burns** of the extremities on pillows above the level of the heart to reduce dependent edema if no obvious fractures are present; diuretics increase the risk of hypovolemia and are generally avoided as a means of decreasing edema.

p. Monitor pulses and capillary refill of the affected extremities and assess perfusion of the distal extremity with a circumferential **burn**.

q. Prepare to obtain chest x-rays and other radiographs to rule out fractures or associated trauma.

r. Keep the room temperature warm.

s. Place the client on an air-fluidized bed or other special mattress and use a bed cradle to keep sheets off the client's skin.

3. Pain management

a. Administer opioid analgesics as prescribed by the IV route.

b. Avoid administering medication by the oral route because of the possibility of gastrointestinal dysfunction.

c. Medicate the client as prescribed and before painful procedures.

⚠ Avoid the intramuscular or subcutaneous medication routes for medication administration because absorption through the soft tissue is unreliable when hypovolemia and large fluid shifts occur.

4. Nutrition

a. Proper nutrition is essential to promote wound healing and prevent infection.

b. The basal metabolic rate is 40 to 100 times higher than normal with a **burn** injury.

c. Maintain an NPO status until the bowel sounds are heard, and then advance to clear liquids as prescribed.

d. Nutrition may be provided via enteral tube feeding or parenteral nutrition through a central line.

e. Provide a diet high in protein, carbohydrates, fats, and vitamins.

f. Monitor calorie intake.

5. Escharotomy

a. A lengthwise incision is made through the **burn** eschar to relieve constriction and pressure and to improve circulation.

b. Escharotomy is performed for circulatory compromise caused by circumferential **burns**.

c. Escharotomy is performed at the bedside without anesthesia because nerve endings have been destroyed by the **burn** injury.

d. Escharotomy can be performed on the thorax to improve ventilation.

e. Following the escharotomy, assess pulses, color, movement, and sensation of affected extremity and control any bleeding with pressure.

f. Pack the incision gently with fine mesh gauze as prescribed after escharotomy.

g. Apply topical antimicrobial agents to the area as prescribed.

TABLE 50-6 Open Method Versus Closed Method of Wound Care

Method	Advantages	Disadvantages
OPEN Antimicrobial cream is applied as prescribed, and wound is left open to the air without a dressing.	Visualization of the wound Easier mobility and joint range of motion Simplicity in wound care	Increased chance of hypothermia from exposure
CLOSED Gauze dressings are carefully wrapped from the distal to the proximal area of the extremity to ensure that circulation is not compromised. No two burn surfaces should be allowed to touch; touching can promote webbing of digits, contractures, and poor cosmetic outcome. Dressings are changed usually every 8 to 12 hr.	Decreases evaporative fluid and heat loss Aids in debridement	Mobility limitations Prevents effective range-of-motion exercises Wound assessment limited

Box 50-4 Debridement

Mechanical
Performed during hydrotherapy; involves use of washcloths or sponges to cleanse and debride eschar and the use of scissors and forceps to lift and trim away loose eschar
May include wet-to-dry or wet-to-wet dressing changes
Painful procedure; may cause bleeding

Enzymatic
Application of topical enzyme agents directly to the wound; the agent digests collagen necrotic tissue

Surgical
Excision of eschar or necrotic tissue via a surgical procedure in the operating room

Tangential Technique
Very thin layers of the necrotic burn surface are excised until bleeding occurs (bleeding indicates that a healthy dermis or subcutaneous fat has been reached).

Fascial Technique
The burn wound is excised to the level of superficial fascia; this technique is usually reserved for very deep and extensive burns.

6. Fasciotomy
   a. An incision is made extending through the subcutaneous tissue and fascia.
   b. The procedure is performed if adequate tissue perfusion does not return following an escharotomy.
   c. Fasciotomy is performed in the operating room with the client under general anesthesia.
   d. Following the procedure, assess pulses, color, movement, and sensation of affected extremity and control any bleeding with pressure.
   e. Apply topical antimicrobial agents and dressings to the area, as prescribed.

 C. Acute phase (see Table 50-4)
   1. Continue with protective isolation techniques.
   2. Provide wound care as prescribed and prepare for wound closure.
   3. Provide pain management.
   4. Provide adequate nutrition as prescribed.
   5. Prepare the client for rehabilitation.

D. Wound care (Table 50-6)
   1. Description: Cleansing, debridement, and dressing of **burn** wounds
   2. Hydrotherapy

   a. Wounds are cleansed by immersion, showering, or spraying.
   b. Hydrotherapy occurs for 30 minutes or less to prevent increased sodium loss through the **burn** wound, heat loss, pain, and stress.
   c. Client should be premedicated before procedure.
   d. Hydrotherapy generally is not used for clients who are hemodynamically unstable or those with new skin grafts.
   e. Care is taken to minimize bleeding and maintain body temperature during the procedure.
   f. If hydrotherapy is not used, wounds are washed and rinsed with the client in bed before the application of antimicrobial agents.
   3. Debridement (Box 50-4)
   a. Debridement is removal of eschar or necrotic tissue to prevent bacterial proliferation under the eschar and to promote wound healing.
   b. Debridement may be mechanical, enzymatic, or surgical.
   c. **Deep partial-thickness burns** or **deep full-thickness burns**: Wound is cleansed and debrided, and topical antimicrobial agents are applied once or twice daily.

Box 50-5 Wound Coverings

Biological

Amniotic Membranes

Amniotic membranes from human placenta are used; adheres to the wound

Effective as a dressing until epithelial cell regrowth occurs

Requires frequent changes because it does not develop a blood supply and disintegrates in about 48 hours

Allograft or Homograft (Human Tissue)

Donated human cadaver skin provided through a skin bank

Monitor for wound exudate and signs of infection

Rejection—can occur within 24 hours

Risk of transmitting bloodborne infection exists when used

Xenograft or Heterograft (Animal Tissue)

Pigskin harvested after slaughter is preserved for storage and use.

Monitor for infection and wound adherence

Placed over granulation tissue; replaced every 2 to 5 days until wound heals naturally or until closure with autograft is complete.

Cultured Skin

Grown in laboratory from a small specimen of epidermal cells from an unburned portion of client's body

Cell sheets are grafted on the client to generate permanent skin surface

Cell sheets are not durable; care must be taken when applying to ensure adherence, and prevent sloughing

Artificial Skin

Consists of two layers—Silastic epidermis and porous dermis made from bovine hide collagen and shark cartilage

After application, fibroblasts move into the collagen part of the artificial skin and create a structure similar to normal dermis

Artificial dermis then dissolves; it is then replaced with normal blood vessels and connective tissue called *neodermis*

Neodermis supports the standard autograph placed over it when Silastic layer is removed

Biosynthetic

Combination of biosynthetic and synthetic materials

Placed in contact with the wound surface; forms an adherent bond until epithelialization occurs

Porous substance allows exudate to pass through

Monitor for wound exudate and signs of infection

Synthetic

Applied directly to the surface of clean or a surgically prepared wound; remains in place until it falls off or is removed

Covering is transparent or translucent; therefore wound can be inspected without removing dressing

Pain at the wound site is reduced because covering prevents contact of the wound with air

Autograft

Skin taken from a remote unburned area of client's own body; transplanted to cover burn wound

Graft placed on a clean granulated bed or over surgically excised area of the burn

Provides for permanent skin coverage

E. Wound closure
   1. Description
      a. Wound closure prevents infection and loss of fluid.
      b. Closure promotes healing.
      c. Closure prevents contractures.
      d. Wound closure is performed usually on day 5 to 21 following the injury, depending on the extent of the **burn**.
   2. Wound coverings (Box 50-5)
   3. Autografting (see Box 50-5)
      a. Autografting provides permanent wound coverage.
      b. Autografting is the surgical removal of a thin layer of the client's own unburned skin, which then is applied to the excised **burn** wound.
      c. Autografting is performed in the operating room under anesthesia.
      d. Monitor for bleeding following the graft because bleeding beneath an autograft can prevent adherence.
      e. If prescribed, small amounts of blood or serum can be removed by gently rolling the

fluid from the center of the graft to the periphery with a sterile gauze pad, where it can be absorbed.
      f. For large accumulations of blood, the physician may aspirate the blood using a small-gauge needle and syringe.
      g. Autografts are immobilized following surgery for 3 to 7 days to allow time to adhere and attach to the wound bed.
      h. Position the client for immobilization and elevation of the graft site to prevent movement and shearing of the graft.
   4. Care of the graft site
      a. Elevate and immobilize the graft site.
      b. Keep the site free from pressure.
      c. Avoid weight-bearing.
      d. When the graft takes, if prescribed, roll a cotton-tipped applicator over the graft to remove exudate, because exudate can lead to infection and prevent graft adherence.
      e. Monitor for foul-smelling drainage, increased temperature, increased white blood cell count, hematoma formation, and fluid accumulation.

f. Instruct the client to avoid using fabric softeners and harsh detergents in the laundry.

g. Instruct the client to lubricate the healing skin with prescribed agents.

h. Instruct the client to protect the affected area from sunlight.

i. Instruct the client to use splints and support garments as prescribed.

5. Care of the donor site
   a. Method of care varies, depending on the physician's preference
   b. A moist gauze dressing may be applied at the time of the surgery to maintain pressure and stop any oozing.
   c. The physician may prescribe site treatment with gauze impregnated with petrolatum or with a biosynthetic dressing.
   d. Keep the donor site clean, dry, and free from pressure.
   e. Prevent the client from scratching the donor site.
   f. Apply lubricating lotions to soften the area and reduce the itching after the donor site is healed.
   g. Donor site can be reused once healing has occurred (heals spontaneously within 7 to 14 days with proper care).

F. Physical therapy
   1. An individualized program of splinting, positioning, exercises, ambulation, and activities of daily living is implemented early in the acute phase of recovery to maximize functional and cosmetic outcomes.
   2. Perform range-of-motion exercises as prescribed to reduce edema and maintain strength and joint function.
   3. Ambulate the client as prescribed to maintain the strength of the lower extremities.
   4. Apply splints as prescribed to maintain proper joint position and prevent contractures.
      a. Static splints immobilize the joint and are applied for periods of immobilization, during sleeping, and for clients who cannot maintain proper positioning.
      b. Dynamic splints exercise the affected joint.
      c. Avoid pressure to skin areas when applying splints, which could lead to further tissue and nerve damage.
   5. Scarring is controlled by elastic wraps and bandages that apply continuous pressure to the healing skin during the time in which the skin is vulnerable to shearing.
   6. Anti–**burn** scar support garments are usually prescribed to be worn 23 hours a day until the **burn** scar tissue has matured, which takes 18 to 24 months.

G. Rehabilitative phase (see Table 50-4)
   1. Description: Rehabilitation is the final phase of **burn** care.

2. Goals
   a. Promote wound healing.
   b. Minimize deformities.
   c. Increase strength and function.
   d. Provide emotional support.

MORE QUESTIONS ON THE CD!

Practice Questions

500. The nurse is conducting a session about the principles of first aid and is discussing the interventions for a snakebite to an extremity. The nurse should inform those attending the session that the first priority intervention in the event of this occurrence is which of the following?
1. Immobilize the affected extremity.
2. Remove jewelry and constricting clothing from the victim.
3. Place the extremity in a position so that it is below the level of the heart.
4. Move the victim to a safe area away from the snake and encourage the victim to rest.

501. A client calls the emergency department and tells the nurse that he had been cleaning a wooded area in the backyard and came directly into contact with poison ivy shrubs. The client tells the nurse that he cannot see anything on the skin and asks the nurse what to do. Which of the following is the appropriate nursing response?
1. "Come to the emergency department."
2. "Apply calamine lotion immediately to the exposed skin areas."
3. "Take a shower immediately, lathering and rinsing several times."
4. "It is not necessary to do anything if you cannot see anything on your skin."

502. The client is being admitted to the hospital for treatment of acute cellulitis of the lower left leg. The client asks the admitting nurse to explain what cellulitis means. The nurse bases the response on the understanding that the characteristics of cellulitis include:
1. An inflammation of the epidermis only
2. A skin infection into the dermis and subcutaneous tissue
3. An acute superficial infection of the dermis and lymphatics
4. An epidermal and lymphatic infection caused by *Staphylococcus*

503. The clinic nurse assesses the skin of a client with a diagnosis of psoriasis. The nurse understands that

which characteristic is associated with this skin disorder?
1. Clear, thin nail beds
2. Red-purplish scaly lesions
3. Oily skin and no episodes of pruritus
4. Silvery-white scaly patches on the scalp, elbows, knees, and sacral regions

504. The clinic nurse notes that the physician has documented a diagnosis of herpes zoster (shingles) in the client's chart. Based on an understanding of the cause of this disorder, the nurse determines that this definitive diagnosis was made following which diagnostic test?
1. Patch test
2. Skin biopsy
3. Culture of the lesion
4. Wood's light examination

505. A client returns to the clinic for follow-up treatment following a skin biopsy of a suspicious lesion performed 1 week ago. The biopsy report indicates that the lesion is a melanoma. The nurse understands that which of the following describes a characteristic of this type of a lesion?
1. Metastasis is rare.
2. Melanoma is encapsulated.
3. Melanoma is highly metastatic.
4. Melanoma is characterized by local invasion.

506. When assessing a lesion diagnosed as malignant melanoma, the nurse most likely expects to note which of the following?
1. An irregularly shaped lesion
2. A small papule with a dry, rough scale
3. A firm, nodular lesion topped with crust
4. A pearly papule with a central crater and a waxy border

507. The client arrives at the emergency department and has experienced frostbite to the right hand. Which of the following would the nurse note on assessment of the client's hand?
1. A pink, edematous hand
2. A fiery red skin with edema in the nail beds
3. Black fingertips surrounded by an erythematous rash
4. A white color to the skin, which is insensitive to touch

508. The evening nurse reviews the nursing documentation in the client's chart and notes that the day nurse has documented that the client has a stage II pressure ulcer in the sacral area. Which of the following would the nurse expect to note on assessment of the client's sacral area?

1. Intact skin
2. Full-thickness skin loss
3. Exposed bone, tendon, or muscle
4. Partial-thickness skin loss of the dermis

509. The adult client was burned as a result of an explosion. The burn initially affected the client's entire face (anterior half of the head) and the upper half of the anterior torso, and there were circumferential burns to the lower half of both arms. The client's clothes caught on fire, and the client ran, causing subsequent burn injuries to the posterior surface of the head and the upper half of the posterior torso. Using the rule of nines, what would be the extent of the burn injury?
1. 18%
2. 24%
3. 36%
4. 48%

510. The nurse is preparing to care for a burn client scheduled for an escharotomy procedure being performed for a third-degree circumferential arm burn. The nurse understands that the anticipated therapeutic outcome of the escharotomy is:
1. Return of distal pulses
2. Brisk bleeding from the site
3. Decreasing edema formation
4. Formation of granulation tissue

511. A client is undergoing fluid replacement after being burned on 20% of her body 12 hours ago. The nursing assessment reveals a blood pressure of 90/50 mm Hg, a pulse rate of 110 beats/min, and a urine output of 20 mL over the past hour. The nurse reports the findings to the physician and anticipates which of the following prescriptions?
1. Transfusing 1 unit of packed red blood cells
2. Administering a diuretic to increase urine output
3. Increasing the amount of intravenous (IV) lactated Ringer's solution administered per hour
4. Changing the IV lactated Ringer's solution to one that contains dextrose in water

512. When caring for a client with extensive burns, the nurse anticipates that pain medication will be administered via which route?
1. Oral
2. Intravenous
3. Intramuscular
4. Subcutaneous

513. The nurse is caring for a client who sustained superficial partial-thickness burns on the anterior lower legs and anterior thorax. Which of the following does the nurse expect to note during the resuscitation/emergent phase of the burn injury?

1. Decreased heart rate
2. Increased urinary output
3. Increased blood pressure
4. Elevated hematocrit levels

514. The nurse is caring for a client who suffered an inhalation injury from a wood stove. The carbon monoxide blood report reveals a level of 12%. Based on this level, the nurse would anticipate which of the following signs in the client?
1. Coma
2. Flushing
3. Dizziness
4. Tachycardia

515. The client arrives at the emergency department following a burn injury that occurred in the basement at home and an inhalation injury is suspected. Which of the following would the nurse anticipate to be prescribed for the client?
1. 100% oxygen via an aerosol mask
2. Oxygen via nasal cannula at 15 L/min
3. Oxygen via nasal cannula at 10 L/min
4. 100% oxygen via a tight-fitting, non-rebreather face mask

516. The nurse is administering fluids intravenously as prescribed to a client who sustained superficial partial-thickness burn injuries of the back and legs. In evaluating the adequacy of fluid resuscitation, the nurse understands that which of the following would provide the most reliable indicator for determining the adequacy?
1. Vital signs
2. Urine output
3. Mental status
4. Peripheral pulses

517. The nurse manager is observing a new nursing graduate caring for a burn client in protective isolation. The nurse manager intervenes if the new nursing graduate planned to implement which incorrect component of protective isolation technique?
1. Using sterile sheets and linens
2. Performing strict hand-washing technique
3. Wearing gloves and a gown only when giving direct care to the client
4. Wearing protective garb, including a mask, gloves, cap, shoe covers, gowns, and plastic apron

518. The nurse is caring for a client following an autograft and grafting to a burn wound on the right knee. Which of the following would the nurse anticipate to be prescribed for the client?
1. Out of bed
2. Bathroom privileges
3. Immobilization of the affected leg
4. Placing the affected leg in a dependent position

Alternate Item Format: Multiple Response

519. The nurse manager is planning the clinical assignments for the day. Which staff members can be assigned to care for a client with herpes zoster? **Select all that apply.**
❏ 1. The nurse who never had roseola
❏ 2. The nurse who never had mumps
❏ 3. The nurse who never had chickenpox
❏ 4. The nurse who never had German measles
❏ 5. The nurse who never received the varicella-zoster vaccine

ANSWERS

500. 4
Rationale: In the event of a snakebite, the first priority is to move the victim to a safe area away from the snake and encourage the victim to rest to decrease venom circulation. Next, jewelry and constricting clothing are removed before swelling occurs. Immobilizing the extremity and maintaining the extremity below heart level would be done next; these actions limit the spread of the venom. The victim is kept warm and calm. Alcohol or stimulants such as alcohol or caffeinated beverages are not given to the victim because these products may speed the absorption of the venom. The victim should be transported to an emergency facility as soon as is possible.
Test-Taking Strategy: Note the strategic words *first priority*. Eliminate options 1 and 3 first because they are comparable or alike and relate to care to the affected extremity. For the remaining options think about them and visualize each. Moving the victim to a safe area is the priority to prevent further injury from the snake. Review the priority interventions in the event of a snake bite if you had difficulty with this question.
Level of Cognitive Ability: Applying
Client Needs: Safe and Effective Care Environment
Integrated Process: Teaching and Learning
Content Area: Critical Care
Reference: Ignatavicius, D., & Workman, M. (2010). *Medical-surgical nursing: Patient-centered collaborative care* (6th ed., p. 144). St. Louis: Saunders.

501. 3
Rationale: When an individual comes in contact with a poison ivy plant, the sap from the plant forms an invisible film on the human skin. The client should be instructed to cleanse the area with alcohol and then shower immediately and to lather the skin several times and rinse each time in running water. Calamine lotion may be one product recommended for use if dermatitis develops. The client does not need to be seen in the emergency department at this time.

Test-Taking Strategy: Use the process of elimination. Recalling that dermatitis can develop from contact with an allergen and that contact with poison ivy results in an invisible film will assist in directing you to option 3. Review the immediate treatment for contact with poison ivy if you had difficulty with this question.
Level of Cognitive Ability: Applying
Client Needs: Physiological Integrity
Integrated Process: Nursing Process—Implementation
Content Area: Adult Health—Integumentary
Reference: Perry, S., Hockenberry, M., Lowdermilk, D., & Wilson, D. (2010). *Maternal child nursing care* (4th ed., p. 1647). St. Louis: Mosby.

502. 2

Rationale: Cellulitis is a skin infection into deeper dermal and subcutaneous tissues that results in a deep red erythema without sharp borders and spreads widely throughout tissue spaces. The skin is erythematous, edematous, tender, and sometimes nodular. Erysipelas is an acute, superficial, rapidly spreading inflammation of the dermis and lymphatics.
Test-Taking Strategy: Use the process of elimination. Eliminate options 3 and 4 because they are comparable or alike and address the lymphatics. Eliminate option 1 because of the close-ended word *only*. If you had difficulty with this question, review the characteristics of cellulitis and erysipelas.
Level of Cognitive Ability: Understanding
Client Needs: Physiological Integrity
Integrated Process: Teaching and Learning
Content Area: Adult Health—Integumentary
Reference: Black, J., & Hawks, J. (2009). *Medical-surgical nursing: Clinical management for positive outcomes* (8th ed., p. 1225). St. Louis: Saunders.

503. 4

Rationale: Psoriatic patches are covered with silvery white scales. Affected areas include the scalp, elbows, knees, shins, sacral area, and trunk. Thickening, pitting, and discoloration of the nails occur. Pruritus may occur. The lesions in psoriasis are not red-purplish scaly lesions.
Test-Taking Strategy: Use the process of elimination and knowledge regarding the pathophysiology associated with psoriasis. Recall that psoriasis is associated with the presence of silvery white scaly patches. This will direct you to option 4 and assist in answering questions similar to this one. If you had difficulty with this question, review the manifestations associated with psoriasis.
Level of Cognitive Ability: Understanding
Client Needs: Physiological Integrity
Integrated Process: Nursing Process—Assessment
Content Area: Adult Health—Integumentary
Reference: Ignatavicius, D., & Workman, M. (2010). *Medical-surgical nursing: Patient-centered collaborative care* (6th ed., p. 506). St. Louis: Saunders.

504. 3

Rationale: With the classic presentation of herpes zoster, the clinical examination is diagnostic. A viral culture of the lesion provides the definitive diagnosis. Herpes zoster (shingles) is caused by a reactivation of the varicella-zoster virus, the virus that causes chickenpox. A patch test is a skin test that involves the administration of an allergen to the surface of the skin to identify specific allergies. A biopsy would provide a cytological examination of tissue. In a Wood's light examination, the skin is viewed under ultraviolet light to identify superficial infections of the skin.
Test-Taking Strategy: Use the process of elimination. Recalling that herpes zoster is caused by a virus will assist in directing you to the correct option. Remember that a biopsy will determine tissue type, whereas a culture will identify an organism. Review the diagnostic measures for herpes zoster (shingles) if you had difficulty with this question.
Level of Cognitive Ability: Understanding
Client Needs: Physiological Integrity
Integrated Process: Nursing Process—Assessment
Content Area: Adult Health—Integumentary
References: Black, J., & Hawks, J. (2009). *Medical-surgical nursing: Clinical management for positive outcomes* (8th ed., p. 1227). St. Louis: Saunders.
Copstead-Kirkhorn, L., & Banasik, J. (2010). *Pathophysiology* (4th ed., p. 1118). St. Louis: Mosby.

505. 3

Rationale: Melanomas are pigmented malignant lesions originating in the melanin-producing cells of the epidermis. This skin cancer is highly metastatic, and a person's survival depends on early diagnosis and treatment. Options 1, 2, and 4 are not characteristics of a melanoma.
Test-Taking Strategy: Use the process of elimination. Note that options 1, 2, and 4 are comparable or alike and indicate a localized lesion rather than one that will spread to other areas of the body. Also, recalling that melanomas are highly metastatic will assist in directing you to the correct option. If you had difficulty with this question, review the characteristics of melanomas.
Level of Cognitive Ability: Understanding
Client Needs: Physiological Integrity
Integrated Process: Nursing Process—Assessment
Content Area: Adult Health—Integumentary
Reference: Ignatavicius, D., & Workman, M. (2010). *Medical-surgical nursing: Patient-centered collaborative care* (6th ed., p. 509). St. Louis: Saunders.

506. 1

Rationale: A melanoma is an irregularly shaped pigmented papule or plaque with a red-, white-, or blue-toned color. Basal cell carcinoma appears as a pearly papule with a central crater and rolled waxy border. Squamous cell carcinoma is a firm, nodular lesion topped with a crust or a central area of ulceration. Actinic keratosis, a premalignant lesion, appears as a small macule or papule with a dry, rough, adherent yellow or brown scale.
Test-Taking Strategy: Use the process of elimination. Remembering that irregularly shaped lesions are a cause for concern will assist in directing you to option 1. If you had difficulty with this question, review the characteristics of a malignant melanoma.
Level of Cognitive Ability: Understanding
Client Needs: Physiological Integrity
Integrated Process: Nursing Process—Assessment
Content Area: Adult Health—Integumentary
Reference: Black, J., & Hawks, J. (2009). *Medical-surgical nursing: Clinical management for positive outcomes* (8th ed., pp. 1221–1222). St. Louis: Saunders.

507. 4
Rationale: Assessment findings in frostbite include a white or blue color; the skin will be hard, cold, and insensitive to touch. As thawing occurs, flushing of the skin, the development of blisters or blebs, or tissue edema appears. Options 1, 2, and 3 are incorrect.
Test-Taking Strategy: Focus on the subject, assessment findings in frostbite. Noting the strategic words *insensitive to touch* in option 4 should direct you to this option. If you had difficulty with this question, review the characteristics associated with frostbite.
Level of Cognitive Ability: Analyzing
Client Needs: Physiological Integrity
Integrated Process: Nursing Process—Assessment
Content Area: Adult Health—Integumentary
References: Black, J., & Hawks, J. (2009). *Medical-surgical nursing: Clinical management for positive outcomes* (8th ed., p. 2213). St. Louis: Saunders.
Ignatavicius, D., & Workman, M. (2010). *Medical-surgical nursing: Patient-centered collaborative care* (6th ed., p. 154). St. Louis: Saunders.

508. 4
Rationale: In a stage II pressure ulcer, the skin is not intact. Partial-thickness skin loss of the dermis has occurred. It presents as a shallow open ulcer with a red-pink wound bed, without slough. It may also present as an intact, open or ruptured, serum-filled blister. The skin is intact in stage I. Full-thickness skin loss occurs in stage III. Exposed bone, tendon, or muscle is present in stage IV.
Test-Taking Strategy: Use the process of elimination and visualize the appearance of pressure ulcers. Focus on the strategic words *stage II* to direct you to option 4. If you had difficulty with this question, review the characteristics associated with each stage of pressure ulcers.
Level of Cognitive Ability: Understanding
Client Needs: Physiological Integrity
Integrated Process: Nursing Process—Assessment
Content Area: Adult Health—Integumentary
Reference: Ignatavicius, D., & Workman, M. (2010). *Medical-surgical nursing: Patient-centered collaborative care* (6th ed., p. 489). St. Louis: Saunders.

509. 3
Rationale: According to the rule of nines, with the initial burn, the anterior half of the head equals 4.5%, the upper half of the anterior torso equals 9%, and the lower half of both arms equals 9%. The subsequent burn included the posterior half of head, equaling 4.5%, and the upper half of posterior torso, equaling 9%. This totals 36%.
Test-Taking Strategy: Knowledge regarding the rule of nines is required to answer this question. The entire head equals 9%, each arm equals 9% (both arms equal 18%), anterior or posterior torso each equals 18% (36% for entire torso), each leg equals 18% (both legs equal 36%), and the perineum equals 1%. If you had difficulty with this question, remember that 9 (head), 18 (arms), 36 (torso), 36 (legs), and 1 (perineum) equals 100.
Level of Cognitive Ability: Analyzing
Client Needs: Physiological Integrity
Integrated Process: Nursing Process—Assessment
Content Area: Critical Care

References: Black, J., & Hawks, J. (2009). *Medical-surgical nursing: Clinical management for positive outcomes* (8th ed., p. 1248). St. Louis: Saunders.
Proehl, J. (2009). *Emergency nursing procedures* (4th ed., pp. 710–711). St. Louis: Saunders.

510. 1
Rationale: Escharotomies are performed to relieve the compartment syndrome that can occur when edema forms under nondistensible eschar in a circumferential third-degree burn. Escharotomies are performed through avascular eschar to subcutaneous fat. Although bleeding may occur from the site, it is considered a complication rather than an anticipated therapeutic outcome. Usually, direct pressure with a bulky dressing and elevation control the bleeding, but occasionally an artery is damaged and may require ligation. Formation of granulation tissue is not the intent of an escharotomy. Escharotomy does not affect the formation of edema.
Test-Taking Strategy: Use the ABCs—airway, breathing, and circulation—to answer the question. The only option that addresses circulation is option 1. If you had difficulty with this question, review the purpose of an escharotomy.
Level of Cognitive Ability: Evaluating
Client Needs: Physiological Integrity
Integrated Process: Nursing Process—Evaluation
Content Area: Critical Care
References: Black, J., & Hawks, J. (2009). *Medical-surgical nursing: Clinical management for positive outcomes* (8th ed., p. 1254). St. Louis: Saunders.
Ignatavicius, D., & Workman, M. (2010). *Medical-surgical nursing: Patient-centered collaborative care* (6th ed., pp. 534–535). St. Louis: Saunders.
Proehl, J. (2009). *Emergency nursing procedures* (4th ed., pp. 712–720). St. Louis: Saunders.

511. 3
Rationale: Fluid management during the first 24 hours following a burn injury generally includes the infusion of (usually) lactated Ringer's solution. Fluid resuscitation is determined by urine output and hourly urine output should be at least 30 mL/hr. The client's urine output is indicative of insufficient fluid resuscitation, which places the client at risk for inadequate perfusion of the brain, heart, kidneys, and other body organs. Therefore the physician would prescribe an increase in the amount of IV lactated Ringer's solution administered per hour. Administering a diuretic would not correct the problem because it would not replace needed fluid. Diuretics promote the removal of the circulating volume, thereby further compromising the inadequate tissue perfusion. Dextrose in water is an isotonic solution and an isotonic solution maintains fluid balance. This type of solution may be administered after the first 24 hours following the burn injury, depending on the client's physiological needs. Blood replacement is not used for fluid therapy for burn injuries.
Test-Taking Strategy: Focus on the data in the question and think about the pathophysiology that occurs in a burn injury. Noting that the burn injury occurred 12 hours ago and that the client's urine output is 20 mL and is indicative of insufficient fluid resuscitation will direct you to the correct option. Review fluid resuscitation in a client with a burn injury if you had difficulty with this question.

Level of Cognitive Ability: Analyzing
Client Needs: Physiological Integrity
Integrated Process: Nursing Process—Analysis
Content Area: Critical Care
Reference: Ignatavicius, D., & Workman, M. (2010). *Medical-surgical nursing: Patient-centered collaborative care* (6th ed., pp. 533–534). St. Louis: Saunders.

512. 2

Rationale: An extensive burn injury causes impairment of muscle and subcutaneous tissue. Additionally, the gastrointestinal tract has decreased perfusion related to the burn injury. Medications administered by mouth, intramuscularly, or subcutaneously are not absorbed consistently as a result of the burn injury. The client may not experience pain relief from these routes of administration and may also receive a sudden bolus of medication at some point after administration, when fluid shifts occur. Therefore options 1, 3, and 4 are incorrect.
Test-Taking Strategy: Focus on the data in the question. Noting the word *extensive* in the question will assist in directing you to option 2. Review pain management techniques in a client with a burn injury if you had difficulty with this question.
Level of Cognitive Ability: Applying
Client Needs: Physiological Integrity
Integrated Process: Nursing Process—Planning
Content Area: Critical Care
Reference: Ignatavicius, D., & Workman, M. (2010). *Medical-surgical nursing: Patient-centered collaborative care* (6th ed., p. 537). St. Louis: Saunders.

513. 4

Rationale: The resuscitation/emergent phase begins at the time of injury and ends with the restoration of capillary permeability, usually at 48 to 72 hours following the injury. During the resuscitation/emergent phase, the hematocrit level increases to above normal because of hemoconcentration from the large fluid shifts. Hematocrit levels of 50% to 55% are expected during the first 24 hours after injury, with return to normal by 36 hours after injury. Initially, blood is shunted away from the kidneys, and renal perfusion and glomerular filtration are decreased, resulting in low urine output. Pulse rates are typically higher than normal, and the blood pressure is decreased as a result of the large fluid shifts.
Test-Taking Strategy: Use the process of elimination and think about how the body would react in such a traumatizing event; this eliminates options 1 and 2. Knowledge that the blood pressure would decrease as a result of the decrease in circulating blood volume will direct you to option 4 from the remaining options. Review the pathophysiology related to burn injuries if you had difficulty with this question.
Level of Cognitive Ability: Analyzing
Client Needs: Physiological Integrity
Integrated Process: Nursing Process—Analysis
Content Area: Critical Care
Reference: Ignatavicius, D., & Workman, M. (2010). *Medical-surgical nursing: Patient-centered collaborative care* (6th ed., p. 532). St. Louis: Saunders.

514. 2

Rationale: Carbon monoxide levels between 11% and 20% result in flushing, headache, decreased visual acuity, decreased cerebral functioning, and slight breathlessness;

levels of 21% to 40% result in nausea, vomiting, dizziness, tinnitus, vertigo, confusion, drowsiness, pale to reddish-purple skin, tachycardia; levels of 41% to 60% result in seizure and coma; and levels higher than 60% result in death.
Test-Taking Strategy: Use the process of elimination and focus on the carbon monoxide level presented in the question. Remember that flushing occurs with levels between 11% and 20%; this will assist you in answering questions similar to this one. If you had difficulty with this question, review the effects of an inhalation injury, carbon monoxide levels, and the associated clinical manifestations.
Level of Cognitive Ability: Analyzing
Client Needs: Physiological Integrity
Integrated Process: Nursing Process—Assessment
Content Area: Critical Care
References: Black, J., & Hawks, J. (2009). *Medical-surgical nursing: Clinical management for positive outcomes* (8th ed., p. 1245). St. Louis: Saunders.
  Ignatavicius, D., & Workman, M. (2010). *Medical-surgical nursing: Patient-centered collaborative care* (6th ed., p. 530). St. Louis: Saunders.

515. 4

Rationale: If an inhalation injury is suspected, administration of 100% oxygen via a tight-fitting non-rebreather face mask is prescribed until carboxyhemoglobin levels fall (usually below 15%). In inhalation injuries, the oropharynx is inspected for evidence of erythema, blisters, or ulcerations. The need for endotracheal intubation also is assessed. Options 1, 2, and 3 are incorrect and would not provide the necessary oxygen supply needed for adequate tissue perfusion.
Test-Taking Strategy: Use the process of elimination. Recalling that 100% oxygen is required following an inhalation injury will assist you in eliminating options 2 and 3. From the remaining options, recall that a tight-fitting non-rebreather mask is preferred so that the client will not rebreathe exhaled air. If you had difficulty with this question review care of the client following an inhalation injury and the methods of delivering oxygen to the client.
Level of Cognitive Ability: Analyzing
Client Needs: Physiological Integrity
Integrated Process: Nursing Process—Analysis
Content Area: Critical Care
Reference: Copstead-Kirkhorn, L., & Banasik, J. (2010). *Pathophysiology* (4th ed., p. 1272). St. Louis: Mosby.

516. 2

Rationale: Successful or adequate fluid resuscitation in the client is signaled by stable vital signs, adequate urine output, palpable peripheral pulses, and clear sensorium. However, the most reliable indicator for determining adequacy of fluid resuscitation is the urine output. For an adult, the hourly urine volume should be 30 to 50 mL.
Test-Taking Strategy: Use the process of elimination and note the strategic words *most reliable*. Note the subject of the question, fluid resuscitation. Urine output is most similar to the subject of administering fluids. Review care of the burn client during fluid resuscitation if you had difficulty with this question.
Level of Cognitive Ability: Evaluating
Client Needs: Physiological Integrity
Integrated Process: Nursing Process—Evaluation
Content Area: Critical Care

Reference: Ignatavicius, D., & Workman, M. (2010). *Medical-surgical nursing: Patient-centered collaborative care* (6th ed., p. 534). St. Louis: Saunders.

517. 3
Rationale: Thorough handwashing should be done before and after each contact with the burn-injured client. Sterile sheets and linens are used because of the client's high risk for infection. Protective garb, including gloves, cap, masks, shoe covers, gowns, and plastic apron need to be worn when in the client's room and when directly caring for the client.
Test-Taking Strategy: Use the process of elimination, noting the strategic word *incorrect* in the question. Options 1 and 2 can be eliminated easily. Note the close-ended word *only* in option 3. Also, option 3 identifies the least thorough technique to prevent infection. If you had difficulty with this question, review protective isolation techniques when caring for a burn client.
Level of Cognitive Ability: Applying
Client Needs: Safe and Effective Care Environment
Integrated Process: Nursing Process—Implementation
Content Area: Leadership and Management—Delegating/Prioritizing
Reference: Black, J., & Hawks, J. (2009). *Medical-surgical nursing: Clinical management for positive outcomes* (8th ed., p. 1255). St. Louis: Saunders.

518. 3
Rationale: Autografts placed over joints or on the lower extremities after surgery often are elevated and immobilized for 3 to 7 days. This period of immobilization allows the autograft time to adhere to the wound bed. Options 1, 2, and 4 are incorrect.
Test-Taking Strategy: Use the process of elimination. Eliminate options 1 and 2 first because they are comparable or alike and allow out-of-bed activities. From the remaining options, note that the autograft was placed over a joint. This should direct you to option 3. If you had difficulty with this question, review care of an autograft placed over a joint.
Level of Cognitive Ability: Analyzing
Client Needs: Physiological Integrity
Integrated Process: Nursing Process—Analysis
Content Area: Adult Health—Integumentary
Reference: Black, J., & Hawks, J. (2009). *Medical-surgical nursing: Clinical management for positive outcomes* (8th ed., p. 1265). St. Louis: Saunders.

ALTERNATE ITEM FORMAT: MULTIPLE RESPONSE

519. 1, 2, 4
Rationale: Herpes zoster (shingles) is caused by a reactivation of the varicella-zoster virus, the causative virus of chickenpox. Individuals who have not been exposed to the varicella-zoster virus or who did not receive the varicella-zoster vaccine are susceptible to chickenpox. Health care workers who are unsure of their immune status should have varicella titers done before exposure to a person with herpes zoster.
Test-Taking Strategy: Use the process of elimination. Recalling that herpes zoster is caused by a reactivation of the varicella-zoster virus, the causative virus of chickenpox, will direct you to the correct options 1, 2, and 4. Review the relationship between herpes zoster virus and chickenpox if you had difficulty with this question.
Level of Cognitive Ability: Applying
Client Needs: Safe and Effective Care Environment
Integrated Process: Nursing Process—Planning
Content Area: Leadership and Management—Delegating/Prioritizing
Reference: Black, J., & Hawks, J. (2009). *Medical-surgical nursing: Clinical management for positive outcomes* (8th ed., p. 1227). St. Louis: Saunders.

51

Integumentary Medications

I. POISON IVY TREATMENT (Fig. 51-1; Box 51-1)

A. Treatment of lesions includes calamine lotion and other products that soothe lesions, Burow's solution compresses, and/or Aveeno baths to relieve discomfort.

B. Topical corticosteroids are effective to prevent or relieve inflammation, especially when used before blisters form.

C. Oral corticosteroids may be prescribed for severe reactions and a sedative such as diphenhydramine (Benadryl) may be prescribed.

II. MEDICATIONS TO TREAT ATOPIC DERMATITIS (Box 51-2)

A. Description
  1. A chronic inflammatory skin disease that is also known as *eczema* and is characterized by dry and scaly skin.
  2. May be treated with moisturizer and topical glucocorticoids; systemic immunosuppressants may also be prescribed if topical treatment is ineffective.
  3. Systemic immunosuppressants may include methotrexate, cyclosporine (Sandimmune), or azathioprine (Imuran), and oral glucocorticoids.

B. Topical immunosuppressants
  1. Tacrolimus (Protopic) and pimecrolimus 1% cream (Elidel).
  2. Side effects include redness, burning, and itching; causes sensitization of the skin to sunlight.
  3. Tacrolimus (Protopic) increases the risk of varicella-zoster infection in children.
  4. Tacrolimus (Protopic) may cause **skin cancer** and lymphoma.

III. TOPICAL GLUCOCORTICOIDS

A. Description
  1. Anti-inflammatory, antipruritic, and vasoconstrictive actions
  2. Preparations vary in potency and depend on the concentration and type of preparation, and method of application (occlusive dressings enhance absorption, increasing the effects).
  3. Systemic effects are more likely to occur with prolonged therapy and when extensive skin surfaces are treated.

⚠ Topical glucocorticoids can be absorbed into the systemic circulation; absorption is greater in permeable skin areas (scalp, axilla, face and neck, eyelids, perineum) and less in areas where permeability is poor (palms, soles, back).

B. Contraindications
  1. Clients demonstrating previous sensitivity to corticosteroids
  2. Clients with current systemic fungal, viral, or bacterial infections
  3. Clients with current complications related to glucocorticoid therapy

C. Local adverse effects
  1. Burning, dryness, irritation, itching
  2. Skin atrophy
  3. Thinning of the skin, striae, purpura, telangiectasia
  4. Acneiform eruptions
  5. Hypopigmentation
  6. Overgrowth of bacteria, fungi, and viruses

D. Systemic adverse effects
  1. Growth retardation in children
  2. Adrenal suppression
  3. Cushing's syndrome
  4. Striae, skin atrophy
  5. Ocular effects (glaucoma and cataracts)

E. Interventions
  1. Monitoring plasma cortisol levels may be prescribed if prolonged therapy is necessary.
  2. Wash the area just before application to increase medication penetration.
  3. Apply sparingly in a thin film, rubbing gently.
  4. Avoid use of a dry occlusive dressing unless specifically prescribed by the physician.
  5. Instruct client to report signs of adverse effects to the physician.

⚠ In the adult, intact skin is generally impermeable to most topical medications. However, medications should not be applied to denuded areas unless prescribed because undesired absorption can occur.

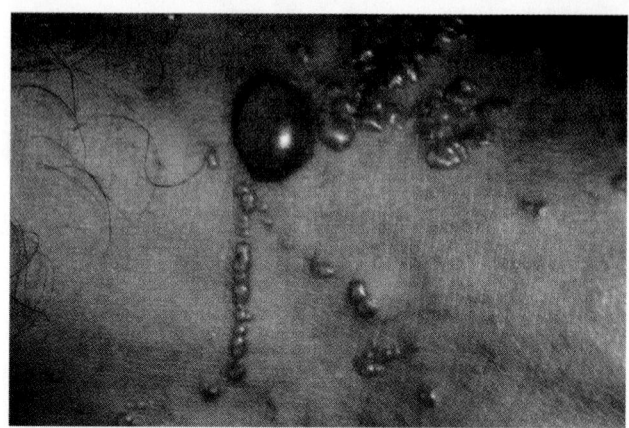

▲ **FIGURE 51-1** Poison ivy. Note "streaked" blisters surrounding one large blister. (From Perry, S., Hockenberry, M., Lowdermilk, D., Wilson, S. [2010]. *Maternal child nursing care* [4th ed.]. St. Louis: Mosby.)

Box 51-1 Poison Ivy Treatment Products

Bentoquatam—for preventive use (Ivy Block)
Calamine lotion (Caladryl lotion)
Hydrocortisone (Ivy Soothe, Ivy Stat)
Isopropanol; cetyl alcohol (Ivy Cleanse)
Zinc acetate; isopropanol (Ivy Dry)
Zinc acetate; isopropanol; benzyl alcohol (Ivy Super Dry)

Box 51-2 Medications to Treat Atopic Dermatitis

Systemic Immunosuppressants
Azathioprine (Imuran)
Cyclosporine (Sandimmune)
Methotrexate
Oral glucocorticoids

Topical Immunosuppressants
Pimecrolimus 1% cream (Elidel)
Tacrolimus (Protopic)

Box 51-3 Medications to Treat Actinic Keratosis

Aminolevulinic acid (Levulan Kerastick)
Diclofenac sodium (Solaraze)
Fluorouracil (Carac, Efudex, Fluoroplex)
Imiquimod 5% cream (Aldara)

IV. MEDICATIONS TO TREAT ACTINIC KERATOSIS (Box 51-3)

A. Description
1. Actinic keratoses are caused by prolonged exposure to the sun and appear as rough, scaly, red or brown lesions usually found on the face, scalp, arms, and back of the hands.
2. Lesions can progress to squamous cell carcinoma.

3. Treatment includes medications and therapies such as excision, cryotherapy, curettage, and laser therapy.

B. Medications include fluorouracil (Carac, Efudex, Fluoroplex), diclofenac sodium (Solaraze), imiquimod 5% cream (Aldara), and aminolevulinic acid (Levulan Kerastick).

1. Fluorouracil (Carac, Efudex, Fluoroplex)
   a. A topical medication that affects DNA and RNA synthesis and causes a sequence of response that results in healing; results are usually seen in 2 to 6 weeks but may take 1 to 2 months longer for complete healing
   b. Side effects include itching, burning, inflammation, rash, and increased sensitivity to sunlight.
2. Diclofenac sodium (Solaraze)
   a. A nonsteroidal anti-inflammatory topical drug; may take 3 months to be effective
   b. Side effects include dry skin, itching, redness, and rash.
3. Imiquimod 5% cream (Aldara)
   a. In addition to treating actinic keratoses, this topical medication has been used to treat venereal warts; it may take up to 4 months to be effective.
   b. Side effects include redness, skin swelling, itching, burning, sores, blisters, scabbing, and crusting of the skin.
4. Aminolevulinic acid (Levulan Kerastick)
   a. A topical medication used in conjunction with blue light photoactivation; the medication is applied and 14 to 18 hours later the medication is activated by exposing the lesions to the blue light.
   b. Side effects include burning, stinging, redness, and swelling of the skin; treated areas need to be protected from sunlight and bright indoor lights.

V. SUNCREENS

A. Ultraviolet (UV) light can damage the skin and can cause premalignant actinic keratoses and some types of **skin cancer**.

B. Sunscreens prevent the penetration of UV light and protect the skin.

C. Organic (chemical) sunscreens absorb UV light; inorganic (physical) reflect and scatter UV light.

D. A sunscreen that protects against both UVB and UVA rays and one that has a sun protection factor (SPF) of at least 15 should be used.

E. Sunscreens are most effective when applied at least 30 minutes before exposure to the sun (sunscreens containing para-aminobenzoic acid [PABA] or padimate O require application 2 hours before sun exposure).

F. Sunscreen should be reapplied every 2 to 3 hours and after swimming or sweating; otherwise, the duration of protection is reduced.

Box 51-4 Medications and Treatments for Psoriasis

Topical Medications
Anthralin (Dritho-Scalp, Psoriatec)
Calcipotriene (Dovonex)
Coal tar
Glucocorticoids
Keratolytics
Tazarotene (Tazorac)

Systemic Medications
Acitretin (Soriatane)
Cyclosporine (Neoral)
Methotrexate

Systemic Biological Medications
Alefacept (Amevive)
Ustekinumab (Stelara)

Phototherapy
Coal tar and ultraviolet B irradiation
Photochemotherapy (PUVA [psoralen and ultraviolet A] therapy)

G. Products containing PABA need to be avoided by individuals allergic to benzocaine, sulfonamides, or thiazides.

H. Sunscreens can cause contact dermatitis and photosensitivity reactions.

⚠ The client should be informed that UV light is greatest between the hours of 10:00 AM and 4:00 PM, and that sunglasses, protective clothing, and a hat should be worn to reduce the risk of skin damage from the sun.

VI. MEDICATIONS TO TREAT PSORIASIS (Box 51-4)

A. Description
  1. Psoriasis is a chronic inflammatory disorder that has varying degrees of severity.
  2. Treatment is based on the severity of symptoms and aims to suppress the proliferation of keratinocytes or suppress the activity of inflammatory cells.

B. Topical medications
  1. Glucocorticoids
    a. Used for mild psoriasis
    b. Should not be applied to the face, groin, axilla, or genitalia because the medication is readily absorbable making the skin vulnerable to glucocorticoid-induced atrophy
  2. Anthralin (Dritho-Scalp, Psoriatec)
    a. Can cause local irritation and skin redness
    b. Is applied to lesions at bedtime and allowed to remain on the skin overnight
    c. Client should be informed that the medication can stain clothing, skin, and hair.
  3. Tazarotene (Tazorac)
    a. Is a vitamin A derivative

b. Local reactions include itching, burning, stinging, dry skin, and redness; other less common effects include rash, desquamation, contact dermatitis, inflammation, fissuring, and bleeding.
    c. Sensitization to sunlight can occur and the client should be instructed to use sunscreen and wear protective clothing.
    d. Medication is usually applied once daily in the evening to dry skin.
  4. Calcipotriene (Dovonex)
    a. Is an analogue of vitamin D
    b. May take up to 1 to 3 weeks to produce a desired effect
    c. Can cause local irritation; high-dose applications may cause hypercalcemia
  5. Coal tar
    a. Suppresses DNA synthesis, miotic activity, and cell proliferation
    b. Has an unpleasant odor and may cause irritation, burning, and stinging; can also stain the skin and hair
  6. Keratolytics
    a. Soften scales and loosen the horny layer of the skin, resulting in minimal peeling to extensive desquamation
    b. Salicylic acid: Can be absorbed systemically and can cause salicylism, which is characterized by dizziness and tinnitus, hyperpnea, and psychological disturbances; salicylic acid is not applied to large surface areas or open wounds because of the risk of systemic effects.
    c. Sulfur: Promotes peeling and drying and is used to treat acne, dandruff, seborrheic dermatitis, and psoriasis

C. Systemic medications
  1. Methotrexate
    a. Reduces proliferation of epidermal cells
    b. Can be toxic; causes gastrointestinal effects such as diarrhea and ulcerative stomatitis and bone marrow depression leading to blood dyscrasias
    c. Can be hepatotoxic; hepatic function should be monitored during therapy
  2. Acitretin (Soriatane)
    a. Inhibits keratinization, proliferation, and differentiation of cells; has anti-inflammatory and immunodulator actions; used for severe psoriasis and reserved for use in those who have not responded to safer medications.
    b. Is embryotoxic and teratogenic: Medication is contraindicated during pregnancy; pregnancy must be ruled out and two reliable forms of contraception need to be implemented before the medication is started (contraception must be implemented at least 1 month before treatment starts and be continued for at least 3 years after treatment is discontinued.)

c. If pregnancy occurs during treatment with the medication, the medication is discontinued immediately and possible termination of the pregnancy is discussed.

d. Dermatological effects include hair loss, skin peeling, dry skin, rash, pruritus, nail disorders; other effects include rhinitis from mucous membrane irritation, inflammation of the lips, dry mouth, dry eyes, nosebleed, gingivitis, stomatitis, bone and joint pain, and spinal disorders.

e. Can be hepatotoxic; can elevate triglyceride levels and reduce levels of high-density lipoprotein cholesterol

f. Medication should be taken with meals to facilitate absorption; alcohol must be avoided.

g. This derivative of vitamin A can cause vitamin A toxicity if taken at the same time as vitamin A supplements.

h. Should not be taken concurrently with tetracycline because it can cause increased intracranial pressure

3. Cyclosporine (Neoral)
   a. An immunosuppressant that inhibits proliferation of B and T cells
   b. Can be toxic and cause kidney damage
   c. Used for severe psoriasis and reserved for use in those who have not responded to safer medications

D. Systemic biological medications
1. Alefacept (Amevive)
   a. The medication reduces the number and activity of memory CD4+ T lymphocytes; therefore the medication is contraindicated in clients with human immunodeficiency virus infection.
   b. CD4 T-cell counts should be monitored before each dose and discontinued if the count falls below 250 cells/mL.
   c. Risk of cancer is increased and the medication should not be administered to a client with a history of malignancy; medication should be discontinued if cancer develops.
   d. Can cause chills, cough, pruritus, myalgia, and inflammation and pain at the intramuscular injection site
2. Ustekinumab (Stelara)
   a. A human monoclonal antibody
   b. Can decrease the activity of the immune system and increase the risk for certain types of cancer
   c. Side effects of the medication include upper respiratory infections, headache, and tiredness.
   d. Contraindicated in clients who have a history of cancer; also contraindicated in clients with infection, or reversible posterior leukoencephalopathy syndrome (rare condition that affects the brain and can cause death)

e. The client should not receive any live virus vaccines because the viruses used in some types of vaccines can cause infection in those with a weakened immune system; additionally the physician needs to be informed if anyone in the household needs a vaccine.

f. The client should not receive the BCG vaccine during the 1 year before taking or 1 year after taking the medication.

g. The client should inform the physician if he or she is receiving phototherapy, has any other medical condition, is pregnant or plans to become pregnant, or is breast-feeding or plans to breast-feed.

E. Phototherapy
1. Coal tar and ultraviolet B irradiation: Treatment that involves the application of coal tar for 8 to 10 hours; coal tar is washed off and the area is exposed to short-wave UV radiation (ultraviolet B, or UVB)
2. Photochemotherapy (PUVA [psoralen and ultraviolet A] therapy)
   a. Combines the use of long-wave radiation (ultraviolet A, or UVA) with oral methoxsalen (photosensitive medication)
   b. Can cause pruritus, nausea, erythema; may accelerate the aging process of the skin; may increase the risk of **skin cancer**

VII. ACNE PRODUCTS (Box 51-5; Fig. 51-2)

A. Description
1. Acne lesions that are mild may be treated with nonpharmacological measures such as gentle

---

Box 51-5 Acne Products

Topical Antibiotics
Benzoyl peroxide
Clindamycin (Cleocin) and erythromycin (Erythroderm)
Dapsone (Aczone)
Fixed dose combinations: clindamycin/benzoyl peroxide (BenzaClin) and erythromycin/benzoyl peroxide (Benzamycin).

Topical Retinoids
Adapalene (Differin)
Azelaic acid (Azelex)
Tazarotene (Tazorac)
Tretinoin (Retin-A, Avita)

Oral Medications
Doxycycline (Vibramycin)
Erythromycin (Ery-Tab)
Isotretinoin (Accutane)
Minocycline (Dynacin, Minocin, Solodyn)
Tetracycline (Sumycin)

Hormonal Medications
Oral contraceptives
Spironolactone (Aldactone)

cleansing two or three times daily (oil-based moisturizing products need to be avoided), dermabrasion, or comedo extraction.
2. Mild acne is usually treated pharmacologically with topical agents (antimicrobials and retinoids).
3. Moderate acne is usually treated with oral antibiotics and comedolytics.
4. Severe acne is usually treated with isotretinoin (Accutane).
5. Hormonal medications such as oral contraceptives and spironolactone (Aldactone) may be prescribed to treat acne in female clients.
6. Combination therapy may be prescribed to treat the acne.
7. Actions of the medications may include suppressing the growth of *Propionibacterium acnes*, reducing inflammation, promoting keratolysis, unplugging existing comedones and preventing their development, normalizing hyperproliferation of epithelial cells within the hair follicles; some medications cause thinning of the skin, which facilitates penetration of other medications.
8. For topical applications: Site should be washed and allowed to completely dry before application; hands should be washed after application.
9. All topical products are kept away from the eyes, inside the nose, lips, mucous membranes, hair, and inflamed or denuded skin.
B. Topical antibiotic products
1. Benzoyl peroxide
   a. Can produce drying and peeling
   b. Severe local irritation (burning, blistering, scaling, swelling) may require reducing the frequency of applications.
   c. Some products may contain sulfites; monitor for allergic reactions.

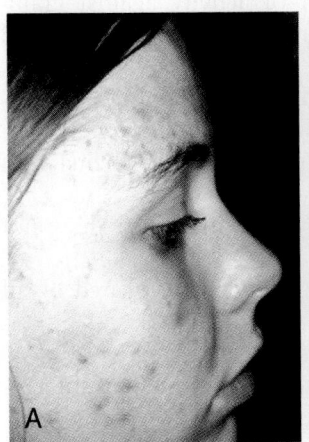 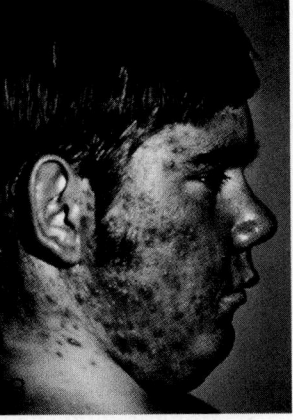

▲ **FIGURE 51-2** Acne vulgaris. **A,** Comedones with a few inflammatory pustules. **B,** Papulopustular acne. (From Wong, D., Hockenberry, M., Wilson, S., Lowdermilk, D., & Wilson, D. [2006]. *Maternal child nursing care* [3rd ed.]. St. Louis: Mosby.)

2. Clindamycin (Cleocin) and erythromycin (Erythroderm)
   a. Both products may be prescribed to prevent emergence of resistance.
   b. Combination therapy with benzoyl peroxide can be prescribed to prevent emergence of resistance; fixed-dose combinations include clindamycin/benzoyl peroxide (BenzaClin) and erythromycin/benzoyl peroxide (Benzamycin).
3. Dapsone (Aczone): Side effects include oiliness, peeling, dryness, and erythema of the skin.
C. Topical retinoids
1. Tretinoin (Retin-A, Avita)
   a. A derivative of vitamin A (vitamin A supplements should be discontinued during therapy)
   b. In addition to treating acne, it may be prescribed to reduce fine wrinkles, skin roughness, mottled hyperpigmentation such as those that occur with age spots (tretinoin [Renova]).
   c. Can cause localized side effects such as blistering, peeling, crusting, burning, and swelling of the skin.
   d. The use of abrasive products and keratolytic products should be discontinued before using tretinoin because they can cause localized side effects.
   e. Medication sensitizes the skin to ultraviolet light (UVL); the client needs to be instructed to apply a sunscreen with a sun protection factor (SPF) of 15 or greater and to wear protective clothing when outdoors because the medication increases susceptibility to sunburn.
2. Adapalene (Differin): Similar to tretinoin and sensitizes the skin to UVL; side effects include burning and itching after application, redness, dryness, and scaling of the skin.
3. Tazarotene (Tazorac)
   a. Is a derivative of vitamin A (vitamin A supplements should be discontinued during therapy)
   b. In addition to acne, it is used to treat wrinkles and psoriasis.
   c. Can cause itching, burning, and dry skin and sensitizes the skin to UVL.
4. Azelaic acid (Azelex) can cause burning, itching, stinging, and redness of the skin; it can also cause hypopigmentation of the skin in clients with a dark complexion.
D. Oral antibiotics
1. Includes doxycycline (Vibramycin); minocycline (Dynacin, Minocin, Solodyn); tetracycline (Sumycin); and erythromycin (Ery-Tab)
2. Improvement develops slowly with the use of oral antibiotics and may take 3 to 6 months for some improvement to be noted; following control of symptoms the client is usually switched to a topical antibiotic.

E. Isotretinoin (Accutane)
1. Derivative of vitamin A (vitamin A supplements should be discontinued during therapy); additionally the use of tetracyclines can increase the risk of adverse effects and should be discontinued before use of isotretinoin
2. Used to treat severe cystic acne; reserved for persons who have not responded to other therapies, including systemic antibiotics
3. Side effects include nosebleeds; inflammation of the lips or eyes; dryness or itching of the skin, nose, or mouth; pain, tenderness, or stiffness in the joints, bones, or muscles; back pain.
4. Less common side effects include rash, hair loss, peeling of the skin, headache, reduction in night vision.
5. Causes sensitization of the skin to UVL
6. The medication elevates triglyceride levels, which should be measured before and during therapy; alcohol consumption should be eliminated during therapy because alcohol could potentiate elevation of serum triglyceride levels.
7. The medication may cause depression in some clients; if depression occurs, the medication should be discontinued.

⚠ Isotretinoin (Accutane) is highly teratogenic and can cause fetal abnormalities. It must not be used if the client is pregnant. The client needs to follow strict rules of the iPLEDGE Program.

F. Hormonal medications
1. Hormonal medications such as oral contraceptives and spironolactone (Aldactone) may be prescribed to treat acne in female clients.
2. These medications decrease androgen activity, resulting in decreased production of sebum (substance that combines with keratin to create a plug within a pore).
3. Spironolactone is teratogenic; therefore contraception during its use is necessary.
4. Adverse effects of spironolactone include breast tenderness, menstrual irregularities, and hyperkalemia.

G. iPLEDGE Program
1. A risk management program that ensures that no woman starting isotretinoin is pregnant or no woman taking this medication becomes pregnant
2. Access to the medication is controlled through a central automated system.
3. Strict rules must be followed by the client, physician prescribing the medication, pharmacist dispensing the medication, and the wholesaler of the medication to ensure safety and to ensure that no woman is pregnant on initiation of therapy or becomes pregnant while taking the medication.

Box 51-6 Burn Products

Mafenide acetate (Sulfamylon)
Nitrofurazone (Furacin)
Silver sulfadiazine (Silvadene)

VIII. BURN PRODUCTS (Box 51-6)

A. Nitrofurazone (Furacin)
1. Applied topically to the **burn** as a solution, ointment, or cream
2. Has a broad spectrum of antibacterial activity
3. Used for **burns** when bacterial resistance to other agents is a problem
4. Topical: Apply 1/16-inch film directly to **burn**.
5. Side effects: Contact dermatitis, rash
6. Less common side effects: Pruritus, local edema

B. Mafenide acetate (Sulfamylon)
1. Water-soluble cream that is bacteriostatic for gram-negative and gram-positive organisms
2. Used to treat **burns** to reduce the bacteria present in avascular tissues
3. Diffuses through the devascularized areas of the skin and may precipitate metabolic acidosis (usually compensated for by hyperventilation)
4. Apply 1/16-inch film directly to the **burn**.
5. Side effects can include local pain and rash.
6. Systemic effects include bone marrow depression, hemolytic anemia, and metabolic acidosis.
7. Keep **burn** covered with mafenide acetate at all times.
8. Notify physician if hyperventilation occurs; if acidosis develops, mafenide acetate is washed off the skin and is usually discontinued for 1 to 2 days.

C. Silver sulfadiazine (Silvadene, Thermazene, SSD Cream)
1. Has broad spectrum of activity against gram-negative bacteria, gram-positive bacteria, and yeast
2. Released slowly from the cream, which is selectively toxic to bacteria
3. Used primarily to prevent sepsis in clients with **burns**
4. Not a carbonic anhydrase inhibitor; does not cause acidosis
5. Apply 1/16-inch film (keep **burn** covered at all times with silver sulfadiazine).
6. Side effects include rash and itching.
7. Systemic effects include leukopenia and interstitial nephritis.
8. Monitor complete blood cell count, particularly the white blood cells, frequently; if leukopenia develops, the physician is notified (medication is usually discontinued).

MORE QUESTIONS ON THE CD!

Practice Questions

520. Salicylic acid is prescribed for a client with a diagnosis of psoriasis. The nurse monitors the client, knowing that which of the following would indicate the presence of systemic toxicity from this medication?
1. Tinnitus
2. Diarrhea
3. Constipation
4. Decreased respirations

521. The camp nurse asks the children preparing to swim in the lake if they have applied sunscreen. The nurse reminds the children that chemical sunscreens are most effective when applied:
1. Immediately before swimming
2. 15 minutes before exposure to the sun
3. Immediately before exposure to the sun
4. At least 30 minutes before exposure to the sun

522. Mafenide acetate (Sulfamylon) is prescribed for the client with a burn injury. When applying the medication, the client complains of local discomfort and burning. Which of the following is the most appropriate nursing action?
1. Notify the physician.
2. Discontinue the medication.
3. Inform the client that this is normal.
4. Apply a thinner film than prescribed to the burn site.

523. The burn client is receiving treatments of topical mafenide acetate (Sulfamylon) to the site of injury. The nurse monitors the client, knowing that which of the following indicates that a systemic effect has occurred?
1. Hyperventilation
2. Elevated blood pressure
3. Local pain at the burn site
4. Local rash at the burn site

524. Isotretinoin (Accutane) is prescribed for a client with severe acne. Before the administration of this medication, the nurse anticipates that which laboratory test will be prescribed?
1. Platelet count
2. Triglyceride level
3. Complete blood count
4. White blood cell count

525. A client with severe acne is seen in the clinic and the physician prescribes isotretinoin (Accutane). The nurse reviews the client's medication record

and would contact the physician if the client is taking which medication?
1. Vitamin A
2. Digoxin (Lanoxin)
3. Furosemide (Lasix)
4. Phenytoin (Dilantin)

526. The nurse is applying a topical corticosteroid to a client with eczema. The nurse would monitor for the potential for increased systemic absorption of the medication if the medication were being applied to which of the following body areas?
1. Back
2. Axilla
3. Soles of the feet
4. Palms of the hands

527. The clinic nurse is performing an admission assessment on a client. The nurse notes that the client is taking azelaic acid (Azelex). Because of the medication prescription, the nurse would suspect that the client is being treated for:
1. Acne
2. Eczema
3. Hair loss
4. Herpes simplex

528. The physician has prescribed silver sulfadiazine (Silvadene) for the client with a partial-thickness burn, which has cultured positive for gram-negative bacteria, and the nurse provides information to the client about the medication. Which statement made by the client indicates a lack of understanding about the treatments?
1. "The medication is an antibacterial."
2. "The medication will help heal the burn."
3. "The medication will permanently stain my skin."
4. "The medication should be applied directly to the wound."

Alternate Item Format: Multiple Response

529. The health education nurse provides instructions to a group of clients regarding measures that will assist in preventing skin cancer. Which instruction(s) should the nurse provide? **Select all that apply.**
- ❏ 1. Use sunscreen when participating in outdoor activities.
- ❏ 2. Wear a hat, opaque clothing, and sunglasses when in the sun.
- ❏ 3. Avoid sun exposure in the late afternoon and early evening hours.
- ❏ 4. Examine your body monthly for any lesions that may be suspicious.
- ❏ 5. Suncreen should be applied every 8 hours.

ANSWERS

520. 1

Rationale: Salicylic acid is absorbed readily through the skin, and systemic toxicity (salicylism) can result. Symptoms include tinnitus, dizziness, hyperpnea, and psychological disturbances. Constipation and diarrhea are not associated with salicylism.

Test-Taking Strategy: Use the process of elimination. Noting the name of the medication will assist in directing you to the correct option if you can recall the toxic effects that occur with acetylsalicylic acid (aspirin). Review the toxic effects of salicylic acid if you are unfamiliar with them.

Level of Cognitive Ability: Analyzing
Client Needs: Physiological Integrity
Integrated Process: Nursing Process—Assessment
Content Area: Pharmacology
Reference: Lehne, R. (2010). *Pharmacology for nursing care* (7th ed., p. 1228). St. Louis: Saunders.

521. 4

Rationale: Sunscreens are most effective when applied at least 30 minutes before exposure to the sun so that they can penetrate the skin. All sunscreens should be reapplied after swimming or sweating.

Test-Taking Strategy: Use the process of elimination. Knowledge that sunscreens need to penetrate the skin will assist in eliminating options 2 and 3. Noting the strategic words *most effective* will assist in directing you to option 4. Review protective skin measures if you had difficulty with this question.

Level of Cognitive Ability: Applying
Client Needs: Physiological Integrity
Integrated Process: Teaching and Learning
Content Area: Pharmacology
Reference: Kee, J., Hayes, E., & McCuistion, L. (2009). *Pharmacology: A nursing process approach* (6th ed., p. 765). St. Louis: Saunders.

522. 3

Rationale: Mafenide acetate is bacteriostatic for gram-negative and gram-positive organisms and is used to treat burns to reduce bacteria present in avascular tissues. The client should be informed that the medication will cause local discomfort and burning and that this is a normal reaction. Therefore options 1, 2, and 4 are incorrect

Test-Taking Strategy: Use the process of elimination. Eliminate options 2 and 4 because it is not within the scope of nursing practice to alter or discontinue a medication therapy. Recalling that this is a normal expected occurrence will direct you to option 3. If you had difficulty with this question, review the effects of this medication.

Level of Cognitive Ability: Applying
Client Needs: Physiological Integrity
Integrated Process: Nursing Process—Implementation
Content Area: Pharmacology
Reference: Kee, J., Hayes, E., & McCuistion, L. (2009). *Pharmacology: A nursing process approach* (6th ed., p. 765). St. Louis: Saunders.

523. 1

Rationale: Mafenide acetate is a carbonic anhydrase inhibitor and can suppress renal excretion of acid, thereby causing acidosis. Clients receiving this treatment should be monitored for signs of an acid-base imbalance (hyperventilation). If this occurs, the medication will probably be discontinued for 1 to 2 days. Options 3 and 4 describe local rather than systemic effects. An elevated blood pressure may be expected from the pain that occurs with a burn injury.

Test-Taking Strategy: Use the process of elimination. Note the strategic words *systemic effect*. Options 3 and 4 can be eliminated because these are local rather than systemic effects. From the remaining options, recall that the client in pain would likely have an elevated blood pressure. This should direct you to option 1. Review the systemic effects of this medication if you had difficulty with this question.

Level of Cognitive Ability: Analyzing
Client Needs: Physiological Integrity
Integrated Process: Nursing Process—Assessment
Content Area: Pharmacology
Reference: Kee, J., Hayes, E., & McCuistion, L. (2009). *Pharmacology: A nursing process approach* (6th ed., p. 765). St. Louis: Saunders.

524. 2

Rationale: Isotretinoin can elevate triglyceride levels. Blood triglyceride levels should be measured before treatment and periodically thereafter until the effect on the triglycerides has been evaluated. Options 1, 3, and 4 do not need to be monitored specifically during this treatment.

Test-Taking Strategy: Use the process of elimination. Eliminate options 3 and 4 first because a complete blood count also measures the white blood cell count. From the remaining options, recall that the medication can affect triglyceride levels in the client. Review this medication if you had difficulty with this question

Level of Cognitive Ability: Analyzing
Client Needs: Physiological Integrity
Integrated Process: Nursing Process—Assessment
Content Area: Pharmacology
Reference: Lehne, R. (2010). *Pharmacology for nursing care* (7th ed., p. 1232). St. Louis: Saunders.

525. 1

Rationale: Isotretinoin is a metabolite of vitamin A and can produce generalized intensification of isotretinoin toxicity. Because of the potential for increased toxicity, vitamin A supplements should be discontinued before isotretinoin therapy. Options 2, 3, and 4 are not contraindicated with the use of isotretinoin.

Test-Taking Strategy: Use the process of elimination. Recalling that isotretinoin is a metabolite of vitamin A will direct you to the correct option. If you are unfamiliar with this medication, review the contraindications associated with its use.

Level of Cognitive Ability: Analyzing
Client Needs: Physiological Integrity
Integrated Process: Nursing Process—Implementation
Content Area: Pharmacology
Reference: Lehne, R. (2010). *Pharmacology for nursing care* (7th ed., p. 1232). St. Louis: Saunders.

526. 2

Rationale: Topical corticosteroids can be absorbed into the systemic circulation. Absorption is higher from regions where the skin is especially permeable (scalp, axilla, face, eyelids,

neck, perineum, genitalia), and lower from regions where permeability is poor (back, palms, soles).
Test-Taking Strategy: Use the process of elimination. Focus on the subject of the question, permeability and the potential for increased systemic absorption. Eliminate options 3 and 4 because these body areas are comparable or alike in terms of skin substance. From the remaining options, think about permeability of the skin area. This should direct you to option 2. Review the principles related to the administration of topical corticosteroids if you had difficulty with this question.
Level of Cognitive Ability: Understanding
Client Needs: Physiological Integrity
Integrated Process: Nursing Process—Assessment
Content Area: Pharmacology
Reference: Black, J., & Hawks, J. (2009). *Medical-surgical nursing: Clinical management for positive outcomes* (8th ed., p. 1204). St. Louis: Saunders.

527. 1
Rationale: Azelaic acid is a topical medication used to treat mild to moderate acne. The acid appears to work by suppressing the growth of *Propionibacterium acnes* and by decreasing the proliferation of keratinocytes. Options 2, 3, and 4 are incorrect.
Test-Taking Strategy: Use the process of elimination. Focusing on the name of the medication, azelaic acid, will direct you to the correct option. Review this medication if you are unfamiliar with it.
Level of Cognitive Ability: Understanding
Client Needs: Physiological Integrity
Integrated Process: Nursing Process—Assessment
Content Area: Pharmacology
Reference: Lehne, R. (2010). *Pharmacology for nursing care* (7th ed., p. 1231). St. Louis: Saunders.

528. 3
Rationale: Silver sulfadiazine (Silvadene) is an antibacterial that has a broad spectrum of activity against gram-negative bacteria, gram-positive bacteria, and yeast. It is applied directly to the wound to assist in healing. It does not stain the skin.
Test-Taking Strategy: Note the strategic words *lack of understanding*. These words indicate a negative event query and ask you to select an option that is an incorrect statement. Recall the characteristics of this medication. Noting the words *permanently stain* in option 3 will direct you to this option. Review this medication if you had difficulty with this question.
Level of Cognitive Ability: Evaluating
Client Needs: Physiological Integrity
Integrated Process: Teaching and Learning
Content Area: Pharmacology
Reference: Lehne, R. (2010). *Pharmacology for nursing care* (7th ed., p. 1027). St. Louis: Saunders.

ALTERNATE ITEM FORMAT: MULTIPLE RESPONSE
529. 1, 2, 4
Rationale: The client should be instructed to avoid sun exposure between the hours of 10 AM and 4 PM. Sunscreen, a hat, opaque clothing, and sunglasses should be worn for outdoor activities. The client should be instructed to examine the body monthly for the appearance of any possible cancerous or any precancerous lesions. Sunscreen should be reapplied every 2 to 3 hours and after swimming or sweating; otherwise, the duration of protection is reduced.
Test-Taking Strategy: Focus on the subject, measures to prevent skin cancer. Read each option carefully. Noting the time frames in options 3 and 5 will assist in eliminating these options. Review client teaching points for the prevention of skin cancer if you had difficulty with this question.
Level of Cognitive Ability: Applying
Client Needs: Health Promotion and Maintenance
Integrated Process: Teaching and Learning
Content Area: Adult Health—Integumentary
Reference: Ignatavicius, D., & Workman, M. (2010). *Medical-surgical nursing: Patient-centered collaborative care* (6th ed., p. 511). St. Louis: Saunders.

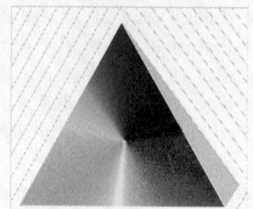

The Adult Client With an Oncological Disorder

PYRAMID TERMS

adenocarcinoma A tumor that arises from glandular epithelial tissue.

benign Usually refers to growths that are encapsulated, remain localized, and are slow growing.

cancer A neoplastic disorder that can involve all body organs. Cells lose their normal growth-controlling mechanism, and the growth of cells is uncontrolled.

carcinogen A physical, chemical, or biological stressor that causes neoplastic changes in normal cells.

carcinoma A new growth or malignant tumor that originates from epithelial cells, the skin, gastrointestinal tract, lungs, uterus, breast, or other organ.

carcinoma in situ A premalignant lesion with all the histological characteristics of cancer except invasion of the basement membrane.

hospice A concept of care for terminally ill clients that includes the idea of intensive caring rather than intensive care. The client and the family are the focus of nursing care, and the goal is to relieve pain and facilitate an optimal quality of life.

lymphoma Neoplasm that originates from lymphoid tissue.

leukemia or myeloma Neoplasm that originates from a blood-forming organ.

malignant Term for growths that are not encapsulated but grow and metastasize. These growths are cancerous lesions having the characteristics of disorderly, uncontrolled, and chaotically proliferating cells.

metastasis The transfer of disease from one organ or part to another not directly connected with it. Secondary malignant lesions, originating from the primary tumor, are located in anatomically distant places.

nadir The period of time during which an antineoplastic medication has its most profound effects on the bone marrow.

neoplasm An abnormal growth, which may be benign or malignant.

sarcoma Neoplasm that originates from muscle, bone, fat, the lymph system, or connective tissue.

staging A method of classifying malignancies based on the presence and extent of the tumor within the body.

tumor marker Specific bodily substances that seem to indicate tumor progression or regression.

undifferentiated cells Cells that have lost the capacity for specialized functions.

PYRAMID TO SUCCESS

Pyramid Points focus on treatment modalities related to an oncological disorder, such as pain management, internal and external radiation, and chemotherapy. Focus for oncological disorders includes disorders such as skin cancer; leukemia; breast cancer; testicular cancer; stomach, bowel, and pancreatic cancer; bladder cancer; prostate cancer; and lung cancer. Specific focus relates to the nursing care related to these treatment modalities and disorders, client adaptation, and the impact of the treatment on the disorder. Specifically, focus on the complications related to chemotherapy and the nursing measures required in monitoring for these complications and preventing life-threatening conditions, such as infection and bleeding.

CLIENT NEEDS

Safe and Effective Care Environment

Discussing oncology-related consultations and referrals
Ensuring advocacy related to the client's decisions
Ensuring ethical practice
Ensuring that advance directives are in the client's medical record

Establishing priorities

Handling hazardous and infectious materials related to radiation and chemotherapy safely

Implementing protective, standard, and other precautions

Maintaining medical and surgical asepsis

Preventing disease related to infection

Providing confidentiality regarding diagnosis

Providing informed consent for treatments and procedures

Upholding the client's rights

Health Promotion and Maintenance

Discussing expected body image changes related to chemotherapy and treatments

Providing the client and family instructions regarding home care

Providing instructions regarding monthly breast or testicular self-examinations

Respecting the client's lifestyle choices

Teaching about health promotion programs regarding risks for cancer

Teaching about health screening measures for cancer

Psychosocial Integrity

Assessing the client's ability to cope, adapt, and/or solve problems during illness or stressful events

Assisting the client and family to cope with the alteration in body image

Discussing end-of-life and grief and loss issues related to death and the dying process

Mobilizing appropriate support and resource systems

Promoting a positive environment to maintain optimal quality of life

Respecting religious and cultural preferences

Assessing the concerns of the client who survived cancer

Physiological Integrity

Administering blood and blood products

Caring for central venous access devices

Caring for the client receiving chemotherapy

Caring for the client receiving radiation therapy

Managing pain

Monitoring diagnostic tests and laboratory values, such as white blood cell and platelet counts

Monitoring for expected and unexpected responses to radiation and chemotherapy

Protecting the client from the life-threatening adverse effects of treatments

Providing basic care and comfort

Providing nutrition

52

Oncological Disorders

I. CANCER

A. Description
 1. **Cancer** is a neoplastic disorder that can involve all body organs with manifestations that vary according to the body system affected and type of tumor cells.
 2. Cells lose their normal growth-controlling mechanism, and the growth of cells is uncontrolled.
 3. **Cancer** produces serious health problems such as impaired immune and hematopoietic (blood-producing) function, altered gastrointestinal tract structure and function, motor and sensory deficits, and decreased respiratory function.

B. **Metastasis** (Box 52-1)
 1. **Cancer** cells move from their original location to other sites.
 2. Routes of **metastasis**
    a. Local seeding: Distribution of shed **cancer** cells occurs in the local area of the primary tumor.
    b. Bloodborne **metastasis**: Tumor cells enter the blood, which is the most common cause of cancer spread.
    c. Lymphatic spread: Primary sites rich in lymphatics are more susceptible to early metastatic spread.

C. **Cancer classification**
 1. Solid tumors: Associated with the organs from which they develop, such as breast **cancer** or lung **cancer**
 2. Hematological **cancers**: Originate from blood cell–forming tissues, such as **leukemias, lymphomas**, and multiple **myeloma**

D. Grading and **staging** (Box 52-2)
 1. Grading and **staging** are methods used to describe the tumor.
 2. These methods describe the extent of the tumor, the extent to which malignancy has increased in size, the involvement of regional nodes, and metastatic development.
 3. Grading a tumor classifies the cellular aspects of the cancer.
 4. **Staging** classifies the clinical aspects of the **cancer** and degree of **metastasis** at diagnosis.

E. Factors that influence **cancer** development
 1. Environmental factors
    a. Chemical **carcinogen**: Factors include industrial chemicals, drugs, and tobacco.
    b. Physical **carcinogen**: Factors include ionizing radiation (diagnostic and therapeutic x-rays) and ultraviolet radiation (sun, tanning beds, and germicidal lights), chronic irritation, and tissue trauma.
    c. Viral **carcinogen**: Viruses capable of causing **cancer** are known as oncoviruses, such as Epstein-Barr virus, hepatitis B virus, and human papillomavirus.
    d. *Helicobacter pylori* infection is associated with an increased risk of gastric **cancer**.
 2. Obesity and dietary factors including preservatives, contaminants, additives, and nitrates
 3. Genetic predisposition: Factors include an inherited predisposition to specific cancers, inherited conditions associated with **cancer**, familial clustering, and chromosomal aberrations.
 4. Age: Advancing age is a significant risk factor for the development of **cancer**.
 5. Immune function: The incidence of **cancer** is higher in immunosuppressed individuals, such as those with acquired immunodeficiency syndrome and organ transplant recipients who are taking immunosuppressive medications.

F. Prevention: Avoidance of known or potential carcinogens and avoidance or modification of the factors associated with the development of cancer cells

G. Early detection (Box 52-3)
 1. Mammography
 2. Papanicolaou's (Pap) test
 3. Stools for occult blood
 4. Sigmoidoscopy, colonoscopy
 5. Breast self-examination and clinical breast examination
 6. Testicular self-examination
 7. Skin inspection

II. BREAST SELF-EXAMINATION

A. Performing breast self-examination (BSE)

Box 52-1 Common Sites of Metastasis

Bladder Cancer
Lung
Bone
Liver
Pelvic, retroperitoneal
    structures

Brain Tumors
Central nervous system

Breast Cancer
Bone
Lung
Brain
Liver

Colorectal Cancer
Liver

Lung Cancer
Brain
Liver

Prostate Cancer
Bone
Spine
Lung
Liver
Kidneys

Testicular Cancer
Lung
Bone
Liver
Adrenal glands
Retroperitoneal lymph
    nodes

Box 52-2 Grading and Staging

Grading
Grade I: Cells differ slightly from normal cells and are well differentiated (mild dysplasia).
Grade II: Cells are more abnormal and are moderately differentiated (moderate dysplasia).
Grade III: Cells are very abnormal and are poorly differentiated (severe dysplasia).
Grade IV: Cells are immature (anaplasia) and undifferentiated; cell of origin is difficult to determine.

Staging
Stage 0: Carcinoma in situ
Stage I: Tumor limited to the tissue of origin; localized tumor growth
Stage II: Limited local spread
Stage III: Extensive local and regional spread
Stage IV: Distant metastasis

Box 52-3 Warning Signs of Cancer

Any sore that does not heal
Change in bowel or bladder habits
Indigestion
Nagging cough or hoarseness
Obvious change in wart or mole
Thickening or lump in breast or elsewhere
Unusual bleeding or discharge

1. Perform monthly 7 to 10 days after menses.
2. Postmenopausal clients or clients who have had a hysterectomy should select a specific day of the month and perform BSE monthly on that day.
B. Client instructions (Fig. 52-1)

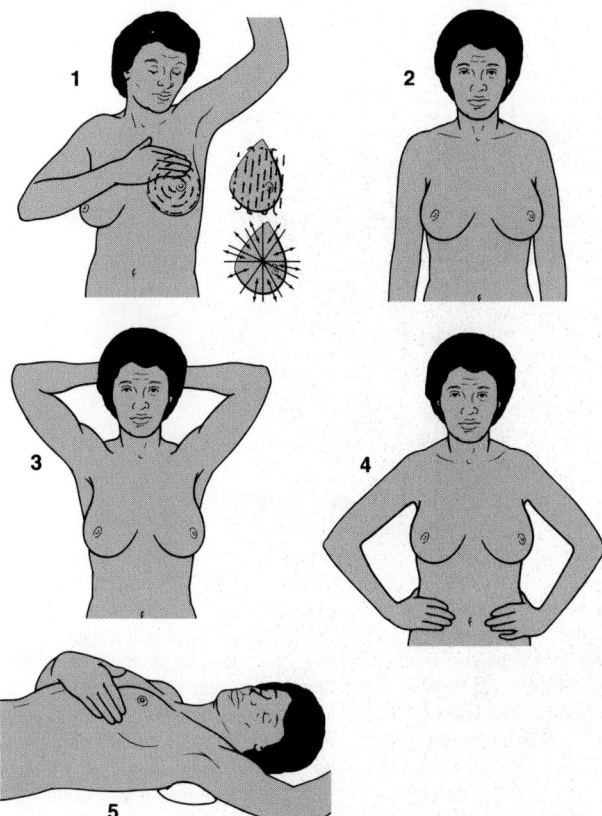

▲ **FIGURE 52-1** Breast self-examination and patient instruction. **1,** While in the shower or bath, when the skin is slippery with soap and water, examine your breasts. Use the pads of your second, third, and fourth fingers to press every part of the breast firmly. Use your right hand to examine your left breast, and use your left hand to examine your right breast. Using the pads of the fingers on your left hand, examine the entire right breast using small circular motions in a spiral or up-and-down motion so that the entire breast area is examined. Repeat the procedure using your right hand to examine your left breast. Repeat the pattern of palpation under the arm. Check for any lump, hard knot, or thickening of the tissue. **2,** Look at your breasts in a mirror. Stand with your arms at your side. **3,** Raise your arms overhead and check for any changes in the shape of your breasts, dimpling of the skin, or any changes in the nipple. **4,** Next, place your hands on your hips and press down firmly, tightening the pectoral muscles. Observe for asymmetry or changes, keeping in mind that your breasts probably do not match exactly. **5,** While lying down, feel your breasts as described in 1. When examining your right breast, place a folded towel under your right shoulder and put your right hand behind your head. Repeat the procedure while examining your left breast. Mark your calendar that you have completed your breast-self-examination; note any changes or unique characteristics you want to check with your health care provider. (From Lewis, S., Heitkemper, M., Dirksen, S., O'Brien, P., and Bucher, L. [2007]. *Medical-surgical nursing: Assessment and management of clinical problems* [7th ed.]. St. Louis: Mosby.)

III. TESTICULAR SELF-EXAMINATION

A. Performing testicular self-examination: Perform monthly; a day of the month is selected and the examination is performed on the same day each month.
B. Client instructions (Fig. 52-2)

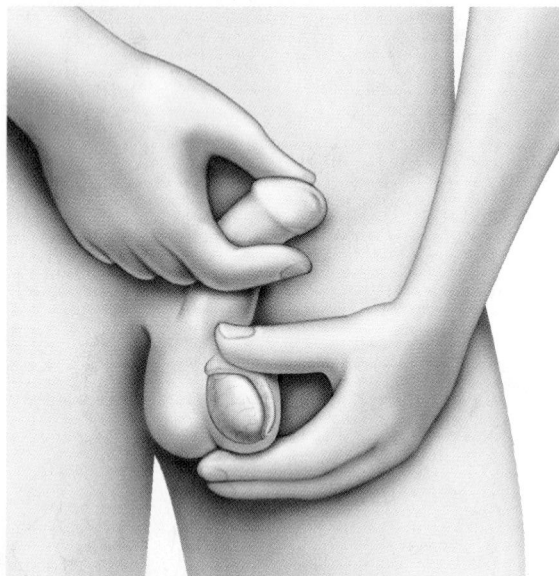

▲ **FIGURE 52-2** Testicular self-examination. The best time to perform this examination is right after a shower when your scrotal skin is moist and relaxed, making the testicles easy to feel. First, gently lift each testicle. Each one should feel like an egg, firm but not hard, and smooth with no lumps. Then, using both hands, place your middle fingers on the underside of each testicle and your thumbs on top. Gently roll the testicle between the thumb and fingers to feel for any lumps, swelling, or mass. If you notice any changes from one month to the next, notify your physician or nurse practitioner. (From Harkreader, H., & Hogan, M. A. [2007]. *Fundamentals of nursing: Caring and clinical judgment* [3rd ed.]. St. Louis: Saunders.)

Box 52-4 Diagnostic Tests

Biopsy
Bone marrow examination (particularly if a hematolymphoid malignancy is suspected)
Chest radiograph
Complete blood count (CBC)
Computed tomography (CT)
Cytological studies (Papanicolaou's smear)
Liver function studies
Magnetic resonance imaging (MRI)
Evaluation of serum tumor markers (e.g., carcinoembryonic antigen and alpha-fetoprotein)
Proctoscopic examination (including guaiac for occult blood)
Radiographic studies (mammography)
Radioisotope scanning (liver, brain, bone, lung)
Tumor markers

IV. DIAGNOSTIC TESTS

A. Diagnostic tests to be performed depend on the suspected primary or metastatic site of the **cancer**; invasive procedures require a signed informed consent (Box 52-4).

B. Biopsy
  1. Description
    a. Biopsy is the definitive means of diagnosing **cancer** and provides histological proof of malignancy.
    b. Biopsy involves the surgical incision of a small piece of tissue for microscopic examination.
  2. Types
    a. Needle: Aspiration of cells
    b. Incisional: Removal of a wedge of suspected tissue from a larger mass
    c. Excisional: Complete removal of the entire lesion
    d. **Staging**: Multiple needle or incisional biopsies in tissues where metastasis is suspected or likely (see Boxes 52-1 and 52-2)
  3. Tissue examination
    a. Following excision, a frozen section or a permanent paraffin section is prepared to examine the specimen.
    b. The advantage of the frozen section is the speed with which the section can be prepared and the diagnosis made, because only minutes are required for this test.
    c. Permanent paraffin section takes about 24 hours; however, it provides clearer details than the frozen section.
  4. Interventions
    a. The procedure usually is performed in an outpatient surgical setting.
    b. Prepare the client for the diagnostic procedure, and provide postprocedure instructions.
    c. Obtain an informed consent.

V. PAIN CONTROL

A. Causes of pain
  1. Bone destruction
  2. Obstruction of an organ
  3. Compression of peripheral nerves
  4. Infiltration, distention of tissue
  5. Inflammation, necrosis
  6. Psychological factors, such as fear or anxiety

B. Interventions
  1. Collaborate with other members of the health care team to develop a pain management program.
  2. Administer oral preparations if possible and if they provide adequate relief of pain; the transdermal route may also be prescribed.
  3. Mild or moderate pain may be treated with salicylates, acetaminophen (Tylenol), and nonsteroidal anti-inflammatory drugs (NSAIDs); drug-drug interactions occur with NSAIDs and anticoagulants, oral hypoglycemics, and antihypertensives.
  4. Severe pain is treated with opioids, such as codeine sulfate, morphine sulfate, methadone, and hydromorphone hydrochloride (Dilaudid). Neuropathic pain is treated with a variety of anticonvulsants and antidepressants, as well as opioids.

5. Subcutaneous injections and continuous intravenous (IV) infusions of opioids provide rapid pain control; equianalgesic comparison charts should be used when switching routes of administration of opioids.
6. Monitor vital signs and for side effects of medications.
7. Monitor for effectiveness of medications.
8. Provide nonpharmacological techniques of pain control, such as relaxation, guided imagery, biofeedback, massage, and heat-cold application.

⚠ Assess the client's pain; pain is what the client describes or says that it is. Do not undermedicate the cancer client who is in pain.

VI. SURGERY

A. Description: Surgery is indicated to diagnose, stage, and treat **cancer**.
B. Prophylactic surgery
  1. Prophylactic surgery is performed in clients with an existing premalignant condition or a known family history that strongly predisposes the person to the development of **cancer**.
  2. An attempt is made to remove the tissue or organ at risk and thus prevent the development of **cancer**.
C. Curative surgery: All gross and microscopic tumor is removed or destroyed.
D. Control (cytoreductive or "debulking") surgery
  1. Control surgery is a debulking procedure that consists of removing a large portion of a locally invasive tumor, such as advanced ovarian **cancer**.
  2. Surgery decreases the number of **cancer** cells; therefore, it may increase the chance that other therapies will be successful.
E. Palliative surgery
  1. Palliative surgery is performed to improve quality of life during the survival time.
  2. Palliative surgery is performed to reduce pain, relieve airway obstruction, relieve obstructions in the gastrointestinal or urinary tract, relieve pressure on the brain or spinal cord, prevent hemorrhage, remove infected or ulcerated tumors, or drain abscesses.
F. Reconstructive or rehabilitative surgery is performed to improve quality of life by restoring maximal function and appearance, such as breast reconstruction after mastectomy.
G. Side effects of surgery
  1. Loss or loss of function of a specific body part
  2. Reduced function as a result of organ loss
  3. Scarring or disfigurement
  4. Grieving about altered body image or imposed change in lifestyle

VII. CHEMOTHERAPY

A. Description
  1. Chemotherapy kills or inhibits the reproduction of neoplastic cells and kills normal cells.

2. The effects are systemic because chemotherapy is usually administered systemically.
3. Normal cells most profoundly affected include those of the skin, hair, and lining of the gastrointestinal tract, spermatocytes, and hematopoietic cells.
4. Cell cycle phase–specific medications affect cells only during a certain phase of the reproductive cycle, and cell cycle phase–nonspecific medications affect cells in any phase of the reproductive cycle.
5. Usually, several chemotherapy and biotherapy agents are used in combination (combination therapy) to increase the therapeutic response.
6. Combination chemotherapy is planned by the physician so that medications with overlapping toxicities and **nadirs** (the time during which bone marrow activity and white blood cell counts are at their lowest) at or near the same time are not administered; this will minimize immunosuppression.
7. Chemotherapy may be combined with other treatments, such as surgery and radiation.
8. The preferred route of administration is intravenously.
B. Common side effects include fatigue, alopecia, nausea and vomiting, mucositis, skin changes, and myelosuppression (neutropenia, anemia, and thrombocytopenia).
C. See Chapter 53 for information regarding the care of the client receiving chemotherapy.

VIII. RADIATION THERAPY

A. Description
  1. Radiation therapy destroys **cancer** cells, with minimal exposure of normal cells to the damaging effects of radiation; the damaged cells die or become unable to divide.
  2. Radiation therapy is effective on tissues directly within the path of the radiation beam.
  3. Side effects include local skin changes and irritation, alopecia (hair loss), fatigue (most common side effect of radiation), and altered taste sensation; the effects vary according to the site of treatment.
  4. External beam radiation (also called teletherapy) and brachytherapy are the types of radiation therapy most commonly used to treat **cancer**.
B. External beam radiation (teletherapy): the actual radiation source is external to the client.
  1. Instruct the client regarding self-care of the skin (Box 52-5).
  2. The client does not emit radiation and does not pose a hazard to anyone else.
C. Brachytherapy
  1. The radiation source comes into direct, continuous contact with tumor tissues for a specific time.
  2. The radiation source is within the client; for a period of time, the client emits radiation and can pose a hazard to others.

Box 52-5 Client Education Guide: Radiation Therapy for Cancer

Wash the irradiated area gently each day with warm water alone or with mild soap and water.

Use the hand rather than a washcloth to wash the area.

Rinse soap thoroughly from the skin.

Take care not to remove the markings that indicate exactly where the beam of radiation is to be focused.

Dry the irradiated area with patting motions rather than rubbing motions; use a clean, soft towel or cloth.

Use no powders, ointments, lotions, or creams on the skin at the radiation site unless they are prescribed by the radiologist.

Wear soft clothing over the skin at the radiation site.

Avoid wearing belts, buckles, straps or any type of clothing that binds or rubs the skin at the radiation site.

Avoid exposure of the irradiated area to the sun.

Avoid heat exposure.

Box 52-6 Care of the Client With a Sealed Radiation Source

Place the client in a private room with a private bath.

Place a caution sign on the client's door.

Organize nursing tasks to minimize exposure to the radiation source.

Nursing assignments to a client with a radiation implant should be rotated.

Limit time to 30 minutes per care provider per shift.

Wear a dosimeter film badge to measure radiation exposure.

Wear a lead shield to reduce the transmission of radiation.

A nurse should never care for more than one client with a radiation implant at one time.

Do not allow a pregnant nurse to care for the client.

Do not allow children younger than 16 years or a pregnant woman to visit the client.

Limit visitors to 30 minutes per day; visitors should be at least 6 feet from the source.

Save bed linens and dressings until the source is removed; then dispose of in the usual manner.

Other equipment can be removed from the room at any time.

3. Brachytherapy includes an unsealed source or a sealed source of radiation.
4. Unsealed radiation source
   a. Administration is via the oral or IV route or by instillation into body cavities.
   b. The source is not confined completely to one body area, and it enters body fluids and eventually is eliminated via various excreta, which are radioactive and harmful to others. Most of the source is eliminated from the body within 48 hours; then neither the client nor the excreta is radioactive or harmful.
5. Sealed radiation source (Box 52-6) (see Priority Nursing Actions)

▰▰▰▰▰ PRIORITY NURSING ACTIONS! ▰▰▰▰▰

Actions to Take If a Sealed Radiation Implant Becomes Dislodged

1. Encourage the client to lie still.
2. Use a long-handled forceps to retrieve the radioactive source.
3. Deposit the radioactive source in a lead container.
4. Contact the radiation oncologist.
5. Document the occurrence and the actions taken.

The client with a sealed radiation implant can emit radiation. Therefore the nurse and any other person who is in contact with the client needs to take special precautions to protect self from radiation exposure. In the event that a radiation source becomes dislodged, the nurse would first encourage the client to lie still until the radioactive source has been placed in a safe closed container. The nurse would never touch the dislodged radiation source with his or her hands and would use a long-handled forceps to place the source in the lead container that should be kept in the client's room. The nurse calls the radiation oncologist and then documents the occurrence and the actions taken. In the event that the radiation source cannot be located, the nurse ensures that no linens or other articles in the client's room are disposed of, prohibits visitors, and notifies the radiation oncologist.

Reference: Ignatavicius, D., & Workman, M. (2010). *Medical-surgical nursing: Patient-centered collaborative care* (6th ed., p. 420). St. Louis: Saunders.

   a. A sealed, temporary or permanent radiation source (solid implant) is implanted within the tumor target tissues.
   b. The client emits radiation while the implant is in place, but the excreta are not radioactive.
6. Removal of sealed radiation sources
   a. The client is no longer radioactive.
   b. Inform the client that cancer is not contagious.
   c. Inform the female client that she may resume sexual intercourse after 7 to 10 days if the implant was cervical or vaginal.
   d. Provide a douche, as prescribed, if the implant was placed into the cervix.
   e. Administer a ready-to-use saline enema if prescribed.
   f. Advise the client who had a cervical or vaginal implant to notify the physician if nausea, vomiting, diarrhea, frequent urination, vaginal or rectal bleeding, hematuria, foul-smelling vaginal discharge, abdominal pain or distention, or fever occurs.

IX. BONE MARROW TRANSPLANTATION

A. Description
1. Bone marrow transplantation (BMT) and peripheral blood stem cell transplantation (PBSCT) are procedures that replace stem cells

that have been destroyed by high doses of chemotherapy and/or radiation therapy.

2. BMT and PBSCT are most commonly used in the treatment of **leukemia** and **lymphoma**, but are also used to treat other cancers, such as neuroblastoma and multiple **myeloma**.

3. The goal of treatment is to rid the client of all leukemic or other **malignant** cells through treatment with high doses of chemotherapy and whole-body irradiation.

4. Because these treatments are damaging to bone marrow cells, without the replacement of blood-forming stem cell function through transplantation, the client would die of infection or hemorrhage.

B. Types of donor stem cells

1. Allogeneic: Stem cell donor is usually a sibling, parent with a similar tissue type, or a person who is not related to the client (unrelated donor).

2. Syngeneic: Stem cell is from an identical twin.

3. Autologous
   a. Autologous donation is the most common type.
   b. The client receives his or her own stem cells.
   c. Stem cells are harvested during disease remission and are stored frozen to be reinfused later.

C. Procedure

1. Harvest
   a. The stem cells used in PBSCT come from the bloodstream in a 4- to 6-hour process called *apheresis* or *leukapheresis* (the blood is removed through a central venous catheter and an apheresis machine removes the stem cells and returns the remainder of the blood to the donor).
   b. In BMT, marrow is harvested through multiple aspirations from the iliac crest to retrieve sufficient bone marrow for the transplant.
   c. Marrow is filtered for residual **cancer** cells.
   d. Allogeneic marrow is transfused immediately; autologous marrow is frozen for later use (cryopreservation).
   e. Harvesting is done before the initiation of the conditioning regimen.

2. Conditioning refers to an immunosuppression therapy regimen used to eradicate all **malignant** cells, provide a state of immunosuppression, and create space in the bone marrow for the engraftment of the new marrow.

3. Transplantation
   a. Stem cells are administered through the client's central line in a manner similar to that for a blood transfusion.
   b. Stem cells may be administered by IV infusion or by IV push directly into the central line.

4. Engraftment
   a. The transfused stem cells move to the marrow-forming sites of the recipient's bones.

   b. Engraftment occurs when the white blood cell, erythrocyte, and platelet counts begin to rise.
   c. When successful, the engraftment process takes 2 to 5 weeks.

D. Post-transplantation period: Infection, bleeding, or neutropenia and thrombocytopenia are major concerns until engraftment occurs.

 During the post-transplantation period, the client remains without any natural immunity until the donor stem cells begin to proliferate and engraftment occurs.

E. Complications

1. Failure to engraft: If the transplanted stem cells fail to engraft, the client will die unless another transplantation is attempted and is successful.

2. Graft-versus-host disease in allogeneic transplants
   a. Although the recipient cannot recognize the donated stem cells as foreign or non-self because of the total immunosuppression, the immune-competent cells of the donor recognize the recipient's cells as foreign and mount an immune offense against them.
   b. Graft-versus-host disease is managed with immunosuppressive agents cautiously to avoid suppressing the new immune system to the extent that the client becomes more susceptible to infection, or the transplanted cells stop engrafting.

3. Veno-occlusive disease
   a. The disease involves occlusion of the hepatic venules by thrombosis or phlebitis.
   b. Signs include right upper quadrant abdominal pain, jaundice, ascites, weight gain, and hepatomegaly.
   c. Early detection is critical because there is no known way to open the hepatic vessels.
   d. The client will be treated with fluids and supportive therapy.

X. SKIN CANCER (see Chapter 50)

XI. LEUKEMIA (Box 52-7)

A. Description

1. **Leukemias** are a group of hematological malignancies involving abnormal overproduction of leukocytes, usually at an immature stage, in the bone marrow.

2. The two major types of **leukemia** are lymphocytic (involving abnormal cells from the lymphoid pathway) and myelocytic or myelogenous (involving abnormal cells from the myeloid pathways).

3. **Leukemia** may be acute, with a sudden onset, or chronic, with a slow onset and persistent symptoms over a period of years.

Box 52-7 Classification of Leukemia

Acute Lymphocytic Leukemia
Mostly lymphoblasts present in bone marrow.
Age of onset is younger than 15 years.

Acute Myelogenous Leukemia
Mostly myeloblasts present in bone marrow.
Age of onset is between 15 and 39 years.

Chronic Myelogenous Leukemia
Mostly granulocytes present in bone marrow.
Age of onset is in the fourth decade.

Chronic Lymphocytic Leukemia
Mostly lymphocytes present in bone marrow.
Age of onset is after 50 years.

Box 52-8 Mouth Care for the Client With Mucositis

Inspect the mouth daily.
Offer complete mouth care before and after every meal and at bedtime.
Brush the teeth and tongue with a soft-bristled toothbrush or sponges.
Provide mouth rinses every 12 hours with the prescribed solution.
Administer topical anesthetic agents to mouth sores as prescribed.
Avoid the use of alcohol- or glycerin-based mouthwashes or swabs because they are irritating to the mucosa.
Offer soft foods that are cool to warm in temperature rather than foods that are hard or spicy.

4. **Leukemia** affects the bone marrow, causing anemia, leukopenia, the production of immature cells, thrombocytopenia, and a decline in immunity.
5. The cause is unknown and appears to involve gene damage of cells, leading to the transformation of cells from a normal state to a **malignant** state.
6. Risk factors include genetic, viral, immunological, and environmental factors and exposure to radiation, chemicals, and medications, such as previous chemotherapy.

B. Assessment
   1. Anorexia, fatigue, weakness, weight loss
   2. Anemia
   3. Overt bleeding (nosebleeds, gum bleeding, rectal bleeding, hematuria, increased menstrual flow) and occult bleeding (e.g., as detected in a fecal occult blood test)
   4. Ecchymosis, petechiae
   5. Prolonged bleeding after minor abrasions or lacerations
   6. Elevated temperature
   7. Enlarged lymph nodes, spleen, liver
   8. Palpitations, tachycardia, orthostatic hypotension
   9. Pallor and dyspnea on exertion
   10. Headache
   11. Bone pain and joint swelling
   12. Normal, elevated, or reduced white blood cell count
   13. Decreased hemoglobin and hematocrit levels
   14. Decreased platelet count
   15. Positive bone marrow biopsy identifying leukemic blast phase cells

C. Infection
   1. Infection can occur through autocontamination or cross-contamination. The WBC count may be extremely low during the period of greatest bone marrow depression, known as the *nadir*.
   2. Common sites of infection are the skin, respiratory tract, and gastrointestinal tract.
   3. Initiate protective isolation procedures.

4. Ensure frequent and thorough hand washing by the client, family, and health care providers.
5. Staff and visitors with known infections or exposure to communicable diseases should avoid contact with the client until risk of infectious spread has passed.
6. Use strict aseptic technique for all procedures.
7. Keep supplies for the client separate from supplies for other clients; keep frequently used equipment in the room for the client's use only.
8. Limit the number of staff entering the client's room; reducing the number of staff who come into contact with the client reduces the risk of cross-infection.
9. Maintain the client in a private room with the door closed.
10. Place the client in a room with high-efficiency particulate air filtration or a laminar airflow system if possible.
11. Reduce exposure to environmental organisms by thoroughly washing or eliminating fresh or raw fruits and vegetables (low-bacteria diet) from the diet; eliminate fresh flowers and live plants from the client's room and avoid leaving standing water in the client's room.
12. Be sure that the client's room is cleaned daily.
13. Assist the client with daily bathing, using an antimicrobial soap.
14. Assist the client to perform oral hygiene frequently.
15. Initiate a bowel program to prevent constipation and prevent rectal trauma.
16. Avoid invasive procedures such as injections, rectal temperatures, and urinary catheterization.
17. Change wound dressings daily, and inspect the wounds for redness, swelling, or drainage.
18. Assess the urine for cloudiness and other characteristics of infection.
19. Assess skin and oral mucous membranes for signs of infection (Box 52-8).

20. Auscultate lung sounds, and encourage the client to cough and deep-breathe.
21. Monitor temperature, pulse, respirations, blood pressure, and for pain.
22. Monitor white blood cell and neutrophil counts.
23. Notify the physician if signs of infection are present, and prepare to obtain specimens for culture of the blood, open lesions, urine, and sputum; chest radiograph may also be prescribed.
24. Administer prescribed antibiotic, antifungal, and antiviral medications.
25. Instruct the client to avoid crowds and those with infections.
26. Instruct the client about a low-bacteria diet.
27. Instruct the client to avoid activities that expose the client to infection, such as changing a pet's litter box or working with house plants or in the garden.
28. Instruct the client that neither they nor their household contacts should receive immunization with a live virus such as measles, mumps, rubella, polio, varicella, shingles, and some influenza, including H1N1 vaccine).

⚠ Infection is a major cause of death in the immunosuppressed client.

D. Bleeding
1. During the period of greatest bone marrow suppression (the **nadir**), the platelet count may be extremely low.
2. The client is at risk for bleeding when the platelet count falls below $50,000/mm^3$, and spontaneous bleeding frequently occurs when the platelet count is fewer than $20,000/mm^3$.
3. Clients with platelet counts lower than $20,000/mm^3$ may need a platelet transfusion.
4. For clients with anemia and fatigue, packed red blood cells may be prescribed.
5. Monitor laboratory values.
6. Examine the client for signs and symptoms of bleeding; examine all body fluids and excrement for the presence of blood.
7. Handle the client gently; use caution when taking blood pressures to prevent skin injury.
8. Monitor for signs of internal hemorrhage (e.g., pain, rapid and weak pulse, increased abdominal girth, and abdomen guarding).
9. Provide soft foods that are cool to warm to avoid oral mucosa damage.
10. Avoid injections, if possible, to prevent trauma to the skin and bleeding; apply firm and gentle pressure to a needle stick site for at least 5 minutes, or longer if needed.
11. Pad side rails and sharp corners of the bed and furniture.
12. Avoid rectal suppositories, enemas, and thermometers.
13. If the female client is menstruating, count the number of pads or tampons used.
14. Administer blood products as prescribed.
15. Instruct the client to use a soft toothbrush and avoid dental floss.
16. Instruct the client to use only an electric razor for shaving.
17. Instruct the client to avoid blowing the nose.
18. Discourage the client from engaging in activities involving the use of sharp objects; contact sports also need to be avoided.
19. Instruct the client to avoid using nonsteroidal anti-inflammatory drugs and products that contain aspirin.

E. Fatigue and nutrition
1. Assist the client in selecting a well-balanced diet.
2. Provide small, frequent meals (high calorie, high protein, high carbohydrate) that require little chewing to reduce energy expenditure at mealtimes.
3. Assist the client in self-care and mobility activities.
4. Allow adequate rest periods during care.
5. Do not perform activities unless they are essential; assist the client in scheduling important or pleasurable activities during periods of highest energy.
6. Administer blood products for anemia as prescribed.

F. Additional interventions
1. Chemotherapy
   a. Induction therapy is aimed at achieving a rapid, complete remission of all manifestations of the disease.
   b. Consolidation therapy is administered early in remission with the aim of cure.
   c. Maintenance therapy may be prescribed for months or years following successful induction and consolidation therapy; the aim is to maintain remission.
2. Administer antibiotic, antibacterial, antiviral, and antifungal medications as prescribed.
3. Administer colony-stimulating factors as prescribed.
4. Administer blood replacements as prescribed.
5. Maintain infection and bleeding precautions.
6. Prepare the client for transplantation if indicated.
7. Instruct the client in appropriate home care measures.
8. Provide psychosocial support and support services for home care.

XII. LYMPHOMA: HODGKIN'S DISEASE

A. Description
1. **Lymphomas**, classified as Hodgkin's and non-Hodgkin's depending on the cell type, are characterized by abnormal proliferation of lymphocytes.

2. Hodgkin's disease is a malignancy of the lymph nodes that originates in a single lymph node or a chain of nodes.
3. **Metastasis** occurs to other adjacent lymph structures and eventually invades nonlymphoid tissue.
4. The disease usually involves lymph nodes, tonsils, spleen, and bone marrow and is characterized by the presence of Reed-Sternberg cells in the nodes.
5. Possible causes include viral infections; clients treated with combination chemotherapy for Hodgkin's disease have a greater risk of developing acute **leukemia** and non-Hodgkin's **lymphoma**, among other secondary malignancies.
6. Prognosis depends on the stage of the disease.

B. Assessment
1. Fever
2. Malaise, fatigue, and weakness
3. Night sweats
4. Loss of appetite and significant weight loss
5. Anemia and thrombocytopenia
6. Enlarged lymph nodes, spleen, and liver
7. Positive biopsy of lymph nodes, with cervical nodes most often affected first
8. Presence of Reed-Sternberg cells in nodes
9. Positive computed tomography (CT) scan of the liver and spleen

C. Interventions
1. For earlier stages (stages I and II), without mediastinal node involvement, the treatment of choice is extensive external radiation of the involved lymph node regions.
2. With more extensive disease, radiation and multiagent chemotherapy are used.
3. Monitor for side effects related to chemotherapy or radiation therapy.
4. Monitor for signs of infection and bleeding.
5. Maintain infection and bleeding precautions.
6. Discuss the possibility of sterility with the male client receiving radiation, and inform the client of fertility options such as sperm banking.

XIII. MULTIPLE MYELOMA

A. Description
1. A **malignant** proliferation of plasma cells within the bone
2. An excessive number of abnormal plasma cells invade the bone marrow and ultimately destroy bone; invasion of the lymph nodes, spleen, and liver occurs.
3. The abnormal plasma cells produce an abnormal antibody (**myeloma** protein or the Bence Jones protein) found in the blood and urine.
4. Multiple **myeloma** causes decreased production of immunoglobulin and antibodies and increased levels of uric acid and calcium, which can lead to renal failure.
5. The disease typically develops slowly and the cause is unknown.

B. Assessment
1. Bone (skeletal) pain, especially in the ribs, spine, and pelvis
2. Weakness and fatigue
3. Recurrent infections
4. Anemia
5. Urinalysis shows Bence Jones proteinuria and elevated total serum protein level.
6. Osteoporosis (bone loss and the development of pathological fractures)
7. Thrombocytopenia and leukopenia
8. Elevated calcium and uric acid levels
9. Renal failure
10. Spinal cord compression and paraplegia
11. Bone marrow aspiration shows an abnormal number of immature plasma cells.

⚠ The client with multiple myeloma is at risk for pathological fractures. Therefore provide skeletal support during moving, turning, and ambulating and provide a hazard-free environment.

C. Interventions
1. Administer chemotherapy as prescribed.
2. Provide supportive care to control symptoms and prevent complications, especially bone fractures, hypercalcemia, renal failure, and infections.
3. Maintain neutropenic and bleeding precautions as necessary.
4. Monitor for signs of bleeding, infection, and skeletal fractures.
5. Encourage at least 2 L of fluids per day to offset potential problems associated with hypercalcemia, hyperuricemia, and proteinuria, and encourage additional fluid as indicated and tolerated.
6. Monitor for signs of renal failure.
7. Encourage ambulation to prevent renal problems and to slow down bone resorption.
8. Administer IV fluids and diuretics as prescribed to increase renal excretion of calcium.
9. Administer blood transfusions as prescribed for anemia.
10. Administer analgesics as prescribed and provide nonpharmacological therapies to control pain.
11. Administer antibiotics as prescribed for infection.
12. Prepare the client for local radiation therapy if prescribed.
13. Instruct the client in home care measures and the signs and symptoms of infection.
14. Administer bisphosphonate medications as prescribed to slow bone damage and reduce pain and risk of fractures.

XIV. TESTICULAR CANCER

A. Description
1. Testicular cancer arises from germinal epithelium from the sperm-producing germ cells or

Box 52-9 Types of Testicular Cancer

Germinal Tumors
Seminomas
Nonseminomas

Nongerminal Tumors
Interstitial cell tumors
Androblastoma

Box 52-10 Premalignant Cancers: Cervical Intraepithelial Neoplasia

Stage I: Mild dysplasia
Stage II: Moderate dysplasia
Stage III: Severe dysplasia to carcinoma in situ

from nongerminal epithelium from other structures in the testicles (Box 52-9).

2. Testicular cancer most often occurs between the ages of 15 and 40 years.

3. The cause of testicular **cancer** is unknown, but a history of undescended testicle (cryptorchidism) and genetic predisposition have been associated with testicular tumor development.

4. **Metastasis** occurs to the lung, liver, bone, and adrenal glands via the blood, and to the retroperitoneal lymph nodes via lymphatic channels.

B. Early detection: Perform monthly testicular self-examination (see Fig. 52-2)

C. Assessment
1. Painless testicular swelling occurs.
2. "Dragging" or "pulling" sensation is experienced in the scrotum.
3. Palpable lymphadenopathy, abdominal masses, and gynecomastia may indicate **metastasis**.
4. Late signs include back or bone pain and respiratory symptoms.

D. Interventions
1. Administer chemotherapy as prescribed.
2. Prepare the client for radiation therapy as prescribed.
3. Prepare the client for unilateral orchiectomy, if prescribed, for diagnosis and primary surgical management or radical orchiectomy (surgical removal of the affected testis, spermatic cord, and regional lymph nodes).
4. Prepare the client for retroperitoneal lymph node dissection, if prescribed, to stage the disease and reduce tumor volume so that chemotherapy and radiation therapy are more effective.
5. Discuss reproduction, sexuality, and fertility information and options with the client.
6. Identify reproductive options such as sperm storage, donor insemination, and adoption.

E. Postoperative interventions
1. Monitor for signs of bleeding and wound infection; antibiotics may be administered to prevent wound infection.
2. Monitor intake and output.
3. Provide and explain pain management methods; to reduce swelling in the first 48 hours, apply an ice pack with an intervening protective layer of cloth.
4. Notify the physician if chills, fever, increasing pain or tenderness at the incision site, or drainage from the incision occurs.

5. After the orchiectomy, instruct the client to avoid heavy lifting and strenuous activity for the length of time prescribed by the physician.

6. Instruct the client to perform a monthly testicular self-examination on the remaining testicle (see Fig. 52-2).

7. Inform the client that sutures will be removed approximately 7 to 10 days after surgery.

XV. **CERVICAL CANCER**

A. Description
1. Preinvasive **cancer** is limited to the cervix (Box 52-10).
2. Invasive **cancer** is in the cervix and other pelvic structures.
3. **Metastasis** usually is confined to the pelvis, but distant **metastasis** occurs through lymphatic spread.
4. Premalignant changes are described on a continuum from dysplasia, which is the earliest premalignancy change, to **carcinoma in situ**, the most advanced premalignant change.

B. Risk factors
1. Human papillomavirus (HPV) infection (vaccination against HPV is effective to avoid HPV infection, and thus cervical **cancer**)
2. Cigarette smoking, both active and passive
3. Reproductive behavior including early first intercourse (before age 17), multiple sex partners, or male partners with multiple sex partners.
4. Screening via regular gynecological examinations and Papanicolaou smear (Pap test), with treatment of precancerous abnormalities, decreases the incidence and mortality of cervical **cancer**.

C. Assessment
1. Painless vaginal postmenstrual and postcoital bleeding
2. Foul-smelling or serosanguineous vaginal discharge
3. Pelvic, lower back, leg, or groin pain
4. Anorexia and weight loss
5. Leakage of urine and feces from the vagina
6. Dysuria
7. Hematuria
8. Cytological changes on Pap test

D. Interventions (Box 52-11)

E. Laser therapy
1. Laser therapy is used when all boundaries of the lesion are visible during colposcopic examination.
2. Energy from the beam is absorbed by fluid in the tissues, causing them to vaporize.

Box 52-11 Treatment for Cervical Cancer

Nonsurgical
Chemotherapy
Cryosurgery
External radiation
Internal radiation implants (intracavitary)
Laser therapy

Surgical
Conization
Hysterectomy
Pelvic exenteration

Box 52-12 Types of Pelvic Exenteration

Anterior
Removal of the uterus, ovaries, fallopian tubes, vagina, bladder, urethra, and pelvic lymph nodes

Posterior
Removal of the uterus, ovaries, fallopian tubes, descending colon, rectum, and anal canal

Total
Combination of anterior and posterior

3. Minimal bleeding is associated with the procedure.
4. Slight vaginal discharge is expected following the procedure, and healing occurs in 6 to 12 weeks.

F. Cryosurgery
1. Cryosurgery involves freezing of the tissues using a probe, with subsequent necrosis and sloughing.
2. No anesthesia is required, although cramping may occur during the procedure.
3. A heavy watery discharge will occur for several weeks following the procedure.
4. Instruct the client to avoid intercourse and the use of tampons while the discharge is present.

G. Conization
1. A cone-shaped area of the cervix is removed.
2. Conization allows the woman to retain reproductive capacity.
3. Long-term follow-up care is needed because new lesions can develop.
4. The risks of the procedure include hemorrhage, uterine perforation, incompetent cervix, cervical stenosis, and preterm labor in future pregnancies.

H. Hysterectomy
1. Description
   a. Hysterectomy is performed for microinvasive cancer if childbearing is not desired.
   b. A vaginal approach is most commonly used.
   c. A radical hysterectomy and bilateral lymph node dissection may be performed for **cancer** that has spread beyond the cervix but not to the pelvic wall.
2. Postoperative interventions
   a. Monitor vital signs
   b. Assist with coughing and deep-breathing exercises.
   c. Assist with range-of-motion exercises and provide early ambulation.
   d. Apply antiembolism stockings or sequential compression devices as prescribed.
   e. Monitor intake and output, Foley catheter drainage, and hydration status.
   f. Monitor bowel sounds.
   g. Assess incision site for signs of infection.

   h. Administer pain medication as prescribed.
   i. Instruct the client to limit stair climbing for 1 month as prescribed and to avoid tub baths and sitting for long periods.
   j. Avoid strenuous activity or lifting anything weighing more than 20 pounds.
   k. Instruct the client to consume foods that promote tissue healing.
   l. Instruct the client to avoid sexual intercourse for 3 to 6 weeks as prescribed.
   m. Instruct the client in the signs associated with complications.

Monitor vaginal bleeding following hysterectomy. More than one saturated pad per hour may indicate excessive bleeding.

I. Pelvic exenteration (Box 52-12)
1. Description
   a. Pelvic exenteration, the removal of all pelvic contents, including bowel, vagina, and bladder, is a radical surgical procedure performed for recurrent **cancer** if no evidence of tumor outside the pelvis and no lymph node involvement exist.
   b. When the bladder is removed, an ileal conduit is created and located on the right side of the abdomen to divert urine.
   c. A colostomy may need to be created on the left side of the abdomen for the passage of feces.
2. Postoperative interventions
   a. Similar to postoperative interventions following hysterectomy.
   b. Monitor for signs of altered respiratory status.
   c. Monitor incision site for infection.
   d. Monitor intake and output and for signs of dehydration.
   e. Monitor for hemorrhage, shock, and deep vein thrombosis.
   f. Apply antiembolism stockings or sequential compression devices as prescribed.
   g. Administer prophylactic heparin as prescribed.
   h. Administer perineal irrigations and sitz baths as prescribed.

i. Instruct the client to avoid strenuous activity for 6 months.

j. Instruct the client that the perineal opening, if present, may drain for several months.

k. Instruct the client in the care of the ileal conduit and colostomy, if created.

l. Provide sexual counseling because vaginal intercourse is not possible after anterior and total pelvic exenteration.

XVI. OVARIAN CANCER

A. Description
1. Ovarian **cancer** grows rapidly, spreads fast, and is often bilateral.
2. **Metastasis** occurs by direct spread to the organs in the pelvis, by distal spread through lymphatic drainage, or by peritoneal seeding.
3. In its early stages, ovarian **cancer** is often asymptomatic; because most women are diagnosed in advanced stages, ovarian **cancer** has more deaths than any other **cancer** of the female reproductive system, particularly white women between 55 and 65 years of age of North American or European descent.
4. An exploratory laparotomy is performed to diagnose and stage the tumor.

B. Assessment
1. Abdominal discomfort or swelling
2. Gastrointestinal disturbances
3. Dysfunctional vaginal bleeding
4. Abdominal mass
5. Elevated **tumor marker** (CA-125)

C. Interventions
1. External radiation may be used if the tumor has invaded other organs; intraperitoneal radioisotopes may be instilled for stage I disease.
2. Chemotherapy is used postoperatively for most stages of ovarian **cancer**.
3. Intraperitoneal chemotherapy involves the instillation of chemotherapy into the abdominal cavity.
4. Total abdominal hysterectomy and bilateral salpingo-oophorectomy with tumor debulking may be necessary.

XVII. ENDOMETRIAL (UTERINE) CANCER

A. Description
1. Endometrial **cancer** is a slow-growing tumor arising from the endometrial mucosa of the uterus, associated with the menopausal years.
2. **Metastasis** occurs through the lymphatic system to the ovaries and pelvis, via the blood to the lungs, liver, and bone, or intra-abdominally to the peritoneal cavity.

B. Risk factors
1. Use of estrogen replacement therapy (ERT)
2. Nulliparity
3. Polycystic ovary disease

4. Increased age
5. Late menopause
6. Family history of uterine **cancer** or hereditary nonpolyposis colorectal **cancer**
7. Obesity
8. Hypertension
9. Diabetes mellitus

C. Assessment
1. Abnormal bleeding, especially in postmenopausal women
2. Vaginal discharge
3. Low back, pelvic, or abdominal pain (pain occurs late in the disease process)
4. Enlarged uterus (in advanced stages)

D. Nonsurgical interventions
1. External or internal radiation is used alone or in combination with surgery, depending on the stage of **cancer**.
2. Chemotherapy is used to treat advanced or recurrent disease.
3. Progestational therapy with medication may be prescribed for estrogen-dependent tumors.
4. Tamoxifen (Nolvadex), an antiestrogen medication, also may be prescribed.

E. Surgical interventions: Total abdominal hysterectomy and bilateral salpingo-oophorectomy

XVIII. BREAST CANCER

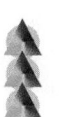

A. Description
1. Breast **cancer** is classified as invasive when it penetrates the tissue surrounding the mammary duct and grows in an irregular pattern.
2. **Metastasis** occurs via lymph nodes.
3. Common sites of **metastasis** are the bone and lungs; **metastasis** may also occur to the brain and liver.
4. Diagnosis is made by breast biopsy through a needle aspiration or by surgical removal of the tumor with microscopic examination for **malignant** cells.

B. Risk factors
1. Age
2. Family history of breast cancer
3. Early menarche and late menopause
4. Previous **cancer** of the breast, uterus, or ovaries
5. Nulliparity, late first birth
6. Obesity
7. High-dose radiation exposure to chest

C. Assessment
1. Mass felt during BSE
2. Mass usually felt in the upper outer quadrant, beneath the nipple, or in axilla
3. A fixed, irregular nonencapsulated mass; typically painless except in the late stages
4. Nipple retraction or elevation
5. Asymmetry, with the affected breast being higher
6. Bloody or clear nipple discharge
7. Skin dimpling, retraction, or ulceration

8. Skin edema or peau d'orange skin
9. Axillary lymphadenopathy
10. Lymphedema of the affected arm
11. Symptoms of bone or lung **metastasis** in late stage
12. Presence of the lesion on mammography
   D. Early detection: Monthly BSE
   E. Nonsurgical interventions
1. Chemotherapy
2. Radiation therapy
3. Hormonal manipulation via the use of medication in postmenopausal women or other medications for estrogen receptor–positive tumors
   F. Surgical interventions: Surgical breast procedures, with possible breast reconstruction (Box 52-13)
   G. Postoperative interventions
1. Monitor vital signs.
2. Position the client in a semi-Fowler's position; turn from the back to the unaffected side, with the affected arm elevated above the level of the heart to promote drainage and prevent lymphedema.
3. Encourage coughing and deep breathing.
4. If a drain (usually a Jackson-Pratt) is in place, maintain suction and record the amount of drainage and drainage characteristics; teach the client about home management of the drain (Fig. 52-3).
5. Assess operative site for infection, swelling, or the presence of fluid collection under the skin flaps or in the arm.
6. Monitor incision site for restriction of dressing, impaired sensation, or color changes of the skin.
7. If breast reconstruction was performed, the client will return from surgery with a surgical brassiere and a prosthesis in place.
8. Provide the use of a pressure sleeve as prescribed if edema is severe.
9. Maintain fluid and electrolyte balance; administer diuretics and provide a low-salt diet as prescribed for severe lymphedema.

10. Consult with the physician and physical therapist regarding the appropriate exercise program and assist client with prescribed exercise.
11. Instruct the client about home care measures (Box 52-14).

⚠ No IVs, no injections, no blood pressure measurements, and no venipunctures should be done in the arm on the side of the mastectomy. The arm on the side of the mastectomy is protected, and any intervention that could traumatize the affected arm is avoided.

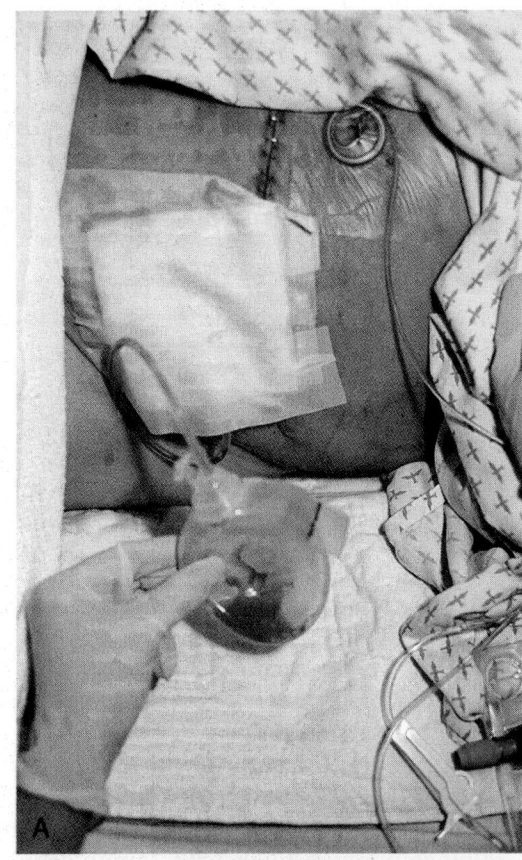

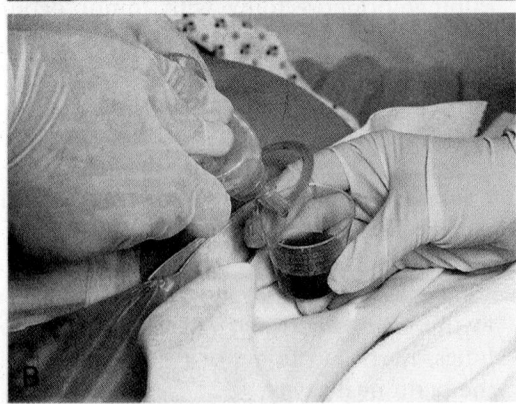

▲ **FIGURE 52-3** Jackson-Pratt device. **A,** Drainage tubes and reservoir. **B,** Emptying drainage reservoir. (From Potter, P., & Perry, A. [2009]. *Fundamentals of nursing* [7th ed.]. St. Louis: Mosby.)

Box 52-13 Surgical Breast Procedures

Lumpectomy
Tumor is excised and removed.
Lymph node dissection may also be performed.

Simple Mastectomy
Breast tissue and the nipple are removed.
Lymph nodes are usually left intact.

Modified Radical Mastectomy
Breast tissue, nipple, and lymph nodes are removed.
Muscles are left intact.

XIX. GASTRIC CANCER

A. Description
1. Gastric **cancer** is a **malignant** growth of the mucosal cells in the inner lining of the stomach, with invasion to the muscle and beyond in advanced disease.
2. No single causative agent has been identified but it is believed that *Helicobacter pylori* infection and a diet of smoked, highly salted, processed, or spiced foods have carcinogenic effects; other risk factors include smoking, alcohol and nitrate ingestion, and a history of gastric ulcers.
3. Complications include hemorrhage, obstruction, **metastasis**, and dumping syndrome.
4. The goal of treatment is to remove the tumor and provide a nutritional program.

B. Assessment
1. Early symptoms of gastric **cancer**
   a. Indigestion
   b. Abdominal discomfort
   c. Full feeling
   d. Epigastric, back, or retrosternal pain
2. Late symptoms of gastric **cancer**
   a. Weakness and fatigue
   b. Anorexia and weight loss
   c. Nausea and vomiting
   d. A sensation of pressure in the stomach
   e. Dysphagia and obstructive symptoms
   f. Iron deficiency anemia
   g. Ascites
   h. Palpable epigastric mass

C. Interventions
1. Monitor vital signs.
2. Monitor hemoglobin and hematocrit and administer blood transfusions as prescribed.
3. Monitor weight.
4. Assess nutritional status; encourage small, bland, easily digestible meals with vitamin and mineral supplements.
5. Administer pain medication as prescribed.
6. Prepare the client for chemotherapy or radiation therapy as prescribed.
7. Prepare the client for surgical resection of the tumor as prescribed (Box 52-15).

D. Postoperative interventions
1. Monitor vital signs.
2. Place in Fowler's position for comfort.
3. Administer analgesics, antiemetics, as prescribed.
4. Monitor intake and output; administer fluids and electrolyte replacement by IV as prescribed; administer parenteral nutrition as indicated.
5. Maintain NPO status as prescribed for 1 to 3 days until peristalsis returns; assess for bowel sounds.
6. Monitor nasogastric suction.
7. Do not irrigate or remove the nasogastric tube (follow agency procedures); assist the physician with irrigation or removal.
8. Advance the diet from NPO to sips of clear water to six small bland meals a day, as prescribed.
9. Monitor for complications such as hemorrhage, dumping syndrome, diarrhea, hypoglycemia, and vitamin B_{12} deficiency.

XX. PANCREATIC CANCER

A. Description
1. Most pancreatic tumors are highly **malignant**, rapidly growing **adenocarcinomas** originating from the epithelium of the ductal system.

Box 52-14 Client Instructions Following Mastectomy

Avoid overuse of the arm during the first few months.
To prevent lymphedema, keep the affected arm elevated; consultation with lymphedema specialist may be prescribed.
Provide incision care with an emollient to soften and prevent wound contracture.
Encourage use of Reach for Recovery volunteers.
Encourage the client to perform breast self-examination on the remaining breast.
Protect the affected hand and arm.
Avoid strong sunlight on the affected arm.
Do not let the affected arm hang dependent.
Do not carry a pocketbook or anything heavy over the affected arm.
Avoid trauma, cuts, bruises, or burns to the affected side.
Avoid wearing constricting clothing or jewelry on the affected side.
Wear gloves when gardening.
Use thick oven mitts when cooking.
Use a thimble when sewing.
Apply hand cream several times daily.
Use cream cuticle remover.
Call the physician if signs of inflammation occur in the affected arm.
Wear a Medic-Alert bracelet stating which arm is lymphedematous.

Box 52-15 Surgical Interventions for Gastric Cancer

Subtotal Gastrectomy

Billroth I
Also called gastroduodenostomy
Partial gastrectomy, with remaining segment anastomosed to the duodenum

Billroth II
Also called gastrojejunostomy
Partial gastrectomy, with remaining segment anastomosed to the jejunum

Total Gastrectomy
Also called esophagojejunostomy
Removal of the stomach, with attachment of the esophagus to the jejunum or duodenum

2. Pancreatic **cancer** is associated with increased age, a history of diabetes mellitus, alcohol use, history of previous pancreatitis, smoking, ingestion of a high-fat diet, and exposure to environmental chemicals.

3. Symptoms usually do not occur until the tumor is large; therefore, the prognosis is poor.

4. Endoscopic retrograde cholangiopancreatography for visualization of the pancreatic duct and biliary system and collection of tissue and secretions may be done.

B. Assessment
1. Nausea and vomiting
2. Jaundice
3. Unexplained weight loss
4. Clay-colored stools
5. Glucose intolerance
6. Abdominal pain

C. Interventions
1. Radiation
2. Chemotherapy
3. Whipple procedure, which involves a pancreaticoduodenectomy with removal of the distal third of the stomach, pancreaticojejunostomy, gastrojejunostomy, and choledochojejunostomy (Fig. 52-4)
4. Postoperative care measures and complications are similar to those for the care of a client with pancreatitis and the client following gastric surgery; monitor blood glucose levels for transient hyperglycemia or hypoglycemia resulting from surgical manipulation of the pancreas.

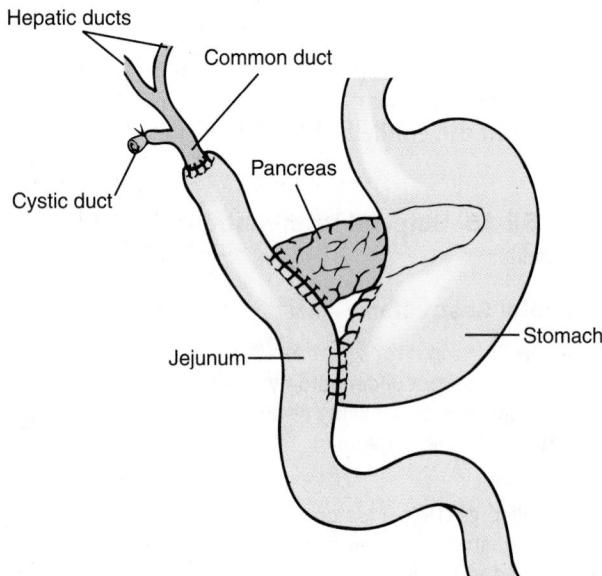

▲ **FIGURE 52-4** Whipple procedure, or radical pancreatico-duodenectomy. (From Lewis, S., Heitkemper, M., Dirksen, S., O'Brien, P., and Bucher, L. [2007]. *Medical-surgical nursing: Assessment and management of clinical problems* [7th ed.]. St. Louis: Mosby.)

XXI. INTESTINAL TUMORS

A. Description
1. Intestinal tumors are **malignant** lesions that develop in the cells lining the bowel wall or develop as adenomatous polyps in the colon or rectum.
2. Tumors spread is by direct invasion and through the lymphatic and circulatory systems.
3. Complications include bowel perforation with peritonitis, abscess and fistula formation, hemorrhage, and complete intestinal obstruction.

B. Risk factors for colorectal cancer
1. Age older than 50 years
2. Familial polyposis, family history of colorectal **cancer**
3. Previous colorectal polyps, history of colorectal **cancer**
4. History of chronic inflammatory bowel disease
5. History of ovarian or breast **cancer**

C. Assessment
1. Blood in stool (most common manifestation)
2. Anorexia, vomiting, and weight loss
3. Anemia
4. Abnormal stools
   a. Ascending colon tumor: Diarrhea
   b. Descending colon tumor: Constipation or some diarrhea, or flat, ribbon-like stool caused by a partial obstruction
   c. Rectal tumor: Alternating constipation and diarrhea
5. Guarding or abdominal distention, abdominal mass (late sign)
6. Cachexia (late sign)
7. Masses noted on barium enema, colonoscopy, CT scan, sigmoidoscopy

D. General interventions
1. Monitor for signs of complications, which include bowel perforation with peritonitis, abscess or fistula formation (fever associated with pain), hemorrhage (signs of shock), and complete intestinal obstruction.
2. Monitor for signs of bowel perforation, which include low blood pressure, rapid and weak pulse, distended abdomen, and elevated temperature.
3. Monitor for signs of intestinal obstruction, which include vomiting (may be fecal contents), pain, constipation, and abdominal distention; provide comfort measures.
4. Note that an early sign of intestinal obstruction is increased peristaltic activity, which produces an increase in bowel sounds; as the obstruction progresses, hypoactive bowel sounds may be heard.
5. Prepare for radiation preoperatively to facilitate surgical resection, and postoperatively to decrease the risk of recurrence or to reduce pain, hemorrhage, bowel obstruction, or **metastasis**.

E. Nonsurgical interventions
1. Preoperative radiation for local control and postoperative radiation for palliation may be prescribed.
2. Postoperative chemotherapy to control symptoms and the spread of disease
F. Surgical interventions: Bowel, local lymph node resection and creation of a colostomy or ileostomy
G. Colostomy, ileostomy
1. Preoperative interventions
   a. Consult with the enterostomal therapist to assist in identifying optimal placement of the ostomy.
   b. Instruct the client to eat a low-fiber diet for 1 to 2 days before surgery and administer bowel preparation (laxatives and enemas), as prescribed.
   c. Administer intestinal antiseptics and antibiotics, as prescribed, to decrease the bacterial content of the colon and to reduce the risk of infection from the surgical procedure.
2. Postoperative: Colostomy
   a. If a pouch system is not in place, apply a petroleum jelly gauze over the stoma to keep it moist, covered with a dry sterile dressing; place a pouch system on the stoma as soon as possible.
   b. Monitor the pouch system for proper fit and signs of leakage; empty the pouch when one-third full.
   c. Monitor the stoma for size, unusual bleeding, color changes, or necrotic tissue.
   d. Note that the normal stoma color is red or pink, indicating high vascularity.
   e. Note that a pale pink stoma indicates low hemoglobin and hematocrit levels.
   f. Assess the functioning of the colostomy.
   g. Expect that stool will be liquid postoperatively but will become more solid, depending on the area of the colostomy.
   h. Expect liquid stool from an ascending colon colostomy, loose to semiformed stool from a transverse colon colostomy, or close to normal stool from a descending colon colostomy.
   i. Fecal matter should not be allowed to remain on the skin.
   j. Administer analgesics and antibiotics as prescribed.
   k. Irrigate perineal wound if present and if prescribed, and monitor for signs of infection; provide comfort measures for perineal itching and pain.
   l. Instruct the client to avoid foods that cause excessive gas formation and odor.
   m. Instruct the client in stoma care and irrigations as prescribed.
   n. Instruct the client on how to resume normal activities, including work, travel, and sexual

intercourse, as prescribed; provide psychosocial support.
3. Postoperative: Ileostomy
   a. Healthy stoma is red; a color change to dark blue or black should be reported to the physician.
   b. Postoperative drainage will be dark green and progress to yellow as the client begins to eat.
   c. Stool is liquid.
   d. Risk for dehydration and electrolyte imbalance exists.
   e. Do not administer medications such as suppositories through an ileostomy.

⚠ Monitor stoma color. A dark blue, purple, or black stoma indicates compromised circulation, requiring physician notification.

XXII. LUNG CANCER

A. Description
1. Lung **cancer**, **malignant** tumor of the bronchi and peripheral lung tissue, is one of the leading causes of **cancer**-related deaths in men and women in the United States.
2. The lungs are a common target for **metastasis** from other organs.
3. Bronchogenic **cancer** (tumors originate in the epithelium of the bronchus) spreads through direct extension and lymphatic dissemination.
4. Classified according to histological cell type, there are two main types of lung **cancer**, small cell lung **cancer** (SCLC) and non–small cell lung **cancer** (NSCLC); epidermal (squamous cell), **adenocarcinoma**, and large cell anaplastic **carcinoma** are classified as NSCLC because of their similar responses to treatment.
5. Diagnosis is made by a chest x-ray study, CT scan, or magnetic resonance imaging (MRI), which shows a lesion or mass, and by bronchoscopy and sputum studies, which demonstrate a positive cytological study for **cancer** cells.
B. Causes
1. Cigarette smoking, also exposure to "passive" tobacco smoke
2. Exposure to environmental and occupational pollutants
C. Assessment
1. Cough
2. Wheezing, dyspnea
3. Hoarseness
4. Hemoptysis, blood-tinged or purulent sputum
5. Chest pain
6. Anorexia and weight loss
7. Weakness
8. Diminished or absent breath sounds, respiratory changes

D. Interventions
  1. Monitor vital signs.
  2. Monitor breathing patterns and breath sounds and for signs of respiratory impairment; monitor for hemoptysis.
  3. Assess for tracheal deviation.
  4. Administer analgesics as prescribed for pain management.
  5. Place in a Fowler's position to help ease breathing.
  6. Administer oxygen as prescribed and humidification to moisten and loosen secretions.
  7. Monitor pulse oximetry.
  8. Provide respiratory treatments as prescribed.
  9. Administer bronchodilators and corticosteroids as prescribed to decrease bronchospasm, inflammation, and edema.
  10. Provide a high-calorie, high-protein, high-vitamin diet.
  11. Provide activity as tolerated, rest periods, and active and passive range-of-motion exercises.
E. Nonsurgical interventions
  1. Radiation therapy may be prescribed for localized intrathoracic lung **cancer** and for palliation of hemoptysis, obstructions, dysphagia, superior vena cava syndrome, and pain.
  2. Chemotherapy may be prescribed for treatment of nonresectable tumors or as adjuvant therapy.
F. Surgical interventions
  1. Laser therapy: To relieve endobronchial obstruction
  2. Thoracentesis and pleurodesis: To remove pleural fluid and relieve hypoxia
  3. Thoracotomy (opening into the thoracic cavity) with pneumonectomy: Surgical removal of one entire lung
  4. Thoracotomy with lobectomy: Surgical removal of one lobe of the lung for tumors confined to a single lobe
  5. Thoracotomy with segmental resection: Surgical removal of a lobe segment
G. Preoperative interventions
  1. Explain the potential postoperative need for chest tubes.
  2. Note that closed chest drainage usually is not used for a pneumonectomy and the serous fluid that accumulates in the empty thoracic cavity eventually consolidates, preventing shifts of the mediastinum, heart, and remaining lung.
H. Postoperative interventions
  1. Monitor vital signs.
  2. Assess cardiac and respiratory status; monitor lung sounds.
  3. Maintain the chest tube drainage system, which drains air and blood that accumulates in the pleural space; monitor for excess bleeding. (See Chapter 21 for care of the client with a chest tube.)
  4. Administer oxygen as prescribed.
  5. Check the physician's prescriptions regarding client positioning; avoid complete lateral turning.
  6. Monitor pulse oximetry.
  7. Provide activity as tolerated.
  8. Encourage active range-of-motion exercises of the operative shoulder as prescribed.
  9. See Chapter 21 for care of the client with a chest tube.

⚠ Airway is the priority for a client with lung or laryngeal cancer.

XXIII. LARYNGEAL CANCER

A. Description
  1. Laryngeal **cancer** is a **malignant** tumor of the larynx (Fig. 52-5).
  2. Laryngeal **cancer** presents as **malignant** ulcerations with underlying infiltration and is spread by local extension to adjacent structures in the throat and neck, and by the lymphatic system.
  3. Diagnosis is made by laryngoscopy and biopsy showing a positive cytological study for **cancer** cells.
  4. Laryngoscopy allows for evaluation of the throat and biopsy of tissues; chest radiography, CT, and MRI are used for **staging**.
B. Risk factors
  1. Cigarette smoking
  2. Heavy alcohol use and the combined use of tobacco and alcohol

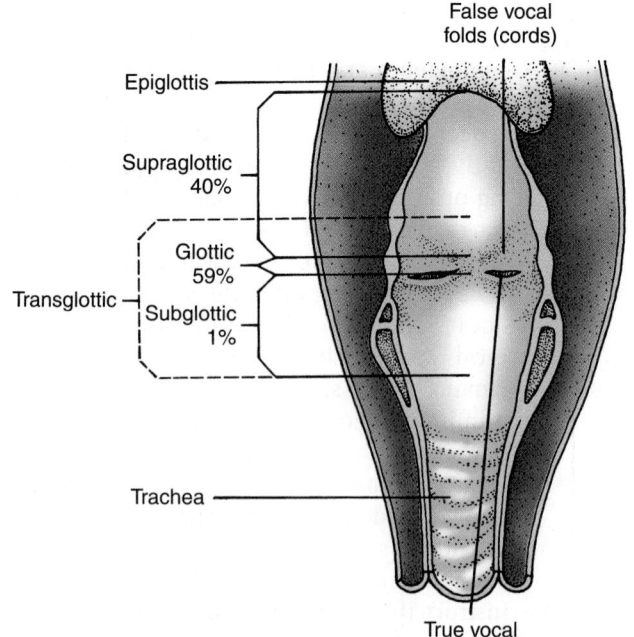

▲ **FIGURE 52-5** Sites and incidence of primary laryngeal tumors. (From Ignatavicius, D., & Workman, M. [2006]. *Medical-surgical nursing: Critical thinking for collaborative care* [5th ed.]. St. Louis: Saunders.)

3. Exposure to environmental pollutants (e.g., asbestos, wood dust)
4. Exposure to radiation

C. Assessment
1. Persistent hoarseness or sore throat
2. Painless neck mass
3. Feeling of a lump in the throat
4. Burning sensation in the throat
5. Dysphagia
6. Change in voice quality
7. Dyspnea
8. Weakness and weight loss
9. Hemoptysis
10. Foul breath odor

D. Interventions
1. Place in Fowler's position to promote optimal air exchange.
2. Monitor respiratory status.
3. Monitor for signs of aspiration of food and fluid.
4. Administer oxygen as prescribed.
5. Provide respiratory treatments as prescribed.
6. Provide activity as tolerated.
7. Provide a high-calorie and high-protein diet.
8. Provide nutritional support via parenteral nutrition, nasogastric tube feedings, or gastrostomy or jejunostomy tube, as prescribed.
9. Administer analgesics as prescribed for pain.

E. Nonsurgical interventions
1. Radiation therapy if the **cancer** is limited to a small area in one vocal cord
2. Chemotherapy, which may be given in combination with radiation and surgery

F. Surgical interventions
1. The goal is to remove the **cancer** while preserving as much normal function as possible.
2. Surgical intervention depends on the tumor size, location, and amount of tissue to be resected.
3. Types of resection include cordal stripping, cordectomy, partial laryngectomy, and total laryngectomy.
4. A tracheostomy is performed with a total laryngectomy; this airway opening is permanent and is referred to as a laryngectomy stoma.

G. Preoperative interventions
1. Discuss self-care of the airway, alternate methods of communication, suctioning, pain control methods, the critical care environment, and nutritional support.
2. Encourage the client to express feelings about changes in body image and loss of voice.
3. Describe the rehabilitation program and information about the tracheostomy and suctioning.

H. Postoperative interventions
1. Monitor vital signs.
2. Monitor respiratory status; monitor airway patency and provide frequent suctioning to remove bloody secretions.

3. Place the client in a high Fowler's position.
4. Maintain mechanical ventilator support or a tracheostomy collar with humidification, as prescribed.
5. Monitor pulse oximetry.
6. Maintain surgical drains in the neck area if present.
7. Observe for hemorrhage and edema in the neck.
8. Monitor IV fluids or parenteral nutrition until nutrition is administered via a nasogastric, gastrostomy, or jejunostomy tube.
9. Provide oral hygiene.
10. Assess gag and cough reflexes and the ability to swallow.
11. Increase activity as tolerated.
12. Assess the color, amount, and consistency of sputum.
13. Provide stoma and laryngectomy care (Box 52-16).
14. Provide consultation with speech and language pathologist as prescribed.
15. Reinforce method of communication established preoperatively.
16. Prepare the client for rehabilitation and speech therapy (Box 52-17).

XXIV. PROSTATE CANCER

A. Description
1. Prostate **cancer**, a slow-growing malignancy of the prostate gland, is a common **cancer** in American men; most prostate tumors are **adenocarcinomas** arising from androgen-dependent epithelial cells.
2. The risk increases in men with each decade after the age of 50 years.

Box 52-16 Stoma Care Following Laryngectomy

Protect the neck from injury.
Instruct the client in how to clean the incision and provide stoma care.
Instruct the client to wear a stoma guard to shield the stoma.
Demonstrate ways to prevent debris from entering the stoma.
Advise the client to wear loose-fitting, high-collared clothing to cover the stoma.
Avoid swimming, showering, and using aerosol sprays.
Teach the client clean suctioning technique.
Advise the client to increase humidity in the home.
Increase fluid intake to 3000 mL/day as prescribed.
Avoid exposure to persons with infections.
Alternate rest periods with activity.
Instruct the client in range-of-motion exercises for the arms, shoulders, and neck as prescribed.
Advise the client to wear a Medic-Alert bracelet.

Box 52-17 Speech Rehabilitation Following Laryngectomy

Esophageal Speech

The client produces esophageal speech by "burping" the air swallowed.

The voice produced is monotone, cannot be raised or lowered, and carries no pitch.

The client must have adequate hearing because his or her mouth shapes words as they are heard.

Mechanical Devices

The devices are known as an electrolarynx.

The device is placed against the side of the neck; the air inside the neck and pharynx is vibrated, and the client articulates.

Other devices consist of a plastic tube placed inside the client's mouth that vibrates on articulation.

Tracheoesophageal Fistula

A fistula is created surgically between the trachea and the esophagus, with eventual placement of a prosthesis to produce speech.

The prosthesis provides the client with a means to divert air from the trachea into the esophagus, and out of the mouth.

Lip and tongue movement produce the speech.

3. Prostate **cancer** can spread via direct invasion of surrounding tissues or by **metastasis** through the bloodstream and lymphatics, to the bony pelvis and spine.

4. Bone **metastasis** is a concern, as is spread to the lungs, liver, and kidneys.

5. The cause of prostate **cancer** is unclear, but advancing age, heavy metal exposure, smoking, and history of sexually transmitted disease are contributing factors.

B. Assessment

1. Asymptomatic in early stages

2. Hard, pea-sized nodule or irregularities palpated on rectal examination

3. Gross, painless hematuria

4. Late symptoms such as weight loss, urinary obstruction, and bone pain radiating from the lumbosacral area down the leg

5. The prostate-specific antigen level is elevated in various noncancerous conditions; therefore, it should not be used as a screening test without a digital rectal examination. It is routinely used to monitor response to therapy.

6. Diagnosis is made through biopsy of the prostate gland.

C. Nonsurgical interventions

1. Prepare the client for hormone manipulation therapy as prescribed.

2. Luteinizing hormone may be prescribed to slow the rate of growth of the tumor.

3. Pain medication, radiation therapy, corticosteroids, and bisphosphonates may be prescribed for palliation of advanced prostate **cancer**.

4. Prepare the client for external beam radiation or brachytherapy, which may be prescribed alone or with surgery, preoperatively or postoperatively, to reduce the lesion and limit **metastasis**.

5. Prepare the client for the administration of chemotherapy in cases of hormone-resistant tumors.

D. Surgical interventions

1. Prepare the client for orchiectomy (palliative), if prescribed, which will limit the production of testosterone.

2. Prepare the client for prostatectomy, if prescribed.

3. The radical prostatectomy can be performed via a retropubic, perineal, or suprapubic approach.

4. Cryosurgical ablation is a minimally invasive procedure that may be an alternative to radical prostatectomy; liquid nitrogen freezes the gland, and the dead cells are absorbed by the body.

E. Transurethral resection of the prostate (TURP) may be performed for palliation in prostate **cancer** clients.

1. The procedure involves insertion of a scope into the urethra to excise prostatic tissue.

2. Monitor for hemorrhage; bleeding is common following TURP.

3. Postoperative continuous bladder irrigation (CBI) may be prescribed, which prevents catheter obstruction from clots.

4. Assess for signs of transurethral resection syndrome, which include signs of cerebral edema and increased intracranial pressure, such as increased blood pressure, bradycardia, confusion, disorientation, muscle twitching, visual disturbances, and nausea and vomiting.

5. Antispasmodics may be prescribed for bladder spasm.

6. Instruct the client to monitor and report dribbling or incontinence postoperatively and teach perineal exercises.

7. Sterility is possible following the surgical procedure.

F. Suprapubic prostatectomy

1. Suprapubic prostatectomy is removal of the prostate gland by an abdominal incision with a bladder incision.

2. The client will have an abdominal dressing that may drain copious amounts of urine, and the abdominal dressing will need to be changed frequently.

3. Severe hemorrhage is possible, and monitoring for blood loss is an important nursing intervention.

4. Antispasmodics may be prescribed for bladder spasms.

5. CBI is prescribed and carried out to maintain pink-colored urine.

6. Sterility occurs with this procedure.

Box 52-18 Continuous Bladder Irrigation

Description
A three-way (lumen) irrigation is used to decrease bleeding and to keep the bladder free from clots—one lumen is for inflating the balloon (30 mL); one lumen is for instillation (inflow); one lumen is for outflow.

Interventions
Maintain traction on the catheter, if applied, to prevent bleeding by pulling the catheter taut and taping it to the abdomen or thigh.

Instruct the client to keep the leg straight if traction is applied to the catheter and it is taped to the thigh.

Catheter traction is not released without a physician's prescription; it usually is released after any bright red drainage has diminished.

Use only sterile bladder irrigation solution or prescribed solution to prevent water intoxication.

Run the solution at a rate, as prescribed, to keep the urine pink. Run the solution rapidly if bright red drainage or clots are present; monitor output closely. Run the solution at about 40 gtt/min when the bright red drainage clears.

If the urinary catheter becomes obstructed, turn off the CBI and irrigate the catheter with 30 to 50 mL of normal saline, if prescribed; notify the physician if obstruction does not resolve.

Discontinue CBI and the Foley catheter as prescribed, usually 24 to 48 hours after surgery.

Monitor for continence and urinary retention when the catheter is removed. Inform the client that some burning, frequency, and dribbling may occur following catheter removal.

Inform the client that he should be voiding 150 to 200 mL of clear yellow urine every 3 to 4 hours by 3 days after surgery.

Inform the client that he may pass small clots and tissue debris for several days.

Teach the client to avoid heavy lifting, stressful exercise, driving, Valsalva maneuver, and sexual intercourse for 2 to 6 weeks to prevent strain, and to call the physician if bleeding occurs or if there is a decrease in urinary stream.

Instruct the client to drink 2400 to 3000 mL of fluid each day, preferably before 8 PM to avoid nocturia.

Instruct the client to avoid alcohol, caffeinated beverages, and spicy foods, and overstimulation of the bladder.

Instruct the client that if the urine becomes bloody, to rest and increase fluid intake and, if the bleeding does not subside, to notify the physician.

G. Retropubic prostatectomy
1. Retropubic prostatectomy is removal of the prostate gland by a low abdominal incision without opening the bladder.
2. Less bleeding occurs with this procedure compared with the suprapubic procedure, and the client experiences fewer bladder spasms.
3. Abdominal drainage is minimal.
4. CBI may be used.
5. Sterility occurs with this procedure.

H. Perineal prostatectomy
1. The prostate gland is removed through an incision made between the scrotum and anus.
2. Minimal bleeding occurs with this procedure.
3. The client needs to be monitored closely for infection, because the risk of infection is increased with this type of prostatectomy.
4. Urinary incontinence is common.
5. The procedure causes sterility.
6. Teach the client how to perform perineal exercises.

I. Postoperative interventions
1. Monitor vital signs.
2. Monitor urinary output and urine for hemorrhage or clots.
3. Increase fluids to 2400 to 3000 mL/day, unless contraindicated.
4. Monitor for arterial bleeding as evidenced by bright red urine with numerous clots; if it occurs, increase CBI and notify the physician immediately.
5. Monitor for venous bleeding as evidenced by burgundy-colored urine output; if it occurs,

inform the physician, who may apply traction on the catheter.
6. Monitor hemoglobin and hematocrit levels.
7. Expect red to light pink urine for 24 hours, turning to amber in 3 days.
8. Ambulate the client as early as possible and as soon as urine begins to clear in color.
9. Inform the client that a continuous feeling of an urge to void is normal.
10. Instruct the client to avoid attempts to void around the catheter because this will cause bladder spasms.
11. Administer antibiotics, analgesics, stool softeners, and antispasmodics as prescribed.
12. Monitor the three-way Foley catheter, which usually has a 30- to 45-mL retention balloon.
13. Maintain CBI with sterile bladder irrigation solution as prescribed to keep the catheter free of obstruction and maintain the urine pink in color (Box 52-18).

Following TURP, monitor for transurethral resection syndrome or severe hyponatremia (water intoxication) caused by the excessive absorption of bladder irrigation during surgery. (Signs include altered mental status, bradycardia, increased blood pressure, and confusion.)

J. Postoperative interventions: Suprapubic prostatectomy
1. Monitor suprapubic and Foley catheter drainage.
2. Monitor CBI if prescribed.

3. Note that the Foley catheter will be removed 2 to 4 days postoperatively if the client has a suprapubic catheter.

4. If prescribed, clamp the suprapubic catheter after the Foley catheter is removed, and instruct the client to attempt to void; after the client has voided, assess the residual urine in the bladder by unclamping the suprapubic catheter and measuring the output.

5. Prepare for removal of the suprapubic catheter when the client consistently empties the bladder and residual urine is 75 mL or less.

6. Monitor the suprapubic incision dressing, which may become saturated with urine, until the incision heals; dressing may need to be changed frequently.

K. Postoperative interventions: Retropubic prostatectomy
1. Note that because the bladder is not entered, there is no urinary drainage on the abdominal dressing.
2. Assess for urinary or purulent drainage on the dressing; if this occurs, notify the physician.
3. Monitor for fever and increased pain, which may indicate an infection.

L. Postoperative interventions: Perineal prostatectomy
1. Note that the client will have an incision, which may or may not have a drain.
2. Avoid the use of rectal thermometers, rectal tubes, and enemas because they may cause trauma and bleeding.

XXV. BLADDER CANCER

A. Description
1. Bladder **cancer** is papillomatous growths in the bladder urothelium that undergo **malignant** changes and that may infiltrate the bladder wall.
2. Predisposing factors include cigarette smoking, exposure to industrial chemicals, and exposure to radiation.
3. Common sites of **metastasis** include the liver, bones, and lungs.
4. As the tumor progresses, it can extend into the rectum, vagina, other pelvic soft tissues, and retroperitoneal structures.

B. Assessment
1. Gross or microscopic, painless hematuria
2. Frequency, urgency, dysuria
3. Clot-induced obstruction
4. Bladder wash specimens and biopsy confirms diagnosis

C. Radiation
1. Radiation therapy is indicated for advanced disease that cannot be eradicated by surgery; palliative radiation may be used to relieve pain and bowel obstruction and control potential hemorrhage and leg edema caused by venous or lymphatic obstruction.
2. Intracavitary radiation may be prescribed, which protects adjacent tissue.

3. External beam radiation combined with chemotherapy or surgery may be prescribed to improve survival.
4. Complications of radiation
   a. Abacterial cystitis
   b. Proctitis
   c. Fistula formation
   d. Ileitis or colitis
   e. Bladder ulceration and hemorrhage

D. Chemotherapy
1. Intravesical instillation
   a. An alkylating chemotherapeutic agent is instilled into the bladder.
   b. This method provides a concentrated topical treatment with little systemic absorption.
   c. The medication is injected into a urethral catheter and retained for 2 hours.
   d. Following instillation, the client's position is rotated every 15 to 30 minutes, starting in the supine position, to avoid lying on a full bladder.
   e. After 2 hours, the client voids in a sitting position and is instructed to increase fluids to flush the bladder.
   f. Treat the urine as a biohazard and send to the radioisotope laboratory for monitoring.
   g. For 6 hours following intravesical chemotherapy, disinfect the toilet with household bleach after the client has voided.
2. Systemic chemotherapy: Used to treat inoperable tumors or distant **metastasis**.
3. Complications of chemotherapy
   a. Bladder irritation
   b. Hemorrhagic cystitis

E. Surgical interventions
1. Transurethral resection of bladder tumor
   a. Local resection and fulguration (destruction of tissue by electrical current through electrodes placed in direct contact with the tissue)
   b. Performed for early tumors for cure or for inoperable tumors for palliation
2. Partial cystectomy
   a. Partial cystectomy is the removal of up to half the bladder.
   b. The procedure is done for early-stage tumors and for clients who cannot tolerate a radical cystectomy.
   c. During the initial postoperative period, bladder capacity is reduced greatly to about 60 mL; however, as the bladder tissue expands, the capacity increases to 200 to 400 mL.
   d. Maintenance of a continuous output of urine following surgery is critical to prevent bladder distention and stress on the suture line.
   e. A urethral catheter and a suprapubic catheter may be in place, and the suprapubic catheter

may be left in place for 2 weeks until healing occurs.

3. Cystectomy and urinary diversion (Fig. 52-6)
   a. Various surgical procedures performed to create alternate pathways for urine collection and excretion
   b. Urinary diversion may be performed with or without cystectomy (bladder removal).
   c. The surgery may be performed in two stages if the tumor is extensive, with the creation of the urinary diversion first and the cystectomy several weeks later.
   d. If a radical cystectomy is performed, lower extremity lymphedema may occur as a result of lymph node dissection, and male impotence may occur.

Ureterostomies divert urine directly to the skin surface through a ureteral-skin opening (stoma). After ureterostomy, the client must wear a pouch.

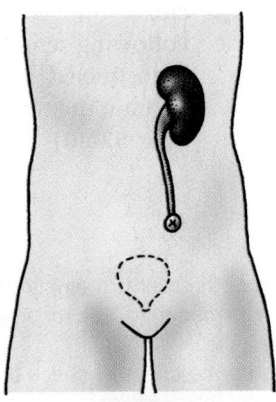
Cutaneous ureterostomy

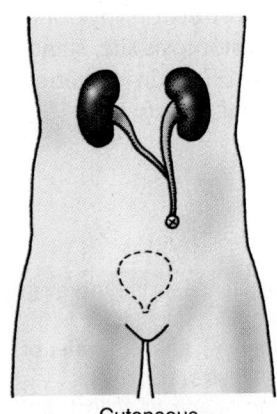
Cutaneous ureteroureterostomy

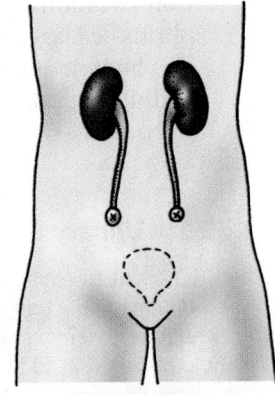
Bilateral cutaneous ureterostomy

Conduits collect urine in a portion of the intestine, which is then opened onto the skin surface as a stoma. After the creation of a conduit, the client must wear a pouch.

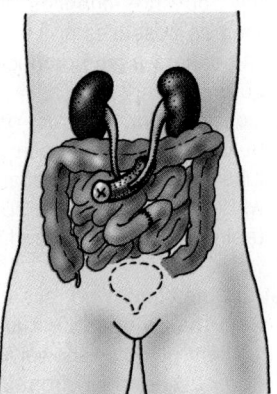
Ileal (Bricker's) conduit

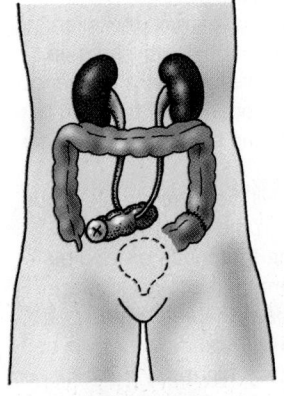
Colon conduit

Ileal reservoirs divert urine into a surgically created pouch, or pocket, that functions as a bladder. The stoma is continent, and the client removes urine by regular self-catheterization.

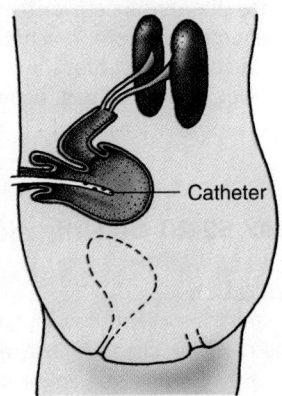
Catheter

Continent internal ileal reservoir (Kock's pouch)

Sigmoidostomies divert urine to the large intestine, so no stoma is required. The client excretes urine with bowel movements, and bowel incontinence may result.

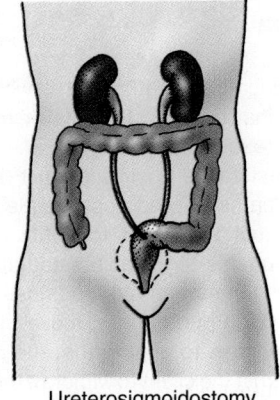
Ureterosigmoidostomy

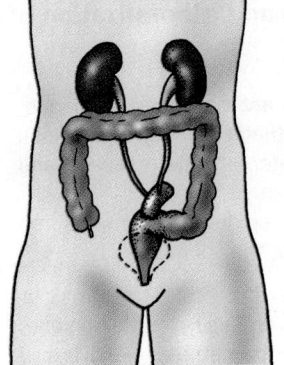
Ureteroiliosigmoidostomy

▲ **FIGURE 52-6** Urinary diversion procedures used in the treatment of bladder cancer. (From Ignatavicius, D., & Workman, M. [2010]. *Medical-surgical nursing: Patient-centered collaborative care* [6th ed.]. St. Louis: Saunders.)

4. Ileal conduit
   a. The ileal conduit also is called ureteroileostomy, or Bricker's procedure.
   b. Ureters are implanted into a segment of the ileum, with the formation of an abdominal stoma.
   c. The urine flows into the conduit and is propelled continuously out through the stoma by peristalsis.
   d. The client is required to wear an appliance over the stoma to collect the urine (Box 52-19).
   e. Complications include obstruction, pyelonephritis, leakage at the anastomosis site, stenosis, hydronephrosis, calculi, skin irritation and ulceration, and stomal defects.
5. Kock pouch
   a. The Kock pouch is a continent internal ileal reservoir created from a segment of the ileum and ascending colon.
   b. The ureters are implanted into the side of the reservoir, and a special nipple valve is constructed to attach the reservoir to the skin.
   c. Postoperatively, the client will have a Foley catheter in place to drain urine continuously until the pouch has healed.
   d. The catheter is irrigated gently with normal saline to prevent obstruction from mucus or clots.
   e. Following removal of the catheter, the client is instructed in how to self-catheterize and to drain the reservoir at 4- to 6-hour intervals (Box 52-20).

Box 52-19 Urinary Stoma Care

Instruct the client to change the appliance in the morning, when urinary production is slowest.

Collect equipment, remove collection bag, and use water or commercial solvent to loosen adhesive.

Hold a rolled gauze pad against the stoma to collect and absorb urine during the procedure.

Cleanse the skin around stoma and under the drainage bag with mild nonresidue soap and water.

Inspect the skin for excoriation, and instruct the client to prevent urine from coming into contact with the skin.

After the skin is dry, apply skin adhesive around the appliance.

Instruct the client to cut the stoma opening of the skin barrier just large enough to fit over the stoma (no more than 3 mm larger than the stoma).

Instruct the client that the stoma will begin to shrink, requiring a smaller stoma opening on the skin barrier.

Apply skin barrier before attaching the pouch or face plate.

Place the appliance over the stoma and secure in place.

Encourage self-care; teach the client to use a mirror.

Instruct the client that the pouch may be drained by a bedside bag or leg bag, especially at night.

Instruct the client to empty the urinary collection bag when it is one-third full to prevent pulling of the appliance and leakage.

Instruct the client to check the appliance seal if perspiring occurs.

Instruct the client to leave the urinary pouch in place as long as it is not leaking and to change it every 5 to 7 days.

During appliance changes, leave the skin open to air as long as possible.

Use a nonkaraya gum product, because urine erodes karaya gum.

To control odor, instruct the client to drink adequate fluids, wash the appliance thoroughly with soap and lukewarm water, and soak the collection pouch in dilute white vinegar for 20 to 30 minutes; a special deodorant tablet can also be placed into the pouch while it is being worn.

Instruct the client who takes baths to keep the level of the water below the stoma and to avoid oily soaps.

If the client plans to shower, instruct the client to direct the flow of water away from the stoma.

Box 52-20 Self-Irrigation and Catheterization of Stoma

Irrigation

Instruct the client to wash hands and use clean technique.

Instruct the client to use a catheter and syringe, instill 60 mL of normal saline or water into the reservoir, and aspirate gently or allow to drain.

Instruct the client to irrigate until the drainage remains free of mucus but to be careful not to overirrigate.

Catheterization

Instruct the client to wash hands and use clean technique.

Initially, instruct the client to insert a catheter every 2 to 3 hours to drain the reservoir; during each week thereafter, increase the interval by 1 hour until catheterization is done every 4 to 6 hours.

Lubricate the catheter well with water-soluble lubricant, and instruct the client never to force the catheter into the reservoir.

If resistance is met, instruct the client to pause, rotate the catheter, and apply gentle pressure to insert.

Instruct the client to notify the physician if the client is unable to insert the catheter.

When urine has stopped, instruct the client to take several deep breaths and move the catheter in and out 2 to 3 inches to ensure that the pouch is empty.

Instruct the client to withdraw the catheter slowly and pinch the catheter when withdrawn so that it does not leak urine.

Instruct the client to carry catheterization supplies with him or her.

6. Indiana pouch
   a. A continent reservoir is created from the ascending colon and terminal ileum, making a pouch larger than the Kock pouch (additional continent reservoirs include the Mainz and Florida pouch systems)
   b. Postoperatively, care is similar as with the Koch pouch.
7. Creation of a neobladder
   a. Creation of a neobladder is similar to the creation of an internal reservoir, with the difference being that instead of emptying through an abdominal stoma, the bladder empties through a pelvic outlet into the urethra.
   b. The client empties the neobladder by relaxing the external sphincter and creating abdominal pressure or by intermittent self-catheterization.
8. Percutaneous nephrostomy or pyelostomy
   a. These procedures are used to prevent or treat obstruction.
   b. The procedures involve a percutaneous or surgical insertion of a nephrostomy tube into the kidney for drainage.
   c. Nursing interventions involve stabilizing the tube to prevent dislodgment and monitoring output.
9. Ureterostomy
   a. Ureterostomy may be performed as a palliative procedure if the ureters are obstructed by the tumor.
   b. The ureters are attached to the surface of the abdomen, where the urine flows directly into a drainage appliance without a conduit.
   c. Potential problems include infection, skin irritation, and obstruction to urinary flow as a result of strictures at the opening.
10. Vesicostomy
   a. The bladder is sutured to the abdomen, and a stoma is created in the bladder wall.
   b. The bladder empties through the stoma.
F. Preoperative interventions
   1. Instruct the client in preoperative, operative, and postoperative management including diet, medications, nasogastric tube placement, IV lines, NPO status, pain control, coughing and deep breathing, leg exercises, and postoperative activity.
   2. Demonstrate appliance application and use for those clients who will have a stoma.
   3. Arrange an enterostomal nurse consult and for a visit with a person who has had urinary diversion.
   4. Administer antimicrobials for bowel preparation as prescribed.
   5. Encourage discussion of feelings including the effects on sexual activities.

G. Postoperative interventions

⚠ Monitor urinary output closely following bladder surgery. Irrigate the ureteral catheter (if present and if prescribed) gently to prevent obstruction. Follow the physician's prescriptions and agency policy regarding irrigation.

   1. Monitor vital signs.
   2. Assess incision site.
   3. Assess stoma (should be red and moist) every hour for the first 24 hours.
   4. Monitor for edema in the stoma, which may be present in the immediate postoperative period.
   5. Notify the physician if the stoma appears dark and dusky (indicates necrosis).
   6. Monitor for prolapse or retraction of the stoma.
   7. Assess bowel function; monitor for expected return of peristalsis in 3 to 4 days.
   8. Maintain NPO status as prescribed until bowel sounds return.
   9. Monitor continuous urine flow (30 to 60 mL/hr).
   10. Notify the physician if the urine output is less than 30 mL/hr or if no urine output occurs for more than 15 minutes.
   11. Ureteral stents or catheters, if present, may be in place for 2 to 3 weeks or until healing occurs; maintain stability with catheters to prevent dislodgment.
   12. Monitor for hematuria.
   13. Monitor for signs of peritonitis.
   14. Monitor for bladder distention following a partial cystectomy.
   15. Monitor for shock, hemorrhage, thrombophlebitis, and lower extremity lymphedema after a radical cystectomy.
   16. Monitor the urinary drainage pouch for leaks, and check skin integrity (see Box 52-20).
   17. Monitor the pH of the urine (do not place the dipstick in the stoma) because strongly alkaline urine can cause skin irritation and facilitate crystal formation.
   18. Instruct the client regarding the potential for urinary tract infection or the development of calculi.
   19. Instruct the client to assess the skin for irritation, monitor the urinary drainage pouch, and report any leakage.
   20. Encourage the client to express feelings about changes in body image, embarrassment, and sexual dysfunction.

XXVI. ONCOLOGICAL EMERGENCIES

A. Sepsis and disseminated intravascular coagulation (DIC)
   1. Description: The client with **cancer** is at increased risk for infection, particularly gram-negative organisms, in the bloodstream (sepsis

or septicemia) and DIC, a life-threatening problem frequently associated with sepsis.
2. Interventions
   a. Prevent the complication through early identification of clients at high risk for sepsis and DIC.
   b. Maintain strict aseptic technique with the immunocompromised client and monitor closely for infection.
   c. Administer antibiotics intravenously as prescribed.
   d. Administer anticoagulants as prescribed during the early phase of DIC.
   e. Administer cryoprecipitated clotting factors, as prescribed, when DIC progresses and hemorrhage is the primary problem.

⚠ Notify the physician immediately if signs of an oncological emergency occur.

B. Syndrome of inappropriate antidiuretic hormone (SIADH)
1. Description
   a. Tumors can produce, secrete, or stimulate substances that mimic antidiuretic hormone.
   b. Mild symptoms include weakness, muscle cramps, loss of appetite, and fatigue; serum sodium levels range from 115 to 120 mEq/L.
   c. More serious signs and symptoms relate to water intoxication and include weight gain, personality changes, confusion, and extreme muscle weakness.
   d. As the serum sodium level approaches 110 mEq/L, seizures, coma, and eventually death will occur, unless the condition is treated rapidly.
2. Interventions
   a. Initiate fluid restriction and increased sodium intake as prescribed.
   b. As prescribed, administer an antagonist to antidiuretic hormone.
   c. Monitor serum sodium levels.
   d. Treat the underlying cause with chemotherapy or radiation to reduce the tumor.
C. Spinal cord compression
1. Description
   a. Spinal cord compression occurs when a tumor directly enters the spinal cord or when the vertebral column collapses from tumor entry, impinging on the spinal cord.
   b. Spinal cord compression causes back pain, usually before neurological deficits occur.
   c. Neurological deficits relate to the spinal level of compression and include numbness, tingling, loss of urethral, vaginal, and rectal sensation, and muscle weakness.

2. Interventions
   a. Early recognition: Assess for back pain and neurological deficits.
   b. Administer high-dose corticosteroids to reduce swelling around the spinal cord and relieve symptoms.
   c. Prepare the client for immediate radiation and/or chemotherapy to reduce the size of the tumor and relieve compression.
   d. Surgery may need to be performed to remove the tumor and relieve the pressure on the spinal cord.
   e. Instruct the client in the use of neck or back braces if they are prescribed.
D. Hypercalcemia
1. Description
   a. Hypercalcemia is a late manifestation of extensive malignancy that occurs most often with bone **metastasis**, when the bone releases calcium into the bloodstream.
   b. Decreased physical mobility contributes to or worsens hypercalcemia.
   c. Early signs include fatigue, anorexia, nausea, vomiting, constipation, and polyuria.
   d. More serious signs and symptoms include severe muscle weakness, diminished deep tendon reflexes, paralytic ileus, dehydration, and changes in the electrocardiogram.
2. Interventions
   a. Monitor serum calcium level and electrocardiographic changes.
   b. Administer oral or parenteral fluids as prescribed.
   c. Administer medications that lower the calcium level as prescribed.
   d. Prepare the client for dialysis if the condition becomes life-threatening or is accompanied by renal impairment.
E. Superior vena cava syndrome
1. Description
   a. Superior vena cava (SVC) syndrome occurs when the SVC is compressed or obstructed by tumor growth (commonly associated with lung **cancer** and **lymphoma**).
   b. Signs and symptoms result from blockage of blood flow in the venous system of the head, neck, and upper trunk.
   c. Early signs and symptoms generally occur in the morning and include edema of the face, especially around the eyes, and tightness of the shirt or blouse collar (Stokes' sign).
   d. As the condition worsens, edema in the arms and hands, dyspnea, erythema of the upper body, and epistaxis occur.
   e. Life-threatening signs and symptoms include airway obstruction, hemorrhage, cyanosis, mental status changes, decreased cardiac output, and hypotension.

2. Interventions
   a. Assess for early signs and symptoms of superior vena cava syndrome.
   b. Prepare the client for high-dose radiation therapy to the mediastinal area, and possible surgery to insert a metal stent in the vena cava.

F. Tumor lysis syndrome
1. Description
   a. Tumor lysis syndrome occurs when large quantities of tumor cells are destroyed rapidly and intracellular components such as potassium and uric acid are released into the bloodstream faster than the body can eliminate them.
   b. Tumor lysis syndrome can indicate that **cancer** treatment is destroying tumor cells; however, if left untreated, it can cause severe tissue damage and death.
   c. Hyperkalemia, hyperphosphatemia with resultant hypocalcemia, and hyperuricemia occur; hyperuricemia can lead to acute renal failure.

2. Interventions
   a. Encourage oral hydration; IV hydration may be prescribed for the client experiencing nausea; monitor renal function.
   b. Administer diuretics to increase the urine flow through the kidneys as prescribed.
   c. Administer medications that increase the excretion of purines, such as allopurinol (Zyloprim), as prescribed.
   d. Prepare to administer IV infusion of glucose and insulin to treat hyperkalemia.
   e. Prepare the client for dialysis if hyperkalemia and hyperuricemia persist despite treatment.

MORE QUESTIONS ON THE CD!

Practice Questions

530. The nurse is reviewing the laboratory results of a client diagnosed with multiple myeloma. Which would the nurse expect to note specifically in this disorder?
1. Increased calcium level
2. Increased white blood cells
3. Decreased blood urea nitrogen level
4. Decreased number of plasma cells in the bone marrow

531. The nurse is developing a plan of care for the client with multiple myeloma and includes which priority intervention in the plan?
1. Encouraging fluids
2. Providing frequent oral care
3. Coughing and deep breathing
4. Monitoring the red blood cell count

532. The nurse is caring for a client with an internal radiation implant. When caring for the client, the nurse should observe which principle?
1. Limit the time with the client to 1 hour per shift.
2. Do not allow pregnant women into the client's room.
3. Remove the dosimeter film badge when entering the client's room.
4. Individuals younger than 16 years old may be allowed to go in the room as long as they are 6 feet away from the client.

533. The client is hospitalized for insertion of an internal cervical radiation implant. While giving care, the nurse finds the radiation implant in the bed. The initial action by the nurse is to:
1. Call the physician.
2. Reinsert the implant into the vagina immediately.
3. Pick up the implant with gloved hands and flush it down the toilet.
4. Pick up the implant with long-handled forceps and place it in a lead container.

534. The nurse is caring for a client experiencing neutropenia as a result of chemotherapy and develops a plan of care for the client. The nurse plans to:
1. Restrict all visitors.
2. Restrict fluid intake.
3. Teach the client and family about the need for hand hygiene.
4. Insert an indwelling urinary catheter to prevent skin breakdown.

535. The home health care nurse is caring for a client with cancer and the client is complaining of acute pain. The most appropriate nursing assessment of the client's pain would include which of the following?
1. The client's pain rating
2. Nonverbal cues from the client
3. The nurse's impression of the client's pain
4. Pain relief after appropriate nursing intervention

536. The nurse is caring for a client who is postoperative following a pelvic exenteration and the physician changes the client's diet from NPO status to clear liquids. The nurse makes which priority assessment before administering the diet?
1. Bowel sounds
2. Ability to ambulate
3. Incision appearance
4. Urine specific gravity

537. The client is admitted to the hospital with a suspected diagnosis of Hodgkin's disease. Which assessment finding would the nurse expect to note specifically in the client?

1. Fatigue
2. Weakness
3. Weight gain
4. Enlarged lymph nodes

538. During the admission assessment of a client with advanced ovarian cancer, the nurse recognizes which symptom as typical of the disease?
1. Diarrhea
2. Hypermenorrhea
3. Abnormal bleeding
4. Abdominal distention

539. When assessing the laboratory results of the client with bladder cancer and bone metastasis, the nurse notes a calcium level of 12 mg/dL. The nurse recognizes that this is consistent with which oncological emergency?
1. Hyperkalemia
2. Hypercalcemia
3. Spinal cord compression
4. Superior vena cava syndrome

540. The female client who has been receiving radiation therapy for bladder cancer tells the nurse that it feels as if she is voiding through the vagina. The nurse interprets that the client may be experiencing:
1. Rupture of the bladder
2. The development of a vesicovaginal fistula
3. Extreme stress caused by the diagnosis of cancer
4. Altered perineal sensation as a side effect of radiation therapy

541. The nurse is instructing the client to perform a testicular self-examination. The nurse tells the client:
1. To examine the testicles while lying down
2. That the best time for the examination is after a shower
3. To gently feel the testicle with one finger to feel for a growth
4. That testicular self-examinations should be done at least every 6 months

542. A client is diagnosed with multiple myeloma and the client asks the nurse about the diagnosis. The nurse bases the response on which description of this disorder?
1. Altered red blood cell production
2. Altered production of lymph nodes
3. Malignant exacerbation in the number of leukocytes
4. Malignant proliferation of plasma cells within the bone

543. A gastrectomy is performed on a client with gastric cancer. In the immediate postoperative period, the nurse notes bloody drainage from the nasogastric tube. Which of the following is the appropriate nursing intervention?
1. Notify the physician.
2. Measure abdominal girth.
3. Irrigate the nasogastric tube.
4. Continue to monitor the drainage.

544. The nurse is teaching a client about the risk factors associated with colorectal cancer. The nurse determines that further teaching related to colorectal cancer is necessary if the client identifies which of the following as an associated risk factor?
1. Age younger than 50 years
2. History of colorectal polyps
3. Family history of colorectal cancer
4. Chronic inflammatory bowel disease

545. The nurse is assessing the perineal wound in a client who has returned from the operating room following an abdominal perineal resection and notes serosanguineous drainage from the wound. Which nursing intervention is appropriate?
1. Notify the physician.
2. Clamp the Penrose drain.
3. Change the dressing as prescribed.
4. Remove and replace the perineal packing.

546. The nurse is assessing the colostomy of a client who has had an abdominal perineal resection for a bowel tumor. Which of the following assessment findings indicates that the colostomy is beginning to function?
1. Absent bowel sounds
2. The passage of flatus
3. The client's ability to tolerate food
4. Bloody drainage from the colostomy

547. The nurse is reviewing the history of a client with bladder cancer. The nurse expects to note documentation of which most common symptom of this type of cancer?
1. Dysuria
2. Hematuria
3. Urgency on urination
4. Frequency of urination

548. The nurse is assessing the stoma of a client following a ureterostomy. Which of the following should the nurse expect to note?
1. A dry stoma
2. A pale stoma
3. A dark-colored stoma
4. A red and moist stoma

549. The nurse is caring for a client following a mastectomy. Which nursing intervention would assist in preventing lymphedema of the affected arm?
1. Placing cool compresses on the affected arm
2. Elevating the affected arm on a pillow above heart level
3. Avoiding arm exercises in the immediate postoperative period
4. Maintaining an intravenous site below the antecubital area on the affected side

550. A nurse is monitoring a client for signs and symptoms related to superior vena cava syndrome. Which of the following is an early sign of this oncological emergency?
1. Cyanosis
2. Arm edema
3. Periorbital edema
4. Mental status changes

551. A nurse manager is teaching the nursing staff about signs and symptoms related to hypercalcemia in a client with metastatic prostate cancer and tells the staff that which of the following is a serious late sign of this oncological emergency?
1. Headache
2. Dysphagia
3. Constipation
4. Electrocardiographic changes

552. As part of chemotherapy education, the nurse teaches a female client about the risk for bleeding and self-care during the period of the greatest bone marrow suppression (the nadir). The nurse understands that further teaching is needed when the client states:
1. "I should avoid blowing my nose."
2. "I may need a platelet transfusion if my platelet count is too low."

3. "I'm going to take aspirin for my headache as soon as I get home."
4. "I will count the number of pads and tampons I use when menstruating."

553. The community health nurse is instructing a group of female clients about breast self-examination. The nurse instructs the clients to perform the examination:
1. At the onset of menstruation
2. Every month during ovulation
3. Weekly at the same time of day
4. 1 week after menstruation begins

554. The client is diagnosed as having a bowel tumor and several diagnostic tests are prescribed. The nurse understands that which test will confirm the diagnosis of malignancy?
1. Biopsy of the tumor
2. Abdominal ultrasound
3. Magnetic resonance imaging
4. Computed tomography scan

Alternate Item Format: Multiple Response

555. A client with carcinoma of the lung develops syndrome of inappropriate antidiuretic hormone (SIADH) as a complication of the cancer. The nurse anticipates that which of the following may be prescribed? **Select all that apply.**
- ❑ 1. Radiation
- ❑ 2. Chemotherapy
- ❑ 3. Increased fluid intake
- ❑ 4. Serum sodium levels
- ❑ 5. Decreased oral sodium intake
- ❑ 6. Medication that is antagonistic to antidiuretic hormone

ANSWERS
530. 1
Rationale: Findings indicative of multiple myeloma are an increased number of plasma cells in the bone marrow, anemia, hypercalcemia caused by the release of calcium from the deteriorating bone tissue, and an elevated blood urea nitrogen level. An increased white blood cell count may or may not be present and is not related specifically to multiple myeloma.
Test-Taking Strategy: Use the process of elimination. Noting the name of the disorder and recalling the pathophysiology of the disease and that proliferation of plasma cells in the bone occurs will direct you to option 1. Review this information if you are unfamiliar with this oncological disorder.
Level of Cognitive Ability: Analyzing

Client Needs: Physiological Integrity
Integrated Process: Nursing Process—Assessment
Content Area: Adult Health—Oncology
References: Copstead-Kirkhorn, L., & Banasik, J. (2010). *Pathophysiology* (4th ed., p. 1193). St. Louis: Mosby.
    Ignatavicius, D., & Workman, M. (2010). *Medical-surgical nursing: Patient-centered collaborative care* (6th ed., p. 915). St. Louis: Saunders.

531. 1
Rationale: Hypercalcemia caused by bone destruction is a priority concern in the client with multiple myeloma. The nurse should administer fluids in adequate amounts to maintain a urine output of 1.5 to 2 L/day; this requires about 3 L of fluid intake per day. The fluid is needed not only to dilute

the calcium overload but also to prevent protein from precipitating in the renal tubules. Options 2, 3, and 4 may be components of the plan of care but are not the priority in this client.

Test-Taking Strategy: Use the process of elimination. Recalling the pathophysiology of this disorder and that hypercalcemia can occur will direct you to option 1. Review the specific manifestations of this disorder if you had difficulty with this question.

Level of Cognitive Ability: Applying
Client Needs: Physiological Integrity
Integrated Process: Nursing Process—Planning
Content Area: Adult Health—Oncology
References: Black, J., & Hawks, J. (2009). *Medical-surgical nursing: Clinical management for positive outcomes* (8th ed., pp. 162, 296). St. Louis: Saunders.

Ignatavicius, D., & Workman, M. (2010). *Medical-surgical nursing: Patient-centered collaborative care* (6th ed., p. 436). St. Louis: Saunders.

532. 2

Rationale: The time that the nurse spends in a room of a client with an internal radiation implant is 30 minutes per 8-hour shift. The dosimeter film badge must be worn when in the client's room. Children younger than 16 years of age and pregnant women are not allowed in the client's room.

Test-Taking Strategy: Use the process of elimination. Option 3 can be eliminated first. Recalling the time frame related to exposure to the client will assist in eliminating option 1. From the remaining options, select option 2 because of the possible risks associated with exposure to the mother and fetus. Review these safety principles if you had difficulty with this question.

Level of Cognitive Ability: Applying
Client Needs: Safe and Effective Care Environment
Integrated Process: Nursing Process—Implementation
Content Area: Adult Health—Oncology
Reference: Ignatavicius, D., & Workman, M. (2010). *Medical-surgical nursing: Patient-centered collaborative care* (6th ed., p. 420). St. Louis: Saunders.

533. 4

Rationale: A lead container and long-handled forceps should be kept in the client's room at all times during internal radiation therapy. If the implant becomes dislodged, the nurse should pick up the implant with long-handled forceps and place it in the lead container. Options 1, 2, and 3 are inaccurate interventions.

Test-Taking Strategy: Use the process of elimination and note the strategic word *initial* in the question. Option 2 is not an appropriate action. Eliminate option 3 next because the implant would not be discarded. Although the physician would be notified, the initial action is option 4. Review the initial measures related to a dislodged radiation implant if you had difficulty with this question.

Level of Cognitive Ability: Applying
Client Needs: Safe and Effective Care Environment
Integrated Process: Nursing Process—Implementation
Content Area: Fundamental Skills—Safety/Infection Control
Reference: Ignatavicius, D., & Workman, M. (2010). *Medical-surgical nursing: Patient-centered collaborative care* (6th ed., p. 420). St. Louis: Saunders.

534. 3

Rationale: In the neutropenic client, meticulous hand hygiene education is implemented for the client, family, visitors, and staff. Not all visitors are restricted, but the client is protected from persons with known infections. Fluids should be encouraged. Invasive measures such as an indwelling urinary catheter should be avoided to prevent infections.

Test-Taking Strategy: Use the process of elimination. Eliminate option 1 because of the word *all*. Next, eliminate option 2 because it is not reasonable to restrict fluids in a client receiving chemotherapy who is at risk for fluid and electrolyte imbalances. Eliminate option 4 because of the risk of infection that exists with this measure. Review interventions for the client with neutropenia if you had difficulty with this question.

Level of Cognitive Ability: Applying
Client Needs: Safe and Effective Care Environment
Integrated Process: Teaching and Learning
Content Area: Fundamental Skills—Safety/Infection Control
Reference: Ignatavicius, D., & Workman, M. (2010). *Medical-surgical nursing: Patient-centered collaborative care* (6th ed., p. 426). St. Louis: Saunders.

535. 1

Rationale: The client's self-report is a critical component of pain assessment. The nurse should ask the client about the description of the pain and listen carefully to the client's words used to describe the pain. The nurse's impression of the client's pain is not appropriate in determining the client's level of pain. Nonverbal cues from the client are important but are not the most appropriate pain assessment measure. Assessing pain relief is an important measure, but this option is not related to the subject of the question.

Test-Taking Strategy: Use the process of elimination. Noting the subject of the question will assist in eliminating option 4. Eliminate option 3 because the nurse is not the client of the question. From the remaining options, the subjective data from the client will provide the most accurate description of the pain. Review pain assessment techniques if the question was difficult.

Level of Cognitive Ability: Analyzing
Client Needs: Physiological Integrity
Integrated Process: Caring
Content Area: Adult Health—Oncology
Reference: Ignatavicius, D., & Workman, M. (2010). *Medical-surgical nursing: Patient-centered collaborative care* (6th ed., pp. 43, 416). St. Louis: Saunders.

536. 1

Rationale: The client is kept NPO until peristalsis returns, usually in 4 to 6 days. When signs of bowel function return, clear fluids are given to the client. If no distention occurs, the diet is advanced as tolerated. The most important assessment is to assess bowel sounds before feeding the client. Options 2, 3, and 4 are unrelated to the subject of the question.

Test-Taking Strategy: Use the process of elimination and note the strategic word *priority* and the strategic words *NPO to clear liquids* in the question. Option 1 is the only option that relates to gastrointestinal function, which is the subject of the question. Review care of the client following pelvic exenteration if you had difficulty with this question.

Level of Cognitive Ability: Applying
Client Needs: Physiological Integrity

Integrated Process: Nursing Process—Assessment
Content Area: Fundamental Skills—Perioperative Care
Reference: Ignatavicius, D., & Workman, M. (2010). *Medical-surgical nursing: Patient-centered collaborative care* (6th ed., pp. 1704–1705). St. Louis: Saunders.

537. 4

Rationale: Hodgkin's disease is a chronic progressive neoplastic disorder of lymphoid tissue characterized by the painless enlargement of lymph nodes with progression to extralymphatic sites, such as the spleen and liver. Weight loss is most likely to be noted. Fatigue and weakness may occur but are not related significantly to the disease.
Test-Taking Strategy: Use the process of elimination. Options 1 and 2 are comparable or alike and are rather vague symptoms that can occur in many disorders. Option 3 can be eliminated because, in such a disorder, weight loss is most likely to occur. Also, recalling that Hodgkin's disease affects the lymph nodes will direct you to option 4. Review the manifestations associated with Hodgkin's disease if you had difficulty with this question.
Level of Cognitive Ability: Analyzing
Client Needs: Physiological Integrity
Integrated Process: Nursing Process—Assessment
Content Area: Adult Health—Oncology
Reference: Black, J., & Hawks, J. (2009). *Medical-surgical nursing: Clinical management for positive outcomes* (8th ed., p. 2125). St. Louis: Saunders.

538. 4

Rationale: Clinical manifestations of ovarian cancer include abdominal distention, urinary frequency and urgency, pleural effusion, malnutrition, pain from pressure caused by the growing tumor and the effects of urinary or bowel obstruction, constipation, ascites with dyspnea, and ultimately general severe pain. Abnormal bleeding, often resulting in hypermenorrhea, is associated with uterine cancer.
Test-Taking Strategy: Use the process of elimination. Eliminate options 2 and 3 first because they are comparable or alike. From the remaining options, consider the anatomical location of the cancer. This will assist in directing you to option 4. Review the manifestations associated with ovarian cancer if you had difficulty with this question.
Level of Cognitive Ability: Analyzing
Client Needs: Physiological Integrity
Integrated Process: Nursing Process—Assessment
Content Area: Adult Health—Oncology
Reference: Ignatavicius, D., & Workman, M. (2010). *Medical-surgical nursing: Patient-centered collaborative care* (6th ed., p. 1706). St. Louis: Saunders.

539. 2

Rationale: Hypercalcemia is a serum calcium level higher than 10 mg/dL, most often occurs in clients who have bone metastasis, and is a late manifestation of extensive malignancy. The presence of cancer in the bone causes the bone to release calcium into the bloodstream.
Test-Taking Strategy: Use the process of elimination. Recalling the normal calcium level will direct you easily to option 2. Also note the relationship of *calcium level* in the question and

hypercalcemia in the correct option. Review oncological emergencies if you had difficulty with this question.
Level of Cognitive Ability: Understanding
Client Needs: Physiological Integrity
Integrated Process: Nursing Process—Assessment
Content Area: Adult Health—Oncology
References: Black, J., & Hawks, J. (2009). *Medical-surgical nursing: Clinical management for positive outcomes* (8th ed., pp. 162, 296). St. Louis: Saunders.
  Copstead-Kirkhorn, L., & Banasik, J. (2010). *Pathophysiology* (4th ed., p. 607). St. Louis: Mosby.
  Ignatavicius, D., & Workman, M. (2010). *Medical-surgical nursing: Patient-centered collaborative care* (6th ed., p. 436). St. Louis: Saunders.

540. 2

Rationale: A vesicovaginal fistula is a genital fistula that occurs between the bladder and vagina. The fistula is an abnormal opening between these two body parts and, if this occurs, the client may experience drainage of urine through the vagina. The client's complaint is not associated with options 1, 3, or 4.
Test-Taking Strategy: Use the process of elimination. Noting the strategic words *voiding through the vagina* should direct you to option 2. Review the symptoms associated with vesicovaginal fistula if you had difficulty with this question.
Level of Cognitive Ability: Analyzing
Client Needs: Physiological Integrity
Integrated Process: Nursing Process—Analysis
Content Area: Adult Health—Oncology
Reference: Ignatavicius, D., & Workman, M. (2010). *Medical-surgical nursing: Patient-centered collaborative care* (6th ed., p. 1694). St. Louis: Saunders.

541. 2

Rationale: The testicular-self examination is recommended monthly after a warm bath or shower when the scrotal skin is relaxed. The client should stand to examine the testicles. Using both hands, with fingers under the scrotum and thumbs on top, the client should gently roll the testicles, feeling for any lumps.
Test-Taking Strategy: Use the process of elimination. Eliminate option 4 first because of the words *6 months*. Next, eliminate option 3 because of the word *one*. From the remaining options, eliminate option 1 by trying to visualize the process of the self-examination. If you had difficulty with this question, review the procedure for this self-examination.
Level of Cognitive Ability: Applying
Client Needs: Health Promotion and Maintenance
Integrated Process: Teaching and Learning
Content Area: Adult Health—Health Assessment/Physical Exam
Reference: Ignatavicius, D., & Workman, M. (2010). *Medical-surgical nursing: Patient-centered collaborative care* (6th ed., p. 1726). St. Louis: Saunders.

542. 4

Rationale: Multiple myeloma is a B-cell neoplastic condition characterized by abnormal malignant proliferation of plasma cells and the accumulation of mature plasma cells in the bone

marrow. Options 1 and 2 are not characteristics of multiple myeloma. Option 3 describes the leukemic process.
Test-Taking Strategy: Use the process of elimination. Focusing on the name of the disorder, *multiple myeloma*, will direct you to option 4. Review the characteristics of multiple myeloma if you are unfamiliar with this oncological disorder.
Level of Cognitive Ability: Understanding
Client Needs: Physiological Integrity
Integrated Process: Teaching and Learning
Content Area: Adult Health—Oncology
Reference: Copstead-Kirkhorn, L., & Banasik, J. (2010). *Pathophysiology* (4th ed., p. 1193). St. Louis: Mosby.

543. 4

Rationale: Following gastrectomy, drainage from the nasogastric tube is normally bloody for 24 hours postoperatively, changes to brown-tinged, and is then to yellow or clear. Because bloody drainage is expected in the immediate postoperative period, the nurse should continue to monitor the drainage. The nurse does not need to notify the physician at this time. Measuring abdominal girth is performed to detect the development of distention. Following gastrectomy, a nasogastric tube should not be irrigated unless there are specific physician prescriptions to do so.
Test-Taking Strategy: Use the process of elimination and note the strategic words *immediate postoperative period*. This should direct you to option 4. Remember that drainage from the nasogastric tube is normally bloody for 24 hours postoperatively, changes to brown-tinged and then to yellow or clear. If you had difficulty with this question, review the postoperative expected findings following gastrectomy.
Level of Cognitive Ability: Applying
Client Needs: Physiological Integrity
Integrated Process: Nursing Process—Implementation
Content Area: Adult Health—Oncology
Reference: Ignatavicius, D., & Workman, M. (2010). *Medical-surgical nursing: Patient-centered collaborative care* (6th ed., pp. 1282, 1285). St. Louis: Saunders.

544. 1

Rationale: Colorectal cancer risk factors include age older than 50 years, a family history of the disease, colorectal polyps, and chronic inflammatory bowel disease.
Test-Taking Strategy: Use the process of elimination and note the strategic words *further teaching is necessary*. These words indicate a negative event query and ask you to select an option that is an incorrect statement. Noting the words *younger than* in option 1 will direct you to this option. Review the risk factors associated with colorectal cancer if you had difficulty with this question.
Level of Cognitive Ability: Evaluating
Client Needs: Health Promotion and Maintenance
Integrated Process: Teaching and Learning
Content Area: Adult Health—Oncology
Reference: Black, J., & Hawks, J. (2009). *Medical-surgical nursing: Clinical management for positive outcomes* (8th ed., pp. 266–267). St. Louis: Saunders.

545. 3

Rationale: Immediately after surgery, profuse serosanguineous drainage from the perineal wound is expected. The nurse does

not need to notify the physician at this time. A Penrose drain should not be clamped because this action will cause the accumulation of drainage within the tissue. Penrose drains and packing are removed gradually over a period of 5 to 7 days as prescribed. The nurse should not remove the perineal packing.
Test-Taking Strategy: Use the process of elimination. Eliminate options 2 and 4, knowing that these are inappropriate interventions. Recalling that serosanguineous drainage is expected following this type of surgery will assist in directing you to option 3. Review postoperative nursing care following abdominal perineal resection if you had difficulty with this question.
Level of Cognitive Ability: Applying
Client Needs: Physiological Integrity
Integrated Process: Nursing Process—Implementation
Content Area: Adult Health—Oncology
References: Black, J., & Hawks, J. (2009). *Medical-surgical nursing: Clinical management for positive outcomes* (8th ed., p. 706). St. Louis: Saunders.
    Ignatavicius, D., & Workman, M. (2010). *Medical-surgical nursing: Patient-centered collaborative care* (6th ed., p. 292). St. Louis: Saunders.

546. 2

Rationale: Following abdominal perineal resection, the nurse would expect the colostomy to begin to function within 72 hours after surgery, although it may take up to 5 days. The nurse should assess for a return of peristalsis, listen for bowel sounds, and check for the passage of flatus. Absent bowel sounds would not indicate the return of peristalsis. The client would remain NPO until bowel sounds return and the colostomy is functioning. Bloody drainage is not expected from a colostomy.
Test-Taking Strategy: Use the process of elimination and note the strategic words *beginning to function*. These should assist in eliminating option 1. Knowledge of general postoperative measures will assist in eliminating option 3. Focus on the subject of the question to assist in eliminating option 4 as a correct option. Review postoperative care of a client following abdominal perineal resection if you had difficulty with this question.
Level of Cognitive Ability: Analyzing
Client Needs: Physiological Integrity
Integrated Process: Nursing Process—Assessment
Content Area: Adult Health—Oncology
Reference: Black, J., & Hawks, J. (2009). *Medical-surgical nursing: Clinical management for positive outcomes* (8th ed., p. 706). St. Louis: Saunders.

547. 2

Rationale: The most common symptom in clients with cancer of the bladder is hematuria. The client also may experience irritative voiding symptoms such as frequency, urgency, and dysuria, and these symptoms often are associated with carcinoma in situ.
Test-Taking Strategy: Focus on the subject, bladder cancer, and note the strategic words *most common* in the question. Options 1, 3, and 4 are symptoms that are associated most often with bladder infection. Review the clinical manifestations associated with bladder cancer if you had difficulty with this question.
Level of Cognitive Ability: Analyzing
Client Needs: Physiological Integrity

Integrated Process: Nursing Process—Assessment
Content Area: Adult Health—Oncology
Reference: Black, J., & Hawks, J. (2009). *Medical-surgical nursing: Clinical management for positive outcomes* (8th ed., p. 737). St. Louis: Saunders.

548. 4
Rationale: Following ureterostomy, the stoma should be red and moist. A pale stoma may indicate an inadequate amount of vascular supply. A dry stoma may indicate a body fluid deficit. Any sign of darkness or duskiness in the stoma may indicate a loss of vascular supply and must be reported immediately or necrosis can occur.
Test-Taking Strategy: Use the process of elimination. You should be able to eliminate options 2 and 3 easily. From the remaining options, note the strategic word *moist* in option 4. This should indicate that this is an expected and positive assessment. If you had difficulty with this question, review expected and unexpected findings following ureterostomy.
Level of Cognitive Ability: Analyzing
Client Needs: Physiological Integrity
Integrated Process: Nursing Process—Assessment
Content Area: Adult Health—Oncology
References: Black, J., & Hawks, J. (2009). *Medical-surgical nursing: Clinical management for positive outcomes* (8th ed., p. 708). St. Louis: Saunders.
　Ignatavicius, D., & Workman, M. (2010). *Medical-surgical nursing: Patient-centered collaborative care* (6th ed., p. 1299). St. Louis: Saunders.

549. 2
Rationale: Following mastectomy, the arm should be elevated above the level of the heart. Simple arm exercises should be encouraged. No blood pressure readings, injections, intravenous lines, or blood draws should be performed on the affected arm. Cool compresses are not a suggested measure to prevent lymphedema from occurring.
Test-Taking Strategy: Note the strategic words *assist in preventing.* Use the process of elimination and note the relationship between *lymphedema* in the question and *elevating* in the correct option. Also using general principles related to gravity will direct you to the correct option. Review postoperative care measures following mastectomy if you had difficulty with this question.
Level of Cognitive Ability: Applying
Client Needs: Physiological Integrity
Integrated Process: Nursing Process—Implementation
Content Area: Adult Health—Oncology
References: Black, J., & Hawks, J. (2009). *Medical-surgical nursing: Clinical management for positive outcomes* (8th ed., p. 957). St. Louis: Saunders.
　Ignatavicius, D., & Workman, M. (2010). *Medical-surgical nursing: Patient-centered collaborative care* (6th ed., p. 1674). St. Louis: Saunders.

550. 3
Rationale: Superior vena cava syndrome occurs when the superior vena cava is compressed or obstructed by tumor growth. Early signs and symptoms generally occur in the morning and include edema of the face, especially around the eyes, and client complaints of tightness of a shirt or blouse collar. As the compression worsens, the client experiences edema of the hands and arms. Mental status changes and cyanosis are late signs.
Test-Taking Strategy: Use the process of elimination and note the strategic word *early* in the question. Think about the pathophysiology associated with this disorder and focus on the strategic word to assist in eliminating options 1, 2, and 4. If you are unfamiliar with vena cava syndrome, review this oncological emergency.
Level of Cognitive Ability: Analyzing
Client Needs: Physiological Integrity
Integrated Process: Nursing Process—Assessment
Content Area: Adult Health—Oncology
Reference: Ignatavicius, D., & Workman, M. (2010). *Medical-surgical nursing: Patient-centered collaborative care* (6th ed., pp. 436–437). St. Louis: Saunders.

551. 4
Rationale: Hypercalcemia is a late manifestation of bone metastasis in late-stage cancer. Headache and dysphagia are not associated with hypercalcemia. Constipation may occur early in the process. Electrocardiogram changes include shortened ST segment and a widened T wave.
Test-Taking Strategy: Use the process of elimination. Focus on the name of the oncological emergency, *hypercalcemia,* to direct you to option 4. Eliminate options 1 and 2 because they are not signs of hypercalcemia. Eliminate option 3 because it is an early sign of hypercalcemia. Also, noting the strategic words *serious* and *late sign* in the question will direct you to option 4. Review the early and late signs of hypercalcemia if you had difficulty with this question.
Level of Cognitive Ability: Applying
Client Needs: Physiological Integrity
Integrated Process: Teaching and Learning
Content Area: Adult Health—Oncology
References: Copstead-Kirkhorn, L., & Banasik, J. (2010). *Pathophysiology* (4th ed., p. 607). St. Louis: Mosby.
　Ignatavicius, D., & Workman, M. (2010). *Medical-surgical nursing: Patient-centered collaborative care* (6th ed., pp. 194, 722). St. Louis: Saunders.

552. 3
Rationale: During the period of greatest bone marrow suppression (the nadir), the platelet count may be low, less than 20,000 cells/mm³. Option 3 describes an incorrect statement by the client. Aspirin and nonsteroidal anti-inflammatory drugs and products that contain aspirin should be avoided because of their antiplatelet activity. Options 1, 2 and 4 are correct statements by the client to prevent and monitor bleeding.
Test-Taking Strategy: Note the strategic words *risk for bleeding* and *nadir.* Also note the strategic words *further teaching is needed.* Recalling the causes of thrombocytopenia will direct you to option 3. Review this information if you are unfamiliar with thrombocytopenia precautions.
Level of Cognitive Ability: Evaluating
Client Needs: Physiological Integrity
Integrated Process: Teaching and Learning
Content Area: Adult Health—Oncology
References: Black, J., & Hawks, J. (2009). *Medical-surgical nursing: Clinical management for positive outcomes* (8th ed., p. 291). St. Louis: Saunders.

Ignatavicius, D., & Workman, M. (2010). *Medical-surgical nursing: Patient-centered collaborative care* (6th ed., pp. 423, 910). St. Louis: Saunders.

553. 4

Rationale: The breast self-examination should be performed monthly 7 days after the onset of the menstrual period. Performing the examination weekly is not recommended. At the onset of menstruation and during ovulation, hormonal changes occur that may alter breast tissue.

Test-Taking Strategy: Use the process of elimination. Option 3 can be eliminated easily because of the word *weekly*. Eliminate options 1 and 2 next because of the similarity that exists regarding the hormonal changes that occur during these times. Review the procedure for performing breast self-examination if you had difficulty with this question.

Level of Cognitive Ability: Applying
Client Needs: Health Promotion and Maintenance
Integrated Process: Teaching and Learning
Content Area: Adult Health—Health Assessment/Physical Exam
Reference: Ignatavicius, D., & Workman, M. (2010). *Medical-surgical nursing: Patient-centered collaborative care* (6th ed., p. 1666). St. Louis: Saunders.

554. 1

Rationale: A biopsy is done to determine whether a tumor is malignant or benign. Magnetic resonance imaging, computed tomography scan, and ultrasound will visualize the presence of a mass but will not confirm a diagnosis of malignancy.

Test-Taking Strategy: Use the process of elimination and note the strategic word *confirm*. This strategic word should direct you easily to option 1. Review the purpose of the tests identified in the options if you had difficulty with this question.

Level of Cognitive Ability: Understanding
Client Needs: Physiological Integrity
Integrated Process: Nursing Process—Assessment
Content Area: Adult Health—Oncology

References: Black, J., & Hawks, J. (2009). *Medical-surgical nursing: Clinical management for positive outcomes* (8th ed., p. 2090). St. Louis: Saunders.

Chernecky, C., & Berger, B. (2008). *Laboratory tests and diagnostic procedures* (5th ed., pp. 201–203). St. Louis: Saunders.

Ignatavicius, D., & Workman, M. (2010). *Medical-surgical nursing: Patient-centered collaborative care* (6th ed., pp. 915, 1293–1294). St. Louis: Saunders.

ALTERNATE ITEM FORMAT: MULTIPLE RESPONSE

555. 1, 2, 4, 6

Rationale: Cancer is a common cause of syndrome of inappropriate antidiuretic hormone (SIADH). In SIADH, excessive amounts of water are reabsorbed by the kidney and put into the systemic circulation. The increased water causes hyponatremia (decreased serum sodium levels) and some degree of fluid retention. The syndrome is managed by treating the condition and cause and usually includes fluid restriction, increased sodium intake, and medication with a mechanism of action that is antagonistic to antidiuretic hormone. Sodium levels are monitored closely because hypernatremia can develop suddenly as a result of treatment. The immediate institution of appropriate cancer therapy, usually radiation or chemotherapy, can cause tumor regression so that antidiuretic hormone synthesis and release processes return to normal.

Test-Taking Strategy: Focusing on the client's diagnosis and recalling that in SIADH excessive amounts of water are reabsorbed by the kidney and put into the systemic circulation will assist in answering this question. Review the treatment for SIADH if you had difficulty with this question.

Level of Cognitive Ability: Analyzing
Client Needs: Physiological Integrity
Integrated Process: Nursing Process—Analysis
Content Area: Adult Health—Oncology
Reference: Ignatavicius, D., & Workman, M. (2010). *Medical-surgical nursing: Patient-centered collaborative care* (6th ed., pp. 435–436). St. Louis: Saunders.

Antineoplastic Medications

I. ANTINEOPLASTIC MEDICATIONS

A. Description

1. Antineoplastic medications kill or inhibit the reproduction of neoplastic cells.
2. Antineoplastic medications are used to cure, increase survival time, and decrease life-threatening complications.
3. The effect of antineoplastic medications may not be limited to neoplastic cells; normal cells also are affected by the medication.
4. Cell cycle phase–specific medications affect cells only during a certain phase of the reproductive cycle (Fig. 53-1).
5. Cell cycle phase–nonspecific medications affect cells in any phase of the reproductive cycle (see Fig. 53-1).
6. Usually, several medications are used in combination to increase the therapeutic response.
7. Antineoplastic medications may be combined with other treatments, such as surgery and radiation.
8. Although the intravenous (IV) route is most common for administration, antineoplastic medication may be given by the oral, intra-arterial, isolated limb perfusion, or intracavitary route; dosing is usually based on the client's body surface area (BSA) and type of **cancer**.
9. Chemotherapy dosing is usually based on total BSA, which requires a current, accurate height and weight for BSA calculation (before each medication administration) to ensure that the client receives optimal doses of chemotherapy medications.

⚠ Side effects from chemotherapy result from the effects of the antineoplastic medication on normal cells.

B. Side effects

1. Mucositis
2. Alopecia
3. Anorexia, nausea, and vomiting
4. Diarrhea
5. Anemia
6. Low white blood cell count (neutropenia)
7. Thrombocytopenia
8. Infertility, sexual alterations

C. General interventions

1. Physiological integrity
   a. Monitor complete blood cell count, white blood cell count, platelet count, uric acid level, and electrolytes.
   b. Initiate bleeding precautions if thrombocytopenia occurs.
   c. When the platelet count is less than 50,000 cells/mm^3, minor trauma can lead to episodes of prolonged bleeding; when less than 20,000 cells/mm^3, spontaneous and uncontrollable bleeding can occur.
   d. Monitor for petechiae, ecchymosis, bleeding of the gums, and nosebleeds because the decreased platelet count can precipitate bleeding tendencies.
   e. Avoid intramuscular injections and venipunctures as much as possible to prevent bleeding.
   f. Initiate neutropenic precautions if the white blood cell count decreases.
   g. Monitor for fever, sore throat, unusual bleeding, or signs and symptoms of infection.
   h. Inform the client that loss of appetite also may be the result of taste changes or a bitter taste in the mouth from the medications.
   i. Monitor for nausea and vomiting and provide a high-calorie diet with protein supplements.
   j. Administer antiemetics several hours before chemotherapy and for 12 to 48 hours after as prescribed, because antineoplastic medications stimulate the vomiting center in the brain.
   k. Encourage hydration; IV fluids are administered before and during therapy.
   l. Promote a fluid intake of at least 2000 mL/day to maintain adequate renal function.

⚠ Antineoplastic medication causes the rapid destruction of cells, resulting in the release of uric acid. Allopurinol (Zyloprim) may be prescribed to lower the serum uric acid level.

2. Safe and effective care environment
   a. Prepare IV chemotherapy in an air-vented space (biohazard cabinet area).

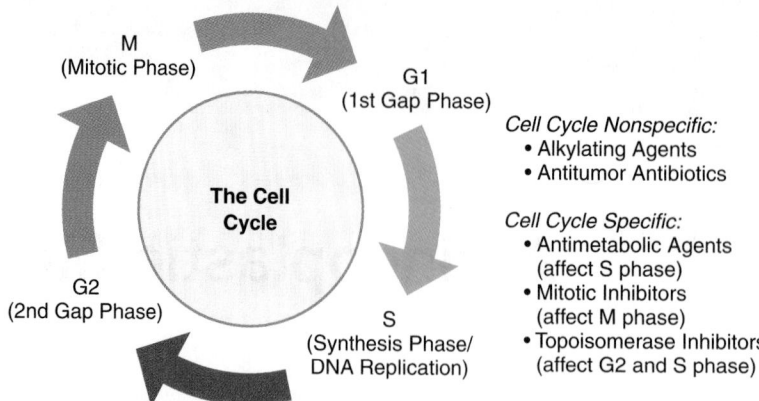

▲ **FIGURE 53-1** The cell cycle. *G1*, The cell is preparing for division; *S* (synthesis phase, DNA replication), the cell doubles its DNA content through DNA synthesis; *G2*, the cell produces proteins to be used in cell division and in normal physiological function after cell division is complete; and *M* (mitotic phase), the single cell splits apart into two cells.

    b. Wear gloves, gown, eye protectors, and mask when handling IV medications.

    c. Nurses who are pregnant should avoid chemotherapy preparation or the administration of chemotherapy.

    d. Discard IV equipment in designated (biohazard) containers.

    e. Administer antineoplastic medication precisely as prescribed to maximize antineoplastic effects while allowing normal cells to recover.

    f. Monitor for phlebitis with IV administration because these medications may irritate the veins.

    g. Monitor for extravasation (leakage of medication into surrounding skin and subcutaneous tissue, which causes tissue necrosis) and notify the physician if this occurs; heat or ice is applied depending on the medication, and an antidote may be injected into the site.

  3. Psychosocial integrity

    a. Instruct the client about the possibility of hair loss and that varying degrees of hair loss may occur after the first or second treatment.

    b. Discuss the purchase of a wig before treatment starts.

    c. Inform the client that new hair growth will occur several months after the final treatment.

    d. Instruct the client about the need for contraception because these medications have teratogenic effects.

    e. Discuss the potential effect of infertility, which may be irreversible.

    f. Encourage pretreatment counseling.

  4. Health promotion and maintenance

    a. Instruct the client, if diarrhea is a problem, to avoid hot foods and high-fiber foods, which increase peristalsis.

    b. Instruct the client to inspect the oral mucosa frequently for erythema and ulcers, rinse the mouth after meals, and carry out good oral hygiene.

    c. Instruct the client to use mouth rinses as prescribed for mouth sores if necessary.

    d. Instruct the client in the use of antifungal agents for mouth sores, if prescribed, for the development of a fungal infection.

    e. Instruct the client to avoid crowds and persons with infections and to report signs of infection such as a low-grade fever, chills, or sore throat.

    f. Instruct individuals with colds or infections to wear a mask when visiting or to avoid visiting the client.

    g. Instruct the client to use a soft toothbrush and electric razor to minimize the risk of bleeding.

    h. Instruct the client to avoid aspirin-containing products to minimize the risk of bleeding.

    i. Instruct the client to consult the physician before receiving vaccinations (live vaccines should not be administered).

D. Anaphylactic reactions

  1. Precautions

    a. Obtain an allergy history.

    b. Administer a test dose when prescribed by the physician.

    c. Stay with the client during the administration of medication.

    d. Monitor vital signs.

    e. Have emergency equipment and medications readily available.

    f. Provide an IV line for the administration of emergency medications if needed.

  2. Signs of an anaphylactic reaction

    a. Dyspnea

    b. Chest tightness or pain

    c. Pruritus or urticaria

    d. Tachycardia

    e. Dizziness

    f. Anxiety or agitation

    g. Flushed appearance

    h. Hypotension

    i. Decreased sensorium

    j. Cyanosis

  3. Interventions for an anaphylactic reaction (see Priority Nursing Actions)

▌▬▬▬▌ PRIORITY NURSING ACTIONS! ▌▬▬▬▌

Actions to Take If an Anaphylactic Reaction Occurs From Medication

1. Assess respiratory status.
2. Stop the medication.
3. Contact the physician and the Rapid Response Team if necessary.
4. Administer oxygen.
5. Maintain the IV access with normal saline.
6. Raise the client's feet and legs, if not contraindicated.
7. Administer prescribed emergency medications.
8. Monitor vital signs.
9. Document the event, actions taken, and the client's response.

If anaphylaxis occurs, the nurse immediately assesses the client's respiratory status. The medication is also immediately stopped. If the client's airway needs to be established or stabilized the Rapid Response Team is called. Additionally the physician is contacted. The IV line is not removed because IV access is needed to administer emergency medications such as diphenhydramine (Benadryl) or epinephrine. The client is positioned appropriately. The legs and feet are elevated. The head of the bed is elevated to improve ventilation; elevate the head of the bed 10 degrees if hypotension is present and 45 degrees or higher if the blood pressure is normal. The nurse stays with the client and monitors the client's status, including the vital signs. The nurse documents the event, actions taken, and the client's response.

Reference: Ignatavicius, D., & Workman, M. (2010). *Medical-surgical nursing: Patient-centered collaborative care.* (6th ed., p. 392). St. Louis: Saunders.

II. ALKYLATING MEDICATIONS (Box 53-1)

A. Description
  1. Breaks DNA helix, thereby interfering with DNA replication
  2. Cell cycle phase–nonspecific medications
B. Side effects
  1. Anorexia, nausea, and vomiting may occur.
  2. Stomatitis may occur.
  3. Rash may occur.
  4. Client may feel IV site pain during IV administration.
  5. Busulfan (Myleran, Busulfex) may cause hyperuricemia.
  6. Chlorambucil (Leukeran) and mechlorethamine (Mustargen) may cause gonadal suppression and hyperuricemia.
  7. Cisplatin (Platinol-AQ), a platinum compound, may cause ototoxicity, tinnitus, hypokalemia, hypocalcemia, hypomagnesemia, and nephrotoxicity.
  8. Cyclophosphamide (Cytoxan, Neosar) may cause alopecia, gonadal suppression, hemorrhagic cystitis, and hematuria.

Box 53-1 Alkylating Medications

Nitrogen Mustards
Bendamustine (Treanda)
Chlorambucil (Leukeran)
Cyclophosphamide (Cytoxan, Neosar)
Ifosfamide (Ifex)
Mechlorethamine (Mustargen)
Melphalan (Alkeran)

Nitrosoureas
Carmustine (BiCNU, Gliadel)
Lomustine (CeeNu)
Streptozocin (Zanosar)

Alkylating-Like Medications
Altretamine (Hexalen)
Busulfan (Myleran, Busulfex)
Carboplatin (Paraplatin)
Cisplatin (Platinol-AQ)
Dacarbazine (DTIC-Dome)
Oxaliplatin (Eloxatin)
Temozolomide (Temodar)
Thiotepa (Thioplex)

C. Interventions: Refer to general interventions section under Antineoplastic Medications.
  1. Withhold medication if the platelet count is less than $75,000/mm^3$ or the neutrophil count is less than $2000/mm^3$, and notify the physician (depending on alkylating agent and agency policy).
  2. Assess results of pulmonary function tests.
  3. Assess results of chest radiography and renal and liver function studies.
  4. Hydrate the client with IV and/or oral fluids before administering the antineoplastic medication as prescribed.
  5. As prescribed, reduce IV site pain by altering IV rates or warming the injection site to distend the vein and increase blood flow.
  6. When administering cisplatin assess the client for dizziness, tinnitus, hearing loss, incoordination, and numbness or tingling of extremities.
  7. Mesna (Mesnex) may be administered with ifosfamide to reduce the potential of ifosfamide-induced cystitis.
  8. Instruct the client that cyclophosphamide, when prescribed orally, is administered without food.
  9. Instruct the client to follow a diet low in purines to alkalinize the urine and lower uric acid blood levels.
  10. Instruct the client how to avoid infection.
  11. Instruct the client to report signs of infection or bleeding.
  12. Instruct the client about good oral hygiene and the use of a soft toothbrush.

⚠ Cyclophosphamide (Cytoxan, Neosar) and ifosfamide (Ifex) are medications that can cause hemorrhagic cystitis. Encourage the client to drink increased fluids (2 to 3 L per day) during therapy, unless contraindicated.

III. ANTITUMOR ANTIBIOTIC MEDICATIONS (Box 53-2)

A. Description
1. Interfere with DNA and RNA synthesis
2. Cell cycle phase–nonspecific medications

B. Side effects
1. Nausea and vomiting
2. Fever
3. Bone marrow depression
4. Rash
5. Alopecia
6. Stomatitis
7. Gonadal suppression
8. Hyperuricemia
9. Vesication (blistering of tissue at IV site)
10. Daunorubicin (DaunoXome) may cause congestive heart failure and dysrhythmias.
11. Doxorubicin (Adriamycin, Doxil) and idarubicin (Idamycin) may cause cardiotoxicity, cardiomyopathy, and electrocardiographic changes (Dexrazoxane [Zinecard] may be administered with doxorubicin to reduce cardiomyopathy).
12. Pulmonary toxicity can occur with bleomycin (Blenoxane).

C. Interventions: Refer to general interventions section under Antineoplastic Medications.
1. Withhold medication if the platelets are lower than 75,000/mm³ or the neutrophil count is lower than 2000/mm³, and notify physician (this may vary depending on antitumor antibiotic agent and agency policy).
2. Assess results of pulmonary function tests.
3. Monitor for electrocardiographic changes.
4. Assess lung sounds for crackles.
5. Assess for signs of congestive heart failure, including dyspnea, crackles, peripheral edema, and weight gain.
6. Assess results of chest radiography and renal and liver function studies.

Box 53-2 Antitumor Antibiotic Medications

Bleomycin sulfate (Blenoxane)
Dactinomycin (Cosmegen)
Daunorubicin (DaunoXome)
Doxorubicin (Adriamycin, Doxil)
Epirubicin (Ellence)
Idarubicin (Idamycin)
Mitomycin (Mutamycin)
Mitoxantrone (Novantrone)

7. Hydrate the client with IV and/or oral fluids before the antineoplastic medication.
8. As prescribed, reduce IV site pain by altering IV rates or warming injection site to distend vein and increase blood flow.
9. Monitor IV site for irritation, phlebitis, and vesication, change site as needed.
10. Assess for myocardial toxicity, dyspnea, dysrhythmias, hypotension, and weight gain when administering doxorubicin (Adriamycin, Doxil) or idarubicin
11. Monitor pulmonary status when administering bleomycin (Blenoxane).

IV. ANTIMETABOLITE MEDICATIONS (Box 53-3)

A. Description
1. Antimetabolite medications halt the synthesis of cell protein; their presence impairs cell division
2. Antimetabolite medications are cell cycle phase–specific and affect the S phase.

B. Side effects
1. Anorexia, nausea, and vomiting
2. Diarrhea
3. Alopecia
4. Stomatitis
5. Depression of bone marrow
6. Cytarabine (Cytosar-U, DepoCyt, Tarabine PFS) may cause alopecia, stomatitis, hyperuricemia, and hepatotoxicity.
7. Fluorouracil (Adrucil) may cause alopecia, stomatitis, diarrhea, phototoxicity reactions, and cerebellar dysfunction.
8. Mercaptopurine (Purinethol) may cause hyperuricemia and hepatotoxicity.
9. Methotrexate (Rheumatrex, Trexall) may cause alopecia, stomatitis, hyperuricemia, photosensitivity, hepatotoxicity, and hematological, gastrointestinal, and skin toxicity.

C. Interventions: Refer to general interventions section under Antineoplastic Medications

Box 53-3 Antimetabolite Medications

Capecitabine (Xeloda)
Cladribine (Leustatin)
Clofarabine (Clolar)
Cytarabine (Cytosar-U, DepoCyt, Tarabine PFS)
Floxuridine (FUDR)
Fludarabine (Fludara)
Fluorouracil (Adrucil)
Gemcitabine (Gemzar)
Hydroxyurea (Hydrea, Mylocel)
Mercaptopurine (Purinethol)
Methotrexate (Rheumatrex, Trexall)
Pemetrexed (Alimta)
Pentostatin (Nipent)
Thioguanine (Tabloid)

1. Hold medication if the neutrophil count is less than 2000 cells/mm^3 or the platelet count is less than 75,000 cells/mm^3, and notify the physician (depending on the antimetabolite medication and agency policy).
2. Monitor renal function studies.
3. Monitor for cerebellar dysfunction.
4. Assess for photosensitivity.
5. Monitor IV site for extravasation.
6. Encourage fluid intake of 2 to 3 L/day.
7. Encourage good oral hygiene.
8. Instruct the client how to avoid infections and bleeding.
9. When administering fluorouracil, assess for signs of cerebellar dysfunction, such as dizziness, weakness, and ataxia, and assess for stomatitis and diarrhea, which may necessitate medication discontinuation.
10. When administering fluorouracil or methotrexate, instruct the client to use sunscreen and wear protective clothing to prevent photosensitivity reactions.

⚠ When administering methotrexate in large doses, prepare to administer leucovorin (folinic acid or citrovorum factor) as prescribed to prevent toxicity. This is known as *leucovorin rescue*.

V. MITOTIC INHIBITOR MEDICATIONS (VINCA ALKALOIDS) (Box 53-4)

A. Description
1. Mitotic inhibitors prevent mitosis, causing cell death; mitotic inhibitors prevent cell division.
2. Mitotic inhibitors are cell cycle phase–specific and act on the M phase.

B. Side effects
1. Leukopenia
2. Neurotoxicity with vincristine (Oncovin, Vincasar) manifested as numbness and tingling in the fingers and toes, constipation, paralytic ileus.
3. Ptosis
4. Hoarseness
5. Motor instability
6. Anorexia, nausea, and vomiting
7. Peripheral neuropathy
8. Alopecia

Box 53-4 Mitotic Inhibitors

Vinca Alkaloids
Vinblastine sulfate (Velban)
Vincristine sulfate (Oncovin, Vincasar)
Vinorelbine (Navelbine)

Taxanes
Docetaxel (Taxotere)
Paclitaxel (Abraxane, Taxol, Onxol)

9. Stomatitis
10. Hyperuricemia
11. Phlebitis at IV site

C. Interventions: Refer to general interventions section under Antineoplastic Medications.
1. Monitor for hoarseness.
2. Assess eyes for ptosis.
3. Assess motor stability and initiate safety precautions as necessary.
4. Monitor for neurotoxicity with vincristine sulfate manifested as numbness and tingling in the fingers and toes.
5. Monitor for constipation and paralytic ileus.

VI. TOPOISOMERASE INHIBITORS (Box 53-5)

A. Description
1. Block the enzyme needed for DNA synthesis and cell division
2. Cell cycle phase–specific; act on the G2 and S phases

B. Side effects
1. Leukopenia, thrombocytopenia, anemia
2. Anorexia, nausea, and vomiting
3. Diarrhea
4. Alopecia
5. Orthostatic hypotension
6. Hypersensitivity reaction

C. Interventions: Refer to general interventions section under Antineoplastic Medications.

VII. HORMONAL MEDICATIONS AND ENZYMES (Box 53-6)

A. Description
1. Suppress the immune system and block normal hormones in hormone-sensitive tumors
2. Change the hormonal balance and slow the growth rates of certain tumors

B. Side effects
1. Anorexia, nausea, and vomiting
2. Leukopenia
3. Impaired pancreatic function with asparaginase (Elspar)
4. Sex characteristic alterations
   a. Masculinizing effect in women: Chest and facial hair, menses stops (androgens, antiestrogen receptor drugs)
   b. Feminine manifestations in men: Gynecomastia (estrogens, progestins, antiestrogen receptors)
5. Breast swelling
6. Hot flashes
7. Weight gain

Box 53-5 Topoisomerase Inhibitors

Etoposide (VePesid, Toposar, Etopophos)
Irinotecan (Camptosar)
Teniposide (Vumon)
Topotecan (Hycamtin)

Box 53-6 Hormonal Medications and Enzymes

Estrogens
Diethylstilbestrol
Estramustine (Emcyt)
Ethinyl estradiol (Estinyl)

Antiestrogens
Anastrozole (Arimidex)
Exemestane (Aromasin)
Fulvestrant (Faslodex)
Letrozole (Femara)
Raloxifene (Evista)
Tamoxifen citrate (Nolvadex)
Toremifene (Fareston)

Antiandrogens
Bicalutamide (Casodex)
Flutamide (Eulexin)
Goserelin acetate (Zoladex)
Nilutamide (Nilandron)
Triptorelin (Trelstar)

Progestins
Medroxyprogesterone (Depo-Provera)
Megestrol acetate (Megace)

Other Hormonal Antagonists and Enzymes
Asparaginase (Elspar)
Leuprolide acetate (Lupron)
Mitotane (Lysodren)

Box 53-7 Immunomodulator Agents

Aldesleukin (Proleukin, interleukin-2)
Interferon alfa-2a
Interferon alfa-2b
Interferon alfa-n3 (Alferon N)
Recombinant interferon alfa-2a (Intron A)
Recombinant interferon alfa-2b (Roferon-A)

Common Monoclonal Antibodies
Alemtuzumab (Campath)
Gemtuzumab ozogamicin (Mylotarg)
Ibritumomab (Zevalin)
Rituximab (Rituxan)
Trastuzumab (Herceptin)

Box 53-8 Colony-Stimulating Factors

Granulocyte-Macrophage Colony-Stimulating Factor
Sargramostim (Leukine)

Granulocyte Colony-Stimulating Factor
Filgrastim (Neupogen)
Pegfilgrastim (Neulasta)

Erythropoietin
Epoetin alfa (Epogen)
Darbepoetin alfa (Aranesp)

Thrombopoietic Growth Factor
Oprelvekin (Interleukin-11)

---

8. Hemorrhagic cystitis, hypouricemia, and hypercholesterolemia, with mitotane (Lysodren)
9. Hypertension
10. Thromboembolic disorders
11. Edema
12. Electrolyte imbalances
13. Tamoxifen citrate (Nolvadex) may cause edema, hypercalcemia, and elevated cholesterol and triglyceride levels.
14. Tamoxifen citrate decreases the effects of estrogen.
15. Diethylstilbestrol may cause impotence and gynecomastia in men.
16. Diethylstilbestrol may alter effects of insulin, orally administered anticoagulants, and orally administered hypoglycemic agents.

C. Interventions
1. Monitor vital signs.
2. Assess medications that the client is taking currently.
3. Monitor serum calcium levels with androgens.
4. Monitor for signs of alterations in sexual characteristics.
5. Monitor pancreatic function with asparaginase
6. Encourage an oral intake of 2 to 3 L of fluids per day.
7. Monitor uric acid and cholesterol levels.
8. Monitor for signs of hemorrhagic cystitis.

VIII. IMMUNOMODULATOR AGENTS: BIOLOGICAL RESPONSE MODIFIERS (Box 53-7)

A. Description
1. Immunomodulators stimulate the immune system to recognize **cancer** cells and take action to eliminate or destroy them.
2. Interleukins help different immune system cells recognize and destroy abnormal body cells.
3. Interferons slow tumor cell division, stimulate proliferation, and cause **cancer** cells to differentiate into nonproliferative forms.

B. Colony-stimulating factors induce more rapid bone marrow recovery after suppression by chemotherapy (Box 53-8).

IX. TARGETED THERAPY

A. Description
1. Medications used as targeted therapies are monoclonal antibodies that target a cellular element of the **cancer** cell or antisense medications that work at the gene level.
2. Examples of monoclonal antibodies are rituximab (Rituxan), tositumomab (Bexxar), trastuzumab (Herceptin), alemtuzumab (Campath), and cetuximab (Erbitux).

Box 53-9 Other Antineoplastic Medications

Asparaginase (Elspar)
Arsenic trioxide (Trisenox)
Bexarotene (Targretin)
Bortezomib (Velcade)
Imatinib (Gleevec)
Temozolomide (Temodar)

B. Side effects: Allergic reactions (monoclonal antibodies)

X. OTHER ANTINEOPLASTIC MEDICATIONS
(Box 53-9)

A. Altretamine (Hexalen): Cytotoxic agent used to treat ovarian **cancer**

B. Denileukin diftitox (Ontak): Recombinant DNA-derived medication used to treat cutaneous T-cell **lymphoma**

C. Gemcitabine (Gemzar): Used to treat non–small cell lung **cancer** and adenocarcinoma of the pancreas, as well as metastatic breast **cancer** and lung cancer (in combination with paclitaxel [Abraxane, Taxol, Onxol])

D. Irinotecan (Camptosar): Used to treat colorectal or rectal **cancer**

E. Paclitaxel (Abraxane, Taxol, Onxol): Used to treat ovarian or metastatic breast **cancer**

F. Pegaspargase (Oncaspar): Used in combination chemotherapies for acute lymphoblastic **leukemia** in clients unable to take asparaginase (Elspar)

G. Topotecan (Hycamtin): Indicated for the treatment of relapsed or refractory metastatic ovarian **cancer** after other therapies have failed

H. Trastuzumab (Herceptin): Used in combination chemotherapy to treat breast **cancer**

I. Bexarotene (Targretin): Use to treat advanced stage cutaneous T-cell **lymphoma**

 MORE QUESTIONS ON THE CD!

Practice Questions

556. Chemotherapy dosage is frequently based on total body surface area (BSA), so it is important for the nurse to do which of the following before administering chemotherapy?
1. Measure abdominal girth.
2. Calculate body mass index.
3. Ask the client about his or her height and weight.
4. Weigh and measure the client on the day of medication administration.

557. The client with squamous cell carcinoma of the larynx is receiving bleomycin (Blenoxane) intravenously. The nurse caring for the client anticipates that which diagnostic study will be prescribed?

1. Echocardiography
2. Electrocardiography
3. Cervical radiography
4. Pulmonary function studies

558. The client with acute myelocytic leukemia is being treated with busulfan (Myleran, Busulfex). Which laboratory value would the nurse specifically monitor during treatment with this medication?
1. Clotting time
2. Blood glucose level
3. Uric acid level
4. Potassium level

559. The client with small cell lung cancer is being treated with etoposide (VePesid). The nurse monitors the client during administration, knowing that which side effect is specifically associated with this medication?
1. Alopecia
2. Chest pain
3. Pulmonary fibrosis
4. Orthostatic hypotension

560. The clinic nurse prepares a teaching plan for the client receiving an antineoplastic medication. When implementing the plan, the nurse tells the client:
1. To take aspirin (acetylsalicylic acid) as needed for headache
2. To drink beverages containing alcohol in moderate amounts each evening
3. To consult with health care providers before receiving immunizations
4. That it is not necessary to consult health care providers before receiving a flu vaccine at the local health fair

561. The client with ovarian cancer is being treated with vincristine (Oncovin, Vincasar). The nurse monitors the client, knowing that which of the following indicates a side effect specific to this medication?
1. Diarrhea
2. Hair loss
3. Chest pain
4. Numbness and tingling in the fingers and toes

562. The nurse is reviewing the history and physical examination of a client who will be receiving asparaginase (Elspar), an antineoplastic agent. The nurse contacts the physician before administering the medication if which of the following is documented in the client's history?
1. Pancreatitis
2. Diabetes mellitus
3. Myocardial infarction
4. Chronic obstructive pulmonary disease

563. Tamoxifen (Nolvadex) is prescribed for the client with metastatic breast carcinoma. The nurse administering the medication understands that the primary action of this medication is to:
1. Increase DNA and RNA synthesis.
2. Promote the biosynthesis of nucleic acids.
3. Increase estrogen concentration and estrogen response.
4. Compete with estradiol for binding to estrogen in tissues containing high concentrations of receptors.

564. The client with metastatic breast cancer is receiving tamoxifen (Nolvadex). The nurse specifically monitors which laboratory value while the client is taking this medication?
1. Glucose level
2. Calcium level
3. Potassium level
4. Prothrombin time

565. Megestrol acetate (Megace), an antineoplastic medication, is prescribed for the client with metastatic endometrial carcinoma. The nurse reviews the client's history and contacts the physician if which diagnosis is documented in the client's history?
1. Gout
2. Asthma
3. Thrombophlebitis
4. Myocardial infarction

566. The nurse is monitoring the laboratory results of a client receiving an antineoplastic medication by the intravenous route. The nurse plans to initiate bleeding precautions if which laboratory result is noted?
1. A clotting time of 10 minutes
2. An ammonia level of 20 mcg/dL
3. A platelet count of 50,000/mm^3
4. A white blood cell count of 5,000/mm^3

567. The nurse is analyzing the laboratory results of a client with leukemia who has received a regimen of chemotherapy. Which laboratory value would the nurse specifically note as a result of the massive cell destruction that occurred from the chemotherapy?
1. Anemia
2. Decreased platelets
3. Increased uric acid level
4. Decreased leukocyte count

568. The nurse is providing medication instructions to a client with breast cancer who is receiving cyclophosphamide (Cytoxan, Neosar). The nurse tells the client to:
1. Take the medication with food.
2. Increase fluid intake to 2000 to 3000 mL daily.
3. Decrease sodium intake while taking the medication.
4. Increase potassium intake while taking the medication.

569. The client with non–Hodgkin's lymphoma is receiving daunorubicin (DaunoXome). Which of the following would indicate to the nurse that the client is experiencing an adverse effect related to the medication?
1. Fever
2. Diarrhea
3. Complaints of nausea and vomiting
4. Crackles on auscultation of the lungs

Alternate Item Format: Multiple Response

570. The nurse is monitoring the intravenous (IV) infusion of an antineoplastic medication. During the infusion, the client complains of pain at the insertion site. On inspection of the site, the nurse notes redness and swelling and that the infusion of the medication has slowed in rate. The nurse should take which actions? **Select all that apply.**
❏ 1. Stop the infusion.
❏ 2. Notify the physician.
❏ 3. Prepare to apply ice or heat to the site.
❏ 4. Restart the IV at a distal part of the same vein.
❏ 5. Prepare to administer a prescribed antidote into the site.
❏ 6. Increase the flow rate of the solution to flush the skin and subcutaneous tissue.

ANSWERS

556. 4
Rationale: To ensure that the client receives optimal doses of chemotherapy, dosing is usually based on the total body surface area (BSA), which requires a current accurate height and weight for BSA calculation (before each medication administration). Asking the client about his or her height and weight may lead to inaccuracies in determining a true BSA and dosage. Calculating body mass index and measuring abdominal girth will not provide the data needed.
Test-Taking Strategy: Use the process of elimination, recalling the basis for dosing chemotherapy. Recalling that a current accurate height and weight need to be obtained for BSA calculation and chemotherapy dosing will direct you to option 4. Eliminate option 3 because it is an unreliable way of obtaining the information, and options 1 and 2 do not

relate to chemotherapy dosing. If you are unfamiliar with BSA and chemotherapy dosing, review these concepts.
Level of Cognitive Ability: Analyzing
Client Needs: Physiological Integrity
Integrated Process: Nursing Process—Implementation
Content Area: Pharmacology
References: Edmunds, M. (2010). *Introduction to clinical pharmacology* (6th ed., p. 86). St. Louis: Mosby.

Kee, J., Hayes, E., & McCuistion, L. (2009). *Pharmacology: A nursing process approach* (6th ed., pp. 59, 74). St. Louis: Saunders.

557. 4
Rationale: Bleomycin (Blenoxane) is an antineoplastic medication that can cause interstitial pneumonitis, which can progress to pulmonary fibrosis. Pulmonary function studies along with hematological, hepatic, and renal function tests need to be monitored. The nurse needs to monitor lung sounds for dyspnea and crackles, which indicate pulmonary toxicity. The medication needs to be discontinued immediately if pulmonary toxicity occurs. Options 1, 2, and 3 are unrelated to the specific use of this medication.
Test-Taking Strategy: Use the process of elimination. Eliminate options 1 and 2 first because they are cardiac-related and are therefore comparable or alike. From the remaining options, use the ABCs—airway, breathing, and circulation—to direct you to option 4. If you had difficulty with this question, review the toxic effects of this medication.
Level of Cognitive Ability: Analyzing
Client Needs: Physiological Integrity
Integrated Process: Nursing Process—Analysis
Content Area: Pharmacology
Reference: Gahart, B., & Nazareno, A. (2010). *2010 Intravenous medications* (26th ed., pp. 203–204). St. Louis: Mosby.

558. 3
Rationale: Busulfan (Myleran, Busulfex) can cause an increase in the uric acid level. Hyperuricemia can produce uric acid nephropathy, renal stones, and acute renal failure. Options 1, 2, and 4 are not specifically related to this medication.
Test-Taking Strategy: Focus on the medication addressed in the question. It is necessary to know the adverse effects associated with this medication. Recalling that busulfan increases the uric acid level will direct you to the correct option. If you had difficulty with this question, review the effects of busulfan.
Level of Cognitive Ability: Analyzing
Client Needs: Physiological Integrity
Integrated Process: Nursing Process—Assessment
Content Area: Pharmacology
References: Kee, J., Hayes, E., & McCuistion, L. (2009). *Pharmacology: A nursing process approach* (6th ed., p. 538). St. Louis: Saunders.

Skidmore-Roth, L. (2010). *Mosby's nursing drug reference* (23rd ed., p. 216). St. Louis: Mosby.

559. 4
Rationale: A side effect specific to etoposide is orthostatic hypotension. Etoposide should be administered slowly over 30 to 60 minutes to avoid hypotension. The client's blood pressure is monitored during the infusion. Hair loss occurs with nearly all the antineoplastic medications.

Chest pain and pulmonary fibrosis are unrelated to this medication.
Test-Taking Strategy: Use the process of elimination. Eliminate option 1 first because this side effect is associated with many of the antineoplastic agents. Eliminate options 2 and 3 next because they are unrelated to etoposide. Note that the question asks for the side effect *specific* to this medication. Correlate hypotension with etoposide. Review the side effects of this medication if you had difficulty with this question.
Level of Cognitive Ability: Analyzing
Client Needs: Physiological Integrity
Integrated Process: Nursing Process—Assessment
Content Area: Pharmacology
Reference: Gahart, B., & Nazareno, A. (2010). *2010 Intravenous medications* (26th ed., p. 566). St. Louis: Mosby.

560. 3
Rationale: Because antineoplastic medications lower the resistance of the body, clients must be informed not to receive immunizations without a physician's or health care provider's approval. Clients also need to avoid contact with individuals who have recently received a live virus vaccine. Clients need to avoid aspirin and aspirin-containing products to minimize the risk of bleeding, and they need to avoid alcohol to minimize the risk of toxicity and side effects.
Test-Taking Strategy: Think about the adverse effects of antineoplastic medications. Recalling that antineoplastic medications lower the resistance of the body will direct you to option 3. Review the client teaching points regarding these medications if you had difficulty with this question.
Level of Cognitive Ability: Applying
Client Needs: Health Promotion and Maintenance
Integrated Process: Teaching and Learning
Content Area: Pharmacology
Reference: Kee, J., Hayes, E., & McCuistion, L. (2009). *Pharmacology: A nursing process approach* (6th ed., p. 541). St. Louis: Saunders.

561. 4
Rationale: A side effect specific to vincristine is peripheral neuropathy, which occurs in almost every client. Peripheral neuropathy can be manifested as numbness and tingling in the fingers and toes. Depression of the Achilles tendon reflex may be the first clinical sign indicating peripheral neuropathy. Constipation rather than diarrhea is most likely to occur with this medication, although diarrhea may occur occasionally. Hair loss occurs with nearly all the antineoplastic medications. Chest pain is unrelated to this medication.
Test-Taking Strategy: Use the process of elimination. Eliminate options 1 and 2 first because these side effects are associated with many of the antineoplastic agents. Note that the question asks for the side effect *specific* to this medication. Correlate peripheral neuropathy with vincristine. Review the side effects of this medication if you had difficulty with this question.
Level of Cognitive Ability: Analyzing
Client Needs: Physiological Integrity
Integrated Process: Nursing Process—Assessment
Content Area: Pharmacology
Reference: Hodgson, B., & Kizior, R. (2010). *Saunders nursing drug handbook 2010* (p. 1184). St. Louis: Saunders.

562. 1

Rationale: Asparaginase (Elspar) is contraindicated if hypersensitivity exists, in pancreatitis, or if the client has a history of pancreatitis. The medication impairs pancreatic function and pancreatic function tests should be performed before therapy begins and when a week or more has elapsed between dose administrations. The client needs to be monitored for signs of pancreatitis, which include nausea, vomiting, and abdominal pain. The conditions noted in options 2, 3, and 4 are not contraindicated with this medication.

Test-Taking Strategy: Focus on the medication addressed in the question. It is necessary to know the contraindications associated with this medication. Recalling that this medication affects pancreatic function will direct you to option 1. Review this medication if you had difficulty answering this question.

Level of Cognitive Ability: Analyzing
Client Needs: Physiological Integrity
Integrated Process: Nursing Process—Assessment
Content Area: Pharmacology
Reference: Hodgson, B., & Kizior, R. (2010). *Saunders nursing drug handbook 2010* (p. 86). St. Louis: Saunders.

563. 4

Rationale: Tamoxifen (Nolvadex) is an antineoplastic medication that competes with estradiol for binding to estrogen in tissues containing high concentrations of receptors. Tamoxifen is used to treat metastatic breast carcinoma in women and men. Tamoxifen is also effective in delaying the recurrence of cancer following mastectomy. Tamoxifen reduces DNA synthesis and estrogen response.

Test-Taking Strategy: Use the process of elimination. Eliminate options 1 and 2 first because they are comparable or alike. Nucleic acids include DNA and RNA. From this point, select option 4, because it is unlikely that treatment of metastatic breast carcinoma would focus on increasing estrogen concentration and estrogen response. If you had difficulty with this question, review the action of this medication.

Level of Cognitive Ability: Understanding
Client Needs: Physiological Integrity
Integrated Process: Nursing Process—Implementation
Content Area: Pharmacology
Reference: Hodgson, B., & Kizior, R. (2010). *Saunders nursing drug handbook 2010* (p. 1072). St. Louis: Saunders.

564. 2

Rationale: Tamoxifen (Nolvadex) may increase calcium, cholesterol, and triglyceride levels. Before the initiation of therapy, a complete blood count, platelet count, and serum calcium levels should be assessed. These blood levels, along with cholesterol and triglyceride levels, should be monitored periodically during therapy. The nurse should assess for hypercalcemia while the client is taking this medication. Signs of hypercalcemia include increased urine volume, excessive thirst, nausea, vomiting, constipation, hypotonicity of muscles, and deep bone and flank pain.

Test-Taking Strategy: Focus on the medication addressed in the question. It is necessary to know the adverse effects associated with this medication. Recalling that this medication causes hypercalcemia will direct you to option 2. Review this medication if you had difficulty answering this question.

Level of Cognitive Ability: Analyzing
Client Needs: Physiological Integrity
Integrated Process: Nursing Process—Assessment
Content Area: Pharmacology
Reference: Hodgson, B., & Kizior, R. (2010). *Saunders nursing drug handbook 2010* (p. 1073). St. Louis: Saunders.

565. 3

Rationale: Megestrol acetate (Megace) suppresses the release of luteinizing hormone from the anterior pituitary by inhibiting pituitary function and regressing tumor size. Megestrol is used with caution if the client has a history of thrombophlebitis. Options 1, 2, and 4 are not contraindications for this medication.

Test-Taking Strategy: Focus on the medication addressed in the question. It is necessary to know the adverse effects associated with this medication. Recalling that megestrol acetate is a hormonal antagonist enzyme and that an adverse effect is thrombotic disorders will direct you to option 3. Review this medication if you had difficulty answering this question.

Level of Cognitive Ability: Analyzing
Client Needs: Physiological Integrity
Integrated Process: Nursing Process—Implementation
Content Area: Pharmacology
Reference: Hodgson, B., & Kizior, R. (2010). *Saunders nursing drug handbook 2010* (p. 708). St. Louis: Saunders.

566. 3

Rationale: Bleeding precautions need to be initiated when the platelet count decreases. The normal platelet count is 150,000 to 450,000/mm^3. When the platelets are lower than 50,000/mm^3, any small trauma can lead to episodes of prolonged bleeding. The normal white blood cell count is 4500 to 11,000/mm^3. When the white blood cell count drops, neutropenic precautions need to be implemented. The normal clotting time is 8 to 15 minutes. The normal ammonia value is 10 to 80 mcg/dL.

Test-Taking Strategy: Use the process of elimination and knowledge regarding normal laboratory values. Options 1, 2, and 4 identify normal laboratory values. Remember to correlate a low platelet count with the need for bleeding precautions and a low white blood cell count with the need for neutropenic precautions. Review the indications to implement bleeding precautions in a client receiving chemotherapy if you had difficulty with this question.

Level of Cognitive Ability: Analyzing
Client Needs: Safe and Effective Care Environment
Integrated Process: Nursing Process—Planning
Content Area: Fundamental Skills—Safety/Infection Control
References: Ignatavicius, D., & Workman, M. (2010). *Medical-surgical nursing: Patient-centered collaborative care* (6th ed., pp. 426, 428). St. Louis: Saunders.

Kee, J., Hayes, E., & McCuistion, L. (2009). *Pharmacology: A nursing process approach* (6th ed., p. 534). St. Louis: Saunders.

567. 3

Rationale: Hyperuricemia is especially common following treatment for leukemias and lymphomas because chemotherapy results in massive cell kill. Although options 1, 2, and 4 also may be noted, an increased uric acid level is related specifically to cell destruction.

Test-Taking Strategy: Note the strategic words *massive cell destruction* in the question. Recalling the cell response to destruction when administering chemotherapy will assist in directing you to option 3. Review the effects of chemotherapy if you had difficulty with this question.
Level of Cognitive Ability: Analyzing
Client Needs: Physiological Integrity
Integrated Process: Nursing Process—Assessment
Content Area: Pharmacology
References: Kee, J., Hayes, E., & McCuistion, L. (2009). *Pharmacology: A nursing process approach* (6th ed., p. 645). St. Louis: Saunders.
   Lehne, R. (2010). *Pharmacology for nursing care* (7th ed., p. 1177). St. Louis: Saunders.

568. 2
Rationale: Hemorrhagic cystitis is an adverse effect that can occur with the use of cyclophosphamide (Cytoxan, Neosar). The client needs to be instructed to drink copious amounts of fluid during the administration of this medication. Clients also should monitor urine output for hematuria. The medication should be taken on an empty stomach, unless gastrointestinal upset occurs. Hyperkalemia can result from the use of the medication; therefore, the client would not be told to increase potassium intake. The client would not be instructed to alter sodium intake.
Test-Taking Strategy: Use the process of elimination. Recalling the adverse effects of cyclophosphamide and that it can cause hemorrhagic cystitis will direct you to option 2. If you had difficulty with this question, review the adverse effects associated with this medication.
Level of Cognitive Ability: Applying
Client Needs: Physiological Integrity
Integrated Process: Teaching and Learning
Content Area: Pharmacology
Reference: Hodgson, B., & Kizior, R. (2010). *Saunders nursing drug handbook 2010* (p. 287). St. Louis: Saunders.

569. 4
Rationale: Cardiotoxicity noted by abnormal electrocardiographic findings or cardiomyopathy manifested as congestive heart failure is an adverse effect of daunorubicin. Bone marrow depression is also a toxic effect. Nausea and vomiting is a frequent side effect associated with the medication that begins a few hours after administration and lasts 24 to 48 hours. Fever is a frequent side effect and diarrhea can occur occasionally. Options 1, 2, and 3, however, are not adverse effects.
Test-Taking Strategy: Use the process of elimination, keeping in mind that the question is asking about an adverse effect. Use of the ABCs—airway, breathing, and circulation—will direct you easily to option 4. If you had difficulty with this question, review the adverse effects associated with daunorubicin.
Level of Cognitive Ability: Analyzing
Client Needs: Physiological Integrity
Integrated Process: Nursing Process—Analysis
Content Area: Pharmacology
Reference: Lehne, R. (2010). *Pharmacology for nursing care* (7th ed., p. 1192). St. Louis: Saunders.

ALTERNATE ITEM FORMAT: MULTIPLE RESPONSE
570. 1, 2, 3, 5
Rationale: Redness and swelling and a slowed infusion indicate signs of extravasation. If extravasation occurs during the intravenous administration of an antineoplastic medication, the infusion is stopped and the physician is notified. Ice or heat may be prescribed for application to the site and an antidote may be prescribed to be administered into the site. Increasing the flow rate can increase damage to the tissues. Restarting an IV in the same vein can increase damage to the site and vein.
Test-Taking Strategy: Focus on the assessment signs in the question. Visualize the situation to identify the nursing actions. Think about the actions that will cause further damage. This will assist in eliminating options 4 and 6. Review nursing actions if extravasation occurs if you had difficulty with this question.
Level of Cognitive Ability: Applying
Client Needs: Physiological Integrity
Integrated Process: Nursing Process—Implementation
Content Area: Pharmacology
Reference: Ignatavicius, D., & Workman, M. (2010). *Medical-surgical nursing: Patient-centered collaborative care* (6th ed., pp. 226, 423–424). St. Louis: Saunders.

UNIT X

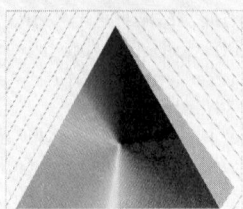

The Adult Client With an Endocrine Disorder

PYRAMID TERMS

addisonian crisis A life-threatening disorder caused by adrenal hormone insufficiency. Crisis is precipitated by infection, trauma, stress, or surgery. Death can occur from shock, vascular collapse, or hyperkalemia.

Addison's disease Hyposecretion of adrenal cortex hormones (glucocorticoids and mineralocorticoids) from the adrenal gland, resulting in deficiency of the corticosteroid hormones. The condition is fatal if left untreated.

adrenalectomy The surgical removal of an adrenal gland. Lifelong replacement of glucocorticoids and mineralocorticoids is necessary with a bilateral adrenalectomy. Temporary replacement may be necessary for up to 2 years for a unilateral adrenalectomy.

Chvostek's sign A spasm of the facial muscles elicited by tapping the facial nerve just anterior to the ear. The sign is noted in hypocalcemia.

Cushing's disease A metabolic disorder characterized by abnormally increased secretion (endogenous) of cortisol, caused by increased amounts of adrenocorticotropic hormone (ACTH) secreted by the pituitary gland.

Cushing's syndrome A metabolic disorder resulting from the chronic and excessive production of cortisol by the adrenal cortex or by the administration of glucocorticoids in large doses for several weeks or longer (exogenous or iatrogenic).

dawn phenomenon A nocturnal release of growth hormone, which may cause blood glucose level elevations before breakfast in the client with diabetes mellitus. Treatment includes administering an evening dose of intermediate-acting insulin at 10 PM.

diabetes insipidus The hyposecretion of antidiuretic hormone from the posterior pituitary gland, resulting in failure of tubular reabsorption of water in the kidneys and diuresis.

diabetic ketoacidosis A life-threatening complication of diabetes mellitus that develops when a severe insulin deficiency occurs. Hyperglycemia progresses to ketoacidosis over a period of several hours to several days. Acidosis occurs in clients with type 1 diabetes mellitus, persons with undiagnosed diabetes, and persons who stop prescribed treatment for diabetes.

diabetes mellitus A chronic disorder of glucose intolerance and impaired carbohydrate, protein, and lipid metabolism caused by a deficiency of insulin or resistance to the action of insulin. A deficiency of effective insulin results in hyperglycemia.

hyperglycemia Elevated blood glucose level greater than 250 mg/dL.

hyperglycemic hyperosmolar nonketotic syndrome Extreme hyperglycemia without acidosis. A complication of type 2 diabetes mellitus, which may result in dehydration or vascular collapse but does not include the acidosis component of diabetic ketoacidosis. Onset is usually slow, taking from hours to days.

hyperthyroidism A condition that occurs as a result of excessive thyroid hormone secretion.

hypoglycemia Low blood glucose level (lower than 70 mg/dL) that results from too much insulin, not enough food, or excess activity.

hypophysectomy The removal of the pituitary gland.

hypothyroidism A hypothyroid state resulting from a hyposecretion of thyroid hormone. The condition occurs in adulthood.

myxedema The most severe form of hypothyroidism characterized by swelling of the hands, face, feet, and periorbital tissues. At this stage, the disease may lead to coma and death.

myxedema coma A rare but serious disorder that results from persistently low thyroid production. Coma can be precipitated by acute illness, rapid withdrawal of thyroid medication, anesthesia and surgery, hypothermia, and the use of sedatives and opioid analgesics.

Somogyi phenomenon A rebound phenomenon that occurs in clients with type 1 diabetes mellitus. Normal or elevated blood glucose levels are present at bedtime; hypoglycemia occurs at about 2 to 3 AM. Counterregulatory hormones, produced to prevent further hypoglycemia, result in hyperglycemia (evident in the prebreakfast blood glucose level). Treatment includes decreasing the evening (predinner or bedtime) dose of intermediate-acting insulin or increasing the bedtime snack.

thyroidectomy Surgical removal of the thyroid gland to treat persistent hyperthyroidism or thyroid tumors.

thyroid storm An acute, potentially fatal exacerbation of hyperthyroidism that may result from manipulation of the thyroid gland during surgery, severe infection, or stress.

Trousseau's sign A sign of hypocalcemia. Carpal spasm can be elicited by compressing the brachial artery with a blood pressure cuff for 3 minutes.

 PYRAMID TO SUCCESS

The endocrine system is made up of organs or glands that secrete hormones and release them directly into the circulation. The endocrine system can be understood easily if you remember that basically one of two situations can occur—hypersecretion or hyposecretion of hormones from the organ or gland. When an excess of the hormone occurs, treatment is aimed at blocking the hormone release through medication or surgery. When a deficit of the hormone exists, treatment is aimed at replacement therapy. Pyramid Points focus on diabetes mellitus, including its prevention, the prevention and treatment of complications, insulin therapy, hypoglycemic and hyperglycemic reactions, and diabetic ketoacidosis; Addison's disease and addisonian crisis; Cushing's disease or Cushing's syndrome; thyroid disorders and thyroid storm; and care of the client after thyroidectomy or adrenalectomy.

 CLIENT NEEDS

Safe and Effective Care Environment

Acting as a client advocate
Collaborating with multidisciplinary team regarding treatment
Consulting with appropriate care providers
Delegating care activities to others
Establishing priorities of care

Handling hazardous and infectious materials
Informed consent for treatments and procedures
Maintaining confidentiality related to the disorder
Preventing accidents and client injury
Using medical and surgical asepsis to prevent infection

Health Promotion and Maintenance

Discussing expected body image changes
Identifying lifestyle choices related to treatment
Performing physical assessment of the endocrine system
Preventing disease
Providing health screening
Teaching about self-care measures

Psychosocial Integrity

Discussing grief and loss issues related to complications of the disorder
Discussing situational role changes related to the disorder
Discussing unexpected body image changes
Identifying coping mechanisms
Monitoring for sensory and perceptual alterations as a result of the disorder
Using support systems

Physiological Integrity

Administering medications safely
Monitoring for alterations in body systems as a result of the disorder
Monitoring for expected outcomes and effects of pharmacological therapy
Monitoring for fluid and electrolyte imbalances that can occur
Monitoring laboratory values
Monitoring for complications of diagnostic tests, treatments, procedures
Monitoring for complications from surgical procedures and health alterations
Monitoring for problems with elimination as a result of the disorder
Monitoring for unexpected response to therapies
Performing dosage calculation related to medication administration
Preparing the client for diagnostic tests
Providing nonpharmacological comfort interventions
Providing nutrition and oral hydration measures
Providing emergency care to the client

54

Endocrine System

I. ANATOMY AND PHYSIOLOGY OF ENDOCRINE GLANDS (Box 54-1)

A. Functions
1. Maintenance and regulation of vital functions
2. Response to stress and injury
3. Growth and development
4. Energy metabolism
5. Reproduction
6. Fluid, electrolyte, and acid-base balance

B. Risk factors (Box 54-2)

C. Hypothalamus (Box 54-3)
1. Portion of the diencephalon of the brain, forming the floor and part of the lateral wall of the third ventricle
2. Activates, controls, and integrates the peripheral autonomic nervous system, endocrine processes, and many somatic functions, such as body temperature, sleep, and appetite

D. Pituitary gland (Box 54-4; Fig. 54-1)
1. The master gland; located at the base of the brain
2. Influenced by the hypothalamus; directly affects the function of the other endocrine glands
3. Promotes growth of body tissue, influences water absorption by the kidney, and controls sexual development and function

E. Adrenal gland
1. One adrenal gland is on top of each kidney.
2. Regulates sodium and electrolyte balance; affects carbohydrate, fat, and protein metabolism; influences the development of sexual characteristics; and sustains the fight-or-flight response
3. Adrenal cortex
   a. The cortex is the outer shell of the adrenal gland.
   b. The cortex synthesizes glucocorticoids and mineralocorticoids and secretes small amounts of sex hormones (androgens, estrogens; Box 54-5).
4. Adrenal medulla
   a. The medulla is the inner core of the adrenal gland.
   b. The medulla works as part of the sympathetic nervous system and produces epinephrine and norepinephrine.

F. Thyroid gland
1. Located in the anterior part of the neck
2. Controls the rate of body metabolism and growth and produces thyroxine (T_4), triiodothyronine (T_3), and thyrocalcitonin

G. Parathyroid glands
1. Located on the thyroid gland
2. Control calcium and phosphorus metabolism; produce parathyroid hormone

H. Pancreas
1. Located posteriorly to the stomach
2. Influences carbohydrate metabolism, indirectly influences fat and protein metabolism, and produces insulin and glucagon

I. Ovaries and testes
1. The ovaries are located in the pelvic cavity and produce estrogen and progesterone.
2. The testes are located in the scrotum, control the development of the secondary sex characteristics, and produce testosterone.

J. Negative-feedback loop
1. Regulates hormone secretion by the hypothalamus and pituitary gland
2. Increased amounts of target gland hormones in the bloodstream decrease secretion of the same hormone and other hormones that stimulate its release.

II. DIAGNOSTIC TESTS

A. Stimulation and suppression tests
1. Stimulation testing
   a. In the client with suspected underactivity of an endocrine gland, a stimulus may be provided to determine whether the gland is capable of normal hormone production.
   b. Measured amounts of selected hormones or substances are administered to stimulate the target gland to produce its hormone.
   c. Hormone levels produced by the target gland are measured.
   d. Failure of the hormone level to increase with stimulation indicates hypofunction.

Box 54-1 Endocrine Glands

Adrenal	Parathyroid
Hypothalamus	Pituitary
Ovaries	Testes
Pancreas	Thyroid

Box 54-2 Risk Factors for Endocrine Disorders

Age	Environmental factors
Heredity	Consequence of other
Congenital factors	disorders
Trauma	

Box 54-3 Hypothalamus Hormones

Corticotropin-releasing hormone (CRH)
Gonadotropin-releasing hormone (GnRH)
Growth hormone-inhibiting hormone (GHIH)
Growth hormone-releasing hormone (GHRH)
Melanocyte-inhibiting hormone (MIH)
Prolactin-inhibiting hormone (PIH)
Thyrotropin-releasing hormone (TRH)

Box 54-4 Pituitary Gland Hormones

Anterior Lobe Production
Adrenocorticotropic hormone (ACTH)
Follicle-stimulating hormone (FSH)
Growth hormone (GH)
Luteinizing hormone (LH)
Melanocyte-stimulating hormone (MSH)
Prolactin (PRL)
Somatotrophic growth-stimulating hormone
Thyroid-stimulating hormone (TSH)

Posterior Lobe
These hormones are produced by the hypothalamus, stored in the posterior lobe, and secreted into the blood when needed:
Oxytocin
Vasopressin, antidiuretic hormone (ADH)

---

    a. T_3: 80 to 230 ng/dL
    b. T_4: 5 to 12 mcg/dL
    c. Thyroxine, free (FT_4): 0.8 to 2.4 ng/dL
  4. The T_3 level is elevated in **hyperthyroidism**, decreases with the aging process, and may be decreased in **hypothyroidism**.
  5. The T_4 level is elevated in **hyperthyroidism** and decreased in **hypothyroidism**.

D. Thyroid-stimulating hormone
  1. Blood test is used to differentiate the diagnosis of primary **hypothyroidism**.
  2. Normal value is 0.2 to 5.4 microunits/mL (normal findings vary among laboratories).
  3. Elevated values indicate primary **hypothyroidism**.
  4. Decreased values indicate **hyperthyroidism** or secondary **hypothyroidism**.

E. Thyroid scan
  1. A thyroid scan is performed to identify nodules or growths in the thyroid gland.
  2. A radioisotope of iodine or technetium is administered before scanning the thyroid gland.
  3. Reassure the client that the level of radioactive medication is not dangerous to self or others.
  4. Determine whether the client has received radiographic contrast agents within the past 3 months, because these may invalidate the scan.
  5. Check with the physician regarding discontinuing medications containing iodine for 14 days before the test and the need to discontinue thyroid medication before the test.
  6. Instruct the client to maintain an NPO status after midnight on the day before the test; if iodine is used, the client will fast for an additional 45 minutes after ingestion of the oral isotope and the scan will be performed in 24 hours.
  7. If technetium is used, it is administered by the intravenous (IV) route 30 minutes before the scan.

  2. Suppression tests
    a. Suppression tests are used when hormone levels are high or in the upper range of normal.
    b. Agents that normally induce a suppressed response are administered to determine whether normal negative feedback is intact.
    c. Failure of hormone production to be suppressed during standardized testing indicates hyperfunction.

B. Radioactive iodine uptake
  1. This thyroid function test measures the absorption of the iodine isotope to determine how the thyroid gland is functioning.
  2. A small dose of radioactive iodine is given by mouth or intravenously; the amount of radioactivity is measured in 2 to 4 hours and again at 24 hours.
  3. Normal values are 3% to 10% at 2 to 4 hours, and 5% to 30% in 24 hours.
  4. Elevated values indicate **hyperthyroidism**, decreased iodine intake, or increased iodine excretion.
  5. Decreased values indicate a low T_4 level, the use of antithyroid medications, thyroiditis, **myxedema**, or **hypothyroidism**.
  6. The test is contraindicated in pregnancy.

C. T_3 and T_4 resin uptake test
  1. Blood tests are used to diagnose thyroid disorders.
  2. T_3 and T_4 regulate thyroid-stimulating hormone.
  3. Normal values (normal findings vary between laboratory settings)

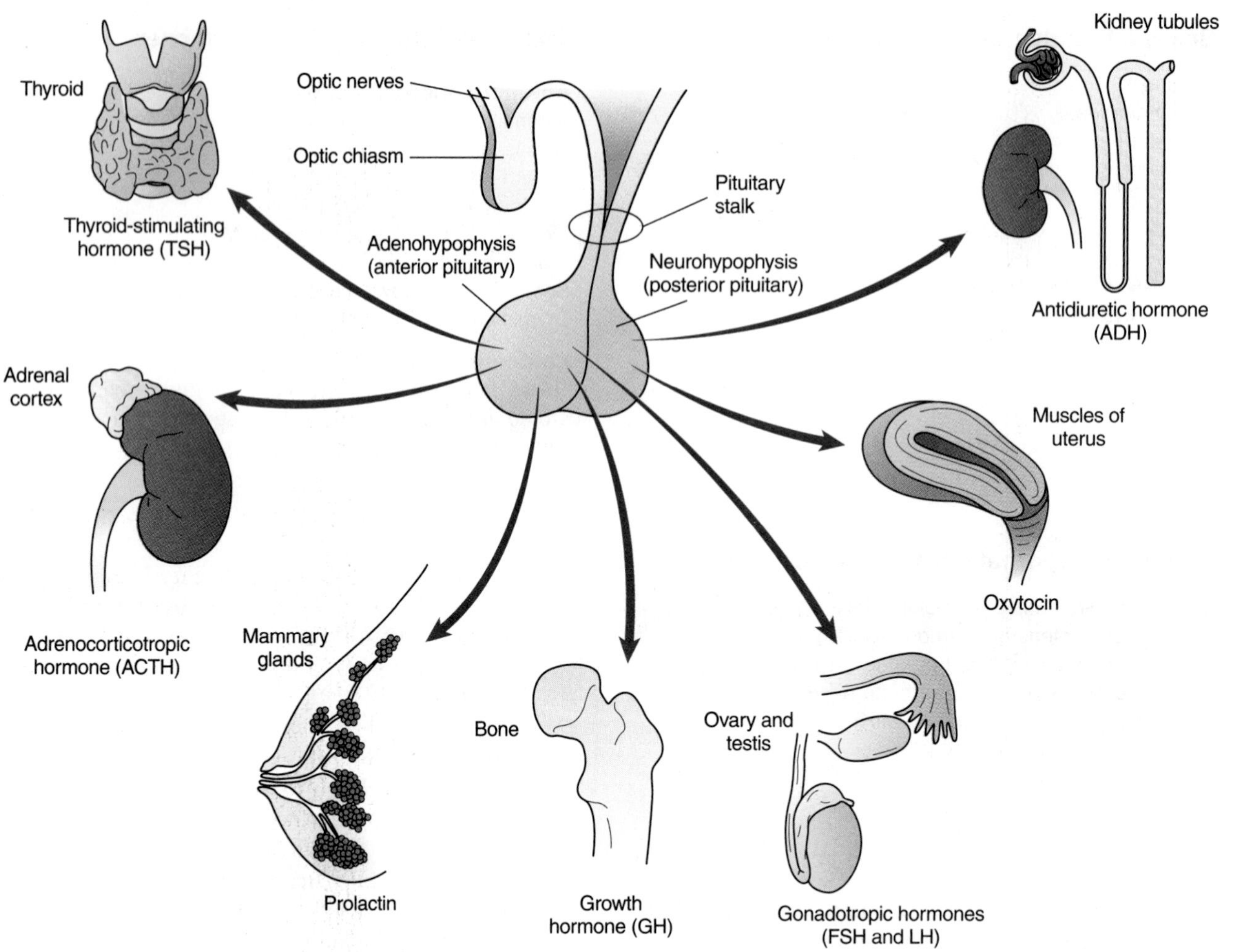

▲ FIGURE 54-1 Pituitary hormones. (From Lilley, L., Harrington, S., & Snyder, J. [2008]. *Pharmacology and the nursing process* [5th ed.]. St. Louis: Mosby.)

Box 54-5 Adrenal Cortex

Glucocorticoids: Cortisol, Cortisone, Corticosterone
Responsible for glucose metabolism, protein metabolism, fluid and electrolyte balance, suppression of the inflammatory response to injury, protective immune response to invasion by infectious agents, and resistance to stress

Mineralocorticoids: Aldosterone
Regulation of electrolyte balance by promoting sodium retention and potassium excretion

8. The test is contraindicated in pregnancy.
F. Needle aspiration of thyroid tissue
   1. Aspiration of thyroid tissue is done for cytological examination.
   2. No client preparation is necessary.
   3. Light pressure is applied to the aspiration site after the procedure.

G. Glucose tolerance test
   1. The glucose tolerance test aids in the diagnosis of **diabetes mellitus**.
   2. A 2-hour postload glucose level (2 hours after injection or ingestion of glucose) higher than 200 mg/dL confirms the diagnosis of **diabetes mellitus**.
   3. Client preparation (Box 54-6)
   4. Many factors can alter the results and therefore it is not always a reliable test.
H. Glycosylated hemoglobin
   1. Description
      a. Glycosylated hemoglobin is blood glucose bound to hemoglobin.
      b. Glycosylated hemoglobin A_{1c} (HbA_{1c}) indicates how well blood glucose levels have been controlled for the prior 3 to 4 months.

⚠ Hyperglycemia in a client with diabetes mellitus is usually the cause of an increase in the HbA_{1c} value.

Box 54-6 Client Preparation: Glucose Tolerance Test

Eat a diet with at least 150 g of carbohydrates for 3 days before the test.
Avoid alcohol, coffee, and smoking for 36 hours before testing.
Fast for 10 to 12 hours before the test.
Avoid strenuous exercise for 8 hours before and after the test.
Withhold morning insulin or oral hypoglycemic medication (client with diabetes mellitus).
A sample is drawn for determination of the fasting blood glucose level and then the client will be given a high-glucose drink.
Blood samples will be drawn at 30-minute intervals for a minimum of 2 hours.

---

2. Values
   a. Values are expressed as a percentage of the total hemoglobin.
   b. The goal for clients with **diabetes mellitus** is 7% or lower.
   c. For clients without **diabetes mellitus**, the normal range is 4% to 6%.
3. Nursing consideration: Fasting is not required.
I. Glycosylated serum albumin (fructosamine)
   1. Reflects average serum glucose levels over a period of 2 to 3 weeks
   2. More sensitive to recent changes than the HbA_{1c} value
   3. Normal ranges vary according to the method of testing used; nondiabetic client, 1.5 to 2.7 mmol/L; diabetic client, 2.0 to 5.0 mmol/L

III. PITUITARY GLAND DISORDERS (Box 54-7)

A. Hypopituitarism
   1. Description: Hyposecretion of one or more of the pituitary hormones caused by tumors, trauma, encephalitis, autoimmunity, or stroke
   2. Hormones most often affected are growth hormone (GH) and gonadotropic hormones (luteinizing hormone, follicle-stimulating hormone), but thyroid-stimulating hormone (TSH), adrenocorticotropic hormone (ACTH), or antidiuretic hormone (ADH) may be involved.
   3. Assessment
      a. Mild to moderate obesity (GH, TSH)
      b. Reduced cardiac output (GH, ADH)
      c. Infertility, sexual dysfunction (gonadotropins, ACTH)
      d. Fatigue, low blood pressure (TSH, ADH, ACTH, GH)
      e. Tumors of the pituitary also may cause headaches and visual defects (pituitary is located near the optic nerve).
   4. Interventions
      a. Provide emotional support to the client and family.

Box 54-7 Pituitary Gland Disorders

Anterior Pituitary
Hyperpituitarism
Hypopituitarism

Posterior Pituitary
These disorders can be caused by damage to the posterior pituitary or hypothalamus.
Diabetes insipidus
Syndrome of inappropriate antidiuretic hormone (SIADH)

---

   b. Encourage the client and family to express feelings related to disturbed body image or sexual dysfunction.
   c. Client may need hormone replacement for the specific deficient hormones.
   d. Client education is needed regarding the signs and symptoms of hypofunction and hyperfunction related to insufficient or excess hormone replacement
B. Hyperpituitarism
   1. Description
      a. Hypersecretion of growth hormone by the anterior pituitary gland in an adult; caused primarily by pituitary tumors
      b. Leads to conditions such as acromegaly and **Cushing's disease**
   2. Assessment
      a. Large hands and feet
      b. Thickening and protrusion of the jaw
      c. Arthritic changes and joint pain
      d. Visual disturbances
      e. Diaphoresis
      f. Oily, rough skin
      g. Organomegaly
      h. Hypertension
      i. Dysphagia
      j. Deepening of the voice
   3. Interventions
      a. Provide emotional support to the client and family, and encourage the client and family to express feelings related to disturbed body image.
      b. Provide frequent skin care.
      c. Provide pharmacological and nonpharmacological interventions for joint pain.
      d. Prepare the client for radiation of the pituitary gland if prescribed.
      e. Prepare the client for **hypophysectomy** if planned.
C. **Hypophysectomy** (pituitary adenectomy, transsphenoidal pituitary surgery)
   1. Description
      a. Removal of the pituitary tumor via craniotomy or transsphenoidal (endoscopic

transnasal) approach (latter approach is preferred because it is associated with fewer complications)

b. Complications for craniotomy include increased intracranial pressure, bleeding, meningitis, and hypopituitarism.

c. Complications for the transsphenoidal surgery include cerebrospinal fluid leak, infection, and hypopituitarism.

2. Postoperative interventions

a. Initiate postoperative care similar to craniotomy care.

b. Monitor vital signs, neurological status, and level of consciousness.

c. Elevate the head of the bed.

d. Monitor for increased intracranial pressure.

e. Monitor for bleeding.

f. Instruct the client to avoid sneezing, coughing, and blowing the nose.

g. Monitor for signs of temporary **diabetes insipidus** or syndrome of inappropriate antidiuretic hormone resulting from ADH disturbances.

h. Monitor intake and output, and avoid water intoxication.

i. Administer glucocorticoids and other hormone replacements as prescribed.

j. Administer antibiotics, analgesics, and antipyretics as prescribed.

k. Instruct the client in the administration of prescribed medications.

⚠ Following transsphenoidal hypophysectomy, monitor for any postnasal drip or nasal drainage, which might indicate leakage of cerebrospinal fluid (check the nasal drainage for glucose).

D. Diabetes insipidus

1. Description

a. Hyposecretion of ADH caused by stroke or trauma, or may be idiopathic

b. Kidney tubules fail to reabsorb water.

2. Assessment

a. Polyuria of 4 to 24 L/day

b. Polydipsia

c. Dehydration (decreased skin turgor and dry mucous membranes)

d. Inability to concentrate urine

e. Low urinary specific gravity, 1.006 or lower

f. Fatigue

g. Muscle pain and weakness

h. Headache

i. Postural hypotension that may progress to vascular collapse without rehydration

j. Tachycardia

3. Interventions

a. Monitor vital signs and neurological and cardiovascular status.

b. Provide a safe environment, particularly for the client with postural hypotension.

c. Monitor electrolyte values and for signs of dehydration.

d. Maintain client intake of adequate fluids.

e. Monitor intake and output, weight, serum osmolality, and specific gravity of urine.

f. Instruct the client to avoid foods or liquids that produce diuresis.

g. Vasopressin tannate (Pitressin) or desmopressin acetate (DDAVP, Stimate) may be prescribed; these are used when the ADH deficiency is severe or chronic.

h. Instruct the client in the administration of medications as prescribed; DDAVP may be administered by injection, intranasally, or orally.

i. Instruct the client to wear a Medic-Alert bracelet.

E. Syndrome of inappropriate antidiuretic hormone (SIADH)

1. Description

a. Excess ADH is released, but not in response to the body's need for it.

b. Causes include trauma, stroke, malignancies (often in the lungs or pancreas), medications, and stress.

c. The syndrome results in water intoxication and hyponatremia.

2. Assessment

a. Signs of fluid volume overload

b. Changes in level of consciousness and mental status changes

c. Weight gain

d. Hypertension

e. Tachycardia

f. Anorexia, nausea, and vomiting

g. Hyponatremia

3. Interventions

a. Monitor vital signs and cardiac and neurological status.

b. Provide a safe environment, particularly for the client with changes in level of consciousness or mental status.

c. Monitor intake and output and obtain weight daily.

d. Monitor fluid and electrolyte balance.

e. Monitor serum and urine osmolality.

f. Restrict fluid intake as prescribed.

g. Administer diuretics and IV fluids (usually normal saline or hypertonic saline) as prescribed; monitor IV fluids carefully because of the risk for fluid volume overload (IV solutions containing water are contraindicated because of the risk of water intoxication).

h. Medications that inhibit ADH-induced water reabsorption and produce water diuresis may be prescribed.

IV. ADRENAL GLAND DISORDERS (Box 54-8)

A. Addison's disease
  1. Description
     a. Hyposecretion of adrenal cortex hormones (glucocorticoids and mineralocorticoids)
     b. Can be primary or secondary
     c. The condition is fatal if left untreated.
  2. Assessment (Table 54-1)
  3. Interventions
     a. Monitor vital signs, particularly blood pressure, weight, and intake and output.
     b. Monitor white blood cell (WBC) count, blood glucose, and potassium, sodium, and calcium levels.
     c. Administer glucocorticoid or mineralocorticoid medications as prescribed.
     d. Observe for **addisonian crisis** caused by stress, infection, trauma, or surgery.
  4. Client education
     a. Avoid individuals with an infection.
     b. Diet: High protein and high carbohydrate, normal sodium intake
     c. Avoid strenuous exercise and stressful situations.
     d. Need for lifelong glucocorticoid therapy
     e. Avoid over-the-counter medications.
     f. Wear a Medic-Alert bracelet.
     g. Signs and symptoms of complications such as underreplacement and overreplacement of hormones

B. Addisonian crisis
  1. Description (Box 54-9)
  2. Assessment
     a. Severe headache
     b. Severe abdominal, leg, and lower back pain
     c. Generalized weakness
     d. Irritability and confusion
     e. Severe hypotension
     f. Shock
  3. Interventions
     a. Prepare to administer glucocorticoids intravenously as prescribed; hydrocortisone sodium succinate (Solu-Cortef) usually is prescribed initially.
     b. Following resolution of the crisis, administer glucocorticoid and mineralocorticoid orally as prescribed.
     c. Monitor vital signs, particularly blood pressure.
     d. Monitor neurological status, noting irritability and confusion.
     e. Monitor intake and output.
     f. Monitor laboratory values, particularly the sodium, potassium, and blood glucose levels.
     g. Administer IV fluids as prescribed to restore electrolyte balance.
     h. Protect the client from infection.
     i. Maintain bedrest and provide a quiet environment.

Addison's disease is characterized by the hyposecretion of adrenal cortex hormones (glucocorticoids and mineralocorticoids), whereas Cushing's disease is characterized by a hypersecretion of glucocorticoids.

Box 54-8 Adrenal Gland Disorders

Adrenal Cortex
Addison's disease
Primary hyperaldosteronism (Conn's syndrome)
Cushing's disease
Cushing's syndrome

Adrenal Medulla
Pheochromocytoma

Box 54-9 Addisonian Crisis

A life-threatening disorder caused by acute adrenal insufficiency
Precipitated by stress, infection, trauma, surgery, or abrupt withdrawal of exogenous corticosteroid use
Can cause hyponatremia, hyperkalemia, hypoglycemia, and shock

TABLE 54-1 Assessment: Addison's Disease and Cushing's Disease (Cushing's Syndrome)

Addison's Disease	Cushing's Disease and Syndrome
Lethargy, fatigue, and muscle weakness	Generalized muscle wasting and weakness
Gastrointestinal disturbances	Moon face, buffalo hump
Weight loss	Truncal obesity with thin extremities, supraclavicular fat pads; weight gain
Menstrual changes in women; impotence in men	Hirsutism (masculine characteristics in female)
Hypoglycemia, hyponatremia	Hyperglycemia, hypernatremia
Hyperkalemia, hypercalcemia	Hypokalemia, hypocalcemia
Postural hypotension	Hypertension
Hyperpigmentation of skin (bronzed) with primary disease	Fragile skin that easily bruises
	Reddish-purple striae on the abdomen and upper thighs

C. Cushing's disease and **Cushing's syndrome** (hypercortisolism)

1. Description
   a. Characterized by a hypersecretion of glucocorticoids from the adrenal cortex
   b. **Cushing's disease** is a metabolic disorder characterized by abnormally increased secretion (endogenous) of cortisol, caused by increased amounts of ACTH secreted by the pituitary gland.
   c. **Cushing's syndrome** is a metabolic disorder resulting from the chronic and excessive production of cortisol by the adrenal cortex or by the administration of glucocorticoids in large doses for several weeks or longer (exogenous or iatrogenic).

2. Assessment (Fig. 54-2; see Table 54-1)

3. Interventions
   a. Monitor vital signs, particularly blood pressure.
   b. Monitor intake and output and weight.
   c. Monitor laboratory values, particularly the white blood cell count, and serum glucose, sodium, potassium, and calcium levels.
   d. Provide meticulous skin care.
   e. Allow the client to discuss feelings related to body appearance.
   f. Administer chemotherapeutic agents as prescribed for inoperable adrenal tumors.
   g. Prepare the client for radiation as prescribed if the condition results from a pituitary adenoma.
   h. Prepare the client for removal of pituitary tumor (**hypophysectomy**, transsphenoidal adenectomy) if the condition results from increased pituitary secretion of ACTH.

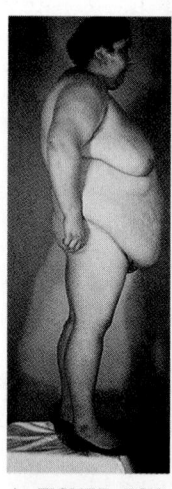
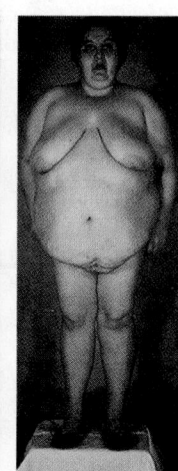
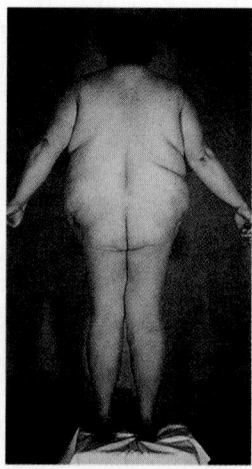

▲ **FIGURE 54-2** Typical appearance of a client with Cushing's syndrome. Note truncal obesity, moon face, buffalo hump, thinner arms and legs, and abdominal striae. (From Ignatavicius, D., & Workman, M. [2010]. *Medical-surgical nursing: Patient-centered collaborative care* [6th ed.]. St. Louis: Saunders.)

   i. Prepare the client for **adrenalectomy** if the condition results from an adrenal adenoma; glucocorticoid replacement may be required following **adrenalectomy**.

D. Primary hyperaldosteronism (Conn's syndrome)

1. Description
   a. Hypersecretion of mineralocorticoids (aldosterone) from the adrenal cortex of the adrenal gland
   b. Most commonly caused by an adenoma

2. Assessment
   a. Symptoms related to hypokalemia, hypernatremia, and hypertension
   b. Headache, fatigue, muscle weakness, nocturia
   c. Polydipsia and polyuria
   d. Paresthesias
   e. Visual changes
   f. Low urine specific gravity and increased urinary aldosterone level
   g. Elevated serum aldosterone levels
   h. Metabolic alkalosis

3. Interventions
   a. Monitor vital signs, particularly blood pressure.
   b. Monitor for signs of hypokalemia and hypernatremia.
   c. Monitor intake and output and urine for specific gravity.
   d. Spironolactone (Aldactone) may be prescribed to promote fluid balance and control hypertension; this is a potassium-sparing diuretic and aldosterone antagonist, and clients need to be monitored for hyperkalemia, particularly those with impaired renal function or excessive potassium intake.
   e. Administer potassium supplements as prescribed.
   f. Prepare the client for **adrenalectomy**.
   g. Maintain sodium restriction, if prescribed, preoperatively.
   h. Administer glucocorticoids preoperatively, as prescribed, to prevent adrenal hypofunction.
   i. Monitor the client for adrenal insufficiency postoperatively.
   j. Instruct the client regarding the need for glucocorticoid therapy following **adrenalectomy**.
   k. Instruct the client about the need to wear a Medic-Alert bracelet.

E. Pheochromocytoma

1. Description
   a. Catecholamine-producing tumor usually found in the adrenal medulla, but extra-adrenal locations include the chest, bladder, abdomen, and brain; typically is a benign tumor but can be malignant
   b. Excessive amounts of epinephrine and norepinephrine are secreted.

c. Diagnostic tests include a 24-hour urine collection for vanillylmandelic acid (VMA), a product of catecholamine metabolism, metanephrine, and catecholamines, all of which are elevated in the presence of pheochromocytoma; the normal range of urinary catecholamines is up to 14 mcg/100 mL of urine, with higher levels occurring in pheochromocytoma.

d. Surgical removal of the adrenal gland is the primary treatment.

e. Symptomatic treatment is initiated if surgical removal is not possible.

f. The complications associated with pheochromocytoma include hypertensive crisis, including hypertensive retinopathy and nephropathy, cardiac enlargement, and dysrhythmias, congestive heart failure, myocardial infarction, increased platelet aggregation, and stroke.

g. Death can occur from shock, stroke, renal failure, dysrhythmias, or dissecting aortic aneurysm.

2. Assessment
   a. Paroxysmal or sustained hypertension
   b. Severe headaches
   c. Palpitations
   d. Flushing and profuse diaphoresis
   e. Pain in the chest or abdomen with nausea and vomiting
   f. Heat intolerance
   g. Weight loss
   h. Tremors
   i. **Hyperglycemia**

3. Interventions
   a. Monitor vital signs, particularly the blood pressure and heart rate.
   b. Monitor for hypertensive crisis; monitor for complications that can occur with hypertensive crisis, such as stroke, cardiac dysrhythmias, myocardial infarction.
   c. Instruct the client not to smoke, drink caffeine-containing beverages, or change position suddenly.
   d. Prepare to administer a β-adrenergic blocking agent as prescribed to control hypertension.
   e. Monitor serum glucose level.
   f. Promote rest and a nonstressful environment.
   g. Provide a diet high in calories, vitamins, and minerals.
   h. Prepare the client for **adrenalectomy**.

⚠ For the client with pheochromocytoma, avoid stimuli that can precipitate a hypertensive crisis, such as increased abdominal pressure and vigorous abdominal palpation.

F. Adrenalectomy
   1. Description (Box 54-10)

Box 54-10 Adrenalectomy

Surgical removal of an adrenal gland
Lifelong glucocorticoid and mineralocorticoid replacement are necessary with bilateral adrenalectomy
Temporary glucocorticoid replacement, usually up to 2 years, is necessary after a unilateral adrenalectomy.
Catecholamine levels drop as a result of surgery, which can result in cardiovascular collapse, hypotension, and shock, and the client needs to be monitored closely.
Hemorrhage also can occur because of the high vascularity of the adrenal glands.

2. Preoperative interventions
   a. Monitor electrolyte levels and correct electrolyte imbalances.
   b. Assess for dysrhythmias.
   c. Monitor for **hyperglycemia**.
   d. Protect the client from infections.
   e. Administer glucocorticoids as prescribed.

3. Postoperative interventions
   a. Monitor vital signs.
   b. Monitor intake and output; if the urinary output is lower than 30 mL/hr, notify the physician, because this may indicate renal failure and impending shock.
   c. Monitor weight daily.
   d. Monitor electrolyte and serum glucose levels.
   e. Monitor for signs of hemorrhage and shock, particularly during the first 24 to 48 hours.
   f. Monitor for manifestations of adrenal insufficiency.
   g. Assess the dressing for drainage.
   h. Monitor for paralytic ileus, as manifested by abdominal distention and pain, nausea, vomiting, and diminished or absent bowel sounds (paralytic ileus can develop from internal bleeding, anesthesia effects, and bowel manipulation).
   i. Administer IV fluids as prescribed to maintain blood volume.
   j. Administer glucocorticoids and mineralocorticoids as prescribed.
   k. Administer pain medication as prescribed.
   l. Provide pulmonary interventions to prevent atelectasis (cough and deep breathing, incentive spirometry, splinting of incision).
   m. Instruct the client in the importance of hormone replacement therapy following surgery.
   n. Instruct the client regarding signs and symptoms of complications such as underreplacement and overreplacement of hormones.
   o. Instruct the client regarding the need to wear a Medic-Alert bracelet.

Box 54-11 Thyroid Gland Disorders

Hyperthyroidism
Hypothyroidism

V. THYROID GLAND DISORDERS (Box 54-11)

A. Hypothyroidism

1. Description
   a. Hypothyroid state resulting from hyposecretion of thyroid hormones T_3 and T_4.
   b. Characterized by a decreased rate of body metabolism
2. Assessment
   a. Lethargy and fatigue
   b. Weakness, muscle aches, paresthesias
   c. Intolerance to cold
   d. Weight gain
   e. Dry skin and hair and loss of body hair
   f. Bradycardia
   g. Constipation
   h. Generalized puffiness and edema around the eyes and face (**myxedema**)
   i. Forgetfulness and loss of memory
   j. Menstrual disturbances
   k. Cardiac enlargement, tendency to develop congestive heart failure
   l. Goiter may or may not be present.
3. Interventions
   a. Monitor vital signs, including heart rate and rhythm.
   b. Administer thyroid replacement; levothyroxine sodium (Synthroid) is most commonly prescribed.
   c. Instruct the client about thyroid replacement therapy and about the clinical manifestations of both **hypothyroidism** and **hyperthyroidism** related to underreplacement or overreplacement of the hormone.
   d. Instruct the client in low-calorie, low-cholesterol, low–saturated fat diet.
   e. Assess the client for constipation; provide roughage and fluids to prevent constipation.
   f. Provide a warm environment for the client.
   g. Avoid sedatives and opioid analgesics because of increased sensitivity to these medications.
   h. Monitor for overdose of thyroid medications, characterized by tachycardia, chest pain, restlessness, nervousness, and insomnia.
   i. Instruct the client to report episodes of chest pain or other signs of overdose immediately.

B. Myxedema coma

1. Description (Box 54-12)
2. Assessment
   a. Hypotension
   b. Bradycardia

Box 54-12 Myxedema Coma

This rare but serious disorder results from persistently low thyroid production.
Coma can be precipitated by acute illness, rapid withdrawal of thyroid medication, anesthesia and surgery, hypothermia, or the use of sedatives and opioid analgesics.

   c. Hypothermia
   d. Hyponatremia
   e. **Hypoglycemia**
   f. Generalized edema
   g. Respiratory failure
   h. Coma
3. Interventions
   a. Maintain a patent airway.
   b. Institute aspiration precautions.
   c. Administer IV fluids (normal or hypertonic saline) as prescribed.
   d. Administer levothyroxine sodium intravenously as prescribed.
   e. Administer glucose intravenously as prescribed.
   f. Administer corticosteroids as prescribed.
   g. Assess client's temperature hourly.
   h. Monitor blood pressure frequently.
   i. Keep the client warm.
   j. Monitor for changes in mental status.
   k. Monitor electrolyte and glucose levels.

C. Hyperthyroidism

1. Description
   a. Hyperthyroid state resulting from hypersecretion of thyroid hormones (T_3 and T_4)
   b. Characterized by an increased rate of body metabolism
   c. A common cause is Graves' disease, also known as toxic diffuse goiter.
   d. Clinical manifestations are referred to as *thyrotoxicosis*.
2. Assessment for **hyperthyroidism** caused by Graves' disease
   a. Enlarged thyroid gland (goiter)
   b. Palpitations, cardiac dysrhythmias, such as tachycardia or atrial fibrillation
   c. Protruding eyeballs (exophthalmos) may be present (Fig. 54-3)
   d. Hypertension
   e. Heat intolerance
   f. Diaphoresis
   g. Weight loss
   h. Diarrhea
   i. Smooth, soft skin and hair
   j. Nervousness and fine tremors of the hands
   k. Personality changes such as irritability, agitation, and mood swings

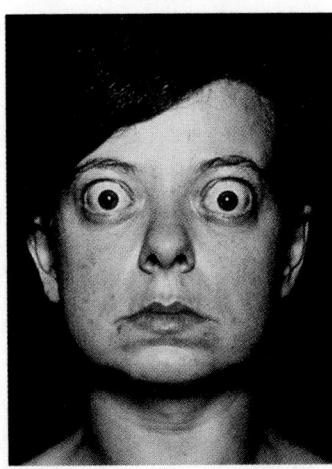

▲ **FIGURE 54-3** Exophthalmos. (From Ignatavicius, D., & Workman, M. [2010]. *Medical-surgical nursing: Patient-centered collaborative care* [6th ed.]. St. Louis: Saunders.)

3. Interventions
   a. Provide adequate rest.
   b. Administer sedatives as prescribed.
   c. Provide a cool and quiet environment.
   d. Obtain weight daily.
   e. Provide a high-calorie diet.
   f. Avoid the administration of stimulants.
   g. Administer antithyroid medications (propylthiouracil, PTU) that block thyroid synthesis as prescribed.
   h. Administer iodine preparations that inhibit the release of thyroid hormone as prescribed.
   i. Administer propranolol (Inderal) for tachycardia as prescribed.
   j. Prepare the client for radioactive iodine therapy, as prescribed, to destroy thyroid cells.
   k. Prepare the client for **thyroidectomy** if prescribed.

D. **Thyroid storm**
   1. Description (Box 54-13)
   2. Assessment
      a. Elevated temperature (fever)
      b. Tachycardia
      c. Systolic hypertension
      d. Nausea, vomiting, and diarrhea
      e. Agitation, tremors, anxiety
      f. Irritability, agitation, restlessness, confusion, and seizures as the condition progresses
      g. Delirium and coma
   3. Interventions
      a. Maintain a patent airway and adequate ventilation.
      b. Administer antithyroid medications, sodium iodide solution, propranolol, and glucocorticoids as prescribed.
      c. Monitor vital signs.
      d. Monitor continually for cardiac dysrhythmias.

Box 54-13 Thyroid Storm

This acute and life-threatening condition occurs in a client with uncontrollable hyperthyroidism.

It can be caused by manipulation of the thyroid gland during surgery and the release of thyroid hormone into the bloodstream; it also can occur from severe infection and stress.

Antithyroid medications, β-blockers, glucocorticoids, and iodides may be administered to the client before thyroid surgery to prevent its occurrence.

   e. Administer nonsalicylate antipyretics as prescribed (salicylates increase free thyroid hormone levels).
   f. Use a cooling blanket to decrease temperature as prescribed.

E. **Thyroidectomy**
   1. Description
      a. Removal of the thyroid gland
      b. Performed when persistent **hyperthyroidism** exists
   2. Preoperative interventions
      a. Obtain vital signs and weight.
      b. Assess electrolyte levels.
      c. Assess for **hyperglycemia**.
      d. Instruct the client in how to perform coughing and deep-breathing exercises and how to support the neck in the postoperative period when coughing and moving.
      e. Administer antithyroid medications, sodium iodide solution, propranolol, and glucocorticoids as prescribed to prevent the occurrence of **thyroid storm**.
   3. Postoperative interventions
      a. Monitor for respiratory distress.
      b. Have a tracheotomy set, oxygen, and suction at the bedside.
      c. Limit client talking, and assess level of hoarseness.
      d. Monitor for laryngeal nerve damage, as evidenced by respiratory obstruction, dysphonia, high-pitched voice, stridor, dysphagia, and restlessness.
      e. Monitor for signs of hypocalcemia and tetany, which can be caused by trauma to the parathyroid gland (Box 54-14).
      f. Prepare to administer calcium gluconate as prescribed for tetany.
      g. Monitor for **thyroid storm**.

⚠ Following thyroidectomy, maintain the client in a semi-Fowler's position. Monitor the surgical site for edema and for signs of bleeding and check the dressing anteriorly and at the back of the neck.

Box 54-14 Signs of Tetany

Cardiac dysrhythmias
Carpopedal spasm
Dysphagia
Muscle and abdominal cramps
Numbness and tingling of the face and extremities
Positive Chvostek's sign
Positive Trousseau's sign
Visual disturbances (photophobia)
Wheezing and dyspnea (bronchospasm, laryngospasm)
Seizures

Box 54-15 Parathyroid Gland Disorders

Hyperparathyroidism
Hypoparathyroidism

VI. PARATHYROID GLAND DISORDERS (Box 54-15)

A. Hypoparathyroidism
  1. Description
     a. Condition caused by hyposecretion of parathyroid hormone by the parathyroid gland
     b. Can occur following **thyroidectomy** because of removal of parathyroid tissue
  2. Assessment
     a. Hypocalcemia and hyperphosphatemia
     b. Numbness and tingling in the face
     c. Muscle cramps and cramps in the abdomen or in the extremities
     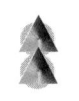
     d. Positive **Trousseau's sign** or **Chvostek's sign**
     e. Signs of overt tetany, such as bronchospasm, laryngospasm, carpopedal spasm, dysphagia, photophobia, cardiac dysrhythmias, seizures
     f. Hypotension
     g. Anxiety, irritability, depression
  3. Interventions
     a. Monitor vital signs.

     b. Monitor for signs of hypocalcemia and tetany.
     c. Initiate seizure precautions.
     d. Place a tracheotomy set, oxygen, and suctioning at the bedside.

     e. Prepare to administer calcium gluconate intravenously for hypocalcemia.

     f. Provide a high-calcium, low-phosphorus diet.

     g. Instruct the client in the administration of calcium supplements as prescribed.
     h. Instruct the client in the administration of vitamin D supplements as prescribed; vitamin D enhances the absorption of calcium from the gastrointestinal tract.
     i. Instruct the client in the administration of phosphate binders as prescribed to promote the excretion of phosphate through the gastrointestinal tract.
     j. Instruct the client to wear a Medic-Alert bracelet.

B. Hyperparathyroidism
  1. Description: Condition caused by hypersecretion of parathyroid hormone by the parathyroid gland
  2. Assessment
     a. Hypercalcemia and hypophosphatemia
     b. Fatigue and muscle weakness
     c. Skeletal pain and tenderness
     d. Bone deformities that result in pathological fractures
     e. Anorexia, nausea, vomiting, epigastric pain
     f. Weight loss
     g. Constipation
     h. Hypertension
     i. Cardiac dysrhythmias
     j. Renal stones
  3. Interventions
     a. Monitor vital signs, particularly the blood pressure.
     b. Monitor for cardiac dysrhythmias.
     c. Monitor intake and output and for signs of renal stones.
     d. Monitor for skeletal pain; move the client slowly and carefully.
     e. Encourage fluid intake.
     f. Administer furosemide (Lasix) as prescribed to lower calcium levels.
     g. Administer normal saline intravenously as prescribed to maintain hydration.
     h. Administer phosphates as prescribed, which interfere with calcium resorption.
     i. Administer calcitonin (Calcimar) as prescribed to decrease skeletal calcium release and increase renal excretion of calcium.
     j. Monitor calcium and phosphorus levels.
     k. Prepare the client for parathyroidectomy as prescribed.

⚠ For the client with hyperparathyroidism, notify the physician immediately if a precipitous drop in the calcium level occurs; assess for tingling and numbness in the face and extremities and for other signs of hypocalcemia.

C. Parathyroidectomy
  1. Description: Removal of one or more of the parathyroid glands
  2. Preoperative interventions
     a. Monitor electrolytes, calcium, phosphate, and magnesium levels.
     b. Ensure that calcium levels are decreased to near-normal values.
     c. Inform the client that talking may be painful for the first day or two after surgery.

Box 54-16 Major Types of Diabetes Mellitus

Type 1: Primary beta cell destruction leading to absolute insulin deficiency

Type 2: Ranges from insulin resistance with an insulin deficiency to secretory deficit with insulin resistance

3. Postoperative interventions
   a. Monitor for respiratory distress.
   b. Place a tracheotomy set, oxygen, and suctioning at the bedside.
   c. Monitor vital signs.
   d. Position the client in a semi-Fowler's position.
   e. Assess neck dressing for bleeding.
   f. Monitor for hypocalcemic crisis, as evidenced by tingling and twitching in the extremities and face.
   g. Assess for positive **Trousseau's sign** or **Chvostek's sign**, which signals the potential for tetany.
   h. Monitor for changes in voice pattern and hoarseness.
   i. Monitor for laryngeal nerve damage.
   j. Instruct the client in the administration of calcium and vitamin D supplements as prescribed.

VII. DISORDERS OF THE PANCREAS

A. Diabetes mellitus (Box 54-16)
   1. Description
      a. Chronic disorder of impaired carbohydrate, protein, and lipid metabolism caused by a deficiency of insulin
      b. An absolute or relative deficiency of insulin results in **hyperglycemia**.
      c. Type 1 **diabetes mellitus** is a nearly absolute deficiency of insulin; if insulin is not given, fats are metabolized for energy, resulting in ketonemia (acidosis).
      d. Type 2 **diabetes mellitus** is a relative lack of insulin or resistance to the action of insulin; usually, insulin is sufficient to stabilize fat and protein metabolism but not carbohydrate metabolism.
      e. Metabolic syndrome is also known as syndrome X and the individual has coexisting risk factors for developing type 2 **diabetes mellitus**; these risk factors include abdominal obesity, **hyperglycemia**, hypertension, high triglyceride level, and a lowered HDL (high-density lipoprotein) cholesterol level.
      f. **Diabetes mellitus** can lead to chronic health problems and early death as a result of complications that occur in the large and small blood vessels in tissues and organs.
      g. Macrovascular complications include coronary artery disease, cardiomyopathy, hypertension, cerebrovascular disease, and peripheral vascular disease. (Refer to Chapter 60 for information on cardiovascular disorders.)
      h. Microvascular complications include retinopathy, nephropathy, and neuropathy.
      i. Infection is also a concern because of reduced healing ability.
      j. Male erectile dysfunction can also occur as a result of the disease.

Obesity is a major risk factor for diabetes mellitus.

   2. Assessment
      a. Polyuria, polydipsia, polyphagia (more common in type 1 **diabetes mellitus**)
      b. **Hyperglycemia**
      c. Weight loss (common in type 1 **diabetes mellitus**, rare in type 2 **diabetes mellitus**)
      d. Blurred vision
      e. Slow wound healing
      f. Vaginal infections
      g. Weakness and paresthesias
      h. Signs of inadequate circulation to the feet
      i. Signs of accelerated atherosclerosis (renal, cerebral, cardiac, peripheral)
   3. Diet
      a. The total number of calories is individualized based on the client's current or desired weight and the presence of other existing health problems.
      b. Day-to-day consistency in timing and amount of food intake helps control the blood glucose level.
      c. As prescribed by the physician, the client may be advised to follow the food exchange recommendations of the American Diabetic Association diet or U.S. dietary guidelines (MyPyramid) issued by the U.S. Departments of Agriculture and Health and Human Services.
      d. Carbohydrate counting may be a simpler approach for some clients; it focuses on the total grams of carbohydrates eaten per meal. The client may be more compliant with carbohydrate counting, resulting in better glycemic control; it is usually necessary for clients undergoing intense insulin therapy.
      e. Incorporate the diet into individual client needs, lifestyle, and cultural and socioeconomic patterns.
   4. Exercise
      a. Exercise lowers the blood glucose level, encourages weight loss, reduces cardiovascular risks, improves circulation and muscle tone, decreases total cholesterol and triglyceride levels, and decreases insulin resistance and glucose intolerance.
      b. Instruct the client in dietary adjustments when exercising; dietary adjustments are individualized.

c. If the client requires extra food during exercise to prevent **hypoglycemia**, it need not be deducted from the regular meal plan.

d. If the blood glucose level is higher than 250 mg/dL and urinary ketones (type 1 **diabetes mellitus**) are present, the client is instructed not to exercise until the blood glucose level is closer to normal and urinary ketones are absent.

⚠ Instruct the client with diabetes mellitus to monitor the blood glucose level before, during, and after exercising.

5. Oral hypoglycemic medications
   a. Oral medications are prescribed for clients with **diabetes mellitus** type 2 when diet and weight control therapy have failed to maintain satisfactory blood glucose levels.
   b. Assess the client's knowledge of **diabetes mellitus** and the use of oral hypoglycemic agents.
   c. Assess vital signs and blood glucose levels.
   d. Assess the medications that the client is currently taking.
   e. Aspirin, alcohol, sulfonamides, oral contraceptives, and monoamine oxidase inhibitors increase the hypoglycemic effect, causing a decrease in blood glucose levels.
   f. Glucocorticoids, thiazide diuretics, and estrogen increase blood glucose levels.
   g. Teach the client to recognize the signs and symptoms of **hypoglycemia** and **hyperglycemia**.
   h. Teach the client to avoid over-the-counter medications unless prescribed by the physician.
   i. Inform the client with type 2 **diabetes mellitus** that insulin may be needed during stress, surgery, or infection.
   j. Teach the client about the importance of compliance with the prescribed medication.
   k. Advise the client to wear a Medic-Alert bracelet.

⚠ To prevent a serious reaction, inform the client taking a sulfonylurea to avoid consuming alcohol.

6. Insulin
   a. Insulin is used to treat types 1 and 2 **diabetes mellitus** when diet, weight control therapy, and oral hypoglycemic agents have failed to maintain satisfactory blood glucose levels.
   b. Aspirin, alcohol, oral anticoagulants, oral hypoglycemic medications, β-blockers, tricyclic antidepressants, tetracycline, and monoamine oxidase inhibitors increase the hypoglycemic effect of insulin, causing a further decrease in the blood glucose level.
   c. Glucocorticoids, thiazide diuretics, thyroid agents, oral contraceptives, and estrogen increase the blood glucose level.

d. Illness, infection, and stress increase the blood glucose level and the need for insulin; insulin should not be withheld during illness, infection, or stress because **hyperglycemia** and **ketoacidosis** can result.

e. Instruct the client to recognize the signs and symptoms of **hypoglycemia** and **hyperglycemia**.

f. The peak action time of insulin is important to explain to the client because of the possibility of hypoglycemic reactions occurring during this time.

⚠ Regular insulin is the only insulin that can be administered intravenously. It is used in the emergency treatment of diabetic ketoacidosis.

B. Complications of insulin therapy
   1. Local allergic reactions
      a. Redness, swelling, tenderness, and induration or a wheal at the site of injection may occur 1 to 2 hours after administration.
      b. Reactions usually occur during the early stages of insulin therapy.
      c. Instruct the client to cleanse the skin with alcohol before injection.
   2. Insulin lipodystrophy
      a. Lipoatrophy is loss of subcutaneous fat and appears as slight dimpling or more serious pitting of subcutaneous fat; the use of human insulin helps prevent this complication (Fig. 54-4).
      b. Lipohypertrophy is the development of fibrous fatty masses at the injection site and is caused by repeated use of an injection site (Fig. 54-5).
      c. Instruct the client to avoid injecting insulin into affected sites.

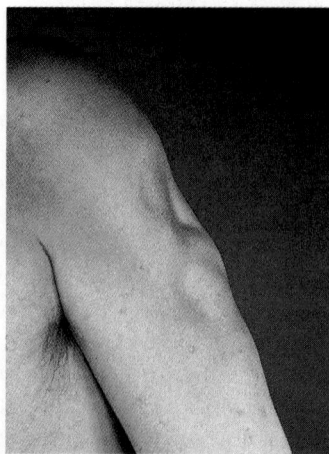

▲ **FIGURE 54-4** Lipoatrophy at insulin injection site. (From Mosby. [2009]. *Mosby's dictionary of medicine, nursing, and health professions* [8th ed.]. St. Louis: Mosby.)

d. Instruct the client about the importance of rotating insulin injection at one anatomical site.

3. Insulin resistance
a. The client receiving insulin develops immune antibodies that bind the insulin, thereby decreasing the insulin available for use in the body.
b. Treatment consists of administering a purer insulin preparation.
c. Insulin resistance is also the term used for lack of tissue sensitivity to the insulin from the body, which results in **hyperglycemia**.

4. **Dawn phenomenon**
a. **Dawn phenomenon** results from reduced tissue sensitivity to insulin that usually develops between 5 and 8 AM (prebreakfast hyperglycemia occurs); it may be caused by nocturnal release of growth hormone.
b. Treatment includes administering an evening dose (or increasing the amount of a current dose) of intermediate-acting insulin at about 10 PM.

5. **Somogyi phenomenon**
a. Normal or elevated blood glucose levels are present at bedtime; **hypoglycemia** occurs at about 2 to 3 AM, which causes an increase in the production of counterregulatory hormones.
b. By about 7 AM, in response to the counterregulatory hormones, the blood glucose rebounds significantly to the hyperglycemic range.
c. Treatment includes decreasing the evening (predinner or bedtime) dose of intermediate-acting insulin or increasing the bedtime snack.

C. Insulin administration
1. Subcutaneous injections and mixing insulin: See Chapter 55.
2. Insulin pumps
a. Continuous subcutaneous insulin infusion is administered by an externally worn device that contains a syringe attached to a long, thin, narrow-lumen tube with a needle or Teflon catheter attached to the end.

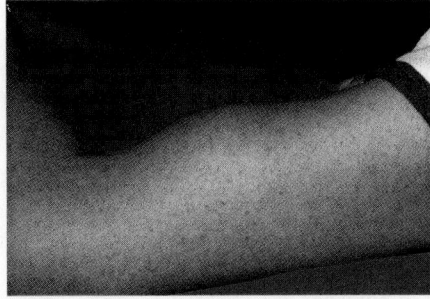

▲ **FIGURE 54-5** Lipohypertrophy at insulin injection site. (From Mosby. [2009]. *Mosby's dictionary of medicine, nursing, and health professions* [8th ed.]. St. Louis: Mosby.)

b. The client inserts the needle or Teflon catheter into the subcutaneous tissue (usually on the abdomen) and secures it with tape or a transparent dressing; the pump is worn on a belt or in a pocket; the needle or Teflon catheter is changed at least every 2 to 3 days.
c. A continuous basal rate of insulin infuses; in addition, based on the blood glucose level, the anticipated food intake, and the activity level, the client delivers a bolus of insulin before each meal.
d. Both rapid-acting and regular insulin (buffered to prevent the precipitation of insulin crystals within the catheter) are appropriate for use in these pumps.

3. Insulin pump and skin sensor
a. A skin sensor device that monitors the client's blood glucose continuously; the information is transmitted to the pump, determines the need for insulin, and then the insulin is injected.
b. The pump holds up to a 3-day supply of insulin and can be easily disconnected for activities such as bathing.

4. Jet injectors
a. A jet injector is a needleless device that delivers insulin through the skin under pressure in an extremely fine stream.
b. Insulin administered by this device usually absorbs faster.
c. The injector can cause bruising at the site of insulin delivery.

5. Pancreas transplants
a. The goal of pancreatic transplantation is to halt or reverse the complications of **diabetes mellitus**.
b. Transplantations are performed on a limited number of clients (generally, these are clients who are undergoing kidney transplantation simultaneously).
c. Immunosuppressive therapy is prescribed to prevent and treat rejection.

D. Self-monitoring of blood glucose level
1. Self-monitoring provides the client with the current blood glucose level and information to maintain good glycemic control.
2. Monitoring requires a finger prick to obtain a drop of blood for testing.
3. Alternative site testing (obtaining blood from the forearm, upper arm, abdomen, thigh, or calf) is now available using specific measurement devices.
4. Tests must be used with caution in clients with diabetic neuropathy.
5. Client instructions (Box 54-17)

E. Urine testing
1. Urine testing for glucose is not a reliable indicator of the blood glucose level and is not used for monitoring purposes.
2. Instruct the client in the procedure for testing for urine ketones.

3. The presence of ketones may indicate impending **ketoacidosis**.
4. Urine ketone testing should be performed during illness and whenever the client with type 1 **diabetes mellitus** has persistently elevated blood glucose levels (higher than 240 mg/dL for two consecutive testing periods).

VIII. ACUTE COMPLICATIONS OF DIABETES MELLITUS

 A. Hypoglycemia (see Priority Nursing Actions)

■■■■ PRIORITY NURSING ACTIONS! ■■■■

Actions to Take If the Client Experiences a Hypoglycemic Reaction
1. Check the client's blood glucose level.
2. Give the client a 10 to 15 g carbohydrate item such as ½ cup of fruit juice to drink.
3. Take the client's vital signs.
4. Retest the blood glucose level
5. Give the client a small snack of carbohydrate and protein.
6. Document the client's complaints, actions taken, and outcome.

If the client experiences symptoms of a hypoglycemic reaction such as hunger, irritability, shakiness, or weakness, the nurse first would check the client's blood glucose level to verify that the client is experiencing hypoglycemia. Once this is verified, the nurse would give the client 10 to 15 g of carbohydrates. The nurse would retest the blood glucose level in 15 minutes. In the meantime, the nurse would check the client's vital signs. The nurse would give the client another 10- to 15-g carbohydrate food item if the client's symptoms do not resolve. Otherwise, the nurse would provide a small snack of carbohydrates and protein if the client's next scheduled meal is more than an hour away from the time of the occurrence. Following treatment and resolution of the hypoglycemic event, the nurse would document the occurrence, actions taken, and outcome.

Reference: Ignatavicius, D., & Workman, M. (2010). *Medical-surgical nursing: Patient-centered collaborative care* (6th ed., pp. 1507-1508). St. Louis: Saunders.

Box 54-17 Client Instructions: Monitoring of Blood Glucose Level

Use the proper procedure for obtaining the sample for determining the blood glucose level.
Perform the procedure precisely to obtain accurate results.
Follow the manufacturer's instructions for the glucometer.
Wash hands before and after performing the procedure to prevent infection.
Calibrate the monitor as instructed by the manufacturer.
Check the expiration date on the test strips.
If the blood glucose level results do not seem reasonable, reread the instructions, reassess technique, check the expiration date of the test strips, and perform the procedure again to verify results.

---

1. Description
   a. **Hypoglycemia** occurs when the blood glucose level falls below 70 mg/dL or when the blood glucose level drops rapidly from an elevated level.
   b. **Hypoglycemia** is caused by too much insulin or oral hypoglycemic agents, too little food, or excessive activity.
   c. The client needs to be instructed always to carry some form of fast-acting simple carbohydrate with him or her.
   d. If the client has a hypoglycemic reaction and does not have any of the recommended emergency foods available, any available food should be eaten; high-fat foods slow the absorption of glucose and the hypoglycemic symptoms may not resolve quickly.
2. Assessment (Box 54-18)
   a. Mild **hypoglycemia**: The client remains fully awake but displays adrenergic symptoms; the blood glucose level is usually lower than 60 mg/dL.
   b. Moderate **hypoglycemia**: The client displays symptoms of worsening **hypoglycemia**; the blood glucose level is usually lower than 40 mg/dL.
   c. Severe **hypoglycemia**: The client displays severe neuroglycopenic symptoms; the blood glucose level is usually lower than 20 mg/dL.

Box 54-18 Assessment of Hypoglycemia

Mild
Hunger
Nervousness
Palpitations
Sweating
Tachycardia
Tremor

Moderate
Confusion
Double vision
Drowsiness
Emotional changes
Headache
Impaired coordination
Inability to concentrate
Irrational or combative behavior
Light-headedness
Numbness of the lips and tongue
Slurred speech

Severe
Difficulty arousing
Disoriented behavior
Loss of consciousness
Seizures

3. Interventions: Mild **hypoglycemia**
   a. Give 10 to 15 g of a fast-acting simple carbohydrate (Box 54-19).
   b. Retest the blood glucose level in 15 minutes and repeat the treatment if symptoms do not resolve.
   c. Once symptoms resolve, a snack containing protein and carbohydrates, such as low-fat milk or cheese and crackers, is recommended unless the client plans to eat a regular meal within 60 minutes.
4. Interventions: Moderate **hypoglycemia**
   a. Administer 15 to 30 g of a fast-acting simple carbohydrate.
   b. Administer additional food such as low-fat milk or cheese and crackers after 10 to 15 minutes.

Box 54-19 Simple Carbohydrates to Treat Hypoglycemia

Commercially prepared glucose tablets
6 to 10 Life Savers or hard candy
4 tsp of sugar
4 sugar cubes
1 Tbsp of honey or syrup
½ cup of fruit juice or regular (nondiet) soft drink
8 oz low-fat milk
6 saltine crackers
3 graham crackers

---

5. Interventions: Severe **hypoglycemia**
   a. If the client is unconscious and cannot swallow, an injection of glucagon is administered subcutaneously or intramuscularly.
   b. Administer a second dose in 10 minutes if the client remains unconscious.
   c. A small meal is given to the client when the client awakens as long as the client is not nauseated.
   d. The physician is notified if a severe hypoglycemic reaction occurs.
   e. Family members need to be instructed about the administration of glucagon.

⚠ Do not attempt to administer oral food or fluids to the client experiencing a severe hypoglycemic reaction who is semiconscious or unconscious and is unable to swallow. This client is at risk for aspiration. For this client, an injection of glucagon is administered subcutaneously or intramuscularly. In the hospital or emergency department, the client may be treated with an IV injection of 25 to 50 mL of 50% dextrose in water.

B. **Diabetic ketoacidosis** (DKA)
   1. Description (Fig. 54-6)
      a. **Diabetic ketoacidosis** is a life-threatening complication of type 1 **diabetes mellitus** that develops when a severe insulin deficiency occurs.

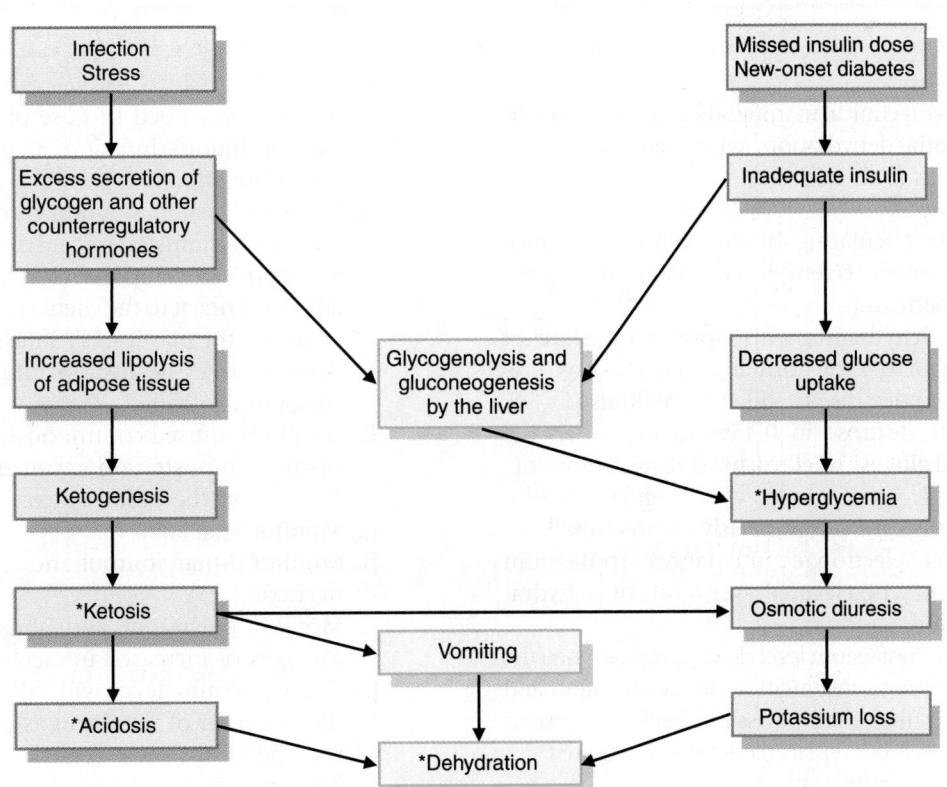

*Hallmarks of DKA

▲ **FIGURE 54-6** Pathophysiology of diabetic ketoacidosis (DKA). (From Black, J., & Hawks, J., [2009]. *Medical-surgical nursing: Clinical management for positive outcomes* [8th ed.]. St. Louis: Saunders.)

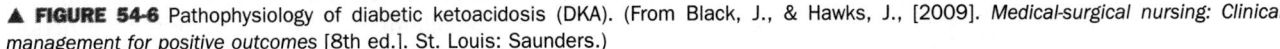

TABLE 54-2 Differences Between Diabetic Ketoacidosis and Hyperglycemic-Hyperosmolar Nonketotic Syndrome

	Diabetic Ketoacidosis (DKA)	Hyperglycemic-Hyperosmolar Nonketotic Syndrome (HHNS)
Onset	Sudden	Gradual
Precipitating factors	Infection	Infection
	Other stressors	Other stressors
	Inadequate insulin dose	Poor fluid intake
Manifestations	Ketosis: Kussmaul's respiration, "fruity" breath, nausea, abdominal pain	Altered central nervous system function with neurologic symptoms
	Dehydration or electrolyte loss: Polyuria, polydipsia, weight loss, dry skin, sunken eyes, soft eyeballs, lethargy, coma	Dehydration or electrolyte loss: Same as for DKA
Laboratory Findings		
Serum glucose	>300 mg/dL (16.7 mmol/L)	>800 mg/dL (44.5 mmol/L)
Osmolarity	Variable	>350 mOsm/L
Serum ketones	Positive at 1:2 dilution	Negative
Serum pH	<7.35	>7.4
Serum HCO_3	<15 mEq/L	>20 mEq/L
Serum Na	Low, normal, or high	Normal or low
Serum K	Normal; elevated with acidosis, low following dehydration	Normal or low
BUN	>20 mg/dL; elevated because of dehydration	Elevated
Creatinine	>1.5 mg/dL; elevated because of dehydration	Elevated
Urine ketones	Positive	Negative

BUN, Blood urea nitrogen; *HCO₃*, bicarbonate.
From Ignatavicius, D., & Workman, M. (2010). *Medical-surgical nursing: Patient-centered collaborative care* (5th ed., p. 1510). St. Louis: Saunders.

b. The main clinical manifestations include **hyperglycemia**, dehydration, ketosis, and acidosis.
2. Assessment (Table 54-2)
3. Interventions
   a. Restore circulating blood volume and protect against cerebral, coronary, and renal hypoperfusion.
   b. Treat dehydration with rapid IV infusions of 0.9% or 0.45% normal saline (NS) as prescribed; dextrose is added to IV fluids (D₅NS, or 5% dextrose in 0.45% saline) when the blood glucose level reaches 250 to 300 mg/dL.
   c. Treat **hyperglycemia** with regular insulin administered intravenously as prescribed.
   d. Correct electrolyte imbalances (potassium level may be elevated as a result of dehydration and acidosis).
   e. Monitor potassium level closely because when the client receives treatment for the dehydration and acidosis, the serum potassium level will decrease and potassium replacement may be required.
4. Insulin IV administration
   a. Use regular insulin only.
   b. An IV bolus dose of regular insulin (usually 5 to 10 units) may be prescribed before a continuous infusion is begun.

c. Mix the prescribed IV dose of regular insulin for continuous infusion in 0.9% or 0.45% NS as prescribed.
d. Flush the insulin solution through the entire intravenous infusion set and discard the first 50 to 100 mL of solution before connecting and administering it to the client (insulin molecules adhere to the plastic of IV infusion sets)
e. Always place the insulin infusion on an IV infusion controller.
f. Insulin is infused continuously until subcutaneous administration resumes to prevent a rebound of the blood glucose level.
g. Monitor vital signs.
h. Monitor urinary output and for signs of fluid overload.
i. Monitor potassium and glucose levels and for signs of increased intracranial pressure.
j. The potassium level will fall rapidly within the first hour of treatment as the dehydration and the acidosis are treated.
k. Potassium is administered intravenously in a diluted solution as prescribed when the potassium reaches a normal level to prevent hypokalemia; ensure adequate renal function before administering potassium.

Box 54-20 Client Education: Guidelines During Illness

Take insulin or oral antidiabetic medications as prescribed.
Test blood glucose level and test the urine for ketones every 3 to 4 hours.
If the usual meal plan cannot be followed, substitute soft foods six to eight times a day.
If vomiting, diarrhea, or fever occurs, consume liquids every 30 to 60 minutes to prevent dehydration and to provide calories.
Notify the physician if vomiting, diarrhea, or fever persists, if blood glucose levels are higher than 250 to 300 mg/dL, when ketonuria is present for more than 24 hours, when unable to take food or fluids for a period of 4 hours, or when illness persists for more than 2 days.

5. Client education (Box 54-20)

⚠ Monitor the client being treated for DKA closely for signs of increased intracranial pressure. If the blood glucose level falls too far or too fast before the brain has time to equilibrate, water is pulled from the blood to the cerebrospinal fluid and the brain, causing cerebral edema and increased intracranial pressure.

C. **Hyperglycemic hyperosmolar nonketotic syndrome** (HHNS)
  1. Description
     a. Extreme **hyperglycemia** occurs without ketosis or acidosis.
     b. The syndrome occurs most often in individuals with type 2 **diabetes mellitus**.
     c. The major difference between HHNS and DKA is that ketosis and acidosis do not occur with HHNS; enough insulin is present with HHNS to prevent breakdown of fats for energy, thus preventing ketosis.
  2. Assessment (see Table 54-2)
  3. Interventions
     a. Treatment is similar to that for DKA.
     b. Treatment includes fluid replacement, correction of electrolyte imbalances, and insulin administration.
     c. Fluid replacement in the older client must be done very carefully because of the potential for heart failure.
     d. Insulin plays a less critical role in the treatment of HHNS than it does for the treatment of DKA because ketosis and acidosis do not occur; rehydration alone may decrease glucose levels.

IX. **CHRONIC COMPLICATIONS OF DIABETES MELLITUS**

A. Diabetic retinopathy
  1. Description
     a. Chronic and progressive impairment of the retinal circulation that eventually causes hemorrhage
     b. Permanent vision changes and blindness can occur.
     c. The client has difficulty with carrying out the daily tasks of blood glucose testing and insulin injections.
  2. Assessment
     a. A change in vision is caused by the rupture of small microaneurysms in retinal blood vessels.
     b. Blurred vision results from macular edema.
     c. Sudden loss of vision results from retinal detachment.
     d. Cataracts result from lens opacity.
  3. Interventions
     a. Maintain safety.
     b. Early prevention via the control of hypertension and blood glucose levels
     c. Photocoagulation (laser therapy) may be done to remove hemorrhagic tissue to decrease scarring and prevent progression of the disease process.
     d. Vitrectomy may be done to remove vitreous hemorrhages and thus decrease tension on the retina, preventing detachment.
     e. Cataract removal with lens implantation improves vision.

B. Diabetic nephropathy
  1. Description: Progressive decrease in kidney function
  2. Assessment
     a. Microalbuminuria
     b. Thirst
     c. Fatigue
     d. Anemia
     e. Weight loss
     f. Signs of malnutrition
     g. Frequent urinary tract infections
     h. Signs of a neurogenic bladder
  3. Interventions
     a. Early prevention measures include the control of hypertension and blood glucose levels.
     b. Assess vital signs.
     c. Monitor intake and output.
     d. Monitor the blood urea nitrogen and creatinine and urine albumin levels.
     e. Restrict dietary protein, sodium, and potassium intake as prescribed.
     f. Avoid nephrotoxic medications.
     g. Prepare the client for dialysis procedures if planned.
     h. Prepare the client for kidney transplant if planned.
     i. Prepare the client for pancreas transplant if planned.

C. Diabetic neuropathy
  1. Description
     a. General deterioration of the nervous system throughout the body

b. Complications include the development of nonhealing ulcers of the feet, gastric paresis, and erectile dysfunction.

2. Classifications
   a. Focal neuropathy or mononeuropathy: Involves a single nerve or group of nerves, most frequently cranial nerves III (oculomotor) and VI (abducens), resulting in diplopia
   b. Sensory or peripheral neuropathy: Affects distal portion of nerves, most frequently in the lower extremities
   c. Autonomic neuropathy: Symptoms vary according to organ system involved
   d. Cardiovascular: Cardiac denervation syndrome (heart rate does not respond to changes in oxygenation needs) and orthostatic hypotension occur.
   e. Pupillary: Pupil does not dilate in response to decreased light.
   f. Gastric: Decreased gastric emptying (gastroparesis)
   g. Urinary: Neurogenic bladder
   h. Sudomotor: Decreased sweating
   i. Adrenal: Hypoglycemic unawareness
   j. Reproductive: Impotence (male), painful intercourse (female)

3. Assessment: findings depend on the classification
   a. Paresthesias
   b. Decreased or absent reflexes
   c. Decreased sensation to vibration or light touch
   d. Pain, aching, and burning in the lower extremities
   e. Poor peripheral pulses
   f. Skin breakdown and signs of infection
   g. Weakness or loss of sensation in cranial nerves III (oculomotor), IV (trochlear), V (trigeminal), VI (abducens)
   h. Dizziness and postural hypotension
   i. Nausea and vomiting
   j. Diarrhea or constipation
   k. Incontinence
   l. Dyspareunia
   m. Impotence
   n. Hypoglycemic unawareness

4. Interventions
   a. Early prevention measures include the control of hypertension and blood glucose levels.
   b. Careful foot care is required to prevent trauma (Box 54-21).
   c. Administer medications as prescribed for pain relief.
   d. Initiate bladder training programs.
   e. Instruct in the use of estrogen-containing lubricants for women with dyspareunia.
   f. Prepare the male client with impotence for penile injections for possible treatment options as prescribed.

Box 54-21 Preventive Foot Care Instructions

Provide meticulous skin care and proper foot care.

Inspect feet daily and monitor feet for redness, swelling, or break in skin integrity.

Notify the physician if redness or a break in the skin occurs.

Avoid thermal injuries from hot water, heating pads, and baths.

Wash feet with warm (not hot) water and dry thoroughly (avoid foot soaks).

Avoid treating corns, blisters, or ingrown toenails.

Do not cross legs or wear tight garments that may constrict blood flow.

Apply moisturizing lotion to the feet but not between the toes.

Prevent moisture from accumulating between the toes.

Wear loose socks and well-fitting (not tight) shoes, and instruct the client not to go barefoot.

Wear clean cotton socks to keep the feet warm and change the socks daily.

Avoid wearing the same pair of shoes 2 days in a row.

Avoid wearing open-toed shoes or shoes with a strap that goes between the toes.

Check shoes for cracks or tears in the lining and for foreign objects before putting them on.

Break in new shoes gradually.

Cut toenails straight across and smooth nails with an emery board.

Avoid smoking.

---

g. Prepare for surgical decompression of compression lesions related to the cranial nerves as prescribed.

X. CARE OF THE DIABETIC CLIENT UNDERGOING SURGERY

A. Preoperative care
   1. Check with physician regarding withholding oral hypoglycemic medications or insulin.
   2. Some long-acting oral antidiabetic medications are discontinued 24 to 48 hours before surgery.
   3. Metformin (Glucophage) may need to be discontinued 48 hours before surgery and may not be restarted until renal function is normal postoperatively.
   4. All other oral antidiabetic medications are usually withheld the day of surgery.
   5. Insulin dose may be adjusted or withheld if IV insulin administration during surgery is planned.
   6. Monitor blood glucose level.
   7. Administer IV fluids as prescribed.

B. Intraoperative care
   1. Monitor blood glucose levels frequently.
   2. Administer IV short- or rapid-acting insulin as prescribed to maintain the blood glucose level lower than 200 mg/dL.

C. Postoperative care
   1. Administer IV glucose and regular insulin infusions as prescribed until the client can tolerate oral feedings.

2. Administer supplemental short-acting insulin as prescribed based on blood glucose results.

3. Monitor blood glucose levels frequently if the client is receiving parenteral nutrition.

4. When the client is tolerating food, ensure that the client receives an adequate amount of carbohydrates daily to prevent **hypoglycemia**.

5. Client is at higher risk for cardiovascular and renal complications postoperatively.

6. Client is also at risk for impaired wound healing.

💿 MORE QUESTIONS ON THE CD!

Practice Questions

571. A client is brought to the emergency department in an unresponsive state, and a diagnosis of hyperglycemic hyperosmolar nonketotic syndrome is made. The nurse would immediately prepare to initiate which of the following anticipated physician's prescriptions?
1. Endotracheal intubation
2. 100 units of NPH insulin
3. Intravenous infusion of normal saline
4. Intravenous infusion of sodium bicarbonate

572. An external insulin pump is prescribed for a client with diabetes mellitus and the client asks the nurse about the functioning of the pump. The nurse bases the response on the information that the pump:
1. Is timed to release programmed doses of regular or NPH insulin into the bloodstream at specific intervals
2. Continuously infuses small amounts of NPH insulin into the bloodstream while regularly monitoring blood glucose levels
3. Is surgically attached to the pancreas and infuses regular insulin into the pancreas, which in turn releases the insulin into the bloodstream
4. Gives a small continuous dose of regular insulin subcutaneously, and the client can self-administer a bolus with an additional dose from the pump before each meal

573. A client with a diagnosis of diabetic ketoacidosis (DKA) is being treated in an emergency department. Which finding would a nurse expect to note as confirming this diagnosis?
1. Comatose state
2. Decreased urine output
3. Increased respirations and an increase in pH
4. Elevated blood glucose level and low plasma bicarbonate level

574. A nurse teaches a client with diabetes mellitus about differentiating between hypoglycemia and ketoacidosis. The client demonstrates an understanding of the teaching by stating that a form of glucose should be taken if which of the following symptoms develops?
1. Polyuria
2. Shakiness
3. Blurred vision
4. Fruity breath odor

575. A client with diabetes mellitus demonstrates acute anxiety when first admitted for the treatment of hyperglycemia. The appropriate intervention to decrease the client's anxiety is to:
1. Administer a sedative.
2. Convey empathy, trust, and respect toward the client.
3. Ignore the signs and symptoms of anxiety so that they will soon disappear.
4. Make sure that the client knows all the correct medical terms to understand what is happening.

576. A nurse provides instructions to a client newly diagnosed with type 1 diabetes mellitus. The nurse recognizes accurate understanding of measures to prevent diabetic ketoacidosis when the client states:
1. "I will stop taking my insulin if I'm too sick to eat."
2. "I will decrease my insulin dose during times of illness."
3. "I will adjust my insulin dose according to the level of glucose in my urine."
4. "I will notify my physician if my blood glucose level is higher than 250 mg/dL."

577. A client is admitted to a hospital with a diagnosis of diabetic ketoacidosis (DKA). The initial blood glucose level was 950 mg/dL. A continuous intravenous infusion of regular insulin is initiated, along with intravenous rehydration with normal saline. The serum glucose level is now 240 mg/dL. The nurse would next prepare to administer which of the following?
1. Ampule of 50% dextrose
2. NPH insulin subcutaneously
3. Intravenous fluids containing 5% dextrose
4. Phenytoin (Dilantin) for the prevention of seizures

578. A nurse is monitoring a client newly diagnosed with diabetes mellitus for signs of complications. Which of the following, if exhibited in the client, would indicate hyperglycemia and warrant physician notification?
1. Polyuria
2. Diaphoresis
3. Hypertension
4. Increased pulse rate

579. A nurse is preparing a plan of care for a client with diabetes mellitus who has hyperglycemia. The priority nursing diagnosis would be:
1. Deficient knowledge
2. Deficient fluid volume
3. Compromised family coping
4. Imbalanced nutrition, less than body requirements

580. A home health nurse visits a client with a diagnosis of type 1 diabetes mellitus. The client relates a history of vomiting and diarrhea and tells the nurse that no food has been consumed for the last 24 hours. Which additional statement by the client indicates a need for further teaching?
1. "I need to stop my insulin."
2. "I need to increase my fluid intake."
3. "I need to monitor my blood glucose every 3 to 4 hours."
4. "I need to call the physician because of these symptoms."

581. A nurse is caring for a client after hypophysectomy. The nurse notices clear nasal drainage from the client's nostril. The initial nursing action would be to:
1. Lower the head of the bed.
2. Test the drainage for glucose.
3. Obtain a culture of the drainage.
4. Continue to observe the drainage.

582. After several diagnostic tests, a client is diagnosed with diabetes insipidus. A nurse performs an assessment on the client, knowing that which symptom is most indicative of this disorder?
1. Fatigue
2. Diarrhea
3. Polydipsia
4. Weight gain

583. A client is admitted to an emergency department, and a diagnosis of myxedema coma is made. Which action would the nurse prepare to carry out initially?
1. Warm the client.
2. Maintain a patent airway.
3. Administer thyroid hormone.
4. Administer fluid replacement.

584. A nurse is caring for a client admitted to the emergency department with diabetic ketoacidosis (DKA). In the acute phase, the priority nursing action is to prepare to:
1. Correct the acidosis.
2. Administer 5% dextrose intravenously.
3. Administer regular insulin intravenously.
4. Apply a monitor for an electrocardiogram.

585. A client with type 1 diabetes mellitus calls the nurse to report recurrent episodes of hypoglycemia with exercising. Which statement by the client indicates an inadequate understanding of the peak action of NPH insulin and exercise?
1. "The best time for me to exercise is after I eat."
2. "The best time for me to exercise is after breakfast."
3. "The best time for me to exercise is mid- to late afternoon."
4. "The best time for me to exercise is after my morning snack."

586. A nurse is completing an assessment on a client who is being admitted for a diagnostic workup for primary hyperparathyroidism. Which client complaint would be characteristic of this disorder?
1. Diarrhea
2. Polyuria
3. Polyphagia
4. Weight gain

587. A nurse is caring for a postoperative parathyroidectomy client. Which client complaint would indicate that a serious, life-threatening complication may be developing, requiring immediate notification of the physician?
1. Laryngeal stridor
2. Abdominal cramps
3. Difficulty in voiding
4. Mild to moderate incisional pain

588. A client is diagnosed with pheochromocytoma. A nurse prepares a plan of care for the client; while planning, the nurse understands that pheochromocytoma is a condition that:
1. Causes profound hypotension
2. Is manifested by severe hypoglycemia
3. Is not curable and is treated symptomatically
4. Causes the release of excessive amounts of catecholamines

589. A nurse is caring for a client with pheochromocytoma who is scheduled for adrenalectomy. In the preoperative period, the priority nursing action would be to monitor:
1. Vital signs
2. Intake and output
3. Blood urea nitrogen results
4. Urine for glucose and ketones

590. A nurse is performing an assessment on a client with pheochromocytoma. Which of the following assessment data would indicate a potential complication associated with this disorder?
1. A coagulation time of 5 minutes

2. A urinary output of 50 mL per hour
3. A blood urea nitrogen level of 20 mg/dL
4. A heart rate that is 90 beats/min and irregular

591. A nursing instructor asks a student to describe the pathophysiology that occurs in Cushing's disease. Which statement by the student indicates an accurate understanding of this disorder?
1. "Cushing's disease results from an oversecretion of insulin."
2. "Cushing's disease results from an undersecretion of corticotropic hormones."
3. "Cushing's disease results from an undersecretion of mineralocorticoid hormones."
4. "Cushing's disease results from an increased pituitary secretion of adrenocorticotropic hormone."

592. A nurse performs a physical assessment on a client with type 2 diabetes mellitus. Findings include a fasting blood glucose of 120 mg/dL, temperature of 101 ° F, pulse of 88 beats/min, respirations of 22 breaths/min, and blood pressure of 100/72 mm Hg. Which finding would be of most concern to the nurse?
1. Pulse
2. Respiration
3. Temperature
4. Blood pressure

593. A nurse is interviewing a client with type 2 diabetes mellitus. Which statement by the client indicates an understanding of the treatment for this disorder?
1. "I take oral insulin instead of shots."
2. "By taking these medications, I am able to eat more."
3. "When I become ill, I need to increase the number of pills I take."
4. "The medications I'm taking help release the insulin I already make."

594. A nurse is providing discharge instructions to a client who has Cushing's syndrome. Which client statement indicates that instructions related to dietary management are understood?

1. "I can eat foods that have a lot of potassium in them."
2. "I will need to limit the amount of protein in my diet."
3. "I am fortunate that I can eat all the salty foods I enjoy."
4. "I am fortunate that I do not need to follow any special diet."

595. The nurse is caring for a client who is 2 days postoperative following an abdominal hysterectomy. The client has a history of diabetes mellitus and has been receiving regular insulin according to capillary blood glucose testing four times a day. A carbohydrate-controlled diet has been prescribed but the client has been complaining of nausea and is not eating. On entering the client's room, the nurse finds the client to be confused and diaphoretic. Which action is appropriate at this time?
1. Call a code to obtain needed assistance immediately.
2. Obtain a capillary blood glucose level and perform a focused assessment.
3. Stay with the client and ask the nursing assistant to call the physician for a prescription for intravenous 50% dextrose.
4. Ask the nursing assistant to stay with the client while obtaining 15 to 30 g of a carbohydrate snack for the client to eat.

Alternate Item Format: Multiple Response

596. A nurse is monitoring a client who was diagnosed with type 1 diabetes mellitus and is being treated with NPH and regular insulin. Which client complaint(s) would alert the nurse to the presence of a possible hypoglycemic reaction? **Select all that apply.**
❑ 1. Tremors
❑ 2. Anorexia
❑ 3. Irritability
❑ 4. Nervousness
❑ 5. Hot, dry skin
❑ 6. Muscle cramps

ANSWERS

571. 3

Rationale: The primary goal of treatment in hyperglycemic hyperosmolar nonketotic syndrome (HHNS) is to rehydrate the client to restore fluid volume and to correct electrolyte deficiency. Intravenous fluid replacement is similar to that administered in diabetic ketoacidosis (DKA) and begins with IV infusion of normal saline. Regular insulin, not NPH insulin, would be administered. The use of sodium bicarbonate to correct acidosis is avoided because it can precipitate a further drop in serum potassium levels. Intubation and mechanical ventilation are not required to treat HHNS.

Test-Taking Strategy: Use the process of elimination. If you can recall the treatment for DKA, you will be able to answer this question easily. Treatment for HHNS is similar to the treatment for DKA and begins with rehydration. Review the treatment for HHNS if you had difficulty with this question.

Level of Cognitive Ability: Analyzing
Client Needs: Physiological Integrity
Integrated Process: Nursing Process—Planning
Content Area: Adult Health—Endocrine
Reference: Black, J., & Hawks, J. (2009). *Medical-surgical nursing: Clinical management for positive outcomes* (8th ed., pp. 1093–1094). St. Louis: Saunders.

572. 4
Rationale: An insulin pump provides a small continuous dose of regular insulin subcutaneously throughout the day and night, and the client can self-administer a bolus with an additional dose from the pump before each meal as needed. Regular insulin is used in an insulin pump. An external pump is not attached surgically to the pancreas.
Test-Taking Strategy: Use the process of elimination. Recalling that regular insulin is used in an insulin pump will assist in eliminating options 1 and 2. Noting the word *external* in the question will assist in eliminating option 3. Review the use of the insulin pump if you are unfamiliar with it.
Level of Cognitive Ability: Applying
Client Needs: Physiological Integrity
Integrated Process: Teaching and Learning
Content Area: Adult Health—Endocrine
Reference: Black, J., & Hawks, J. (2009). *Medical-surgical nursing: Clinical management for positive outcomes* (8th ed., pp. 1074–1075). St. Louis: Saunders.

573. 4
Rationale: In DKA, the arterial pH is lower than 7.35, plasma bicarbonate is lower than 15 mEq/L, the blood glucose level is higher than 250 mg/dL, and ketones are present in the blood and urine. The client would be experiencing polyuria, and Kussmaul's respirations would be present. A comatose state may occur if DKA is not treated, but coma would not confirm the diagnosis.
Test-Taking Strategy: Use the process of elimination and note the strategic word *confirming* in the question. Eliminate option 1 because a comatose state can exist in many conditions. Eliminate option 3 because in acidosis the pH would be low. Remember that polyuria exists in DKA. Review the clinical manifestations of DKA if you had difficulty with this question.
Level of Cognitive Ability: Analyzing
Client Needs: Physiological Integrity
Integrated Process: Nursing Process—Assessment
Content Area: Adult Health—Endocrine
References: Copstead-Kirkhorn, L., & Banasik, J. (2010). *Pathophysiology* (4th ed., p. 949). St. Louis: Mosby.
   Ignatavicius, D., & Workman, M. (2010). *Medical-surgical nursing: Patient-centered collaborative care* (6th ed., pp. 1510–1511). St. Louis: Saunders.
   Swearingen, P. (2008). *All-in-one care planning resource: Medical-surgical, pediatric, maternity, & psychiatric nursing care plans* (2nd ed., pp. 387–388). St. Louis: Mosby.

574. 2
Rationale: Shakiness is a sign of hypoglycemia and would indicate the need for food or glucose. A fruity breath odor, blurred vision, and polyuria are signs of hyperglycemia.
Test-Taking Strategy: Focus on the subject of the question, the treatment of hypoglycemia, and think about its

pathophysiology and the manifestations that occur. Recalling the signs of hypoglycemia will direct you to option 2. Review these signs if you had difficulty with this question.
Level of Cognitive Ability: Evaluating
Client Needs: Physiological Integrity
Integrated Process: Nursing Process—Evaluation
Content Area: Adult Health—Endocrine
Reference: Ignatavicius, D., & Workman, M. (2010). *Medical-surgical nursing: Patient-centered collaborative care* (6th ed., pp. 1507–1508, 1510). St. Louis: Saunders.

575. 2
Rationale: The appropriate intervention is to address the client's feelings related to the anxiety. Administering a sedative is not the most appropriate intervention. The nurse should not ignore the client's anxious feelings. A client will not relate to medical terms, particularly when anxiety exists.
Test-Taking Strategy: Use therapeutic communication techniques to answer the question. Remember that the client's feelings are the priority. Keeping this in mind will direct you easily to option 2. Review therapeutic communication techniques if you had difficulty with this question.
Level of Cognitive Ability: Applying
Client Needs: Psychosocial Integrity
Integrated Process: Caring
Content Area: Adult Health—Endocrine
Reference: Ignatavicius, D., & Workman, M. (2010). *Medical-surgical nursing: Patient-centered collaborative care* (6th ed., p. 1475). St. Louis: Saunders.

576. 4
Rationale: During illness, the client should monitor blood glucose levels and should notify the physician if the level is higher than 250 mg/dL. Insulin should never be stopped. In fact, insulin may need to be increased during times of illness. Doses should not be adjusted without the physician's advice and are usually adjusted based on blood glucose levels, not urinary glucose readings.
Test-Taking Strategy: Use the process of elimination. Note that options 1, 2, and 3 are comparable or alike and all relate to adjustment of insulin doses. Review diabetic management during illness if you had difficulty with this question.
Level of Cognitive Ability: Evaluating
Client Needs: Physiological Integrity
Integrated Process: Nursing Process—Evaluation
Content Area: Adult Health—Endocrine
Reference: Ignatavicius, D., & Workman, M. (2010). *Medical-surgical nursing: Patient-centered collaborative care* (6th ed., p. 1512). St. Louis: Saunders.

577. 3
Rationale: During management of DKA, when the blood glucose level falls to 250 to 300 mg/dL, the infusion rate is reduced and a 5% dextrose in 0.45% saline is added to maintain a blood glucose level of about 250 mg/dL, or until the client recovers from ketosis. NPH insulin is not used to treat DKA. Fifty percent dextrose is used to treat hypoglycemia. Phenytoin (Dilantin) is not a usual treatment measure for DKA.
Test-Taking Strategy: Use the process of elimination. Eliminate option 2 first, knowing that regular insulin is used in

the management of DKA. Eliminate option 1 next, knowing that this is the treatment for hypoglycemia. Note the strategic words *the serum glucose level is now 240 mg/dL*. This should indicate that the IV solution containing 5% dextrose is the next step in the management of care. Review care of the client with DKA if you had difficulty with this question.
Level of Cognitive Ability: Analyzing
Client Needs: Physiological Integrity
Integrated Process: Nursing Process—Planning
Content Area: Adult Health—Endocrine
Reference: Black, J., & Hawks, J. (2009). *Medical-surgical nursing: Clinical management for positive outcomes* (8th ed., pp. 1093–1094). St. Louis: Saunders.

578. 1
Rationale: Classic symptoms of hyperglycemia include polydipsia, polyuria, and polyphagia. Options 2, 3, and 4 are not signs of hyperglycemia.
Test-Taking Strategy: Use the process of elimination. Remember the three P's associated with hyperglycemia—polyuria, polydipsia, polyphagia. Learn the signs of hyperglycemia if you had difficulty with this question.
Level of Cognitive Ability: Understanding
Client Needs: Physiological Integrity
Integrated Process: Nursing Process—Assessment
Content Area: Adult Health—Endocrine
Reference: Copstead-Kirkhorn, L., & Banasik, J. (2010). *Pathophysiology* (4th ed., p. 952). St. Louis: Mosby.

579. 2
Rationale: An increased blood glucose level will cause the kidneys to excrete the glucose in the urine. This glucose is accompanied by fluids and electrolytes, causing an osmotic diuresis leading to dehydration. This fluid loss must be replaced when it becomes severe. Options 1, 3, and 4 are not related specifically to the subject of the question.
Test-Taking Strategy: Use Maslow's Hierarchy of Needs theory to answer this question. Option 2 indicates a physiological need and is the priority. Options 1, 3, and 4 are nursing diagnoses that may need to be addressed after providing for the high-priority physiological needs. Review the priority concerns for the client with hyperglycemia if you had difficulty with this question.
Level of Cognitive Ability: Analyzing
Client Needs: Physiological Integrity
Integrated Process: Nursing Process—planning
Content Area: Adult Health—Endocrine
Reference: Ignatavicius, D., & Workman, M. (2010). *Medical-surgical nursing: Patient-centered collaborative care* (6th ed., p. 1475). St. Louis: Saunders.

580. 1
Rationale: When a client with diabetes mellitus is unable to eat normally because of illness, the client still should take the prescribed insulin or oral medication. The client should consume additional fluids and should notify the physician. The client should monitor the blood glucose level every 3 to 4 hours. The client should also monitor the urine for ketones.
Test-Taking Strategy: Note the strategic words *need for further teaching*. These words indicate a negative event query and the need to select the incorrect statement. Remembering that the client needs to take insulin will direct you easily to option 1.

Review the sick rule guidelines for the client with diabetes mellitus if you had difficulty with this question.
Level of Cognitive Ability: Evaluating
Client Needs: Physiological Integrity
Integrated Process: Teaching and Learning
Content Area: Adult Health—Endocrine
Reference: Ignatavicius, D., & Workman, M. (2010). *Medical-surgical nursing: Patient-centered collaborative care* (6th ed., p. 1512). St. Louis: Saunders.

581. 2
Rationale: After hypophysectomy, the client should be monitored for rhinorrhea, which could indicate a cerebrospinal fluid leak. If this occurs, the drainage should be collected and tested for the presence of cerebrospinal fluid. The head of the bed should not be lowered to prevent increased intracranial pressure. Clear nasal drainage would not indicate the need for a culture. Continuing to observe the drainage without taking action could result in a serious complication.
Test-Taking Strategy: Use the process of elimination and note the strategic word *initial*. This indicates that an action is required. Option 1 can be eliminated first recalling that this action can increase intracranial pressure. Option 3 can be eliminated also because the drainage is clear. Because an action is required, eliminate option 4. Review the complications following hypophysectomy if you had difficulty with this question.
Level of Cognitive Ability: Applying
Client Needs: Physiological Integrity
Integrated Process: Nursing Process—Implementation
Content Area: Adult Health—Endocrine
Reference: Ignatavicius, D., & Workman, M. (2010). *Medical-surgical nursing: Patient-centered collaborative care* (6th ed., p. 1431). St. Louis: Saunders.

582. 3
Rationale: Diabetes insipidus is characterized by a hyposecretion of the antidiuretic hormone and the kidney tubules fail to reabsorb water. Polydipsia and polyuria are classic symptoms of diabetes insipidus. The urine is pale, and the specific gravity is low. Anorexia and weight loss occur. Option 1 is a vague symptom. Options 2 and 4 are not specific to this disorder.
Test-Taking Strategy: Note the strategic words *most indicative*. Eliminate option 1 first because this symptom is rather vague and occurs in many conditions. Knowledge of the pathophysiology and manifestations of diabetes insipidus will assist you in eliminating options 2 and 4. If you had difficulty with this question, review the clinical manifestations associated with diabetes insipidus.
Level of Cognitive Ability: Analyzing
Client Needs: Physiological Integrity
Integrated Process: Nursing Process—Assessment
Content Area: Adult Health—Endocrine
Reference: Swearingen, P. (2008). *All-in-one care planning resource: Medical-surgical, pediatric, maternity, & psychiatric nursing care plans* (2nd ed., p. 373). St. Louis: Mosby.

583. 2
Rationale: The initial nursing action would be to maintain a patent airway. Oxygen would be administered, followed by

fluid replacement, keeping the client warm, monitoring vital signs, and administering thyroid hormones by the intravenous route.

Test-Taking Strategy: Use the process of elimination and note the strategic word *initially*. All the options are appropriate interventions, but use the ABCs—airway, breathing, and circulation—in selecting the correct option. Review the initial interventions for myxedema coma if you had difficulty with this question.

Level of Cognitive Ability: Applying
Client Needs: Physiological Integrity
Integrated Process: Nursing Process—Implementation
Content Area: Adult Health—Endocrine
Reference: Black, J., & Hawks, J. (2009). *Medical-surgical nursing: Clinical management for positive outcomes* (8th ed., p. 1022). St. Louis: Saunders.

584. 3

Rationale: Lack (absolute or relative) of insulin is the primary cause of DKA. Treatment consists of insulin administration (regular insulin), intravenous fluid administration (normal saline initially), and potassium replacement, followed by correcting acidosis. Applying an electrocardiogram monitor is not a priority action.

Test-Taking Strategy: Use the process of elimination and focus on the client's diagnosis. Note the strategic word *priority*. Remember that in DKA, the initial treatment is regular insulin. Normal saline is administered initially; therefore, option 2 is incorrect. Options 1 and 4 may be components of the treatment plan but are not the priority. Review the initial treatment for DKA if you had difficulty with this question.

Level of Cognitive Ability: Applying
Client Needs: Physiological Integrity
Integrated Process: Nursing Process—Implementation
Content Area: Adult Health—Endocrine
Reference: Black, J., & Hawks, J. (2009). *Medical-surgical nursing: Clinical management for positive outcomes* (8th ed., p. 1092). St. Louis: Saunders.

585. 3

Rationale: A hypoglycemic reaction may occur in response to increased exercise. Clients should avoid exercise during the peak time of insulin. NPH insulin peaks at 4 to 12 hours; therefore, afternoon exercise takes place during the peak of the medication. Options 1, 2, and 4 do not address peak action times.

Test-Taking Strategy: Use the process of elimination and note the strategic words *inadequate understanding*. Focus on the subject, peak action of NPH. Recalling that NPH peaks at 4 to 12 hours will direct you to option 3. Review the peak action time of NPH insulin if you had difficulty with this question.

Level of Cognitive Ability: Evaluating
Client Needs: Physiological Integrity
Integrated Process: Teaching and Learning
Content Area: Adult Health—Endocrine
References: Black, J., & Hawks, J. (2009). *Medical-surgical nursing: Clinical management for positive outcomes* (8th ed., p. 1079). St. Louis: Saunders.
Ignatavicius, D., & Workman, M. (2010). *Medical-surgical nursing: Patient-centered collaborative care* (6th ed., p. 1497). St. Louis: Saunders.

Kee, J., Hayes, E., & McCuistion, L. (2009). *Pharmacology: A nursing process approach* (6th ed., p. 795). St. Louis: Saunders.

586. 2

Rationale: Hypercalcemia is the hallmark of hyperparathyroidism. Elevated serum calcium levels produce osmotic diuresis and thus polyuria. This diuresis leads to dehydration (weight loss rather than weight gain). Options 1, 3, and 4 are gastrointestinal symptoms and are not associated with the common gastrointestinal symptoms typical of hyperparathyroidism (nausea, vomiting, anorexia, constipation).

Test-Taking Strategy: Use the process of elimination and think about the pathophysiology associated with hyperparathyroidism. Note that options 1, 3, and 4 are gastrointestinal symptoms and are comparable or alike. Review the clinical manifestations of hyperparathyroidism if you had difficulty with this question.

Level of Cognitive Ability: Analyzing
Client Needs: Physiological Integrity
Integrated Process: Nursing Process—Assessment
Content Area: Adult Health—Endocrine
References: Black, J., & Hawks, J. (2009). *Medical-surgical nursing: Clinical management for positive outcomes* (8th ed., pp. 1033–1034). St. Louis: Saunders.
Copstead-Kirkhorn, L., & Banasik, J. (2010). *Pathophysiology* (4th ed., p. 937). St. Louis: Mosby.

587. 1

Rationale: During the postoperative period, the nurse carefully observes the client for signs of hemorrhage, which causes swelling and compression of adjacent tissue. Laryngeal stridor is a harsh, high-pitched sound heard on inspiration and expiration; stridor is caused by compression of the trachea, leading to respiratory distress. Stridor is an acute emergency situation that requires immediate attention to avoid complete obstruction of the airway. Options 2, 3, and 4 do not identify signs of a life-threatening complication.

Test-Taking Strategy: Consider the anatomical location of the surgical procedure and use the ABCs—airway, breathing, and circulation—to select the correct option. Options 2, 3, and 4 are usual postoperative findings that are not life-threatening. Option 1 addresses the airway. Review postoperative care of the parathyroidectomy client if you had difficulty with this question.

Level of Cognitive Ability: Analyzing
Client Needs: Physiological Integrity
Integrated Process: Nursing Process—Assessment
Content Area: Adult Health—Endocrine
References: Black, J., & Hawks, J. (2009). *Medical-surgical nursing: Clinical management for positive outcomes* (8th ed., p. 1035). St. Louis: Saunders.
Ignatavicius, D., & Workman, M. (2010). *Medical-surgical nursing: Patient-centered collaborative care* (6th ed., p. 1463). St. Louis: Saunders.

588. 4

Rationale: Pheochromocytoma is a catecholamine-producing tumor and causes secretion of excessive amounts of epinephrine and norepinephrine. Hypertension is the principal manifestation, and the client has episodes of high blood pressure accompanied by pounding headaches. The excessive release of catecholamine

also results in excessive conversion of glycogen into glucose in the liver. Consequently, hyperglycemia and glucosuria occur during attacks. Pheochromocytoma is curable. The primary treatment is surgical removal of one or both of the adrenal glands, depending on whether the tumor is unilateral or bilateral.
Test-Taking Strategy: Use the process of elimination and knowledge of the manifestations of pheochromocytoma to answer this question. Remember that pheochromocytoma is a catecholamine-producing tumor. If you are unfamiliar with this disorder, review this content.
Level of Cognitive Ability: Understanding
Client Needs: Physiological Integrity
Integrated Process: Nursing Process—Planning
Content Area: Adult Health—Endocrine
Reference: Black, J., & Hawks, J. (2009). *Medical-surgical nursing: Clinical management for positive outcomes* (8th ed., p. 1051). St. Louis: Saunders.

589. 1
Rationale: Pheochromocytoma is a catecholamine-producing tumor. Hypertension is the hallmark of pheochromocytoma. Severe hypertension can precipitate a stroke or sudden blindness. Although all the options are accurate nursing interventions for the client with pheochromocytoma, the priority nursing action is to monitor the vital signs, particularly the blood pressure.
Test-Taking Strategy: Use the process of elimination and note the strategic words *priority nursing action.* Use the ABCs—airway, breathing, and circulation. Monitoring vital signs is the nursing action that would assess airway, breathing, and circulation. Also, options 2, 3, and 4 refer to the assessment of the renal system, whereas option 1 does not. Review preoperative care of the client with pheochromocytoma if you had difficulty with this question.
Level of Cognitive Ability: Applying
Client Needs: Physiological Integrity
Integrated Process: Nursing Process—Implementation
Content Area: Adult Health—Endocrine
Reference: Black, J., & Hawks, J. (2009). *Medical-surgical nursing: Clinical management for positive outcomes* (8th ed., p. 1053). St. Louis: Saunders.

590. 4
Rationale: The complications associated with pheochromocytoma include hypertensive retinopathy and nephropathy, myocarditis, increased platelet aggregation, and stroke. Death can occur from shock, stroke, renal failure, dysrhythmias, or dissecting aortic aneurysm. An irregular heart rate indicates the presence of a dysrhythmia. A urinary output of 50 mL/hr is an adequate output. A blood urea nitrogen level of 20 mg/dL is a normal finding. A coagulation time of 5 minutes is normal.
Test-Taking Strategy: Use the process of elimination and the ABCs—airway, breathing, and circulation. An irregular heart rate is associated with circulation. In addition, if you knew the normal hourly expectations associated with urinary output and the normal laboratory values for coagulation time and blood urea nitrogen level, you would be easily directed to option 4. Review the complications associated with pheochromocytoma if you had difficulty with this question.
Level of Cognitive Ability: Analyzing

Client Needs: Physiological Integrity
Integrated Process: Nursing Process—Analysis
Content Area: Adult Health—Endocrine
Reference: Copstead-Kirkhorn, L., & Banasik, J. (2010). *Pathophysiology* (4th ed., p. 936). St. Louis: Mosby.

591. 4
Rationale: Cushing's disease is a metabolic disorder characterized by abnormally increased secretion (endogenous) of cortisol, caused by increased amounts of adrenocorticotropic hormone (ACTH) secreted by the pituitary gland. Addison's disease is characterized by the hyposecretion of adrenal cortex hormones (glucocorticoids and mineralocorticoids) from the adrenal gland, resulting in deficiency of the corticosteroid hormones. Options 1, 2, and 3 are inaccurate regarding Cushing's disease.
Test-Taking Strategy: Use the process of elimination. Options 2 and 3 can be eliminated easily if you remember that in Cushing's (up) disease there is an oversecretion and in Addison's disease there is an undersecretion. Next, eliminate option 1 because this disease is unrelated to insulin. Review the pathophysiology associated with Cushing's disease if you had difficulty with this question.
Level of Cognitive Ability: Evaluating
Client Needs: Physiological Integrity
Integrated Process: Teaching and Learning
Content Area: Adult Health—Endocrine
References: Black, J., & Hawks, J. (2009). *Medical-surgical nursing: Clinical management for positive outcomes* (8th ed., p. 1049). St. Louis: Saunders.
Ignatavicius, D., & Workman, M. (2010). *Medical-surgical nursing: Patient-centered collaborative care* (6th ed., p. 1440). St. Louis: Saunders.

592. 3
Rationale: An elevated temperature may indicate infection. Infection is a leading cause of hyperglycemic hyperosmolar nonketotic syndrome or diabetic ketoacidosis. The other findings noted in the question are within normal limits.
Test-Taking Strategy: Use the process of elimination and knowledge of the normal values of vital signs to direct you to option 3. The client's temperature is the only abnormal value. Remember that an elevated temperature can indicate an infectious process that can lead to complications in the client with diabetes mellitus. Review normal and abnormal findings in the client with diabetes mellitus if you had difficulty with this question.
Level of Cognitive Ability: Understanding
Client Needs: Physiological Integrity
Integrated Process: Nursing Process—Assessment
Content Area: Adult Health—Endocrine
References: Ignatavicius, D., & Workman, M. (2010). *Medical-surgical nursing: Patient-centered collaborative care* (6th ed., p. 1475). St. Louis: Saunders.
Swearingen, P. (2008). *All-in-one care planning resource: Medical-surgical, pediatric, maternity, & psychiatric nursing care plans* (2nd ed., p. 397). St. Louis: Mosby.

593. 4
Rationale: Clients with type 2 diabetes mellitus have decreased or impaired insulin secretion. Oral hypoglycemic

agents are given to these clients to facilitate glucose uptake. Insulin injections may be given during times of stress-induced hyperglycemia. Oral insulin is not available because of the breakdown of the insulin by digestion. Options 1, 2, and 3 are incorrect.

Test-Taking Strategy: Use the process of elimination, focusing on the subject, type 2 diabetes mellitus. Eliminate option 1 because *oral insulin* is not available. Treatment with medication does not mean that the client can eat more; therefore, eliminate option 2. Recalling that during times of illness insulin may be required will eliminate option 3. Review treatment measures for type 2 diabetes mellitus if you had difficulty with this question.

Level of Cognitive Ability: Evaluating
Client Needs: Physiological Integrity
Integrated Process: Nursing Process—Evaluation
Content Area: Adult Health—Endocrine
References: Black, J., & Hawks, J. (2009). *Medical-surgical nursing: Clinical management for positive outcomes* (8th ed., p. 1069). St. Louis: Saunders.

Ignatavicius, D., & Workman, M. (2010). *Medical-surgical nursing: Patient-centered collaborative care* (6th ed., p. 1472). St. Louis: Saunders.

594. 1
Rationale: A diet low in carbohydrates and sodium but ample in protein and potassium is encouraged for a client with Cushing's syndrome. Such a diet promotes weight loss, reduction of edema and hypertension, control of hypokalemia, and rebuilding of wasted tissue.

Test-Taking Strategy: Use the process of elimination. Eliminate option 4 because it reflects that no dietary change is necessary. Eliminate option 2 next because protein most likely is limited in liver or renal disorders (not in Cushing's syndrome). From the remaining options, eliminate option 3 because excess sodium is not normally healthy. Review dietary management in Cushing's syndrome if you had difficulty with this question.

Level of Cognitive Ability: Evaluating
Client Needs: Physiological Integrity
Integrated Process: Nursing Process—Evaluation
Content Area: Adult Health—Endocrine
References: Ignatavicius, D., & Workman, M. (2010). *Medical-surgical nursing: Patient-centered collaborative care* (6th ed., p. 1444). St. Louis: Saunders.

Nix, S. (2009). *Williams' basic nutrition and diet therapy* (13th ed., p. 388). St. Louis: Mosby.

595. 2
Rationale: Diaphoresis and confusion are signs of moderate hypoglycemia. A likely cause of the client's change in condition could be related to the administration of insulin without the client eating enough food. However, an assessment is necessary to confirm the presence of hypoglycemia. The nurse would obtain a capillary blood glucose level to confirm the hypoglycemia and perform a focused assessment to determine the extent and cause of the client's condition. Once hypoglycemia is confirmed, the nurse stays with the client and asks the nursing assistant to obtain the appropriate carbohydrate snack. A code is called if the client is not breathing or if the heart is not beating.

Test-Taking Strategy: Focus on the data in the question and note the strategic words *at this time*. Eliminate option 1 because there are no data in the question indicating the need to call a code. Eliminate option 3 next because it is inappropriate to ask a nursing assistant to call a physician for a prescription. To select from the remaining options, use the steps of the nursing process, recalling that assessment is the first step. Review care of the client experiencing a hypoglycemic reaction if you had difficulty with this question.

Level of Cognitive Ability: Applying
Client Needs: Physiological Integrity
Integrated Process: Nursing Process—Implementation
Content Area: Adult Health—Endocrine
Reference: Swearingen, P. (2008). *All-in-one care planning resource: Medical-surgical, pediatric, maternity, & psychiatric nursing care plans* (2nd ed., p. 387). St. Louis: Mosby.

ALTERNATE ITEM FORMAT: MULTIPLE RESPONSE
596. 1, 3, 4
Rationale: Decreased blood glucose levels produce autonomic nervous system symptoms, which are manifested classically as nervousness, irritability, and tremors. Option 5 is more likely to occur with hyperglycemia. Options 2 and 6 are unrelated to the signs of hypoglycemia.

Test-Taking Strategy: Focus on the subject, a hypoglycemic reaction. Think about the manifestations that occur in this complication. Recalling the signs of this type of reaction will direct you easily to the correct options. Review the signs of hypoglycemia if you had difficulty with this question.

Level of Cognitive Ability: Analyzing
Client Needs: Physiological Integrity
Integrated Process: Nursing Process—Assessment
Content Area: Adult Health—Endocrine
Reference: Ignatavicius, D., & Workman, M. (2010). *Medical-surgical nursing: Patient-centered collaborative care* (6th ed., p. 1507). St. Louis: Saunders.

Endocrine Medications

I. PITUITARY MEDICATIONS

A. Description
1. The anterior pituitary gland secretes growth hormone (GH), thyroid-stimulating hormone (TSH), adrenocorticotropic hormone (ACTH), prolactin, melanocyte-stimulating hormone (MSH), and gonadotropins (follicle-stimulating hormone [FSH] and luteinizing hormone [LH]).
2. The posterior pituitary gland secretes antidiuretic hormone (vasopressin) and oxytocin.

B. Growth hormones and related medications (Box 55-1)
1. Uses
   a. Growth hormones are used to treat pediatric or adult growth hormone deficiency.
   b. Growth hormone receptor antagonists are used to treat acromegaly.
   c. Growth hormone releasing factor is used to evaluate anterior pituitary function.
2. Side effects
   a. May vary depending on the medication
   b. Development of antibodies to growth hormone
   c. Headache, muscle pain, weakness, vertigo
   d. Diarrhea, nausea, abdominal discomfort
   e. Mild **hyperglycemia**
   f. Hypertension
   g. Weight gain
   h. Allergic reaction (rash, swelling), pain at injection site
   i. Elevated aspartate aminotransferase (AST) and alanine aminotransferase (ALT)
3. Interventions
   a. Assess the child's physical growth and compare growth with standards.
   b. Recommend annual bone age determinations for children receiving growth hormones.
   c. Monitor vital signs, blood glucose levels, AST and ALT levels, and thyroid function tests.
   d. Teach the client and family about the clinical manifestations of **hyperglycemia** and about other side effects of therapy and the importance of follow-up regarding periodic blood tests.

II. ANTIDIURETIC HORMONES (Box 55-2)

A. Description
1. Antidiuretic hormones enhance reabsorption of water in the kidneys, promoting an antidiuretic effect and regulating fluid balance.
2. Antidiuretic hormones are used in **diabetes insipidus.**

B. Side effects
1. Flushing
2. Headache
3. Nausea and abdominal cramps
4. Water intoxication
5. Hypertension with water intoxication
6. Nasal congestion with nasal administration

C. Interventions
1. Monitor weight.
2. Monitor intake and output and urine osmolality.
3. Monitor electrolyte levels.
4. Monitor for signs of dehydration, indicating the need to increase the dosage.
5. Monitor for signs of water intoxication (drowsiness, listlessness, shortness of breath, and headache), indicating need to decrease dosage.
6. Monitor blood pressure.
7. Instruct the client in how to use the intranasal medication.
8. Instruct the client to weigh themselves daily to identify weight gain.
9. Instruct the client to report signs of water intoxication or symptoms of headache or shortness of breath.

III. THYROID HORMONES (Box 55-3)

A. Description
1. Thyroid hormones control the metabolic rate of tissues and accelerate heat production and oxygen consumption.
2. Thyroid hormones are used to replace the thyroid hormone deficit in conditions such as **hypothyroidism** and **myxedema.**
3. Thyroid hormones enhance the action of oral anticoagulants, sympathomimetics, and antidepressants and decrease the action of insulin, oral hypoglycemics, and digitalis preparations; the

Box 55-1 Growth Hormones and Related Medications

Growth Hormones
Somatropin (Humatrope)
Mecasermin (Increlex)

Growth Hormone Receptor Antagonists
Octreotide acetate (Sandostatin)
Pegvisomant (Somavert)

Growth Hormone Releasing Factor
Sermorelin (Geref)

Box 55-2 Antidiuretic Hormones

Desmopressin acetate (DDAVP, Stimate, Minirin)
Vasopressin (Pitressin)

Box 55-3 Thyroid Hormones

Levothyroxine sodium (Synthroid, Levothroid, Levoxyl, Thyro-Tabs, Unithroid)
Liothyronine sodium (Cytomel, Triostat)
Liotrix (Thyrolar)
Thyroid (Armour Thyroid, Bio-Throid, Nature-Throid, Thyroid USP, Westhroid)

action of thyroid hormones is decreased by phenytoin (Dilantin) and carbamazepine (Tegretol).
4. Thyroid hormones should be given at least 4 hours apart from multivitamins, aluminum hydroxide and magnesium hydroxide, simethicone, calcium carbonate, bile acid sequestrants, iron, and sucralfate (Carafate) because these medications decrease the absorption of thyroid replacements.
B. Side effects
1. Nausea and decreased appetite
2. Abdominal cramps and diarrhea
3. Weight loss
4. Nervousness and tremors
5. Insomnia
6. Sweating and heat intolerance
7. Tachycardia, dysrhythmias, palpitations, chest pain
8. Hypertension
9. Headache
10. Toxicity: **Hyperthyroidism**
C. Interventions
1. Assess the client for a history of medications currently being taken.
2. Monitor vital signs.
3. Monitor weight.

Box 55-4 Antithyroid Medications

Methimazole (Tapazole)
Propylthiouracil (PTU)
Strong iodine solution (Lugol's solution)
Potassium iodide
Iodide I 131 (Iodotope)

4. Monitor triiodothyronine, thyroxine, and thyroid-stimulating hormone levels.
5. Instruct the client to take the medication at the same time each day, in the morning without food.
6. Instruct the client in how to monitor the pulse rate.
7. Instruct the client to avoid foods that can inhibit thyroid secretion, such as strawberries, peaches, pears, cabbage, turnips, spinach, kale, Brussels sprouts, cauliflower, radishes, and peas.
8. Advise the client to avoid over-the-counter medications.
9. Instruct the client to wear a Medic-Alert bracelet.

⚠ Advise the client taking a thyroid hormone to report symptoms of hyperthyroidism, such as tachycardia, chest pain, palpitations, and excessive sweating. These indicate signs of toxicity.

IV. ANTITHYROID MEDICATIONS (Box 55-4)
A. Description
1. Antithyroid medications inhibit the synthesis of thyroid hormone.
2. Antithyroid medications are used for **hyperthyroidism,** or Graves' disease.
B. Side effects
1. Nausea and vomiting
2. Diarrhea
3. Drowsiness, headache, fever
4. Hypersensitivity with rash
5. Agranulocytosis with leukopenia and thrombocytopenia
6. Alopecia and hyperpigmentation
7. Toxicity: **Hypothyroidism**
8. Iodism: Characterized by vomiting, abdominal pain, metallic or brassy taste in the mouth, rash, and sore gums and salivary glands
C. Interventions
1. Monitor vital signs.
2. Monitor triiodothyronine, thyroxine, and thyroid-stimulating hormone levels.
3. Monitor weight.
4. Instruct the client to take medication with meals to avoid gastrointestinal upset.
5. Instruct the client in how to monitor the pulse rate.
6. Inform the client of side effects and when to notify the physician.

Box 55-5 Medications to Treat Calcium Disorders

Oral Calcium Supplements
Calcium acetate (PhosLo)
Calcium carbonate (Rolaids, Tums, others)
Calcium chloride
Calcium citrate (Citracal)
Calcium glubionate (Calcionate, calciquid)
Calcium gluconate
Calcium lactate (Cal-lac)
Tribasic calcium phosphate (Posture)

Vitamin D Supplements
Cholecalciferol (Vitamin D$_3$)
Ergocalciferol (Vitamin D$_2$)

Biphosphonates and Calcium Regulators
Alendronate sodium (Fosamax)

Calcitonin salmon (Calcimar, Cibacalcin, Fortical)
Etidronate disodium (Didronel)
Ibandronate (Boniva)
Pamidronate disodium (Aredia)
Risedronate sodium (Actonel)
Tiludronate disodium (Skelid)
Zoledronate (Reclast)
Zoledronate (Zometa)

Medications to Treat Hypercalcemia
Cinacalcet hydrochloride (Sensipar)
Doxercalciferol (Hectorol)
Gallium nitrate (Ganite)
Paricalcitol (Zemplar)

---

7. Instruct the client in the signs of **hypothyroidism.**
8. Instruct the client regarding the importance of medication compliance and that abruptly stopping the medication could cause **thyroid storm.**
9. Instruct the client to monitor for signs and symptoms of **thyroid storm** (fever, flushed skin, confusion and behavioral changes, tachycardia, dysrhythmias, and signs of heart failure).
10. Instruct the client to monitor for signs of iodism.
11. Advise the client to consult physician before eating iodized salt and iodine-rich foods.
12. Instruct the client to avoid acetylsalicylic acid (aspirin) and medications containing iodine.

⚠ Propylthiouracil (PTU) causes agranulocytosis. Therefore, advise the client to contact the physician if a fever or sore throat develops.

V. PARATHYROID MEDICATIONS (Box 55-5)

A. Description
1. Parathyroid hormone regulates serum calcium levels.
2. Low serum levels of calcium stimulate parathyroid hormone release.
3. Hyperparathyroidism results in a high serum calcium level and bone demineralization; medication is used to lower the serum calcium level.
4. Hypoparathyroidism results in a low serum calcium level, which increases neuromuscular excitability; treatment includes calcium and vitamin D supplements.
5. Calcium salts administered with digoxin (Lanoxin) increases the risk of digoxin toxicity.
6. Oral calcium salts reduce the absorption of tetracycline hydrochloride.

B. Interventions

Box 55-6 Corticosteroid: Mineralocorticoid

Fludrocortisone acetate

1. Monitor electrolyte and calcium levels.
2. Assess for signs and symptoms of hypocalcemia and hypercalcemia.
3. Assess for symptoms of tetany in the client with hypocalcemia.
4. Assess for renal calculi in the client with hypercalcemia
5. Instruct the client in the signs and symptoms of hypercalcemia and hypocalcemia.
6. Instruct the client to check over-the-counter medication labels for the possibility of calcium content.
7. Instruct the client receiving oral calcium supplements to maintain an adequate intake of vitamin D because vitamin D enhances absorption of calcium.
8. Instruct the client receiving calcium regulators such as alendronate sodium (Fosamax) to swallow the tablet whole with water at least 30 minutes before breakfast and not to lie down for at least 30 minutes.
9. Instruct the client using nasal spray of calcitonin (Calcimar) to alternate nares.
10. Instruct the client using antihypercalcemic agents to avoid foods rich in calcium such as green, leafy vegetables, dairy products, shellfish, and soy.
11. Instruct the client not to take other medications within 1 hour of taking a calcium salt.
12. Instruct the client to increase fluid and fiber in diet to prevent constipation associated with calcium supplements.

VI. CORTICOSTEROIDS (MINERALOCORTICOIDS) (Box 55-6)

A. Description
1. Mineralocorticoids are steroid hormones that enhance the reabsorption of sodium and chloride and promote the excretion of potassium and hydrogen from the renal tubules, thereby helping maintain fluid and electrolyte balance.
2. Mineralocorticoids are used for replacement therapy in primary and secondary adrenal insufficiency in **Addison's disease.**

B. Side effects
1. Sodium and water retention (hypernatremia and edema), hypertension
2. Hypokalemia
3. Hypocalcemia
4. Osteoporosis, compression fractures
5. Weight gain
6. Heart failure

C. Interventions
1. Monitor vital signs.
2. Monitor intake and output and weight and for edema.
3. Monitor electrolyte and calcium levels.
4. Instruct the client to take medication with food or milk.
5. Instruct the client to consume a high-potassium diet.
7. Instruct the client to report illness, such as severe diarrhea, vomiting, and fever.
8. Instruct the client to notify the physician if low blood pressure, weakness, cramping, palpitations, or changes in mental status occur.
9. Instruct the client to wear a Medic-Alert bracelet.

⚠ Instruct the client taking a corticosteroid not to stop the medication abruptly because this could result in adrenal insufficiency.

VII. CORTICOSTEROIDS (GLUCOCORTICOIDS) (Box 55-7)

A. Description
1. Glucocorticoids affect glucose, protein, and bone metabolism, alter the normal immune response and suppress inflammation, and produce anti-inflammatory, antiallergic, and antistress effects.
2. Glucocorticoids may be used as a replacement in adrenocortical insufficiency.

Box 55-7 Corticosteroids: Glucocorticoids

Betamethasone
Cortisone acetate
Dexamethasone
Hydrocortisone
Methylprednisolone
Prednisolone
Prednisone
Triamcinolone

B. Side effects
1. **Hyperglycemia**
2. Hypokalemia
3. Hypocalcemia, osteoporosis
4. Sodium and fluid retention
5. Weight gain
6. Mood swings
7. Moon face, buffalo hump, truncal obesity
8. Increased susceptibility to infection and masking of the signs and symptoms of infection
9. Cataracts
10. Hirsutism, acne, fragile skin, bruising
11. Growth retardation in children
12. Gastrointestinal (GI) irritation, peptic ulcer, pancreatitis
13. Seizures, psychosis

C. Contraindications and cautions
1. Contraindicated in clients with hypersensitivity, psychosis, and fungal infections
2. Should be used with caution in clients with **diabetes mellitus**
3. Used with extreme caution in clients with infections because they mask the signs and symptoms of an infection
4. Increase the potency of medications taken concurrently, such as aspirin, and nonsteroidal anti-inflammatory drugs, thus increasing the risk of gastrointestinal bleeding and ulceration.
5. Use of potassium-wasting diuretics increases potassium loss, resulting in hypokalemia.
6. Dexamethasone decreases the effects of orally administered anticoagulants and antidiabetic agents.
7. Barbiturates, phenytoin (Dilantin), and rifampin (Rifadin) decrease the effect of prednisone.

D. Interventions
1. Monitor vital signs.
2. Monitor serum electrolyte and blood glucose levels.
3. Monitor for hypokalemia and **hyperglycemia.**
4. Monitor intake and output and weight and for edema.
5. Monitor for hypertension.
6. Assess medical history for glaucoma, cataracts, peptic ulcer, mental health disorders, or **diabetes mellitus.**
7. Monitor the older client for signs and symptoms of increased osteoporosis.
8. Assess for changes in muscle strength.
9. Prepare a schedule for the client with information on short-term tapered doses.
10. Instruct the client that it is best to take medication in the early morning.
11. Advise the client to eat foods high in potassium.
12. Instruct the client to avoid individuals with respiratory infections.
13. Advise the client to inform all health care providers of the medication regimen.

14. Instruct the client to report signs and symptoms of a medication overdose or **Cushing's syndrome,** including a moon face, puffy eyelids, edema in the feet, increased bruising, dizziness, bleeding, and menstrual irregularities.
15. Note that the client may need additional doses during periods of stress, such as surgery.
16. Instruct the client not to stop the medication abruptly because abrupt withdrawal can result in severe adrenal insufficiency.
17. Advise the client to consult with the physician before receiving vaccinations.
18. Advise the client to wear a Medic-Alert bracelet.

VIII. ANDROGENS (Box 55-8)

A. Description
1. Used to replace deficient hormones or to treat hormone-sensitive disorders
2. Can cause bleeding if the client is taking oral anticoagulants (increase the effect of anticoagulants)
3. Can cause decreased serum glucose concentration, thereby reducing insulin requirements in the client with **diabetes mellitus**
4. Hepatotoxic medications are avoided with the use of androgens because of the risk of additive damage to the liver.
5. Androgens usually are avoided in men with known prostate or breast carcinoma because androgens often stimulate growth of these tumors.

B. Side effects
1. Masculine secondary sexual characteristics (body hair growth, lowered voice, muscle growth)
2. Bladder irritation and urinary tract infections
3. Breast tenderness
4. Gynecomastia
5. Priapism
6. Menstrual irregularities
7. Virilism
8. Sodium and water retention with edema
9. Nausea, vomiting, or diarrhea
10. Acne
11. Changes in libido
12. Hepatotoxicity, jaundice
13. Hypercalcemia

C. Interventions
1. Monitor vital signs.
2. Monitor for edema, weight gain, and skin changes.
3. Assess mental status and neurological function.
4. Assess for signs of liver dysfunction, including right upper quadrant abdominal pain, malaise, fever, jaundice, and pruritus.
5. Assess for the development of secondary sexual characteristics.
6. Instruct the client to take medication with meals or a snack.
7. Instruct the client to notify the physician if priapism develops.
8. Instruct the client to notify the physician if fluid retention occurs.
9. Instruct women to use a nonhormonal contraceptive while on therapy.
10. For women, monitor for menstrual irregularities and decreased breast size.

IX. ESTROGENS AND PROGESTINS

A. Description
1. Estrogens are steroids that stimulate female reproductive tissue.
2. Progestins are steroids that specifically stimulate the uterine lining.
3. Estrogen and progestin preparations may be used to stimulate the endogenous hormones to restore hormonal balance or to treat hormone-sensitive tumors (suppress tumor growth) or for contraception (Boxes 55-9 and 55-10).

B. Contraindications and cautions
1. Estrogens
   a. Estrogens are contraindicated in clients with breast cancer, endometrial hyperplasia,

Box 55-9 Estrogens

Esterified estrogens (Menest)
Estradiol (Estrace, Femtrace)
Estrogens, conjugated (Premarin, Cenestin, Enjuvia)
Ethinyl estradiol (Estinyl)

Box 55-10 Progestins

Estradiol/drospirenone (Angeliq)
Estradiol/norgestimate (Prefest)
Estradiol/norethindrone (Femhrt)
Medroxyprogesterone acetate (Depo-Provera, Provera)
Medroxyprogesterone and conjugated estrogens (Premphase, Prempro)
Megestrol acetate (Megace)
Norethindrone acetate (Aygestin)
Norgestrel (Ovrette)
Progesterone (Prometrium)

Box 55-8 Androgens

Fluoxymesterone
Methyltestosterone (Testred)
    Testosterone preparations
    Testosterone, pellets (Testopel)
    Testosterone, transdermal (Androderm)
    Testosterone cypionate (Depo-Testosterone)
    Testosterone enanthate (Delatestryl)
    Testerone (Striant)

endometrial cancer, history of thromboembolism, known or suspected pregnancy, or lactation.
  b. Use estrogens with caution in clients with hypertension, gallbladder disease, or liver or kidney dysfunction.
  c. Estrogens increase the risk of toxicity when used with hepatotoxic medications.
  d. Barbiturates, phenytoin (Dilantin), and rifampin (Rifadin) decrease the effectiveness of estrogen.
  2. Progestins are contraindicated in clients with thromboembolic disorders and should be avoided in clients with breast tumors or hepatic disease.
C. Side effects
  1. Breast tenderness, menstrual changes
  2. Nausea, vomiting, and diarrhea
  3. Malaise, depression, excessive irritability
  4. Weight gain
  5. Edema and fluid retention
  6. Atherosclerosis
  7. Hypertension, stroke, myocardial infarction
  8. Thromboembolism (estrogen)
  9. Migraine headaches and vomiting (estrogen)
D. Interventions
  1. Monitor vital signs.
  2. Monitor for hypertension.
  3. Assess for edema and weight gain.
  4. Advise the client not to smoke.
  5. Advise the client to undergo routine breast and pelvic examinations.

X. CONTRACEPTIVES

A. Description
  1. These medications contain a combination of estrogen and a progestin or a progestin alone.
  2. Estrogen-progestin combinations suppress ovulation and change the cervical mucus, making it difficult for sperm to enter.
  3. Medications that contain only progestins are less effective than the combined medications.
  4. Contraceptives usually are taken for 21 consecutive days and stopped for 7 days; the administration cycle is then repeated.
  5. Contraceptives provide reversible prevention of pregnancy.
  6. Contraceptives are useful in controlling irregular or excessive menstrual cycles.
  7. Risk factors associated with the development of complications related to the use of contraceptives include smoking, obesity, and hypertension.
  8. Contraceptives are contraindicated in women with hypertension, thromboembolic disease, cerebrovascular or coronary artery disease, estrogen-dependent cancers, and pregnancy.
  9. Contraceptives should be avoided with the use of hepatotoxic medications.

  10. Contraceptives interfere with the activity of bromocriptine mesylate (Parlodel) and anticoagulants and increase the toxicity of tricyclic antidepressants.
  11. Contraceptives may alter blood glucose levels.
  12. Antibiotics may decrease the absorption and effectiveness of oral contraceptives.
B. Side effects
  1. Breakthrough bleeding
  2. Excessive cervical mucus formation
  3. Breast tenderness
  4. Hypertension
  5. Nausea, vomiting
C. Interventions
  1. Monitor vital signs and weight.
  2. Instruct the client in the administration of the medication (it may take up to 1 week for full contraceptive effect to occur when the medication is begun).
  3. Instruct the client with **diabetes mellitus** to monitor blood glucose levels carefully.
  4. Instruct the client to report signs of thromboembolic complications.
  5. Instruct the client to notify the physician if vaginal bleeding or menstrual irregularities occur or if pregnancy is suspected.
  6. Advise the client to use an alternate method of birth control when taking antibiotics because these may decrease absorption of the oral contraceptive.
  7. Instruct the client to perform breast self-examination monthly and about the importance of annual physical examinations.
  8. Contraceptive patches
    a. Designed to be worn for 3 weeks and removed for a 1-week period
    b. Applied on clean, dry, intact skin on the buttocks, abdomen, upper outer arm, or upper torso
    c. Instruct the client to peel away half of backing on patch, apply the sticky surface to the skin, remove the other half of the backing, and then press down on the patch with the palm for 10 seconds.
    d. Instruct the client to change the patch weekly, using a new location for each patch.
    e. If the patch falls off and remains off for less than 24 hours (such as when the client is sleeping or is unaware that it has fallen off), it can be reapplied if still sticky, or it can be replaced with a new patch.
    f. If the patch is off for more than 24 hours, a new 4-week cycle must be started immediately.
  9. Vaginal ring
    a. Inserted into the vagina by the client, left in place for 3 weeks, and removed for 1 week
    b. The medication is absorbed through mucous membranes of the vagina.
    c. Removed rings should be wrapped in a foil pouch and discarded, not flushed down the toilet.

Box 55-11 Fertility Medications

Chorionic gonadotropin (Profasi)
Clomiphene citrate (Clomid)
Follitropin alfa (Gonal-f)
Follitropin beta (Follistim AQ)
Menotropins (Pergonal, Repronex, Menopur)
Urotropin alfa (Bravelle, Fertinex, Metrodin)
Lutropin alfa (Luveris)

10. Implants and depot injections provide long-acting forms of birth control, from 3 months to 5 years in duration.

⚠ If the client decides to discontinue the contraceptive to become pregnant, recommend that the client use an alternative form of birth control for 2 months after discontinuation to ensure more complete excretion of hormonal agents before conception.

XI. FERTILITY MEDICATIONS (Box 55-11)

A. Description
1. Fertility medications act to stimulate follicle development and ovulation in functioning ovaries and are combined with human chorionic gonadotropin to maintain the follicles once ovulation has occurred.
2. Fertility medications are contraindicated in the presence of primary ovarian dysfunction, thyroid or adrenal dysfunction, ovarian cysts, pregnancy, or idiopathic uterine bleeding.
3. Fertility medications should be used with caution in clients with thromboembolic or respiratory disease.

B. Side effects
1. Risk of multiple births and birth defects
2. Ovarian overstimulation (abdominal pain, distention, ascites, pleural effusion)
3. Headache, irritability
4. Fluid retention and bloating
5. Nausea, vomiting
6. Uterine bleeding
7. Ovarian enlargement
8. Gynecomastia
9. Rash
10. Orthostatic hypotension
11. Febrile reactions

C. Interventions
1. Instruct the client regarding administration of the medication.
2. Provide a calendar of treatment days and instructions on when intercourse should occur to increase therapeutic effectiveness of the medication.
3. Provide information about the risks and hazards of multiple births.

4. Instruct the client to notify the physician if signs of ovarian overstimulation occur.
5. Inform the client about the need for regular follow-up for evaluation.

XII. MEDICATIONS FOR ERECTILE DYSFUNCTION

A. Description
1. Alprostadil (Caverject, Edex) is a prostaglandin that relaxes smooth muscle and promotes blood flow when injected directly into the corpus cavernosum.
2. Sildenafil (Viagra), tadalafil (Cialis), and vardenafil (Levitra) cause smooth muscle relaxation and allow blood flow into the corpus cavernosum.
3. Erectile dysfunction medications are contraindicated in the presence of any anatomical obstruction or condition that might predispose to priapism and in clients with penile implants.
4. Caution should be used in clients with bleeding disorders.
5. Sildenafil, tadalafil, and vardenafil are used cautiously in clients with coronary artery disease, active peptic ulcer disease, bleeding disorders, or retinitis pigmentosa.
6. Sildenafil, tadalafil, and vardenafil cannot be administered to clients taking nitrates, nitroprusside, or β-blockers.

B. Side effects
1. Alprostadil: Pain at the injection site, infection, priapism, penile fibrosis, rash
2. Sildenafil, tadalafil, and vardenafil: Headache, flushing, dyspepsia, urinary tract infection, diarrhea, hypotension, dizziness, rash, neuralgia, insomnia
3. Blurred vision and changes in color vision

C. Interventions
1. Perform a thorough assessment of health and medication history.
2. Instruct the client regarding administration of the medication; alprostadil is injected intracavernously; sildenafil, tadalafil, and vardenafil are taken orally.
3. Inform the client of side effects necessitating the need to notify the physician.

XIII. MEDICATIONS FOR DIABETES MELLITUS

A. Insulin and oral hypoglycemic medications
1. Description
   a. Insulin increases glucose transport into cells and promotes conversion of glucose to glycogen, decreasing serum glucose levels.
   b. Oral hypoglycemic agents stimulate the pancreas to produce more insulin, increase the sensitivity of peripheral receptors to insulin, decrease hepatic glucose output, or delay intestinal absorption of glucose, thus decreasing serum glucose levels.

2. Contraindications and concerns
   a. Insulin is contraindicated in clients with hypersensitivity.
   b. Oral hypoglycemic agents are contraindicated in type 1 **diabetes mellitus**.
   c. β-Adrenergic blocking agents may mask signs and symptoms of **hypoglycemia** associated with hypoglycemic medications.
   d. Anticoagulants, chloramphenicol (Chloromycetin), salicylates, propranolol (Inderal), monoamine oxidase inhibitors, pentamidine (Pentam 300), and sulfonamides may cause **hypoglycemia**.
   e. Corticosteroids, sympathomimetics, thiazide diuretics, phenytoin (Dilantin), thyroid preparations, oral contraceptives, and estrogen compounds may cause **hyperglycemia**.
   f. Side effects of the sulfonylureas include gastrointestinal symptoms and dermatological reactions; **hypoglycemia** can occur when an excessive dose is administered or when meals are omitted or delayed, food intake is decreased, or activity is increased.

⚠ Sulfonylureas can cause a disulfiram (Antabuse) type of reaction when alcohol is ingested.

B. Oral hypoglycemic medications
   1. Prescribed for clients with type 2 **diabetes mellitus**
   2. Sulfonylureas (Box 55-12)
      a. Sulfonylureas may be classified as first- or second-generation sulfonylureas.
      b. Sulfonylureas stimulate the beta cells to produce more insulin.
   3. Biguanides (see Box 55-12)
      a. May be used alone or in combination with a sulfonylurea
      b. Suppresses hepatic production of glucose and increases insulin sensitivity
      c. Side effects: Diarrhea (most common), lactic acidosis (most serious)
   4. Alpha-glucosidase inhibitors (see Box 55-12)
      a. Delay absorption of ingested carbohydrates (sucrose and complex carbohydrates), resulting in smaller increase in blood glucose level after meals.
      b. Do not increase insulin production
      c. Can be given alone or in combination with sulfonylureas
      d. Will not cause **hypoglycemia** when given alone
      e. Given with first bite of meal
   5. Thiazolidinediones (see Box 55-12)
      a. Insulin-sensitizing agents that lower blood glucose by decreasing hepatic glucose production and improving target cell response to insulin
      b. May cause liver toxicity

Box 55-12 Sulfonylureas and Nonsulfonylureas

Sulfonylureas
Acetohexamide (Dymelor)
Chlorpropamide (Diabinese)
Glimepiride (Amaryl)
Glipizide (Glucotrol)
Glyburide (DiaBeta, Micronase)
Tolazamide (Tolinase)
Tolbutamide (Orinase)

Biguanide
Metformin (Glucophage)

Alpha-Glucosidase Inhibitors
Acarbose (Precose)
Miglitol (Glyset)

Thiazolidinediones
Pioglitazone (Actos)
Rosiglitazone (Avandia)

Meglitinides
Nateglinide (Starlix)
Repaglinide (Prandin)

Gliptins
Sitagliptin (Januvia)

---

6. Meglitinides (see Box 55-12)
   a. Stimulate pancreatic insulin secretion
   b. Quicker and shorter duration of action; therefore, less chance of **hypoglycemia** because blood glucose–lowering effect wears off quickly
   c. Very fast onset of action allows client to take the medication with meals and skip a dose when a meal is skipped
7. Interventions
   a. Assess the client's knowledge of **diabetes mellitus** and the use of oral antidiabetic agents.
   b. Obtain a medication history regarding the medications that the client is taking currently.
   c. Assess vital signs and blood glucose levels.
   d. Instruct the client to recognize the signs and symptoms of **hypoglycemia** and **hyperglycemia**.
   e. Instruct the client to avoid over-the-counter medications unless prescribed by the health care provider.
   f. Instruct the client not to ingest alcohol with sulfonylureas.
   g. Inform the client that insulin may be needed during stress, surgery, or infection.
   h. Instruct the client in the necessity of compliance with prescribed medication.
   i. Instruct the client on how to take each specific medication, such as with the first bite of the meal for meglitinides and alpha-glucosidase inhibitors.
   j. Advise the client to wear a Medic-Alert bracelet.

C. Insulin
1. Insulin primarily acts in the liver, muscle, and adipose tissue by attaching to receptors on cellular membranes and facilitating the passage of glucose, potassium, and magnesium.
2. Insulin is prescribed for clients with type 1 **diabetes mellitus** and type 2 **diabetes mellitus** in clients whose blood glucose level is not controlled with oral hypoglycemic agents.
3. The onset, peak, and duration of action depend on the insulin type (Table 55-1).
4. Storing of insulin (Box 55-13)
5. Insulin injection sites
   a. The main areas for injections are the abdomen, arms (posterior surface), thighs (anterior surface), and hips (Fig. 55-1).
   b. Insulin injected into the abdomen may absorb more evenly and rapidly than at other sites.
   c. Systematic rotation within one anatomical area is recommended to prevent lipodystrophy; client should be instructed not to use the same site more than once in a 2- to 3-week period.
   d. Injections should be 1½ inches apart within the anatomical area.
   e. Heat, massage, and exercise of the injected area can increase absorption rates and may result in **hypoglycemia.**

Box 55-13 Storing Insulin

Avoid exposing insulin to extremes in temperature.
Insulin should not be frozen or kept in direct sunlight or a hot car.
Before injection, insulin should be at room temperature.
If a vial of insulin will be used up in 1 month, it may be kept at room temperature; otherwise, the vial should be refrigerated.

TABLE 55-1 Time Activity of Pharmacological Insulin*

Preparation	Brand	Onset (hr)	Peak (hr)	Duration (hr)
RAPID-ACTING INSULIN				
Insulin aspart	NovoLog	0.25	1-3	3-5
Insulin glulisine	Apidra	0.3	0.5-1.5	3-4
Human lispro injection	Humalog	0.25	0.5-1.5	5
SHORT-ACTING INSULIN				
Regular human insulin injection	Humulin R	0.5	2-4	5-7
	Novolin R	0.5	2.5-5	8
	ReliOn R			
Humulin R (concentrated U-500)	Humulin R (U 500)	1.5	4-12	24
INTERMEDIATE-ACTING INSULIN				
Isophane insulin NPH injection	Humulin N	1.5	4-12	16-24+
	Novolin N	1.5	4-12	16-24+
	ReliOn N			
Insulin detemir injection	Levemir	1	6-8	5.7-24
70% human insulin isophane suspension/30% human insulin injection	Humulin 70/30	0.5	2-12	24
	Novolin 70/30			
	ReliOn 70/30			
50% human insulin isophane suspension/50% human insulin injection	Humulin 50/50	0.5	3-5	24
70% insulin aspart protamine suspension/30% insulin aspart injection	NovoLog Mix 70/30	0.25	1-4	24
75% insulin lispro protamine suspension/25% insulin lispro injection	Humalog Mix 75/25	0.25	1-2	24
LONG-ACTING INSULIN				
Insulin glargine injection	Lantus	2-4	None	24

*Time acivity may be dose related.
From Ignatavicius, D., & Workman, M. (2010). *Medical surgical nursing: Patient centered collaborative care* (6th ed., p. 1485). St. Louis: Saunders.

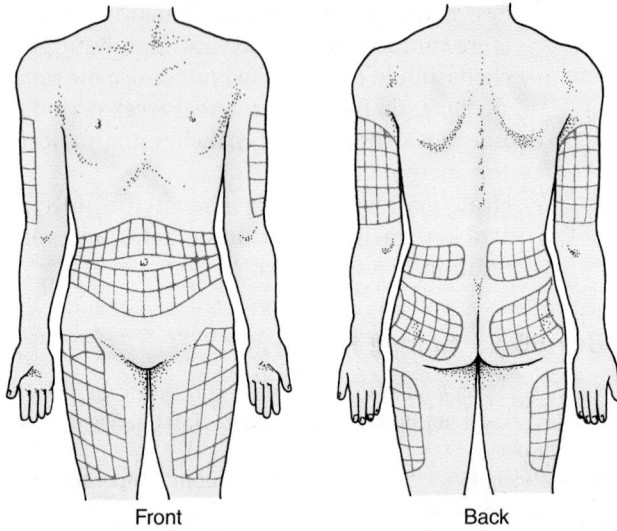

▲ **FIGURE 55-1** Common insulin injection sites. (From Ignatavicius, D., & Workman, M. [2010]. *Medical surgical nursing: Patient-centered collaborative care* [6th ed.]. St. Louis: Saunders.)

1 Wash hands.
2 Gently rotate NPH insulin bottle.
3 Wipe off tops of insulin vials with alcohol sponge.
4 Draw back amount of air into the syringe that equals total dose.

5 Inject air equal to NPH dose into NPH vial. Remove syringe from vial.

6 Inject air equal to regular dose into regular vial.

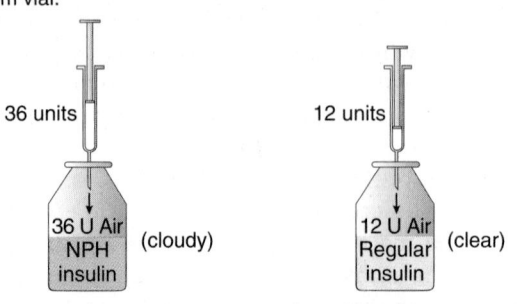

7 Invert regular insulin bottle and withdraw regular insulin dose.

8 Without adding more air to NPH vial, carefully withdraw NPH dose.

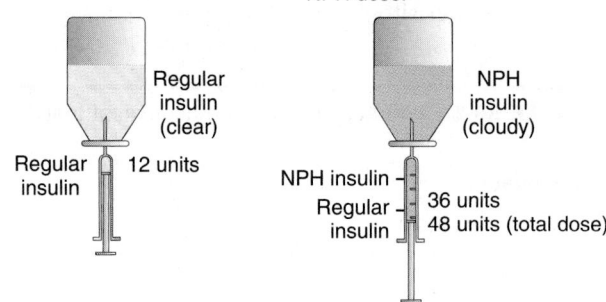

▲ **FIGURE 55-2** Steps for mixing insulins. (From Lewis, S., Heitkemper, M., Dirksen, S., O'Brien, P., & Bucher, L. [2007]. *Medical-surgical nursing: Assessment and management of clinical problems* [7th ed.]. St. Louis: Mosby.)

    f. Injection into scar tissue may delay absorption of insulin.

6. Administering insulin

⚠ Insulin glargine *cannot* be mixed with any other types of insulin.

    a. To prevent dosage errors, be certain that there is a match between the insulin concentration noted on the vial and the calibration of units on the insulin syringe; the usual concentration of insulin is U 100 (100 units/mL).

    b. Most insulin syringes have a 27- to 29-gauge needle that is about ½-inch long.

    c. Before use, swirl insulin vial gently or rotate between palms to ensure that the insulin and ingredients are mixed well; otherwise, an inaccurate dose will be drawn; vigorously shaking the bottle will cause bubbles to form.

    d. Premixed insulins (NPH and regular insulin) are available as 70/30 (most commonly used) and 50/50 (premixed insulin lispro protamine and insulin lispro 75/25 are also available).

    e. Inject air into the insulin bottle (a vacuum makes it difficult to draw up the insulin).

    f. When mixing insulins, draw up the regular (shorter acting) insulin first (Fig. 55-2).

    g. Regular insulin may be mixed with NPH or Lente insulin.

    h. Lispro insulin may be mixed with Humulin N or Humulin-U (Ultralente)

    i. Insulin aspart protamine may be mixed with NPH insulin only.

    j. Insulin zinc suspensions may be mixed only with each other and regular insulin, not with other types of insulin.

    k. Administer a mixed dose of insulin within 5 to 15 minutes of preparation; after this time, the regular insulin binds with the NPH insulin and its action is reduced.

    l. Aspiration generally is not recommended with self-injection of insulin.

    m. Administer insulin at a 45- to 90-degree angle in clients with normal subcutaneous mass and at a 45- to 60-degree angle in thin persons or those with a decreased amount of subcutaneous mass.

⚠ Regular insulin is the only type of insulin that can be administered intravenously.

D. Exenatide (Byetta)

    1. A synthetic hormone classified as an incretin mimetic that is administered subcutaneously.

    2. Used for clients with type 2 **diabetes mellitus** (not recommended for clients taking insulin nor should clients be taken off of insulin and given exenatide)

    3. Restores first-phase insulin response (first 10 minutes after food ingestion), lowers the production of glucagon after meals, slows gastric emptying (which limits the rise in the blood glucose level after a meal), reduces fasting and postprandial blood glucose levels, and reduces caloric intake, resulting in weight loss

4. Packaged in premeasured doses (pen) that require refrigeration (cannot be frozen)
5. Administered as a subcutaneous injection in the thigh, abdomen, or upper arm within 60 minutes before morning and evening meals; not taken after meals; if a dose is missed, the treatment regimen is resumed as prescribed with the next scheduled dose.
6. Can cause mild to moderate nausea that abates with use.

E. Pramlintide (Symlin)
1. Synthetic form of amylin, a naturally occurring hormone secreted by the pancreas
2. Used for clients with types 1 and 2 **diabetes mellitus** who use insulin; given before meals to lower blood glucose level after meals, leading to less fluctuation during the day and better long-term glucose control
3. Associated with an increased risk of insulin-induced severe **hypoglycemia**, particularly in clients with type 1 **diabetes mellitus**
4. Gastrointestinal side effects including nausea can occur.
5. Unopened vials are refrigerated; opened vials can be refrigerated or kept at room temperature for up to 28 days.

F. Glucagon
1. Hormone secreted by the alpha cells of the islets of Langerhans in the pancreas
2. Increases blood glucose level by stimulating glycogenolysis in the liver
3. Can be administered subcutaneously, intramuscularly, or intravenously
4. Used to treat insulin-induced **hypoglycemia** when the client is semiconscious or unconscious and is unable to ingest liquids
5. The blood glucose level begins to increase within 5 to 20 minutes after administration.
6. Instruct the family in the procedure for administration.
7. See Chapter 54 for additional information regarding interventions for severe **hypoglycemia.**

🔘 **MORE QUESTIONS ON THE CD!**

Practice Questions

597. A nurse is teaching a client how to mix regular insulin and NPH insulin in the same syringe. Which of the following actions, if performed by the client, indicates the need for further teaching?

1. Withdraws the NPH insulin first
2. Withdraws the regular insulin first
3. Injects air into NPH insulin vial first
4. Injects an amount of air equal to the desired dose of insulin into the vial

598. A home care nurse visits a client recently diagnosed with diabetes mellitus who is taking Humulin NPH insulin daily. The client asks the nurse how to store the unopened vials of insulin. The nurse tells the client to:
1. Freeze the insulin.
2. Refrigerate the insulin.
3. Store the insulin in a dark, dry place.
4. Keep the insulin at room temperature.

599. Glimepiride (Amaryl) is prescribed for a client with diabetes mellitus. A nurse instructs the client to avoid which of the following while taking this medication?
1. Alcohol
2. Organ meats
3. Whole-grain cereals
4. Carbonated beverages

600. Sildenafil (Viagra) is prescribed to treat a client with erectile dysfunction. A nurse reviews the client's medical record and would question the prescription if which of the following is noted in the client's history?
1. Neuralgia
2. Insomnia
3. Use of nitroglycerin
4. Use of multivitamins

601. The health care provider prescribes exenatide (Byetta) for a client with type 1 diabetes mellitus who takes insulin. The nurse plans to take which appropriate intervention?
1. Administer the medication within 60 minutes before the morning and evening meal.
2. Hold the medication and call the health care provider, questioning the prescription for the client.
3. Monitor the client for gastrointestinal side effects after administering the medication.
4. Withdraw the insulin from the prefilled pen into an insulin syringe to prepare for administration.

602. A client is taking Humulin NPH insulin daily every morning. The nurse instructs the client that the most likely time for a hypoglycemic reaction to occur is:
1. 2 to 4 hours after administration
2. 4 to 12 hours after administration
3. 16 to 18 hours after administration
4. 18 to 24 hours after administration

603. A client with diabetes mellitus visits a health care clinic. The client's diabetes mellitus previously had been well controlled with glyburide (DiaBeta) daily, but recently the fasting blood glucose level has been 180 to 200 mg/dL. Which medication, if added to the client's regimen, may have contributed to the hyperglycemia?
1. Prednisone
2. Phenelzine (Nardil)
3. Atenolol (Tenormin)
4. Allopurinol (Zyloprim)

604. A community health nurse visits a client at home. Prednisone 10 mg orally daily, has been prescribed for the client and the nurse teaches the client about the medication. Which statement, if made by the client, indicates that further teaching is necessary?
1. "I can take aspirin or my antihistamine if I need it."
2. "I need to take the medication every day at the same time."
3. "I need to avoid coffee, tea, cola, and chocolate in my diet."
4. "If I gain more than 5 pounds a week, I will call my doctor."

605. Desmopressin acetate (DDAVP) is prescribed for the treatment of diabetes insipidus. The nurse administering the medication monitors the client for which therapeutic response?
1. Decreased urinary output
2. Decreased blood pressure
3. Decreased peripheral edema
4. Decreased blood glucose level

606. A nurse is monitoring a client receiving desmopressin acetate (DDAVP) for adverse effects to the medication. Which of the following indicates the presence of an adverse effect?
1. Insomnia
2. Drowsiness
3. Weight loss
4. Increased urination

607. A nurse provides instructions to a client who is taking levothyroxine (Synthroid). The nurse tells the client to take the medication:
1. With food
2. At lunchtime
3. On an empty stomach
4. At bedtime with a snack

608. A nurse provides medication instructions to a client who is taking levothyroxine (Synthroid). The nurse instructs the client to notify the physician if which of the following occurs?

1. Fatigue
2. Tremors
3. Cold intolerance
4. Excessively dry skin

609. A nurse performs an admission assessment on a client who visits a health care clinic for the first time. The client tells the nurse that propylthiouracil (PTU) is taken daily. The nurse continues to collect data from the client, suspecting that the client has a history of:
1. Myxedema
2. Graves' disease
3. Addison's disease
4. Cushing's syndrome

610. A nurse is instructing a client regarding intranasal desmopressin (DDAVP). The nurse tells the client that which of the following is a side effect of the medication?
1. Headache
2. Vulval pain
3. Runny nose
4. Flushed skin

611. A daily dose of prednisone is prescribed for a client. A nurse provides instructions to the client regarding administration of the medication and instructs the client that the best time to take this medication is:
1. At noon
2. At bedtime
3. Early morning
4. Any time, at the same time, each day

612. Prednisone is prescribed for a client with diabetes mellitus who is taking Humulin NPH insulin daily. Which of the following prescription changes does the nurse anticipate during therapy with the prednisone?
1. An additional dose of prednisone daily
2. A decreased amount of daily Humulin NPH insulin
3. An increased amount of daily Humulin NPH insulin
4. The addition of an oral hypoglycemic medication daily

Alternate Item Format: Multiple Response

613. The home health care nurse is visiting a client who was recently diagnosed with type 2 diabetes mellitus. The client is prescribed repaglinide (Prandin) and metformin (Glucophage) and asks the nurse to explain these medications. The nurse should provide which instructions to the client? **Select all that apply.**

☐ 1. Diarrhea may occur secondary to the metformin.
☐ 2. The repaglinide is not taken if a meal is skipped.
☐ 3. The repaglinide is taken 30 minutes before eating.
☐ 4. Candy or another simple sugar is carried and used to treat mild hypoglycemia episodes.

☐ 5. Metformin increases hepatic glucose production to prevent hypoglycemia associated with repaglinide.
☐ 6. Muscle pain is an expected side effect of metformin and may be treated with acetaminophen (Tylenol).

ANSWERS

597. 1
Rationale: When preparing a mixture of regular insulin with another insulin preparation, the regular insulin is drawn into the syringe first. This sequence will avoid contaminating the vial of regular insulin with insulin of another type. Options 2, 3, and 4 identify the correct actions for preparing NPH and regular insulin.
Test-Taking Strategy: Use the process of elimination, noting the strategic words *need for further teaching*. These words indicate a negative event query and ask you to select an option that is an incorrect action. Remember *RN*—draw up the *Reg*ular insulin before the *N*PH insulin. Review the procedure for preparing NPH and regular insulin if you had difficulty with this question.
Level of Cognitive Ability: Evaluating
Client Needs: Physiological Integrity
Integrated Process: Teaching and Learning
Content Area: Pharmacology
Reference: Kee, J., Hayes, E., & McCuistion, L. (2009). *Pharmacology: A nursing process approach* (6th ed., p. 797). St. Louis: Saunders.

598. 2
Rationale: Insulin in unopened vials should be stored under refrigeration until needed. Vials should not be frozen. When stored unopened under refrigeration, insulin can be used up to the expiration date on the vial. Options 1, 3, and 4 are incorrect.
Test-Taking Strategy: Use the process of elimination and note the strategic words *store the unopened vials*. Remembering that insulin should not be frozen will assist in eliminating option 1. Options 3 and 4 are comparable or alike and should be eliminated. Review client teaching points related to insulin if you had difficulty with this question.
Level of Cognitive Ability: Applying
Client Needs: Physiological Integrity
Integrated Process: Teaching and Learning
Content Area: Pharmacology
Reference: Kee, J., Hayes, E., & McCuistion, L. (2009). *Pharmacology: A nursing process approach* (6th ed., p. 793). St. Louis: Saunders.

599. 1
Rationale: When alcohol is combined with glimepiride (Amaryl), a disulfiram-like reaction may occur. This syndrome includes flushing, palpitations, and nausea. Alcohol can also potentiate the hypoglycemic effects of the medication. Clients need to be instructed to avoid alcohol consumption while taking this medication. The items in options 2, 3, and 4 do not need to be avoided.

Test-Taking Strategy: Use the process of elimination. Eliminate options 2, 3, and 4 because these food items are allowed in a diabetic diet. Remembering that alcohol can affect the action of many medications will assist in directing you to option 1. Review this medication if you had difficulty with this question.
Level of Cognitive Ability: Applying
Client Needs: Physiological Integrity
Integrated Process: Teaching and Learning
Content Area: Pharmacology
References: Kee, J., Hayes, E., & McCuistion, L. (2009). *Pharmacology: A nursing process approach* (6th ed., p. 802). St. Louis: Saunders.
 Lehne, R. (2010). *Pharmacology for nursing care* (7th ed., p. 687). St. Louis: Saunders.

600. 3
Rationale: Sildenafil (Viagra) enhances the vasodilating effect of nitric oxide in the corpus cavernosum of the penis, thus sustaining an erection. Because of the effect of the medication, it is contraindicated with concurrent use of organic nitrates and nitroglycerin. Sildenafil is not contraindicated with the use of vitamins. Neuralgia and insomnia are side effects of the medication.
Test-Taking Strategy: Use the process of elimination, noting the strategic words *would question the prescription*. Recalling the action of the medication will direct you to option 3. If you had difficulty with this question, review the contraindications associated with the use of this medication.
Level of Cognitive Ability: Analyzing
Client Needs: Physiological Integrity
Integrated Process: Nursing Process—Analysis
Content Area: Pharmacology
Reference: Hodgson, B., & Kizior, R. (2010). *Saunders nursing drug handbook 2010* (p. 1034). St. Louis: Saunders.

601. 2
Rationale: Exenatide (Byetta) is an incretin mimetic used for type 2 diabetes mellitus only. It is not recommended for clients taking insulin. Hence, the nurse should hold the medication and question the health care provider regarding this prescription. Although options 1 and 3 are correct statements about the medication, in this situation the medication should not be administered. The medication is packaged in prefilled pens ready for injection without the need for drawing it up into another syringe.
Test-Taking Strategy: Use the process of elimination. Eliminate option 4 because the medication is packaged in prefilled pens ready for injection without the need for drawing it up into another syringe. From the remaining options, focus on the data in the question. Although options 1 and 3 are appropriate when administering this medication, this client should not receive the medication. Review this medication if you had difficulty with this question.

Level of Cognitive Ability: Applying
Client Needs: Physiological Integrity
Integrated Process: Nursing Process—Planning
Content Area: Pharmacology
References: The Diabetes Monitor. (2007). *Exenatide (Byetta)*. Available at http://www.diabetesmonitor.com/byetta.htm. Retrieved February 2, 2010.

Lehne, R. (2010). *Pharmacology for nursing care* (7th ed., p. 680). St. Louis: Saunders.

602. 2
Rationale: Humulin NPH is an intermediate-acting insulin. The onset of action is 1.5 hours, it peaks in 4 to 12 hours, and its duration of action is 24 hours. Hypoglycemic reactions most likely occur during peak time.
Test-Taking Strategy: Use the process of elimination and knowledge regarding the onset, peak, and duration of action for NPH insulin. Remember that NPH peaks in 4 to 12 hours. If you had difficulty with this question, review the characteristics of NPH insulin.
Level of Cognitive Ability: Applying
Client Needs: Physiological Integrity
Integrated Process: Teaching and Learning
Content Area: Adult Health—Endocrine
References: Edmunds, M. (2010). *Introduction to clinical pharmacology* (6th ed., p. 335). St. Louis: Mosby.

Kee, J., Hayes, E., & McCuistion, L. (2009). *Pharmacology: A nursing process approach* (6th ed., p. 795). St. Louis: Saunders.

603. 1
Rationale: Prednisone may decrease the effect of oral hypoglycemics, insulin, diuretics, and potassium supplements. Option 2, a monoamine oxidase inhibitor, and option 3, a β-blocker, have their own intrinsic hypoglycemic activity. Option 4 decreases urinary excretion of sulfonylurea agents, causing increased levels of the oral agents, which can lead to hypoglycemia.
Test-Taking Strategy: Use the process of elimination and focus on the subject, an increase in the blood glucose level. Recalling that prednisone decreases the effects of oral hypoglycemics will direct you to the correct option. Review medication interactions with hypoglycemics if you had difficulty with this question.
Level of Cognitive Ability: Analyzing
Client Needs: Physiological Integrity
Integrated Process: Nursing Process—Analysis
Content Area: Adult Health—Endocrine
Reference: Lehne, R. (2010). *Pharmacology for nursing care* (7th ed., p. 855). St. Louis: Saunders.

604. 1
Rationale: Aspirin and other over-the-counter medications should not be taken unless the client consults with the physician. The client needs to take the medication at the same time every day and should be instructed not to stop the medication. A slight weight gain as a result of an improved appetite is expected, but after the dosage is stabilized, a weight gain of 5 pounds or more weekly should be reported to the physician. Caffeine-containing foods and fluids need to be avoided because they may contribute to steroid-ulcer development.
Test-Taking Strategy: Use the process of elimination, noting the strategic words *further teaching is necessary*. These words indicate a negative event query and ask you to select an

option that is an incorrect statement. Remember that a client should not take other medications, especially over-the-counter medications, without first consulting with his or her physician. Review teaching points for the client taking prednisone if you had difficulty with this question.
Level of Cognitive Ability: Evaluating
Client Needs: Physiological Integrity
Integrated Process: Teaching and Learning
Content Area: Adult Health—Endocrine
Reference: Lehne, R. (2010). *Pharmacology for nursing care* (7th ed., p. 855). St. Louis: Saunders.

605. 1
Rationale: Desmopressin promotes renal conservation of water. The hormone carries out this action by acting on the collecting ducts of the kidney to increase their permeability to water, which results in increased water reabsorption. The therapeutic effect of this medication would be manifested by a decreased urine output. Options 2, 3, and 4 are unrelated to the effects of this medication.
Test-Taking Strategy: Use the process of elimination. Focus on the diagnosis in the question to assist in answering the question. Recalling the manifestations related to the loss of large volumes of urine in this disorder will help direct you to option 1. Review diabetes insipidus and the action of desmopressin if you had difficulty with this question.
Level of Cognitive Ability: Evaluating
Client Needs: Physiological Integrity
Integrated Process: Nursing Process—Evaluation
Content Area: Pharmacology
References: Hodgson, B., & Kizior, R. (2010). *Saunders nursing drug handbook 2010* (p. 323). St. Louis: Saunders.

Lehne, R. (2010). *Pharmacology for nursing care* (7th ed., p. 709). St. Louis: Saunders.

606. 2
Rationale: Water intoxication (overhydration) or hyponatremia is an adverse reaction to desmopressin. Early signs include drowsiness, listlessness, and headache. Decreased urination, rapid weight gain, confusion, seizures, and coma also may occur in overhydration.
Test-Taking Strategy: Use the process of elimination. Recalling that this medication is used to treat diabetes insipidus will assist you in eliminating options 3 and 4. Also, recalling the action of the medication will assist you in determining that water intoxication is an adverse reaction. This will direct you to option 2. Review the adverse effects related to this medication if you had difficulty with this question.
Level of Cognitive Ability: Analyzing
Client Needs: Physiological Integrity
Integrated Process: Nursing Process—Assessment
Content Area: Pharmacology
Reference: Lehne, R. (2010). *Pharmacology for nursing care* (7th ed., p. 709). St. Louis: Saunders.

607. 3
Rationale: Oral doses of levothyroxine (Synthroid) should be taken on an empty stomach to enhance absorption. Dosing should be done in the morning before breakfast.
Test-Taking Strategy: Use the process of elimination. Note that options 1, 2, and 4 are comparable or alike in that these

options address administering the medication with food. Review client teaching points regarding the administration of levothyroxine if you had difficulty with this question.
Level of Cognitive Ability: Applying
Client Needs: Physiological Integrity
Integrated Process: Teaching and Learning
Content Area: Pharmacology
Reference: Hodgson, B., & Kizior, R. (2010). *Saunders nursing drug handbook 2010* (p. 672). St. Louis: Saunders.

608. 2
Rationale: Excessive doses of levothyroxine (Synthroid) can produce signs and symptoms of hyperthyroidism. These include tachycardia, chest pain, tremors, nervousness, insomnia, hyperthermia, heat intolerance, and sweating. The client should be instructed to notify the physician if these occur. Options 1, 3, and 4 are signs of hypothyroidism.
Test-Taking Strategy: Use the process of elimination, recalling the symptoms associated with hypothyroidism, the purpose of administering levothyroxine, and the effects of the medication. Options 1, 3, and 4 are symptoms related to hypothyroidism. Review the adverse effects of this medication if you are unfamiliar with them.
Level of Cognitive Ability: Applying
Client Needs: Physiological Integrity
Integrated Process: Teaching and Learning
Content Area: Pharmacology
Reference: Hodgson, B., & Kizior, R. (2010). *Saunders nursing drug handbook 2010* (p. 673). St. Louis: Saunders.

609. 2
Rationale: Propylthiouracil (PTU) inhibits thyroid hormone synthesis and is used to treat hyperthyroidism, or Graves' disease. Myxedema indicates hypothyroidism. Cushing's syndrome and Addison's disease are disorders related to adrenal function.
Test-Taking Strategy: Use the process of elimination and knowledge regarding the action of the medication and treatment measures for Graves' disease to answer the question. Remember that propylthiouracil is used to treat Graves' disease. Review this medication and Graves' disease if you had difficulty with this question.
Level of Cognitive Ability: Analyzing
Client Needs: Physiological Integrity
Integrated Process: Nursing Process—Assessment
Content Area: Pharmacology
References: Hodgson, B., & Kizior, R. (2010). *Saunders nursing drug handbook 2010* (p. 957). St. Louis: Saunders.
Lehne, R. (2010). *Pharmacology for nursing care* (7th ed., p. 699). St. Louis: Saunders.

610. 3
Rationale: Desmopressin administered by the intranasal route can cause a runny or stuffy nose. Options 1, 2, and 4 are side effects if the medication is administered by the intravenous route.
Test-Taking Strategy: Note the relationship between the words *intranasal* in the question and *runny nose* in option 3. Review this medication if you are unfamiliar with it.
Level of Cognitive Ability: Applying
Client Needs: Physiological Integrity
Integrated Process: Teaching and Learning
Content Area: Pharmacology
Reference: Hodgson, B., & Kizior, R. (2010). *Saunders nursing drug handbook 2010* (p. 323). St. Louis: Saunders.

611. 3
Rationale: Corticosteroids (glucocorticoids) should be administered before 9 AM. Administration at this time helps minimize adrenal insufficiency and mimics the burst of glucocorticoids released naturally by the adrenal glands each morning. Options 1, 2, and 4 are incorrect.
Test-Taking Strategy: Use the process of elimination. Note the suffix -*sone* and recall that medication names that end with these letters are corticosteroids. This will direct you to option 3. If you had difficulty with this question, review the administration of glucocorticoids.
Level of Cognitive Ability: Applying
Client Needs: Physiological Integrity
Integrated Process: Teaching and Learning
Content Area: Pharmacology
Reference: Hodgson, B., & Kizior, R. (2010). *Saunders nursing drug handbook 2010* (p. 934). St. Louis: Saunders.

612. 3
Rationale: Glucocorticoids can elevate blood glucose levels. Clients with diabetes mellitus may need their dosages of insulin or oral hypoglycemic medications increased during glucocorticoid therapy. Therefore, options 1, 2, and 4 are incorrect.
Test-Taking Strategy: Use the process of elimination. Recalling that glucocorticoids can increase blood glucose levels will direct you to option 3. Review the effects of glucocorticoids if you had difficulty with this question.
Level of Cognitive Ability: Analyzing
Client Needs: Physiological Integrity
Integrated Process: Nursing Process—Analysis
Content Area: Pharmacology
Reference: Lehne, R. (2010). *Pharmacology for nursing care* (7th ed., p. 855). St. Louis: Saunders.

ALTERNATE ITEM FORMAT: MULTIPLE RESPONSE
613. 1, 2, 3, 4
Rationale: Repaglinide is a rapid-acting oral hypoglycemic agent that stimulates pancreatic insulin secretion that should be taken before meals, and that should be held if the client does not eat. Hypoglycemia is a side effect of repaglinide and the client should always be prepared by carrying a simple sugar with her or him at all times. Metformin is an oral hypoglycemic given in combination with repaglinide and works by decreasing hepatic glucose production. A common side effect of metformin is diarrhea. Muscle pain may occur as an adverse effect from metformin but it might signify a more serious condition that warrants physician notification, not the use of acetaminophen.
Test-Taking Strategy: Focus on the data in the question and the client's diagnosis to assist in answering the question. Also, recalling the actions and effects of these medications will assist in answering correctly. Review these medications if you are not familiar with them.
Level of Cognitive Ability: Applying
Client Needs: Physiological Integrity
Integrated Process: Nursing Process—Implementation
Content Area: Pharmacology
Reference: Lehne, R. (2010). *Pharmacology for nursing care* (7th ed., pp. 674, 676). St. Louis: Saunders.

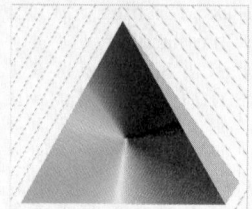

UNIT XI

The Adult Client With a Gastrointestinal Disorder

PYRAMID TERMS

ascites The accumulation of fluid within the peritoneal cavity that results from venous congestion of the hepatic capillaries, which leads to plasma leaking directly from the liver surface and portal vein.

asterixis A coarse tremor characterized by rapid, nonrhythmic extensions and flexions in the wrist and fingers; also termed *liver flap.*

Billroth I Partial gastrectomy with the remaining segment being anastomosed to duodenum; also termed *gastroduodenostomy.*

Billroth II Partial gastrectomy with the remaining segment being anastomosed to the jejunum; also termed *gastrojejunostomy.*

cholecystectomy Removal of the gallbladder.

cholecystitis An inflammation of the gallbladder that may occur as an acute or chronic process. Acute inflammation is associated with gallstones (cholelithiasis). Chronic cholecystitis results when inefficient bile emptying and gallbladder muscle wall disease causes a fibrotic and contracted gallbladder.

choledocholithotomy Incision into the common bile duct to remove a gallstone.

cirrhosis A chronic progressive disease of the liver characterized by diffuse degeneration and destruction of hepatocytes. Repeated destruction of hepatic cells causes the formation of scar tissue.

Crohn's disease An inflammatory disease that can occur anywhere in the gastrointestinal tract but most often affects the terminal ileum; leads to thickening and scarring, narrowed lumen, fistulas, ulcerations, and abscesses. The disease is characterized by remissions and exacerbations.

Cullen's sign Bluish discoloration of the abdomen and periumbilical area seen in acute hemorrhagic pancreatitis.

diverticulitis Inflammation of one or more diverticula from penetration of fecal matter through the thin-walled diverticula, resulting in local abscess formation. A perforated diverticulum can progress to intra-abdominal perforation with generalized peritonitis.

diverticulosis Outpouching or herniations of the intestinal mucosa that can occur in any part of the intestine but is most common in the sigmoid colon.

dumping syndrome Rapid emptying of the gastric contents into the small intestine, which occurs following gastric resection.

esophageal varices Dilated and tortuous veins in the submucosa of the esophagus caused by portal hypertension, often associated with liver cirrhosis; at high risk for rupture if portal circulation pressure rises.

fetor hepaticus The fruity, musty breath odor associated with severe chronic liver disease.

gastrectomy Removal of the stomach with attachment of the esophagus to the jejunum or duodenum; also termed *esophagojejunostomy* or *esophagoduodenostomy.*

gastric resection Removal of the lower half of the stomach, usually including a vagotomy; also termed *antrectomy.*

hepatitis Inflammation of the liver caused by a virus, bacteria, or exposure to medications or hepatotoxins.

hiatal hernia A portion of the stomach that herniates through the diaphragm and into the thorax. Herniation results from weakening of the muscles of the diaphragm and is aggravated by factors that increase abdominal pressure, such as pregnancy, ascites, obesity, tumors, and heavy lifting; also termed *esophageal* or *diaphragmatic hernia.*

Kock ileostomy (continent ileostomy) An intraabdominal pouch constructed from the terminal ileum. The pouch is connected to the stoma with a nipple-like valve constructed from a portion of the ileum. The stoma is flush with the skin.

Murphy's sign A sign of gallbladder disease consisting of pain on taking a deep breath when the examiner's fingers are on the approximate location of the gallbladder.

pancreatitis An acute or chronic inflammation of the pancreas, with associated escape of pancreatic enzymes into surrounding tissue. Acute pancreatitis can occur suddenly as one attack or can be recurrent with resolution. Chronic pancreatitis is a continual inflammation and destruction of the pancreas, with scar tissue replacing pancreatic tissue.

peristalsis Wave-like rhythmic contractions that propel material through the gastrointestinal tract.

portal hypertension A persistent increase in pressure within the portal vein that develops as a result of obstruction to flow.

pyloroplasty Enlarging the pylorus to prevent or decrease pyloric obstruction, thereby enhancing gastric emptying.

Turner's sign A gray-blue discoloration of the flanks seen in acute hemorrhagic pancreatitis.

ulcerative colitis Ulcerative and inflammatory disease of the bowel that results in poor absorption of nutrients. Acute ulcerative colitis results in vascular congestion, hemorrhage, edema, and ulceration of the bowel mucosa. Chronic ulcerative colitis causes muscular hypertrophy, fat deposits, and fibrous tissue with bowel thickening, shortening, and narrowing.

vagotomy Surgical division of the vagus nerve to eliminate the vagal impulses that stimulate hydrochloric acid secretion in the stomach.

PYRAMID TO SUCCESS

Pyramid Points focus on diagnostic tests and nursing care related to the various gastric or intestinal tubes, gastric surgery, cirrhosis, hepatitis, pancreatitis, and colostomy care. Focus on preprocedure and postprocedure care of the client undergoing a gastrointestinal diagnostic test. Remember that an informed consent is required for any invasive procedure. Focus on diet restrictions before and after the diagnostic test and remember that the gag reflex or bowel sounds must return before allowing a client to consume food or fluids. Pyramid Points include instructions to the client and family regarding the prevention of gastrointestinal disorders and the complications associated with the disorder. Focus on teaching the client and family about diet and nutrition specific to the disorder, tube and wound care, preventing the transmission of infection such as with hepatitis, and care of a colostomy or ileostomy. Remember that body image disturbances can occur in clients with a gastrointestinal disorder. Specific focus relates to the client with a diversion, such as an ileostomy or colostomy, the social isolation issues that can occur, and effective coping strategies.

CLIENT NEEDS

Safe and Effective Care Environment

Consulting with other health care professionals regarding the client's nutritional status

Ensuring that confidentiality issues related to the gastrointestinal disorder are maintained

Establishing priorities of care

Handling infectious drainage and secretions safely

Maintaining standard precautions and other precautions as appropriate

Obtaining informed consent for treatments and surgical procedures

Obtaining referrals for home care and community services

Preventing disease transmission

Health Promotion and Maintenance

Performing physical assessment techniques of the gastrointestinal system

Preventing disease related to the gastrointestinal system

Providing health screening and health promotion programs related to gastrointestinal disorders

Teaching related to colostomy or ileostomy care

Teaching related to preventing the transmission of disease

Teaching related to prescribed dietary and other treatment measures

Psychosocial Integrity

Assessing coping mechanisms

Considering end-of-life and grief and loss issues

Identifying available support systems

Monitoring for expected body image changes

Physiological Integrity

Administering medications as prescribed specific to the gastrointestinal disorder

Assessing for signs and symptoms of infectious diseases of the gastrointestinal tract

Assisting with personal hygiene

Monitoring elimination patterns

Monitoring for complications related to tests, procedures, and surgical interventions

Monitoring for fluid and electrolyte imbalances

Monitoring laboratory values related to gastrointestinal disorders

Monitoring parenterally administered fluids, including parenteral nutrition

Providing adequate nutrition and oral hydration

Providing care for gastrointestinal tubes

Providing nonpharmacological and pharmacological comfort measures

Providing preprocedure and postprocedure care for diagnostic tests related to the gastrointestinal system

56

Gastrointestinal System

I. ANATOMY AND PHYSIOLOGY

A. Functions of the gastrointestinal system
1. Process food substances
2. Absorb the products of digestion into the blood
3. Excrete unabsorbed materials
4. Provide an environment for microorganisms to synthesize nutrients, such as vitamin K
5. For risk factors associated with the gastrointestinal system, see Box 56-1.

B. Mouth
1. Contains the lips, cheeks, palate, tongue, teeth, salivary glands, muscles, and maxillary bones
2. Saliva contains the enzyme amylase (ptyalin), which aids in digestion.

C. Esophagus
1. Collapsible muscular tube about 10 inches long
2. Carries food from the pharynx to the stomach

D. The stomach
1. Contains the cardia, fundus, the body, and the pylorus
2. Mucous glands are located in the mucosa and prevent autodigestion by providing an alkaline protective covering.
3. The lower esophageal (cardiac) sphincter prevents reflux of gastric contents into the esophagus.
4. The pyloric sphincter regulates the rate of stomach emptying into the small intestine.
5. Hydrochloric acid kills microorganisms, breaks food into small particles, and provides a chemical environment that facilitates gastric enzyme activation.
6. Pepsin is the chief coenzyme of gastric juice, which converts proteins into proteases and peptones.
7. Intrinsic factor is necessary for the absorption of vitamin B_{12}.
8. Gastrin controls gastric acidity.

E. Small intestine
1. The duodenum contains the openings of the bile and pancreatic ducts.
2. The jejunum is about 8 feet long.
3. The ileum is about 12 feet long.
4. The small intestine terminates in the cecum.

F. Pancreatic intestinal juice enzymes
1. Amylase digests starch to maltose.
2. Maltase reduces maltose to monosaccharide glucose.
3. Lactase splits lactose into galactose and glucose.
4. Sucrase reduces sucrose to fructose and glucose.
5. Nucleases split nucleic acids to nucleotides.
6. Enterokinase activates trypsinogen to trypsin.

G. Large intestine
1. About 5 feet long
2. Absorbs water and eliminates wastes
3. Intestinal bacteria play a vital role in the synthesis of some B vitamins and vitamin K.
4. Colon: Includes the ascending, transverse, descending, and sigmoid colons and rectum
5. The ileocecal valve prevents contents of the large intestine from entering the ileum.
6. The anal sphincters control the anal canal.

H. Peritoneum: Lines the abdominal cavity and forms the mesentery that supports the intestines and blood supply

I. Liver
1. The largest gland in the body, weighing 3 to 4 pounds
2. Contains Kupffer's cells, which remove bacteria in the portal venous blood
3. Removes excess glucose and amino acids from the portal blood
4. Synthesizes glucose, amino acids, and fats
5. Aids in the digestion of fats, carbohydrates, and proteins
6. Stores and filters blood (200 to 400 mL of blood stored)
7. Stores vitamins A, D, and B and iron
8. The liver secretes bile to emulsify fats (500 to 1000 mL of bile/day).
9. Hepatic ducts
   a. Deliver bile to the gallbladder via the cystic duct and to the duodenum via the common bile duct.
   b. The common bile duct opens into the duodenum, with the pancreatic duct at the ampulla of Vater.

Box 56-1 Risk Factors Associated With the Gastrointestinal System

Allergic reactions to food or medications
Cardiac, respiratory, and endocrine disorders that may lead to slowed gastrointestinal (GI) movement or constipation
Chronic alcohol use
Chronic high stress levels
Chronic laxative use
Chronic use of aspirin or nonsteroidal anti-inflammatory drugs
Diabetes mellitus, which may predispose to oral candidal infections or other GI disorders
Family history of GI disorders
Long-term GI conditions, such as ulcerative colitis, that may predispose to colorectal cancer
Neurological disorders that can impair movement, particularly with chewing and swallowing
Previous abdominal surgery or trauma, which may lead to adhesions
Tobacco use

Box 56-2 Gastrointestinal System Diagnostic Studies*

Anoscopy, proctoscopy, and sigmoidoscopy
Cholecystography
Defecography
Endoscopic retrograde cholangiopancreatography
Fiberoptic colonoscopy
Gastric analysis
Gastrointestinal motility studies
Hydrogen and urea breath test
Laparoscopy (peritoneoscopy)
Liver and pancreas laboratory studies
Liver biopsy
Lower gastrointestinal tract study (barium enema)
Paracentesis
Percutaneous transhepatic cholangiography
Stool specimens
Upper gastrointestinal fiberoscopy or esophagogastro-duodenoscopy
Upper gastrointestinal tract study (barium swallow)

*Informed consent is obtained for a diagnostic study that is invasive.

c. The sphincter prevents the reflux of intestinal contents into the common bile duct and pancreatic duct.
J. Gallbladder
1. Stores and concentrates bile and contracts to force bile into the duodenum during the digestion of fats
2. The cystic duct joins the hepatic duct to form the common bile duct.
3. The sphincter of Oddi is located at the entrance to the duodenum.
4. The presence of fatty materials in the duodenum stimulates the liberation of cholecystokinin, which causes contraction of the gallbladder and relaxation of the sphincter of Oddi.
K. Pancreas
1. Exocrine gland
a. Secretes sodium bicarbonate to neutralize the acidity of the stomach contents that enter the duodenum
b. Pancreatic juices contain enzymes for digesting carbohydrates, fats, and proteins.
2. Endocrine gland
a. Secretes glucagon to raise blood glucose levels and secretes somatostatin to exert a hypoglycemic effect
b. The islets of Langerhans secrete insulin.
c. Insulin is secreted into the bloodstream and is important for carbohydrate metabolism.

II. DIAGNOSTIC PROCEDURES (Box 56-2)

A. Upper gastrointestinal tract study (barium swallow)
1. Description: Examination of the upper gastrointestinal tract under fluoroscopy after the client drinks barium sulfate

2. Preprocedure: NPO after midnight the day of the test
3. Postprocedure
a. A laxative may be prescribed.
b. Instruct the client to increase oral fluid intake to help pass the barium.
c. Monitor stools for the passage of barium (stools will appear chalky white) because barium can cause a bowel obstruction.
B. Lower gastrointestinal tract study (barium enema)
1. Description
a. A fluoroscopic and radiographic examination of the large intestine is performed after rectal instillation of barium sulfate.
b. The study may be done with or without air.
2. Preprocedure
a. A low-fiber diet is given for 1 to 2 days before the test.
b. A clear liquid diet and laxative are given the evening before the test.
c. NPO after midnight the day of the test
d. Cleansing enemas may be prescribed on the morning of the test.
3. Postprocedure
a. Instruct the client to increase oral fluid intake to help pass the barium.
b. Administer a mild laxative as prescribed to facilitate emptying of the barium.
c. Monitor stools for the passage of barium.
d. Notify the physician if a bowel movement does not occur within 2 days.
C. Gastric analysis
1. Description
a. Gastric analysis requires the passage of a nasogastric tube into the stomach to aspirate gastric

contents for the analysis of acidity (pH), appearance, and volume; the entire gastric contents are aspirated, and then specimens are collected every 15 minutes for 1 hour.

b. Histamine or pentagastrin may be administered subcutaneously to stimulate gastric secretions; these medications may produce a flushed feeling.

c. Esophageal reflux of gastric acid may be diagnosed by ambulatory pH monitoring; a probe is placed just above the lower esophageal sphincter and connected to an external recording device. It provides a computer analysis and graphic display of results.

2. Preprocedure
   a. Fasting for 8 to 12 hours is required before the test.
   b. Use of tobacco and chewing gum are avoided for 6 hours before the test.
   c. Medications that stimulate gastric secretions are withheld for 24 to 48 hours.

3. Postprocedure
   a. Client may resume normal activities.
   b. Refrigerate gastric samples if not tested within 4 hours.

D. Upper gastrointestinal fiberoscopy
1. Description
   a. Also known as esophagogastroduodenoscopy
   b. Following sedation, an endoscope is passed down the esophagus to view the gastric wall, sphincters, and duodenum; tissue specimens can be obtained.

2. Preprocedure
   a. The client must be NPO for 6 to 12 hours before the test.
   b. A local anesthetic (spray or gargle) is administered along with medication that provides conscious sedation and relieves anxiety, such as intravenous (IV) midazolam (Versed), just before the scope is inserted.
   c. Atropine sulfate may be administered to reduce secretions, and glucagon may be administered to relax smooth muscle.
   d. Client is positioned on the left side to facilitate saliva drainage and to provide easy access of the endoscope.
   e. Airway patency is monitored during the test and pulse oximetry is used to monitor oxygen saturation; emergency equipment should be readily available.

3. Postprocedure
   a. Client must be NPO until the gag reflex returns (1 to 2 hours).
   b. Monitor for signs of perforation (pain, bleeding, unusual difficulty swallowing, elevated temperature).
   c. Maintain bedrest for the sedated client until alert.

d. Lozenges, saline gargles, or oral analgesics can relieve a minor sore throat (not given to the client until the gag reflex returns).

E. Anoscopy, proctoscopy, and sigmoidoscopy
1. Description
   a. Anoscopy requires the use of a rigid scope to examine the anal canal; the client is placed in the knee-chest or left lateral position.
   b. Proctoscopy and sigmoidoscopy require the use of a flexible scope to examine the rectum and sigmoid colon; the client is placed on the left side with the right leg bent and placed anteriorly.
   c. Biopsies and polypectomies can be performed.

2. Preprocedure: Enemas are administered to cleanse the bowel.

3. Postprocedure: Monitor for rectal bleeding and signs of perforation and peritonitis (Box 56-3).

F. Fiberoptic colonoscopy
1. Description
   a. Colonoscopy is a fiberoptic endoscopy study in which the lining of the large intestine is visually examined; biopsies and polypectomies can be performed.
   b. Cardiac and respiratory function are monitored continuously during the test.
   c. Colonoscopy is performed with the client lying on the left side with the knees drawn up to the chest; position may be changed during the test to facilitate passing of the scope.

2. Preprocedure
   a. Adequate cleansing of the colon is necessary, as prescribed by the physician.
   b. A clear liquid diet is started at noon on the day before the test.
   c. Consult with the physician regarding medications that must be withheld before the test.
   d. Client is NPO after midnight on the day of the test.
   e. A mild sedative is administered intravenously.
   f. Glucagon may be administered to relax smooth muscle.

3. Postprocedure
   a. Provide bedrest until alert.
   b. Monitor for signs of bowel perforation and peritonitis (see Box 56-3).

Box 56-3 Signs of Bowel Perforation and Peritonitis

Guarding of the abdomen
Increased fever and chills
Pallor
Progressive abdominal distention and abdominal pain
Restlessness
Tachycardia and tachypnea

c. Instruct the client to report any bleeding to the physician.

⚠ The client receiving enemas is at risk for fluid and electrolyte imbalances.

G. Laparoscopy (peritoneoscopy) is performed with a fiberoscopic laparoscope that allows direct visualization of organs and structures within the abdomen; biopsies may be obtained.

H. Cholecystography
1. Description: Performed to detect gallstones and assess the ability of the gallbladder to fill, concentrate its contents, contract, and empty
2. Preprocedure
   a. Assess for allergies to iodine or seafood.
   b. Contrast agents may be administered 10 to 12 hours (evening before) before the test.
   c. Client is NPO after the contrast agent is administered.
   d. Instruct the client that if a rash, itching, hives, or difficulty in breathing occurs after taking the contrast agent to report to the emergency department.
3. Postprocedure
   a. Inform the client that dysuria is common because the contrast agent is excreted in the urine.
   b. A normal diet may be resumed (a fatty meal may enhance excretion of the contrast agent).

I. Endoscopic retrograde cholangiopancreatography (ERCP)
1. Description
   a. Examination of the hepatobiliary system is performed via a flexible endoscope inserted into the esophagus to the descending duodenum; multiple positions are required during the procedure to pass the endoscope.
   b. If medication is administered before the procedure, the client is monitored closely for signs of respiratory and central nervous system depression, hypotension, oversedation, and vomiting.
2. Preprocedure
   a. Client is NPO for several hours before the procedure.
   b. Sedation is administered before the procedure.
3. Postprocedure
   a. Monitor vital signs.
   b. Monitor for the return of the gag reflex.
   c. Monitor for signs of perforation (see Box 56-3) or peritonitis.

J. Endoscopic ultrasonography
1. Description: provides images of the GI wall and digestive organs.
2. Preprocedure and postprocedure: Care is similar to that implemented for endoscopy.

⚠ Following endoscopic procedures, monitor for the return of a gag reflex before giving the client any oral substance. If the gag reflex has not returned, the client could aspirate.

K. Percutaneous transhepatic cholangiography
1. Description
   a. The examination involves the injection of dye directly into the biliary tree.
   b. The hepatic ducts within the liver, the entire length of the common bile duct, the cystic duct, and the gallbladder are outlined clearly.
2. Preprocedure
   a. Client is NPO.
   b. Sedating medication is administered.
3. Postprocedure
   a. Monitor vital signs.
   b. Monitor for signs of bleeding, peritonitis (see Box 56-3), and septicemia; report the presence of pain immediately.
   c. Administer antibiotics as prescribed to reduce the risk of sepsis.

L. Paracentesis (see Priority Nursing Actions)
1. Description: Transabdominal removal of fluid from the peritoneal cavity for analysis
2. Preprocedure
   a. Have the client void before the start of procedure to empty the bladder and to move the bladder out of the way of the paracentesis needle.
   b. Measure abdominal girth, weight, and baseline vital signs.
   c. Note that the client is positioned upright on the edge of the bed, with the back supported and the feet resting on a stool (or Fowler's position in bed).

⚠ The rapid removal of fluid from the abdominal cavity during paracentesis leads to decreased abdominal pressure, which can cause vasodilation and resultant shock.

3. Postprocedure
   a. Monitor vital signs.
   b. Measure fluid collected, describe, and record.
   c. Label fluid samples and send to the laboratory for analysis.
   d. Apply a dry sterile dressing to the insertion site; monitor site for bleeding.
   e. Measure abdominal girth and weight.
   f. Monitor for hypovolemia, electrolyte loss, mental status changes, or encephalopathy.
   g. Monitor for hematuria caused by bladder trauma.
   h. Instruct the client to notify the physician if the urine becomes bloody, pink, or red.

PRIORITY NURSING ACTIONS!

Actions to Take in Caring for a Client With a Paracentesis

1. Ensure that the client understands the procedure and that informed consent has been obtained.
2. Obtain vital signs, including weight.
3. Have the client void.
4. Position the client upright.
5. Assist the physician, monitor vital signs, and provide comfort and support during the procedure.
6. Apply a dressing to the site of puncture.
7. Monitor vital signs, weigh the client, and maintain the client on bedrest.
8. Measure the amount of fluid removed.
9. Label and send the fluid for laboratory analysis.
10. Document the event, client's response, appearance and amount of fluid removed.

Paracentesis is the transabdominal removal of fluid from the peritoneal cavity. The nurse first ensures that the client understands the procedure and that informed consent has been obtained because the procedure is invasive. The nurse next obtains preprocedure vital signs, including weight so that a baseline is obtained. Weight is taken before and after the procedure to provide an indication of the effectiveness of the procedure in fluid removal. The client is positioned upright on the edge of the bed with the back supported and the feet resting on a stool or in a Fowler's position in bed. The nurse assists the physician, monitors vital signs per protocol, and provides comfort and support to the client during the procedure. Once the procedure is complete the nurse applies a dressing to the site of puncture and monitors for leakage or bleeding. The client is placed in a position of comfort, bedrest is maintained as prescribed, and vital signs are monitored to assess for complications. The fluid removed from the client is measured, labeled and sent to the laboratory for analysis. The nurse documents the event, the client's response, the appearance and amount of fluid removed, and any additional pertinent data.

Reference: Ignatavicius, D., & Workman, M. (2010). *Medical-surgical nursing: Patient-centered collaborative care.* (6th ed., p. 1352). St. Louis: Saunders.

M. Liver biopsy
1. Description: A needle is inserted through the abdominal wall to the liver to obtain a tissue sample for biopsy and microscopic examination.
2. Preprocedure
   a. Assess results of coagulation tests (prothrombin time, partial thromboplastin time, platelet count).
   b. Administer a sedative as prescribed.
   c. Note that the client is placed in the supine or left lateral position during the procedure to expose the right side of the upper abdomen.
3. Postprocedure
   a. Assess vital signs.
   b. Assess biopsy site for bleeding.

c. Monitor for peritonitis (see Box 56-3).
d. Maintain bedrest for several hours.
e. Place the client on the right side with a pillow under the costal margin to decrease the risk of hemorrhage, and instruct the client to avoid coughing and straining.
f. Instruct the client to avoid heavy lifting and strenuous exercise for 1 week.

⚠ Following a liver biopsy, place the client on the right side with a pillow under the costal margin at the anatomical location of the liver to decrease the risk of hemorrhage.

N. Stool specimens
1. Testing of stool specimens includes inspecting the specimen for consistency and color and testing for occult blood.
2. Tests for fecal urobilinogen, fat, nitrogen, parasites, pathogens, food substances, and other substances may be performed; these tests require that the specimen be sent to the laboratory.
3. Random specimens are sent promptly to the laboratory.
4. Quantitative 24- to 72-hour collections must be kept refrigerated until they are taken to the laboratory.
5. Some specimens require that a certain diet be followed or that certain medications be withheld; check agency guidelines regarding specific procedures.

O. Urea breath test
1. The urea breath test detects the presence of *Helicobacter pylori,* the bacteria that cause peptic ulcer disease.
2. The client consumes a capsule of carbon-labeled urea and provides a breath sample 10 to 20 minutes later.
3. Certain medications may need to be avoided before testing; these may include antibiotics or bismuth subsalicylate (Pepto-Bismol) for 1 month before the test; sucralfate (Carafate) and omeprazole (Prilosec) for 1 week before the test; and cimetidine (Tagamet), famotidine (Pepcid), ranitidine (Zantac), or nizatidine (Axid) for 24 hours before breath testing.
4. *H. pylori* can also be detected by assessing serum antibody levels.

P. Liver and pancreas laboratory studies (see Chapter 11)
1. Alkaline phosphatase is released during liver damage or biliary obstruction.
2. Prothrombin time is prolonged with liver damage.
3. The serum ammonia level assesses the ability of the liver to deaminate protein by-products.
4. Liver enzyme levels (transaminase studies) are elevated with liver damage.
5. An increase in cholesterol level indicates **pancreatitis** or biliary obstruction.

6. An increase in bilirubin level indicates liver damage or biliary obstruction.
7. Increased values for amylase and lipase levels indicate **pancreatitis**.

III. ASSESSMENT (See Chapter 34 for abdominal assessment techniques.)

IV. GASTROINTESTINAL TUBES (See Chapter 21 for information regarding these tubes.)

V. GASTROESOPHAGEAL REFLUX DISEASE

A. Description
1. Gastroesophageal reflux is the backflow of gastric and duodenal contents into the esophagus.
2. The reflux is caused by an incompetent lower esophageal sphincter, pyloric stenosis, or motility disorder.
B. Assessment
1. Heartburn
2. Epigastric pain
3. Dyspepsia
4. Regurgitation
5. Pain and difficulty with swallowing
6. Hypersalivation
C. Interventions
1. Instruct the client to avoid factors that decrease lower esophageal sphincter pressure or cause esophageal irritation such as peppermint, chocolate, coffee, fried or fatty foods, carbonated beverages, alcoholic beverages, and cigarette smoking.
2. Instruct the client to eat a low-fat, high-fiber diet and to avoid eating and drinking 2 hours before bedtime, and wearing tight clothes; also, elevate the head of the bed on 6- to 8-inch blocks.
3. Avoid the use of anticholinergics, which delay stomach emptying; also, nonsteroidal anti-inflammatory medications and other medications that contain acetylsalicylic acid need to be avoided.
4. Instruct the client regarding prescribed medications, such as antacids, H_2-receptor antagonists, or proton pump inhibitors.
5. Instruct the client regarding the administration of prokinetic medications, if prescribed, which accelerate gastric emptying.
6. If medical management is unsuccessful, surgery may be required; this involves a fundoplication (wrapping a portion of the gastric fundus around the sphincter area of the esophagus); surgery may be performed by laparoscopy.

VI. GASTRITIS

A. Description
1. Inflammation of the stomach or gastric mucosa
2. Acute gastritis is caused by the ingestion of food contaminated with disease-causing

microorganisms or food that is irritating or too highly seasoned, the overuse of aspirin or other nonsteroidal anti-inflammatory drugs (NSAIDs), excessive alcohol intake, bile reflux, or radiation therapy.
3. Chronic gastritis is caused by benign or malignant ulcers or by the bacteria *H. pylori*, and also may be caused by autoimmune diseases, dietary factors, medications, alcohol, smoking, or reflux.
B. Assessment (Box 56-4)
C. Interventions
1. Acute gastritis: Food and fluids may be withheld until symptoms subside; afterward, ice chips can be given, followed by clear liquids, and then solid food.
2. Monitor for signs of hemorrhagic gastritis such as hematemesis, tachycardia, and hypotension, and notify the physician if these signs occur.
3. Instruct the client to avoid irritating foods, fluids, and other substances, such as spicy and highly seasoned foods, caffeine, alcohol, and nicotine.
4. Instruct the client in the use of prescribed medications, such as antibiotics and antacids.
5. Provide the client with information about the importance of vitamin B_{12} injections if a deficiency is present.

VII. PEPTIC ULCER DISEASE

A. Description
1. A peptic ulcer is an ulceration in the mucosal wall of the stomach, pylorus, duodenum, or esophagus in portions accessible to gastric secretions; erosion may extend through the muscle.
2. The ulcer may be referred to as gastric, duodenal, or esophageal, depending on its location.
3. The most common peptic ulcers are gastric ulcers and duodenal ulcers.
B. Gastric ulcers
1. Description
a. A gastric ulcer involves ulceration of the mucosal lining that extends to the submucosal layer of the stomach.
b. Predisposing factors include stress, smoking, the use of corticosteroids, NSAIDs, alcohol,

Box 56-4 Assessment Findings in Acute and Chronic Gastritis

Acute	Chronic
Abdominal discomfort	Anorexia, nausea, and vomiting
Anorexia, nausea, and vomiting	Belching
Headache	Heartburn after eating
Hiccupping	Sour taste in the mouth
	Vitamin B_{12} deficiency

Box 56-5 Assessment: Gastric and Duodenal Ulcers

Gastric
Gnawing, sharp pain in or left of the midepigastric region occurs 30 to 60 minutes after a meal (food ingestion accentuates the pain).
Hematemesis is more common than melena.

Duodenal
Burning pain occurs in the midepigastric area 1½ to 3 hours after a meal and during the night (often awakens the client).
Melena is more common than hematemesis.
Pain is often relieved by the ingestion of food.

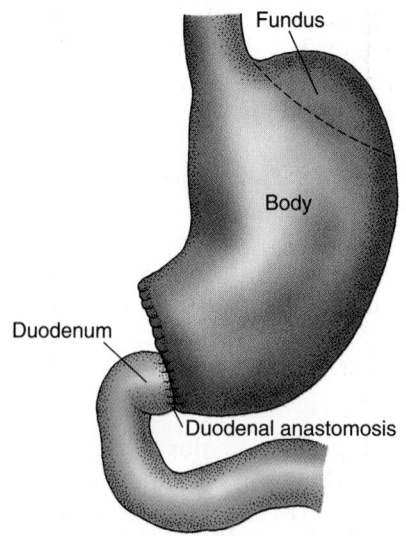

▲ **FIGURE 56-1** The Billroth I procedure (gastroduodenostomy). The distal portion of the stomach is removed, and the remainder is anastomosed to the duodenum. (From Ignatavicius, D., & Workman, M. [2006]. *Medical-surgical nursing: Critical thinking for collaborative care* [5th ed.]. St. Louis: Saunders.)

history of gastritis, family history of gastric ulcers, or infection with *H. pylori*.
  c. Complications include hemorrhage, perforation, and pyloric obstruction.
2. Assessment (Box 56-5)
3. Interventions
  a. Monitor vital signs and for signs of bleeding.
  b. Administer small, frequent bland feedings during the active phase.
  c. Administer H₂-receptor antagonists or proton pump inhibitors as prescribed to decrease the secretion of gastric acid.
  d. Administer antacids as prescribed to neutralize gastric secretions.
  e. Administer anticholinergics as prescribed to reduce gastric motility.
  f. Administer mucosal barrier protectants as prescribed 1 hour before each meal.
  g. Administer prostaglandins as prescribed for their protective and antisecretory actions.
4. Client education
  a. Avoid consuming alcohol and substances that contain caffeine or chocolate.
  b. Avoid smoking.
  c. Avoid aspirin or NSAIDs.
  d. Obtain adequate rest and reduce stress.
5. Interventions during active bleeding
  a. Monitor vital signs closely.
  b. Assess for signs of dehydration, hypovolemic shock, sepsis, and respiratory insufficiency.
  c. Maintain NPO status and administer IV fluid replacement as prescribed; monitor intake and output.
  d. Monitor hemoglobin and hematocrit.
  e. Administer blood transfusions as prescribed.
  f. Prepare to assist with administering medications as prescribed to induce vasoconstriction and reduce bleeding.
6. Surgical interventions
  a. Total **gastrectomy**: Removal of the stomach with attachment of the esophagus to the jejunum or duodenum; also called *esophagojejunostomy* or *esophagoduodenostomy*
  b. **Vagotomy**: Surgical division of the vagus nerve to eliminate the vagal impulses that stimulate hydrochloric acid secretion in the stomach
  c. **Gastric resection**: Removal of the lower half of the stomach and usually includes a **vagotomy**; also called *antrectomy*
  d. **Billroth I**: Partial **gastrectomy**, with the remaining segment anastomosed to the duodenum; also called *gastroduodenostomy* (Fig. 56-1)
  e. **Billroth II**: Partial **gastrectomy**, with the remaining segment anastomosed to the jejunum; also called *gastrojejunostomy* (Fig. 56-2)
  f. **Pyloroplasty**: Enlargement of the pylorus to prevent or decrease pyloric obstruction, thereby enhancing gastric emptying
7. Postoperative interventions
  a. Monitor vital signs.
  b. Place in a Fowler's position for comfort and to promote drainage.
  c. Administer fluids and electrolyte replacements intravenously as prescribed; monitor intake and output.
  d. Assess bowel sounds.
  e. Monitor nasogastric suction as prescribed.
  f. Maintain NPO status as prescribed for 1 to 3 days until **peristalsis** returns.
  g. Progress the diet from NPO to sips of clear water to six small bland meals a day, as prescribed when bowel sounds return.
  h. Monitor for postoperative complications of hemorrhage, **dumping syndrome**, diarrhea, hypoglycemia, and vitamin B₁₂ deficiency.

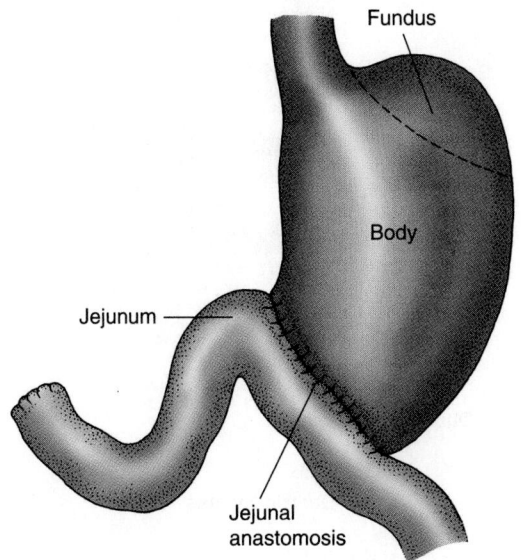

▲ **FIGURE 56-2** The Billroth II procedure (gastrojejunostomy). The lower portion of the stomach is removed, and the remainder is anastomosed to the jejunum. (From Ignatavicius, D., & Workman, M. [2006]. *Medical-surgical nursing: Critical thinking for collaborative care* [5th ed.]. St. Louis: Saunders.)

⚠ Following gastric surgery, do not irrigate or remove the nasogastric (NG) tube unless specifically prescribed because of the risk for disruption of the gastric sutures. Monitor closely to ensure proper functioning of the NG tube to prevent strain on the anastomosis site. Contact the physician if the tube is not functioning properly.

C. Duodenal ulcers
1. Description
    a. A duodenal ulcer is a break in the mucosa of the duodenum.
    b. Risk factors and causes include infection with *H. pylori*; alcohol intake; smoking; stress; caffeine; the use of aspirin, corticosteroids, and NSAIDs.
    c. Complications include bleeding, perforation, gastric outlet obstruction, and intractable disease.
2. Assessment (see Box 56-5)
3. Interventions
    a. Monitor vital signs.
    b. Instruct the client about a bland diet, with small frequent meals.
    c. Provide for adequate rest.
    d. Encourage the cessation of smoking.
    e. Instruct the client to avoid alcohol intake, caffeine, the use of aspirin, corticosteroids, and NSAIDs.
    f. Administer medications to treat *H. pylori* and antacids to neutralize acid secretions as prescribed.

Box 56-6 Client Education: Preventing Dumping Syndrome

Avoid sugar, salt, and milk.
Eat a high-protein, high-fat, low-carbohydrate diet.
Eat small meals and avoid consuming fluids with meals.
Lie down after meals.
Take antispasmodic medications as prescribed to delay gastric emptying.

---

    g. Administer H_2-receptor antagonists or proton pump inhibitors as prescribed to block the secretion of acid.
4. Surgical interventions: Surgery is performed only if the ulcer is unresponsive to medications or if hemorrhage, obstruction, or perforation occurs.

D. Dumping syndrome
1. Description: The rapid emptying of the gastric contents into the small intestine that occurs following **gastric resection**
2. Assessment
    a. Symptoms occurring 30 minutes after eating
    b. Nausea and vomiting
    c. Feelings of abdominal fullness and abdominal cramping
    d. Diarrhea
    e. Palpitations and tachycardia
    f. Perspiration
    g. Weakness and dizziness
    h. Borborygmi (loud gurgles indicating hyperperistalsis)
3. Client education (Box 56-6)

VIII. VITAMIN B$_{12}$ DEFICIENCY

A. Description
1. Vitamin B_{12} deficiency results from an inadequate intake of vitamin B_{12} or a lack of absorption of ingested vitamin B_{12} from the intestinal tract.
2. Pernicious anemia results from a deficiency of intrinsic factor, necessary for intestinal absorption of vitamin B_{12}; gastric disease or surgery can result in a lack of intrinsic factor.

B. Assessment
1. Severe pallor
2. Fatigue
3. Weight loss
4. Smooth, beefy red tongue
5. Slight jaundice
6. Paresthesias of the hands and feet
7. Disturbances with gait and balance

C. Interventions
1. Increase dietary intake of foods rich in vitamin B_{12} if the anemia is the result of a dietary deficiency (Box 56-7).

Box 56-7 Foods Rich in Vitamin B₁₂

Brewer's yeast   Liver
Citrus fruits   Nuts
Dried beans   Organ meats
Green, leafy vegetables

Box 56-8 Community Resources Following Bariatric Surgery

American Obesity Association
American Society of Bariatric Surgery
Overeaters Anonymous

2. Administer vitamin B₁₂ injections as prescribed weekly initially and then monthly for maintenance (lifelong) if the anemia is the result of a deficiency of intrinsic factor or disease or surgery of the ileum.

IX. BARIATRIC SURGERY

A. Description
  1. Surgical reduction of gastric capacity that may be performed on a client with morbid obesity to produce permanent weight loss
  2. Surgery may be performed by laparoscope; the decision is based on the client's weight, body build, history of abdominal surgery, and current medical disorders.
  3. Obese clients are at increased postoperative risk for pulmonary and thromboembolic complications and death.
  4. Surgery can prevent the complications of obesity, such as diabetes mellitus, hypertension and other cardiovascular disorders, depression, or sleep apnea.
  5. The client needs to agree to modify his or her lifestyle, lose weight and keep the weight off, and obtain support from available community resources (Box 56-8).
B. Types (Fig. 56-3)
  1. Gastric restrictive surgery
     a. Allows for normal digestion without the risk of nutritional deficiency
     b. A vertical banded gastroplasty may be performed; the surgeon places a vertical line of staples to create a small stomach pouch to which the band is connected to provide an outlet to the small intestine.
     c. A circumgastric banding may be performed; an inflatable band is placed around the stomach to limit stomach size; the band can be inflated or deflated through a subcutaneous port to change the size of the stomach as the client loses weight.
  2. Gastric restriction combined with malabsorption surgery

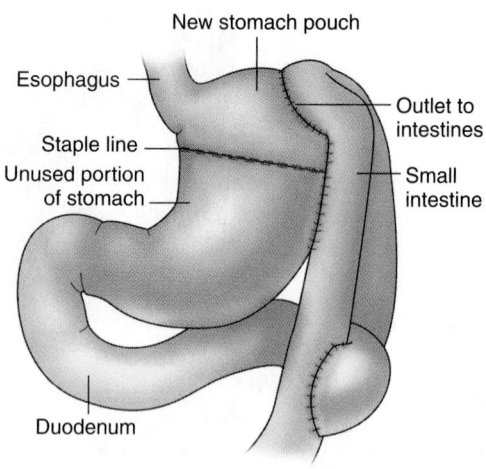

Gastric Bypass

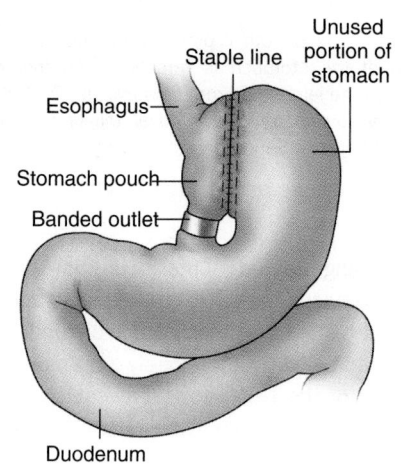

Vertical Banded Gastroplasty

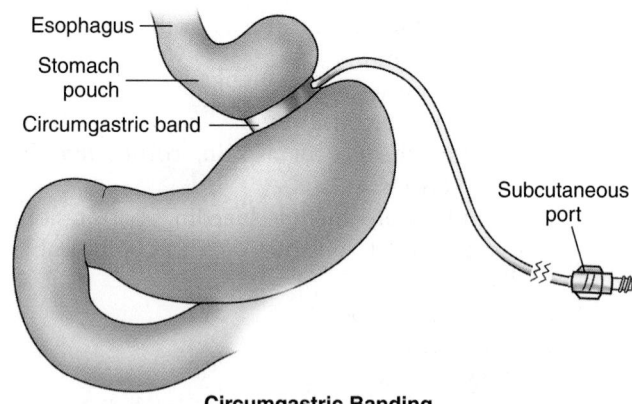

Circumgastric Banding

▲ **FIGURE 56-3** Bariatric surgical procedures. (From Ignatavicius, D., & Workman, M. [2006]. *Medical-surgical nursing: Critical thinking for collaborative care* [5th ed.]. St. Louis: Saunders.)

     a. Known as a gastric bypass or Roux-en-Y gastric bypass
     b. In addition to stapling, the stomach, duodenum, and part of the ileum are bypassed so that fewer calories can be absorbed.

Box 56-9 Dietary Measures for the Client Following Bariatric Surgery

Avoid alcohol, high-protein foods, and foods high in sugar and fat.
Eat slowly and chew food well.
Progress food types and amounts as prescribed.
Take nutritional supplements as prescribed, which may include calcium, iron, multivitamins, and vitamin B_{12}.
Monitor and report signs and symptoms of complications, such as dehydration.

C. Postoperative interventions
1. Care is similar to that for the client undergoing abdominal surgery.
2. Clear liquids are introduced slowly once bowel sounds have returned and the client passes flatus (1-oz cups are used for each serving).
3. Clear fluids are followed by puréed foods, juices, thin soups, and milk 24 to 48 hours after clear fluids are tolerated (the diet is usually limited to liquids or puréed foods for 6 weeks); then the diet is progressed to nutrient-dense regular food.

D. Client teaching points about diet (Box 56-9)

X. GASTRIC CANCER (see Chapter 52)

XI. HIATAL HERNIA

A. Description
1. A **hiatal hernia** is also known as esophageal or diaphragmatic hernia.
2. A portion of the stomach herniates through the diaphragm and into the thorax.
3. Herniation results from weakening of the muscles of the diaphragm and is aggravated by factors that increase abdominal pressure such as pregnancy, **ascites**, obesity, tumors, and heavy lifting.
4. Complications include ulceration, hemorrhage, regurgitation and aspiration of stomach contents, strangulation, and incarceration of the stomach in the chest with possible necrosis, peritonitis, and mediastinitis.

B. Assessment
1. Heartburn
2. Regurgitation or vomiting
3. Dysphagia
4. Feeling of fullness

C. Interventions
1. Medical and surgical management are similar to those for gastroesophageal reflux disease.
2. Provide small frequent meals and limit the amount of liquids taken with meals.
3. Advise the client not to recline for 1 hour after eating.
4. Avoid anticholinergics, which delay stomach emptying.

XII. CHOLECYSTITIS

A. Description
1. Inflammation of the gallbladder that may occur as an acute or chronic process
2. Acute inflammation is associated with gallstones (cholelithiasis).
3. Chronic **cholecystitis** results when inefficient bile emptying and gallbladder muscle wall disease cause a fibrotic and contracted gallbladder.
4. Acalculous **cholecystitis** occurs in the absence of gallstones and is caused by bacterial invasion via the lymphatic or vascular system.

B. Assessment
1. Nausea and vomiting
2. Indigestion
3. Belching
4. Flatulence
5. Epigastric pain that radiates to the scapula 2 to 4 hours after eating fatty foods and may persist for 4 to 6 hours
6. Pain localized in right upper quadrant
7. Guarding, rigidity, and rebound tenderness
8. Mass palpated in the right upper quadrant
9. **Murphy's sign** (cannot take a deep breath when the examiner's fingers are passed below the hepatic margin because of pain)
10. Elevated temperature
11. Tachycardia
12. Signs of dehydration

C. Biliary obstruction
1. Jaundice
2. Dark orange and foamy urine
3. Steatorrhea and clay-colored feces
4. Pruritus

D. Interventions
1. Maintain NPO status during nausea and vomiting episodes.
2. Maintain nasogastric decompression as prescribed for severe vomiting.
3. Administer antiemetics as prescribed for nausea and vomiting.
4. Administer analgesics as prescribed to relieve pain and reduce spasm.
5. Administer antispasmodics (anticholinergics) as prescribed to relax smooth muscle.
6. Instruct the client with chronic **cholecystitis** to eat small, low-fat meals.
7. Instruct the client to avoid gas-forming foods.
8. Prepare the client for nonsurgical and surgical procedures as prescribed.

E. Surgical interventions
1. **Cholecystectomy** is the removal of the gallbladder.
2. **Choledocholithotomy** requires incision into the common bile duct to remove the stone.
3. Surgical procedures may be performed by laparoscopy.

Box 56-10 Care of a T-Tube

Purpose and Description
A T-tube is placed after surgical exploration of the common bile duct. The tube preserves the patency of the duct and ensures drainage of bile until edema resolves and bile is effectively draining into the duodenum. A gravity drainage bag is attached to the T-tube to collect the drainage.

Interventions
Position the client in a semi-Fowler's position to facilitate drainage.
Monitor the amount, color, consistency, and odor of the drainage.
Report sudden increases in bile output to the physician.
Monitor for inflammation and protect the skin from irritation.
Keep the drainage system below the level of the gallbladder.
Monitor for foul odor and purulent drainage and report its presence to the physician.
Avoid irrigation, aspiration, or clamping of the T-tube without a physician's prescription.
As prescribed, clamp the tube before a meal and observe for abdominal discomfort and distention, nausea, chills, or fever; unclamp the tube if nausea or vomiting occurs.

Box 56-11 Types of Cirrhosis

Laënnec's Cirrhosis
Cirrhosis is alcohol-induced, nutritional, or portal.
Cellular necrosis causes eventual widespread scar tissue, with fibrotic infiltration of the liver.

Postnecrotic Cirrhosis
Cirrhosis occurs after massive liver necrosis.
Cirrhosis results as a complication of hepatitis or exposure to hepatotoxins.
Scar tissue causes destruction of liver lobules and entire lobes.

Biliary Cirrhosis
Cirrhosis develops from chronic biliary obstruction, bile stasis, and inflammation, resulting in severe obstructive jaundice.

Cardiac Cirrhosis
Cirrhosis is associated with severe, right-sided congestive heart failure and results in an enlarged, edematous, congested liver.
The liver becomes anoxic, resulting in liver cell necrosis and fibrosis.

F. Postoperative interventions
1. Monitor for respiratory complications caused by pain at the incisional site.
2. Encourage coughing and deep breathing.
3. Encourage early ambulation.
4. Instruct the client about splinting the abdomen to prevent discomfort during coughing.
5. Administer antiemetics as prescribed for nausea and vomiting.
6. Administer analgesics as prescribed for pain relief.
7. Maintain NPO status and nasogastric tube suction as prescribed.
8. Advance diet from clear liquids to solids when prescribed and as tolerated by the client.
9. Maintain and monitor drainage from the T-tube, if present (Box 56-10).

XIII. CIRRHOSIS (Box 56-11)

A. Description
1. A chronic, progressive disease of the liver characterized by diffuse degeneration and destruction of hepatocytes
2. Repeated destruction of hepatic cells causes the formation of scar tissue.

B. Complications
1. **Portal hypertension**: A persistent increase in pressure in the portal vein that develops as a result of obstruction to flow
2. **Ascites**
   a. Accumulation of fluid in the peritoneal cavity that results from venous congestion of the hepatic capillaries

   b. Capillary congestion leads to plasma leaking directly from the liver surface and portal vein.
3. Bleeding **esophageal varices**: Fragile, thin-walled, distended esophageal veins that become irritated and rupture
4. Coagulation defects
   a. Decreased synthesis of bile fats in the liver prevents the absorption of fat-soluble vitamins.
   b. Without vitamin K and clotting factors II, VII, IX, and X, the client is prone to bleeding.
5. Jaundice: Occurs because the liver is unable to metabolize bilirubin and because the edema, fibrosis, and scarring of the hepatic bile ducts interfere with normal bile and bilirubin secretion
6. Portal systemic encephalopathy: End-stage hepatic failure characterized by altered level of consciousness, neurological symptoms, impaired thinking, and neuromuscular disturbances; caused by failure of the diseased liver to detoxify neurotoxic agents such as ammonia.
7. Hepatorenal syndrome
   a. Progressive renal failure associated with hepatic failure
   b. Characterized by a sudden decrease in urinary output, elevated blood urea nitrogen and creatinine levels, decreased urine sodium excretion, and increased urine osmolarity

C. Assessment (Fig. 56-4)

D. Interventions
1. Elevate the head of the bed to minimize shortness of breath.
2. If **ascites** and edema are absent and the client does not exhibit signs of impending coma, a

NEUROLOGIC FINDINGS
Asterixis
Paresthesias of feet
Peripheral nerve degeneration
Portal-systemic encephalopathy
Reversal of sleep-wake pattern
Sensory disturbances

GASTROINTESTINAL (GI)
FINDINGS
Abdominal pain
Anorexia
Ascites
Clay-colored stools
Diarrhea
Esophageal varices
Fetor hepaticus
Gallstones
Gastritis
Gastrointestinal bleeding
Hemorrhoidal varices
Hepatomegaly
Hiatal hernia
Hypersplenism
Malnutrition
Nausea
Small nodular liver
Vomiting

RENAL FINDINGS
Hepatorenal syndrome
Increased urine bilirubin

ENDOCRINE FINDINGS
Increased aldosterone
Increased antidiuretic hormone
Increased circulating estrogens
Increased glucocorticoids
Gynecomastia

IMMUNE SYSTEM DISTURBANCES
Increased susceptibility to infection
Leukopenia

CARDIOVASCULAR FINDINGS
Cardiac dysrhythmias
Development of collateral circulation
Fatigue
Hyperkinetic circulation
Peripheral edema
Portal hypertension
Spider angiomas

PULMONARY FINDINGS
Dyspnea
Hydrothorax
Hyperventilation
Hypoxemia

HEMATOLOGIC FINDINGS
Anemia
Disseminated intravascular
  coagulation
Impaired coagulation
Splenomegaly
Thrombocytopenia

DERMATOLOGIC FINDINGS
Axillary and pubic hair changes
Caput medusae (dilated abdominal veins)*
Ecchymosis; petechiae*
Increased skin pigmentation
Jaundice
Palmar erythema*
Pruritus
Spider angiomas (chest and thorax)*

FLUID AND ELECTROLYTE
DISTURBANCES
Ascites
Decreased effective blood volume
Dilutional hyponatremia or
  hypernatremia
Hypocalcemia
Hypokalemia
Peripheral edema
Water retention

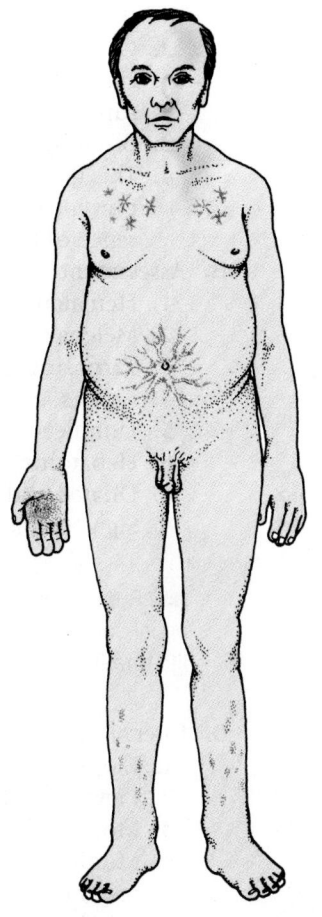

▲ **FIGURE 56-4** Clinical picture of a client with liver dysfunction. Manifestations vary according to the progression of the disease. Some dermatologic manifestations are noted in color (and marked with asterisks). (From Ignatavicius, D., & Workman, M. [2010]. *Medical-surgical nursing: Patient-centered collaborative care* [6th ed.]. St. Louis: Saunders.)

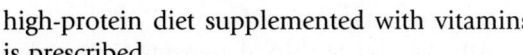

high-protein diet supplemented with vitamins is prescribed.

3. Provide supplemental vitamins (B complex, vitamins A, C, and K, folic acid, and thiamine) as prescribed.

4. Restrict sodium intake and fluid intake as prescribed.

5. Initiate enteral feedings or parenteral nutrition as prescribed.

6. Administer diuretics as prescribed to treat **ascites**.

7. Monitor intake and output and electrolyte balance.

8. Weigh client and measure abdominal girth daily (Fig. 56-5).

9. Monitor level of consciousness; assess for pre-coma state (tremors, delirium).

10. Monitor for **asterixis**, a coarse tremor characterized by rapid, nonrhythmic extensions and flexions in the wrist and fingers (Fig. 56-6).

11. Monitor for **fetor hepaticus**, the fruity, musty breath odor of severe chronic liver disease.

12. Maintain gastric intubation to assess bleeding or esophagogastric balloon tamponade to control bleeding varices if prescribed.

13. Administer blood products as prescribed.

14. Monitor coagulation laboratory results; administer vitamin K if prescribed.

15. Administer antacids as prescribed.

16. Administer lactulose (Constulose, Enulose) as prescribed, which decreases the pH of the bowel, decreases production of ammonia by bacteria in the bowel, and facilitates the excretion of ammonia.

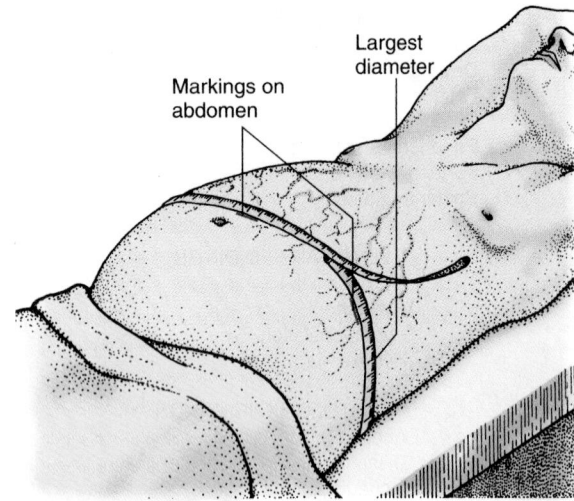

▲ **FIGURE 56-5** How to measure abdominal girth. With the client supine, bring the tape measure around the client and take a measurement at the level of the umbilicus. Before removing the tape, mark the client's abdomen along the sides of tape on the client's flanks (sides) and midline to ensure that later measurements are taken at the same place. (From Ignatavicius, D., & Workman, M. [2010]. *Medical-surgical nursing: Patient-centered collaborative care* [6th ed.]. St. Louis: Saunders.)

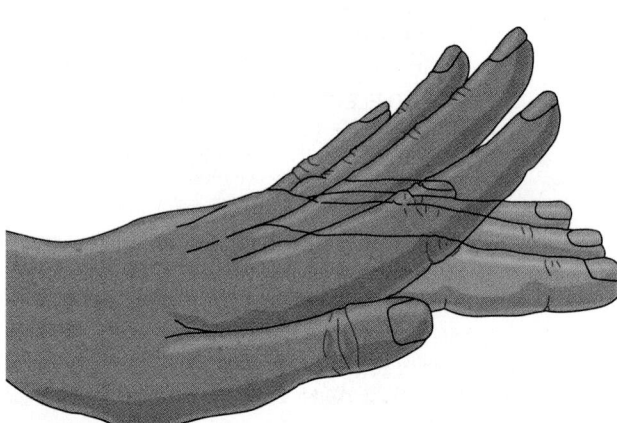

▲ **FIGURE 56-6** Eliciting asterixis (flapping tremor). Have the client extend the arm, dorsiflex the wrist, and extend the fingers. Observe for rapid, nonrhythmic extensions and flexions. (From Ignatavicius, D., & Workman, M. [2006]. *Medical-surgical nursing: Critical thinking for collaborative care* [5th ed.]. St. Louis: Saunders.)

 17. Administer antibiotics as prescribed to inhibit protein synthesis in bacteria and decrease the production of ammonia.

 18. Avoid medications such as opioids, sedatives, and barbiturates and any hepatotoxic medications or substances.

19. Instruct the client about the importance of abstinence of alcohol intake.

20. Prepare the client for paracentesis to remove abdominal fluid.

21. Prepare the client for surgical shunting procedures if prescribed to divert fluid from **ascites** into the venous system.

XIV. ESOPHAGEAL VARICES

A. Description
1. Dilated and tortuous veins in the submucosa of the esophagus.
2. Caused by **portal hypertension**, often associated with liver **cirrhosis**; are at high risk for rupture if portal circulation pressure rises
3. Bleeding varices are an emergency.
4. The goal of treatment is to control bleeding, prevent complications, and prevent the recurrence of bleeding.

B. Assessment
1. Hematemesis
2. Melena
3. Tarry stools
4. **Ascites**
5. Jaundice
6. Hepatomegaly and splenomegaly
7. Dilated abdominal veins
8. Signs of shock

⚠ Rupture and resultant hemorrhage of the esophageal varices is the primary concern because it is a life-threatening situation.

C. Interventions
1. Monitor vital signs.
2. Elevate the head of the bed.
3. Monitor for orthostatic hypotension.
4. Monitor lung sounds and for the presence of respiratory distress.
5. Administer oxygen as prescribed to prevent tissue hypoxia.
6. Monitor level of consciousness.
7. Maintain NPO status.
8. Administer fluids intravenously as prescribed to restore fluid volume and electrolyte imbalances; monitor intake and output.
9. Monitor hemoglobin and hematocrit values and coagulation factors.
10. Administer blood transfusions or clotting factors as prescribed.
11. Assist in inserting a nasogastric tube or a balloon tamponade as prescribed; balloon tamponade is not used frequently because it is very uncomfortable for the client and its use is associated with complications.
12. Prepare to assist with administering medications to induce vasoconstriction and reduce bleeding.
13. Instruct the client to avoid activities that will initiate vasovagal responses.
14. Prepare the client for endoscopic procedures or surgical procedures as prescribed.

D. Endoscopic injection (sclerotherapy)
1. The procedure involves the injection of a sclerosing agent into and around bleeding varices.

NORMAL HEPATIC CIRCULATION   PORTACAVAL (END-TO-SIDE) SHUNT   SPLENORENAL (END-TO-SIDE) SHUNT

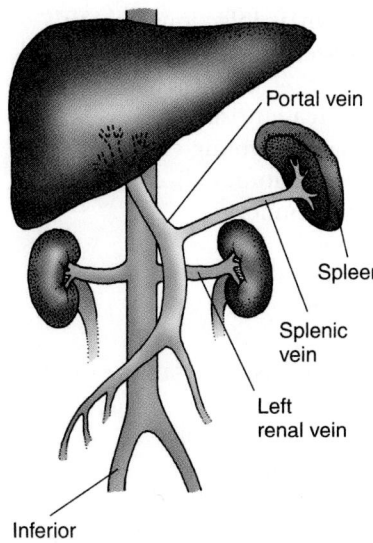
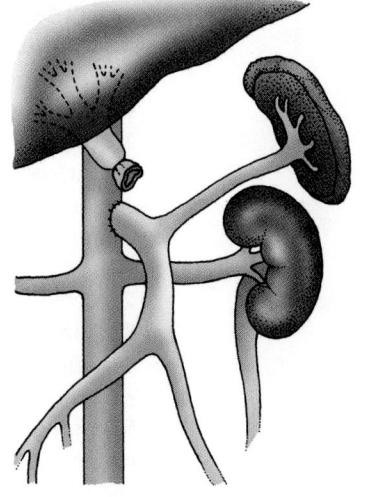
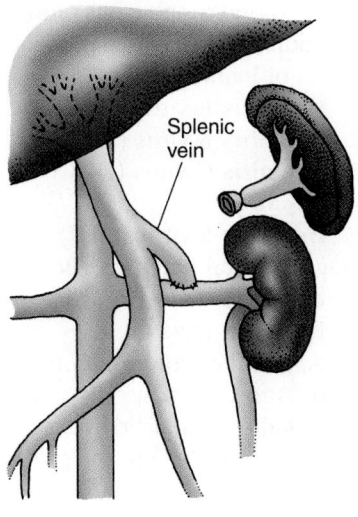

Portal vein

Spleen

Splenic vein

Left renal vein

Inferior vena cava

Splenic vein

▲ **FIGURE 56-7** Surgical shunting diverts portal venous blood flow from the liver to decrease portal and esophageal pressure. (From Ignatavicius, D., & Workman, M. [2006]. *Medical-surgical nursing: Critical thinking for collaborative care* [5th ed.]. St. Louis: Saunders.)

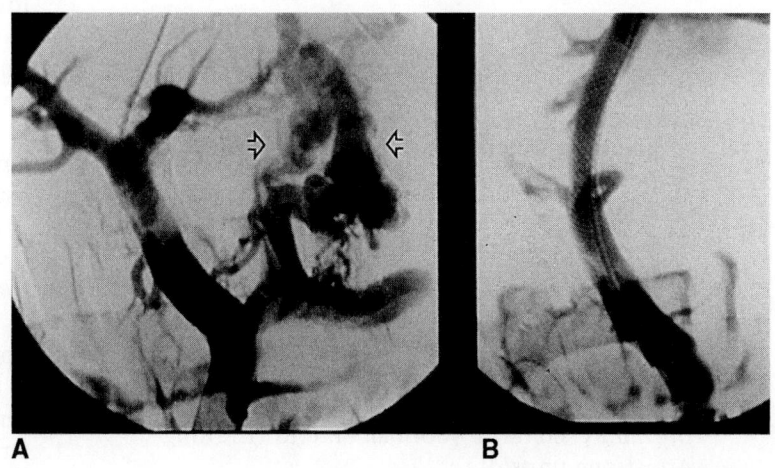

▲ **FIGURE 56-8** Total portal diversion after transjugular intrahepatic portosystemic shunt (TIPS). **A,** Portal venogram before TIPS shows filling of large esophageal varices *(arrows).* **B,** After insertion of a TIPS, flow to varices is eliminated. Intrahepatic portal vein flow is now reversed, with the direction of intrahepatic flow toward the TIPS. (From Lewis, S., Heitkemper, M., Dirksen, S., O'Brien, P., & Bucher, L. [2007]. *Medical-surgical nursing: Assessment and management of clinical problems* [7th ed.]. St. Louis: Mosby.)

A   B

2. Complications include chest pain, pleural effusion, aspiration pneumonia, esophageal stricture, and perforation of the esophagus.
E. Endoscopic variceal ligation
1. The procedure involves ligation of the varices with an elastic rubber band.
2. Sloughing, followed by superficial ulceration, occurs in the area of ligation within 3 to 7 days.
F. Shunting procedures
1. Description: Shunt blood away from the **esophageal varices**
2. Portacaval shunt involves anastomosis of the portal vein to the inferior vena cava, diverting blood from the portal system to the systemic circulation (Fig. 56-7)
3. Distal splenorenal shunt (see Fig. 56-7)
    a. The shunt involves anastomosis of the splenic vein to the left renal vein.

    b. The spleen conducts blood from the high pressure varices to the low pressure renal vein.
4. Mesocaval shunting involves a side anastomosis of the superior mesenteric vein to the proximal end of the inferior vena cava.
5. Transjugular intrahepatic portosystemic shunt (TIPS; Fig. 56-8)
    a. The nonsurgical procedure uses the normal vascular anatomy of the liver to create a shunt with the use of a metallic stent.
    b. The shunt is between the portal and systemic venous system in the liver and is aimed at relieving **portal hypertension**.

XV. HEPATITIS

A. Description
1. Inflammation of the liver caused by a virus, bacteria, or exposure to medications or hepatotoxins

2. The goals of treatment include resting the inflamed liver to reduce metabolic demands and increasing the blood supply, thus promoting cellular regeneration and preventing complications.

B. Types of **hepatitis**
1. **Hepatitis** A virus (HAV)
2. **Hepatitis** B virus (HBV)
3. **Hepatitis** C virus (HCV)
4. **Hepatitis** D virus (HDV)
5. **Hepatitis** E virus (HEV)

C. Stages of viral **hepatitis** (Box 56-12)

D. Assessment
1. Preicteric stage
   a. Flu-like symptoms—malaise, fatigue
   b. Anorexia, nausea, vomiting, diarrhea
   c. Pain—headache, muscle aches, polyarthritis
   d. Serum bilirubin and enzyme levels are elevated.
2. Icteric stage
   a. Jaundice
   b. Pruritus
   c. Dark or tea-colored urine
   d. Clay colored stools
   e. Decrease in preicteric-phase symptoms
3. Posticteric stage
   a. Increased energy levels
   b. Subsiding of pain
   c. Minimal to absent gastrointestinal symptoms
   d. Serum bilirubin and enzyme levels return to normal.

E. Laboratory assessment
1. Alanine aminotransferase level: Elevated into the thousands (normal, 4 to 36 international units/L)
2. Aspartate aminotransferase level: Elevated into the thousands (normal, 8 to 33 units/L).
3. Alkaline phosphatase levels: May be normal or mildly elevated (normal, 4.5 to 13 King-Armstrong units/dL).
4. Total bilirubin levels: Elevated in the serum and urine (normal, lower than 1.5 mg/dL)

Box 56-12 Stages of Viral Hepatitis

Preicteric Stage
The first stage of hepatitis preceding the appearance of jaundice; includes flu-like symptoms

Icteric Stage
The second stage of hepatitis; includes the appearance of jaundice and associated symptoms such as elevated bilirubin levels, dark or tea-colored urine, and clay-colored stools

Posticteric Stage
The convalescent stage of hepatitis, in which the jaundice decreases and the color of the urine and stool return to normal

---

XVI. HEPATITIS A

A. Description
1. Formerly known as infectious **hepatitis**
2. Commonly seen during the fall and early winter

B. Individuals at increased risk
1. Commonly seen in young children
2. Individuals in institutionalized settings
3. Health care personnel

C. Transmission
1. Fecal-oral route
2. Person-to-person contact
3. Parenteral
4. Contaminated fruits, vegetables, or uncooked shellfish
5. Contaminated water or milk
6. Poorly washed utensils

D. Incubation and infectious period
1. Incubation period is 2 to 6 weeks.
2. Infectious period is 2 to 3 weeks before and 1 week after development of jaundice.

E. Testing
1. Infection is established by the presence of HAV antibodies (anti-HAV) in the blood.
2. Immunoglobulin M (IgM) and IgG are normally present in the blood, and increased levels indicate infection and inflammation.
3. Ongoing inflammation of the liver is evidenced by the presence of elevated levels of IgM antibodies, which persist in the blood for 4 to 6 weeks.
4. Previous infection is indicated by the presence of elevated levels of IgG antibodies.

F. Complication: Fulminant (severe acute and often fatal) **hepatitis**

G. Prevention
1. Strict handwashing
2. Stool precautions
3. Treatment of municipal water supplies
4. Serological screening of food handlers
5. **Hepatitis** A vaccine (Havrix VAQTA)
6. Immune globulin: For individuals exposed to HAV who have never received the **hepatitis** A vaccine; administer immune globulin during the period of incubation and within 2 weeks of exposure.
7. Immune globulin and **hepatitis** A vaccine are recommended for household members and sexual contacts of individuals with **hepatitis** A.
8. Preexposure prophylaxis with immunoglobulin is recommended to individuals traveling to countries with poor or uncertain sanitation conditions.

⚠ Strict and frequent handwashing is key to preventing the spread of all types of hepatitis.

XVII. HEPATITIS B

A. Description
1. **Hepatitis** B is nonseasonal.
2. All age groups are affected.

B. Individuals at increased risk
1. IV drug user
2. Clients undergoing long-term hemodialysis
3. Health care personnel

C. Transmission
1. Blood or body fluid contact
2. Infected blood products
3. Infected saliva or semen
4. Contaminated needles
5. Sexual contact
6. Parenteral
7. Perinatal period
8. Blood or body fluids contact at birth

D. Incubation period: 6 to 24 weeks

E. Testing
1. Infection is established by the presence of **hepatitis** B antigen-antibody systems in the blood.
2. Presence of **hepatitis** B surface antigen (HBsAg) is the serological marker to establish the diagnosis of **hepatitis** B.
3. The client is considered infectious if these antigens are present in the blood.
4. If the serological marker (HBsAg) is present after 6 months, it indicates a carrier state or chronic **hepatitis**.
5. Normally, the serological marker (HBsAg) level declines and disappears after the acute **hepatitis** B episode.
6. The presence of antibodies to HBsAg (anti-HBs) indicates recovery and immunity to **hepatitis** B.
7. **Hepatitis** B early antigen (HBeAg) is detected in the blood about 1 week after the appearance of HBsAg and its presence determines the infective state of the client.

F. Complications
1. Fulminant **hepatitis**
2. Chronic liver disease
3. **Cirrhosis**
4. Primary hepatocellular carcinoma

G. Prevention
1. Strict handwashing
2. Screening blood donors
3. Testing of all pregnant women
4. Needle precautions
5. Avoiding intimate sexual contact if test for **hepatitis** B surface antigen (HBsAg) is positive.
6. **Hepatitis** B vaccine: Engerix-B (adult), Recombivax HB (pediatric);there is also an adult vaccine that protects against **hepatitis** A and B known as Twinrix.
7. **Hepatitis** B immune globulin is for individuals exposed to HBV through sexual contact or through the percutaneous or transmucosal routes who have never had **hepatitis** B and have never received **hepatitis** B vaccine.

XVIII. HEPATITIS C

A. Description
1. **Hepatitis** C virus infection occurs year-round.
2. Infection can occur in any age group.
3. Infection with HCV is common among IV drug users and is the major cause of post-transfusion **hepatitis**.
4. Risk factors are similar to those for HBV because **hepatitis** C is also transmitted parenterally.

B. Individuals at increased risk
1. Parenteral drug users
2. Clients receiving frequent transfusions
3. Health care personnel

C. Transmission: Same as for HBV, primarily through blood

D. Incubation period: 5 to 10 weeks

E. Testing: Anti-HCV is the antibody to HCV and is measured to detect chronic states of **hepatitis** C.

F. Complications
1. Chronic liver disease
2. **Cirrhosis**
3. Primary hepatocellular carcinoma

G. Prevention
1. Strict handwashing
2. Needle precautions
3. Screening of blood donors

XIX. HEPATITIS D

A. Description
1. **Hepatitis** D is common in the Mediterranean and Middle Eastern areas.
2. **Hepatitis** D occurs with **hepatitis** B and causes infection only in the presence of active HBV infection.
3. Coinfection with the delta agent (HDV) intensifies the acute symptoms of **hepatitis** B.
4. Transmission and risk of infection are the same as for HBV via contact with blood and blood products.
5. Prevention of HBV infection with vaccine also prevents HDV infection, because HDV depends on HBV for replication.

B. High-risk individuals
1. Drug users
2. Clients receiving hemodialysis
3. Clients receiving frequent blood transfusions

C. Transmission: Same as for HBV

D. Incubation period: 7 to 8 weeks

E. Testing: Serological HDV determination is made by detection of the **hepatitis** D antigen (HDAg) early in the course of the infection and by detection of anti-HDV antibody in the later disease stages.

> **Box 56-13 Home Care Instructions About Hepatitis**
>
> Handwashing must be strict and frequent.
> Do not share bathrooms unless the client strictly adheres to personal hygiene measures.
> Individual washcloths, towels, drinking and eating utensils, and toothbrushes and razors must be labeled and identified.
> The client must not prepare food for other family members.
> The client should avoid alcohol and over-the-counter medications, particularly acetaminophen (Tylenol) and sedatives, because these medications are hepatotoxic.
> The client should increase activity gradually to prevent fatigue.
> The client should consume small, frequent meals consisting of high-carbohydrate, low-fat foods.
> The client is not to donate blood.
>
> The client may maintain normal contact with persons as long as proper personal hygiene is maintained.
> Close personal contact such as kissing should be discouraged until hepatitis B surface antigen test results are negative.
> The client is to avoid sexual activity until hepatitis B surface antigen results are negative.
> The client needs to carry a Medic-Alert card noting the date of hepatitis onset.
> The client needs to inform other health professionals, such as medical or dental personnel, of the onset of hepatitis.
> The client needs to keep follow-up appointments with the health care provider.

F. Complications
　　1. Chronic liver disease
　　2. Fulminant **hepatitis**
G. Prevention: Because **hepatitis** D must coexist with **hepatitis B**, the precautions that help prevent **hepatitis** B are also useful in preventing delta **hepatitis**.

XX. HEPATITIS E

A. Description
　　1. **Hepatitis** E is a waterborne virus.
　　2. **Hepatitis** E is prevalent in areas where sewage disposal is inadequate or where communal bathing in contaminated rivers is practiced.
　　3. Risk of infection is the same as for HAV.
　　4. Infection with HEV presents as a mild disease except in infected women in the third trimester of pregnancy, who have a high mortality rate.
B. Individuals with increased risk
　　1. Travelers to countries that have a high incidence of **hepatitis** E such as India, Burma (Myanmar), Afghanistan, Algeria, and Mexico
　　2. Eating or drinking of food or water contaminated with the virus
C. Transmission: Same as for HAV
D. Incubation period: 2 to 9 weeks
E. Testing: Specific serological tests for HEV include detection of IgM and IgG antibodies to **hepatitis** E (anti-HEV).
F. Complications
　　1. High mortality rate in pregnant women
　　2. Fetal demise
G. Prevention
　　1. Strict handwashing
　　2. Treatment of water supplies and sanitation measures

XXI. HEPATITIS G

A. **Hepatitis** G is non-A, non-B, non-C **hepatitis**.
B. Autoantibodies are absent.

C. Risk factors are similar to those for **hepatitis** C.
D. **Hepatitis** G virus has been found in some blood donors, IV drug users, hemodialysis clients, and clients with hemophilia; however, **hepatitis** G virus does not appear to cause significant liver disease.

XXII. CLIENT AND FAMILY HOME CARE INSTRUCTIONS FOR HEPATITIS
(Box 56-13)

XXIII. PANCREATITIS

A. Description
　　1. Acute or chronic inflammation of the pancreas, with associated escape of pancreatic enzymes into surrounding tissue
　　2. Acute **pancreatitis** occurs suddenly as one attack or can be recurrent, with resolutions.
　　3. Chronic **pancreatitis** is a continual inflammation and destruction of the pancreas, with scar tissue replacing pancreatic tissue.
　　4. Precipitating factors include trauma, the use of alcohol, biliary tract disease, viral or bacterial disease, hyperlipidemia, hypercalcemia, cholelithiasis, hyperparathyroidism, ischemic vascular disease, and peptic ulcer disease.
B. Acute **pancreatitis**
　　1. Assessment
　　　　a. Abdominal pain, including a sudden onset at a midepigastric or left upper quadrant location with radiation to the back
　　　　b. Pain aggravated by a fatty meal, alcohol, or lying in a recumbent position
　　　　c. Abdominal tenderness and guarding
　　　　d. Nausea and vomiting
　　　　e. Weight loss
　　　　f. Absent or decreased bowel sounds
　　　　g. Elevated white blood cell count, and glucose, bilirubin, alkaline phosphatase, and urinary amylase levels
　　　　h. Elevated serum lipase and amylase levels

Cullen's sign is the discoloration of the abdomen and periumbilical area. Turner's sign is the bluish discoloration of the flanks. Both signs are indicative of pancreatitis.

2. Interventions
   a. Maintain NPO status and maintain hydration with IV fluids as prescribed.
   b. Administer parenteral nutrition for severe nutritional depletion.
   c. Administer supplemental preparations and vitamins and minerals to increase caloric intake if prescribed.
   d. Maintain nasogastric tube to decrease gastric distention and suppress pancreatic secretion.
   e. Administer meperidine hydrochloride (Demerol) as prescribed for pain because it causes less incidence of smooth muscle spasm of the pancreatic ducts and sphincter of Oddi than some other medications.
   f. Administer antacids as prescribed to neutralize gastric secretions.
   g. Administer H_2-receptor antagonists or proton pump inhibitors as prescribed to decrease hydrochloric acid production and prevent activation of pancreatic enzymes.
   h. Administer anticholinergics as prescribed to decrease vagal stimulation, decrease gastrointestinal motility, and inhibit pancreatic enzyme secretion.
   i. Instruct the client in the importance of avoiding alcohol.
   j. Instruct the client in the importance of follow-up visits with the physician.
   k. Instruct the client to notify the physician if acute abdominal pain, jaundice, clay-colored stools, or dark-colored urine develops.
C. Chronic **pancreatitis**
   1. Assessment
      a. Abdominal pain and tenderness
      b. Left upper quadrant mass
      c. Steatorrhea and foul-smelling stools that may increase in volume as pancreatic insufficiency increases
      d. Weight loss
      e. Muscle wasting
      f. Jaundice
      g. Signs and symptoms of diabetes mellitus
   2. Interventions
      a. Instruct the client in the prescribed dietary measures (fat and protein intake may be limited).
      b. Instruct the client to avoid heavy meals.
      c. Instruct the client about the importance of avoiding alcohol.
      d. Provide supplemental preparations and vitamins and minerals to increase caloric intake.

   e. Administer pancreatic enzymes as prescribed to aid in the digestion and absorption of fat and protein.
   f. Administer insulin or oral hypoglycemic medications as prescribed to control diabetes mellitus, if present.
   g. Instruct the client in the use of pancreatic enzyme medications.
   h. Instruct the client in the treatment plan for glucose management.
   i. Instruct the client to notify the physician if increased steatorrhea, abdominal distention or cramping, or skin breakdown develops.
   j. Instruct the client in the importance of follow-up visits.

XXIV. PANCREATIC TUMORS, INTESTINAL TUMORS, AND BOWEL OBSTRUCTIONS (See Chapter 52)

XXV. ULCERATIVE COLITIS

A. Description
   1. An ulcerative and inflammatory disease of the bowel that results in poor absorption of nutrients.
   2. Commonly begins in the rectum and spreads upward toward the cecum
   3. The colon becomes edematous and may develop bleeding lesions and ulcers; the ulcers may lead to perforation.
   4. Scar tissue develops and causes loss of elasticity and loss of the ability to absorb nutrients.
   5. Colitis is characterized by various periods of remissions and exacerbations.
   6. Acute **ulcerative colitis** results in vascular congestion, hemorrhage, edema, and ulceration of the bowel mucosa.
   7. Chronic **ulcerative colitis** causes muscular hypertrophy, fat deposits, and fibrous tissue, with bowel thickening, shortening, and narrowing.
B. Assessment
   1. Anorexia
   2. Weight loss
   3. Malaise
   4. Abdominal tenderness and cramping
   5. Severe diarrhea that may contain blood and mucus
   6. Malnutrition, dehydration, and electrolyte imbalances
   7. Anemia
   8. Vitamin K deficiency
C. Interventions
   1. Acute phase: Maintain NPO status and administer fluids and electrolytes intravenously or via parenteral nutrition as prescribed.
   2. Restrict the client's activity to reduce intestinal activity.
   3. Monitor bowel sounds and for abdominal tenderness and cramping.

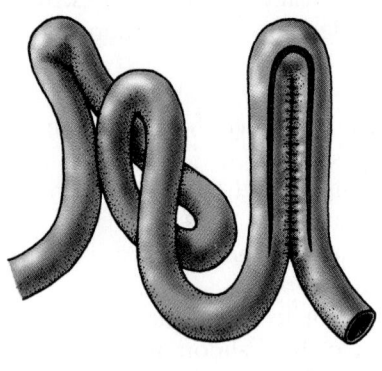 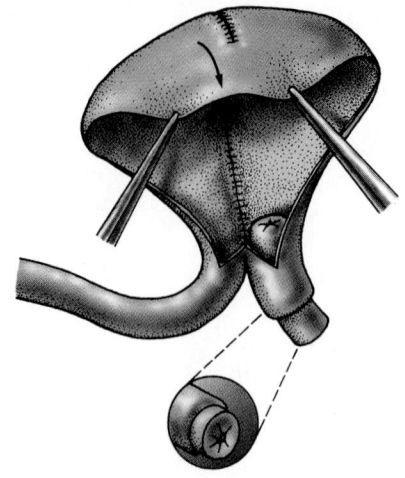 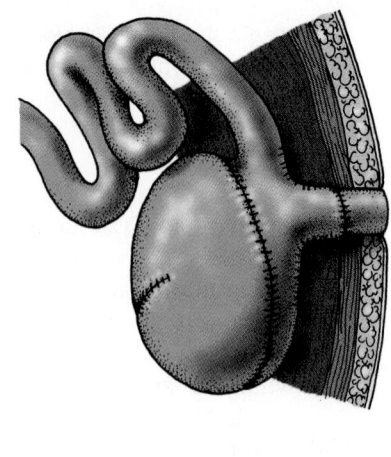

1. A reservoir, in which the client will retain stool until draining it, is constructed from a loop of ileum folded and sutured together, then cut.

2. A portion of the ileum is intussuscepted to form a nipple valve, and the upper part of the stitched and cut ileum is pulled down and sutured to form a pouch.

3. The nipple valve, which shuts tight against pressure from a filled pouch, is pulled through the stoma and sutured flush with the abdomen.

▲ **FIGURE 56-9** Creation of a Kock (continent) ileostomy. (From Ignatavicius, D., & Workman, M. [2010]. *Medical-surgical nursing: Patient-centered collaborative care* [5th ed.]. St. Louis: Saunders.)

4. Monitor stools, noting color, consistency, and the presence or absence of blood.
5. Monitor for bowel perforation, peritonitis (see Box 56-3), and hemorrhage.
6. Following the acute phase, the diet progresses from clear liquids to a low-fiber diet as tolerated.
7. Instruct the client about diet; usually a low-fiber, high-protein diet with vitamins and iron supplements are prescribed.
8. Instruct the client to avoid gas-forming foods, milk products, and foods such as whole wheat grains, nuts, raw fruits and vegetables, pepper, alcohol, and caffeine-containing products.
9. Instruct the client to avoid smoking.
10. Administer medications as prescribed, which may include a combination of medications such as salicylate compounds, corticosteroids, immunosuppressants, and antidiarrheals.

D. Surgical interventions
1. Total proctocolectomy with permanent ileostomy
   a. The procedure is curative and involves the removal of the entire colon (colon, rectum, and anus, with anal closure).
   b. The end of the terminal ileum forms the stoma, which is located in the right lower quadrant.
2. **Kock ileostomy** (continent ileostomy) (Fig. 56-9)
   a. The **Kock ileostomy** is an intra-abdominal pouch that stores the feces and is constructed from the terminal ileum.
   b. The pouch is connected to the stoma with a nipple-like valve constructed from a portion of the ileum; the stoma is flush with the skin.

   c. A catheter is used to empty the pouch, and a small dressing or adhesive bandage is worn over the stoma between emptyings.
3. Ileoanal reservoir (Fig. 56-10)
   a. Creation of an ileoanal reservoir is a two-stage procedure that involves the excision of the rectal mucosa, an abdominal colectomy, construction of a reservoir to the anal canal, and a temporary loop ileostomy.
   b. The ileostomy is closed in 3 to 4 months after the capacity of the reservoir is increased and has had time to heal.
4. Ileoanal anastomosis (ileorectostomy)
   a. Ileorectostomy does not require an ileostomy.
   b. A 12- to 15-cm rectal stump is left after the colon is removed, and the small intestine is inserted into this rectal sleeve and anastomosed.
   c. Ileorectostomy requires a large, compliant rectum.
5. Preoperative colostomy and ileostomy interventions
   a. Consult with the enterostomal therapist to help identify optimal placement of the ostomy.
   b. Instruct the client to eat a low-fiber diet for 1 to 2 days before surgery as prescribed.
   c. Administer intestinal antiseptics and antibiotics as prescribed to cleanse the bowel and to decrease the bacterial content of the colon.
   d. Administer laxatives and enemas as prescribed.
6. Postoperative colostomy interventions
   a. Place a petrolatum gauze over the stoma as prescribed to keep it moist, followed by a dry sterile dressing if a pouch (external) system is not in place.

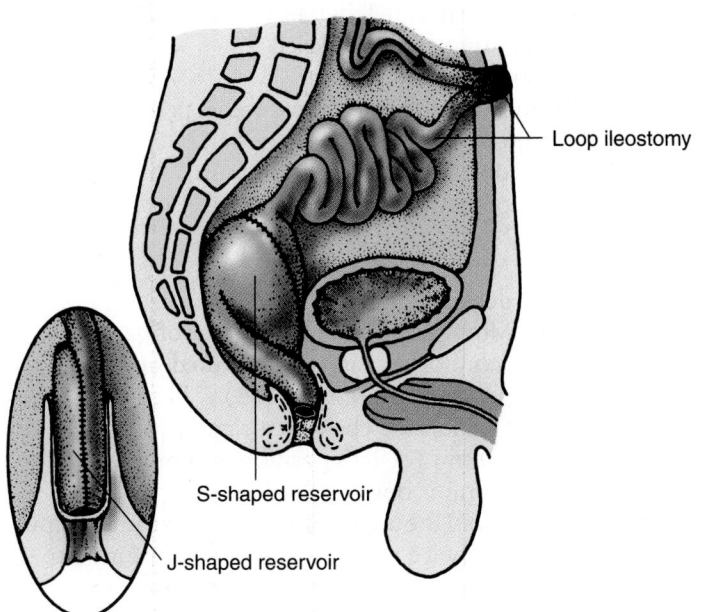
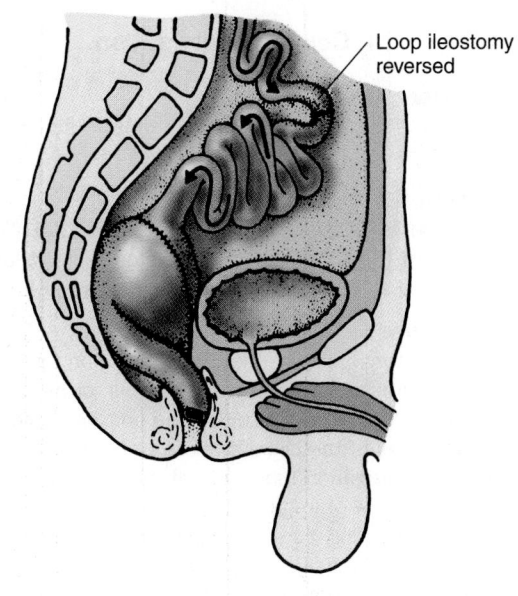

Stage 1.
After removal of the colon, a temporary loop ileostomy is created and an ileoanal reservoir is formed. The reservoir is created in an S-shaped reservoir (using three loops of ileum) or a J-shaped reservoir (suturing a portion of ileum to the rectal cuff, with an upward loop).

Stage 2.
After the reservoir has had time to heal—usually several months—the temporary loop ileostomy is reversed, and stool is allowed to drain into the reservoir.

▲ **FIGURE 56-10** Creation of an ileoanal reservoir. (From Ignatavicius, D., & Workman, M. [2010]. *Medical-surgical nursing: Patient-centered collaborative care* [6th ed.]. St. Louis: Saunders.)

b. Place a pouch system on the stoma as soon as possible.
c. Monitor the stoma for size, unusual bleeding, or necrotic tissue.
d. Monitor for color changes in the stoma.
e. Note that the normal stoma color is pink to bright red and shiny, indicating high vascularity.
f. Note that a pale pink stoma indicates low hemoglobin and hematocrit levels and a purple-black stoma indicates compromised circulation, requiring physician notification.
g. Assess the functioning of the colostomy.
h. Expect that stool is liquid in the immediate postoperative period but becomes more solid depending on the area of the colostomy—ascending colon, liquid; transverse colon, loose to semiformed; and descending colon, close to normal.
i. Monitor the pouch system for proper fit and signs of leakage.
j. Empty the pouch when it is one-third full.
k. Fecal matter should not be allowed to remain on the skin.
l. Administer analgesics and antibiotics as prescribed.
m. Irrigate the perineal wound (if present) as prescribed and monitor for signs of infection.

n. Instruct the client to avoid foods that cause excess gas formation and odor.
o. Instruct the client about stoma care and irrigations as prescribed (Box 56-14).
p. Instruct the client that normal activities may be resumed when approved by the physician.
7. Postoperative ileostomy interventions
a. Note that normal stool is liquid.
b. Monitor for dehydration and electrolyte imbalance.

⚠ A stoma that is purple-black in color indicates compromised circulation, requiring immediate physician notification.

XXVI. CROHN'S DISEASE

A. Description
1. An inflammatory disease that can occur anywhere in the gastrointestinal tract but most often affects the terminal ileum and leads to thickening and scarring, a narrowed lumen, fistulas, ulcerations, and abscesses
2. Characterized by remissions and exacerbations
B. Assessment
1. Fever
2. Cramp-like and colicky pain after meals

Box 56-14 Colostomy Irrigation

Purpose

An enema is given through the stoma to stimulate bowel emptying.

Description

Irrigation is performed by instilling 500 to 1000 mL of lukewarm tap water through the stoma and allowing the water and stool to drain into a collection bag.

Procedure

If ambulatory, position the client sitting on the toilet.

If on bedrest, position the client on his or her side.

Hang the irrigation bag so that the bottom of the bag is at the level of the client's shoulder or slightly higher.

Insert the irrigation tube carefully without force.

Begin the flow of irrigation.

Clamp the tubing if cramping occurs; release the tubing as cramping subsides.

Avoid frequent irrigations, which can lead to loss of fluids and electrolytes.

Perform irrigation at about the same time each day.

Perform irrigation preferably 1 hour after a meal.

To enhance effectiveness of the irrigation, massage the abdomen gently.

---

   3. Diarrhea (semisolid), which may contain mucus and pus
   4. Abdominal distention
   5. Anorexia, nausea, and vomiting
   6. Weight loss
   7. Anemia
   8. Dehydration
   9. Electrolyte imbalances
   10. Malnutrition (may be worse than that seen in **ulcerative colitis**)
C. Interventions: Care is similar to that for the client with **ulcerative colitis**; however, surgery may be necessary but is avoided for as long possible because recurrence of the disease process in the same region is likely to occur.

XXVII. APPENDICITIS

A. Description
   1. Inflammation of the appendix.
   2. When the appendix becomes inflamed or infected, rupture may occur within a matter of hours, leading to peritonitis and sepsis.
B. Assessment
   1. Pain in the periumbilical area that descends to the right lower quadrant
   2. Abdominal pain that is most intense at McBurney's point
   3. Rebound tenderness and abdominal rigidity
   4. Low-grade fever
   5. Elevated white blood cell count
   6. Anorexia, nausea, and vomiting

   7. Client in side-lying position, with abdominal guarding and legs flexed
   8. Constipation or diarrhea
C. Peritonitis: Inflammation of the peritoneum (see Box 56-3)
D. Appendectomy: Surgical removal of the appendix
   1. Preoperative interventions
     a. Maintain NPO status.
     b. Administer fluids intravenously to prevent dehydration.
     c. Monitor for changes in level of pain.
     d. Monitor for signs of ruptured appendix and peritonitis (see Box 56-3).
     e. Position the client in a right side-lying or low to semi-Fowler's position to promote comfort.
     f. Monitor bowel sounds.
     g. Avoid the application of heat to the abdomen.
     h. Apply ice packs to the abdomen for 20 to 30 minutes every hour as prescribed.
     i. Administer antibiotics as prescribed.
     j. Avoid laxatives or enemas.

⚠ Avoid the application of heat to the abdomen of a client with appendicitis. Heat can cause rupture of the appendix leading to peritonitis, a life-threatening condition.

   2. Postoperative interventions
     a. Monitor temperature for signs of infection.
     b. Assess incision for signs of infection such as redness, swelling, and pain.
     c. Maintain NPO status until bowel function has returned.
     d. Advance diet gradually as tolerated and as prescribed, when bowel sounds return.
     e. If rupture of the appendix occurred, expect a Penrose drain to be inserted, or the incision may be left open to heal from the inside out.
     f. Expect that drainage from the Penrose drain may be profuse for the first 12 hours.
     g. Position the client in a right side-lying or low to semi-Fowler's position, with legs flexed, to facilitate drainage.
     h. Change the dressing as prescribed and record the type and amount of drainage.
     i. Perform wound irrigations if prescribed.
     j. Maintain nasogastric suction and patency of the nasogastric tube if present.
     k. Administer antibiotics and analgesics as prescribed.

XXVIII. DIVERTICULOSIS AND DIVERTICULITIS

A. Description
   1. **Diverticulosis**
     a. **Diverticulosis** is an outpouching or herniation of the intestinal mucosa.

b. The disorder can occur in any part of the intestine but is most common in the sigmoid colon.

2. **Diverticulitis**
   a. **Diverticulitis** is the inflammation of one or more diverticula that occurs from penetration of fecal matter through the thin-walled diverticula; it can result in local abscess formation and perforation.
   b. A perforated diverticulum can progress to intra-abdominal perforation with generalized peritonitis.

B. Assessment
   1. Left lower quadrant abdominal pain that increases with coughing, straining, or lifting
   2. Elevated temperature
   3. Nausea and vomiting
   4. Flatulence
   5. Cramp-like pain
   6. Abdominal distention and tenderness
   7. Palpable, tender rectal mass may be present.
   8. Blood in the stools

C. Interventions
   1. Provide bedrest during the acute phase.
   2. Maintain NPO status or provide clear liquids during the acute phase as prescribed.
   3. Introduce a fiber-containing diet gradually, when the inflammation has resolved.
   4. Administer antibiotics, analgesics, and anticholinergics to reduce bowel spasms as prescribed.
   5. Instruct the client to refrain from lifting, straining, coughing, or bending to avoid increased intra-abdominal pressure.
   6. Monitor for perforation (see Box 56-3), hemorrhage, fistulas, and abscesses.
   7. Instruct the client to increase fluid intake to 2500 to 3000 mL daily, unless contraindicated.
   8. Instruct the client to eat soft high-fiber foods, such as whole grains; the client should avoid high-fiber foods when inflammation occurs because these foods will irritate the mucosa further.
   9. Instruct the client to avoid gas-forming foods or foods containing indigestible roughage, seeds, or nuts because these food substances become trapped in diverticula and cause inflammation.
   10. Instruct the client to consume a small amount of bran daily and to take bulk-forming laxatives as prescribed to increase stool mass.

D. Surgical interventions
   1. Colon resection with primary anastomosis may be an option.
   2. Temporary or permanent colostomy may be required for increased bowel inflammation.

XXIX. HEMORRHOIDS

A. Description
   1. Dilated varicose veins of the anal canal
   2. May be internal, external, or prolapsed

3. Internal hemorrhoids lie above the anal sphincter and cannot be seen on inspection of the perianal area.
4. External hemorrhoids lie below the anal sphincter and can be seen on inspection.
5. Prolapsed hemorrhoids can become thrombosed or inflamed.
6. Hemorrhoids are caused from **portal hypertension**, straining, irritation, or increased venous or abdominal pressure.

B. Assessment
   1. Bright red bleeding with defecation
   2. Rectal pain
   3. Rectal itching

C. Interventions
   1. Apply cold packs to the anal-rectal area followed by sitz baths as prescribed.
   2. Apply witch hazel soaks and topical anesthetics as prescribed.
   3. Encourage a high-fiber diet and fluids to promote bowel movements without straining.
   4. Administer stool softeners as prescribed.

D. Surgical interventions: May include ultrasound, sclerotherapy, circular stapling, band ligation, or simple resection of the hemorrhoids (hemorrhoidectomy)

E. Postoperative interventions following hemorrhoidectomy
   1. Assist the client to a prone or side-lying position to prevent bleeding.
   2. Maintain ice packs over the dressing as prescribed until the packing is removed by the physician.
   3. Monitor for urinary retention.
   4. Administer stool softeners as prescribed.
   5. Instruct the client to increase fluids and high-fiber foods.
   6. Instruct the client to limit sitting to short periods of time.
   7. Instruct the client in the use of sitz baths three or four times a day as prescribed.

💿 MORE QUESTIONS ON THE CD!

Practice Questions

614. The nurse is monitoring a client admitted to the hospital with a diagnosis of appendicitis who is scheduled for surgery in 2 hours. The client begins to complain of increased abdominal pain and begins to vomit. On assessment, the nurse notes that the abdomen is distended and bowel sounds are diminished. Which is the appropriate nursing intervention?
   1. Notify the physician.
   2. Administer the prescribed pain medication.
   3. Call and ask the operating room team to perform the surgery as soon as possible.
   4. Reposition the client and apply a heating pad on warm setting to the client's abdomen.

615. The client has been admitted to the hospital with a diagnosis of acute pancreatitis and the nurse is assessing the client's pain. What type of pain is consistent with this diagnosis?
1. Burning and aching, located in the left lower quadrant and radiating to the hip
2. Severe and unrelenting, located in the epigastric area and radiating to the back
3. Burning and aching, located in the epigastric area and radiating to the umbilicus
4. Severe and unrelenting, located in the left lower quadrant and radiating to the groin

616. The nurse is assessing a client who is experiencing an acute episode of cholecystitis. Where should the nurse anticipate the location of the pain?
1. Right lower quadrant, radiating to the back
2. Right lower quadrant, radiating to the umbilicus
3. Right upper quadrant, radiating to the left scapula and shoulder
4. Right upper quadrant, radiating to the right scapula and shoulder

617. The client is admitted to the hospital with viral hepatitis, complaining of "no appetite" and "losing my taste for food." What instruction should the nurse give the client to provide adequate nutrition?
1. Select foods high in fat.
2. Increase intake of fluids, including juices.
3. Eat a good supper when anorexia is not as severe.
4. Eat less often, preferably only three large meals daily.

618. A client has developed hepatitis A after eating contaminated oysters. The nurse assesses the client for which of the following?
1. Malaise
2. Dark stools
3. Weight gain
4. Left upper quadrant discomfort

619. A client has just had a hemorrhoidectomy. What nursing intervention is appropriate for this client?
1. Instruct the client to limit fluid intake to avoid urinary retention.
2. Instruct the client to eat low-fiber foods to decrease the bulk of the stool.
3. Apply and maintain ice packs over the dressing until the packing is removed.
4. Help the client to a Fowler's position to place pressure on the rectal area and decrease bleeding.

620. The nurse is planning to teach the client with gastroesophageal reflux disease about substances that will increase the lower esophageal sphincter pressure. Which item should the nurse include on this list?

1. Coffee
2. Chocolate
3. Fatty foods
4. Nonfat milk

621. The client has undergone esophagogastroduodenoscopy. The nurse places highest priority on which item as part of the client's care plan?
1. Monitoring the temperature
2. Monitoring complaints of heartburn
3. Giving warm gargles for a sore throat
4. Assessing for the return of the gag reflex

622. The nurse has taught the client about an upcoming endoscopic retrograde cholangiopancreatography procedure. The nurse determines that the client needs further information if the client makes which statement?
1. "I know I must sign the consent form."
2. "I hope the throat spray keeps me from gagging."
3. "I'm glad I don't have to lie still for this procedure."
4. "I'm glad some IV medication will be given to relax me."

623. The physician has determined that the client with hepatitis has contracted the infection from contaminated food. The nurse understands that this client is most likely experiencing what type of hepatitis?
1. Hepatitis A
2. Hepatitis B
3. Hepatitis C
4. Hepatitis D

624. The nurse is caring for a client with a diagnosis of chronic gastritis. The nurse monitors the client knowing that this client is at risk for which vitamin deficiency?
1. Vitamin A
2. Vitamin B_{12}
3. Vitamin C
4. Vitamin E

625. The nurse is assessing a client 24 hours following a cholecystectomy. The nurse notes that the T-tube has drained 750 mL of green-brown drainage since the surgery. Which nursing intervention is appropriate?
1. Clamp the T-tube.
2. Irrigate the T-tube.
3. Notify the physician.
4. Document the findings.

626. The nurse is monitoring a client with a diagnosis of peptic ulcer. Which assessment finding would most likely indicate perforation of the ulcer?

1. Bradycardia
2. Numbness in the legs
3. Nausea and vomiting
4. A rigid, board-like abdomen

627. The nurse is caring for a client following a Billroth II procedure. Which postoperative prescription should the nurse question and verify?
1. Leg exercises
2. Early ambulation
3. Irrigating the nasogastric tube
4. Coughing and deep-breathing exercises

628. The nurse is providing discharge instructions to a client following gastrectomy and instructs the client to take which measure to assist in preventing dumping syndrome?
1. Ambulate following a meal.
2. Eat high carbohydrate foods.
3. Limit the fluids taken with meals.
4. Sit in a high Fowler's position during meals.

629. The nurse is monitoring a client for the early signs and symptoms of dumping syndrome. Which of the following indicate this occurrence?
1. Sweating and pallor
2. Bradycardia and indigestion
3. Double vision and chest pain
4. Abdominal cramping and pain

630. The nurse is reviewing the record of a client with Crohn's disease. Which stool characteristic should the nurse expect to note documented in the client's record?
1. Diarrhea
2. Chronic constipation
3. Constipation alternating with diarrhea
4. Stool constantly oozing from the rectum

631. The nurse is reviewing the record of a client with a diagnosis of cirrhosis and notes that there is documentation of the presence of asterixis. How should the nurse assess for its presence?
1. Dorsiflex the client's foot.
2. Measure the abdominal girth.
3. Ask the client to extend the arms.
4. Instruct the client to lean forward.

632. The nurse is reviewing the laboratory results in a client with cirrhosis and notes that the ammonia level is elevated. Which diet does the nurse anticipate to be prescribed for this client?
1. Low-protein diet
2. High-protein diet
3. Moderate-fat diet
4. High-carbohydrate diet

633. The nurse is doing an admission assessment on a client with a history of duodenal ulcer. To determine whether the problem is currently active, the nurse should assess the client for which symptom(s) of duodenal ulcer?
1. Weight loss
2. Nausea and vomiting
3. Pain relieved by food intake
4. Pain radiating down the right arm

634. The client with hiatal hernia chronically experiences heartburn following meals. The nurse plans to teach the client to avoid which action because it is contraindicated with a hiatal hernia?
1. Lying recumbent following meals
2. Taking in small, frequent, bland meals
3. Raising the head of bed on 6-inch blocks
4. Taking H_2-receptor antagonist medication

635. The nurse is assessing for stoma prolapse in a client with a colostomy. What should the nurse observe if stoma prolapse occurs?
1. Protruding stoma
2. Sunken and hidden stoma
3. Narrowed and flattened stoma
4. Dark- and bluish-colored stoma

636. The client had a new colostomy created 2 days earlier and is beginning to pass malodorous flatus from the stoma. What is the correct interpretation by the nurse?
1. This is a normal, expected event.
2. The client is experiencing early signs of ischemic bowel.
3. The client should not have the nasogastric tube removed.
4. This indicates inadequate preoperative bowel preparation.

637. The client has just had surgery to create an ileostomy. The nurse assesses the client in the immediate postoperative period for which most frequent complication of this type of surgery?
1. Folate deficiency
2. Malabsorption of fat
3. Intestinal obstruction
4. Fluid and electrolyte imbalance

638. The nurse is doing preoperative teaching with the client who is about to undergo creation of a Kock pouch. The nurse interprets that the client has the best understanding of the nature of the surgery if the client makes which statement?
1. "I will be able to pass stool by the rectum eventually."
2. "The drainage from this type of ostomy will be formed."

3. "I will need to drain the pouch regularly with a catheter."
4. "I will need to wear a drainage bag for the rest of my life."

Alternate Item Format: Multiple Response

639. A nurse is reviewing the prescription for a client admitted to the hospital with a diagnosis of acute pancreatitis. Which of the following interventions would the nurse expect to be prescribed for the client? **Select all that apply.**

❑ 1. Administer antacids as prescribed.
❑ 2. Encourage coughing and deep breathing.
❑ 3. Administer anticholinergics as prescribed.
❑ 4. Give small, frequent high-calorie feedings.
❑ 5. Maintain the client in a supine and flat position.
❑ 6. Give Meperidine (Demerol) as prescribed for pain.

ANSWERS

614. 1

Rationale: Based on the signs and symptoms presented in the question, the nurse should suspect peritonitis and notify the physician. Administering pain medication is not an appropriate intervention. Heat should never be applied to the abdomen of a client with suspected appendicitis because of the risk of rupture. Scheduling surgical time is not within the scope of nursing practice, although the physician probably would perform the surgery earlier than the prescheduled time.

Test-Taking Strategy: Use the process of elimination. Options 3 and 4 can be eliminated easily. Focus on the signs and symptoms in the question and consider the complications that can occur with appendicitis. Noting that the signs presented in the question indicate a complication will assist in directing you to option 1. Review care of the client with appendicitis if you had difficulty with this question.

Level of Cognitive Ability: Applying
Client Needs: Physiological Integrity
Integrated Process: Nursing Process—Implementation
Content Area: Adult Health—Gastrointestinal
Reference: Swearingen, P. (2008). *All-in-one care planning resource: Medical-surgical, pediatric, maternity, & psychiatric nursing care plans* (2nd ed., pp. 430–431). St. Louis: Mosby.

615. 2

Rationale: The pain associated with acute pancreatitis is often severe and unrelenting, is located in the epigastric region, and radiates to the back. The other options are incorrect.

Test-Taking Strategy: Use the process of elimination. Noting the strategic word *acute* will assist in eliminating options 1 and 3. From the remaining options, recalling the anatomical location of the pancreas will direct you to option 2. Review the manifestations in acute pancreatitis if you had difficulty with this question.

Level of Cognitive Ability: Understanding
Client Needs: Physiological Integrity
Integrated Process: Nursing Process—Assessment
Content Area: Adult Health—Gastrointestinal
Reference: Swearingen, P. (2008). *All-in-one care planning resource: Medical-surgical, pediatric, maternity, & psychiatric nursing care plans* (2nd ed., p. 469). St. Louis: Mosby.

616. 4

Rationale: During an acute episode of cholecystitis, the client may complain of severe right upper quadrant pain that radiates to the right scapula and shoulder. This is determined by the pattern of dermatomes in the body. The other options are incorrect.

Test-Taking Strategy: Use the process of elimination. Recalling the anatomical location of the gallbladder will direct you to option 4. Review the characteristics of the pain associated with cholecystitis if you had difficulty with this question.

Level of Cognitive Ability: Understanding
Client Needs: Physiological Integrity
Integrated Process: Nursing Process—Assessment
Content Area: Adult Health—Gastrointestinal
References: Ignatavicius, D., & Workman, M. (2010). *Medical-surgical nursing: Patient-centered collaborative care* (6th ed., p. 1368). St. Louis: Saunders.

Swearingen, P. (2008). *All-in-one care planning resource: Medical-surgical, pediatric, maternity, & psychiatric nursing care plans* (2nd ed., p. 433). St. Louis: Mosby.

617. 2

Rationale: Although no special diet is required to treat viral hepatitis, it is generally recommended that clients consume a low-fat diet because fat may be tolerated poorly because of decreased bile production. Small frequent meals are preferable and may even prevent nausea. Frequently, appetite is better in the morning, so it is easier to eat a good breakfast. An adequate fluid intake of 2500 to 3000 mL/day that includes nutritional juices is also important.

Test-Taking Strategy: Use the process of elimination. Knowledge regarding the nutritional problems associated with hepatitis and focusing on the client's complaints will assist in directing you to the correct option. Review measures to provide adequate nutrition in the client with hepatitis if you had difficulty with this question.

Level of Cognitive Ability: Applying
Client Needs: Physiological Integrity
Integrated Process: Teaching and Learning
Content Area: Adult Health—Gastrointestinal
References: Ignatavicius, D., & Workman, M. (2010). *Medical-surgical nursing: Patient-centered collaborative care* (6th ed., p. 1360). St. Louis: Saunders.

Swearingen, P. (2008). *All-in-one care planning resource: Medical-surgical, pediatric, maternity, & psychiatric nursing care plans* (2nd ed., p. 464). St. Louis: Mosby.

618. 1

Rationale: Hepatitis causes gastrointestinal symptoms such as anorexia, nausea, right upper quadrant discomfort, and weight loss. Fatigue and malaise are common. Stools will be light- or clay-colored if conjugated bilirubin is unable to flow out of the liver because of inflammation or obstruction of the bile ducts.

Test-Taking Strategy: Use the process of elimination. Recalling the function of the liver will easily direct you to option 1. Remember that fatigue and malaise are common. If you had difficulty with this question, review the signs and symptoms of hepatitis.

Level of Cognitive Ability: Analyzing
Client Needs: Physiological Integrity
Integrated Process: Nursing Process—Assessment
Content Area: Adult Health—Gastrointestinal
Reference: Ignatavicius, D., & Workman, M. (2010). *Medical-surgical nursing: Patient-centered collaborative care* (6th ed., p. 1359). St. Louis: Saunders.

619. 3

Rationale: Nursing interventions after a hemorrhoidectomy are aimed at management of pain and avoidance of bleeding. An ice pack will increase comfort and decrease bleeding. Options 1, 2, and 4 are incorrect interventions.

Test-Taking Strategy: Use the process of elimination. Decreasing fluid intake and avoiding high-fiber foods will cause difficulty with defecation because of hard stool, eliminating options 1 and 2. Fowler's position will increase pressure in the rectal area, causing increased bleeding and increased pain, eliminating option 4. Knowing that an ice pack will decrease swelling and cause vasoconstriction leads you to option 3. Review care of the client following hemorrhoidectomy if you had difficulty with this question.

Level of Cognitive Ability: Applying
Client Needs: Physiological Integrity
Integrated Process: Nursing Process—Implementation
Content Area: Adult Health—Gastrointestinal
Reference: Black, J., & Hawks, J. (2009). *Medical-surgical nursing: Clinical management for positive outcomes* (8th ed., p. 722). St. Louis: Saunders.

620. 4

Rationale: Foods that increase lower esophageal sphincter (LES) pressure will decrease reflux and lessen the symptoms of gastroesophageal reflux disease (GERD). The food that will increase LES pressure is nonfat milk. The other substances listed decrease LES pressure, thus increasing reflux symptoms. Aggravating substances include chocolate, coffee, fatty foods, and alcohol.

Test-Taking Strategy: Use the process of elimination and knowledge of the effect of various foods on LES pressure and GERD. However, if you were unsure, select the option that identifies the most healthful food item. Review the dietary regimen for a client with GERD if you had difficulty with this question.

Level of Cognitive Ability: Applying
Client Needs: Physiological Integrity
Integrated Process: Teaching and Learning
Content Area: Adult Health—Gastrointestinal
References: Ignatavicius, D., & Workman, M. (2010). *Medical-surgical nursing: Patient-centered collaborative care* (6th ed., p. 1244). St. Louis: Saunders.

Nix, S. (2009). *Williams' basic nutrition and diet therapy* (13th ed., p. 342). St. Louis: Mosby.

621. 4

Rationale: The nurse places highest priority on assessing for return of the gag reflex. This assessment addresses the client's airway. The nurse also monitors the client's vital signs and for a sudden increase in temperature, which could indicate perforation of the gastrointestinal tract. This complication would be accompanied by other signs as well, such as pain. Monitoring for sore throat and heartburn are also important; however, the client's airway is the priority.

Test-Taking Strategy: Use the ABCs—airway, breathing, and circulation. Note the strategic words *highest priority*. Option 4 addresses the airway. Review care of the client following esophagogastroduodenoscopy if you had difficulty with this question.

Level of Cognitive Ability: Applying
Client Needs: Safe and Effective Care Environment
Integrated Process: Nursing Process—Planning
Content Area: Adult Health—Gastrointestinal
References: Ignatavicius, D., & Workman, M. (2010). *Medical-surgical nursing: Patient-centered collaborative care* (6th ed., p. 1227). St. Louis: Saunders.

Pagana, K., & Pagana, T. (2009). *Mosby's diagnostic and laboratory test reference* (9th ed., p. 407). St. Louis: Mosby.

622. 3

Rationale: The client does have to lie still for endoscopic retrograde cholangiopancreatography (ERCP), which takes about 1 hour to perform. The client also has to sign a consent form. Intravenous sedation is given to relax the client, and an anesthetic spray is used to help keep the client from gagging as the endoscope is passed.

Test-Taking Strategy: Note the strategic words *needs further information*. These words indicate a negative event query and ask you to select an option that is incorrect. Invasive procedures require consent, so option 1 can be eliminated. Noting the name of the procedure and considering the anatomical location will assist you in eliminating options 2 and 4. Review this procedure if you had difficulty with this question.

Level of Cognitive Ability: Evaluating
Client Needs: Physiological Integrity
Integrated Process: Teaching and Learning
Content Area: Adult Health—Gastrointestinal
References: Ignatavicius, D., & Workman, M. (2010). *Medical-surgical nursing: Patient-centered collaborative care* (6th ed., p. 1227). St. Louis: Saunders.

Pagana, K., & Pagana, T. (2009). *Mosby's diagnostic and laboratory test reference* (9th ed., pp. 389-392). St. Louis: Mosby.

623. 1

Rationale: Hepatitis A is transmitted by the fecal-oral route via contaminated food or infected food handlers. Hepatitis B, C, and D are transmitted most commonly via infected blood or body fluids.

Test-Taking Strategy: Knowledge regarding the modes of transmission of the various types of hepatitis is required to answer this question. Remember that hepatitis A is transmitted by the fecal-oral route. Review the methods of transmission of hepatitis if you had difficulty with this question.

Level of Cognitive Ability: Understanding
Client Needs: Safe and Effective Care Environment
Integrated Process: Nursing Process—Assessment

Content Area: Adult Health—Gastrointestinal
References: Copstead-Kirkhorn, L., & Banasik, J. (2010). *Pathophysiology* (4th ed., pp. 885–886). St. Louis: Mosby.
Ignatavicius, D., & Workman, M. (2010). *Medical-surgical nursing: Patient-centered collaborative care* (6th ed., pp. 1356–1357). St. Louis: Saunders.

624. 2
Rationale: Chronic gastritis causes deterioration and atrophy of the lining of the stomach, leading to the loss of the function of the parietal cells. The source of the intrinsic factor is lost, which results in the inability to absorb vitamin B_{12}. This leads to the development of pernicious anemia. The client is not at risk for vitamin A, C, or E deficiency.
Test-Taking Strategy: Recalling the pathophysiology related to pernicious anemia and vitamin B_{12} deficiency will direct you to option 2. If you are unfamiliar with vitamin B_{12} deficiency and its relationship to gastric disorders, review this content.
Level of Cognitive Ability: Understanding
Client Needs: Physiological Integrity
Integrated Process: Nursing Process—Assessment
Content Area: Adult Health—Gastrointestinal
Reference: Ignatavicius, D., & Workman, M. (2010). *Medical-surgical nursing: Patient-centered collaborative care* (6th ed., p. 1268). St. Louis: Saunders.

625. 4
Rationale: Following cholecystectomy, drainage from the T-tube is initially bloody and then turns to a greenish-brown color. The drainage is measured as output. The amount of expected drainage will range from 500 to 1000 mL/day. The nurse would document the output.
Test-Taking Strategy: Use the process of elimination. Options 1 and 2 can be eliminated because a T-tube is not irrigated and would not be clamped with this amount of drainage. From the remaining options, you must know normal expected findings following this surgical procedure. Review postoperative assessment findings following cholecystectomy if you had difficulty with this question.
Level of Cognitive Ability: Applying
Client Needs: Physiological Integrity
Integrated Process: Nursing Process—Implementation
Content Area: Adult Health—Gastrointestinal
Reference: Ignatavicius, D., & Workman, M. (2010). *Medical-surgical nursing: Patient-centered collaborative care* (6th ed., p. 1370). St. Louis: Saunders.

626. 4
Rationale: Perforation of an ulcer is a surgical emergency and is characterized by sudden, sharp, intolerable severe pain beginning in the midepigastric area and spreading over the abdomen, which becomes rigid and board-like. Nausea and vomiting may occur. Tachycardia may occur as hypovolemic shock develops. Numbness in the legs is not an associated finding.
Test-Taking Strategy: Use the process of elimination and note the strategic words *most likely.* Option 2 can be eliminated easily because it is not related to perforation. Eliminate option 1 next because tachycardia rather than bradycardia would develop if perforation occurs. From the remaining

options, focusing on the strategic words will help direct you to option 4. Review the signs of a perforated ulcer if you had difficulty with this question.
Level of Cognitive Ability: Analyzing
Client Needs: Physiological Integrity
Integrated Process: Nursing Process—Assessment
Content Area: Adult Health—Gastrointestinal
References: Black, J., & Hawks, J. (2009). *Medical-surgical nursing: Clinical management for positive outcomes* (8th ed., p. 633). St. Louis: Saunders.
Ignatavicius, D., & Workman, M. (2010). *Medical-surgical nursing: Patient-centered collaborative care* (6th ed., p. 1272). St. Louis: Saunders.

627. 3
Rationale: In a Billroth II procedure, the proximal remnant of the stomach is anastomosed to the proximal jejunum. Patency of the nasogastric tube is critical for preventing the retention of gastric secretions. The nurse should never irrigate or reposition the gastric tube after gastric surgery, unless specifically prescribed by the physician. In this situation, the nurse should clarify the prescription. Options 1, 2, and 4 are appropriate postoperative interventions.
Test-Taking Strategy: Note the strategic words *question and verify.* Eliminate options 1, 2, and 4 because they are general postoperative measures. Consider the anatomical location of the surgical procedure to assist in directing you to option 3. Review postoperative measures following a Billroth II procedure if you had difficulty with this question.
Level of Cognitive Ability: Analyzing
Client Needs: Physiological Integrity
Integrated Process: Nursing Process—Analysis
Content Area: Adult Health—Gastrointestinal
References: Black, J., & Hawks, J. (2009). *Medical-surgical nursing: Clinical management for positive outcomes* (8th ed., p. 639). St. Louis: Saunders.
Ignatavicius, D., & Workman, M. (2010). *Medical-surgical nursing: Patient-centered collaborative care* (6th ed., p. 1285). St. Louis: Saunders.

628. 3
Rationale: Dumping syndrome is a term that refers to a constellation of vasomotor symptoms that occurs after eating, especially following a Billroth II procedure. Early manifestations usually occur within 30 minutes of eating and include vertigo, tachycardia, syncope, sweating, pallor, palpitations, and the desire to lie down. The nurse should instruct the client to decrease the amount of fluid taken at meals and to avoid high-carbohydrate foods, including fluids such as fruit nectars; to assume a low Fowler's position during meals; to lie down for 30 minutes after eating to delay gastric emptying; and to take antispasmodics as prescribed.
Test-Taking Strategy: Use the process of elimination. Eliminate options 1 and 4 first because these measures will promote gastric emptying. From the remaining options, select option 3 because this measure will delay gastric emptying. If you are unfamiliar with this syndrome, review the important client teaching points.
Level of Cognitive Ability: Applying
Client Needs: Physiological Integrity

Integrated Process: Teaching and Learning
Content Area: Adult Health—Gastrointestinal
References: Black, J., & Hawks, J. (2009). *Medical-surgical nursing: Clinical management for positive outcomes* (8th ed., p. 637). St. Louis: Saunders.

Ignatavicius, D., & Workman, M. (2010). *Medical-surgical nursing: Patient-centered collaborative care* (6th ed., p. 1285). St. Louis: Saunders.

629. 1
Rationale: Early manifestations of dumping syndrome occur 5 to 30 minutes after eating. Symptoms include vertigo, tachycardia, syncope, sweating, pallor, palpitations, and the desire to lie down.
Test-Taking Strategy: Use the process of elimination and recall the pathophysiology associated with dumping syndrome. Focus on the strategic word *early* to direct you to option 1. Review the early manifestations of this syndrome if you had difficulty with this question.
Level of Cognitive Ability: Analyzing
Client Needs: Physiological Integrity
Integrated Process: Nursing Process—Assessment
Content Area: Adult Health—Gastrointestinal
References: Black, J., & Hawks, J. (2009). *Medical-surgical nursing: Clinical management for positive outcomes* (8th ed., p. 637). St. Louis: Saunders.

Ignatavicius, D., & Workman, M. (2010). *Medical-surgical nursing: Patient-centered collaborative care* (6th ed., p. 1285). St. Louis: Saunders.

630. 1
Rationale: Crohn's disease is characterized by nonbloody diarrhea of usually not more than four to five stools daily. Over time, the diarrhea episodes increase in frequency, duration, and severity. Options 2, 3, and 4 are not characteristics of Crohn's disease.
Test-Taking Strategy: Use the process of elimination. Eliminate option 4 first as the most unlikely occurrence. From the remaining options, think about the pathophysiology associated with Crohn's disease to direct you to option 1. If you are unfamiliar with this disorder, review this content.
Level of Cognitive Ability: Analyzing
Client Needs: Physiological Integrity
Integrated Process: Nursing Process—Assessment
Content Area: Adult Health—Gastrointestinal
Reference: Swearingen, P. (2008). *All-in-one care planning resource: Medical-surgical, pediatric, maternity, & psychiatric nursing care plans* (2nd ed., p. 445). St. Louis: Mosby.

631. 3
Rationale: Asterixis is irregular flapping movements of the fingers and wrists when the hands and arms are outstretched, with the palms down, wrists bent up, and fingers spread. Asterixis is the most common and reliable sign that hepatic encephalopathy is developing. Options 1, 2, and 4 are incorrect.
Test-Taking Strategy: Use the process of elimination and knowledge regarding the procedure for this assessment to answer this question. Remember that asterixis is irregular flapping movements of the fingers and wrists. This will direct you to the correct option. Review this assessment procedure if you had difficulty with this question.

Level of Cognitive Ability: Applying
Client Needs: Health Promotion and Maintenance
Integrated Process: Nursing Process—Assessment
Content Area: Adult Health—Gastrointestinal
References: Black, J., & Hawks, J. (2009). *Medical-surgical nursing: Clinical management for positive outcomes* (8th ed., pp. 1166–1167). St. Louis: Saunders.

Ignatavicius, D., & Workman, M. (2010). *Medical-surgical nursing: Patient-centered collaborative care* (6th ed., p. 1349). St. Louis: Saunders.

Swearingen, P. (2008). *All-in-one care planning resource: Medical-surgical, pediatric, maternity, & psychiatric nursing care plans* (2nd ed., p. 437). St. Louis: Mosby.

632. 1
Rationale: Cirrhosis is a chronic, progressive disease of the liver characterized by diffuse degeneration and destruction of hepatocytes. Most of the ammonia in the body is found in the gastrointestinal tract. Protein provided by the diet is transported to the liver by the portal vein. The liver breaks down protein, which results in the formation of ammonia. If the client has hepatic encephalopathy, a low-protein diet would be prescribed.
Test-Taking Strategy: Recall the physiology of the liver in answering this question. You should be directed easily to option 1. Also, note that options 1 and 2 are opposite, which should provide you with the clue that one of these options is correct. Review dietary measures for the client with a high ammonia level if you had difficulty with this question.
Level of Cognitive Ability: Understanding
Client Needs: Physiological Integrity
Integrated Process: Nursing Process—Planning
Content Area: Adult Health—Gastrointestinal
Reference: Black, J., & Hawks, J. (2009). *Medical-surgical nursing: Clinical management for positive outcomes* (8th ed., p. 1153). St. Louis: Saunders.

633. 3
Rationale: A frequent symptom of duodenal ulcer is pain that is relieved by food intake. These clients generally describe the pain as a burning, heavy, sharp, or "hungry" pain that often localizes in the midepigastric area. The client with duodenal ulcer usually does not experience weight loss or nausea and vomiting. These symptoms are more typical in the client with a gastric ulcer.
Test-Taking Strategy: Use the process of elimination. To answer this question accurately, you must be able to discriminate between symptoms of duodenal and gastric ulcer. This will allow you to eliminate options 1 and 2 first. Choose option 3 over option 4, knowing that the pain does not radiate down the right arm and that a pattern of pain-food-relief occurs with duodenal ulcer. Review the clinical manifestations of a duodenal ulcer if you had difficulty with this question.
Level of Cognitive Ability: Analyzing
Client Needs: Physiological Integrity
Integrated Process: Nursing Process—Assessment
Content Area: Adult Health—Gastrointestinal
References: Black, J., & Hawks, J. (2009). *Medical-surgical nursing: Clinical management for positive outcomes* (8th ed., pp. 629, 631). St. Louis: Saunders.

Ignatavicius, D., & Workman, M. (2010). *Medical-surgical nursing: Patient-centered collaborative care* (6th ed., p. 1273). St. Louis: Saunders.

634. 1

Rationale: Hiatal hernia is caused by a protrusion of a portion of the stomach above the diaphragm where the esophagus usually is positioned. The client usually experiences pain from reflux caused by ingestion of irritating foods, lying flat following meals or at night, and eating large or fatty meals. Relief is obtained with the intake of small, frequent, and bland meals, use of H_2-receptor antagonists and antacids, and elevation of the thorax following meals and during sleep.

Test-Taking Strategy: Use the process of elimination noting the strategic word *contraindicated*. Thinking about the pathophysiology that occurs in hiatal hernia will direct you to option 1. Review this pathophysiology if you had difficulty with this question.

Level of Cognitive Ability: Applying
Client Needs: Physiological Integrity
Integrated Process: Teaching and Learning
Content Area: Adult Health—Gastrointestinal
References: Black, J., & Hawks, J. (2009). *Medical-surgical nursing: Clinical management for positive outcomes* (8th ed., p. 610). St. Louis: Saunders.

Ignatavicius, D., & Workman, M. (2010). *Medical-surgical nursing: Patient-centered collaborative care* (6th ed., p. 1254). St. Louis: Saunders.

635. 1

Rationale: A prolapsed stoma is one in which the bowel protrudes through the stoma. A stoma retraction is characterized by sinking of the stoma. Ischemia of the stoma would be associated with a dusky or bluish color. A stoma with a narrowed opening at the level of the skin or fascia is said to be *stenosed*.

Test-Taking Strategy: Focus on the subject and the strategic word *prolapse*. This will direct you to option 1. If this question was difficult, review the complications associated with a colostomy stoma.

Level of Cognitive Ability: Analyzing
Client Needs: Physiological Integrity
Integrated Process: Nursing Process—Assessment
Content Area: Adult Health—Gastrointestinal
References: Ignatavicius, D., & Workman, M. (2010). *Medical-surgical nursing: Patient-centered collaborative care* (6th ed., p. 1299). St. Louis: Saunders.

Perry, A., & Potter, P. (2010). *Clinical nursing skills & techniques* (7th ed., p. 925). St. Louis: Mosby.

636. 1

Rationale: As peristalsis returns following creation of a colostomy, the client begins to pass malodorous flatus. This indicates returning bowel function and is an expected event. Within 72 hours of surgery, the client should begin passing stool via the colostomy. Options 2, 3, and 4 are incorrect.

Test-Taking Strategy: Use the process of elimination. Recalling the normal progression of bowel activity following ostomy formation will direct you to option 1. Review the expected findings following creation of a colostomy if you had difficulty with this question.

Level of Cognitive Ability: Analyzing
Client Needs: Physiological Integrity
Integrated Process: Nursing Process—Assessment
Content Area: Adult Health—Gastrointestinal

References: Black, J., & Hawks, J. (2009). *Medical-surgical nursing: Clinical management for positive outcomes* (8th ed., p. 706). St. Louis: Saunders.

Swearingen, P. (2008). *All-in-one care planning resource: Medical-surgical, pediatric, maternity, & psychiatric nursing care plans* (2nd ed., p. 458). St. Louis: Mosby.

637. 4

Rationale: A frequent complication that occurs following ileostomy is fluid and electrolyte imbalance. The client requires constant monitoring of intake and output to prevent this from occurring. Losses require replacement by intravenous infusion until the client can tolerate a diet orally. Intestinal obstruction is a less frequent complication. Fat malabsorption and folate deficiency are complications that could occur later in the postoperative period.

Test-Taking Strategy: Use the process of elimination and note the strategic words *ileostomy, immediate postoperative period,* and *complication.* This tells you that the correct option occurs early in the postoperative course, with relative frequency. Remember that ileostomy drainage is liquid, placing the client at risk for fluid and electrolyte imbalance. If you had difficulty with this question, review the postoperative complications following this surgical procedure.

Level of Cognitive Ability: Analyzing
Client Needs: Physiological Integrity
Integrated Process: Nursing Process—Assessment
Content Area: Adult Health—Gastrointestinal
Reference: Ignatavicius, D., & Workman, M. (2010). *Medical-surgical nursing: Patient-centered collaborative care* (6th ed., p. 1323). St. Louis: Saunders.

638. 3

Rationale: A Kock pouch is a continent ileostomy. As the ileostomy begins to function, the client drains it every 3 to 4 hours and then decreases the draining to about three times a day, or as needed when full. The client does not need to wear a drainage bag but should wear an absorbent dressing to absorb mucous drainage from the stoma. Ileostomy drainage is liquid. The client would be able to pass stool only from the rectum if an ileal-anal pouch or anastomosis were created. This type of operation is a two-stage procedure.

Test-Taking Strategy: Use the process of elimination. Focusing on the strategic word *pouch* will assist in directing you to option 3. If this question was difficult, review this content.

Level of Cognitive Ability: Evaluating
Client Needs: Physiological Integrity
Integrated Process: Nursing Process—Evaluation
Content Area: Adult Health—Gastrointestinal
Reference: Ignatavicius, D., & Workman, M. (2010). *Medical-surgical nursing: Patient-centered collaborative care* (6th ed., p. 1326). St. Louis: Saunders.

ALTERNATE ITEM FORMAT: MULTIPLE RESPONSE

639. 1, 2, 3, 6

Rationale: The client with acute pancreatitis normally is placed on NPO status to rest the pancreas and suppress gastrointestinal secretions. Because abdominal pain is a prominent symptom of pancreatitis, pain medication such as meperidine is prescribed. Some clients experience lessened pain by assuming positions that flex the trunk, with the knees drawn up to the chest. A side-lying position with the head elevated 45 degrees decreases tension on the abdomen and may help ease the pain. The client is susceptible to respiratory infections because the retroperitoneal fluid raises the diaphragm, which causes the client to take shallow, guarded abdominal breaths. Therefore measures such as turning, coughing, and deep breathing are instituted. Antacids and anticholinergics may be prescribed to suppress gastrointestinal secretions.

Test-Taking Strategy: Focus on the pathophysiology associated with pancreatitis and note the strategic word *acute*. This will assist in answering the question. Review treatment measures for acute pancreatitis if you had difficulty with this question.

Level of Cognitive Ability: Analyzing
Client Needs: Physiological Integrity
Integrated Process: Nursing Process—Analysis
Content Area: Adult Health—Gastrointestinal
References: Ignatavicius, D., & Workman, M. (2010). *Medical-surgical nursing: Patient-centered collaborative care* (6th ed., pp. 1375–1376). St. Louis: Saunders.

Swearingen, P. (2008). *All-in-one care planning resource: Medical-surgical, pediatric, maternity, & psychiatric nursing care plans* (2nd ed., p. 472). St. Louis: Mosby.

Gastrointestinal Medications

I. ANTACIDS (Table 57-1; Fig. 57-1)

A. React with gastric acid to produce neutral salts or salts of low acidity

B. Inactivate pepsin and enhance mucosal protection but do not coat the ulcer crater.

C. These medications are used for peptic ulcer disease and gastroesophageal reflux disease.

D. These medications should be taken on a regular schedule; some are prescribed to be taken 1 and 3 hours after each meal and at bedtime.

E. To provide maximum benefit, treatment should elevate the gastric pH above 5.

F. Antacid tablets should be chewed thoroughly and followed with a glass of water or milk.

G. Liquid preparations should be shaken before dispensing.

▲ To prevent interactions with other medications and the interference with the action of other medications, allow 1 hour between antacid administration and the administration of other medications.

II. GASTRIC PROTECTANTS (Box 57-1)

A. Misoprostol (Cytotec)
   1. An antisecretory medication that enhances mucosal defenses
   2. Suppresses secretion of gastric acid and maintains submucosal blood flow by promoting vasodilation
   3. Used to prevent gastric ulcers caused by nonsteroidal anti-inflammatory drugs and aspirin.
   4. Administered with meals
   5. Causes diarrhea and abdominal pain
   6. Contraindicated for use in pregnancy

B. Sucralfate (Carafate)
   1. Creates a protective barrier against acid and pepsin.
   2. Administered orally; should be taken on an empty stomach
   3. May cause constipation
   4. May impede absorption of warfarin sodium (Coumadin), phenytoin (Dilantin), theophylline, digoxin (Lanoxin), and some antibiotics; should be administered at least 2 hours apart from these medications.

III. MUSCARINIC ANTAGONIST

A. Description: Suppresses acid secretion by blocking muscarinic cholinergic receptors

B. Medication: Pirenzepine (Gastrozepine)

IV. HISTAMINE 2 (H₂)-RECEPTOR ANTAGONISTS (Box 57-2)

A. Description
   1. Suppress secretion of gastric acid
   2. Alleviate symptoms of heartburn and assist in preventing complications of peptic ulcer disease
   3. Prevent stress ulcers and reduce the recurrence of all ulcers
   4. Promote healing in gastroesophageal reflux disease
   5. Are contraindicated in hypersensitive clients
   6. Should be used with caution in clients with impaired renal or hepatic function

B. Cimetidine (Tagamet)
   1. Can be administered orally, intramuscularly, or intravenously
   2. Food reduces the rate of absorption; if taken with meals, absorption will be slowed.
   3. Intravenous administration can cause hypotension and dysrhythmias.
   4. Antacids can decrease the absorption of oral cimetidine.
   5. Cimetidine and antacids should be administered at least 1 hour apart from each other.
   6. Cimetidine passes the blood-brain barrier, and central nervous system side effects can occur; it may cause mental confusion, agitation, psychosis, depression, anxiety, and disorientation.
   7. Dosage should be reduced in clients with renal impairment.
   8. If cimetidine is administered with warfarin sodium (Coumadin), phenytoin (Dilantin), theophylline, or lidocaine, the dosages of these medications should be reduced.

C. Ranitidine (Zantac)
   1. Can be administered orally, intramuscularly, or intravenously

TABLE 57-1 Classification of Antacids and Considerations

Classification	Consideration
Aluminum compounds	Aluminum hydroxide is used to treat hyperphosphatemia; therefore it can cause hypophosphatemia. Aluminum hydroxide can reduce the effects of tetracyclines, warfarin sodium (Coumadin), and digoxin (Lanoxin) and can reduce phosphate absorption and thereby cause hypophosphatemia. Aluminum compounds contain significant amounts of sodium; they should be used with caution in clients with hypertension and heart failure The most common side effect is constipation.
Magnesium compounds	Magnesium hydroxide is also a saline laxative and the most prominent side effect is diarrhea; it is usually administered in combination with aluminum hydroxide, an antacid that assists in preventing diarrhea. Magnesium compounds are contraindicated in clients with intestinal obstruction, appendicitis, or undiagnosed abdominal pain. In clients with renal impairment, magnesium can accumulate to high levels, causing signs of toxicity.
Calcium compounds	Calcium carbonate can cause acid rebound. Calcium compounds are rapid-acting and release carbon dioxide in the stomach, causing belching and flatulence A common side effect is constipation. Milk-alkali syndrome (headache, urinary frequency, anorexia, nausea/vomiting, fatigue) can occur (the client should avoid milk products and vitamin D supplements).
Sodium bicarbonate	Sodium bicarbonate has a rapid onset, liberates carbon dioxide, increases intra-abdominal pressure, and promotes flatulence. Sodium bicarbonate should be used with caution in clients with hypertension and heart failure. Sodium bicarbonate can cause systemic alkalosis in clients with renal impairment. Sodium bicarbonate is useful for treating acidosis and elevating urinary pH to promote excretion of acidic medications following overdose.

Gastric Ulcer

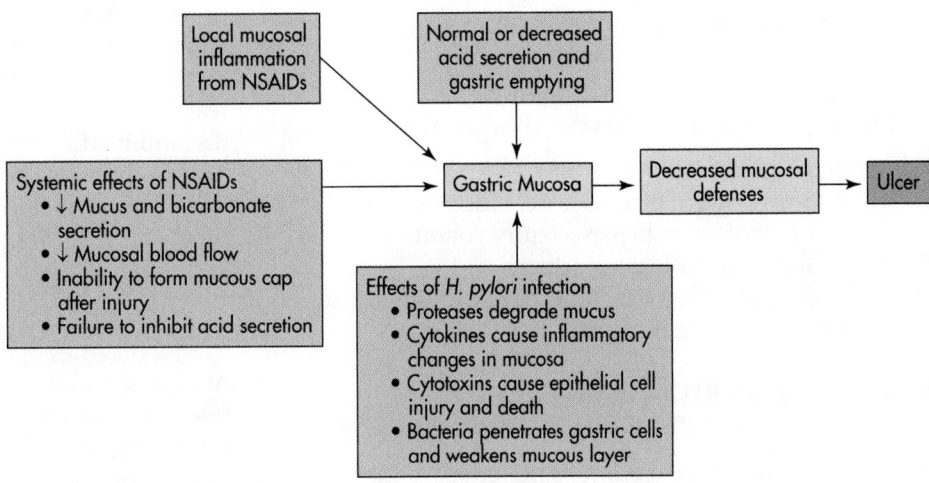

Duodenal Ulcer

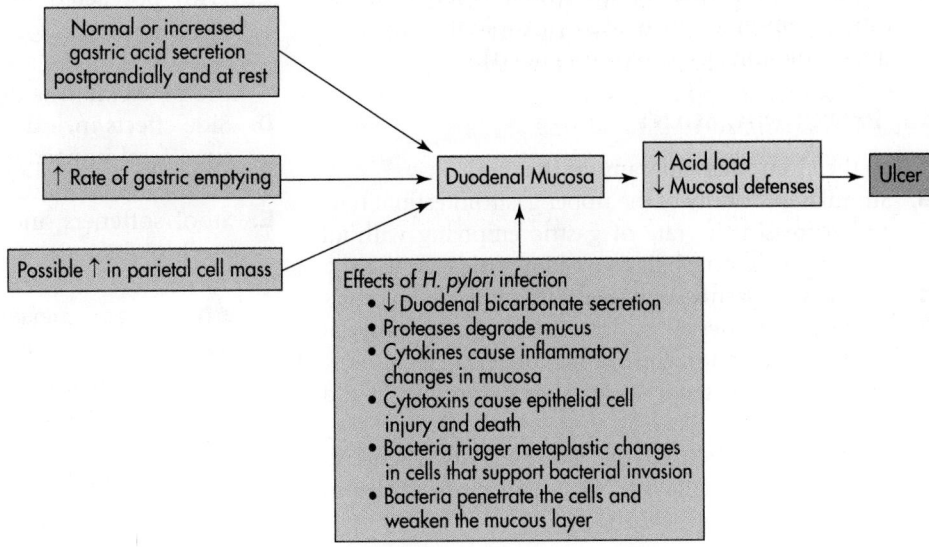

▲ **FIGURE 57-1** Pathophysiological components of peptic ulcer. (From Monahan, F., Sands, J., Neighbors, M., Marek, J., & Green, C. [2007] *Phipps' medical-surgical nursing: Health and illness perspectives* [8th ed.]. St. Louis: Mosby.)

Box 57-1 Gastric Protectants

Misoprostol (Cytotec)   Sucralfate (Carafate)

Box 57-2 H₂-Receptor Antagonists

Cimetidine (Tagamet)   Nizatidine (Axid)
Famotidine (Pepcid)   Ranitidine (Zantac)

Box 57-3 Proton Pump Inhibitors

Esomeprazole (Nexium)   Pantoprazole (Protonix)
Lansoprazole (Prevacid)   Rabeprazole (Aciphex)
Omeprazole (Prilosec)

---

2. Side effects are uncommon and does not penetrate the blood-brain barrier as cimetidine does.
3. Ranitidine is not affected by food.

D. Famotidine (Pepcid) and nizatidine (Axid)
1. Famotidine and nizatidine are similar to ranitidine and cimetidine.
2. These medications do not need to be administered with food.

V. PROTON PUMP INHIBITORS (Box 57-3)

A. Suppress gastric acid secretion
B. Used to treat active ulcer disease, erosive esophagitis, and pathological hypersecretory conditions
C. Contraindicated in hypersensitivity
D. Common side effects include headache, diarrhea, abdominal pain, and nausea

VI. MEDICATION REGIMENS TO TREAT HELICOBACTER PYLORI INFECTIONS (Box 57-4)

A. An antibacterial agent alone is not effective for eradicating *Helicobacter pylori* because the bacterium readily becomes resistant to the agent.
B. Triple or quadruple therapy with a variety of medication combinations is used (if triple therapy fails, quadruple therapy is recommended).

VII. PROKINETIC AGENT

A. Medication: Metoclopramide (Reglan)
B. Stimulates motility of the upper gastrointestinal tract and increases the rate of gastric emptying without stimulating gastric, biliary, or pancreatic secretions
C. Used to treat gastroesophageal reflux and paralytic ileus
D. May cause restlessness, drowsiness, extrapyramidal reactions, dizziness, insomnia, and headache
E. Usually administered 30 minutes before meals and at bedtime
F. Contraindicated in clients with sensitivity and in clients with mechanical obstruction, perforation, or gastrointestinal hemorrhage

---

Box 57-4 Medication Regimens for Treating *Helicobacter Pylori* Infections

Triple Therapy
Esomeprazole (Nexium), amoxicillin (Amoxil), clarithromycin (Biaxin)

Quadruple Therapies
Esomeprazole (Nexium), metronidazole (Flagyl), tetracycline, bismuth subsalicylate
Ranitidine (Zantac), metronidazole (Flagyl), tetracycline, bismuth subsalicylate
Additional medications may be prescribed for each level of therapy.

Box 57-5 Bile Acid Sequestrants

Colesevelam (Welchol)
Cholestyramine (Questran, Prevalite)
Colestipol (Colestid)

G. Can precipitate hypertensive crisis in clients with pheochromocytoma
H. Safety in pregnancy is not established
I. Metoclopramide (Reglan) can cause parkinsonian reactions; if this occurs, the medication will be discontinued by the physician.
J. Anticholinergics and opioid analgesics antagonize the effects of metoclopramide.
K. Alcohol, sedatives, cyclosporine (Sandimmune), and tranquilizers produce an additive effect.

VIII. BILE ACID SEQUESTRANTS (Box 57-5)

A. Act by absorbing and combining with intestinal bile salts, which then are secreted in the feces, preventing intestinal reabsorption
B. Used to treat hypercholesterolemia in adults, biliary obstruction, and pruritus associated with biliary disease
C. With powdered forms, taste and palatability are often reasons for noncompliance and can be improved by the use of flavored products or mixing the medication with various juices.
D. Side effects include nausea, bloating, and constipation; fecal impaction and intestinal obstruction can result.
E. Stool softeners and other sources of fiber can be used to abate the gastrointestinal side effects.

⚠ Bile acid sequestrants should be used cautiously in clients with suspected bowel obstruction or severe constipation because they can worsen these conditions.

IX. TREATING HEPATIC ENCEPHALOPATHY

A. Medication: Lactulose (Constulose, Enulose)

Box 57-6 Pancreatic Enzyme Replacements

Pancreatin
Pancrelipase (Pancrease MT, Viokase, Lipram, Pancrecarb MS)

Box 57-7 Medications to Treat Inflammatory Bowel Disease

Antimicrobials
Ciprofloxacin (Cipro)
Metronidazole (Flagyl)

5-Aminosalicylates
Balsalazide (Colazal)
Mesalamine (Rowasa, Asacol, Pentasa, Canasa)
Olsalazine (Dipentum)
Sulfasalazine (Azulfidine)

Corticosteroids
Budesonide (Entocort-EC)
Prednisone

Immunosuppressants
Azathioprine (Imuran)
Cyclosporine (Sandimmune, Neoral, Gengraf)
Mercaptopurine (Purinethol)

Immunomodulators
Adalimumab (Humira)
Certolizumab (Cimzia)
Infliximab (Remicade)
Natalizumab (Tysabri)

B. Used in the prevention and treatment of portal systemic encephalopathy including hepatic precoma and coma; also used in the treatment of chronic constipation
C. Promotes increased **peristalsis** and bowel evacuation, expelling ammonia from the colon and thus lowering the ammonia level
D. Improves protein tolerance in clients with advanced hepatic **cirrhosis**
E. Administered orally in the form of a syrup or rectally

X. PANCREATIC ENZYME REPLACEMENTS (Box 57-6)

A. Used to supplement or replace pancreatic enzymes and thus improve nutritional status and reduce the amount of fatty stools (a deficiency of pancreatic enzymes can compromise digestion, especially the digestion of fats).
B. Should be taken with all meals and snacks
C. Side effects include abdominal cramps or pain, nausea, and diarrhea.
D. Products that contain calcium carbonate or magnesium hydroxide interfere with the action of the medication.

XI. TREATMENT FOR INFLAMMATORY BOWEL DISEASE (Box 57-7)

A. Inflammatory bowel disease has two forms including **Crohn's disease** and **ulcerative colitis**.

B. Antimicrobials: may be prescribed to prevent or treat secondary infection (see Chapter 71 for information on antimicrobials)
C. 5-Aminosalicylates (5-ASA): Decrease gastrointestinal inflammation; adverse effects include nausea, rash, arthralgia, and hematological disorders.
D. Corticosteroids: Act as an anti-inflammatory to decrease gastrointestinal inflammation (see Chapter 55 for information on glucocorticocoids and corticosteroids).
E. Immunosuppressants: Suppress the immune system; can cause **pancreatitis** and neutropenia secondary to bone marrow depression and their use is reserved for those who have not responded to other traditional therapies (see Chapter 71 for information on immunosuppressants).
F. Immunomodulators: Monoclonal antibodies that modulate the immune response to induce and maintain remission

XII. TREATMENT FOR IRRITABLE BOWEL SYNDROME (IBS)

A. Irritable bowel syndrome is a gastrointestinal disorder that is characterized by crampy abdominal pain accompanied by diarrhea, constipation, or both.
B. Symptomatic relief is sometimes provided with the use of antispasmodics that relax the smooth muscle of the gastrointestinal tract, bulk-forming medications, antidiarrheals, and antidepressants.
C. Alosetron (Lotronex)
　1. Used for severe IBS.
　2. Can cause severe adverse effects such as constipation, impaction, bowel obstruction, perforation of the bowel, and ischemic colitis.
　3. A strict risk management procedure must be followed by both the prescriber of the medication and the client, which includes several guidelines that must be followed including monitoring for serious adverse effects, reporting them, and immediate discontinuation of the medication if they arise.
D. Lubiprostone (Amitiza)
　1. Increases intestinal motility and increases the passage of stool, thereby, reducing abdominal pain
　2. Side effects include nausea, headache, diarrhea, flatulence; adverse effects include urinary tract infection and upper respiratory tract infection.
E. Tegaserod (Zelnorm)
　1. Decreases visceral sensation and increases gastrointestinal motility and secretions.
　2. Most serious adverse effect is diarrhea and cardiovascular events such as myocardial infarction and stroke.
　3. Use of the medication is restricted; only those who do not have cardiovascular disease and have not responded to an alternative treatment may be eligible for treatment with this medication.

Box 57-8 Commonly Administered Antiemetics

Serotonin Antagonists
Dolasetron (Anzemet)
Granisetron (Kytril)
Ondansetron (Zofran)
Palonosetron (Aloxi)

Glucocorticoids
Dexamethasone (Decadron)
Methylprednisolone (Solu-Medrol)

Substance P/Neurokinin 1 Antagonists
Aprepitant (Emend)
Fosaprepitant (Emend)

Benzodiazepines
Lorazepam (Ativan)
Diazepam (Valium)

Dopamine Antagonists
Phenothiazines
Chlorpromazine (Thorazine)
Perphenazine (Trilafon)
Prochlorperazine (Compazine)
Promethazine (Phenergan)

Butyrophenones
Haloperidol (Haldol)
Droperidol (Inapsine)

Others
Metoclopramide (Reglan)
Domperidone (Motilium)

Cannabinoids
Dronabinol (Marinol)
Nabilone (Cesamet)

Anticholinergics
Antihistamines
Cyclizine (Marezine)
Dimenhydrinate (Dramamine)
Diphenhydramine (Benadryl)
Hydroxyzine (Vistaril, Atarax)
Meclizine hydrochloride (Bonine, Antivert)

Others
Scopolamine transdermal (Transderm Scop)

Modified from Lehne, R. (2010). *Pharmacology for nursing care* (7th ed., p. 937). St. Louis: Saunders.

XIII. ANTIEMETICS (Box 57-8)

A. Medications used to control vomiting and motion sickness.
B. The choice of the antiemetic is determined by the cause of the nausea and vomiting.
C. Monitor for drowsiness and protect the client from injury.
D. Monitor vital signs and intake and output.
E. Limit odors in the client's room when the client is nauseated or vomiting.
F. Limit oral intake to clear liquids when the client is nauseated or vomiting.

⚠ Antiemetics can cause drowsiness; therefore a priority intervention is to protect the client from injury.

XIV. LAXATIVES (Box 57-9)

A. Bulk-forming
  1. Description
     a. Absorb water into the feces and increase bulk to produce large and soft stools
     b. Contraindicated in bowel obstruction
     c. Dependency can occur with long-term use.
  2. Side effects include gastrointestinal disturbances, dehydration, and electrolyte imbalances.
B. Stimulants: Stimulate motility of large intestine
C. Surfactants
  1. Inhibit absorption of water so fecal mass remains large and soft
  2. Used to avoid straining

Box 57-9 Laxatives

Bulk-Forming
Methylcellulose (Citrucel)
Polycarbophil (FiberCon)
Psyllium (Metamucil, others)

Stimulants
Bisacodyl (Correctol, Dulcolax, Feen-a-mint, Fleet laxative, others)
Senna (Senokot Ex-Lax, others), Cascara sagrada

Surfactant
Docusate sodium (Colace, others)

Osmotics
Magnesium hydroxide (Milk of Magnesia)
Magnesium citrate (Citrate of Magnesia)
Sodium phosphates (Fleet enema, Fleet Phospho-Soda)
Polyethylene glycol and electrolytes (GoLYTELY)

Lubricant
Mineral oil

D. Osmotics: Attract water into the large intestine to produce bulk and stimulate **peristalsis**
E. Lubricants
  1. Act to soften the feces, ease the strain of passing stool, and lessen irritation to hemorrhoids
  2. Mineral oil: Interferes with absorption of the fat-soluble vitamins A, D, E, and K and can cause lipid pneumonia if accidentally aspirated

Box 57-10 Medications to Control Diarrhea

Opioids and Related Medications
Difenoxin with atropine sulfate (Motofen)
Diphenoxylate with atropine sulfate (Lomotil)
Loperamide (Imodium)
Paregoric (camphorated tincture of opium)
Tincture of opium

Other Antidiarrheals
Bismuth subsalicylate (Pepto-Bismol, Kaopectate, Kapectolin)
Bulk-forming medications
Anticholinergic antispasmodics

 The client receiving a laxative needs to increase fluid intake to prevent dehydration.

XV. MEDICATIONS TO CONTROL DIARRHEA
(Box 57-10)

A. Goals: Identify and treat the underlying cause, treat dehydration, replace fluids and electrolytes, relieve abdominal discomfort and cramping, and reduce the passage of stool
B. Opioids
1. Opioids are effective antidiarrheal medications that decrease intestinal motility and peristalsis.
2. When poisons, infections, or bacterial toxins are the cause of the diarrhea, opioids worsen the condition by delaying the elimination of toxins.
3. Tincture of opium has an unpleasant taste and can be diluted with 15 to 30 mL of water for administration.
C. Other antidiarrheals: See Box 57-10.

💿 MORE QUESTIONS ON THE CD!

Practice Questions

640. A client with Crohn's disease is scheduled to receive an infusion of infliximab (Remicade). What intervention by the nurse will determine the effectiveness of treatment?
1. Monitoring the leukocyte count for 2 days after the infusion
2. Checking the frequency and consistency of bowel movements
3. Checking serum liver enzyme levels before and after the infusion
4. Carrying out a Hematest on gastric fluids after the infusion is completed

641. The client has a PRN prescription for loperamide hydrochloride (Imodium). For which condition should the nurse plan to administer this medication?

1. Constipation
2. Abdominal pain
3. An episode of diarrhea
4. Hematest-positive nasogastric tube drainage

642. The client has a PRN prescription for ondansetron (Zofran). For which condition should the nurse administer this medication to the postoperative client?
1. Paralytic ileus
2. Incisional pain
3. Urinary retention
4. Nausea and vomiting

643. The client has begun medication therapy with pancrelipase (Pancrease). The nurse evaluates that the medication is having the optimal intended benefit if which effect is observed?
1. Weight loss
2. Relief of heartburn
3. Reduction of steatorrhea
4. Absence of abdominal pain

644. An older client recently has been taking cimetidine (Tagamet). The nurse monitors the client for which most frequent central nervous system side effect of this medication?
1. Tremors
2. Dizziness
3. Confusion
4. Hallucinations

645. The client with a gastric ulcer has a prescription for sucralfate (Carafate), 1 g by mouth 4 times daily. The nurse schedules the medication for which times?
1. With meals and at bedtime
2. Every 6 hours around the clock
3. One hour after meals and at bedtime
4. One hour before meals and at bedtime

646. The client who chronically uses nonsteroidal anti-inflammatory drugs (NSAIDs) has been taking misoprostol (Cytotec). The nurse determines that the medication is having the intended therapeutic effect if which of the following is noted?
1. Resolved diarrhea
2. Relief of epigastric pain
3. Decreased platelet count
4. Decreased white blood cell count

647. The client has been taking omeprazole (Prilosec) for 4 weeks. The ambulatory care nurse evaluates that the client is receiving optimal intended effect of the medication if the client reports the absence of which symptom?

1. Diarrhea
2. Heartburn
3. Flatulence
4. Constipation

648. A client with a peptic ulcer is diagnosed with a *Helicobacter pylori* infection. The nurse is teaching the client about the medications prescribed, including clarithromycin (Biaxin), esomeprazole (Nexium), and amoxicillin (Amoxil). Which statement by the client indicates the best understanding of the medication regimen?
1. "My ulcer will heal because these medications will kill the bacteria."
2. "These medications are only taken when I have pain from my ulcer."
3. "The medications will kill the bacteria and stop the acid production."
4. "These medications will coat the ulcer and decrease the acid production in my stomach."

649. The client has a new prescription for metoclopramide (Reglan). On review of the chart, the nurse identifies that this medication can be safely administered with which condition?
1. Intestinal obstruction
2. Peptic ulcer with melena

3. Diverticulitis with perforation
4. Vomiting following cancer chemotherapy

650. The nurse has given instructions to a client who has just been prescribed cholestyramine (Questran). Which statement by the client indicates a need for further instructions?
1. I will continue taking vitamin supplements.
2. This medication will help lower my cholesterol.
3. This medication should only be taken with water.
4. A high-fiber diet is important while taking this medication.

Alternate Item Format: Multiple Response

651. A histamine (H_2)-receptor antagonist will be prescribed for a client. The nurse understands that which medications are H_2-receptor antagonists? **Select all that apply**.
❑ 1. Nizatidine (Axid)
❑ 2. Ranitidine (Zantac)
❑ 3. Famotidine (Pepcid)
❑ 4. Cimetidine (Tagamet)
❑ 5. Esomeprazole (Nexium)
❑ 6. Lansoprazole (Prevacid)

ANSWERS
640. 2
Rationale: The principal manifestations of Crohn's disease are diarrhea and abdominal pain. Infliximab (Remicade) is an immunomodulator that reduces the degree of inflammation in the colon, thereby reducing the diarrhea. Options 1, 3, and 4 are unrelated to this medication.
Test-Taking Strategy: Focus on the client's diagnosis, Crohn's disease. Eliminate option 4 because gastric bleeding is not a characteristic of Crohn's disease. Monitoring the leukocyte count and liver enzyme levels is appropriate when infliximab (Remicade) is given but not to evaluate the effectiveness of treatment, eliminating options 1 and 3. Review the manifestations of Crohn's disease and the actions of this medication if you had difficulty with this question.
Level of Cognitive Ability: Evaluating
Client Needs: Physiological Integrity
Integrated Process: Nursing Process—Evaluation
Content Area: Pharmacology
References: Gahart, B., & Nazareno, A. (2010). *2010 Intravenous medications* (26th ed., p. 748). St. Louis: Mosby.
Hodgson, B., & Kizior, R. (2010). *Saunders nursing drug handbook 2010* (pp. 597–599). St. Louis: Saunders.

641. 3
Rationale: Loperamide is an antidiarrheal agent. It is used to manage acute and chronic diarrhea in conditions such as inflammatory bowel disease. Loperamide also can be used

to reduce the volume of drainage from an ileostomy. It is not used for the conditions in options 1, 2, and 4.
Test-Taking Strategy: Focus on the name of the medication. Recalling that this medication is an antidiarrheal agent will direct you to option 3. Review the action of this medication if you had difficulty with this question.
Level of Cognitive Ability: Applying
Client Needs: Physiological Integrity
Integrated Process: Nursing Process—Planning
Content Area: Pharmacology
Reference: Lehne, R. (2010). *Pharmacology for nursing care* (7th ed., p. 941). St. Louis: Saunders.

642. 4
Rationale: Ondansetron is an antiemetic used to treat postoperative nausea and vomiting, as well as nausea and vomiting associated with chemotherapy. The other options are incorrect.
Test-Taking Strategy: Use the process of elimination. Recalling that this medication is an antiemetic will direct you to option 4. Review this medication if you had difficulty with this question.
Level of Cognitive Ability: Applying
Client Needs: Physiological Integrity
Integrated Process: Nursing Process—Implementation
Content Area: Pharmacology
Reference: Lehne, R. (2010). *Pharmacology for nursing care* (7th ed., pp. 937–938). St. Louis: Saunders.

643. 3

Rationale: Pancrelipase (Pancrease) is a pancreatic enzyme used in clients with pancreatitis as a digestive aid. The medication should reduce the amount of fatty stools (steatorrhea). Another intended effect could be improved nutritional status. It is not used to treat abdominal pain or heartburn. Its use could result in weight gain but should not result in weight loss if it is aiding in digestion.

Test-Taking Strategy: Use the process of elimination and focus on the name of the medication. Use knowledge of physiology of the pancreas to assist in directing you to the correct option. Review this medication if you had difficulty with this question.

Level of Cognitive Ability: Evaluating
Client Needs: Physiological Integrity
Integrated Process: Nursing Process—Evaluation
Content Area: Pharmacology
References: Hodgson, B., & Kizior, R. (2010). *Saunders nursing drug handbook 2010* (p. 876). St. Louis: Saunders.
　　Lehne, R. (2010). *Pharmacology for nursing care* (7th ed., p. 949). St. Louis: Saunders.

644. 3

Rationale: Cimetidine is a histamine 2 (H_2)-receptor antagonist. Older clients are especially susceptible to central nervous system side effects of cimetidine. The most frequent of these is confusion. Less common central nervous system side effects include headache, dizziness, drowsiness, and hallucinations.

Test-Taking Strategy: Use the process of elimination and note the strategic words *most frequent.* Use knowledge of the older client and medication effects to direct you to option 3. Review the side effects of cimetidine if you had difficulty with this question.

Level of Cognitive Ability: Applying
Client Needs: Physiological Integrity
Integrated Process: Nursing Process—Assessment
Content Area: Pharmacology
Reference: Hodgson, B., & Kizior, R. (2010). *Saunders nursing drug handbook 2010* (p. 236). St. Louis: Saunders.

645. 4

Rationale: Sucralfate is a gastric protectant. The medication should be scheduled for administration 1 hour before meals and at bedtime. The medication is timed to allow it to form a protective coating over the ulcer before food intake stimulates gastric acid production and mechanical irritation. The other options are incorrect.

Test-Taking Strategy: Use the process of elimination. Focusing on the client's diagnosis and thinking about the pathophysiology associated with a gastric ulcer will assist in directing you to option 4. Review the administration of this medication if you had difficulty with this question.

Level of Cognitive Ability: Applying
Client Needs: Physiological Integrity
Integrated Process: Nursing Process—Implementation
Content Area: Pharmacology
Reference: Hodgson, B., & Kizior, R. (2010). *Saunders nursing drug handbook 2010* (p. 1061). St. Louis: Saunders.

646. 2

Rationale: The client who chronically uses nonsteroidal antiinflammatory drugs (NSAIDs) is prone to gastric mucosal injury. Misoprostol is a gastric protectant and is given specifically to prevent this occurrence. Diarrhea can be a side effect of the medication but is not an intended effect. Options 3 and 4 are incorrect.

Test-Taking Strategy: The strategic words in this question are *intended therapeutic effect.* This tells you that the medication is being given to prevent the occurrence of specific symptoms. Recalling that NSAIDs can cause gastric mucosal injury will direct you to option 2. Review this medication and the side effects of NSAIDs if you had difficulty with this question.

Level of Cognitive Ability: Evaluating
Client Needs: Physiological Integrity
Integrated Process: Nursing Process—Evaluation
Content Area: Pharmacology
Reference: Hodgson, B., & Kizior, R. (2010). *Saunders nursing drug handbook 2010* (pp. 762–763). St. Louis: Saunders.

647. 2

Rationale: Omeprazole is a proton pump inhibitor classified as an antiulcer agent. The intended effect of the medication is relief of pain from gastric irritation, often called heartburn by clients. Omeprazole is not used to treat the conditions identified in options 1, 3, and 4.

Test-Taking Strategy: Use the process of elimination. Recalling that this medication is a proton pump inhibitor will direct you to option 2. Review the action of this medication if you had difficulty with this question.

Level of Cognitive Ability: Evaluating
Client Needs: Physiological Integrity
Integrated Process: Nursing Process—Evaluation
Content Area: Pharmacology
Reference: Hodgson, B., & Kizior, R. (2010). *Saunders nursing drug handbook 2010* (pp. 848–849). St. Louis: Saunders.

648. 3

Rationale: Triple therapy for *Helicobacter pylori* infection usually includes two antibacterial drugs and a proton pump inhibitor. Clarithromycin and amoxicillin are antibacterials. Esomeprazole is a proton pump inhibitor. These medications will kill the bacteria and decrease acid production.

Test-Taking Strategy: Focus on the name of the medications and their actions. Eliminate option 1 because the medications do more than kill the bacteria. These medications are taken not only when there is pain but continually until gone, usually for 1 to 2 weeks. This will eliminate option 2. These medications do not coat the ulcer, eliminating option 4. Review the medication regimens for treatment of *H. pylori* and their actions if you had difficulty with this question.

Level of Cognitive Ability: Evaluating
Client Needs: Physiological Integrity
Integrated Process: Nursing Process—Evaluation
Content Area: Pharmacology
References: Ignatavicius, D., & Workman, M. (2010). *Medical-surgical nursing: Patient-centered collaborative care* (6th ed., pp. 1274–1275). St. Louis: Saunders.
　　Kee, J., Hayes, E., & McCuistion, L. (2009). *Pharmacology: A nursing process approach* (6th ed., p. 724). St. Louis: Saunders.

649. 4

Rationale: Metoclopramide is a gastrointestinal stimulant and antiemetic. Because it is a gastrointestinal stimulant, it is contraindicated with gastrointestinal obstruction, hemorrhage, or perforation. It is used in the treatment of emesis after surgery, chemotherapy, and radiation.

Test-Taking Strategy: Use the process of elimination. Recalling the classification and action of this medication and that it is an antiemetic will direct you to option 4. Review the action of this medication if you had difficulty with this question.

Level of Cognitive Ability: Analyzing
Client Needs: Physiological Integrity
Integrated Process: Nursing Process—Analysis
Content Area: Pharmacology
References: Hodgson, B., & Kizior, R. (2010). *Saunders nursing drug handbook 2010* (pp. 741–743). St. Louis: Saunders.

Lehne, R. (2010). *Pharmacology for nursing care* (7th ed., p. 947). St. Louis: Saunders.

650. 3

Rationale: Cholestyramine (Questran) is a bile acid sequestrant used to lower the cholesterol level and client compliance is a problem because of its taste and palatability. The use of flavored products or fruit juices can improve the taste. Some side effects of bile acid sequestrants include constipation and decreased vitamin absorption.

Test-Taking Strategy: Use the process of elimination and note the strategic words *need for further instructions.* These words indicate a negative event query and ask you to select an option that is an incorrect statement. Noting the close-ended word *only* in option 3 will direct you to this option. Review the action and side effects of this class of medications if you had difficulty with this question.

Level of Cognitive Ability: Evaluating
Client Needs: Physiological Integrity

Integrated Process: Teaching and Learning
Content Area: Pharmacology
Reference: Hodgson, B., & Kizior, R. (2010). *Saunders nursing drug handbook 2010* (p. 229). St. Louis: Saunders.

ALTERNATE ITEM FORMAT: MULTIPLE RESPONSE
651. 1, 2, 3, 4

Rationale: H_2-receptor antagonists suppress secretion of gastric acid, alleviate symptoms of heartburn, and assist in preventing complications of peptic ulcer disease. These medications also suppress gastric acid secretions and are used in active ulcer disease, erosive esophagitis, and pathological hypersecretory conditions. The other medications listed are proton pump inhibitors.

Test-Taking Strategy: Focus on the subject, H_2-receptor antagonists. Recalling that these medication names end with *-dine* will assist in answering this question. Also, recall that proton pump inhibitor medication names end with *-zole*. Review the H_2-receptor antagonists if you had difficulty with this question.

Level of Cognitive Ability: Analyzing
Client Needs: Physiological Integrity
Integrated Process: Nursing Process—Analysis
Content Area: Pharmacology
References: Kee, J., Hayes, E., & McCuistion, L. (2009). *Pharmacology: A nursing process approach* (6th ed., p. 731). St. Louis: Saunders.

Lehne, R. (2010). *Pharmacology for nursing care* (7th ed., pp. 919–920). St. Louis: Saunders.

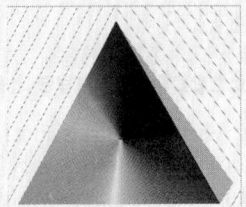

The Adult Client With a Respiratory Disorder

PYRAMID TERMS

asthma A chronic inflammatory disorder of the airways marked by airway hyperresponsiveness. Asthma causes recurrent episodes of wheezing, breathlessness, chest tightness, and coughing associated with airflow obstruction that is often reversible with treatment.

bacille Calmette-Guérin vaccine A vaccine containing attenuated tubercle bacilli that may be given to persons in foreign countries or to those traveling to foreign countries to produce increased resistance to tuberculosis.

chronic obstructive pulmonary disease A disease state characterized by pulmonary airflow obstruction that is usually progressive, not fully reversible, and sometimes accompanied by airway hyperreactivity. Airflow obstruction may be caused by chronic bronchitis and/or emphysema. In chronic hypercapnia, the stimulus to breathe is a low Po_2 instead of an increased Pco_2.

emphysema Abnormal permanent enlargement of air spaces distal to the terminal bronchioles, with destruction of alveolar walls without obvious fibrosis.

Mantoux skin test The most reliable determinant of infection with tuberculosis. A small amount (0.1 mL) of intermediate-strength purified protein derivative containing 5 tuberculin units is given intradermally in the forearm. An area of induration measuring 10 mm or more in diameter, 48 to 72 hours after injection, indicates that the individual has been exposed to tuberculosis.

mechanical ventilation The use of a ventilator to move room air or oxygen-enriched air into and out of the lungs mechanically to maintain proper levels of oxygen and carbon dioxide in the blood. Types of ventilators include negative-pressure and positive-pressure ventilators. Various ventilator modes are adjusted to the client's individual needs.

multidrug-resistant strain A multidrug-resistant strain of tuberculosis (MDR-TB) can occur as a result of improper or noncompliant use of treatment programs and the development of mutations in the tubercle bacilli.

Mycobacterium tuberculosis The causative organism (bacillus) of tuberculosis; an aerobic bacterium that is a nonmotile, nonsporulating, acid-fast rod that secretes niacin.

pneumothorax The accumulation of atmospheric air in the pleural space caused by a rupture in the visceral or parietal pleura. The loss of negative intrapleural pressure results in collapse of the lung. Diagnosis of pneumothorax is made by chest radiography.

suctioning A sterile procedure involving the removal of respiratory secretions that accumulate in the tracheobronchial airway when the client is unable to expectorate secretions; performed to maintain a patent airway.

tuberculosis A highly communicable disease caused by *Mycobacterium tuberculosis*. Tuberculosis is transmitted by the airborne route via droplet infection.

PYRAMID TO SUCCESS

The Pyramid to Success focuses on respiratory acid-base imbalances and reading arterial blood gas results, infectious diseases, particularly tuberculosis, and respiratory care in relation to oxygen delivery systems and mechanical ventilation. Pyramid Points focus on the client with pneumonia, respiratory failure, chronic obstructive pulmonary disease, pneumothorax, influenza, and tuberculosis. The Pyramid to Success includes the care of the client with tuberculosis, especially regarding the importance of the medication regimen, providing adequate nutrition and adequate rest to promote the healing process, and prevention of the progression of the disease. Focus on assisting the client to cope with the social isolation issues that exist during the period of illness and on teaching the client and family the critical measures of screening and of preventing respiratory disease and the transmission of disease.

 CLIENT NEEDS

Safe and Effective Care Environment

Collaborating with the multidisciplinary team in the management of the respiratory disorder

Discussing consultations and referrals related to the respiratory disorder

Establishing priorities

Handling infectious materials such as sputum or body fluids safely

Maintaining asepsis when caring for wounds or tracheostomy sites and during mechanical ventilation or suctioning

Maintaining confidentiality related to the respiratory disorder

Maintaining respiratory precautions, standard precautions, and other precautions

Obtaining informed consent related to diagnostic and surgical procedures

Upholding client rights

Health Promotion and Maintenance

Educating the client about adequate fluid and nutritional intake

Educating the client about breathing exercises and respiratory therapy and care

Educating the client about medication administration

Educating the client about the need for follow-up care

Educating the client about the prevention of transmission of infection

Informing the client about health promotion programs

Performing respiratory assessment techniques

Preventing respiratory disorders and infectious diseases

Providing health screening related to risks for respiratory disorders

Psychosocial Integrity

Considering religious, cultural, and spiritual influences when providing care

Discussing body image changes related to tracheostomy if performed

Discussing end-of-life and grief and loss issues

Discussing situational role changes

Identifying coping mechanisms

Identifying support systems

Informing the client about community resources

Physiological Integrity

Administering medications

Caring for the client on mechanical ventilation

Caring for the client receiving respiratory care and oxygen

Managing illnesses

Monitoring for acid-base imbalances

Monitoring for alterations in body systems

Monitoring for infectious diseases

Providing comfort

Providing nutrition and oral hygiene

Providing personal hygiene and promoting rest and sleep

Reading arterial blood gas results

Respiratory System

I. ANATOMY AND PHYSIOLOGY

A. Primary functions of the respiratory system
  1. Provides oxygen for metabolism in the tissues
  2. Removes carbon dioxide, the waste product of metabolism

B. Secondary functions of the respiratory system
  1. Facilitates sense of smell
  2. Produces speech
  3. Maintains acid-base balance
  4. Maintains body water levels
  5. Maintains heat balance

C. Upper respiratory tract
  1. Nose: Humidifies, warms, and filters inspired air
  2. Sinuses: Air-filled cavities within the hollow bones that surround the nasal passages and provide resonance during speech
  3. Pharynx
    a. Passageway for the respiratory and digestive tracts located behind the oral and nasal cavities
    b. Divided into the nasopharynx, oropharynx, and laryngopharynx
  4. Larynx
    a. Located above the trachea, just below the pharynx at the root of the tongue; commonly called the voice box
    b. Contains two pairs of vocal cords, the false and true cords
    c. The opening between the true vocal cords is the glottis.
    d. The glottis plays an important role in coughing, which is the most fundamental defense mechanism of the lungs.
  5. Epiglottis
    a. Leaf-shaped elastic structure attached along one end to the top of the larynx
    b. Prevents food from entering the tracheobronchial tree by closing over the glottis during swallowing

D. Lower respiratory tract
  1. Trachea: Located in front of the esophagus; branches into the right and left mainstem bronchi at the carina

  2. Mainstem bronchi
    a. Begin at the carina
    b. The right bronchus is slightly wider, shorter, and more vertical than the left bronchus.
    c. The mainstem bronchi divide into secondary or lobar bronchi that enter each of the five lobes of the lung.
    d. The bronchi are lined with cilia, which propel mucus up and away from the lower airway to the trachea, where it can be expectorated or swallowed.
  3. Bronchioles
    a. Branch from the secondary bronchi and subdivide into the small terminal and respiratory bronchioles
    b. The bronchioles contain no cartilage and depend on the elastic recoil of the lung for patency.
    c. The terminal bronchioles contain no cilia and do not participate in gas exchange.
  4. Alveolar ducts and alveoli
    a. *Acinus* (plural acini) is a term used to indicate all structures distal to the terminal bronchiole.
    b. Alveolar ducts branch from the respiratory bronchioles.
    c. Alveolar sacs, which arise from the ducts, contain clusters of alveoli, which are the basic units of gas exchange.
    d. Type II alveolar cells in the walls of the alveoli secrete surfactant, a phospholipid protein that reduces the surface tension in the alveoli; without surfactant, the alveoli would collapse.
  5. Lungs
    a. Located in the pleural cavity in the thorax
    b. Extend from just above the clavicles to the diaphragm, the major muscle of inspiration
    c. The right lung, which is larger than the left, is divided into three lobes: the upper, middle, and lower lobes.
    d. The left lung, which is narrower than the right lung to accommodate the heart, is divided into two lobes.

e. The respiratory structures are innervated by the phrenic nerve, the vagus nerve, and the thoracic nerves.

f. The parietal pleura lines the inside of the thoracic cavity, including the upper surface of the diaphragm.

g. The visceral pleura covers the pulmonary surfaces.

h. A thin fluid layer, which is produced by the cells lining the pleura, lubricates the visceral pleura and the parietal pleura, allowing them to glide smoothly and painlessly during respiration.

i. Blood flows through the lungs via the pulmonary system and the bronchial system.

6. Accessory muscles of respiration include the scalene muscles, which elevate the first two ribs, the sternocleidomastoid muscles, which raise the sternum, and the trapezius and pectoralis muscles, which fix the shoulders.

7. The respiratory process

a. The diaphragm descends into the abdominal cavity during inspiration, causing negative pressure in the lungs.

b. The negative pressure draws air from the area of greater pressure, the atmosphere, into the area of lesser pressure, the lungs.

c. In the lungs, air passes through the terminal bronchioles into the alveoli to oxygenate the body tissues.

d. At the end of inspiration, the diaphragm and intercostal muscles relax and the lungs recoil.

e. As the lungs recoil, pressure within the lungs becomes higher than atmospheric pressure, causing the air, which now contains the cellular waste products carbon dioxide and water, to move from the alveoli in the lungs to the atmosphere.

f. Effective gas exchange depends on distribution of gas (ventilation) and blood (perfusion) in all portions of the lungs.

II. DIAGNOSTIC TESTS

A. Risk factors for respiratory disorders (Box 58-1)

B. Chest x-ray film (radiograph)

1. Description: Provides information regarding the anatomical location and appearance of the lungs

2. Preprocedure

a. Remove all jewelry and other metal objects from the chest area.

b. Assess the client's ability to inhale and hold his or her breath.

3. Postprocedure: Help the client get dressed.

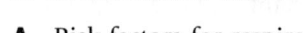 Question women regarding pregnancy or the possibility of pregnancy before performing radiography studies.

Box 58-1 Risk Factors for Respiratory Disorders

Allergies
Chest injury
Crowded living conditions
Exposure to chemicals and environmental pollutants
Family history of infectious disease
Frequent respiratory illnesses
Geographic residence and travel to foreign countries
Smoking
Surgery
Use of chewing tobacco
Viral syndromes

C. Sputum specimen

1. Description: Specimen obtained by expectoration or tracheal **suctioning** to assist in the identification of organisms or abnormal cells (see Priority Nursing Actions)

▰▰▰▰ PRIORITY NURSING ACTIONS! ▰▰▰▰

Actions to Take to Perform Respiratory Suctioning

1. Explain the procedure to the client.
2. Assist the client to an upright position.
3. Perform hand hygiene and don protective garb.
4. Prepare suctioning equipment and turn on the suction.
5. Hyperoxygenate the client.
6. Insert the catheter without suction applied.
7. Once inserted, apply suction intermittently while rotating and withdrawing the catheter.
8. Hyperoxygenate the client.
9. Listen to breath sounds.
10. Document the procedure, client response, and effectiveness.

Once the nurse has assessed the client, the nurse would explain the procedure. The client is assisted to a sitting upright position such as semi-Fowler's with the head hyperextended (unless contraindicated). The nurse next performs hand hygiene and applies appropriate protective garb using aseptic technique. The nurse prepares the needed suctioning equipment, turns on the suction device, and sets it to the appropriate pressure. The nurse hyperoxygenates the client by a resuscitation bag, increasing the oxygen flow rate, or asking the client to take deep breaths. The nurse next lubricates the catheter with sterile water or water-soluble lubricant (per agency procedure), inserts the catheter without the application of suction, and then applies intermittent suction for up to 10 seconds while rotating and withdrawing the catheter. After suctioning, the nurse hyperoxygenates the client and encourages the client to take deep breaths if possible. During the procedure the nurse monitors the client for toleration of the procedure and the presence of complications. Finally, the nurse listens to breath sounds to assist in determining effectiveness and documents the procedure, the client's response, and effectiveness.

Reference: Perry, A., & Potter, P. (2006). *Clinical nursing skills & techniques* (6th ed., pp. 824-828). St. Louis: Mosby.

2. Preprocedure
   a. Determine specific purpose of collection and check with institutional policy for appropriate method for collection of a specimen.
   b. Obtain an early morning sterile specimen from **suctioning** or expectoration after a respiratory treatment if a treatment is prescribed.
   c. Instruct the client to rinse the mouth with water before collection.
   d. Obtain 15 mL of sputum.
   e. Instruct the client to take several deep breaths and then cough deeply to obtain sputum.
   f. Always collect the specimen before the client begins antibiotic therapy.
3. Postprocedure
   a. If a culture of sputum is prescribed, transport the specimen to the laboratory immediately.
   b. Assist the client with mouth care.

D. Laryngoscopy and bronchoscopy
1. Description: Direct visual examination of the larynx, trachea, and bronchi with a fiberoptic bronchoscope
2. Preprocedure
   a. Obtain informed consent.
   b. Maintain NPO status for the client from midnight before the procedure.
   c. Obtain vital signs.
   d. Assess the results of coagulation studies.
   e. Remove dentures and eyeglasses.
   f. Prepare suction equipment.
   g. Establish an intravenous (IV) access as necessary and administer medication for sedation as prescribed.
   h. Have emergency resuscitation equipment readily available.
3. Postprocedure
   a. Monitor vital signs.
   b. Maintain the client in a semi-Fowler's position.
   c. Assess for the return of the gag reflex.
   d. Maintain NPO status until the gag reflex returns.
   e. Have an emesis basin readily available for the client to expectorate sputum.
   f. Monitor for bloody sputum.
   g. Monitor respiratory status, particularly if sedation has been administered.
   h. Monitor for complications, such as bronchospasm or bronchial perforation, indicated by facial or neck crepitus, dysrhythmias, hemorrhage, hypoxemia, and **pneumothorax**.
   i. Notify the physician if fever, difficulty in breathing, or other signs of complications occur following the procedure.

E. Mediastinoscopy
1. Insertion of a flexible tube through the chest wall above the sternum into the area of the upper chest between the lungs.
2. Performed in the operating room under general anesthesia.
3. Done to look for the presence of tumors and to obtain tissue samples for biopsy and culture.
4. Complications relate to anesthetic mediations and bleeding.

F. Pulmonary angiography
1. Description
   a. An invasive fluoroscopic procedure in which a catheter is inserted through the antecubital or femoral vein into the pulmonary artery or one of its branches
   b. Involves an injection of iodine or radiopaque contrast material
2. Preprocedure
   a. Obtain informed consent.
   b. Assess for allergies to iodine, seafood, or other radiopaque dyes.
   c. Maintain NPO status of the client for 8 hours before the procedure.
   d. Monitor vital signs.
   e. Assess results of coagulation studies.
   f. Establish an intravenous access.
   g. Administer sedation as prescribed.
   h. Instruct the client to lie still during the procedure.
   i. Instruct the client that he or she may feel an urge to cough, flushing, nausea, or a salty taste following injection of the dye.
   j. Have emergency resuscitation equipment available.
3. Postprocedure
   a. Monitor vital signs.
   b. Avoid taking blood pressures for 24 hours in the extremity used for the injection.
   c. Monitor peripheral neurovascular status of the affected extremity.
   d. Assess insertion site for bleeding.
   e. Monitor for delayed reaction to the dye.

G. Thoracentesis
1. Description: Removal of fluid or air from the pleural space via a transthoracic aspiration
2. Preprocedure
   a. Obtain informed consent.
   b. Obtain vital signs.
   c. Prepare the client for ultrasound or chest radiograph, if prescribed, before procedure.
   d. Assess results of coagulation studies.
   e. Note that the client is positioned sitting upright, with the arms and shoulders supported by a table at the bedside during the procedure (Fig. 58-1).

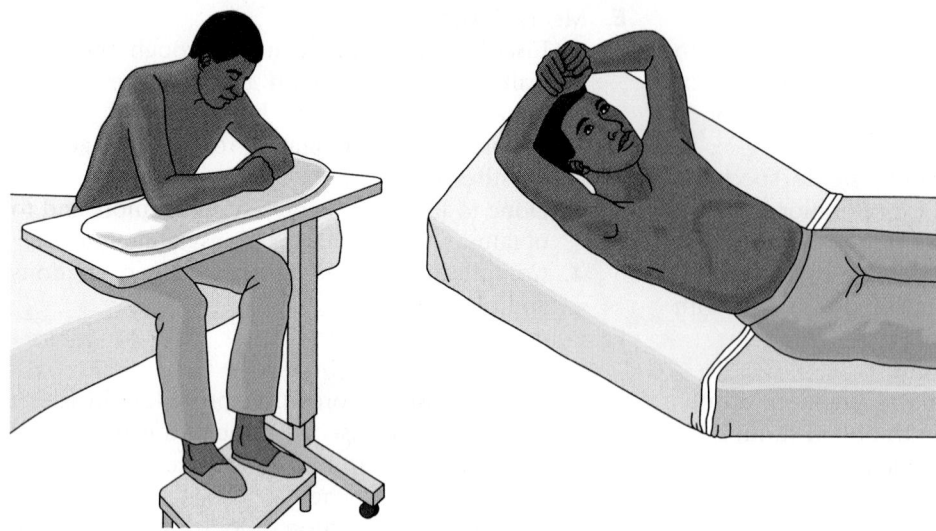

▲ **FIGURE 58-1** Positions for thoracentesis. (From Ignatavicius, D., & Workman, M. [2006]. *Medical-surgical nursing: Critical thinking for collaborative care* [5th ed.]. St. Louis: Saunders.)

    f. If the client cannot sit up, the client is placed lying in bed toward the unaffected side, with the head of the bed elevated.

    g. Instruct the client not to cough, breathe deeply, or move during the procedure.

  3. Postprocedure

    a. Monitor vital signs.

    b. Monitor respiratory status.

    c. Apply a pressure dressing, and assess the puncture site for bleeding and crepitus.

    d. Monitor for signs of **pneumothorax**, air embolism, and pulmonary edema.

H. Pulmonary function tests

  1. Description: Tests used to evaluate lung mechanics, gas exchange, and acid-base disturbance through spirometric measurements, lung volumes, and arterial blood gas levels.

  2. Preprocedure

    a. Determine whether an analgesic that may depress the respiratory function is being administered.

    b. Consult with the physician regarding holding bronchodilators before testing.

    c. Instruct the client to void before the procedure and to wear loose clothing.

    d. Remove dentures.

    e. Instruct the client to refrain from smoking or eating a heavy meal for 4 to 6 hours before the test.

  3. Postprocedure: Client may resume normal diet and any bronchodilators and respiratory treatments that were held before the procedure.

I. Lung biopsy

  1. Description

    a. A transbronchial biopsy and a transbronchial needle aspiration may be performed to obtain tissue for analysis by culture or cytological examination.

    b. An open lung biopsy is performed in the operating room.

  2. Preprocedure

    a. Obtain informed consent.

    b. Maintain NPO status of the client before the procedure.

    c. Inform the client that a local anesthetic will be used for a needle biopsy but a sensation of pressure during needle insertion and aspiration may be felt.

    d. Administer analgesics and sedatives as prescribed.

  3. Postprocedure

    a. Monitor vital signs.

    b. Apply a dressing to the biopsy site and monitor for drainage or bleeding.

    c. Monitor for signs of respiratory distress, and notify the physician if they occur.

    d. Monitor for signs of **pneumothorax** and air emboli, and notify the physician if they occur.

    e. Prepare the client for chest radiography if prescribed.

J. Ventilation-perfusion lung scan

  1. Description

    a. The perfusion scan evaluates blood flow to the lungs.

    b. The ventilation scan determines the patency of the pulmonary airways and detects abnormalities in ventilation.

    c. A radionuclide may be injected for the procedure.

  2. Preprocedure

    a. Obtain informed consent.

    b. Assess the client for allergies to dye, iodine, or seafood.

    c. Remove jewelry around the chest area.

    d. Review breathing methods that may be required during testing.

e. Establish an intravenous access.
f. Administer sedation if prescribed.
g. Have emergency resuscitation equipment available.
3. Postprocedure
a. Monitor client for reaction to the radionuclide.
b. Instruct the client that the radionuclide clears from the body in about 8 hours.
K. Skin tests: A skin test uses an intradermal injection to help diagnose various infectious diseases (Box 58-2)
L. Arterial blood gases (ABGs) (Box 58-3)
1. Description: Measurement of the dissolved oxygen and carbon dioxide in the arterial blood helps indicate the acid-base state and how well oxygen is being carried to the body.
2. Preprocedure
a. Perform Allen's test before drawing radial artery specimens.
b. Have the client rest for 30 minutes before specimen collection to ensure accurate measurement of body oxygenation.
c. Do not turn off oxygen unless the ABG sample is prescribed to be drawn with the client breathing room air.

⚠ Avoid suctioning the client before drawing an ABG sample because the suctioning procedure will deplete the client's oxygen resulting in inaccurate ABG results.

Box 58-2 Skin Test Procedure

Determine hypersensitivity or previous reactions to skin tests.
Use a skin site that is free of excessive body hair, dermatitis, and blemishes.
Apply the injection at the upper third of the inner surface of the left arm.
Circle and mark the injection test site.
Document the date, time, and test site.
Advise the client not to scratch the test site to prevent infection and possible abscess formation.
Instruct the client to avoid washing the test site.
Interpret the reaction at the injection site 24 to 72 hours after administration of the test antigen.
Assess the test site for the amount of induration (hard swelling) in millimeters and for the presence of erythema and vesiculation (small blister-like elevations).

Box 58-3 Normal Arterial Blood Gas Values

pH: 7.35 to 7.45
Pco_2: 35 to 45 mm Hg
HCO_3: 22 to 27 mEq/L
Po_2: 80 to 100 mm Hg
O_2 saturation: 96% to 100%
Oxyhemoglobin dissociation curve: No shift

3. Postprocedure
a. Place the specimen on ice.
b. Note the client's temperature on the laboratory form.
c. Note the oxygen and type of ventilation that the client is receiving on the laboratory form.
d. Apply pressure to the puncture site for 5 to 10 minutes or longer if the client is receiving anticoagulant therapy or has a bleeding disorder.
e. Transport the specimen to the laboratory within 15 minutes.
f. See Chapter 10 for discussion of the analysis of ABG results.
M. Pulse oximetry
1. Description
a. Pulse oximetry is a noninvasive test that registers the oxygen saturation of the client's hemoglobin.
b. The capillary oxygen saturation (Sao_2) is recorded as a percentage.
c. The normal value is 96% to 100%.
d. After a hypoxic client uses up the readily available oxygen (measured as the arterial oxygen pressure, Pao_2, on ABG testing), the reserve oxygen, that oxygen attached to the hemoglobin (Sao_2), is drawn on to provide oxygen to the tissues.
e. A pulse oximeter reading can alert the nurse to hypoxemia before clinical signs occur.
2. Procedure
a. A sensor is placed on the client's finger, toe, nose, ear lobe, or forehead to measure oxygen saturation, which then is displayed on a monitor.
b. Maintain the transducer at heart level.
c. Do not select an extremity with an impediment to blood flow.

⚠ A pulse oximetry reading lower than 91% necessitate physician notification; if the reading is lower than 85%, oxygenation to body tissues is compromised, and a reading lower than 70% is life-threatening.

III. RESPIRATORY TREATMENTS

A. Breathing retraining (Box 58-4)
B. Chest physiotherapy (CPT) (Fig. 58-2)
1. Description: Percussion, vibration, and postural drainage techniques are performed over the thorax to loosen secretions in the affected area of the lungs and move them into more central airways.
2. Interventions (Box 58-5)
3. Contraindications
a. Unstable vital signs
b. Increased intracranial pressure
c. Bronchospasm

Box 58-4 Client Education: Breathing Retraining and Huff Coughing

Breathing Retraining

This includes exercises to decrease the use of accessory muscles of breathing, to decrease fatigue, and to promote CO_2 elimination.

The main types of exercises include pursed-lip breathing and diaphragmatic breathing.

The client should inhale slowly through the nose.

The client should place the hand over the abdomen while inhaling; the abdomen should expand with inhalation and contract during exhalation.

The client should exhale three times longer than inhalation by blowing through pursed lips.

Huff Coughing

This is an effective coughing technique that conserves energy, reduces fatigue, and facilitates mobilization of secretions.

The client should take three or four deep breaths using pursed-lip and diaphragmatic breathing. Leaning slightly forward, the client should cough three to four times during exhalation.

The client may need to splint the thorax or abdomen to achieve a maximum cough.

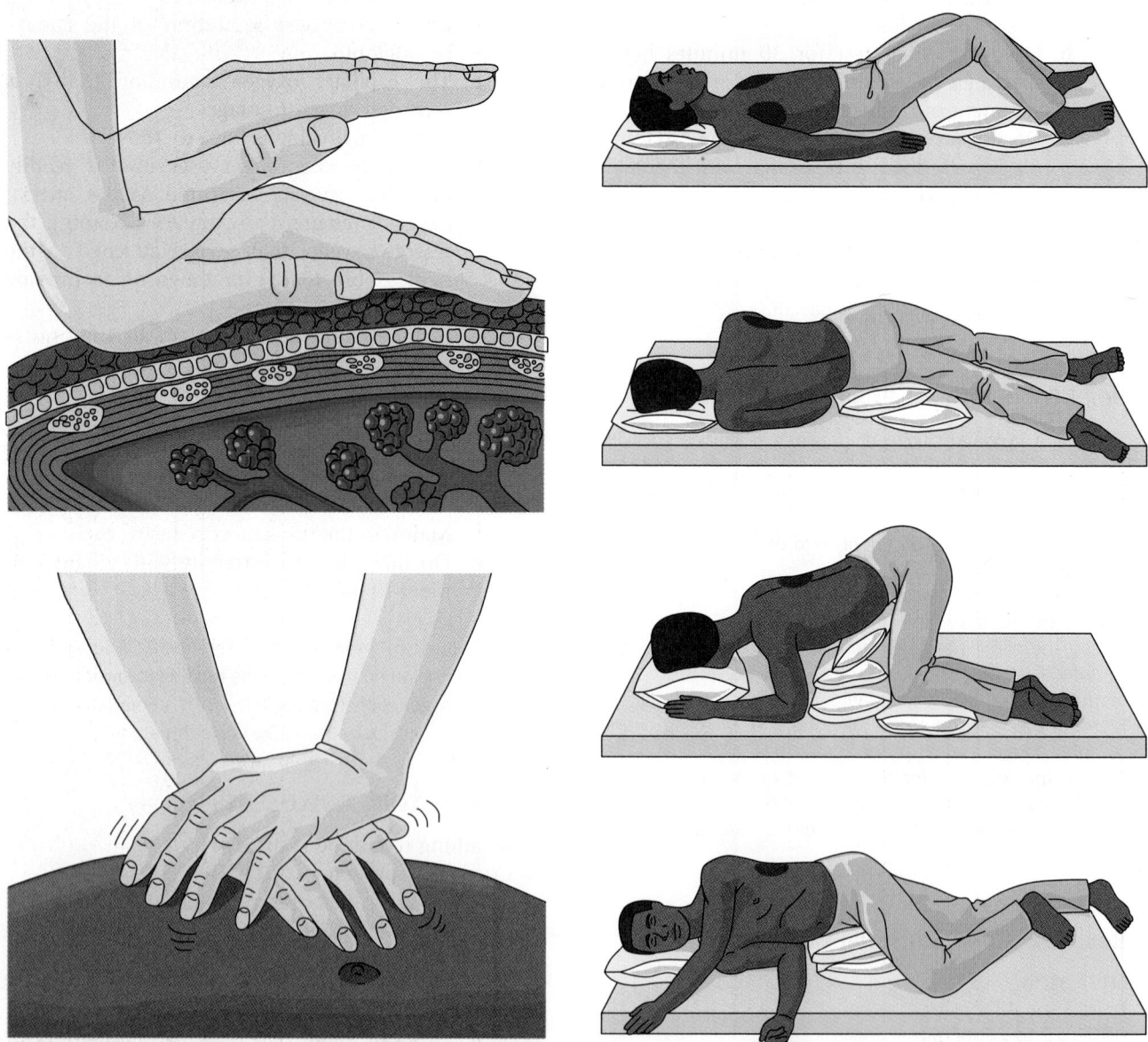

▲ **FIGURE 58-2** Chest physiotherapy (CPT) and postural drainage. *Left*, Percussion and vibration techniques. The nurse may use one or two hands with vibration, which is performed when the client exhales or coughs. *Right*, Positions for postural drainage of respiratory secretions. (From Ignatavicius, D., & Workman, M. [2010]. *Medical-surgical nursing: Patient-centered collaborative care* [6th ed.]. St. Louis: Saunders.)

Box 58-5 Chest Physiotherapy Procedure

Perform chest physiotherapy (CPT) in the morning on arising, 1 hour before meals, or 2 to 3 hours after meals.

Stop CPT if pain occurs.

If the client is receiving a tube feeding, stop the feeding and aspirate the residual before beginning CPT.

Administer the bronchodilator (if prescribed) 15 minutes before the procedure.

Place a layer of material (gown or pajamas) between the hands or percussion device and the client's skin.

Position the client for postural drainage based on assessment.

Percuss the area for 1 to 2 minutes.

Vibrate the same area while the client exhales four or five deep breaths.

Monitor for respiratory tolerance to the procedure.

Stop the procedure if cyanosis or exhaustion occurs.

Maintain the position for 5 to 20 minutes after the procedure.

Repeat in all necessary positions until the client no longer expectorates mucus.

Dispose of sputum properly.

Provide mouth care after the procedure.

Box 58-6 Client Instructions for Incentive Spirometry

Instruct the client to assume a sitting or upright position.

Instruct the client to place the mouth tightly around the mouthpiece of the device.

Instruct the client to inhale slowly to raise and maintain the flow rate indicator between the 600 and 900 marks.

Instruct the client to hold the breath for 5 seconds and then to exhale through pursed lips.

Instruct the client to repeat this process 10 times every hour.

d. History of pathological fractures
e. Rib fractures
f. Chest incisions
C. Incentive spirometry (Box 58-6)

IV. OXYGEN

A. Interventions
1. Assess color and vital signs before and during treatment.
2. Place an *Oxygen in Use* sign at the client's bedside.
3. Assess for the presence of chronic lung problems.
4. Humidify the oxygen if indicated.
B. Nasal cannula (nasal prongs) (Box 58-7 and Fig. 58-3)
1. Description
   a. A nasal cannula is used at a flow rate of 1 to 6 L/min, providing approximate oxygen concentrations of 24% (at 1 L/min) to 44% (at 6 L/min).

Box 58-7 Fraction of Inspired Oxygen Delivered via Nasal Cannula

24% at 1 L/min	36% at 4 L/min
28% at 2 L/min	40% at 5 L/min
32% at 3 L/min	44% at 6 L/min

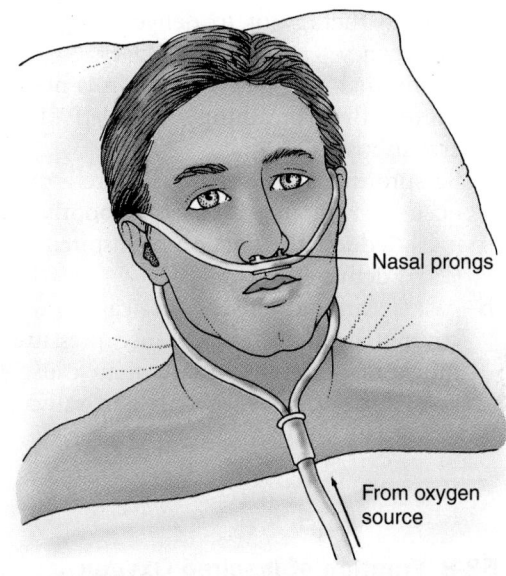

▲ **FIGURE 58-3** A nasal cannula (prongs). (From Ignatavicius, D., & Workman, M. [2006]. *Medical-surgical nursing: Critical thinking for collaborative care* [5th ed.]. St. Louis: Saunders.)

   b. Flow rates higher than 6 L/min do not significantly increase oxygenation because the anatomical reserve or dead space (oral and nasal cavities) is full.
   c. A nasal cannula is used for the client with chronic airflow limitation and for long-term oxygen use.
   d. Effective oxygen concentration can be delivered to nose breathers and mouth breathers with the use of a nasal cannula.

⚠ A client who is hypoxemic and has chronic hypercapnia requires low levels of oxygen delivery at 1 to 2 L/min because a low arterial oxygen level is the client's primary drive for breathing.

2. Interventions
   a. Place the nasal prongs in the nostrils, with the openings facing the client.
   b. Add humidification as prescribed when a flow rate higher than 2 L/min is prescribed.
   c. Check the water level and change the humidifier as needed.
   d. Assess the client for changes in respiratory rate or depth.

e. Assess the nasal mucosa because high flow rates have a drying effect and increase mucosal irritation.

f. Assess skin integrity because the oxygen tubing can irritate the skin.

C. Simple face mask (Box 58-8 and Fig. 58-4)

1. Description

a. A face mask is used to deliver oxygen concentrations of 40% to 60% for short-term oxygen therapy or to deliver oxygen in an emergency.

b. A minimal flow rate of 5 L/min is needed to prevent the rebreathing of exhaled air.

2. Interventions

a. Be sure that the mask fits securely over the nose and mouth because a poorly fitting mask reduces the fraction of inspired oxygen (FIO_2) delivered.

b. Assess skin and provide skin care to the area covered by the mask because pressure and moisture under the mask may cause skin breakdown (remove mucus and saliva from the mask).

c. Monitor the client closely for the risk of aspiration because the mask limits the client's ability to clear the mouth, especially if vomiting occurs.

d. Provide emotional support to decrease anxiety in the client who feels claustrophobic.

e. Consult with the physician regarding switching the client from a mask to a nasal cannula during eating.

D. Partial rebreather mask (Box 58-9 and Fig. 58-5)

1. Description

a. A partial rebreather mask consists of a mask with a reservoir bag that provides an oxygen concentration of 70% to 90% with flow rates of 6 to 15 L/min.

b. The client rebreathes one third of the exhaled tidal volume, which is high in oxygen, thus providing a high FIO_2.

2. Interventions

a. Make sure that the reservoir does not twist, kink, or become deflated.

b. Adjust the flow rate to keep the reservoir bag inflated two-thirds full during inspiration

---

Box 58-8 Fraction of Inspired Oxygen Delivered via Simple Face Mask

40% at 5 L/min
45% to 50% at 6 L/min
55% to 60% at 8 L/min
Pyramid Point: Flow rate must be set to at least 5 L/min to flush the mask of carbon dioxide.

Box 58-9 Fraction of Inspired Oxygen Delivered via Partial Rebreather Mask

70% to 90% FIO_2 delivered at 6 to 15 L/min
Pyramid Point: A flow rate high enough to maintain the bag two-thirds full during inspiration is needed.

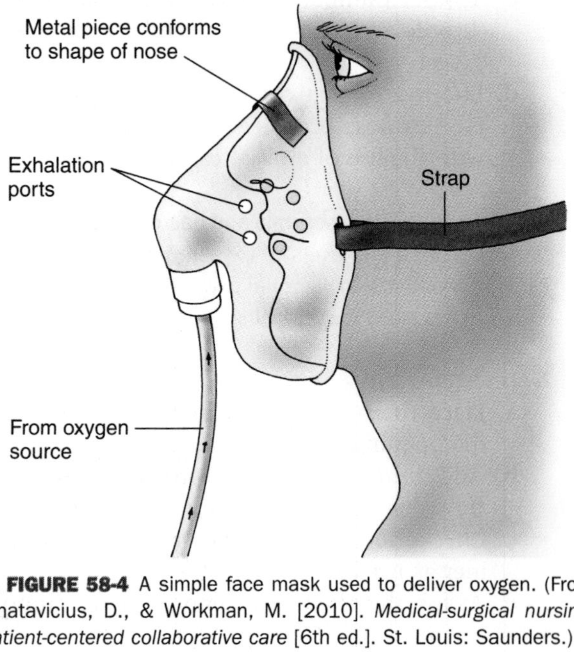

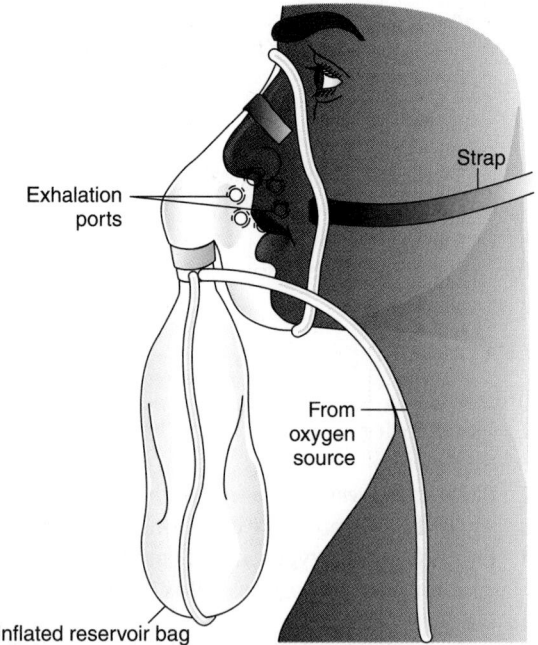

▲ **FIGURE 58-4** A simple face mask used to deliver oxygen. (From Ignatavicius, D., & Workman, M. [2010]. *Medical-surgical nursing: Patient-centered collaborative care* [6th ed.]. St. Louis: Saunders.)

▲ **FIGURE 58-5** A partial rebreather mask. (From Ignatavicius, D., & Workman, M. [2010]. *Medical-surgical nursing: Patient-centered collaborative care* [6th ed.]. St. Louis: Saunders.)

because deflation results in decreased oxygen delivered and rebreathing of exhaled air.
E. Nonrebreather mask (Fig. 58-6)
 1. Description
  a. Of the low-flow systems, a nonrebreather mask provides the highest concentration of oxygen and can deliver an FIO_2 higher than 90%, depending on the client's ventilatory pattern.
  b. A nonrebreather mask most frequently is used in the client with a deteriorating respiratory status who might require intubation.
  c. The nonrebreather mask has a one-way valve between the mask and the reservoir and two flaps over the exhalation ports.
  d. The valve allows the client to draw the entire quantity of oxygen from the reservoir bag.
  e. The flaps prevent room air from entering through the exhalation ports.
  f. During exhalation, air leaves through these exhalation ports while the one-way valve prevents exhaled air from reentering the reservoir bag.
 2. FIO_2 delivered: 60% to 100% FIO_2 at a rate of flow that maintains the bag two-thirds full
 3. Interventions
  a. Remove mucus or saliva from the mask.
  b. Assess the client closely.
  c. Ensure that the valve and flaps are intact and functional during each breath.
  d. Valves should open during expiration and close during inhalation.
  e. Suffocation can occur if the reservoir bag kinks or if the oxygen source disconnects.
F. Face tent
 1. A face tent fits over the client's chin, with the top extending halfway across the face.
 2. The oxygen concentration varies, but the face tent is useful instead of a tight-fitting mask for the client who has facial trauma or burns.
G. Aerosol mask: Used for the client who requires high humidity after extubation or upper airway surgery, or for the client who has thick secretions
H. Tracheostomy collar and T-piece (Fig. 58-7)
 1. The tracheostomy collar can be used to deliver high humidity and the desired oxygen to the client with a tracheostomy.
 2. A special adapter, called the T-piece, can be used to deliver any desired FIO_2 to the client with a tracheostomy, laryngectomy, or endotracheal tube.
 3. See Chapter 21 for information on endotracheal and tracheostomy tubes.
I. Interventions for face tent, aerosol mask, tracheostomy collar, and T-piece
 1. Change delivery system to a nasal cannula during mealtime if indicated for the client with a face mask or aerosol mask.
 2. Assess that the aerosol mist escapes from the vents of the delivery system during inspiration and expiration.
 3. Empty condensation from the tubing to prevent the client from being lavaged with water and to

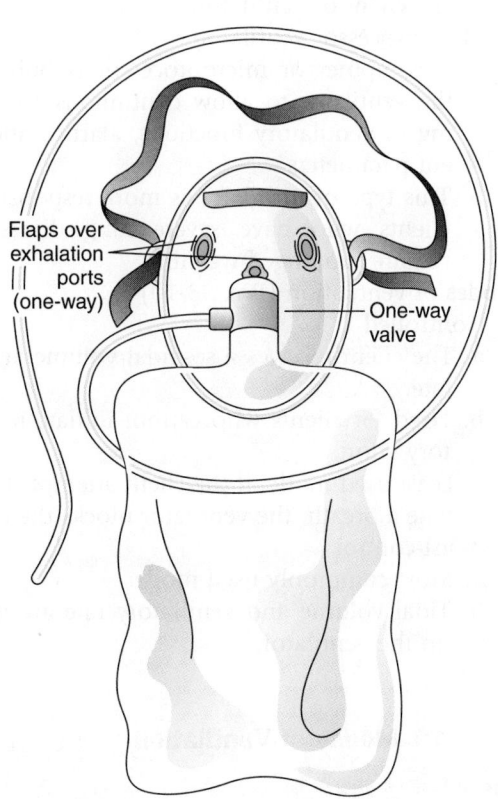

▲ **FIGURE 58-6** A nonrebreather mask. (From Ignatavicius, D., & Workman, M. [2010]. *Medical-surgical nursing: Patient-centered collaborative care* [6th ed.]. St. Louis: Saunders.)

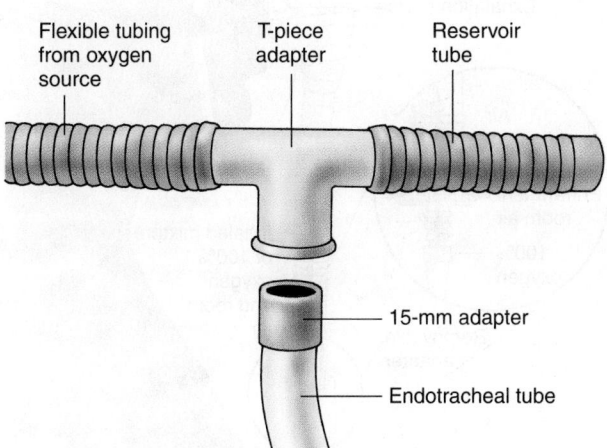

▲ **FIGURE 58-7** A T-piece apparatus for attachment to an endotracheal tube or tracheostomy tube. (From Ignatavicius, D., & Workman, M. [2010]. *Medical-surgical nursing: Patient-centered collaborative care* [6th ed.]. St. Louis: Saunders.)

promote an adequate oxygen flow rate; remove and clean the tubing at least every 4 hours.

4. Ensure that sufficient water is in the aerosol water container and change the container as needed.

5. Keep the exhalation port on the T-piece open and uncovered (if the port is occluded, the client can suffocate).

6. Position the T-piece so that it does not pull on the tracheostomy or endotracheal tube and cause erosion of the skin at the tracheostomy insertion site.

7. Make sure that the humidifier creates enough mist; a mist should be seen during inspiration and expiration.

J. Venturi mask (Fig. 58-8)
   1. Description
      a. High-flow oxygen delivery system
      b. Operation of the Venturi mask is based on a mechanism that pulls in a specific proportional amount of room air for each liter of oxygen delivered.
      c. An adapter is located between the bottom of the mask and the oxygen source; the adapter contains holes of different sizes that allow only specific amounts of air to mix with the oxygen.
      d. The adapter allows selection of the amount of oxygen desired.
   2. FIO_2 delivered: 24% to 55% FIO_2, with flow rates of 4 to 10 L/min

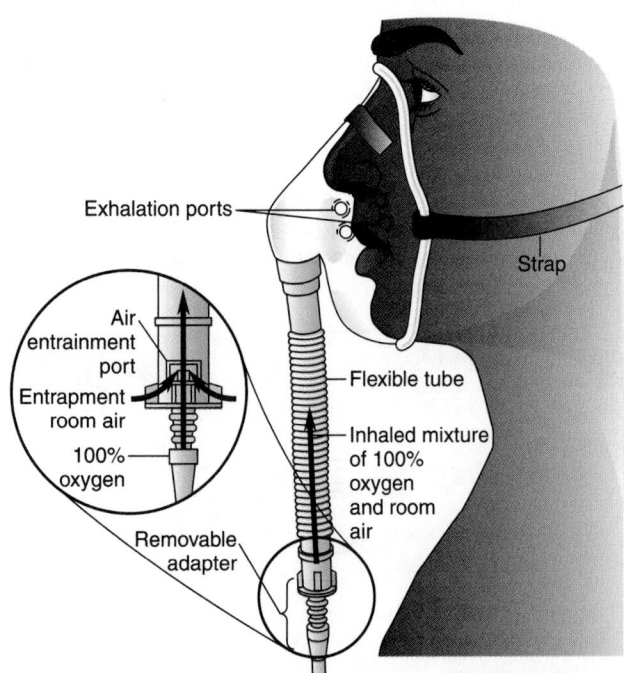

▲ **FIGURE 58-8** A Venturi mask for precise oxygen delivery. (From Ignatavicius, D., & Workman, M. [2010]. *Medical-surgical nursing: Patient-centered collaborative care* [6th ed.]. St. Louis: Saunders.)

3. Interventions
   a. Monitor the client closely to ensure an accurate flow rate for a specific FIO_2.
   b. Keep the air entrapment port for the Venturi adapter open and uncovered to ensure adequate oxygen delivery.
   c. Ensure that the mask fits snugly and that the tubing is free of kinks, because the FIO_2 is altered if kinking occurs or if the mask fits poorly.
   d. Assess the client for dry mucous membranes; humidity or aerosol can be added to the system.

V. MECHANICAL VENTILATION

A. Types
   1. Pressure-cycled ventilator: The ventilator pushes air into the lungs until a specific airway pressure is reached; it is used for short periods, as in the postanesthesia care unit.
   2. Time-cycled ventilator: The ventilator pushes air into the lungs until a preset time has elapsed; it is used for the pediatric or neonatal client.
   3. Volume-cycled ventilator
      a. The ventilator pushes air into the lungs until a preset volume is delivered.
      b. A constant tidal volume is delivered regardless of the changing compliance of the lungs and chest wall or the airway resistance in the client or ventilator.
   4. Microprocessor ventilator
      a. A computer or microprocessor is built into the ventilator to allow continuous monitoring of ventilatory functions, alarms, and client parameters.
      b. This type of ventilator is more responsive to clients who have severe lung disease or require prolonged weaning.

B. Modes of ventilation (Box 58-10)
   1. Controlled
      a. The client receives a set tidal volume at a set rate.
      b. Used for clients who cannot initiate respiratory effort.
      c. Least used mode; if the client attempts to initiate a breath, the ventilator blocks the effort.
   2. Assist-control
      a. Most commonly used mode
      b. Tidal volume and ventilatory rate are preset on the ventilator.

Box 58-10 Modes of Ventilation

Controlled
Assist-control
Synchronized intermittent mandatory ventilation

c. The ventilator takes over the work of breathing for the client.

d. The ventilator is programmed to respond to the client's inspiratory effort if the client does initiate a breath.

e. The ventilator delivers the preset tidal volume when the client initiates a breath while allowing the client to control the rate of breathing.

f. If the client's spontaneous ventilatory rate increases, the ventilator continues to deliver a preset tidal volume with each breath, which may cause hyperventilation and respiratory alkalosis.

3. Synchronized intermittent mandatory ventilation (SIMV)

a. Similar to assist-control ventilation in that the tidal volume and ventilatory rate are preset on the ventilator.

b. Allows the client to breath spontaneously at her or his own rate and tidal volume between the ventilator breaths

c. Can be used as a primary ventilatory mode or as a weaning mode.

d. When SIMV is used as a weaning mode, the number of SIMV breaths is decreased gradually, and the client gradually resumes spontaneous breathing.

C. Ventilator controls and settings (Table 58-1)

D. Interventions

⚠ For a client receiving mechanical ventilation, always assess the client first and then assess the ventilator.

1. Assess vital signs, lung sounds, respiratory status, and breathing patterns (the client will never breathe at a rate lower than the rate set on the ventilator).

2. Monitor skin color, particularly in the lips and nail beds.

3. Monitor the chest for bilateral expansion.

4. Obtain pulse oximetry readings.

5. Monitor ABG results.

6. Assess the need for **suctioning** and observe the type, color, and amount of secretions.

7. Assess ventilator settings.

8. Assess the level of water in the humidifier and the temperature of the humidification system because extremes in temperature can damage the mucosa in the airway.

9. Ensure that the alarms are set.

10. If a cause for an alarm cannot be determined, ventilate the client manually with a resuscitation bag until the problem is corrected.

11. Empty the ventilator tubing when moisture collects.

TABLE 58-1 Ventilator Controls and Settings and Descriptions

Controls and Settings	Descriptions
Tidal volume	The volume of air that the client receives with each breath.
Rate	The number of ventilator breaths delivered per minute.
Sighs	The volumes of air that are 1.5 to 2 times the set tidal volume, delivered 6 to 10 times per hour; may be used to prevent atelectasis.
Fraction of inspired oxygen (Fio_2)	The oxygen concentration delivered to the client; determined by the client's condition and ABG levels.
Peak airway inspiratory pressure	The pressure needed by the ventilator to deliver a set tidal volume at a given compliance. Monitoring peak airway inspiratory pressure reflects changes in compliance of the lungs and resistance in the ventilator or client.
Continuous positive airway pressure	The application of positive airway pressure throughout the entire respiratory cycle for spontaneously breathing clients. Keeps the alveoli open during inspiration and prevents alveolar collapse; used primarily as a weaning modality. No ventilator breaths are delivered, but the ventilator delivers oxygen and provides monitoring and an alarm system; the respiratory pattern is determined by the client's efforts.
Positive end-expiratory pressure (PEEP)	Positive pressure is exerted during the expiratory phase of ventilation, which improves oxygenation by enhancing gas exchange and preventing atelectasis. The need for PEEP indicates a severe gas exchange disturbance. Higher amounts of PEEP (more than 15) increase the chance of complications, such as barotrauma tension pneumothorax.
Pressure support	The application of positive pressure on inspiration that eases the workload of breathing. May be used in combination with PEEP as a weaning method. As the weaning process continues, the amount of pressure applied to inspiration is gradually decreased.

Box 58-11 Causes of Ventilator Alarms

High-Pressure Alarm
Increased secretions are in the airway.
Wheezing or bronchospasm causes decreased airway size.
The endotracheal tube is displaced.
The ventilator tube is obstructed because of water or a kink in the tubing.
Client coughs, gags, or bites on the oral endotracheal tube.
Client is anxious or fights the ventilator.

Low-Pressure Alarm
Disconnection or leak in the ventilator or in the client's airway cuff occurs.
The client stops spontaneous breathing.

12. Turn the client at least every 2 hours or get the client out of bed, as prescribed, to prevent complications of immobility.
13. Have resuscitation equipment available at the bedside.

E. Causes of alarms (Box 58-11)

⚠ Never set ventilator alarm controls to the off position.

F. Complications
1. Hypotension caused by the application of positive pressure, which increases intrathoracic pressure and inhibits blood return to the heart
2. Respiratory complications such as **pneumothorax** or subcutaneous **emphysema** as a result of positive pressure
3. Gastrointestinal alterations such as stress ulcers
4. Malnutrition if nutrition is not maintained
5. Infections
6. Muscular deconditioning
7. Ventilator dependence or inability to wean

G. Weaning: Process of going from ventilator dependence to spontaneous breathing
1. SIMV
   a. The client breathes between the preset breaths per minute rate of the ventilator.
   b. The SIMV rate is decreased gradually until the client is breathing on his or her own without the use of the ventilator.
2. T-piece
   a. The client is taken off the ventilator and the ventilator is replaced with a T-piece or continuous positive airway pressure, which delivers humidified oxygen.
   b. The client is taken off the ventilator for short periods initially and allowed to breathe spontaneously.
   c. Weaning progresses as the client is able to tolerate progressively longer periods off the ventilator.

3. Pressure support
   a. Pressure support is a predetermined pressure set on the ventilator to assist the client in respiratory effort.
   b. As weaning continues, the amount of pressure is decreased gradually.
   c. With pressure support, pressure may be maintained while the preset breaths per minute of the ventilator gradually are decreased.

VI. CHEST INJURIES

A. Rib fracture
1. Description
   a. Results from direct blunt chest trauma and causes a potential for intrathoracic injury, such as **pneumothorax** or pulmonary contusion
   b. Pain with movement and chest splinting result in impaired ventilation and inadequate clearance of secretions.
2. Assessment
   a. Pain at the injury site that increases with inspiration
   b. Tenderness at the site
   c. Shallow respirations
   d. Client splints chest
   e. Fractures noted on chest x-ray
3. Interventions
   a. Note that the ribs usually unite spontaneously.
   b. Place the client in a Fowler's position.
   c. Administer pain medication as prescribed to maintain adequate ventilatory status.
   d. Monitor for increased respiratory distress.
   e. Instruct the client to self-splint with the hands and arms.
   f. Prepare the client for an intercostal nerve block as prescribed if the pain is severe.

B. Flail chest
1. Description
   a. Occurs from blunt chest trauma associated with accidents, which may result in hemothorax and rib fractures.
   b. The loose segment of the chest wall becomes paradoxical to the expansion and contraction of the rest of the chest wall.
2. Assessment
   a. Paradoxical respirations (inward movement of a segment of the thorax during inspiration with outward movement during expiration)
   b. Severe pain in the chest
   c. Dyspnea
   d. Cyanosis
   e. Tachycardia
   f. Hypotension
   g. Tachypnea, shallow respirations
   h. Diminished breath sounds
3. Interventions
   a. Place the client in a Fowler's position.

b. Administer humidified oxygen as prescribed.

c. Monitor for increased respiratory distress.

d. Encourage coughing and deep breathing.

e. Administer pain medication as prescribed.

f. Maintain bed rest and limit activity to reduce oxygen demands.

g. Prepare for intubation with **mechanical ventilation**, with positive end-expiratory pressure (PEEP) for severe flail chest associated with respiratory failure and shock.

C. Pulmonary contusion

1. Description

   a. Characterized by interstitial hemorrhage associated with intra-alveolar hemorrhage, resulting in decreased pulmonary compliance

   b. The major complication is acute respiratory distress syndrome.

2. Assessment

   a. Dyspnea

   b. Hypoxemia

   c. Increased bronchial secretions

   d. Hemoptysis

   e. Restlessness

   f. Decreased breath sounds

   g. Crackles and wheezes

3. Interventions

   a. Maintain a patent airway and adequate ventilation.

   b. Place the client in a Fowler's position.

   c. Administer oxygen as prescribed.

   d. Monitor for increased respiratory distress.

   e. Maintain bed rest and limit activity to reduce oxygen demands.

   f. Prepare for **mechanical ventilation** with PEEP if required.

D. Pneumothorax (Fig. 58-9)

1. Description

a. Accumulation of atmospheric air in the pleural space, which results in a rise in intrathoracic pressure and reduced vital capacity

b. The loss of negative intrapleural pressure results in collapse of the lung.

c. A spontaneous **pneumothorax** occurs with the rupture of a pulmonary bleb.

d. An open **pneumothorax** occurs when an opening through the chest wall allows the entrance of positive atmospheric air pressure into the pleural space.

e. A tension **pneumothorax** occurs from a blunt chest injury or from **mechanical ventilation** with PEEP when a buildup of positive pressure occurs in the pleural space.

f. Diagnosis of **pneumothorax** is made by chest x-ray.

2. Assessment (Box 58-12)

3. Interventions

   a. Apply a dressing over an open chest wound.

   b. Administer oxygen as prescribed.

   c. Place the client in a Fowler's position.

   d. Prepare for chest tube placement, which will remain in place until the lung has expanded fully.

   e. Monitor the chest tube drainage system.

   f. Monitor for subcutaneous **emphysema**.

   g. See Chapter 21 for information on caring for a client with chest tubes.

⚠ Clients with a respiratory disorder should be positioned with the head of the bed elevated.

VII. ACUTE RESPIRATORY FAILURE

A. Description

1. Occurs when insufficient oxygen is transported to the blood or inadequate carbon dioxide is removed from the lungs and the client's compensatory mechanisms fail

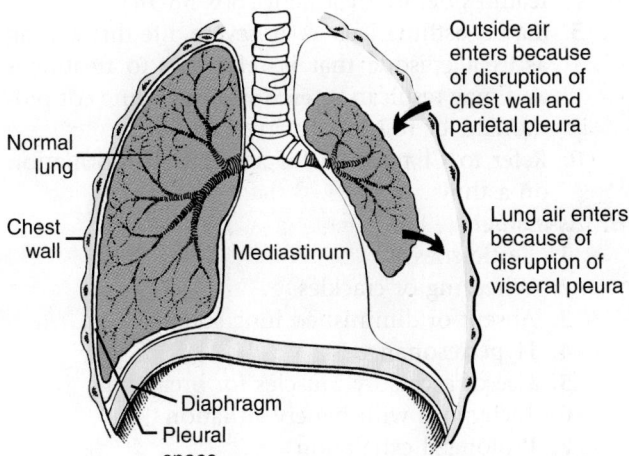

▲ **FIGURE 58-9** Pneumothorax. Air in the pleural space causes the lungs to collapse around the hilus and may push the mediastinal contents (heart and great vessels) toward the other lung. (From McCance, K., & Huether, S. [2010]. *Pathophysiology: The biologic basis for disease in adults and children* [6th ed.]. St. Louis: Mosby.)

Box 58-12 Assessment Findings: Pneumothorax

Absent breath sounds on affected side

Cyanosis

Decreased chest expansion unilaterally

Dyspnea

Hypotension

Sharp chest pain

Subcutaneous emphysema as evidenced by crepitus on palpation

Sucking sound with open chest wound

Tachycardia

Tachypnea

Tracheal deviation to the unaffected side with tension pneumothorax

2. Causes include a mechanical abnormality of the lungs or chest wall, a defect in the respiratory control center in the brain, or an impairment in the function of the respiratory muscles.
3. In oxygenation failure, or hypoxemic respiratory failure, oxygen may reach the alveoli but cannot be absorbed or used properly, resulting in a Pao_2 lower than 60 mm Hg, arterial oxygen saturation (Sao_2) lower than 90%, or partial pressure of arterial carbon dioxide ($Paco_2$) greater than 50 mm Hg occurring with acidemia.
4. Many clients experience both hypoxemic and hypercapnic respiratory failure and retained carbon dioxide in the alveoli displaces oxygen, contributing to the hypoxemia.
5. Manifestations of respiratory failure are related to the extent and rapidity of change in Pao_2 and $Paco_2$.

B. Assessment
   1. Dyspnea
   2. Headache
   3. Restlessness
   4. Confusion
   5. Tachycardia
   6. Hypertension
   7. Dysrhythmias
   8. Decreased level of consciousness
   9. Alterations in respirations and breath sounds

C. Interventions
   1. Identify and treat the cause of the respiratory failure
   2. Administer oxygen to maintain the Pao_2 level higher than 60 to 70 mm Hg.
   3. Place the client in a Fowler's position.
   4. Encourage deep breathing.
   5. Administer bronchodilators as prescribed.
   6. Prepare the client for **mechanical ventilation** if supplemental oxygen cannot maintain acceptable Pao_2 and $Paco_2$ levels.

VIII. ACUTE RESPIRATORY DISTRESS SYNDROME

A. Description
   1. A form of acute respiratory failure that occurs as a complication of some other condition; it is caused by a diffuse lung injury and leads to extravascular lung fluid.
   2. The major site of injury is the alveolar capillary membrane.
   3. The interstitial edema causes compression and obliteration of the terminal airways and leads to reduced lung volume and compliance.
   4. The ABG levels identify respiratory acidosis and hypoxemia that do not respond to an increased percentage of oxygen.
   5. The chest x-ray shows bilateral interstitial and alveolar infiltrates; interstitial edema may not be noted until there is a 30% increase in fluid content.

6. Causes include sepsis, fluid overload, shock, trauma, neurological injuries, burns, disseminated intravascular coagulation, drug ingestion, aspiration, and inhalation of toxic substances.

B. Assessment
   1. Tachypnea
   2. Dyspnea
   3. Decreased breath sounds
   4. Deteriorating ABG levels
   5. Hypoxemia despite high concentrations of delivered oxygen
   6. Decreased pulmonary compliance
   7. Pulmonary infiltrates

C. Interventions
   1. Identify and treat the cause of the acute respiratory distress syndrome.
   2. Administer oxygen as prescribed.
   3. Place the client in a Fowler's position.
   4. Restrict fluid intake as prescribed.
   5. Provide respiratory treatments as prescribed.
   6. Administer diuretics, anticoagulants, or corticosteroids as prescribed.
   7. Prepare the client for intubation and **mechanical ventilation** using PEEP.

IX. ASTHMA (Fig. 58-10)

A. Description
   1. Chronic inflammatory disorder of the airways that causes varying degrees of obstruction in the airways
   2. **Asthma** is marked by airway inflammation and hyperresponsiveness to a variety of stimuli or triggers (Box 58-13).
   3. **Asthma** causes recurrent episodes of wheezing, breathlessness, chest tightness, and coughing associated with airflow obstruction that may resolve spontaneously; it is often reversible with treatment.
   4. **Asthma** severity is classified based on the clinical features before treatment (Box 58-14).
   5. Status asthmaticus is a severe life-threatening **asthma** episode that is refractory to treatment and may result in **pneumothorax**, acute cor pulmonale, or respiratory arrest.
   6. Refer to Chapter 38 for additional information on asthma.

B. Assessment
   1. Restlessness
   2. Wheezing or crackles
   3. Absent or diminished lung sounds
   4. Hyperresonance
   5. Use of accessory muscles for breathing
   6. Tachypnea with hyperventilation
   7. Prolonged exhalation
   8. Tachycardia
   9. Pulsus paradoxus
   10. Diaphoresis
   11. Cyanosis

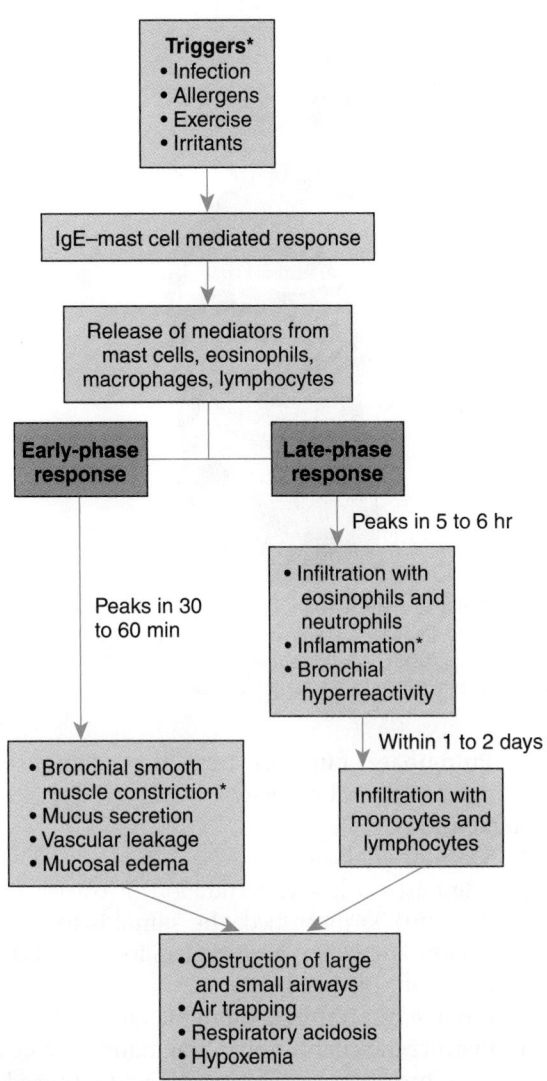

Triggers*
- Infection
- Allergens
- Exercise
- Irritants

↓

IgE–mast cell mediated response

↓

Release of mediators from mast cells, eosinophils, macrophages, lymphocytes

Early-phase response / **Late-phase response**

Peaks in 5 to 6 hr

- Infiltration with eosinophils and neutrophils
- Inflammation*
- Bronchial hyperreactivity

Peaks in 30 to 60 min

Within 1 to 2 days

- Bronchial smooth muscle constriction*
- Mucus secretion
- Vascular leakage
- Mucosal edema

Infiltration with monocytes and lymphocytes

- Obstruction of large and small airways
- Air trapping
- Respiratory acidosis
- Hypoxemia

▲ **FIGURE 58-10** Pathophysiology in asthma. Stems with asterisks are primary processes. (From Lewis, S., Heitkemper, M., & Dirksen, S. [2007]. *Medical-surgical nursing: Assessment and management of clinical problems* [7th ed.]. St. Louis: Mosby.)

12. Decreased oxygen saturation
13. Pulmonary function test results that demonstrate decreased air flow rates
C. Interventions
 1. Monitor vital signs.
 2. Monitor pulse oximetry.
 3. Monitor peak flow.
 4. During an acute **asthma** episode, provide interventions to assist with breathing (Box 58-15).
D. Client education
 1. Instruct the client on the intermittent nature of symptoms and need for long-term management.
 2. Instruct the client to identify possible triggers and measures to prevent episodes.
 3. Instruct the client on the management of medication and proper administration.
 4. Instruct the client on the correct use of a peak flowmeter.

Box 58-13 Asthma Triggers

Environmental Factors
Animal dander
Cockroaches
Dust
Exhaust fumes
Fireplaces
Molds
Perfumes or other products with aerosol sprays
Pollen
Smoke, including cigarette or cigar smoke
Sudden weather changes

Physiological Factors
Gastroesophageal reflux disease (GERD)
Hormonal changes
Sinusitis
Stress
Viral upper respiratory infection

Medications
Acetylsalicylic acid (Aspirin)
β-Adrenergic blockers
Nonsteroidal anti-inflammatory drugs

Occupational Exposure Factors
Metal salts
Wood and vegetable dusts
Industrial chemicals and plastics

Food Additives
Sulfites (bisulfites and metabisulfites)
Beer, wine, dried fruit, shrimp, processed potatoes
Monosodium glutamate

Modified from Lewis, S., Heitkemper, M., & Dirksen, S. (2007). *Medical-surgical nursing: Assessment and management of clinical problems* (7th ed.). St. Louis: Mosby.

 5. Help the client develop an **asthma** action plan with the primary provider and teach the client what to do if an **asthma** episode occurs.

X. CHRONIC OBSTRUCTIVE PULMONARY DISEASE

A. Description
 1. Also known as chronic obstructive lung disease and chronic airflow limitation
 2. **Chronic obstructive pulmonary** disease is a disease state characterized by airflow obstruction caused by **emphysema** or chronic bronchitis.
 3. Progressive airflow limitation occurs, associated with an abnormal inflammatory response of the lungs that is not completely reversible.
 4. **Chronic obstructive pulmonary disease** leads to pulmonary insufficiency, pulmonary hypertension, and cor pulmonale.
B. Assessment
 1. Cough
 2. Exertional dyspnea

Box 58-14 Classification of Asthma Severity

Severe Persistent
Symptoms are continuous.
Physical activity requires limitations.
Frequent exacerbations occur.
Nocturnal symptoms occur frequently.

Moderate Persistent
Daily symptoms occur.
Daily use of inhaled short-acting β agonist is needed.
Exacerbations affect activity.
Exacerbations occur at least twice weekly and may last for days.
Nocturnal symptoms occur more frequently than once weekly.

Mild Persistent
Symptoms occur more frequently than twice weekly but less often than once daily.
Exacerbations may affect activity.
Nocturnal symptoms occur more frequently than twice a month.

Mild Intermittent
Symptoms occur twice weekly or less.
Client is asymptomatic between exacerbations.
Exacerbations are brief (hours to days).
Intensity of exacerbations varies.
Nocturnal symptoms occur twice a month or less.

Modified from Ignatavicius, D., & Workman, M. (2010). *Medical-surgical nursing: Patient-centered collaborative care* (6th ed.). St. Louis: Saunders.

Box 58-15 Nursing Interventions During an Acute Asthma Episode

Position the client in a high Fowler's position or sitting to aid in breathing.
Administer oxygen as prescribed.
Stay with the client to decrease anxiety.
Administer bronchodilators as prescribed.
Record the color, amount, and consistency of sputum, if any.
Administer corticosteroids as prescribed.
Auscultate lung sounds before, during, and after treatments.

3. Wheezing and crackles
4. Sputum production
5. Weight loss
6. Barrel chest (**emphysema**) (Fig. 58-11)
7. Use of accessory muscles for breathing
8. Prolonged expiration
9. Orthopnea
10. Cardiac dysrhythmias
11. Congestion and hyperinflation seen on chest x-ray (Fig. 58-12)
12. ABG levels that indicate respiratory acidosis and hypoxemia

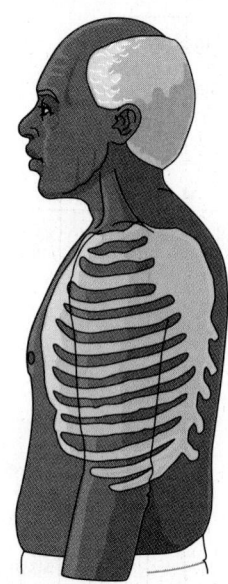

▲ **FIGURE 58-11** Typical barrel chest in a client with chronic obstructive pulmonary disease. (From Ignatavicius, D., & Workman, M. [2006]. *Medical-surgical nursing: Critical thinking for collaborative care* [5th ed.]. St. Louis: Saunders.)

13. Pulmonary function tests that demonstrate decreased vital capacity
C. Interventions
   1. Monitor vital signs.
   2. Administer a low concentration of oxygen (1 to 2 L/min) as prescribed; the stimulus to breathe is a low arterial Po_2 instead of an increased Pco_2.
   3. Monitor pulse oximetry.
   4. Provide respiratory treatments and CPT.
   5. Instruct the client in diaphragmatic or abdominal breathing techniques and pursed-lip breathing techniques.
   6. Record the color, amount, and consistency of sputum.
   7. Suction fluids from the client's lungs, if necessary, to clear the airway and prevent infection.
   8. Monitor weight.
   9. Encourage small frequent meals to maintain nutrition and prevent dyspnea.
   10. Provide a high-calorie, high-protein diet with supplements.
   11. Encourage fluid intake up to 3000 mL/day to keep secretions thin, unless contraindicated.
   12. Place the client in a Fowler's position and leaning forward to aid in breathing (Fig. 58-13).
   13. Allow activity as tolerated.
   14. Administer bronchodilators as prescribed, and instruct the client in the use of oral and inhalant medications.
   15. Administer corticosteroids as prescribed for exacerbations.
   16. Administer mucolytics as prescribed to thin secretions.
   17. Administer antibiotics for infection if prescribed.

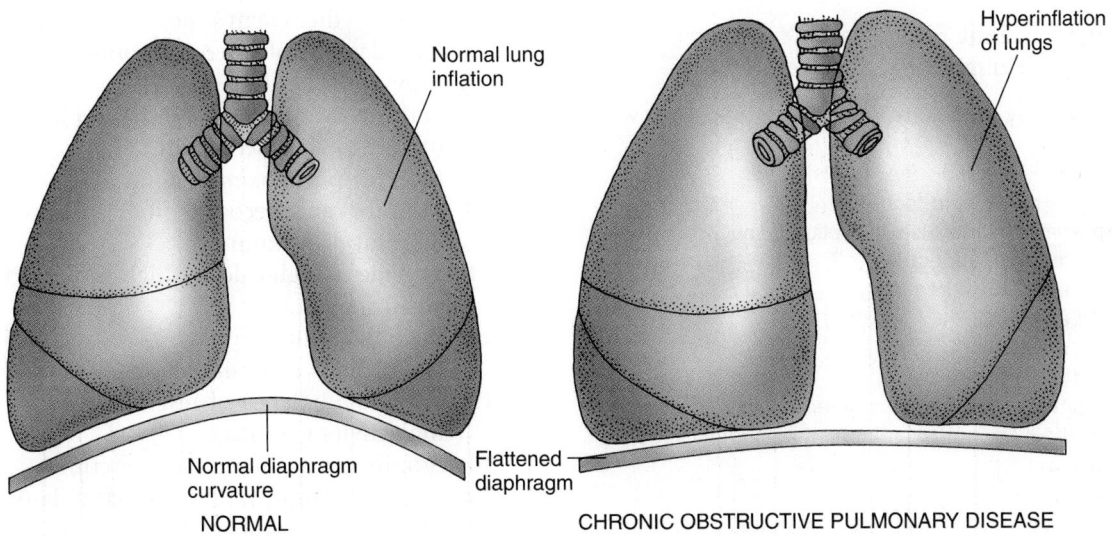

▲ **FIGURE 58-12** Diaphragm shape and lung inflation in the normal client and in the client with chronic obstructive pulmonary disease. (From Ignatavicius, D., & Workman, M. [2010]. *Medical-surgical nursing: Patient-centered collaborative care* [6th ed.]. St. Louis: Saunders.)

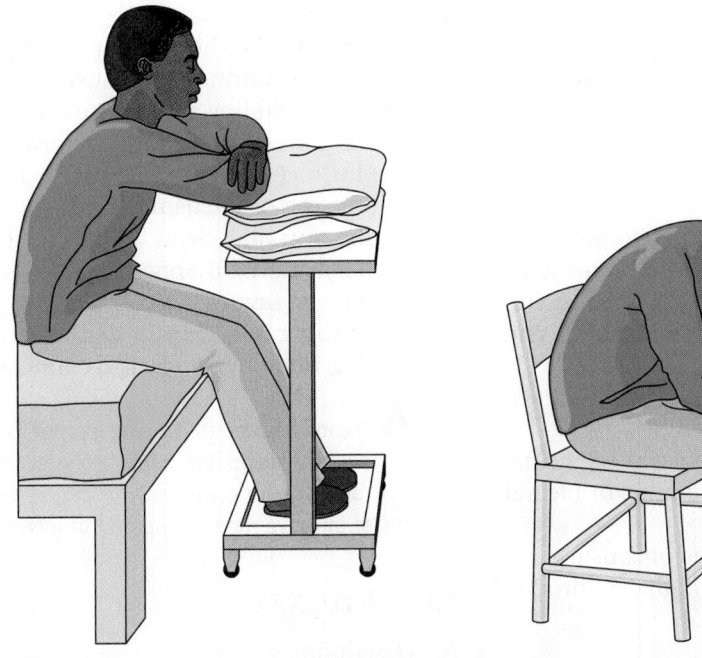

Sitting on the edge of a bed with the arms folded and placed on two or three pillows positioned over a nightstand.

Sitting in a chair with the feet spread shoulder-width apart and leaning forward with the elbows on the knees. Arms and hands are relaxed.

▲ **FIGURE 58-13** Orthopnea positions that clients with chronic obstructive pulmonary disease can assume to ease the work of breathing. (From Ignatavicius, D., & Workman, M. [2010]. *Medical-surgical nursing: Patient-centered collaborative care* [6th ed.]. St. Louis: Saunders.)

D. Client education (Box 58-16)

XI. SEVERE ACUTE RESPIRATORY SYNDROME (SARS)

A. Respiratory illness caused by the coronavirus, called *SARS-associated coronavirus*

B. The syndrome begins with a fever, an overall feeling of discomfort, body aches, and mild respiratory symptoms.

C. After 2 to 7 days, the client may develop a dry cough and dyspnea.

D. Infection is spread by close person-to-person contact by direct contact with infectious material (respiratory secretions or contact with persons or objects infected with infectious droplets).

E. Prevention includes avoiding contact with those suspected of having SARS, avoiding travel to countries where an outbreak of SARS exists, avoiding close

Box 58-16 Client Education: Chronic Obstructive Pulmonary Disease

Adhere to activity limitations, alternating rest periods with activity.

Avoid eating gas-producing foods, spicy foods, and extremely hot or cold foods.

Avoid exposure to individuals with infections and avoid crowds.

Avoid extremes in temperature.

Avoid fireplaces, pets, feather pillows, and other environmental allergens.

Avoid powerful odors.

Meet nutritional requirements.

Receive immunizations as recommended.

Recognize the signs and symptoms of respiratory infection and hypoxia.

Stop smoking.

Use medications and inhalers as prescribed.

Use oxygen therapy as prescribed.

Use pursed-lip and diaphragmatic or abdominal breathing.

When dusting, use a wet cloth.

contact with crowds in areas where SARS exists, and frequent hand washing if in an area where SARS exists.

XII. PNEUMONIA

A. Description
1. Infection of the pulmonary tissue, including the interstitial spaces, the alveoli, and the bronchioles.
2. The edema associated with inflammation stiffens the lung, decreases lung compliance and vital capacity, and causes hypoxemia.
3. Pneumonia can be community-acquired or hospital-acquired.
4. The chest x-ray film shows lobar or segmental consolidation, pulmonary infiltrates, or pleural effusions.
5. A sputum culture identifies the organism.
6. The white blood cell count and the erythrocyte sedimentation rate are elevated.

B. Assessment
1. Chills
2. Elevated temperature
3. Pleuritic pain
4. Tachypnea
5. Rhonchi and wheezes
6. Use of accessory muscles for breathing
7. Mental status changes
8. Sputum production

C. Interventions
1. Administer oxygen as prescribed.
2. Monitor respiratory status.
3. Monitor for labored respirations, cyanosis, and cold and clammy skin.
4. Encourage coughing and deep breathing and use of the incentive spirometer.
5. Place the client in a semi-Fowler's position to facilitate breathing and lung expansion.

6. Change the client's position frequently and ambulate as tolerated to mobilize secretions.
7. Provide CPT.
8. Perform nasotracheal **suctioning** if the client is unable to clear secretions.
9. Monitor pulse oximetry.
10. Monitor and record color, consistency, and amount of sputum.
11. Provide a high-calorie, high-protein diet with small frequent meals.
12. Encourage fluids, up to 3 L/day, to thin secretions unless contraindicated.
13. Provide a balance of rest and activity, increasing activity gradually.
14. Administer antibiotics as prescribed.
15. Administer antipyretics, bronchodilators, cough suppressants, mucolytic agents, and expectorants as prescribed.
16. Prevent the spread of infection by hand washing and the proper disposal of secretions.

D. Client education
1. Instruct the client about the importance of rest, proper nutrition, and adequate fluid intake.
2. Avoid chilling and exposure to individuals with respiratory infections or viruses.
3. Instruct the client regarding medications and the use of inhalants as prescribed.
4. Instruct the client to notify the physician if chills, fever, dyspnea, hemoptysis, or increased fatigue occurs.
5. Instruct the client in the importance of receiving immunizations as recommended.

⚠ Teach clients that using proper hand washing techniques, disposing respiratory secretions properly, and receiving vaccines (if one is available) will assist in preventing the spread of infection.

XIII. INFLUENZA

A. Description
1. Also known as the flu; highly contagious acute viral respiratory infection
2. May be caused by several viruses, usually known as types A, B, and C
3. Yearly vaccination is recommended to prevent the disease, especially for those older than 50 years of age, individuals with chronic illness or who are immunocompromised, those living in institutions, and health care personnel providing direct care to clients (the vaccination is contraindicated in the individual with egg allergies).
4. Additional prevention measures include avoiding those who developed influenza, frequent and proper hand washing, and cleaning and disinfecting surfaces that have become contaminated with secretions.

5. Avian influenza A (H5N1)
   a. Affects birds; does not usually affect humans; however, human cases have been reported in some countries.
   b. An H5N1 vaccine has been developed for use if a pandemic virus were to emerge.
   c. Reported symptoms are similar to those associated with influenza types A, B, and C.
   d. Prevention measures include thorough cooking of poultry products, avoiding contact with wild animals, frequent and proper hand washing and cleaning and disinfecting surfaces that have become contaminated with secretions.
6. Swine (H1N1) influenza
   a. It is a new strain of flu that consists of genetic materials from swine, avian, and human influenza viruses.
   b. Signs and symptoms are similar to those that present with seasonal flu; additionally vomiting and diarrhea commonly occur.
   c. Prevention measures and treatment are the same as for the seasonal flu.
   d. Refer to Chapter 48 for additional information on swine flu and Chapter 59 for information on H1N1 vaccines.
B. Assessment
   1. Acute onset of fever and muscle aches
   2. Headache
   3. Fatigue, weakness, anorexia
   4. Sore throat, cough, and rhinorrhea
C. Interventions
   1. Encourage rest.
   2. Encourage fluids to prevent pulmonary complications (unless contraindicated).
   3. Monitor lung sounds.
   4. Provide supportive therapy such as antipyretics or antitussives as indicated.
   5. Administer antiviral medications as prescribed for current strain of influenza (see Chapter 59).

XIV. LEGIONNAIRE'S DISEASE

A. Description
   1. Acute bacterial infection caused by *Legionella pneumophila*
   2. Sources of the organism include contaminated cooling tower water and warm stagnant water supplies, including water vaporizers, water sonicators, whirlpool spas, and showers.
   3. Person-to-person contact does not occur; the risk for infection is increased by the presence of other conditions.
B. Assessment: Influenza-like symptoms with a high fever, chills, muscle aches, and headache that may progress to dry cough, pleurisy, and sometimes diarrhea.
C. Interventions: Treatment is supportive and antibiotics may be prescribed.

XV. PLEURAL EFFUSION

A. Description
   1. Pleural effusion is the collection of fluid in the pleural space.
   2. Any condition that interferes with secretion or drainage of this fluid will lead to pleural effusion.
B. Assessment
   1. Pleuritic pain that is sharp and increases with inspiration
   2. Progressive dyspnea with decreased movement of the chest wall on the affected side
   3. Dry, nonproductive cough caused by bronchial irritation or mediastinal shift
   4. Tachycardia
   5. Elevated temperature
   6. Decreased breath sounds over affected area
   7. Chest x-ray film that shows pleural effusion and a mediastinal shift away from the fluid if the effusion is more than 250 mL
C. Interventions
   1. Identify and treat the underlying cause.
   2. Monitor breath sounds.
   3. Place the client in a Fowler's position.
   4. Encourage coughing and deep breathing.
   5. Prepare the client for thoracentesis.
   6. If pleural effusion is recurrent, prepare the client for pleurectomy or pleurodesis as prescribed.
D. Pleurectomy
   1. Consists of surgically stripping the parietal pleura away from the visceral pleura
   2. This produces an intense inflammatory reaction that promotes adhesion formation between the two layers during healing.
E. Pleurodesis
   1. Involves the instillation of a sclerosing substance into the pleural space via a thoracotomy tube
   2. The substance creates an inflammatory response that scleroses tissues together.

XVI. EMPYEMA

A. Description
   1. Collection of pus within the pleural cavity
   2. The fluid is thick, opaque, and foul-smelling.
   3. The most common cause is pulmonary infection and lung abscess caused by thoracic surgery or chest trauma, in which bacteria are introduced directly into the pleural space.
   4. Treatment focuses on treating the infection, emptying the empyema cavity, reexpanding the lung, and controlling the infection.
B. Assessment
   1. Recent febrile illness or trauma
   2. Chest pain
   3. Cough
   4. Dyspnea
   5. Anorexia and weight loss
   6. Malaise

7. Elevated temperature and chills
8. Night sweats
9. Pleural exudate on chest x-ray
C. Interventions
1. Monitor breath sounds.
2. Place the client in a semi-Fowler's or high Fowler's position.
3. Encourage coughing and deep breathing.
4. Administer antibiotics as prescribed.
5. Instruct the client to splint the chest as necessary.
6. Assist with thoracentesis or chest tube insertion to promote drainage and lung expansion.
7. If marked pleural thickening occurs, prepare the client for decortication, if prescribed; this surgical procedure involves removal of the restrictive mass of fibrin and inflammatory cells.

XVII. PLEURISY

A. Description
1. Inflammation of the visceral and parietal membranes; may be caused by pulmonary infarction or pneumonia
2. The visceral and parietal membranes rub together during respiration and cause pain.
3. Pleurisy usually occurs on one side of the chest, usually in the lower lateral portions in the chest wall.
B. Assessment
1. Knife-like pain aggravated on deep breathing and coughing
2. Dyspnea
3. Pleural friction rub heard on auscultation
4. Apprehension
C. Interventions
1. Identify and treat the cause.
2. Monitor lung sounds.
3. Administer analgesics as prescribed.
4. Apply hot or cold applications as prescribed.
5. Encourage coughing and deep breathing.
6. Instruct the client to lie on the affected side to splint chest.

XVIII. PULMONARY EMBOLISM

A. Description
1. Occurs when a thrombus forms (most commonly in a deep vein), detaches, travels to the right side of the heart, and then lodges in a branch of the pulmonary artery
2. Clients prone to pulmonary embolism are those at risk for deep vein thrombosis, including those with prolonged immobilization, surgery, obesity, pregnancy, congestive heart failure, advanced age, or a history of thromboembolism.
3. Fat emboli can occur as a complication following fracture of a long bone and can cause pulmonary emboli.
4. Treatment is aimed at prevention through risk factor recognition and elimination.

B. Assessment (Box 58-17)
C. Interventions (see Priority Nursing Actions)

XIX. LUNG CANCER AND LARYNGEAL CANCER
(see Chapter 52)

XX. CARBON MONOXIDE POISONING
(see Chapter 50)

Box 58-17 Assessment Findings: Pulmonary Embolism

Apprehension and restlessness
Blood-tinged sputum
Chest pain
Cough
Crackles and wheezes on auscultation
Cyanosis
Distended neck veins
Dyspnea accompanied by anginal and pleuritic pain, exacerbated by inspiration
Feeling of impending doom
Hypotension
Petechiae over the chest and axilla
Shallow respirations
Tachypnea and tachycardia

▬▬▬ PRIORITY NURSING ACTIONS! ▬▬▬

Actions to Take If a Pulmonary Embolism is Suspected
1. Notify the Rapid Response Team.
2. Reassure the client and elevate the head of the bed.
3. Prepare to administer oxygen.
4. Obtain vital signs and check lung sounds.
5. Prepare to obtain an arterial blood gas.
6. Prepare for the administration of heparin therapy or other therapies.
7. Document the event, interventions taken, and the client's response to treatment.

Signs and symptoms of a pulmonary embolism include the sudden onset of dyspnea, apprehension and restlessness, a feeling of impending doom, cough, hemoptysis, tachypnea, crackles, petechiae over the chest and axillae, and a decreased arterial oxygen saturation. If suspected, the nurse immediately notifies the Rapid Response Team. The nurse stays with the client, reassures the client, and elevates the head of the bed. The nurse prepares to administer oxygen and obtains the vital signs and checks lung sounds. The nurse continues to monitor the client closely, prepares the client for tests prescribed to confirm the diagnosis, and prepares to obtain an arterial blood gas. When prescribed, the client is prepared for the administration of heparin therapy or other therapies such as embolectomy or placement of a vena cava filter if necessary. Finally, the nurse documents the event, interventions taken, and the client's response to treatment.

Reference: Ignatavicius, D., & Workman, M. (2010). *Medical-surgical nursing: Patient-centered collaborative care* (6th ed., p. 680). St. Louis: Saunders.

XXI. HISTOPLASMOSIS

A. Description
1. Pulmonary fungal infection caused by spores of *Histoplasma capsulatum*
2. Transmission occurs by the inhalation of spores, which commonly are found in contaminated soil.
3. Spores also are usually found in bird droppings.

B. Assessment
1. Similar to pneumonia
2. Positive skin test for histoplasmosis
3. Positive agglutination test
4. Splenomegaly, hepatomegaly

C. Interventions
1. Administer oxygen as prescribed.
2. Monitor breath sounds.
3. Administer antiemetics, antihistamines, antipyretics, and corticosteroids as prescribed.
4. Administer fungicidal medications as prescribed.
5. Encourage coughing and deep breathing.
6. Place the client in a semi-Fowler's position.
7. Monitor vital signs.
8. Monitor for nephrotoxicity from fungicidal medications.
9. Instruct the client to spray the floor with water before sweeping barn and chicken coops.

XXII. SARCOIDOSIS

A. Description
1. Presence of epithelioid cell tubercles in the lung
2. The cause is unknown, but a high titer of Epstein-Barr virus may be noted.
3. Viral incidence is highest in Blacks and young adults.

B. Assessment
1. Night sweats
2. Fever
3. Weight loss
4. Cough and dyspnea
5. Skin nodules
6. Polyarthritis
7. Kveim test: Sarcoid node antigen is injected intradermally and causes a local nodular lesion in about 1 month.

C. Interventions
1. Administer corticosteroids to control symptoms.
2. Monitor temperature.
3. Increase fluid intake.
4. Provide frequent periods of rest.
5. Encourage small, nutritious meals.

XXIII. OCCUPATIONAL LUNG DISEASE

A. Description
1. Caused by exposure to environmental or occupational fumes, dust, vapors, gases, bacterial or fungal antigens, and allergens; can result in acute reversible effects or chronic lung disease

2. Common disease classifications include occupational **asthma** pneumoconiosis (silicosis or coal miner's [black lung] disease), diffuse interstitial fibrosis (asbestosis, talcosis, berylliosis), or extrinsic allergic alveolitis (farmer's lung, bird fancier's lung, or machine operator's lung).

B. Assessment: Manifestations depend on the type of disease and respiratory symptoms.

C. Interventions
1. Prevention through the use of respiratory protective devices
2. Treatment is based on the symptoms experienced by the client.

XXIV. TUBERCULOSIS

A. Description
1. Highly communicable disease caused by **Mycobacterium tuberculosis**
2. **M. tuberculosis** is a nonmotile, nonsporulating, acid-fast rod that secrets niacin; when the bacillus reaches a susceptible site, it multiplies freely.
3. Because **M. tuberculosis** is an aerobic bacterium, it primarily affects the pulmonary system, especially the upper lobes, where the oxygen content is highest, but also can affect other areas of the body, such as the brain, intestines, peritoneum, kidney, joints, and liver.
4. An exudative response causes a nonspecific pneumonitis and the development of granulomas in the lung tissue.
5. **Tuberculosis** has an insidious onset, and many clients are not aware of symptoms until the disease is well advanced.
6. Improper or noncompliant use of treatment programs may cause the development of mutations in the tubercle bacilli, resulting in a **multidrug-resistant strain** of **tuberculosis** (MDR-TB).
7. The goal of treatment is to prevent transmission, control symptoms, and prevent progression of the disease.

B. Risk factors (Box 58-18)

Box 58-18 Risk Factors for Tuberculosis

Child younger than 5 years of age
Drinking unpasteurized milk if the cow is infected with bovine tuberculosis
Homeless individuals or those from a lower socioeconomic group, minority group, or refugee group
Individuals in constant, frequent contact with an untreated or undiagnosed individual
Individuals living in crowded areas, such as long-term care facilities, prisons, and mental health facilities
Older client
Individuals with malnutrition, infection, immune dysfunction or human immunodeficiency virus infection, or immunosuppressed as a result of medication therapy
Individual who abuses alcohol or is an intravenous drug user

C. Transmission
1. Transmission of **tuberculosis** is via the airborne route by droplet infection.
2. When an infected individual coughs, laughs, sneezes, or sings, droplet nuclei containing **tuberculosis** bacteria enter the air and may be inhaled by others.
3. Identification of those in close contact with the infected individual is important so that they can be tested and treated as necessary.
4. When contacts have been identified, these persons are assessed with a tuberculin skin test and chest x-rays to determine infection with **tuberculosis**.
5. After the infected individual has received **tuberculosis** medication for 2 to 3 weeks, the risk of transmission is reduced greatly.

D. Disease progression
1. Droplets enter the lungs, and the bacteria form a tubercle lesion.
2. The defense systems of the body encapsulate the tubercle, leaving a scar.
3. If encapsulation does not occur, bacteria may enter the lymph system, travel to the lymph nodes, and cause an inflammatory response termed granulomatous inflammation.
4. Primary lesions form; the primary lesions may become dormant but can be reactivated and become a secondary infection when reexposed to the bacterium.
5. In an active phase, **tuberculosis** can cause necrosis and cavitation in the lesions, leading to rupture, the spread of necrotic tissue, and damage to various parts of the body.

E. Client history
1. Past exposure to **tuberculosis**
2. Client's country of origin and travel to foreign countries in which the incidence of **tuberculosis** is high
3. Recent history of influenza, pneumonia, febrile illness, cough, or foul-smelling sputum production
4. Previous tests for **tuberculosis**; results of the testing
5. Recent **bacille Calmette-Guérin vaccine** (a vaccine containing attenuated tubercle bacilli that may be given to persons in foreign countries or to persons traveling to foreign countries to produce increased resistance to **tuberculosis**).

⚠ An individual who has received a bacille Calmette-Guérin vaccine will have a positive tuberculin skin test result and should be evaluated for tuberculosis with a chest x-ray.

F. Clinical manifestations
1. May be asymptomatic in primary infection
2. Fatigue
3. Lethargy
4. Anorexia
5. Weight loss
6. Low-grade fever
7. Chills
8. Night sweats
9. Persistent cough and the production of mucoid and mucopurulent sputum, which is occasionally streaked with blood
10. Chest tightness and a dull, aching chest pain may accompany the cough.

G. Chest assessment
1. A physical examination of the chest does not provide conclusive evidence of **tuberculosis**.
2. A chest x-ray is not definitive, but the presence of multinodular infiltrates with calcification in the upper lobes suggests **tuberculosis**.
3. If the disease is active, caseation and inflammation may be seen on the chest x-ray.
4. Advanced disease
   a. Dullness with percussion over involved parenchymal areas, bronchial breath sounds, rhonchi, and crackles indicate advanced disease.
   b. Partial obstruction of a bronchus caused by endobronchial disease or compression by lymph nodes may produce localized wheezing and dyspnea.

H. QuantiFERON-TB Gold test
1. A blood analysis test by an enzyme-linked immunosorbent assay.
2. A sensitive and rapid test (results can be available in 24 hours) that assists in diagnosing the client.

I. Sputum cultures
1. Sputum specimens are obtained for an acid-fast smear.
2. A sputum culture identifying **M. tuberculosis** confirms the diagnosis.
3. After medications are started, sputum samples are obtained again to determine the effectiveness of therapy.
4. Most clients have negative cultures after 3 months of treatment.

J. **Mantoux skin test**
1. A positive Mantoux reaction does not mean that active disease is present but indicates previous exposure to **tuberculosis** or the presence of inactive (dormant) disease.
2. Once the test result is positive, it will be positive in any future tests.
3. Purified protein derivative containing 5 tuberculin units is administered intradermally in the forearm.
4. An area of induration measuring 10 mm or more in diameter, 48 to 72 hours after injection, indicates that the individual has been exposed to **tuberculosis**.

Box 58-19 Client Education: Tuberculosis

Provide the client and family with information about tuberculosis and allay concerns about the contagious aspect of the infection.

Instruct the client to follow the medication regimen exactly as prescribed and always to have a supply of the medication on hand.

Advise the client of the side effects of the medication and ways of minimizing them to ensure compliance.

Reassure the client that after 2 to 3 weeks of medication therapy, it is unlikely that the client will infect anyone.

Inform the client to resume activities gradually.

Instruct the client about the need for adequate nutrition and a well-balanced diet to promote healing and to prevent recurrence of the infection.

Instruct the client to increase intake of foods rich in iron, protein, and vitamin C.

Inform the client and family that respiratory isolation is not necessary because family members already have been exposed.

Instruct the client to cover the mouth and nose when coughing or sneezing and to put used tissues into plastic bags.

Instruct the client and family about thorough hand washing.

Inform the client that a sputum culture is needed every 2 to 4 weeks once medication therapy is initiated.

Inform the client that when the results of three sputum cultures are negative, the client is no longer considered infectious and usually can return to former employment.

Advise the client to avoid excessive exposure to silicone or dust because these substances can cause further lung damage.

Instruct the client regarding the importance of compliance with treatment, follow-up care, and sputum cultures, as prescribed.

5. For individuals with human immunodeficiency virus infection or who are immunosuppressed, a reaction of 5 mm or more is considered positive.
6. Once an individual's skin test is positive, a chest x-ray is necessary to rule out active **tuberculosis** or to detect old healed lesions.

K. The hospitalized client
1. The client with active **tuberculosis** is placed in respiratory isolation precautions in a negative-pressure room; to maintain negative pressure, the door of the room must be tightly closed.
2. The room should have at least six exchanges of fresh air per hour and should be ventilated to the outside environment, if possible.
3. The nurse wears a particulate respirator (a special individually fitted mask) when caring for the client and a gown when the possibility of clothing contamination exists.
4. Thorough handwashing is required before and after caring for the client.

5. If the client needs to leave the room for a test or procedure, the client is required to wear a mask.
6. Respiratory isolation is discontinued when the client is no longer considered infectious.
7. After the infected individual has received **tuberculosis** medication for 2 to 3 weeks, the risk of transmission is reduced greatly.

L. Client education (Box 58-19)
M. Medications (see Chapter 59)

 MORE QUESTIONS ON THE CD!

Practice Questions

652. An emergency department nurse is assessing a client who has sustained a blunt injury to the chest wall. Which of these signs would indicate the presence of a pneumothorax in this client?
1. A low respiratory rate
2. Diminished breath sounds
3. The presence of a barrel chest
4. A sucking sound at the site of injury

653. A nurse is caring for a client hospitalized with acute exacerbation of chronic obstructive pulmonary disease. Which of the following would the nurse expect to note on assessment of this client?
1. Hypocapnia
2. A hyperinflated chest noted on the chest x-ray
3. Increased oxygen saturation with exercise
4. A widened diaphragm noted on the chest x-ray

654. A nurse instructs a client to use the pursed-lip method of breathing and the client asks the nurse about the purpose of this type of breathing. The nurse responds, knowing that the primary purpose of pursed-lip breathing is to:
1. Promote oxygen intake.
2. Strengthen the diaphragm.
3. Strengthen the intercostal muscles.
4. Promote carbon dioxide elimination.

655. The low-pressure alarm sounds on a ventilator. A nurse assesses the client and then attempts to determine the cause of the alarm. The nurse is unsuccessful in determining the cause of the alarm and takes what initial action?
1. Administers oxygen
2. Checks the client's vital signs
3. Ventilates the client manually
4. Starts cardiopulmonary resuscitation

656. A nurse is caring for a client after a bronchoscopy and biopsy. Which of the following signs, if noted in the client, should be reported immediately to the physician?

1. Dry cough
2. Hematuria
3. Bronchospasm
4. Blood-streaked sputum

657. A nurse is suctioning fluids from a client via a tracheostomy tube. When suctioning, the nurse must limit the suctioning time to a maximum of:
1. 1 minute
2. 5 seconds
3. 10 seconds
4. 30 seconds

658. A nurse is suctioning fluids from a client through an endotracheal tube. During the suctioning procedure, the nurse notes on the monitor that the heart rate is decreasing. Which of the following is the appropriate nursing intervention?
1. Continue to suction.
2. Notify the physician immediately.
3. Stop the procedure and reoxygenate the client.
4. Ensure that the suction is limited to 15 seconds.

659. A nurse is assessing the respiratory status of a client who has suffered a fractured rib. The nurse would expect to note which of the following?
1. Slow deep respirations
2. Rapid deep respirations
3. Paradoxical respirations
4. Pain, especially with inspiration

660. A client with a chest injury has suffered flail chest. A nurse assesses the client for which most distinctive sign of flail chest?
1. Cyanosis
2. Hypotension
3. Paradoxical chest movement
4. Dyspnea, especially on exhalation

661. A client has been admitted with chest trauma after a motor vehicle accident and has undergone subsequent intubation. A nurse checks the client when the high-pressure alarm on the ventilator sounds, and notes that the client has absence of breath sounds in the right upper lobe of the lung. The nurse immediately assesses for other signs of:
1. Right pneumothorax
2. Pulmonary embolism
3. Displaced endotracheal tube
4. Acute respiratory distress syndrome

662. A nurse is assessing a client with multiple trauma who is at risk for developing acute respiratory distress syndrome. The nurse assesses for which earliest sign of acute respiratory distress syndrome?
1. Bilateral wheezing
2. Inspiratory crackles

3. Intercostal retractions
4. Increased respiratory rate

663. A nurse is assessing a client with chronic airflow limitation and notes that the client has a "barrel chest." The nurse interprets that this client has which of the following forms of chronic airflow limitation?
1. Emphysema
2. Bronchial asthma
3. Chronic obstructive bronchitis
4. Bronchial asthma and bronchitis

664. A nurse has conducted discharge teaching with a client diagnosed with tuberculosis. The client has been taking medication for 1½ weeks. The nurse evaluates that the client has understood the information if the client makes which of the following statements?
1. "I need to continue drug therapy for 2 months."
2. "I can't shop at the mall for the next 6 months."
3. "I can return to work if a sputum culture comes back negative."
4. "I should not be contagious after 2 to 3 weeks of medication therapy."

665. A nurse is preparing to give a bed bath to an immobilized client with tuberculosis. The nurse should wear which of the following items when performing this care?
1. Surgical mask and gloves
2. Particulate respirator, gown, and gloves
3. Particulate respirator and protective eyewear
4. Surgical mask, gown, and protective eyewear

666. A client has experienced pulmonary embolism. A nurse assesses for which symptom, which is most commonly reported?
1. Hot, flushed feeling
2. Sudden chills and fever
3. Chest pain that occurs suddenly
4. Dyspnea when deep breaths are taken

667. A client who is human immunodeficiency virus–positive has had a Mantoux skin test. The nurse notes a 7-mm area of induration at the site of the skin test. The nurse interprets the results as:
1. Positive
2. Negative
3. Inconclusive
4. Indicating the need for repeat testing

668. A client with acquired immunodeficiency syndrome has histoplasmosis. A nurse assesses the client for which of the following signs and symptoms?

1. Dyspnea
2. Headache
3. Weight gain
4. Hypothermia

669. A nurse is giving discharge instructions to a client with pulmonary sarcoidosis. The nurse concludes that the client understands the information if the client reports which of the following early signs of exacerbation?
1. Fever
2. Fatigue
3. Weight loss
4. Shortness of breath

670. A nurse is taking the history of a client with silicosis. The nurse assesses whether the client wears which of the following items during periods of exposure to silica particles?
1. Mask
2. Gown
3. Gloves
4. Eye protection

671. An oxygen delivery system is prescribed for a client with chronic obstructive pulmonary disease to deliver a precise oxygen concentration. Which oxygen delivery system would the nurse anticipate to be prescribed?
1. Face tent
2. Venturi mask
3. Aerosol mask
4. Tracheostomy collar

672. A nurse is instructing a hospitalized client with a diagnosis of emphysema about measures that will enhance the effectiveness of breathing during dyspneic periods. Which of the following positions will the nurse instruct the client to assume?
1. Sitting up in bed
2. Side-lying in bed
3. Sitting in a recliner chair
4. Sitting on the side of the bed and leaning on an overbed table

673. A community health nurse is conducting an educational session with community members regarding tuberculosis. The nurse tells the group that one of the first symptoms associated with tuberculosis is:
1. Dyspnea
2. Chest pain
3. A bloody, productive cough
4. A cough with the expectoration of mucoid sputum

674. A nurse performs an admission assessment on a client with a diagnosis of tuberculosis. The nurse reviews the results of which diagnostic test that will confirm this diagnosis?
1. Chest x-ray
2. Bronchoscopy
3. Sputum culture
4. Tuberculin skin test

Alternate Item Format: Multiple Response

675. The nurse is preparing a list of home care instructions for the client who has been hospitalized and treated for tuberculosis. Of the following instructions, which will the nurse include on the list? **Select all that apply.**
❏ 1. Activities should be resumed gradually.
❏ 2. Avoid contact with other individuals, except family members, for at least 6 months.
❏ 3. A sputum culture is needed every 2 to 4 weeks once medication therapy is initiated.
❏ 4. Respiratory isolation is not necessary because family members already have been exposed.
❏ 5. Cover the mouth and nose when coughing or sneezing and put used tissues in plastic bags.
❏ 6. When one sputum culture is negative, the client is no longer considered infectious and usually can return to former employment.

ANSWERS

652. 2

Rationale: This client has sustained a blunt or a closed chest injury. Basic symptoms of a closed pneumothorax are shortness of breath and chest pain. A larger pneumothorax may cause tachypnea, cyanosis, diminished breath sounds, and subcutaneous emphysema. Hyperresonance also may occur on the affected side. A sucking sound at the site of injury would be noted with an open chest injury.

Test-Taking Strategy: Use the process of elimination and note the strategic word *blunt* in the question. This will assist in eliminating option 4, sucking chest wound injury. Knowing that in a respiratory injury increased respirations will occur will assist you in eliminating option 1. Option 3 can be eliminated because a barrel chest is a characteristic finding in a client with chronic obstructive pulmonary disease. Review the signs of pneumothorax if you had difficulty with this question.

Level of Cognitive Ability: Analyzing
Client Needs: Physiological Integrity
Integrated Process: Nursing Process—Assessment
Content Area: Adult Health—Respiratory

Reference: Ignatavicius, D., & Workman, M. (2010). *Medical-surgical nursing: Patient-centered collaborative care* (6th ed., p. 699). St. Louis: Saunders.

653. 2

Rationale: Clinical manifestations of chronic obstructive pulmonary disease (COPD) include hypoxemia, hypercapnia, dyspnea on exertion and at rest, oxygen desaturation with exercise, and the use of accessory muscles of respiration. Chest x-rays reveal a hyperinflated chest and a flattened diaphragm if the disease is advanced.

Test-Taking Strategy: Use the process of elimination. Eliminate option 1 because in the client with COPD, hypercapnia would be noted. Next, eliminate option 3 because oxygen desaturation rather than saturation would occur. From the remaining options, reading carefully will assist in directing you to option 2. If you are unfamiliar with the manifestations associated with COPD, review this content.

Level of Cognitive Ability: Analyzing
Client Needs: Physiological Integrity
Integrated Process: Nursing Process—Assessment
Content Area: Adult Health—Respiratory
Reference: Ignatavicius, D., & Workman, M. (2010). *Medical-surgical nursing: Patient-centered collaborative care* (6th ed., pp. 623, 627). St. Louis: Saunders.

654. 4

Rationale: Pursed-lip breathing facilitates maximal expiration for clients with obstructive lung disease. This type of breathing allows better expiration by increasing airway pressure that keeps air passages open during exhalation. Options 1, 2, and 3 are not the purposes of this type of breathing.

Test-Taking Strategy: Visualize the use of this procedure to assist you in answering correctly. Knowledge regarding the respiratory conditions in which this type of breathing is helpful also will assist in directing you to option 4. Review the purpose of this breathing technique if you had difficulty with this question.

Level of Cognitive Ability: Understanding
Client Needs: Physiological Integrity
Integrated Process: Teaching and Learning
Content Area: Adult Health—Respiratory
References: Ignatavicius, D., & Workman, M. (2010). *Medical-surgical nursing: Patient-centered collaborative care* (6th ed., pp. 630–631). St. Louis: Saunders.
Potter, P., & Perry, A. (2009) *Fundamentals of nursing* (7th ed., pp. 960, 963). St. Louis: Mosby.

655. 3

Rationale: If at any time an alarm is sounding and the nurse cannot quickly ascertain the problem, the client is disconnected from the ventilator and manual resuscitation is used to support respirations until the problem can be corrected. No reason is given to begin cardiopulmonary resuscitation. Checking vital signs is not the initial action. Although oxygen is helpful, it will not provide ventilation to the client.

Test-Taking Strategy: Read the question carefully, and note that the subject relates to adequate ventilation of the client. Also note that the nurse is unsuccessful in determining the cause of the alarm. This will direct you to option 3. If you are unfamiliar with the management of ventilators and alarms, review this content.

Level of Cognitive Ability: Applying

Client Needs: Physiological Integrity
Integrated Process: Nursing Process—Implementation
Content Area: Adult Health—Respiratory
Reference: Black, J., & Hawks, J. (2009). *Medical-surgical nursing: Clinical management for positive outcomes* (8th ed., p. 1643). St. Louis: Saunders.

656. 3

Rationale: If a biopsy was performed during a bronchoscopy, blood-streaked sputum is expected for several hours. Frank blood indicates hemorrhage. A dry cough may be expected. The client should be assessed for signs of complications, which would include cyanosis, dyspnea, stridor, bronchospasm, hemoptysis, hypotension, tachycardia, and dysrhythmias. Hematuria is unrelated to this procedure.

Test-Taking Strategy: Use the process of elimination. Eliminate option 2 first because it is unrelated to the procedure. Next, eliminate option 1 because a dry cough may be expected. Noting that a biopsy has been performed will assist in eliminating option 4, because blood-streaked sputum would be expected. Note that option 3, the correct option, relates to the airway. If you had difficulty with this question, review postprocedure care following bronchoscopy with biopsy.

Level of Cognitive Ability: Analyzing
Client Needs: Physiological Integrity
Integrated Process: Nursing Process—Implementation
Content Area: Adult Health—Respiratory
Reference: Chernecky, C., & Berger, B. (2008). *Laboratory tests and diagnostic procedures* (5th ed., p. 262). St. Louis: Saunders.

657. 3

Rationale: Hypoxemia can be caused by prolonged suctioning, which stimulates the pacemaker cells in the heart. A vasovagal response may occur, causing bradycardia. The nurse must preoxygenate the client before suctioning and limit the suctioning pass to 10 seconds.

Test-Taking Strategy: Use the process of elimination. Recall that during suctioning, the client's airway is blocked; therefore you should be able to eliminate options 1 and 4 easily. From the remaining options, eliminate option 2 because of the short time frame. Five seconds does not seem reasonable to achieve removal of secretions. Review the procedure for suctioning if you had difficulty with this question.

Level of Cognitive Ability: Applying
Client Needs: Physiological Integrity
Integrated Process: Nursing Process—Implementation
Content Area: Adult Health—Respiratory
Reference: Ignatavicius, D., & Workman, M. (2010). *Medical-surgical nursing: Patient-centered collaborative care* (6th ed., p. 584). St. Louis: Saunders.

658. 3

Rationale: During suctioning, the nurse should monitor the client closely for side effects, including hypoxemia, cardiac irregularities such as a decrease in heart rate resulting from vagal stimulation, mucosal trauma, hypotension, and paroxysmal coughing. If side effects develop, especially cardiac irregularities, the procedure is stopped and the client is reoxygenated.

Test-Taking Strategy: Use the process of elimination, recalling that suctioning can cause cardiac irregularities. Noting the strategic words *heart rate is decreasing* should direct you to option 3. If you had difficulty with this question, review

the complications and interventions associated with suctioning procedures.
Level of Cognitive Ability: Applying
Client Needs: Physiological Integrity
Integrated Process: Nursing Process—Implementation
Content Area: Adult Health—Respiratory
Reference: Black, J., & Hawks, J. (2009). *Medical-surgical nursing: Clinical management for positive outcomes* (8th ed., pp. 1647, 1799). St. Louis: Saunders.

659. 4
Rationale: Rib fractures are a common injury, especially in the older client, and result from a blunt injury or a fall. Typical signs and symptoms include pain and tenderness localized at the fracture site and exacerbated by inspiration and palpation, shallow respirations, splinting or guarding the chest protectively to minimize chest movement, and possible bruising at the fracture site. Paradoxical respirations are seen with flail chest.
Test-Taking Strategy: Use the process of elimination. Focusing on the anatomical location of the injury will direct you to option 4. Review the assessment findings in rib fractures if you had difficulty with this question.
Level of Cognitive Ability: Analyzing
Client Needs: Physiological Integrity
Integrated Process: Nursing Process—Assessment
Content Area: Adult Health—Respiratory
Reference: Black, J., & Hawks, J. (2009). *Medical-surgical nursing: Clinical management for positive outcomes* (8th ed., pp. 1658-1659). St. Louis: Saunders.

660. 3
Rationale: Flail chest results from multiple rib fractures. This results in a "floating" section of ribs. Because this section is unattached to the rest of the bony rib cage, this segment results in paradoxical chest movement. This means that the force of inspiration pulls the fractured segment inward, while the rest of the chest expands. Similarly, during exhalation, the segment balloons outward while the rest of the chest moves inward. This is a characteristic sign of flail chest.
Test-Taking Strategy: Use the process of elimination, focusing on the strategic words *most distinctive*. Cyanosis and hypotension occur with many different disorders, so eliminate options 1 and 2 first. From the remaining options, choose paradoxical chest movement over dyspnea on exhalation by remembering that a flail chest has broken rib segments that move independently of the rest of the rib cage. Review the assessment findings in flail chest if you had difficulty with this question.
Level of Cognitive Ability: Applying
Client Needs: Physiological Integrity
Integrated Process: Nursing Process—Assessment
Content Area: Adult Health—Respiratory
Reference: Black, J., & Hawks, J. (2009). *Medical-surgical nursing: Clinical management for positive outcomes* (8th ed., pp. 1659-1660). St. Louis: Saunders.

661. 1
Rationale: Pneumothorax is characterized by restlessness, tachycardia, dyspnea, pain with respiration, asymmetrical chest expansion, and diminished or absent breath sounds on the affected side. Pneumothorax can cause increased airway pressure because of resistance to lung inflation. Acute respiratory distress syndrome and pulmonary embolism are not characterized by absent breath sounds. An endotracheal tube that is inserted too far can cause absent breath sounds, but the lack of breath sounds most likely would be on the left side because of the degree of curvature of the right and left main stem bronchi.
Test-Taking Strategy: Use the process of elimination. Focus on the symptoms presented in the question and note the relationship between *right* upper lobe and *right* pneumothorax in option 1. Review the manifestations associated with pneumothorax if you had difficulty with this question.
Level of Cognitive Ability: Analyzing
Client Needs: Physiological Integrity
Integrated Process: Nursing Process—Assessment
Content Area: Adult Health—Respiratory
Reference: Ignatavicius, D., & Workman, M. (2010). *Medical-surgical nursing: Patient-centered collaborative care* (6th ed., pp. 569, 698-699). St. Louis: Saunders.

662. 4
Rationale: The earliest detectable sign of acute respiratory distress syndrome is an increased respiratory rate, which can begin from 1 to 96 hours after the initial insult to the body. This is followed by increasing dyspnea, air hunger, retraction of accessory muscles, and cyanosis. Breath sounds may be clear or consist of fine inspiratory crackles or diffuse coarse crackles.
Test-Taking Strategy: Use the process of elimination, noting the strategic word *earliest*. Eliminate option 3 first because intercostal retraction is a later sign of respiratory distress. Of the remaining options, recall that adventitious breath sounds (options 1 and 2) would occur later than an increased respiratory rate. Review the early signs of acute respiratory distress syndrome if you had difficulty with this question.
Level of Cognitive Ability: Analyzing
Client Needs: Physiological Integrity
Integrated Process: Nursing Process—Assessment
Content Area: Adult Health—Respiratory
Reference: Ignatavicius, D., & Workman, M. (2010). *Medical-surgical nursing: Patient-centered collaborative care* (6th ed., p. 687). St. Louis: Saunders.

663. 1
Rationale: The client with emphysema has hyperinflation of the alveoli and flattening of the diaphragm. These lead to increased anteroposterior diameter, referred to as *barrel chest*. The client also has dyspnea with prolonged expiration and has hyperresonant lungs to percussion.
Test-Taking Strategy: Use the process of elimination. Recall that the barrel chest is a result of long-term hyperinflation of the lungs and air trapping. Knowing that a barrel chest occurs in emphysema will direct you to option 1. Review the characteristics of emphysema if you had difficulty with this question.
Level of Cognitive Ability: Analyzing
Client Needs: Physiological Integrity
Integrated Process: Nursing Process—Assessment
Content Area: Adult Health—Respiratory
Reference: Copstead-Kirkhorn, L., & Banasik, J. (2010). *Pathophysiology* (4th ed., p. 553). St. Louis: Mosby.

664. 4

Rationale: The client is continued on medication therapy for 6 to 12 months, depending on the situation. The client generally is considered not to be contagious after 2 to 3 weeks of medication therapy. The client is instructed to wear a mask if there will be exposure to crowds until the medication is effective in preventing transmission. The client is allowed to return to work when the results of three sputum cultures are negative.

Test-Taking Strategy: Use the process of elimination. Knowing that the medication therapy lasts for at least 6 months helps you eliminate option 1 first. Knowing that three sputum cultures must be negative helps you to eliminate option 3 next. From the remaining options, recalling that the client is not contagious after 2 to 3 weeks of therapy will direct you to option 4. If you had difficulty with this question, review the infectious period of tuberculosis.

Level of Cognitive Ability: Evaluating
Client Needs: Physiological Integrity
Integrated Process: Nursing Process—Evaluation
Content Area: Adult Health—Respiratory
Reference: Ignatavicius, D., & Workman, M. (2010). *Medical-surgical nursing: Patient-centered collaborative care* (6th ed., pp. 672–673). St. Louis: Saunders.

665. 2

Rationale: The nurse who is in contact with a client with tuberculosis should wear an individually fitted particulate respirator. The nurse also would wear gloves as per standard precautions. The nurse wears a gown when the possibility exists that the clothing could become contaminated, such as when giving a bed bath.

Test-Taking Strategy: Use the process of elimination. Knowing that the nurse should wear a particulate respirator eliminates options 1 and 4. Knowledge of basic standard precautions directs you to option 2 from the remaining options. Review precautions related to the care of a client with tuberculosis if you had difficulty with this question.

Level of Cognitive Ability: Applying
Client Needs: Safe and Effective Care Environment
Integrated Process: Nursing Process—Implementation
Content Area: Adult Health—Respiratory
References: Ignatavicius, D., & Workman, M. (2010). *Medical-surgical nursing: Patient-centered collaborative care* (6th ed., pp. 670, 672). St. Louis: Saunders.

Perry, A., & Potter, P. (2010). *Clinical nursing skills & techniques* (7th ed., p. 185). St. Louis: Mosby.

666. 3

Rationale: The most common initial symptom in pulmonary embolism is chest pain that is sudden in onset. The next most commonly reported symptom is dyspnea, which is accompanied by an increased respiratory rate. Other typical symptoms of pulmonary embolism include apprehension and restlessness, tachycardia, cough, and cyanosis.

Test-Taking Strategy: Use the process of elimination. Because pulmonary embolism does not result from an infectious process or an allergic reaction, eliminate options 1 and 2 first. To select between options 3 and 4, look at them closely. Option 4 states dyspnea when deep breaths are taken. Although dyspnea commonly occurs with pulmonary embolism, dyspnea is not associated only with deep breathing. Therefore eliminate option 4. Review the signs of pulmonary embolism if you had difficulty with this question.

Level of Cognitive Ability: Analyzing
Client Needs: Physiological Integrity
Integrated Process: Nursing Process—Assessment
Content Area: Adult Health—Respiratory
Reference: Swearingen, P. (2008). *All-in-one care planning resource: Medical-surgical, pediatric, maternity, & psychiatric nursing care plans* (2nd ed., p. 137). St. Louis: Mosby.

667. 1

Rationale: The client with human immunodeficiency virus (HIV) infection is considered to have positive results on Mantoux skin testing with an area larger than 5 mm of induration. The client without HIV is positive with an induration larger than 10 mm. The client with HIV is immunosuppressed, making a smaller area of induration positive for this type of client. It is possible for the client infected with HIV to have false-negative readings because of the immunosuppression factor. Options 2, 3, and 4 are incorrect interpretations.

Test-Taking Strategy: Use the process of elimination. Eliminate options 3 and 4 first because they are comparable or alike. From the remaining options, recalling that the client with HIV is immunosuppressed will assist in determining the interpretation of the area of induration. Review results of tuberculosis skin testing in an immunosuppressed client if you had difficulty with this question.

Level of Cognitive Ability: Analyzing
Client Needs: Physiological Integrity
Integrated Process: Nursing Process—Analysis
Content Area: Adult Health—Respiratory
Reference: Ignatavicius, D., & Workman, M. (2010). *Medical-surgical nursing: Patient-centered collaborative care* (6th ed., p. 669). St. Louis: Saunders.

668. 1

Rationale: Histoplasmosis is an opportunistic fungal infection that can occur in the client with acquired immunodeficiency syndrome (AIDS). The infection begins as a respiratory infection and can progress to disseminated infection. Typical signs and symptoms include fever, dyspnea, cough, and weight loss. Enlargement of the client's lymph nodes, liver, and spleen may occur as well.

Test-Taking Strategy: Use the process of elimination. Recalling that histoplasmosis is an infectious process will help you eliminate option 4. Because the client has AIDS and another infection, weight gain is an unlikely symptom and can be eliminated next. Knowing that histoplasmosis begins as a respiratory infection helps you choose dyspnea over headache as the correct option. Review the signs of histoplasmosis if you had difficulty with this question.

Level of Cognitive Ability: Applying
Client Needs: Physiological Integrity
Integrated Process: Nursing Process—Assessment
Content Area: Adult Health—Respiratory
Reference: Ignatavicius, D., & Workman, M. (2010). *Medical-surgical nursing: Patient-centered collaborative care* (6th ed., p. 371). St. Louis: Saunders.

669. 4

Rationale: Dry cough and dyspnea are typical signs and symptoms of pulmonary sarcoidosis. Others include night sweats, fever, weight loss, and skin nodules.

Test-Taking Strategy: Use the process of elimination and note the strategic word *early*. Because sarcoidosis is a pulmonary problem, eliminate options 1 and 3 first. Select option 4 over option 2 because the shortness of breath (and impaired ventilation) appears first and would cause the fatigue as a secondary symptom. Review the early signs of exacerbation in sarcoidosis if you had difficulty with this question.
Level of Cognitive Ability: Evaluating
Client Needs: Physiological Integrity
Integrated Process: Nursing Process—Evaluation
Content Area: Adult Health—Respiratory
Reference: Ignatavicius, D., & Workman, M. (2010). *Medical-surgical nursing: Patient-centered collaborative care* (6th ed., p. 639). St. Louis: Saunders.

670. 1

Rationale: Silicosis results from chronic, excessive inhalation of particles of free crystalline silica dust. The client should wear a mask to limit inhalation of this substance, which can cause restrictive lung disease after years of exposure. Options 2, 3, and 4 are not necessary.
Test-Taking Strategy: Use the process of elimination. Recalling that exposure to silica dust causes the illness and that the dust is inhaled into the respiratory tract will direct you to option 1. If you had difficulty with this question, review the protective measures associated with silicosis.
Level of Cognitive Ability: Understanding
Client Needs: Safe and Effective Care Environment
Integrated Process: Nursing Process—Assessment
Content Area: Adult Health—Respiratory
References: Black, J., & Hawks, J. (2009). *Medical-surgical nursing: Clinical management for positive outcomes* (8th ed., pp. 1625–1626). St. Louis: Saunders.

Ignatavicius, D., & Workman, M. (2010). *Medical-surgical nursing: Patient-centered collaborative care* (6th ed., p. 640). St. Louis: Saunders.

Potter, P., & Perry, A. (2009) *Fundamentals of nursing* (7th ed., pp. 662–663). St. Louis: Mosby.

671. 2

Rationale: The Venturi mask delivers the most accurate oxygen concentration. It is the best oxygen delivery system for the client with chronic airflow limitation because it delivers a precise oxygen concentration. The face tent, aerosol mask, and tracheostomy collar are also high-flow oxygen delivery systems but most often are used to administer high humidity.
Test-Taking Strategy: Use the process of elimination and note the strategic words *precise oxygen concentration*. Eliminate options 1, 3, and 4 because they are comparable or alike in that they are used to provide high humidity. Review the various types of oxygen delivery systems if you had difficulty with this question.
Level of Cognitive Ability: Understanding
Client Needs: Physiological Integrity
Integrated Process: Nursing Process—Planning
Content Area: Adult Health—Respiratory
Reference: Ignatavicius, D., & Workman, M. (2010). *Medical-surgical nursing: Patient-centered collaborative care* (6th ed., p. 628). St. Louis: Saunders.

672. 4

Rationale: Positions that will assist the client with emphysema with breathing include sitting up and leaning on an overbed table, sitting up and resting the elbows on the knees, and standing and leaning against the wall.
Test-Taking Strategy: Use the process of elimination. Eliminate options 1 and 3 first because they are comparable or alike. Next, eliminate option 2 because this position will not enhance breathing. If you had difficulty with this question, review the positions that will decrease the work of breathing in a client with emphysema.
Level of Cognitive Ability: Applying
Client Needs: Physiological Integrity
Integrated Process: Teaching and Learning
Content Area: Adult Health—Respiratory
Reference: Ignatavicius, D., & Workman, M. (2010). *Medical-surgical nursing: Patient-centered collaborative care* (6th ed., p. 624). St. Louis: Saunders.

673. 4

Rationale: One of the first pulmonary symptoms of tuberculosis is a slight cough with the expectoration of mucoid sputum. Options 1, 2, and 3 are late symptoms and signify cavitation and extensive lung involvement.
Test-Taking Strategy: Use the process of elimination and note the strategic word *first* in the question. Next focusing on the diagnosis should direct you to option 4. If you are unfamiliar with the signs associated with tuberculosis, review this content.
Level of Cognitive Ability: Applying
Client Needs: Physiological Integrity
Integrated Process: Teaching and Learning
Content Area: Adult Health—Respiratory
References: Copstead-Kirkhorn, L., & Banasik, J. (2010). *Pathophysiology* (4th ed., pp. 586–587). St. Louis: Mosby.

Swearingen, P. (2008). *All-in-one care planning resource: Medical-surgical, pediatric, maternity, & psychiatric nursing care plans* (2nd ed., p. 143). St. Louis: Mosby.

674. 3

Rationale: Tuberculosis is definitively diagnosed through culture and isolation of *Mycobacterium tuberculosis*. A presumptive diagnosis is made based on a tuberculin skin test, a sputum smear that is positive for acid-fast bacteria, a chest x-ray, and histological evidence of granulomatous disease on biopsy.
Test-Taking Strategy: Note the strategic word *confirm* in the question. Confirmation is made by identifying *M. tuberculosis*. If you had difficulty with this question, review the diagnostic procedures related to tuberculosis.
Level of Cognitive Ability: Analyzing
Client Needs: Physiological Integrity
Integrated Process: Nursing Process—Assessment
Content Area: Adult Health—Respiratory
References: Black, J., & Hawks, J. (2009). *Medical-surgical nursing: Clinical management for positive outcomes* (8th ed., pp. 1605–1606). St. Louis: Saunders.

Ignatavicius, D., & Workman, M. (2010). *Medical-surgical nursing: Patient-centered collaborative care* (6th ed., p. 669). St. Louis: Saunders.

Swearingen, P. (2008). *All-in-one care planning resource: Medical-surgical, pediatric, maternity, & psychiatric nursing care plans* (2nd ed., p. 144). St. Louis: Mosby.

ALTERNATE ITEM FORMAT: MULTIPLE RESPONSE

675. 1, 3, 4, 5

Rationale: The nurse should provide the client and family with information about tuberculosis and allay concerns about the contagious aspect of the infection. Instruct the client to follow the medication regimen exactly as prescribed and always to have a supply of the medication on hand. Advise the client of the side effects of the medication and ways of minimizing them to ensure compliance. Reassure the client that after 2 to 3 weeks of medication therapy, it is unlikely that the client will infect anyone. Inform the client that activities should be resumed gradually and about the need for adequate nutrition and a well-balanced diet that is rich in iron, protein, and vitamin C to promote healing and prevent recurrence of infection. Inform the client and family that respiratory isolation is not necessary because family members already have been exposed. Instruct the client about thorough hand washing and to cover the mouth and nose when coughing or sneezing and to put used tissues into plastic bags. Inform the client that a sputum culture is needed every 2 to 4 weeks once medication therapy is initiated. When the results of three sputum cultures are negative, the client is no longer considered infectious and can usually return to former employment.

Test-Taking Strategy: Knowledge regarding the pathophysiology, transmission, and treatment of tuberculosis is needed to answer this question. Read each option carefully to answer correctly. Review home care instructions for the client with tuberculosis if you had difficulty with this question.

Level of Cognitive Ability: Applying
Client Needs: Safe and Effective Care Environment
Integrated Process: Teaching and Learning
Content Area: Adult Health—Respiratory

References: Black, J., & Hawks, J. (2009). *Medical-surgical nursing: Clinical management for positive outcomes* (8th ed., p. 1608). St. Louis: Saunders.

Ignatavicius, D., & Workman, M. (2010). *Medical-surgical nursing: Patient-centered collaborative care* (6th ed., pp. 670, 672). St. Louis: Saunders.

Respiratory Medications

I. USE OF AN INHALER

A. Client instructions for use of a metered-dose inhaler (MDI; Figs. 59-1 and 59-2)

B. If two different inhaled medications are prescribed and one of the medications contains a glucocorticoid (corticosteroid), administer the bronchodilator first and the corticosteroid second.

⚠ If two different inhaled medications are prescribed, instruct the client to wait 5 minutes following administration of the first before inhaling the second.

II. BRONCHODILATORS (Box 59-1)

A. Description

1. Sympathomimetic bronchodilators relax the smooth muscle of the bronchi and dilate the airways of the respiratory tree, making air exchange and respiration easier for the client.
2. Methylxanthine bronchodilators stimulate the central nervous system and respiration, dilate coronary and pulmonary vessels, cause diuresis, and relax smooth muscle.
3. Bronchodilators are used to treat allergic rhinitis and sinusitis, acute bronchospasm, acute and chronic **asthma**, bronchitis, **chronic obstructive pulmonary disease**, **emphysema**, and other restrictive airway diseases.
4. Bronchodilators are contraindicated in individuals with hypersensitivity, peptic ulcer disease, severe cardiac disease and cardiac dysrhythmias, hyperthyroidism, or uncontrolled seizure disorders.
5. Bronchodilators should be used with caution in clients with hypertension, diabetes mellitus, or narrow-angle glaucoma.
6. Theophylline increases the risk of digoxin toxicity and decreases the effects of lithium and phenytoin (Dilantin).
7. If theophylline and a β_2-adrenergic agonist are administered together, cardiac dysrhythmias may result.
8. β-Blockers, cimetidine (Tagamet), and erythromycin increase the effects of theophylline.

9. Barbiturates and carbamazepine (Tegretol) decrease the effects of theophylline.

B. Side effects

1. Palpitations and tachycardia
2. Dysrhythmias
3. Restlessness, nervousness, tremors
4. Anorexia, nausea, and vomiting
5. Headaches and dizziness
6. Hyperglycemia
7. Decreased clotting time
8. Mouth dryness and throat irritation with inhalers
9. Tolerance and paradoxical bronchoconstriction with inhalers

C. Interventions

1. Assess vital signs and lung sounds.
2. Monitor for cardiac dysrhythmias.
3. Assess for cough, wheezing, decreased breath sounds, and sputum production.
4. Monitor for restlessness and confusion.
5. Provide adequate hydration.
6. Administer the medication at regular intervals around the clock to maintain a sustained therapeutic level.
7. Administer oral medications with or after meals to decrease gastrointestinal irritation.
8. Instruct the client not to crush enteric-coated or sustained-release tablets or capsules.
9. Instruct the client to avoid caffeine-containing products such as coffee, tea, cola, and chocolate.
10. Instruct the client in the side effects of bronchodilators.
11. Instruct the client in how to monitor the pulse and to report any abnormalities to the physician.
12. Instruct the client in how to use an inhaler or nebulizer and how to monitor the amount of medication remaining in an inhaler canister; how to use a spacer (a device that enhances the delivery of medication) is also taught (see Figs. 59-1 and 59-2)
13. Instruct the client to avoid over-the-counter medications.
14. Instruct the client to stop smoking and provide information regarding support resources.

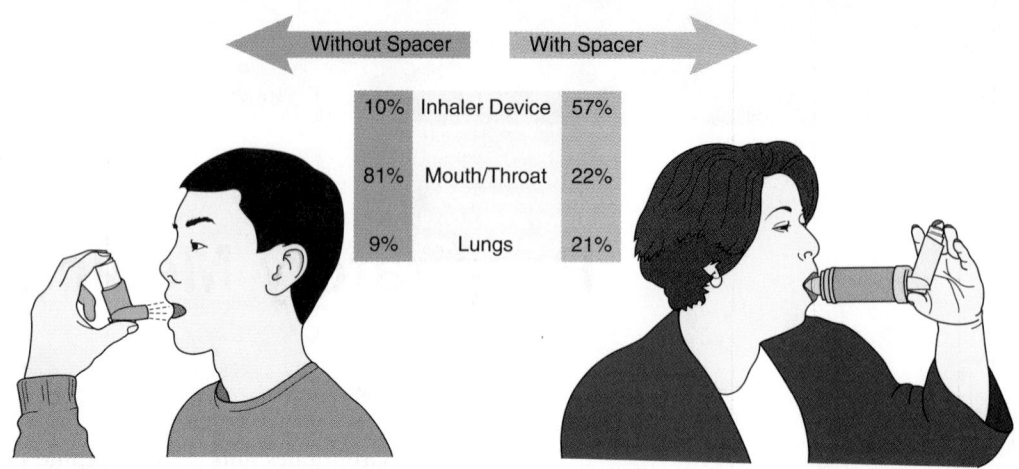

▲ **FIGURE 59-1** Distribution of medication with and without a spacer. (From Kee, J., & Marshall, S. [2009]. *Clinical calculations: With applications to general and specialty areas* [6th ed.]. St. Louis: Saunders.)

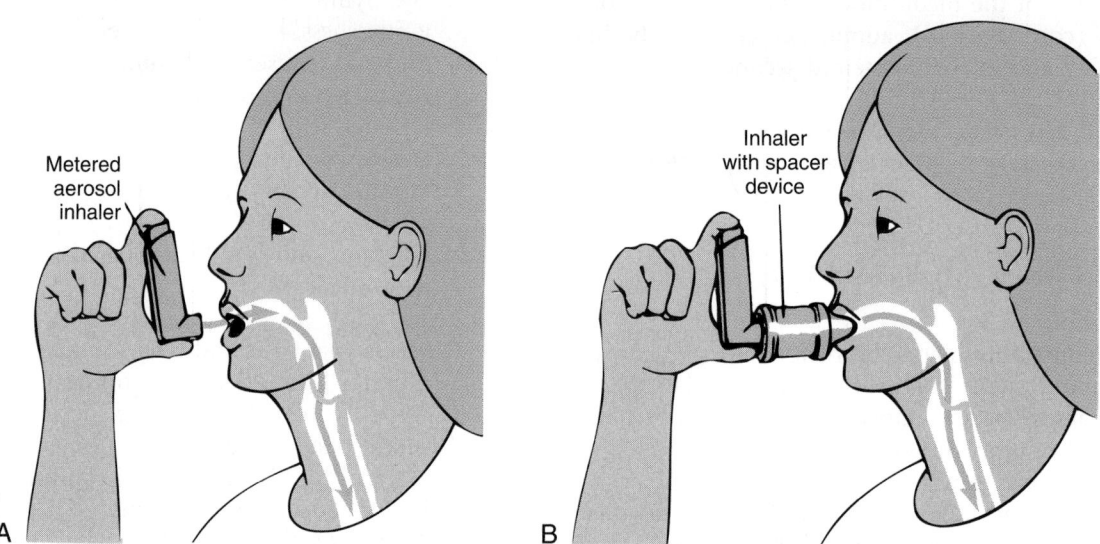

▲ **FIGURE 59-2** Inhaled drugs commonly used in asthma treatment include β-adrenergic bronchodilators, cromolyn sodium, and aerosol glucocorticoids. **A,** The metered-dose inhaler should not be put in the mouth but held about two fingerwidths (1½ inches) in front of the mouth. **B,** Alternatively, an inhaler with a spacer device can be used. Patients should breathe deeply once before activating the inhaler and then continue breathing in for about 5 seconds. Patients then should hold their breath for 10 to 15 seconds before breathing out slowly. If a second dose is needed, patients should wait 1 to 2 minutes before taking another dose. (From Clark, J., Queener, S., & Karb, V. [2000]. *Pharmacologic basis of nursing practice* [6th ed.]. St. Louis: Mosby.)

15. Instruct the client with diabetes mellitus to monitor blood glucose levels.
16. Instruct the client with **asthma** to wear a Medic-Alert bracelet.
17. Monitor for a therapeutic serum theophylline level of 10 to 20 mcg/mL.
18. Intravenously administered theophylline preparations should be administered slowly and always via an infusion pump.

 Theophylline toxicity is likely to occur when the serum level is higher than 20 mcg/mL. Early signs of toxicity include restlessness, nervousness, tremors, palpitations, and tachycardia.

III. ANTICHOLINERGICS (see Box 59-1)

A. Inhaled medications that improve lung function by blocking muscarinic receptors in the bronchi, which results in bronchodilation.
B. Effective for treating **chronic obstructive pulmonary disease**, allergy-induced **asthma**, and exercise-induced bronchospasm.
C. Side effects include dry mouth and irritation of the pharynx; sucking on sugarless candy will help to relieve symptoms.
D. Systemic anticholinergic effects rarely occur but can include increased intraocular pressure, blurred vision, tachycardia, cardiovascular events, urinary retention, and constipation.

Box 59-1 Medications to Treat Restrictive Airway Disorders

Bronchodilators

β₂-Adrenergic Agonists

Inhaled

Albuterol (Proventil HFA, AccuNeb, ProAir HFA, Ventolin HFA)

Arformoterol (Brovana)

Formoterol (Foradil Aerolizer, Perforomist)

Levalbuterol (Xopenex, Xopenex HFA)

Pirbuterol (Maxair Autohaler)

Salmeterol (Serevent Diskus)

Oral

Albuterol (VoSpire)

Terbutaline (Brethine)

Methylxanthines

Theophylline, oral (Theo-24, Theochron, Uniphyl, Elixophyllin)

Anticholinergics

Ipratropium, inhaled (Atrovent, Atrovent HFA)

Ipratropium/albuterol, inhaled (Combivent)

Tiotropium, inhaled (Spiriva)

Glucocorticoids (Corticosteroids)

Inhaled

Beclomethasone dipropionate (Qvar)

Budesonide (Pulmicort Turbohaler, Pulmicort Respules)

Ciclesonide (Alvesco)

Flunisolide (AeroBid)

Fluticasone propionate (Flovent HFA, Flovent Diskus)

Mometasone furoate (Asmanex Twisthaler)

Triamcinolone acetonide (Azmacort)

Oral

Prednisone

Prednisolone

Leukotriene Modifiers

Montelukast, oral (Singulair)

Zafirlukast, oral (Accolate)

Zileuton, oral (Zyflo, Zyflo CR)

Inhaled Nonsteroidal Antiallergy Agent

Cromolyn sodium, inhaled (Intal)

Monoclonal Antibody

Omalizumab (Xolair)

Modified from Lehne, R. (2010). *Pharmacology for nursing care* (7th ed., p. 890). St. Louis: Saunders.

⚠ The client with a peanut allergy should not take ipratropium (Atrovent HFA and Combivent) because the product contains soy lecithin, which is in the same plant family as peanuts.

IV. GLUCOCORTICOIDS (CORTICOSTEROIDS)
(see Box 59-1)

A. Glucocorticoids act as anti-inflammatory agents and reduce edema of the airways; they are used to treat **asthma** and other inflammatory respiratory conditions.

B. See Chapter 55 for information on glucocorticoids.

V. LEUKOTRIENE MODIFIERS (see Box 59-1)

A. Description
1. Used in the prophylaxis and treatment of chronic bronchial **asthma** (not used for acute **asthma** episodes)
2. Inhibit bronchoconstriction caused by specific antigens and reduce airway edema and smooth muscle constriction
3. Contraindicated in clients with hypersensitivity and in breast-feeding mothers
4. Should be used with caution in clients with impaired hepatic function
5. Coadministration of inhaled glucocorticoids increases the risk of upper respiratory infection.

B. Side effects
1. Headache
2. Nausea and vomiting
3. Dyspepsia
4. Diarrhea

5. Generalized pain, myalgia
6. Fever
7. Dizziness

C. Interventions
1. Monitor vital signs.
2. Assess lung sounds for rhonchi and wheezing.
3. Assess liver function laboratory values.
4. Monitor for cyanosis.
5. Instruct the client to take medication 1 hour before or 2 hours after meals.
6. Instruct the client to increase fluid intake.
7. Instruct the client not to discontinue the medication and to take as prescribed, even during symptom-free periods.

VI. INHALED NONSTEROIDAL ANTIALLERGY AGENT (see Box 59-1)

A. Description
1. Antiasthmatic, antiallergic, and mast cell stabilizers inhibit mast cell release after exposure to antigens.
2. This medication is used to treat allergic rhinitis, bronchial **asthma**, and exercise-induced bronchospasm (see Box 59-1).
3. It is contraindicated in clients with known hypersensitivity.
4. Orally administered cromolyn sodium (Intal) is used with caution in clients with impaired hepatic or renal function.

B. Side effects
1. Cough or bronchospasm following inhalation
2. Nasal sting or sneezing following inhalation
3. Unpleasant taste in the mouth

C. Interventions
 1. Monitor vital signs.
 2. Monitor respirations and assess lung sounds for rhonchi or wheezing.
 3. Administer oral capsules at least 30 minutes before meals.
 4. Instruct the client not to discontinue the medication abruptly because a rebound asthmatic attack can occur.

⚠ Instruct the client taking inhaled medications to drink a few sips of water before and after inhalation to prevent a cough and an unpleasant taste in the mouth.

VII. MONOCLONAL ANTIBODY

A. Description
 1. Omalizumab (Xolair) is a recombinant DNA-derived humanized immunoglobulin G (IgG) murine monoclonal antibody that selectively binds to IgE to limit the release of mediators in the allergic response.
 2. Used to treat allergy-related **asthma**; administered subcutaneously every 2 to 4 weeks
 3. Dose is titrated based on the serum IgE level and body weight.
 4. Contraindicated in those with hypersensitivity to the medication

B. Side effects
 1. Injection site reactions
 2. Viral infections
 3. Upper respiratory infections
 4. Sinusitis
 5. Headache
 6. Pharyngitis
 7. Anaphylaxis
 8. Malignancies

C. Interventions
 1. Assess respiratory rate, rhythm, and depth and auscultate lung fields bilaterally.
 2. Assess for allergies and/or allergic reaction symptoms such as rash or urticaria.
 3. Instruct the client that respiratory improvement will not be immediate.
 4. Instruct the client not to stop taking or decrease the currently prescribed **asthma** medications unless instructed.
 5. Avoid live virus vaccines for the duration of treatment.
 6. Have medications for the treatment of severe hypersensitivity reactions available during initial administration in case anaphylaxis occurs.

VIII. ANTIHISTAMINES (Box 59-2)

A. Description
 1. Antihistamines are called histamine antagonists or H_1 blockers; these medications compete with histamine for receptor sites, thus preventing a histamine response.

Box 59-2 Antihistamines

Cetirizine (Zyrtec)
Chlorpheniramine (Chlor-Trimeton, others)
Desloratadine (Clarinex)
Dimenhydrinate (Dramamine)
Diphenhydramine (Benadryl)
Fexofenadine (Allegra)
Levocetirizine (Xyzal)
Loratadine (Claritin, Alavert)
Olopatadine (Patanase)

---

 2. When the H_1 receptor is stimulated, the extravascular smooth muscles, including those lining the nasal cavity, are constricted.
 3. Antihistamines decrease nasopharyngeal, gastrointestinal, and bronchial secretions by blocking the H_1 receptor.
 4. Antihistamines are used for the common cold, rhinitis, nausea and vomiting, motion sickness, urticaria, and as a sleep aid.
 5. Can cause central nervous system (CNS) depression if taken with alcohol, opioids, hypnotics, or barbiturates
 6. Should be used with caution in clients with **chronic obstructive pulmonary disease** because of their drying effect
 7. Diphenhydramine (Benadryl) has an anticholinergic effect and should be avoided in clients with narrow-angle glaucoma.

B. Side effects
 1. Drowsiness and fatigue
 2. Dizziness
 3. Urinary retention
 4. Blurred vision
 5. Wheezing
 6. Constipation
 7. Dry mouth
 8. Gastrointestinal irritation
 9. Hypotension
 10. Hearing disturbances
 11. Photosensitivity
 12. Nervousness and irritability
 13. Confusion
 14. Nightmares

C. Interventions
 1. Monitor vital signs.
 2. Monitor for signs of urinary dysfunction.
 3. Administer with food or milk.
 4. Avoid subcutaneous injection, and administer by intramuscular injection in a large muscle if the intramuscular route is prescribed.
 5. Instruct the client to avoid hazardous activities, alcohol, and other CNS depressants.
 6. Instruct the client taking the medication for motion sickness to take it 30 minutes before the event and then before meals and at bedtime during the event as prescribed.

Box 59-3 Nasal Decongestants

Nonglucocorticoids
Naphazoline (Privine)
Oxymetazoline (Afrin 12-Hour, others)
Phenylephrine hydrochloride (Neo-Synephrine, others)
Pseudoephedrine hydrochloride (Sudafed)
Tetrahydrozoline (Tyzine)
Xylometazoline (Natru-Vent, Otrivin)

Glucocorticoids
Beclomethasone (Beconase AQ)
Budesonide (Rhinocort Aqua)
Ciclesonide (Omnaris)
Flunisolide (Nasarel)
Fluticasone propionate (Flonase)
Fluticasone furoate (Veramyst)
Mometasone (Nasonex)
Triamcinolone (Nasacort AQ)

Box 59-4 Expectorants and Mucolytic Agents

Expectorants   **Mucolytic**
Guaifenesin (Humibid,   Acetylcysteine (Mucomyst)
Mucinex)

Box 59-5 Antitussives

Opioids
Codeine phosphate, codeine sulfate
Hydrocodone

Nonopioids
Benzonatate (Tessalon)
Dextromethorphan
Diphenhydramine hydrochloride (Benadryl)

7. Instruct the client to suck on hard candy or ice chips for dry mouth.

IX. NASAL DECONGESTANTS (Box 59-3)

A. Description
   1. Nasal decongestants include adrenergic, anticholinergic, and corticosteroid medications.
   2. These medications shrink nasal mucosal membranes and reduce fluid secretion.
   3. Are used for allergic rhinitis, hay fever, and acute coryza (profuse nasal discharge).
   4. Contraindicated or used with extreme caution in clients with hypertension, cardiac disease, hyperthyroidism, or diabetes mellitus
B. Side effects
   1. Frequent use of decongestants, especially nasal sprays or drops, can result in tolerance and rebound nasal congestion (vasodilation) caused by irritation of the nasal mucosa.
   2. Nervousness
   3. Restlessness, insomnia
   4. Hypertension
   5. Hyperglycemia

⚠ Nasal decongestants can cause tolerance and rebound nasal congestion (vasodilation) caused by irritation of the nasal mucosa. Therefore, the client needs to be informed that these medications should not be used for longer than 48 hours.

C. Interventions
   1. Assess the client for existing medical disorders.
   2. Monitor for cardiac dysrhythmias.
   3. Monitor blood glucose levels.
   4. Instruct the client to avoid consuming caffeine in large amounts because it can increase restlessness and palpitations.
   5. Instruct the client in the importance of limiting the use of nasal sprays and drops.

X. EXPECTORANTS AND MUCOLYTIC AGENTS (Box 59-4)

A. Description
   1. Expectorants loosen bronchial secretions so that they can be eliminated with coughing; they are used for a dry unproductive cough and to stimulate bronchial secretions.
   2. Mucolytic agents thin mucous secretions to help make the cough more productive.
   3. Mucolytic agents with dextromethorphan should not be used by clients with **chronic obstructive pulmonary disease** because they suppress the cough.
   4. Acetylcysteine (Mucomyst) can increase airway resistance and should not be used in clients with **asthma**.
B. Side effects
   1. Gastrointestinal irritation
   2. Rash
   3. Oropharyngeal irritation
C. Interventions
   1. Instruct the client to take the medication with a full glass of water to loosen mucus.
   2. Instruct the client to maintain an adequate fluid intake.
   3. Encourage the client to cough and deep breathe.
   4. Acetylcysteine (Mucomyst), administered by nebulization, should not be mixed with another medication.
   5. If acetylcysteine is administered with a bronchodilator, the bronchodilator should be administered 5 minutes before the acetylcysteine.
   6. Monitor for side effects of acetylcysteine such as nausea and vomiting, stomatitis, and runny nose.

XI. ANTITUSSIVES (Box 59-5)

A. Description: Act on the cough control center in the medulla to suppress the cough reflex; used for a cough that is nonproductive and irritating

Box 59-6 Opioid Antagonists

Alvimopan (Entereg)
Methylnaltrexone (Relistor)
Nalmefene (Revex)
Naloxone (Narcan)
Naltrexone (ReVia, Depade)

Box 59-7 First-Line and Second-Line Medications for Tuberculosis

First-Line Agents
Isoniazid (INH, Nydrazid)
Rifampin (Rifadin)
Ethambutol (Myambutol)
Pyrazinamide
Rifabutin (Mycobutin)
Rifapentine (Priftin)

Second-Line Agents
Amikacin (Amikin)
Capreomycin sulfate (Capastat Sulfate)
Cycloserine (Seromycin)
Ethionamide (Trecator)
Kanamycin (Kantrex)
Levofloxacin (Levaquin)
Moxifloxacin (Avelox)
p-Aminosalicylic acid (Paser)
Streptomycin

B. Side effects
  1. Dizziness, drowsiness, sedation
  2. Gastrointestinal irritation, nausea
  3. Dry mouth
  4. Constipation
  5. Respiratory depression
C. Interventions
  1. Instruct the client that if the cough lasts longer than 1 week and a fever or rash occurs to notify the physician.
  2. Encourage the client to take adequate fluids with the medication.
  3. Encourage the client to sleep with the head of the bed elevated.
  4. Instruct the client to avoid hazardous activities.
  5. Note that drug dependency can occur.
  6. Avoid administration to the client with a head injury or a postoperative cranial surgery client.
  7. Avoid administration to the client using opioids, sedative-hypnotics, barbiturates, or antidepressants because CNS depression can occur.
  8. Instruct the client to avoid the use of alcohol.

XII. OPIOID ANTAGONISTS (Box 59-6)

A. Description
  1. An opioid antagonist reverses respiratory depression in opioid overdose.
  2. Avoid its use for non-opioid respiratory depression.
B. Side effects
  1. CNS depression
  2. Nausea, vomiting
  3. Tremors
  4. Sweating
  5. Increased blood pressure
  6. Tachycardia
C. Interventions
  1. Assess vital signs, especially respirations.
  2. For intravenous administration, the dose is titrated every 2 to 5 minutes as prescribed.
  3. Have oxygen and resuscitative equipment available during administration.

XIII. TUBERCULOSIS MEDICATIONS (Box 59-7)

A. Description
  1. **Tuberculosis** medications offer the most effective method for treating the disease and preventing transmission.
  2. Treatment of identified lesions depends on whether the individual has active disease or has only been exposed to the disease.
  3. Treatment is difficult because the bacterium has a waxy substance on the capsule that makes penetration and destruction difficult.
  4. The use of a multidrug regimen destroys organisms as quickly as possible and minimizes the emergence of drug-resistant organisms.
  5. Active **tuberculosis** is treated with a combination of medications to which the organism is susceptible.
  6. Individuals with active **tuberculosis** are treated for 6 to 9 months; however, clients with human immunodeficiency virus (HIV) infection are treated for a longer period of time.
  7. After the infected individual has received medication for 2 to 3 weeks, the risk of transmission is greatly reduced.
  8. Most clients have negative sputum cultures after 3 months of compliance with medication therapy.
  9. Individuals who have been exposed to active **tuberculosis** are treated with preventive isoniazid (INH) for 9 to 12 months.
B. First-line or second-line medications
  1. First-line medications provide the most effective antituberculosis activity.
  2. Second-line medications are used in combination with first-line medications but are more toxic.
  3. Current infecting organisms are proving resistant to standard first-line medications; the resistant organisms develop because individuals with the disease fail to complete the course of treatment, so surviving bacteria adapt to the medication and become resistant.

4. Multidrug therapies are instituted because of the resistant organisms.

C. Multidrug-resistant strain of **tuberculosis** (MDR-TB)

1. Resistance occurs when a client receiving two medications (first-line and second-line medications) discontinues one of the medications.
2. The client briefly experiences some response from the single medication but then large numbers of resistant organisms begin to grow.
3. The client, infectious again, transmits the drug-resistant organism to other individuals.
4. As this event is repeated, an organism develops that is resistant to many of the first-line **tuberculosis** medications.

XIV. FIRST-LINE MEDICATIONS FOR TUBERCULOSIS (see Box 59-7)

A. Isoniazid (INH)

1. Description
   a. Isoniazid is bactericidal.
   b. It inhibits the synthesis of mycolic acids and acts to kill actively growing organisms in the extracellular environment.
   c. It inhibits the growth of dormant organisms in the macrophages and caseating granulomas.
   d. It is active only during cell division and is used in combination with other antitubercular medications.
2. Contraindications and cautions
   a. Isoniazid is contraindicated in clients with hypersensitivity or with acute liver disease.
   b. Use with caution in clients with chronic liver disease, alcoholism, or renal impairment.
   c. Use with caution in clients taking nicotinic acid (niacin).
   d. Use with caution in clients taking hepatotoxic medications because the risk for hepatotoxicity increases.
   e. Alcohol increases the risk of hepatotoxicity.
   f. Isoniazid may increase the risk of toxicity of carbamazepine (Tegretol) and phenytoin (Dilantin).
   g. Isoniazid may decrease ketoconazole (Nizoral) concentrations.
3. Side effects
   a. Hypersensitivity reactions
   b. Peripheral neuritis
   c. Neurotoxicity
   d. Hepatotoxicity; increased liver function test levels
   e. Pyridoxine (vitamin B_6) deficiency
   f. Irritation at injection site with intramuscular administration
   g. Nausea and vomiting
   h. Dry mouth
   i. Dizziness
   j. Hyperglycemia
   k. Vision changes
   l. Hepatitis

4. Interventions
   a. Assess for hypersensitivity.
   b. Assess for hepatic dysfunction.
   c. Assess for sensitivity to nicotinic acid.
   d. Monitor liver function test results.
   e. Monitor for signs of hepatitis, such as anorexia, nausea, vomiting, weakness, fatigue, dark urine, or jaundice; if these symptoms occur, withhold the medication and notify the physician.
   f. Monitor for tingling, numbness, or burning of the extremities.
   g. Assess mental status.
   h. Monitor for visual changes, and notify the physician if they occur.
   i. Assess for dizziness and initiate safety precautions.
   j. Monitor complete blood count (CBC) and blood glucose levels.
   k. Administer isoniazid 1 hour before or 2 hours after a meal because food may delay absorption.
   l. Administer isoniazid at least 1 hour before antacids, especially those antacids that contain aluminum.
   m. Administer pyridoxine as prescribed to reduce the risk of neurotoxicity.

⚠ Many tuberculosis medications can cause toxic effects such as hepatotoxicity, nephrotoxicity, neurotoxicity, optic neuritis, or ototoxicity. Teach the client about the signs of toxicity and inform the client that the physician needs to be notified if any signs arise.

5. Client education
   a. Instruct the client not to skip doses and to take the medication for the full length of the prescribed therapy.
   b. Instruct the client not to take any other medication without consulting the physician.
   c. Advise the client of the importance of follow-up physician visits, vision testing, and laboratory tests.
   d. Instruct the client to avoid alcohol.
   e. Advise the client to take medication on an empty stomach with 8 oz of water 1 hour before or 2 hours after meals and to avoid taking antacids with the medication.
   f. Instruct the client to avoid tyramine-containing foods because they may cause a reaction such as red and itching skin, a pounding heartbeat, lightheadedness, a hot or clammy feeling, or a headache; if this does occur, the client should notify the physician.
   g. Instruct the client in the signs of neurotoxicity, hepatitis, and hepatotoxicity.
   h. Instruct the client to notify the physician if signs of neurotoxicity, hepatitis and hepatotoxicity, or visual changes occur.

B. Rifampin (Rifadin)
1. Description
   a. Rifampin inhibits bacterial RNA synthesis.
   b. It binds to DNA-dependent RNA polymerase and blocks RNA transcription.
   c. It is used with at least one other antitubercular medication.
2. Contraindications and cautions
   a. Rifampin is contraindicated in clients with hypersensitivity.
   b. It should be used with caution in clients with hepatic dysfunction or alcoholism.
   c. Use of alcohol or hepatotoxic medications may increase the risk of hepatotoxicity.
   d. Rifampin decreases the effects of several medications, including oral anticoagulants, oral hypoglycemics, chloramphenicol (Chloromycetin), digoxin (Lanoxin), disopyramide phosphate (Norpace), mexiletine (Mexitil), quinidine polygalacturonate, tocainide hydrochloride, fluconazole (Diflucan), methadone hydrochloride (Dolophine), phenytoin (Dilantin), and verapamil hydrochloride (Calan).
3. Side effects
   a. Hypersensitivity reaction, including fever, chills, shivering, headache, muscle and bone pain, and dyspnea
   b. Heartburn, nausea, vomiting, diarrhea
   c. Red-orange–colored body secretions
   d. Vision changes
   e. Hepatotoxicity and hepatitis
   f. Increased uric acid levels
   g. Blood dyscrasias
   h. Colitis
4. Interventions
   a. Assess for hypersensitivity.
   b. Evaluate CBC, uric acid, and liver function test results.
   c. Assess for signs of hepatitis; if they occur, withhold the medication and notify the physician.
   d. Monitor stools for signs of colitis.
   e. Monitor mental status.
   f. Assess for visual changes.
5. Client education
   a. Instruct the client not to skip doses and to take medication for the full length of the prescribed therapy.
   b. Instruct the client not to take any other medication without consulting the physician.
   c. Advise the client of the importance of follow-up physician visits and laboratory tests.
   d. Instruct the client to avoid alcohol.
   e. Advise the client to take medication on an empty stomach with 8 oz of water 1 hour before or 2 hours after meals and to avoid taking antacids with the medication.

   f. Instruct the client that urine, feces, sweat, and tears will be red-orange and that soft contact lens can become permanently discolored.
   g. Instruct the client to notify the physician if jaundice (yellow eyes or skin) develops or if weakness, fatigue, nausea, vomiting, sore throat, fever, or unusual bleeding occurs.

C. Ethambutol (Myambutol)
1. Description
   a. Ethambutol is bacteriostatic.
   b. It interferes with cell metabolism and multiplication by inhibiting one or more metabolites in susceptible organisms.
   c. It inhibits bacterial RNA synthesis and is active only during cell division.
   d. Ethambutol is slow-acting and must be used with other bactericidal agents.
2. Contraindications and cautions
   a. Ethambutol is contraindicated in clients with hypersensitivity or optic neuritis and in children younger than 13 years.
   b. Use with caution in clients with renal dysfunction, gout, ocular defects, diabetic retinopathy, cataracts, or ocular inflammatory conditions.
   c. Use with caution in clients taking neurotoxic medications because the risk for neurotoxicity increases.
3. Side effects
   a. Hypersensitivity reactions
   b. Anorexia, nausea, vomiting
   c. Dizziness
   d. Malaise
   e. Mental confusion
   f. Joint pain
   g. Dermatitis
   h. Optic neuritis
   i. Peripheral neuritis
   j. Thrombocytopenia
   k. Increased uric acid levels
   l. Anaphylactoid reaction
4. Interventions
   a. Assess the client for hypersensitivity.
   b. Evaluate results of CBC, uric acid, and renal and liver function tests.
   c. Obtain baseline visual acuity and color discrimination, especially to green.
   d. Monitor for visual changes such as altered color perception and decreased visual acuity; if changes occur, withhold the medication and notify the physician.
   e. Administer once every 24 hours and administer with food to decrease gastrointestinal upset.
   f. Monitor uric acid concentration and assess for painful or swollen joints or signs of gout.
   g. Monitor intake and output and for adequate renal function.
   h. Assess mental status.

i. Monitor for dizziness and initiate safety precautions.

j. Assess for peripheral neuritis (numbness, tingling or burning of the extremities); if it occurs, notify the physician.

5. Client education
   a. Inform the client that he or she can prevent nausea related to the medication by taking the daily dose at bedtime or by taking the prescribed antinausea medications.
   b. Instruct the client not to skip doses and to take the medication for the full length of the prescribed therapy.
   c. Instruct the client not to take any other medication without consulting the physician.
   d. Advise the client of the importance of follow-up physician visits, vision testing, and laboratory tests.
   e. Instruct the client to notify the physician immediately if any visual problems occur or a rash, swelling and pain in the joints, or numbness, tingling, or burning in the hands or feet occurs.

D. Pyrazinamide
1. Description
   a. The exact mechanism of action of pyrazinamide is unknown.
   b. Pyrazinamide may be bacteriostatic or bactericidal, depending on its concentration at the infection site and susceptibility of infecting organism.
   c. It is used with at least one other antitubercular medication after failure or ineffectiveness of the primary medication(s).
2. Contraindications and cautions
   a. Pyrazinamide is contraindicated in clients with hypersensitivity.
   b. Use pyrazinamide with caution in clients with diabetes mellitus, renal impairment, or gout, and in children.
   c. Pyrazinamide may decrease the effects of allopurinol (Zyloprim), colchicine, probenecid (Benemid), and sulfinpyrazone (Anturane).
   d. Cross-sensitivity is possible with isoniazid (INH), ethionamide (Trecator), or nicotinic acid.
3. Side effects
   a. Increases liver function tests and uric acid levels
   b. Arthralgia, myalgia
   c. Photosensitivity
   d. Hepatotoxicity
   e. Thrombocytopenia
4. Interventions
   a. Assess for hypersensitivity.
   b. Evaluate CBC, liver function test results, and uric acid levels.
   c. Observe for hepatotoxic effects; if they occur, withhold the medication and notify the physician.

d. Assess for painful or swollen joints.

e. Evaluate blood glucose level because diabetes mellitus may be difficult to control while client is taking the medication.

5. Client education
   a. Instruct the client to take the medication with food to reduce gastrointestinal distress.
   b. Instruct the client to avoid sunlight or ultraviolet light until photosensitivity is determined.
   c. Instruct the client to notify the physician if any side effects occur.
   d. Instruct the client not to skip doses and to take the medication for the full length of the prescribed therapy.
   e. Instruct the client not to take any other medication without consulting the physician.
   f. Advise the client of the importance of follow-up physician visits and laboratory tests.

E. Rifabutin (Mycobutin)
1. Description
   a. Inhibits mycobacterial DNA-dependent RNA polymerase and suppresses protein synthesis
   b. Used to prevent disseminated *Mycobacterium avium* complex (MAC) disease in clients with advanced HIV infection
   c. Used to treat active MAC disease and **tuberculosis** in clients with HIV infection
2. Cautions
   a. Can affect blood levels of some medications, including oral contraceptives and some medications used to treat HIV infection
   b. A nonhormonal method of birth control should be used instead of an oral contraceptive.
3. Side effects
   a. Rash
   b. GI disturbances
   c. Neutropenia
   d. Red-orange–colored body secretions
   e. Uveitis
   f. Myositis
   g. Arthralgia
   h. Hepatitis
   i. Chest pain with dyspnea
   j. Flu-like syndrome
4. Interventions
   a. Assess medication history of the client.
   b. Observe for hepatotoxic effects; if they occur, withhold the medication and notify the physician.
   c. Assess for painful or swollen joints.
   d. Assess for ocular pain or blurred vision.
5. Client education
   a. Instruct the client that the medication can be taken without regard to food.
   b. Instruct the client to notify the physician if any side effects occur.

c. Instruct the client not to skip doses and to take the medication for the full length of the prescribed therapy.

d. Instruct the client not to take any other medication without consulting the physician.

e. Advise the client of the importance of follow-up physician visits and laboratory tests.

F. Rifapentine (Priftin)

1. Description: Used only for pulmonary **tuberculosis**

2. Cautions: Can affect blood levels of some medications, including oral contraceptives and warfarin (Coumadin), and some medications used to treat HIV infection

3. Side effects
   a. Red-orange–colored body secretions
   b. Hepatotoxicity

4. Interventions
   a. Assess medication history of the client.
   b. Obtain baseline liver function studies and assess throughout therapy.
   c. Observe for hepatotoxic effects; if they occur, withhold the medication and notify the physician.

5. Client education
   a. Instruct the client that the medication can be taken without regard to food.
   b. Instruct the client to avoid sunlight or ultraviolet light until photosensitivity is determined.
   c. Instruct the client to notify the physician if any side effects occur
   d. Instruct the client not to skip doses and to take the medication for the full length of the prescribed therapy.
   e. Instruct the client not to take any other medication without consulting the physician.
   f. Advise the client of the importance of follow-up physician visits and laboratory tests.

⚠ Some tuberculosis medications can cause red-orange colored body secretions. Inform the client that this is not a harmful effect but that the secretions can stain and permanently discolor items.

XV. SECOND-LINE MEDICATIONS FOR TUBERCULOSIS (see Box 59-7)

A. Capreomycin sulfate (Capastat Sulfate)

1. Description
   a. Mechanism of action for capreomycin is unknown.
   b. Used to treat MDR-TB when significant resistance to other medications is expected
   c. Capreomycin must be given intramuscularly.

2. Contraindications and cautions
   a. The risk of nephrotoxicity, ototoxicity, and neuromuscular blockade is increased with the use of aminoglycosides or loop diuretics.

b. Use capreomycin with caution in clients with renal insufficiency, acoustic nerve impairment, hepatic disorder, myasthenia gravis, or parkinsonism.
   c. Do not administer to clients receiving streptomycin.

3. Side effects
   a. Nephrotoxicity
   b. Ototoxicity
   c. Neuromuscular blockade

4. Interventions
   a. Perform baseline audiometric testing.
   b. Assess renal, hepatic, and electrolyte levels before administration.
   c. Monitor intake and output.
   d. Reconstituted medication may be stored for 48 hours at room temperature.
   e. Administer intramuscularly deep into a large muscle mass.
   f. Rotate injection sites.
   g. Observe injection site for redness, excessive bleeding, and inflammation.

5. Client education
   a. Instruct the client not to perform tasks that require mental alertness.
   b. Instruct the client to report any hearing loss, balance disturbances, respiratory difficulty, weakness, or signs of hypersensitivity reactions.

B. Antibiotics

1. Description
   a. Aminoglycoside antibiotics (kanamycin [Kantrex]; amikacin [Amikin]) or fluoroquinolones (levofloxacin [Levaquin]; moxifloxacin [Avelox]) are given with at least one other antitubercular medication.
   b. These medications are bactericidal because of receptor-binding action interfering with protein synthesis in susceptible microorganisms.
   c. Gastrointestinal disturbances are the most common side effect.
   d. Fluoroquinolones are not recommended for use in children.

2. Contraindications and cautions
   a. Contraindicated in clients with hypersensitivity, neuromuscular disorders, or eighth cranial nerve damage
   b. Used with caution in the older client, in neonates because of renal insufficiency and immaturity, and in young infants because it may cause CNS depression.
   c. The risk of toxicity increases if taken with other aminoglycosides or nephrotoxicity- or ototoxicity-producing medications.

3. Side effects
   a. Hypersensitivity
   b. Pain and irritation at the injection site

c. Nephrotoxicity is indicated by increased blood urea nitrogen and serum creatinine levels.

d. Ototoxicity is indicated by tinnitus, dizziness, ringing or roaring in the ears, and reduced hearing.

e. Neurotoxicity is indicated by headache, dizziness, lethargy, tremors, and visual disturbances.

f. Superinfections

4. Interventions
   a. Assess for hypersensitivity.
   b. Monitor for ototoxic, neurotoxic, and nephrotoxic reactions.
   c. Monitor liver and renal function test results.
   d. Obtain baseline audiometric test and repeat every 1 to 2 months because the medication impairs the eighth cranial nerve.
   e. Assess acuteness of hearing.
   f. Monitor for visual changes.
   g. Assess hydration status and maintain adequate hydration during therapy.
   h. Monitor intake and output.
   i. Assess urinalysis.
   j. Monitor for superinfection.

5. Client education
   a. Instruct the client not to skip doses and to take the medication for the full length of the prescribed therapy.
   b. Instruct the client not to take any other medication without consulting the physician.
   c. Advise the client of the importance of follow-up physician visits and laboratory tests.
   d. Instruct the client to notify the physician if hearing loss, changes in vision, or urinary problems occur.

C. Ethionamide (Trecator)
1. Description
   a. Mechanism of action of ethionamide is unknown.
   b. Ethionamide is used to treat MDR-TB when significant resistance to other medications is expected.

2. Contraindications and cautions
   a. Ethionamide is contraindicated in clients with hypersensitivity.
   b. Use ethionamide with caution in clients with diabetes mellitus or renal dysfunction.

3. Side effects
   a. Anorexia, nausea, vomiting
   b. Metallic taste in the mouth
   c. Orthostatic hypotension
   d. Jaundice
   e. Mental changes
   f. Peripheral neuritis
   g. Rash

4. Interventions
   a. Assess liver and renal function test results.

b. Monitor glucose levels in the client with diabetes mellitus.
c. Administer pyridoxine as prescribed to reduce the risk of neurotoxicity.

5. Client education
   a. Instruct the client to take medication with food or meals to minimize gastrointestinal irritation.
   b. Instruct the client to change positions slowly.
   c. Instruct the client to report signs of a rash, which can progress to exfoliative dermatitis if the medication is not discontinued.
   d. Instruct the client to avoid alcohol.
   e. Instruct the client to report signs of jaundice and other side effects of the medication if they occur.

D. Aminosalicylic acid (Paser)
1. Description
   a. Aminosalicylic acid inhibits folic acid metabolism in mycobacteria.
   b. It is used to treat MDR-TB when significant resistance to other medications is expected.

2. Contraindications and cautions
   a. Contraindicated with hypersensitivity to aminosalicylates, salicylates, or compounds containing the para-aminophenol group.
   b. Aminobenzoates block the absorption of aminosalicylate sodium.

3. Side effects
   a. Hypersensitivity
   b. Bitter taste in the mouth
   c. Gastrointestinal tract irritation
   d. Exfoliative dermatitis
   e. Blood dyscrasias
   f. Crystalluria
   g. Changes in thyroid function

4. Interventions
   a. Assess for hypersensitivity.
   b. Offer clear water to rinse the mouth and chewing gum or hard candy to alleviate the bitter taste.
   c. Encourage fluid intake to prevent crystalluria.
   d. Monitor intake and output.

5. Client education
   a. Instruct the client to discard the medication and obtain a new supply if a purplish-brown discoloration occurs.
   b. Instruct the client to take the medication with food.
   c. Inform the client that urine may turn red on contact with hypochlorite bleach if bleach was used to clean a toilet.
   d. Instruct the client not to take aspirin or over-the-counter medications without the physician's approval.
   e. Instruct the client to report signs of a blood dyscrasia, such as sore throat or mouth, malaise, fatigue, bruising, or bleeding.

E. Cycloserine (Seromycin)
1. Description
   a. Cycloserine interferes with cell wall biosynthesis.
   b. It is used to treat MDR-TB when significant resistance to other medications is expected.
2. Contraindications and cautions
   a. Use of alcohol or ethionamide increases the risk of seizures.
   b. Use cycloserine with caution in clients with epilepsy, depression, severe anxiety, psychosis, or renal insufficiency, or the client who uses alcohol.
3. Side effects
   a. Hypersensitivity
   b. CNS reactions
   c. Neurotoxicity
   d. Seizures
   e. Congestive heart failure
   f. Headache
   g. Vertigo
   h. Altered level of consciousness
   i. Irritability, nervousness, anxiety
   j. Confusion
   k. Mood changes, depression, thoughts of suicide
4. Interventions
   a. Monitor level of consciousness.
   b. Monitor for changes in mental status and thought processes.
   c. Monitor renal and hepatic function tests.
   d. Monitor serum drug level to avoid the risk of neurotoxicity; the peak concentration, measured 2 hours after dosing, should be 25 to 35 mcg/mL.
5. Client education
   a. Instruct the client to take the medication after meals to prevent gastrointestinal upset.
   b. Instruct the client to avoid alcohol.
   c. Instruct the client to report signs of a rash or signs of CNS toxicity.
   d. Instruct the client to avoid driving or performing tasks that require alertness until the reaction to the medication has been determined.
   e. Advise the client of the need for monitoring serum drug levels weekly, as prescribed.
F. Streptomycin
1. Description
   a. Streptomycin is an aminoglycoside antibiotic used with at least one other antitubercular medication.
   b. It is bactericidal because of receptor-binding action that interferes with protein synthesis in susceptible organisms.
2. Contraindications and cautions
   a. Streptomycin is contraindicated in clients with hypersensitivity, myasthenia gravis, parkinsonism, or eighth cranial nerve damage.

Box 59-8 Side Effects of Streptomycin

Nephrotoxicity
Changes in urine output
Decreased appetite
Increased thirst
Nausea, vomiting

Neurotoxicity
Muscle numbness
Seizures
Tingling
Twitching

Vestibular Ototoxicity
Clumsiness
Dizziness
Unsteadiness

Auditory Ototoxicity
A full feeling in the ears
Ringing in the ears
Loss of hearing

   b. Use streptomycin with caution in the older client, in neonates because of renal insufficiency and immaturity, and in young infants because the medication may cause CNS depression.
   c. The risk of toxicity increases when streptomycin is taken with other aminoglycosides or nephrotoxicity- or ototoxicity-producing medications.
3. Side effects (Box 59-8)
   a. Hypersensitivity
   b. Visual changes
   c. Increased liver and renal function studies
   d. Peripheral neuritis, such as burning of the face or mouth
4. Interventions
   a. Assess for hypersensitivity.
   b. Monitor liver and renal function test results.
   c. Monitor for ototoxic, neurotoxic, and nephrotoxic reactions.
   d. Perform baseline audiometric testing and repeat every 1 to 2 months because the medication impairs the eighth cranial nerve.
   e. Assess hearing acuity.
   f. Monitor for visual changes.
   g. Assess hydration status and maintain adequate hydration during therapy.
   h. Monitor intake and output.
   i. Assess urinalysis results.
   j. Monitor for signs of peripheral neuritis.
5. Client education
   a. Instruct the client not to skip doses and to take medication for the full length of the prescribed therapy.
   b. Instruct the client not to take any other medication without consulting the physician.
   c. Advise the client of the importance of follow-up physician visits and laboratory tests.
   d. Instruct the client to notify the physician if hearing loss, changes in vision, or urinary problems occur.

XVI. INFLUENZA MEDICATIONS

A. Vaccines (Box 59-9)

1. Description
   a. Because the strain of influenza virus is different every year, annual vaccination is recommended (usually in October or November).
   b. Vaccine is available as inactivated influenza vaccine administered intramuscularly or as a live attenuated influenza vaccine, which is administered nasally.
   c. Future influenza vaccines will contain both seasonal and H1N1 vaccines in the same preparation.

⚠ Seasonal flu and the H1N1 (swine) flu vaccines are recommended for all individuals unless a contraindication to receiving them exists.

2. Swine flu and the H1N1 vaccine
   a. Refer to Chapter 48 for additional information on the swine flu and its vaccine.
   b. The nasal spray (live) vaccine is approved only for healthy people ages 2 through 49.
   c. The nasal spray vaccine is not approved for pregnant women.
   d. The flu shots (inactivated vaccine) depending on the manufacturer, are approved for children as young as 6 months of age and are safe for pregnant women.
   e. The nasal spray contains a live flu virus that has been weakened to the point that it can't cause the flu; its advantage is that it may elicit a stronger immune response than the shot in children who have never had the flu or a flu vaccine before.
   f. The disadvantage of the nasal spray is that it may not be quite as protective as the flu shot for older people who have had the flu or flu vaccines before.
   g. All individuals should receive a H1N1 vaccine; high priority individuals include: pregnant woman, household contacts and caregivers of children younger than 6 months of age; people ages 6 months to 24 years; health care workers and emergency medical personnel; and adults aged 25 through 64 with a chronic medical condition, such as **asthma**, or a weakened immune system, which increases risk of flu complications.

3. Contraindications and cautions
   a. Contraindications of the inactivated vaccine include hypersensitivity, chicken egg allergy, active infection, Guillain-Barré syndrome, active febrile illness, and children younger than 6 months.
   b. Contraindications of the live attenuated vaccine include age younger than 2 years or adults 50 years or older, pregnant women, children or adolescents on long-term aspirin therapy, and those with severe nasal congestion or long-term conditions such as **asthma**, diabetes mellitus, anemia or blood disorders, or heart, kidney, or lung disease.
4. Side effects
   a. Side effects of the inactivated vaccine include localized pain and swelling at the injection site, general body aches and pains, malaise, fever.
   b. Side effects of the attenuated vaccine include runny nose or nasal congestion, cough, headache, and sore throat.
5. Interventions
   a. The intramuscular route is recommended for the inactivated vaccine; adults and older children should be vaccinated in the deltoid muscle.
   b. Monitor for side effects of the vaccine.
   c. Monitor for hypersensitivity reactions in clients receiving vaccination for the first time.
6. Client education
   a. Instruct the client about the importance of an annual vaccination.
   b. Instruct the client that the inactivated vaccine contains noninfectious killed viruses and cannot cause influenza.
   c. Instruct the client that any respiratory disease unrelated to influenza can occur after the vaccination.
   d. Instruct the client who has received the attenuated vaccine that the virus may be shed in secretion up to 2 days after vaccination.
   e. Instruct the client that development of antibodies in adults takes approximately 2 weeks.
7. Visit the Centers for Disease Control and Prevention for updates at www.cdc.gov/flu.
B. Antiviral medications (Box 59-10)
   1. Description
      a. Antiviral medication use during outbreaks of influenza depends on the current strain of influenza.
      b. Diagnosis of influenza should include rapid diagnostic tests because symptoms of infection from other pathogens may cause symptoms similar to those of influenza infection.
      c. Influenza antivirals may also be administered as prophylaxis against infection but should not replace vaccination.

Box 59-10 Antiviral Influenza Medications

Amantadine (Symmetrel)
Oseltamivir (Tamiflu)
Rimantadine (Flumadine)
Zanamivir (Relenza)

TABLE 59-1 Side Effects of Antiviral Influenza Medications

Antiviral Medication	Side Effects
Amantadine (Symmetrel)	Drowsiness, anxiety, psychosis, depression, hallucinations, tremors, confusion, insomnia, orthostatic hypotension, heart failure, blurred vision, constipation, dry mouth, urinary frequency and retention, leukopenia, photosensitivity, dermatitis
Oseltamivir (Tamiflu)	Insomnia, diarrhea, abdominal pain, cough
Rimantadine (Flumadine)	Depression, hallucinations, tremors, seizures, insomnia, poor concentration, asthenia, gait abnormalities, anxiety, confusion, pallor, palpitations, hypotension, edema, tinnitus, eye pain, constipation, dry mouth, anorexia, abdominal pain, diarrhea, dyspepsia, rash
Zanamivir (Relenza)	Ear, nose, throat infections, diarrhea, nasal symptoms, cough, sinusitis, bronchitis

2. Contraindication and cautions: Antiviral medications are contraindicated in hypersensitive clients.
3. Side effects
   a. Common side effects include headache, dizziness, fatigue, nausea and vomiting.
   b. Some side effects depend on the medication (Table 59-1)
4. Interventions
   a. Administer within 2 days of onset of symptoms and continue for the entire prescription.
   b. Monitor for side effects of specific medications.
5. Client education
   a. Teach the client that the medication may not prevent the transmission of influenza to others.
   b. Adjust activities if dizziness or fatigue occur.
   c. Instruct the client about management of side effects of various medications.
   d. Instruct the client to take medication exactly as prescribed and for the duration of prescription.

XVII. PNEUMOCOCCAL CONJUGATE VACCINE

A. Pneumococcal conjugate vaccine (PCV, Prevnar) is used for the prevention of invasive pneumococcal disease in infants and children

B. Pneumococcal polysaccharide vaccine (Pneumovax 23) is used for adults and high-risk children older than 2 years.
C. Side effects may include erythema, swelling, pain, and tenderness at the injection site, fever, irritability, drowsiness, and reduced appetite.
D. See Chapter 48 for additional information about vaccines for pneumonia.

 MORE QUESTIONS ON THE CD!

Practice Questions

676. A client has a prescription to take guaifenesin (Mucinex). The nurse determines that the client understands the proper administration of this medication if the client states that he or she will:
1. Take an extra dose if fever develops.
2. Take the medication with meals only.
3. Take the tablet with a full glass of water.
4. Decrease the amount of daily fluid intake.

677. A nurse is preparing to administer a dose of naloxone hydrochloride (Narcan) intravenously to a client with an intravenous opioid overdose. Which supportive medical equipment would the nurse plan to have at the client's bedside if needed?
1. Nasogastric tube
2. Paracentesis tray
3. Resuscitation equipment
4. Central line insertion tray

678. A nurse teaches a client about the effects of diphenhydramine (Benadryl), which has been prescribed as a cough suppressant. The nurse determines that the client needs further instructions if the client states that he or she will:
1. Take the medication on an empty stomach.
2. Avoid using alcohol while taking this medication.
3. Use sugarless gum, candy, or oral rinses to decrease dry mouth.
4. Avoid activities requiring mental alertness while taking this medication.

679. A cromolyn sodium (Intal) inhaler is prescribed for a client with allergic asthma. A nurse provides instructions regarding the side effects of this medication. The nurse tells that client that which undesirable effect is associated with this medication?
1. Insomnia
2. Constipation
3. Hypotension
4. Bronchospasm

680. Terbutaline (Brethine) is prescribed for a client with bronchitis. A nurse understands that this

medication should be used with caution if which of the following medical conditions is present in the client?
1. Osteoarthritis
2. Hypothyroidism
3. Diabetes mellitus
4. Polycystic disease

681. Zafirlukast (Accolate) is prescribed for a client with bronchial asthma. Which laboratory test does the nurse expect to be prescribed before the administration of this medication?
1. Platelet count
2. Neutrophil count
3. Liver function tests
4. Complete blood count

682. A client has been taking isoniazid (INH) for 1½ months. The client complains to a nurse about numbness, paresthesias, and tingling in the extremities. The nurse interprets that the client is experiencing:
1. Hypercalcemia
2. Peripheral neuritis
3. Small blood vessel spasm
4. Impaired peripheral circulation

683. A client is to begin a 6-month course of therapy with isoniazid (INH). A nurse plans to teach the client to:
1. Use alcohol in small amounts only.
2. Report yellow eyes or skin immediately.
3. Increase intake of Swiss or aged cheeses.
4. Avoid vitamin supplements during therapy.

684. A client has been started on long-term therapy with rifampin (Rifadin). A nurse teaches the client that the medication:
1. Should always be taken with food or antacids
2. Should be double-dosed if one dose is forgotten
3. Causes orange discoloration of sweat, tears, urine, and feces
4. May be discontinued independently if symptoms are gone in 3 months

685. A nurse has given a client taking ethambutol (Myambutol) information about the medication. The nurse determines that the client understands the instructions if the client states to report immediately:
1. Impaired sense of hearing
2. Gastrointestinal side effects
3. Orange-red discoloration of body secretions
4. Difficulty in discriminating the color red from green

686. A client with tuberculosis is being started on anti-tuberculosis therapy with isoniazid (INH). Before giving the client the first dose, a nurse ensures that which of the following baseline studies has been completed?
1. Electrolyte levels
2. Liver enzyme levels
3. Serum creatinine level
4. Coagulation times

687. A nurse has an order to give a client salmeterol (Serevent Diskus), two puffs, and beclomethasone dipropionate (Qvar), two puffs, by metered-dose inhaler. The nurse administers the medication by giving the:
1. Beclomethasone first and then the salmeterol
2. Salmeterol first and then the beclomethasone
3. Alternating a single puff of each, beginning with the salmeterol
4. Alternating a single puff of each, beginning with the beclomethasone

688. The nurse is caring for a client with a diagnosis of influenza who first began to experience symptoms yesterday. Antiviral therapy is prescribed and the nurse provides instructions to the client about the therapy. Which statement by the client indicates an understanding of the instructions?
1. "I must take the medication exactly as prescribed."
2. "Once I start the medication, I will no longer be contagious."
3. "I will not get any colds or infections while taking this medication."
4. "This medication has minimal side effects and I can return to normal activities."

689. A client has begun therapy with theophylline (Theo-24). A nurse plans to teach the client to limit the intake of which of the following while taking this medication?
1. Coffee, cola, and chocolate
2. Oysters, lobster, and shrimp
3. Melons, oranges, and pineapple
4. Cottage cheese, cream cheese, and dairy creamers

690. The nurse has just administered the first dose of omalizumab (Xolair) to a client. Which statement by the client would alert the nurse that the client may be experiencing a life threatening adverse reaction?
1. "I have a severe headache."
2. "My feet are quite swollen."
3. "I am nauseated and may vomit."
4. "My lips and tongue are swollen."

Alternate Item Format: Multiple Response

691. Rifabutin (Mycobutin) is prescribed for a client with active *Mycobacterium avium* complex (MAC) disease and tuberculosis. For which of the following side effects of the medication should the nurse monitor? **Select all that apply.**

❑ 1. Signs of hepatitis
❑ 2. Flu-like syndrome
❑ 3. Low neutrophil count
❑ 4. Vitamin B$_6$ deficiency
❑ 5. Ocular pain or blurred vision
❑ 6. Tingling and numbness of the fingers

ANSWERS

676. 3

Rationale: Guaifenesin (Mucinex) is an expectorant and should be taken with a full glass of water to decrease the viscosity of secretions. Extra doses should not be taken. The client should contact the physician if the cough lasts longer than 1 week or is accompanied by fever, rash, sore throat, or persistent headache. Fluids are needed to decrease the viscosity of secretions. The medication does not have to be taken with meals.

Test-Taking Strategy: Use the process of elimination. Begin to answer this question by eliminating option 1 first recalling that *extra doses* of medication should not be taken. Next eliminate option 2 because of the close-ended word *only*. From the remaining options, knowing that increased fluids helps liquefy secretions for more effective coughing directs you to option 3 as correct. If you had difficulty with this question, review this medication.

Level of Cognitive Ability: Evaluating
Client Needs: Physiological Integrity
Integrated Process: Nursing Process—Evaluation
Content Area: Pharmacology
References: Edmunds, M. (2010). *Introduction to clinical pharmacology* (6th ed., p. 154). St. Louis: Mosby.

Kee, J., Hayes, E., & McCuistion, L. (2009). *Pharmacology: A nursing process approach* (6th ed., p. 599). St. Louis: Saunders.

677. 3

Rationale: The nurse administering naloxone for suspected opioid overdose should have resuscitation equipment readily available to support naloxone therapy if it is needed. Other adjuncts that may be needed include oxygen, mechanical ventilator, and vasopressors.

Test-Taking Strategy: Use the process of elimination. Note the strategic words *intravenous opioid overdose*. Recalling the effects of these medications will direct you to option 3. Option 3 is also the umbrella response. Review this medication if you had difficulty with this question.

Level of Cognitive Ability: Applying
Client Needs: Physiological Integrity
Integrated Process: Nursing Process—Planning
Content Area: Critical Care
References: Gahart, B., & Nazareno, A. (2010). *Intravenous medications* (26th ed., p. 956). St. Louis: Mosby.

Skidmore-Roth, L. (2010). *Mosby's nursing drug reference* (23rd ed., p. 759). St. Louis: Mosby.

678. 1

Rationale: Diphenhydramine (Benadryl) has several uses, including antihistamine, antitussive, antidyskinetic, and sedative-hypnotic. Instructions for use include taking with food or milk to decrease gastrointestinal upset and using oral rinses or sugarless gum or hard candy to minimize dry mouth. Because the medication causes drowsiness, the client should avoid use of alcohol or central nervous system depressants, operating a car, or engaging in other activities requiring mental awareness during use.

Test-Taking Strategy: Use the process of elimination, noting the strategic words *needs further instructions*. These words indicate a negative event query and ask you to select an option that is incorrect. Knowing that the medication has a sedative effect helps you eliminate options 2 and 4 first. Recalling that the medication causes a dry mouth helps you choose option 1 as the answer to the question, according to the way the question is stated. If you had difficulty with this question, review client education related to this medication.

Level of Cognitive Ability: Evaluating
Client Needs: Physiological Integrity
Integrated Process: Teaching and Learning
Content Area: Pharmacology
References: Hodgson, B., & Kizior, R. (2010). *Saunders nursing drug handbook 2010* (p. 356). St. Louis: Saunders.

Lehne, R. (2010). *Pharmacology for nursing care* (7th ed., p. 827). St. Louis: Saunders.

679. 4

Rationale: Cromolyn sodium (Intal) is an inhaled nonsteroidal antiallergy agent and a mast cell stabilizer. Undesirable side effects associated with inhalation therapy of cromolyn sodium are bronchospasm, cough, nasal congestion, throat irritation, and wheezing. Clients receiving this medication orally may experience pruritus, nausea, diarrhea, and myalgia.

Test-Taking Strategy: Use the process of elimination and note the strategic words *undesirable effect*. This should assist in directing you to option 4. In addition, use the ABCs—airway, breathing, and circulation—to select the correct option. Option 4 addresses the airway. Review the undesirable effects of this medication if you had difficulty with this question.

Level of Cognitive Ability: Applying
Client Needs: Physiological Integrity
Integrated Process: Teaching and Learning
Content Area: Pharmacology
Reference: Hodgson, B., & Kizior, R. (2010). *Saunders nursing drug handbook 2010* (p. 282). St. Louis: Saunders.

680. 3

Rationale: Terbutaline (Brethine) is a bronchodilator and is contraindicated in clients with hypersensitivity to sympathomimetics. It should be used with caution in clients with impaired cardiac function, diabetes mellitus, hypertension, hyperthyroidism, or a history of seizures. The medication may increase blood glucose levels.

Test-Taking Strategy: Knowledge regarding the contraindications and cautions associated with the use of this medication is needed to answer this question. Remember that terbutaline is used with caution in the client with diabetes mellitus. Review the contraindications and cautions associated with this medication if you are unfamiliar with them.

Level of Cognitive Ability: Understanding
Client Needs: Physiological Integrity
Integrated Process: Nursing Process—Planning
Content Area: Pharmacology
Reference: Hodgson, B., & Kizior, R. (2010). *Saunders nursing drug handbook 2010* (p. 1090). St. Louis: Saunders.

681. 3

Rationale: Zafirlukast (Accolate) is a leukotriene receptor antagonist used in the prophylaxis and long-term treatment of bronchial asthma. Zafirlukast is used with caution in clients with impaired hepatic function. Liver function laboratory tests should be performed to obtain a baseline, and the levels should be monitored during administration of the medication.

Test-Taking Strategy: Use the process of elimination, eliminating options 2 and 4 first because a complete blood count would include a neutrophil count. From the remaining options, you would need to know that this medication would affect hepatic function. If you had difficulty with this question, review this medication.

Level of Cognitive Ability: Analyzing
Client Needs: Physiological Integrity
Integrated Process: Nursing Process—Planning
Content Area: Pharmacology
Reference: Hodgson, B., & Kizior, R. (2010). *Saunders nursing drug handbook 2010* (p. 1199). St. Louis: Saunders.

682. 2

Rationale: Isoniazid (INH) is an antitubercular medication. A common side effect of isoniazid is peripheral neuritis, manifested by numbness, tingling, and paresthesias in the extremities. This can be minimized with pyridoxine (vitamin B_6) intake. Options 1, 3, and 4 are incorrect.

Test-Taking Strategy: Use the process of elimination. Options 3 and 4 would not cause the symptoms presented in the question but instead would cause pallor and coolness. From the remaining options, you should know that peripheral neuritis is a side effect of the medication or that these signs and symptoms do not correlate with hypercalcemia. Review the side effects associated with isoniazid if you had difficulty with this question.

Level of Cognitive Ability: Analyzing
Client Needs: Physiological Integrity
Integrated Process: Nursing Process—Analysis
Content Area: Pharmacology
References: Hodgson, B., & Kizior, R. (2010). *Saunders nursing drug handbook 2010* (p. 620). St. Louis: Saunders.

Lehne, R. (2010). *Pharmacology for nursing care* (7th ed., pp. 1049–1050). St. Louis: Saunders.

683. 2

Rationale: Isoniazid (INH) is hepatotoxic, and therefore the client is taught to report signs and symptoms of hepatitis immediately, which include yellow skin and sclera. For the same reason, alcohol should be avoided during therapy. The client should avoid intake of Swiss cheese, fish such as tuna, and foods containing tyramine because they may cause a reaction characterized by redness and itching of the skin, flushing, sweating, tachycardia, headache, or lightheadedness. The client can avoid developing peripheral neuritis by increasing the intake of pyridoxine (vitamin B_6) during the course of isoniazid therapy.

Test-Taking Strategy: Use the process of elimination. Because alcohol intake is prohibited with the use of many medications, eliminate option 1 first. Because the client receiving this medication typically is given supplements of vitamin B_6, option 4 is incorrect and is eliminated next. Recalling that the medication is hepatotoxic will direct you to option 2. If you had difficulty with this question, review this medication.

Level of Cognitive Ability: Applying
Client Needs: Physiological Integrity
Integrated Process: Teaching and Learning
Content Area: Pharmacology
Reference: Lehne, R. (2010). *Pharmacology for nursing care* (7th ed., p. 1050). St. Louis: Saunders.

684. 3

Rationale: Rifampin should be taken exactly as directed. Doses should not be doubled or skipped. The client should not stop therapy until directed to do so by a physician. The medication should be administered on an empty stomach unless it causes gastrointestinal upset, and then it may be taken with food. Antacids, if prescribed, should be taken at least 1 hour before the medication. Rifampin causes orange-red discoloration of body secretions and will stain soft contact lenses permanently.

Test-Taking Strategy: Use the process of elimination. Options 2 and 4 are inaccurate in general and are eliminated first. Eliminate option 1 next because of the close-ended word *always*. If you had difficulty with this question, review the side effects associated with this medication.

Level of Cognitive Ability: Applying
Client Needs: Physiological Integrity
Integrated Process: Teaching and Learning
Content Area: Pharmacology
Reference: Hodgson, B., & Kizior, R. (2010). *Saunders nursing drug handbook 2010* (p. 997). St. Louis: Saunders.

685. 4

Rationale: Ethambutol causes optic neuritis, which decreases visual acuity and the ability to discriminate between the colors red and green. This poses a potential safety hazard when a client is driving a motor vehicle. The client is taught to report this symptom immediately. The client also is taught to take the medication with food if gastrointestinal upset occurs. Impaired hearing results from antitubercular therapy with streptomycin. Orange-red discoloration of secretions occurs with rifampin (Rifadin).

Test-Taking Strategy: Use the process of elimination. Option 2 is the least likely symptom to report; instead, it should be managed by taking the medication with food. To select among the other options, you must know that this medication causes optic neuritis, resulting in difficulty with red-green discrimination. If this question was difficult, review antitubercular medications because the incorrect options for this question are typical side effects of other antitubercular medications.
Level of Cognitive Ability: Evaluating
Client Needs: Physiological Integrity
Integrated Process: Nursing Process—Evaluation
Content Area: Pharmacology
References: Hodgson, B., & Kizior, R. (2010). *Saunders nursing drug handbook 2010* (p. 441). St. Louis: Saunders.
   Lehne, R. (2010). *Pharmacology for nursing care* (7th ed., p. 1051). St. Louis: Saunders.

686. 2
Rationale: Isoniazid (INH) therapy can cause an elevation of hepatic enzyme levels and hepatitis. Therefore, liver enzyme levels are monitored when therapy is initiated and during the first 3 months of therapy. They may be monitored longer in the client who is older than 50 or abuses alcohol. The laboratory tests in options 1, 3, and 4 are not necessary.
Test-Taking Strategy: Use the process of elimination. Recalling that this medication can be toxic to the liver will direct you to the correct option. Review the adverse effects of the various antituberculosis medications if this is an area that is unfamiliar to you.
Level of Cognitive Ability: Applying
Client Needs: Physiological Integrity
Integrated Process: Nursing Process—Implementation
Content Area: Pharmacology
References: Edmunds, M. (2010). *Introduction to clinical pharmacology* (6th ed., p. 174). St. Louis: Mosby.
   Lehne, R. (2010). *Pharmacology for nursing care* (7th ed., p. 1050). St. Louis: Saunders.

687. 2
Rationale: Salmeterol (Serevent Diskus) is an adrenergic type of bronchodilator and beclomethasone dipropionate is a glucocorticoid. Bronchodilators are always administered before glucocorticoids when both are to be given on the same time schedule. This allows for widening of the air passages by the bronchodilator, which then makes the glucocorticoid more effective.
Test-Taking Strategy: To answer this question correctly, you must know two different things. First, you must know that a bronchodilator is always given before a glucocorticoid. This would allow you to eliminate options 3 and 4 because you would not alternate the medications. To select between options 1 and 2, you must know that salmeterol is a bronchodilator, whereas beclomethasone is a glucocorticoid. Review these medications if you had difficulty with this question.
Level of Cognitive Ability: Applying
Client Needs: Physiological Integrity
Integrated Process: Nursing Process—Implementation
Content Area: Pharmacology
References: Kee, J., Hayes, E., & McCuistion, L. (2009). *Pharmacology: A nursing process approach* (6th ed., p. 607). St. Louis: Saunders.

   Lehne, R. (2010). *Pharmacology for nursing care* (7th ed., p. 895). St. Louis: Saunders.

688. 1
Rationale: Antiviral medications for influenza must be taken exactly as prescribed. These medications do not prevent the spread of influenza and clients are usually contagious for up to 2 days after the initiation of antiviral medications. Secondary bacterial infections may occur despite antiviral treatment. Side effects occur with these medications and may necessitate change in activities, especially when driving or operating machinery if dizziness occurs.
Test-Taking Strategy: Use process of elimination and note the strategic words *indicates an understanding*. Using general medication guidelines will direct you to option 1. Review these medications if you had difficulty with this question.
Level of Cognitive Ability: Evaluating
Client Needs: Physiological Integrity
Integrated Process: Nursing Process—Evaluation
Content Area: Pharmacology
Reference: Edmunds, M. (2010). *Introduction to clinical pharmacology* (6th ed., pp. 189–190). St. Louis: Mosby.

689. 1
Rationale: Theophylline (Theo-24) is a methylxanthine bronchodilator. The nurse teaches the client to limit the intake of xanthine-containing foods while taking this medication. These foods include coffee, cola, and chocolate.
Test-Taking Strategy: Use the process of elimination. Recall that theophylline is a xanthine bronchodilator and that intake of excessive amounts of foods naturally high in xanthines should be curtailed. Also recalling that these medications cause cardiac and central nervous system stimulation will direct you to option 1. Review the foods naturally high in xanthines if you had difficulty with this question.
Level of Cognitive Ability: Applying
Client Needs: Physiological Integrity
Integrated Process: Teaching and Learning
Content Area: Pharmacology
References: Edmunds, M. (2010). *Introduction to clinical pharmacology* (6th ed., p. 148). St. Louis: Mosby.
   Hodgson, B., & Kizior, R. (2010). *Saunders nursing drug handbook 2010* (p. 1102). St. Louis: Saunders.

690. 4
Rationale: Omalizumab is an anti-inflammatory used for long-term control of asthma. Anaphylactic reactions can occur with the administration of omalizumab. The nurse administering the medication should monitor for adverse reactions of the medication. Swelling of the lips and tongue are an indication of an adverse reaction. The client statements in options 1, 2, and 3 are not indicative of an adverse reaction.
Test-Taking Strategy: Use the process of elimination. Recall that anaphylactic reactions can occur with the administration of omalizumab. Knowing the signs of a reaction will direct you to the correct option. Review this medication if you had difficulty with this question.
Level of Cognitive Ability: Evaluating
Client Needs: Physiological Integrity
Integrated Process: Nursing Process—Evaluation

Content Area: Pharmacology
Reference: Lehne, R. (2010). *Pharmacology for nursing care* (7th ed., p. 895). St. Louis: Saunders.

ALTERNATE ITEM FORMAT: MULTIPLE RESPONSE

691. 1, 2, 3, 5

Rationale: Rifabutin (Mycobutin) may be prescribed for a client with active *Mycobacterium avium* complex (MAC) disease and tuberculosis. It inhibits mycobacterial DNA-dependent RNA polymerase and suppresses protein synthesis. Side effects include rash, gastrointestinal disturbances, neutropenia (low neutrophil count), red-orange–colored body secretions, uveitis (blurred vision and eye pain), myositis, arthralgia, hepatitis, chest pain with dyspnea, and flu-like syndrome. Vitamin B_6 deficiency and numbness and tingling in the extremities is associated with the use of isoniazid (INH). Ethambutol (Myambutol) also causes peripheral neuritis.

Test-Taking Strategy: Focus on the name of the medication to assist in answering the question and use the process of elimination. Recalling that vitamin B_6 deficiency and numbness and tingling in the extremities is associated with the use of isoniazid will assist in answering. Review the side effects associated with rifabutin if you had difficulty with this question.

Level of Cognitive Ability: Analyzing
Client Needs: Physiological Integrity
Integrated Process: Nursing Process—Assessment
Content Area: Pharmacology
Reference: Lehne, R. (2010). *Pharmacology for nursing care* (7th ed., pp. 1045, 1050). St. Louis: Saunders.

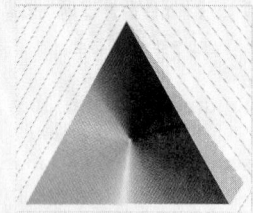

The Adult Client With a Cardiovascular Disorder

PYRAMID TERMS

afterload The force against which the heart has to pump (peripheral resistance) to eject blood from the left ventricle. Factors and conditions that would impede blood flow increase left ventricular afterload.

arterial pressure The pressure of the blood against the arterial walls. Pressure can be measured indirectly by sphygmomanometer or directly by arterial catheter. Readings are expressed as systolic over diastolic. Arterial pressure increases when the cardiac output, peripheral resistance, or blood volume increases.

automaticity The ability of cardiac cells to initiate an impulse spontaneously and repetitively without external neurohormonal control. The pacemaker cells have the highest rate of automaticity of all cardiac cells.

baroreceptors Specialized nerve endings (also called pressoreceptors) located in the walls of the aortic arch and carotid sinuses. They are affected by changes in the arterial blood pressure (BP). Increases in arterial pressure stimulate baroreceptors and the heart rate and arterial pressure decrease. Decreases in arterial pressure lead to a lessened stimulation of the baroreceptors, vasoconstriction occurs, and the heart rate increases.

blood pressure (BP) The force exerted by the blood against the walls of the blood vessels. If the blood pressure falls too low, blood flow to the tissues, heart, brain, and other organs becomes inadequate. If the blood pressure becomes too high, the risk of vessel rupture and damage increases.

capillary pressure or hydrostatic pressure The pressure exerted by the blood against the capillary wall. Normal capillary pressure is 25 to 30 mm Hg at the arterial end of the capillaries, and 10 to 15 mm Hg at the venous end.

cardiac output The total volume of blood pumped through the heart in 1 minute. The normal cardiac output is 4 to 7 L/min. Cardiac output equals stroke volume multiplied by heart rate. Cardiac output can be calculated via the thermodilution method when the client has a pulmonary artery catheter (Swan-Ganz catheter).

chemoreceptors Nerve endings located in the aortic arch and carotid bodies that are stimulated by hypoxemia and that subsequently transmit impulses to the central nervous system.

conductivity The ability of the heart muscle fibers to propagate electrical impulses along and across cell membranes.

contractility The inherent ability of the myocardium to alter contractile force and velocity. Sympathetic stimulation increases myocardial contractility, so stroke volume increases. Conditions that decrease myocardial contractility reduce stroke volume.

diastole The phase of the cardiac cycle in which the heart relaxes between contractions. Diastole represents the period of time when the two ventricles are dilated by the blood flowing into them.

diastolic pressure The force of the blood exerted against the artery walls when the heart relaxes or fills.

excitability The ability of cardiac muscle cells to depolarize in response to a stimulus. Excitability is influenced by hormones, electrolytes, nutrition, oxygen supply, medication, infections, and nerve characteristics.

mean arterial pressure (MAP) An approximation of the average pressure in the systemic circulation throughout the cardiac cycle; used in hemodynamic monitoring. Mean arterial pressure must be at least 60 mm Hg for adequate organ perfusion.

paradoxical blood pressure An exaggerated decrease in systolic pressure by more than 10 mm Hg during the inspiratory phase of the respiratory cycle. Normal value is 3 to 10 mm Hg.

postural (orthostatic) hypotension A blood pressure decrease of more than 10 to 15 mm Hg of the systolic pressure or a decrease of more than 10 mm Hg of the diastolic pressure and a 10% to 20% increase in heart rate. Postural hypotension occurs when the client's blood pressure is not maintained adequately when moving from a lying to a sitting or standing position.

preload The volume of blood stretching the left ventricle at the end of diastole. Preload is determined by the total circulating blood volume and is increased by an increase in venous return to the heart.

pulmonary capillary wedge pressure (PCWP) The measurement obtained during momentary balloon inflation of a pulmonary artery catheter; it is reflective of left ventricular end-diastolic pressure. The PCWP normally ranges between 6 and 12 mm Hg. Decreased PCWP indicates hypovolemia, whereas increased PCWP indicates hypervolemia, left ventricular failure, or mitral regurgitation.

pulse pressure The difference between the systolic and diastolic pressure. Normal pulse pressure is 30 to 40 mm Hg.

refractoriness A property of excitable tissue. Refractoriness prevents uncontrolled rapid cardiac contractions and helps preserve the heart rhythm.

stretch receptors Nerve endings located in the vena cava and the right atrium that respond to pressure changes affecting circulatory blood volume. When the blood pressure decreases because of hypovolemia, a sympathetic response occurs, causing an increased heart rate and blood vessel constriction. When the blood pressure increases because of hypervolemia, an opposite effect occurs.

stroke volume The amount of blood ejected from the left ventricle with each contraction. The normal stroke volume is 70 to 130 mL/heartbeat. The stroke volume can be affected by preload, afterload, contractility, and the Frank-Starling law.

systole The phase of contraction of the heart, especially of the ventricles, during which blood is forced into the aorta and pulmonary artery.

systolic pressure The maximum pressure of blood exerted against the artery walls when the heart contracts.

venous pressure The force exerted by the blood against the vein walls. Normal venous pressures are highest in the extremities (5 to 14 cm H_2O in the arm), and lowest closest to the heart (6 to 8 cm H_2O in the inferior vena cava).

 PYRAMID TO SUCCESS

Pyramid Points focus on assessment data related to cardiovascular risks, health screening and promotion, complications of the various cardiovascular disorders, emergency implementation measures, and client education. Focus on the assessment findings in angina, myocardial infarction, congestive heart failure and pulmonary edema, pericarditis, aneurysms, hypertension, and arterial and venous disorders. You must be able to identify the most common dysrhythmias and determine the appropriate interventions for these dysrhythmias, including the use of a pacemaker. Focus also on the care of the client following diagnostic treatments and surgical procedures. Note appropriate and therapeutic client positions, particularly with arterial and venous disorders of the extremities. Focus on treatments and medications prescribed for the various cardiovascular disorders and client teaching related to prescribed treatment plans. Be familiar with the components related to cardiac rehabilitation.

CLIENT NEEDS

Safe and Effective Care Environment

Consulting with members of the health care team
Establishing priorities
Initiating cardiovascular consultations and referrals
Maintaining asepsis
Maintaining standard and other precautions
Obtaining informed consent related to treatments and procedures
Upholding client rights

Health Promotion and Maintenance

Discussing alterations in lifestyle
Implementing cardiovascular assessment techniques
Mobilizing appropriate community resources
Promoting cardiac rehabilitation
Providing health screening and health promotion programs
Preventing cardiovascular disease
Teaching related to diet therapy, exercise, and medications

Psychosocial Integrity

Assisting the client to accept lifestyle changes
Considering religious, spiritual, and cultural influences on health
Discussing grief and loss and end-of-life issues
Discussing situational role changes
Discussing unexpected body image changes
Identifying coping mechanisms
Identifying fear, anxiety, and denial
Identifying support systems

Physiological Integrity

Administering intravenous medications
Assisting with basic care measures
Discussing activity limitations and promoting rest and sleep

Monitoring hemodynamics

Monitoring for complications related to cardiovascular disorders

Monitoring for therapeutic effects of medications

Monitoring of cardiac enzyme and troponin levels and other laboratory values related to the cardiovascular system

Providing interventions required in emergencies

Providing nonpharmacological and pharmacological comfort interventions

Responding to medical emergencies

Cardiovascular Disorders

I. ANATOMY AND PHYSIOLOGY

A. Heart and heart wall layers
  1. The heart is located in the left side of the mediastinum.
  2. The heart consists of three layers.
     a. The epicardium is the outermost layer of the heart.
     b. The myocardium is the middle layer and is the actual contracting muscle of the heart.
     c. The endocardium is the innermost layer and lines the inner chambers and heart valves.

B. Pericardial sac
  1. Encases and protects the heart from trauma and infection
  2. Has two layers
     a. The parietal pericardium is the tough, fibrous outer membrane that attaches anteriorly to the lower half of the sternum, posteriorly to the thoracic vertebrae, and inferiorly to the diaphragm.
     b. The visceral pericardium is the thin, inner layer that closely adheres to the heart.
  3. The pericardial space is between the parietal and visceral layers; it holds 5 to 20 mL of pericardial fluid, lubricates the pericardial surfaces, and cushions the heart.

C. There are four heart chambers
  1. The right atrium receives deoxygenated blood from the body via the superior and inferior vena cava.
  2. The right ventricle receives blood from the right atrium and pumps it to the lungs via the pulmonary artery.
  3. The left atrium receives oxygenated blood from the lungs via four pulmonary veins.
  4. The left ventricle is the largest and most muscular chamber; it receives oxygenated blood from the lungs via the left atrium and pumps blood into the systemic circulation via the aorta.

D. There are four valves in the heart.
  1. There are two atrioventricular valves, the tricuspid and the mitral, which lie between the atria and ventricles.

  a. The tricuspid valve is located on the right side of the heart.
  b. The bicuspid (mitral) valve is located on the left side of the heart.
  c. The atrioventricular valves close at the beginning of ventricular contraction and prevent blood from flowing back into the atria from the ventricles; these valves open when the ventricle relaxes.
  2. There are two semilunar valves, the pulmonic and the aortic.
     a. The pulmonic semilunar valve lies between the right ventricle and the pulmonary artery.
     b. The aortic semilunar valve lies between the left ventricle and the aorta.
     c. The semilunar valves prevent blood from flowing back into the ventricles during relaxation; they open during ventricular contraction and close when the ventricles begin to relax.

E. Sinoatrial (SA) node
  1. The main pacemaker that initiates each heartbeat
  2. It is located at the junction of the superior vena cava and the right atrium.
  3. The sinoatrial node generates electrical impulses at 60 to 100 times per minute and is controlled by the sympathetic and parasympathetic nervous systems.

F. Atrioventricular (AV) node
  1. Located in the lower aspect of the atrial septum
  2. Receives electrical impulses from the sinoatrial node
  3. If the sinoatrial node fails, the atrioventricular node can initiate and sustain a heart rate of 40 to 60 beats/min.

G. The bundle of His
  1. A continuation of the AV node; located at the interventricular septum
  2. It branches into the right bundle branch, which extends down the right side of the interventricular septum, and the left bundle branch, which extends into the left ventricle.
  3. The right and left bundle branches terminate into Purkinje fibers.

H. Purkinje fibers
1. Purkinje fibers are a diffuse network of conducting strands located beneath the ventricular endocardium.
2. These fibers spread the wave of depolarization through the ventricles.
3. Purkinje fibers can act as the pacemaker with a rate between 20 and 40 beats/min when higher pacemakers (such as the sinoatrial nerve) fail.

I. Coronary arteries (Fig. 60-1)
1. The right coronary artery supplies the right atrium and ventricle, the inferior portion of the left ventricle, the posterior septal wall, and the sinoatrial and atrioventricular nodes.
2. The left main coronary artery consists of two major branches, the left anterior descending and the circumflex arteries.
3. The left anterior descending artery supplies blood to the anterior wall of the left ventricle, the anterior ventricular septum, and the apex of the left ventricle.
4. The circumflex artery supplies blood to the left atrium and the lateral and posterior surfaces of the left ventricle.

⚠ The coronary arteries supply the capillaries of the myocardium with blood. If blockage occurs in these arteries, the client is at risk for myocardial infarction.

J. Heart sounds
1. The first heart sound (S_1) is heard as the atrioventricular valves close and is heard loudest at the apex of the heart.
2. The second heart sound (S_2) is heard when the semilunar valves close and is heard loudest at the base of the heart.

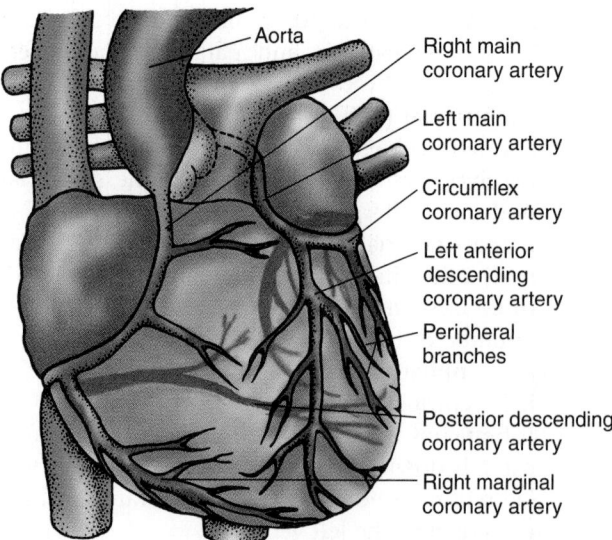

▲ **FIGURE 60-1** Coronary arterial system. (From Ignatavicius, D., & Workman, M. [2010]. *Medical-surgical nursing: Patient-centered collaborative care* [6th ed.]. St. Louis: Saunders.)

3. A third heart sound (S_3) may be heard if ventricular wall compliance is decreased and structures in the ventricular wall vibrate; this can occur in conditions such as congestive heart failure or valvular regurgitation. However, a third heart sound may be normal in individuals younger than 30 years.
4. A fourth heart sound (S_4) may be heard on atrial **systole** if resistance to ventricular filling is present; this is an abnormal finding, and the causes include cardiac hypertrophy, disease, or injury to the ventricular wall.

K. Heart rate
1. The faster the heart rate, the less time the heart has for filling, and the **cardiac output** decreases.
2. An increase in heart rate increases oxygen consumption.
3. The normal sinus heart rate is 60 to 100 beats/min.
4. Sinus tachycardia is a rate more than 100 beats/min.
5. Sinus bradycardia is a rate less than 60 beats/min.

L. Autonomic nervous system
1. Stimulation of sympathetic nerve fibers releases the neurotransmitter norepinephrine, producing an increased heart rate, increased conduction speed through the atrioventricular node, increased atrial and ventricular **contractility**, and peripheral vasoconstriction. Stimulation occurs when a decrease in pressure is detected.
2. Stimulation of the parasympathetic nerve fibers releases the neurotransmitter acetylcholine, which decreases the heart rate and lessens atrial and ventricular **contractility** and **conductivity**. Stimulation occurs when an increase in pressure is detected.

M. Blood pressure (BP) control
1. **Baroreceptors**, also called *pressoreceptors*, are located in the walls of the aortic arch and carotid sinuses.
2. **Baroreceptors** are specialized nerve endings affected by changes in the arterial **BP**.
3. Increases in **arterial pressure** stimulate **baroreceptors**, and the heart rate and **arterial pressure** decrease.
4. Decreases in **arterial pressure** reduce stimulation of the **baroreceptors** and vasoconstriction occurs, as does an increase in heart rate.
5. **Stretch receptors**, located in the vena cava and the right atrium, respond to pressure changes that affect circulatory blood volume.
6. When the **BP** decreases as a result of hypovolemia, a sympathetic response occurs, causing an increased heart rate and blood vessel constriction; when the **BP** increases as a result of hypervolemia, an opposite effect occurs.
7. Antidiuretic hormone (vasopressin) influences **BP** indirectly by regulating vascular volume.
8. Increases in blood volume result in decreased antidiuretic hormone release, increasing

diuresis, decreasing blood volume, and thus decreasing **BP**.
9. Decreases in blood volume result in increased antidiuretic hormone release; this promotes an increase in blood volume and therefore **BP**.
10. Renin, a potent vasoconstrictor, causes the **BP** to increase.
11. Renin converts angiotensinogen to angiotensin I; angiotensin I is then converted to angiotensin II in the lungs.
12. Angiotensin II stimulates the release of aldosterone, which promotes water and sodium retention by the kidneys; this action increases blood volume and **BP**.

N. The vascular system
1. Arteries are vessels through which the blood passes away from the heart to various parts of the body; they convey highly oxygenated blood from the left side of heart to the tissues.
2. Arterioles control the blood flow into the capillaries.
3. Capillaries allow the exchange of fluid and nutrients between the blood and the interstitial spaces.
4. Venules receive blood from the capillary bed and move blood into the veins.
5. Veins transport deoxygenated blood from the tissues back to the right heart and then to the lungs for oxygenation.
6. Valves help return blood to the heart against the force of gravity.
7. The lymphatics drain the tissues and return the tissue fluid to the blood.

II. DIAGNOSTIC TESTS AND PROCEDURES

A. Cardiac enzymes
1. CK-MB (creatine kinase, myocardial muscle)
   a. An elevation in value indicates myocardial damage.
   b. An elevation occurs within hours and peaks at 18 hours following an acute ischemic attack.
   c. Normal value is 0% to 5% of total; total CK is 26 to 174 units/L.
2. Lactate dehydrogenase (LDH)
   a. Elevations in LDH levels occur 24 hours following myocardial infarction and peak in 48 to 72 hours.
   b. Normally, LDH1 is lower than LDH2; when the serum concentration of LDH1 is higher than LDH2, the pattern is indicated as "flipped," signifying myocardial necrosis.
   c. The normal value of LDH in conventional units is 140 to 280 international units/L.
3. Troponin
   a. Troponin is composed of three proteins—troponin C, cardiac troponin I, and cardiac troponin T.

   b. Troponin I especially has a high affinity for myocardial injury; it rises within 3 hours and persists for up to 7 to 10 days.
   c. Normal values are low, with troponin I being lower than 0.6 ng/mL and troponin T normally ranging from 0 to 0.2 ng/mL; thus, any rise can indicate myocardial cell damage.
4. Myoglobin
   a. Myoglobin is an oxygen-binding protein found in cardiac and skeletal muscle.
   b. The level rises within 2 hours after cell death, with a rapid decline in the level after 7 hours.

B. Complete blood count
1. The red blood cell count decreases in rheumatic heart disease and infective endocarditis and increases in conditions characterized by inadequate tissue oxygenation.
2. The white blood cell count increases in infectious and inflammatory diseases of the heart and after myocardial infarction (MI) because large numbers of white blood cells are needed to dispose of the necrotic tissue resulting from the infarction.
3. An elevated hematocrit level can result from vascular volume depletion.
4. Decreases in hemoglobin and hematocrit levels can indicate anemia.

C. Blood coagulation factors: An increase in coagulation factors can occur during and after MI, which places the client at greater risk for thrombophlebitis and extension of clots in the coronary arteries.

D. Serum lipids
1. The lipid profile measures serum cholesterol, triglyceride, and lipoprotein levels.
2. The lipid profile is used to assess the risk of developing coronary artery disease.
3. The desirable range for serum cholesterol is lower than 200 mg/dL, with low-density lipoprotein cholesterol lower than 130 mg/dL and high-density lipoprotein cholesterol at 30 to 70 mg/dL.
4. Lipoprotein-*a* or *Lp(a)*, a modified form of LDL, increases atherosclerotic plaques and increases clots; value should be less than 30 mg/dL.

E. Homocysteine: elevated levels may increase the risk of cardiovascular disease; level should be less than 14 mmol/dL.

F. Highly sensitive C-reactive protein (hsCRP): Detects an inflammatory process such as that associated with the development of atherothrombosis; a level less than 1 mg/dL is considered low risk and a level over 3 mg/dL places the client at high risk for heart disease.

G. Microalbuminuria: A small amount of protein in the urine has been a marker for endothelial dysfunction in cardiovascular disease.

H. Electrolytes

▲

1. Potassium

a. Hypokalemia causes increased cardiac electrical instability, ventricular dysrhythmias, and increased risk of digoxin toxicity.

b. In hypokalemia, the electrocardiogram shows flattening and inversion of the T wave, the appearance of a U wave, and ST depression.

c. Hyperkalemia causes asystole and ventricular dysrhythmias.

d. In hyperkalemia, the electrocardiogram may show tall peaked T waves, widened QRS complexes, prolonged PR intervals, or flat P waves.

2. Sodium

a. The serum sodium level decreases with the use of diuretics.

b. The serum sodium level decreases in heart failure, indicating water excess.

I. Calcium

1. Hypocalcemia can cause ventricular dysrhythmias, prolonged ST and QT intervals, and cardiac arrest.

2. Hypercalcemia can cause a shortened ST segment and widened T wave, atrioventricular block, tachycardia or bradycardia, digitalis hypersensitivity, and cardiac arrest.

J. Phosphorus level: Phosphorus levels should be interpreted with calcium levels because the kidneys retain or excrete one electrolyte in an inverse relationship to the other.

K. Magnesium

1. A low magnesium level can cause ventricular tachycardia and fibrillation.

2. Electrocardiographic changes that may be observed with hypomagnesemia include tall T waves and depressed ST segments.

3. A high magnesium level can cause muscle weakness, hypotension, and bradycardia.

4. Electrocardiographic changes that may be observed with hypermagnesemia include a prolonged PR interval and widened QRS complex.

▲ Electrolyte and mineral imbalances can cause cardiac electrical instability that can result in life-threatening dysrhythmias.

L. Blood urea nitrogen: The blood urea nitrogen level is elevated in heart disorders that adversely affect renal circulation, such as heart failure and cardiogenic shock.

M. Blood glucose: An acute cardiac episode can elevate the blood glucose level.

N. B-type natriuretic peptide (BNP)

▲

1. BNP is released in response to atrial and ventricular stretch; it serves as a marker for congestive heart failure (CHF).

2. BNP levels should be lower than 100 pg/mL; the higher the level, the more severe the CHF.

O. Chest x-ray

1. Description

a. Radiography of the chest is done to determine the size, silhouette, and position of the heart.

b. Specific pathological changes are difficult to determine on x-rays, but anatomical changes can be seen.

2. Interventions

a. Prepare the client for radiography, explaining the purpose and procedure.

b. Remove jewelry.

c. Ensure that the client is not pregnant.

P. Electrocardiography (Box 60-1)

1. Description: This common noninvasive diagnostic test records the electrical activity of the heart and is useful for detecting cardiac dysrhythmias, location and extent of MI, and cardiac hypertrophy and for evaluation of the effectiveness of cardiac medications.

2. Interventions

a. Determine the client's ability to lie still; advise the client to lie still, breathe normally, and refrain from talking during the test.

b. Reassure the client that an electrical shock will not occur.

c. Document any cardiac medications the client is taking.

Q. Holter monitoring

1. Description

a. In this noninvasive test, the client wears a Holter monitor and an electrocardiographic tracing is recorded continuously over a period of 24 hours or more while the client performs his or her activities of daily living.

b. The Holter monitor identifies dysrhythmias if they occur and evaluates the effectiveness of antidysrhythmics or pacemaker therapy.

2. Interventions

a. Instruct the client to resume normal daily activities and to maintain a diary documenting activities and any symptoms that may develop for correlation with the electrocardiographic tracing.

b. Instruct the client to avoid tub baths or showers because they will interfere with the electrocardiographic recorder device.

R. Echocardiography

1. Description

a. This noninvasive procedure is based on the principles of ultrasound and evaluates structural and functional changes in the heart.

b. Heart chamber size is measured, ejection fraction is calculated, and flow gradient across the valves is determined.

Box 60-1 Basics of Electrocardiography

An electrocardiogram (ECG) reflects the electrical activity of cardiac cells and records electrical activity at a speed of 25 mm/sec.

An electrocardiographic strip consists of horizontal lines representing seconds and vertical lines representing voltage.

Each small square represents 0.04 second.

Each large square represents 0.20 second.

The P wave represents atrial depolarization.

The PR interval represents the time it takes an impulse to travel from the atria through the atrioventricular node, bundle of His, and bundle branches to the Purkinje fibers.

Normal PR interval duration ranges from 0.12 to 0.2 second.

The PR interval is measured from the beginning of the P wave to the end of the PR segment.

The QRS complex represents ventricular depolarization.

Normal QRS complex duration ranges from 0.04 to 0.1 second.

The Q wave appears as the first negative deflection in the QRS complex and reflects initial ventricular septal depolarization.

The R wave is the first positive deflection in the QRS complex.

The S wave appears as the second negative deflection in the QRS complex.

The J point marks the end of the QRS complex and the beginning of the ST segment.

The QRS duration is measured from the end of the PR segment to the J point.

The ST segment represents early ventricular repolarization.

The T wave represents ventricular repolarization and ventricular diastole.

The U wave may follow the T wave.

A prominent U wave may indicate an electrolyte abnormality, such as hypokalemia.

The QT interval represents ventricular refractory time or the total time required for ventricular depolarization and repolarization.

The QT interval is measured from the beginning of the QRS complex to the end of the T wave.

The QT interval normally lasts 0.32 to 0.4 second but varies with the client's heart rate, age, and gender.

---

c. Transesophageal echocardiography may be performed in which the echocardiogram is done through the esophagus; this is an invasive exam and requires pre- and postprocedure preparation and care similar to endoscopy procedures.

2. Interventions: Determine the client's ability to lie still, and advise the client to lie still, breathe normally, and refrain from talking during the test.

S. Exercise electrocardiography testing (stress test)

1. Description

    a. This noninvasive test studies the heart during activity and detects and evaluates coronary artery disease.

    b. Treadmill testing is the most commonly used mode of stress testing.

    c. Stress testing may be used with myocardial radionuclide testing (perfusion imaging), at which point the procedure becomes invasive because a radionuclide must be injected.

    d. If the client is unable to tolerate exercise, an intravenous (IV) infusion of dipyridamole (Persantine), dobutamine hydrochloride, or adenosine (Adenocard) is given to dilate the coronary arteries and simulate the effect of exercise.

    e. An informed consent is required if a radionuclide is injected.

2. Preprocedure interventions

    a. Obtain an informed consent if required.

    b. Provide adequate rest the night before the procedure.

c. Instruct the client to eat a light meal 1 to 2 hours before the procedure.

d. Instruct the client to avoid smoking, alcohol, and caffeine before the procedure.

e. Instruct the client to ask the physician about taking prescribed medication on the day of the procedure; theophylline products are usually withheld 12 hours before the test and calcium channel blockers and β-blockers are usually held for 24 hours.

f. Instruct the client to wear nonconstrictive, comfortable clothing and supportive rubber-soled shoes for the exercise stress test.

g. Instruct the client to notify the physician if any chest pain, dizziness, or shortness of breath occurs during the procedure.

3. Postprocedure interventions: Instruct the client to avoid taking a hot bath or shower for at least 1 to 2 hours.

T. Digital subtraction angiography

1. Description

    a. This test combines x-ray techniques and a computerized subtraction technique with fluoroscopy for visualization of the cardiovascular system.

    b. A contrast medium (dye) is injected.

2. Preprocedure interventions

    a. Assess for allergies to seafood, iodine, or radiopaque dyes. If allergic, the client may be premedicated with antihistamines and corticosteroids to prevent a reaction.

    b. Obtain informed consent.

3. Postprocedure interventions

    a. Monitor vital signs.

    b. Assess injection site for bleeding or discomfort.

U. Myocardial nuclear perfusion imaging (MNPI)

  1. Description

    a. Nuclear cardiology is the use of radionuclide techniques and scanning for cardiovascular assessment.

    b. The most common tests include technetium pyrophosphate scanning, thallium imaging, and multigated cardiac blood pool imaging; can evaluate cardiac motion and calculate the ejection fraction.

  2. Preprocedure interventions

    a. Obtain informed consent.

    b. Inform the client that a small amount of radioisotope will be injected and that the radiation exposure and risks are minimal.

  3. Postprocedure interventions

    a. Assess vital signs.

    b. Assess injection site for bleeding or discomfort.

    c. Inform the client that fatigue is possible.

V. Magnetic resonance imaging (MRI)

  1. Description

    a. This is a noninvasive diagnostic test that produces an image of the heart or great vessels through interaction of magnetic fields, radio waves, and atomic nuclei.

    b. It provides information on chamber size and thickness, valve and ventricular function, and blood flow through the great vessels and coronary arteries.

  2. Preprocedure interventions

    a. Evaluate the client for the presence of a pacemaker or other implanted items that present a contraindication to the test.

    b. Ensure that the client has removed all metallic objects such as a watch, other jewelry, clothing with metal fasteners, and metal hair fasteners.

    c. Inform the client that she or he may experience claustrophobia while in the scanner.

W. Electrophysiologic studies: An invasive procedure in which a programmed electrical stimulation of the heart is induced to cause dysrhythmias and conduction defects; assists in finding an accurate diagnosis and aids in determining treatment.

X. Electronic-beam computer tomography scan (EBCT): determines whether calcifications are present in the arteries; coronary artery calcium (CAC) score is provided (a score higher than 400 requires intensive preventive treatment).

Y. Cardiac catheterization (Fig. 60-2)

  1. Description

    a. An invasive test involving insertion of a catheter into the heart and surrounding vessels

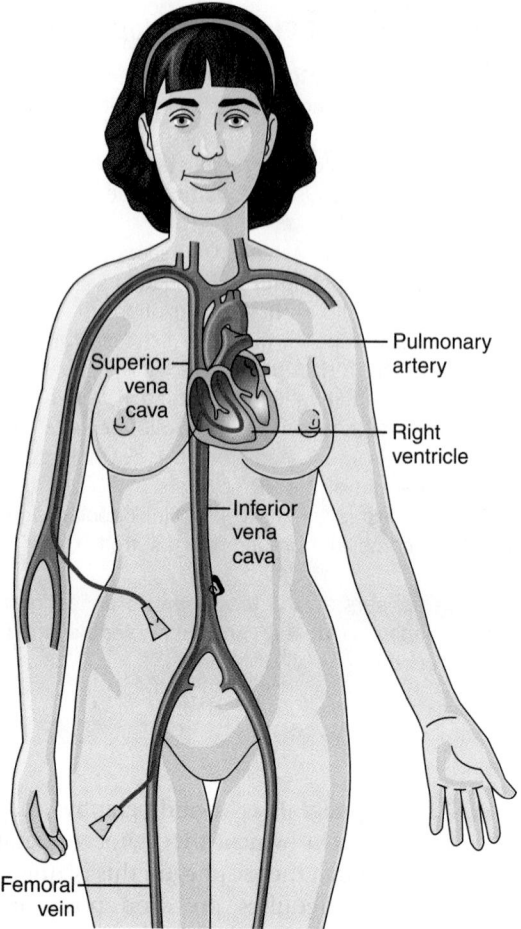

▲ **FIGURE 60-2** Right-sided heart catheterization. The catheter is inserted into the femoral vein and advanced into the inferior vena cava (or, if into an antecubital or basilic vein, through the superior vena cava), right atrium, and right ventricle and into the pulmonary artery. (From Ignatavicius, D., & Workman, M. [2010]. *Medical-surgical nursing: Patient-centered collaborative care* [6th ed.]. St. Louis: Saunders.)

    b. Obtains information about the structure and performance of the heart chambers and valves and the coronary circulation

  2. Preprocedure interventions

    a. Obtain informed consent.

    b. Assess for allergies to seafood, iodine, or radiopaque dyes; if allergic, the client may be premedicated with antihistamines and corticosteroids to prevent a reaction.

    c. Withhold solid food for 6 to 8 hours and liquids for 4 hours as prescribed to prevent vomiting and aspiration during the procedure.

    d. Document the client's height and weight because these data will be needed to determine the amount of dye to be administered.

    e. Document baseline vital signs and note the quality and presence of peripheral pulses for postprocedure comparison.

    f. Inform the client that a local anesthetic will be administered before catheter insertion.

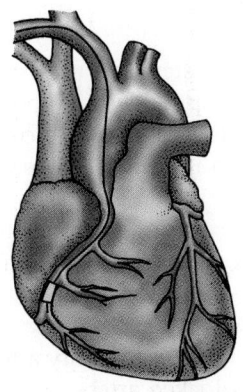 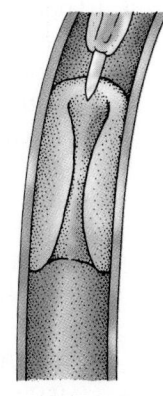 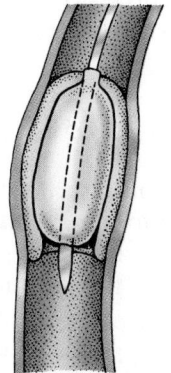 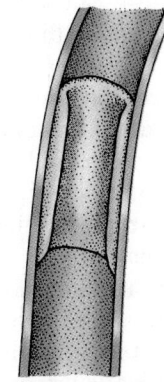

1. The balloon-tipped catheter is positioned in the artery.

2. The uninflated balloon is centered in the obstruction.

3. The balloon is inflated, which flattens plaque against the artery wall.

4. The balloon is removed, and the artery is left unoccluded.

▲ **FIGURE 60-3** Percutaneous transluminal coronary angioplasty. (From Ignatavicius, D., & Workman, M. [2010]. *Medical-surgical nursing: Patient-centered collaborative care* [6th ed.]. St. Louis: Saunders.)

g. Inform the client that he or she may feel fatigued because of the need to lie still and quiet on a hard table for up to 2 hours.

h. Inform the client that he or she may feel a fluttery feeling as the catheter passes through the heart, a flushed, warm feeling when the dye is injected, a desire to cough, and palpitations caused by heart irritability.

i. Prepare the insertion site by shaving and cleaning with an antiseptic solution if prescribed.

j. Administer preprocedure medications such as sedatives if prescribed.

k. Insert an IV line if prescribed.

⚠ If a client taking metformin (Glucophage) is scheduled to undergo a procedure requiring the administration of iodine dye, the metformin is withheld 48 hours prior because of the risk of lactic acidosis. The medication is not resumed until directed to do so by the physician (usually 48 hours after the procedure or after renal function studies are done and the results are evaluated).

3. Postprocedure interventions

a. Monitor vital signs and cardiac rhythm for dysrhythmias at least every 30 minutes for 2 hours initially.

b. Assess for chest pain and, if dysrhythmias or chest pain occurs, notify the physician.

c. Monitor peripheral pulses and the color, warmth, and sensation of the extremity distal to the insertion site at least every 30 minutes for 2 hours initially.

d. Notify the physician if the client complains of numbness and tingling, if the extremity becomes cool, pale, or cyanotic, or if loss of the peripheral pulses occurs.

e. Monitor the pressure dressing for bleeding or hematoma formation.

f. Apply a sandbag or compression device (if prescribed) to the insertion site to provide additional pressure if required.

g. Monitor for bleeding; if bleeding occurs, apply manual pressure immediately and notify the physician.

h. Monitor for hematoma; if a hematoma develops, notify the physician.

i. Keep extremity extended for 4 to 6 hours, as prescribed, keeping the leg straight to prevent arterial occlusion.

j. Maintain strict bed rest for 6 to 12 hours, as prescribed; however, the client may turn from side to side. Do not elevate the head of the bed more than 15 degrees.

k. If the antecubital vessel was used, immobilize the arm with an armboard.

l. Encourage fluid intake, if not contraindicated, to promote renal excretion of the dye and to replace fluid loss caused by the osmotic diuretic effect of the dye.

m. Monitor for nausea, vomiting, rash, or other signs of hypersensitivity to the dye.

III. THERAPEUTIC MANAGEMENT

A. Percutaneous transluminal coronary angioplasty (PTCA)

1. Description (Fig. 60-3)

a. An invasive, nonsurgical technique in which one or more arteries is (are) dilated with a balloon catheter to open the vessel lumen and improve arterial blood flow

b. PTCA may be used for clients with an evolving myocardial infarction (MI), alone or in combination with medications to achieve reperfusion.

c. The client can experience reocclusion after the procedure; thus, the procedure may need to be repeated.

d. Complications can include arterial dissection or rupture, embolization of plaque fragments, spasm, and acute MI.

e. Firm commitment is needed on the client's part to stop smoking, adhere to diet restrictions, lose weight, alter his or her exercise pattern, and stop any behaviors that lead to progression of artery occlusion.

2. Preprocedure interventions
   a. Maintain NPO status after midnight.
   b. Obtain informed consent, allergy assessment to iodine, and hold metformin (as for cardiac catheterization).
   c. Prepare the groin area with antiseptic soap and shave per institutional procedure and as prescribed.
   d. Assess baseline vital signs and peripheral pulses.
   e. Instruct the client that chest pain may occur during balloon inflation and to report it if it does occur.

3. Postprocedure interventions
   a. Monitor vital signs closely.
   b. Assess distal pulses in both extremities.
   c. Maintain bed rest as prescribed, keeping the limb straight for 6 to 8 hours.
   d. Administer anticoagulants such as intravenous heparin and antiplatelet agents as prescribed to prevent thrombus formation.
   e. Intravenous nitroglycerin may be prescribed to prevent coronary artery vasospasm.
   f. Encourage fluids, if not contraindicated, to enhance renal excretion of dye.
   g. Instruct the client in the administration of nitrates, calcium channel blockers, antiplatelet agents, and anticoagulants as prescribed.
   h. Instruct the client to take acetylsalicylic acid (aspirin) daily permanently if prescribed.
   i. Assist the client with planning lifestyle modifications.

B. Laser-assisted angioplasty
   1. Description
      a. A laser probe is advanced through a cannula similar to that used for PTCA.
      b. Laser-assisted angioplasty is used also for clients with small occlusions in the distal superficial femoral, proximal popliteal, and common iliac arteries, and in coronary arteries.
      c. Heat from the laser vaporizes the plaque to open the occluded artery.
   2. Preprocedure and postprocedure interventions
      a. Care is similar to that for PTCA.
      b. Monitor for complications of coronary dissection, acute occlusion, perforation, embolism, and MI.

C. Coronary artery stents
   1. Description
      a. Coronary artery stents are used in conjunction with PTCA to provide a supportive scaffold to eliminate the risk of acute coronary vessel closure and to improve long-term patency of the vessel.
      b. A balloon catheter bearing the stent is inserted into the coronary artery and positioned at the site of occlusion; balloon inflation deploys the stent.
      c. When placed in the coronary artery, the stent reopens the blocked artery.
   2. Preprocedure and postprocedure interventions
      a. Care is similar to that for PTCA.
      b. Acute thrombosis is a major concern following the procedure; the client is placed on antiplatelet therapy such as clopidogrel (Plavix) and acetylsalicylic acid (aspirin) for several months following the procedure.
      c. Monitor for complications of the procedure such as stent migration or occlusion, coronary artery dissection, and bleeding resulting from anticoagulation.

D. Atherectomy
   1. Description
      a. Atherectomy removes plaque from a coronary artery by the use of a cutting chamber on the inserted catheter or a rotating blade that pulverizes the plaque.
      b. Atherectomy is also used to improve blood flow to ischemic limbs in individuals with peripheral arterial disease.
   2. Preprocedure and postprocedure interventions
      a. Care is similar to that for PTCA.
      b. Monitor for complications of perforation, embolus, and reocclusion.

E. Transmyocardial revascularization
   1. May be used for clients with widespread atherosclerosis involving vessels that are too small and numerous for replacement or balloon catheterization; performed through a small chest incision
   2. Transmyocardial revascularization uses a high-powered laser that creates 20 to 24 channels through the ventricular muscle of the left ventricle; blood enters these small channels, providing the affected region of the heart with oxygenated blood.
   3. The opening on the surface of the heart heals; however, the main channels remain and perfuse the myocardium.

F. Arterial revascularization
   1. Description
      a. Performed to increase arterial blood flow to the affected limb
      b. Inflow procedures involve bypassing the arterial occlusion above the superficial femoral arteries

c. Outflow procedures involve bypassing the arterial occlusions at or below the superficial femoral arteries.

d. Graft material is sutured above and below the occlusion to facilitate blood flow around the occlusion.

2. Preoperative interventions
   a. Assess baseline vital signs and peripheral pulses.
   b. Insert an IV line and urinary catheter as prescribed.
   c. Maintain a central venous catheter and/or arterial line if inserted.

3. Postoperative interventions
   a. Assess vital signs.
   b. Monitor the **BP** and notify the physician if changes occur.
   c. Monitor for hypotension, which may indicate hypovolemia.
   d. Monitor for hypertension, which may place stress on the graft and cause clot formation.
   e. Maintain bed rest for 24 hours as prescribed.
   f. Instruct the client to keep the affected extremity straight, limit movement, and avoid bending the knee and hip.
   g. Monitor for warmth, redness, and edema, which often are expected outcomes because of increased blood flow.
   h. Monitor for graft occlusion, which often occurs within the first 24 hours.
   i. Assess peripheral pulses and for adverse changes in color and temperature of the extremity.
   j. Encourage coughing, deep breathing, and the use of incentive spirometry.
   k. Maintain NPO status, with progression to clear liquids as prescribed.
   l. Use strict aseptic technique when in contact with the incision.
   m. Assess the incision for drainage, warmth, or swelling.
   n. Monitor for excessive bleeding (a small amount of bloody drainage is expected).
   o. Monitor the area over the graft for hardness, tenderness, and warmth, which may indicate infection; if this occurs, notify the physician immediately.
   p. Instruct the client about proper foot care and measures to prevent ulcer formation.
   q. Instruct the client to take medications as prescribed.
   r. Instruct the client in how to care for incision.
   s. Assist the client in modifying lifestyle to prevent further plaque formation.

⚠ Following arterial revascularization, monitor for a sharp increase in pain because pain is frequently the first indicator of postoperative graft occlusion. If signs of graft occlusion occur, notify the physician immediately.

G. Coronary artery bypass grafting (Fig. 60-4)
1. Description
   a. The occluded coronary arteries are bypassed with the client's own venous or arterial blood vessels.
   b. The saphenous vein, internal mammary artery, or other arteries may be used to bypass lesions in the coronary arteries.
   c. Coronary artery bypass grafting is performed when the client does not respond to medical management of coronary artery disease or when vessels are severely occluded.

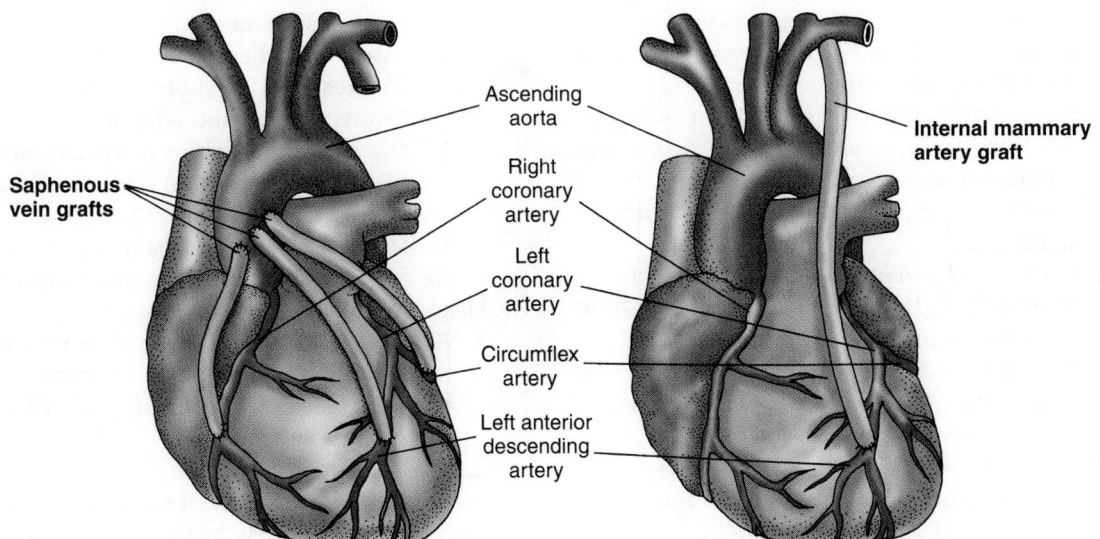

Saphenous vein grafts

Ascending aorta

Right coronary artery

Left coronary artery

Circumflex artery

Left anterior descending artery

Internal mammary artery graft

▲ **FIGURE 60-4** Two methods of coronary artery bypass grafting. The procedure used depends on the nature of the coronary disease, the condition of the vessels available for grafting, and the client's health status. (From Ignatavicius, D., & Workman, M. [2010]. *Medical-surgical nursing: Patient-centered collaborative care* [6th ed.]. St. Louis: Saunders.)

2. Preoperative interventions
   a. Familiarize the client and family with the cardiac surgical critical care unit.
   b. Inform the client to expect a sternal incision, possible arm or leg incision(s), one or two chest tubes, a Foley catheter, and several IV fluid catheters.
   c. Inform the client that an endotracheal tube will be in place and that he or she will be unable to speak.
   d. Advise the client that he or she will be on mechanical ventilation and to breathe with the ventilator and not fight it.
   e. Instruct the client to inform the nurse of any postoperative pain because pain medication will be available.
   f. Instruct the client in how to splint the chest incision, cough and deep-breathe, use the incentive spirometer, and perform arm and leg exercises.
   g. Encourage the client and family to discuss anxieties and fears related to surgery.
   h. Note that prescribed medications may be discontinued preoperatively (usually, diuretics 2 to 3 days before surgery, digoxin 12 hours before surgery, and aspirin and anticoagulants 1 week before surgery).
   i. Administer medications as prescribed, which may include potassium chloride, antihypertensives, antidysrhythmics, and antibiotics.
3. Cardiac surgical unit postoperative interventions
   a. Maintain mechanical ventilation for 6 to 24 hours as prescribed.
   b. Monitor heart rate and rhythm, pulmonary artery and **arterial pressures**, urinary output, and neurological status.
   c. Maintain mediastinal and pleural chest tubes to the water seal drainage system with prescribed suction and report drainage exceeding 100 to 150 mL/hr.
   d. Epicardial pacing wires should be covered by sterile caps or connected to a temporary pacemaker generator; all equipment in use must be properly grounded to prevent microshock.
   e. Assess fluid and electrolyte balance.
   f. Restrict fluids, as prescribed, to 1500 to 2000 mL because the client usually has edema.
   g. Monitor for hypotension, which can cause collapse of a vein graft; determine the cause and provide intervention.
   h. Monitor for hypertension because increased pressure promotes leakage from the suture line and may cause bleeding.
   i. Monitor the temperature and initiate rewarming procedures using warm or thermal blankets if the temperature drops below

96.8° F; rewarm the client no faster than 1.8° F/hr to prevent shivering, and discontinue rewarming procedures when the temperature approaches 98.6° F.
   j. Administer potassium intravenously as prescribed to maintain the potassium level between 4 and 5 mEq/L to prevent dysrhythmias.
   k. Monitor for signs of cardiac tamponade, which will include sudden cessation of previously heavy mediastinal drainage, jugular vein distention with clear lung sounds, equalization of right atrial pressure and pulmonary artery wedge pressure, and pulsus paradoxus.
   l. Monitor pain, differentiating sternotomy pain from anginal pain, which would indicate graft failure.
4. Transfer of the client from the cardiac surgical unit
   a. Monitor vital signs, level of consciousness, and peripheral perfusion.
   b. Monitor for dysrhythmias.
   c. Auscultate lungs and assess respiratory status.
   d. Encourage the client to splint the incision, cough, deep-breathe, and use the incentive spirometer to raise secretions and prevent atelectasis.
   e. Monitor temperature and white blood cell count, which, if elevated after 3 to 4 days, indicate infection.
   f. Provide adequate fluids and hydration as prescribed to liquefy secretions.
   g. Assess suture line and chest tube insertion sites for redness, purulent discharge, and signs of infection.
   h. Assess sternal suture line for instability, which may indicate an infection.
   i. Guide the client to gradually resume activity.
   j. Assess the client for tachycardia, **postural (orthostatic) hypotension**, and fatigue before, during, and after activity.
   k. Discontinue activities if the **BP** drops more than 10 to 20 mm Hg or if the pulse increases more than 10 beats/min.
   l. Monitor episodes of pain closely.
   m. See Box 60-2 for home care instructions.
H. Heart transplantation
1. A donor heart from an individual with a comparable body weight and ABO compatibility is transplanted into a recipient within less than 6 hours of procurement.
2. The surgeon removes the diseased heart, leaving the posterior portion of the atria to serve as an anchor for the new heart.
3. Because a remnant of the client's atria remains, two unrelated P waves are noted on the electrocardiogram.

4. The transplanted heart is denervated and unresponsive to vagal stimulation; because the heart is denervated, clients do not experience angina.
5. Symptoms of heart rejection include hypotension, dysrhythmias, weakness, fatigue, and dizziness.
6. Endomyocardial biopsies are performed at regular scheduled intervals and whenever rejection is suspected.
7. The client requires lifetime immunosuppressive therapy.
8. Strict aseptic technique and vigilant hand washing must be maintained when caring for the post-transplantation client because of increased risk for infection from immunosuppression.
9. The heart rate approximates 100 beats/min and responds slowly to exercise or stress with regard to increases in heart rate, **contractility**, and **cardiac output**.

IV. CARDIAC DYSRHYTHMIAS

A. Normal sinus rhythm (Fig. 60-5)

Box 60-2 Home Care Instructions Following Cardiac Surgery

Progressive return to activities at home

Limiting of pushing or pulling activities for 6 weeks following discharge

Maintenance of incisional care and recording signs of redness, swelling, or drainage

Sternotomy incision heals in about 6 to 8 weeks

Avoidance of crossing legs; wearing elastic hose as prescribed until edema subsides, and elevating the surgical limb (if used to obtain the graft) when sitting in a chair

Use of prescribed medications

Dietary measures, including the avoidance of saturated fats and cholesterol and the use of salt

Resumption of sexual intercourse on the advice of the physician after exercise tolerance is assessed (if client can walk one block or climb two flights of stairs without symptoms, he or she can resume sexual activity safely)

---

1. Rhythm originates from the sinoatrial node.
2. Description
   a. Atrial and ventricular rhythms are regular.
   b. Atrial and ventricular rates are 60 to 100 beats/min (Fig. 60-6 and Box 60-3).
   c. PR interval and QRS width are within normal limits.
B. Sinus bradycardia
1. Description
   a. Atrial and ventricular rhythms are regular.
   b. Atrial and ventricular rates are less than 60 beats/min.
   c. PR interval and QRS width are within normal limits.
   d. Treatment may be necessary if the client is symptomatic (signs of decreased **cardiac output**).
   e. Note that a low heart rate may be normal for some individuals.
2. Interventions
   a. Attempt to determine the cause of sinus bradycardia; if a medication is suspected of causing the bradycardia, withhold the medication and notify the physician.
   b. Administer oxygen as prescribed.
   c. Administer atropine sulfate as prescribed to increase the heart rate to 60 beats/min.
   d. Be prepared to apply a noninvasive (transcutaneous) pacemaker initially as prescribed if the atropine sulfate does not increase the heart rate sufficiently.
   e. Avoid additional doses of atropine sulfate because this will induce tachycardia.
   f. Monitor for hypotension and administer fluids intravenously as prescribed.
   g. Depending on the cause of the bradycardia, the client may need a permanent pacemaker.
C. Sinus tachycardia
1. Description
   a. Atrial and ventricular rates are 100 to 180 beats/min.

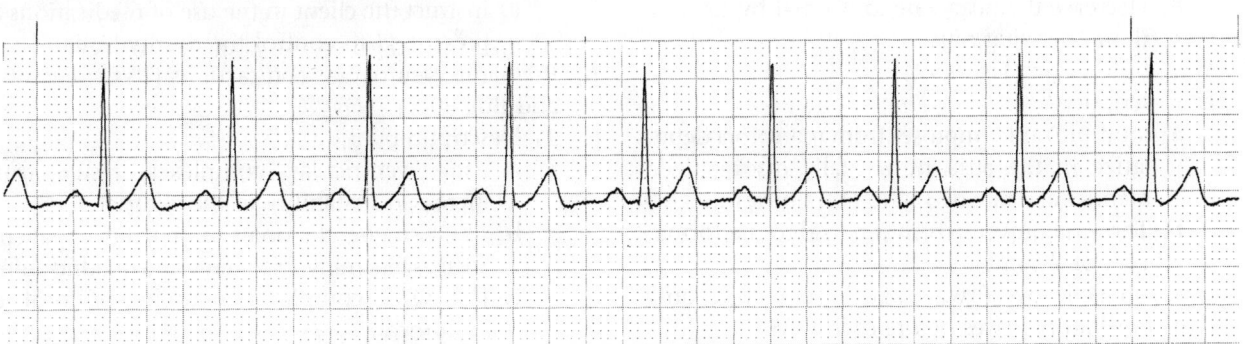

▲ **FIGURE 60-5** Normal sinus rhythm. Both atrial and ventricular rhythms are essentially regular (a slight variation in rhythm is normal). Atrial and ventricular rates are both 83 beats/min. There is one P wave before each QRS complex, and all the P waves are of a consistent morphology, or shape. The PR interval measures 0.18 second and is constant; the QRS complex measures 0.06 second and is constant. (From Ignatavicius, D., & Workman, M. [2010]. *Medical-surgical nursing: Patient-centered collaborative care* [6th ed.]. St. Louis: Saunders.)

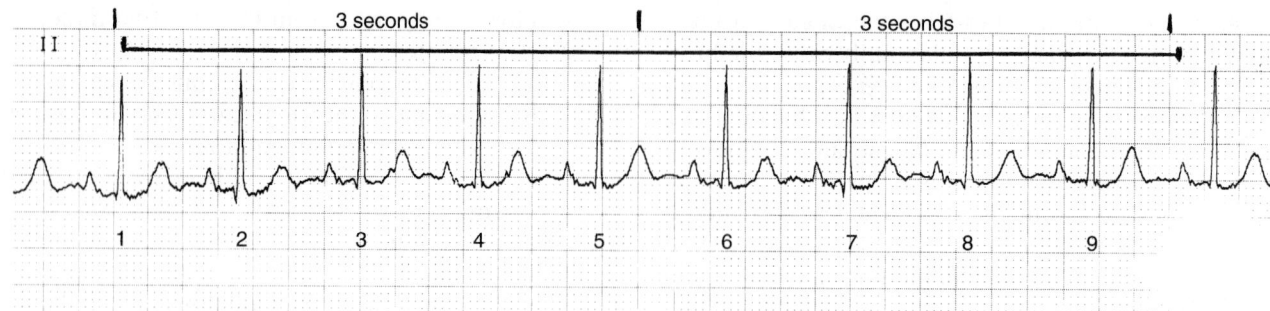

▲ **FIGURE 60-6** Each segment between the dark lines (above the monitor strip) represents 3 seconds when the monitor is set at a speed of 25 mm/sec. To estimate the ventricular rate, count the QRS complexes in a 6-second strip and then multiply that number by 10 to estimate the heart rate for 1 minute. In this example, there are 9 QRS complexes in 6 seconds. Therefore the heart rate can be estimated as 90 beats/min. (From Ignatavicius, D., & Workman, M. [2010]. *Medical-surgical nursing: Patient-centered collaborative care* [6th ed.]. St. Louis: Saunders.)

Box 60-3 Determination of Heart Rate Using 6-Second Strip Method

The method can be used to determine heart rate for regular and irregular rhythms.

To determine atrial rate, count the number of P waves in 6 seconds and multiply by 10 to obtain a full minute rate.

To determine ventricular rate, count the number of R waves or QRS complexes in 6 seconds and multiply by 10 to obtain a full minute rate.

For accuracy, timing should begin on the P wave or the QRS complex and end exactly at 30 large blocks later.

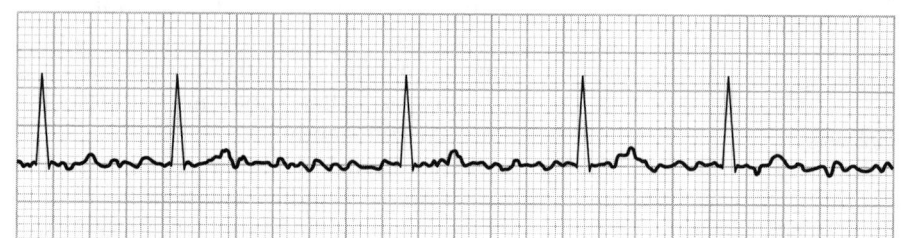

▲ **FIGURE 60-7** Atrial dysrhythmias—atrial fibrillation. (From Ignatavicius, D., & Workman, M. [2010]. *Medical-surgical nursing: Patient-centered collaborative care* [6th ed.]. St. Louis: Saunders.)

---

b. Atrial and ventricular rhythms are regular.
c. PR interval and QRS width are within normal limits.

2. Interventions
  a. Identify the cause of the tachycardia.
  b. Decrease the heart rate to normal by treating the underlying cause.

D. Atrial fibrillation (Fig. 60-7)
  1. Description
    a. Multiple rapid impulses from many foci depolarize in the atria in a totally disorganized manner at a rate of 350 to 600 times/min.
    b. The atria quiver, which can lead to the formation of thrombi.
    c. No definitive P wave can be observed, only fibrillatory waves before each QRS.
  2. Interventions
    a. Administer oxygen.
    b. Administer anticoagulants as prescribed because of the risk of emboli.

c. Administer cardiac medications as prescribed to control the ventricular rhythm and assist in the maintenance of **cardiac output**.
d. Prepare the client for cardioversion as prescribed.
e. Instruct the client in the use of medications as prescribed to control the dysrhythmia.

E. Premature ventricular contractions (PVCs; Fig. 60-8 and Box 60-4)
  1. Description
    a. Early ventricular complexes result from increased irritability of the ventricles.
    b. PVCs frequently occur in repetitive patterns such as bigeminy, trigeminy, and quadrigeminy.
    c. The QRS complexes may be unifocal or multifocal.
  2. Interventions
    a. Notify the physician if PVCs occur.
    b. Identify the cause and treat based on the cause.

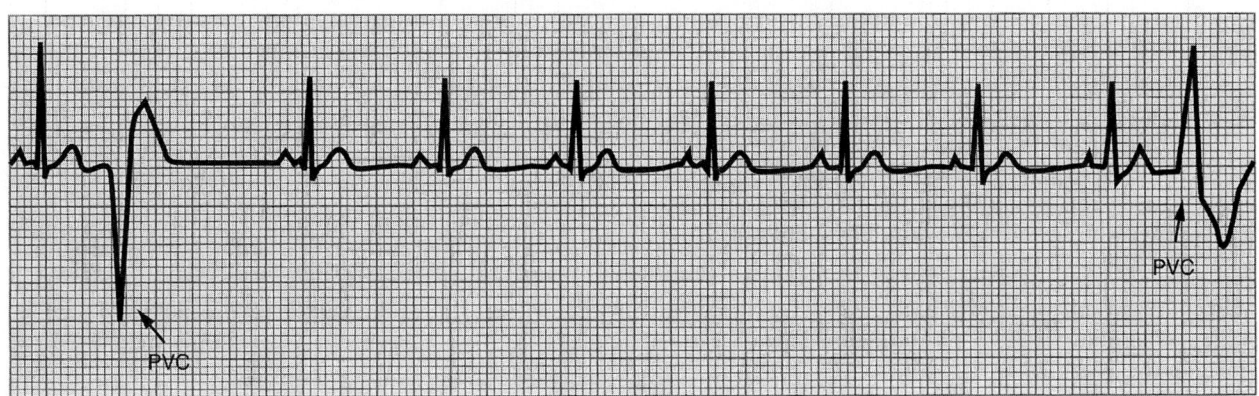

▲ **FIGURE 60-8** Ventricular dysrhythmias—normal sinus rhythm with multifocal premature ventricular complexes (PVCs; one negative and the other positive). (From Ignatavicius, D., & Workman, M. [2010]. *Medical-surgical nursing: Patient-centered collaborative care* [6th ed.]. St. Louis: Saunders.)

Box 60-4 Premature Ventricular Contractions

Bigeminy: Premature ventricular contraction (PVC) every other heartbeat

Trigeminy: PVC every third heartbeat

Quadrigeminy: PVC every fourth heartbeat

Couplet or pair: Two sequential PVCs

Unifocal: Uniform upward or downward deflection, arising from the same ectopic focus

Multifocal: Different shapes, with the impulse generation from different sites

R-on-T phenomenon: PVC falls on the T wave of the preceding beat; may precipitate ventricular fibrillation

---

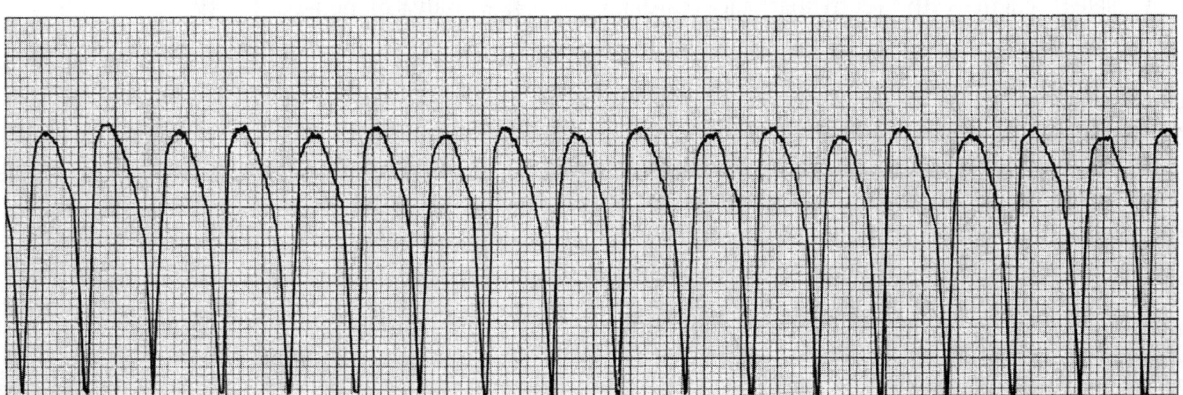

▲ **FIGURE 60-9** Ventricular dysrhythmias—sustained ventricular tachycardia at a rate of 166 beats/min. (From Ignatavicius, D., & Workman, M. [2010]. *Medical-surgical nursing: Patient-centered collaborative care* [6th ed.]. St. Louis: Saunders.)

---

c. Evaluate oxygen saturation to assess for hypoxemia, which can cause PVCs.

d. Administer oxygen as prescribed.

e. Evaluate electrolytes, particularly the potassium level, because hypokalemia can cause PVCs.

f. Lidocaine (Xylocaine) may be prescribed.

⚠ For the client experiencing PVCs, notify the physician if the client complains of chest pain or if the PVCs increase in frequency, are multifocal, occur on the T wave (R on T), or occur in runs of ventricular tachycardia.

F. Ventricular tachycardia (VT; Fig. 60-9)

1. Description

   a. Ventricular tachycardia occurs because of a repetitive firing of an irritable ventricular ectopic focus at a rate of 140 to 250 beats/min or more.

   b. Ventricular tachycardia may present as a paroxysm of three self-limiting beats or more or may be a sustained rhythm.

   c. Ventricular tachycardia can lead to cardiac arrest.

2. Stable client with sustained VT (with pulse and no signs or symptoms of decreased **cardiac output**)

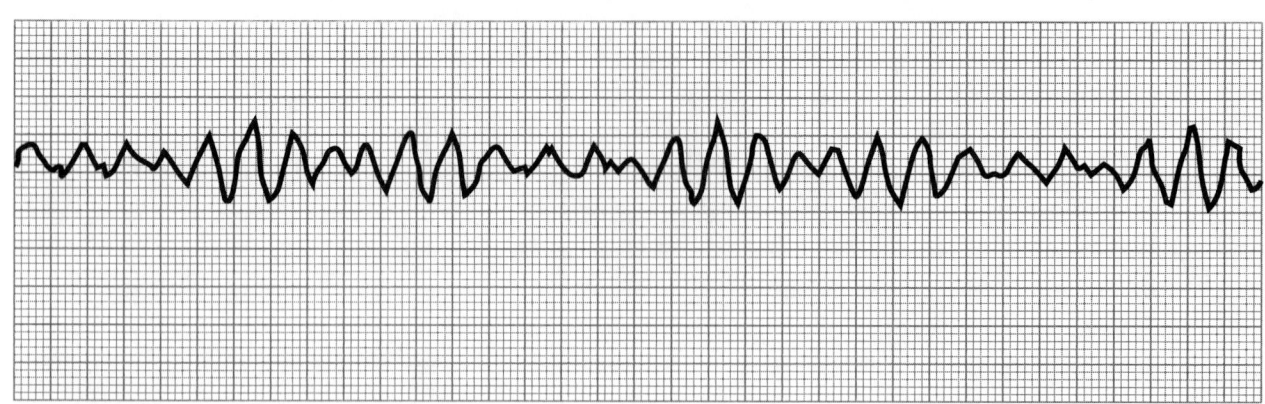

▲ **FIGURE 60-10** Ventricular dysrhythmias—coarse ventricular fibrillation. (From Ignatavicius, D., & Workman, M. [2010]. *Medical-surgical nursing: Patient-centered collaborative care* [6th ed.]. St. Louis: Saunders.)

    a. Administer oxygen as prescribed.
    b. Administer antidysrhythmics as prescribed.
  3. Unstable client with VT (with pulse and signs and symptoms of decreased **cardiac output**)
    a. Administer oxygen and antidysrhythmic therapy as prescribed.
    b. Prepare for synchronized cardioversion if the client is unstable.
    c. Attempt cough cardiopulmonary resuscitation (CPR) by asking the client to cough hard every 1 to 3 seconds.
  4. Pulseless client with ventricular tachycardia: defibrillation and CPR

G. Ventricular fibrillation (VF; Fig. 60-10)
  1. Description
    a. Impulses from many irritable foci in the ventricles fire in a totally disorganized manner.
    b. VF is a chaotic rapid rhythm in which the ventricles quiver and there is no **cardiac output**.
    c. VF is fatal if not successfully terminated within 3 to 5 minutes.
    d. Client lacks a pulse, **BP**, respirations, and heart sounds.
  2. Interventions
    a. Defibrillate the client immediately, up to 3 times consecutively at 200, 300, and 360 joules (J).
    b. Initiate CPR.
    c. Administer oxygen as prescribed.
    d. Administer antidysrhythmic therapy as prescribed.

V. MANAGEMENT OF DYSRHYTHMIAS

A. Vagal maneuvers
  1. Description: Vagal maneuvers induce vagal stimulation of the cardiac conduction system and are used to terminate supraventricular tachydysrhythmias.
  2. Carotid sinus massage
    a. The physician instructs the client to turn the head away from the side to be massaged.

    b. The physician massages over one carotid artery for a few seconds to determine whether a change in cardiac rhythm occurs.
    c. The client should be on a cardiac monitor; an electrocardiographic rhythm strip before, during, and after the procedure should be documented on the chart.
    d. Have a defibrillator and resuscitative equipment available.
    e. Monitor vital signs, cardiac rhythm, and level of consciousness following the procedure.
  3. Valsalva maneuver
    a. The physician instructs the client to bear down or induces a gag reflex in the client to stimulate a vagal response
    b. Monitor the heart rate, rhythm, and **BP**.
    c. Observe the cardiac monitor for a change in rhythm.
    d. Record an electrocardiographic rhythm strip before, during, and after the procedure.
    e. Provide an emesis basin if the gag reflex is stimulated, and initiate precautions to prevent aspiration.
    f. Have a defibrillator and resuscitative equipment available.

B. Cardioversion
  1. Description
    a. Cardioversion is synchronized countershock to convert an undesirable rhythm to a stable rhythm.
    b. Cardioversion can be an elective procedure performed by the physician for stable tachydysrhythmias resistant to medical therapies or an emergent procedure for hemodynamically unstable ventricular or supraventricular tachydysrhythmias.
    c. A lower amount of energy is used than with defibrillation.
    d. The defibrillator is synchronized to the client's R wave to avoid discharging the shock during the vulnerable period (T wave).

e. If the defibrillator were not synchronized, it could discharge on the T wave and cause VF.

2. Preprocedure interventions
   a. Obtain an informed consent if an elective procedure.
   b. Administer sedation as prescribed.
   c. If an elective procedure, hold digoxin (Lanoxin) 48 hours preprocedure as prescribed to prevent postcardioversion ventricular irritability.
   d. If an elective procedure for atrial fibrillation or atrial flutter, the client should receive anticoagulant therapy for 4 to 6 weeks preprocedure.

3. During the procedure
   a. Ensure that the skin is clean and dry in the area where the electrode paddles will be placed.
   b. Stop the oxygen during the procedure to avoid the hazard of fire.
   c. Be sure that no one is touching the bed or the client when delivering the countershock.

4. Postprocedure interventions
   a. Priority assessment includes ability of the client to maintain the airway and breathing.
   b. Resume oxygen administration as prescribed.
   c. Assess vital signs.
   d. Assess level of consciousness.
   e. Monitor cardiac rhythm.
   f. Monitor for indications of successful response, such as conversion to sinus rhythm, strong peripheral pulses, an adequate **BP**, and adequate urine output.
   g. Assess the skin on the chest for evidence of burns from the edges of the paddles.

C. Defibrillation
   1. Defibrillation is an asynchronous countershock used to terminate pulseless ventricular tachycardia (VT) or VF.
   2. Monophasic defibrillators deliver energy in one direction; includes an initial shock at 360 joules followed by immediate CPR beginning with chest compressions.
   3. Biphasic defibrillators deliver energy in two directions and delivers the first and any other successive shocks at 120 to 200 joules.

⚠ Before defibrillating a client be sure that the oxygen is shut off to avoid the hazard of fire and be sure that no one is touching the bed or the client.

D. Use of paddle electrodes
   1. Apply conductive pads.
   2. One paddle is placed at the third intercostal space to the right of the sternum; the other is placed at the fifth intercostal space on the left midaxillary line.
   3. Apply firm pressure of at least 25 lb to each of the paddles.
   4. Be sure that no one is touching the bed or the client when delivering the countershock.

E. Automatic external defibrillator
   1. An automatic external defibrillator is used by laypersons and emergency medical technicians for prehospital cardiac arrest.
   2. Place the client on a firm dry surface.
   3. Stop CPR.
   4. Ensure that no one is touching the client to avoid motion artifact during rhythm analysis.
   5. Place the electrode patches in the correct position on the client's chest.
   6. Press the analyzer button to identify the rhythm, which may take 30 seconds; the machine will advise whether a shock is necessary.
   7. Shocks are recommended for pulseless VT or VF only.
   8. If shock is recommended, the shock initially is delivered at an energy of 200 J.
   9. If unsuccessful, the shock is repeated at 200 to 300 J.
   10. The third and subsequent shock will be 360 J.
   11. If unsuccessful, CPR is continued for 1 minute and then another series of three shocks is delivered, each at 360 J.

F. Implantable cardioverter-defibrillator (ICD)
   1. Description
      a. An ICD monitors cardiac rhythm and detects and terminates episodes of VT and VF.
      b. The ICD senses VT or VF and delivers 25 to 30 J up to four times, if necessary.
      c. An ICD is used in clients with episodes of spontaneous sustained VT or VF unrelated to an MI or in clients whose medication therapy has been unsuccessful in controlling life-threatening dysrhythmias.
      d. Transvenous electrode leads are placed in the right atrium and ventricle in contact with the endocardium; leads are used for sensing, pacing, and delivery of cardioversion or defibrillation.
      e. The generator is most commonly implanted in the left pectoral region.
   2. Client education
      a. Instruct the client in the basic functions of the ICD.
      b. Know the rate cutoff of the ICD and the number of consecutive shocks that it will deliver.
      c. Wear loose-fitting clothing over the ICD generator site.
      d. Avoid contact sports to prevent trauma to the ICD generator and lead wires.
      e. Report any fever, redness, swelling, or drainage from the insertion site.
      f. Report symptoms of fainting, nausea, weakness, blackouts, and rapid pulse rates to the physician.
      g. During shock discharge, the client may feel faint or short of breath.

h. Instruct the client to sit or lie down if he or she feels a shock and to notify the physician.

i. Advise the client to maintain a log of the date, time, and activity preceding the shock, the symptoms preceding the shock, and postshock sensations.

j. Instruct the client and family in how to access emergency medical system.

k. Encourage the family to learn CPR.

l. Instruct the client to avoid electromagnetic fields directly over the ICD because they can inactivate the device.

m. Instruct the client to move away from the magnetic field immediately if beeping tones are heard, and to notify the physician.

n. Keep an ICD identification card in the wallet and obtain and wear a Medic-Alert bracelet.

o. Inform all health care providers that an ICD has been inserted; certain diagnostic tests, such as an MRI, and procedures using diathermy or electrocautery interfere with ICD function.

p. Advise the client of restrictions on activities such as driving and operating dangerous equipment.

VI. PACEMAKERS

A. Description: Temporary or permanent device that provides electrical stimulation and maintains the heart rate when the client's intrinsic pacemaker fails to provide a perfusing rhythm

B. Settings
1. A synchronous (demand) pacemaker senses the client's rhythm and paces only if the client's intrinsic rate falls below the set pacemaker rate for stimulating depolarization.

2. An asynchronous (fixed rate) pacemaker paces at a preset rate regardless of the client's intrinsic rhythm and is used when the client is asystolic or profoundly bradycardic.

3. Overdrive pacing suppresses the underlying rhythm in tachydysrhythmias so that the sinus node will regain control of the heart.

C. Spikes
1. When a pacing stimulus is delivered to the heart, a spike (straight vertical line) is seen on the monitor or electrocardiogram strip.

2. Spikes precede the chamber being paced; a spike preceding a P wave indicates that the atrium is paced and a spike preceding the QRS indicates that the ventricle is being paced.

3. An atrial spike followed by a P wave indicates atrial depolarization and a ventricular spike followed by a QRS complex represents ventricular depolarization; this is referred to as *capture*.

4. If the electrode is in the atrium, the spike is before the P wave; if the electrode is in the ventricle, the spike is before the QRS complex.

D. Temporary pacemakers
1. Noninvasive transcutaneous pacing
   a. Noninvasive transcutaneous pacing is used as a temporary emergency measure in the profoundly bradycardic or asystolic client until invasive pacing can be initiated.
   b. Large electrode pads are placed on the client's chest and back and connected to an external pulse generator.
   c. Wash the skin with soap and water before applying electrodes.
   d. It is not necessary to shave the hair or apply alcohol or tinctures to the skin.
   e. Place the posterior electrode between the spine and left scapula behind the heart, avoiding placement over bone (Fig. 60-11).

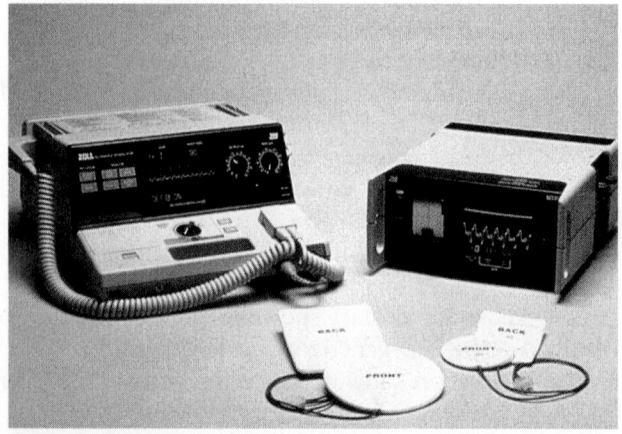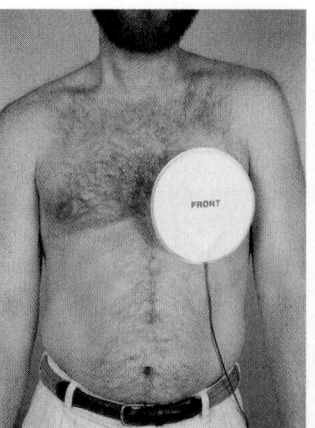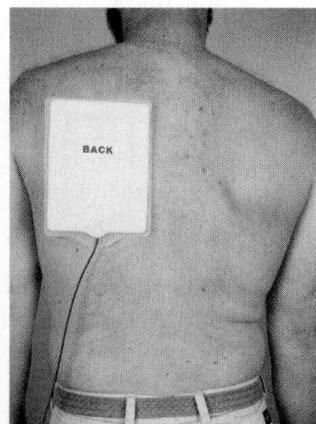

▲ **FIGURE 60-11** Equipment and electrode placement for transcutaneous external pacing. (From Ignatavicius, D., & Workman, M. [2006]. *Medical-surgical nursing: Critical thinking for collaborative care* [5th ed.]. St. Louis: Saunders. Courtesy of ZOLL Medical Corporation, Chelmsford, MA.)

f. Place the anterior electrode between V2 and V5 positions over the heart (see Fig. 60-11).

g. Do not place the anterior electrode over female breast tissue; rather, displace breast tissue and place under the breast.

h. Do not take the pulse or **BP** on the left side; the results will not be accurate because of the muscle twitching and electrical current.

i. Ensure that electrodes are in good contact with the skin.

j. Set pacing rate as prescribed; establish stimulation threshold to ensure capture.

k. If loss of capture occurs, assess the skin contact of the electrodes and increase the current until capture is regained.

l. Evaluate the client for discomfort from cutaneous and muscle stimulation; administer analgesics as needed.

2. Invasive transvenous pacing

a. Pacing lead wire is placed through the antecubital, femoral, jugular, or subclavian vein into the right atrium or right ventricle; so that it is in direct contact with the endocardium.

b. Monitor cardiac rhythm continuously.

c. Monitor vital signs.

d. Monitor the pacemaker insertion site.

e. Restrict client movement to prevent lead wire displacement.

3. Invasive epicardial pacing—applied by using a transthoracic approach; the lead wires are threaded loosely on the epicardial surface of the heart after cardiac surgery

4. Reducing the risk of microshock

a. Use only inspected and approved equipment.

b. Insulate the exposed portion of wires with plastic or rubber material (fingers of rubber gloves) when wires are not attached to the pulse generator; cover with nonconductive tape.

c. Ground all electrical equipment using a three-pronged plug.

d. Wear gloves when handling exposed wires.

e. Keep dressings dry.

E. Permanent pacemakers

1. Pulse generator is internal and surgically implanted in a subcutaneous pocket below the clavicle.

2. The leads are passed transvenously via the cephalic or subclavian vein to the endocardium on the right side of the heart; postoperatively, limitation of arm movement on the operative side is required to prevent lead wire dislodgement.

3. Permanent pacemakers may be single-chambered, in which the lead wire is placed in the chamber to be paced, or dual-chambered, with lead wires placed in both the right atrium and ventricle.

4. Biventricular pacing of the ventricles allows for synchronized depolarization and is used for moderate to severe heart failure to improve **cardiac output**.

5. A permanent pacemaker is programmed when inserted and can be reprogrammed if necessary by noninvasive transmission from an external programmer to the implanted generator.

6. Pacemakers may be powered by a lithium battery with an average life span of 10 years, nuclear-powered with a life span of 20 years or longer, or designed to be recharged externally.

7. Pacemaker function can be checked in the physician's office or clinic by a pacemaker interrogator or programmer or from home using a special telephone transmitter device.

8. The client may be provided with a device placed over the pacemaker battery generator with an attachment to the telephone; the heart rate then can be transmitted to the clinic.

9. Provide client teaching (Box 60-5).

Box 60-5 Pacemakers: Client Education

Instruct the client about the pacemaker, including the programmed rate.

Instruct the client in the signs of battery failure and when to notify the physician.

Instruct the client to report any fever, redness, swelling, or drainage from the insertion site.

Report signs of dizziness, weakness or fatigue, swelling of the ankles or legs, chest pain, or shortness of breath.

Keep a pacemaker identification card in the wallet and obtain and wear a Medic-Alert bracelet.

Instruct the client in how to take the pulse, to take the pulse daily, and to maintain a diary of pulse rates.

Wear loose-fitting clothing over the pulse generator site.

Avoid contact sports.

Inform all health care providers that a pacemaker has been inserted.

Instruct the client to inform airport security that he or she has a pacemaker because the pacemaker may set off the security detector.

Instruct the client that most electrical appliances can be used without any interference with the functioning of the pacemaker; however, advise the client not to operate electrical appliances directly over the pacemaker site.

Avoid transmitter towers and antitheft devices in stores.

Instruct the client that if any unusual feelings occur when near any electrical devices to move 5 to 10 feet away and check the pulse.

Instruct the client about the methods of monitoring the function of the device.

Emphasize the importance of follow-up with the physician.

Use cell phones on the side opposite the pacemaker.

VII. CORONARY ARTERY DISEASE

A. Description
1. Coronary artery disease is a narrowing or obstruction of one or more coronary arteries as a result of atherosclerosis, which is an accumulation of lipid-containing plaque in the arteries (Fig. 60-12).
2. The disease causes decreased perfusion of myocardial tissue and inadequate myocardial oxygen supply leading to hypertension, angina, dysrhythmias, MI, heart failure, and death.
3. Collateral circulation, more than one artery supplying a muscle with blood, is normally present in the coronary arteries, especially in older persons.
4. The development of collateral circulation takes time and develops when chronic ischemia occurs to meet the metabolic demands; therefore an occlusion of a coronary artery in a younger individual is more likely to be lethal than in an older individual.
5. Symptoms occur when the coronary artery is occluded to the point that inadequate blood supply to the muscle occurs, causing ischemia.
6. Coronary artery narrowing is significant if the lumen diameter of the left main artery is reduced at least 50%, or if any major branch is reduced at least 75%.
7. The goal of treatment is to alter the atherosclerotic progression.

B. Assessment
1. Possibly normal findings during asymptomatic periods
2. Chest pain
3. Palpitations
4. Dyspnea
5. Syncope
6. Cough or hemoptysis
7. Excessive fatigue

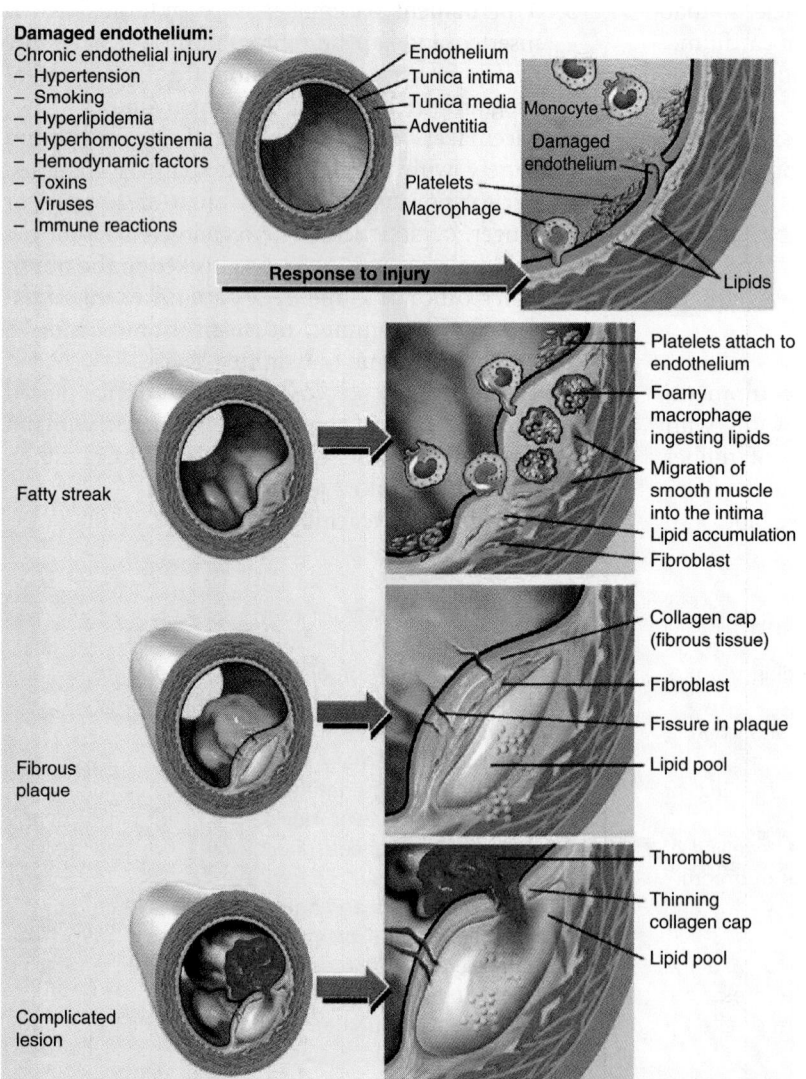

▲ FIGURE 60-12 Cross section of an atherosclerotic coronary artery. (From Ignatavicius, D., & Workman, M. [2010]. *Medical-surgical nursing: Patient-centered collaborative care* [6th ed.]. St. Louis: Saunders.)

C. Diagnostic studies
1. Electrocardiography
   a. When blood flow is reduced and ischemia occurs, ST-segment depression, T-wave inversion, or both is noted; the ST segment returns to normal when the blood flow returns.
   b. With infarction, cell injury results in ST segment elevation, followed by T wave inversion and an abnormal Q wave.
2. Cardiac catheterization
   a. Cardiac catheterization provides the most definitive source for diagnosis.
   b. Cardiac catheterization shows the presence of atherosclerotic lesions.
3. Blood lipid levels
   a. Blood lipid levels may be elevated.
   b. Cholesterol-lowering medications may be prescribed to reduce the development of atherosclerotic plaques.

D. Interventions
1. Instruct the client regarding the purpose of diagnostic medical and surgical procedures and preprocedure and postprocedure expectations.
2. Assist the client to identify risk factors that can be modified.
3. Assist the client to set goals to promote lifestyle changes to reduce the impact of risk factors.
4. Assist the client to identify barriers to compliance with the therapeutic plan and to identify methods to overcome barriers.
5. Instruct the client regarding a low-calorie, low-sodium, low-cholesterol, and low-fat diet, with an increase in dietary fiber.
6. Stress to the client that dietary changes are not temporary and must be maintained for life; instruct the client regarding prescribed medications.
7. Provide community resources to the client regarding exercise, smoking cessation, and stress reduction as appropriate.

E. Surgical procedures
1. PTCA to compress the plaque against the walls of the artery and dilate the vessel
2. Laser angioplasty to vaporize the plaque
3. Atherectomy to remove the plaque from the artery
4. Vascular stent to prevent the artery from closing and to prevent restenosis
5. Coronary artery bypass grafting to improve blood flow to the myocardial tissue at risk for ischemia or infarction because of the occluded artery

F. Medications
1. Nitrates to dilate the coronary arteries and decrease **preload** and **afterload**
2. Calcium channel blockers to dilate coronary arteries and reduce vasospasm
3. Cholesterol-lowering medications to reduce the development of atherosclerotic plaques
4. β-Blockers to reduce the **BP** in individuals who are hypertensive

VIII. ANGINA

A. Description
1. Angina is chest pain resulting from myocardial ischemia caused by inadequate myocardial blood and oxygen supply.
2. Angina is caused by an imbalance between oxygen supply and demand.
3. Causes include obstruction of coronary blood flow resulting from atherosclerosis, coronary artery spasm, or conditions increasing myocardial oxygen consumption.

⚠ The goal of treatment for angina is to provide relief of the acute attack, correct the imbalance between myocardial oxygen supply and demand, and prevent the progression of the disease and further attacks to reduce the risk of MI.

B. Patterns of angina
1. Stable angina
   a. Also called *exertional angina*
   b. Occurs with activities that involve exertion or emotional stress; relieved with rest or nitroglycerin
   c. Usually has a stable pattern of onset, duration, severity, and relieving factors
2. Unstable angina
   a. Also called *preinfarction angina*
   b. Occurs with an unpredictable degree of exertion or emotion and increases in occurrence, duration, and severity over time
   c. Pain may not be relieved with nitroglycerin.
3. Variant angina
   a. Also called *Prinzmetal's* or *vasospastic angina*
   b. Results from coronary artery spasm
   c. May occur at rest
   d. Attacks may be associated with ST segment elevation noted on the electrocardiogram (ECG).
4. Intractable angina is a chronic, incapacitating angina unresponsive to interventions.
5. Preinfarction angina
   a. Associated with acute coronary insufficiency
   b. Lasts longer than 15 minutes
   c. Symptom of worsening cardiac ischemia
   d. Occurs after an MI, when residual ischemia may cause episodes of angina

C. Assessment
1. Pain
   a. Pain can develop slowly or quickly.
   b. Pain usually is described as mild or moderate.

c. Substernal, crushing, squeezing pain may occur.
d. Pain may radiate to the shoulders, arms, jaw, neck, or back.
e. Pain intensity is unaffected by inspiration and expiration.
f. Pain usually lasts less than 5 minutes; however, pain can last up to 15 to 20 minutes.
g. Pain is relieved by nitroglycerin or rest.
2. Dyspnea
3. Pallor
4. Sweating
5. Palpitations and tachycardia
6. Dizziness and faintness
7. Hypertension
8. Digestive disturbances
D. Diagnostic studies
1. Electrocardiography: Readings are normal during rest, with ST depression, or T-wave inversion during an episode of pain.
2. Stress testing: Chest pain or changes in the electrocardiogram or vital signs during testing may indicate ischemia.
3. Cardiac enzyme and troponin levels: Findings are normal in angina.
4. Cardiac catheterization: Catheterization provides a definitive diagnosis by providing information about the patency of the coronary arteries.
E. Interventions
1. Immediate management
a. Assess pain; institute pain relief measures.
b. Administer oxygen at 3 L/min by nasal cannula as prescribed.
c. Assess vital signs and provide continuous cardiac monitoring and nitroglycerin as prescribed to dilate the coronary arteries, reduce the oxygen requirements of the myocardium, and relieve the chest pain.
d. Ensure bed rest is maintained, place the client in semi-Fowler's position, and stay with the client.
e. Obtain a 12-lead ECG.
f. Establish an IV access route.
2. Following the acute episode
a. Instruct the client regarding the purpose of diagnostic medical and surgical procedures and the preprocedure and postprocedure expectations.
b. Assist the client to identify angina-precipitating events.
c. Instruct the client to stop activity and rest if chest pain occurs and to take nitroglycerin as prescribed.
d. Instruct the client to seek medical attention if pain persists.
e. Instruct the client regarding prescribed medications.

f. Provide diet instructions to the client, stressing that dietary changes are not temporary and must be maintained for life.
g. Assist the client to identify risk factors that can be modified.
h. Assist the client to set goals that will promote changes in lifestyle to reduce the impact of risk factors.
i. Assist the client to identify barriers to compliance with the therapeutic plan and to identify methods to overcome barriers.
j. Provide community resources to the client regarding exercise, smoking cessation, and stress reduction.
F. Surgical procedures: See Section VII, Coronary Artery Disease.
G. Medications
1. See Section VII, Coronary Artery Disease.
2. Antiplatelet therapy may be prescribed; it inhibits platelet aggregation and reduces the risk of developing an acute MI.

IX. MYOCARDIAL INFARCTION

A. Description
1. Myocardial infarction occurs when myocardial tissue is abruptly and severely deprived of oxygen.
2. Ischemia can lead to necrosis of myocardial tissue if blood flow is not restored.
3. Infarction does not occur instantly but evolves over several hours.
4. Obvious physical changes do not occur in the heart until 6 hours after the infarction, when the infarcted area appears blue and swollen.
5. After 48 hours, the infarct turns gray, with yellow streaks developing as neutrophils invade the tissue.
6. By 8 to 10 days after infarction, granulation tissue forms.
7. Over 2 to 3 months, the necrotic area develops into a scar; scar tissue permanently changes the size and shape of the entire left ventricle.
8. Not all clients experience the classic symptoms of an MI.
9. Women may experience atypical discomfort, shortness of breath, or fatigue and often present with NSTEMI (non–ST elevation myocardial infarction) or T-wave inversion.
10. An older client may experience shortness of breath, pulmonary edema, dizziness, altered mental status, or a dysrhythmia.
B. Location of MI (see Fig. 60-1)
1. Obstruction of the left anterior descending artery results in anterior wall or septal MI, or both.

2. Obstruction of the circumflex artery results in posterior wall MI or lateral wall MI.
3. Obstruction of the right coronary artery results in inferior wall MI.
C. Risk factors
  1. Atherosclerosis
  2. Coronary artery disease
  3. Elevated cholesterol levels
  4. Smoking
  5. Hypertension
  6. Obesity
  7. Physical inactivity
  8. Impaired glucose tolerance
  9. Stress
D. Diagnostic studies
  1. Troponin level
    a. Level rises within 3 hours.
    b. Level remains elevated for up to 7 to 10 days.
  2. Total creatine kinase level
    a. Level rises within 6 hours after the onset of chest pain.
    b. Level peaks within 18 hours after damage and death of cardiac tissue.
  3. CK-MB isoenzyme
    a. Peak elevation occurs 18 hours after the onset of chest pain.
    b. Level returns to normal 48 to 72 hours later.
  4. Myoglobin: Level rises within 2 hours after cell death, with a rapid decline in the level after 7 hours.
  5. LDH level
    a. Level rises 24 hours after MI.
    b. Level peaks between 48 and 72 hours and falls to normal in 7 to 14 days.
    c. Serum level of LDH1 isoenzyme rises higher than serum level of LDH2.
  6. White blood cell count: An elevated white blood cell count of 10,000 to 20,000 /mm^3 appears on the second day following the MI and lasts up to 1 week.
  7. Electrocardiogram
    a. Electrocardiogram shows either ST elevation MI (STEMI), T wave inversion, or non-ST elevation MI (NSTEMI); an abnormal Q wave may also present.
    b. Hours to days after the MI, ST and T wave changes will return to normal but the Q wave changes usually remain permanently.
  8. Diagnostic tests following the acute stage
    a. Exercise tolerance test or stress test may be prescribed to assess for electrocardiographic changes and ischemia and to evaluate for medical therapy or identify clients who may need invasive therapy.

Box 60-6 Complications of Myocardial Infarction

Dysrhythmias
Heart failure
Pulmonary edema
Cardiogenic shock
Thrombophlebitis
Pericarditis
Mitral valve insufficiency
Postinfarction angina
Ventricular rupture
Dressler's syndrome (a combination of pericarditis, pericardial effusion, and pleural effusion, which can occur several weeks to months following a myocardial infarction)

---

    b. Thallium scans may be prescribed to assess for ischemia or necrotic muscle tissue.
    c. Multigated cardiac blood pool imaging scans may be used to evaluate left ventricular function.
    d. Cardiac catheterization is performed to determine the extent and location of obstructions of the coronary arteries.
E. Assessment
  1. Pain
    a. Client may experience crushing substernal pain.
    b. Pain may radiate to the jaw, back, and left arm.
    c. Pain may occur without cause, primarily early in the morning.
    d. Pain is unrelieved by rest or nitroglycerin and is relieved only by opioids.
    e. Pain lasts 30 minutes or longer.
  2. Nausea and vomiting
  3. Diaphoresis
  4. Dyspnea
  5. Dysrhythmias
  6. Feelings of fear and anxiety
  7. Pallor, cyanosis, coolness of extremities
F. Complications of MI (Box 60-6)
G. Interventions, acute stage

⚠ Pain relief increases oxygen supply to the myocardium; administer morphine as a priority in managing pain in the client having an MI.

  1. Obtain a description of the chest discomfort.
  2. Administer oxygen by nasal cannula as prescribed and institute pain relief measures (morphine, nitroglycerin as prescribed).
  3. Assess vital signs and cardiovascular status and maintain cardiac monitoring.

4. Ensure bedrest and place the client in a semi-Fowler's position to enhance comfort and tissue oxygenation; stay with the client.
5. Establish an IV access route.
6. Obtain a 12-lead ECG.
7. Administer antidysrhythmics as prescribed.
8. Administer thrombolytic therapy, which may be prescribed within the first 6 hours of the coronary event.
9. Monitor for signs of bleeding if the client is receiving thrombolytic therapy.
10. Monitor laboratory values as prescribed.
11. Administer β-blockers as prescribed to slow the heart rate and increase myocardial perfusion while reducing the force of myocardial contraction.
12. Monitor for complications related to the MI.
13. Monitor for cardiac dysrhythmias because tachycardia and PVCs frequently occur in the first few hours after MI.
14. Assess distal peripheral pulses and skin temperature because poor **cardiac output** may be identified by cool diaphoretic skin and diminished or absent pulses.
15. Monitor intake and output.
16. Assess respiratory rate and breath sounds for signs of heart failure, as indicated by the presence of crackles or wheezes or dependent edema.
17. Monitor the **BP** closely after the administration of medications; if the **BP** is lower than 100 mm Hg systolic or 25 mm Hg lower than the previous reading, lower the head of the bed and notify the physician.
18. Provide reassurance to the client and family.

H. Interventions following the acute episode
1. Maintain bed rest for the first 24 to 36 hours as prescribed.
2. Allow the client to stand to void or use a bedside commode if prescribed.
3. Provide range-of-motion exercises to prevent thrombus formation and maintain muscle strength.
4. Progress to dangling legs at the side of the bed or out of bed to the chair for 30 minutes three times a day as prescribed.
5. Progress to ambulation in the client's room and to the bathroom and then in the hallway three times a day.
6. Monitor for complications.
7. Encourage the client to verbalize feelings regarding the MI.

I. Cardiac rehabilitation: Process of actively assisting the client with cardiac disease to achieve and maintain a vital and productive life within the limitations of the heart disease.

X. HEART FAILURE

A. Description
1. Heart failure is the inability of the heart to maintain adequate **cardiac output** to meet the metabolic needs of the body because of impaired pumping ability.
2. Diminished **cardiac output** results in inadequate peripheral tissue perfusion.
3. Congestion of the lungs and periphery may occur; the client can develop acute pulmonary edema.

B. Classification
1. Acute heart failure occurs suddenly.
2. Chronic heart failure develops over time; however, a client with chronic heart failure can develop an acute episode.

C. Types of heart failure
1. Right ventricular failure, left ventricular failure
   a. Because the two ventricles of the heart represent two separate pumping systems, it is possible for one to fail alone for a short period.
   b. Most heart failure begins with left ventricular failure and progresses to failure of both ventricles.
   c. Acute pulmonary edema, a medical emergency, results from left ventricular failure.
   d. If pulmonary edema is not treated, death will occur from suffocation because the client literally drowns in his or her own fluids.
2. Forward failure, backward failure
   a. In forward failure, an inadequate output of the affected ventricle causes decreased perfusion to vital organs.
   b. In backward failure, blood backs up behind the affected ventricle, causing increased pressure in the atrium behind the affected ventricle.
3. Low output, high output
   a. In low-output failure, not enough **cardiac output** is available to meet the demands of the body.
   b. High-output failure occurs when a condition causes the heart to work harder to meet the demands of the body.
4. Systolic failure, diastolic failure
   a. Systolic failure leads to problems with contraction and ejection of blood.
   b. Diastolic failure leads to problems with the heart relaxing and filling with blood.

D. Compensatory mechanisms
1. Compensatory mechanisms act to restore **cardiac output** to near-normal levels.
2. Initially, these mechanisms increase **cardiac output**; however, they eventually have a damaging effect on pump action.

TABLE 60-1 Clinical Manifestations of Right-Sided and Left-Sided Heart Failure

Right-Sided Heart Failure	Left-Sided Heart Failure
Dependent edema (legs and sacrum)	Signs of pulmonary congestion
Jugular venous distention	Dyspnea
Abdominal distention	Tachypnea
Hepatomegaly	Crackles in the lungs
Splenomegaly	Dry, hacking cough
Anorexia and nausea	Paroxysmal nocturnal dyspnea
Weight gain	Increased blood pressure (from fluid volume excess)
Nocturnal diuresis	or decreased BP (from pump failure)
Swelling of the fingers and hands	
Increased BP (from fluid volume excess) or decreased BP (from pump failure)	

BP, Blood pressure.

3. Compensatory mechanisms contribute to an increase in myocardial oxygen consumption; when this occurs, myocardial reserve is exhausted and clinical manifestations of heart failure develop.
4. Compensatory mechanisms include increased heart rate, improved **stroke volume**, arterial vasoconstriction, sodium and water retention, and myocardial hypertrophy.

E. Assessment (Table 60-1)

1. Right- and left-sided heart failure

⚠ Signs of left ventricular failure are evident in the pulmonary system. Signs of right ventricular failure are evident in the systemic circulation.

2. Acute pulmonary edema
   a. Severe dyspnea and orthopnea
   b. Pallor
   c. Tachycardia
   d. Expectoration of large amounts of blood-tinged, frothy sputum
   e. Wheezing and crackles on auscultation
   f. Bubbling respirations
   g. Acute anxiety, apprehension, restlessness
   h. Profuse sweating
   i. Cold, clammy skin
   j. Cyanosis
   k. Nasal flaring
   l. Use of accessory breathing muscles
   m. Tachypnea
   n. Hypocapnia, evidenced by muscle cramps, weakness, dizziness, and paresthesias

F. Immediate management of acute episode (see Priority Nursing Actions)

■■■■■ **PRIORITY NURSING ACTIONS!** ■■■■■

Actions to Take If a Client Develops Pulmonary Edema

1. Place the client in a high Fowler's position.
2. Administer oxygen.
3. Assess the client quickly, including assessing lung sounds.
4. Ensure an intravenous access device is in place.
5. Prepare for the administration of a diuretic and morphine sulfate.
6. Insert a Foley catheter as prescribed.
7. Prepare for intubation and ventilator support, if required.
8. Document the event, actions taken, and the client's response.

Pulmonary edema is a life-threatening event that can result from severe heart failure. In pulmonary edema, the left ventricle fails to eject sufficient blood, and pressure increases in the lungs because of the accumulated blood. The client is immediately placed in a high Fowler's position, with the legs in a dependent position, to reduce pulmonary congestion and relieve edema. Oxygen is always prescribed, usually in high concentrations by mask or cannula to improve gas exchange and pulmonary function; the goal is to keep the oxygen saturation above 90%. The client is then assessed quickly, including checking the lung sounds. Next it is important to ensure that an IV access device is in place for the administration of a diuretic and morphine sulfate. Furosemide, a rapid-acting diuretic, will eliminate accumulated fluid. Morphine sulfate reduces venous return (preload), decreases anxiety, and also reduces the work of breathing. A Foley catheter is inserted to measure output accurately. The nurse then prepares for intubation and ventilator support, if required. The nurse stays with the client and provides reassurance. Vital signs are monitored and a cardiac monitor is used to monitor the heart rate and for dysrhythmias. The lung sounds are monitored for crackles, decreased breath sounds, and for a response to treatment. A weight measurement will also determine a response to treatment. Other interventions may include the administration of digoxin to increase ventricular contractility and improve cardiac output, bronchodilators for severe bronchospasm or bronchoconstriction, medications to facilitate myocardial contractility and enhance stroke volume, and vasodilators to reduce afterload, increase the capacity of the systemic venous bed, and decrease venous return to the heart. The nurse finally documents the event, actions taken, and the client's response.

Reference: Ignatavicius, D., & Workman, M. (2010). *Medical-surgical nursing: Patient-centered collaborative care* (6th ed., p. 775). St. Louis: Saunders.

G. Following the acute episode
   1. Encourage the client to verbalize feelings about the lifestyle changes required as a result of the heart failure.

2. Assist the client to identify precipitating risk factors of heart failure and methods of eliminating these risk factors.

3. Instruct the client in the prescribed medication regimen, which may include digoxin, a diuretic, angiotensin-converting enzyme (ACE) inhibitors, low-dose β-blockers, and vasodilators.

4. Advise the client to notify the physician if side effects occur from the medications.

5. Advise the client to avoid over-the-counter medications.

6. Instruct the client to contact the physician if he or she is unable to take medications because of illness.

7. Instruct the client to avoid large amounts of caffeine, found in coffee, tea, cocoa, chocolate, and some carbonated beverages.

8. Instruct the client about the prescribed low-sodium, low-fat, and low-cholesterol diet.

9. Provide the client with a list of potassium-rich foods because diuretics can cause hypokalemia (except for potassium-sparing diuretics).

10. Instruct the client regarding fluid restriction, if prescribed, advising the client to spread the fluid out during the day and to suck on hard candy to reduce thirst.

11. Instruct the client to balance periods of activity and rest.

12. Advise the client to avoid isometric activities, which increase pressure in the heart.

13. Instruct the client to monitor daily weight.

14. Instruct the client to report signs of fluid retention such as edema or weight gain.

XI. CARDIOGENIC SHOCK

A. Description
1. Cardiogenic shock is failure of the heart to pump adequately, thereby reducing **cardiac output** and compromising tissue perfusion.
2. Necrosis of more than 40% of the left ventricle occurs, usually as a result of occlusion of major coronary vessels.
3. The goal of treatment is to maintain tissue oxygenation and perfusion and improve the pumping ability of the heart.

B. Assessment
1. Hypotension: **BP** lower than 90 mm Hg systolic or 30 mm Hg lower than the client's baseline
2. Urine output lower than 30 mL/hr
3. Cold, clammy skin
4. Poor peripheral pulses
5. Tachycardia
6. Pulmonary congestion
7. Tachypnea
8. Disorientation, restlessness, and confusion
9. Continuing chest discomfort

C. Interventions
1. Administer morphine sulfate intravenously as prescribed to decrease pulmonary congestion and relieve pain.
2. Administer oxygen as prescribed.
3. Prepare for intubation and mechanical ventilation.
4. Administer diuretics and nitrates as prescribed while monitoring the **BP** constantly.
5. Administer vasopressors and positive inotropics as prescribed to maintain organ perfusion.
6. Prepare the client for insertion of an intra-aortic balloon pump, if prescribed, to improve coronary artery perfusion and improve **cardiac output**.
7. Prepare the client for immediate reperfusion procedures such as PTCA or coronary artery bypass graft.
8. Monitor arterial blood gas levels and prepare to treat imbalances.
9. Monitor urinary output.
10. Assist with the insertion of a pulmonary artery (Swan-Ganz) catheter to assess degree of heart failure; readings obtained from the catheter correlating to cardiogenic shock include an increased **pulmonary capillary wedge pressure (PCWP)** and a decreased **cardiac output** (Fig. 60-13).
11. Monitor distal pulses and maintain the transducer at the level of the right atrium if the client has a Swan-Ganz catheter.

D. Hemodynamic monitoring (see Fig. 60-13)
1. Central **venous pressure** (CVP)
    a. The CVP is the pressure within the superior vena cava; it reflects the pressure under which blood is returned to the superior vena cava and right atrium.
    b. The CVP is measured with a central venous line in the superior vena cava.
    c. Normal CVP pressure is about 3 to 8 mm Hg.
    d. An elevated CVP indicates an increase in blood volume as a result of sodium and water retention, excessive IV fluids, alterations in fluid balance, or renal failure.
    e. A decreased CVP indicates a decrease in circulating blood volume and may be a result of fluid imbalances, hemorrhage, or severe vasodilation, with pooling of blood in the extremities that limits venous return.
2. Measuring CVP
    a. The right atrium is located at the midaxillary line at the fourth intercostal space; the zero point on the transducer needs to be at the level of the right atrium.
    b. The client needs to be supine, with the head of the bed at 45 degrees.
    c. The client needs to be relaxed; note that activity that increases intrathoracic pressure,

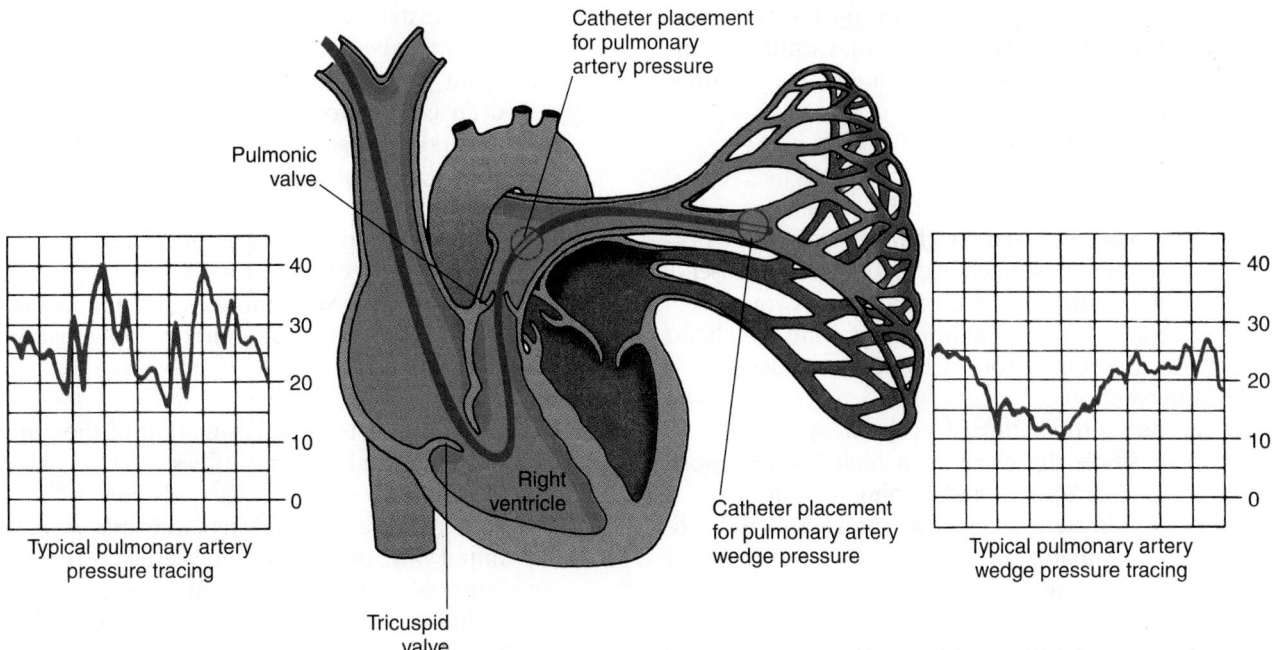

Catheter placement
for pulmonary
artery pressure

Pulmonic
valve

Right
ventricle

Catheter placement
for pulmonary artery
wedge pressure

Tricuspid
valve

Typical pulmonary artery
pressure tracing

Typical pulmonary artery
wedge pressure tracing

▲ **FIGURE 60-13** Cardiac pressure waveforms can be visualized on the monitor. (From Ignatavicius, D., & Workman, M. [2010]. *Medical-surgical nursing: Patient-centered collaborative care* [6th ed.]. St. Louis: Saunders.)

such as coughing or straining, will cause false increases in the readings.
  d. If the client is on a ventilator, the reading should be taken at the point of end-expiration.
  e. To maintain patency of the line, a constant small amount of fluid is delivered under pressure.
3. Pulmonary artery pressures
  a. A pulmonary artery catheter is used to measure right atrial and indirect left atrial pressures or pulmonary artery wedge pressure (PAWP), which is also known as pulmonary artery occlusive pressure (PAOP).
  b. Pulmonary artery wedge pressure (PAWP) normally ranges between 4 and 12 mm Hg; elevations may indicate left ventricular failure, hypervolemia, mitral regurgitation, or intracardiac shunt whereas decreases may indicate hypovolemia or **afterload** reduction.
  c. Normal right atrial (RA) pressure ranges from 1 to 8 mm Hg; increases occur with right ventricular failure, whereas decreases may indicate hypovolemia.
  d. Normal pulmonary artery pressure (PAP) ranges from 15 to 26 mm Hg systolic/5 to 15 mm Hg diastolic.
4. **Mean arterial pressure (MAP)**
  a. An approximation of the average pressure in the systemic circulation throughout the cardiac cycle; used in hemodynamic monitoring.
  b. **MAP** must be at least 60 mm Hg for adequate organ perfusion.

5. **Pulmonary capillary wedge pressure (PCWP)**
  a. The measurement obtained during momentary balloon inflation of a pulmonary artery catheter; it is reflective of left ventricular end-diastolic pressure.
  b. The **PCWP** normally ranges between 6 and 12 mm Hg; decreased **PCWP** indicates hypovolemia, whereas increased **PCWP** indicates hypervolemia, left ventricular failure, or mitral regurgitation.

XII. INFLAMMATORY DISEASES OF THE HEART

A. Pericarditis
  1. Description
    a. Pericarditis is an acute or chronic inflammation of the pericardium.
    b. Chronic pericarditis, a chronic inflammatory thickening of the pericardium, constricts the heart, causing compression.
    c. The pericardial sac becomes inflamed.
    d. Pericarditis can result in loss of pericardial elasticity or an accumulation of fluid within the sac.
    e. Heart failure or cardiac tamponade may result.
  2. Assessment
    a. Precordial pain in the anterior chest that radiates to the left side of the neck, shoulder, or back
    b. Pain is grating and is aggravated by breathing (particularly inspiration), coughing, and swallowing
    c. Pain is worse when in the supine position and may be relieved by leaning forward.

d. Pericardial friction rub (scratchy, high-pitched sound) is heard on auscultation and is produced by the rubbing of the inflamed pericardial layers.

e. Fever and chills

f. Fatigue and malaise

g. Elevated white blood cell count

h. Electrocardiographic changes with acute pericarditis; ST segment elevation with the onset of inflammation; atrial fibrillation is common.

i. Signs of right ventricular failure in clients with chronic constrictive pericarditis

3. Interventions

a. Assess the nature of the pain.

b. Position the client in a high Fowler's position, or upright and leaning forward.

c. Administer analgesics, nonsteroidal anti-inflammatory drugs, or corticosteroids for pain as prescribed.

d. Auscultate for a pericardial friction rub.

e. Check results of blood culture to identify causative organism.

f. Administer antibiotics for bacterial infection as prescribed.

g. Administer diuretics and digoxin as prescribed to the client with chronic constrictive pericarditis; surgical incision of the pericardium (pericardiectomy) may be necessary.

h. Monitor for signs of cardiac tamponade, including pulsus paradoxus, jugular vein distention with clear lung sounds, muffled heart sounds, narrowed **pulse pressure**, tachycardia, and decreased **cardiac output**.

i. Notify the physician if signs of cardiac tamponade occur.

B. Myocarditis

1. Description: Acute or chronic inflammation of the myocardium as a result of pericarditis, systemic infection, or allergic response

2. Assessment

a. Fever

b. Pericardial friction rub

c. Gallop rhythm

d. Murmur that sounds like fluid passing an obstruction

e. Pulsus alternans

f. Signs of heart failure

g. Fatigue

h. Dyspnea

i. Tachycardia

j. Chest pain

3. Interventions

a. Assist the client to a position of comfort, such as sitting up and leaning forward.

b. Administer analgesics, salicylates, and nonsteroidal anti-inflammatory drugs as prescribed to reduce fever and pain.

c. Administer oxygen as prescribed.

d. Provide adequate rest periods.

e. Limit activities to avoid overexertion and decrease the workload of the heart.

f. Administer digoxin as prescribed, and monitor for signs of digoxin toxicity.

g. Administer antidysrhythmics as prescribed.

h. Administer antibiotics as prescribed to treat the causative organism.

i. Monitor for complications, which can include thrombus, heart failure, and cardiomyopathy.

C. Endocarditis

1. Description

a. Endocarditis is an inflammation of the inner lining of the heart and valves.

b. Occurs primarily in clients who are IV drug abusers, have had valve replacements, or have mitral valve prolapse or other structural defects

c. Ports of entry for the infecting organism include the oral cavity (especially if the client has had a dental procedure in the previous 3 to 6 months), cutaneous invasion, infections, invasive procedures, or surgery.

2. Assessment

a. Fever

b. Anorexia

c. Weight loss

d. Fatigue

e. Cardiac murmurs

f. Heart failure

g. Embolic complications from vegetation fragments traveling through the circulation

h. Petechiae

i. Splinter hemorrhages in the nail beds

j. Osler's nodes (reddish tender lesions) on the pads of the fingers, hands, and toes

k. Janeway lesions (nontender hemorrhagic lesions) on the fingers, toes, nose, or earlobes

l. Splenomegaly

m. Clubbing of the fingers

3. Interventions

a. Provide adequate rest balanced with activity to prevent thrombus formation.

b. Maintain antiembolism stockings.

c. Monitor cardiovascular status.

d. Monitor for signs of heart failure.

e. Monitor for signs of emboli.

f. Monitor for splenic emboli, as evidenced by sudden abdominal pain radiating to the left shoulder and the presence of rebound abdominal tenderness on palpation.

g. Monitor for renal emboli, as evidenced by flank pain radiating to the groin, hematuria, and pyuria.

h. Monitor for confusion, aphasia, or dysphasia, which may indicate central nervous system emboli.

i. Monitor for pulmonary emboli as evidenced by pleuritic chest pain, dyspnea, and cough.

j. Assess skin, mucous membranes, and conjunctiva for petechiae.

k. Assess nail beds for splinter hemorrhages.

l. Assess for Osler's nodes on the pads of the fingers, hands, and toes.

m. Assess for Janeway lesions on the fingers, toes, nose, or earlobes.

n. Assess for clubbing of the fingers.

o. Evaluate blood culture results.

p. Administer antibiotics intravenously as prescribed.

q. Plan and arrange for discharge, providing resources required for the continued administration of IV antibiotics.

4. Client education (Box 60-7)

XIII. CARDIAC TAMPONADE

A. Description

1. A pericardial effusion occurs when the space between the parietal and visceral layers of the pericardium fills with fluid.

2. Pericardial effusion places the client at risk for cardiac tamponade, an accumulation of fluid in the pericardial cavity.

3. Tamponade restricts ventricular filling, and cardiac output drops.

⚠ Acute cardiac tamponade can occur when small volumes (20 to 50 mL) of fluid accumulate rapidly in the pericardium.

Box 60-7 Home Care Instructions for the Client With Infective Endocarditis

Teach the client to maintain aseptic technique during setup and administration of intravenous antibiotics.

Instruct the client to administer intravenous antibiotics at scheduled times to maintain the blood level.

Instruct the client to monitor intravenous catheter sites for signs of infection and report this immediately to the physician.

Instruct the client to record the temperature daily for up to 6 weeks and report fever.

Encourage oral hygiene at least twice a day with a soft toothbrush and rinse well with water after brushing.

Client should avoid use of oral irrigation devices and flossing to avoid bacteremia.

Teach the client to cleanse any skin lacerations thoroughly and apply an antibiotic ointment as prescribed.

Client should inform all health care providers of history of endocarditis and request prophylactic antibiotics prior to every invasive procedure, including dentistry.

Teach the client to observe for signs and symptoms of embolic phenomena and heart failure.

B. Assessment

1. Pulsus paradoxus
2. Increased CVP
3. Jugular venous distention with clear lungs
4. Distant, muffled heart sounds
5. Decreased **cardiac output**

C. Interventions

1. The client needs to be placed in a critical care unit for hemodynamic monitoring.

2. Administer fluids intravenously as prescribed to manage decreased **cardiac output**.

3. Prepare the client for chest x-ray or echocardiography.

4. Prepare the client for pericardiocentesis to withdraw pericardial fluid if prescribed.

5. Monitor for recurrence of tamponade following pericardiocentesis.

6. If the client experiences recurrent tamponade or recurrent effusions or develops adhesions from chronic pericarditis, a portion (pericardial window) or all of the pericardium (pericardiectomy) may be removed to allow adequate ventricular filling and contraction.

XIV. VALVULAR HEART DISEASE

A. Description

1. Valvular heart disease occurs when the heart valves cannot fully open (stenosis) or close completely (insufficiency or regurgitation).

2. Valvular heart disease prevents efficient blood flow through the heart.

B. Types

1. Mitral stenosis: Valvular tissue thickens and narrows the valve opening, preventing blood from flowing from the left atrium to the left ventricle.

2. Mitral insufficiency, regurgitation: Valve is incompetent, preventing complete valve closure during **systole**.

3. Mitral valve prolapse: Valve leaflets protrude into the left atrium during **systole**.

4. Aortic stenosis: Valvular tissue thickens and narrows the valve opening, preventing blood from flowing from the left ventricle into the aorta.

5. Aortic insufficiency: Valve is incompetent, preventing complete valve closure during **diastole**.

C. Repair procedures

1. Balloon valvuloplasty

a. Balloon valvuloplasty is an invasive nonsurgical procedure.

b. A balloon catheter is passed from the femoral vein through the atrial septum to the mitral valve or through the femoral artery to the aortic valve.

c. The balloon is inflated to enlarge the orifice.

d. Institute precautions for arterial puncture if appropriate.

e. Monitor for bleeding from the catheter insertion site.

f. Monitor for signs of systemic emboli.

g. Monitor for signs of a regurgitant valve by monitoring cardiac rhythm, heart sounds, and **cardiac output**.

2. Mitral annuloplasty: Tightening and suturing the malfunctioning valve annulus to eliminate or greatly reduce regurgitation

3. Commissurotomy, valvotomy
   a. The procedure is accomplished with cardiopulmonary bypass during open heart surgery.
   b. The valve is visualized, thrombi are removed from the atria, fused leaflets are incised, and calcium is debrided from the leaflets, thus widening the orifice.

D. Valve replacement procedures
1. Mechanical prosthetic valves: These prosthetic valves are durable.

⚠ Thromboembolism is a problem following the valve replacement with a mechanical prosthetic valve, and lifetime anticoagulant therapy is required.

2. Bioprosthetic valves
   a. Biological grafts are xenografts (valves from other species)—porcine valves (pig), bovine valves (cow), or homografts (human cadavers).
   b. The risk of clot formation is small; therefore long-term anticoagulation may not be indicated.

3. Preoperative interventions: Consult with the physician regarding discontinuing anticoagulants 72 hours before surgery.

4. Postoperative interventions
   a. Monitor closely for signs of bleeding.
   b. Monitor **cardiac output** and for signs of heart failure.
   c. Administer digoxin as prescribed to maintain **cardiac output** and prevent atrial fibrillation.
   d. Provide client teaching (Box 60-8).

E. Mitral stenosis
1. Assessment
   a. Asymptomatic initially
   b. Symptoms occur when the orifice is reduced by 50%.
   c. Dyspnea
   d. Orthopnea
   e. Paroxysmal nocturnal dyspnea
   f. Dry cough
   g. Rumbling apical diastolic murmur
   h. Right ventricular failure
   i. Hepatomegaly
   j. Neck vein distention
   k. Pitting peripheral edema
   l. Hemoptysis and pulmonary edema as pulmonary hypertension and congestion progress
   m. Development of atrial fibrillation, indicating that the client may decompensate (notify physician immediately)

2. Interventions
   a. Administer prescribed treatment for heart failure.
   b. Administer oxygen as prescribed.
   c. Provide a low-sodium diet.
   d. Administer diuretics and digoxin as prescribed.
   e. Administer antibiotics as prescribed if infective endocarditis is present.
   f. Administer antidysrhythmics and anticoagulants for atrial fibrillation as prescribed.
   g. Prepare the client for commissurotomy or valve replacement as indicated.

F. Mitral valve prolapse
1. Assessment
   a. Fatigue
   b. Atypical chest pain
   c. Palpitations
   d. Dizziness and syncope
   e. Tachycardia
   f. Systolic click

2. Interventions
   a. Administer β-blockers for chest pain and antidysrhythmics as prescribed.
   b. Administer prophylactic antibiotics as prescribed prior to invasive procedures.

G. Mitral insufficiency
1. Assessment
   a. Dyspnea
   b. Orthopnea

Box 60-8 Client Instructions Following Valve Replacement

Adequate rest is important, and fatigue is usual.

Anticoagulant therapy is necessary if a mechanical prosthetic valve has been inserted.

Instruct the client concerning hazards related to anticoagulant therapy and to notify the physician if bleeding or excessive bruising occurs.

Instruct the client concerning the importance of good oral hygiene to reduce the risk of infective endocarditis.

Brush teeth twice daily with a soft toothbrush, followed by oral rinses.

Avoid irrigation devices, electric toothbrushes, and flossing because these activities can cause the gums to bleed, allowing bacteria to enter the mucous membranes and bloodstream.

Monitor incision and report any drainage or redness.

Avoid any dental procedures for 6 months.

Heavy lifting (more than 10 lb) is to be avoided, and exercise caution when in an automobile to prevent injury to the sternal incision.

If a prosthetic valve was inserted, a soft, audible, clicking sound may be heard.

Instruct the client concerning the importance of prophylactic antibiotics before any invasive procedure and the importance of informing all health care professionals of the valvular disease history.

Obtain and wear a Medic-Alert bracelet.

c. Fatigue

d. Dizziness

e. Palpitations

f. Signs of right ventricular failure

g. Atrial fibrillation

h. Neck vein distention

i. Pitting peripheral edema

j. High-pitched systolic murmur

2. Interventions: Refer to interventions for mitral stenosis.

H. Aortic stenosis

1. Assessment

a. Dyspnea on exertion

b. Angina

c. Syncope on exertion

d. Fatigue

e. Orthopnea

f. Paroxysmal nocturnal dyspnea

g. Harsh systolic crescendo-decrescendo murmur

2. Interventions

a. Refer to interventions for mitral stenosis.

b. Prepare the client for valve replacement as indicated.

I. Aortic insufficiency

1. Assessment

a. Dyspnea

b. Orthopnea

c. Paroxysmal nocturnal dyspnea

d. Fatigue

e. Angina

f. Tachycardia

g. Blowing decrescendo diastolic murmur

2. Interventions

a. Refer to interventions for mitral stenosis.

b. Prepare the client for valve replacement as indicated.

J. Tricuspid stenosis

1. Assessment

a. Easily fatigued

b. Effort intolerance

c. Complaints of fluttering sensations in the neck (obstructed venous flow)

d. Cyanosis

e. Signs of right ventricular failure

f. Symptoms of decreased **cardiac output**

g. Ascites

h. Hepatomegaly

i. Peripheral edema

j. Rumbling diastolic murmur

k. Jugular vein distention with clear lung fields

2. Interventions

a. Refer to interventions for mitral stenosis.

b. Prepare the client for valve replacement as indicated.

K. Tricuspid insufficiency

1. Assessment

a. Asymptomatic in mild situations

b. Signs of right ventricular failure

c. Ascites

d. Hepatomegaly

e. Pleural effusion

f. Peripheral edema

g. Systolic murmur heard at the left sternal border, fourth intercostal space

2. Interventions

a. Refer to interventions for mitral stenosis.

b. Prepare the client for valve replacement as indicated.

L. Pulmonary stenosis

1. Assessment

a. Asymptomatic in a mild condition

b. Dyspnea

c. Fatigue

d. Syncope

e. Signs of right ventricular failure

f. Ascites

g. Hepatomegaly

h. Peripheral edema

i. Systolic thrill heard at left sternal border

2. Interventions

a. Refer to interventions for mitral stenosis.

b. Prepare the client for pulmonary valve commissurotomy as indicated.

M. Pulmonary insufficiency

1. Assessment

a. Asymptomatic in mild condition

b. Dyspnea

c. Fatigue

d. Syncope

e. Signs of right ventricular failure

f. Ascites

g. Hepatomegaly

h. Peripheral edema

i. Systolic thrill heard at the left sternal border

2. Interventions

a. Refer to interventions for mitral stenosis.

b. Prepare the client for valve replacement as indicated.

XV. CARDIOMYOPATHY

A. Description

1. Cardiomyopathy is a subacute or chronic disorder of the heart muscle.

2. Treatment is palliative, not curative, and the client needs to deal with numerous lifestyle changes and a shortened life span.

B. Types, signs and symptoms, and treatment (Table 60-2)

XVI. VASCULAR DISORDERS

A. Venous thrombosis

1. Description

a. Thrombus can be associated with an inflammatory process.

TABLE 60-2 Pathophysiology, Signs and Symptoms, and Treatment of Cardiomyopathies

| Dilated Cardiomyopathy | Hypertrophic Cardiomyopathy | | Restrictive Cardiomyopathy |
	Nonobstructed	Obstructed	
Pathophysiology			
Fibrosis of myocardium and endocardium Dilated chambers Mural wall thrombi prevalent	Hypertrophy of the walls Hypertrophied septum Relatively small chamber size	Same as for nonobstructed except for obstruction of left ventricular outflow tract associated with the hypertrophied septum and mitral valve incompetence	Mimics constrictive pericarditis Fibrosed walls cannot expand or contract Chambers narrowed; emboli common
Signs and Symptoms			
Fatigue and weakness Heart failure (left side) Dysrhythmias or heart block Systemic or pulmonary emboli S_3 and S_4 gallops Moderate to severe cardiomegaly	Dyspnea Angina Fatigue, syncope, palpitations Mild cardiomegaly S_4 gallop Ventricular dysrhythmias Sudden death common Heart failure	Same as for nonobstructed except with mitral regurgitation murmur Atrial fibrillation	Dyspnea and fatigue Heart failure (right sided) Mild to moderate cardiomegaly S_3 and S_4 gallops Heart block Emboli
Treatment			
Symptomatic treatment of heart failure Vasodilators Control of dysrhythmias Surgery: Heart transplant	For both: Symptomatic treatment β-Blockers Conversion of atrial fibrillation Surgery: ventriculomyotomy or muscle resection with mitral valve replacement Digoxin, nitrates, and other vasodilators contraindicated with the obstructed form		Supportive treatment of symptoms Treatment of hypertension Conversion from dysrhythmias Exercise restrictions Emergency treatment of acute pulmonary edema

From Ignatavicius, D., & Workman, M. (2010). *Medical-surgical nursing: Patient-centered collaborative care* (6th ed.). St. Louis: Saunders.

b. When a thrombus develops, inflammation occurs, thickening the vein wall and leading to embolization.
2. Types
 a. Thrombophlebitis: Thrombus associated with inflammation
 b. Phlebothrombus: Thrombus without inflammation
 c. Phlebitis: Vein inflammation associated with invasive procedures, such as IV lines

d. Deep vein thrombophlebitis: More serious than a superficial thrombophlebitis because of the risk for pulmonary embolism
3. Risks factors for thrombus formation
 a. Venous stasis from varicose veins, heart failure, immobility
 b. Hypercoaguability disorders
 c. Injury to the venous wall from IV injections; administration of vessel irritants (chemotherapy, hypertonic solutions)

d. Following surgery, particularly orthopedic and abdominal surgery
e. Pregnancy
f. Ulcerative colitis
g. Use of oral contraceptives
h. Certain malignancies
i. Fractures or other injuries of the pelvis or lower extremities

B. Phlebitis
1. Assessment
   a. Red, warm area radiating up the vein and extremity
   b. Pain and soreness
   c. Swelling
2. Interventions
   a. Apply warm moist soaks as prescribed to dilate the vein and promote circulation (assess temperature of soak before applying).
   b. Assess for signs of complications such as tissue necrosis, infection, or pulmonary embolus.

C. Deep vein thrombophlebitis
1. Assessment
   a. Calf or groin tenderness or pain with or without swelling
   b. Positive Homans' sign may be noted; however, false-positive results are common.
   c. Warm skin that is tender to touch
2. Interventions
   a. Provide bed rest as prescribed.
   b. Elevate the affected extremity above the level of the heart as prescribed.
   c. Avoid using the knee gatch or a pillow under the knees.
   d. Do not massage the extremity.
   e. Provide thigh-high or knee-high antiembolism stockings as prescribed to reduce venous stasis and assist in the venous return of blood to the heart.
   f. Administer intermittent or continuous warm, moist compresses as prescribed.
   g. Palpate the site gently, monitoring for warmth and edema.
   h. Measure and record the circumferences of the thighs and calves.
   i. Monitor for shortness of breath and chest pain, which can indicate pulmonary emboli.
   j. Administer thrombolytic therapy (tissue plasminogen activator) if prescribed, which must be initiated within 5 days after the onset of symptoms.
   k. Administer heparin therapy as prescribed to prevent enlargement of the existing clot and prevent the formation of new clots.
   l. Monitor activated partial thromboplastin time during heparin therapy.
   m. Administer warfarin (Coumadin) as prescribed following heparin therapy when the

symptoms of deep vein thrombophlebitis have resolved.
   n. Monitor prothrombin time and international normalized ratio during warfarin (Coumadin) therapy.
   o. Monitor for the hazards and side effects associated with anticoagulant therapy.
   p. Administer analgesics as prescribed to reduce pain.
   q. Administer diuretics as prescribed to reduce lower extremity edema.
   r. Provide client teaching (Box 60-9).

D. Venous insufficiency
1. Description
   a. Venous insufficiency results from prolonged venous hypertension, which stretches the veins and damages the valves.
   b. The resultant edema and venous stasis cause venous stasis ulcers, swelling, and cellulitis.
   c. Treatment focuses on decreasing edema and promoting venous return from the affected extremity.
   d. Treatment for venous stasis ulcers focuses on healing the ulcer and preventing stasis and ulcer recurrence.
2. Assessment
   a. Stasis dermatitis or brown discoloration along the ankles, extending up to the calf
   b. Edema
   c. Ulcer formation: Edges are uneven, ulcer bed is pink, and granulation is present.
3. Interventions

⚠ For venous insufficiency, leg elevation is usually prescribed to assist with the return of blood to the heart.

Box 60-9 Instructions for the Client With Deep Vein Thrombophlebitis

Instruct the client concerning the hazards of anticoagulation therapy.
Recognize the signs and symptoms of bleeding.
Avoid prolonged sitting or standing, constrictive clothing, or crossing legs when seated.
Elevate the legs for 10 to 20 minutes every few hours each day.
Plan a progressive walking program.
Inspect the legs for edema, and measure the circumference of the legs.
Wear antiembolism stockings as prescribed.
Avoid smoking.
Avoid any medications unless prescribed by the physician.
Instruct the client concerning the importance of follow-up physician visits and laboratory studies.
Obtain and wear a Medic-Alert bracelet.

a. Instruct the client to wear elastic or compression stockings during the day and evening as prescribed (instruct the client to put on elastic stockings on awakening, before getting out of bed).

b. Advise the client to put on a clean pair of elastic stockings each day; it will probably be necessary to wear the stockings for the remainder of life.

c. Instruct the client to avoid prolonged sitting or standing, constrictive clothing, or crossing legs when seated.

d. Instruct the client to elevate the legs for 10 to 20 minutes every few hours each day.

e. Instruct the client to elevate the legs above the level of the heart when in bed.

f. Instruct the client in the use of an intermittent sequential pneumatic compression system, if prescribed; instruct the client to apply the compression system twice daily for 1 hour in the morning and evening.

g. Advise the client with an open ulcer that the compression system is applied over a dressing.

4. Wound care
   a. Provide care to the wound as prescribed by the physician.
   b. Assess the client's ability to care for the wound, and initiate home care resources as necessary.
   c. If an Unna boot (dressing constructed of gauze moistened with zinc oxide) is prescribed, the physician will change it weekly.
   d. The wound is cleansed with normal saline before application of the Unna boot; povidone-iodine (Betadine) and hydrogen peroxide are not used because they destroy granulation tissue.
   e. The Unna boot is covered with an elastic wrap that hardens to promote venous return and prevent stasis.
   f. Monitor for signs of arterial occlusion from an Unna boot that may be too tight.
   g. Keep tape off the client's skin.
   h. Occlusive dressings such as polyethylene film or a hydrocolloid dressing may be used to cover the ulcer.

5. Medications
   a. Apply topical agents to wound as prescribed to debride the ulcer, eliminate necrotic tissue, and promote healing.
   b. When applying topical agents, apply an oil-based agent such as petroleum jelly (Vaseline) on surrounding skin, because debriding agents can injure healthy tissue.
   c. Administer antibiotics as prescribed if infection or cellulitis occurs.

E. Varicose veins
   1. Description
      a. Distended, protruding veins that appear darkened and tortuous are evident.

b. Vein walls weaken and dilate, and valves become incompetent.

2. Assessment
   a. Pain in the legs with dull aching after standing
   b. A feeling of fullness in the legs
   c. Ankle edema

3. Trendelenburg's test
   a. Place the client in a supine position with the legs elevated.
   b. When the client sits up, if varicosities are present, veins fill from the proximal end; veins normally fill from the distal end.

4. Interventions
   a. Assist with Trendelenburg's test.
   b. Emphasize the importance of antiembolism stockings as prescribed.
   c. Instruct the client to elevate the legs as much as possible.
   d. Instruct the client to avoid constrictive clothing and pressure on the legs.
   e. Prepare the client for sclerotherapy or vein stripping as prescribed.

5. Sclerotherapy
   a. A solution is injected into the vein, followed by the application of a pressure dressing.
   b. Incision and drainage of the trapped blood in the sclerosed vein is performed 14 to 21 days after the injection, followed by the application of a pressure dressing for 12 to 18 hours.

6. Vein stripping
   a. Varicose veins are removed if they are larger than 4 mm in diameter or if they are in clusters.
   b. Preoperatively assist the physician with vein marking.
   c. Evaluate pulses as a baseline for comparison postoperatively.
   d. Maintain elastic (Ace) bandages on the client's legs postoperatively.
   e. Monitor the groin and leg for bleeding through the elastic bandages.
   f. Monitor the extremity for edema, warmth, color, and pulses.
   g. Assess for paresthesias, which could include saphenous nerve damage.
   h. Elevate the legs above the level of the heart postoperatively.
   i. Encourage range-of-motion exercises of the legs.
   j. Instruct the client to avoid leg dangling or chair sitting.
   k. Instruct the client to elevate the legs when sitting.
   l. Emphasize the importance of wearing elastic stockings after bandage removal.

7. Laser therapy: A laser fiber is used to heat and close the main vessel contributing to the varicosity.

XVII. ARTERIAL DISORDERS

A. Peripheral arterial disease

1. Description
   a. Chronic disorder in which partial or total arterial occlusion deprives the lower extremities of oxygen and nutrients
   b. Tissue damage occurs below the level of the arterial occlusion.
   c. Atherosclerosis is the most common cause of peripheral arterial disease.

2. Assessment
   a. Intermittent claudication (pain in the muscles resulting from an inadequate blood supply)
   b. Rest pain, characterized by numbness, burning, or aching in the distal portion of the lower extremities, which awakens the client at night and is relieved by placing the extremity in a dependent position
   c. Lower back or buttock discomfort
   d. Loss of hair and dry scaly skin on the lower extremities
   e. Thickened toenails
   f. Cold and gray-blue color of skin in the lower extremities
   g. Elevational pallor and dependent rubor in the lower extremities
   h. Decreased or absent peripheral pulses
   i. Signs of arterial ulcer formation occurring on or between the toes or on the upper aspect of the foot that are characterized as painful
   j. **BP** measurements at the thigh, calf, and ankle are lower than the brachial pressure (normally, **BP** readings in the thigh and calf are higher than those in the upper extremities).

3. Interventions

   ⚠ Because swelling in the extremities prevents arterial blood flow, the client with peripheral arterial disease is instructed to elevate the feet at rest but to refrain from elevating them above the level of the heart because extreme elevation slows arterial blood flow to the feet. In severe cases of peripheral arterial disease, clients with edema may sleep with the affected limb hanging from the bed or they may sit upright (without leg elevation) in a chair for comfort.

   a. Assess pain.
   b. Monitor the extremities for color, motion and sensation, and pulses.
   c. Obtain **BP** measurements.
   d. Assess for signs of ulcer formation or signs of gangrene.
   e. Assist in developing an individualized exercise program, which is initiated gradually and slowly increased.
   f. Encourage prescribed exercise, which will improve arterial flow through the development of collateral circulation.
   g. Instruct the client to walk to the point of claudication, stop and rest, and then walk a little farther.
   h. Instruct the client with peripheral arterial disease to avoid crossing the legs, which interferes with blood flow.
   i. Instruct the client to avoid exposure to cold (causes vasoconstriction) to the extremities and to wear socks or insulated shoes for warmth at all times.
   j. Instruct the client never to apply direct heat to the limb, such as with a heating pad or hot water, because the decreased sensitivity in the limb will cause burning.
   k. Instruct the client to inspect the skin on the extremities daily and to report any signs of skin breakdown.
   l. Instruct the client to avoid tobacco and caffeine because of their vasoconstrictive effects.
   m. Instruct the client in the use of hemorheological and antiplatelet medications as prescribed.
   n. Inform the client of the importance of taking all medications prescribed by the physician.

4. Procedures to improve arterial blood flow
   a. Percutaneous transluminal angioplasty, with or without intravascular stent
   b. Laser-assisted angioplasty
   c. Atherectomy
   d. Bypass surgery: Inflow procedures bypass the occlusion above the superficial femoral arteries and include aortoiliac, aortofemoral, and axillofemoral bypasses; outflow procedures bypass the occlusion at or below the superficial femoral arteries and include femoropopliteal and femorotibial bypass (Fig. 60-14).

B. Raynaud's disease

1. Description
   a. Raynaud's disease is vasospasm of the arterioles and arteries of the upper and lower extremities.
   b. Vasospasm causes constriction of the cutaneous vessels.
   c. Attacks are intermittent and occur with exposure to cold or stress.
   d. Affects primarily fingers, toes, ears, and cheeks

2. Assessment
   a. Blanching of the extremity, followed by cyanosis during vasoconstriction
   b. Reddened tissue when the vasospasm is relieved
   c. Numbness, tingling, swelling, and a cold temperature at the affected body part

3. Interventions
   a. Monitor pulses.
   b. Administer vasodilators as prescribed.

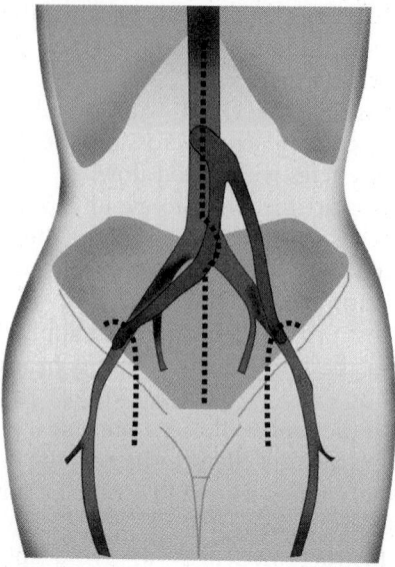

▲ **FIGURE 60-14** In aortoiliac and aortofemoral bypass surgery, a midline incision into the abdominal cavity is required, with an additional incision in each groin. (From Ignatavicius, D., & Workman, M. [2010]. *Medical-surgical nursing: Patient-centered collaborative care* [6th ed.]. St. Louis: Saunders.)

    c. Instruct the client regarding medication therapy.
    d. Assist the client to identify and avoid precipitating factors such as cold and stress.
    e. Instruct the client to avoid smoking.
    f. Instruct the client to wear warm clothing, socks, and gloves in cold weather.
    g. Advise the client to avoid injuries to fingers and hands.

C. Buerger's disease (thromboangiitis obliterans)
  1. Description
    a. Buerger's disease is an occlusive disease of the median and small arteries and veins.
    b. The distal upper and lower limbs are affected most commonly.
  2. Assessment
    a. Intermittent claudication
    b. Ischemic pain occurring in the digits while at rest
    c. Aching pain that is more severe at night
    d. Cool, numb, or tingling sensation
    e. Diminished pulses in the distal extremities
    f. Extremities that are cool and red in the dependent position
    g. Development of ulcerations in the extremities
  3. Interventions
    a. Instruct the client to stop smoking.
    b. Monitor pulses.
    c. Instruct the client to avoid injury to the upper and lower extremities.
    d. Administer vasodilators as prescribed.
    e. Instruct the client regarding medication therapy.

XVIII. AORTIC ANEURYSMS

A. Description
  1. An aortic aneurysm is an abnormal dilation of the arterial wall caused by localized weakness and stretching in the medial layer or wall of an artery.
  2. The aneurysm can be located anywhere along the abdominal aorta.
  3. The goal of treatment is to limit the progression of the disease by modifying risk factors, controlling the **BP** to prevent strain on the aneurysm, recognizing symptoms early, and preventing rupture.

B. Types of aortic aneurysm
  1. Fusiform: Diffuse dilation that involves the entire circumference of the arterial segment
  2. Saccular: Distinct localized outpouching of the artery wall
  3. Dissecting: Created when blood separates the layers of the artery wall, forming a cavity between them
  4. False (pseudoaneurysm)
    a. Pseudoaneurysm occurs when the clot and connective tissue are outside the arterial wall.
    b. Pseudoaneurysm occurs as a result of vessel injury or trauma to all three layers of the arterial wall.

C. Assessment
  1. Thoracic aneurysm
    a. Pain extending to neck, shoulders, lower back, or abdomen
    b. Syncope
    c. Dyspnea
    d. Increased pulse
    e. Cyanosis
    f. Weakness
    g. Hoarseness, difficulty swallowing because of pressure from the aneurysm
  2. Abdominal aneurysm
    a. Prominent, pulsating mass in abdomen, at or above the umbilicus
    b. Systolic bruit over the aorta
    c. Tenderness on deep palpation
    d. Abdominal or lower back pain
  3. Rupturing aneurysm
    a. Severe abdominal or back pain
    b. Lumbar pain radiating to the flank and groin
    c. Hypotension
    d. Increased pulse rate
    e. Signs of shock
    f. Hematoma at flank area
  4. Diagnostic tests
    a. Diagnostic tests are done to confirm the presence, size, and location of the aneurysm.
    b. Tests includes abdominal ultrasound, computed tomography scan, and arteriography.
  5. Interventions
    a. Monitor vital signs.
    b. Assess risk factors for the arterial disease process.

c. Obtain information regarding back or abdominal pain.

d. Question the client regarding the sensation of pulsation in the abdomen.

e. Inspect the skin for the presence of vascular disease or breakdown.

f. Check peripheral circulation, including pulses, temperature, and color.

g. Observe for signs of rupture.

h. Note any tenderness over the abdomen.

i. Monitor for abdominal distention.

6. Nonsurgical interventions

a. Modify risk factors.

b. Instruct the client regarding the procedure for monitoring **BP**.

c. Instruct the client on the importance of regular physician visits to follow the size of the aneurysm.

d. Instruct the client that if severe back or abdominal pain or fullness, soreness over the umbilicus, sudden development of discoloration in the extremities, or a persistent elevation of **BP** occurs to notify the physician immediately.

⚠ Instruct the client with an aortic aneurysm to report immediately the occurrence of chest or back pain, shortness of breath, difficulty swallowing, or hoarseness.

D. Pharmacological interventions

1. Administer antihypertensives to maintain the **BP** within normal limits and to prevent strain on the aneurysm.

2. Instruct the client about the purpose of the medications.

3. Instruct the client about the side effects and schedule of the medication.

E. Abdominal aortic aneurysm resection

1. Description: Surgical resection or excision of the aneurysm; the excised section is replaced with a graft that is sewn end to end (Fig. 60-15).

2. Preoperative interventions

a. Assess all peripheral pulses as a baseline for postoperative comparison.

b. Instruct the client in coughing and deep-breathing exercises.

c. Administer bowel preparation as prescribed.

3. Postoperative interventions

a. Monitor vital signs.

b. Monitor peripheral pulses distal to the graft site.

c. Monitor for signs of graft occlusion, including changes in pulses, cool to cold extremities below the graft, white or blue extremities or flanks, severe pain, or abdominal distention.

d. Limit elevation of the head of the bed to 45 degrees to prevent flexion of the graft.

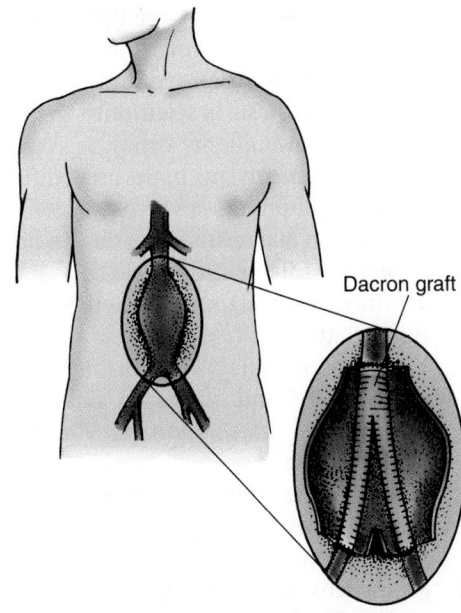

▲ **FIGURE 60-15** Surgical repair of an abdominal aortic aneurysm with a woven Dacron graft. (From Ignatavicius, D., & Workman, M. [2006]. *Medical-surgical nursing: Critical thinking for collaborative care* [5th ed.]. St. Louis: Saunders.)

e. Monitor for hypovolemia and renal failure resulting from significant blood loss during surgery.

f. Monitor urine output hourly, and notify the physician if it is lower than 30 to 50 mL/hr.

g. Monitor serum creatinine and blood urea nitrogen levels daily.

h. Monitor respiratory status and auscultate breath sounds to identify respiratory complications.

i. Encourage turning, coughing and deep breathing, and splinting the incision.

j. Ambulate as prescribed.

k. Maintain nasogastric tube to low suction until bowel sounds return.

l. Assess for bowel sounds and report their return to the physician

m. Monitor for pain and administer medication as prescribed.

n. Assess incision site for bleeding or signs of infection.

o. Prepare the client for discharge by providing instructions regarding pain management, wound care, and activity restrictions.

p. Instruct the client not to lift objects heavier than 15 to 20 lb for 6 to 12 weeks.

q. Advise the client to avoid activities requiring pushing, pulling, or straining.

r. Instruct the client not to drive a vehicle until approved by the physician.

F. Thoracic aneurysm repair

1. Description

a. A thoracotomy or median sternotomy approach is used to enter the thoracic cavity.

b. The aneurysm is exposed and excised, and a graft or prosthesis is sewn onto the aorta.

c. Total cardiopulmonary bypass is necessary for excision of aneurysms in the ascending aorta.

d. Partial cardiopulmonary bypass is used for clients with an aneurysm in the descending aorta.

2. Postoperative interventions

a. Monitor vital signs and neurological and renal status.

b. Monitor for signs of hemorrhage, such as a drop in **BP** and increased pulse rate and respirations, and report to the physician immediately.

c. Monitor chest tubes for an increase in chest drainage, which may indicate bleeding or separation at the graft site.

d. Assess sensation and motion of all extremities and notify the physician if deficits are noted, which can occur because of a lack of blood supply to the spinal cord during surgery.

e. Monitor respiratory status and auscultate breath sounds to identify respiratory complications.

f. Encourage turning, coughing, and deep breathing while splinting the incision.

g. Monitor cardiac status for dysrhythmias.

h. Monitor for pain and administer medication as prescribed.

i. Assess the incision site for bleeding or signs of infection.

j. Prepare the client for discharge by providing instructions regarding pain management, wound care, and activity restrictions.

k. Instruct the client not to lift objects heavier than 15 to 20 lb for 6 to 12 weeks.

l. Advise the client to avoid activities requiring pushing, pulling, or straining.

m. Instruct the client not to drive a vehicle until approved by the physician.

XIX. EMBOLECTOMY

A. Description

1. Embolectomy is removal of an embolus from an artery using a catheter.

2. A patch graft may be required to close the artery.

B. Preoperative interventions

1. Obtain a baseline vascular assessment.

2. Administer anticoagulants as prescribed.

3. Administer thrombolytics as prescribed.

4. Place a bed cradle on the bed.

5. Avoid bumping or jarring the bed.

6. Maintain the extremity in a slightly dependent position.

C. Postoperative interventions

1. Assess cardiac, respiratory, and neurological status.

2. Monitor affected extremity for color, temperature, and pulse.

3. Assess sensory and motor function of the affected extremity.

4. Monitor for signs and symptoms of new thrombi or emboli.

5. Administer oxygen as prescribed.

6. Monitor pulse oximetry.

7. Monitor for complications caused by reperfusion of the artery, such as spasms and swelling of the skeletal muscles.

8. Monitor for signs of swollen skeletal muscles such as edema, pain on passive movement, poor capillary refill, numbness, and muscle tenseness.

9. Maintain bed rest initially, with the client in a semi-Fowler's position.

10. Place a bed cradle on the bed.

11. Check the incision site for bleeding or hematoma.

12. Administer anticoagulants as prescribed.

13. Monitor laboratory values related to anticoagulant therapy.

14. Instruct the client to recognize the signs and symptoms of infection and edema.

15. Instruct the client to avoid prolonged sitting or crossing the legs when sitting.

16. Instruct the client to elevate the legs when sitting.

17. Instruct the client to wear antiembolism stockings as prescribed and how to remove and reapply the stockings

18. Instruct the client to ambulate daily.

19. Instruct the client about anticoagulant therapy and the hazards associated with anticoagulants.

XX. VENA CAVAL FILTER AND LIGATION OF INFERIOR VENA CAVA

A. Vena caval filter: Insertion of an intracaval filter (umbrella) that partially occludes the inferior vena cava and traps emboli to prevent pulmonary emboli (Fig. 60-16)

B. Ligation: Suturing or placing clips on the inferior vena cava to prevent pulmonary emboli; done via abdominal laparotomy

C. Preoperative interventions: If the client has been taking an anticoagulant, consult with the physician regarding discontinuation of the medication to prevent hemorrhage.

D. Postoperative interventions

1. Monitor vital signs.

2. Assess cardiac, respiratory, neurological, and renal status.

3. Administer oxygen as prescribed.

4. Monitor pulse oximetry.

5. Maintain a semi-Fowler's position.

6. Avoid hip flexion.

7. Provide activity as prescribed.

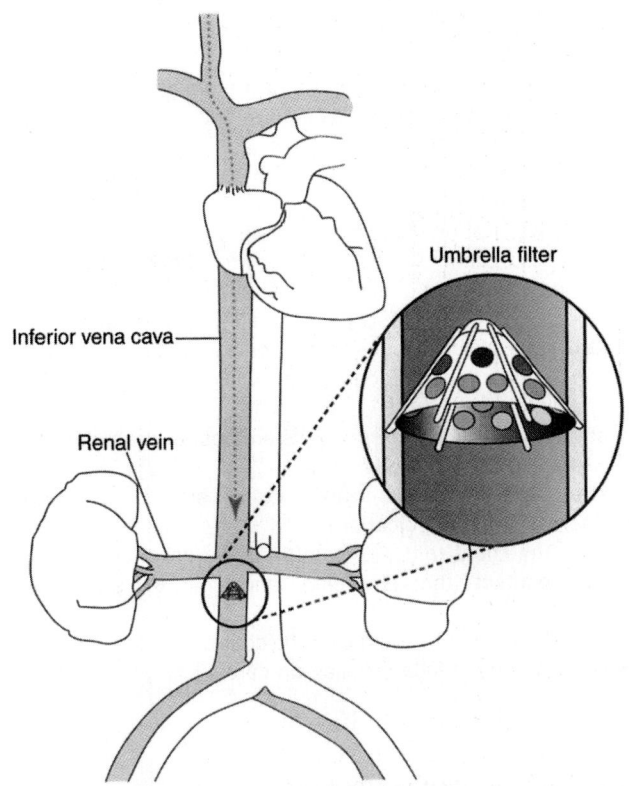

Umbrella filter

Inferior vena cava

Renal vein

▲ **FIGURE 60-16** An inferior vena caval filter. (From Ignatavicius, D., & Workman, M. [2006]. *Medical-surgical nursing: Critical thinking for collaborative care* [5th ed.]. St. Louis: Saunders.)

8. Check the insertion site for bleeding or hematoma and signs or symptoms of infection.
9. Assess for peripheral edema.
10. Maintain antiembolism stockings as prescribed.
11. Monitor laboratory values related to anticoagulant therapy.
12. Instruct the client to recognize the signs and symptoms of infection and edema.
13. Instruct the client to avoid prolonged sitting or crossing the legs when sitting.
14. Instruct the client to elevate the legs when sitting.
15. Instruct the client to wear antiembolism stockings as prescribed and how to remove and reapply the stockings.
16. Instruct the client to ambulate daily.
17. Instruct the client about anticoagulant therapy and the hazards associated with anticoagulants.

XXI. HYPERTENSION

A. Description
1. For an adult (ages 18 and older), a normal **BP** is a systolic **BP** below 120 mm Hg and a diastolic below 80 mm Hg.
2. An individual classified with prehypertension has a systolic **BP** between 120 and 139 mm Hg or a **diastolic pressure** between 80 and 89 mm Hg.

Table 60-3 Hypertension

Organ Involvement	Complications
Eyes	Visual changes
Brain	Stroke
Cardiovascular system	Heart failure, hypertensive crisis
Kidneys	Renal failure

3. Stage 1 hypertension can be classified as a systolic **BP** between 140 and 159 mm Hg or a **diastolic pressure** between 90 and 99 mm Hg.
4. Stage 2 hypertension can be classified as a systolic **BP** equal to or greater than 160 mm Hg or a **diastolic pressure** equal to or greater than 100 mm Hg.
5. Hypertension is a major risk factor for coronary, cerebral, renal, and peripheral vascular disease.
6. The disease is initially asymptomatic.
7. The goals of treatment include reduction of the **BP** and preventing or lessening the extent of organ damage (Table 60-3).
8. Nonpharmacological approaches, such as lifestyle changes, may be prescribed initially; if the **BP** cannot be decreased after a reasonable time period (1 to 3 months), the client may require pharmacological treatment.

B. Primary or essential hypertension
1. No known cause
2. Risk factors
   a. Aging
   b. Family history
   c. Black race, with higher prevalence in males
   d. Obesity
   e. Smoking
   f. Stress
   g. Excessive alcohol
   h. Hyperlipidemia
   i. Increased intake of salt or caffeine

C. Secondary hypertension
1. Treatment depends on the cause and the organs involved.
2. Secondary hypertension occurs as a result of other disorders or conditions.
3. Precipitating disorders or conditions
   a. Cardiovascular disorders
   b. Renal disorders
   c. Endocrine system disorders
   d. Pregnancy
   e. Medications (e.g., estrogens, glucocorticoids, mineralocorticoids)

D. Assessment
1. May be asymptomatic
2. Headache
3. Visual disturbances
4. Dizziness
5. Chest pain
6. Tinnitus

Box 60-10 Client Education for Hypertension

Describe the importance of compliance with the treatment plan.

Describe the disease process, explaining that symptoms usually do not develop until organs have suffered damage.

Initiate and assist the client in planning a regular exercise program, avoiding heavy weight-lifting and isometric exercises.

Emphasize the importance of beginning the exercise program gradually.

Encourage the client to express feelings about daily stress.

Assist the client to identify ways to reduce stress.

Teach relaxation techniques.

Instruct the client in how to incorporate relaxation techniques into the daily living pattern.

Instruct the client and family in the technique for monitoring blood pressure.

Instruct the client to maintain a diary of blood pressure readings.

Emphasize the importance of lifelong medication and the need for follow-up treatment.

Instruct the client and family about the dietary restrictions, which may include sodium, fat, calories, and cholesterol.

Instruct the client in how to shop for and prepare low-sodium meals.

Provide a list of products that contain sodium.

Instruct the client to read labels of products to determine sodium content, focusing on substances listed as sodium, NaCl, or MSG (monosodium glutamate).

Instruct the client to bake, roast, or boil foods, avoid salt in preparation of foods, and avoid using salt at the table.

Instruct the client that fresh foods are best to consume and to avoid canned foods.

Instruct the client about the actions, side effects, and scheduling of medications.

Advise the client that if uncomfortable side effects occur to contact the physician and not to stop the medication.

Instruct the client to avoid over-the-counter medications.

Stress the importance of follow-up care.

---

7. Flushed face
8. Epistaxis

E. Interventions

1. Goals
   a. One treatment goal is to reduce the **BP**.
   b. Another treatment goal is to prevent or lessen the extent of organ damage.
2. Question the client regarding the signs and symptoms indicative of hypertension.
3. Obtain the **BP** two or more times on both arms, with the client supine and standing.
4. Compare the **BP** with prior documentation.
5. Determine family history of hypertension.
6. Identify current medication therapy.
7. Obtain weight.
8. Evaluate dietary patterns and sodium intake.
9. Assess for visual changes or retinal damage.
10. Assess for cardiovascular changes such as distended neck veins, increased heart rate, and dysrhythmias.
11. Evaluate chest x-ray for heart enlargement.
12. Assess the neurological system.
13. Evaluate renal function.
14. Evaluate results of diagnostic and laboratory studies.

F. Nonpharmacological interventions

1. Weight reduction, if necessary, or maintenance of ideal weight
2. Dietary sodium restriction to 2 g daily as prescribed
3. Moderate intake of alcohol and caffeine-containing products
4. Initiation of a regular exercise program

5. Avoidance of smoking
6. Relaxation techniques and biofeedback therapy
7. Elimination of unnecessary medications that may contribute to the hypertension

G. Pharmacological interventions

1. Medication therapy is individualized for each client and the selection of the medication is based on such factors as the client's age, culture, presence of coexisting conditions, severity of the hypertension, and client's preferences.
2. See Chapter 61 for medications to treat hypertension.

H. See Box 60-10 for client education.

XXII. HYPERTENSIVE CRISIS

A. Description

1. A hypertensive crisis is any clinical condition requiring immediate reduction in **BP**.
2. A hypertensive crisis is an acute and life-threatening condition.
3. The accelerated hypertension requires emergency treatment because target organ damage (brain, heart, kidneys, retina of the eye) can occur quickly.
4. Death can be caused by stroke, renal failure, or cardiac disease.

B. Assessment

1. An extremely high **BP**; usually the **diastolic pressure** is higher than 120 mm Hg
2. Headache
3. Drowsiness and confusion
4. Blurred vision
5. Changes in neurological status
6. Tachycardia and tachypnea

7. Dyspnea
8. Cyanosis
9. Seizures

C. Interventions
1. Maintain a patent airway.
2. Administer antihypertensive medications intravenously as prescribed.
3. Monitor vital signs, assessing the **BP** every 5 minutes.
4. Maintain bed rest, with the head of the bed elevated at 45 degrees.
5. Assess for hypotension during the administration of antihypertensives; place the client in a supine position if hypotension occurs.
6. Have emergency medications and resuscitation equipment readily available.
7. Monitor IV therapy, assessing for fluid overload.
8. Monitor intake and output.
9. Insert a Foley catheter as prescribed.
10. Monitor urinary output; if oliguria or anuria occurs, notify the physician.

 MORE QUESTIONS ON THE CD!

Practice Questions

692. A client is admitted to an emergency department with chest pain that is being ruled out for myocardial infarction. Vital signs are as follows: at 11 AM, pulse (P), 92 beats/min, respiratory rate (RR), 24 breaths/min, blood pressure (BP), 140/88 mm Hg; 11:15 AM, P, 96 beats/min, RR, 26 breaths/min, BP, 128/82 mm Hg; 11:30 AM, P, 104 beats/min, RR, 28 breaths/min, BP, 104/68 mm Hg; 11:45 AM, P, 118 beats/min, RR, 32 breaths/min, BP, 88/58 mm Hg. The nurse should alert the physician because these changes are most consistent with which of the following complications?
1. Cardiogenic shock
2. Cardiac tamponade
3. Pulmonary embolism
4. Dissecting thoracic aortic aneurysm

693. A client admitted to the hospital with chest pain and history of type 2 diabetes mellitus is scheduled for cardiac catheterization. Which of the following medications would need to be withheld for 48 hours before and after the procedure?
1. Regular insulin
2. Glipizide (Glucotrol)
3. Repaglinide (Prandin)
4. Metformin (Glucophage)

694. A client is in sinus bradycardia with a heart rate of 45 beats/min, complains of dizziness, and

has a blood pressure of 82/60 mm Hg. Which of the following should the nurse anticipate will be prescribed?
1. Defibrillate the client.
2. Administer digoxin (Lanoxin).
3. Continue to monitor the client.
4. Prepare for transcutaneous pacing.

695. A nurse notes that a client with sinus rhythm has a premature ventricular contraction that falls on the T wave of the preceding beat. The client's rhythm suddenly changes to one with no P waves, no definable QRS complexes, and coarse wavy lines of varying amplitude. How would the nurse correctly interpret this rhythm?
1. Asystole
2. Atrial fibrillation
3. Ventricular fibrillation
4. Ventricular tachycardia

696. A client with myocardial infarction suddenly becomes tachycardic, shows signs of air hunger, and begins coughing frothy, pink-tinged sputum. Which of the following would the nurse anticipate when auscultating the client's breath sounds?
1. Stridor
2. Crackles
3. Scattered rhonchi
4. Diminished breath sounds

697. A client with myocardial infarction is developing cardiogenic shock. Because of the risk of myocardial ischemia, for which of the following should the nurse carefully assess the client?
1. Bradycardia
2. Ventricular dysrhythmias
3. Rising diastolic blood pressure
4. Falling central venous pressure

698. A client who had cardiac surgery 24 hours ago has a urine output averaging 20 mL/hr for 2 hours. The client received a single bolus of 500 mL of intravenous fluid. Urine output for the subsequent hour was 25 mL. Daily laboratory results indicate that the blood urea nitrogen level is 45 mg/dL and the serum creatinine level is 2.2 mg/dL. Based on these findings, the nurse would anticipate that the client is at risk for which of the following?
1. Hypovolemia
2. Acute renal failure
3. Glomerulonephritis
4. Urinary tract infection

699. The nurse is reviewing an electrocardiogram rhythm strip. The P waves and QRS complexes are regular. The PR interval is 0.16 second, and

QRS complexes measure 0.06 second. The overall heart rate is 64 beats/min. Which of the following would be a correct interpretation based on these characteristics?
1. Sinus bradycardia
2. Sick sinus syndrome
3. Normal sinus rhythm
4. First-degree heart block

700. A client is wearing a continuous cardiac monitor, which begins to sound its alarm. A nurse sees no electrocardiographic complexes on the screen. Which of the following should be the priority action of the nurse?
1. Call a code blue.
2. Call the physician.
3. Check the client status and lead placement.
4. Press the recorder button on the electrocardiogram console.

701. A nurse is watching the cardiac monitor and notices that the rhythm suddenly changes. There are no P waves, the QRS complexes are wide, and the ventricular rate is regular but more than 100 beats/min. The nurse determines that the client is experiencing which of the following dysrhythmias?
1. Sinus tachycardia
2. Ventricular fibrillation
3. Ventricular tachycardia
4. Premature ventricular contractions

702. A client has frequent bursts of ventricular tachycardia on the cardiac monitor. What should the nurse be most concerned about with this dysrhythmia?
1. It can develop into ventricular fibrillation at any time.
2. It is almost impossible to convert to a normal rhythm.
3. It is uncomfortable for the client, giving a sense of impending doom.
4. It produces a high cardiac output that quickly leads to cerebral and myocardial ischemia.

703. A client is having frequent premature ventricular contractions. A nurse would place priority on assessment of which of the following?
1. Sensation of palpitations
2. Causative factors, such as caffeine
3. Precipitating factors, such as infection
4. Blood pressure and oxygen saturation

704. A client has developed atrial fibrillation, with a ventricular rate of 150 beats/min. The nurse should assess the client for which associated signs or symptoms?

1. Flat neck veins
2. Nausea and vomiting
3. Hypotension and dizziness
4. Hypertension and headache

705. A nurse is watching the cardiac monitor, and a client's rhythm suddenly changes. There are no P waves; instead, there are fibrillatory waves before each QRS complex. How should the nurse correctly interpret the client's heart rhythm?
1. Atrial fibrillation
2. Sinus tachycardia
3. Ventricular fibrillation
4. Ventricular tachycardia

706. A nurse is preparing to defibrillate a client in ventricular fibrillation. After placing the paddles on the client's chest and before discharging them, which of the following should be done?
1. Ensure that the client has been intubated.
2. Set the defibrillator to the "synchronize" mode.
3. Administer lidocaine hydrochloride (Xylocaine).
4. Confirm that the rhythm is actually ventricular fibrillation.

707. A client in ventricular fibrillation is about to be defibrillated. A nurse knows that to convert this rhythm effectively, the biphasic defibrillator should be set at which of the following energy levels (in joules, J)?
1. 50 J
2. 80 J
3. 200 J
4. 360 J

708. A nurse would evaluate that defibrillation of a client was most successful if which of the following observations was made?
1. Arousable, sinus rhythm, BP 116/72 mm Hg
2. Arousable, marked bradycardia, BP 86/54 mm Hg
3. Nonarousable, supraventricular tachycardia, BP 122/60 mm Hg
4. Nonarousable, sinus rhythm, BP 88/60 mm Hg

709. A nurse is evaluating a client's response to cardioversion. Which of the following observations would be of highest priority to the nurse?
1. Blood pressure
2. Status of airway
3. Oxygen flow rate
4. Level of consciousness

710. A nurse is caring for a client who has just had implantation of an automatic internal cardioverter-defibrillator. The nurse immediately would

assess which of the following items based on priority?
1. Anxiety level of the client and family
2. Presence of a Medic-Alert card for the client to carry
3. Knowledge of restrictions of postdischarge physical activity
4. Activation status of the device, heart rate cut-off, and number of shocks it is programmed to deliver

711. A client's electrocardiogram strip shows atrial and ventricular rates of 110 beats/min. The PR interval is 0.14 second, the QRS complex measures 0.08 second, and the PP and RR intervals are regular. How should the nurse correctly interpret this rhythm?
1. Sinus dysrhythmia
2. Sinus tachycardia
3. Sinus bradycardia
4. Normal sinus rhythm

712. A nurse is assessing the neurovascular status of a client who returned to the surgical nursing unit 4 hours ago after undergoing aortoiliac bypass graft. The affected leg is warm, and the nurse notes redness and edema. The pedal pulse is palpable and unchanged from admission. How would the nurse correctly interpret the client's neurovascular status?
1. The neurovascular status is normal because of increased blood flow through the leg.
2. The neurovascular status is moderately impaired, and the surgeon should be called.
3. The neurovascular status is slightly deteriorating and should be monitored for another hour.
4. The neurovascular status is adequate from an arterial approach, but venous complications are arising.

713. A nurse is evaluating the condition of a client after pericardiocentesis performed to treat cardiac tamponade. Which of the following observations would indicate that the procedure was unsuccessful?
1. Rising blood pressure
2. Clearly audible heart sounds
3. Client expressions of relief
4. Rising central venous pressure

714. A nurse is caring for a client who had a resection of an abdominal aortic aneurysm yesterday. The client has an intravenous infusion with a rate of 150 mL/hr, unchanged for the last 10 hours. The client's urine output for the last 3 hours was 90, 50, and 28 mL (28 mL most recent). The client's blood urea nitrogen level is 35 mg/dL and serum creatinine level is 1.8 mg/dL, measured this morning. Which of the following actions should the nurse take next?
1. Call the physician.
2. Check the urine specific gravity.
3. Check to see if the client had a sample for serum albumin level drawn.
4. Put the intravenous line on a pump so that the infusion rate is sure to stay stable.

715. A client with angina complains that the anginal pain is prolonged and severe and occurs at the same time each day, most often at rest in the absence of precipitating factors. How would the nurse best describe this type of anginal pain?
1. Stable angina
2. Variant angina
3. Unstable angina
4. Nonanginal pain

Alternate Item Format: Multiple Response

716. A nurse in a medical unit is caring for a client with heart failure. The client suddenly develops extreme dyspnea, tachycardia, and lung crackles and the nurse suspects pulmonary edema. The nurse immediately asks another nurse to contact the physician and prepares to implement which priority interventions? **Select all that apply.**
❑ 1. Administering oxygen
❑ 2. Inserting a Foley catheter
❑ 3. Administering furosemide (Lasix)
❑ 4. Administering morphine sulfate intravenously
❑ 5. Transporting the client to the coronary care unit
❑ 6. Placing the client in a low Fowler's side-lying position

ANSWERS

692. 1

Rationale: Cardiogenic shock occurs with severe damage (more than 40%) to the left ventricle. Classic signs include hypotension, a rapid pulse that becomes weaker, decreased urine output, and cool, clammy skin. Respiratory rate increases as the body develops metabolic acidosis from shock.

Cardiac tamponade is accompanied by distant, muffled heart sounds and prominent neck vessels. Pulmonary embolism presents suddenly with severe dyspnea accompanying the chest pain. Dissecting aortic aneurysms usually are accompanied by back pain.

Test-Taking Strategy: Use the process of elimination. Recalling that the early serious complications of myocardial infarction

include dysrhythmias, cardiogenic shock, and sudden death will direct you to option 1. No information in the question is associated with options 2, 3, or 4. Review the complications of myocardial infarction if you had difficulty with this question.
Level of Cognitive Ability: Analyzing
Client Needs: Physiological Integrity
Integrated Process: Nursing Process—Analysis
Content Area: Critical Care
References: Copstead-Kirkhorn, L., & Banasik, J. (2010). *Pathophysiology* (4th ed., pp. 494–495). St. Louis: Mosby.
　Ignatavicius, D., & Workman, M. (2010). *Medical-surgical nursing: Patient-centered collaborative care* (6th ed., pp. 828, 830). St. Louis: Saunders.

693. 4
Rationale: Metformin (Glucophage) needs to be withheld 48 hours before and after cardiac catheterization because of the injection of contrast medium during the procedure. If the contrast medium affects kidney function, with metformin in the system, the client would be at increased risk for lactic acidosis. The medications in options 1, 2, and 3 do not need to be withheld 48 hours before or after cardiac catheterization.
Test-Taking Strategy: Use the process of elimination. Eliminate options 2 and 3 first. Although these medications may be withheld on the morning of the procedure because of the client's NPO status, there is no indication for withholding the medication the day prior to and the day postprocedure. Regular insulin may be administered if elevated blood glucose levels from infused intravenous solutions occur on the day of the procedure. Review preprocedure and postprocedure interventions if you had difficulty with this question.
Level of Cognitive Ability: Analyzing
Client Needs: Physiological Integrity
Integrated Process: Nursing Process—Planning
Content Area: Adult Health—Cardiovascular
References: Pagana, K., & Pagana, T. (2009). *Mosby's diagnostic and laboratory test reference* (9th ed., p. 225). St. Louis: Mosby.
　Perry, A., & Potter, P. (2010). *Clinical nursing skills & techniques* (7th ed., p. 1172). St. Louis: Mosby.

694. 4
Rationale: Hypotension and dizziness are signs of decreased cardiac output. Transcutaneous pacing provides a temporary measure to increase the heart rate and thus perfusion in the symptomatic client. Digoxin will further decrease the client's heart rate. Defibrillation is used for treatment of pulseless ventricular tachycardia and ventricular fibrillation. Continuing to monitor the client delays necessary intervention.
Test-Taking Strategy: Use the process of elimination. Eliminate option 3 because the client is symptomatic and requires intervention. Option 2 is eliminated because digoxin will further decrease the client's heart rate. Defibrillation is used for treatment of pulseless ventricular tachycardia and ventricular fibrillation; therefore eliminate option 1. Review the indications for transcutaneous pacing if you had difficulty with this question.
Level of Cognitive Ability: Analyzing
Client Needs: Physiological Integrity
Integrated Process: Nursing Process—Planning
Content Area: Critical Care

Reference: Black, J., & Hawks, J. (2009). *Medical-surgical nursing: Clinical management for positive outcomes* (8th ed., p. 1474). St. Louis: Saunders.

695. 3
Rationale: Ventricular fibrillation is characterized by irregular chaotic undulations of varying amplitudes. Ventricular fibrillation has no measurable rate and no visible P waves or QRS complexes and results from electrical chaos in the ventricles.
Test-Taking Strategy: Use the process of elimination and knowledge regarding the characteristics of ventricular fibrillation. The lack of visible QRS complexes eliminates atrial fibrillation and ventricular tachycardia. Recalling that asystole is lack of any electrical activity of the heart will direct you to option 3. Review the characteristics of ventricular fibrillation if you had difficulty with this question.
Level of Cognitive Ability: Analyzing
Client Needs: Physiological Integrity
Integrated Process: Nursing Process—Assessment
Content Area: Critical Care
Reference: Black, J., & Hawks, J. (2009). *Medical-surgical nursing: Clinical management for positive outcomes* (8th ed., pp. 1467–1468). St. Louis: Saunders.

696. 2
Rationale: Pulmonary edema is characterized by extreme breathlessness, dyspnea, air hunger, and the production of frothy, pink-tinged sputum. Auscultation of the lungs reveals crackles. Rhonchi and diminished breath sounds are not associated with pulmonary edema. Stridor is a crowing sound associated with laryngospasm or edema of the upper airway.
Test-Taking Strategy: Use the process of elimination. Recalling that fluid produces sounds that are called *crackles* will assist you in eliminating options 1, 3, and 4. If you had difficulty with this question, review the manifestations found in pulmonary edema.
Level of Cognitive Ability: Analyzing
Client Needs: Physiological Integrity
Integrated Process: Nursing Process—Assessment
Content Area: Adult Health—Cardiovascular
Reference: Ignatavicius, D., & Workman, M. (2010). *Medical-surgical nursing: Patient-centered collaborative care* (6th ed., p. 775). St. Louis: Saunders.

697. 2
Rationale: Classic signs of cardiogenic shock as they relate to this question include low blood pressure and tachycardia. The central venous pressure would rise as the backward effects of the severe left ventricular failure became apparent. Dysrhythmias commonly occur as a result of decreased oxygenation and severe damage to greater than 40% of the myocardium.
Test-Taking Strategy: Use the process of elimination and focus on the strategic words *myocardial ischemia*. Recall that ischemia makes the myocardium irritable, producing dysrhythmias. Also, knowledge of the classic signs of shock helps eliminate the incorrect options. Review the clinical manifestations associated with cardiogenic shock if you had difficulty with this question.
Level of Cognitive Ability: Analyzing
Client Needs: Physiological Integrity

Integrated Process: Nursing Process—Assessment
Content Area: Critical Care
Reference: Copstead, L., & Banasik, J. (2010). *Pathophysiology* (4th ed., pp. 494–495). St. Louis: Mosby.

698. 2

Rationale: The client who undergoes cardiac surgery is at risk for renal injury from poor perfusion, hemolysis, low cardiac output, or vasopressor medication therapy. Renal insult is signaled by decreased urine output and increased blood urea nitrogen and creatinine levels. The client may need medications to increase renal perfusion and possibly could need peritoneal dialysis or hemodialysis. No data in the question indicate the presence of hypovolemia, urinary tract infection, or glomerulonephritis.
Test-Taking Strategy: Use the process of elimination. Eliminate options 3 and 4 first because no data indicate infection or inflammation. Noting that the urine output is inadequate will assist you in eliminating option 1. Review the complications associated with cardiac surgery if you had difficulty with this question.
Level of Cognitive Ability: Analyzing
Client Needs: Physiological Integrity
Integrated Process: Nursing Process—Analysis
Content Area: Critical Care
Reference: Black, J., & Hawks, J. (2009). *Medical-surgical nursing: Clinical management for positive outcomes* (8th ed., p. 1426). St. Louis: Saunders.

699. 3

Rationale: Normal sinus rhythm is defined as a regular rhythm, with an overall rate of 60 to 100 beats/min. The PR and QRS measurements are normal, measuring 0.12 to 0.20 second and 0.04 to 0.10 second, respectively.
Test-Taking Strategy: A baseline knowledge of normal electrocardiographic measurements is needed to answer this question. Focusing on the data in the question and recalling the characteristics of normal sinus rhythm will direct you to option 3. Review this content if you are unfamiliar with it.
Level of Cognitive Ability: Analyzing
Client Needs: Physiological Integrity
Integrated Process: Nursing Process—Assessment
Content Area: Adult Health—Cardiovascular
Reference: Ignatavicius, D., & Workman, M. (2010). *Medical-surgical nursing: Patient-centered collaborative care* (6th ed., p. 737). St. Louis: Saunders.

700. 3

Rationale: Sudden loss of electrocardiographic complexes indicates ventricular asystole or possibly electrode displacement. Accurate assessment of the client and equipment is necessary to determine the cause and identify the appropriate intervention. Options 1, 2, and 4 are unnecessary.
Test-Taking Strategy: Use the steps of the nursing process. Always assess the client directly before taking any action. Option 3 is the only option that addresses assessment. Review care of the client on a cardiac monitor if you had difficulty with this question.
Level of Cognitive Ability: Applying
Client Needs: Physiological Integrity
Integrated Process: Nursing Process—Implementation

Content Area: Adult Health—Cardiovascular
References: Ignatavicius, D., & Workman, M. (2010). *Medical-surgical nursing: Patient-centered collaborative care* (6th ed., pp. 749–750). St. Louis: Saunders.
    Perry, A., & Potter, P. (2010). *Clinical nursing skills & techniques* (7th ed., p. 1192). St. Louis: Mosby.

701. 3

Rationale: Ventricular tachycardia is characterized by the absence of P waves, wide QRS complexes (longer than 0.12 second), and typically a rate between 140 and 180 impulses/min. The rhythm is regular.
Test-Taking Strategy: Focus on the data in the question. Eliminate option 1 first because there are no P waves. Premature ventricular contractions are isolated ectopic beats superimposed on an underlying rhythm, so option 4 is eliminated next. Recalling that there are no true QRS complexes with ventricular fibrillation will direct you to option 3 from the remaining options. Review the characteristics of ventricular tachycardia if you are unfamiliar with it.
Level of Cognitive Ability: Analyzing
Client Needs: Physiological Integrity
Integrated Process: Nursing Process—Assessment
Content Area: Critical Care
Reference: Ignatavicius, D., & Workman, M. (2010). *Medical-surgical nursing: Patient-centered collaborative care* (6th ed., p. 748). St. Louis: Saunders.

702. 1

Rationale: Ventricular tachycardia is a life-threatening dysrhythmia that results from an irritable ectopic focus that takes over as the pacemaker for the heart. The low cardiac output that results can lead quickly to cerebral and myocardial ischemia. Clients frequently experience a feeling of impending doom. Ventricular tachycardia is treated with antidysrhythmic medications, cardioversion (client awake), or defibrillation (loss of consciousness). Ventricular tachycardia can deteriorate into ventricular fibrillation at any time.
Test-Taking Strategy: Use the process of elimination and note the strategic words *most concerned*. Option 2 is incorrect and is eliminated first. From the remaining options, focusing on the strategic words will direct you to option 1 because this option identifies the life-threatening condition. Review the concerns associated with ventricular tachycardia if you had difficulty with this question.
Level of Cognitive Ability: Understanding
Client Needs: Physiological Integrity
Integrated Process: Nursing Process—Planning
Content Area: Adult Health—Cardiovascular
Reference: Ignatavicius, D., & Workman, M. (2010). *Medical-surgical nursing: Patient-centered collaborative care* (6th ed., p. 748). St. Louis: Saunders.

703. 4

Rationale: Premature ventricular contractions can cause hemodynamic compromise. The shortened ventricular filling time with the ectopic beat leads to decreased stroke volume and, if frequent enough, to decreased cardiac output. The client may be asymptomatic or may feel palpitations. Premature ventricular contractions can be caused by cardiac disorders, states of hypoxemia, or by any number of physiological stressors, such as infection, illness, surgery, or trauma, and by intake of caffeine, nicotine, or alcohol.

Test-Taking Strategy: Note the strategic words *priority on assessment.* Use the ABCs—airway, breathing, and circulation—to direct you to option 4. Review the effects of premature ventricular contractions if you had difficulty with this question.

Level of Cognitive Ability: Analyzing
Client Needs: Physiological Integrity
Integrated Process: Nursing Process—Assessment
Content Area: Adult Health—Cardiovascular
References: Black, J., & Hawks, J. (2009). *Medical-surgical nursing: Clinical management for positive outcomes* (8th ed., pp. 1464–1465). St. Louis: Saunders.

Ignatavicius, D., & Workman, M. (2010). *Medical-surgical nursing: Patient-centered collaborative care* (6th ed., pp. 747–748). St. Louis: Saunders.

704. 3
Rationale: The client with uncontrolled atrial fibrillation with a ventricular rate more than 100 beats/min is at risk for low cardiac output because of loss of atrial kick. The nurse assesses the client for palpitations, chest pain or discomfort, hypotension, pulse deficit, fatigue, weakness, dizziness, syncope, shortness of breath, and distended neck veins.

Test-Taking Strategy: Use the process of elimination. Flat neck veins are normal or indicate hypovolemia, so eliminate option 1. Nausea and vomiting (option 2) are associated with vagus nerve activity and do not correlate with a tachycardic state. From the remaining options, think of the consequences of falling cardiac output to direct you to option 3. Review the effects of atrial fibrillation if you had difficulty with this question.

Level of Cognitive Ability: Analyzing
Client Needs: Physiological Integrity
Integrated Process: Nursing Process—Assessment
Content Area: Critical Care
Reference: Ignatavicius, D., & Workman, M. (2010). *Medical-surgical nursing: Patient-centered collaborative care* (6th ed., p. 745). St. Louis: Saunders.

705. 1
Rationale: Atrial fibrillation is characterized by a loss of P waves and fibrillatory waves before each QRS complex. The atria quiver, which can lead to thrombus formation.

Test-Taking Strategy: Focus on the data in the question. Noting the strategic words *there are no P waves* should direct you to option 1. Loss of P waves is characteristic of this dysrhythmia. Review the characteristics of atrial fibrillation if you had difficulty with this question.

Level of Cognitive Ability: Analyzing
Client Needs: Physiological Integrity
Integrated Process: Nursing Process—Assessment
Content Area: Critical Care
References: Black, J., & Hawks, J. (2009). *Medical-surgical nursing: Clinical management for positive outcomes* (8th ed., pp. 1457–1458). St. Louis: Saunders.

Ignatavicius, D., & Workman, M. (2010). *Medical-surgical nursing: Patient-centered collaborative care* (6th ed., p. 745). St. Louis: Saunders.

706. 4
Rationale: Until the defibrillator is attached and charged, the client is resuscitated by using cardiopulmonary resuscitation.

Once the defibrillator has been attached, the electrocardiogram is checked to verify that the rhythm is ventricular fibrillation or pulseless ventricular tachycardia. Leads also are checked for any loose connections. A nitroglycerin patch, if present, is removed. The client does not have to be intubated to be defibrillated. Lidocaine may be given subsequently but is not required before defibrillation. The machine is not set to the synchronous mode because there is no underlying rhythm with which to synchronize.

Test-Taking Strategy: Use the process of elimination, focusing on the subject, ventricular fibrillation. Note that option 4 directly addresses this subject and also addresses assessment of the client. Review the procedure for defibrillation if you had difficulty with this question.

Level of Cognitive Ability: Applying
Client Needs: Physiological Integrity
Integrated Process: Nursing Process—Implementation
Content Area: Critical Care
Reference: Ignatavicius, D., & Workman, M. (2010). *Medical-surgical nursing: Patient-centered collaborative care* (6th ed., p. 749). St. Louis: Saunders.

707. 3
Rationale: A biphasic defibrillator delivers energy in two directions and delivers the first and any successive shocks at 120 to 200 joules. A monophasic defibrillator delivers energy in one direction and includes an initial shock at 360 joules followed by immediate CPR beginning with chest compressions. Options 1 and 2 are low energy levels and would be ineffective.

Test-Taking Strategy: Focus on the strategic words *biphasic defibrillator.* Recalling that this type of defibrillator delivers energy in two directions will assist in answering correctly. Review the procedure for defibrillation if you had difficulty with this question.

Level of Cognitive Ability: Applying
Client Needs: Physiological Integrity
Integrated Process: Nursing Process—implementation
Content Area: Critical Care
Reference: Lewis, S., Dirksen, S., Heitkemper, M., Bucher, L., & Camera, I., (2011). *Medical-surgical nursing: Assessment and managemant of clinical problems* (8th ed., p. 833). St. Louis: Mosby.

708. 1
Rationale: After defibrillation, the client requires continuous monitoring of electrocardiographic rhythm, hemodynamic status, and neurological status. Respiratory and metabolic acidosis develop during ventricular fibrillation because of lack of respiration and cardiac output. These can cause cerebral and cardiopulmonary complications. Arousable status, adequate blood pressure, and a sinus rhythm indicate successful response to defibrillation.

Test-Taking Strategy: Use the process of elimination and note the strategic words *most successful.* Eliminate options 3 and 4 first because of the word *nonarousable.* From the remaining options, select option 1 because a sinus rhythm is a more successful response compared with marked bradycardia. Review the expected effects of defibrillation if you had difficulty with this question.

Level of Cognitive Ability: Evaluating
Client Needs: Physiological Integrity
Integrated Process: Nursing Process—Evaluation

Content Area: Critical Care
Reference: Black, J., & Hawks, J. (2009). *Medical-surgical nursing: Clinical management for positive outcomes* (8th ed., p. 1471). St. Louis: Saunders.

709. 2
Rationale: Nursing responsibilities after cardioversion include maintenance first of a patent airway, and then oxygen administration, assessment of vital signs and level of consciousness, and dysrhythmia detection.
Test-Taking Strategy: Use the process of elimination, noting the strategic words *highest priority*. Use the ABCs—airway, breathing, and circulation—to direct you to option 2. Review care of the client following cardioversion if you had difficulty with this question.
Level of Cognitive Ability: Evaluating
Client Needs: Physiological Integrity
Integrated Process: Nursing Process—Evaluation
Content Area: Critical Care
Reference: Ignatavicius, D., & Workman, M. (2010). *Medical-surgical nursing: Patient-centered collaborative care* (6th ed., p. 756). St. Louis: Saunders.

710. 4
Rationale: The nurse who is caring for the client after insertion of an automatic internal cardioverter-defibrillator needs to assess device settings, similar to after insertion of a permanent pacemaker. Specifically, the nurse needs to know whether the device is activated, the heart rate cutoff above which it will fire, and the number of shocks it is programmed to deliver. Options 1, 2, and 3 are also nursing interventions but are not the priority.
Test-Taking Strategy: Note the strategic word *priority*. Use Maslow's Hierarchy of Needs theory. Option 4 is the option that identifies the physiological need. Review care to the client following insertion of an automatic internal cardioverter-defibrillator if you had difficulty with this question.
Level of Cognitive Ability: Applying
Client Needs: Physiological Integrity
Integrated Process: Nursing Process—Assessment
Content Area: Critical Care
Reference: Black, J., & Hawks, J. (2009). *Medical-surgical nursing: Clinical management for positive outcomes* (8th ed., pp. 1472-1473). St. Louis: Saunders.

711. 2
Rationale: Sinus tachycardia has the characteristics of normal sinus rhythm, including a regular PP interval and normal-width PR and QRS intervals; however, the rate is the differentiating factor. In sinus tachycardia, the atrial and ventricular rates are greater than 100 beats/min.
Test-Taking Strategy: Use the process of elimination. Eliminate options 3 and 4 because they do not meet the rate criteria (ventricular rate is 110 beats/min). Eliminate option 1 because sinus dysrhythmia is an irregular rhythm, with changing PP and RR intervals. Review the characteristics of sinus tachycardia if you had difficulty with this question.
Level of Cognitive Ability: Analyzing
Client Needs: Physiological Integrity
Integrated Process: Nursing Process—Assessment
Content Area: Critical Care
Reference: Copstead, L., & Banasik, J. (2010). *Pathophysiology* (4th ed., p. 477). St. Louis: Mosby.

712. 1
Rationale: An expected outcome of aortoiliac bypass graft surgery is warmth, redness, and edema in the surgical extremity because of increased blood flow. Therefore options 2, 3, and 4 are incorrect interpretations.
Test-Taking Strategy: Use the process of elimination. Option 2 can be eliminated because the pedal pulse is unchanged from admission. Venous complications from immobilization resulting from surgery would not be apparent within 4 hours, so eliminate option 4. From the remaining options, think about the effects of sudden reperfusion in an ischemic limb. There would be redness from new blood flow and edema from the sudden change in pressure in the blood vessels. Review the expected assessment findings following this surgical procedure if you had difficulty with this question.
Level of Cognitive Ability: Analyzing
Client Needs: Physiological Integrity
Integrated Process: Nursing Process—Assessment
Content Area: Adult Health—Cardiovascular
Reference: Ignatavicius, D., & Workman, M. (2010). *Medical-surgical nursing: Patient-centered collaborative care* (6th ed., pp. 808-809). St. Louis: Saunders.

713. 4
Rationale: Following pericardiocentesis, a rise in blood pressure and a fall in central venous pressure are expected. The client usually expresses immediate relief. Heart sounds are no longer muffled or distant.
Test-Taking Strategy: Use the process of elimination and note the strategic word *unsuccessful*. Successful therapy is measured by the disappearance of the original signs and symptoms of cardiac tamponade. Therefore look for the option that identifies a sign consistent with continued tamponade. Review signs of cardiac tamponade and the expected effects of pericardiocentesis if you had difficulty with this question.
Level of Cognitive Ability: Evaluating
Client Needs: Physiological Integrity
Integrated Process: Nursing Process—Evaluation
Content Area: Critical Care
References: Ignatavicius, D., & Workman, M. (2010). *Medical-surgical nursing: Patient-centered collaborative care* (6th ed., p. 786). St. Louis: Saunders.
Pagana, K., & Pagana, T. (2009). *Mosby's diagnostic and laboratory test reference* (9th ed., pp. 714-715). St. Louis: Mosby.

714. 1
Rationale: Following abdominal aortic aneurysm resection or repair, the nurse monitors the client for signs of renal failure. Renal failure can occur because often much blood is lost during the surgery and, depending on the aneurysm location, the renal arteries may be hypoperfused for a short period during surgery. The nurse monitors hourly intake and output and notes the results of daily blood urea nitrogen and creatinine levels. Urine output lower than 30 to 50 mL/hr is reported to the physician.
Test-Taking Strategy: Focus on the information in the question and the abnormal assessment data. This question indicates elevations in blood urea nitrogen and creatinine levels and a significant drop in hourly urine output. These assessment findings should direct you to option 1. Review the

complications associated with this surgical procedure if you had difficulty with this question.

Level of Cognitive Ability: Applying
Client Needs: Physiological Integrity
Integrated Process: Nursing Process—Implementation
Content Area: Critical Care
References: Black, J., & Hawks, J. (2009). *Medical-surgical nursing: Clinical management for positive outcomes* (8th ed., pp. 1327–1328). St. Louis: Saunders.

Ignatavicius, D., & Workman, M. (2010). *Medical-surgical nursing: Patient-centered collaborative care* (6th ed., p. 811). St. Louis: Saunders.

715. 2

Rationale: Variant angina, or Prinzmetal's angina, is prolonged and severe and occurs at the same time each day, most often at rest. Stable angina is induced by exercise and relieved by rest or nitroglycerin tablets. Unstable angina occurs at lower and lower levels of activity or at rest, is less predictable, and is often a precursor of myocardial infarction.

Test-Taking Strategy: Use the process of elimination, focusing on the data in the question. Noting the strategic words *at rest* will direct you to option 2. If you had difficulty with this question, review the characteristics of the various types of angina.

Level of Cognitive Ability: Understanding
Client Needs: Physiological Integrity
Integrated Process: Nursing Process—Assessment
Content Area: Adult Health—Cardiovascular
Reference: Black, J., & Hawks, J. (2009). *Medical-surgical nursing: Clinical management for positive outcomes* (8th ed., pp. 1485–1486). St. Louis: Saunders.

ALTERNATE ITEM FORMAT: MULTIPLE RESPONSE

716. 1, 2, 3, 4

Rationale: Pulmonary edema is a life-threatening event that can result from severe heart failure. In pulmonary edema, the left ventricle fails to eject sufficient blood, and pressure increases in the lungs because of the accumulated blood. Oxygen is always prescribed, and the client is placed in a high Fowler's position to ease the work of breathing. Furosemide, a rapid-acting diuretic, will eliminate accumulated fluid. A Foley catheter is inserted to measure output accurately. Intravenously administered morphine sulfate reduces venous return (preload), decreases anxiety, and also reduces the work of breathing. Transporting the client to the coronary care unit is not a priority intervention. In fact, this may not be necessary at all if the client's response to treatment is successful.

Test-Taking Strategy: Note the strategic words *priority interventions* and focus on the client's diagnosis. Recall the pathophysiology associated with pulmonary edema and use the ABCs—airway, breathing, and circulation—to help determine priority interventions. Review priority interventions for the client with pulmonary edema if you had difficulty with this question.

Level of Cognitive Ability: Applying
Client Needs: Physiological Integrity
Integrated Process: Nursing Process—Implementation
Content Area: Critical Care
Reference: Ignatavicius, D., & Workman, M. (2010). *Medical-surgical nursing: Patient-centered collaborative care* (6th ed., pp. 775–776). St. Louis: Saunders.

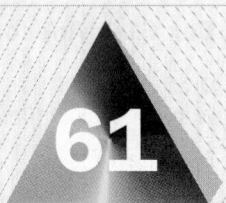

Cardiovascular Medications

I. ANTICOAGULANTS (Box 61-1)

A. Description (Box 61-2)
1. Anticoagulants prevent the extension and formation of clots by inhibiting factors in the clotting cascade and decreasing blood coagulability.
2. Anticoagulants are administered when there is evidence of or likelihood of clot formation—myocardial infarction, unstable angina, atrial fibrillation, deep vein thrombosis, pulmonary embolism, and the presence of mechanical heart valves.
3. Anticoagulants are contraindicated with active bleeding (except for disseminated intravascular coagulation), bleeding disorders or blood dyscrasias, ulcers, liver and kidney disease, and hemorrhagic brain injuries.

B. Side effects
1. Hemorrhage
2. Hematuria
3. Epistaxis
4. Ecchymosis
5. Bleeding gums
6. Thrombocytopenia
7. Hypotension

C. Heparin sodium
1. Description
   a. Heparin prevents thrombin from converting fibrinogen to fibrin.
   b. Heparin prevents thromboembolism.
   c. The therapeutic dose does not dissolve clots but prevents new thrombus formation.
2. Blood levels
   a. The normal activated partial thromboplastin time (aPTT) is 20 to 36 seconds in most laboratories but may be as high as 40 seconds.
   b. To maintain a therapeutic level of anticoagulation when the client is receiving a continuous infusion of heparin, the aPTT should be 1.5 to 2.5 times the normal value.
   c. Activated partial thromboplastin time therapy should be measured every 4 to 6 hours during initial continuous infusion therapy and then daily.
   d. If the aPTT is too long, longer than 80 seconds, the dosage should be lowered.
   e. If aPTT is too short, less than 60 seconds, the dosage should be increased.
3. Interventions
   a. Monitor aPTT.
   b. Monitor platelet count.
   c. Observe for bleeding gums, bruises, nosebleeds, hematuria, hematemesis, occult blood in the stool, and petechiae.
   d. When administering heparin subcutaneously, inject into the abdomen with a ⅝-inch needle (25 to 28 gauge) at a 90-degree angle and do not aspirate or rub the injection site.
   e. Continuous infusions must be run on an infusion pump to ensure precise rate of delivery.
   f. Instruct the client regarding measures to prevent bleeding.
   g. The antidote to heparin is protamine sulfate.

D. Enoxaparin (Lovenox)—low-molecular-weight heparin
1. Description: Enoxaparin has the same mechanism of action and use as heparin but is not interchangeable; has a longer half-life than heparin.
2. Interventions
   a. Administer by subcutaneous injection only to the recumbent client in the anterolateral or posterolateral abdominal wall; do not expel the air bubble from the prefilled syringe or aspirate during injection.
   b. Monitor the same laboratory values as for heparin and observe for bleeding.
   c. The antidote to enoxaparin is protamine sulfate.

E. Warfarin sodium (Coumadin)
1. Description
   a. Warfarin suppresses coagulation by acting as an antagonist of vitamin K by inhibiting four dependent clotting factors (X, IX, VII, and II).
   b. Warfarin prolongs clotting time and is monitored by the prothrombin time (PT) and the international normalized ratio (INR).

831

Box 61-1 Anticoagulants

Oral
Warfarin sodium (Coumadin)

Parenteral
Argatroban (Acova)
Bivalirudin (Angiomax)
Dalteparin (Fragmin)
Desirudin (Iprivask)
Enoxaparin (Lovenox)
Fondaparinux (Arixtra)
Heparin sodium
Tinzaparin (Innohep)
Lepirudin (Refludan)

Box 61-2 Substances to Avoid With Anticoagulants

Allopurinol (Zyloprim)
Cimetidine (Tagamet)
Corticosteroids
Green leafy vegetables and foods high in vitamin K
Nonsteroidal anti-inflammatory drugs
Oral hypoglycemic agents
Phenytoin (Dilantin)
Salicylates
Sulfonamides
Ginkgo and ginseng (herbs)

Box 61-3 Thrombolytic Medications

Alteplase (Activase, tPA)
Reteplase (Retavase)
Streptokinase (Streptase)
Tenecteplase (TNKase)

    f. If the INR is above the recommended range, warfarin sodium should be reduced.
  4. Interventions
    a. Monitor PT and INR.
    b. Observe for bleeding gums, bruises, nose-bleeds, hematuria, hematemesis, occult blood in the stool, and petechiae.
    c. Instruct the client regarding measures to prevent bleeding.

II. THROMBOLYTIC MEDICATIONS (Box 61-3)

A. Description
  1. Thrombolytic medications activate plasminogen; plasminogen generates plasmin (the enzyme that dissolves clots).
  2. Thrombolytic medications are used early in the course of myocardial infarction (within 4 to 6 hours of the onset of the infarct) to restore blood flow, limit myocardial damage, preserve left ventricular function, and prevent death.
  3. Thrombolytics are also used in arterial thrombosis, deep vein thrombosis, occluded shunts or catheters, and pulmonary emboli.
B. Contraindications
  1. Active internal bleeding
  2. History of hemorrhagic brain attack (stroke)
  3. Intracranial problems, including trauma
  4. Intracranial or intraspinal surgery within the previous 2 months
  5. History of thoracic, pelvic, or abdominal surgery in the previous 10 days
  6. History of hepatic or renal disease
  7. Uncontrolled hypertension
  8. Recently required, prolonged cardiopulmonary resuscitation
  9. Known allergy to the specific product or any of its preservatives
C. Side effects
  1. Bleeding
  2. Dysrhythmias
  3. Allergic reactions
D. Interventions
  1. Determine aPTT, PT, fibrinogen level, hematocrit, and platelet count.
  2. Monitor vital signs.
  3. Assess pulses.
  4. Monitor for bleeding.
  5. Monitor all excretions for occult blood.

    c. It is used for long-term anticoagulation and is used mainly to prevent thromboembolic conditions such as thrombophlebitis, pulmonary embolism, and embolism formation caused by atrial fibrillation, thrombosis, myocardial infarction, or heart valve damage.
  2. Blood levels
    a. The normal PT is 9.6 to 11.8 seconds.
    b. Warfarin sodium prolongs the PT; the therapeutic range is 1.5 to 2 times the control value.
  3. International normalized ratio (INR)
    a. The normal INR is 1.3 to 2.0.
    b. The INR is determined by multiplying the observed PT ratio (the ratio of the client's PT to a control PT) by a correction factor specific to a particular thromboplastin preparation used in the testing.
    c. The treatment goal is to raise the INR to an appropriate value.
    d. An INR of 2 to 3 is appropriate for most clients, although for some clients the target INR is 3 to 4.5.
    e. If the INR is below the recommended range, warfarin sodium should be increased.

Box 61-4 Antiplatelet Medications

Abciximab (ReoPro)
Aspirin (acetylsalicylic acid, ASA)
Cilostazol (Pletal)
Clopidogrel (Plavix)
Dipyridamole (Persantine)
Dipyridamole; aspirin (Aggrenox)
Eptifibatide (Integrilin)
Ticlopidine (Ticlid)
Tirofiban (Aggrastat)

6. Monitor for neurological changes such as slurred speech, lethargy, confusion, and hemiparesis.
7. Monitor for hypotension and tachycardia.
8. Avoid injections if possible.
9. Apply direct pressure over a puncture site for 20 to 30 minutes.
10. Handle the client as little as possible when moving.
11. Instruct the client to use an electric razor for shaving and to brush teeth gently.
12. Withhold the medication if bleeding develops, and notify the physician.
13. Antidote
    a. Aminocaproic acid (Amicar) is the antidote for streptokinase.
    b. Used only in acute, life-threatening conditions

⚠ Bleeding is the primary concern for a client taking an anticoagulant, thrombolytic, or antiplatelet medication.

III. ANTIPLATELET MEDICATIONS (Box 61-4)

A. Description
1. Antiplatelet medications inhibit the aggregation of platelets in the clotting process, thereby prolonging the bleeding time.
2. Antiplatelet medications may be used with anticoagulants.
3. Used in the prophylaxis of long-term complications following myocardial infarction, coronary revascularization, stents, and brain attacks (stroke).
4. These medications are contraindicated in those with bleeding disorders and known sensitivity.

B. Side effects
1. Gastrointestinal bleeding
2. Bruising
3. Hematuria
4. Tarry stools

C. Interventions
1. Determine sensitivity before administration.
2. Monitor vital signs.
3. Instruct the client to take medication with food if gastrointestinal upset occurs.

Box 61-5 Positive Inotropic/Cardiotonic Medications

Dopamine
Used as a short-term rescue measure for clients with severe, acute cardiac failure
Increases myocardial contractility, thereby improving cardiac performance
Dilates renal blood vessels and increases renal blood flow and urine output

Dobutamine
Used for short-term management of heart failure
Increases myocardial contractility, thereby improving cardiac performance

Inamrinone Lactate
Used for short-term management of congestive heart failure in those who have not responded adequately to cardiac glycosides, diuretics, and vasodilators

Milrinone (Primacor)
Used for short-term management of congestive heart failure; may be given before heart transplantation

4. Monitor bleeding time.
5. Monitor for side effects related to bleeding.
6. Instruct the client in the use of the medication.
7. Instruct the client to monitor for side effects related to bleeding and in the measures to prevent bleeding.

IV. POSITIVE INOTROPIC AND CARDIOTONIC MEDICATIONS (Box 61-5)

A. Description
1. These medications stimulate myocardial **contractility** and produce a positive inotropic effect.
2. These are used for short-term management of advanced heart failure; the increase in myocardial **contractility** improves cardiac, peripheral, and kidney function by increasing **cardiac output**, decreasing **preload**, improving blood flow to the periphery and kidneys, decreasing edema, and increasing fluid excretion. As a result, fluid retention in the lungs and extremities is decreased (Fig. 61-1).

B. Side effects
1. Dysrhythmias
2. Hypotension
3. Thrombocytopenia

C. Toxic and adverse reactions
1. Hepatotoxicity manifested by elevated liver enzyme levels
2. Hypersensitivity manifested by wheezing, shortness of breath, pruritus, urticaria, clammy skin, and flushing

D. Interventions
1. Positive inotropic and cardiotonic medications are used for intravenous (IV) administration.

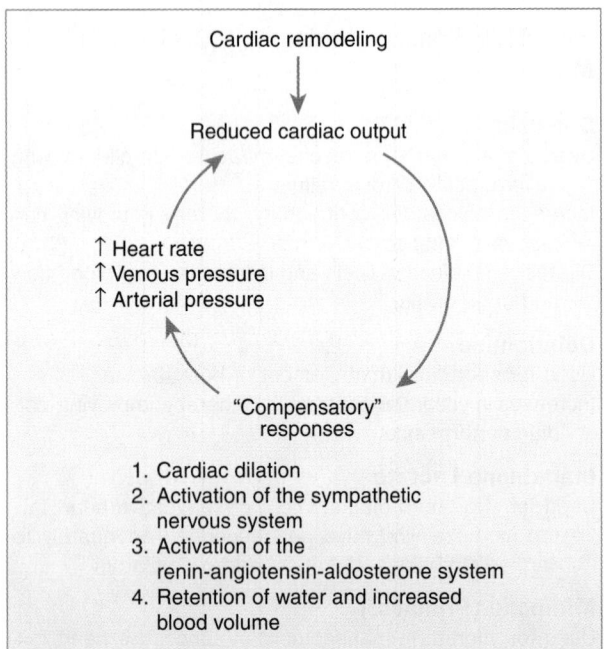

Cardiac remodeling

↓

Reduced cardiac output

↑ Heart rate
↑ Venous pressure
↑ Arterial pressure

"Compensatory"
responses

1. Cardiac dilation
2. Activation of the sympathetic nervous system
3. Activation of the renin-angiotensin-aldosterone system
4. Retention of water and increased blood volume

▲ **FIGURE 61-1** The vicious cycle of maladaptive compensatory responses to a failing heart. (From Lehne, R. [2010]. *Pharmacology for nursing care* [7th ed.]. St. Louis: Saunders.)

a. Should not be diluted with dextrose-containing solutions (follow physician prescription and agency procedure).
b. For continuous IV infusion, administer with an infusion pump.
c. Stop the infusion if the client's **blood pressure (BP)** drops or dysrhythmias occur.
2. Monitor the apical pulse and **BP**.
3. Monitor for hypersensitivity.
4. Assess lung sounds for wheezing and crackles.
5. Monitor for edema.
6. Monitor for relief of heart failure as noted by reduction in edema, lessening of dyspnea, orthopnea, and fatigue.
7. Monitor electrolyte and liver enzyme levels, platelet count, and renal function studies; the medications may decrease potassium and increase liver enzyme levels; continuous electrocardiographic monitoring is done during administration.

V. CARDIAC GLYCOSIDES (Box 61-6)

A. Description
1. Cardiac glycosides inhibit the sodium-potassium pump, thus increasing intracellular calcium, which causes the heart muscle fibers to contract more efficiently.
2. Cardiac glycosides produce a positive inotropic action, which increases the force of myocardial contractions.
3. Cardiac glycosides produce a negative chronotropic action, which slows the heart rate.

Box 61-6 Cardiac Glycoside

Digoxin (Lanoxicaps, Lanoxin)

4. Cardiac glycosides produce a negative dromotropic action that slows conduction velocity through the atrioventricular (AV) node.
5. The increase in myocardial **contractility** increases cardiac, peripheral, and kidney function by increasing **cardiac output**, decreasing **preload**, improving blood flow to the periphery and kidneys, decreasing edema, and increasing fluid excretion; as a result, fluid retention in the lungs and extremities is decreased.
6. Cardiac glycosides are used for heart failure and cardiogenic shock, atrial tachycardia, atrial fibrillation, and atrial flutter.
7. These medications are contraindicated in those with ventricular dysrhythmias and second- or third-degree heart block and should be used with caution in clients with renal disease, hypothyroidism, and hypokalemia.

B. Side effects and toxic effects
1. Anorexia, nausea, vomiting, diarrhea
2. Headache
3. Visual disturbances: Diplopia, blurred vision, yellow-green halos, photophobia
4. Drowsiness
5. Bradycardia
6. Fatigue, weakness

⚠ Early signs of digoxin toxicity present as gastrointestinal manifestations (anorexia, nausea, vomiting, diarrhea); then, heart rate abnormalities and visual disturbances appear.

C. Interventions
1. Monitor for toxicity as evidenced by anorexia, nausea, vomiting, visual disturbances, confusion, bradycardia, heart block, premature ventricular contractions, and tachydysrhythmias.
2. Monitor serum digoxin level, electrolyte levels, and renal function test results.
3. Therapeutic digoxin range is 0.5 to 2 ng/mL; levels above 2 ng/mL are toxic.
4. An increased risk of toxicity exists in clients with hypercalcemia, hypokalemia, hypomagnesemia, or hypothyroidism.
5. Monitor the potassium level; if hypokalemia occurs (potassium lower than 3.5 mEq/L), notify the physician.
6. Instruct the client to avoid over-the-counter medications.
7. Monitor the client taking a potassium-wasting diuretic or corticosteroids closely for hypokalemia

Box 61-7 Classifications of Diuretics

Loop diuretics
Osmotic diuretics
Potassium-sparing diuretics
Thiazide diuretics

Box 61-8 Thiazide and Thiazide-like Diuretics

Bendroflumethiazide
Benzthiazide
Chlorothiazide (Diuril)
Chlorthalidone (Hygroton, Thalitone)
Hydrochlorothiazide (HydroDIURIL)
Hydroflumethiazide (Saluron)
Indapamide (Lozol)
Methyclothiazide (Enduron)
Metolazone (Zaroxolyn)
Polythiazide
Quinethazone
Trichlormethiazide

because the hypokalemia can cause digoxin toxicity.
8. Note that older clients are more sensitive to digoxin toxicity.
9. Advise the client to eat foods high in potassium, such as fresh and dried fruits, fruit juices, vegetables, and potatoes.
10. Monitor the apical pulse.
11. If the apical pulse rate is lower than 60 beats/min, the medication should be held and the physician notified.
12. Teach the client how to measure the pulse.
13. Teach the client to notify physician if the pulse rate is lower than 60 or more than 100 beats/min.
14. Teach the client the signs and symptoms of toxicity.
15. Antidote: Digoxin immune Fab (Digibind) is used in extreme toxicity.

VI. ANTIHYPERTENSIVE MEDICATIONS (Box 61-7)

A. Thiazide diuretics (Box 61-8)
   1. Description
      a. Thiazide diuretics increase sodium and water excretion by inhibiting sodium reabsorption in the distal tubule of the kidney.
      b. Used for hypertension and peripheral edema
      c. Not effective for immediate diuresis
      d. Used in clients with normal renal function (contraindicated in clients with renal failure)
      e. Thiazide diuretics should be used with caution in the client taking lithium because lithium toxicity can occur and in the client

Box 61-9 Loop Diuretics

Bumetanide (Bumex)
Ethacrynic acid (Edecrin)
Furosemide (Lasix)
Torsemide (Demadex)

taking digoxin, corticosteroids, or hypoglycemic medications.
   2. Side effects
      a. Hypercalcemia, hyperglycemia, hyperuricemia
      b. Hypokalemia, hyponatremia
      c. Hypovolemia
      d. Hypotension
      e. Headaches
      f. Nausea, vomiting
      g. Constipation
      h. Rashes
      i. Photosensitivity
      j. Blood dyscrasias
   3. Interventions
      a. Monitor vital signs.
      b. Monitor weight.
      c. Monitor urine output.
      d. Monitor electrolytes, glucose, calcium, blood urea nitrogen (BUN), creatinine, and uric acid levels.
      e. Check peripheral extremities for edema.
      f. Instruct the client to take the medication in the morning to avoid nocturia and sleep interruption.
      g. Instruct the client in how to record the **BP**.
      h. Instruct the client to eat foods high in potassium.
      i. Instruct the client in how to take potassium supplements if prescribed.
      j. Instruct the client to take medication with food to avoid gastrointestinal upset.
      k. Instruct the client to change positions slowly to prevent **orthostatic hypotension**.
      l. Instruct the client to use sunscreen when in direct sunlight because of increased photosensitivity.
      m. Instruct the client with diabetes mellitus to have the blood glucose level checked periodically.

B. Loop diuretics (Box 61-9)
   1. Description
      a. Loop diuretics inhibit sodium and chloride reabsorption from the loop of Henle and the distal tubule.
      b. Loop diuretics have little effect on the blood glucose level; however, they cause depletion of water and electrolytes, increased uric acid levels, and the excretion of calcium.
      c. Loop diuretics are more potent than thiazide diuretics, causing rapid diuresis, and thus decreasing vascular fluid volume, **cardiac output**, and **BP**.

d. Used for hypertension, pulmonary edema, edema associated with heart failure, hypercalcemia, and renal disease
e. Use loop diuretics with caution in the client taking digoxin or lithium and the client on aminoglycosides, anticoagulants, corticosteroids, or amphotericin B.
2. Side effects
   a. Hypokalemia, hyponatremia, hypocalcemia, hypomagnesemia
   b. Hypochloremia
   c. Thrombocytopenia
   d. Hyperuricemia
   e. **Orthostatic hypotension**
   f. Skin disturbances
   g. Ototoxicity and deafness
   h. Thiamine deficiency
   i. Dehydration
3. Interventions
   a. Monitor vital signs.
   b. Monitor weight.
   c. Monitor urine output.
   d. Monitor electrolytes, calcium, magnesium, BUN, creatinine, and uric acid levels.
   e. Check the peripheral extremities for edema.
   f. Monitor for signs of digoxin or lithium toxicity if the client is on these medications.
   g. Instruct the client to take the medication in the morning to avoid nocturia and sleep interruption.
   h. Instruct the client in how to record the **BP**.
   i. Instruct the client to eat foods high in potassium.
   j. Instruct the client in how to take potassium supplements if prescribed.
   k. Instruct the client to take medication with food to avoid gastrointestinal upset.
   l. Instruct the client to change positions slowly to prevent **orthostatic hypotension**.
   m. Administer IV furosemide (Lasix) slowly because hearing loss can occur if injected rapidly.
C. Osmotic diuretics
   1. See Chapter 67 for information regarding osmotic diuretics.
   2. Box 61-10 lists osmotic diuretics.
D. Potassium-sparing diuretics (Box 61-11)
   1. Description
      a. Potassium-sparing diuretics act on the distal tubule to promote sodium and water excretion and potassium retention.
      b. Used for edema and hypertension, to increase urine output, and to treat fluid retention and overload associated with heart failure, ascites resulting from cirrhosis or nephrotic syndrome, and diuretic-induced hypokalemia.

Box 61-10 Osmotic Diuretics

Glycerin (Osmoglyn)
Isosorbide (Ismotic)
Mannitol (Osmitrol)
Urea (Ureaphil)

Box 61-11 Potassium-Sparing Diuretics

Amiloride (Midamor)
Amiloride hydrochloride; hydrochlorothiazide (Moduretic)
Spironolactone (Aldactone)
Spironolactone; hydrochlorothiazide (Aldactazide)
Triamterene (Dyrenium)

   c. Potassium-sparing diuretics are contraindicated in severe kidney or hepatic disease and in severe hyperkalemia.
   d. Potassium-sparing diuretics should be used with caution in the client with diabetes mellitus, taking antihypertensives or lithium, or taking angiotensin-converting enzyme inhibitors or potassium supplements because hyperkalemia can result.

⚠ The primary concern with administering potassium-sparing diuretics is hyperkalemia.

2. Side effects
   a. Hyperkalemia
   b. Nausea, vomiting, diarrhea
   c. Rash
   d. Dizziness, weakness
   e. Headache
   f. Dry mouth
   g. Photosensitivity
   h. Anemia
   i. Thrombocytopenia
3. Interventions
   a. Monitor vital signs.
   b. Monitor urine output.
   c. Monitor for signs and symptoms of hyperkalemia such as nausea, diarrhea, abdominal cramps, tachycardia followed by bradycardia, tall peaked T waves on the electrocardiogram, and oliguria.
   d. Monitor for a potassium level greater than 5.1 mEq/L, which indicates hyperkalemia.
   e. Instruct the client to avoid foods high in potassium.
   f. Instruct the client to avoid exposure to direct sunlight.
   g. Instruct the client to monitor for signs of hyperkalemia.
   h. Instruct the client to avoid salt substitutes because they contain potassium.

Box 61-12 Peripherally Acting α-Adrenergic Blockers

Doxazosin (Cardura)
Prazosin (Minipress)
Terazosin (Hytrin)

Box 61-13 Centrally Acting Sympatholytics

Clonidine (Catapres)
Guanabenz (Wytensin)
Guanfacine (Tenex)
Methyldopa (Aldomet)

    i. Instruct the client to take with or after meals to decrease gastrointestinal irritation.

VII. PERIPHERALLY ACTING α-ADRENERGIC BLOCKERS (Box 61-12)

A. Description
1. These medications decrease sympathetic vasoconstriction by reducing the effects of norepinephrine at peripheral nerve endings, resulting in vasodilation and decreased **BP**.
2. These medications are used to maintain renal blood flow.
3. These medications are used to treat hypertension.

B. Side effects
1. **Orthostatic hypotension**
2. Reflex tachycardia
3. Sodium and water retention
4. Gastrointestinal disturbances
5. Nausea
6. Drowsiness
7. Nasal congestion
8. Edema
9. Weight gain

C. Interventions
1. Monitor vital signs.
2. Monitor for fluid retention and edema.
3. Instruct the client to change positions slowly to prevent **orthostatic hypotension**.
4. Instruct the client in how to monitor the **BP**.
5. Instruct the client to monitor for edema.
6. Instruct the client to decrease salt intake.
7. Instruct the client to avoid over-the-counter medications.

VIII. CENTRALLY ACTING SYMPATHOLYTICS (ADRENERGIC BLOCKERS) (Box 61-13)

A. Description
1. Centrally acting sympatholytics stimulate alpha receptors in the central nervous system to inhibit vasoconstriction, thus reducing peripheral resistance.

Box 61-14 Angiotensin-Converting Enzyme Inhibitors and Angiotensin Receptor Blockers

Angiotensin-Converting Enzyme Inhibitors
Benazepril (Lotensin)
Captopril (Capoten)
Enalapril (Vasotec)
Fosinopril (Monopril)
Lisinopril (Prinivil, Zestril)
Moexipril (Univasc)
Perindopril (Aceon)
Quinapril (Accupril)
Ramipril (Altace)
Trandolapril (Mavik)

Angiotensin II Receptor Blockers
Candesartan (Atacand)
Eprosartan (Teveten)
Irbesartan (Avapro)
Losartan (Cozaar)
Olmesartan (Benicar)
Telmisartan (Micardis)
Valsartan (Diovan)

2. Used to treat hypertension
3. Contraindicated in impaired liver function

B. Side effects
1. Sodium and water retention
2. Drowsiness, dizziness
3. Dry mouth
4. Bradycardia
5. Edema
6. Impotence
7. Hypotension
8. Depression

C. Interventions
1. Monitor vital signs.
2. Instruct the client not to discontinue medication because abrupt withdrawal can cause severe rebound hypertension.
3. Monitor liver function tests.

IX. ANGIOTENSIN-CONVERTING ENZYME (ACE) INHIBITORS AND ANGIOTENSIN II RECEPTOR BLOCKERS (ARBs) (Box 61-14)

A. Description
1. ACE inhibitors prevent peripheral vasoconstriction by blocking conversion of angiotensin I to angiotensin II (AII).
2. ARBs prevent peripheral vasoconstriction and secretion of aldosterone and block the binding of AII to type 1 AII receptors.
3. These medications are used to treat hypertension and heart failure; also, ACE inhibitors are administered for their cardioprotective effect after myocardial infarction.
4. Avoid use with potassium supplements and potassium-sparing diuretics.

B. Side effects

1. Nausea, vomiting, diarrhea
2. Persistent dry cough (ACE inhibitors only)
3. Hypotension
4. Hyperkalemia
5. Tachycardia
6. Headache
7. Dizziness, fatigue
8. Insomnia
9. Hypoglycemic reaction in the client with diabetes mellitus
10. Bruising, petechiae, bleeding
11. Diminished taste (ACE inhibitors)

⚠ A persistent dry cough is a common complaint for those taking an ACE inhibitor. Instruct the client to contact the physician if this side effect occurs and persists.

C. Interventions

1. Monitor vital signs.
2. Monitor white blood cells, and protein, albumin, BUN, creatinine, and potassium levels.
3. Monitor for hypoglycemic reactions in the client with diabetes mellitus.
4. Instruct the client to take captopril (Capoten) 20 to 60 minutes before a meal.
5. Monitor for bruising, petechiae, or bleeding with captopril.
6. Instruct the client not to discontinue medications because rebound hypertension can occur.
7. Instruct the client not to take over-the-counter medications.
8. Instruct the client in how to take the **BP**.
9. Instruct the client that if dizziness or any other side effects occur and persist to notify the physician.
10. Inform the client that the taste of food may be diminished during the first month of therapy.
11. Instruct the client to report the side effect of angioedema (dermal, subcutaneous, or submucosal swelling) immediately to the health care provider.

X. ANTIANGINAL MEDICATIONS (Box 61-15)

A. Nitrates (see Priority Nursing Actions)

1. Description
   a. Nitrates produce vasodilation.
   b. Nitrates decrease **preload** and **afterload** and reduce myocardial oxygen consumption.
   c. Contraindicated in the client with significant hypotension, increased intracranial pressure, or severe anemia
   d. Should be used with caution with severe renal or hepatic disease
   e. Avoid abrupt withdrawal of long-acting preparations to prevent the rebound effect of severe pain from myocardial ischemia.

■■■■ PRIORITY NURSING ACTIONS! ■■■■

Actions to Take If a Client With Cardiac Disease Complains of Chest Pain

1. Quickly assess the client, specifically characteristics of pain, heart rate and rhythm, and blood pressure (BP).
2. Administer a nitroglycerin tablet.
3. Stay with the client.
4. Reassess in 5 minutes.
5. Administer another nitroglycerin tablet if pain is not relieved and the BP is stable.
6. Reassess in 5 minutes.
7. Administer a third nitroglycerin tablet if pain is not relieved and the BP is stable.
8. Reassess in 5 minutes; contact the physician if the third nitroglycerin tablet does not relieve the pain.
9. Document the event, actions taken, and the client's response to treatment.

The usual guidelines for administering nitroglycerin tablets for chest pain include administering 1 tablet every 5 minutes PRN for chest pain, for a total dose of 3 tablets. If the client does not obtain relief after taking a third dose of nitroglycerin, the physician is notified. Before administering the first dose of nitroglycerin, the nurse quickly assesses the client, specifically the characteristics of the pain, the heart rate and rhythm, and BP. The nurse always stays with the client during the event to provide reassurance and to relieve anxiety. Additionally the nurse needs to be present if a life-threatening situation develops. The nurse assesses the client before administering each subsequent dose of nitroglycerin and pays particular attention to the BP because nitroglycerin causes hypotension. The nurse needs to lower the head of the bed and contact the physician before administering another nitroglycerin if hypotension occurs. Agency protocols for this type of event should also be followed. The nurse documents the event, actions taken, and the client's response to treatment.

References: Ignatavicius, D., & Workman, M. (2010). *Medical-surgical nursing: Patient-centered collaborative care* (6th ed., p. 856). St. Louis: Saunders.

Kee, J., Hayes, E., & McCuistion, L. (2009). *Pharmacology: A nursing process approach* (6th ed., p. 926). St. Louis: Saunders.

Box 61-15 Antianginal Medications (Organic Nitrates)

Amyl nitrate inhalant
Isosorbide dinitrate (Isordil, Isordil Titradose, Dilatrate-SR)
Isosorbide mononitrate (Imdur, Monoket, ISMO, Isotrate ER)
Nitroglycerin, sublingual (Nitrostat, NitroQuick, Nitrotab)
Nitroglycerin, translingual (Nitrolingual Pumpspray)
Nitroglycerin, transmucosal (Nitrogard)
Nitroglycerin, transdermal patches (Minitran, Nitro-Dur, Nitrodisc, Nitrek, Transderm-Nitro)
Nitroglycerin ointment (Nitro-Bid)
Intravenous nitroglycerin (Nitro-Bid IV, Tridil)

2. Side effects
   a. Headache
   b. **Orthostatic hypotension**
   c. Dizziness, weakness
   d. Faintness
   e. Nausea, vomiting
   f. Flushing or pallor
   g. Confusion
   h. Rash
   i. Dry mouth
   j. Reflex tachycardia
3. Sublingual medications
   a. Monitor vital signs.
   b. Offer sips of water before giving because dryness may inhibit medication absorption.
   c. Instruct the client to place under the tongue and leave until fully dissolved.
   d. Instruct the client not to swallow the medication.
   e. Instruct the client to take one tablet and if the pain does not subside to call emergency medical services (911).
   f. While waiting for emergency medical services, the client should take a second nitroglycerin tablet and if the pain is still unrelieved in 5 minutes, take a third nitroglycerin tablet.
   g. Inform the client that a stinging or burning sensation may indicate that the tablet is fresh.
   h. Instruct the client to store medication in a dark, tightly closed bottle.
   i. Instruct the client to take acetaminophen (Tylenol) for a headache.
4. Translingual medications (spray)
   a. Instruct the client to direct the spray against the oral mucosa.
   b. Instruct the client to avoid inhaling the spray.
5. Sustained-released medications: Instruct the client to swallow and not to chew or crush the medication.
6. Transmucosal-buccal medications
   a. Instruct the client to place the medication between the upper lip and gum or in the buccal area between the cheek and gum.
   b. Inform the client that the medication will adhere to the oral mucosa and slowly dissolve.
7. Transdermal patch
   a. Instruct the client to apply the patch to a hairless area, using a new patch and different site each day.
   b. As prescribed, instruct the client to remove the patch after 12 to 14 hours, allowing 10 to 12 "patch-free" hours each day to prevent tolerance.
8. Topical ointments
   a. Instruct the client to remove the ointment on the skin from the previous dose.
   b. Instruct the client to squeeze a ribbon of ointment of the prescribed length onto the applicator paper.

Box 61-16 β-Adrenergic Blockers

Nonselective (Block β₁ and β₂)
Carteolol (Cartrol Filmtabs)
Carvedilol (Coreg Tiltab)
Labetalol (Trandate)
Nadolol (Corgard)
Nebivolol (Bystolic)
Penbutolol (Levatol)
Pindolol (Visken)
Propranolol (Inderal)
Sotalol (Betapace)
Timolol (Blocadren)

Cardioselective (Block β₁)
Acebutolol (Sectral)
Atenolol (Tenormin)
Betaxolol (Kerlone)
Bisoprolol (Zebeta)
Metoprolol (Lopressor, Toprol-XL)

---

   c. Instruct the client to spread the ointment over a 6×6–inch area, using the chest, back, abdomen, upper arm, or anterior thigh (avoiding hairy areas), and cover with a plastic wrap.
   d. Instruct the client to rotate sites and to avoid touching the ointment when applying.
9. Patches and ointments
   a. Wear gloves when applying.
   b. Do not apply on the chest in the area of defibrillator-cardioverter paddle placement because skin burns can result if the paddles need to be used.

⚠ Instruct the client using nitroglycerin tablets to check the expiration date on the medication bottle because expiration may occur within 6 months of obtaining the medication. The tablets will not relieve the chest pain if they have expired.

XI. β-ADRENERGIC BLOCKERS (Box 61-16)

A. Description
1. β-Adrenergic blockers inhibit response to β-adrenergic stimulation, thus decreasing **cardiac output**.
2. β-Adrenergic blockers block the release of catecholamines, epinephrine, and norepinephrine, thus decreasing the heart rate and **BP**.
3. β-Adrenergic blockers decrease the workload of the heart and decrease oxygen demands.
4. Used for angina, dysrhythmias, hypertension, migraine headaches, prevention of myocardial infarction, and glaucoma
5. β-Adrenergic blockers are contraindicated in the client with asthma, bradycardia, heart failure (with exceptions), severe renal or hepatic disease, hyperthyroidism, or brain attack (stroke); carvedilol,

metoprolol and bisoprolol have been approved for use in heart failure once the client has been stabilized with ACE inhibitor and diuretic therapy.

6. β-Adrenergic blockers should be used with caution in the client with diabetes mellitus because the medication may mask symptoms of hypoglycemia.

7. β-Adrenergic blockers should be used with caution in the client taking antihypertensive medications.

B. Side effects
1. Bradycardia
2. Bronchospasm
3. Hypotension
4. Weakness, fatigue
5. Nausea, vomiting
6. Dizziness
7. Hyperglycemia
8. Agranulocytosis
9. Behavioral or psychotic response
10. Depression
11. Nightmares

C. Interventions
1. Monitor vital signs.
2. Withhold the medication if the pulse or **BP** is not within the prescribed parameters.
3. Monitor for signs of heart failure or worsening heart failure.
4. Assess for respiratory distress and for signs of wheezing and dyspnea.
5. Instruct the client to report dizziness, light-headedness, or nasal congestion.
6. Instruct the client not to stop the medication because rebound hypertension, rebound tachycardia, or an anginal attack can occur.
7. Advise the client taking insulin that the β-adrenergic blocker can mask early signs of hypoglycemia, such as tachycardia and nervousness.
8. Instruct the client taking insulin to monitor the blood glucose level.
9. Instruct the client in how to take pulse and **BP**.
10. Instruct the client to change positions slowly to prevent **orthostatic hypotension**.
11. Instruct the client to avoid over-the-counter medications, especially cold medications and nasal decongestants.

XII. CALCIUM CHANNEL BLOCKERS (Box 61-17)

A. Description
1. Calcium channel blockers decrease cardiac **contractility** (negative inotropic effect by relaxing smooth muscle) and the workload of the heart, thus decreasing the need for oxygen.
2. Calcium channel blockers promote vasodilation of the coronary and peripheral vessels.
3. Used for angina, dysrhythmias, or hypertension

Box 61-17 Calcium Channel Blockers

Amlodipine (Norvasc)
Clevidipine (Cleviprex)
Diltiazem (Cardizem, Dilacor XR, others)
Felodipine (Plendil)
Isradipine (DynaCirc)
Nicardipine (Cardene)
Nifedipine (Adalat, Nifedical, Nifediac, Procardia)
Nimodipine (Nimotop)
Nisoldipine (Sular)
Verapamil (Calan, Isoptin SR, Covera-HS, Verelan)

---

4. Should be used with caution in the client with CHF, bradycardia, or atrioventricular block

B. Side effects
1. Bradycardia
2. Hypotension
3. Reflex tachycardia as a result of hypotension
4. Headache
5. Dizziness, light-headedness
6. Fatigue
7. Peripheral edema
8. Constipation
9. Flushing of the skin
10. Changes in liver and kidney function

C. Interventions
1. Monitor vital signs.
2. Monitor for signs of heart failure.
3. Monitor liver enzyme levels.
4. Monitor kidney function tests.
5. Instruct the client not to discontinue the medication.
6. Instruct the client in how to take the pulse.
7. Instruct the client to notify the physician if dizziness or fainting occurs.
8. Instruct the client not to crush or chew sustained-release tablets.

XIII. PERIPHERAL VASODILATORS (Box 61-18)

A. Description
1. Peripheral vasodilators decrease peripheral resistance by exerting a direct action on the arteries or on the arteries and the veins.
2. Peripheral vasodilators increase blood flow to the extremities and are used in peripheral vascular disorders of venous and arterial vessels.
3. Peripheral vasodilators are most effective for disorders resulting from vasospasm (Raynaud's disease).
4. These medications may decrease some symptoms of cerebral vascular insufficiency.

B. Side effects
1. Light-headedness, dizziness
2. **Orthostatic hypotension**
3. Tachycardia
4. Palpitations

Box 61-18 Peripheral Vasodilators

α-Adrenergic Blockers
Prazosin (Minipress)
Terazosin (Hytrin)

Calcium Channel Blockers
Diltiazem (Cardizem, Dilacor XR, others)
Nifedipine (Adalat, Nifedical, Nifediac, Procardia)
Nimodipine (Nimotop)
Verapamil (Calan, Isoptin SR, Covera-HS, Verelan)

Hemorheological
Pentoxifylline (Trental; increases microcirculation and tissue perfusion)

Box 61-19 Direct-Acting Vasodilators

Diazoxide (Hyperstat)
Fenoldopam (Corlopam)
Hydralazine (Apresoline)
Minoxidil (Loniten)
Nitroglycerin
Sodium nitroprusside (Nitropress)

5. Flushing
6. Gastrointestinal distress
C. Interventions
   1. Monitor vital signs, especially the **BP** and the heart rate.
   2. Monitor for **orthostatic hypotension** and tachycardia.
   3. Monitor for signs of inadequate blood flow to the extremities, such as pallor, feeling cold, and pain.
   4. Instruct the client that it may take up to 3 months for a desired therapeutic response.
   5. Advise the client not to smoke because smoking increases vasospasm.
   6. Instruct the client to avoid aspirin or aspirin-like compounds unless approved by the physician.
   7. Instruct the client to take the medication with meals if gastrointestinal disturbances occur.
   8. Instruct the client to avoid alcohol because it may cause a hypotensive reaction.
   9. Encourage the client to change positions slowly to avoid **orthostatic hypotension**.

XIV. DIRECT-ACTING ARTERIOLAR VASODILATORS
(Box 61-19)

A. Description
   1. Direct-acting vasodilators relax the smooth muscles of the blood vessels, mainly the arteries, causing vasodilation.
   2. Direct-acting vasodilators promote an increase in blood flow to the brain and kidneys.

3. With vasodilation, the **BP** drops and sodium and water are retained, resulting in peripheral edema.
4. Diuretics may be given to decrease the edema.
5. Direct-acting vasodilators are used in the client with moderate to severe hypertension.
6. Direct-acting vasodilators are used during acute hypertensive emergencies.

B. Side effects
   1. Hypotension
   2. Reflex tachycardia caused by vasodilation and the drop in **BP**
   3. Palpitations
   4. Edema
   5. Dizziness
   6. Headaches
   7. Nasal congestion
   8. Gastrointestinal bleeding
   9. Neurological symptoms
   10. Confusion
   11. Excess hair growth with minoxidil (Loniten)
   12. With sodium nitroprusside, cyanide toxicity and thiocyanate toxicity can occur.

C. Interventions
   1. Monitor vital signs, especially **BP**.
   2. Sodium nitroprusside
      a. Monitor cyanide and thiocyanate levels.
      b. Protect from light because the medication decomposes.
      c. When administering, solution must be covered by a dark bag provided by the manufacturer and is stable for 24 hours.
      d. Discard if the medication is red, green, or blue.

⚠ Vasodilators cause orthostatic hypotension. Instruct the client about safety measures when taking these medications, such as the need to rise from a lying to a sitting or standing position slowly.

XV. MISCELLANEOUS VASODILATOR

A. Description
   1. Nesiritide (Natrecor)
      a. Recombinant version of human B-type natriuretic peptide that vasodilates arteries and veins
      b. Used for the treatment of decompensated heart failure
   2. Side effects
      a. Hypotension
      b. Confusion
      c. Dizziness
      d. Dysrhythmias
   3. Interventions
      a. Administer by continuous intravenous infusion via pump
      b. Monitor **BP**, cardiac rhythm, urine output, and body weight.
      c. Monitor for signs of resolving heart failure.

XVI. ANTIDYSRHYTHMIC MEDICATIONS

A. Description: Antidysrhythmic medications suppress dysrhythmias by inhibiting abnormal pathways of electrical conduction through the heart.

B. Class I antidysrhythmics are sodium channel blockers, class II are β-blockers, class III are potassium channel blockers (medications that delay repolarization), and class IV are calcium channel blockers.

C. Class IA antidysrhythmics
1. Disopyramide (Norpace)
2. Procainamide (Procanbid)
3. Quinidine sulfate

D. Class IB antidysrhythmics
1. Lidocaine (Xylocaine)
2. Mexiletine hydrochloride (Mexitil)
3. Phenytoin (Dilantin)

E. Class IC antidysrhythmics
1. Flecainide acetate (Tambocor)
2. Propafenone hydrochloride (Rythmol)
3. Other Class I medication: Moricizine (Ethmozine)
4. Side effects: Class I antidysrhythmics
   a. Hypotension
   b. Heart failure
   c. Worsened or new dysrhythmias
   d. Nausea, vomiting, or diarrhea

F. Class II antidysrhythmics
1. Acebutolol (Sectral)
2. Esmolol (Brevibloc)
3. Propranolol (Inderal)
4. Side effects: Class II antidysrhythmics
   a. Dizziness
   b. Fatigue
   c. Hypotension
   d. Bradycardia
   e. Heart failure
   f. Dysrhythmias
   g. Heart block
   h. Bronchospasms
   i. Gastrointestinal distress

G. Class III antidysrhythmics
1. Amiodarone (Cordarone, Pacerone)
2. Bretylium
3. Dofetilide (Tikosyn)
4. Ibutilide (Corvert)
5. Sotalol (Betapace)
6. Side effects: Class III antidysrhythmics
   a. Hypotension
   b. Bradycardia
   c. Nausea, vomiting
   d. Amiodarone hydrochloride may cause pulmonary fibrosis, photosensitivity, bluish skin discoloration, corneal deposits, peripheral neuropathy, tremor, poor coordination, abnormal gait, and hypothyroidism.
   e. Bretylium may cause vertigo, syncope, and dizziness.

Box 61-20 Adrenergic Agonists

Dobutamine
Dopamine
Epinephrine (Adrenalin)
Isoproterenol (Isuprel)
Norepinephrine (Levophed)

H. Class IV antidysrhythmics
1. Verapamil (Isoptin, Calan, Verelan)
2. Diltiazem (Cardizem)
3. Side effects: Class IV antidysrhythmics
   a. Dizziness
   b. Hypotension
   c. Bradycardia
   d. Edema
   e. Constipation

I. Other antidysrhythmics
1. Adenosine (Adenocard)
2. Digoxin (Lanoxin)

J. Interventions for antidysrhythmics
1. Monitor heart rate, respiratory rate, and **BP**.
2. Monitor electrocardiogram.
3. Provide continuous cardiac monitoring.
4. Maintain therapeutic serum drug levels.
5. Before administering lidocaine, always check the vial label to prevent administering a form that contains epinephrine or preservatives because these solutions are used for local anesthesia only.
6. Do not administer antidysrhythmics with food because food may affect absorption.
7. Mexiletine may be administered with food or antacids to reduce gastrointestinal distress.
8. Always administer IV antidysrhythmics via an infusion pump.
9. Monitor for signs of fluid retention such as weight gain, peripheral edema, or shortness of breath.
10. Advise the client to limit fluid and salt intake to minimize fluid retention.
11. Monitor respiratory, thyroid, and neurological functions.
12. After administering bretylium, keep the client supine and monitor for hypotension.
13. Instruct the client to change positions slowly to minimize **orthostatic hypotension**.
14. Instruct the client taking amiodarone to use sunscreen and protective clothing to prevent photosensitivity reactions.
15. Encourage the client to increase fiber intake to prevent constipation.

XVII. ADRENERGIC AGONISTS (Box 61-20)

A. Dobutamine
1. Increases myocardial force and **cardiac output** through stimulation of beta receptors

2. Used in clients with heart failure and for clients undergoing cardiopulmonary bypass surgery

B. Dopamine
1. Increases **BP** and **cardiac output** through positive inotropic action and increases renal blood flow through its action on alpha and beta receptors
2. Used to treat mild renal failure caused by low **cardiac output**

C. Epinephrine (Adrenalin)
1. Used for cardiac stimulation in cardiac arrest
2. Used for bronchodilation in asthma or allergic reactions
3. Produces mydriasis
4. Produces local vasoconstriction when combined with local anesthetics and prolongs anesthetic action by decreasing blood flow to the site

D. Isoproterenol (Isuprel)
1. Stimulates beta receptors
2. Used for cardiac stimulation and bronchodilation

E. Norepinephrine (Levophed)
1. Stimulates the heart in cardiac arrest
2. Vasoconstricts and increases the **BP** in hypotension and shock

F. Side effects
1. Dysrhythmias
2. Tachycardia
3. Angina
4. Restlessness
5. Urgency or urinary incontinence

G. Interventions
1. Monitor vital signs.
2. Monitor lung sounds.
3. Monitor urinary output.
4. Monitor electrocardiogram.
5. Administer the medication through a large vein.

XVIII. ANTILIPEMIC MEDICATIONS

A. Description
1. Antilipemic medications reduce serum levels of cholesterol, triglycerides, or low-density lipoprotein.
2. When cholesterol, triglyceride, and low-density lipoprotein levels are elevated, the client is at increased risk for coronary artery disease.
3. In many cases, diet alone will not lower blood lipid levels; therefore antilipemic medications will be prescribed.

B. Bile sequestrants (Box 61-21)
1. Description
   a. Bind with acids in the intestines, which prevents reabsorption of cholesterol
   b. Should not be used as the only therapy in clients with elevated triglyceride levels because they may raise triglyceride levels.
2. Side effects
   a. Constipation
   b. Gastrointestinal disturbances: Heartburn, nausea, belching, bloating

Box 61-21 Bile Acid Sequestrants

Cholestyramine (Questran)
Colesevelam (WelChol)
Colestipol (Colestid)

Box 61-22 HMG-CoA Reductase Inhibitors

Atorvastatin (Lipitor)
Fluvastatin (Lescol)
Lovastatin (Mevacor)
Pravastatin (Pravachol)
Rosuvastatin (Crestor)
Simvastatin (Zocor)

3. Interventions
   a. Cholestyramine (Questran) comes in a gritty powder that must be mixed thoroughly in juice or water before administration.
   b. Monitor the client for early signs of peptic ulcer such as nausea and abdominal discomfort followed by abdominal pain and distention.
   c. Instruct the client that the medication must be taken with and followed by sufficient fluids.

C. HMG-CoA reductase inhibitors (Box 61-22)
1. Description
   a. Lovastatin (Mevacor) is highly protein-bound and should not be administered with anticoagulants.
   b. Lovastatin should not be administered with gemfibrozil (Lopid).
   c. Administer lovastatin with caution to the client taking immunosuppressive medications.
2. Side effects
   a. Nausea
   b. Diarrhea or constipation
   c. Abdominal pain or cramps
   d. Flatulence
   e. Dizziness
   f. Headache
   g. Blurred vision
   h. Rash
   i. Pruritus
   j. Elevated liver enzyme levels
   k. Muscle cramps and fatigue
3. Interventions
   a. Monitor serum liver enzyme levels.
   b. Instruct the client to receive an annual eye examination because the medications can cause cataract formation.
   c. If lovastatin is not effective in lowering the lipid level after 3 months, it should be discontinued.

Box 61-23 Other Antilipemic Medications

Ezetimibe (Zetia)
Ezetimibe; simvastatin (Vytorin)
Fenofibrate
Gemfibrozil (Lopid)
Nicotinic acid (Niacin)
Probucol

⚠ Instruct the client who is taking an antilipemic medication to report any unexplained muscular pain to the health care provider immediately.

D. Other antilipemic medications (Box 61-23)

  1. Description

    a. Gemfibrozil should not be taken with anticoagulants because they compete for protein sites; if the client is taking an anticoagulant, the anticoagulant dose should be reduced during antilipemic therapy and the INR should be monitored closely.

    b. Do not administer gemfibrozil with HMG-CoA reductase inhibitors because it increases the risk for myositis, myalgias, and rhabdomyolysis.

    c. Fish oil supplements have been associated with a decreased risk for cardiovascular heart disease; plant stanol and sterol esters and cholestin have been associated with reducing cholesterol levels.

  2. Interventions

    a. Monitor vital signs.

    b. Monitor liver enzyme levels.

    c. Monitor serum cholesterol and triglyceride levels.

    d. Instruct the client to restrict intake of fats, cholesterol, carbohydrates, and alcohol.

    e. Instruct the client to follow an exercise program.

    f. Instruct the client that it will take several weeks before the lipid level declines.

    g. Instruct the client to have an annual eye examination and to report any changes in vision.

    h. Instruct the client with diabetes mellitus who is taking gemfibrozil to monitor blood glucose levels regularly.

    i. Instruct the client to increase fluid intake.

    j. Note that nicotinic acid has numerous side effects, including gastrointestinal disturbances, flushing of the skin, elevated liver enzyme levels, hyperglycemia, and hyperuricemia.

    k. Instruct the client that aspirin or nonsteroidal anti-inflammatory drugs taken 30 minutes before may assist in reducing the side effect of cutaneous flushing from nicotinic acid.

    l. Instruct the client to take nicotinic acid with meals to reduce gastrointestinal discomfort.

 MORE QUESTIONS ON THE CD!

Practice Questions

717. A client with atrial fibrillation is receiving a continuous heparin infusion at 1000 units/hr. The nurse would determine that the client is receiving the therapeutic effect based on which of the following results?

  1. Prothrombin time of 12.5 seconds

  2. Activated partial thromboplastin time of 60 seconds

  3. Activated partial thromboplastin time of 28 seconds

  4. Activated partial thromboplastin time longer than 120 seconds

718. A nurse provides discharge instructions to a postoperative client who is taking warfarin sodium (Coumadin). Which statement, if made by the client, reflects the need for further teaching?

  1. "I will take my pills every day at the same time."

  2. "I will avoid alcohol consumption."

  3. "I have already called my family to pick up a Medic-Alert bracelet."

  4. "I will take Ecotrin (enteric-coated aspirin) for my headaches because it is coated."

719. A client who is receiving digoxin (Lanoxin) daily has a serum potassium level of 3 mEq/L and is complaining of anorexia. A physician prescribes a digoxin level to rule out digoxin toxicity. A nurse checks the results, knowing that which of the following is the therapeutic serum level (range) for digoxin?

  1. 0.5 to 2 ng/mL

  2. 1.2 to 2.8 ng/mL

  3. 3 to 5 ng/mL

  4. 3.5 to 5.5 ng/mL

720. A client is being treated with procainamide (Procanbid) for a cardiac dysrhythmia. Following intravenous administration of the medication, the client complains of dizziness. What intervention should the nurse take first?

  1. Administer prescribed nitroglycerin tablets.

  2. Measure the heart rate on the rhythm strip.

  3. Obtain a 12-lead electrocardiogram immediately.

  4. Auscultate the client's apical pulse and obtain a blood pressure.

721. A nurse is monitoring a client who is taking propranolol (Inderal). Which assessment data would indicate a potential serious complication associated with propranolol?

  1. The development of complaints of insomnia

  2. The development of audible expiratory wheezes

3. A baseline blood pressure of 150/80 mm Hg followed by a blood pressure of 138/72 mm Hg after two doses of the medication
4. A baseline resting heart rate of 88 beats/min followed by a resting heart rate of 72 beats/min after two doses of the medication

722. A nurse is caring for a client receiving a heparin intravenous (IV) infusion. The nurse anticipates that which laboratory study will be prescribed to monitor the therapeutic effect of heparin?
1. Hematocrit
2. Hemoglobin
3. Prothrombin time
4. Activated partial thromboplastin time

723. A client is diagnosed with an acute myocardial infarction and is receiving tissue plasminogen activator, alteplase (Activase, tPA). Which of the following is a priority nursing intervention?
1. Monitor for renal failure.
2. Monitor psychosocial status.
3. Monitor for signs of bleeding.
4. Have heparin sodium available.

724. A nurse is planning to administer hydrochlorothiazide (HydroDIURIL) to a client. The nurse understands that which of the following are concerns related to the administration of this medication?
1. Hypouricemia, hyperkalemia
2. Increased risk of osteoporosis
3. Hypokalemia, hyperglycemia, sulfa allergy
4. Hyperkalemia, hypoglycemia, penicillin allergy

725. A home health care nurse is visiting a client with elevated triglyceride levels and a serum cholesterol level of 398 mg/dL. The client is taking cholestyramine (Questran). Which of the following statements, if made by the client, indicates the need for further education?
1. "Constipation and bloating might be a problem."
2. "I'll continue to watch my diet and reduce my fats."
3. "Walking a mile each day will help the whole process."
4. "I'll continue my nicotinic acid from the health food store."

726. A client is on nicotinic acid (niacin) for hyperlipidemia and the nurse provides instructions to the client about the medication. Which statement by the client would indicate an understanding of the instructions?
1. "It is not necessary to avoid the use of alcohol."
2. "The medication should be taken with meals to decrease flushing."

3. "Clay-colored stools are a common side effect and should not be of concern."
4. "Ibuprofen (Motrin) taken 30 minutes before the nicotinic acid should decrease the flushing."

727. A 66-year-old client complaining of not feeling well is seen in a clinic. The client is taking several medications for the control of heart disease and hypertension. These medications include atenolol (Tenormin), digoxin (Lanoxin), and chlorothiazide (Diuril). A tentative diagnosis of digoxin toxicity is made. Which of the following assessment data would support this diagnosis?
1. Dyspnea, edema, and palpitations
2. Chest pain, hypotension, and paresthesia
3. Double vision, loss of appetite, and nausea
4. Constipation, dry mouth, and sleep disorder

728. A client is being treated for acute congestive heart failure with intravenously administered bumetanide (Bumex). The vital signs are as follows: blood pressure, 100/60 mm Hg; pulse, 96 beats/min; and respirations, 24 breaths/min. After the initial dose, which of the following is the priority assessment?
1. Monitoring weight loss
2. Monitoring urine output
3. Monitoring blood pressure
4. Monitoring potassium level

729. Intravenous heparin therapy is prescribed for a client. While implementing this prescription, a nurse ensures that which of the following medications is available on the nursing unit?
1. Protamine sulfate
2. Potassium chloride
3. Aminocaproic acid (Amicar)
4. Vitamin K (AquaMEPHYTON)

730. A client is receiving thrombolytic therapy with a continuous infusion of streptokinase (Streptase). The client suddenly becomes extremely anxious and complains of itching. A nurse hears stridor and on examination of the client notes generalized urticaria and hypotension. Which of the following should be the priority action of the nurse?
1. Administer oxygen and protamine sulfate.
2. Stop the infusion and call the physician.
3. Cut the infusion rate in half and sit the client up in bed.
4. Administer diphenhydramine (Benadryl) and continue the infusion.

731. A client is admitted with pulmonary embolism and is to be treated with streptokinase (Streptase). A nurse would report which of the following assessments to the physician before initiating this therapy?

1. Adventitious breath sounds
2. Temperature of 99.4° F orally
3. Blood pressure of 198/110 mm Hg
4. Respiratory rate of 28 breaths/min

Alternate Item Format: Multiple Response

732. The nurse is monitoring a client who is taking digoxin (Lanoxin) for adverse effects. Which findings are characteristic of digoxin toxicity. **Select all that apply**.

❑ 1. Tremors
❑ 2. Diarrhea
❑ 3. Irritability
❑ 4. Blurred vision
❑ 5. Nausea and vomiting

ANSWERS

717. 2

Rationale: Common laboratory ranges for activated partial thromboplastin time are 20 to 36 seconds. Because the activated partial thromboplastin time should be 1.5 to 2.5 times the normal value, the client's activated partial thromboplastin time would be considered therapeutic if it was 60 seconds.

Test-Taking Strategy: Use the process of elimination. Option 1 is eliminated because the prothrombin time assesses response to warfarin (Coumadin) therapy. Eliminate option 3 because at 28 seconds the client is receiving no therapeutic effect from the continuous heparin infusion. Eliminate option 4 because this value is beyond the therapeutic range and the client is at risk for bleeding. Review laboratory tests to monitor the effectiveness of heparin therapy if you had difficulty with this question.

Level of Cognitive Ability: Evaluating
Client Needs: Physiological Integrity
Integrated Process: Nursing Process—Evaluation
Content Area: Pharmacology
References: Kee, J., Hayes, E., & McCuistion, L. (2009). *Pharmacology: A nursing process approach* (6th ed., pp. 682–683). St. Louis: Saunders.

   Lehne, R. (2010). *Pharmacology for nursing care* (7th ed., p. 600). St. Louis: Saunders.

718. 4

Rationale: Ecotrin is an aspirin-containing product and should be avoided. Alcohol consumption should be avoided by a client taking warfarin sodium. Taking prescribed medication at the same time each day increases client compliance. The Medic-Alert bracelet provides health care personnel emergency information.

Test-Taking Strategy: Use the process of elimination and note the strategic words *need for further teaching*. These words indicate a negative event query and ask you to select an option that is an incorrect statement. Recalling that warfarin (Coumadin) is an anticoagulant and that Ecotrin is an aspirin-containing product will direct you to option 4. Review client teaching points related to warfarin if you had difficulty with this question.

Level of Cognitive Ability: Evaluating
Client Needs: Physiological Integrity
Integrated Process: Teaching and Learning
Content Area: Pharmacology
References: Hodgson, B., & Kizior, R. (2010). *Saunders nursing drug handbook 2010* (p. 1197). St. Louis: Saunders.

   Lehne, R. (2010). *Pharmacology for nursing care* (7th ed., p. 606). St. Louis: Saunders.

719. 1

Rationale: Therapeutic levels for digoxin range from 0.5 to 2 ng/mL. Therefore options 2, 3, and 4 are incorrect.

Test-Taking Strategy: Knowledge of the therapeutic serum digoxin level will direct you to option 1. If you had difficulty with this question, learn the therapeutic level for digoxin.

Level of Cognitive Ability: Understanding
Client Needs: Physiological Integrity
Integrated Process: Nursing Process—Assessment
Content Area: Pharmacology
Reference: Kee, J., Hayes, E., & McCuistion, L. (2009). *Pharmacology: A nursing process approach* (6th ed., p. 624). St. Louis: Saunders.

720. 4

Rationale: Signs of toxicity from procainamide include confusion, dizziness, drowsiness, decreased urination, nausea, vomiting, and tachydysrhythmias. If the client complains of dizziness, the nurse should assess the vital signs first. Although options 2 and 3 may be interventions, these would be done after the vital signs are taken. Nitroglycerin is a vasodilator and will lower the blood pressure.

Test-Taking Strategy: Use the steps of the nursing process to eliminate options 1 and 3. From the remaining options, remember always to assess the client first, not the monitoring devices. Therefore option 4 is correct. Review the signs of toxicity and the nursing interventions if you had difficulty with this question.

Level of Cognitive Ability: Applying
Client Needs: Physiological Integrity
Integrated Process: Nursing Process—Implementation
Content Area: Pharmacology
References: Gahart, B., & Nazareno, A. (2010). *2010 Intravenous medications* (26th ed., p. 1115). St. Louis: Mosby.

   Lehne, R. (2010). *Pharmacology for nursing care* (7th ed., p. 551). St. Louis: Saunders.

721. 2

Rationale: Audible expiratory wheezes may indicate a serious adverse reaction, bronchospasm. β-Blockers may induce this reaction, particularly in clients with chronic obstructive pulmonary disease or asthma. Normal decreases in blood pressure and heart rate are expected. Insomnia is a frequent mild side effect and should be monitored.

Test-Taking Strategy: Use the process of elimination, eliminating options 3 and 4 because these are expected effects from

the medication. Note the strategic words *potential serious complication.* These strategic words will direct you to option 2. Review the adverse effects of this medication if you had difficulty with this question.
Level of Cognitive Ability: Analyzing
Client Needs: Physiological Integrity
Integrated Process: Nursing Process—Assessment
Content Area: Pharmacology
Reference: Hodgson, B., & Kizior, R. (2010). *Saunders nursing drug handbook 2010* (pp. 955–957). St. Louis: Saunders.

722. 4
Rationale: The prothrombin time will assess for the therapeutic effect of warfarin sodium (Coumadin), and the activated partial thromboplastin time (aPTT) will assess the therapeutic effect of heparin. Hematocrit and hemoglobin values assess red blood cell concentrations. Baseline assessment, including an aPTT value, should be completed, as well as ongoing daily aPTT values while the client is taking heparin. Heparin doses are determined based on the result of the aPTT.
Test-Taking Strategy: Use the process of elimination. Eliminate options 1 and 2 because they are comparable or alike and are unrelated to heparin therapy. From the remaining options, recall the relationship between the prothrombin time and warfarin and the aPTT and heparin. Review care of a client on heparin infusion if you had difficulty with this question.
Level of Cognitive Ability: Evaluating
Client Needs: Physiological Integrity
Integrated Process: Nursing Process—Assessment
Content Area: Pharmacology
Reference: Gahart, B., & Nazareno, A. (2010). *2010 Intravenous medications* (26th ed., p. 680). St. Louis: Mosby.

723. 3
Rationale: Tissue plasminogen activator is a thrombolytic. Hemorrhage is a complication of any type of thrombolytic medication. The client is monitored for bleeding. Monitoring for renal failure and monitoring the client's psychosocial status are important but are not the most critical interventions. Heparin is given after thrombolytic therapy, but the question is not asking about follow-up medications.
Test-Taking Strategy: Use the process of elimination and note the strategic word *priority.* Remember, bleeding is a priority. Review care of the client on tissue plasminogen activator if you had difficulty with this question.
Level of Cognitive Ability: Applying
Client Needs: Physiological Integrity
Integrated Process: Nursing Process—Implementation
Content Area: Pharmacology
Reference: Hodgson, B., & Kizior, R. (2010). *Saunders nursing drug handbook 2010* (p. 42). St. Louis: Saunders.

724. 3
Rationale: Thiazide diuretics such as hydrochlorothiazide are sulfa-based medications, and a client with a sulfa allergy is at risk for an allergic reaction. Also, clients are at risk for hypokalemia, hyperglycemia, hypercalcemia, hyperlipidemia, and hyperuricemia.
Test-Taking Strategy: Use the process of elimination. Recalling that thiazide diuretics carry a sulfa ring will direct you to option 3. Review the nursing considerations related to administering this medication if you had difficulty with this question.

Level of Cognitive Ability: Analyzing
Client Needs: Physiological Integrity
Integrated Process: Nursing Process—Analysis
Content Area: Pharmacology
References: Hodgson, B., & Kizior, R. (2010). *Saunders nursing drug handbook 2010* (pp. 558–559). St. Louis: Saunders.
Lehne, R. (2010). *Pharmacology for nursing care* (7th ed., pp. 453–454). St. Louis: Saunders.

725. 4
Rationale: Nicotinic acid, even an over-the-counter form, should be avoided because it may lead to liver abnormalities. All lipid-lowering medications also can cause liver abnormalities, so a combination of nicotinic acid and cholestyramine resin is to be avoided. Constipation and bloating are the two most common side effects. Walking and the reduction of fats in the diet are therapeutic measures to reduce cholesterol and triglyceride levels.
Test-Taking Strategy: Use the process of elimination and note the strategic words *need for further education.* These words indicate a negative event query and ask you to select an option that is an incorrect statement. Remembering that over-the-counter medications should be avoided when a client is taking a prescription medication will direct you to option 4. Review client teaching points related to this medication if you had difficulty with this question.
Level of Cognitive Ability: Evaluating
Client Needs: Physiological Integrity
Integrated Process: Teaching and Learning
Content Area: Pharmacology
Reference: Lehne, R. (2010). *Pharmacology for nursing care* (7th ed., pp. 577–578). St. Louis: Saunders.

726. 4
Rationale: Flushing is a side effect of this medication. Aspirin or a nonsteroidal anti-inflammatory drug can be taken 30 minutes prior to taking the medication to decrease flushing. Alcohol consumption needs to be avoided because it will enhance this side effect. The medication should be taken with meals but this will decrease gastrointestinal upset; taking the medication with meals has no effect on the flushing. Clay-colored stools are a sign of hepatic dysfunction and should be immediately reported to the physician.
Test-Taking Strategy: Use the process of elimination. Option 1 can be eliminated because alcohol must be abstained from. Option 2 can be eliminated because taking the medication with meals helps decrease the gastrointestinal symptoms. The clay-colored stools in option 3 is a sign of hepatic dysfunction and should be immediately reported to the physician. Review the client teaching points related to this medication if you had difficulty with this question.
Level of Cognitive Ability: Evaluating
Client Needs: Physiological Integrity
Integrated Process: Nursing Process—Evaluation
Content Area: Pharmacology
Reference: Lehne, R. (2010). *Pharmacology for nursing care* (7th ed., p. 578). St. Louis: Saunders.

727. 3
Rationale: Double vision, loss of appetite, and nausea are early signs of digoxin toxicity. Additional signs of digoxin toxicity

include bradycardia, difficulty reading, other visual alterations such as green and yellow vision or seeing spots or halos, confusion, vomiting, diarrhea, decreased libido, and impotence.
Test-Taking Strategy: Use the process of elimination. Recalling that gastrointestinal and visual disturbances occur with digoxin toxicity will direct you to option 3. If you had difficulty with this question, review the signs of digoxin toxicity.
Level of Cognitive Ability: Analyzing
Client Needs: Physiological Integrity
Integrated Process: Nursing Process—Assessment
Content Area: Pharmacology
References: Kee, J., Hayes, E., & McCuistion, L. (2009). *Pharmacology: A nursing process approach* (6th ed., p. 624). St. Louis: Saunders.
   Lehne, R. (2010). *Pharmacology for nursing care* (7th ed., pp. 531–532). St. Louis: Saunders.

728. 3
Rationale: Hypotension is a common side effect associated with the use of this medication. Options 1, 2, and 4 also require assessment but are not the priority.
Test-Taking Strategy: Use the process of elimination and note the strategic word *priority*. Also, note that blood pressure is mentioned in the question and in option 3. Use of the ABCs—airway, breathing, and circulation—also will direct you to option 3. Review care of the client receiving this medication by the intravenous route if you had difficulty with this question.
Level of Cognitive Ability: Applying
Client Needs: Physiological Integrity
Integrated Process: Nursing Process—Implementation
Content Area: Pharmacology
References: Gahart, B., & Nazareno, A. (2010). *2010 Intravenous medications* (26th ed., p. 215). St. Louis: Mosby.
   Hodgson, B., & Kizior, R. (2010). *Saunders nursing drug handbook 2010* (p. 150). St. Louis: Saunders.

729. 1
Rationale: The antidote to heparin is protamine sulfate; it should be readily available for use if excessive bleeding or hemorrhage should occur. Vitamin K is an antidote for warfarin sodium. Aminocaproic acid is the antidote for thrombolytic therapy. Potassium chloride is administered for a potassium deficit.
Test-Taking Strategy: Knowledge regarding the various antidotes is needed to answer this question. Remember the antidote to heparin is protamine sulfate. Learn these antidotes if you had difficulty with this question.
Level of Cognitive Ability: Applying
Client Needs: Physiological Integrity
Integrated Process: Nursing Process—Planning
Content Area: Pharmacology
Reference: Gahart, B., & Nazareno, A. (2010). *2010 Intravenous medications* (26th ed., p. 682). St. Louis: Mosby.

730. 2
Rationale: The client is experiencing an anaphylactic reaction to streptokinase, which is allergenic. The infusion should be stopped, the physician notified, and the client treated with epinephrine, antihistamines, and corticosteroids.
Test-Taking Strategy: Recall that an allergic reaction and possible anaphylaxis are risks associated with streptokinase therapy. Also, focusing on the signs and symptoms in the question will assist in answering the question. When a severe allergic reaction

occurs, the offending substance should be stopped, and lifesaving treatment should begin. Review the adverse effects of this medication if you had difficulty with this question.
Level of Cognitive Ability: Applying
Client Needs: Physiological Integrity
Integrated Process: Nursing Process—Implementation
Content Area: Pharmacology
Reference: Kee, J., Hayes, E., & McCuistion, L. (2009). *Pharmacology: A nursing process approach* (6th ed., p. 688). St. Louis: Saunders.

731. 3
Rationale: Thrombolytic therapy is contraindicated in a number of preexisting conditions in which there is a risk of uncontrolled bleeding, similar to the case in anticoagulant therapy. Thrombolytic therapy also is contraindicated in severe uncontrolled hypertension because of the risk of cerebral hemorrhage. Therefore the nurse would report the results of the blood pressure to the physician before initiating therapy.
Test-Taking Strategy: Use the process of elimination and focus on the client's diagnosis. Options 1, 2, and 4 may be present in the client with pulmonary embolism but are not necessarily signs that warrant reporting before this therapy is initiated. Review the contraindications associated with the administration of this medication if you had difficulty with this question.
Level of Cognitive Ability: Analyzing
Client Needs: Physiological Integrity
Integrated Process: Nursing Process—Implementation
Content Area: Pharmacology
Reference: Ignatavicius, D., & Workman, M. (2010). *Medical-surgical nursing: Patient-centered collaborative care* (6th ed., pp. 858–859). St. Louis: Saunders.

ALTERNATE ITEM FORMAT: MULTIPLE RESPONSE
732. 2, 4, 5
Rationale: Digoxin (Lanoxin) is a cardiac glycoside. The risk of toxicity can occur with the use of this medication. Toxicity can lead to life-threatening events and the nurse needs to monitor the client closely for signs of toxicity. Early signs of toxicity include gastrointestinal manifestations such as anorexia, nausea, vomiting, and diarrhea. Subsequent manifestations include headache, visual disturbances such as diplopia, blurred vision, yellow-green halos, photophobia, drowsiness, fatigue, and weakness. Cardiac rhythm abnormalities can also occur. The nurse also monitors the digoxin level. Therapeutic levels for digoxin range from 0.5 to 2 ng/mL.
Test-Taking Strategy: Specific knowledge regarding the characteristics of digoxin toxicity is needed to answer this question. Recall that the early signs are gastrointestinal manifestations. Next, recall that visual disturbances occur. If you had difficulty with this question review the manifestations associated with digoxin toxicity.
Level of Cognitive Ability: Analyzing
Client Needs: Physiological Integrity
Integrated Process: Nursing Process—Assessment
Content Area: Pharmacology
Reference: Kee, J., Hayes, E., & McCuistion, L. (2009). *Pharmacology: A nursing process approach* (6th ed., p. 624). St. Louis: Saunders.

UNIT XIV

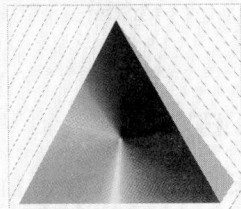

The Adult Client With a Renal System Disorder

PYRAMID TERMS

acute renal failure (ARF) The sudden loss of kidney function caused by renal cell damage from ischemia or toxic substances. Acute renal failure occurs abruptly and can be reversible. Acute renal failure leads to hypoperfusion, cell death, and decompensation in renal function. The prognosis depends on the cause and condition of the client. Near-normal or normal kidney function may resume gradually.

anuria Urine output of less than 100 mL/day.

arterial steal syndrome A syndrome that can develop following the insertion of an arteriovenous fistula when too much blood is diverted to the vein and arterial perfusion to the hand is compromised.

arteriovenous fistula Surgical creation by anastomosis of an opening, or fistula, between a large artery and a large vein. The flow of arterial blood into the venous system causes the vein to become engorged (maturity). Maturity is necessary so that the engorged vein can be punctured using a large-bore needle. This also allows the blood to be returned quickly for effective dialysis.

azotemia The retention of nitrogenous waste products in the blood.

chronic renal failure (CRF) The progressive loss and ongoing deterioration in kidney function. It is characterized by a glomerular filtration rate of less than 60 mL/min for a period of 3 months or longer. Chronic renal failure is irreversible and results in uremia or end-stage renal disease. Chronic renal failure requires dialysis or kidney transplantation to maintain life.

dialysis A blood filtering procedure that is indicated when kidney function deteriorates and the accumulation of water and waste products interferes with life functions. Dialysis is performed via the blood stream (hemodialysis) or through the peritoneal cavity (peritoneal dialysis).

disequilibrium syndrome A rapid change in the composition of the extracellular fluid that occurs during hemodialysis. Solutes are removed from the blood faster than from the cerebrospinal fluid and brain. Fluid is pulled into the brain, causing cerebral edema.

nephrolithiasis The formation of kidney stones. Kidney stones are formed in the renal parenchyma.

oliguria Urine output of less than 400 mL/day.

renal failure The loss of kidney function. The types of renal failure include acute renal failure and chronic renal failure. The signs and symptoms of renal failure are caused by the retention of wastes, the retention of fluids, and the inability of the kidneys to regulate electrolytes.

urolithiasis The formation of urinary stones or calculi. Urinary calculi are formed in the ureter.

PYRAMID TO SUCCESS

Pyramid Points focus on acute renal failure and chronic renal failure, dialysis procedures such as hemodialysis and peritoneal dialysis, urinary diversions, and postoperative care following urinary or renal surgery. Focus on the major problems associated with renal failure and the rationale for the prescribed treatment modalities. Be familiar with the complications associated with hemodialysis and peritoneal dialysis, the specific assessment data related to complications, and the expected treatment. Focus on the care of a peritoneal catheter and hemodialysis access devices, the complications associated with these access devices, and the appropriate nursing interventions if a complication is suspected. Review preoperative and postoperative care related to renal transplantation and the assessment data indicating rejection. Be familiar with urinary diversions, care to the client following prostatectomy, and treatment measures for the client with urinary or renal calculi.

 CLIENT NEEDS

Safe and Effective Care Environment

Consulting with members of the health care team

Establishing priorities

Identifying the guidelines related to renal organ donation

Maintaining confidentiality related to the renal disorder

Maintaining asepsis related to wound care and dialysis access devices

Obtaining informed consent related to diagnostic and surgical procedures

Preventing injury related to complications of the disorder

Maintaining standard and other precautions related to care of the client

Upholding client rights

Health Promotion and Maintenance

Discussing expected body image changes

Performing urinary and renal physical assessment techniques

Providing client instructions regarding care of a urinary diversion, dialysis access device, and dialysis procedures

Providing client instructions regarding postoperative management

Providing client instructions regarding prescribed treatments related to urinary or renal disorder

Providing client instructions regarding the prevention of the recurrence of a urinary or renal disorder

Psychosocial Integrity

Assisting the client to use appropriate coping mechanisms

Discussing body image disturbances

Discussing the loss of renal function

Identifying appropriate community resources

Identifying grief and loss and end-of-life issues

Identifying religious and spiritual influences on health

Identifying support systems

Physiological Integrity

Ensuring elimination measures

Informing the client about diagnostic tests and laboratory results

Monitoring for fluid and electrolyte imbalances and acid-base disorders

Obtaining assessment data indicating rejection of renal transplant

Preventing complications arising as a result of dialysis

Providing adequate rest and sleep

Providing care related to dialysis access devices

Providing care related to hemodialysis and peritoneal dialysis

Providing care to the client following prostatectomy

Providing comfort interventions

Providing pharmacological therapy

Providing preoperative and postoperative care related to renal transplantation

Providing treatment measures for the client with urinary or renal calculi or the client with a urinary diversion

Teaching the client about the prescribed nutrition and fluid measures

Renal System

I. ANATOMY AND PHYSIOLOGY

A. Kidney anatomy
1. Each person has two kidneys; one is attached to the left abdominal wall at the level of the last thoracic and first three lumbar vertebrae and the other is on the right.
2. The kidneys are enclosed in the renal capsule.
3. The renal cortex is the outer layer of the renal capsule, which contains blood-filtering mechanisms (glomeruli).
4. The renal medulla is the inner region, which contains the renal pyramids and renal tubules.
5. Together the renal cortex, pyramids, and medulla constitute the parenchyma, or functional unit of the kidneys.
6. Nephrons
   a. Located within the parenchyma
   b. Composed of glomerulus and tubules
   c. Selectively secretes and reabsorbs ions and filtrates, including fluid, wastes, electrolytes, acids, and bases

⚠ The nephrons are the functional units of the kidney.

7. Glomerulus
   a. Each nephron contains tufts of capillaries, which filter large plasma proteins and blood cells.
   b. Blood flows into the glomerular capillaries from the afferent arteriole and flows out of the glomerular capillaries into the efferent arteriole.
8. Bowman's capsule
   a. Thin double-walled capsule that surrounds the glomerulus
   b. Fluid and particles from the blood such as electrolytes, glucose, amino acids, and metabolic waste (glomerular filtrate) are filtered through the glomerular membrane into a fluid-filled space in Bowman's capsule (Bowman's space) and then enters the proximal convoluted tubule (PCT).
9. Tubules
   a. The tubules include the PCT, Henle's loop, and the distal convoluted tubule (DCT).
   b. The PCT receives filtrate from the glomerular capsule and reabsorbs water and electrolytes through active and passive transport.
   c. The descending loop of Henle passively reabsorbs water from the filtrate.
   d. The ascending loop of Henle passively reabsorbs sodium and chloride from the filtrate and helps maintain osmolality.
   e. The DCT actively and passively removes sodium and water.
   f. The filtered fluid is converted to urine in the tubules, and then the urine moves to the pelvis of the kidney.
   g. The urine flows from the pelvis of the kidneys through the ureters and empties into the bladder.

B. Functions of kidneys
1. Maintain acid-base balance
2. Excrete end products of body metabolism
3. Control fluid and electrolyte balance
4. Excrete bacterial toxins, water-soluble drugs, and drug metabolites
5. Secrete renin to regulate the blood pressure and erythropoietin to stimulate the bone marrow to produce red blood cells.
6. Synthesize vitamin D for calcium absorption and regulation of the parathyroid hormones.

C. Urine production
1. As fluid flows through the tubules, water, electrolytes, and solutes are reabsorbed and other solutes such as creatinine, hydrogen ions, and potassium are secreted.
2. Water and solutes that are not reabsorbed become urine.
3. The process of selective reabsorption determines the amount of water and solutes to be secreted.

D. Homeostasis of water
1. Antidiuretic hormone (ADH) is primarily responsible for the reabsorption of water by the kidneys.
2. ADH is produced by the hypothalamus and secreted from the posterior lobe of the pituitary gland.
3. Secretion of ADH is stimulated by dehydration or high sodium intake and by a decrease in blood volume.

4. ADH makes the distal convoluted tubules and collecting duct permeable to water.
5. Water is drawn out of the tubules by osmosis and returns to the blood; concentrated urine remains in the tubule to be excreted.
6. When ADH is lacking, the client develops diabetes insipidus (DI).
7. Clients with DI produce large amounts of dilute urine; treatment is necessary because the client cannot drink sufficient water to survive.

E. Homeostasis of sodium
1. When the amount of sodium increases, extra water is retained to preserve osmotic pressure.
2. An increase in sodium and water produces an increase in blood volume and blood pressure (BP).
3. When the BP increases, glomerular filtration increases, and extra water and sodium are lost; blood volume is reduced, returning the BP to normal.
4. Reabsorption of sodium in the distal convoluted tubules is controlled by the renin-angiotensin system.
5. Renin, an enzyme, is released from the nephron when the BP or fluid concentration in the distal convoluted tubule is low.
6. Renin catalyzes the splitting of angiotensin I from angiotensinogen; angiotensin I converts to angiotensin II as blood flows through the lung.
7. Angiotensin II, a potent vasoconstrictor, stimulates the secretion of aldosterone.
8. Aldosterone stimulates the distal convoluted tubules to reabsorb sodium and secrete potassium.
9. The additional sodium increases water reabsorption and increases blood volume and BP, returning the BP to normal; the stimulus for the secretion of renin then is removed.

F. Homeostasis of potassium
1. Increases in the serum potassium level stimulate the secretion of aldosterone.
2. Aldosterone stimulates the distal convoluted tubules to secrete potassium; this action returns the serum potassium concentration to normal.

G. Homeostasis of acidity (pH)
1. Blood pH is controlled by maintaining the concentration of buffer systems.
2. Carbonic acid and sodium bicarbonate form the most important buffers for neutralizing acids in the plasma.
3. The concentration of carbonic acid is controlled by the respiratory system.
4. The concentration of sodium bicarbonate is controlled by the kidneys.
5. Normal arterial pH is 7.35 to 7.45, maintained by keeping the ratio of concentrations of sodium bicarbonate to carbon dioxide constant at 20:1.
6. Strong acids are neutralized by sodium bicarbonate to produce carbonic acid and the sodium

salts of the strong acid; this process quickly restores the ratio and thus blood pH.
7. The carbonic acid dissociates into carbon dioxide and water; because the concentration of carbon dioxide is maintained at a constant level by the respiratory system, the excess carbonic acid is rapidly excreted.
8. Sodium combined with the strong acid is actively reabsorbed in the distal convoluted tubules in exchange for hydrogen or potassium ions. The strong acid is neutralized by ammonia and is excreted as ammonia or potassium salts.

H. Adrenal glands (see Chapter 54 for information about the adrenal glands)
1. One adrenal gland is on top of each kidney.
2. The adrenal glands influence blood pressure and sodium and water retention.

I. Bladder
1. The bladder detrusor muscle, composed of smooth muscle, distends during bladder filling and contracts during bladder emptying.
2. The ureterovesical sphincter prevents reflux of urine from the bladder to the ureter.
3. The total bladder capacity is 1 L; normal adult urine output is 1500 mL/day.

J. Prostate gland
1. The prostate gland surrounds the male urethra.
2. The prostate gland contains a duct that opens into the prostatic portion of the urethra and secretes the alkaline portion of seminal fluid, which protects passing sperm.

K. Risk factors associated with renal disorders (Box 62-1)

II. DIAGNOSTIC TESTS

A. See Chapter 11 and Box 62-2 for information regarding normal values for renal function studies.

Box 62-1 Risk Factors Associated With Renal Disorders

Chemical or environmental toxin exposure
Contact sports
Diabetes mellitus
Family history of renal disease
Frequent urinary tract infections
Heart failure
High-sodium diet
Hypertension
Medications
Trauma
Urolithiasis or nephrolithiasis

Box 62-2 Normal Renal Function Values

Blood urea nitrogen level, 8 to 25 mg/dL
Serum creatinine level, 0.6 to 1.3 mg/dL
Serum uric acid level, 2.5 to 8.0 mg/dL

B. Determination of serum creatinine level
   1. Description: A test that measures the amount of creatinine in the serum. Creatinine is an end product of protein and muscle metabolism.
   2. Analysis
      a. Creatinine level reflects glomerular filtration rate.
      b. Renal disease is the only pathological condition that increases the serum creatinine level.
      c. Serum creatinine level increases only when at least 50% of renal function is lost.
C. Determination of blood urea nitrogen (BUN) level
   1. Description: A serum test that measures the amount of nitrogenous urea, a byproduct of protein metabolism in the liver.
   2. Analysis
      a. BUN levels indicate the extent of renal clearance of urea nitrogenous waste products.
      b. An elevation does not always mean that renal disease is present.
      c. Some factors that can elevate the BUN level include dehydration, poor renal perfusion, intake of a high-protein diet, infection, stress, corticosteroid use, gastrointestinal (GI) bleeding, and factors that cause muscle breakdown.
      d. When the BUN and serum creatinine levels increase at the same rate, the ratio of the BUN to creatinine remains constant; elevated serum creatinine and BUN levels suggest renal dysfunction.
D. Urinalysis
   1. Description: A urine test for evaluation of the renal system and renal disease
   2. Interventions
      a. Wash perineal area and use a clean container for collection.
      b. Obtain 10 to 15 mL of the first morning voiding if possible.
      c. Refrigerated samples may alter the specific gravity.
      d. If the client is menstruating, note this on the laboratory requisition form.
E. Specific gravity determination
   1. Description: A urine test that measures the ability of the kidneys to concentrate urine
   2. Interventions
      a. Specific gravity can be measured by a multiple-test dipstick method (most common method), refractometer (an instrument used in the laboratory setting), or urinometer (least accurate method).
      b. Factors that interfere with an accurate reading include radiopaque contrast agents, glucose, and proteins.
      c. Cold specimens may produce a false high reading.
      d. Normal value is 1.016 to 1.022 (may vary depending on the laboratory).

   e. An increase in specific gravity (more concentrated urine) occurs with insufficient fluid intake, decreased renal perfusion, or increased ADH.
   f. A decrease in specific gravity (less concentrated urine) occurs with increased fluid intake or diabetes insipidus; it may also indicate renal disease or the kidneys inability to concentrate urine.
F. Urine culture and sensitivity testing
   1. Description: A urine test that identifies the presence of microorganisms (culture) and determines the specific antibiotics to treat the existing microorganism (sensitivity) appropriately
   2. Interventions
      a. Clean the perineal area and urinary meatus with a bacteriostatic solution.
      b. Collect the midstream sample in a sterile container.
      c. Send the collected specimen to the laboratory immediately.
      d. Identify any sources of potential contaminants during the collection of the specimen, such as the hands, skin, clothing, hair, or vaginal or rectal secretions.
      e. Urine from the client who drank a very large amount of fluids may be too dilute to provide a positive culture.
G. Creatinine clearance test
   1. Description
      a. The creatinine clearance test evaluates how well the kidneys remove creatinine from the blood.
      b. The test includes obtaining a blood sample and timed urine specimens.
      c. Blood is drawn when the urine specimen collection is complete.
      d. The urine specimen for the creatinine clearance is usually collected for 24 hours, but shorter periods such as 8 or 12 hours could be prescribed.

   ⚠ The creatinine clearance test provides the best estimate of the glomerular filtration rate (GFR) and the normal GFR is 125 mL/min.

   2. Interventions
      a. Encourage fluids before and during the test.
      b. Instruct the client to avoid caffeinated beverages during testing.
      c. Check with the physician regarding the administration of any prescribed medications during testing.
      d. Instruct the client about the urine collection.
      e. At the start time, ask the client to void (or empty the tubing and drainage bag if the client has a Foley catheter) and discard the first sample.

f. Collect all urine for the prescribed time.

g. Keep the urine specimen on ice or refrigerated and check with the laboratory regarding adding a preservative to the specimen during collection.

h. At the end of the prescribed time, ask the client to empty the bladder (or empty the tubing and drainage bag if the client has a Foley catheter) and add that final urine to the collection container.

i. Send the labeled urine specimen to the laboratory in a biohazard bag along with the requisition.

j. Document specimen collection, time started and completed, and pertinent assessments.

H. Uric acid test

1. Description: A 24-hour urine collection sample is tested to diagnose gout and kidney disease.

2. Interventions

a. Encourage fluid intake and a regular diet during testing.

b. Follow the same procedure for urine collection as with the creatinine clearance test.

I. Vanillylmandelic acid (VMA) test

1. Description

a. The test is a 24-hour urine collection to diagnose pheochromocytoma, a tumor of the adrenal gland.

b. The test determines catecholamine levels in the urine.

2. Interventions

a. Check with the laboratory regarding medication restrictions.

b. Instruct the client to avoid foods such as caffeine, cocoa, vanilla, cheese, gelatin, licorice, and fruits for at least 2 days before and during urine collection and to check with the physician regarding the administration of any prescribed medications before or during testing.

c. Instruct the client to avoid stress; encourage adequate food and fluid intake during the test.

d. Follow the same procedure for urine collection as for the creatinine clearance test.

J. KUB (kidneys, ureters, and bladder) radiography

1. Description: An x-ray of the urinary system and adjacent structures to detect urinary calculi.

2. Interventions: No specific preparation is necessary.

K. Bladder ultrasonography (bladder scanning)

1. Bladder ultrasonography is a noninvasive method for measuring the volume of urine in the bladder.

2. Bladder ultrasonography may be performed for evaluating urinary frequency, inability to urinate, or amount of residual urine (the amount of urine remaining in the bladder after voiding).

L. Computed tomography (CT) and magnetic resonance imaging (MRI)

1. Description: These imaging methods provide cross-sectional views of the kidney and urinary tract.

2. Interventions: See Chapter 66.

M. Intravenous pyelography

1. Description: An x-ray procedure in which an intravenous injection of a radiopaque dye is used to visualize and identify abnormalities in the renal system.

2. Preprocedure interventions

a. Obtain an informed consent.

b. Assess the client for allergies to iodine, seafood, and radiopaque dyes.

c. Withhold food and fluids after midnight on the night before the test.

d. Administer laxatives if prescribed.

e. Inform the client about possible throat irritation, flushing of the face, warmth, or a salty or metallic taste during the test.

3. Postprocedure interventions

a. Monitor vital signs.

b. Instruct the client to drink at least 1 L of fluid unless contraindicated.

c. Assess the venipuncture site for bleeding.

d. Monitor urinary output.

e. Monitor for signs of a possible allergic reaction to the dye used during the test and instruct the client to notify the physician if any signs of an allergic reaction occur.

N. Renal angiography

1. Description: An injection of a radiopaque dye through a catheter inserted into the femoral artery to examine the renal blood vessels and renal arterial supply

2. Preprocedure interventions

a. Obtain an informed consent.

b. Assess the client for allergies to iodine, seafood, and radiopaque dyes.

c. Inform the client about a possible feeling of burning or heat along the vessel when the dye is injected.

d. Withhold food and fluids after midnight on the night before the test.

e. Instruct the client to void immediately before the procedure.

f. Administer enemas if prescribed.

g. Shave injection sites as prescribed.

h. Assess and mark the peripheral pulses.

3. Postprocedure interventions

a. Assess vital signs and peripheral pulses frequently as prescribed

b. Maintain bed rest and apply a sandbag or other device that will provide pressure to prevent bleeding, if prescribed, at the insertion site for 4 to 8 hours.

c. Instruct the client to maintain a supine position with the leg straight (the head of the bed should not be elevated greater than 20 degrees for 8 hours, or as prescribed).

d. Assess the temperature, color, movement, and sensation (CMS) of the toes of the involved extremity with each vital sign check.

e. Inspect the catheter insertion site for bleeding or swelling with each vital sign check.

⚠ The dye used in a renal angiography may be nephrotoxic; therefore encourage increased fluids unless contraindicated and monitor urinary output.

O. Renal scanning

1. Description: An intravenous (IV) injection of a radioisotope for visual imaging of renal blood flow, glomerular filtration, tubular function, and excretion

2. Preprocedure interventions
   a. Obtain an informed consent.
   b. Assess for allergies.
   c. Inform the client that the test requires no dietary or activity restrictions.
   d. Assist with administering the radioisotope as necessary.
   e. Instruct the client to remain motionless during the test.
   f. Instruct the client that imaging may be repeated at various intervals before the test is complete.

3. Postprocedure interventions
   a. Encourage fluid intake unless contraindicated.
   b. Assess the client for signs of delayed allergic reaction such as itching and hives.
   c. The radioisotope is eliminated in 24 hours; wear gloves for excretion precautions.
   d. Follow standard precautions when caring for incontinent clients and double-bag client linens per agency policy.

P. Cystoscopy and biopsy of the bladder

1. Description: The bladder mucosa is examined for inflammation, calculi, or tumors by means of a cystoscope; a sample for biopsy may be obtained.

2. Preprocedure interventions
   a. Obtain an informed consent.
   b. If a biopsy is planned, withhold food and fluids after midnight the night before the test.
   c. If a cystoscopy alone is planned, no special preparation is necessary, and the procedure may be performed in the physician's office; postprocedure interventions include increasing fluid intake.

3. Postprocedure interventions following biopsy
   a. Monitor vital signs.
   b. Increase fluid intake as prescribed.

c. Monitor intake and output.

d. Encourage deep-breathing exercises to relieve bladder spasms.

e. Administer analgesics as prescribed.

f. Administer sitz or tub baths for back and abdominal pain.

g. Note that leg cramps are common because of the lithotomy position maintained during the procedure.

h. Assess the urine for color and consistency.

i. Inform the client that burning on urination, pink-tinged or tea-colored urine, and urinary frequency are common after cystoscopy and resolve in a few days.

j. Monitor for bright red urine or clots, and notify the physician if this occurs.

Q. Renal biopsy

1. Description: Insertion of a needle into the kidney to obtain a sample of tissue for examination; usually done percutaneously

2. Preprocedure interventions
   a. Assess vital signs.
   b. Assess baseline coagulation studies; notify the physician if abnormal results are noted.
   c. Obtain an informed consent.
   d. Withhold food and fluids after midnight the night before the test.

3. Interventions during the procedure: Position the client prone with a pillow under the abdomen and shoulders.

4. Postprocedure interventions
   a. Monitor vital signs, especially for hypotension and tachycardia, which could indicate bleeding.
   b. Provide pressure to the biopsy site for 30 minutes.
   c. Monitor the hemoglobin and hematocrit levels for decreases, which could indicate bleeding.
   d. Place the client in the supine position and on bed rest for 8 hours as prescribed.
   e. Check the biopsy site and under the client for bleeding.
   f. Encourage fluid intake of 1500 to 2000 mL as prescribed.
   g. Observe the urine for gross and microscopic bleeding.
   h. Instruct the client to avoid heavy lifting and strenuous activity for 2 weeks.
   i. Instruct the client to notify the physician if either a temperature greater than 100° F or hematuria occurs after the first 24 hours postprocedure.

III. ACUTE RENAL FAILURE

A. Description

1. **Acute renal failure (ARF)** is the rapid loss of kidney function from renal cell damage.

Box 62-3 Potentially Nephrotoxic Substances

Medications
Antibiotics—Anti-Infectives
Amphotericin B
Colistimethate
Methicillin
Polymyxin B
Rifampin
Sulfonamides
Tetracycline hydrochloride
Vancomycin

Aminoglycoside Antibiotics
Gentamicin
Kanamycin
Neomycin
Netilmicin sulfate
Tobramycin

Antineoplastics
Cisplatin
Cyclophosphamide
Methotrexate

Nonsteroidal Anti-Inflammatory Drugs (NSAIDs)
Celecoxib
Flurbiprofen
Ibuprofen
Indomethacin
Ketorolac
Meclofenamate
Meloxicam
Nabumetone

Naproxen
Oxaprozin
Rofecoxib
Tolmetin

Other Medications
Acetaminophen
Captopril
Cyclosporine
Fluorinate anesthetics
D-Penicillamine
Phenazopyridine hydrochloride
Quinine

Other Substances
Organic Solvents
Carbon tetrachloride
Ethylene glycol

Nonpharmacological Chemical Agents
Radiographic contrast dye
Pesticides
Fungicides
Myoglobin (from breakdown of skeletal muscle)

Heavy Metals and Ions
Arsenic
Bismuth
Copper sulfate
Gold salts
Lead
Mercuric chloride

From Ignatavicius, D., & Workman, M. (2010). *Medical-surgical nursing: Patient-centered collaborative care* (6th ed., p. 1603). St. Louis: Saunders.

2. Occurs abruptly and can be reversible
3. **ARF** leads to cell hypoperfusion, cell death, and decompensation of renal function.
4. The prognosis depends on the cause and the condition of the client.
5. Near-normal or normal kidney function may resume gradually.
B. Causes
   1. Prerenal: Outside the kidney; caused by intravascular volume depletion, dehydration, decreased cardiac output, decreased peripheral vascular resistance, decreased renovascular blood flow, and prerenal infection or obstruction.
   2. Intrarenal: Within the parenchyma of the kidney; caused by tubular necrosis, prolonged pre renal ischemia, intrarenal infection or obstruction, and nephrotoxicity (Box 62-3).
   3. Postrenal: Between the kidney and urethral meatus, such as bladder neck obstruction, bladder cancer, calculi, and postrenal infection
C. Phases of **ARF** and interventions (Box 62-4)
   1. Onset: Begins with precipitating event
   2. Oliguric phase

a. For some clients, **oliguria** does not occur and the urine output is normal; otherwise the duration of **oliguria** is 8 to 15 days; the longer the duration, the less chance of recovery.
b. Sudden decrease in urine output; urine output is less than 400 mL/day.
c. Signs of excess fluid volume: Hypertension, edema, pleural and pericardial effusions, dysrhythmias, congestive heart failure (CHF), and pulmonary edema
d. Signs of uremia: Anorexia, nausea, vomiting, and pruritus
e. Signs of metabolic acidosis: Kussmaul's respirations
f. Signs of neurological changes: Tingling of extremities, drowsiness progressing to disorientation, and then coma
g. Signs of pericarditis: Friction rub, chest pain with inspiration, and low-grade fever
h. Laboratory analysis (see Box 62-4)
i. Restrict fluid intake; if hypertension is present, daily fluid allowances may be 400 mL

Box 62-4 Acute Renal Failure: Phases and Laboratory Findings

Onset
Begins with precipitating event

Oliguric Phase
Elevated blood urea nitrogen and serum creatinine levels
Decreased urine specific gravity (prerenal causes) or normal (intrarenal causes)
Decreased glomerular filtration rate and creatinine clearance
Hyperkalemia
Normal or decreased serum sodium level
Hypervolemia
Hypocalcemia
Hyperphosphatemia

Diuretic Phase
Gradual decline in blood urea nitrogen and serum creatinine levels, but still elevated
Continued low creatinine clearance with improving glomerular filtration rate
Hypokalemia
Hyponatremia
Hypovolemia

Recovery Phase (Convalescent)
Increased glomerular filtration rate
Stabilization or continual decline in blood urea nitrogen and serum creatinine levels toward normal
Complete recovery—may take 1 to 2 years

⚠ The signs and symptoms of acute renal failure are primarily caused by the retention of nitrogenous wastes, the retention of fluids, and the inability of the kidneys to regulate electrolytes.

D. Assessment: Assess objective and subjective data noted in the phases of **ARF** (see Box 62-4).
E. Other interventions
1. Monitor vital signs, especially for signs of hypertension, tachycardia, tachypnea, and an irregular heart rate.
2. Monitor urine and intake and output (hourly in **ARF**) and urine color and characteristics.
3. Monitor daily weight (same scale, same clothes, same time of the day), noting that an increase of ½ to 1 lb/day indicates fluid retention.
4. Monitor for changes in the BUN, serum creatinine, and serum electrolyte levels.
5. Monitor for acidosis (may be treated with sodium bicarbonate).
6. Monitor urinalysis for protein level, hematuria, casts, and specific gravity.
7. Monitor for altered level of consciousness caused by uremia.
8. Monitor for signs of infection because the client may not exhibit an elevated temperature or an increased white blood cell count.
9. Monitor the lungs for wheezes and rhonchi and monitor for edema, which can indicate fluid overload.
10. Administer a prescribed diet, which is usually a low- to moderate-protein (to decrease the workload on the kidneys) and high-carbohydrate diet.
11. Restrict potassium and sodium intake as prescribed based on the electrolyte level.
12. Administer medications as prescribed; be alert to the mechanism for metabolism and excretion of all prescribed medications.
13. Be alert to nephrotoxic medications, which may be prescribed (see Box 62-3).
14. Be alert to the health care provider's adjustment of medication dosages for **renal failure**.
15. Prepare the client for **dialysis** if prescribed; continuous renal replacement therapy may be used in **ARF** to treat fluid volume overload or rapidly developing **azotemia** and metabolic acidosis.
16. Provide emotional support by allowing opportunities for the client to express concerns and fears and by encouraging family interactions.
17. Promote consistency in caregivers.
18. Also refer to the section in this chapter on special problems in **renal failure** and interventions.

to 1000 mL plus the measured urinary output.
   j. Administer medications as prescribed, such as diuretics (furosemide [Lasix]), to increase renal blood flow and diuresis.
  3. Diuretic phase
   a. Urine output rises slowly, followed by diuresis (4 to 5 L/day).
   b. Excessive urine output indicates that damaged nephrons are recovering their ability to excrete wastes.
   c. Dehydration, hypovolemia, hypotension, and tachycardia can occur.
   d. Level of consciousness improves.
   e. Laboratory analysis (see Box 62-4)
   f. Administer IV fluids as prescribed, which may contain electrolytes to replace losses.
  4. Recovery phase (convalescent)
   a. Recovery is a slow process; complete recovery may take 1 to 2 years.
   b. Urine volume returns to normal.
   c. Memory improves.
   d. Strength increases.
   e. The older adult is less likely than a younger adult to regain full kidney function.
   f. Laboratory analysis (see Box 62-4)
   g. **ARF** can progress to **chronic renal failure (CRF)**.

TABLE 62-1 Progression of Chronic Kidney Disease

Stage of CKD	Estimated GFR
At risk; normal kidney function (early kidney disease may or may not be present)	>90 mL/min
Mild CKD	60-89 mL/min
Moderate CKD	30-59 mL/mim
Severe CKD	15-29 mL/niin
ESKD	<15 mL/min

CDK, chronic kidney disease; *ESKD*, end-stage kidney disease; *GFR*, glomular filtration rate.
From Ignatavicius, D., & Workman, M. (2010). *Medical-surgical nursing: Patient-centered collaborative care* (6th ed., p. 1609). St. Louis: Saunders.

IV. CHRONIC RENAL FAILURE

A. Description
   1. **CRF** is a slow, progressive, irreversible loss in kidney function, with a GFR less than or equal to 60 mL/min for 3 months or longer.
   2. It occurs in stages and results in uremia or end-stage renal disease (Table 62-1).
   3. Hypervolemia can occur because of the kidneys' inability to excrete sodium and water; hypovolemia can occur because of the kidneys' inability to conserve sodium and water.

   ⚠ Chronic renal failure affects all major body systems and requires dialysis or kidney transplantation to maintain life.

B. Primary causes
   1. May follow **ARF**
   2. Diabetes mellitus and other metabolic disorders
   3. Hypertension
   4. Chronic urinary obstruction
   5. Recurrent infections
   6. Renal artery occlusion
   7. Autoimmune disorders

C. Assessment
   1. Assess body systems for the manifestations of **CRF** (Box 62-5).
   2. Assess psychological changes, which could include emotional lability, withdrawal, depression, anxiety, suicidal behavior, denial, dependence-independence conflict, and changes in body image.

D. Interventions
   1. Same as the interventions for **ARF**
   2. Administer a prescribed diet, which is usually a moderate-protein (to decrease the workload on the kidneys) and high-carbohydrate, low-potassium, and low-phosphorus diet.
   3. Provide oral care to prevent stomatitis and reduce discomfort from mouth sores.
   4. Provide skin care to prevent pruritus.
   5. Teach the client about fluid and dietary restrictions and the importance of daily weights.
   6. Provide support to promote acceptance of the chronic illness and prepare the client for long-term **dialysis** and transplantation, or explain to the client about his or her choice to decline **dialysis** or transplantation.

E. Special problems in **renal failure** and interventions (Box 62-6)
   1. Activity intolerance and insomnia
      a. Fatigue results from anemia and the buildup of wastes from the diseased kidneys.
      b. Provide adequate rest periods.
      c. Teach the client to plan activities to avoid fatigue.
      d. Administer mild central nervous system depressants as prescribed to promote rest.
   2. Anemia
      a. Anemia results from the decreased secretion of erythropoietin by damaged nephrons resulting in decreased production of red blood cells.
      b. Monitor for decreased hemoglobin and hematocrit levels.
      c. Administer epoetin alfa (Epogen, Procrit) or darbepoetin alfa (Aranesp), hematopoietics, as prescribed to promote maturity of the red blood cells.
      d. Administer folic acid (vitamin B_9) as prescribed.
      e. Administer iron orally as prescribed, but not at the same time as phosphate binders.
      f. Administer stool softeners as prescribed because of the constipating effects of iron.
      g. Note that oral iron is not well absorbed by the gastrointestinal tract in **CRF** and causes nausea and vomiting; parenteral iron (iron sucrose [Venofer] or sodium ferric gluconate complex [Ferrlecit]) may be used if iron deficiencies persist despite folic acid or oral iron administration.
      h. Administer blood transfusions if prescribed; blood transfusions are prescribed only when necessary (acute blood loss, symptomatic anemia) because they decrease the stimulus to produce red blood cells; note that certain clients' religious beliefs (e.g., Jehovah's Witness) may refuse blood and blood products.
      i. Blood transfusions also cause the development of antibodies against human tissues, which can make matching for organ transplantation difficult.
   3. Gastrointestinal bleeding
      a. Urea is broken down by the intestinal bacteria to ammonia; ammonia irritates the gastrointestinal mucosa, causing ulceration and bleeding.

Box 62-5 Key Features of Chronic Renal Failure

Neurological Manifestations
Asterixis
Ataxia (alteration in gait)
Coma
Inability to concentrate or decreased attention span
Lethargy and daytime drowsiness
Myoclonus
Paresthesias
Seizures
Slurred speech
Tremors, twitching, or jerky movements

Cardiovascular Manifestations
Cardiac tamponade
Cardiomyopathy
Heart failure
Hypertension
Pericardial effusion
Pericardial friction rub
Peripheral edema
Uremic pericarditis

Respiratory Manifestations
Crackles
Deep sighing, yawning
Depressed cough reflex
Kussmaul's respirations
Pleural effusion
Pulmonary edema
Shortness of breath
Tachypnea
Uremic halitosis
Uremic pneumonia

Hematological Manifestations
Abnormal bleeding and bruising
Anemia

Gastrointestinal Manifestations
Anorexia

Changes in taste acuity and sensation
Constipation
Diarrhea
Metallic taste in the mouth
Nausea
Stomatitis
Uremic colitis (diarrhea)
Uremic fetor
Uremic gastritis (possible gastrointestinal bleeding)
Vomiting

Urinary Manifestations
Diluted, straw-colored appearance
Hematuria
Oliguria, anuria (later)
Polyuria, nocturia (early)
Proteinuria

Integumentary Manifestations
Decreased skin turgor
Dry skin
Ecchymosis
Pruritus
Purpura
Soft tissue calcifications
Uremic frost (late, premorbid)
Yellow-gray pallor

Musculoskeletal Manifestations
Bone pain
Muscle weakness and cramping
Pathological fractures
Renal osteodystrophy

Reproductive Manifestations
Decreased fertility
Decreased libido
Impotence
Infrequent or absent menses

From Ignatavicius, D., & Workman, M. (2010). *Medical-surgical nursing: Patient-centered collaborative care* (6th ed., p. 1613). St. Louis: Saunders.

Box 62-6 Special Problems in Renal Failure

Activity intolerance and insomnia	Hypovolemia
	Infection
Anemia	Metabolic acidosis
Gastrointestinal bleeding	Muscle cramps
Hyperkalemia	Neurological changes
Hypermagnesemia	Ocular irritation
Hyperphosphatemia	Potential for injury
Hypertension	Pruritus
Hypervolemia	Psychosocial problems
Hypocalcemia	

b. Monitor for decreasing hemoglobin and hematocrit levels.
c. Monitor stools for occult blood.
d. Instruct the client to use a soft toothbrush.

e. Avoid the administration of acetylsalicylic acid (aspirin) because it is excreted by the kidneys; if administered, aspirin toxicity can occur and prolong the bleeding time.
4. Hyperkalemia
   a. Monitor vital signs for hypertension or hypotension and the apical heart rate; an irregular heart rate could indicate dysrhythmias.
   b. Monitor the serum potassium level; an elevated serum potassium level can cause tall, peaked T waves, flat P waves, a widened QRS complex, and a prolonged PR interval; decreased cardiac output; heart blocks; fibrillation; or asystole (Fig. 62-1).
   c. Provide a low-potassium diet, avoiding foods high in potassium (see Chapter 9 for a listing of foods that are high in potassium).

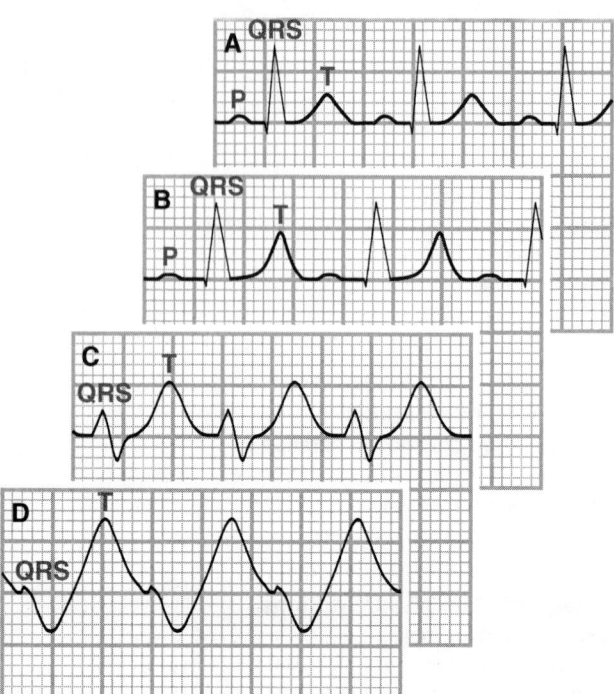

Serum Potassium Levels

A. Normal (3.5-5.1 mEq/L)
B. About 7.0 mEq/L
C. 8.0-9.0 mEq/L
D. >10.0 mEq/L

▲ **FIGURE 62-1** Cardiac rhythm changes with hyperkalemia. *ECG,* Electrocardiogram. (From Huszar, R. [2002]. *Basic dysrhythmias: Interpretation and management* [3rd ed.]. St. Louis: Mosby. Developed by Kathleen Ohman.)

d. Administer electrolyte-binding and electrolyte-excreting medications such as oral or rectal sodium polystyrene sulfonate (Kayexalate) as prescribed to lower the serum potassium level.

e. Administer prescribed medications: 50% dextrose and insulin may be prescribed to shift potassium into the cell; calcium gluconate IV may be prescribed to reduce myocardial irritability from hyperkalemia; and sodium bicarbonate IV may be prescribed to correct acidosis.

f. Administer prescribed loop diuretics to excrete potassium.

g. Avoid potassium-sparing medications such as spironolactone (Aldactone) and triamterene (Dyrenium) because these medications will increase the potassium level.

h. Prepare the client for peritoneal **dialysis** or hemodialysis as prescribed.

⚠ Place the client with renal failure on continuous cardiac monitoring. The client can develop hyperkalemia resulting in the risk for dysrhythmias.

5. Hypermagnesemia
   a. Results from decreased renal excretion of magnesium.
   b. Monitor for cardiac manifestations such as bradycardia, peripheral vasodilation, and hypotension.
   c. Monitor central nervous system (CNS) manifestations of decreased nerve impulse transmission, such as drowsiness or lethargy.
   d. Monitor neuromuscular manifestations, such as reduced or absent deep tendon reflexes or weak or absent voluntary skeletal muscle contractions.
   e. Administer loop diuretics as prescribed, such as furosemide (Lasix).
   f. Administer calcium as prescribed for resulting cardiac problems.
   g. Avoid medications that contain magnesium, such as antacids, laxatives, or enemas.
   h. During severe elevations, avoid foods that increase magnesium levels (see Chapter 9 for a listing of foods that are high in magnesium).

6. Hyperphosphatemia
   a. As the phosphorus level rises, the calcium level drops; this leads to the stimulation of parathyroid hormone, causing bone demineralization.
   b. Treatment is aimed at lowering the serum phosphorus level.
   c. Administer phosphate binders such as calcium carbonate (TUMS), calcium acetate (PhosLo), or sevelamer (Renagel) as prescribed with meals to lower serum phosphate levels.
   d. Avoid the use of aluminum hydroxide preparations to bind phosphates because they are associated with dementia and osteomalacia.
   e. Administer stool softeners and laxatives as prescribed because phosphate binders are constipating.
   f. Teach the client about the need to limit the intake of foods high in phosphorus (see Chapter 9 for a listing of foods that are high in phosphorus).

7. Hypertension
   a. Caused by failure of the kidneys to maintain BP homeostasis
   b. Monitor vital signs for elevated blood pressure.
   c. Maintain fluid and sodium restrictions as prescribed.
   d. Administer diuretics and antihypertensives as prescribed.
   e. Administer propranolol (Inderal), a β-blocker, as prescribed; propranolol decreases renin release (renin causes vasoconstriction and subsequent hypertension).

8. Hypervolemia
   a. Monitor vital signs for an elevated blood pressure.

b. Monitor intake and output and daily weight for indications of fluid retention.

c. Monitor for periorbital, sacral, and peripheral edema.

d. Monitor the serum electrolyte levels.

e. Monitor for hypertension and notify the health care provider for sustained elevations.

f. Monitor for signs of CHF and pulmonary edema, such as restlessness, heightened anxiety, tachycardia, dyspnea, basilar lung crackles, and blood-tinged sputum; notify the physician immediately if signs occur.

g. Maintain fluid restriction.

h. Avoid the administration of large amounts of IV fluids.

i. Administer diuretics such as furosemide (Lasix) as prescribed.

j. Teach the client to maintain a low-sodium diet.

k. Teach the client to avoid antacids, cold remedies, or other products containing sodium bicarbonate.

9. Hypocalcemia

a. Results from the high phosphorus level and the inability of the diseased kidney to activate vitamin D

b. The absence of vitamin D causes poor calcium absorption from the intestinal tract.

c. Monitor the serum calcium level.

d. Administer calcium supplements as prescribed.

e. Administer activated vitamin D as prescribed.

f. See Chapter 9 for a listing of foods that are high in calcium.

10. Hypovolemia

a. Monitor the vital signs for hypotension and tachycardia.

b. Monitor for decreasing intake and output and a reduction in the daily weight.

c. Monitor for dehydration.

d. Monitor electrolyte levels.

e. Provide replacement therapy based on the serum electrolyte level values.

f. Provide sodium supplements as prescribed, based on the serum electrolyte level.

11. Infection

a. The client is at risk for infection caused by a suppressed immune system, **dialysis** access site, and possible malnutrition.

b. Monitor for signs of infection.

c. Avoid urinary catheters when possible; if used, provide catheter care.

d. Provide strict asepsis during urinary catheter insertion and other invasive procedures.

e. Instruct the client to avoid fatigue, which decreases body resistance.

f. Instruct the client to avoid persons with infections.

g. Administer antibiotics as prescribed, monitoring for nephrotoxic effects.

12. Metabolic acidosis

a. The kidneys are unable to excrete hydrogen ions or manufacture bicarbonate, resulting in acidosis.

b. Administer alkalizers such as sodium bicarbonate as prescribed.

c. Note that clients with **CRF** adjust to low bicarbonate levels and as a result do not become acutely ill.

13. Muscle cramps

a. Occur from electrolyte imbalances and the effects of uremia on peripheral nerves

b. Monitor serum electrolyte levels.

c. Administer electrolyte replacements and medications to control muscle cramps as prescribed.

d. Administer heat and massage as prescribed.

14. Neurological changes

a. The buildup of active particles and fluids causes changes in the brain cells and leads to confusion and impairment in decision-making ability.

b. Peripheral neuropathy results from the effects of uremia on peripheral nerves.

c. Monitor the level of consciousness and for confusion.

d. Monitor for restless leg syndrome, which is also common during **dialysis** treatments.

e. Teach the client to examine areas of decreased sensation for signs of injury.

15. Ocular irritation

a. Calcium deposits in the conjunctivae cause burning and watering of the eyes.

b. Administer medications to control the calcium and phosphate levels as prescribed.

c. Administer lubricating eye drops.

d. Protect the client from injury.

e. Provide a safe and hazard-free environment.

f. Use side rails as needed.

16. Potential for injury

a. The client is at risk for fractures caused by alterations in the absorption of calcium, excretion of phosphate, and vitamin D metabolism.

b. Provide for a safe environment.

c. Avoid injury; tissue breakdown causes increased serum potassium levels.

17. Pruritus

a. To rid the body of excess wastes, urate crystals are excreted through the skin, causing pruritus.

b. The deposit of urate crystals (uremic frost) occurs in advanced stages of **renal failure**.

c. Monitor for skin breakdown, rash, and uremic frost.

d. Provide meticulous skin care and oral hygiene.

e. Avoid the use of soaps.

f. Administer antihistamines and antipruritics as prescribed to relieve itching.

g. Teach the client to keep the nails trimmed to prevent local infection from scratching.
18. Psychosocial problems
   a. Listen to the client's concerns to determine how the client is handling the situation.
   b. Allow the client time to mourn the loss of kidney function.
   c. With client permission, include the family members in discussions of the client's concerns.
   d. Provide education about treatment options and support their decision.
   e. Offer information about support groups.
   f. Provide end-of-life care for the client with end-stage renal disease.

V. UREMIC SYNDROME

A. Description
   1. Accumulation of nitrogenous waste products in the blood caused by the kidneys' inability to filter out these waste products
   2. Uremic syndrome may occur as a result of **ARF** or **CRF**.
B. Assessment
   1. **Oliguria**
   2. Presence of protein, red blood cells, and casts in the urine
   3. Elevated levels of urea, uric acid, potassium, and magnesium in the urine
   4. Hypotension or hypertension
   5. Alterations in the level of consciousness
   6. Electrolyte imbalances
   7. Stomatitis
   8. Nausea or vomiting
   9. Diarrhea or constipation
C. Interventions
   1. Monitor vital signs for hypertension, tachycardia, and an irregular heart rate.
   2. Monitor serum electrolyte levels.
   3. Monitor intake and output and for **oliguria**.
   4. Provide a limited but high-quality protein diet as prescribed.
   5. Provide a limited sodium, nitrogen, potassium, and phosphate diet as prescribed.
   6. Assist the client to cope with body image disturbances caused by uremic syndrome.

VI. HEMODIALYSIS

A. Description
   1. Hemodialysis is the process of cleansing the client's blood.
   2. It involves the diffusion of dissolved particles from one fluid compartment into another across a semipermeable membrane; the client's blood flows through one fluid compartment of a **dialysis** filter, and the dialysate is in another fluid compartment.
B. Functions of hemodialysis
   1. Cleanses the blood of accumulated waste products

2. Removes the byproducts of protein metabolism such as urea, creatinine, and uric acid from the blood
3. Removes excess body fluids
4. Maintains or restores the buffer system of the body
5. Corrects electrolyte levels in the body
C. Principles of hemodialysis
   1. The semipermeable membrane is made of a thin, porous cellophane.
   2. The pore size of the membrane allows small particles to pass through, such as urea, creatinine, uric acid, and water molecules.
   3. Proteins, bacteria, and some blood cells are too large to pass through the membrane.
   4. The client's blood flows into the dialyzer; the movement of substances occurs from the blood to the dialysate by the principles of osmosis, diffusion, and ultrafiltration.
   5. Diffusion is the movement of particles from an area of higher concentration to one of lower concentration.
   6. Osmosis is the movement of fluids across a semipermeable membrane from an area of lower concentration of particles to an area of higher concentration of particles.
   7. Ultrafiltration is the movement of fluid across a semipermeable membrane as a result of an artificially created pressure gradient.
D. Dialysate bath
   1. A dialysate bath is composed of water and major electrolytes.
   2. The dialysate need not be sterile because bacteria and viruses are too large to pass through the pores of the semipermeable membrane; however, the dialysate must meet specific standards, and water is treated to ensure a safe water supply.
E. Interventions
   1. Monitor vital signs before, during, and after **dialysis**; the client's temperature may elevate because of slight warming of the blood from the **dialysis** machine (notify the physician about excessive temperature elevations because this could indicate sepsis; obtain samples for blood culture as prescribed for excessive temperature elevations).
   2. Monitor laboratory values before, during, and after **dialysis**.
   3. Assess the client for fluid overload before **dialysis** and fluid volume deficit following **dialysis**.
   4. Weigh the client before and after **dialysis** to determine fluid loss.
   5. Assess the patency of the blood access device before, during, and after **dialysis**.
   6. Monitor for bleeding; heparin is added to the **dialysis** bath to prevent clots from forming in the dialyzer or the blood tubing.
   7. Monitor for hypovolemia and shock during **dialysis**, which can occur from blood loss or excess fluid and electrolyte removal.

8. Provide adequate nutrition; the client may eat before or during **dialysis**.
9. Identify the client's reactions to the treatment and support coping mechanisms; encourage independence and involvement in care.

⚠ Withhold antihypertensives and other medications that can affect the blood pressure or result in hypotension until after the hemodialysis treatment. Also withhold medications that could be removed by dialysis, such as water-soluble vitamins, certain antibiotics, and digoxin (Lanoxin).

VII. ACCESS FOR HEMODIALYSIS

A. Subclavian and femoral catheter
1. Description
   a. A subclavian (subclavian vein) or femoral (femoral vein) catheter may be inserted for short-term or temporary use in **ARF**.
   b. The catheter is used until a fistula or graft matures or develops, which is typically 6 weeks, or may be required when the client's fistula or graft access has failed because of infection or clotting.
2. Interventions
   a. Assess insertion site for hematoma, bleeding, catheter dislodgement, and infection.
   b. These catheters should only be used for **dialysis** treatments.
   c. Maintain an occlusive dressing over the catheter insertion site.

3. Subclavian vein catheter
   a. The catheter is usually filled with heparin and capped to maintain patency between **dialysis** treatments.
   b. The catheter should not be uncapped except for **dialysis** treatments.
   c. The catheter may be left in place for up to 6 weeks if no complications occur.
4. Femoral vein catheter
   a. Assess the extremity for circulation, temperature, and pulses.
   b. Prevent pulling or disconnecting of the catheter when giving care.
   c. Because the groin is not a clean site, meticulous perineal care is required.
   d. Use an IV infusion pump or controller with microdrip tubing if a heparin infusion through the catheter to maintain patency is prescribed.

⚠ The client with a femoral vein catheter should not sit up more than 45 degrees or lean forward, because the catheter may kink and occlude.

B. External arteriovenous shunt (Fig. 62-2)
1. Description
   a. Two Silastic cannulas are surgically inserted into an artery and vein in the forearm or leg to form an external blood path.
   b. The cannulas are connected to form a U shape; blood flows from the client's artery through the shunt into the vein.

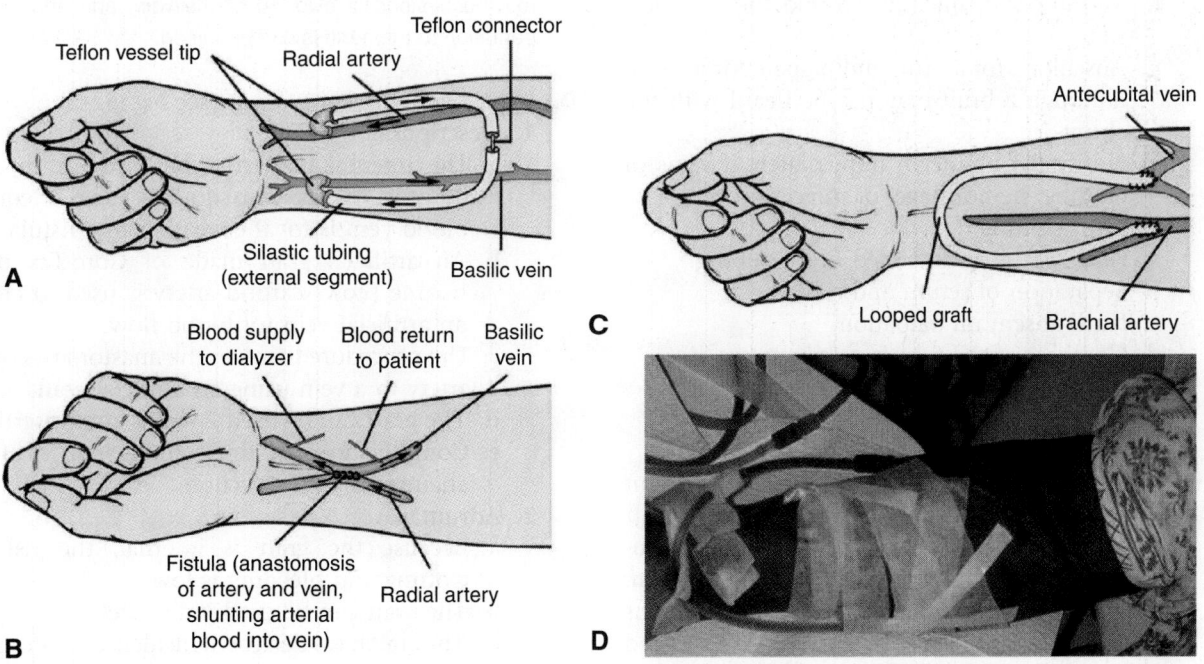

A Teflon vessel tip • Teflon connector • Radial artery • Silastic tubing (external segment) • Basilic vein

B Blood supply to dialyzer • Blood return to patient • Basilic vein • Fistula (anastomosis of artery and vein, shunting arterial blood into vein) • Radial artery

C Antecubital vein • Looped graft • Brachial artery

D

▲ **FIGURE 62-2** Vascular access for hemodialysis. **A,** External shunt. **B,** Internal arteriovenous fistula. **C,** Internal arteriovenous graft. **D,** A hemodialysis graft while connected to a hemodialysis machine. (From Lewis, S., Heitkemper, M., Dirksen, S., O'Brien, P., & Bucher, L. [2007]. *Medical-surgical nursing: Assessment and management of clinical problems* [7th ed.]. St. Louis: Mosby.)

c. A tube leading to the membrane compartment of the dialyzer is connected to the arterial cannula.

d. Blood fills the membrane compartment, passes through the dialyzer, and is returned back to the client through a tube connected to the venous cannula.

e. When **dialysis** is complete, the cannulas are clamped and reattached, reforming the U shape.

2. Advantages
   a. The external arteriovenous shunt can be used immediately following its creation.
   b. No venipuncture is necessary for **dialysis**.

3. Disadvantages
   a. Disconnection or dislodgment of the external shunt
   b. Risk of hemorrhage, infection, or clotting
   c. Potential for skin erosion around the catheter site

4. Interventions
   a. Avoid getting the shunt wet.
   b. Wrap a dressing completely around the shunt and keep it dry and intact.
   c. Keep cannula clamps at the client's bedside or attached to the arteriovenous dressing for use in case of accidental disconnection.
   d. Teach the client that the shunt extremity should not be used for monitoring BP, drawing blood, placing IV lines, or administering injections.
   e. Fold back the dressing to expose the shunt tubing and assess for signs of hemorrhage, infection, or clotting.
   f. Monitor skin integrity around the insertion site.
   g. Auscultate for a bruit and palpate for a thrill, although a bruit may not be heard with the shunt.
   h. Notify the physician immediately if signs of clotting, hemorrhage, or infection occur.

5. Signs of clotting
   a. Fibrin-white flecks noted in the tubing
   b. Separation of serum and cells
   c. Thrill absent on palpation
   d. Coolness of the tubing or extremity
   e. Tingling sensation at site or in extremity

C. Internal **arteriovenous fistula** (see Fig. 62-2)
   1. Description
      a. A permanent access of choice for the client with **CRF** requiring **dialysis**
      b. The fistula is created surgically by anastomosis of a large artery and large vein in the arm.
      c. The flow of arterial blood into the venous system causes the vein to become engorged (matured or developed).
      d. Maturity takes about 4 to 6 weeks, depending on the client's ability to do hand-flexing exercises such as ball squeezing, which help the fistula mature.
      e. The fistula is required to be mature before it can be used because the engorged vein is punctured with a large-bore needle for the **dialysis** procedure.
      f. Subclavian or femoral catheters, peritoneal **dialysis**, or an external arteriovenous shunt can be used for **dialysis** while the fistula is maturing or developing.

   2. Advantages
      a. Because the fistula is internal, the risk of clotting and bleeding is low.
      b. The fistula can be used indefinitely.
      c. Fistulas have a decreased incidence of infection because it is internal and is not exposed.
      d. Once healing has occurred, no external dressing is required.
      e. The fistula allows freedom of movement.

   3. Disadvantages
      a. The fistula cannot be used immediately after insertion so planning ahead for an alternate access for **dialysis** is important.
      b. Needle insertions through the skin and tissues to the fistula are required for **dialysis**.
      c. Infiltration of the needles during **dialysis** can occur and cause hematomas.
      d. An aneurysm can form in the fistula.
      e. Congestive heart failure can occur from the increased blood flow in the venous system.

⚠ Arterial steal syndrome can develop in a client with an internal arteriovenous fistula. In this complication, too much blood is diverted to the vein, and arterial perfusion to the hand is compromised.

D. Internal arteriovenous graft (see Fig. 62-2)
   1. Description
      a. The internal graft may be used for chronic **dialysis** clients who do not have adequate blood vessels for the creation of a fistula.
      b. An artificial graft made of Gore-Tex or a bovine (cow) carotid artery is used to create an artificial vein for blood flow.
      c. The procedure involves the anastomosis of an artery to a vein using an artificial graft.
      d. The graft can be used 2 weeks after insertion.
      e. Complications of the graft include clotting, aneurysms, and infection.

   2. Advantages
      a. Because the graft is internal, the risk of clotting and bleeding is low.
      b. The graft can be used indefinitely.
      c. The graft has a decreased incidence of infection.
      d. Once healing has occurred, no external dressing is required.
      e. The graft allows freedom of movement.

3. Disadvantages
   a. The graft cannot be used immediately after insertion.
   b. Needle insertions through the skin and tissues to the graft are required for **dialysis**.
   c. Infiltration of the needles during **dialysis** can occur and cause hematomas.
   d. An aneurysm can form in the graft; additionally, grafts clot more frequently than **arteriovenous fistulas**.
   e. **Arterial steal syndrome** can develop (too much blood is diverted to the vein, and arterial perfusion to the hand is compromised).
   f. Congestive heart failure can occur from the increased blood flow in the venous system.

E. Interventions for an **arteriovenous fistula** and arteriovenous graft
   1. Teach the client that the extremity should not be used for monitoring blood pressure, drawing blood, placing IV lines, or administering injections.
   2. Teach the client with an **arteriovenous fistula** hand-flexing exercises such as ball squeezing (if prescribed) to promote graft maturity.
   3. Note the temperature and capillary refill of the extremity.
   4. Palpate pulses below the fistula or graft, and monitor for hand swelling as an indication of ischemia.
   5. Monitor for clotting.
      a. Complaints of tingling or discomfort in the extremity.
      b. Inability to palpate a thrill or auscultate a bruit over the fistula or graft.
   6. Monitor for **arterial steal syndrome**.
   7. Monitor for infection.
   8. Monitor lung and heart sounds for signs of CHF.
   9. Notify the physician immediately if signs of clotting, infection, or **arterial steal syndrome** occur.

⚠ To ensure patency, palpate for a thrill or auscultate for a bruit over the fistula or graft. Notify the physician if a thrill or bruit is absent.

VIII. COMPLICATIONS OF HEMODIALYSIS (Box 62-7)

A. Air embolus
   1. Description
      a. Introduction of air into the circulatory system
      b. Results in cardiopulmonary complications
   2. Assessment
      a. Dyspnea and tachypnea
      b. Chest pain
      c. Hypotension
      d. Reduced oxygen saturation
      e. Cyanosis
      f. Anxiety
      g. Changes in sensorium
   3. Interventions (see Priority Nursing Actions box)

Box 62-7 Complications of Hemodialysis

Air embolus	Hepatitis
Disequilibrium syndrome	Hypotension
Electrolyte alterations	Sepsis
Encephalopathy	Shock
Hemorrhage	

▰▰▰▰ PRIORITY NURSING ACTIONS! ▰▰▰▰

Actions to Take If a Client Receiving Hemodialysis Develops an Air Embolism
1. Stop the hemodialysis.
2. Turn the client on the left side, with the head down (Trendelenburg's).
3. Notify the physician.
4. Administer oxygen.
5. Assess vital signs and pulse oximetry.
6. Document the event, actions taken, and the client's response.

Air embolism occurs when air enters the catheter system and is a complication of hemodialysis. The signs of air embolism include dyspnea, tachypnea, chest pain, hypotension, reduced oxygen saturation, cyanosis, anxiety, and changes in sensorium. Air embolism is a critical situation and if it is suspected, hemodialysis is stopped immediately and the client should be placed in a left side-lying position with the head lower than the feet. This position is used to try to prevent the air from traveling as a bolus to the lungs by trapping it in the right side of the heart. The physician is notified immediately and oxygen is administered. Vital signs are assessed including the pulse oximetry and other prescribed interventions are done. The event, actions taken, and the client's response are documented.

References: Ignatavicius, D., & Workman, M. (2010). *Medical-surgical nursing: Patient-centered collaborative care* (6th ed., p. 231). St. Louis: Saunders.

Perry, A., & Potter, P. (2010). *Clinical nursing skills & techniques* (7th ed., p. 850). St. Louis: Mosby.

B. **Disequilibrium syndrome**
   1. Description
      a. A rapid change in the composition of the extracellular fluid occurs during hemodialysis.
      b. Solutes are removed from the blood faster than from the cerebrospinal fluid and brain; fluid is pulled into the brain, causing cerebral edema.
      c. Occurs more frequently in a new client during the initial onset of hemodialysis.
   2. Assessment
      a. Nausea and vomiting
      b. Headache
      c. Hypertension
      d. Restlessness and agitation
      e. Muscle cramps
      f. Confusion
      g. Seizures

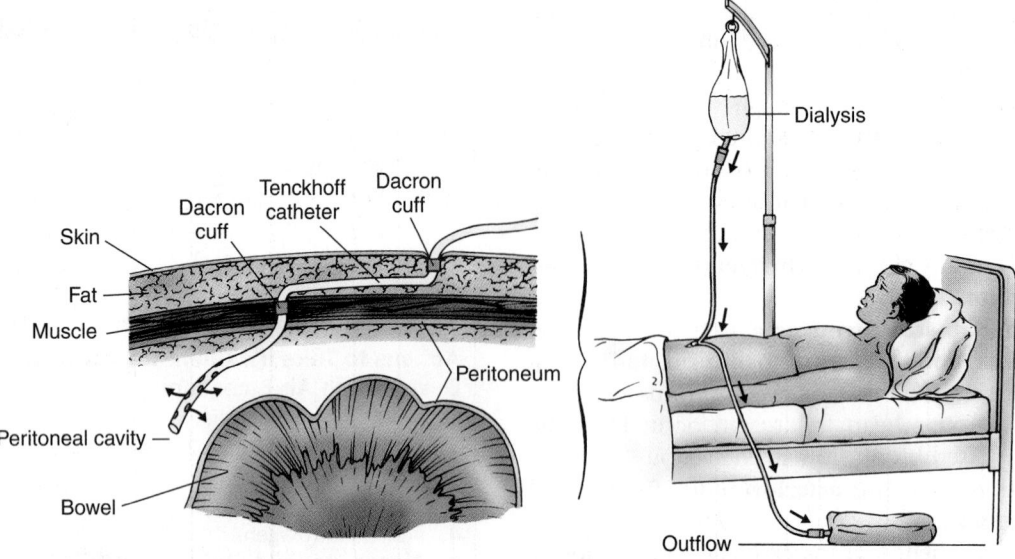

▲ **FIGURE 62-3** Manual peritoneal dialysis via an implanted abdominal catheter (Tenckhoff catheter). (From Ignatavicius, D., & Workman, M. [2010]. *Medical-surgical nursing: Patient-centered collaborative care* [6th ed.]. St. Louis: Saunders.)

3. Interventions
   a. Slow or stop the **dialysis**.
   b. Notify the physician if signs of **disequilibrium syndrome** occur.
   c. Reduce environmental stimuli.
   d. Prepare to administer intravenous hypertonic saline solution, albumin, or mannitol (Osmitrol) if prescribed.
   e. Prepare to dialyze the client for a shorter period of time at reduced flow rates to prevent its occurrence.
C. Dialysis encephalopathy
   1. Description: An aluminum toxicity from dialysate water sources containing aluminum; also can occur from ingestion of aluminum-containing antacids (phosphate binders). This is not a common occurrence.
   2. Assessment
      a. Progressive neurological impairment
      b. Mental cloudiness
      c. Speech disturbances
      d. Dementia
      e. Muscle incoordination
      f. Bone pain
      g. Seizures
   3. Interventions
      a. Monitor for the signs of **dialysis** encephalopathy.
      b. Notify the physician if signs of **dialysis** encephalopathy occur.
      c. Administer aluminum-chelating agents as prescribed so that the aluminum is released and dialyzed from the body.

IX. PERITONEAL DIALYSIS

A. Description
   1. The peritoneum acts as the dialyzing membrane (semipermeable membrane) to achieve **dialysis** during kidney failure.

2. Peritoneal **dialysis** (PD) works on the principles of osmosis, diffusion and ultrafiltration; PD occurs via the transfer of fluid and solute from the bloodstream through the peritoneum into the dialysate solution.
3. The peritoneal membrane is large and porous, allowing solutes and fluid to move via osmosis from an area of higher concentration in the body to an area of lower concentration in the dialyzing fluid.
4. The peritoneal cavity is rich in capillaries; therefore it provides a ready access to the blood supply.
B. Contraindications to peritoneal **dialysis**
   1. Peritonitis
   2. Recent abdominal surgery
   3. Abdominal adhesions
   4. Other gastrointestinal problems such as diverticulosis
C. Access for peritoneal **dialysis** (Fig. 62-3)
   1. A siliconized rubber catheter such as a Tenckhoff catheter is surgically inserted into the client's peritoneal cavity to allow infusion of **dialysis** fluid.
   2. The preferred insertion site is 3 to 5 cm below the umbilicus; this area is relatively avascular and has less fascial resistance.
   3. The catheter is tunneled under the skin, through the fat and muscle tissue to the peritoneum; it is stabilized with inflatable Dacron cuffs in the muscle and under the skin.
   4. Over a period of 1 to 2 weeks following insertion, fibroblasts and blood vessels grow around the cuffs, fixing the catheter in place and providing an extra barrier against dialysate leakage and bacterial invasion.
   5. If the client is scheduled for transplant surgery, the peritoneal **dialysis** catheter may either be

removed or left in place if the need for **dialysis** is suspected post-transplantation.

D. Dialysate solution

1. The solution is sterile.
2. All **dialysis** solutions are prescribed by the physician; the solution contains electrolytes and minerals and has a specific osmolarity, specific glucose concentration, and other medication additives as prescribed.
3. The higher the glucose concentration, the greater the hypertonicity and the amount of fluid removed during a peritoneal **dialysis** exchange.
4. Increasing the glucose concentration increases the concentration of active particles that cause osmosis, increases the rate of ultrafiltration, and increases the amount of fluid removed.
5. If hyperkalemia is not a problem, potassium may be added to each bag of dialysate solution.
6. Heparin is added to the dialysate solution to prevent clotting of the catheter.
7. Prophylactic antibiotics may be added to the dialysate solution to prevent peritonitis.
8. Insulin may be added to the dialysate solution for the client with diabetes mellitus.

E. Peritoneal **dialysis** infusion

1. Description
   a. One infusion (fill), dwell, and drain is considered one exchange.
   b. Fill: The infusion of 1 to 2 L of dialysate as prescribed is infused by gravity into the peritoneal space, which usually takes 10 to 20 minutes.
   c. Dwell time: The amount of time that the dialysate solution remains in the peritoneal cavity is prescribed by the physician and can last 20 to 30 minutes to 8 or more hours, depending on the type of **dialysis** used.
   d. Drain (outflow): Fluid drains out of body by gravity into the drainage bag.
2. Interventions before treatment
   a. Monitor vital signs.
   b. Obtain weight.
   c. Have the client void, if possible.
   d. Assess electrolyte and glucose levels.
3. Interventions during treatment
   a. Monitor vital signs.
   b. Monitor for respiratory distress, pain, or discomfort.
   c. Monitor for signs of pulmonary edema.
   d. Monitor for hypotension and hypertension.
   e. Monitor for malaise, nausea, vomiting.
   f. Assess the catheter site dressing for wetness or bleeding.
   g. Monitor dwell time as prescribed by the physician.
   h. Do not allow dwell time to extend beyond the physician's prescription because this increases the risk for hyperglycemia.
   i. Initiate outflow; turn the client from side to side if the outflow is slow to start.
   j. Monitor outflow, which should be a continuous stream after the clamp is opened.
   k. Monitor outflow for color and clarity.
   l. Monitor intake and output accurately; if outflow is less than inflow, the difference is equal to the amount absorbed or retained by the client during **dialysis** and should be counted as intake.
   m. An outflow greater than inflow should be reported to the physician as well as the appearance of frank blood or cloudiness in the outflow.

F. Types of peritoneal **dialysis**

1. Continuous ambulatory peritoneal **dialysis** (CAPD)
   a. Closely resembles renal function because it is a continuous process
   b. Does not require a machine for the procedure
   c. Promotes client independence
   d. The client performs self-**dialysis** 24 hours a day, 7 days a week.
   e. Four **dialysis** cycles are usually administered in a 24-hour period, including an overnight 8-hour dwell time.
   f. Dialysate, 1½ to 2 L, is instilled into the abdomen four times daily and allowed to dwell as prescribed.
   g. After dwell, the bag is placed lower than the insertion site so that fluid drains by gravity flow.
   h. After fluid is drained, the bag is changed, new dialysate is instilled into the abdomen, and the process continues.
   i. Between exchanges, the catheter is clamped.
2. Automated peritoneal **dialysis** (Box 62-8)
   a. Automated **dialysis** requires a peritoneal cycling machine.
   b. Automated **dialysis** can be done as intermittent peritoneal **dialysis**, continuous cycling peritoneal **dialysis**, or nightly peritoneal **dialysis**.
   c. The exchanges are automated instead of manual

X. COMPLICATIONS OF PERITONEAL DIALYSIS (Box 62-9)

⚠ Infection is a concern with peritoneal dialysis; sites of infection are either the catheter insertion site or in the peritoneum causing peritonitis.

A. Peritonitis

1. Monitor for symptoms of peritonitis: Fever, cloudy outflow, rebound abdominal tenderness, abdominal pain, general malaise, nausea, and vomiting.

Box 62-8 Types of Automated Peritoneal Dialysis

Continuous Cycling Peritoneal Dialysis
Dialysis requires a peritoneal cycling machine.
Dialysis usually consists of three cycles done at night and one cycle with an 8-hour dwell done in the morning.
The sterile catheter system is opened only for the on-and-off procedures, which reduces the risk of infection.
The client does not need to do exchanges during the day.

Intermittent Peritoneal Dialysis
Dialysis requires a peritoneal cycling machine.
Dialysis is not a continuous procedure.
Dialysis is performed for 10 to 14 hours, three or four times a week.

Nightly Peritoneal Dialysis
Dialysis requires a cycling machine.
Dialysis is performed 8 to 12 hours each night, with no daytime exchanges or dwells.

Box 62-9 Complications of Peritoneal Dialysis

Abdominal pain
Bladder or bowel perforation
Insufficient outflow
Leakage around the catheter site
Peritonitis

2. Cloudy or opaque outflow is an early sign of peritonitis.
3. If peritonitis is suspected, obtain a sample for culture and sensitivity of the outflow to determine the infective organism.
4. Administer antibiotics as prescribed.
5. Avoid infections by maintaining meticulous sterile technique when connecting and disconnecting PD solution bags and when caring for the catheter insertion site.
6. Prevent the catheter insertion site dressing from becoming wet during care of the client or the **dialysis** procedure; change the dressing if wet or soiled.
7. Follow institutional procedure for connecting and disconnecting PD solution bags, which may include scrubbing the connection sites with an antiseptic solution.
B. Abdominal pain
   1. Peritoneal irritation during inflow commonly causes pain during the first few exchanges; the pain usually disappears after 1 to 2 weeks of **dialysis** treatments.
   2. Warm the dialysate before administration using a special dialysate warmer pad, because the cold temperature of the dialysate can cause discomfort.

C. Abnormal outflow characteristics indicative of complications
   1. Bloody outflow after the first few exchanges indicates vascular complications (the outflow should be clear after the initial exchanges).
   2. Brown outflow indicates bowel perforation.
   3. Urine-colored outflow indicates bladder perforation.
   4. Cloudy outflow indicates peritonitis.
D. Insufficient outflow
   1. The main cause of insufficient outflow is a full colon; encourage a high-fiber diet, because constipation can cause inflow and outflow problems. Administer stool softeners as prescribed.
   2. Insufficient outflow may also be caused by catheter migration out of the peritoneal area; if this occurs, an x-ray will be prescribed to evaluate catheter position.
   3. Maintain the drainage bag below the client's abdomen.
   4. Check for kinks in the tubing.
   5. Check for fibrin clots in the tubing and milk the tubing to dislodge the clot as prescribed.
   6. Change the client's outflow position by turning the client to a side-lying position or ambulating the client.
E. Leakage around the catheter site
   1. Clear fluid that leaks from the catheter exit site will be noted.
   2. It takes 1 to 2 weeks following insertion of the catheter before fibroblasts and blood vessels grow into the catheter cuffs, which fix it in place and provide an extra barrier against dialysate leakage and bacterial invasion.
   3. Smaller amounts of dialysate need to be used; it may take up to 2 weeks for the client to tolerate a full 2-L exchange without leaking around the catheter site.

XI. CONTINUOUS RENAL REPLACEMENT THERAPY

A. Continuous renal replacement therapy (CRRT) provides continuous ultrafiltration of extracellular fluid and clearance of urinary toxins over a period of 8 to 24 hours; used primarily for clients in **ARF** or critically ill clients with **CRF** who cannot tolerate hemodialysis.
B. Water, electrolytes, and other solutes are removed as the client's blood passes through a hemofilter.
C. Because rapid shifts in fluids and electrolytes typically do not occur, hemofiltration is usually better tolerated by critically ill clients.
D. There are five variations of CRRT (Box 62-10), some requiring a hemodialysis machine and others that rely on the client's blood pressure to power the system.
E. If CRRT does not require a hemodialysis machine, the client's mean arterial blood pressure needs to be

maintained above 60 mm Hg and arterial and venous access sites are necessary.

XII. KIDNEY TRANSPLANTATION (Fig. 62-4)

A. Description
1. A human kidney from a compatible donor is implanted into a recipient.
2. Kidney transplantation is performed for irreversible kidney failure; specific criteria is established for eligibility for a transplant.
3. The recipient must take immunosuppressive medications for life.

B. Living related donors
1. The most desirable source of kidneys for transplantation is living related donors who closely match the client.
2. Donors are screened for ABO blood group, tissue-specific antigen, human leukocyte antigen suitability, mixed lymphocyte culture index (histocompatibility); donors are also screened for the presence of any communicable diseases and undergo a complete medical evaluation as well as a nephrology consultation.

Box 62-10 Types of Continuous Renal Replacement Therapy

Continuous venovenous hemofiltration (CVVH)
Continuous arteriovenous hemofiltration (CAVH)
Continuous venovenous hemodialysis (CVVHD)
Continuous arteriovenous hemodialysis (CAVHD)
Slow continuous ultrafiltration (SCUF)

3. The donor must be in excellent health, with two properly functioning kidneys.
4. The emotional well-being of the donor is determined.
5. Complete understanding of the donation process and outcome by the donor is necessary.

C. Cadaver donors
1. Cadaver donors must meet the institution's criteria of brain death.
2. Cadaver donors usually need to be younger than 70 years.
3. Cadaver donors must have normal renal function, although "marginal" donor organs have been used with the consent of the recipient.
4. No malignant disease outside the central nervous system can be present.
5. No generalized infection or communicable disease can be present.
6. No renal trauma can be present.
7. The potential donor must be negative for communicable diseases at the time of donation.
8. Once cerebral death has been established for a potential donor, restoration of intravascular volume, weaning from vasopressors, and establishing diuresis are crucial; management of the donor is determined by organ bank personnel.
9. Continuous ventilation, and normal blood pressure and heart rate are maintained until the kidneys and other organs are surgically removed.

D. Cold ischemic time
1. Cold ischemic time is the time elapsed between the cessation of blood flow to the kidney and the time required for anastomosis of the kidney in the recipient.

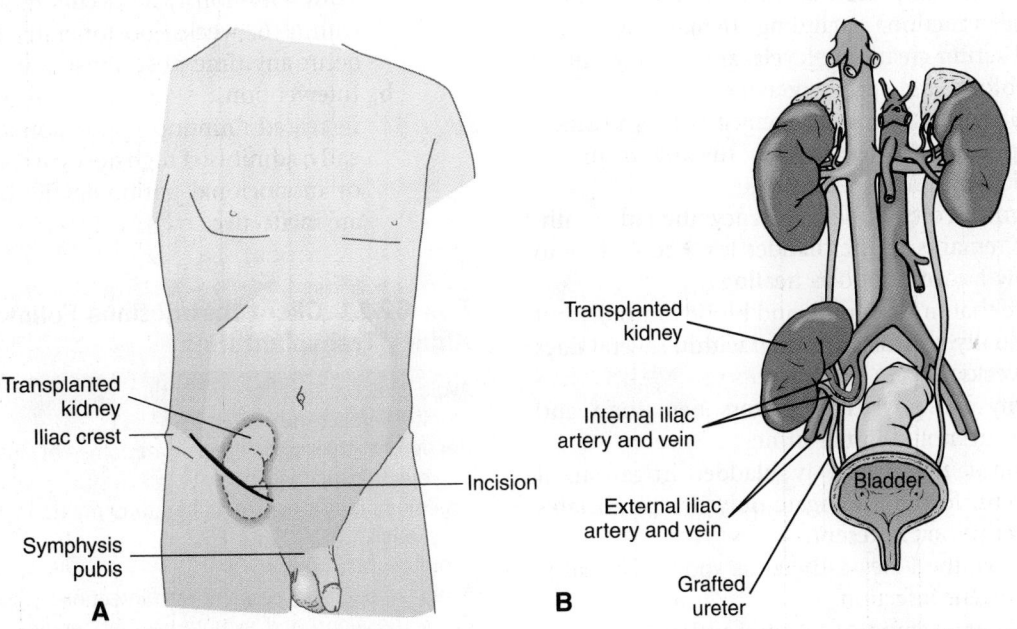

▲ **FIGURE 62-4 A,** Surgical incision for renal transplantation. **B,** Surgical placement of transplanted kidney. (From Lewis, S., Heitkemper, M., Dirksen, S., O'Brien, P., & Bucher, L. [2007]. *Medical-surgical nursing: Assessment and management of clinical problems* [7th ed.]. St. Louis: Mosby.)

2. The maximum transplantation time is up to 72 hours.

E. Preoperative interventions

1. Verify histocompatibility tests of donor, which will be done by organ bank personnel.
2. Administer immunosuppressive medications to the recipient for 2 days before the transplantation, as prescribed.
3. Maintain strict aseptic technique for the recipient.
4. Verify that hemodialysis of the recipient was completed 24 hours before transplantation.
5. Ensure that the recipient is free of any infections.
6. Assess renal function studies.
7. Encourage discussion of feelings of the donor and the recipient.
8. Provide psychological support to the live donor or cadaver donor family and the recipient.

F. Postoperative interventions for the recipient

1. Urine output usually begins immediately if the donor was a living donor; it may be delayed for a few days or more with a cadaver kidney.
2. Hemodialysis may be performed until adequate kidney function is established.
3. Monitor vital signs, central venous pressure (CVP), and pulse oximetry for signs of complications.
4. Monitor urine output hourly; immediately report a urine output less than 100 mL/hr.
5. Monitor IV fluids closely; for the first 12 to 24 hours, IV fluid replacement is based on hourly urine output.
6. Administer prescribed diuretics and osmotic agents.
7. Monitor daily weight to evaluate fluid status.
8. Monitor daily laboratory results to evaluate renal function, including hematocrit, BUN, and serum creatinine levels, and monitor urine for blood and specific gravity.
9. Position the client in a semi-Fowler's position to promote gas exchange, turning from the back to the nonoperative side.
10. Monitor Foley catheter patency; the Foley catheter remains in the bladder for 3 to 5 days to allow for anastomosis healing.
11. Note that urine is pink and bloody initially but gradually returns to normal within several days to weeks.
12. Notify the physician if gross hematuria and clots are noted in the urine.
13. Monitor the three-way bladder irrigation, if present, for clots; irrigate only if a physician's prescription is present.
14. Remove the Foley catheter as soon as possible to prevent infection.
15. Maintain aseptic technique and monitor for infection; infection is the primary cause of death in the first year post-transplant.
16. Maintain strict aseptic technique with wound care.
17. Monitor for bowel sounds and for the passage of flatus; initiate a specific diet and oral fluids as prescribed when flatus and bowel sounds return (usually, fluids, sodium, and potassium are restricted if the client is oliguric).
18. Maintain good oral hygiene, monitoring for stomatitis and bacterial and fungal infections.
19. Encourage coughing and deep-breathing exercises.
20. Administer medications as prescribed, which may include antifungal medications, antibiotics, immunosuppressive agents, and corticosteroids.
21. The client is usually ambulated after 24 hours.
22. Assess for organ rejection by monitoring of laboratory values closely.
23. Promote live donor and recipient relationship.
24. Monitor both the donor and recipient for depression.
25. Provide the recipient with instructions following the kidney transplantation (Box 62-11).
26. Assist the recipient to cope with the body image disturbances that occur from long-term use of immunosuppressants.
27. Advise the recipient of available support groups.

G. Graft rejection

1. Assessment (Box 62-12)
2. Hyperacute rejection
   a. Hyperacute rejection occurs at the time of anastomosis of the organ.
   b. Interventions: Removal of rejected kidney
3. Acute rejection
   a. Most common type; occurs most frequently within 6 weeks postoperatively, but can occur any time post-transplant.
   b. Interventions: Potentially reversible with increased immunosuppression and if treated early; administer high doses of corticosteroids, or monoclonal antibodies if corticosteroids are ineffective.

Box 62-11 Client Instructions Following Kidney Transplantation

Avoid prolonged periods of sitting.

Monitor intake and output.

Recognize the signs and symptoms of infection and rejection.

Use medications as prescribed, and maintain immunosuppressive therapy for life.

Avoid contact sports.

Avoid exposure to persons with infections.

Know the signs and symptoms that require the need to contact the physician.

Ensure follow-up care.

Box 62-12 Clinical Signs of Renal Transplant (Graft) Rejection

Temperature higher than 100° F (37.7° C)
Pain or tenderness over the grafted kidney
2- to 3-lb weight gain in 24 hours
Edema
Hypertension
Malaise
Elevated blood urea nitrogen and serum creatinine levels
Decreased creatinine clearance
Elevated white blood cell count
Rejection indicated by ultrasound or biopsy

Box 62-13 Causes of Cystitis

Allergens or irritants, such as soaps, sprays, bubble bath, perfumed sanitary napkins
Bladder distention
Calculus
Hormonal changes, influencing alterations in vaginal flora
Indwelling urinary catheters
Invasive urinary tract procedures
Loss of bactericidal properties of prostatic secretions in the male
Microorganisms
Poor-fitting vaginal diaphragms
Sexual intercourse
Synthetic underwear and pantyhose
Urinary stasis
Use of spermicides
Wet bathing suits

4. Chronic rejection
   a. Occurs slowly months to years after transplant and mimics **CRF**.
   b. Interventions: Immunosuppressive medications and retransplantation if necessary.

⚠ Except for identical twin donors and recipients, the major postoperative complication following renal transplant is graft rejection.

⚠ Altered mentation is a sign of a urinary tract infection in older adults; frequency and urgency may not be specific symptoms of UTI because of urinary elimination changes that occur with aging.

XIII. CYSTITIS—URINARY TRACT INFECTION

A. Description
   1. Cystitis (urinary tract infection, UTI) is an inflammation of the bladder from an infection, obstruction of the urethra, or other irritants (Box 62-13).
   2. The most common causative organisms are *Escherichia coli* and *Enterobacter*, *Pseudomonas*, and *Serratia* species.
   3. Cystitis is more common in women because women have a shorter urethra than men and the urethra in the woman is located close to the rectum.
   4. Sexually active and pregnant women are most vulnerable to cystitis.

B. Assessment
   1. Frequency and urgency
   2. Burning on urination
   3. Voiding in small amounts
   4. Inability to void
   5. Incomplete emptying of the bladder
   6. Lower abdominal discomfort or back discomfort
   7. Cloudy, dark, foul-smelling urine
   8. Hematuria
   9. Bladder spasms
   10. Malaise, chills, fever
   11. Nausea and vomiting
   12. WBC count greater than 100,000 cells/mm^3 on urinalysis
   13. An elevated specific gravity and pH may be noted on urinalysis.

C. Interventions
   1. Before administering prescribed antibiotics, obtain a urine specimen for culture and sensitivity, if prescribed, to identify bacterial growth.
   2. Encourage the client to increase fluids up to 3000 mL/day, especially if the client is taking a sulfonamide; sulfonamides can form crystals in concentrated urine.
   3. Administer prescribed medications, which may include analgesics, antiseptics, antispasmodics, antibiotics, and antimicrobials.
   4. Maintain an acid urine pH (5.5); instruct the client about foods to consume to maintain acidic urine.
   5. Provide heat to the abdomen or sitz baths for complaints of discomfort.
   6. Note that if the client is prescribed an aminoglycoside, sulfonamide, or nitrofurantoin (Macrodantin), the actions of these medications are decreased by acidic urine.
   7. Use sterile technique when inserting a urinary catheter.
   8. Maintain closed urinary drainage systems for the client with an indwelling catheter and avoid elevating the urinary drainage bag above the level of the bladder.
   9. Provide meticulous perineal care for the client with an indwelling catheter.
   10. Discourage caffeine products such as coffee, tea, and cola.
   11. Client education
       a. Avoid alcohol.
       b. Take medications as prescribed.

Box 62-14 Teaching for Prevention of Cystitis

Use good perineal care, wiping front to back.
Avoid bubble baths, tub baths, and vaginal deodorants or sprays.
Void every 2 to 3 hours.
Wear cotton pants and avoid wearing tight clothes or pantyhose with slacks.
Avoid sitting in a wet bathing suit for prolonged periods of time.
If pregnant, void every 2 hours.
If menopausal, use estrogen vaginal creams to restore pH.
Use water-soluble lubricants for intercourse, especially after menopause.
Void and drink a glass of water after intercourse.

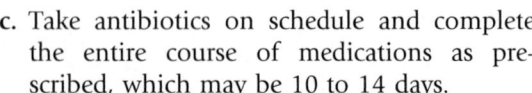

   c. Take antibiotics on schedule and complete the entire course of medications as prescribed, which may be 10 to 14 days.
   d. Repeat the urine culture following treatment.
   e. Prevent recurrence of cystitis (Box 62-14).

XIV. UROSEPSIS

A. Description
  1. Urosepsis is a gram-negative bacteremia originating in the urinary tract.
  2. The most common causative organism is *Escherichia coli*.
  3. In a client who is immunocompromised, the most common cause is infection from an indwelling urinary catheter or an untreated UTI.
  4. The major problem is the ability of this bacterium to develop resistant strains.
  5. Urosepsis can lead to septic shock if not treated aggressively.

B. Assessment: Fever is the most common and earliest manifestation.

C. Interventions
  1. Obtain a urine specimen for urine culture and sensitivity before administering antibiotics.
  2. Administer antibiotics intravenously as prescribed, usually until the client has been afebrile for 3 to 5 days.
  3. Administer oral antibiotics as prescribed after the 3- to 5-day afebrile period.

XV. URETHRITIS

A. Description
  1. Inflammation of the urethra commonly associated with a sexually transmitted disease; may occur with cystitis.
  2. In men, urethritis most often is caused by gonorrhea or chlamydial infection.
  3. In women, urethritis most often is caused by feminine hygiene sprays, perfumed toilet paper or sanitary napkins, spermicidal jelly, UTI, or changes in the vaginal mucosal lining.

B. Assessment
  1. Pain or burning on urination
  2. Frequency and urgency
  3. Nocturia
  4. Difficulty voiding
  5. Males may have clear to mucopurulent discharge from the penis.
  6. Females may have lower abdominal discomfort.

C. Interventions
  1. Encourage fluid intake.
  2. Prepare the client for testing to determine whether a sexually transmitted infection (STI) is present.
  3. Administer antibiotics as prescribed.
  4. Instruct the client in the administration of sitz or tub baths.
  5. If stricture occurs, prepare the client for dilation of the urethra and instillation of an antiseptic solution.
  6. Instruct the female client to avoid the use of perfumed toilet paper or sanitary napkins and feminine hygiene sprays.
  7. Instruct the client to avoid intercourse until the symptoms subside or treatment of the STI is complete.
  8. Instruct the client about STIs if this is the cause.
    a. Prevent STIs by the use of latex condoms or abstinence.
    b. All sexual partners during the 30 days before diagnosis with chlamydial infection should be notified, examined, and treated if indicated.
    c. Chlamydial infection often coexists with gonorrhea; diagnostic testing is done for both STIs.
    d. Treatment for STIs includes antibiotics as prescribed to treat the causative organism.
    e. The most serious complication of chlamydial infection is sterility.
    f. Follow-up culture may be requested in 4 to 7 days to evaluate the effectiveness of medications.

XVI. URETERITIS

A. Description: An inflammation of the ureter commonly associated with bacterial or viral infections and pyelonephritis

B. Assessment
  1. Dysuria
  2. Frequent urination
  3. Clear to mucopurulent penile discharge in males

C. Interventions
  1. Treatment includes identifying and treating the underlying cause and providing symptomatic relief.
  2. Administer metronidazole (Flagyl) or clotrimazole (Mycelex) as prescribed for treating *Trichomonas* infection.
  3. Administer nystatin (Mycostatin) or fluconazole (Diflucan) as prescribed for treating yeast infections.

4. Doxycycline (Vibramycin) or azithromycin (Zithromax) may be prescribed for treating chlamydial infections.

XVII. PYELONEPHRITIS

A. Description
  1. An inflammation of the renal pelvis and the parenchyma commonly caused by bacterial invasion
  2. Acute pyelonephritis often occurs after bacterial contamination of the urethra or following an invasive procedure of the urinary tract.
  3. Chronic pyelonephritis most commonly occurs following chronic urinary flow obstruction with reflux.
  4. *Escherichia coli* is the most common causative bacterial organism.

B. Acute pyelonephritis
  1. Acute pyelonephritis occurs as a new infection or recurs as a relapse of a previous infection.
  2. It can progress to bacteremia or chronic pyelonephritis.
  3. Assessment
     a. Fever and chills
     b. Nausea
     c. Flank pain on the affected side
     d. Costovertebral angle tenderness
     e. Headache
     f. Dysuria
     g. Frequency and urgency
     h. Cloudy, bloody, or foul-smelling urine
     i. Increased white blood cells in the urine

C. Chronic pyelonephritis
  1. A slow, progressive disease usually associated with recurrent acute attacks
  2. Causes contraction of the kidney and dysfunctioning of the nephrons, which are replaced by scar tissue
  3. Causes the ureter to become fibrotic and narrowed by strictures
  4. Can lead to **renal failure**
  5. Assessment
     a. Frequently diagnosed incidentally when a client is being evaluated for hypertension
     b. Poor urine-concentrating ability
     c. Pyuria
     d. **Azotemia**
     e. Proteinuria

D. Interventions
  1. Monitor vital signs, especially for elevated temperature.
  2. Encourage fluid intake up to 3000 mL/day to reduce fever and prevent dehydration.
  3. Monitor intake and output (ensure that output is a minimum of 1500 mL/24 hr).
  4. Monitor weight.
  5. Encourage adequate rest.

6. Instruct the client in a high-calorie, low-protein diet.
7. Provide warm, moist compresses to the flank area to help relieve pain.
8. Encourage the client to take warm baths for pain relief.
9. Administer analgesics, antipyretics, antibiotics, urinary antiseptics, and antiemetics as prescribed.
10. Monitor for signs of **renal failure**.
11. Encourage follow-up urine culture.

XVIII. GLOMERULONEPHRITIS

A. Description
  1. Term that includes a variety of disorders, most of which are caused by an immunological reaction
  2. Results in proliferative and inflammatory changes within the glomerular structure
  3. Destruction, inflammation, and sclerosis of the glomeruli of both kidneys occur.
  4. The inflammation of the glomeruli results from an antigen-antibody reaction produced from an infection or autoimmune process elsewhere in the body.
  5. Loss of kidney function occurs.

B. Causes
  1. Immunological or autoimmune diseases
  2. Group A beta-hemolytic streptococcal infection
  3. History of pharyngitis or tonsillitis 2 to 3 weeks before symptoms

C. Types
  1. Acute glomerulonephritis occurs 5 to 21 days after a streptococcal infection.
  2. Chronic glomerulonephritis can occur after the acute phase or slowly over time.

D. Assessment
  1. Gross hematuria
  2. Dark, smoky, cola-colored or red-brown urine
  3. Proteinuria that produces a persistent and excessive foam in the urine
  4. Urinary debris
  5. Moderately elevated to high urine specific gravity
  6. Low urinary pH
  7. Urinalysis shows large numbers of erythrocytes
  8. **Oliguria** or **anuria**
  9. Headache
  10. Chills and fever
  11. Fatigue and weakness
  12. Anorexia, nausea, and vomiting
  13. Pallor
  14. Edema in the face, periorbital area, feet, or generalized
  15. Shortness of breath, ascites, pleural effusion, and CHF
  16. Abdominal or flank pain
  17. Hypertension
  18. Reduced visual acuity

19. Increased blood urea nitrogen and serum creatinine levels
20. Increased antistreptolysin O titer (used to diagnose disorders caused by streptococcal infections)

E. Interventions
1. Monitor vital signs, especially for hypertension and temperature elevations.
2. Monitor intake and output and urine characteristics closely.
3. Monitor daily weight.
4. Monitor for edema.
5. Monitor for fluid overload, ascites, pulmonary edema, and CHF.
6. Restrict fluid intake as prescribed.
7. Provide a high-calorie, low-protein, low-sodium, and low-potassium diet to prevent worsening **azotemia**, fluid retention, and hyperkalemia.
8. Provide bed rest and limit activity.
9. Administer diuretics, antihypertensives, and antibiotics as prescribed.
10. Monitor for signs of **renal failure**, cardiac failure, and hypertensive encephalopathy.
11. Instruct the client to report signs of bloody urine, headache, or edema.
12. Instruct the client to obtain treatment for infections, especially sore throats, skin lesions, and upper respiratory infections.

F. Complications
1. Heart failure
2. Hypertensive encephalopathy
3. Pulmonary edema
4. **Renal failure**
5. Nephrotic syndrome

XIX. NEPHROTIC SYNDROME

A. Description: A set of clinical manifestations arising from protein wasting caused by diffuse glomerular damage
B. Assessment
1. Proteinuria
2. Hematuria
3. Hypoalbuminemia
4. Edema (periorbital that is most notable in the morning, and dependent, such as in the ankles when sitting and in the sacrum or scrotum when lying)
5. Hyperlipidemia
6. Anemia
7. Waxy pallor to the skin
8. Anorexia
9. Malaise
10. Irritability
11. Amenorrhea or abnormal menses
C. Interventions
1. Monitor vital signs, especially for signs of hypertension from fluid excess or hypotension from fluid shifting into the tissues.

2. Monitor intake and output.
3. Bed rest is necessary if severe edema is present.
4. Monitor daily weights.
5. Measure abdominal girth or extremity size.
6. Provide a low- to moderate-protein and -sodium diet that is adequate in carbohydrates and calories as prescribed to prevent worsening **azotemia** and fluid retention.
7. Monitor the serum potassium level; potassium may be restricted from the diet if the serum potassium level rises.
8. Administer antihypertensives, diuretics, and lipid-lowering agents as prescribed.
9. Administer corticosteroids and cytotoxic medications as prescribed.
10. Administer plasma volume expanders, such as albumin, plasma, and dextran, to increase the osmotic pressure.
11. Administer anticoagulants as prescribed for clients who develop renal vein thrombosis.
12. Avoid trauma to edematous tissues.
13. Instruct the client to keep the nails trimmed to avoid tissue trauma.

XX. POLYCYSTIC KIDNEY DISEASE

A. Description
1. A cystic formation and hypertrophy of the kidneys, which leads to cystic rupture, infection, formation of scar tissue, and damaged nephrons
2. There is no specific treatment to arrest the progress of the destructive cysts.
3. The ultimate result of this disease is **renal failure**.
B. Types
1. Infantile polycystic disease: An inherited autosomal recessive trait that results in the death of the infant within a few months after birth
2. Adult polycystic disease: An autosomal dominant trait that manifests between 30 and 40 years of age and results in end-stage renal disease
C. Assessment
1. Often asymptomatic until the ages of 30 to 40 years
2. Flank, lumbar, or abdominal pain that worsens with activity and is relieved when lying
3. Fever and chills
4. Recurrent urinary tract infections
5. Hematuria, proteinuria, pyuria
6. Calculi
7. Hypertension
8. Palpable abdominal masses and enlarged kidneys
D. Interventions
1. Monitor for gross hematuria, which indicates cyst rupture.
2. Increase sodium and water intake because sodium loss rather than retention occurs.
3. Provide bed rest if ruptured cysts and bleeding occur.

4. Prepare the client for percutaneous cyst puncture for relief of obstruction or for draining an abscess.
5. Administer antihypertensives as prescribed.
6. Prevent and/or treat urinary tract infections.
7. Prepare the client for **dialysis** or renal transplantation.
8. Encourage the client to seek genetic counseling.
9. Provide psychological support to the client and family.
10. Provide psychosocial support and genetic counseling for family who may want to donate a kidney.

XXI. HYDRONEPHROSIS

A. Description (Fig. 62-5)
1. Distention of the renal pelvis and calices caused by an obstruction of normal urine flow
2. The urine becomes trapped proximal to the obstruction.
3. The causes include calculus, tumors, scar tissue, ureter obstructions, and hypertrophy of the prostate.

B. Assessment
1. Hypertension
2. Headache
3. Colicky or dull flank pain that radiates to the groin

C. Interventions
1. Monitor vital signs frequently.
2. Monitor for fluid and electrolyte imbalances, including dehydration after the obstruction is relieved.
3. Monitor for diuresis, which can lead to fluid depletion.
4. Monitor weights daily.
5. Monitor urine for specific gravity and albumin and glucose levels.
6. Administer fluid replacement as prescribed.
7. Prepare the client for insertion of a nephrostomy tube or a surgical procedure to relieve the obstruction if prescribed.

XXII. RENAL CALCULI

A. Description
1. Calculi are stones that can form anywhere in the urinary tract; however, the most frequent site is the kidneys.
2. Problems resulting from calculi are pain, obstruction, tissue trauma, secondary hemorrhage, and infection.
3. The stone can be located through radiography of the kidneys, ureters, and bladder; intravenous pyelography; CT scanning; and renal ultrasonography.
4. A stone analysis will be done after passage to determine the type of stone and assist in determining treatment.
5. **Urolithiasis** refers to the formation of urinary calculi; these form in the ureters.

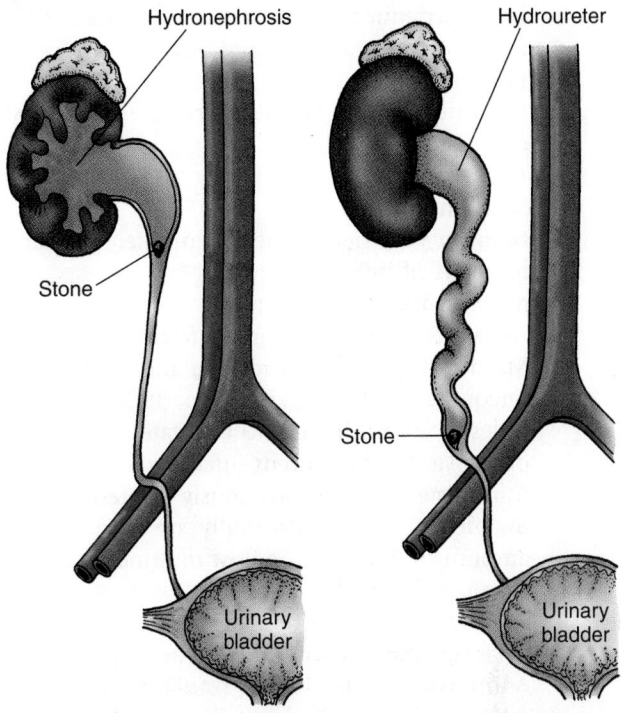

▲ **FIGURE 62-5** Hydronephrosis and hydroureter. (From Ignatavicius, D., & Workman, M. [2010]. *Medical-surgical nursing: Patient-centered collaborative care* [6th ed.]. St. Louis: Saunders.)

6. **Nephrolithiasis** refers to the formation of kidney calculi; these form in the renal parenchyma.
7. When a calculus occludes the ureter and blocks the flow of urine, the ureter dilates, producing hydroureter (see Fig. 62-5).
8. If the obstruction is not removed, urinary stasis results in infection, impairment of renal function on the side of the blockage, hydronephrosis (see Fig. 62-5), and irreversible kidney damage.

B. Causes
1. Family history of stone formation
2. Diet high in calcium, vitamin D, protein, oxalate, purines, or alkali
3. Obstruction and urinary stasis
4. Dehydration
5. Use of diuretics, which can cause volume depletion
6. Urinary tract infections and prolonged urinary catheterization
7. Immobilization
8. Hypercalcemia and hyperparathyroidism
9. Elevated uric acid level, such as in gout

C. Assessment
1. Renal colic, which originates in the lumbar region and radiates around the side and down to the testicles in men and to the bladder in women
2. Ureteral colic, which radiates toward the genitalia and thighs
3. Sharp, severe pain of sudden onset
4. Dull, aching pain in the kidney
5. Nausea and vomiting, pallor, and diaphoresis during acute pain

6. Urinary frequency, with alternating retention
7. Signs of a urinary tract infection
8. Low-grade fever
9. High numbers of red blood cells, white blood cells, and bacteria noted in the urinalysis report
10. Gross hematuria
D. Interventions
1. Monitor vital signs, especially the temperature, for signs of infection.
2. Monitor intake and output.
3. Assess for fever, chills, and infection.
4. Monitor for nausea, vomiting, and diarrhea.
5. Encourage fluid intake up to 3000 mL/day, unless contraindicated, to facilitate the passage of the stone and prevent infection.
6. Administer fluids intravenously as prescribed if unable to take fluids orally or in adequate amounts to increase the flow of urine and facilitate passage of the stone.
7. Provide warm baths and heat to the flank area (massage therapy should be avoided).
8. Administer analgesics at regularly scheduled intervals as prescribed to relieve pain.
9. Assess the client's response to pain medication.
10. Assist the client in performing relaxation techniques to assist in relieving pain.
11. Encourage client ambulation, if stable, to promote the passage of the stone.
12. Turn and reposition the immobilized client to promote passage of the stone.
13. Instruct the client in the diet restrictions specific to the stone composition if prescribed.
14. Prepare the client for surgical procedures if prescribed

⚠ For the client with renal calculi, strain all urine for the presence of stones and send the stones to the laboratory for analysis.

E. Stone composition
1. A special diet, such as an alkaline-ash or acid-ash diet, may be prescribed, depending on the physician's preference (Boxes 62-15 and 62-16).
2. Calcium phosphate stones
   a. Caused by supersaturation of urine with calcium and phosphate
   b. Diet includes acid-ash foods because calcium stones are alkaline.
   c. Dietary prescription may include decreasing intake of foods high in calcium and phosphate to reduce urinary calcium content and avoiding excess vitamin D intake to prevent stones from forming.
   d. Medications prescribed for calcium stones may include phosphates, thiazide diuretics, and allopurinol (Zyloprim).

Box 62-15 Alkaline-Ash Diet

Outcome
Diet increases the pH of the urine.
Diet reduces the acidity of the urine.

Foods to Include
Fruits except cranberries, plums, prunes, and tomatoes
Milk
Most vegetables
Rhubarb
Small amounts of beef, halibut, veal, trout, and salmon

Box 62-16 Acid-Ash Diet

Outcome
Diet decreases the pH of the urine.
Diet makes the urine more acidic.

Foods to Include
Bread, cereal, whole grains
Cheese, eggs
Corn and legumes
Cranberries, prunes, plums, tomatoes
Meat, fish, oysters, poultry

---

3. Calcium oxalate stones
   a. Caused by supersaturation of urine with calcium and oxalate
   b. Diet includes acid-ash foods because calcium stones are alkaline.
   c. Dietary prescription may include decreasing the intake of foods high in calcium and avoiding oxalate food sources to reduce urinary oxalate content and stone formation.
   d. Oxalate-rich food sources include tea, almonds, cashews, chocolate, cocoa, beans, spinach, and rhubarb.
   e. Allopurinol, pyridoxine (vitamin B_6), or magnesium oxide may be prescribed for clients with oxalate stones.
4. Struvite stones
   a. Composed of magnesium and ammonium phosphate
   b. Struvite stones are caused by urea-splitting bacteria and tend to form in alkaline urine.
   c. Diet includes acid-ash foods and includes limiting high-phosphate foods such as dairy products, red and organ meats, and whole grains to reduce urinary phosphate content.
   d. Treatment includes controlling infection with antibiotics (long-term antibiotic use may be prescribed).
5. Uric acid stones
   a. Caused by excess dietary purine or from gout
   b. Tend to form in acidic urine

c. Dietary prescription to reduce urinary purine content may include alkaline-ash foods and decreased intake of high-purine foods such as organ meats, gravies, red wines, and sardines.

d. Allopurinol may be prescribed to lower uric acid levels.

6. Cystine stones

a. Caused by cystine crystal formation; tend to form in acidic urine

b. Diet includes alkaline-ash foods; dietary prescription also may include a low intake of methionine, an essential amino acid that forms cystine. Therefore, the client would be instructed to avoid meat, milk, cheese, and eggs.

c. Dietary measures also focus on encouraging fluid intake up to 3 L/day, unless contraindicated, to help dilute the urine and prevent cystine crystals from forming.

d. Long-term antibiotic use may be prescribed for clients with cystine stones.

XXIII. TREATMENT OPTIONS FOR RENAL CALCULI (Fig. 62-6)

A. Cystoscopy

1. Cystoscopy may be done for stones in the bladder or lower ureter.

2. No incision is made.

3. One or two ureteral catheters are inserted past the stone; the stone may be manipulated and dislodged by the procedure and the catheters may guide the stones mechanically downward as they are removed.

4. The catheters are left in place for 24 hours to drain the urine trapped proximal to the stone and to dilate the ureter.

5. A continuous chemical irrigation may be prescribed to dissolve the stone.

B. Extracorporeal shock wave lithotripsy (ESWL)

1. A noninvasive mechanical procedure for breaking up stones located in the kidney or upper ureter so that they can pass spontaneously or be removed by other methods

2. No incision is made and no drains are placed; a stent may be placed to facilitate passing stone fragments.

3. Fluoroscopy is used to visualize the stone and ultrasonic waves are delivered to the area of the stone to disintegrate it.

4. The stones are passed in the urine within a few days.

5. Preprocedure: Maintain the client on an NPO status for 8 hours before the procedure.

6. Postprocedure

a. Monitor vital signs, especially for hypotension and tachycardia, which could indicate bleeding.

b. Monitor intake and output.

c. Monitor for bleeding.

d. Monitor for pain and signs of urinary obstruction.

e. Instruct the client that if a ureteral stent is placed to help the stone pass, it is usually removed in 1 to 2 weeks.

f. Instruct the client to increase fluid intake to flush out the stone fragments.

g. Inform the client that ambulation is important.

C. Percutaneous lithotripsy

1. Performed for stones in the bladder, ureter, or kidney

2. An invasive procedure in which a guide is inserted under fluoroscopy near the area of the stone; an ultrasonic wave is aimed at the stone to break it into fragments.

3. Percutaneous lithotripsy may be performed via cystoscopy or nephroscopy.

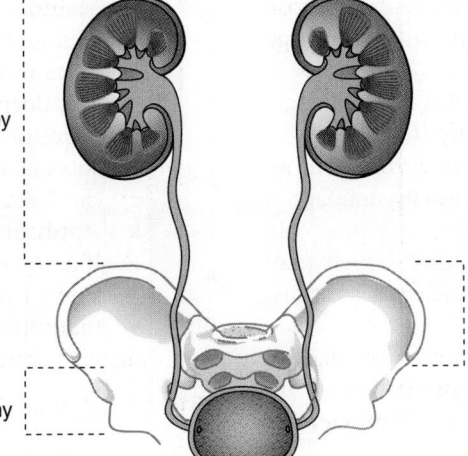

PROXIMAL URETER
• ESWL
• Retrograde ureteroscopy
• Antegrade nephrostoureterolithotomy
• Stenting alone
• Percutaneous ureterolithotomy or nephrolithotomy

DISTAL URETER
• ESWL/ureteroscopy
• Antegrade nephrostoureterolithotomy
• Stenting alone
• Open ureterolithotomy

MIDURETER
• Retrograde ureteroscopy
• ESWL
• Antegrade nephrostoureterolithotomy
• Open ureterolithotomy

▲ **FIGURE 62-6** Treatment options for ureteral stones. *ESWL,* extracorporeal shock wave lithotrips. (From Ignatavicius, D., & Workman, M. [2010]. *Medical-surgical nursing: Patient-centered collaborative care* [6th ed.]. St. Louis: Saunders.)

4. No incision is required for cystoscopy; a small flank incision is needed for nephroscopy.
5. The client might have an indwelling bladder catheter.
6. A nephrostomy tube may be placed to administer chemical irrigations to break up the stone; the nephrostomy tube may remain in place for 1 to 5 days.
7. Encourage the client to drink 3000 to 4000 mL of fluid/day following the procedure.
8. Monitor for and instruct the client to monitor for complications of infection, hemorrhage, and extravasation of fluid into the retroperitoneal cavity.

D. Ureterolithotomy
1. An open surgical procedure performed if lithotripsy is not effective for removal of a stone in the ureter
2. An incision is made through the lower abdomen or flank and then into the ureter to remove the stone.
3. The client may have a Penrose drain, ureteral stent catheter, and/or indwelling bladder catheter.

E. Pyelolithotomy and nephrolithotomy
1. Pyelolithotomy is an incision into the renal pelvis to remove a stone; a large flank incision is required and the client may have a Penrose drain and indwelling bladder catheter.
2. Nephrolithotomy is an incision into the kidney made to remove a stone; a large flank incision is required, and the client may have a nephrostomy tube and an indwelling bladder catheter.

F. Partial or total nephrectomy
1. Performed for extensive kidney damage, renal infection, severe obstruction from stones or tumors, and prevention of stone recurrence
2. Postoperative interventions
   a. The plan of care depends on the incision location and the type of drainage tubes present.
   b. Monitor the incision, particularly if a Penrose drain is in place, because it will drain large amounts of urine.
   c. Protect the skin from urinary drainage, changing dressings frequently if necessary.
   d. Place an ostomy pouch over the Penrose drain to protect the skin if urinary drainage is excessive.
   e. Monitor the nephrostomy tube, which may be attached to a drainage bag, for a continuous flow of urine.
   f. Do not irrigate the nephrostomy or bladder catheters unless specifically prescribed.
   g. Monitor the indwelling bladder catheter for drainage.
   h. Encourage fluid intake to ensure a urine output of 2500 to 3000 mL/day or more.
   i. Measure intake and output accurately.

j. If a stone was removed, determine its composition from laboratory analysis.

XXIV. KIDNEY TUMORS

A. Description
1. Kidney tumors may be benign or malignant, bilateral or unilateral.
2. Common sites of metastasis of malignant tumors include bone, lungs, liver, spleen, and other kidney.
3. The exact cause of renal carcinoma is unknown.

B. Assessment
1. Dull flank pain
2. Palpable renal mass
3. Painless gross hematuria

C. Radical nephrectomy
1. Description
   a. Surgical removal of the entire kidney, adjacent adrenal gland, and renal artery and vein.
   b. Radiation therapy and possibly chemotherapy may follow radical nephrectomy.
   c. Before surgery, radiation may be used to embolize (occlude) the arteries supplying the kidney to reduce bleeding during nephrectomy.
2. Postoperative interventions
   a. Monitor vital signs for signs of bleeding (hypotension and tachycardia).
   b. Monitor for abdominal distention, decreases in urinary output, and alterations in level of consciousness as signs of bleeding; check the bed linens under the client for bleeding.
   c. Monitor for signs of adrenal insufficiency, which include a large urinary output followed by hypotension and subsequent **oliguria**.
   d. Administer fluids and packed red blood cells intravenously as prescribed.
   e. Monitor intake and output and daily weight.
   f. Monitor for a urinary output of 30 to 50 mL/hr to ensure adequate renal function.
   g. Monitor urine specific gravity.
   h. Maintain the client in a semi-Fowler's position.
   i. Monitor for signs of respiratory complications related to surgery; encourage coughing and deep-breathing exercises.
   j. Monitor for passing of flatus and bowel sounds (lack of flatus and bowel sounds can be indicative of paralytic ileus).
   k. Apply antiembolism stockings as prescribed.
   l. If a nephrostomy tube is in place, do not irrigate (unless specifically prescribed) or manipulate the tube.
   m. Administer pain medications as prescribed.

XXV. EPIDIDYMITIS

A. Description
1. Acute or chronic inflammation of the epididymis that occurs as a result of a UTI, STI, prostatitis, or long-term use of a bladder catheter

2. The infective organism travels upward through the urethra and ejaculatory duct and along the vas deferens to the epididymis.

B. Assessment
   1. Scrotal pain
   2. Groin pain
   3. Swelling in the scrotum and groin
   4. Pus and bacteria in the urine
   5. Fever and chills
   6. Abscess development

C. Interventions
   1. Encourage fluid intake.
   2. Encourage bed rest with the scrotum elevated to prevent traction on the spermatic cord, facilitate drainage, and relieve pain.
   3. Instruct the client in the intermittent application of cold compresses to the scrotum.
   4. Instruct the client in the use of tub or sitz baths.
   5. Instruct the client in the administration of antibiotics for self and sexual partner if the cause is chlamydial or gonorrheal infection.
   6. Instruct the client to avoid lifting, straining, and sexual contact until the infection subsides.
   7. Instruct the client to limit the force of the stream because organisms can be forced into the vas deferens and epididymis from strain or pressure during voiding.
   8. Teach the client that condom use can help prevent urethritis and epididymitis.
   9. Teach the client measures to prevent UTI or STI recurrence.

XXVI. PROSTATITIS

A. Description
   1. Inflammation of the prostate gland commonly caused by an infectious agent; may be acute or chronic.
   2. The bacterial type occurs as a result of the organism reaching the prostate via the urethra, bladder, bloodstream, or lymphatic channels.
   3. The abacterial type usually occurs following a viral illness or a decrease in sexual activity.

B. Assessment
   1. Bacterial prostatitis
      a. Client becomes acutely ill
      b. Fever and chills
      c. Frequency and urgency of urination; dysuria
      d. Perineal and low back pain
      e. Urethral discharge
      f. Prostate is tender, indurated, and warm to the touch.
      g. Urethral discharge on palpation of prostate
      h. White blood cells are found in prostatic secretions.
      i. Urine culture is usually positive for gram negative bacteria, especially after prostate massage.

   2. Abacterial prostatitis (most common form of chronic prostatitis)
      a. Backache
      b. Dysuria
      c. Perineal pain
      d. Frequency
      e. Hematuria
      f. Irregularly enlarged, firm, and tender prostate

C. Interventions
   1. Encourage adequate fluid intake.
   2. Instruct the client in the use of tub or sitz baths to promote comfort.
   3. Administer antibiotics, analgesics, antispasmodics, and stool softeners as prescribed.
   4. Inform the client of activities to drain the prostate, such as intercourse, masturbation, and prostatic massage.
   5. Instruct the client to avoid spicy foods, coffee, alcohol, prolonged automobile rides, and sexual intercourse during an acute inflammation.

XXVII. BENIGN PROSTATIC HYPERTROPHY (HYPERPLASIA)

A. Description
   1. Benign prostatic hypertrophy (benign prostatic hyperplasia; BPH) is a slow enlargement of the prostate gland, with hypertrophy and hyperplasia of normal tissue.
   2. Enlargement compresses the urethra, resulting in partial or complete obstruction.
   3. Usually occurs in men older than 50 years

B. Assessment
   1. Diminished size and force of urinary stream (early sign of BPH)
   2. Urinary urgency and frequency
   3. Nocturia
   4. Inability to start (hesitancy) or continue a urinary stream
   5. Feelings of incomplete bladder emptying
   6. Postvoid dribbling from overflow incontinence (later sign)
   7. Urinary retention and bladder distention
   8. Hematuria
   9. Urinary stasis
   10. Dysuria and bladder pain
   11. UTIs

C. Interventions
   1. Encourage fluid intake of up to 2000 to 3000 mL/day unless contraindicated.
   2. Prepare for urinary catheterization to drain the bladder and prevent distention.
   3. Avoid administering medications that cause urinary retention, such as anticholinergics, antihistamines, decongestants, and antidepressants.

Box 62-17 Surgical and Invasive Procedures for Prostatic Hyperplasia

Laser prostatectomy: Ablation of the enlarged prostate using laser instead of radiofrequency waves.

Perineal prostatectomy: Removal of prostatic tissue (may be performed for prostatic cancer) low in the pelvic region through an incision between the scrotum and rectum; impotence and incontinence usually result.

Retropubic prostatectomy: Removal of hypertrophied prostatic tissue high in the pelvic region through a low abdominal incision; the bladder is not incised.

Suprapubic prostatectomy: Removal of prostatic tissue mass through a low midline incision; an incision is made into the bladder and urethral mucosa to the anterior aspect of the prostate.

Transurethral electrovaporization of the prostate: Placement of a special metal instrument that emits a high-frequency electrical current that cuts and vaporizes excess tissue and seals the remaining tissue to prevent bleeding; this is especially useful for men on anticoagulants and those at risk for complications.

Transurethral incision of the prostate (TUIP): Removal of prostatic tissue through an incision made in the bladder neck.

Transurethral microwave thermotherapy: Application of heat to destroy the hypertrophied tissue.

Transurethral needle ablation of the prostate (TUNA): Placement of interstitial radiofrequency needles through the urethra and into the lateral lobes of the prostate, causing heat-induced coagulation necrosis of the prostate for treating benign prostatic hypertrophy (BPH).

Transurethral resection of the prostate (TURP): Removal of benign prostatic tissue surrounding the urethra with use of a resectoscope introduced through the urethra; there is little risk of impotence and it is most commonly used for BPH.

Urethral stents: Application of stents or coils in the urethra where it is narrowed by the prostate.

4. Administer medications as prescribed to shrink the prostate gland and improve urine flow.

5. Administer medications as prescribed to relax prostatic smooth muscle and improve urine flow.

6. Instruct the client to decrease intake of caffeine and artificial sweeteners and limit spicy or acidic foods.

7. Instruct the client to follow a timed voiding schedule.

8. Prepare the client for surgery or invasive procedures as prescribed (Box 62-17; Figs. 62-7 and 62-8).

D. Surgical interventions and postoperative care (see Chapter 52)

XXVIII. BLADDER TRAUMA

A. Description
1. Occurs following a blunt or penetrating injury to the lower abdomen
2. Blunt trauma causes compression of the abdominal wall and bladder.
3. Penetrating wounds occur as a result of a stabbing, gunshot wound, or other objects piercing the abdominal wall.
4. A fractured pelvis that causes bone fragments to puncture the bladder is a common cause of bladder trauma.

B. Assessment
1. **Anuria**
2. Hematuria
3. Pain below the level of the umbilicus; can radiate to the shoulders
4. Nausea and vomiting

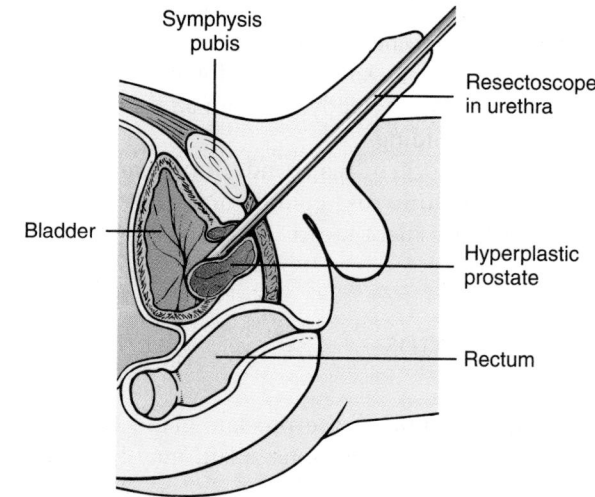

▲ **FIGURE 62-7** Transurethral resection of the prostate. (From Lewis, S., Heitkemper, M., Dirksen, S., O'Brien, P., & Bucher, L. [2007]. *Medical-surgical nursing: Assessment and management of clinical problems* [7th ed.]. St. Louis: Mosby.)

C. Interventions
1. Monitor vital signs.
2. Monitor for hematuria, bleeding, and signs of shock.
3. Promote bed rest.
4. Monitor pain level.
5. If blood is seen at the meatus, avoid urinary catheterization until a retrograde ureterogram can be obtained.
6. Prepare the client for insertion of a suprapubic catheter to aid in urinary drainage if prescribed.
7. Prepare the client for surgical repair of the laceration if indicated.

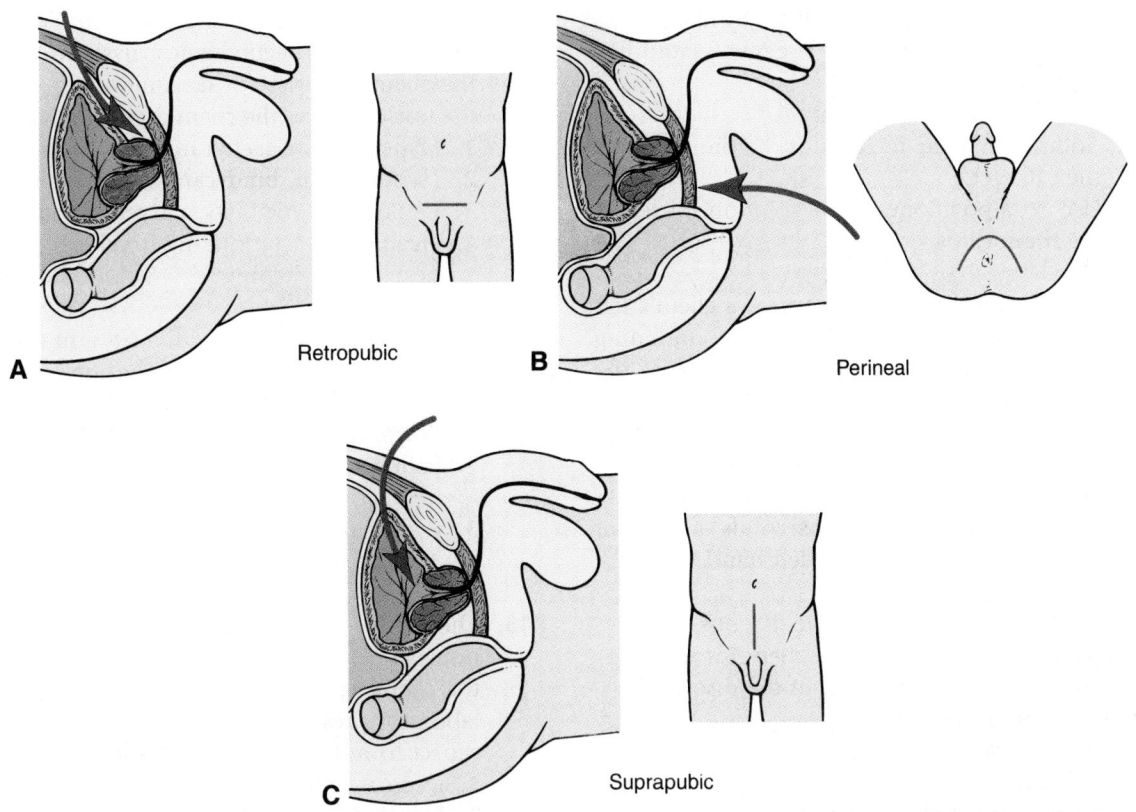

▲ FIGURE 62-8 Surgical approaches for prostatectomy. **A,** Retropubic approach involves a low abdominal incision. **B,** Perineal approach involves an incision between the scrotum and anus. **C,** Suprapubic approach involves a midline abdominal incision. (From Lewis, S., Heitkemper, M., Dirksen, S., O'Brien, P., & Bucher, L. [2007]. *Medical-surgical nursing: Assessment and management of clinical problems* [7th ed.]. St. Louis: Mosby.)

MORE QUESTIONS ON THE CD!

Practice Questions

733. The client with acute renal failure has a serum potassium level of 6.0 mEq/L. The nurse would plan which of the following as a priority action?
1. Check the sodium level.
2. Place the client on a cardiac monitor.
3. Encourage increased vegetables in the diet.
4. Allow an extra 500 mL of fluid intake to dilute the electrolyte concentration.

734. The client being hemodialyzed suddenly becomes short of breath and complains of chest pain. The client is tachycardic, pale, and anxious. The nurse suspects air embolism. The priority action for the nurse is to:
1. Discontinue dialysis and notify the physician.
2. Monitor vital signs every 15 minutes for the next hour.
3. Continue dialysis at a slower rate after checking the lines for air.
4. Bolus the client with 500 mL of normal saline to break up the air embolus.

735. The client arrives at the emergency department with complaints of low abdominal pain and hematuria. The client is afebrile. The nurse next assesses the client to determine a history of:
1. Pyelonephritis
2. Glomerulonephritis
3. Trauma to the bladder or abdomen
4. Renal cancer in the client's family

736. The client is admitted to the emergency department following a motor vehicle accident. The client was wearing a lap seat belt when the accident occurred and now the client has hematuria and lower abdominal pain. To assess further whether the pain is caused by bladder trauma, the nurse asks the client if the pain is referred to which of the following areas?
1. Hip
2. Shoulder
3. Umbilicus
4. Costovertebral angle

737. The female client is admitted to the emergency department following a fall from a horse and the physician prescribes insertion of a Foley catheter.

While preparing for the procedure, the nurse notes blood at the urinary meatus. The nurse should:
1. Notify the physician.
2. Use a small-sized catheter.
3. Administer pain medication before inserting the catheter.
4. Use extra povidone-iodine solution in cleansing the meatus.

738. A nurse is assessing the patency of a client's left arm arteriovenous fistula prior to initiating hemodialysis. Which finding indicates that the fistula is patent?
1. Palpation of a thrill over the fistula
2. Presence of a radial pulse in the left wrist
3. Absence of a bruit on auscultation of the fistula
4. Capillary refill less than 3 seconds in the nail beds of the fingers on the left hand

739. The male client has a tentative diagnosis of urethritis. The nurse assesses the client for which of the following manifestations of the disorder?
1. Hematuria and pyuria
2. Dysuria and proteinuria
3. Hematuria and urgency
4. Dysuria and penile discharge

740. The nurse is assessing the client with epididymitis. The nurse anticipates which of the following findings on physical examination?
1. Fever, diarrhea, groin pain, and ecchymosis
2. Nausea, vomiting, scrotal edema, and ecchymosis
3. Fever, nausea, vomiting, and painful scrotal edema
4. Diarrhea, groin pain, testicular torsion, and scrotal edema

741. The client complains of fever, perineal pain, and urinary urgency, frequency, and dysuria. To assess whether the client's problem is related to bacterial prostatitis, the nurse would look at the results of the prostate examination, which should reveal that the prostate gland is:
1. Soft and swollen
2. Reddened, swollen, and boggy
3. Tender and edematous with ecchymosis
4. Tender, indurated, and warm to the touch

742. The nurse is taking the history of a client who has had benign prostatic hyperplasia in the past. To determine whether the client currently is experiencing difficulty, the nurse asks the client about the presence of which early symptom?
1. Nocturia
2. Urinary retention
3. Urge incontinence
4. Decreased force in the stream of urine

743. The client newly diagnosed with chronic renal failure recently has begun hemodialysis. Knowing that the client is at risk for disequilibrium syndrome, the nurse assesses the client during dialysis for:
1. Hypertension, tachycardia, and fever
2. Hypotension, bradycardia, and hypothermia
3. Restlessness, irritability, and generalized weakness
4. Headache, deteriorating level of consciousness, and twitching

744. The hemodialysis client with a left arm fistula is at risk for arterial steal syndrome. The nurse assesses this client for which of the following manifestations?
1. Warmth, redness, and pain in the left hand
2. Pallor, diminished pulse, and pain in the left hand
3. Edema and reddish discoloration of the left arm
4. Aching pain, pallor, and edema of the left arm

745. The nurse is reviewing the client's record and notes that the physician has documented that the client has a renal disorder. On review of the laboratory results, the nurse most likely would expect to note which of the following?
1. Decreased hemoglobin level
2. Elevated creatinine level
3. Decreased red blood cell count
4. Decreased white blood cell count

746. The client with chronic renal failure returns to the nursing unit following a hemodialysis treatment. On assessment, the nurse notes that the client's temperature is 100.2° F. Which of the following is the appropriate nursing action?
1. Encourage fluids.
2. Notify the physician.
3. Continue to monitor vital signs.
4. Monitor the site of the shunt for infection.

747. The nurse is performing an assessment on a client who has returned from the dialysis unit following hemodialysis. The client is complaining of headache and nausea and is extremely restless. Which of the following is the most appropriate nursing action?
1. Monitor the client.
2. Notify the physician.
3. Elevate the head of the bed.
4. Medicate the client for nausea.

748. A client newly diagnosed with renal failure has just been started on peritoneal dialysis. During the infusion of the dialysate, the client complains of abdominal pain. Which action by the nurse is appropriate?
1. Stop the dialysis.
2. Slow the infusion.

3. Decrease the amount to be infused.
4. Explain that the pain will subside after the first few exchanges.

749. The nurse is instructing a client with diabetes mellitus about peritoneal dialysis. The nurse tells the client that it is important to maintain the prescribed dwell time for the dialysis because of the risk of:
1. Infection
2. Hyperglycemia
3. Hypophosphatemia
4. Disequilibrium syndrome

750. A week after kidney transplantation, the client develops a temperature of 101° F, the blood pressure is elevated, and the kidney is tender. The x-ray indicates that the transplanted kidney is enlarged. Based on these assessment findings, the nurse would suspect which of the following complications?
1. Acute rejection
2. Kidney infection
3. Chronic rejection
4. Kidney obstruction

751. The client is admitted to the hospital with a diagnosis of benign prostatic hyperplasia, and a transurethral resection of the prostate is performed. Four hours after surgery, the nurse takes the client's vital signs and empties the urinary drainage bag. Which of the following assessment findings would indicate the need to notify the physician?
1. Red bloody urine
2. Pain related to bladder spasms
3. Urinary output of 200 mL higher than intake
4. Blood pressure, 100/50 mm Hg; pulse, 130 beats/min

Alternate Item Format: Multiple Response

752. The nurse monitoring a client receiving peritoneal dialysis notes that the client's outflow is less than the inflow. Which nursing actions should the nurse take? **Select all that apply.**
❏ 1. Contact the physician.
❏ 2. Check the level of the drainage bag.
❏ 3. Reposition the client to his or her side.
❏ 4. Place the client in good body alignment.
❏ 5. Check the peritoneal dialysis system for kinks.
❏ 6. Increase the flow rate of the peritoneal dialysis solution.

ANSWERS

733. 2

Rationale: The client with hyperkalemia is at risk of developing cardiac dysrhythmias and cardiac arrest. Because of this, the client should be placed on a cardiac monitor. Fluid intake is not increased because it contributes to fluid overload and would not affect the serum potassium level significantly. Vegetables are a natural source of potassium in the diet, and their use would not be increased. The nurse also may assess the sodium level because sodium is another electrolyte commonly measured with the potassium level. However, this is not a priority action of the nurse.

Test-Taking Strategy: First, note that the potassium level is elevated. Next, use the ABCs—airway, breathing, and circulation—to direct you to option 2. Review care of the client with hyperkalemia if you had difficulty with this question.

Level of Cognitive Ability: Applying
Client Needs: Physiological Integrity
Integrated Process: Nursing Process—Planning
Content Area: Adult Health—Renal
Reference: Ignatavicius, D., & Workman, M. (2010). *Medical-surgical nursing: Patient-centered collaborative care* (6th ed., pp. 191, 1610). St. Louis: Saunders.

734. 1

Rationale: If the client experiences air embolus during hemodialysis, the nurse should terminate dialysis immediately, notify the physician, and administer oxygen as needed. Options 2, 3, and 4 are incorrect.

Test-Taking Strategy: Use the process of elimination. Recalling that air embolism is an emergency situation that affects the cardiopulmonary system suddenly and profoundly will direct you to option 1. Review the emergency care of a client who develops air embolism if you had difficulty with this question.

Level of Cognitive Ability: Applying
Client Needs: Physiological Integrity
Integrated Process: Nursing Process—Implementation
Content Area: Adult Health—Renal
References: Black, J., & Hawks, J. (2009). *Medical-surgical nursing: Clinical management for positive outcomes* (8th ed., p. 828). St. Louis: Saunders.

Swearingen, P. (2008). *All-in-one care planning resource: Medical-surgical, pediatric, maternity, & psychiatric nursing care plans* (2nd ed., p. 225). St. Louis: Mosby.

735. 3

Rationale: Bladder trauma or injury should be considered or suspected in the client with low abdominal pain and hematuria. Glomerulonephritis and pyelonephritis would be accompanied by fever and are thus not applicable to the client described in this question. Renal cancer would not cause pain that is felt in the low abdomen; rather pain would be in the flank area.

Test-Taking Strategy: Use the process of elimination. Eliminate options 1 and 2, knowing that any inflammatory disease or infection is accompanied by fever. Because this client is afebrile, these are not possible options. Use knowledge of

anatomy and pain assessment to select option 3. Pain from renal cancer is a later finding and is localized in the flank area. Review renal assessment techniques and findings if you had difficulty with this question.
Level of Cognitive Ability: Analyzing
Client Needs: Physiological Integrity
Integrated Process: Nursing Process—Assessment
Content Area: Adult Health—Renal
Reference: Ignatavicius, D., & Workman, M. (2010). *Medical-surgical nursing: Patient-centered collaborative care* (6th ed., p. 1578). St. Louis: Saunders.

736. 2

Rationale: Bladder trauma or injury is characterized by lower abdominal pain that may radiate to one of the shoulders due to phrenic nerve irritation. Bladder injury pain does not radiate to the umbilicus, costovertebral angle, or hip.
Test-Taking Strategy: Use the process of elimination. Recalling the concepts related to dermatomes of the body and pain characteristics of bladder trauma will direct you to option 2. Review the characteristics of bladder trauma if you had difficulty with this question.
Level of Cognitive Ability: Applying
Client Needs: Physiological Integrity
Integrated Process: Nursing Process—Assessment
Content Area: Adult Health—Renal
References: Black, J., & Hawks, J. (2009). *Medical-surgical nursing: Clinical management for positive outcomes* (8th ed., p. 774). St. Louis: Saunders.

Ignatavicius, D., & Workman, M. (2010). *Medical-surgical nursing: Patient-centered collaborative care* (6th ed., p. 1578). St. Louis: Saunders.

737. 1

Rationale: The presence of blood at the urinary meatus may indicate urethral trauma or disruption. The nurse notifies the physician, knowing that the client should not be catheterized until the cause of the bleeding is determined by diagnostic testing. Therefore options 2, 3, and 4 are incorrect.
Test-Taking Strategy: Use the process of elimination. Noting the strategic words *blood at the urinary meatus* will direct you to option 1. Review the assessment findings in a client with trauma to the urinary tract if you had difficulty with this question.
Level of Cognitive Ability: Applying
Client Needs: Physiological Integrity
Integrated Process: Nursing Process—Implementation
Content Area: Adult Health—Renal
Reference: Black, J., & Hawks, J. (2009). *Medical-surgical nursing: Clinical management for positive outcomes* (8th ed., pp. 775–776). St. Louis: Saunders.

738. 1

Rationale: The nurse assesses the patency of the fistula by palpating for the presence of a thrill or auscultating for a bruit. The presence of a thrill and bruit indicate patency of the fistula. Although the presence of a radial pulse in the left wrist and capillary refill shorter than 3 seconds in the nail beds of the fingers on the left hand are normal findings, they do not assess fistula patency.
Test-Taking Strategy: Use the process of elimination. Eliminate options 2 and 4 first because they are comparable or alike and assess for adequate circulation in the distal portion of the extremity (not the fistula). From the remaining options, focusing on the subject (patency) and noting the word *absence* in option 3 will assist you in eliminating this option. Review the expected findings when assessing an arteriovenous fistula if you had difficulty with this question.
Level of Cognitive Ability: Analyzing
Client Needs: Physiological Integrity
Integrated Process: Nursing Process—Assessment
Content Area: Adult Health—Renal
References: Ignatavicius, D., & Workman, M. (2010). *Medical-surgical nursing: Patient-centered collaborative care* (6th ed., pp. 1623, 1625). St. Louis: Saunders.

Swearingen, P. (2008). *All-in-one care planning resource: Medical-surgical, pediatric, maternity, & psychiatric nursing care plans* (2nd ed., p. 226). St. Louis: Mosby.

739. 4

Rationale: Urethritis in the male client often results from chlamydial infection and is characterized by dysuria, which is accompanied by a clear to mucopurulent discharge. Because this disorder often coexists with gonorrhea, diagnostic tests are done for both and include culture and rapid assays.
Test-Taking Strategy: Use the process of elimination. Recalling that urethritis generally is accompanied by dysuria in the male client will assist you in eliminating options 1 and 3. Knowing that the problem originates in the urethra, not the kidney, will assist you in eliminating option 2, because proteinuria indicates a problem with kidney function. Review the clinical manifestations of urethritis if you had difficulty with this question.
Level of Cognitive Ability: Applying
Client Needs: Physiological Integrity
Integrated Process: Nursing Process—Assessment
Content Area: Adult Health—Renal
Reference: Ignatavicius, D., & Workman, M. (2010). *Medical-surgical nursing: Patient-centered collaborative care* (6th ed., p. 1747). St. Louis: Saunders.

740. 3

Rationale: Typical signs and symptoms of epididymitis include scrotal pain and edema, which often are accompanied by fever, nausea and vomiting, and chills. Epididymitis most often is caused by infection, although sometimes it can be caused by trauma. Epididymitis needs to be distinguished correctly from testicular torsion.
Test-Taking Strategy: Use the process of elimination. Any disorder that ends in *-itis* results from inflammation or infection. Therefore an expected finding would be elevated temperature. With this in mind, eliminate options 2 and 4 because they do not contain fever as part of the option. Knowing that ecchymosis results from bleeding, which is not part of this clinical picture, directs you to option 3. Review the clinical manifestations of epididymitis if you had difficulty with this question.
Level of Cognitive Ability: Analyzing
Client Needs: Physiological Integrity
Integrated Process: Nursing Process—Assessment
Content Area: Adult Health—Renal
Reference: Copstead, L., & Banasik, J. (2010). *Pathophysiology* (4th ed., p. 745). St. Louis: Mosby.

741. 4
Rationale: The client with prostatitis has a swollen and tender prostate gland that is also warm to the touch, firm, and indurated. Systemic symptoms include fever with chills, perineal and low back pain, and signs of urinary tract infection, which often accompany the disorder.
Test-Taking Strategy: Use the process of elimination. Begin to answer this question by reasoning that inflammation of the prostate gland would cause the area to be tender. This would allow you to eliminate options 1 and 2. Recalling that inflammation is accompanied by local warmth will direct you to option 4. Review the signs of prostatitis if you had difficulty with this question.
Level of Cognitive Ability: Analyzing
Client Needs: Physiological Integrity
Integrated Process: Nursing Process—Assessment
Content Area: Adult Health—Renal
Reference: Ignatavicius, D., & Workman, M. (2010). *Medical-surgical nursing: Patient-centered collaborative care* (6th ed., p. 1733). St. Louis: Saunders.

742. 4
Rationale: Decreased force in the stream of urine is an early sign of benign prostatic hyperplasia. The stream later becomes weak and dribbling. The client then may develop hematuria, frequency, urgency, urge incontinence, and nocturia. If untreated, complete obstruction and urinary retention can occur.
Test-Taking Strategy: Use the process of elimination and note the strategic word *early*. If you know that benign prostatic hyperplasia can lead to urinary obstruction, look for the option that identifies the least severe symptom. Review early signs of benign prostatic hyperplasia if you had difficulty with this question.
Level of Cognitive Ability: Applying
Client Needs: Physiological Integrity
Integrated Process: Nursing Process—Assessment
Content Area: Adult Health—Renal
Reference: Black, J., & Hawks, J. (2009). *Medical-surgical nursing: Clinical management for positive outcomes* (8th ed., p. 876). St. Louis: Saunders.

743. 4
Rationale: Disequilibrium syndrome is characterized by headache, mental confusion, decreasing level of consciousness, nausea, vomiting, twitching, and possible seizure activity. Disequilibrium syndrome is caused by rapid removal of solutes from the body during hemodialysis. At the same time, the blood-brain barrier interferes with the efficient removal of wastes from brain tissue. As a result, water goes into cerebral cells because of the osmotic gradient, causing increased intracranial pressure and onset of symptoms. The syndrome most often occurs in clients who are new to dialysis and is prevented by dialyzing for shorter times or at reduced blood flow rates.
Test-Taking Strategy: Use the process of elimination. Focus on the name, disequilibrium syndrome, to assist in directing you to option 4. Review the manifestations of this syndrome if you had difficulty with this question.
Level of Cognitive Ability: Applying
Client Needs: Physiological Integrity
Integrated Process: Nursing Process—Assessment
Content Area: Adult Health—Renal

Reference: Black, J., & Hawks, J. (2009). *Medical-surgical nursing: Clinical management for positive outcomes* (8th ed., p. 828). St. Louis: Saunders.

744. 2
Rationale: Steal syndrome results from vascular insufficiency after creation of a fistula. The client exhibits pallor and a diminished pulse distal to the fistula. The client also complains of pain distal to the fistula, caused by tissue ischemia. Warmth and redness probably would characterize a problem with infection. The manifestations described in options 3 and 4 are incorrect.
Test-Taking Strategy: You must understand steal syndrome and know the signs and symptoms to answer this question. Recalling that steal syndrome results from vascular insufficiency after creation of a fistula will direct you to option 2. Review this syndrome and associated signs and symptoms if you had difficulty with this question.
Level of Cognitive Ability: Applying
Client Needs: Physiological Integrity
Integrated Process: Nursing Process—Assessment
Content Area: Adult Health—Renal
References: Ignatavicius, D., & Workman, M. (2010). *Medical-surgical nursing: Patient-centered collaborative care* (6th ed., p. 1623). St. Louis: Saunders.
Swearingen, P. (2008). *All-in-one care planning resource: Medical-surgical, pediatric, maternity, & psychiatric nursing care plans* (2nd ed., p. 225). St. Louis: Mosby.

745. 2
Rationale: Measuring the creatinine level is a frequently used laboratory test to determine renal function. The creatinine level increases when at least 50% of renal function is lost. A decreased hemoglobin level and red blood cell count may be noted if bleeding from the urinary tract occurs or if erythropoietic function by the kidney is impaired. An increased white blood cell count is most likely to be noted in renal disease.
Test-Taking Strategy: Use the process of elimination. Recalling the relationship between the creatinine level and renal function will direct you to option 2. Review significant laboratory tests related to renal function if you had difficulty with this question.
Level of Cognitive Ability: Analyzing
Client Needs: Physiological Integrity
Integrated Process: Nursing Process—Assessment
Content Area: Adult Health—Renal
Reference: Ignatavicius, D., & Workman, M. (2010). *Medical-surgical nursing: Patient-centered collaborative care* (6th ed., p. 1604). St. Louis: Saunders.

746. 3
Rationale: The client may have an elevated temperature following dialysis because the dialysis machine warms the blood slightly. If the temperature is elevated excessively and remains elevated, sepsis would be suspected and a blood sample would be obtained as prescribed for culture and sensitivity determinations.
Test-Taking Strategy: Use the process of elimination and focus on the data in the question. Recalling that an elevation in temperature is expected following dialysis will direct you to

option 3. Review the normal expected findings following dialysis if you had difficulty with this question.
Level of Cognitive Ability: Applying
Client Needs: Physiological Integrity
Integrated Process: Nursing Process—Implementation
Content Area: Adult Health—Renal
Reference: Ignatavicius, D., & Workman, M. (2010). *Medical-surgical nursing: Patient-centered collaborative care* (6th ed., pp. 1621, 1625–1626). St. Louis: Saunders.

747. 2
Rationale: Disequilibrium syndrome may be caused by the rapid decreases in the blood urea nitrogen level during hemodialysis. These changes can cause cerebral edema that leads to increased intracranial pressure. The client is exhibiting early signs of disequilibrium syndrome and appropriate treatments with anticonvulsive medications and barbiturates may be necessary to prevent a life-threatening situation. The physician must be notified.
Test-Taking Strategy: Use the process of elimination and focus on the client's signs and symptoms. Recalling the complications associated with hemodialysis will direct you to option 2. Review the signs and symptoms of disequilibrium syndrome if you had difficulty with this question.
Level of Cognitive Ability: Applying
Client Needs: Physiological Integrity
Integrated Process: Nursing Process—Implementation
Content Area: Adult Health—Renal
Reference: Black, J., & Hawks, J. (2009). *Medical-surgical nursing: Clinical management for positive outcomes* (8th ed., p. 828). St. Louis: Saunders.

748. 4
Rationale: Pain during the inflow of dialysate is common during the first few exchanges because of peritoneal irritation; however, the pain usually disappears after 1 to 2 weeks of treatment. The infusion amount should not be decreased, and the infusion should not be slowed or stopped.
Test-Taking Strategy: Use the process of elimination. Eliminate options 1, 2, and 3 because they are comparable or alike actions. Review the complications associated with peritoneal dialysis and the appropriate nursing actions if you had difficulty with this question.
Level of Cognitive Ability: Applying
Client Needs: Physiological Integrity
Integrated Process: Nursing Process—Implementation
Content Area: Adult Health—Renal
Reference: Ignatavicius, D., & Workman, M. (2010). *Medical-surgical nursing: Patient-centered collaborative care* (6th ed., p. 1629). St. Louis: Saunders.

749. 2
Rationale: An extended dwell time increases the risk of hyperglycemia in the client with diabetes mellitus as a result of absorption of glucose from the dialysate and electrolyte changes. Diabetic clients may require extra insulin when receiving peritoneal dialysis.
Test-Taking Strategy: Use the process of elimination. Noting the client's diagnosis and recalling that the dialysate solution contains glucose will direct you to option 2. Review the

complications associated with peritoneal dialysis if you had difficulty with this question.
Level of Cognitive Ability: Understanding
Client Needs: Physiological Integrity
Integrated Process: Teaching and Learning
Content Area: Adult Health—Renal
Reference: Black, J., & Hawks, J. (2009). *Medical-surgical nursing: Clinical management for positive outcomes* (8th ed., p. 823). St. Louis: Saunders.

750. 1
Rationale: Acute rejection most often occurs in the first 2 weeks after transplantation. Clinical manifestations include fever, malaise, elevated white blood cell count, acute hypertension, graft tenderness, and manifestations of deteriorating renal function. Chronic rejection occurs gradually over a period of months to years. Although kidney infection or obstruction can occur, the symptoms presented in the question do not relate specifically to these disorders.
Test-Taking Strategy: Use the process of elimination and note the strategic words *a week after kidney transplantation*. These words should direct you easily to option 1, *acute rejection*. Review the signs of acute rejection if you had difficulty with this question.
Level of Cognitive Ability: Analyzing
Client Needs: Physiological Integrity
Integrated Process: Nursing Process—Analysis
Content Area: Adult Health—Renal
References: Ignatavicius, D., & Workman, M. (2010). *Medical-surgical nursing: Patient-centered collaborative care* (6th ed., pp. 1632–1633). St. Louis: Saunders.
Swearingen, P. (2008). *All-in-one care planning resource: Medical-surgical, pediatric, maternity, & psychiatric nursing care plans* (2nd ed., p. 239). St. Louis: Mosby.

751. 4
Rationale: Frank bleeding (arterial or venous) may occur during the first day after surgery. Some hematuria is usual for several days after surgery. A urinary output of 200 mL more than intake is adequate. Bladder spasms are expected to occur following surgery. A rapid pulse with a low blood pressure is a potential sign of excessive blood loss. The physician should be notified.
Test-Taking Strategy: Use the process of elimination and focus on the subject, need to notify the physician. Think about the expected findings following this procedure and note that the vital signs presented in option 4 indicate excessive blood loss. Review the expected findings following transurethral resection of the prostate if you had difficulty with this question.
Level of Cognitive Ability: Analyzing
Client Needs: Physiological Integrity
Integrated Process: Nursing Process—Analysis
Content Area: Adult Health—Renal
References: Black, J., & Hawks, J. (2009). *Medical-surgical nursing: Clinical management for positive outcomes* (8th ed., p. 882). St. Louis: Saunders.
Ignatavicius, D., & Workman, M. (2010). *Medical-surgical nursing: Patient-centered collaborative care* (6th ed., p. 1718). St. Louis: Saunders.

ALTERNATE ITEM FORMAT: MULTIPLE RESPONSE
752. 2, 3, 4, 5
Rationale: If outflow drainage is inadequate, the nurse attempts to stimulate outflow by changing the client's position. Turning the client to the other side or making sure that the client is in good body alignment may assist with outflow drainage. The drainage bag needs to be lower than the client's abdomen to enhance gravity drainage. The connecting tubing and peritoneal dialysis system are also checked for kinks or twisting and the clamps on the system are checked to ensure that they are open. There is no reason to contact the physician. Increasing the flow rate is an inappropriate action and is not associated with the amount of outflow solution.

Test-Taking Strategy: Use the principles related to gravity flow and preventing obstruction to flow to answer this question. This will assist in determining the correct interventions. Review the nursing interventions related to insufficient flow of dialysate if you had difficulty with this question.
Level of Cognitive Ability: Applying
Client Needs: Physiological Integrity
Integrated Process: Nursing Process—Implementation
Content Area: Adult Health—Renal
Reference: Ignatavicius, D., & Workman, M. (2010). *Medical-surgical nursing: Patient-centered collaborative care* (6th ed., p. 1630). St. Louis: Saunders.

63

Renal Medications

I. URINARY TRACT ANTISEPTICS

A. Description
1. Urinary tract antiseptics inhibit the growth of bacteria in the urine (Fig. 63-1; Box 63-1).
2. Act as disinfectants within the urinary tract
3. Used to treat acute cystitis or urinary tract infections (UTIs)
4. Urinary tract antiseptics do not achieve effective antibacterial concentrations in blood or tissues and therefore cannot be used for infections outside the urinary tract.

B. Side effects and nursing considerations
1. Cinoxacin (Cinobac)
   a. Side effects are similar to those of nalidixic acid.
   b. Dosage should be reduced in clients with renal impairment; failure to do so could result in accumulation of the medication to toxic levels.
2. Methenamine (Mandelamine, Hiprex, Urex)
   a. Used to treat chronic UTIs, but not recommended for acute infections
   b. Administer after meals and at bedtime to minimize gastric distress.
   c. Chronic high-dose therapy can cause bladder irritation.
   d. Methenamine can cause crystalluria and should not be used in clients with renal impairment.
   e. Decomposition of the medication generates ammonia; therefore, it should not be used for clients with liver dysfunction.
   f. Methenamine requires acidic urine with a pH of 5.5 or lower.
   g. Increasing fluid intake reduces antibacterial effects by diluting the medication and raising urine pH.
   h. Methenamine should not be combined with sulfonamides because of the risk of crystalluria and urinary tract injury.
   i. Clients taking this medication should avoid alkalinizing agents, including over-the-counter antacids containing sodium bicarbonate or sodium carbonate.

3. Nalidixic acid (NegGram)
   a. Gastrointestinal side effects include anorexia, nausea, vomiting, and diarrhea.
   b. Integumentary side effects include rash and photosensitivity.
   c. Central nervous system (CNS) side effects include visual disturbances and insomnia.
   d. Nalidixic acid may produce intracranial hypertension in pediatric clients and should not be administered to children younger than 3 months.
   e. When nalidixic acid is used for more than 2 weeks, complete blood cell counts and liver function tests should be performed.
   f. Nalidixic acid can intensify the effects of orally administered anticoagulants.
   g. Nalidixic acid is contraindicated in clients with a history of convulsive disorders.
4. Nitrofurantoin (Furadantin, Macrodantin, Macrobid)
   a. Gastrointestinal side effects include anorexia, nausea, vomiting, and diarrhea; administration with milk or meals minimizes gastrointestinal distress.
   b. Pulmonary reactions include dyspnea, chest pain, chills, fever, cough, and alveolar infiltrates; these resolve in 2 to 4 days following cessation of treatment.
   c. Hematological side effects include agranulocytosis, leukopenia, thrombocytopenia, and megaloblastic anemia.
   d. Peripheral neuropathy side effects include muscle weakness, tingling sensations, and numbness.
   e. Neurological side effects include headache, vertigo, drowsiness, and nystagmus.
   f. Allergic reactions include anaphylaxis, hives, rash, and tingling sensations around the mouth.
   g. Nitrofurantoin may produce a harmless brown color to the urine.
   h. Nitrofurantoin is contraindicated in clients with renal impairment.

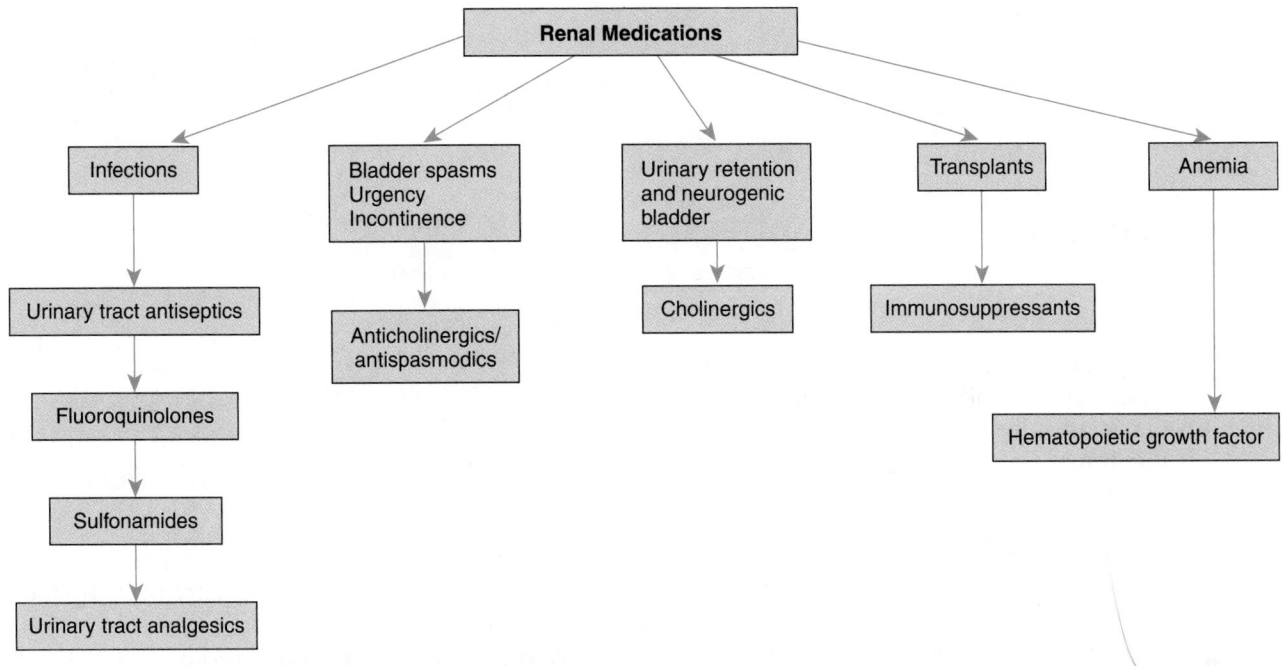

▲ **FIGURE 63-1** Renal conditions and medications. (Developed by Kathleen Ohman).

Box 63-1 Urinary Tract Antiseptics

Cinoxacin (Cinobac)
Methenamine (Mandelamine, Hiprex, Urex)
Nalidixic acid (NegGram)
Nitrofurantoin (Furadantin, Macrodantin, Macrobid)

Box 63-2 Fluoroquinolones

Ciprofloxacin (Cipro)	Moxifloxacin (Avelox)
Enoxacin	Norfloxacin (Noroxin)
Gemifloxacin (Factive)	Ofloxacin (Floxin)
Levofloxacin (Levaquin)	Sparfloxacin
Lomefloxacin (Maxaquin)	Trovafloxacin (Trovan)

    i. Instruct the client in expected side effects, signs warranting notification of the physician, and not to take nitrofurantoin with antacids.

II. FLUOROQUINOLONES (Box 63-2)

A. Description: Suppress bacterial growth by inhibiting an enzyme necessary for DNA synthesis; active against a broad spectrum of microbes

B. Side effects and nursing considerations
  1. Side effects include dizziness, drowsiness, gastric distress, diarrhea, vaginitis (trovafloxacin), nausea, and vomiting.
  2. Adverse effects include psychoses, hallucinations, confusion, tremors, hypersensitivity, and interstitial nephritis.
  3. Fluoroquinolones should be used with caution in clients with hepatic, renal, or CNS disorders.
  4. Monitor client for side effects or signs of adverse reactions.
  5. Enoxacin and norfloxacin (Noroxin) are to be taken on an empty stomach.
  6. Ciprofloxacin (Cipro), lomefloxacin (Maxaquin), and ofloxacin (Floxin) may be taken with or without food.
  7. Intravenously administered ciprofloxacin and ofloxacin are infused slowly over 60 minutes to minimize discomfort and vein irritation.

  8. Advise the client to report dizziness, lightheadedness, visual disturbances, increased light sensitivity, and feelings of depression, because these signs could indicate CNS toxicity.
  9. Inform the client of signs of hepatic and renal toxicity and the importance of reporting these signs to the physician.

⚠ Administer fluoroquinolones with a full glass of water and ensure that the client maintains a urine output of at least 1200 to 1500 mL daily to minimize the development of crystalluria.

III. SULFONAMIDES (Box 63-3)

A. Description: Suppress bacterial growth by inhibiting the synthesis of folic acid; active against a broad spectrum of microbes; used primarily to treat acute urinary tract infections

B. Side effects and nursing considerations
  1. Hypersensitivity reactions include rash, fever, and photosensitivity.
  2. Stevens-Johnson syndrome, the most severe hypersensitivity response, produces symptoms that include widespread lesions of the skin and mucous membranes, fever, malaise, and toxemia.

Box 63-3 Sulfonamides

Sulfadiazine
Sulfamethizole
Sulfamethoxazole
Sulfisoxazole
Trimethoprim (Proloprim, Trimpex)
Trimethoprim-sulfamethoxazole (TMP/SMZ) (Bactrim, Cotrim)

Box 63-4 Urinary Tract Analgesic

Phenazopyridine (Pyridium, Azo-Standard, Pyridiate, Urogesic)

Box 63-5 Anticholinergics—Antispasmodics

Darifenacin (Enablex)
Oxybutynin chloride (Ditropan, Ditropan XL)
Solifenacin (VESIcare)
Tolterodine (Detrol, Detrol LA)
Trospium (Sanctura, Sanctura XR)

3. Sulfonamides can cause hemolytic anemia, agranulocytosis, leukopenia, and thrombocytopenia; instruct the client to notify the physician if sore throat or fever occurs.
4. Administer sulfonamides with caution in clients with renal impairment.
5. Sulfonamides are contraindicated if a hypersensitivity exists to sulfonamides, sulfonylureas, or thiazide or loop diuretics.
6. Sulfonamides are contraindicated in infants younger than 2 months and in pregnant women or mothers who are breast-feeding.
7. Sulfonamides can potentiate the effects of warfarin sodium (Coumadin), phenytoin (Dilantin), and orally administered hypoglycemics such as tolbutamide (Orinase); when combined with sulfonamides, these medications may require a reduction in dosage.
8. Instruct the client to take the medication on an empty stomach with a full glass of water.
9. Instruct the client to complete the entire course of the prescribed medication.
10. Instruct the client to avoid prolonged exposure to sunlight, wear protective clothing, and apply a sunscreen to exposed skin.
11. Adults should maintain a daily urine output of 1200 mL by consuming 8 to 10 glasses of water each day to minimize the risk of renal damage from the medication.
12. Inform the client that some combination medications of sulfonamides can cause the urine to turn dark brown or red.
13. The sulfonamide combination of trimethoprim-sulfamethoxazole (TMP-SMZ; Bactrim, Cotrim) is more effective than either medication alone because it inhibits the sequential steps in bacterial folic acid synthesis.
14. TMP-SMZ is used cautiously with clients experiencing impaired kidney function, folate deficiency, severe allergy, or bronchial asthma.
15. An intravenous dose of TMP-SMZ is administered over 60 to 90 minutes and is not mixed with other medications.

⚠ Sulfonamides should be withheld if a rash is noted. Inform the client to contact the physician if a rash appears.

IV. URINARY TRACT ANALGESIC (Box 63-4)

A. Description
1. Phenazopyridine is a urinary tract analgesic used to treat pain from urinary tract irritation or infection.
2. A urinary tract analgesic is administered with an antibiotic because the analgesic only treats pain, not the infection.
B. Side effects
1. Nausea
2. Headache
3. Vertigo
C. Nursing considerations
1. Instruct the client that the urine will turn red or orange and stain clothing.
2. A urinary tract analgesic is contraindicated in clients with renal or hepatic disease.
3. The medication interferes with accurate urine testing for glucose and ketones.

V. ANTICHOLINERGICS—ANTISPASMODICS (Box 63-5)

A. Description: Used for overactive bladder (urge incontinence)
B. Side effects
1. Anorexia, nausea, vomiting, and dry mouth
2. Blurred vision
3. Confusion in older clients
4. Constipation
5. Decreased sweating
6. Dizziness
7. Drowsiness
8. Dry eyes
9. Gastric distress
10. Headache
11. Tachycardia
12. Urinary retention
C. Nursing considerations
1. Extended-release capsules should not be split, chewed, or crushed
2. Detrol LA should be used cautiously in clients with narrow-angle glaucoma.

Box 63-6 Cholinergic

Bethanechol chloride (Urecholine)

3. Do not administer oxybutynin to clients with known hypersensitivity, gastrointestinal or genitourinary obstruction, glaucoma, severe colitis, or myasthenia gravis.
4. Do not administer propantheline bromide to clients with narrow-angle glaucoma, obstructive uropathy, gastrointestinal disease, or ulcerative colitis.
5. Instruct the client to avoid hazardous activities because of the side effects of dizziness and drowsiness.
6. Monitor intake and output.
7. Provide gum or hard candy for dry mouth.
8. Monitor for signs of toxicity (CNS stimulation) such as hypotension, hypertension, confusion, tachycardia, flushed or red face, signs of respiratory depression, nervousness, restlessness, hallucinations, and irritability.

VI. CHOLINERGIC (Box 63-6)

A. Description: Bethanechol chloride (Urecholine) is a cholinergic used to increase bladder tone and function and to treat nonobstructive urinary retention and neurogenic bladder.
B. Side effects
   1. Headache
   2. Hypotension
   3. Flushing and sweating
   4. Increased salivation
   5. Abdominal cramps
   6. Nausea and vomiting
   7. Diarrhea
   8. Urinary urgency
   9. Bronchoconstriction
   10. Transient complete heart block
C. Nursing considerations
   1. Administer on an empty stomach, 1 hour before or 2 hours after meals to lessen nausea and vomiting.
   2. Never administer by the intramuscular or intravenous (IV) route.
   3. Monitor intake and output.
   4. Monitor for increased bladder tone and function.
   5. Monitor for cholinergic overdose (excessive salivation, sweating, involuntary urination and defecation, bradycardia, and severe hypotension).
   6. Have atropine sulfate (antidote) readily available for IV or subcutaneous administration.

⚠ A cholinergic such as bethanechol chloride (Urecholine) is not given to a client who has a urinary stricture or obstruction.

Box 63-7 Preventing Organ Rejection

Immunosuppressants
Cyclosporine (Sandimmune, Gengraf, Neoral)
Sirolimus (Rapamune)
Tacrolimus (Prograf)

Glucocorticoid
Prednisone

Cytotoxic Medications
Azathioprine (Imuran)
Mycophenolate mofetil (CellCept)

Antibodies
Antithymocyte globulin, equine (Atgam)
Basiliximab (Simulect)
Daclizumab (Zenapax)
Muromonab-CD3 (Orthoclone OKT3)

VII. MEDICATIONS FOR PREVENTING ORGAN REJECTION (Box 63-7)

A. Medications include immunosuppressants, corticosteroids, cytotoxic medications, and antibodies.
B. Some medications may be used in combination with one another to produce different actions on the immune system; combination therapy also allows for administration of the medications in lower doses, reducing the possibility of side effects.
C. Cyclosporine (Sandimmune, Gengraf, Neoral)
   1. Cyclosporine inhibits calcineurin and acts on T lymphocytes to suppress the production of interleukin-2, interferon-γ, and other cytokines.
   2. Cyclosporine may be used to prevent rejection of allogeneic kidney, liver, and heart transplants.
   3. Prednisone may be administered concurrently.
   4. Oral administration of cyclosporine is preferred; intravenous administration is reserved for clients who cannot take the medication orally.
   5. Blood levels of the medication should be measured regularly because of its nephrotoxic effects.
   6. The most common adverse effects are nephrotoxicity, infection, hypertension, tremor, and hirsutism.
   7. Assure the client that hirsutism is reversible; instruct on the use of a depilatory.
   8. Other adverse effects include neurotoxicity, gastrointestinal effects, hyperkalemia, and hyperglycemia.
   9. The risk of infection and lymphomas is increased with the use of cyclosporine.
   10. Cyclosporine is contraindicated in the presence of hypersensitivity, pregnancy and breastfeeding, recent inoculation with live virus vaccines, and recent contact with an active infection such as chickenpox or herpes zoster.

11. Cyclosporine is embryotoxic, and women of childbearing age should use a mechanical form of contraception and avoid oral contraceptives.

12. The client should be informed about the possibility of renal damage and liver damage and the need for periodic liver function tests and determination of coagulation factors and blood urea nitrogen, serum creatinine, serum potassium, and blood glucose levels.

13. The client should be instructed to monitor for early signs of infection and to report these signs immediately.

14. Available in a pill form; if the client is unable to swallow the pill, instruct the client to dispense the oral liquid medication into a glass container by using a specially calibrated pipette, mix well, and drink immediately; rinse the glass container with diluent and drink it to ensure ingestion of the complete dose; dry the outside of the pipette and return to its cover for storage.

15. To promote palatability, instruct the client to mix the liquid medication with milk, chocolate milk, or orange juice just before administration.

16. Consuming grapefruit juice is prohibited because it raises cyclosporine levels and increases the risk of toxicity.

17. Ketoconazole (Nizoral), erythromycin, and amphotericin B (Abelcet, Amphotec, AmBisome) can elevate cyclosporine levels.

18. Phenytoin (Dilantin), phenobarbital, rifampin (Rifadin), and TMP-SMX can decrease cyclosporine levels.

19. Renal damage can be intensified by the concurrent use of other nephrotoxic medications.

D. Sirolimus (Rapamune)
1. Sirolimus is used for the prevention of renal transplant rejection by inhibiting the response of helper T lymphocytes and B lymphocytes to cytokinesis.
2. It may be used with cyclosporine or tacrolimus (CellCept) and corticosteroids.
3. Increases the risk of infection, increases the risk of renal injury, increases the risk of lymphocele (a complication of renal transplant surgery), and raises cholesterol and triglyceride levels
4. Side effects include rash, acne, anemia, thrombocytopenia, joint pain, diarrhea, and hypokalemia.

E. Tacrolimus (Prograf)
1. Tacrolimus inhibits calcineurin and thereby prevents T cells from producing interleukin-2, interferon-γ, and other cytokines.
2. Tacrolimus is more effective than cyclosporine, but is more toxic.
3. Adverse effects are similar to those of cyclosporine and include nephrotoxicity, infection, hypertension, tremor, hirsutism, neurotoxicity,

gastrointestinal effects, hyperkalemia, and hyperglycemia.
4. Tacrolimus should be used cautiously in immunosuppressed clients and those with renal, hepatic, or pancreatic impairment.
5. Tacrolimus is contraindicated for clients hypersensitive to cyclosporine.
6. Monitor blood glucose levels and administer prescribed insulin or oral hypoglycemics.

F. Prednisone
1. Prednisone is a glucocorticoid that inhibits accumulation of inflammatory cells at inflammation sites.
2. Hyperglycemia and hypokalemia can occur with prednisone use; monitor glucose and serum potassium levels.
3. See Chapter 55 for additional information about prednisone.

G. Azathioprine (Imuran)
1. Azathioprine suppresses cell-mediated and humoral immune responses by inhibiting the proliferation of B and T lymphocytes.
2. Not used routinely since the advent of newer medications that prevent transplant rejection.
3. Can cause neutropenia and thrombocytopenia from bone marrow suppression
4. Contraindicated in pregnancy; associated with an increased incidence of neoplasms
5. Monitor hematocrit, white blood cell count, platelet count, liver enzyme levels, and coagulation factors.

H. Mycophenolate mofetil (CellCept)
1. Mycophenolate mofetil causes selective inhibition of B- and T-lymphocyte proliferation.
2. May be used with cyclosporine or tacrolimus and glucocorticoids for prophylaxis against organ rejection
3. Adverse effects include diarrhea, severe neutropenia, vomiting, and sepsis.
4. Mycophenolate mofetil is associated with an increased risk of infection and malignancies.
5. Absorption is decreased by the use of magnesium and aluminum antacids and by cholestyramine (Questran, Prevalite).
6. It is contraindicated in pregnancy and during breast-feeding.
7. Instruct the client to take the medication on an empty stomach and not to open or crush capsules.
8. Instruct the client to contact the physician for unusual bleeding or bruising, sore throat, mouth sores, abdominal pain, or fever.

I. Daclizumab (Zenapax) and basiliximab (Simulect)
1. Daclizumab and basiliximab bind to interleukin-2 receptors on lymphocytes, resulting in diminished cell-mediated immune reactions.
2. Used primarily as an induction agent at the time of transplantation; may be used with other

Box 63-8 Hematopoietic Growth Factors

Erythropoietic Growth Factors
Epoetin alfa (Epogen, Procrit)
Darbepoetin alfa (Aranesp)
MPEG-epoetin beta (Mircera)

Leukopoietic Growth Factors
Filgrastim (Neupogen)
Pegfilgrastim (Neulasta)
Sargramostim (Leukine)

Thrombopoietic Growth Factor
Oprelvekin (Neumega)

immunosuppressants to prevent acute rejection of transplanted kidneys

3. Administered by the intravenous route
4. Daclizumab (Zenapax)
   a. Initial dose is administered within 24 hours before transplantation.
   b. Side effects include chest pain, gastrointestinal distress, edema, shortness of breath, pain in the joints, and slow wound healing.
5. Basiliximab (Simulect)
   a. Initial dose is administered within 2 hours before transplantation.
   b. Side effects are similar to those for daclizumab; in addition, headache, insomnia, dizziness, and tremors can occur.

J. Antithymocyte globulin, equine (Atgam)
1. Antithymocyte globulin, equine, causes a decrease in the number and activity of thymus-derived lymphocytes and is used to suppress organ rejection following renal, liver, bone marrow, and heart transplantation.
2. It is used primarily to treat acute rejection episodes.
3. Before the first infusion, the client should undergo intradermal skin testing to determine hypersensitivity.
4. Because this product is made using equine and human blood components, it may carry a risk of transmitting infectious agents, such as viruses.
5. Monitor the platelet count and report it if below 100,000/mm^3.
6. Arrange for outpatient referral for repeated infusions after discharge.

K. Muromonab-CD3 (Orthoclone OKT3)
1. Blocks all T-cell functions; used to prevent acute allograft rejection of kidney transplants
2. Adverse reactions include fever, chills, dyspnea, chest pain, and nausea and vomiting.
3. Administered via the IV route; the client is pretreated with IV glucocorticoid.

VIII. HEMATOPOIETIC GROWTH FACTORS (Box 63-8)

A. Erythropoietic growth factors
1. Stimulate the production of red blood cells

2. Used to treat anemia of **chronic renal failure**, chemotherapy-induced anemia, anemia caused by zidovudine (AZT), and anemia in clients requiring surgery
3. Initial effects can be seen within 1 to 2 weeks, and the hematocrit reaches normal levels (30% to 33%) in 2 to 3 months.
4. Side effect: Major side effect is hypertension.
5. Adverse effects can include heart failure, thrombotic effects such as stroke or myocardial infarction, and cardiac arrest.

B. Leukopoietic growth factors
1. Stimulate the production of white blood cells (leukocytes)
2. Used for clients undergoing myelosuppressive chemotherapy or bone marrow transplantation and those with severe chronic neutropenia
3. Can cause bone pain, leukocytosis, and elevation of plasma uric acid, lactate dehydrogenase, and alkaline phosphatase levels; long-term therapy has caused splenomegaly

C. Thrombopoietic growth factor
1. Stimulates the production of platelets
2. Used for clients undergoing myelosuppressive chemotherapy to minimize thrombocytopenia and to decrease the need for platelet transfusions
3. Adverse effects include fluid retention, cardiac dysrhythmias, conjunctival infection, visual blurring, and papilledema.

● MORE QUESTIONS ON THE CD!

Practice Questions

753. The client who has a cold is seen in the emergency department with an inability to void. Because the client has a history of benign prostatic hyperplasia, the nurse determines that the client should be questioned about the use of which of the following medications?
1. Diuretics
2. Antibiotics
3. Antitussives
4. Decongestants

754. Nalidixic acid (NegGram) is prescribed for a client with a urinary tract infection. On review of the client's record, the nurse notes that the client is taking warfarin sodium (Coumadin) daily. Which prescription should the nurse anticipate for this client?
1. Discontinuation of warfarin sodium (Coumadin)
2. A decrease in the warfarin sodium (Coumadin) dosage
3. An increase in the warfarin sodium (Coumadin) dosage
4. A decrease in the usual dose of nalidixic acid (NegGram)

755. A nurse is providing discharge instructions to a client receiving sulfisoxazole. Which of the following would be included in the list of instructions?
1. Restrict fluid intake.
2. Maintain a high fluid intake.
3. If the urine turns dark brown, call the physician immediately.
4. Decrease the dosage when symptoms are improving to prevent an allergic response.

756. Trimethoprim-sulfamethoxazole (TMP-SMZ; Bactrim) is prescribed for a client. A nurse would instruct the client to report which symptom if it developed during the course of this medication therapy?
1. Nausea
2. Diarrhea
3. Headache
4. Sore throat

757. Phenazopyridine hydrochloride (Pyridium) is prescribed for a client for symptomatic relief of pain resulting from a lower urinary tract infection. The nurse teaches the client:
1. To take the medication at bedtime
2. To take the medication before meals
3. To discontinue the medication if a headache occurs
4. That a reddish orange discoloration of the urine may occur

758. Bethanechol chloride (Urecholine) is prescribed for a client with urinary retention. Which disorder would be a contraindication to the administration of this medication?
1. Gastric atony
2. Urinary strictures
3. Neurogenic atony
4. Gastroesophageal reflux

759. A nurse who is administering bethanechol chloride (Urecholine) is monitoring for acute toxicity associated with the medication. The nurse checks the client for which sign of toxicity?
1. Dry skin
2. Dry mouth
3. Bradycardia
4. Signs of dehydration

760. Oxybutynin chloride (Ditropan) is prescribed for a client with neurogenic bladder. Which sign would indicate a possible toxic effect related to this medication?
1. Pallor
2. Drowsiness
3. Bradycardia
4. Restlessness

761. Following kidney transplantation, cyclosporine (Sandimmune) is prescribed for a client. Which laboratory result would indicate an adverse effect from the use of this medication?
1. Decreased creatinine level
2. Decreased hemoglobin level
3. Elevated blood urea nitrogen level
4. Decreased white blood cell count

762. A nurse is providing dietary instructions to a client who has been prescribed cyclosporine (Sandimmune). Which food item would the nurse instruct the client to avoid?
1. Red meats
2. Orange juice
3. Grapefruit juice
4. Green leafy vegetables

763. Tacrolimus (Prograf) is prescribed for a client. Which disorder, if noted in the client's record, would indicate that the medication needs to be administered with caution?
1. Pancreatitis
2. Ulcerative colitis
3. Diabetes insipidus
4. Coronary artery disease

764. A nurse is reviewing the laboratory results for a client receiving tacrolimus (Prograf). Which laboratory result would indicate to the nurse that the client is experiencing an adverse effect of the medication?
1. Blood glucose of 200 mg/dL
2. Potassium level of 3.8 mEq/L
3. Platelet count of 300,000 cells/mm^3
4. White blood cell count of 6000 cells/mm^3

765. The nurse receives a call from a client concerned about eliminating brown-colored urine after taking nitrofurantoin (Furadantin) for a urinary tract infection. Which of the following is the appropriate response from the nurse?
1. "Discontinue taking the medication and make an appointment for a urine culture."
2. "Continue taking the medication because the urine is discolored from the medication."
3. "Decrease your medication to half the dose because your urine is too concentrated."
4. "Take magnesium hydroxide (Maalox) with your medication to lighten the urine color."

766. A client with chronic renal failure is receiving epoetin alfa (Epogen, Procrit). Which laboratory result would indicate a therapeutic effect of the medication?

1. Hematocrit of 32%
2. Platelet count of 400,000 cells/mm^3
3. Blood urea nitrogen level of 15 mg/dL
4. White blood cell count of 6000 cells/mm^3

Alternate Item Format: Chart/Exhibit

767. Cinoxacin (Cinobac), a urinary antiseptic, is prescribed for the client. The nurse reviews the client's medical record and would contact the physician regarding which documented finding to verify the prescription?
1. Renal insufficiency
2. Chest x-ray: normal
3. Blood glucose, 102 mg/dL
4. Folic acid (vitamin B$_6$) 0.5 mg, orally daily

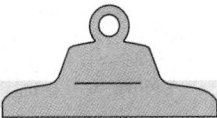

CHART/EXHIBIT
CLIENT'S MEDICAL RECORD

Laboratory Test Result: Blood glucose, 102 mg/dL
Diagnostic Test Result: Chest x-ray: normal
Client's History: Renal Insufficiency
Medication History: Folic acid (vitamin B$_6$) 0.5 mg, orally daily

ANSWERS

753. 4

Rationale: In the client with benign prostatic hyperplasia, episodes of urinary retention can be triggered by certain medications, such as decongestants, anticholinergics, and antidepressants. The client should be questioned about the use of these medications if the client has urinary retention. Retention also can be precipitated by other factors, such as alcoholic beverages, infection, bed rest, and becoming chilled.

Test-Taking Strategy: Use the process of elimination. The question is asking about medications that could exacerbate or contribute to urinary retention in the client with benign prostatic hyperplasia. Diuretics should help voiding; therefore, eliminate option 1. Antibiotics should have no effect at all, and thus eliminate option 2. From the remaining options, recalling that medications that contain anticholinergics may cause urinary retention will direct you to option 4. Review the factors that can precipitate urinary retention in the client with benign prostatic hyperplasia if you had difficulty with this question.

Level of Cognitive Ability: Analyzing
Client Needs: Physiological Integrity
Integrated Process: Nursing Process—Assessment
Content Area: Adult Health—Renal
Reference: Black, J., & Hawks, J. (2009). *Medical-surgical nursing: Clinical management for positive outcomes* (8th ed., p. 878). St. Louis: Saunders.

754. 2

Rationale: Nalidixic acid can intensify the effects of oral anticoagulants by displacing these agents from binding sites on plasma protein. When an oral anticoagulant is combined with nalidixic acid, a decrease in the anticoagulant dosage may be needed.

Test-Taking Strategy: Knowledge about the medication interactions associated with the use of nalidixic acid is needed to answer this question. Remember that nalidixic acid can intensify the effects of oral anticoagulants. Review these interactions if you had difficulty with this question.

Level of Cognitive Ability: Analyzing
Client Needs: Physiological Integrity
Integrated Process: Nursing Process—Analysis

Content Area: Pharmacology
References: Kee, J., Hayes, E., & McCuistion, L. (2009). *Pharmacology: A nursing process approach* (6th ed., p. 490). St. Louis: Saunders.

Lehne, R. (2010). *Pharmacology for nursing care* (7th ed., p. 1036). St. Louis: Saunders.

755. 2

Rationale: Each dose of sulfisoxazole should be administered with a full glass of water, and the client should maintain a high fluid intake. The medication is more soluble in alkaline urine. The client should not be instructed to taper or discontinue the dose. Some forms of sulfisoxazole cause urine to turn dark brown or red. This does not indicate the need to notify the physician.

Test-Taking Strategy: Use the process of elimination. Recalling that this medication is used to treat urinary tract infections will direct you to option 2. Review client instructions regarding this medication if you had difficulty with this question.

Level of Cognitive Ability: Applying
Client Needs: Physiological Integrity
Integrated Process: Teaching and Learning
Content Area: Pharmacology
Reference: Lehne, R. (2010). *Pharmacology for nursing care* (7th ed., p. 1030). St. Louis: Saunders.

756. 4

Rationale: Clients taking trimethoprim (TMP)-sulfamethoxazole (SMZ) should be informed about early signs of blood disorders that can occur from this medication. These include sore throat, fever, and pallor, and the client should be instructed to notify the physician if these symptoms occur. The other options do not require physician notification.

Test-Taking Strategy: Use the process of elimination. Knowledge that this medication can cause blood dyscrasias will direct you to option 4. If you are unfamiliar with this medication, review this content.

Level of Cognitive Ability: Applying
Client Needs: Physiological Integrity
Integrated Process: Teaching and Learning

Content Area: Pharmacology
Reference: Hodgson, B., & Kizior, R. (2010). *Saunders nursing drug handbook 2010* (p. 1156). St. Louis: Saunders.

757. 4

Rationale: The nurse should instruct the client that a reddish-orange discoloration of urine may occur. The nurse also should instruct the client that this discoloration can stain fabric. The medication should be taken after meals to reduce the possibility of gastrointestinal upset. A headache is an occasional side effect of the medication and does not warrant discontinuation of the medication.
Test-Taking Strategy: Use the process of elimination. Eliminate options 1 and 2 first because they are comparable or alike in that they address time schedules for the administration of the medication. From the remaining options, eliminate option 3 because the nurse would not advise the client to discontinue this medication. Review client instructions regarding this medication if you had difficulty with this question.
Level of Cognitive Ability: Applying
Client Needs: Physiological Integrity
Integrated Process: Teaching and Learning
Content Area: Pharmacology
Reference: Hodgson, B., & Kizior, R. (2010). *Saunders nursing drug handbook 2010* (p. 900). St. Louis: Saunders.

758. 2

Rationale: Bethanechol chloride (Urecholine) can be hazardous to clients with urinary tract obstruction or weakness of the bladder wall. The medication has the ability to contract the bladder and thereby increase pressure within the urinary tract. Elevation of pressure within the urinary tract could rupture the bladder in clients with these conditions.
Test-Taking Strategy: Use the process of elimination. Noting that the medication is used for urinary retention may assist in directing you to option 2. Review the contraindications associated with this medication if you had difficulty with this question.
Level of Cognitive Ability: Analyzing
Client Needs: Physiological Integrity
Integrated Process: Nursing Process—Analysis
Content Area: Pharmacology
References: Hodgson, B., & Kizior, R. (2010). *Saunders nursing drug handbook 2010* (p. 125). St. Louis: Saunders.
    Kee, J., Hayes, E., & McCuistion, L. (2009). *Pharmacology: A nursing process approach* (6th ed., p. 288). St. Louis: Saunders.

759. 3

Rationale: Toxicity (overdose) of bethanechol chloride produces manifestations of excessive muscarinic stimulation such as salivation, sweating, involuntary urination and defecation, bradycardia, and severe hypotension. Treatment includes supportive measures and the administration of atropine sulfate subcutaneously or intravenously.
Test-Taking Strategy: Use the process of elimination. Noting the similarity in options 1, 2, and 4 will assist in eliminating these options. Review the signs of toxicity if you had difficulty with this question.
Level of Cognitive Ability: Analyzing
Client Needs: Physiological Integrity

Integrated Process: Nursing Process—Assessment
Content Area: Pharmacology
References: Hodgson, B., & Kizior, R. (2010). *Saunders nursing drug handbook 2010* (p. 125). St. Louis: Saunders.
    Kee, J., Hayes, E., & McCuistion, L. (2009). *Pharmacology: A nursing process approach* (6th ed., p. 285). St. Louis: Saunders.
    Lehne, R. (2010). *Pharmacology for nursing care* (7th ed., pp. 122, 130). St. Louis: Saunders.

760. 4

Rationale: Toxicity (overdosage) of oxybutynin chloride produces central nervous system excitation, such as nervousness, restlessness, hallucinations, and irritability. Other signs of toxicity include hypotension or hypertension, confusion, tachycardia, flushed or red face, and signs of respiratory depression. Drowsiness is a frequent side effect of the medication but does not indicate overdosage.
Test-Taking Strategy: Knowledge regarding the manifestations related to toxicity is required to answer this question. Remember restlessness is a sign of toxicity. Review the signs that indicate toxicity if you had difficulty with this question.
Level of Cognitive Ability: Analyzing
Client Needs: Physiological Integrity
Integrated Process: Nursing Process—Assessment
Content Area: Pharmacology
Reference: Hodgson, B., & Kizior, R. (2007). *Saunders nursing drug handbook 2007* (p. 861). St. Louis: Saunders.

761. 3

Rationale: Nephrotoxicity can occur from the use of cyclosporine (Sandimmune). Nephrotoxicity is evaluated by monitoring for elevated blood urea nitrogen and serum creatinine levels. Cyclosporine does not depress the bone marrow.
Test-Taking Strategy: Use the process of elimination. Eliminate options 2 and 4 first because they are unrelated to renal function. Next, eliminate option 1 because the creatinine level would be elevated, not decreased. Option 3 is the only option that indicates an increased level of a renal function test. Review the adverse effects related to this medication if you had difficulty with this question.
Level of Cognitive Ability: Analyzing
Client Needs: Physiological Integrity
Integrated Process: Nursing Process—Analysis
Content Area: Pharmacology
Reference: Lehne, R. (2010). *Pharmacology for nursing care* (7th ed., pp. 815, 820). St. Louis: Saunders.

762. 3

Rationale: A compound present in grapefruit juice inhibits metabolism of cyclosporine. As a result, consumption of grapefruit juice can raise cyclosporine levels by 50% to 100%, thereby greatly increasing the risk of toxicity.
Test-Taking Strategy: Use the process of elimination, noting the strategic word *avoid*. Use of general pharmacology guidelines will direct you to option 3. If you had difficulty with this question, review this medication and the client instructions regarding its use.
Level of Cognitive Ability: Applying
Client Needs: Physiological Integrity
Integrated Process: Teaching and Learning
Content Area: Pharmacology

Reference: Lehne, R. (2010). *Pharmacology for nursing care* (7th ed., pp. 815, 820). St. Louis: Saunders.

763. 1

Rationale: Tacrolimus (Prograf) is used with caution in immunosuppressed clients and in clients with renal, hepatic, or pancreatic function impairment. Tacrolimus is contraindicated in clients with hypersensitivity to this medication or hypersensitivity to cyclosporine.

Test-Taking Strategy: Use the process of elimination. Many medications affect renal, hepatic, and pancreatic function. If you had to select an option and were unsure, select the option that addresses these body systems. Review the cautions and contraindications associated with the administration of this medication if you had difficulty with this question.

Level of Cognitive Ability: Analyzing
Client Needs: Physiological Integrity
Integrated Process: Nursing Process—Analysis
Content Area: Pharmacology
Reference: Lehne, R. (2010). *Pharmacology for nursing care* (7th ed., p. 816). St. Louis: Saunders.

764. 1

Rationale: A blood glucose level of 200 mg/dL is significantly elevated above the normal range of 70 to 110 mg/dL and suggests an adverse reaction. Other adverse reactions include neurotoxicity evidenced by headache, tremor, and insomnia; gastrointestinal effects such as diarrhea, nausea, and vomiting; hypertension; and hyperkalemia.

Test-Taking Strategy: Use the process of elimination, noting that options 2, 3, and 4 represent normal values. Option 1 is the only abnormal value, reflecting an elevation. Review the adverse effects related to this medication and normal laboratory values if you had difficulty with this question.

Level of Cognitive Ability: Analyzing
Client Needs: Physiological Integrity
Integrated Process: Nursing Process—Analysis
Content Area: Pharmacology
References: Ignatavicius, D., & Workman, M. (2010). *Medical-surgical nursing: Patient-centered collaborative care* (6th ed., p. 1498). St. Louis: Saunders.

Lehne, R. (2010). *Pharmacology for nursing care* (7th ed., p. 816). St. Louis: Saunders.

765. 2

Rationale: Nitrofurantoin (Furadantin) produces a harmless brown color to the urine and the medication should not be discontinued until the prescribed dose is completed. Magnesium hydroxide (Maalox) will not affect urine color. Additionally, antacids should be avoided because they interfere with medication effectiveness.

Test-Taking Strategy: Use the process of elimination. Option 1 can be eliminated because the client should not need a urine culture at this time. These are done before treatment is initiated, if treatment is ineffective, and during follow-up appointment. Option 3 can be eliminated, because the nurse cannot change a medication dosage without a physician's prescription. Additionally, there is no data in the question to indicate that the urine is concentrated. Option 4 can be

eliminated because antacids should be avoided as a result of their interference with the effectiveness of nitrofurantoin. Additionally, magnesium hydroxide will not have an effect on urine color. Review the effects of nitrofurantoin if you had difficulty with this question.

Level of Cognitive Ability: Applying
Client Needs: Physiological Integrity
Integrated Process: Nursing Process—Implementation
Content Area: Pharmacology
Reference: Hodgson, B., & Kizior, R. (2010). *Saunders nursing drug handbook 2010* (p. 824). St. Louis: Saunders.

766. 1

Rationale: Epoetin alfa is used to reverse anemia associated with chronic renal failure. Therapeutic effect is seen when the hematocrit is between 30% and 33%. Options 2, 3, and 4 are not associated with the action of this medication.

Test-Taking Strategy: Use the process of elimination. Relate the name of the medication, erythropoietin, to the potential action or effect. The only laboratory test that would reflect the effect of this medication is option 1. Review the therapeutic effect of this medication and normal serum laboratory results if you had difficulty with this question.

Level of Cognitive Ability: Evaluating
Client Needs: Physiological Integrity
Integrated Process: Nursing Process—Evaluation
Content Area: Pharmacology
Reference: Hodgson, B., & Kizior, R. (2010). *Saunders nursing drug handbook 2010* (p. 417). St. Louis: Saunders.

ALTERNATE ITEM FORMAT: CHART/EXHIBIT

767. 1

Rationale: Cinoxacin should be administered with caution in clients with renal impairment. The dosage should be reduced, and failure to do so could result in accumulation of cinoxacin to toxic levels. Therefore, the nurse would verify the prescription with the physician if the client had a documented history of renal insufficiency. The laboratory and diagnostic test results are normal findings. Folic acid (vitamin B_6) may be prescribed for a client with renal insufficiency to prevent anemia.

Test-Taking Strategy: Focus on the subject, the need to contact the physician. Eliminate options 2 and 3 because the laboratory and diagnostic test results are normal findings. From the remaining options, note the disorder in the client's history. This directs you to option 1. Review the contraindications associated with this medication if you had difficulty with this question.

Level of Cognitive Ability: Analyzing
Client Needs: Physiological Integrity
Integrated Process: Nursing Process—Analysis
Content Area: Pharmacology
References: Kee, J., Hayes, E., & McCuistion, L. (2009). *Pharmacology: A nursing process approach* (6th ed., pp. 488–489). St. Louis: Saunders.

Lehne, R. (2010). *Pharmacology for nursing care* (7th ed., p. 1036). St. Louis: Saunders.

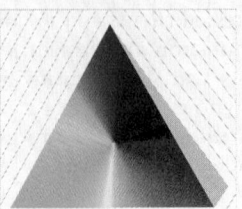

The Adult Client With an Eye or Ear Disorder

PYRAMID TERMS

accommodation Process whereby a clear visual image is maintained as the gaze is shifted from a distant to a near point.

astigmatism Visual distortion that results from an uneven curvature of the cornea or lens in which light rays focus on two different points on the retina.

cataract An opacity of the lens that distorts the image projected onto the retina and that can progress to blindness.

conductive hearing loss A mechanical dysfunction or blockage of sound waves to the inner ear fibers because of external ear or middle ear disorders. The blockage can be caused by impacted cerumen, foreign bodies, pus, or serum in the middle ear. Disorders often can be corrected with no damage to hearing or minimal permanent hearing loss.

cycloplegia The paralysis of the ciliary muscles by medications that block muscarinic receptors. Cycloplegia causes blurred vision because the shape of the lens can no longer be adjusted to near-vision.

fenestration Removal of the stapes with a small hole drilled in the footplate and connection of a prosthesis between the incus and foot plate. Sounds cause the prosthesis to vibrate in the same manner as the stapes.

glaucoma Increased intraocular pressure as a result of inadequate drainage of aqueous humor from the canal of Schlemm or from overproduction of aqueous humor. The condition damages the optic nerve and can result in blindness.

hyperopia Farsightedness; objects converge to a point behind the retina. Vision beyond 20 feet is normal, but near-vision is poor. The condition is corrected by a convex lens.

legally blind The best visual acuity with corrective lenses in the better eye of 20/200 or less, or the visual field is no greater than 20 degrees in its widest diameter in the better eye.

macular degeneration A blurred central vision caused by progressive degeneration of the center of the retina. The condition may be atrophic or age-related, or dry or exudative (wet).

Meniere's syndrome Also called endolymphatic hydrops, this syndrome involves dilation of the endolymphatic system by overproduction or decreased reabsorption of endolymphatic fluid. It is characterized by tinnitus, unilateral sensorineural hearing loss, and vertigo.

miosis A constricted pupil that occurs primarily by stimulation of the muscarinic receptors of the sphincter muscles. It is seen with the use of pilocarpine drops when treating glaucoma, when using opioids, or when there is brain damage of the pons.

miotic Medication that causes contraction of the pupil.

mydriasis A dilated pupil that occurs because of blockage of the muscarinic receptors of the sphincter muscles or by stimulation of the alpha receptors of the dilator muscles. Enlarged pupils occur with stimulation of the sympathetic nervous system, use of dilating drops, acute glaucoma, or past or recent trauma.

mydriatic Medication that dilates the pupil.

myopia Nearsightedness; rays coming from an object are focused in front of the retina. Near-vision is normal, but distant vision is defective. A biconcave lens is used for correction.

otosclerosis Disease of the labyrinthine capsule of the middle ear that results in a bony overgrowth of tissue surrounding the ossicles. Otosclerosis causes the development of irregular areas of new bone formation and causes fixation of the bones, leading to a conductive hearing loss.

presbycusis Gradual nerve degeneration associated with aging; a common cause of sensorineural hearing loss.

retinal detachment Separation of the layers of the retina because of the accumulation of fluid between them or because both retinal layers elevate away from the choroid as a result of a tumor. Partial separation becomes complete if untreated. When detachment becomes complete, blindness occurs.

sensorineural hearing loss A pathological process of the inner ear or of the sensory fibers that lead to the cerebral cortex. Such hearing loss often is permanent, and measures must be taken to reduce further damage or to attempt to amplify sound as a means of improving hearing to some degree.

▲ PYRAMID TO SUCCESS

Pyramid Points focus on nursing interventions for clients with impairment of sight or hearing and on the nursing care related to disorders such as cataracts, glaucoma, and retinal detachment. Pyramid Points also focus on emergency interventions for eye and ear disorders and injuries. Review nursing care related to tissue (corneal) donation for the donor and the recipient. Pyramid Points also focus on client instructions related to medication administration, sensory perceptual alterations and safety issues, and available support systems.

▲ CLIENT NEEDS

Safe and Effective Care Environment

Caring for the recipient of a tissue (corneal) donation
Consulting with members of the health care team
Establishing priorities
Maintaining asepsis with procedures and treatments
Maintaining standard and other precautions
Obtaining informed consent for invasive procedures
Preventing accidents that can occur as a result of sensory impairments
Upholding client rights

Health Promotion and Maintenance

Changes that occur with the aging process
Discussing expected body image changes and self-care deficits
Implementing measures for the prevention and early detection of health problems and diseases related to the eye and the ear
Performing physical assessments of eye and ear disorders
Providing home care instructions following procedures related to the eye and ear
Providing instructions regarding the administration of eye and ear medications
Providing instructions regarding activity limitations or postoperative activities
Teaching regarding the importance of compliance with the prescribed therapy

Psychosocial Integrity

Assessing the client's ability to cope with feelings of isolation, fear or anxiety regarding a possible change in vision and/or hearing status, and loss of independence
Discussing role changes
Identifying family support systems
Informing the client about available community resources
Monitoring for sensory perceptual alterations
Using appropriate communication techniques for impaired vision and hearing

Physiological Integrity

Monitoring for complications related to procedures
Monitoring for expected responses to therapy
Providing care for assistive devices such as eyeglasses, contact lenses, and hearing aids
Taking action in medical emergencies

The Eye and the Ear

I. ANATOMY AND PHYSIOLOGY OF THE EYE

A. The eye
1. The eye is 1 inch in diameter and is located in the anterior portion of the orbit.
2. The orbit is the bony structure of the skull that surrounds the eye and offers protection to the eye.

B. Layers of the eye
1. External layer
   a. The fibrous coat that supports the eye
   b. Contains the cornea, the dense transparent outer layer
   c. Contains the sclera, the fibrous "white of the eye"
2. Middle layer
   a. Called the uveal tract
   b. Consists of the choroid, ciliary body, and iris
   c. The choroid is the dark brown membrane located between the sclera and the retina that has dark pigmentation to prevent light from reflecting internally.
   d. The choroid lines most of the sclera and is attached to the retina but can detach easily from the sclera.
   e. The choroid contains many blood vessels and supplies nutrients to the retina.
   f. The ciliary body connects the choroid with the iris and secretes aqueous humor that helps give the eye its shape; the muscles of the ciliary body control the thickness of the lens.
   g. The iris is the colored portion of the eye, located in front of the lens, and it has a central circular opening called the pupil. The pupil controls the amount of light admitted into the retina (darkness produces dilation and light produces constriction).
3. Internal layer
   a. Consists of the retina, a thin, delicate structure in which the fibers of the optic nerve are distributed
   b. The retina is bordered externally by the choroid and sclera and internally by the vitreous.
   c. The retina is the visual receptive layer of the eye in which light waves are changed into nerve impulses; it contains blood vessels and photoreceptors called rods and cones.

C. Vitreous body
1. Contains a gelatinous substance that occupies the vitreous chamber, the space between the lens and the retina
2. The vitreous body transmits light and gives shape to the posterior eye.

D. Vitreous
1. Gel-like substance that maintains the shape of the eye
2. Provides additional physical support to the retina

E. Rods and cones
1. Rods are responsible for peripheral vision and function at reduced levels of illumination.
2. Cones function at bright levels of illumination and are responsible for color vision and central vision.

F. Optic disc
1. The optic disc is a creamy pink to white depressed area in the retina.
2. The optic nerve enters and exits the eyeball at this area.
3. This area is called the blind spot because it contains only nerve fibers, lacks photoreceptor cells, and is insensitive to light.

G. Macula lutea
1. Small, oval, yellowish-pink area located laterally and temporally to the optic disc
2. The central depressed part of the macula is the fovea centralis, the area of sharpest and keenest vision, where most acute vision occurs.

H. Aqueous humor
1. The aqueous humor is a clear watery fluid that fills the anterior and posterior chambers of the eye.
2. The aqueous humor is produced by the ciliary processes, and the fluid drains into the canal of Schlemm.
3. The anterior chamber lies between the cornea and the iris.
4. The posterior chamber lies between the iris and the lens.

I. Canal of Schlemm: Passageway that extends completely around the eye; it permits fluid to drain out of the eye into the systemic circulation so a constant intraocular pressure is maintained.

J. Lens
   1. Transparent convex structure behind the iris and in front of the vitreous body
   2. The lens bends rays of light so that the light falls on the retina.
   3. The curve of the lens changes to focus on near or distant objects.

K. Conjunctivae: Thin transparent mucous membranes of the eye that line the posterior surface of each eyelid, located over the sclera

L. Lacrimal gland
   1. The lacrimal gland produces tears.
   2. Tears are drained through the punctum into the lacrimal duct and sac.

M. Eye muscles
   1. Muscles do not work independently but work with the muscle that produces the opposite movement.
   2. Rectus muscles exert their pull when the eye turns temporally.
   3. Oblique muscles exert their pull when the eye turns nasally.

N. Nerves (Fig. 64-1)
   1. Cranial nerve II: Optic nerve (nerve of sight)
   2. Cranial nerve III: Oculomotor
   3. Cranial nerve IV: Trochlear
   4. Cranial nerve VI: Abducens

O. Blood vessels
   1. The ophthalmic artery is the major artery supplying the structures in the eye.
   2. The ophthalmic veins drain the blood from the eye.

II. ASSESSMENT OF VISION (also see Chapter 34)

A. Acuity
   1. Visual acuity tests measure the client's distance and near vision
   2. Snellen chart—"eye chart"
      a. The chart is a simple tool to measure distance vision.

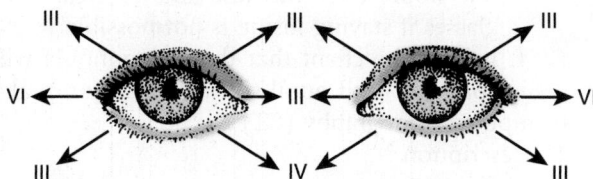

▲ FIGURE 64-1 Checking extraocular muscles in the six cardinal positions. This indicates the functioning of cranial nerves III, IV, and VI. (From Ignatavicius, D., & Workman, M. [2010]. *Medical-surgical nursing: Patient-centered collaborative care* [6th ed.]. St. Louis: Saunders.)

b. The client stands 20 feet from the chart, covers one eye, and uses the other eye to read the line that appears most clearly.
      c. If the client is able to do this accurately, the client reads the next lower line.
      d. This sequence is repeated until the client is unable to identify correctly more than half the characters on the line.
      e. The procedure is repeated for the other eye, and then both eyes together may be tested.
      f. The findings are recorded as a comparison between what the client can read at 20 feet and the distance at which an individual with normal vision can read the same line.
      g. A result of 20/50 means that the client is able to read at 20 feet from the chart what a healthy eye can read at 50 feet.
      h. Clients who wear corrective lenses other than for reading should have their vision tested with the lens in place.

B. Confrontational test
   1. The confrontational test is performed to examine visual fields or peripheral vision.
   2. The examiner and the client sit facing each other.
   3. The client is asked to look directly into the eyes of the examiner throughout the test.
   4. The examiner covers his or her right eye while the client covers his or her left eye (the client covers the eye directly opposite to the examiner's covered eye).
   5. The examiner moves a finger from a nonvisible area into the client's line of vision.
   6. The examiner and client should see the object at approximately the same time.
   7. When the client sees the object coming into the line of vision, the client informs the examiner.
   8. The procedure is repeated on the opposite eye.
   9. The test assumes that the examiner has normal peripheral vision.

C. Extraocular muscle function (see Fig. 64-1)
   1. The six muscles that attach the eyeball to its orbit and serve to direct the eye to points of interest are tested.
   2. Six cardinal positions of gaze include the following:
      a. Client's right (lateral position)
      b. Upward and right (temporal position)
      c. Down and right
      d. Client's left (lateral position)
      e. Upward and left (temporal position)
      f. Down and left
   3. Client holds head still and is asked to move his or her eyes and follow a small object.
   4. The examiner notes for any parallel movements of the eye or for nystagmus, an involuntary, rhythmic, rapid twitching of the eyeballs.

D. Color vision
1. Tests for color vision involve picking numbers or letters out of a complex and colorful picture.
2. Ishihara chart
   a. The Ishihara chart consists of numbers composed of colored dots located within a circle of colored dots.
   b. The client is asked to read the numbers on the chart.
   c. Each eye is tested separately.
   d. Reading the numbers correctly indicates normal color vision
   e. The test is sensitive for the diagnosis of red-green blindness but cannot detect discrimination of blue.

 The first slide on the Ishihara chart is one that everyone can discriminate; failure to identify numbers on this slide suggests a problem with performing the test, not a problem with color vision.

E. Pupils
1. The pupils are round and of equal size.
2. Increasing light causes pupillary constriction.
3. Decreasing light causes pupillary dilation.
4. Constriction of both pupils is a normal response to direct light.
5. The client is asked to look straight ahead while the examiner quickly brings a beam of light (flashlight) in from the side and directs it onto the eye.
6. The constriction of the eye is a direct response to shining a light into that eye; constriction of the opposite eye is known as a consensual response.

F. Sclera and cornea
1. Normal sclera color is white.
2. A yellow color to the sclera may indicate jaundice or systemic problems.
3. In a dark-skinned person, the sclera may normally appear yellow; pigmented dots may be present.
4. The cornea is transparent, smooth, shiny, and bright.
5. Cloudy areas or specks on the cornea may be the result of an accident or eye injury.

G. Ophthalmoscopy
1. The ophthalmoscope is an instrument used to examine the external structures and the interior of the eye.
2. The room is darkened so that the pupil will dilate.
3. The instrument is held with the right hand when examining the right eye and with the left hand when examining the left eye.
4. The client is asked to look straight ahead at an object on the wall.
5. The examiner should approach the client's eye from about 12 to 15 inches away and 15 degrees lateral to the client's line of vision.
6. As the instrument is directed at the pupil, a red glare (red reflex) is seen in the pupil.
7. The red reflex is the reflection of light on the vascular retina.
8. Absence of the red reflex may indicate opacity of the lens.
9. The retina, optic disc, optic vessels, fundus, and macula can be examined.

III. DIAGNOSTIC TESTS FOR THE EYE

A. Fluorescein angiography
1. Description
   a. A detailed imaging and recording of ocular circulation by a series of photographs after the administration of a dye
   b. This test is useful for assessing problems with retinal circulation, such as those that occur in diabetic retinopathy, retinal bleeding, and **macular degeneration**, or to rule out intraocular tumors.
2. Preprocedure interventions
   a. Assess the client for allergies and previous reactions to dyes.
   b. Obtain informed consent.
   c. A **mydriatic** medication, which causes pupil dilation, is instilled into the eye 1 hour before the test.
   d. The dye is injected into a vein of the client's arm.
   e. Inform the client that the dye may cause the skin to appear yellow for several hours after the test and is eliminated gradually through the urine.
   f. The client may experience nausea, vomiting, sneezing, paresthesia of the tongue, or pain at the injection site.
   g. If hives appear, antihistamines such as diphenhydramine (Benadryl) are administered as prescribed.
3. Postprocedure interventions
   a. Encourage rest.
   b. Encourage fluid intake to assist in eliminating the dye from the client's system.
   c. Remind the client that the yellow skin appearance will disappear.
   d. Inform the client that the urine will appear bright green until the dye is excreted.
   e. Advise the client to avoid direct sunlight for a few hours after the test and to wear sunglasses if staying inside is not possible.
   f. Inform the client that the photophobia will continue until pupil size returns to normal.

B. Computed tomography (CT)
1. Description
   a. The test is performed to examine the eyes, bony structures around the eye, and extraocular muscles.
   b. A beam of x-rays scans the skull and orbits of the eye.

c. A cross-sectional image is formed by the use of a computer.

d. Contrast material may be used unless eye trauma is suspected.

2. Interventions

a. No special client preparation or follow-up care is required.

b. Instruct the client that he or she will be positioned in a confined space and will need to keep the head still during the procedure.

C. Slit lamp

1. Description

a. A slit lamp allows examination of the anterior ocular structures under microscopic magnification.

b. The client leans on a chin rest to stabilize the head while a narrowed beam of light is aimed so that it illuminates only a narrow segment of the eye.

2. Interventions

a. Explain the procedure to the client.

b. Advise the client about the brightness of the light and the need to look forward at a point over the examiner's ear.

D. Corneal staining

1. Description

a. A topical dye is instilled into the conjunctival sac to outline irregularities of the corneal surface that are not easily visible.

b. The eye is viewed through a blue filter, and a bright green color indicates areas of a nonintact corneal epithelium.

2. Interventions

a. If the client wears contact lenses, the lenses must be removed.

b. The client is instructed to blink after the dye has been applied to distribute the dye evenly across the cornea.

E. Tonometry

1. Description: The test is used primarily to assess for an increase of intraocular pressure and potential **glaucoma**.

2. Noncontact tonometry

a. No direct contact with the client's cornea is needed and no topical eye anesthetic is needed.

b. A puff of air is directed at the cornea to indent the cornea, which can be unpleasant and may startle the client.

c. It is a less accurate method of measurement as compared with contact tonometry.

3. Contact tonometry

a. Requires a topical anesthetic

b. A flattened cone is brought into contact with the cornea and the amount of pressure needed to flatten the cornea is measured.

c. The client must be instructed to avoid rubbing the eye following the examination if

Box 64-1 Risk Factors for Eye Disorders

Aging process	Hereditary
Congenital	Medications
Diabetes mellitus	Trauma

the eye has been anesthetized because of the potential for scratching the cornea.

⚠ Normal intraocular pressure is 10 to 21 mm Hg; intraocular pressure varies throughout the day and is normally higher in the morning (always document the time of intraocular pressure measurement).

F. Ultrasound: Procedure is similar to an ultrasound procedure done in other parts of the body and is done to detect lesions or tumors in the eye.

G. Magnetic resonance imaging (MRI): Similar to an MRI done in other parts of the body; refer to Chapter 66 for additional information on MRI.

IV. DISORDERS OF THE EYE

A. Risk factors related to eye disorders (Box 64-1)

B. Refractive errors

1. Description

a. Refraction is the bending of light rays; any problem associated with eye length or refraction can lead to refractive errors.

b. **Myopia** (nearsightedness): Refractive ability of the eye is too strong for the eye length; images are bent and fall in front of, not on, the retina.

c. **Hyperopia** (farsightedness): Refractive ability of the eye is too weak; images are focused behind the retina.

d. Presbyopia: Loss of lens elasticity because of aging; less able to focus the eye for close work and images fall behind the retina.

e. **Astigmatism**: Occurs because of the irregular curvature of the cornea; image focuses at two different points on the retina.

2. Assessment

a. Refractive errors are diagnosed through a process called refraction.

b. The client views an eye chart while various lenses of different strengths are systematically placed in front of the eye and is asked whether the lenses sharpen or worsen the vision.

3. Nonsurgical interventions: Eyeglasses or contact lenses

4. Surgical interventions

a. Radial keratotomy: Incisions are made through the peripheral cornea to flatten the cornea, which allows the image to be focused closer to the retina; used to treat **myopia**.

b. Photorefractive keratotomy: A laser beam is used to remove small portions of the corneal surface to reshape the cornea to focus an image properly on the retina; used to treat **myopia** and **astigmatism**.

c. Laser-assisted in-situ keratomileusis (LASIK): The superficial layers of the cornea are lifted as a flap, a laser reshapes the deeper corneal layers, and then the corneal flap is replaced; used to treat **hyperopia**, **myopia**, and **astigmatism**.

d. Corneal ring: The shape of the cornea is changed by placing a flexible ring in the outer edges of the cornea; used to treat **myopia**.

C. Legally blind

1. Description: The best visual acuity with corrective lenses in the better eye of 20/200 or less, or the visual field is no greater than 20 degrees in its widest diameter in the better eye

2. Interventions

a. When speaking to the client who has limited sight or is blind, the nurse uses a normal tone of voice.

b. Alert the client when approaching.

c. Orient the client to the environment.

d. Use a focal point and provide further orientation to the environment from that focal point.

e. Allow the client to touch objects in the room.

f. Use the clock placement of foods on the meal tray to orient the client.

g. Promote independence as much as is possible.

h. Provide radios, televisions, and clocks that give the time orally, or provide a Braille watch.

i. When ambulating, allow the client to grasp the nurse's arm at the elbow; the nurse keeps his or her arm close to the body so that the client can detect the direction of movement.

j. Instruct the client to remain one step behind the nurse when ambulating.

k. Instruct the client in the use of the cane for the blind, which is differentiated from other canes by its straight shape and white color with red tip.

l. Instruct the client that the cane is held in the dominant hand several inches off the floor.

m. Instruct the client that the cane sweeps the ground where the client's foot will be placed next to determine the presence of obstacles.

D. Cataracts (Fig. 64-2)

1. Description

a. A **cataract** is an opacity of the lens that distorts the image projected onto the retina and that can progress to blindness.

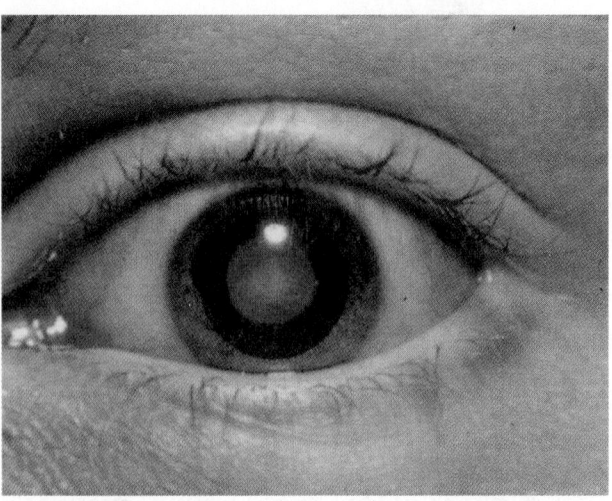

▲ FIGURE 64-2 The cloudy appearance of a lens affected by cataract. (From Black, J., & Hawks, J. [2009]. *Medical-surgical nursing: Clinical management for positive outcomes* [8th ed.]. St. Louis: Saunders. Courtesy of Ophthalmic Photography at the University of Michigan, W.K. Kellogg Eye Center, Ann Arbor, MI.)

b. Causes include the aging process (senile **cataracts**), inherited (congenital **cataracts**), and injury (traumatic **cataracts**); **cataracts** also can result from another eye disease (secondary **cataracts**).

c. Causes of secondary **cataracts** include diabetes mellitus, maternal rubella, severe **myopia**, ultraviolet light exposure, and medications such as corticosteroids.

d. Intervention is indicated when visual acuity has been reduced to a level that the client finds to be unacceptable or adversely affects his or her lifestyle.

2. Assessment

a. Blurred vision and decreased color perception are early signs

b. Diplopia, reduced visual acuity, absence of the red reflex, and the presence of a white pupil are late signs. Pain or eye redness is associated with age-related **cataract** formation.

c. Loss of vision is gradual.

3. Interventions

a. Surgical removal of the lens, one eye at a time, is performed.

b. With extracapsular extraction, the lens is lifted out without removing the lens capsule; the procedure may be performed by phacoemulsification, in which the lens is broken up by ultrasonic vibrations and extracted.

c. With intracapsular extraction, the lens and capsule are removed completely.

d. A partial iridectomy may be performed with the lens extraction to prevent acute secondary **glaucoma**.

e. A lens implantation may be performed at the time of the surgical procedure.

Box 64-2 Client Education Following Cataract Surgery

Avoid eye straining.

Avoid rubbing or placing pressure on the eyes.

Avoid rapid movements, straining, sneezing, coughing, bending, vomiting, or lifting objects heavier than 5 lb.

Take measures to prevent constipation.

Follow instructions for dressing changes and prescribed eye drops and medications.

Wipe excess drainage or tearing with a sterile wet cotton ball from the inner to the outer canthus.

Use an eye shield at bedtime.

If lens implantation is not performed, accommodation is affected and glasses must be worn at all times.

Cataract glasses act as magnifying glasses and replace central vision only.

Because cataract glasses magnify, objects will appear closer; therefore, the client needs to accommodate, judge distance, and climb stairs carefully.

Contact lenses provide sharp visual acuity but dexterity is needed to insert them.

Contact the physician about any decrease in vision, severe eye pain, or increase in eye discharge.

4. Preoperative interventions
   a. Instruct the client regarding the postoperative measures to prevent or decrease intraocular pressure, such as bending over, coughing, straining, and rubbing the eye.
   b. Stress to the client that care after surgery requires instillation of different types of eye drops several times a day for 2 to 4 weeks.
   c. Administer eye medications preoperatively, including **mydriatics** and cycloplegics as prescribed.
5. Postoperative interventions
   a. Elevate the head of the bed 30 to 45 degrees.
   b. Turn the client to the back or nonoperative side.
   c. Maintain an eye patch as prescribed; orient the client to the environment.
   d. Position the client's personal belongings to the nonoperative side.
   e. Use side rails for safety.
   f. Assist with ambulation.
6. Client education (Box 64-2)

E. Glaucoma

1. Description
   a. A group of ocular diseases resulting in increased intraocular pressure
   b. Intraocular pressure is the fluid (aqueous humor) pressure within the eye (normal intraocular pressure is 10 to 21 mm Hg).
   c. Increased intraocular pressure results from inadequate drainage of aqueous humor from the canal of Schlemm or overproduction of aqueous humor.
   d. The condition damages the optic nerve and can result in blindness.
   e. The gradual loss of visual fields may go unnoticed because central vision is unaffected.
2. Types
   a. Primary open-angle **glaucoma** (POAG) results from obstruction to outflow of aqueous humor and is the most common type.
   b. Primary angle-closure **glaucoma** (PACG) results from blocking the outflow of aqueous humor into the trabecular meshwork; causes include lens or pupil dilation from medications or sympathetic stimulation.
3. Assessment
   a. Early signs include diminished **accommodation** and increased intraocular pressure.
   b. Primary open-angle **glaucoma** (POAG): Painless, and vision changes are slow; results in "tunnel" vision.
   c. Primary angle-closure **glaucoma** (PACG): Blurred vision, halos around lights, and ocular erythema.
4. Interventions for acute angle-closure **glaucoma**

⚠ Acute angle-closure glaucoma is a medical emergency that causes sudden eye pain and possible nausea and vomiting.

   a. Treat acute angle-closure **glaucoma** as a medical emergency.
   b. Administer medications as prescribed to lower intraocular pressure.
   c. Prepare the client for peripheral iridectomy, which allows aqueous humor to flow from the posterior to the anterior chamber.
5. Interventions for the client with **glaucoma**
   a. Instruct the client on the importance of medications to constrict the pupils (**miotics**), to decrease the production of aqueous humor (carbonic anhydrase inhibitors), and to decrease the production of aqueous humor and intraocular pressure (β-blockers).
   b. Instruct the client of the need for lifelong medication use.
   c. Instruct the client to wear a Medic-Alert bracelet.
   d. Instruct the client to avoid anticholinergic medications.
   e. Instruct the client to report eye pain, halos around the eyes, and changes in vision to the physician.
   f. Instruct the client that when maximal medical therapy has failed to halt the progression of visual field loss and optic nerve damage, surgery will be recommended.

g. Instruct the client to contact the physician before taking medications, including over-the-counter medications.

h. Prepare the client for trabeculoplasty as prescribed to facilitate aqueous humor drainage.

i. Prepare the client for trabeculectomy as prescribed, which allows drainage of aqueous humor into the conjunctival spaces by the creation of an opening.

F. Retinal detachment

1. Description

a. Detachment or separation of the retina from the epithelium

b. **Retinal detachment** occurs when the layers of the retina separate because of the accumulation of fluid between them, or when both retinal layers elevate away from the choroid as a result of a tumor.

c. Partial detachment becomes complete if untreated.

d. When detachment becomes complete, blindness occurs.

2. Assessment

a. Flashes of light

b. Floaters or black spots (signs of bleeding)

c. Increase in blurred vision

d. Sense of a curtain being drawn over the eye

e. Loss of a portion of the visual field; painless loss of central or peripheral vision

3. Immediate interventions

a. Provide bedrest.

b. Cover both eyes with patches as prescribed to prevent further detachment.

c. Speak to the client before approaching.

d. Position the client's head as prescribed.

e. Protect the client from injury.

f. Avoid jerky head movements.

g. Minimize eye stress.

h. Prepare the client for a surgical procedure as prescribed.

4. Surgical procedures

a. Draining fluid from the subretinal space so that the retina can return to the normal position

b. Sealing retinal breaks by cryosurgery, a cold probe applied to the sclera, to stimulate an inflammatory response leading to adhesions

c. Diathermy, the use of an electrode needle and heat through the sclera, to stimulate an inflammatory response

d. Laser therapy, to stimulate an inflammatory response and seal small retinal tears before the detachment occurs

e. Scleral buckling, to hold the choroid and retina together with a splint until scar tissue forms, closing the tear (Fig. 64-3)

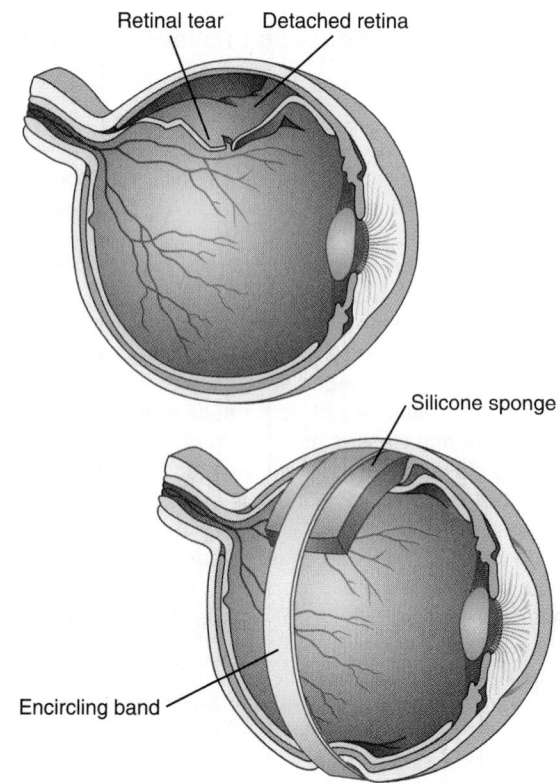

▲ **FIGURE 64-3** The scleral buckling procedure for repair of retinal detachment. (From Ignatavicius, D., & Workman, M. [2010]. *Medical-surgical nursing: Patient-centered collaborative care* [6th ed.]. St. Louis: Saunders.)

f. Insertion of gas or silicone oil to promote reattachment; these agents float against the retina to hold it in place until healing occurs.

5. Postoperative interventions

a. Maintain eye patches as prescribed.

b. Monitor for hemorrhage.

c. Prevent nausea and vomiting and monitor for restlessness, which can cause hemorrhage.

d. Monitor for sudden, sharp eye pain (notify the physician).

e. Encourage deep breathing but avoid coughing.

f. Provide bedrest for 1 to 2 days as prescribed.

g. Position the client as prescribed (positioning depends on the location of the detachment).

h. Administer eye medications as prescribed.

i. Assist the client with activities of daily living.

j. Avoid sudden head movements or anything that increases intraocular pressure.

k. Instruct the client to limit reading for 3 to 5 weeks.

l. Instruct the client to avoid squinting, straining and constipation, lifting heavy objects, and bending from the waist.

m. Instruct the client to wear dark glasses during the day and an eye patch at night.

n. Encourage follow-up care because of the danger of recurrence or occurrence in the other eye.

G. Macular degeneration
1. A deterioration of the macula, the area of central vision
2. Can be atrophic (age-related or dry) or exudative (wet)
3. Age-related: Caused by gradual blocking of retinal capillaries leading to an ischemic and necrotic macula; rods and cones photoreceptors die.
4. Exudative: Serous detachment of pigment epithelium in the macula occurs; fluid and blood collect under the macula, resulting in scar formation and visual distortion.
5. Interventions are aimed at maximizing the remaining vision.
6. Assessment
   a. A decline in central vision
   b. Blurred vision and distortion
7. Interventions
   a. Initiate strategies to assist in maximizing remaining vision and maintaining independence.
   b. Provide referrals to community organizations.
   c. Laser therapy, photodynamic therapy, or other therapies may be prescribed to seal the leaking blood vessels in or near the macula.

H. Ocular melanoma
1. Most common malignant eye tumor in adults
2. Tumor usually found in the uveal tract and can spread easily because of the rich blood supply
3. Assessment
   a. Tumor can be discovered during routine examination.
   b. If macular area is invaded, blurring of vision occurs.
   c. Increased intraocular pressure (IOP) is present if the canal of Schlemm is invaded.
   d. Change of iris color is noted if the tumor invades the iris.
   e. Ultrasonography may be performed to determine tumor size and location.
4. Interventions
   a. Enucleation: The entire eyeball is removed surgically and a ball implant is inserted to provide a base for a socket prosthesis.
   b. Radiation is given via a radioactive plaque that is sutured to the sclera; the radioactive plaque remains in place until the prescribed radiation dose is delivered.

I. Enucleation and exenteration
1. Description
   a. Enucleation is the removal of the entire eyeball.
   b. Exenteration is the removal of the eyeball and surrounding tissues and bone.
   c. The procedures are performed for the removal of ocular tumors.
   d. After the eye is removed, a ball implant is inserted to provide a firm base for a socket

prosthesis and to facilitate the best cosmetic result.
   e. A prosthesis is fitted about 1 month after surgery.
2. Preoperative interventions
   a. Provide emotional support to the client.
   b. Encourage the client to verbalize feelings related to loss.
3. Postoperative interventions
   a. Monitor vital signs.
   b. Assess a pressure patch or dressing as prescribed.
   c. Report changes in vital signs or the presence of bright red drainage on the pressure patch or dressing.

J. Hyphema
1. Description
   a. Presence of blood in the anterior chamber that occurs as a result of an injury
   b. The condition usually resolves in 5 to 7 days.
2. Interventions
   a. Encourage rest with the client in a semi-Fowler's position.
   b. Avoid sudden eye movements for 3 to 5 days to decrease the likelihood of bleeding.
   c. Administer cycloplegic eye drops as prescribed to relax the eye muscles and place the eye at rest.
   d. Instruct the client in the use of eye shields or eye patches as prescribed.
   e. Instruct the client to restrict reading and limit watching television.

K. Contusions
1. Description
   a. Bleeding into the soft tissue as a result of an injury.
   b. A contusion causes a black eye; the discoloration disappears in about 10 days.
   c. Pain, photophobia, edema, and diplopia may occur.
2. Interventions
   a. Place ice on the eye immediately.
   b. Instruct the client to receive a thorough eye examination.

L. Foreign bodies
1. Description: An object such as dust or dirt that enters the eye and causes irritation
2. Interventions
   a. Have the client look upward, expose the lower lid, wet a cotton-tipped applicator with sterile normal saline, gently twist the swab over the particle, and remove it.
   b. If the particle cannot be seen, have the client look downward, place a cotton applicator horizontally on the outer surface of the upper eye lid, grasp the lashes, and pull the upper

lid outward and over the cotton applicator; if the particle is seen, gently twist a swab over it to remove.

M. Penetrating objects
1. Description: An eye injury in which an object penetrates the eye
2. Interventions
   a. Never remove the object because it may be holding ocular structures in place; the object must be removed by the physician.
   b. Cover the object with a cup.
   c. Do not allow the client to bend over or lie flat; these positions may move the object.
   d. Do not place pressure on the eye.
   e. Client is to be seen by a physician immediately.
   f. X-rays and CT scans of the orbit are usually obtained.
   g. Magnetic resonance imaging (MRI) is contraindicated because of the possibility of metal-containing projectile movement during the procedure.

N. Chemical burns (see Priority Nursing Actions)
1. Description: An eye injury in which a caustic substance enters the eye
2. Interventions

⚠ If a chemical splash to the eye occurs, treatment should begin immediately; immediately flush the eyes at the scene of the injury with water for at least 15 to 20 minutes.

   a. At the scene of the injury, obtain a sample of the chemical involved.
   b. At the emergency department, the eye is irrigated with normal saline solution or an ophthalmic irrigation solution for at least 10 minutes or longer as prescribed; the pH is then checked.
   c. The solution is directed across the cornea and toward the lateral canthus.
   d. Prepare for visual acuity assessment.
   e. Apply an antibiotic ointment as prescribed.
   f. Cover the eye with a patch as prescribed.

O. Eye (tissue) donation
1. Donor eyes
   a. Donor eyes are obtained from cadavers.
   b. Donor eyes must be enucleated soon after death because of rapid endothelial cell death.
   c. Donor eyes must be stored in a preserving solution.
   d. Storage, handling, and coordination of donor tissue with surgeons is provided by a network of state eye bank associations.
2. Care to the deceased client as a potential eye donor
   a. Discuss the option of eye donation with the physician and family.

Box 64-3 Signs of Graft Rejection Following Corneal Transplantation: RSVP

Redness	**V**isual acuity decreased
Swelling	**P**ain

---

   b. Raise the head of the bed 30 degrees.
   c. Instill antibiotic eye drops as prescribed.
   d. Close the eyes and apply a small ice pack to the closed eyes.
3. Preoperative care to the recipient of the cornea
   a. Recipient may be told of the tissue (cornea) availability only several hours to 1 day before the surgery.
   b. Assist in alleviating client anxiety.
   c. Assess the recipient's eye for signs of infection.
   d. Report the presence of any redness, watery or purulent drainage, or edema around the recipient's eye to the physician.
   e. Instill antibiotic drops into the recipient's eye as prescribed to reduce the number of microorganisms present.
   f. Administer fluids and medications intravenously as prescribed.
4. Postoperative care to the recipient
   a. Eye is covered with a pressure patch and protective shield that is left in place for 1 day.
   b. Do not remove or change the dressing without a physician's prescription.
   c. Monitor vital signs.
   d. Monitor level of consciousness.
   e. Assess the eye dressing.
   f. Position the client with the head elevated and on the nonoperative side to reduce intraocular pressure.
   g. Orient the client frequently.
   h. Monitor for complications of bleeding, wound leakage, infection, and tissue rejection.
   i. Instruct the client how to apply a patch and eye shield.
   j. Instruct the client to wear the eye shield at night for 1 month and whenever around small children or pets.
   k. Advise the client not to rub the eye.
5. Graft rejection (Box 64-3; Fig. 64-4)
   a. Rejection can occur at any time.
   b. Inform the client of the signs of rejection.
   c. Signs include *r*edness, *s*welling, *d*ecreased vision, and *p*ain (RSVP).
   d. The eye is treated with topical corticosteroids.

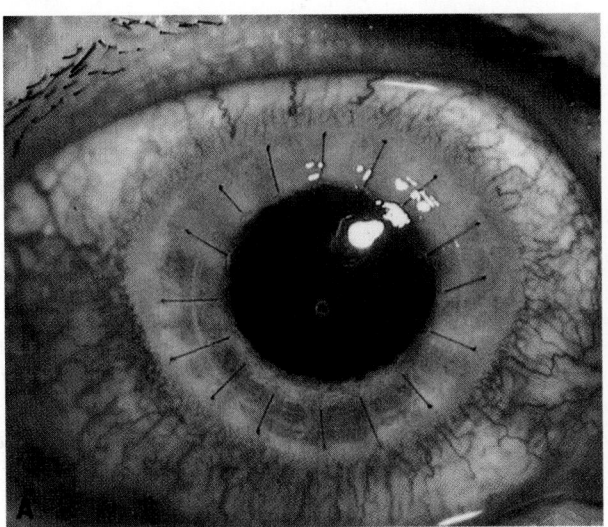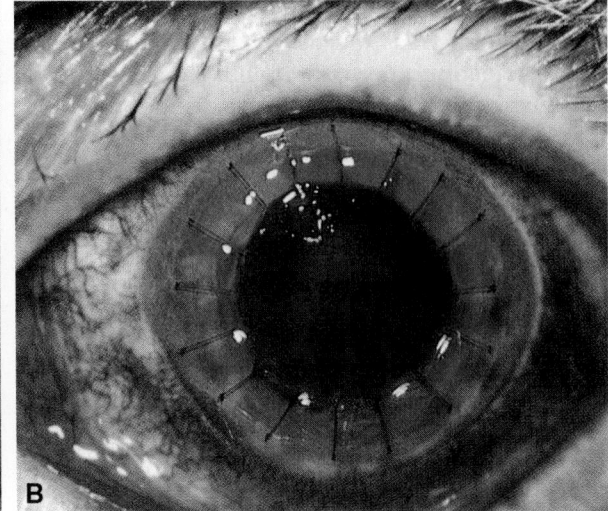

▲ **FIGURE 64-4** Graft rejection. **A,** Clinical appearance of the eye after keratoplasty. **B,** Acute graft rejection. (From Black, J., & Hawks, J. [2009]. *Medical-surgical nursing: Clinical management for positive outcomes* [8th ed.]. St. Louis: Saunders. Courtesy of Ophthalmic Photography at the University of Michigan, W.K. Kellogg Eye Center, Ann Arbor, MI.)

▬▬▬ PRIORITY NURSING ACTIONS! ▬▬▬

Actions to Take if a Client Sustains a Chemical Eye Injury

1. Irrigate the eye.
2. Check the pH of the eye.
3. Assess visual acuity.
4. Document the event, actions taken, and the client's response.

Emergency care following a chemical burn to the eye includes irrigating the eye immediately with sterile normal saline or ocular irrigating solution. If the injury occurred outside the hospital, the eye is irrigated immediately with tap water and then the client is brought to the emergency department. In the emergency department, the irrigation should be maintained for at least 10 minutes (and at least 1 liter should be used to irrigate). After irrigation, the pH of the eye is checked and, if a pH of 6 to 7 has not returned, the irrigation should be continued. Some physician's prefer the use of lactated Ringer's solution for irrigation because its pH is 6 to 7.5, which is closer to the pH of tears (7.1) than that of normal saline, which may range from 4.5 to 7.

Following this emergency treatment, visual acuity is assessed. It is also important for the nurse to find out what chemical splashed into the eye.

Finally, the event is documented, as well as the actions taken and the client's response.

References: Black, J., & Hawks, J. (2009). *Medical-surgical nursing: Clinical management for positive outcomes* (8th ed., pp. 1252, 2206). St. Louis: Saunders.
Proehl, J. (2009). *Emergency nursing procedures* (4th ed., p. 756). St. Louis: Saunders.

V. ANATOMY AND PHYSIOLOGY OF THE EAR

A. Functions
   1. Hearing
   2. Maintenance of balance
B. External ear (pinna)
   1. The external ear is embedded in the temporal bone bilaterally at the level of the eyes.
   2. The external ear extends from the auricle through the external canal to the tympanic membrane or eardrum.
   3. The external ear includes the mastoid process, the bony ridge located over the temporal bone.
C. Middle ear
   1. The middle ear consists of the medial side of the tympanic membrane.
   2. The middle ear contains three bony ossicles.
      a. Malleus
      b. Incus
      c. Stapes
   3. Functions of the middle ear
      a. Conduct sound vibrations from the outer ear to the central hearing apparatus in the inner ear
      b. Protect the inner ear by reducing the amplitude of loud sounds
      c. The auditory canal (eustachian tube) allows equalization of air pressure on each side of the tympanic membrane so that the membrane does not rupture.
D. Inner ear
   1. The inner ear contains the semicircular canals, cochlea, and distal end of the eighth cranial nerve.

2. The semicircular canals contain fluid and hair cells connected to sensory nerve fibers of the vestibular portion of the eighth cranial nerve.
3. The inner ear maintains sense of balance or equilibrium.
4. The cochlea is the spiral-shaped organ of hearing.
5. The organ of Corti (within the cochlea) is the receptor and organ of hearing.
6. Eighth cranial nerve
   a. The cochlear branch of the nerve transmits neuroimpulses from the cochlea to the brain, where they are interpreted as sound.
   b. The vestibular branch maintains balance and equilibrium.
E. Hearing and equilibrium
1. The external ear conducts sound waves to the middle ear.
2. The middle ear, also called the tympanic cavity, conducts sound waves to the inner ear.
3. The middle ear is filled with air, which is kept at atmospheric pressure by the opening of the auditory canal.
4. The inner ear contains sensory receptors for sound and for equilibrium.
5. The receptors in the inner ear transmit sound waves and changes in body position to the nerve impulses.

VI. ASSESSMENT OF THE EAR (also see Chapter 34)

A. Otoscopic examination
1. The client's head is tilted slightly away and the otoscope is held upside down as if it were a large pen; this permits the examiner's hand to lay against the client's head for support.
2. In an adult, pull the pinna up and back to straighten the external canal.
3. Visualize the external canal while slowly inserting the speculum.
4. The normal external canal is pink and intact, without lesions and with varying amounts of cerumen and fine little hairs.
5. Assess the tympanic membrane for intactness; the normal tympanic membrane is intact, without perforations, and should be free from lesions.
6. The tympanic membrane is transparent, opaque, pearly gray, and slightly concave.
7. A fluid line or the presence of air bubbles is not normally visible.
8. If the tympanic membrane is bulging or retracting, the edges of the light reflex will be fuzzy (diffuse) and may spread over the tympanic membrane.

⚠ The otoscope is never introduced blindly into the external canal because of the risk of perforating the tympanic membrane.

B. Auditory assessment
1. Sound is transmitted by air conduction and bone conduction.
2. Air conduction takes two or three times longer than bone conduction.
3. Hearing loss is categorized as **conductive**, **sensorineural**, or mixed **conductive** and **sensorineural**.
4. **Conductive hearing loss** is caused by any physical obstruction to the transmission of sound waves.
5. **Sensorineural hearing loss** is caused by a defect in the cochlea, eighth cranial nerve, or the brain itself.
6. A mixed **conductive-sensorineural hearing loss** results in profound hearing loss.

C. Voice test
1. Ask the client to block one external canal.
2. The examiner stands 1 to 2 feet away and whispers a statement.
3. The client is asked to repeat the whispered statement.
4. Each ear is tested separately.

D. Watch test
1. A ticking watch is used to test for high-frequency sounds.
2. The examiner holds a ticking watch about 5 inches from each ear and asks the client if the ticking is heard.

E. Tuning fork tests
1. Weber's tuning fork test
   a. Place the vibrating tuning fork stem in the middle of the client's head, at the midline of the forehead, or above the upper lip over the teeth.
   b. Hold the fork by the stem only.
   c. The client is asked whether the sound is heard equally in both ears or whether the sound is louder in one ear.
   d. Normal test result is hearing the sound equally in both ears.
   e. If the client hears the sound louder in one ear, the term *lateralization* is applied to the side that hears the loudest.
   f. Such a finding may indicate that the client has a **conductive hearing loss** in the ear to which the sound is lateralized or that **sensorineural hearing loss** has occurred in the opposite ear.
2. Rinne tuning fork test
   a. The test compares the client's hearing by air conduction and bone conduction.
   b. Air conduction is two or three times longer than bone conduction.
   c. The vibrating tuning fork stem is placed on the client's mastoid process and the client is asked to indicate when he or she no longer hears the sound.

d. The examiner quickly brings the tuning fork in front of the pinna without touching the client and asks the client to indicate whether he or she still hears the sound.

e. The client normally continues to hear the sound two times longer in front of the pinna; such results are a positive Rinne test.

f. The examiner records the duration of both phases, bone conduction followed by air conduction, and compares the times.

g. If the client is unable to hear the sound through the ear in front of the pinna, the client may have a **conductive hearing loss** on the side tested; in this situation, the bone conduction is greater than the air conduction (negative Rinne test).

h. Both the Rinne test and the Weber tuning fork test are limited in distinguishing between **conductive** and **sensorineural hearing losses**.

F. Vestibular assessment
   1. Test for falling
      a. The examiner asks the client to stand with the feet together, arms hanging loosely at the side, and eyes closed.
      b. The client normally remains erect, with only slight swaying.
      c. A significant sway is a positive Romberg sign.
   2. Test for past pointing
      a. The client sits in front of the examiner.
      b. The client closes the eyes and extends the arms in front, pointing both index fingers at the examiner.
      c. The examiner holds and touches his or her own extended index fingers under the client's extended index fingers to give the client a point of reference.
      d. The client is instructed to raise both arms and then lower them, attempting to return to the examiner's extended index fingers.
      e. The normal test response is that the client can easily return to the point of reference.
      f. The client with a vestibular function problem lacks a normal sense of position and cannot return the extended fingers to the point of reference; instead, the fingers deviate to the right or left of the reference point.
   3. Gaze nystagmus evaluation
      a. The client's eyes are examined as the client looks straight ahead, 30 degrees to each side, upward and downward.
      b. Any spontaneous nystagmus—an involuntary, rhythmic, rapid twitching of the eyeballs—represents a problem with the vestibular system.
   4. Dix-Hallpike maneuver
      a. The client starts in a sitting position; the examiner lowers the client to the exam table

and rather quickly turns the client's head to 45 degrees position.

b. If after about 30 seconds there is no nystagmus, the client is returned to a sitting position and the test is repeated on the other side.

VII. DIAGNOSTIC TESTS FOR THE EAR

A. Tomography
   1. Description
      a. Tomography may be performed with or without contrast medium.
      b. Tomography assesses the mastoid, middle ear, and inner ear structures.
      c. Multiple radiographs of the head are obtained.
      d. Tomography is especially helpful in the diagnosis of acoustic tumors.
   2. Interventions
      a. All jewelry is removed.
      b. Lead eye shields are used to cover the cornea to diminish the radiation dose to the eyes.
      c. The client must remain still in a supine position.
      d. No follow-up care is required.

B. Audiometry
   1. Description
      a. Audiometry measures hearing acuity.
      b. Audiometry uses two types, pure tone audiometry and speech audiometry.
      c. Pure tone audiometry is used to identify problems with hearing, speech, music, and other sounds in the environment.
      d. In speech audiometry, the client's ability to hear spoken words is measured.
      e. After testing, audiographic patterns are depicted on a graph to determine the type and level of the hearing loss.
   2. Interventions
      a. Inform the client regarding the procedure.
      b. Instruct the client to identify the sounds as they are heard.

C. Electronystagmography (ENG)
   1. Description
      a. Electronystagmography is a vestibular test that evaluates spontaneous and induced eye movements known as nystagmus.
      b. ENG is used to distinguish between normal nystagmus and medication-induced nystagmus, or nystagmus caused by a lesion in the central or peripheral vestibular pathway.
      c. ENG records changing electrical fields with the movement of the eye, as monitored by electrodes placed on the skin around the eye.
   2. Interventions
      a. The client is instructed to remain NPO for 3 hours before testing, avoiding caffeine-containing beverages for 24 to 48 hours before the test.

b. Unnecessary medications are withheld for 24 hours before testing.

c. Instruct the client that this is a long and tiring procedure.

d. The client should bring prescription eyeglasses to the examination.

e. The client sits and is instructed to gaze at lights, focus on a moving pattern, focus on a moving point, and then close the eyes.

f. While sitting in a chair, the client may be rotated to obtain information about vestibular function.

g. In addition, the client's ears are irrigated with cool and warm water, which may cause nausea and vomiting.

h. Following the procedure, the client begins taking clear fluids slowly and cautiously because nausea and vomiting may occur.

i. Assistance with ambulation may also be necessary following the procedure.

D. Magnetic resonance imaging (MRI): Refer to Chapter 66 for information on MRI.

VIII. DISORDERS OF THE EAR

A. Risk factors related to ear disorders (Box 64-4)

B. **Conductive hearing loss**
   1. Description
      a. **Conductive hearing loss** occurs when sound waves are blocked to the inner ear fibers because of external or middle ear disorders.
      b. Disorders often can be corrected with no damage to hearing or minimal permanent hearing loss.
   2. Causes
      a. Any inflammatory process or obstruction of the external or middle ear
      b. Tumors
      c. **Otosclerosis**
      d. A buildup of scar tissue on the ossicles from previous middle ear surgery

C. **Sensorineural hearing loss**
   1. Description
      a. **Sensorineural hearing loss** is a pathological process of the inner ear or of the sensory fibers that lead to the cerebral cortex.
      b. **Sensorineural hearing loss** is often permanent, and measures must be taken to reduce further damage.
   2. Causes
      a. Damage to the inner ear structures
      b. Damage to the eighth cranial nerve or brain itself

c. Prolonged exposure to loud noise
d. Medications
e. Trauma
f. Inherited disorders
g. Metabolic and circulatory disorders
h. Infections
i. Surgery
j. **Meniere's syndrome**
k. Diabetes mellitus
l. Myxedema

D. Mixed hearing loss
   1. Mixed hearing loss also is known as **conductive-sensorineural hearing loss**.
   2. Client has **sensorineural** and **conductive hearing loss**.

E. Central hearing loss: Involves the inability to interpret sound, including speech, due to a problem in the brain.

F. Signs of hearing loss and facilitating communication (Boxes 64-5 and 64-6)

G. Cochlear implantation (Fig. 64-5)
   1. Cochlear implants are used for **sensorineural hearing loss**.
   2. A small computer converts sound waves into electrical impulses.
   3. Electrodes are placed by the internal ear with a computer device attached to the external ear.
   4. Electronic impulses directly stimulate nerve fibers.

H. Hearing aids
   1. Hearing aids are used for the client with **conductive hearing loss**.
   2. Hearing aids have limited value for the client with **sensorineural hearing loss**, because they only make sounds louder, not clearer.
   3. A difficulty that exists in the use of hearing aids is the amplification of background noise and voices.
   4. Client education (Box 64-7)

I. Presbycusis
   1. Description
      a. Presbycusis is a **sensorineural hearing loss** associated with aging.

Box 64-4 Risk Factors for Ear Disorders

Aging process	Ototoxicity
Infection	Trauma
Medications	Tumors

Box 64-5 Signs of Hearing Loss

Frequently asking others to repeat statements
Straining to hear
Turning head or leaning forward to favor one ear
Shouting in conversation
Ringing in the ears
Failing to respond when not looking in the direction of the sound
Answering questions incorrectly
Raising the volume of the television or radio
Avoiding large groups
Better understanding of speech when in small groups
Withdrawing from social interactions

b. **Presbycusis** leads to degeneration or atrophy of the ganglion cells in the cochlea and a loss of elasticity of the basilar membranes.

c. **Presbycusis** leads to compromise of the vascular supply to the inner ear, with changes in several areas of the ear structure.

2. Assessment
   a. Hearing loss is gradual and bilateral.
   b. Client states that he or she has no problem with hearing but cannot understand what the words are.
   c. Client thinks that the speaker is mumbling.

Box 64-6 Facilitating Communication

Using written words if the client is able to see, read, and write

Providing plenty of light in the room

Getting the attention of the client before beginning to speak

Facing the client when speaking

Talking in a room without distracting noises

Moving close to the client and speaking slowly and clearly

Keeping hands and other objects away from the mouth when talking to the client

Talking in normal volume and at a lower pitch because shouting is not helpful and higher frequencies are less easily heard

Rephrasing sentences and repeating information

Validating with the client the understanding of statements made by asking the client to repeat what was said

Reading lips

Encouraging the client to wear glasses when talking to someone to improve vision for lip reading

Using sign language, which combines speech with hand movements that signify letters, words, or phrases

Using telephone amplifiers

Using flashing lights that are activated by ringing of the telephone or doorbell

Using specially trained dogs to help the client be aware of sound and alert the client to potential danger

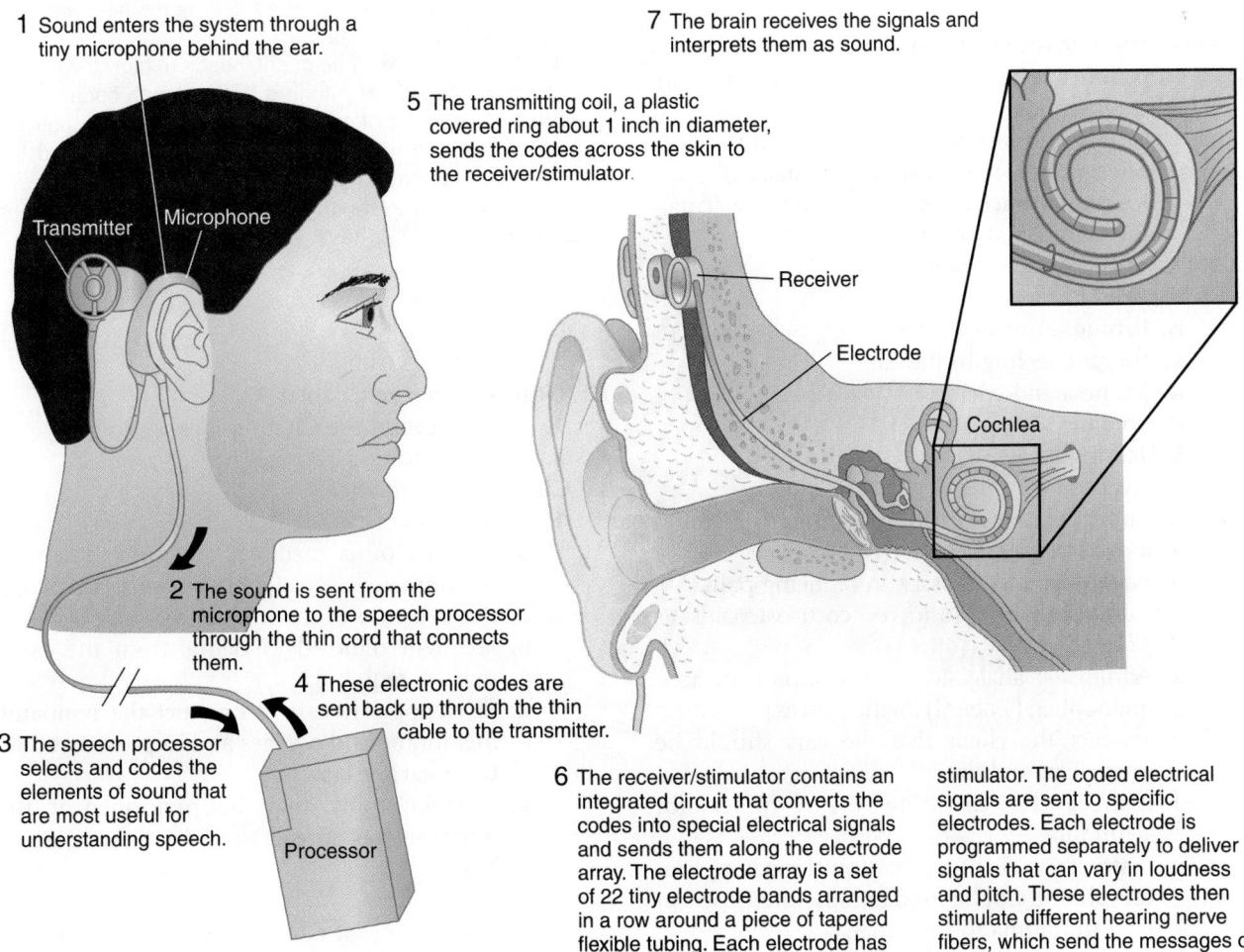

1 Sound enters the system through a tiny microphone behind the ear.

7 The brain receives the signals and interprets them as sound.

5 The transmitting coil, a plastic covered ring about 1 inch in diameter, sends the codes across the skin to the receiver/stimulator.

Transmitter   Microphone

Receiver

Electrode

Cochlea

2 The sound is sent from the microphone to the speech processor through the thin cord that connects them.

4 These electronic codes are sent back up through the thin cable to the transmitter.

3 The speech processor selects and codes the elements of sound that are most useful for understanding speech.

Processor

6 The receiver/stimulator contains an integrated circuit that converts the codes into special electrical signals and sends them along the electrode array. The electrode array is a set of 22 tiny electrode bands arranged in a row around a piece of tapered flexible tubing. Each electrode has a wire connecting it to the receiver/ stimulator. The coded electrical signals are sent to specific electrodes. Each electrode is programmed separately to deliver signals that can vary in loudness and pitch. These electrodes then stimulate different hearing nerve fibers, which send the messages on to the brain.

▲ **FIGURE 64-5** Cochlear implant to restore hearing. (From Black, J., & Hawks, J. [2009]. *Medical-surgical nursing: Clinical management for positive outcomes* [8th ed.]. St. Louis: Saunders.)

Box 64-7 Client Education Regarding a Hearing Aid

Begin using the hearing aid slowly to adjust to the device.
Adjust the volume to the minimal hearing level to prevent feedback squealing.
Concentrate on the sounds that are to be heard and to filter out background noise.
Clean the ear mold with mild soap and water.
Avoid excessive wetting of the hearing aid and try to keep the hearing aid dry.
Clean the ear cannula of the hearing aid with a toothpick or pipe cleaner.

Turn the hearing aid off before removing from the ear to prevent squealing feedback; remove the battery when not in use.
Keep extra batteries on hand.
Keep the hearing aid in a safe place.
Prevent hair sprays, oils, or other hair and face products from coming into contact with the receiver of the hearing aid.

J. External otitis
　1. Description
　　a. External otitis is an infective inflammatory or allergic response involving the structure of the external auditory canal or auricles.
　　b. An irritating or infective agent comes into contact with the epithelial layer of the external ear.
　　c. Contact leads to an allergic response or signs and symptoms of an infection.
　　d. The skin becomes red, swollen, and tender to touch on movement.
　　e. The extensive swelling of the canal can lead to **conductive hearing loss** because of obstruction.
　　f. External otitis is more common in children; it is termed *swimmer's ear* and occurs more often in hot, humid environments.
　　g. Prevention includes the elimination of irritating or infecting agents.
　2. Assessment
　　a. Pain
　　b. Itching
　　c. Plugged feeling in the ear
　　d. Redness and edema
　　e. Exudate
　　f. Hearing loss
　3. Interventions
　　a. Apply heat locally for 20 minutes three times a day.
　　b. Encourage rest to assist in reducing pain.
　　c. Administer antibiotics or corticosteroids as prescribed.
　　d. Administer analgesics such as aspirin or acetaminophen (Tylenol) for the pain as prescribed.
　　e. Instruct the client that the ears should be kept clean and dry.
　　f. Instruct the client to use earplugs for swimming.
　　g. Instruct the client that cotton-tipped applicators should not be used because their use can lead to trauma to the canal.
　　h. Instruct the client that irritating agents such as hair products or headphones should be discontinued.

Box 64-8 Client Education Following Myringotomy

Avoid strenuous activities.
Avoid rapid head movements, bouncing, or bending.
Avoid straining on bowel movement.
Avoid drinking through a straw.
Avoid traveling by air.
Avoid forceful coughing.
Avoid contact with persons with colds.
Avoid washing hair, showering, or getting the head wet for 1 week as prescribed.
Instruct the client that if he or she needs to blow the nose, to blow one side at a time with the mouth open.
Instruct the client to keep ears dry by keeping a ball of cotton coated with petroleum jelly in the ear and to change the cotton ball daily.
Instruct the client to report excessive ear drainage to the physician.

K. Otitis media: See Chapter 37.
　1. Myringotomy: See Chapter 37.
　2. Client education (Box 64-8)
L. Chronic otitis media
　1. Description
　　a. Chronic otitis media is a chronic infective, inflammatory, or allergic response involving the structure of the middle ear.
　　b. Frequent removal of debris from the canal may be required.
　　c. Myringoplasty can reconstruct the tympanic membrane and ossicles and improve **conductive hearing loss**.
　　d. Mastoidectomy may be performed if the infection has spread to involve the mastoid bone.

 Monitor the client with otitis media closely for response to treatment. Otic and systemic antibiotics may be used to treat the infection, but often the organism is resistant.

2. Preoperative interventions
   a. Administer antibiotic drops as prescribed.
   b. Clean the ear of debris as prescribed; irrigate the ear with a solution of equal parts of vinegar and sterile water as prescribed to restore the normal pH of the ear.
   c. Instruct the client to avoid persons with upper respiratory infections.
   d. Instruct the client to obtain adequate rest, eat a balanced diet, and drink adequate fluids.
   e. Instruct the client in deep breathing and coughing; forceful coughing, which increases pressure in the middle ear, is to be avoided postoperatively.
3. Postoperative interventions
   a. Inform the client that initial hearing after surgery is diminished because of the packing in the ear canal; hearing improvement will occur after the ear canal packing is removed.
   b. Keep the dressing clean and dry.
   c. Keep the client flat, with the operative ear up for at least 12 hours.
   d. Administer antibiotics as prescribed.
M. Mastoiditis
   1. Description
      a. Mastoiditis may be acute or chronic and results from untreated or inadequately treated chronic or acute otitis media.
      b. The pain is not relieved by myringotomy.
   2. Assessment
      a. Swelling behind the ear and pain with minimal movement of the head
      b. Cellulitis on the skin or external scalp over the mastoid process
      c. A reddened, dull, thick, immobile tympanic membrane, with or without perforation
      d. Tender and enlarged postauricular lymph nodes
      e. Low-grade fever
      f. Malaise
      g. Anorexia
   3. Interventions
      a. Prepare the client for surgical removal of infected material.
      b. Monitor for complications.
      c. Simple or modified radical mastoidectomy with tympanoplasty is the most common treatment.
      d. Once tissue that is infected is removed, the tympanoplasty is performed to reconstruct the ossicles and tympanic membranes in an attempt to restore normal hearing.
   4. Complications
      a. Damage to the abducens and facial cranial nerves
      b. Damage is exhibited by inability to look laterally (cranial nerve VI, abducens) and a drooping of the mouth on the affected side (cranial nerve VII, facial).

   c. Meningitis
   d. Brain abscess
   e. Chronic purulent otitis media
   f. Wound infections
   g. Vertigo, if the infection spreads into the labyrinth
5. Postoperative interventions
   a. Monitor for dizziness.
   b. Monitor for signs of meningitis, as evidenced by a stiff neck and vomiting.
   c. Prepare for a wound dressing change 24 hours postoperatively.
   d. Monitor the surgical incision for edema, drainage, and redness.
   e. Position the client flat with the operative side up.
   f. Restrict the client to bed with bedside commode privileges for 24 hours as prescribed.
   g. Assist the client with getting out of bed to prevent falling or injuries from dizziness.
   h. With reconstruction of the ossicles via a graft, take precautions to prevent dislodging of the graft.
N. Otosclerosis
   1. Description
      a. **Otosclerosis** is a genetic disorder of the labyrinthine capsule of the middle ear that results in a bony overgrowth of the tissue surrounding the ossicles.
      b. **Otosclerosis** causes the development of irregular areas of new bone formation and causes the fixation of the bones.
      c. Stapes fixation leads to a **conductive hearing loss.**
      d. If the disease involves the inner ear, **sensorineural hearing loss** is present.
      e. Bilateral involvement is common, although hearing loss may be worse in one ear.
      f. It is thought to be a hereditary autosomal dominant disorder and is most commonly seen in young woman.
      g. Nonsurgical intervention promotes the improvement of hearing through amplification.
      h. Surgical intervention involves removal of the bony growth causing the hearing loss.
      i. A partial stapedectomy or complete stapedectomy with prosthesis (**fenestration**) may be performed surgically.
   2. Assessment
      a. Slowly progressing **conductive hearing loss**
      b. Bilateral hearing loss
      c. A ringing or roaring type of constant tinnitus
      d. Loud sounds heard in the ear when chewing
      e. Pinkish discoloration (Schwartze's sign) of the tympanic membrane, which indicates vascular changes within the ear.
      f. Negative Rinne test

g. Weber's test shows lateralization of sound to the ear with the most **conductive hearing loss**.

O. Fenestration

1. Description
   a. **Fenestration** is removal of the stapes, with a small hole drilled in the footplate; a prosthesis is connected between the incus and footplate.
   b. Sounds cause the prosthesis to vibrate in the same manner as the stapes.
   c. Complications include complete hearing loss, prolonged vertigo, infection, or facial nerve damage.
2. Preoperative interventions
   a. Instruct the client in measures to prevent middle ear or external ear infections.
   b. Instruct the client to avoid excessive nose blowing.
   c. Instruct the client not to clean the ear canal with cotton-tipped applicators and to avoid trauma or injury to the ear canal.
3. Postoperative interventions
   a. Inform the client that hearing is initially worse after the surgical procedure because of swelling and that no noticeable improvement in hearing may occur for as long as 6 weeks.
   b. Inform the client that the Gelfoam ear packing (if used) interferes with hearing but is used to decrease bleeding.
   c. Assist with ambulating during the first 1 to 2 days after surgery.
   d. Provide side rails when the client is in bed.
   e. Administer antibiotic, antivertiginous, and pain medications as prescribed.
   f. Assess for facial nerve damage, weakness, changes in tactile sensation and taste sensation, vertigo, nausea, and vomiting.
   g. Instruct the client to move the head slowly when changing positions to prevent vertigo.
   h. Instruct the client to avoid persons with upper respiratory tract infections.
   i. Instruct the client to avoid showering and getting the head and wound wet.
   j. Instruct the client to avoid using small objects (cotton-tipped applicators) to clean the external ear canal.
   k. Instruct the client to avoid rapid extreme changes in pressure caused by quick head movements, sneezing, nose blowing, straining, and changes in altitude.
   l. Instruct the client to avoid changes in middle ear pressure because they could dislodge the graft or prosthesis.

P. Labyrinthitis
1. Description: Infection of the labyrinth that occurs as a complication of acute or chronic otitis media

2. May result from growth of a cholesteatoma—benign overgrowth of squamous cell epithelium
3. Assessment
   a. Hearing loss that may be permanent on the affected side
   b. Tinnitus
   c. Spontaneous nystagmus to the affected side
   d. Vertigo
   e. Nausea and vomiting
4. Interventions
   a. Monitor for signs of meningitis, the most common complication, as evidenced by headache, stiff neck, and lethargy.
   b. Administer systemic antibiotics as prescribed.
   c. Advise the client to rest in bed in a darkened room.
   d. Administer antiemetics and antivertiginous medications as prescribed.
   e. Instruct the client that the vertigo subsides as the inflammation resolves.
   f. Instruct the client that balance problems that persist may require gait training through physical therapy.

Q. Meniere's syndrome
1. Description
   a. **Meniere's syndrome** is also called endolymphatic hydrops; it refers to dilation of the endolymphatic system by overproduction or decreased reabsorption of endolymphatic fluid.
   b. The syndrome is characterized by tinnitus, unilateral **sensorineural hearing loss**, and vertigo.
   c. Symptoms occur in attacks and last for several days, and the client becomes totally incapacitated during the attacks.
   d. Initial hearing loss is reversible but as the frequency of attacks continues, hearing loss becomes permanent.

⚠ A priority nursing intervention in the care of a client with Meniere's syndrome is instituting safety measures.

2. Causes
   a. Any factor that increases endolymphatic secretion in the labyrinth
   b. Viral and bacterial infections
   c. Allergic reactions
   d. Biochemical disturbances
   e. Vascular disturbance, producing changes in the microcirculation in the labyrinth
   f. Long-term stress may be a contributing factor.
3. Assessment
   a. Feelings of fullness in the ear
   b. Tinnitus, as a continuous low-pitched roar or humming sound, that is present much of the

time but worsens just before and during severe attacks

c. Hearing loss that is worse during an attack

d. Vertigo, periods of whirling, that might cause the client to fall to the ground

e. Vertigo that is so intense that even while lying down, the client holds the bed or ground in an attempt to prevent the whirling

f. Nausea and vomiting

g. Nystagmus

h. Severe headaches

4. Nonsurgical interventions

a. Prevent injury during vertigo attacks.

b. Provide bedrest in a quiet environment.

c. Provide assistance with walking.

d. Instruct the client to move the head slowly to prevent worsening of the vertigo.

e. Initiate sodium and fluid restrictions as prescribed.

f. Instruct the client to stop smoking.

g. Instruct the client to avoid watching television because the flickering of lights may exacerbate symptoms.

h. Administer nicotinic acid (niacin) as prescribed for its vasodilatory effect.

i. Administer antihistamines as prescribed to reduce the production of histamine and the inflammation.

j. Administer antiemetics as prescribed.

k. Administer tranquilizers and sedatives as prescribed to calm the client, allow the client to rest, and control vertigo, nausea, and vomiting.

l. Mild diuretics may be prescribed to decrease endolymph volume.

m. Inform the client about vestibular rehabilitation as prescribed.

5. Surgical interventions

a. Surgery is performed when medical therapy is ineffective and the functional level of the client has decreased significantly.

b. Endolymphatic drainage and insertion of a shunt may be performed early in the course of the disease to assist with the drainage of excess fluids.

c. A resection of the vestibular nerve or total removal of the labyrinth or a labyrinthectomy may be performed.

6. Postoperative interventions

a. Assess packing and dressing on the ear.

b. Speak to the client on the side of the unaffected ear.

c. Perform neurological assessments.

d. Maintain safety with the use of side rails.

e. Assist with ambulating.

f. Encourage the client to use a bedside commode rather than ambulating to the bathroom.

g. Administer antivertiginous and antiemetic medications as prescribed.

R. Acoustic neuroma

1. Description

a. An acoustic neuroma is a benign tumor of the vestibular or acoustic nerve.

b. The tumor may cause damage to hearing and to facial movements and sensations.

c. Treatment includes surgical removal of the tumor via craniotomy.

d. Care is taken to preserve the function of the facial nerve.

e. The tumor rarely recurs after surgical removal.

f. Postoperative nursing care is similar to postoperative craniotomy care.

2. Assessment

a. Symptoms usually begin with tinnitus and progress to gradual **sensorineural hearing loss**.

b. As the tumor enlarges, damage to adjacent cranial nerves occurs.

S. Trauma

1. Description

a. The tympanic membrane has a limited stretching ability and gives way under high pressure.

b. Foreign objects placed in the external canal may exert pressure on the tympanic membrane and cause perforation.

c. If the object continues through the canal, the bony structure of the stapes, incus, and malleus may be damaged.

d. A blunt injury to the basal skull and ear can damage the middle ear structures through fractures extending to the middle ear.

e. Excessive nose blowing and rapid changes of pressure that occur with nonpressurized air flights can increase pressure in the middle ear.

f. Depending on the damage to the ossicles, hearing loss may or may not return.

2. Interventions

a. Tympanic membrane perforations usually heal within 24 hours.

b. Surgical reconstruction of the ossicles and tympanic membrane through tympanoplasty or myringoplasty may be performed to improve hearing.

T. Cerumen and foreign bodies

1. Description

a. Cerumen, or wax, is the most common cause of impacted canals.

b. Foreign bodies can include vegetables, beads, pencil erasers, insects, and other objects.

2. Assessment

a. Sensation of fullness in the ear with or without hearing loss

b. Pain, itching, or bleeding

3. Cerumen
   a. Removal of wax by irrigation is a slow process.
   b. Irrigation is contraindicated in clients with a history of tympanic membrane perforation or otitis media.
   c. If prescribed to soften cerumen, glycerin or mineral oil is placed in the ear at bedtime; hydrogen peroxide may also be prescribed.
   d. After several days, the ear is irrigated.
   e. The maximum amount of solution that should be used for irrigation is 50 to 70 mL.

 Inform that client that ear candles should never be used to remove cerumen. Their use can cause burns and a vacuum effect, causing a perforation in the tympanic membrane.

4. Foreign bodies
   a. With a foreign object of vegetable matter, irrigation is used with care because this material expands with hydration.
   b. Insects are killed before removal, unless they can be coaxed out by flashlight or a humming noise; lidocaine may be placed in the ear to relieve pain.
   c. Mineral oil or diluted alcohol is instilled to suffocate the insect, which then is removed using ear forceps.
   d. Use a small ear forceps to remove the object and avoid pushing the object farther into the canal and damaging the tympanic membrane.

MORE QUESTIONS ON THE CD!

Practice Questions

768. During the early postoperative period, the client who has had a cataract extraction complains of nausea and severe eye pain over the operative site. The initial nursing action is to:
1. Call the physician.
2. Reassure the client that this is normal.
3. Turn the client on his or her operative side.
4. Administer the prescribed pain medication and antiemetic.

769. The nurse is developing a teaching plan for the client with glaucoma. Which of the following instructions would the nurse include in the plan of care?
1. Avoid overuse of the eyes.
2. Decrease the amount of salt in the diet.
3. Eye medications will need to be administered for the client's entire life.
4. Decrease fluid intake to control the intra-ocular pressure.

770. The nurse is performing an admission assessment on a client with a diagnosis of detached retina. Which of the following is associated with this eye disorder?
1. Total loss of vision
2. Pain in the affected eye
3. A yellow discoloration of the sclera
4. A sense of a curtain falling across the field of vision

771. The nurse is performing an otoscopic examination on a client with mastoiditis. On examination of the tympanic membrane, which of the following would the nurse expect to observe?
1. A pink-colored tympanic membrane
2. A pearly colored tympanic membrane
3. A transparent and clear tympanic membrane
4. A red, dull, thick, and immobile tympanic membrane

772. The client is diagnosed with a disorder involving the inner ear. Which of the following is the most common client complaint associated with a disorder involving this part of the ear?
1. Pruritus
2. Tinnitus
3. Hearing loss
4. Burning in the ear

773. The nurse is performing an assessment on a client with a suspected diagnosis of cataract. The chief clinical manifestation that the nurse would expect to note in the early stages of cataract formation is:
1. Diplopia
2. Eye pain
3. Floating spots
4. Blurred vision

774. The client arrives in the emergency department following an automobile accident. The client's forehead hit the steering wheel and a hyphema is diagnosed. The nurse places the client in which position?
1. Flat on bedrest
2. Semi-Fowler's on bedrest
3. Lateral on the affected side
4. Lateral on the unaffected side

775. The client sustains a contusion of the eyeball following a traumatic injury with a blunt object. Which intervention is initiated immediately?
1. Notify the physician.
2. Apply ice to the affected eye.
3. Irrigate the eye with cool water.
4. Accompany the client to the emergency department.

776. The client arrives in the emergency department with a penetrating eye injury from wood chips that occurred while cutting wood. The nurse assesses the eye and notes a piece of wood protruding from the eye. What is the initial nursing action?
1. Apply an eye patch.
2. Perform visual acuity tests.
3. Irrigate the eye with sterile saline.
4. Remove the piece of wood using a sterile eye clamp.

777. The nurse is caring for a client following enucleation. The nurse notes the presence of bright red drainage on the dressing. Which nursing action is appropriate?
1. Notify the physician.
2. Document the finding.
3. Continue to monitor the drainage.
4. Mark the drainage on the dressing and monitor for any increase in bleeding.

778. A woman was working in her garden. She accidentally sprayed insecticide into her right eye. She calls the emergency department frantic and screaming for help. The nurse should instruct the woman to take which immediate action?
1. Call the physician.
2. Irrigate the eyes with water.
3. Come to the emergency room.
4. Irrigate the eyes with diluted hydrogen peroxide.

779. The nurse is caring for a hearing-impaired client. Which of the following approaches will facilitate communication?
1. Speak loudly.
2. Speak frequently.
3. Speak at a normal volume.
4. Speak directly into the impaired ear.

780. Tonometry is performed on the client with a suspected diagnosis of glaucoma. The nurse analyzes the test results as documented in the client's chart and understands that normal intraocular pressure is:
1. 2 to 7 mm Hg
2. 10 to 21 mm Hg
3. 22 to 30 mm Hg
4. 31 to 35 mm Hg

781. The nurse is caring for a client following craniotomy for removal of an acoustic neuroma. Assessment of which of the following cranial nerves would identify a complication specifically associated with this surgery?
1. Cranial nerve I, olfactory
2. Cranial nerve IV, trochlear
3. Cranial nerve III, oculomotor
4. Cranial nerve VII, facial nerve

782. The nurse notes that the physician has documented a diagnosis of presbycusis on the client's chart. The nurse plans care knowing that the condition is:
1. Tinnitus that occurs with aging
2. Nystagmus that occurs with aging
3. A conductive hearing loss that occurs with aging
4. A sensorineural hearing loss that occurs with aging

783. A client with Meniere's disease is experiencing severe vertigo. Which instruction should the nurse give to the client to assist in controlling the vertigo?
1. Increase sodium in the diet.
2. Avoid sudden head movements.
3. Lie still and watch the television.
4. Increase fluid intake to 3000 mL a day.

784. The clinic nurse is preparing to test the visual acuity of a client using a Snellen chart. Which of the following identifies the accurate procedure for this visual acuity test?
1. The right eye is tested, followed by the left eye, and then both eyes are tested.
2. Both eyes are assessed together, followed by the assessment of the right and then the left eyes.
3. The client is asked to stand at a distance of 40 feet from the chart and is asked to read the largest line on the chart.
4. The client is asked to stand at a distance of 40 feet from the chart and to read the line that can be read 200 feet away by an individual with unimpaired vision.

785. The client's vision is tested with a Snellen chart. The results of the tests are documented as 20/60. The nurse interprets this as:
1. The client is legally blind.
2. The client's vision is normal.
3. The client can read at a distance of 60 feet what a client with normal vision can read at 20 feet.
4. The client can read only at a distance of 20 feet what a client with normal vision can read at 60 feet.

Alternate Item Format: Multiple Response

786. The nurse is preparing a teaching plan for a client who is undergoing cataract extraction with intraocular implantation. Which home care measures will the nurse include in the plan? **Select all that apply.**
   ❑ 1. Avoid activities that require bending over.
   ❑ 2. Contact the surgeon if eye scratchiness occurs.
   ❑ 3. Place an eye shield on the surgical eye at bedtime.
   ❑ 4. Episodes of sudden severe pain in the eye are expected.
   ❑ 5. Contact the surgeon if a decrease in visual acuity occurs.
   ❑ 6. Take acetaminophen (Tylenol) for minor eye discomfort.

ANSWERS

768. 1

Rationale: Severe pain or pain accompanied by nausea following a cataract extraction is an indicator of increased intraocular pressure and should be reported to the physician immediately. Options 2, 3, and 4 are inappropriate actions.

Test-Taking Strategy: Use the process of elimination. Note the strategic word *severe*. Eliminate option 2 because this is not a normal condition. The client should not be turned to the operative side; therefore, eliminate option 3. From the remaining options, focusing on the strategic word will direct you to option 1. If you had difficulty with this question, review the postoperative complications of cataract surgery requiring physician notification.

Level of Cognitive Ability: Applying
Client Needs: Physiological Integrity
Integrated Process: Nursing Process—Implementation
Content Area: Adult Health—Eye
Reference: Black, J., & Hawks, J. (2009). *Medical-surgical nursing: Clinical management for positive outcomes* (8th ed., p. 1706). St. Louis: Saunders.

769. 3

Rationale: The administration of eye drops is a critical component of the treatment plan for the client with glaucoma. The client needs to be instructed that medications will need to be taken for the rest of his or her life. Options 1, 2, and 4 are not accurate instructions.

Test-Taking Strategy: Use the process of elimination. Recalling that medications are an integral component of the treatment plan will assist in directing you to the correct option. Review the treatment associated with the care of the client with glaucoma if you had difficulty with this question.

Level of Cognitive Ability: Applying
Client Needs: Physiological Integrity
Integrated Process: Nursing Process—Implementation
Content Area: Adult Health—Eye
Reference: Black, J., & Hawks, J. (2009). *Medical-surgical nursing: Clinical management for positive outcomes* (8th ed., p. 1702). St. Louis: Saunders.

770. 4

Rationale: A characteristic manifestation of retinal detachment described by the client is the feeling that a shadow or curtain is falling across the field of vision. No pain is associated with detachment of the retina. Options 1 and 3 are not characteristics of this disorder. A retinal detachment is an ophthalmic emergency and even more so if visual acuity is still normal.

Test-Taking Strategy: Use the process of elimination, focusing on the diagnosis. Thinking about the pathophysiology associated with this disorder will direct you to option 4. Review the manifestations associated with this condition if you had difficulty with this question.

Level of Cognitive Ability: Analyzing
Client Needs: Physiological Integrity
Integrated Process: Nursing Process—Assessment
Content Area: Adult Health—Eye
Reference: Copstead, L., & Banasik, J. (2010). *Pathophysiology* (4th ed., p. 1098). St. Louis: Mosby.

771. 4

Rationale: Otoscopic examination in a client with mastoiditis reveals a red, dull, thick, and immobile tympanic membrane, with or without perforation. Postauricular lymph nodes are tender and enlarged. Clients also have a low-grade fever, malaise, anorexia, swelling behind the ear, and pain with minimal movement of the head.

Test-Taking Strategy: Knowledge regarding the pathophysiology associated with mastoiditis is required to answer this question. Remember that mastoiditis reveals a red, dull, thick, and immobile tympanic membrane. If you had difficulty with this question, review the assessment findings associated with this disorder.

Level of Cognitive Ability: Analyzing
Client Needs: Physiological Integrity
Integrated Process: Nursing Process—Assessment
Content Area: Adult Health—Ear
Reference: Ignatavicius, D., & Workman, M. (2010). *Medical-surgical nursing: Patient-centered collaborative care* (6th ed., p. 1125). St. Louis: Saunders.

772. 2

Rationale: Tinnitus is the most common complaint of clients with otological disorders, especially disorders involving the inner ear. Symptoms of tinnitus range from mild ringing in the ear, which can go unnoticed during the day, to a loud roaring in the ear, which can interfere with the client's thinking process and attention span. Options 1, 3, and 4 are not associated specifically with disorders of the inner ear.

Test-Taking Strategy: Use the process of elimination. Recalling the function of the inner ear will direct you to option 2. Review the manifestations associated with an inner ear disorder if you had difficulty with this question.

Level of Cognitive Ability: Analyzing
Client Needs: Physiological Integrity
Integrated Process: Nursing Process—Assessment
Content Area: Adult Health—Ear
Reference: Ignatavicius, D., & Workman, M. (2010). *Medical-surgical nursing: Patient-centered collaborative care* (6th ed., p. 1126). St. Louis: Saunders.

773. 4
Rationale: A gradual, painless blurring of central vision is the chief clinical manifestation of a cataract. Early symptoms include slightly blurred vision and a decrease in color perception. Options 1, 2, and 3 are not signs of a cataract.
Test-Taking Strategy: Use the process of elimination. Remember the pathophysiology related to cataract development. As a cataract develops, the lens of the eye becomes opaque. This description will assist in directing you to the correct option. If you had difficulty with this question, review the assessment signs associated with cataract development.
Level of Cognitive Ability: Analyzing
Client Needs: Physiological Integrity
Integrated Process: Nursing Process—Assessment
Content Area: Adult Health—Eye
Reference: Black, J., & Hawks, J. (2009). *Medical-surgical nursing: Clinical management for positive outcomes* (8th ed., p. 1704). St. Louis: Saunders.

774. 2
Rationale: A hyphema is the presence of blood in the anterior chamber. Hyphema is produced when a force is sufficient to break the integrity of the blood vessels in the eye and can be caused by direct injury, such as a penetrating injury from a BB or pellet, or indirectly, such as from striking the forehead on a steering wheel during an accident. The client is treated by bedrest in a semi-Fowler's position to assist gravity in keeping the hyphema away from the optical center of the cornea.
Test-Taking Strategy: Use the process of elimination to answer this question. Remember that placing the client flat will produce an increase in pressure at the injured site. Also, note that option 2 is the option that identifies a position different from the other options. Review care of the client with hyphema if you had difficulty with this question.
Level of Cognitive Ability: Applying
Client Needs: Physiological Integrity
Integrated Process: Nursing Process—Implementation
Content Area: Adult Health—Eye
Reference: Ignatavicius, D., & Workman, M. (2010). *Medical-surgical nursing: Patient-centered collaborative care* (6th ed., p. 1103). St. Louis: Saunders.

775. 2
Rationale: Treatment for a contusion begins at the time of injury. Ice is applied immediately. The client then should be seen by a physician and receive a thorough eye examination to rule out the presence of other eye injuries.
Test-Taking Strategy: Note the type of injury sustained. Focus on the strategic word *immediately*. Recalling the principles related to initial treatment of injuries will direct you to option 2. Review emergency treatment of eye injuries if you had difficulty with this question.
Level of Cognitive Ability: Applying

Client Needs: Physiological Integrity
Integrated Process: Nursing Process—Implementation
Content Area: Adult Health—Eye
Reference: Ignatavicius, D., & Workman, M. (2010). *Medical-surgical nursing: Patient-centered collaborative care* (6th ed., p. 1103). St. Louis: Saunders.

776. 2
Rationale: If the eye injury is the result of a penetrating object, the object may be noted protruding from the eye. This object must never be removed except by the ophthalmologist because it may be holding ocular structures in place. Application of an eye patch or irrigation of the eye may disrupt the foreign body and cause further tearing of the cornea.
Test-Taking Strategy: Use the process of elimination to answer this question. Note the strategic word *penetrating*. This should indicate that a laceration has occurred and that interventions are directed at preventing further disruption of the integrity of the eye. The only option that will prevent further disruption is to assess visual acuity. Review emergency eye care if you had difficulty with this question.
Level of Cognitive Ability: Applying
Client Needs: Physiological Integrity
Integrated Process: Nursing Process—Implementation
Content Area: Adult Health—Eye
Reference: Ignatavicius, D., & Workman, M. (2010). *Medical-surgical nursing: Patient-centered collaborative care* (6th ed., pp. 1103-1104). St. Louis: Saunders.

777. 1
Rationale: If the nurse notes the presence of bright red drainage on the dressing, it must be reported to the physician, because this indicates hemorrhage. Options 2, 3, and 4 are inappropriate.
Test-Taking Strategy: Use the process of elimination and note the strategic words *bright red*. Remember that bright red drainage indicates active bleeding. Review postoperative complications associated with an enucleation if you had difficulty with this question.
Level of Cognitive Ability: Applying
Client Needs: Physiological Integrity
Integrated Process: Nursing Process—Implementation
Content Area: Adult Health—Eye
Reference: Black, J., & Hawks, J. (2009). *Medical-surgical nursing: Clinical management for positive outcomes* (8th ed., p. 1714). St. Louis: Saunders.

778. 2
Rationale: In this type of accident, the client is instructed to irrigate the eyes immediately with running water for at least 20 minutes, or until the emergency medical service personnel arrive. In the emergency department, the cleansing agent of choice is usually normal saline. Calling the physician and going to the emergency department delays necessary intervention. Hydrogen peroxide is never placed in the eyes.
Test-Taking Strategy: Use the process of elimination and note the strategic word *immediate*. Focus on the type of injury and eliminate options 1 and 3 because they delay necessary intervention. Next, eliminate option 4 because hydrogen peroxide is never placed in the eyes. Review immediate interventions for a chemical eye injury if you had difficulty with this question.
Level of Cognitive Ability: Applying

Client Needs: Physiological Integrity.
Integrated Process: Nursing Process—Implementation
Content Area: Adult Health—Eye
Reference: Perry, A., & Potter, P. (2010). *Clinical nursing skills and techniques* (7th ed., p. 496). St. Louis: Mosby.

779. 3

Rationale: Speaking in a normal tone to the client with impaired hearing and not shouting are important. The nurse should talk directly to the client while facing the client and speak clearly. If the client does not seem to understand what is said, the nurse should express it differently. Moving closer to the client and toward the better ear may facilitate communication, but the nurse should avoid talking directly into the impaired ear.
Test-Taking Strategy: Use the process of elimination and knowledge regarding effective communication techniques for the hearing impaired to answer this question. Remember that it is important to speak in a normal tone. If you had difficulty with this question, review these techniques.
Level of Cognitive Ability: Applying
Client Needs: Psychosocial Integrity
Integrated Process: Communication and Documentation
Content Area: Adult Health—Ear
Reference: Ignatavicius, D., & Workman, M. (2010). *Medical-surgical nursing: Patient-centered collaborative care* (6th ed., p. 1135). St. Louis: Saunders.

780. 2

Rationale: Tonometry is the method of measuring intraocular fluid pressure using a calibrated instrument that indents or flattens the corneal apex. Pressures between 10 and 21 mm Hg are considered within the normal range.
Test-Taking Strategy: Use the process of elimination and knowledge regarding normal intraocular pressure to answer this question. Remember that normal intraocular pressure is between 10 and 21 mm Hg. If you had difficulty with this question, learn this normal value.
Level of Cognitive Ability: Understanding
Client Needs: Physiological Integrity
Integrated Process: Nursing Process—Assessment
Content Area: Adult Health—Eye
Reference: Ignatavicius, D., & Workman, M. (2010). *Medical-surgical nursing: Patient-centered collaborative care* (6th ed., p. 1080). St. Louis: Saunders.

781. 4

Rationale: Treatment for acoustic neuroma is surgical removal via a craniotomy. Extreme care is taken to preserve remaining hearing and preserve the function of the facial nerve. Acoustic neuromas rarely recur following surgical removal.
Test-Taking Strategy: Use the process of elimination and knowledge regarding the anatomical location of an acoustic neuroma to direct you to option 4. If you had difficulty with this question, review the complications associated with this surgical procedure.
Level of Cognitive Ability: Analyzing
Client Needs: Physiological Integrity
Integrated Process: Nursing Process—Assessment
Content Area: Adult Health—Ear
Reference: Ignatavicius, D., & Workman, M. (2010). *Medical-surgical nursing: Patient-centered collaborative care* (6th ed., p. 1129). St. Louis: Saunders.

782. 4

Rationale: Presbycusis is a type of hearing loss that occurs with aging. Presbycusis is a gradual sensorineural loss caused by nerve degeneration in the inner ear or auditory nerve. Options 1, 2, and 3 are incorrect.
Test-Taking Strategy: Knowledge regarding the description of presbycusis is required to answer this question. Remember that presbycusis is a gradual sensorineural loss. If you are unfamiliar with this condition, review this age-related disorder.
Level of Cognitive Ability: Understanding
Client Needs: Physiological Integrity
Integrated Process: Nursing Process—Planning
Content Area: Adult Health—Ear
Reference: Ignatavicius, D., & Workman, M. (2010). *Medical-surgical nursing: Patient-centered collaborative care* (6th ed., p. 1130). St. Louis: Saunders.

783. 2

Rationale: The nurse instructs the client to make slow head movements to prevent worsening of the vertigo. Dietary changes such as salt and fluid restrictions that reduce the amount of endolymphatic fluid are sometimes prescribed. Lying still and watching television will not control vertigo.
Test-Taking Strategy: Use the process of elimination. Identify the subject, vertigo. Note the relationship between vertigo and avoiding sudden head movements in the correct option. If you had difficulty with this question, review the measures that will reduce vertigo in the client with Meniere's disease.
Level of Cognitive Ability: Applying
Client Needs: Safe and Effective Care Environment
Integrated Process: Nursing Process—Implementation
Content Area: Adult Health—Ear
Reference: Ignatavicius, D., & Workman, M. (2010). *Medical-surgical nursing: Patient-centered collaborative care* (6th ed., pp. 1126-1127). St. Louis: Saunders.

784. 1

Rationale: Visual acuity is assessed in one eye at a time, and then in both eyes together, with the client comfortably standing or sitting. The right eye is tested with the left eye covered; then the left eye is tested with the right eye covered. Both eyes are then tested together. Visual acuity is measured with or without corrective lenses and the client stands at a distance of 20 feet from the chart.
Test-Taking Strategy: Use the process of elimination. Remember that normal visual acuity as measured by a Snellen chart is 20/20 vision. This should assist in eliminating options 3 and 4. From the remaining options, remember that it is best to test each eye separately and then test both eyes together. This method assesses visual acuity most accurately. Review the procedure for testing visual acuity with a Snellen chart if you had difficulty with this question.
Level of Cognitive Ability: Applying
Client Needs: Health Promotion and Maintenance
Integrated Process: Nursing Process—Assessment
Content Area: Adult Health—Health Assessment/Physical Exam
References: Ignatavicius, D., & Workman, M. (2010). *Medical-surgical nursing: Patient-centered collaborative care* (6th ed., pp. 1077-1078). St. Louis: Saunders.

Jarvis, C. (2008). *Physical examination and health assessment* (5th ed, p. 308). St. Louis: Saunders.

785. 4

Rationale: Vision that is 20/20 is normal—that is, the client is able to read from 20 feet what a person with normal vision can read from 20 feet. A client with a visual acuity of 20/60 can only read at a distance of 20 feet what a person with normal vision can read at 60 feet.

Test-Taking Strategy: Use the process of elimination. Focus on the test result, 20/60, to direct you to option 4. If you had difficulty with this question, review interpretation of visual acuity test results.

Level of Cognitive Ability: Understanding
Client Needs: Physiological Integrity
Integrated Process: Nursing Process—Assessment
Content Area: Adult Health—Eye
Reference: Jarvis, C. (2008). *Physical examination and health assessment* (5th ed, p. 309). St. Louis: Saunders.

ALTERNATE ITEM FORMAT: MULTIPLE RESPONSE

786. 1, 3, 5, 6

Rationale: Following eye surgery, some scratchiness and mild eye discomfort may occur in the operative eye and usually is relieved by mild analgesics. If the eye pain becomes severe, the client should notify the surgeon because this may indicate hemorrhage, infection, or increased intraocular pressure. The nurse also would instruct the client to notify the surgeon of increased purulent drainage, increased redness, or any decrease in visual acuity. The client is instructed to place an eye shield over the operative eye at bedtime to protect the eye from injury during sleep and to avoid activities that increase intraocular pressure, such as bending over.

Test-Taking Strategy: Note that the client has had eye surgery. Recalling that the eye needs to be protected and that increased intraocular pressure is a concern will assist in determining the home care measures to be included in the plan. Review these measures if you had difficulty with this question.

Level of Cognitive Ability: Applying
Client Needs: Physiological Integrity
Integrated Process: Teaching and Learning
Content Area: Adult Health—Eye
Reference: Black, J., & Hawks, J. (2009). *Medical-surgical nursing: Clinical management for positive outcomes* (8th ed., p. 1706). St. Louis: Saunders.

65

Ophthalmic and Otic Medications

I. OPHTHALMIC MEDICATION ADMINISTRATION

A. Guidelines for the use of eye medications

1. Eye medications are usually in the form of drops or ointments.
2. To prevent overflow of medication into the nasal and pharyngeal passages, thus reducing systemic absorption, instruct the client to apply pressure over the inner canthus next to the nose for 30 to 60 seconds following administration of the medication; instruct the client to close the eye gently to help distribute the medication.
3. If both an eye drop and eye ointment are scheduled to be administered at the same time, administer the eye drop first.
4. Wash hands and don gloves before administering eye medications to avoid contaminating the eye or medication dropper or applicator.
5. Use a separate bottle or tube of medication for each client to avoid accidental cross-contamination.
6. Place the prescribed dose of eye medication in the lower conjunctival sac, never directly onto the cornea.
7. Avoid touching any part of the eye with the dropper or applicator.
8. Administer glucocorticoid preparations before other medications.
9. Monitor the pulse of the client receiving an ophthalmic β-blocker, and instruct the client to do the same; if the pulse is less than 50 to 60 beats/min (adult), withhold the next dose of eye medication and notify the physician.
10. Instruct the client how to instill medication correctly and supervise instillation until the client can do it safely.
11. Instruct the client to read the medication labels carefully to ensure administration of the correct medication and correct strength.
12. Remind the client to keep these medications out of the reach of children.
13. Instruct the client to avoid driving or operating hazardous equipment if vision is blurred.
14. Inform the client that he or she may be unable to drive home after eye examinations when a medication to dilate the pupil (**mydriatic**) or to paralyze the ciliary muscle (cycloplegic) is used.
15. If photophobia occurs, instruct the client to wear sunglasses and avoid bright lights.
16. Instruct the client to administer a missed dose of the eye medication as soon as it is remembered, unless the next dose is scheduled to be administered in 1 to 2 hours.
17. Inform the client with **glaucoma** that the disorder cannot be cured, only controlled.
18. Reinforce the importance of using medications to treat **glaucoma** as prescribed and not to discontinue these medications without consulting the physician.
19. Inform the client that medications used to treat **glaucoma** may cause pain and blurred vision, especially when therapy is begun.
20. Instruct the client to report the development of any eye irritation.
21. Inform the client using eye gel to store the gel at room temperature or in the refrigerator, but not to freeze it.
22. Instruct the client to discard unused eye gel kept at room temperature as recommended by the physician and/or the pharmacist.
23. Inform the client that soft contact lenses may absorb certain eye medications and that preservatives in eye medications may discolor the contact lenses.
24. Advise the client wearing contact lenses to question the physician carefully about special precautions to observe with eye medications.
25. Inform the parents of infants that atropine sulfate eye drops may contribute to abdominal distention.
26. Instruct the parents to keep a record of the infant's bowel movements if atropine sulfate eye drops are being administered.
27. Auscultate bowel sounds of the infant or child receiving atropine sulfate eye drops.

⚠ Because the timing of medication administration is critical, administer eye medications at frequent, precise intervals; separate the instillation by 3 to 5 minutes if two medications must be administered at the same time.

 B. Instillation of eye medications
1. Drops
   a. Wash hands.
   b. Put gloves on.
   c. Check the name, strength, and expiration date of the medication.
   d. Instruct the client to tilt the head backward, open the eyes, and look up.
   e. Pull the lower lid down against the cheekbone.
   f. Hold the bottle like a pencil, with the tip downward.
   g. Holding the bottle, gently rest the wrist of the hand on the client's cheek.
   h. Squeeze the bottle gently to allow the drop to fall into the conjunctival sac.
   i. Instruct the client to close the eyes gently and not to squeeze the eyes shut.
   j. Wait 3 to 5 minutes before instilling another drop, if more than one drop is prescribed, to promote maximal absorption of the medication.
   k. Do not allow the medication bottle, dropper, or applicator to come into contact with the eyelid or conjunctival sac.
   l. To prevent systemic absorption of the medication, apply gentle pressure with a clean tissue to the client's nasolacrimal duct for 30 to 60 seconds.
2. Ointments
   a. Instruct the client to lie down or tilt head backward and look up.
   b. Hold the ointment tube near, but not touching, the eye or eyelashes.
   c. Squeeze a thin ribbon of ointment along the lining of the lower conjunctival sac, from the inner to the outer canthus.
   d. Instruct the client to close the eyes gently, rolling the eyeball in all directions (increases contact area of medication to eye).
   e. Instruct the client that vision may be blurred by the ointment.
   f. If possible, apply ointment just before bedtime.

II. MYDRIATIC-CYCLOPLEGIC AND ANTICHOLINERGIC MEDICATIONS (Box 65-1)

A. Description (Fig. 65-1)
1. **Mydriatics** and cycloplegics dilate the pupils (**mydriasis**) and relax the ciliary muscles (**cycloplegia**).
2. Anticholinergics block responses of the sphincter muscle in the ciliary body, producing **mydriasis** and **cycloplegia**.

3. These medications are used preoperatively or for eye examinations to produce **mydriasis**.
4. **Mydriatics** are contraindicated in cardiac dysrhythmias and cerebral atherosclerosis and should be used with caution in the older client and in clients with prostatic hypertrophy, diabetes mellitus, or parkinsonism.

B. Side effects
1. Tachycardia
2. Photophobia
3. Conjunctivitis
4. Dermatitis
5. Elevated blood pressure

C. Atropine toxicity
1. Dry mouth
2. Blurred vision
3. Photophobia
4. Tachycardia
5. Fever
6. Urinary retention
7. Constipation
8. Headache, brow pain

Box 65-1 Mydriatic and Cycloplegic Medications

Atropine (Isopto Atropine)
Cyclopentolate (AK-Pentolate, Cyclogyl, Pentolair)
Homatropine (Isopto Homatropine)
Scopolamine (Isopto Hyoscine)
Tropicamide (Mydriacyl, Tropicacyl, Opticyl)

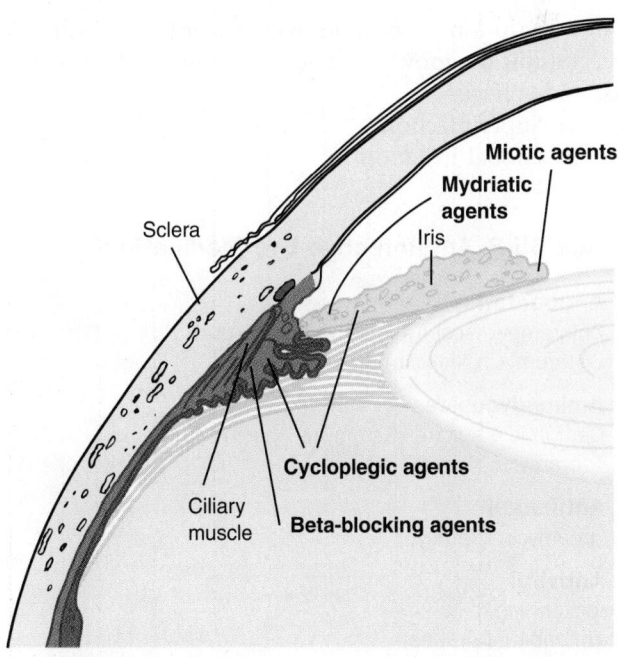

▲ **FIGURE 65-1** Sites of action of mydriatic, β-blocking, cycloplegic, and miotic agents. (From Black, J., & Hawks, J., [2009]. *Medical-surgical nursing: Clinical management for positive outcomes* [8th ed.]. St. Louis: Saunders.)

9. Confusion
10. Hallucinations, delirium
11. Coma
12. Worsening of **glaucoma**
D. Systemic reactions of anticholinergics
1. Dry mouth and skin
2. Fever
3. Thirst
4. Confusion
5. Hyperactivity
E. Interventions
1. Monitor for allergic response.
2. Assess for risk of injury.
3. Assess for constipation and urinary retention.
4. Instruct the client that a burning sensation may occur on instillation.
5. Instruct the client not to drive or perform hazardous activities for 24 hours after instillation of the medication unless otherwise directed by the physician.
6. Instruct the client to wear sunglasses until the effects of the medication wear off.
7. Instruct the client to notify the physician if blurring of vision, loss of sight, difficulty breathing, sweating, or flushing occurs.
8. Instruct the client to report eye pain to the physician.

⚠ Mydriatics are contraindicated in clients with glaucoma because of the risk of increased intraocular pressure.

III. ANTI-INFECTIVE EYE MEDICATIONS (Box 65-2)

A. Description: Anti-infective medications kill or inhibit the growth of bacteria, fungi, and viruses.
B. Side effects
1. Superinfection
2. Global irritation

Box 65-2 Anti-Infective Eye Medications

Antibacterial
Chloramphenicol (Chloromycetin powder)
Erythromycin (Ilotycin)

Aminoglycosides
Gentamicin sulfate (Garamycin, Genoptic)
Tobramycin (Tobrex)

Antifungal
Natamycin (Natacyn)

Antiviral
Idoxuridine
Trifluridine (Viroptic)
Vidarabine (Vira-A)

Sulfonamide
Sulfacetamide (Bleph-10, Sodium Sulamyd)

C. Interventions
1. Assess for risk of injury.
2. Instruct the client how to apply the eye medication; remind the client to clean exudates from the eyes before administering the medication.
3. Reinforce the importance of completing the prescribed medication regimen.
4. Instruct the client to wash the hands thoroughly and frequently.
5. Advise the client that if improvement does not occur to notify the physician.

IV. ANTI-INFLAMMATORY EYE MEDICATIONS (Box 65-3)

A. Description
1. Anti-inflammatory medications control inflammation, thereby reducing vision loss and scarring.
2. Anti-inflammatory medications are used for uveitis, allergic conditions, and inflammation of the conjunctiva, cornea, and lids.
B. Side effects
1. Cataracts
2. Increased intraocular pressure
3. Impaired healing
4. Masking signs and symptoms of infection
C. Interventions
1. Interventions are the same as for anti-infective medications.
2. Note that dexamethasone (Maxidex) should not be used for eye abrasions and wounds.

Box 65-3 Anti-Inflammatory Eye Medications

Antiallergic Agents
Cromolyn sodium (Crolom, Opticrom)
Lodoxamide (Alomide)
Nedocromil sodium (Alocril)
Pemirolast potassium (Alamast)

Corticosteroids
Dexamethasone (Maxidex)
Fluorometholone; sulfacetamide (FML-S eye drop suspension)
Loteprednol etabonate (Alrex, Lotemax)
Prednisolone, gentamicin (Pred-G, Pred Forte)

Nonsteroidal Anti-Inflammatory Agents
Cyclosporine (Restasis)
Diclofenac (Voltaren)
Flurbiprofen sodium (Ocufen)
Ketorolac tromethamine (Acular)

Mast Cell Stabilizers–H_1 Blockers
Azelastine hydrochloride (Optivar)
Epinastine (Elestat)
Ketotifen fumarate (Zaditor, Alaway)
Olopatadine hydrochloride (Patanol)

H_1 Receptor Blocker
Emedastine difumarate (Emadine)

V. TOPICAL EYE ANESTHETICS

A. Description
1. Topical anesthetics produce corneal anesthesia.
2. Topical anesthetics are used for anesthesia for eye examinations and surgery or to remove foreign bodies from the eye.
3. Do not use the solution if it is discolored, and store the bottle tightly closed.
4. Medication: Proparacaine hydrochloride (Ophthetic)

B. Side effects
1. Temporary stinging or burning of the eye
2. Temporary loss of corneal reflex

C. Interventions
1. Assess for risk of injury.
2. Note that the medications should not be given to the client for home use and are not to be self-administered by the client.
3. Instruct the client not to rub or touch the eye while it is anesthetized.
4. Note that the blink reflex is lost temporarily and that the corneal epithelium needs to be protected.
5. Provide an eye patch to protect the eye from injury until the corneal reflex returns.

VI. EYE LUBRICANTS (Box 65-4)

A. Description
1. Eye lubricants replace tears or add moisture to the eyes.
2. Eye lubricants moisten contact lenses or an artificial eye and protect the eyes during surgery or diagnostic procedures.
3. Eye lubricants are used for keratitis, during anesthesia, or for a disorder that results in unconsciousness or decreased blinking.

B. Side effects
1. Burning on instillation
2. Discomfort or pain on instillation

C. Interventions
1. Inform the client that burning may occur on instillation.
2. Be alert to allergic responses to the preservatives in the lubricants.

VII. MEDICATIONS TO TREAT GLAUCOMA
(Box 65-5; see Fig. 65-1)

A. Description
1. These medications reduce intraocular pressure by constricting the pupil and contracting the ciliary muscle, thereby increasing the blood flow to the retina and decreasing retinal damage and loss of vision.
2. These medications open the anterior chamber angle and increase the outflow of aqueous humor.
3. Some may be used to achieve **miosis** during eye surgery.
4. Contraindicated in clients with **retinal detachment**, adhesions between the iris and lens, or inflammatory diseases.
5. Use with caution in clients with asthma, hypertension, corneal abrasion, hyperthyroidism, coronary vascular disease, urinary tract obstruction, gastrointestinal obstruction, ulcer disease, parkinsonism, and bradycardia.

B. Side effects
1. **Myopia**
2. Headache
3. Eye pain
4. Decreased vision in poor light
5. Local irritation
6. Systemic effects
   a. Flushing
   b. Diaphoresis
   c. Gastrointestinal upset and diarrhea

Box 65-5 Medications to Treat Glaucoma

Miotics
Echothiophate
Pilocarpine hydrochloride (Isopto Carpine)

β-Adrenergic Blocking Eye Medications
Betaxolol hydrochloride (Betoptic)
Carteolol hydrochloride (Ocupress)
Levobetaxolol (Betaxon)
Levobunolol hydrochloride (Betagan Liquifilm)
Metipranolol (OptiPranolol)
Timolol maleate (Timoptic)

α-Adrenergic Agonists
Apraclonidine (Iopidine)
Brimonidine (Alphagan P)

Prostaglandin Analogues
Latanoprost (Xalatan)
Travoprost (Travatan)
Bimatoprost (Lumigan)

Cholinergic Agonists
Pilocarpine hydrochloride (Isopto Carpine, others)
Echothiophate iodide (Phospholine Iodide)

Carbonic Anhydrase Inhibitors
Dorzolamide (Trusopt)
Brinzolamide (Azopt)

Nonselective Adrenergic Agonist
Dipivefrin (Propine)

Box 65-4 Eye Lubricants

Hydroxypropyl methylcellulose (Lacril, Isopto Plain)
Petroleum-based ointment (Artificial Tears)
Polyvinyl alcohol (Liquifilm Tears)

  d. Frequent urination
  e. Increased salivation
  f. Muscle weakness
  g. Respiratory difficulty
  7. Toxicity
    a. Vertigo and syncope
    b. Bradycardia
    c. Hypotension
    d. Cardiac dysrhythmias
    e. Tremors
    f. Seizures
C. Interventions
  1. Assess vital signs.
  2. Assess for risk of injury.
  3. Assess the client for the degree of diminished vision.
  4. Monitor for side effects and toxic effects.
  5. Monitor for postural hypotension, and instruct the client to change positions slowly.
  6. Assess breath sounds for wheezes and rhonchi because cholinergic medications can cause bronchospasms and increased bronchial secretions.
  7. Maintain oral hygiene because of the increase in salivation.
  8. Have atropine sulfate available as an antidote for pilocarpine.
  9. Instruct the client or family regarding the correct administration of eye medications.
  10. Instruct the client not to stop the medication suddenly.
  11. Instruct the client to avoid activities such as driving while vision is impaired.

⚠ Instruct the client with glaucoma to read labels on over-the-counter medications and to avoid atropine-like medications because atropine will increase intraocular pressure.

VIII. β-ADRENERGIC BLOCKER EYE MEDICATIONS (Box 65-5)

A. Description (see Fig. 65-1)
  1. These medications reduce intraocular pressure by decreasing sympathetic impulses and decreasing aqueous humor production without affecting **accommodation** or pupil size.
  2. These medications are used to treat **glaucoma**.
  3. These medications are contraindicated in the client with asthma or chronic obstructive pulmonary disease because systemic absorption can cause increased airway resistance.
  4. Use these medications with caution in the client receiving oral β-blockers.
B. Side effects
  1. Ocular irritation
  2. Visual disturbances
  3. Bradycardia

  4. Hypotension
  5. Bronchospasm
C. Interventions
  1. Monitor vital signs, especially blood pressure and pulse, before administering medication.
  2. If the pulse is 60 beats/min or less or if the systolic blood pressure is less than 90 mm Hg, withhold the medication and contact the physician.
  3. Monitor for shortness of breath.
  4. Assess for risk of injury.
  5. Monitor intake and output.
  6. Instruct the client to notify the physician if shortness of breath occurs.
  7. Instruct the client not to discontinue the medication abruptly.
  8. Instruct the client to change positions slowly because of the potential for orthostatic hypotension.
  9. Instruct the client to avoid hazardous activities.
  10. Instruct the client to avoid over-the-counter medications without the physician's approval.
  11. Instruct clients with diabetes mellitus using β-adrenergic blockers to monitor blood glucose levels frequently.

IX. CARBONIC ANHYDRASE INHIBITORS
(see Box 65-5)

A. Description
  1. Carbonic anhydrase inhibitors interfere with the production of carbonic acid, which leads to decreased aqueous humor formation and decreased intraocular pressure.
  2. These medications are used for the long-term treatment of **glaucoma**.
  3. These medications are contraindicated in the client allergic to sulfonamides.
  4. Use with caution for clients with severe renal or liver disease.
B. Side effects
  1. Appetite loss
  2. Gastrointestinal upset
  3. Paresthesias in the fingers, toes, and face
  4. Polyuria
  5. Hypokalemia
  6. Renal calculi
  7. Photosensitivity
  8. Lethargy and drowsiness
  9. Depression
C. Interventions
  1. Monitor vital signs.
  2. Assess visual acuity.
  3. Assess for risk of injury.
  4. Monitor intake and output.
  5. Monitor weight.
  6. Maintain oral hygiene.
  7. Monitor for side effects such as lethargy, anorexia, drowsiness, polyuria, nausea, and vomiting.

8. Monitor electrolyte levels for hypokalemia.
9. Increase fluid intake unless contraindicated.
10. Advise the client to avoid prolonged exposure to sunlight.
11. Encourage the use of artificial tears for dry eyes.
12. Instruct the client not to discontinue the medication abruptly.
13. Instruct the client to avoid hazardous activities while vision is impaired.
14. Teach the client not to wear contact lenses during or within 15 minutes of instilling these medications.

X. OCUSERT SYSTEM

A. Description
1. A thin eye wafer (disk) is impregnated with a time-release dose of pilocarpine (Ocusert Pilo-20, Ocusert Pilo-40).
2. The Ocusert system was devised to overcome the need for frequent instillation of pilocarpine.
3. It is placed in the upper or lower cul-de-sac of the eye.
4. The pilocarpine is released over 1 week.
5. The disk is replaced every 7 days.
6. Drawbacks of its use include sudden leakage of pilocarpine, migration of the system over the cornea, and unnoticed loss of the system.

B. Interventions
1. Assess the client's ability to insert the medication disk.
2. Store the medication in the refrigerator.
3. Instruct the client to discard damaged or contaminated disks.
4. Inform the client that temporary stinging is expected but to notify the physician if blurred vision or brow pain occurs.
5. Instruct the client to check for the presence of the disk in the conjunctival sac daily at bedtime and on arising.
6. Because vision may change in the first few hours after the eye system is inserted, instruct the client to replace the disk at bedtime.

XI. OSMOTIC MEDICATIONS (Box 65-6)

A. Description
1. Osmotic medications lower intraocular pressure.
2. Osmotic medications are used in emergency treatment of **glaucoma**.

3. Osmotic medications are used preoperatively and postoperatively to decrease vitreous humor volume.

B. Side effects
1. Headache
2. Nausea, vomiting, diarrhea, dehydration
3. Disorientation
4. Electrolyte imbalances

C. Interventions
1. Assess vital signs.
2. Assess visual acuity.
3. Assess for risk of injury.
4. Monitor intake and output.
5. Monitor weight.
6. Monitor for electrolyte imbalances.
7. Increase fluid intake unless contraindicated.
8. Monitor for changes in level of orientation.

XII. MEDICATIONS TO TREAT MACULAR DEGENERATION (Box 65-7)

A. Description
1. Age-related macular degeneration (ARMD) can be dry ARMD (atrophic ARMD) or wet ARMD (neovascular)
2. Dry is more common; macular photoreceptors undergo gradual breakdown, leading to gradual blurring of central vision.
3. Wet progresses faster and macular degeneration is caused by the growth of new subretinal blood vessels, which leads to fluid leakage that lifts the macula and causes permanent injury.
4. Characterized by the presence of drusen (yellow deposits under the retina).

B. Side effects
1. Endophthalmitis (eye inflammation caused by bacterial, viral, or fungal infection)
2. Blurred vision
3. Cataracts
4. Corneal edema
5. Eye discomfort and discharge
6. Conjunctival hemorrhage
7. Increased intraocular pressure
8. Reduced visual acuity

C. Interventions
1. Teach the client about administration of the medications.
2. Teach the client about the side effects and the need to notify the physician.

Box 65-6 Osmotic Medications for the Eye

Glycerin (Osmoglyn)
Mannitol (Osmitrol)

Box 65-7 Medications to Treat Macular Degeneration

Pegaptanib (Macugen)   Bevacizumab (Avastin)
Ranibizumab (Lucentis)

XIII. OTIC MEDICATION ADMINISTRATION (Box 65-8)

A. Instillation of eardrops
1. In an adult, pull the pinna up and back to straighten the external canal to instill eardrops.
2. Tilt the client's head in the opposite direction of the affected ear and apply the drops into the ear.
3. With the head tilted, gently move the head back and forth five times.
4. Pull the pinna down and back for infants and children younger than 3 years, up and back for older children.

B. Irrigation of the ear
1. Irrigation of the ear needs to be prescribed by the physician.
2. Ensure direct visualization of the tympanic membrane.
3. Warm the irrigating solution to 98° F because a solution temperature that is not close to the client's body temperature will cause ear injury, nausea, and vertigo.
4. Irrigation must be done gently to avoid damage to the eardrum.
5. When irrigating, do not direct irrigation solution directly toward the eardrum.

⚠ If a perforation of the eardrum is suspected, do not perform an ear irrigation.

XIV. ANTI-INFECTIVE EAR MEDICATIONS (Box 65-9)

A. Description
1. Anti-infective medications kill or inhibit the growth of bacteria and are used for otitis media or otitis externa.
2. Anti-infective medications are contraindicated if a prior hypersensitivity exists.

B. Side effects: Overgrowth of nonsusceptible organisms
C. Interventions
1. Monitor vital signs.
2. Assess for allergies.
3. Assess for pain.
4. Monitor for nephrotoxicity.
5. Instruct the client to report dizziness, fatigue, fever, or sore throat, which may indicate a superimposed infection.
6. Instruct the client to complete the entire course of the medication.
7. Instruct the client to keep ear canals dry.

XV. ANTIHISTAMINES AND DECONGESTANTS (Box 65-10)

A. Description
1. These medications produce vasoconstriction.
2. These medications stimulate the receptors of the respiratory mucosa.
3. These medications reduce respiratory tissue hyperemia and edema to open obstructed eustachian tubes.
4. These medications are used for acute otitis media.
B. Side effects
1. Drowsiness
2. Blurred vision
3. Dry mucous membranes
C. Interventions
1. Inform the client that drowsiness, blurred vision, and a dry mouth may occur.
2. Instruct the client to increase fluid intake unless contraindicated and to suck on hard candy to alleviate the dry mouth.

Box 65-8 Medications That Affect Hearing

Antibiotics
Amikacin (Amikin)
Chloramphenicol
Erythromycin (ERYC, Ery-Tab, PCE Dispertab, Ilotycin)
Gentamicin (Garamycin)
Streptomycin sulfate
Tobramycin sulfate (Nebcin)
Vancomycin (Vancocin)

Diuretics
Ethacrynic acid (Edecrin)
Furosemide (Lasix)

Others
Cisplatin (Platinol)
Nitrogen mustard
Quinine
Quinidine

Box 65-9 Anti-Infective Ear Medications

Acetic acid; aluminum acetate (Domeboro Otic)
Amoxicillin (Amoxil)
Ampicillin (Principen)
Cefaclor (Ceclor)
Chloramphenicol
Clarithromycin (Biaxin)
Clindamycin hydrochloride (Cleocin)
Erythromycin (Ilotycin)
Gentamicin sulfate otic solution (Garamycin)
Penicillin V potassium (Veetids)
Trimethoprim; sulfamethoxazole (Bactrim, Cotrim)

Box 65-10 Antihistamines and Decongestants

Cetirizine (Zyrtec)
Chlorpheniramine (Chlor-Trimeton)
Naphazoline hydrochloride (Allerest)

Box 65-11 Ceruminolytic Medications

Boric acid (Ear-Dry)
Carbamide peroxide (Debrox)
Trolamine polypeptide oleate-condensate (Cerumenex)

3. Instruct the client to avoid hazardous activities if drowsiness occurs.

XVI. LOCAL ANESTHETICS

A. Description
  1. Local anesthetics block nerve conduction at or near the application site to control pain.
  2. Local anesthetics are used for pain associated with ear infections.
B. Medication: Benzocaine-antipyrine-phenylephrine (Tympagesic)
C. Side effects
  1. Allergic reaction
  2. Irritation
D. Interventions
  1. Monitor for effectiveness if used for pain relief.
  2. Assess for irritation or allergic reaction.

XVII. CERUMINOLYTIC MEDICATIONS
  (Box 65-11)

A. Description
  1. Ceruminolytic medications emulsify and loosen cerumen deposits.
  2. Ceruminolytic medications are used to loosen and remove impacted wax from the ear canal.
B. Side effects
  1. Irritation
  2. Redness or swelling of the ear canal
C. Interventions
  1. Instruct the client not to use drops more often than prescribed.
  2. Moisten a cotton plug with medication before insertion.
  3. Keep the container tightly closed and away from moisture.
  4. Avoid touching the ear with the dropper.
  5. Thirty minutes after instillation, gently irrigate the ear as prescribed with warm water, using a soft rubber bulb ear syringe.
  6. Irrigation may be done with hydrogen peroxide solution as prescribed to flush cerumen deposits out of the ear canal.
  7. For a chronic cerumen impaction, one or two drops of mineral oil (if prescribed) will soften the wax.
  8. Instruct the client to notify the physician if redness, pain, or swelling persists.

MORE QUESTIONS ON THE CD!

Practice Questions

787. Betaxolol hydrochloride (Betoptic) eye drops have been prescribed for the client with glaucoma. Which of the following nursing actions is most appropriate related to monitoring for the side effects of this medication?
  1. Monitoring temperature
  2. Monitoring blood pressure
  3. Assessing peripheral pulses
  4. Assessing blood glucose level

788. The nurse prepares the client for an ear irrigation as prescribed by the physician. In performing the procedure, the nurse
  1. Warms the irrigating solution to 98° F
  2. Positions the client with the affected side up following the irrigation
  3. Directs a slow steady stream of irrigation solution toward the eardrum
  4. Assists the client to turn his or her head so that the ear to be irrigated is facing upward

789. In preparation for cataract surgery, the nurse is to administer cyclopentolate (Cyclogyl) eye drops. The nurse administers the eye drops, knowing that the purpose of this medication is to:
  1. Produce miosis of the operative eye.
  2. Dilate the pupil of the operative eye.
  3. Provide lubrication to the operative eye.
  4. Constrict the pupil of the operative eye.

790. The nurse is providing instructions to a client who will be self-administering eye drops. To minimize the systemic effects that eye drops can produce, the nurse instructs the client to:
  1. Eat before instilling the drops.
  2. Swallow several times after instilling the drops.
  3. Blink vigorously to encourage tearing after instilling the drops.
  4. Occlude the nasolacrimal duct with a finger over the inner canthus for 30 to 60 seconds after instilling the drops.

791. The client is receiving an eye drop and an eye ointment to the right eye. The nurse should:
  1. Administer the eye drop first, followed by the eye ointment.
  2. Administer the eye ointment first, followed by the eye drop.
  3. Administer the eye drop, wait 10 minutes, and administer the eye ointment.
  4. Administer the eye ointment, wait 10 minutes, and administer the eye drop.

792. The nurse is caring for a client with glaucoma. Which of the following medications, if prescribed for the client, would the nurse question?
1. Betaxolol (Betoptic)
2. Atropine sulfate (Isopto Atropine)
3. Pilocarpine hydrochloride (Isopto Carpine)
4. Pilocarpine (Ocusert Pilo-20, Ocusert Pilo-40)

793. A miotic medication has been prescribed for the client with glaucoma. The client asks the nurse about the purpose of the medication. The nurse tells the client that:
1. "The medication will help dilate the eye to prevent pressure from occurring."
2. "The medication will relax the muscles of the eyes and prevent blurred vision."
3. "The medication causes the pupil to constrict and will lower the pressure in the eye."
4. "The medication will help block the responses that are sent to the muscles in the eye."

794. A client was just admitted to the hospital to rule out a gastrointestinal (GI) bleed. The client has brought several bottles of medications prescribed by different specialists. During the admission assessment, the client states, "Lately, I have been hearing some roaring sounds in my ears, especially when I am alone." Which medication would the nurse determine could be the cause of the client's complaint?
1. Doxycycline (Vibramycin)
2. Acetylsalicylic acid (aspirin)
3. Atropine sulfate (Isopto Atropine)
4. Diltiazem hydrochloride (Cardizem)

Alternate Item Format: Multiple Response

795. The nurse is preparing to administer eye drops. Select the interventions that the nurse takes to administer the drops. **Select all that apply.**
❑ 1. Wash hands.
❑ 2. Put gloves on.
❑ 3. Place the drop in the conjunctival sac.
❑ 4. Pull the lower lid down against the cheek bone.
❑ 5. Instruct the client to squeeze the eyes shut after instilling the eye drop.
❑ 6. Instruct the client to tilt the head forward, open the eyes, and look down.

ANSWERS

787. 2
Rationale: Hypotension, dizziness, nausea, diaphoresis, headache, fatigue, constipation, and diarrhea are systemic effects of the medication. Nursing interventions include monitoring the blood pressure for hypotension and assessing the pulse for strength, weakness, irregular rate, and bradycardia. Options 1, 3, and 4 are not specifically associated with this medication.
Test-Taking Strategy: Use the ABCs—airway, breathing, and circulation—to direct you to option 2. Although option 3, peripheral pulses, also is related to circulation monitoring, the blood pressure is the umbrella option. Review the side effects of this medication if you had difficulty with this question.
Level of Cognitive Ability: Applying
Client Needs: Physiological Integrity
Integrated Process: Nursing Process—Assessment
Content Area: Adult Health—Eye
Reference: Hodgson, B., & Kizior, R. (2010). *Saunders nursing drug handbook 2010* (p. 124). St. Louis: Saunders.

788. 1
Rationale: Irrigation solutions that are not close to the client's body temperature can be uncomfortable and may cause injury, nausea, and vertigo. The client is positioned so that the ear to be irrigated is facing downward, because this allows gravity to assist in the removal of the ear wax and solution. Following the irrigation, the client is to lie on the affected side to finish draining the irrigating solution. A slow steady stream of solution should be directed toward the upper wall of the ear canal and not toward the eardrum. Too much force could cause the tympanic membrane to rupture.
Test-Taking Strategy: Use the process of elimination. Read each option carefully and remember that the nurse's concern is to prevent damage to the tympanic membrane. Additionally, remember that the client should be positioned with the affected side downward to allow drainage of the irrigation solution. Review the procedure for performing an ear irrigation if you had difficulty with this question.
Level of Cognitive Ability: Applying
Client Needs: Physiological Integrity
Integrated Process: Nursing Process—Implementation
Content Area: Adult Health—Ear
References: Ignatavicius, D., & Workman, M. (2010). *Medical-surgical nursing: Patient-centered collaborative care* (6th ed., p. 1123). St. Louis: Saunders.
  Proehl, J. (2009). *Emergency nursing procedures* (4th ed., pp. 792–795). St. Louis: Saunders.

789. 2
Rationale: Cyclopentolate is a rapidly acting mydriatic and cycloplegic medication. Cyclopentolate is effective in 25 to 75 minutes, and accommodation returns in 6 to 24 hours. Cyclopentolate is used for preoperative mydriasis.
Test-Taking Strategy: Use the process of elimination. Options 1 and 4 are comparable or alike and are eliminated first. Miosis refers to a constricted pupil. Note that the question identifies a client being prepared for eye surgery. The pupil would need to be dilated for the surgical procedure. Review the action and purpose of this medication if you had difficulty with this question.
Level of Cognitive Ability: Understanding
Client Needs: Physiological Integrity
Integrated Process: Nursing Process—Implementation
Content Area: Adult Health—Eye
Reference: Lehne, R. (2010). *Pharmacology for nursing care* (7th ed., pp. 1222–1223). St. Louis: Saunders.

790. 4

Rationale: Applying pressure on the nasolacrimal duct prevents systemic absorption of the medication. Options 1, 2, and 3 will not prevent systemic absorption.

Test-Taking Strategy: Use the process of elimination. Eating and swallowing are comparable options and are not related to the systemic absorption of an eye medication. Blinking vigorously to produce tearing may result in the loss of the administered medication. Review the procedure for administering eye drops to prevent systemic absorption if you had difficulty with this question.

Level of Cognitive Ability: Applying
Client Needs: Physiological Integrity
Integrated Process: Teaching and Learning
Content Area: Adult Health—Eye
References: Kee, J., Hayes, E., & McCuistion, L. (2009). *Pharmacology: A nursing process approach* (6th ed., p. 34). St. Louis: Saunders.
Perry, A., & Potter, P. (2010). *Clinical nursing skills and techniques* (7th ed., pp. 545–549). St. Louis: Mosby.

791. 1

Rationale: When an eye drop and an eye ointment are scheduled to be administered at the same time, the eye drop is administered first. The instillation of 2 medications is separated by 3 to 5 minutes.

Test-Taking Strategy: Use the process of elimination. Recalling the guidelines for administering eye medications will direct you to option 1. Review these guidelines if you had difficulty with this question.

Level of Cognitive Ability: Applying
Client Needs: Physiological Integrity
Integrated Process: Nursing Process—Implementation
Content Area: Adult Health—Eye
Reference: Perry, A., & Potter, P. (2010). *Clinical nursing skills and techniques* (7th ed., p. 549). St. Louis: Mosby.

792. 2

Rationale: Options 1, 3, and 4 are miotic agents used to treat glaucoma. Option 2 is a mydriatic and cycloplegic medication, and its use is contraindicated in clients with glaucoma. Mydriatic medications dilate the pupil and can cause an increase in intraocular pressure in the eye.

Test-Taking Strategy: Use the process of elimination. Knowledge regarding the classifications of the medications identified in the options will assist in answering the question. Remember that mydriatics dilate and that these medications are contraindicated in glaucoma. Review the contraindications related to medications for the client with glaucoma if you had difficulty with this question.

Level of Cognitive Ability: Analyzing
Client Needs: Physiological Integrity
Integrated Process: Nursing Process—Analysis
Content Area: Adult Health—Eye
References: Kee, J., Hayes, E., & McCuistion, L. (2009). *Pharmacology: A nursing process approach* (6th ed., p. 750). St. Louis: Saunders.
Lehne, R. (2010). *Pharmacology for nursing care* (7th ed., pp. 124, 1222–1223). St. Louis: Saunders.

793. 3

Rationale: Miotics cause pupillary constriction and are used to treat glaucoma. They lower the intraocular pressure, thereby increasing blood flow to the retina and decreasing retinal damage and loss of vision. Miotics cause a contraction of the ciliary muscle and a widening of the trabecular meshwork. Options 1, 2, and 4 are incorrect.

Test-Taking Strategy: Use the process of elimination. Note that the client has glaucoma. Recall that prevention of increased intraocular pressure is the goal in the client with glaucoma. Options 1, 2, and 4 describe actions related to mydriatic medications, which primarily dilate the pupils and relax the ciliary muscles. Review the action of a miotic medication if you had difficulty with this question.

Level of Cognitive Ability: Applying
Client Needs: Physiological Integrity
Integrated Process: Nursing Process—Implementation
Content Area: Adult Health—Eye
References: Edmunds, M. (2010). *Introduction to clinical pharmacology* (6th ed., p. 396). St. Louis: Mosby.
Kee, J., Hayes, E., & McCuistion, L. (2009). *Pharmacology: A nursing process approach* (6th ed., pp. 743–744). St. Louis: Saunders.

794. 2

Rationale: Aspirin is contraindicated for gastrointestinal bleeding and is potentially ototoxic. The client should be advised to notify the prescribing physician so the medication can be discontinued and/or a substitute that is less toxic to the ear can be taken instead. Options 1, 3, and 4 do not have side effects that are potentially associated with hearing difficulties.

Test-Taking Strategy: Focus on the client's complaint. Review the classifications and/or therapeutic effects as well as the side effects of each medication in the options. Of the medications identified, only aspirin can cause ototoxicity. Additionally, it is contraindicated for GI bleed as well. Review medications that can cause ototoxicity if you had difficulty with this question.

Level of Cognitive Ability: Analyzing
Client Needs: Physiological Integrity
Integrated Process: Nursing Process—Analysis
Content Area: Adult Health—Ear
Reference: Hodgson, B., & Kizior, R. (2010). *Saunders nursing drug handbook 2010* (p. 89). St. Louis: Saunders.

ALTERNATE ITEM FORMAT: MULTIPLE RESPONSE

795. 1, 2, 3, 4

Rationale: To administer eye medications, the nurse should wash hands and put gloves on. The client is instructed to tilt the head backward, open the eyes, and look up. The nurse pulls the lower lid down against the cheekbone and holds the bottle like a pencil with the tip downward. Holding the bottle, the nurse gently rests the wrist of the hand on the client's cheek and squeezes the bottle gently to allow the drop to fall into the conjunctival sac. The client is instructed to close the eyes gently and not to squeeze the eyes shut to prevent the loss of medication.

Test-Taking Strategy: Use guidelines related to standard precautions and visualize this procedure. This will assist in determining the correct interventions. If you are unfamiliar with the procedure for administering eye medications, review these guidelines.

Level of Cognitive Ability: Applying
Client Needs: Physiological Integrity
Integrated Process: Nursing Process—Implementation
Content Area: Adult Health—Eye
References: Kee, J., Hayes, E., & McCuistion, L. (2009). *Pharmacology: A nursing process approach* (6th ed., p. 34). St. Louis: Saunders.
Perry, A., & Potter, P. (2010). *Clinical nursing skills and techniques* (7th ed., pp. 545–549). St. Louis: Mosby.

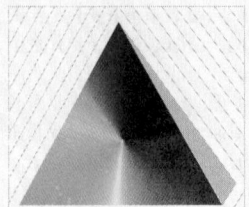

The Adult Client With a Neurological Disorder

PYRAMID TERMS

agnosia The inability to recognize familiar objects or persons.

apraxia Called dyspraxia if the condition is mild; characterized by loss of ability to execute or carry out skilled movements or gestures, despite having the desire and physical ability to perform them.

autonomic dysreflexia Syndrome characterized by paroxysmal hypertension, bradycardia, excessive sweating, facial flushing, nasal congestion, pilomotor responses, and headache. The syndrome occurs with spinal lesions above T6 after the period of spinal shock is complete. Triggers include visceral stimulation from a distended bladder or impacted rectum. The syndrome is a neurological emergency and must be treated immediately to prevent a hypertensive stroke. It is also known as hyperreflexia.

Babinski reflex Dorsiflexion of the big toe with extension; elicited by firmly stroking the lateral aspect of the sole of the foot.

Brudzinski's sign Involuntary flexion of the hip and knee when the neck is passively flexed; indicates meningeal irritation.

decerebrate (extensor) posturing Stiff extension of one or both arms and possibly the legs; indicates a brainstem lesion.

decorticate (flexor) posturing Flexure of one or both arms on the chest and possibly stiff extension of the legs; indicates damaged cortex.

flaccid posturing No motor response display in any extremity.

Glasgow Coma Scale A method of assessing a client's neurological condition. The scoring system is based on a scale of 1 to 15 points. A score of less than 8 indicates that coma is present.

halo traction Insertion of pins or screws into the client's skull and application of a circular fixation device and halo jacket or cast; used to immobilize the cervical spine.

hemianopsia Blindness in half the visual field.

homonymous hemianopsia Loss of half of the field of view on the same side in both eyes.

increased intracranial pressure Increased pressure within the skull caused by trauma, hemorrhage, growths or tumors, hydrocephalus, edema, or inflammation. Increased pressure can impede circulation to the brain and absorption of cerebrospinal fluid and can affect nerve cell functioning, leading to brainstem compression and death.

Kernig's sign Loss of the ability of a supine client to straighten the leg completely when it is fully flexed at the knee and hip; indicates meningeal irritation.

nuchal rigidity Stiff neck; flexion of the neck onto the chest causes intense pain.

skull tongs Tongs inserted into the outer aspect of the client's skull, just above the ears, with application of traction. Types include Gardner-Wells, Barton, and Crutchfield tongs.

spinal shock A sudden depression of reflex activity in the spinal cord below the level of injury (areflexia) that occurs within the first hour of injury and lasts days to months. The muscles become completely paralyzed and flaccid, and reflexes are absent.

Tensilon test Test used to diagnose myasthenia gravis and to differentiate between myasthenic crisis and cholinergic crisis.

unconscious client A state of depressed cerebral functioning with unresponsiveness to sensory and motor function. Causes include head trauma, cerebral toxins, shock, hemorrhage, tumor, or infections.

unilateral neglect An inability to recognize a physical impairment on one side of the body. It occurs most commonly in clients who have had a right cerebral stroke; also known as neglect syndrome.

PYRAMID TO SUCCESS

Pyramid Points related to neurological disorders focus on monitoring for increased intracranial pressure, assessing level of consciousness, positioning clients, head injuries, spinal cord injuries, spinal shock, autonomic dysreflexia, interventions during a seizure, the client with a stroke, Parkinson's disease, myasthenia gravis, and the Tensilon test. Altered body image and psychosocial issues that occur as a result of the neurological disorder are also a focus of the Pyramid to Success.

CLIENT NEEDS

Safe and Effective Care Environment

Acting as a client advocate
Consulting with members of the health care team
Ensuring that advance directives are in the client's medical record
Establishing priorities
Initiating referrals to appropriate services
Maintaining asepsis with procedures and treatments
Maintaining confidentiality
Maintaining standard and other precautions
Obtaining informed consent for invasive procedures
Preventing accidents that can occur as a result of neurological deficits
Upholding client rights

Health Promotion and Maintenance

Discussing expected and unexpected body image changes resulting from neurological deficits

Performing neurological assessment using various techniques
Preventing and detecting health problems associated with neurological deficits
Providing home care instructions regarding care related to the neurological disorder
Teaching about the importance of prescribed therapy

Psychosocial Integrity

Acknowledging end-of-life and grief and loss issues
Assessing the ability to cope with feelings of isolation and loss of independence
Considering the cultural, religious, and spiritual influences of the client when planning care
Identifying sensory and perceptual alterations
Identifying support systems and encouraging the use of community resources
Mobilizing coping mechanisms

Physiological Integrity

Administering pharmacological therapy
Maintaining nutrition
Monitoring for alterations in body systems
Monitoring for complications related to procedures
Monitoring for fluid and electrolyte imbalances
Providing assistive devices for mobility
Providing emergency care
Providing measures to promote comfort
Promoting normal elimination patterns
Promoting self-care measures

Neurological System

I. ANATOMY AND PHYSIOLOGY OF THE BRAIN AND SPINAL CORD

A. Cerebrum
1. The cerebrum consists of the right and left hemispheres.
2. Each hemisphere receives sensory information from the opposite side of the body and controls the skeletal muscles of the opposite side.
3. The cerebrum governs sensory and motor activity and thought and learning.

B. Cerebral cortex (Box 66-1)
1. The cerebral cortex is the outer gray layer; it is divided into five lobes.
2. It is responsible for the conscious activities of the cerebrum.

C. Basal ganglia: Cell bodies in white matter that help the cerebral cortex produce smooth voluntary movements

D. Diencephalon
1. Thalamus
   a. Relays sensory impulses to the cortex
   b. Provides a pain gate
   c. Part of the reticular activating system
2. Hypothalamus
   a. Regulates autonomic responses of the sympathetic and parasympathetic nervous systems
   b. Regulates the stress response, sleep, appetite, body temperature, fluid balance, and emotions
   c. Responsible for the production of hormones secreted by the pituitary gland and the hypothalamus

E. Brainstem
1. Midbrain
   a. Responsible for motor coordination
   b. Contains the visual reflex and auditory relay centers
2. Pons: Contains the respiratory centers and regulates breathing
3. Medulla oblongata
   a. Contains all afferent and efferent tracts and cardiac, respiratory, vomiting, and vasomotor centers
   b. Controls heart rate, respiration, blood vessel diameter, sneezing, swallowing, vomiting, and coughing

F. Cerebellum: Coordinates smooth muscle movement, posture, equilibrium, and muscle tone

G. Spinal cord
1. Provides neuron and synapse networks to produce involuntary responses to sensory stimulation
2. Controls body movement and regulates visceral function
3. Carries sensory information to and motor information from the brain
4. Extends from the first cervical to the second lumbar vertebra
5. Protected by the meninges; cerebrospinal fluid, and adipose tissue
6. Horns
   a. Inner column of gray matter; contains two anterior and two posterior horns
   b. Posterior horns connect with afferent (sensory) nerve fibers.
   c. Anterior horns contain efferent (motor) nerve fibers.
7. Nerve tracts
   a. White matter contains the nerve tract.
   b. Ascending tracts (sensory pathway)
   c. Descending tract (motor pathway)

H. Meninges
1. Dura mater is the tough and fibrous membrane.
2. Arachnoid membrane is the delicate membrane and contains cerebrospinal fluid.
3. Pia mater is the vascular membrane.
4. Subarachnoid space is formed by the arachnoid membrane and the pia mater.

I. Cerebrospinal fluid (CSF)
1. Secreted in the ventricles; circulates in the subarachnoid space and through the ventricles to the subarachnoid layer of the meninges, where it is reabsorbed
2. Acts as a protective cushion; aids in the exchange of nutrients and wastes
3. Normal pressure is 50 to 175 mm H_2O.
4. Normal volume is 125 to 150 mL.

J. Ventricles
1. Four ventricles
2. The ventricles communicate between the subarachnoid spaces and produce and circulate cerebrospinal fluid.

Box 66-1 Cerebral Cortex

Frontal Lobe
Broca's area for speech
Morals, emotions, reasoning and judgment, concentration, and abstraction

Parietal Lobe
Interpretation of taste, pain, touch, temperature, and pressure
Spatial perception

Temporal Lobe
Auditory center
Wernicke's area for sensory and speech

Occipital Lobe
Visual area

Limbic System
Emotional and visceral patterns for survival
Learning and memory

K. Blood supply
1. Right and left internal carotid arteries
2. Right and left vertebral arteries
3. These arteries supply the brain via an anastomosis at the base of the brain called the circle of Willis.

L. Neurotransmitters
1. Acetylcholine
2. Norepinephrine
3. Dopamine
4. Serotonin
5. Amino acids
6. Polypeptides

M. Neurons
1. The neuron consists of the cell body, axons, and dendrites.
2. The cell body contains the nucleus.
3. Neurons carrying impulses to the central nervous system (CNS) are called sensory neurons.
4. Neurons carrying impulses away from the CNS are called motor neurons.
5. Synapse is the chemical transmission of impulses from one neuron to another.

N. Axons and dendrites
1. The axon conducts impulses from the cell body.
2. The dendrites receive stimuli from the body and transmit them to the axon.
3. The neurons are protected and insulated by Schwann cells.
4. The Schwann cell sheath is called the neurolemma.
5. Neurons do not reproduce after the neonatal period.
6. If an axon or dendrite is damaged, it will die and be replaced slowly only if the neurolemma is intact and the cell body has not died.

O. Spinal nerves
1. There are 31 pairs of spinal nerves.
2. Mixed nerve fibers are formed by the joining of the anterior motor and posterior sensory roots.
3. Posterior roots contain afferent (sensory) nerve fibers.
4. Anterior roots contain efferent (motor) nerve fibers.

P. Autonomic nervous system
1. Sympathetic (adrenergic) fibers dilate pupils, increase heart rate and rhythm, contract blood vessels, and relax smooth muscles of the bronchi.
2. Parasympathetic (cholinergic) fibers produce the opposite effect.

II. DIAGNOSTIC TESTS

A. Skull and spinal radiography
1. Description
   a. Radiographs of the skull reveal the size and shape of the skull bones, suture separation in infants, fractures or bony defects, erosion, and calcification.
   b. Spinal radiographs identify fractures, dislocation, compression, curvature, erosion, narrowed spinal cord, and degenerative processes.
2. Preprocedure interventions
   a. Provide nursing support for the confused, combative, or ventilator-dependent client.
   b. Maintain immobilization of the neck if a spinal fracture is suspected.
   c. Remove metal items from body parts.
   d. If the client has thick and heavy hair, this should be documented, because it could affect interpretation of the x-ray film.
3. Postprocedure intervention: Maintain immobilization until results are known.

⚠ Always check with the client about the possibility of pregnancy before any radiographic procedures are done.

B. Computed tomography (CT)
1. Description
   a. Computed tomography is a type of brain scanning that may or may not require injection of a dye.
   b. It is used to detect intracranial bleeding, space-occupying lesions, cerebral edema, infarctions, hydrocephalus, cerebral atrophy, and shifts of brain structures.
2. Preprocedure interventions
   a. Obtain an informed consent if a dye is used.
   b. Assess for allergies to iodine, contrast dyes, or shellfish if a dye is used.
   c. Instruct the client of the need to lie still and flat during the test.

d. Instruct the client to hold his or her breath when requested.

e. Initiate an intravenous line if prescribed.

f. Remove objects from the head, such as wigs, barrettes, earrings, and hairpins.

g. Assess for claustrophobia.

h. Inform the client of possible mechanical noises as the scanning occurs.

i. Inform the client that there may be a hot flushed sensation and a metallic taste in the mouth when the dye is injected.

j. Note that some clients may be given the dye even if they report an allergy; they are treated with an antihistamine and corticosteroids before the injection to reduce the severity of a reaction.

⚠ Assess the need to withhold metformin (Glucophage) if iodinated contrast dye is used for a diagnostic procedure because of the risk for metformin-induced lactic acidosis.

3. Postprocedure interventions

a. Provide replacement fluids because diuresis from the dye is expected.

b. Monitor for an allergic reaction to the dye.

c. Assess dye injection site for bleeding or hematoma, and monitor the extremity for color, warmth, and the presence of distal pulses.

C. Magnetic resonance imaging (MRI)

1. Description

a. Magnetic resonance imaging is a noninvasive procedure that identifies tissues, tumors, and vascular abnormalities.

b. It is similar to CT scanning but provides more detailed pictures.

2. Preprocedure interventions

a. Remove all metal objects from the client.

b. Determine whether the client has a pacemaker, implanted defibrillator, or other metal implants such as a hip prosthesis or vascular clips because these clients cannot have this test performed.

c. Remove intravenous fluid pumps during the test.

d. Provide precautions for the client who is attached to a pulse oximeter because it can cause a burn during testing if coiled around the body or a body part.

e. Provide an assessment of the client with claustrophobia.

f. Administer medication as prescribed for the client with claustrophobia.

g. Determine whether a contrast agent is to be used and follow the prescription related to the administration of food, fluids, and medications.

h. Instruct the client that he or she will need to remain still during the procedure.

⚠ An MRI is contraindicated in a pregnant woman because the increase in amniotic fluid temperature that occurs during the procedure may be harmful to the fetus.

3. Postprocedure interventions

a. Client may resume normal activities.

b. Expect diuresis if a contrast agent is used.

D. Lumbar puncture

1. Description

a. Insertion of a spinal needle through the L3-L4 interspace into the lumbar subarachnoid space to obtain cerebrospinal fluid (CSF), measure CSF fluid or pressure, or instill air, dye, or medications

b. The test is contraindicated in clients with **increased intracranial pressure** because the procedure will cause a rapid decrease in pressure in the CSF around the spinal cord, leading to brain herniation.

2. Preprocedure interventions

a. Obtain an informed consent.

b. Have the client empty the bladder.

3. Interventions during the procedure

a. Position the client in a lateral recumbent position and have the client draw the knees up to the abdomen and the chin onto the chest; the prone position may be required for radiologically guided punctures.

b. Assist with the collection of specimens (label the specimens in sequence).

c. Maintain strict asepsis.

4. Postprocedure interventions

a. Monitor vital signs and neurological signs to check for the presence of leakage of cerebrospinal fluid.

b. Position the client flat as prescribed.

c. Encourage fluids to replace CSF obtained from the specimen collection or from leakage.

d. Monitor intake and output.

E. Myelography

1. Description: Injection of dye or air into the subarachnoid space to detect abnormalities of the spinal cord and vertebrae

2. Preprocedure interventions

a. Obtain an informed consent.

b. Provide hydration for at least 12 hours before the test.

c. Assess for allergies to contrast agents, iodine, or shellfish.

d. If the client is taking a phenothiazine, withhold the medication because this medication lowers the seizure threshold.

e. Premedicate for sedation as prescribed.

3. Postprocedure interventions

a. Assess vital signs and neurological condition frequently as prescribed.

b. Maintain bedrest as prescribed; the head position varies according to the dye used; the head is usually elevated if an oil-based or water-soluble contrast agent is used and usually positioned lower than the trunk if air contrast is used.

c. Administer analgesics for headache or backache as prescribed.

d. Encourage fluids to help excrete the contrast material.

e. Monitor intake and output to ensure adequate fluid intake and to ensure an adequate urine output of at least 30 mL/hr.

F. Cerebral angiography

1. Description: Injection of a contrast material usually through the femoral artery (or another artery) into the carotid arteries to visualize the cerebral arteries and assess for lesions

2. Preprocedure interventions

a. Obtain an informed consent.

b. Assess the client for allergies to iodine and shellfish.

c. Assess for a medication history of anticoagulation therapy.

d. Encourage hydration for 2 days before the test.

e. Maintain the client on NPO status 4 to 6 hours before the test as prescribed.

f. Perform a neurological assessment, which will serve as a baseline for postprocedure assessments.

g. Mark the peripheral pulses.

h. Remove metal items from the hair.

i. Administer premedication as prescribed.

3. Postprocedure interventions

a. Monitor neurological status, vital signs, and neurovascular status of the affected extremity frequently until stable.

b. Monitor for swelling in the neck and for difficulty swallowing; notify the physician if these symptoms occur.

c. Maintain bed rest for 12 hours as prescribed.

d. Elevate the head of the bed 15 to 30 degrees only if prescribed.

e. Keep the bed flat if the femoral artery is used as prescribed.

f. Assess peripheral pulses.

g. Apply sandbags or another device to immobilize the limb and a pressure dressing to the injection site to decrease bleeding as prescribed.

h. Place ice on the puncture site as prescribed.

i. Encourage fluid intake.

G. Electroencephalography

1. Description: Graphic recording of the electrical activity of the superficial layers of the cerebral cortex

2. Preprocedure interventions

a. Wash the client's hair.

b. Inform the client that electrodes are attached to the head and that electricity does not enter the head.

c. Withhold stimulants such as coffee, tea, and caffeine beverages, antidepressants, tranquilizers, and possibly anticonvulsants for 24 to 48 hours before the test as prescribed.

d. Allow the client to have breakfast if prescribed.

e. Premedicate for sedation as prescribed.

3. Postprocedure interventions

a. Wash the client's hair.

b. Maintain side rails and safety precautions, if the client was sedated.

H. Caloric testing (oculovestibular reflex)

1. Description: Caloric testing provides information about the function of the vestibular portion of the eighth cranial nerve and aids in the diagnosis of cerebellar and brainstem lesions.

2. Procedure

a. Patency of the external auditory canal is confirmed.

b. The client is positioned supine with the head of the bed elevated 30 degrees.

c. Water that is warmer or cooler than body temperature is infused into the ear.

d. A normal response is the onset of vertigo and nystagmus (involuntary eye movements) within 20 to 30 seconds

e. Absent or disconjugate eye movements indicate brainstem damage.

III. NEUROLOGICAL ASSESSMENT

(see Chapter 34 for additional information on neurological assessment)

A. Assessment of risk factors

1. Trauma
2. Hemorrhage
3. Tumors
4. Infection
5. Toxicity
6. Metabolic disorders
7. Hypoxic conditions
8. Hypertension
9. Cigarette smoking
10. Stress
11. Aging process
12. Chemicals, either ingestion or environmental exposure

B. Assessment of the cranial nerves (see Chapter 34)

C. Assessment of level of consciousness (LOC)

1. Assessment becomes increasingly invasive as the client is less responsive

a. Speak to the client (auditory)

b. Lightly touch the client (gentle tactile)

Box 66-2 Assessment of Respirations

Cheyne-Stokes
Rhythmic, with periods of apnea
Can indicate a metabolic dysfunction or dysfunction in the cerebral hemisphere or basal ganglia

Neurogenic Hyperventilation
Regular rapid and deep sustained respirations
Indicates a dysfunction in the low midbrain and middle pons

Apneustic
Irregular respirations, with pauses at the end of inspiration and expiration
Indicates a dysfunction in the middle or caudal pons

Ataxic
Totally irregular in rhythm and depth
Indicates a dysfunction in the medulla

Cluster
Clusters of breaths with irregularly spaced pauses
Indicates a dysfunction in the medulla and pons

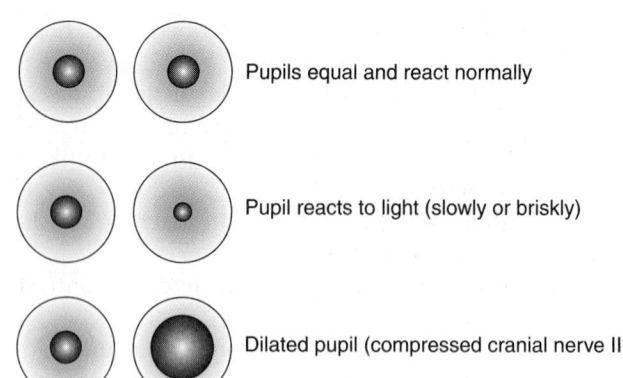
Pupils equal and react normally

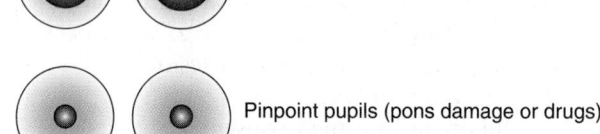
Pupil reacts to light (slowly or briskly)

Dilated pupil (compressed cranial nerve III)

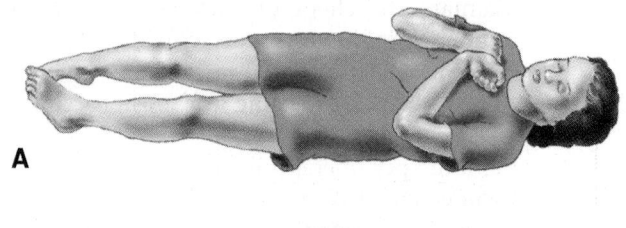
Bilateral dilated, fixed pupils (ominous sign)

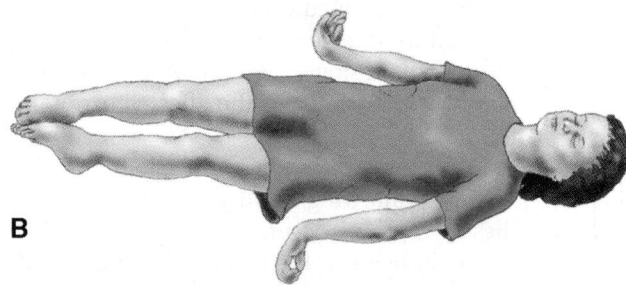
Pinpoint pupils (pons damage or drugs)

▲ **FIGURE 66-1** Pupillary check for size and response. (From Lewis, S., Heitkemper, M., Dirksen, S., O'Brien, P., & Bucher, L. [2007]. *Medical-surgical nursing: Assessment and management of clinical problems* [7th ed.]. St. Louis: Mosby.)

c. Painful stimuli (sternal rub, supraorbital pressure, trapezius squeeze)
2. Assess client behavior to determine level of consciousness, such as confusion, delirium, unconsciousness, stupor, or coma.

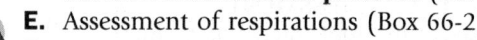 Level of consciousness is the most sensitive indicator of neurological status.

D. Assessment of vital signs: Monitor for blood pressure or pulse changes, which may indicate **increased intracranial pressure (ICP)**.
E. Assessment of respirations (Box 66-2)
F. Assessment of temperature
1. An elevated temperature increases the metabolic rate of the brain.
2. An elevation in temperature may indicate a dysfunction of the hypothalamus or brainstem.
3. A slow rise in temperature may indicate infection.
G. Assessment of pupils (Fig. 66-1)
5. Unilateral pupil dilation indicates compression of the third cranial nerve.
6. Midposition fixed pupil indicates midbrain injury.
7. Pinpoint fixed pupil indicates pontine damage.
H. Assessment of motor function
1. Muscle tone, including strength and equality
2. Voluntary and involuntary movements
3. Purposeful and nonpurposeful movements
I. Assessment for posturing (Fig. 66-2)
1. Posturing indicates a deterioration of the condition.
2. Flexor (**decorticate posturing**)
a. Client flexes one or both arms on the chest and may extend the legs stiffly.
b. Flexor posturing indicates a nonfunctioning cortex.

A

B

▲ **FIGURE 66-2** Posturing. **A,** Decorticate posturing. **B,** Decerebrate posturing. (From Ignatavicius, D., and Workman, M. [2010]. *Medical-surgical nursing: Patient-centered collaborative care* [6th ed.]. St. Louis: Saunders.)

3. Extensor (**decerebrate posturing**)
a. Client stiffly extends one or both arms and possibly the legs.
b. Extensor posturing indicates a brainstem lesion.
4. **Flaccid posturing**: Client displays no motor response in any extremity.
J. Assessment of reflexes (Box 66-3)
K. Assessment of meningeal irritation (Box 66-4)

Box 66-3 Assessment of Reflexes

Babinski Reflex
Dorsiflexion of the big toe, with extension; elicited by firmly stroking the lateral aspect of the sole of the foot

Corneal Reflex
Loss of the blink reflex
Indicates a dysfunction of cranial nerve V

Gag Reflex
Loss of the gag reflex
Indicates a dysfunction of cranial nerves IX and X

Box 66-4 Assessment of Meningeal Irritation

General Findings
Irritability
Nuchal rigidity
Severe, unrelenting headaches
Generalized muscle aches and pains
Nausea and vomiting
Fever and chills
Tachycardia
Photophobia
Nystagmus
Abnormal pupil reaction and eye movement

Brudzinski's Sign
Involuntary flexion of the hip and knee when the neck is passively flexed; indicates meningeal irritation

Kernig's Sign
Loss of the ability of a supine client to straighten the leg completely when it is fully flexed at the knee and hip; indicates meningeal irritation

Motor Response
Hemiparesis, hemiplegia, and decreased muscle tone
Cranial nerve dysfunction, especially cranial nerves III, IV, VI, VII, and VIII

Memory Changes
Short attention span
Personality and behavioral changes
Bewilderment

Box 66-5 Glasgow Coma Scale

Score
The highest possible score is 15 points.

Motor Response Points
Obeys a simple response = 6
Localizes painful stimuli = 5
Normal flexion (withdrawal) = 4
Abnormal flexion (decorticate posturing) = 3
Extensor response (decerebrate posturing) = 2
No motor response to pain = 1

Verbal Response Points
Oriented = 5
Confused conversation = 4
Inappropriate words = 3
Responds with incomprehensible sounds = 2
No verbal response = 1

Eye-Opening Points
Spontaneous = 4
In response to sound = 3
In response to pain = 2
No response, even to painful stimuli = 1

Modified from Ignatavicius, D., & Workman, M. (2010). *Medical-surgical nursing: Patient-centered collaborative care* (6th ed.). St. Louis: Saunders.

   e. Dilated blood vessels
   f. Bladder contraction
M. Assessment of sensory function: Touch, pressure, pain
N. **Glasgow Coma Scale** (Box 66-5)
   1. The scale is a method of assessing a client's neurological condition.
   2. The scoring system is based on a scale of 1 to 15 points.
   3. A score lower than 8 indicates that coma is present.

IV. THE UNCONSCIOUS CLIENT

A. Description
   1. The **unconscious client** is in a state of depressed cerebral functioning with unresponsiveness to stimulation of sensory and motor function.
   2. Some causes include head trauma, cerebral toxins, shock, hemorrhage, tumor, and infection.
B. Assessment
   1. Unarousable
   2. Primitive or no response to painful stimuli
   3. Altered respirations
   4. Decreased cranial nerve and reflex activity
C. Interventions (Box 66-6)

V. INCREASED INTRACRANIAL PRESSURE (ICP)

A. Description
   1. **Increased ICP** may be caused by trauma, hemorrhage, growths or tumors, hydrocephalus, edema, or inflammation.

L. Assessment of the autonomic system
   1. Sympathetic functions, adrenergic responses
      a. Increased pulse and blood pressure
      b. Dilated pupils
      c. Decreased peristalsis
      d. Increased perspiration
   2. Parasympathetic function, cholinergic responses
      a. Decreased pulse and blood pressure
      b. Constricted pupils
      c. Increased salivation
      d. Increased peristalsis

Box 66-6 Care of the Unconscious Client

Assess patency of the airway and keep an airway and emergency equipment at the bedside.

Monitor blood pressure, pulse, and heart sounds.

Assess respiratory and circulatory status.

Maintain a patent airway and ventilation because a high CO_2 level increases intracranial pressure.

Assess lung sounds for the accumulation of secretions.

Suction fluids from the airway as needed.

Assess neurological status, including level of consciousness, pupillary reactions, and motor and sensory function, using the Glasgow Coma Scale.

Place the client in a semi-Fowler's position.

Change position of the client every 2 hours, avoiding injury when turning.

Avoid Trendelenburg's position.

Use side rails unless contraindicated or according to agency protocol.

Assess for edema.

Monitor for dehydration.

Monitor intake and output and daily weight.

Maintain NPO status until consciousness returns.

Maintain nutrition as prescribed, and monitor fluid and electrolyte balance.

Check the gag and swallow reflex before resuming a diet, and begin the diet with ice chips and fluids when the client becomes alert.

Provide intravenous or enteral feedings as prescribed.

Assess bowel sounds.

Monitor elimination patterns.

Monitor for constipation, impaction, and paralytic ileus.

Maintain urinary output to prevent stasis, infection, and calculus formation.

Monitor the status of skin integrity.

Initiate measures to prevent skin breakdown.

Provide frequent mouth care.

Remove dentures and contact lenses.

Assess the eyes for the presence of a corneal reflex and irritation, and instill artificial tears or cover the eyes with eye patches.

Monitor drainage from the ears or nose for the presence of cerebrospinal fluid.

Assume that the unconscious client can hear.

Avoid restraints.

Do not leave the client unattended if unstable.

Initiate seizure precautions if necessary.

Provide range-of-motion exercises to prevent contractures.

Use a footboard or high-topped sneakers to prevent footdrop.

Use splints to prevent wrist deformities.

Initiate physical therapy as appropriate.

---

2. **Increased ICP** can impede circulation to the brain, impede the absorption of CSF, affect the functioning of nerve cells, and lead to brainstem compression and death.

B. Assessment
1. Altered level of consciousness, which is the most sensitive and earliest indication of increasing **ICP**
2. Headache
3. Abnormal respirations (see Box 66-2)
4. Rise in blood pressure with widening pulse pressure
5. Slowing of pulse
6. Elevated temperature
7. Vomiting
8. Pupil changes
9. Late signs of **increased ICP**, including increased systolic blood pressure, widened pulse pressure, and slowed heart rate
10. Other late signs include changes in motor function from weakness to hemiplegia, a positive **Babinski reflex**, **decorticate** or **decerebrate posturing**, and seizures.

C. Interventions
1. Monitor respiratory status and prevent hypoxia.
2. Avoid the administration of morphine sulfate to prevent the occurrence of hypoxia.
3. Maintain mechanical ventilation as prescribed; maintaining the $Paco_2$ at 30 to 35 mm Hg will

result in vasoconstriction of the cerebral blood vessels, decreased blood flow, and therefore decreased ICP.
4. Maintain body temperature.
5. Prevent shivering, which can increase ICP.
6. Decrease environmental stimuli.
7. Monitor electrolyte levels and acid-base balance.
8. Monitor intake and output.
9. Limit fluid intake to 1200 mL/day.
10. Instruct the client to avoid straining activities, such as coughing and sneezing.
11. Instruct the client to avoid Valsalva's maneuver.

⚠ For the client with increased intracranial pressure, elevate the head of the bed 30 to 40 degrees, avoid the Trendelenburg position, and prevent flexion of the neck and hips.

D. Medications (Box 66-7)
E. Surgical intervention: Also see Chapter 36 for additional information on ventriculoperitoneal shunts (Box 66-8)

VI. HYPERTHERMIA

A. Description
1. Temperature higher than 105° F, which increases the cerebral metabolism and increases the risk of hypoxia

Box 66-7 Medications for Increased Intracranial Pressure

Anticonvulsants
Anticonvulsants may be given prophylactically to prevent seizures.
Seizures increase metabolic requirements and cerebral blood flow and volume, thus increasing intracranial pressure.

Antipyretics and Muscle Relaxants
Temperature reduction decreases metabolism, cerebral blood flow, and thus intracranial pressure.
Antipyretics prevent temperature elevations.
Muscle relaxants prevent shivering.

Blood Pressure Medication
Blood pressure medication may be required to maintain cerebral perfusion at a normal level.
Notify the physician if the blood pressure range is lower than 100 or higher than 150 mm Hg systolic.

Corticosteroids
Corticosteroids stabilize the cell membrane and reduce the leakiness in the blood-brain barrier.

Corticosteroids decrease cerebral edema.
A histamine blocker may be administered to counteract the excess gastric secretion that occurs with the corticosteroid.
Clients must be withdrawn slowly from corticosteroid therapy to reduce the risk of adrenal crisis.

Intravenous Fluids
Fluids are administered intravenously via an infusion pump to control the amount administered.
Hypertonic intravenous solutions are avoided because of the risk of promoting additional cerebral edema.

Hyperosmotic Agent
Mannitol (Osmitrol) is a hyperosmotic agent that increases intravascular pressure by drawing fluid from the interstitial spaces and from the brain cells.
Monitor renal function.
Diuresis is expected.

Box 66-8 Surgical Intervention for Chronic Increased Intracranial Pressure: Ventriculoperitoneal Shunt

Description
A ventriculoperitoneal shunt diverts cerebrospinal fluid from the ventricles into the peritoneum.

Postprocedure Interventions
Position the client supine and turn from the back to the nonoperative side.
Monitor for signs of increasing intracranial pressure resulting from shunt failure.
Monitor for signs of infection.

2. Administer medications as prescribed to prevent shivering and to lower body temperature.
3. Monitor neurological status.
4. Monitor for infection and respiratory complications because hyperthermia may mask the signs of infection.
5. Monitor for cardiac dysrhythmias.
6. Monitor intake and output.
7. Prevent trauma to the skin and tissues.
8. Apply lotion to the skin frequently.
9. Inspect for frostbite if a hypothermia blanket is used.

---

2. Causes include infection, heat stroke, exposure to high environmental temperatures, and dysfunction of the thermoregulatory center
  B. Assessment
    1. Temperature higher than 105° F
    2. Shivering
    3. Nausea and vomiting
  C. Interventions
    1. Maintain a patent airway.
    2. Initiate seizure precautions.
    3. Monitor intake and output and assess the skin and mucous membranes for signs of dehydration.
    4. Monitor lung sounds.
    5. Monitor for dysrhythmias.
    6. Assess peripheral pulses for systemic blood flow.
    7. Induce normothermia with fluids, cool baths, fans, or a hypothermia blanket.
  D. Inducement of normothermia
    1. Prevent shivering, which will increase intracranial pressure and oxygen consumption.

VII. HEAD INJURY

A. Description
    1. Head injury is trauma to the skull, resulting in mild to extensive damage to the brain.
    2. Immediate complications include cerebral bleeding, hematomas, uncontrolled **increased ICP**, infections, and seizures.
    3. Changes in personality or behavior, cranial nerve deficits, and any other residual deficits depend on the area of the brain damage and the extent of the damage.
B. Types of head injuries (Box 66-9)
    1. Open
      a. Scalp lacerations
      b. Fractures in the skull
      c. Interruption of the dura mater
    2. Closed
      a. Concussions
      b. Contusions
      c. Fractures

Box 66-9 Types of Head Injuries

Concussion
Concussion is a jarring of the brain within the skull, with no loss of consciousness.

Contusion
Contusion is a bruising type of injury to the brain tissue.
Contusion may occur along with other neurological injuries, such as with subdural or extradural collections of blood.

Skull Fractures
Linear
Depressed
Compound
Comminuted

Epidural Hematoma
The most serious type of hematoma, epidural hematoma forms rapidly and results from arterial bleeding.

Epidural hematoma forms between the dura and skull from a tear in the meningeal artery.
It is often associated with temporary loss of consciousness, followed by a lucid period, that rapidly progresses to coma.
Epidural hematoma is a surgical emergency.

Subdural Hematoma
Subdural hematoma forms slowly and results from a venous bleed.
Subdural hematoma occurs under the dura as a result of tears in the veins crossing the subdural space.

Intracerebral Hemorrhage
Multiple hemorrhages occur around a contused area.

Subarachnoid Hemorrhage
Bleeding occurs directly into the brain, ventricles, or subarachnoid space.

C. Hematoma
  1. Description: Hematoma can occur as a result of a subarachnoid hemorrhage or an intracerebral hemorrhage.
  2. Assessment
      a. Assessment findings depend on the injury.
      b. Clinical manifestations usually result from **increased ICP**.
      c. Changing neurological signs in the client
      d. Changes in level of consciousness
      e. Airway and breathing pattern changes
      f. Vital signs changes reflecting **increased ICP**
      g. Headache, nausea, and vomiting
      h. Visual disturbances, pupillary changes, and papilledema
      i. **Nuchal rigidity** (not tested until spinal cord injury is ruled out)
      j. CSF drainage from the ears or nose
      k. Weakness and paralysis
      l. Posturing
      m. Decreased sensation or absence of feeling
      n. Reflex activity changes
      o. Seizure activity

  ⚠ CSF can be distinguished from other fluids by the presence of concentric rings (yellowish stain surrounded by bloody fluid) when the fluid is placed on a white sterile background, such as a gauze pad. CSF also tests positive for glucose when tested using a strip test.

  3. Interventions
      a. Monitor respiratory status and maintain a patent airway because increased CO_2 levels increase cerebral edema.
      b. Monitor neurological status and vital signs, including temperature.
      c. Monitor for **increased ICP**.
      d. Maintain head elevation to reduce venous pressure.
      e. Prevent neck flexion.
      f. Initiate normothermia measures for increased temperature.
      g. Assess cranial nerve function, reflexes, and motor and sensory function.
      h. Initiate seizure precautions.
      i. Monitor for pain and restlessness.
      j. Morphine sulfate may be prescribed to decrease agitation and control restlessness caused by pain for the head injured client on a ventilator; administer with caution because it is a respiratory depressant and may increase ICP.
      k. Monitor for drainage from the nose or ears because this fluid may be CSF.
      l. Do not attempt to clean the nose, suction, or allow the client to blow his or her nose if drainage occurs.
      m. Do not clean the ear if drainage is noted, but apply a loose, dry sterile dressing.
      n. Check drainage for the presence of CSF.
      o. Notify the physician if drainage from the ears or nose is noted and if the drainage tests positive for CSF.
      p. Instruct the client to avoid coughing because this increases ICP.
      q. Monitor for signs of infection.
      r. Prevent complications of immobility.
      s. Inform the client and family about the possible behavior changes that may occur, including those that are expected and those that need to be reported.

D. Craniotomy
  1. Description

Box 66-10 Nursing Care Following Craniotomy

Monitor vital signs and neurological status every 30 to 60 minutes.

Monitor for increased intracranial pressure.

Monitor for decreased level of consciousness, motor weakness or paralysis, aphasia, visual changes, and personality changes.

Maintain mechanical ventilation and slight hyperventilation for the first 24 to 48 hours as prescribed to prevent increased intracranial pressure.

Assess the physician's prescription regarding client positioning.

Avoid extreme hip or neck flexion, and maintain the head in a midline neutral position.

Provide a quiet environment.

Monitor the head dressing frequently for signs of drainage.

Mark any area of drainage at least once each nursing shift for baseline comparison.

Monitor the Hemovac or Jackson-Pratt drain, which may be in place for 24 hours.

Maintain suction on the Hemovac or Jackson-Pratt drain.

Measure drainage from the Hemovac or Jackson-Pratt drain every 8 hours, and record the amount and color.

Notify the physician if drainage is more than the normal amount of 30 to 50 mL per shift.

Notify the physician immediately of excessive amounts of drainage or a saturated head dressing.

Record strict measurement of hourly intake and output.

Maintain fluid restriction at 1500 mL/day as prescribed.

Monitor electrolyte levels.

Monitor for dysrhythmias, which may occur as a result of fluid or electrolyte imbalance.

Apply ice packs or cool compresses as prescribed; expect periorbital edema and ecchymosis of one or both eyes, which is not an unusual occurrence.

Provide range-of-motion exercises every 8 hours.

Place antiembolism stockings on the client as prescribed.

Administer anticonvulsants, antacids, corticosteroids, and antibiotics as prescribed.

Administer analgesics such as codeine sulfate or acetaminophen (Tylenol) as prescribed for pain.

Box 66-11 Client Positioning Following Craniotomy

Positions prescribed following a craniotomy vary with the type of surgery and the specific postoperative physician's prescription.

Always check the physician's prescription regarding client positioning.

Incorrect positioning may cause serious and possibly fatal complications.

Removal of a Bone Flap for Decompression

To facilitate brain expansion, the client should be turned from the back to the nonoperative side, but not to the side operated on.

Posterior Fossa Surgery

To protect the operative site from pressure and minimize tension on the suture line, position the client on the side, with a pillow under the head for support and not on the back.

Infratentorial Surgery

Infratentorial surgery involves surgery below the tentorium of the brain.

The physician may prescribe a flat position without head elevation or may prescribe the head of the bed to be elevated at 30 to 45 degrees.

Do not elevate the head of the bed in the acute phase of care following surgery without a physician's prescription.

Supratentorial Surgery

Supratentorial surgery involves surgery above the tentorium of the brain.

The physician may prescribe the head of the bed to be elevated at 30 degrees to promote venous outflow through the jugular veins.

Do not lower the head of the bed in the acute phase of care following surgery without a physician's prescription.

---

a. Surgical procedure that involves an incision through the cranium to remove accumulated blood or a tumor

b. Complications of the procedure include **increased ICP** from cerebral edema, hemorrhage, or obstruction of the normal flow of CSF.

c. Additional complications include hematomas, hypovolemic shock, hydrocephalus, respiratory and neurogenic complications, pulmonary edema, and wound infections.

d. Complications related to fluid and electrolyte imbalances include diabetes insipidus and inappropriate secretion of antidiuretic hormone.

2. Preoperative interventions

a. Explain the procedure to the client and family.

b. Ensure that an informed consent has been obtained.

c. Prepare to shave the client's head as prescribed (usually done in the operating room) and cover the head with an appropriate covering.

d. Stabilize the client before surgery.

3. Postoperative interventions (Box 66-10)

4. Postoperative positioning (Box 66-11)

VIII. SPINAL CORD INJURY

A. Description

1. Trauma to the spinal cord causes partial or complete disruption of the nerve tracts and neurons.

2. The injury can involve contusion, laceration, or compression of the cord.
3. Spinal cord edema develops; necrosis of the spinal cord can develop as a result of compromised capillary circulation and venous return.
4. Loss of motor function, sensation, reflex activity, and bowel and bladder control may result.
5. The most common causes include motor vehicle accidents, falls, sporting and industrial accidents, and gunshot or stab wounds.
6. Complications related to the injury include respiratory failure, **autonomic dysreflexia, spinal shock,** further cord damage, and death.

B. Most frequently involved vertebrae
1. Cervical—C5, C6, and C7
2. Thoracic—T12
3. Lumbar—L1

C. Transection of the cord
1. Complete transection of the cord: The spinal cord is severed completely, with total loss of sensation, movement, and reflex activity below the level of injury.
2. Partial transection of the cord
   a. The spinal cord is damaged or severed partially.
   b. The symptoms depend on the extent and location of the damage.
   c. If the cord has not suffered irreparable damage, early treatment is needed to prevent partial damage from developing into total and permanent damage.

D. Spinal cord syndromes in incomplete injury (Fig. 66-3)
1. Central cord syndrome
   a. Central cord syndrome occurs from a lesion in the central portion of the spinal cord.

COMPLETE LESION

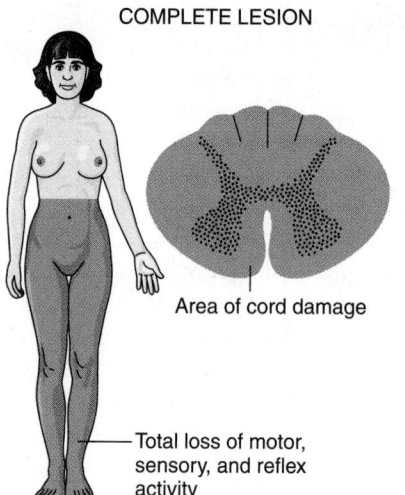

Area of cord damage

Total loss of motor, sensory, and reflex activity

ANTERIOR CORD SYNDROME

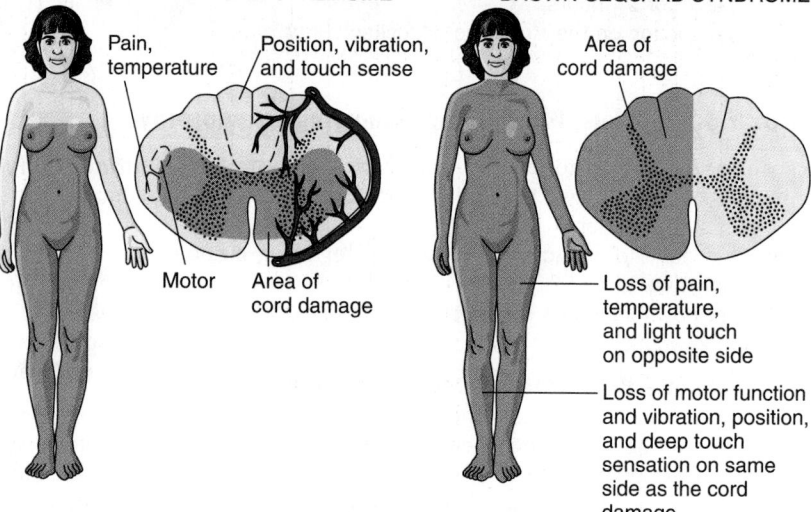

Pain, temperature

Position, vibration, and touch sense

Motor   Area of cord damage

BROWN-SÉQUARD SYNDROME

Area of cord damage

Loss of pain, temperature, and light touch on opposite side

Loss of motor function and vibration, position, and deep touch sensation on same side as the cord damage

CENTRAL CORD SYNDROME

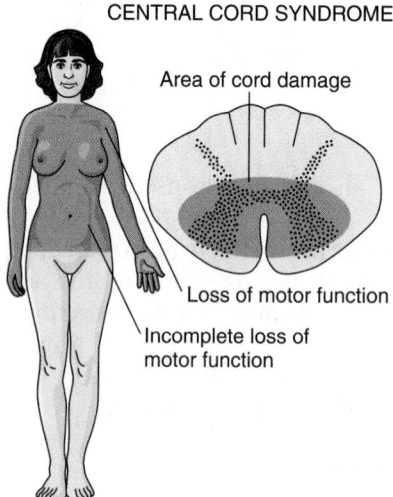

Area of cord damage

Loss of motor function

Incomplete loss of motor function

CONUS MEDULLARIS AND CAUDA EQUINA SYNDROMES

Loss of motor sensory function in various patterns, with potential for recovery of function with regeneration of peripheral nerves; neurogenic bowel and bladder

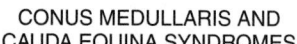
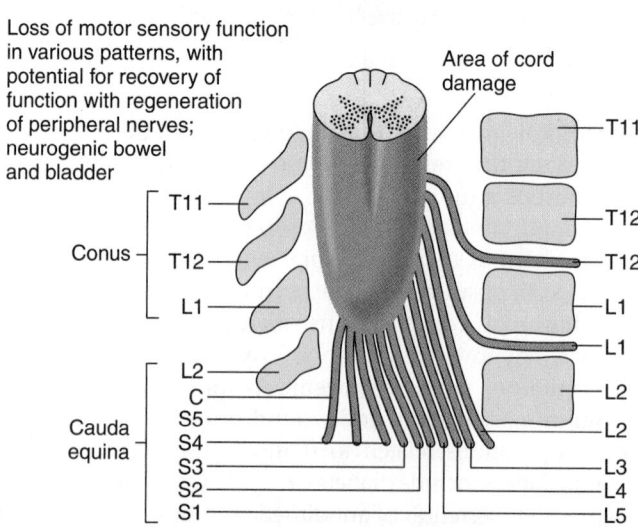

Area of cord damage

Conus — T11, T12, L1

Cauda equina — L2, C, S5, S4, S3, S2, S1

T11, T12, T12, L1, L1, L2, L2, L3, L4, L5

▲ **FIGURE 66-3** Common spinal cord syndromes. (From Ignatavicius, D., and Workman, M. [2010]. *Medical-surgical nursing: Patient-centered collaborative care* [6th ed.]. St. Louis: Saunders.)

b. Loss of motor function is more pronounced in the upper extremities, and varying degrees and patterns of sensation remain intact.

2. Anterior cord syndrome
   a. Anterior cord syndrome is caused by damage to the anterior portion of the gray and white matter of the spinal cord.
   b. Motor function, pain, and temperature sensation are lost below the level of injury; however, the sensations of position, vibration, and touch remain intact.

3. Posterior cord syndrome
   a. Posterior cord syndrome is caused by damage to the posterior portion of the gray and white matter of the spinal cord.
   b. Motor function remains intact, but the client experiences a loss of vibratory sense, crude touch, and position sensation.

4. Brown-Séquard syndrome
   a. Brown-Séquard syndrome results from penetrating injuries that cause hemisection of the spinal cord or injuries that affect half the cord.
   b. Motor function, vibration, proprioception, and deep touch sensations are lost on the same side of the body (ipsilateral) as the lesion or cord damage.
   c. On the opposite side of the body (contralateral) from the lesion or cord damage, the sensations of pain, temperature, and light touch are affected.

5. Conus medullaris syndrome
   a. Conus medullaris syndrome follows damage to the lumbar nerve roots and conus medullaris in the spinal cord.
   b. Client experiences bowel and bladder areflexia and flaccid lower extremities.
   c. If damage is limited to the upper sacral segments of the spinal cord, bulbospongiosus penile (erection) and micturition reflexes will remain.

6. Cauda equina syndrome
   a. Cauda equina syndrome occurs from injury to the lumbosacral nerve roots below the conus medullaris.
   b. The client experiences areflexia of the bowel, bladder, and lower reflexes.

E. Assessment of spinal cord injuries (Box 66-12)
   1. Dependent on the level of the cord injury
   2. Level of spinal cord injury: Lowest spinal cord segment with intact motor and sensory function
   3. Respiratory status changes
   4. Motor and sensory changes below the level of injury
   5. Total sensory loss and motor paralysis below the level of injury
   6. Loss of reflexes below the level of injury

7. Loss of bladder and bowel control
8. Urinary retention and bladder distention
9. Presence of sweat, which does not occur on paralyzed areas

F. Cervical injuries
   1. Injury at C2 to C3 is usually fatal.
   2. C4 is the major innervation to the diaphragm by the phrenic nerve.
   3. Involvement above C4 causes respiratory difficulty and paralysis of all four extremities.
   4. Client may have movement in the shoulder if the injury is at C5 through C8, and may also have decreased respiratory reserve.

G. Thoracic level injuries
   1. Loss of movement of the chest, trunk, bowel, bladder, and legs may occur, depending on the level of injury.
   2. Leg paralysis (paraplegia) may occur.
   3. **Autonomic dysreflexia** with lesions or injuries above T6 and in cervical lesions may occur.
   4. Visceral distention from a noxious stimuli such as a distended bladder or impacted rectum may cause reactions such as sweating, bradycardia, hypertension, nasal stuffiness, and goose flesh.

H. Lumbar and sacral level injuries
   1. Loss of movement and sensation of the lower extremities may occur.
   2. S2 and S3 center on micturition; therefore, below this level, the bladder will contract but not empty (neurogenic bladder).
   3. Injury above S2 in males allows them to have an erection, but they are unable to ejaculate because of sympathetic nerve damage.
   4. Injury between S2 and S4 damages the sympathetic and parasympathetic response, preventing erection or ejaculation.

I. Emergency interventions

   ⚠ Always suspect spinal cord injury when trauma occurs until this injury is ruled out. Immobilize the client on a spinal backboard with the head in a neutral position to prevent an incomplete injury from becoming complete.

   1. Emergency management is critical because improper movement can cause further damage and loss of neurological function.

Box 66-12 Effects of Spinal Cord Injury

Tetraplegia (Quadriplegia)
Injury occurring between C1 and C8
Paralysis involving all four extremities

Paraplegia
Injury occurring between T1 and L4
Paralysis involving only the lower extremities

2. Assess the respiratory pattern and maintain a patent airway.
3. Prevent head flexion, rotation, or extension.
4. During immobilization, maintain traction and alignment on the head by placing hands on both sides of the head by the ears.
5. Maintain an extended position.
6. Logroll the client.
7. No part of the body should be twisted or turned, and the client is not allowed to assume a sitting position.
8. In the emergency department, a client who has sustained a cervical fracture should be placed immediately in skeletal traction via **skull tongs** or **halo traction** to immobilize the cervical spine and reduce the fracture and dislocation (Fig. 66-4).

J. Interventions during hospitalization
1. Respiratory system
   a. Assess respiratory status because paralysis of the intercostal and abdominal muscles occurs with C4 injuries.
   b. Monitor arterial blood gas levels and maintain mechanical ventilation if prescribed to prevent respiratory arrest, especially with cervical injuries.
   c. Encourage deep breathing and the use of an incentive spirometer.
   d. Monitor for signs of infection, particularly pneumonia.
2. Cardiovascular system
   a. Monitor for cardiac dysrhythmias.
   b. Assess for signs of hemorrhage or bleeding around the fracture site.
   c. Assess for signs of shock, such as hypotension, tachycardia, and a weak and thready pulse.

d. Assess the lower extremities for deep vein thrombosis.
e. Measure circumferences of the calf and thigh to identify increases in size.
f. Apply thigh-high antiembolism stockings as prescribed.
g. Remove antiembolism stockings daily to assess the skin.
h. Monitor for orthostatic hypotension when repositioning the client.
3. Neuromuscular system
   a. Assess neurological status.
   b. Assess motor and sensory status to determine the level of injury.
   c. Assess motor ability by testing the client's ability to squeeze hands, spread the fingers, move the toes, and turn the feet.
   d. Assess absence of sensation, hyposensation, or hypersensation by pinching the skin or pricking it with a pin, starting at the shoulders and working down the extremities.
   e. Monitor for signs of **autonomic dysreflexia** and **spinal shock**.
   f. Immobilize the client to promote healing and prevent further injury.
   g. Assess pain.
   h. Initiate measures to reduce pain.
   i. Administer analgesics as prescribed.
   j. Monitor for complications of immobility.
   k. Prepare the client for decompression laminectomy, spinal fusion, or insertion of instrumentation or rods if prescribed.
   l. Collaborate with the physical therapist and occupational therapist to determine appropriate exercise techniques, assess the need for hand and wrist splints, and develop an appropriate plan to prevent footdrop.

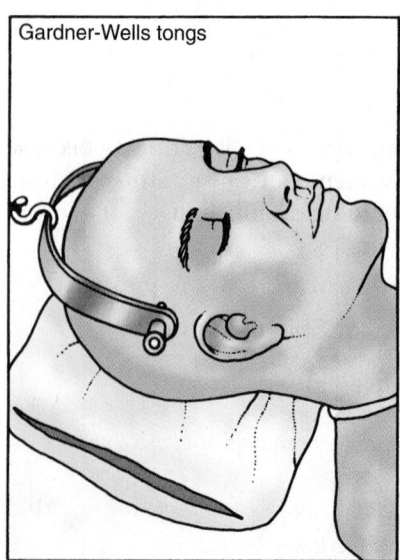

Gardner-Wells tongs

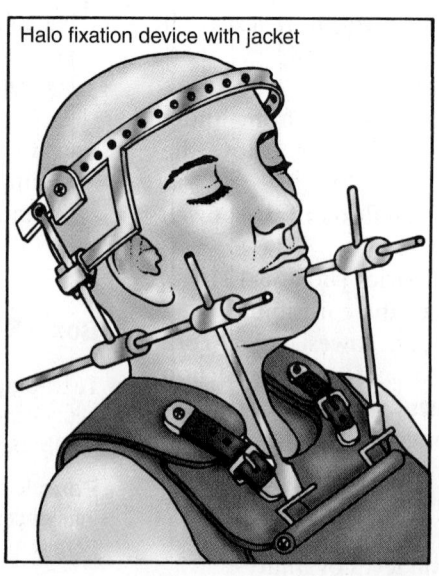

Halo fixation device with jacket

▲ **FIGURE 66-4** Types of cervical spine traction. (From Ignatavicius, D., and Workman, M. [2010]. *Medical-surgical nursing: Patient-centered collaborative care* [6th ed.]. St. Louis: Saunders.)

4. Gastrointestinal system
   a. Assess abdomen for distention and hemorrhage.
   b. Monitor bowel sounds and assess for paralytic ileus.
   c. Prevent bowel retention.
   d. Initiate a bowel control program as appropriate.
   e. Maintain adequate nutrition and a high-fiber diet.
5. Renal system
   a. Prevent urinary retention.
   b. Initiate a bladder control program as appropriate.
   c. Maintain fluid and electrolyte balance.
   d. Maintain adequate fluid intake of 2000 mL/day.
   e. Monitor for urinary tract infection and calculi.
6. Integumentary system
   a. Assess skin integrity.
   b. Turn the client every 2 hours.
7. Psychosocial integrity
   a. Assess psychosocial status.
   b. Encourage the client to express feelings of anger and depression.
   c. Discuss the sexual concerns of the client.
   d. Promote rehabilitation with self-care measures, setting realistic goals based on the client's potential functional level.
   e. Encourage contact with appropriate community resources.

K. Spinal and Neurogenic shock
   1. Description
      a. **Spinal shock** is a transient condition that occurs after the spinal cord injury and is characterized by the absence of all voluntary and reflex activity below the level of the injury; it often lasts less than 48 hours but can last for several weeks.
      b. **Neurogenic shock** is a type of shock that occurs after the spinal cord injury that results in a massive vasodilation leading to pooling of blood in blood vessels, hypoperfusion, and impaired cellular metabolism.
      c. **Neurogenic shock** is an emergency and treatment focuses on restoring the circulatory blood volume.
   2. Assessment (Box 66-13)
   3. Interventions
      a. Monitor for signs of **spinal shock** following a spinal cord injury.
      b. Monitor for hypotension and bradycardia.
      c. Monitor for reflex activity.
      d. Assess bowel sounds.
      e. Monitor for bowel and urinary retention.
      f. Provide supportive measures as prescribed, based on the presence of symptoms.
      g. Monitor for the return of reflexes.

L. Autonomic dysreflexia
   1. Description
      a. **Autonomic dysreflexia** is also known as autonomic hyperreflexia.

      b. **Autonomic dysreflexia** generally occurs after the period of **spinal shock** is resolved and occurs with lesions or injuries above T6 and in cervical lesions.
      c. It is commonly caused by visceral distention from a distended bladder or impacted rectum.
      d. It is a neurological emergency and must be treated immediately to prevent a hypertensive stroke.
   2. Assessment (see Box 66-13)
   3. Interventions (see Priority Nursing Actions)

M. Cervical spine traction for cervical injuries (see Fig. 66-4)
   1. Description
      a. Skeletal traction is used to stabilize fractures or dislocations of the cervical or upper thoracic spine.
      b. Two types of equipment used for cervical traction are skull (cervical) tongs and **halo traction** (halo fixation device).
   2. **Skull tongs**
      a. **Skull tongs** are inserted into the outer aspect of the client's skull, and traction is applied.
      b. Weights are attached to the tongs, and the client is used as countertraction.
      c. Monitor the neurological status of the client.
      d. Determine the amount of weight prescribed to be added to the traction.
      e. Ensure that weights hang securely and freely at all times.
      f. Ensure that the ropes for the traction remain within the pulley.
      g. Maintain body alignment and maintain care of the client on a special bed (such as a RotoRest bed or Stryker or Foster frame) as prescribed.
      h. Turn the client every 2 hours.

Box 66-13 Spinal Shock and Autonomic Dysreflexia

Spinal Shock
Flaccid paralysis
Loss of reflex activity below the level of the injury
Bradycardia
Paralytic ileus
Hypotension

Autonomic Dysreflexia
Sudden onset, severe throbbing headache
Severe hypertension
Flushing above the level of the injury
Pale extremities below the level of the injury
Nasal stuffiness
Nausea
Dilated pupils or blurred vision
Sweating
Piloerection (goose bumps)
Restlessness and a feeling of apprehension

i. Assess insertion site of the tongs for infection.
j. Provide sterile pin site care as prescribed.
3. **Halo traction**
   a. **Halo traction** is a static traction device that consists of a headpiece with four pins, two anterior and two posterior, inserted into the client's skull.
   b. The metal halo ring may be attached to a vest (jacket) or cast when the spine is stable, allowing increased client mobility.

████ PRIORITY NURSING ACTIONS! ████

Actions to Take for a Spinal Cord Injury Client Who Develops Autonomic Dysreflexia
1. Raise the head of the bed.
2. Loosen tight clothing on the client.
3. Check for bladder distention or other noxious stimulus.
4. Administer an antihypertensive medication.
5. Document the occurrence, treatment, and response.

Autonomic dysreflexia is characterized by severe hypertension, bradycardia, severe headache, nasal stuffiness, and flushing. The cause is a noxious stimulus, most often a distended bladder or constipation. Autonomic dysreflexia is a neurological emergency and must be treated promptly to prevent a hypertensive stroke. Immediate nursing actions are to contact the physician and sit the client up in bed in a high Fowler's position and remove the noxious stimulus. The nurse would loosen any tight clothing and then check for bladder distention. If the client has a Foley catheter, the nurse would check for kinks in the tubing. The nurse also would check for a fecal impaction and disimpact the client, if necessary. The nurse assesses the environment to ensure that it is not too cool or too drafty and also monitors vital signs, particularly the blood pressure, every 15 minutes. Antihypertensive medication may be prescribed by the physician to minimize cerebral hypertension. Finally, the nurse documents the occurrence, treatment, and client response.

Reference: Ignatavicius, D., & Workman, M. (2010). *Medical-surgical nursing: Patient-centered collaborative care* (6th ed., p. 998). St. Louis: Saunders.

---

c. Monitor the client's neurological status for changes in movement or decreased strength.
d. Never move or turn the client by holding or pulling on the **halo traction** device.
e. Assess for tightness of the jacket by ensuring that one finger can be placed under the jacket.
f. Assess skin integrity to ensure that the jacket or cast is not causing pressure.
g. Provide sterile pin site care as prescribed.
4. Client education for **halo traction** device (Box 66-14)
5. Initiate interventions in support of the client's self image.
6. Teach the client and family pin care, care of the vest, and signs and symptoms of infection to report to his or her health care provider.

N. Interventions for thoracic, lumbar, and sacral injuries
1. Bed rest
2. Immobilization with a body cast if prescribed
3. Assess for respiratory impairment and paralytic ileus, possible complications of the body cast.
4. Use of a brace or corset when the client is out of bed

O. Surgical interventions for thoracic, lumbar, and sacral injuries
1. Decompressive laminectomy
   a. Removal of one or more laminae
   b. Allows for cord expansion from edema; performed if conventional methods fail to prevent neurological deterioration
2. Spinal fusion
   a. Spinal fusion is used for thoracic spinal injuries.
   b. Bone is grafted between the vertebrae for support and to strengthen the back.
3. Postoperative interventions
   a. Monitor for respiratory impairment.
   b. Monitor vital signs, motor function, sensation, and circulatory status in the lower extremities.
   c. Encourage breathing exercises.

Box 66-14 Client Education for a Halo Fixation Device

Notify the physician if the halo vest (jacket) or ring bolts loosen.
Use fleece or foam inserts to relieve pressure points.
Keep the vest lining dry.
Clean the pin site daily.
Notify the physician if redness, swelling, drainage, open areas, pain, tenderness, or a clicking sound occurs from the pin site.
A sponge bath or tub bath is allowed; showers are prohibited.
Assess the skin under the vest daily for breakdown, using a flashlight.
Do not use any products other than shampoo on the hair.
When shampooing the hair, cover the vest with plastic.

When getting out of bed, roll onto the side and push on the mattress with the arms.
Never use the metal frame for turning or lifting.
Use a rolled towel or pillowcase between the back of the neck and bed or next to the cheek when lying on the side, and raise the head of the bed to increase sleep comfort.
Adapt clothing to fit over the halo device.
Eat foods high in protein and calcium to promote bone healing.
Have the correct-sized wrench available at all times for an emergency (tape the wrench to the vest).
If cardiopulmonary resuscitation is required, the anterior portion of the vest will be loosened and the posterior portion will remain in place to provide stability.

d. Assess for signs of fluid and electrolyte imbalances.

e. Observe for complications of immobility.

f. Keep the client in a flat position as prescribed.

g. Provide cast care if the client is in a full body cast.

h. Turn and reposition frequently by logrolling side to back to side, using turning sheets and pillows between the legs to maintain alignment.

i. Administer pain medication as prescribed.

j. Maintain on NPO status until the client is passing flatus.

k. Monitor bowel sounds.

l. Provide the use of a fracture bedpan.

m. Monitor intake and output.

n. Maintain nutritional status.

P. Medications

1. Dexamethasone (Decadron)

a. Used for its anti-inflammatory and edema-reducing effects

b. May interfere with healing

2. Dextran: Plasma expander used to increase capillary blood flow within the spinal cord and to prevent or treat hypotension

3. Dantrolene (Dantrium), baclofen (Lioresal): These medications are used for clients with upper motor neuron injuries to control muscle spasticity.

IX. CEREBRAL ANEURYSM

A. Description

1. Dilation of the walls of a weakened cerebral artery

2. Aneurysm can lead to rupture.

B. Assessment

1. Headache and pain

2. Irritability

3. Diplopia

4. Blurred vision

5. Tinnitus

6. Hemiparesis

7. **Nuchal rigidity**

8. Seizures

C. Interventions

1. Maintain a patent airway (suction only with a physician's prescription).

2. Administer oxygen as prescribed.

3. Monitor vital signs and for hypertension or dysrhythmias.

4. Avoid taking temperatures via the rectum.

5. Initiate aneurysm precautions (Box 66-15)

X. SEIZURES

A. Description

1. Seizures are an abnormal, sudden, excessive discharge of electrical activity within the brain.

2. Epilepsy is a disorder characterized by chronic seizure activity and indicates brain or CNS irritation.

3. Causes include genetic factors, trauma, tumors, circulatory or metabolic disorders, toxicity, and infections.

4. Status epilepticus involves a rapid succession of epileptic spasms without intervals of consciousness; it is a potential complication that can occur with any type of seizure, and brain damage may result.

B. Types of seizures (Box 66-16)

1. Generalized seizures

2. Partial seizures

C. Assessment

1. Seizure history

2. Type of seizure

3. Occurrences before, during, and after the seizure

4. Prodromal signs, such as mood changes, irritability, and insomnia

5. Aura: Sensation that warns the client of the impending seizure

6. Loss of motor activity or bowel and bladder function or loss of consciousness during the seizure

7. Occurrences during the postictal state, such as headache, loss of consciousness, sleepiness, and impaired speech or thinking

---

Box 66-15 Aneurysm Precautions

Maintain the client on bed rest in a semi-Fowler's or a side-lying position.

Maintain a darkened room (subdued lighting and avoid direct, bright, artificial lights) without stimulation (a private room is optimal).

Provide a quiet environment (avoid activities or startling noises); a telephone in the room is not usually allowed.

Reading, watching television, and listening to music are permitted, provided that they do not overstimulate the client.

Limit visitors.

Maintain fluid restrictions.

Provide diet as prescribed; avoid stimulants in the diet.

Prevent any activities that initiate the Valsalva maneuver (straining at stool, coughing); provide stool softeners to prevent straining.

Administer care gently (such as the bath, back rub, range of motion).

Limit invasive procedures.

Maintain normothermia.

Prevent hypertension.

Provide sedation.

Provide pain control.

Administer prophylactic anticonvulsant medications.

Provide deep vein thrombosis (DVT) prophylaxis as prescribed.

Box 66-16 Types of Seizures

Generalized Seizures

Tonic-Clonic
Tonic-clonic seizures may begin with an aura.
The tonic phase involves the stiffening or rigidity of the muscles of the arms and legs and usually lasts 10 to 20 seconds, followed by loss of consciousness.
The clonic phase consists of hyperventilation and jerking of the extremities and usually lasts about 30 seconds.
Full recovery from the seizure may take several hours.

Absence
A brief seizure that lasts seconds, and the individual may or may not lose consciousness.
No loss or change in muscle tone occurs.
Seizures may occur several times during a day.
The victim appears to be daydreaming.
This type of seizure is more common in children.

Myoclonic
Myoclonic seizures present as a brief generalized jerking or stiffening of extremities.
The victim may fall to the ground from the seizure.

Atonic or Akinetic (Drop Attacks)
An atonic seizure is a sudden momentary loss of muscle tone.
The victim may fall to the ground as a result of the seizure.

Partial Seizures

Simple Partial
The simple partial seizure produces sensory symptoms accompanied by motor symptoms that are localized or confined to a specific area.
The client remains conscious and may report an aura.

Complex Partial
The complex partial seizure is a psychomotor seizure.
The area of the brain most usually involved is the temporal lobe.
The seizure is characterized by periods of altered behavior of which the client is not aware.
The client loses consciousness for a few seconds.

D. Interventions

⚠ If the client is having a seizure, maintain a patent airway. Do not force the jaws open or place anything in the client's mouth.

1. Note the time and duration of the seizure.
2. Assess behavior at the onset of the seizure: If the client has experienced an aura, if a change in facial expression occurred, or if a sound or cry occurred from the client
3. If the client is standing or sitting, place the client on the floor and protect the head and body.
4. Support the ABCs (airway, breathing, and circulation).
5. Administer oxygen.
6. Prepare to suction secretions.
7. Turn the client to the side to allow secretions to drain while maintaining the airway.
8. Prevent injury during the seizure.
9. Remain with the client.
10. Do not restrain the client.
11. Loosen restrictive clothing.
12. Note the type, character, and progression of the movements during the seizure.
13. Monitor for incontinence.
14. Administer intravenous medications as prescribed to stop the seizure.
15. Document the characteristics of the seizure.
16. Provide privacy, if possible.
17. Monitor behavior following the seizure, such as the state of consciousness, motor ability, and speech ability.

18. Instruct the client about the importance of life-long medication and the need for follow-up determination of medication blood levels.
19. Instruct the client to avoid alcohol, excessive stress, fatigue, and strobe lights.
20. Encourage the client to contact available community resources, such as the Epilepsy Foundation of America.
21. Encourage the client to wear a Medic-Alert bracelet.

XI. STROKE (BRAIN ATTACK)

A. Description
1. A stroke or brain attack, formerly known as a cerebrovascular accident (CVA), is a sudden focal neurological deficit caused by cerebrovascular disease.
2. A stroke is a syndrome in which the cerebral circulation is interrupted, causing neurological deficits.
3. Cerebral anoxia lasting longer than 10 minutes causes cerebral infarction with irreversible change.
4. Cerebral edema and congestion cause further dysfunction.
5. Diagnosis is determined by a CT scan, electroencephalography, cerebral arteriography, and MRI.
6. Transient ischemic attack may be a warning sign of an impending stroke
7. The permanent disability cannot be determined until the cerebral edema subsides.
8. The order in which function may return is facial, swallowing, lower limb, speech, and arms.
9. Carotid endarterectomy is a surgical intervention used in stroke management; it is targeted at stroke prevention, especially in clients with symptomatic carotid stenosis.

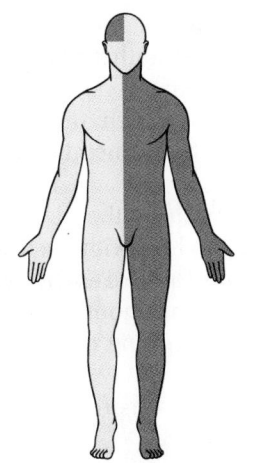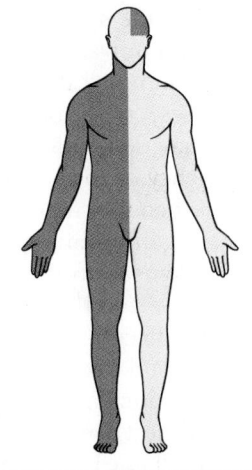

Right-brain damage (stroke on right side of the brain)	**Left-brain damage** (stroke on left side of the brain)
• Paralyzed left side: hemiplegia	• Paralyzed right side: hemiplegia
• Left-sided neglect	• Impaired speech/language aphasias
• Spatial-perceptual deficits	• Impaired right/left discrimination
• Tends to deny or minimize problems	• Slow performance, cautious
• Rapid performance, short attention span	• Aware of deficits: depression, anxiety
• Impulsive, safety problems	• Impaired comprehension related to language, math
• Impaired judgment	
• Impaired time concepts	

▲ **FIGURE 66-5** Manifestations of right brain and left brain stroke. (From Lewis, S., Heitkemper, M., Dirksen, S., O'Brien, P., & Bucher, L. [2007]. *Medical-surgical nursing: Assessment and management of clinical problems* [7th ed.]. St. Louis: Mosby.)

B. Causes
1. Thrombosis
2. Embolism
3. Hemorrhage from rupture of a vessel

C. Risk factors
1. Atherosclerosis
2. Hypertension
3. Anticoagulation therapy
4. Diabetes mellitus
5. Stress
6. Obesity
7. Oral contraceptives

D. Assessment (Fig. 66-5; Boxes 66-17 and 66-18)

⚠ A critical factor in the early intervention and treatment of stroke is the accurate identification of stroke manifestations and establishing the onset of the manifestations. Stroke screening scales may be used to quickly identify stroke manifestations.

1. Assessment findings depend on the area of the brain affected.
2. Lesions in the cerebral hemisphere result in manifestations on the contralateral side, which is the side of the body opposite the stroke.

Box 66-17 Neurological Assessment in Stroke

Changes in level of consciousness
Signs of increasing intracranial pressure
Assessment of cranial nerves V, VII, IX, X, and XII
    Cranial nerve V: Difficulty with chewing
    Cranial nerve VII: Facial paralysis or paresis
    Cranial nerves IX and X: Dysphagia
    Cranial nerve IX: Absent gag reflex
    Cranial nerve XII: Impaired tongue movement

Box 66-18 Assessment Findings in a Stroke (Brain Attack)

Agnosia
The inability to recognize familiar objects or persons

Apraxia
Called dyspraxia if the condition is mild
Characterized by loss of ability to execute or carry out skilled movements or gestures, despite having the desire and physical ability to perform them

Hemianopsia
Blindness in half the visual field

Homonymous Hemianopsia
Loss of half of the field of view on the same side in both eyes.

Neglect Syndrome (Unilateral Neglect)
Client unaware of the existence of his or her paralyzed side

Proprioception Alterations
Altered position sense that places the client at increased risk of injury
Pyramid Point: With visual problems, the client must turn the head to scan the complete range of vision.

---

3. Airway patency is always a priority.
4. Pulse (may be slow and bounding)
5. Respirations (Cheyne-Stokes)
6. Blood pressure (hypertension)
7. Headache, nausea, and vomiting
8. Facial drooping
9. **Nuchal rigidity**
10. Visual changes
11. Ataxia
12. Dysarthria
13. Dysphagia
14. Speech changes
15. Decreased sensation to pressure, heat, and cold
16. Bowel and bladder dysfunctions
17. Paralysis

E. Aphasia
1. Expressive
    a. Damage occurs in Broca's area of the frontal brain.

b. The client understands what is said but is unable to communicate verbally.

2. Receptive
   a. Injury involves Wernicke's area in the temporoparietal area.
   b. The client is unable to understand the spoken and often the written word.

3. Global or mixed: Language dysfunction occurs in expression and reception.

4. Interventions for aphasia
   a. Provide repetitive directions.
   b. Break tasks down to one step at a time.
   c. Repeat names of objects frequently used.
   d. Allow time for the client to communicate.
   e. Use a picture board, communication board, or computer technology.

F. Interventions during the acute phase of stroke
   1. Maintain a patent airway and administer oxygen as prescribed.
   2. Monitor vital signs.
   3. Usually a blood pressure of 150/100 mm Hg is maintained to ensure cerebral perfusion.
   4. Suction secretions as prescribed, but never suction nasally or for longer than 10 seconds to prevent **increased ICP**.
   5. Monitor for **increased ICP** because the client is most at risk during the first 72 hours following the stroke.
   6. Position the client on the side, with the head of bed elevated 15 to 30 degrees as prescribed.
   7. Monitor level of consciousness, pupillary response, motor and sensory response, cranial nerve function, and reflexes.
   8. Maintain a quiet environment.
   9. Insert a Foley catheter as prescribed.
   10. Administer intravenous fluids as prescribed.
   11. Maintain fluid and electrolyte balance.
   12. Prepare to administer anticoagulants, antiplatelets, diuretics, antihypertensives, and anticonvulsants as prescribed.
   13. Establish a form of communication.

G. Interventions in the postacute phase of a stroke
   1. Continue with interventions from the acute phase.
   2. Position the client 2 hours on the unaffected side and 20 minutes on the affected side.
   3. Position the client in the prone position if prescribed, for 30 minutes three times daily.
   4. Provide skin, mouth, and eye care.
   5. Perform passive range-of-motion exercises to prevent contractures.
   6. Place antiembolism stockings on the client; remove daily to check skin.
   7. Measure thighs and calves daily for an increase in size.
   8. Monitor the gag reflex and ability to swallow.
   9. Provide sips of fluids and slowly advance diet to foods that are easy to chew and swallow.

10. Provide soft and semisoft foods and flavored, cool or warm, thickened fluids rather than thin liquids because the stroke client can tolerate these types of food better; speech therapists may do swallow studies to recommend consistency of food and fluids.
11. When the client is eating, position the client sitting in a chair or sitting up in bed, with the head and neck positioned slightly forward and flexed.
12. Place food in the back of the mouth on the unaffected side to prevent trapping of food in the affected cheek.

H. Interventions in the chronic phase of stroke
   1. Neglect syndrome
      a. Client is unaware of the existence of his or her paralyzed side (**unilateral neglect**), which places the client at risk for injury.
      b. Teach the client to touch and use both sides of the body.
   2. **Hemianopsia**
      a. Client has blindness in half the visual field.
      b. **Homonymous hemianopsia** is blindness in the same visual field of both eyes.
      c. Encourage the client to turn the head to scan the complete range of vision; otherwise, he or she does not see half of the visual field.
   3. Approach the client from the unaffected side.
   4. Place the client's personal objects within the visual field.
   5. Provide eye care for visual deficits.
   6. Place a patch over the affected eye if the client has diplopia.
   7. Increase mobility as tolerated.
   8. Encourage fluid intake and a high-fiber diet.
   9. Administer stool softeners as prescribed.
   10. Encourage the client to express her or his feelings.
   11. Encourage independence in activities of daily living.
   12. Assess the need for assistive devices such as a cane, walker, splint, or braces.
   13. Teach transfer technique from bed to chair and from chair to bed.
   14. Provide gait training.
   15. Initiate physical and occupational therapy for assessment and the need for adaptive equipment or other supports for self-care and mobility.
   16. Refer client to a speech and language pathologist as prescribed.
   17. Encourage the client and family to contact available community resources.

XII. MULTIPLE SCLEROSIS

A. Description
   1. Multiple sclerosis is a chronic, progressive, noncontagious, degenerative disease of the CNS characterized by demyelinization of the neurons.

2. It usually occurs between the ages of 20 and 40 years and consists of periods of remissions and exacerbations.
3. The causes are unknown, but the disease is thought to be the result of an autoimmune response or viral infection.
4. Precipitating factors include pregnancy, fatigue, stress, infection, and trauma.
5. Electroencephalographic findings are abnormal.
6. Assessment of a lumbar puncture indicates an increased gamma globulin level, but the serum globulin level is normal.

B. Assessment
1. Fatigue and weakness
2. Ataxia and vertigo
3. Tremors and spasticity of the lower extremities
4. Parasthesias
5. Blurred vision, diplopia, and transient blindness
6. Nystagmus
7. Dysphasia
8. Decreased perception to pain, touch, and temperature
9. Bladder and bowel disturbances, including urgency, frequency, retention, and incontinence
10. Abnormal reflexes, including hyperreflexia, absent reflexes, and a positive **Babinski reflex**
11. Emotional changes such as apathy, euphoria, irritability, and depression
12. Memory changes and confusion

C. Interventions
1. Provide energy conservation measures during exacerbation.
2. Protect the client from injury by providing safety measures.
3. Place an eye patch on the eye for diplopia.
4. Monitor for potential complications such as urinary tract infections, calculi, pressure ulcers, respiratory tract infections, and contractures.
5. Promote regular elimination by bladder and bowel training.
6. Encourage independence.
7. Assist the client to establish a regular exercise and rest program.
8. Instruct the client to balance moderate activity with rest periods.
9. Assess the need for and provide assistive devices.
10. Initiate physical and speech therapy.
11. Instruct the client to avoid fatigue, stress, infection, overheating, and chilling.
12. Instruct the client to increase fluid intake and eat a balanced diet, including low-fat, high-fiber foods and foods high in potassium.
13. Instruct the client in safety measures related to sensory loss, such as regulating the temperature of bath water and avoiding heating pads.

14. Instruct the client in safety measures related to motor loss, such as avoiding the use of scatter rugs and using assistive devices.
15. Instruct the client in the self-administration of prescribed medications.
16. Provide information about the National Multiple Sclerosis Society.

XIII. MYASTHENIA GRAVIS

A. Description
1. Myasthenia gravis is a neuromuscular disease characterized by considerable weakness and abnormal fatigue of the voluntary muscles.
2. A defect in the transmission of nerve impulses at the myoneural junction occurs.
3. Causes include insufficient secretion of acetylcholine, excessive secretion of cholinesterase, and unresponsiveness of the muscle fibers to acetylcholine.

B. Assessment
1. Weakness and fatigue
2. Difficulty chewing
3. Dysphagia
4. Ptosis
5. Diplopia
6. Weak, hoarse voice
7. Difficulty breathing
8. Diminished breath sounds
9. Respiratory paralysis and failure

C. Interventions
1. Monitor respiratory status and ability to cough and deep-breathe adequately.
2. Monitor for respiratory failure.
3. Maintain suctioning and emergency equipment at the bedside.
4. Monitor vital signs.
5. Monitor speech and swallowing abilities to prevent aspiration.
6. Encourage the client to sit up when eating.
7. Assess muscle status.
8. Instruct the client to conserve strength.
9. Plan short activities that coincide with times of maximal muscle strength.
10. Monitor for myasthenic and cholinergic crises.
11. Administer anticholinesterase medications as prescribed.
12. Instruct the client to avoid stress, infection, fatigue, and over-the counter medications.
13. Instruct the client to wear a Medic-Alert bracelet.
14. Inform the client about services from the Myasthenia Gravis Foundation.

D. Anticholinesterase medications: Increase levels of acetylcholine at the myoneural junction (see Chapter 67)

E. Myasthenic crisis
1. Description
   a. Myasthenic crisis is an acute exacerbation of the disease.

    b. The crisis is caused by a rapid, unrecognized progression of the disease, inadequate amount of medication, infection, fatigue, or stress.
2. Assessment
    a. Increased pulse, respirations, and blood pressure
    b. Dyspnea, anoxia, and cyanosis
    c. Bowel and bladder incontinence
    d. Decreased urine output
    e. Absent cough and swallow reflex
3. Interventions
    a. Assess for signs of myasthenic crisis.
    b. Increase anticholinesterase medication, as prescribed.

F. Cholinergic crisis
1. Description
    a. Cholinergic crisis results in depolarization of the motor end plates.
    b. The crisis is caused by overmedication with anticholinesterase.
2. Assessment
    a. Abdominal cramps
    b. Nausea, vomiting, and diarrhea
    c. Blurred vision
    d. Pallor
    e. Facial muscle twitching
    f. Hypotension
    g. Pupillary miosis
3. Interventions
    a. Hold anticholinesterase medication.
    b. Prepare to administer the antidote, atropine sulfate, if prescribed.

G. Tensilon test

⚠ Have atropine sulfate available when performing the Tensilon test.

1. Description
    a. The **Tensilon test** is performed to diagnose myasthenia gravis and to differentiate between myasthenic crisis and cholinergic crisis.
    b. The test places the client at risk for ventricular fibrillation and cardiac arrest; the nurse must be prepared for this possibility.
2. To diagnose myasthenia gravis
    a. Edrophonium (Tensilon) injection is administered to the client.
    b. Positive for myasthenia gravis: Client shows improvement in muscle strength after the administration of Tensilon.
    c. Negative for myasthenia gravis: Client shows no improvement in muscle strength, and strength may even deteriorate after injection of Tensilon.
3. To differentiate crisis
    a. Myasthenic crisis: Tensilon is administered and, if strength improves, the client needs more medication.

    b. Cholinergic crisis: Tensilon is administered and, if weakness is more severe, the client is overmedicated; administer atropine sulfate, the antidote, as prescribed.

XIV. PARKINSON'S DISEASE

A. Description
1. Parkinson's disease is a degenerative disease caused by the depletion of dopamine, which interferes with the inhibition of excitatory impulses, resulting in a dysfunction of the extrapyramidal system.
2. It is a slow, progressive disease that results in a crippling disability.
3. The debilitation can result in falls, self-care deficits, failure of body systems, and depression.
4. Mental deterioration occurs late in the disease.

B. Assessment
1. Bradykinesia, abnormal slowness of movement, and sluggishness of physical and mental responses
2. Akinesia
3. Monotonous speech
4. Handwriting that becomes progressively smaller
5. Tremors in hands and fingers at rest (pill rolling)
6. Tremors increasing when fatigued and decreasing with purposeful activity or sleep
7. Rigidity with jerky movements
8. Restlessness and pacing
9. Blank facial expression; mask-like facies
10. Drooling
11. Difficulty swallowing and speaking
12. Loss of coordination and balance
13. Shuffling steps, stooped position, and propulsive gait

C. Interventions
1. Assess neurological status.
2. Assess ability to swallow and chew.
3. Provide high-calorie, high-protein, high-fiber soft diet with small, frequent feedings.
4. Increase fluid intake to 2000 mL/day.
5. Monitor for constipation.
6. Promote independence along with safety measures.
7. Avoid rushing the client with activities.
8. Assist with ambulation and provide assistive devices.
9. Instruct the client to rock back and forth to initiate movement.
10. Instruct the client to wear low-heeled shoes.
11. Encourage the client to lift feet when walking and to avoid prolonged sitting.
12. Provide a firm mattress and position the client prone, without a pillow, to facilitate proper posture.
13. Instruct in proper posture by teaching the client to hold the hands behind the back to keep the spine and neck erect.

14. Promote physical therapy and rehabilitation.
15. Administer antiparkinsonian medications to increase the level of dopamine in the CNS.
16. Instruct the client to avoid foods high in vitamin B$_6$ because they block the effects of antiparkinsonian medications.
17. Instruct the client to avoid monoamine oxidase inhibitors because they will precipitate hypertensive crisis.
18. See Chapter 67 regarding medication to treat Parkinson's disease.

XV. TRIGEMINAL NEURALGIA

A. Description
1. Trigeminal neuralgia is a sensory disorder of the trigeminal (fifth cranial) nerve.
2. It results in severe, recurrent, sharp, facial pain along the trigeminal nerve.
B. Assessment
1. Client has severe pain on the lips, gums, or nose, or across the cheeks.
2. Situations that stimulate symptoms include cold, washing the face, chewing, or food or fluids of extreme temperatures.
C. Interventions
1. Instruct the client to avoid hot or cold foods and fluids.
2. Provide small feedings of liquid and soft foods.
3. Instruct the client to chew food on the unaffected side.
4. Administer medications as prescribed (see Chapter 67).
D. Surgical interventions
1. Microvascular decompression: Surgical relocation of the artery that compresses the trigeminal nerve as it enters the pons may relieve pain without compromising facial sensation
2. Radiofrequency waveforms: Creates lesions that provides relief of pain without compromising touch or motor function
3. Rhizotomy: Resection of the root of the nerve to relieve pain.
4. Glycerol injection: Destroys the myelinated fibers of the trigeminal nerve (may take up to 3 weeks for pain relief to occur)

XVI. BELL'S PALSY (FACIAL PARALYSIS)

A. Description
1. Bell's palsy is caused by a lower motor neuron lesion of the seventh cranial nerve that may result from infection, trauma, hemorrhage, meningitis, or tumor.
2. It results in paralysis of one side of the face.
3. Recovery usually occurs in a few weeks, without residual effects.

B. Assessment
1. Flaccid facial muscles
2. Inability to raise the eyebrows, frown, smile, close the eyelids, or puff out the cheeks
3. Upward movement of the eye when attempting to close the eyelid
4. Loss of taste
C. Interventions
1. Encourage facial exercises to prevent the loss of muscle tone (a face sling may be prescribed to prevent stretching of weak muscles).
2. Protect the eyes from dryness and prevent injury.
3. Promote frequent oral care.
4. Instruct the client to chew on the unaffected side.

XVII. GUILLAIN-BARRÉ SYNDROME

A. Description
1. Guillain-Barré syndrome is an acute infectious neuronitis of the cranial and peripheral nerves.
2. The immune system overreacts to the infection and destroys the myelin sheath.
3. The syndrome usually is preceded by a mild upper respiratory infection or gastroenteritis.
4. The recovery is a slow process and can take years.

⚠ The major concern in Guillain-Barré syndrome is difficulty breathing; monitor respiratory status closely.

B. Assessment
1. Paresthesias
2. Pain and/or hypersensitivity such as with the weight of bed sheets or other items touching the body
3. Weakness of lower extremities
4. Gradual progressive weakness of the upper extremities and facial muscles
5. Possible progression to respiratory failure
6. Cardiac dysrhythmias
7. CSF that reveals an elevated protein level
8. Abnormal electroencephalogram
C. Interventions
1. Care is directed toward the treatment of symptoms, including pain management.
2. Monitor respiratory status.
3. Provide respiratory treatments.
4. Prepare to initiate respiratory support.
5. Monitor cardiac status.
6. Assess for complications of immobility.
7. Provide the client and family with support.

XVIII. AMYOTROPHIC LATERAL SCLEROSIS

A. Description
1. Amyotrophic lateral sclerosis is also known as Lou Gehrig's disease.
2. It is a progressive degenerative disease involving the motor system.

3. The sensory and autonomic systems are not involved, and mental status changes do not result from the disease.
4. The cause of the disease may be related to an excess of glutamate, a chemical responsible for relaying messages between the motor neurons.
5. As the disease progresses, muscle weakness and atrophy develop until a flaccid tetraplegia develops.
6. Eventually, the respiratory muscles become affected, leading to respiratory compromise, pneumonia, and death.
7. No cure is known, and the treatment is symptomatic.

B. Assessment
1. Respiratory difficulty
2. Fatigue while talking
3. Muscle weakness and atrophy
4. Tongue atrophy
5. Dysphagia
6. Weakness of the hands and arms
7. Fasciculations of the face
8. Nasal quality of speech
9. Dysarthria

C. Interventions
1. Care is directed toward the treatment of symptoms.
2. Monitor respiratory status and institute measures to prevent aspiration.
3. Provide respiratory treatments.
4. Prepare to initiate respiratory support.
5. Assess for complications of immobility.
6. Address advance directives as appropriate
7. Provide the client and family with support.

XIX. ENCEPHALITIS

A. Description
1. Encephalitis is an inflammation of the brain parenchyma and often of the meninges.
2. It affects the cerebrum, brainstem, and cerebellum.
3. It most often is caused by a viral agent, although bacteria, fungi, or parasites also may be involved.
4. Viral encephalitis is almost always preceded by a viral infection.

B. Transmission
1. Arboviruses can be transmitted to human beings through the bite of an infected mosquito or tick.
2. Echovirus, coxsackievirus, poliovirus, herpes zoster virus, and viruses that cause mumps and chickenpox are common enteroviruses associated with encephalitis.
3. Herpes simplex type 1 virus can cause viral encephalitis.
4. The organism that causes amebic meningoencephalitis can enter the nasal mucosa of persons swimming in warm fresh water—for example, in a pond or lake.

C. Assessment
1. Presence of cold sores, lesions, or ulcerations of the oral cavity
2. History of insect bites and swimming in fresh water
3. Exposure to infectious diseases
4. Travel to areas where the disease is prevalent
5. Fever
6. Nausea and vomiting
7. **Nuchal rigidity**
8. Changes in level of consciousness and mental status
9. Signs of **increased ICP**
10. Motor dysfunction and focal neurological deficits

D. Interventions
1. Monitor vital and neurological signs.
2. Assess level of consciousness using the **Glasgow Coma Scale**.
3. Assess for mental status changes and personality and behavior changes.
4. Assess for signs of **increased ICP**.
5. Assess for the presence of **nuchal rigidity** and a positive **Kernig's sign** or **Brudzinski's sign**, indicating meningeal irritation.
6. Assist the client to turn, cough, and deep-breathe frequently.
7. Elevate the head of the bed 30 to 45 degrees.
8. Assess for muscle and neurological deficits.
9. Administer acyclovir (Zovirax) as prescribed (usually is the medication of choice for herpes encephalitis).
10. Initiate rehabilitation as needed for motor dysfunction or neurological deficits.

XX. WEST NILE VIRUS INFECTION

A. Description
1. West Nile virus infection is a potentially serious illness that affects the CNS.
2. The virus is contracted primarily by the bite of an infected mosquito (mosquitoes become carriers when they feed on infected birds).
3. Symptoms typically develop between 3 and 14 days after being bitten by the infected mosquito.
4. Neurological effects can be permanent.

B. Assessment
1. Many individuals will not experience any symptoms.
2. Mild symptoms include fever, headache and body aches, nausea, vomiting, swollen glands, or a rash on the chest, stomach, or back.
3. Severe symptoms include a high fever, headache, neck stiffness, stupor, disorientation, tremors, muscle weakness, vision loss, numbness, paralysis, seizures, or coma.

C. Interventions are supportive; there is no specific treatment for the virus.

D. Prevention
1. Use insect repellents containing DEET (diethyltoluamide) when outdoors and wear long sleeves and pants and light-colored clothing.
2. Stay indoors at dusk and dawn when mosquitoes are most active.
3. Ensure that mosquito breeding sites are eliminated, such as standing water and water in bird baths, and keep wading pools empty and on their sides when not in use.

XXI. MENINGITIS

A. Description
1. Meningitis is inflammation of the arachnoid and pia mater of the brain and spinal cord.
2. It is caused by bacterial and viral organisms, although fungal and protozoal meningitis also occur.
3. Predisposing factors include skull fractures, brain or spinal surgery, sinus or upper respiratory infections, the use of nasal sprays, and a compromised immune system.
4. Cerebrospinal fluid is analyzed to determine the diagnosis and type of meningitis.
B. Transmission: Transmission occurs in areas of high population density, crowded living areas such as college dormitories, and prisons.

⚠ Transmission of meningitis is by direct contact, including droplet spread.

C. Assessment (see Box 66-4)
1. Mild lethargy
2. Photophobia
3. Deterioration in the level of consciousness
4. Signs of meningeal irritation, such as **nuchal rigidity** and a positive **Kernig's sign** and **Brudzinski's sign**
5. Red, macular rash with meningococcal meningitis
6. Abdominal and chest pain with viral meningitis
D. Interventions
1. Monitor vital signs and neurological signs.
2. Assess for signs of **increased ICP**.
3. Initiate seizure precautions.
4. Monitor for seizure activity.
5. Monitor for signs of meningeal irritation.
6. Perform cranial nerve assessment.
7. Assess peripheral vascular status (septic emboli may block circulation).
8. Maintain isolation precautions as necessary with bacterial meningitis.
9. Maintain urine and stool precautions with viral meningitis.
10. Maintain respiratory isolation for the client with pneumococcal meningitis.
11. Elevate the head of the bed 30 degrees, and avoid neck flexion and extreme hip flexion.
12. Prevent stimulation and restrict visitors.
13. Administer analgesics as prescribed.
14. Administer antibiotics as prescribed.

MORE QUESTIONS ON THE CD!

Practice Questions

796. The nurse is assessing the motor function of an unconscious client. The nurse would plan to use which of the following to test the client's peripheral response to pain?
1. Sternal rub
2. Nail bed pressure
3. Pressure on the orbital rim
4. Squeezing of the sternocleidomastoid muscle

797. The nurse is caring for the client with increased intracranial pressure. The nurse would note which of the following trends in vital signs if the intracranial pressure is rising?
1. Increasing temperature, increasing pulse, increasing respirations, decreasing blood pressure
2. Increasing temperature, decreasing pulse, decreasing respirations, increasing blood pressure
3. Decreasing temperature, decreasing pulse, increasing respirations, decreasing blood pressure
4. Decreasing temperature, increasing pulse, decreasing respirations, increasing blood pressure

798. The client recovering from a head injury is arousable and participating in care. The nurse determines that the client understands measures to prevent elevations in intracranial pressure if the nurse observes the client doing which of the following activities?
1. Blowing the nose
2. Isometric exercises
3. Coughing vigorously
4. Exhaling during repositioning

799. The client has clear fluid leaking from the nose following a basilar skull fracture. The nurse assesses that this is cerebrospinal fluid if the fluid:
1. Is clear and tests negative for glucose
2. Is grossly bloody in appearance and has a pH of 6
3. Clumps together on the dressing and has a pH of 7
4. Separates into concentric rings and tests positive for glucose

800. The client with a spinal cord injury is prone to experiencing autonomic dysreflexia. The nurse would avoid which of the following measures to minimize the risk of recurrence?

1. Strict adherence to a bowel retraining program
2. Keeping the linen wrinkle-free under the client
3. Preventing unnecessary pressure on the lower limbs
4. Limiting bladder catheterization to once every 12 hours

801. The nurse is evaluating the neurological signs of a client in spinal shock following spinal cord injury. Which of the following observations by the nurse indicates that spinal shock persists?
1. Hyperreflexia
2. Positive reflexes
3. Reflex emptying of the bladder
4. Flaccid paralysis

802. The nurse is caring for the client who begins to experience seizure activity while in bed. Which of the following actions by the nurse would be contraindicated?
1. Loosening restrictive clothing
2. Restraining the client's limbs
3. Removing the pillow and raising padded side rails
4. Positioning the client to the side, if possible, with the head flexed forward

803. The nurse is assigned to care for a client with complete right-sided hemiparesis. The nurse plans care knowing that in this condition:
1. The client has complete bilateral paralysis of the arms and legs.
2. The client has weakness on the right side of the body, including the face and tongue.
3. The client has lost the ability to move the right arm but is able to walk independently.
4. The client has lost the ability to ambulate independently but is able to feed and bathe himself or herself without assistance.

804. The nurse has instructed the family of a client with brain attack (stroke) who has homonymous hemianopsia about measures to help the client overcome the deficit. The nurse determines that the family understands the measures to use if they state that they will:
1. Place objects in the client's impaired field of vision.
2. Discourage the client from wearing eyeglasses.
3. Approach the client from the impaired field of vision.
4. Remind the client to turn the head to scan the lost visual field.

805. The nurse is assessing the adaptation of the client to changes in functional status after a brain attack

(stroke). The nurse determines that the client is adapting most successfully if the client
1. Gets angry with family if they interrupt a task
2. Experiences bouts of depression and irritability
3. Has difficulty with using modified feeding utensils
4. Consistently uses adaptive equipment in dressing self

806. The nurse is teaching the client with myasthenia gravis about the prevention of myasthenic and cholinergic crises. The nurse tells the client that this is most effectively done by:
1. Eating large, well-balanced meals
2. Doing muscle-strengthening exercises
3. Doing all chores early in the day while less fatigued
4. Taking medications on time to maintain therapeutic blood levels

807. The nurse has given instructions to the client with Parkinson's disease about maintaining mobility. The nurse determines that the client understands the directions if the client states that he or she will:
1. Sit in soft, deep chairs.
2. Exercise in the evening to combat fatigue.
3. Rock back and forth to start movement with bradykinesia.
4. Buy clothes with many buttons to maintain finger dexterity.

808. The nurse has given suggestions to the client with trigeminal neuralgia about strategies to minimize episodes of pain. The nurse determines that the client needs reinforcement of information if the client makes which of the following statements?
1. "I will wash my face with cotton pads."
2. "I'll have to start chewing on my unaffected side."
3. "I'll try to eat my food either very warm or very cold."
4. "I should rinse my mouth if toothbrushing is painful."

809. The client is admitted to the hospital with a diagnosis of Guillain-Barré syndrome. The nurse inquires during the nursing admission interview if the client has a history of:
1. Seizures or trauma to the brain
2. Meningitis during the last 5 years
3. Back injury or trauma to the spinal cord
4. Respiratory or gastrointestinal infection during the previous month

810. The client with Guillain-Barré syndrome has ascending paralysis and is intubated and receiving mechanical ventilation. Which of the following strategies would the nurse incorporate in the plan of care to help the client cope with this illness?

1. Giving client full control over care decisions and restricting visitors
2. Providing positive feedback and encouraging active range of motion
3. Providing information, giving positive feedback, and encouraging relaxation
4. Providing intravenously administered sedatives, reducing distractions, and limiting visitors

811. The client has a neurological deficit involving the limbic system. Which assessment finding is specific to this type of deficit?
1. Is disoriented to person, place, and time
2. Affect is flat, with periods of emotional lability
3. Cannot recall what was eaten for breakfast today
4. Demonstrates inability to add and subtract; does not know who is the president of the United States

812. The nurse is admitting a client with Guillain-Barré syndrome to the nursing unit. The client has an ascending paralysis to the level of the waist. Knowing the complications of the disorder, the nurse brings which of the following essential items into the client's room?
1. Nebulizer and pulse oximeter
2. Blood pressure cuff and flashlight
3. Flashlight and incentive spirometer
4. Electrocardiographic monitoring electrodes and intubation tray

813. The nurse is evaluating the status of the client who had a craniotomy 3 days ago. The nurse

would suspect that the client is developing meningitis as a complication of surgery if the client exhibits:
1. A negative Kernig sign
2. Absence of nuchal rigidity
3. A positive Brudzinski sign
4. A Glasgow Coma Scale score of 15

814. The nurse has completed discharge instructions for the client with application of a halo device. The nurse determines that the client needs further clarification of the instructions if the client states that he or she will:
1. Use a straw for drinking.
2. Drive only during the daytime.
3. Use caution because the device alters balance.
4. Wash the skin daily under the lamb's wool liner of the vest.

Alternate Item Format: Multiple Response

815. The nurse is planning to institute seizure precautions for a client who is being admitted from the emergency department. Which of the following measures would the nurse include in planning for the client's safety? **Select all that apply**.
- ❏ 1. Padding the side rails of the bed
- ❏ 2. Placing an airway at the bedside
- ❏ 3. Placing the bed in the high position
- ❏ 4. Placing oxygen and suction equipment at the bedside
- ❏ 5. Putting a padded tongue blade at the head of the bed
- ❏ 6. Having intravenous equipment ready for insertion of an intravenous catheter

ANSWERS
796. 2
Rationale: Motor testing in the unconscious client can be done only by testing response to painful stimuli. Nail bed pressure tests a basic peripheral response. Cerebral responses to pain are tested using a sternal rub, placing upward pressure on the orbital rim, or squeezing the clavicle or sternocleidomastoid muscle.
Test-Taking Strategy: Note the strategic words *peripheral response.* The nail beds are the most distal of all the options and are therefore the most peripheral. Each of the other options may elicit a generalized response, but not a localized one. Review the process of testing peripheral response to pain if you had difficulty with this question.
Level of Cognitive Ability: Applying
Client Needs: Health Promotion and Maintenance
Integrated Process: Nursing Process—Assessment
Content Area: Adult health—Neurological

Reference: Black, J., & Hawks, J. (2009). *Medical-surgical nursing: Clinical management for positive outcomes* (8th ed., p. 1797). St. Louis: Saunders.

797. 2
Rationale: A change in vital signs may be a late sign of increased intracranial pressure. Trends include increasing temperature and blood pressure and decreasing pulse and respirations. Respiratory irregularities also may arise.
Test-Taking Strategy: This question looks complex but can be answered logically. If you remember that the temperature rises, then you are able to eliminate options 3 and 4. If you know that the client becomes bradycardic, or know that the blood pressure rises, you are able to select the correct option. Review the signs of increased intracranial pressure if you had difficulty with this question.
Level of Cognitive Ability: Analyzing
Client Needs: Physiological Integrity
Integrated Process: Nursing Process—Assessment

Content Area: Adult Health—Neurological
Reference: Black, J., & Hawks, J. (2009). *Medical-surgical nursing: Clinical management for positive outcomes* (8th ed., p. 1923). St. Louis: Saunders.

798. 4
Rationale: Activities that increase intrathoracic and intra-abdominal pressures cause an indirect elevation of the intracranial pressure. Some of these activities include isometric exercises, Valsalva's maneuver, coughing, sneezing, and blowing the nose. Exhaling during activities such as repositioning or pulling up in bed, opens the glottis, which prevents intrathoracic pressure from rising.
Test-Taking Strategy: Use the process of elimination. Evaluate each option in terms of the tension it puts on the body. Doing so will help you eliminate each incorrect option systematically. Review the measures that will reduce or prevent increased intracranial pressure if you had difficulty with this question.
Level of Cognitive Ability: Evaluating
Client Needs: Physiological Integrity
Integrated Process: Nursing Process—Evaluation
Content Area: Adult Health—Neurological
References: Black, J., & Hawks, J. (2009). *Medical-surgical nursing: Clinical management for positive outcomes* (8th ed., p. 1946). St. Louis: Saunders.
Ignatavicius, D., & Workman, M. (2010). *Medical-surgical nursing: Patient-centered collaborative care* (6th ed., p. 1064). St. Louis: Saunders.

799. 4
Rationale: Leakage of cerebrospinal fluid (CSF) from the ears or nose may accompany basilar skull fracture. CSF can be distinguished from other body fluids because the drainage will separate into bloody and yellow concentric rings on dressing material, called a halo sign. The fluid also tests positive for glucose.
Test-Taking Strategy: Use the process of elimination and knowledge regarding the characteristics of CSF. Recall that CSF contains glucose, whereas other secretions, such as mucus, do not. Knowing that CSF separates into rings also will help you answer this question. Review testing for CSF fluid if you had difficulty with this question.
Level of Cognitive Ability: Analyzing
Client Needs: Physiological Integrity
Integrated Process: Nursing Process—Assessment
Content Area: Adult Health—Neurological
Reference: Ignatavicius, D., & Workman, M. (2010). *Medical-surgical nursing: Patient-centered collaborative care* (6th ed., p. 1055). St. Louis: Saunders.

800. 4
Rationale: The most frequent cause of autonomic dysreflexia is a distended bladder. Straight catheterization should be done every 4 to 6 hours, and Foley catheters should be checked frequently to prevent kinks in the tubing. Constipation and fecal impaction are other causes, so maintaining bowel regularity is important. Other causes include stimulation of the skin from tactile, thermal, or painful stimuli. The nurse administers care to minimize risk in these areas.
Test-Taking Strategy: Use the process of elimination. Remember that autonomic dysreflexia is caused by noxious stimuli to the bowel, bladder, or skin. With this in mind, you can eliminate easily each of the incorrect options. Review the measures to minimize the risk of autonomic dysreflexia if you had difficulty with this question.
Level of Cognitive Ability: Applying
Client Needs: Physiological Integrity
Integrated Process: Nursing Process—Implementation
Content Area: Adult Health—Neurological
References: Black, J., & Hawks, J. (2009). *Medical-surgical nursing: Clinical management for positive outcomes* (8th ed., p. 772). St. Louis: Saunders.
Ignatavicius, D., & Workman, M. (2010). *Medical-surgical nursing: Patient-centered collaborative care* (6th ed., p. 998). St. Louis: Saunders.

801. 4
Rationale: Resolution of spinal shock is occurring when there is return of reflexes (especially flexors to noxious cutaneous stimuli), a state of hyperreflexia rather than flaccidity, and reflex emptying of the bladder.
Test-Taking Strategy: Recall that spinal shock is characterized by the loss of movement of skeletal muscles, bowel or bladder wall, and depressed reflex action. Return of any of these indicates that spinal shock is beginning to resolve. Note that options 1, 2, and 3 are comparable or alike, indicating the presence of reflexes. Review signs of spinal shock if you had difficulty with this question.
Level of Cognitive Ability: Evaluating
Client Needs: Physiological Integrity
Integrated Process: Nursing Process—Evaluation
Content Area: Adult Health—Neurological
References: Black, J., & Hawks, J. (2009). *Medical-surgical nursing: Clinical management for positive outcomes* (8th ed., p. 1954). St. Louis: Saunders.
Copstead-Kirkhorn, L., & Banasik, J. (2010). *Pathophysiology* (4th ed., p. 1082). St. Louis: Mosby.

802. 2
Rationale: Nursing actions during a seizure include providing for privacy, loosening restrictive clothing, removing the pillow and raising side rails in the bed, and placing the client on one side with the head flexed forward, if possible, to allow the tongue to fall forward and facilitate drainage. The limbs are never restrained because the strong muscle contractions could cause the client harm. If the client is not in bed when seizure activity begins, the nurse lowers the client to the floor, if possible, protects the head from injury, and moves furniture that may injure the client. Other aspects of care are as described for the client who is in bed.
Test-Taking Strategy: Use the process of elimination and note the strategic word *contraindicated*. Evaluate this question from the perspective of causing possible harm. No harm can come to the client from any of the options except for restraining the limbs. Remember, avoid restraints. Review care of a client during a seizure if you had difficulty with this question.
Level of Cognitive Ability: Applying
Client Needs: Physiological Integrity
Integrated Process: Nursing Process—Implementation
Content Area: Adult Health—Neurological

References: Ignatavicius, D., & Workman, M. (2010). *Medical-surgical nursing: Patient-centered collaborative care* (6th ed., p. 959). St. Louis: Saunders.

Swearingen, P. (2008). *All-in-one care planning resource: Medical-surgical, pediatric, maternity, and psychiatric nursing care plans* (2nd ed., pp. 325–326). St. Louis: Mosby.

803. 2

Rationale: Hemiparesis is a weakness of one side of the body that may occur after a stroke. Complete hemiparesis is weakness of the face and tongue, arm, and leg on one side. Complete bilateral paralysis does not occur in this condition. The client with right-sided hemiparesis has weakness of the right arm and leg and needs assistance with feeding, bathing, and ambulating.

Test-Taking Strategy: Use the process of elimination. Note the strategic words *complete right-sided* and focus on the subject, hemiparesis. Recalling that hemiparesis indicates weakness and focusing on the strategic words will direct you to option 2. Review the description of hemiparesis and care of the client with hemiparesis if you had difficulty with this question.

Level of Cognitive Ability: Understanding

Client Needs: Physiological Integrity

Integrated Process: Nursing Process—Planning

Content Area: Adult Health—Neurological

Reference: Ignatavicius, D., & Workman, M. (2010). *Medical-surgical nursing: Patient-centered collaborative care* (6th ed., p. 1034). St. Louis: Saunders.

804. 4

Rationale: Homonymous hemianopsia is loss of half of the visual field. The client with homonymous hemianopsia should have objects placed in the intact field of vision, and the nurse also should approach the client from the intact side. The nurse instructs the client to scan the environment to overcome the visual deficit and does client teaching from within the intact field of vision. The nurse encourages the use of personal eyeglasses, if they are available.

Test-Taking Strategy: Use the process of elimination. Recalling the definition of homonymous hemianopsia will direct you easily to option 4. Review the concept of homonymous hemianopsia if you are unfamiliar with it.

Level of Cognitive Ability: Evaluating

Client Needs: Safe and Effective Care Environment

Integrated Process: Nursing Process—Evaluation

Content Area: Adult Health—Neurological

Reference: Black, J., & Hawks, J. (2009). *Medical-surgical nursing: Clinical management for positive outcomes* (8th ed., p. 1849). St. Louis: Saunders.

805. 4

Rationale: Clients are evaluated as coping successfully with lifestyle changes after a brain attack (stroke) if they make appropriate lifestyle alterations, use the assistance of others, and have appropriate social interactions. Options 1, 2, and 3 are not adaptive behaviors.

Test-Taking Strategy: Use the process of elimination, focusing on the strategic words *adapting most successfully.* Options 1 and 2 are behaviors that may be expected in the client with a brain attack (stroke), but they are not adaptive responses.

Instead, they are a result of the insult to the brain. Options 3 and 4 indicate that the client is trying to adapt, but option 4 has the best outcome. Review care of the client with a brain attack (stroke) if you had difficulty with this question.

Level of Cognitive Ability: Evaluating

Client Needs: Psychosocial Integrity

Integrated Process: Nursing Process—Evaluation

Content Area: Adult Health—Neurological

Reference: Black, J., & Hawks, J. (2009). *Medical-surgical nursing: Clinical management for positive outcomes* (8th ed., pp. 1861–1862, 1866–1867). St. Louis: Saunders.

806. 4

Rationale: Clients with myasthenia gravis are taught to space out activities over the day to conserve energy and restore muscle strength. Taking medications correctly to maintain blood levels that are not too low or too high is important. Muscle-strengthening exercises are not helpful and can fatigue the client. Overeating is a cause of exacerbation of symptoms, as is exposure to heat, crowds, erratic sleep habits, and emotional stress.

Test-Taking Strategy: Use the process of elimination. Recalling that the common causes of myasthenic and cholinergic crises are undermedication and overmedication, respectively, will assist you in eliminating each of the incorrect options. No other option would prevent both of those complications. Review measures to prevent myasthenic and cholinergic crises if you are unfamiliar with them.

Level of Cognitive Ability: Applying

Client Needs: Physiological Integrity

Integrated Process: Teaching and Learning

Content Area: Adult Health—Neurological

Reference: Black, J., & Hawks, J. (2009). *Medical-surgical nursing: Clinical management for positive outcomes* (8th ed., pp. 1916–1917). St. Louis: Saunders.

807. 3

Rationale: The client with Parkinson's disease should exercise in the morning when energy levels are highest. The client should avoid sitting in soft deep chairs because they are difficult to get up from. The client can rock back and forth to initiate movement. The client should buy clothes with Velcro fasteners and slide-locking buckles to support the ability to dress self.

Test-Taking Strategy: Use the process of elimination. Option 2 is not useful to clients with fatigue from any disorder, so eliminate this option first. Knowing that the client with Parkinson's has difficulty with movement and dexterity helps eliminate options 1 and 4 next. Review client teaching points with Parkinson's disease if you had difficulty with this question.

Level of Cognitive Ability: Evaluating

Client Needs: Physiological Integrity

Integrated Process: Nursing Process—Evaluation

Content Area: Adult Health—Neurological

Reference: Swearingen, P. (2008). *All-in-one care planning resource: Medical-surgical, pediatric, maternity, and psychiatric nursing care plans* (2nd ed., p. 316). St. Louis: Mosby.

808. 3

Rationale: Facial pain can be minimized by using cotton pads to wash the face and using room temperature water. The client should chew on the unaffected side of the mouth, eat a soft diet, and take in foods and beverages at room temperature. If toothbrushing triggers pain, an oral rinse after meals may be helpful instead.

Test-Taking Strategy: Use the process of elimination, and note the strategic words *needs reinforcement of information*. These words indicate a negative event query and ask you to select an option that is incorrect. Recall that the pain of trigeminal neuralgia is triggered by mechanical or thermal stimuli. Very hot or cold foods are likely to trigger the pain, not relieve it. Review client education points if you had difficulty with this question.

Level of Cognitive Ability: Evaluating
Client Needs: Physiological Integrity
Integrated Process: Teaching and Learning
Content Area: Adult Health—Neurological
Reference: Ignatavicius, D., & Workman, M. (2010). *Medical-surgical nursing: Patient-centered collaborative care* (6th ed., pp. 1025–1026). St. Louis: Saunders.

809. 4

Rationale: Guillain-Barré syndrome is a clinical syndrome of unknown origin that involves cranial and peripheral nerves. Many clients report a history of respiratory or gastrointestinal infection in the 1 to 4 weeks before the onset of neurological deficits. Occasionally, the syndrome can be triggered by vaccination or surgery.

Test-Taking Strategy: Use the process of elimination and knowledge regarding the causes related to this disorder. Remember that a recent history of respiratory or gastrointestinal infection are predisposing factors. If you are unfamiliar with Guillain-Barré syndrome, review this disorder.

Level of Cognitive Ability: Analyzing
Client Needs: Physiological Integrity
Integrated Process: Nursing Process—Assessment
Content Area: Adult Health—Neurological
Reference: Swearingen, P. (2008). *All-in-one care planning resource: Medical-surgical, pediatric, maternity, and psychiatric nursing care plans* (2nd ed., p. 287). St. Louis: Mosby.

810. 3

Rationale: The client with Guillain-Barré syndrome experiences fear and anxiety from the ascending paralysis and sudden onset of the disorder. The nurse can alleviate these fears by providing accurate information about the client's condition, giving expert care and positive feedback to the client, and encouraging relaxation and distraction. The family can become involved with selected care activities and provide diversion for the client as well.

Test-Taking Strategy: Use the process of elimination. Option 1 should be eliminated first because it is not practical to think that the client would want full control over all care decisions. The client who is paralyzed cannot participate in active range of motion, which eliminates option 2. From the remaining options, option 3 is more beneficial in helping the client cope than option 4. Review care of the client with Guillain-Barré syndrome if you had difficulty with this question.

Level of Cognitive Ability: Applying
Client Needs: Psychosocial Integrity
Integrated Process: Caring
Content Area: Adult Health—Neurological

References: Ignatavicius, D., & Workman, M. (2010). *Medical-surgical nursing: Patient-centered collaborative care* (6th ed., p. 1016). St. Louis: Saunders.
Swearingen, P. (2008). *All-in-one care planning resource: Medical-surgical, pediatric, maternity, and psychiatric nursing care plans* (2nd ed., p. 290). St. Louis: Mosby.

811. 2

Rationale: The limbic system is responsible for feelings (affect) and emotions. Calculation ability and knowledge of current events relates to function of the frontal lobe. The cerebral hemispheres, with specific regional functions, control orientation. Recall of recent events is controlled by the hippocampus.

Test-Taking Strategy: Use the process of elimination. Recall that the limbic system is responsible for feelings and emotions to direct you to option 2. Review the function of the limbic system if you had difficulty with this question.

Level of Cognitive Ability: Analyzing
Client Needs: Psychosocial Integrity
Integrated Process: Nursing Process—Assessment
Content Area: Adult Health—Neurological
Reference: Copstead, L., & Banasik, J. (2010). *Pathophysiology* (4th ed., p. 996). St. Louis: Mosby.

812. 4

Rationale: The client with Guillain-Barré syndrome is at risk for respiratory failure because of ascending paralysis. An intubation tray should be available for use. Another complication of this syndrome is cardiac dysrhythmias, which necessitates the use of electrocardiographic monitoring. Because the client is immobilized, the nurse should assess for deep vein thrombosis and pulmonary embolism routinely.

Test-Taking Strategy: Note the strategic word *essential*. With an ascending paralysis, the client is at risk for involvement of respiratory muscles and subsequent respiratory failure. Option 4 is the only option that includes an intubation tray, which would be needed if the client's status deteriorated to needing intubation and mechanical ventilation. This option most directly addresses airway. Review care of the client with Guillain-Barré syndrome if you had difficulty with this question.

Level of Cognitive Ability: Applying
Client Needs: Physiological Integrity
Integrated Process: Nursing Process—Implementation
Content Area: Adult Health—Neurological
References: Ignatavicius, D., & Workman, M. (2010). *Medical-surgical nursing: Patient-centered collaborative care* (6th ed., p. 1015). St. Louis: Saunders.
Swearingen, P. (2008). *All-in-one care planning resource: Medical-surgical, pediatric, maternity, and psychiatric nursing care plans* (2nd ed., pp. 288–289). St. Louis: Mosby.

813. 3

Rationale: Signs of meningeal irritation compatible with meningitis include nuchal rigidity, a positive Brudzinski sign, and positive Kernig sign. Nuchal rigidity is characterized by a stiff neck and soreness, which is especially noticeable when the neck is flexed. Kernig's sign is positive when the client feels pain and spasm of the hamstring muscles when the leg is fully flexed at the knee and hip. Brudzinski's sign is positive when the client flexes the hips and knees in response to the nurse gently flexing the head and neck onto the chest. A Glasgow Coma Scale score of 15 is a perfect score and indicates that the client is awake and alert, with no neurological deficits.

Test-Taking Strategy: Use the process of elimination, focusing on the client's diagnosis, meningitis. You can eliminate options 1, 2, and 4 because they are normal findings. Review the signs of meningitis if you had difficulty with this question.

Level of Cognitive Ability: Analyzing
Client Needs: Physiological Integrity
Integrated Process: Nursing Process—Assessment
Content Area: Adult Health—Neurological
Reference: Black, J., & Hawks, J. (2009). *Medical-surgical nursing: Clinical management for positive outcomes* (8th ed., pp. 1835–1836). St. Louis: Saunders.

814. 2

Rationale: The halo device alters balance and can cause fatigue because of its weight. The client should cleanse the skin daily under the vest to protect the skin from ulceration and should use powder or lotions sparingly, or not at all. The liner should be changed if odor becomes a problem. The client should have food cut into small pieces to facilitate chewing and use a straw for drinking. Pin care is done as instructed. The client cannot drive at all because the device impairs the range of vision.

Test-Taking Strategy: Use the process of elimination and note the strategic words *needs further clarification*. These words indicate a negative event query and ask you to select an option that is incorrect. Visualize this device to answer correctly. The inability to turn the head without turning the torso would contraindicate driving. Review client education points related to a halo device if you had difficulty with this question

Level of Cognitive Ability: Evaluating
Client Needs: Physiological Integrity
Integrated Process: Teaching and Learning

Content Area: Adult Health—Neurological
References: Ignatavicius, D., & Workman, M. (2010). *Medical-surgical nursing: Patient-centered collaborative care* (6th ed., p. 996). St. Louis: Saunders.
Perry, A., & Potter, P. (2010). *Clinical nursing skills and techniques* (7th ed., pp. 283–285). St. Louis: Mosby.

ALTERNATE ITEM FORMAT: MULTIPLE RESPONSE
815. 1, 2, 4, 6

Rationale: Seizure precautions may vary from agency to agency, but they generally have some common features. Usually, an airway, oxygen, and suctioning equipment are kept available at the bedside. The side rails of the bed are padded, and the bed is kept in the lowest position. The client has an intravenous access in place to have a readily accessible route if anticonvulsant medications must be administered. The use of padded tongue blades is highly controversial, and they should not be kept at the bedside. Forcing a tongue blade into the mouth during a seizure more likely will harm the client who bites down during seizure activity. Risks include blocking the airway from improper placement, chipping the client's teeth, and subsequent risk of aspirating tooth fragments. If the client has an aura before the seizure, it may give the nurse enough time to place an oral airway before seizure activity begins.

Test-Taking Strategy: Use the process of elimination. Evaluate this question from the perspective of causing possible harm. No harm can come to the client from any of the options except for placing the bed in the high position and using a tongue blade. Review seizure precautions if you had difficulty with this question.

Level of Cognitive Ability: Applying
Client Needs: Safe and Effective Care Environment
Integrated Process: Nursing Process—Planning
Content Area: Adult Health—Neurological
Reference: Swearingen, P. (2008). *All-in-one care planning resource: Medical-surgical, pediatric, maternity, and psychiatric nursing care plans* (2nd ed., p. 325). St. Louis: Mosby.

Neurological Medications

I. ANTIMYASTHENIC MEDICATIONS

A. Description
1. Antimyasthenic, also called anticholinesterase, medications relieve muscle weakness associated with myasthenia gravis by blocking acetylcholine breakdown at the neuromuscular junction.
2. Antimyasthenic medications are used to treat or diagnose myasthenia gravis or to distinguish cholinergic crisis from myasthenic crisis.
3. Neostigmine bromide (Prostigmin), pyridostigmine (Mestinon), and ambenonium chloride (Mytelase) are used to control myasthenic symptoms.
4. Edrophonium chloride (Tensilon) is used to diagnose myasthenia gravis and to distinguish cholinergic crisis from myasthenic crisis.

B. Medications (Box 67-1)

C. Side effects: Cholinergic crisis (Box 67-2)

D. Interventions
1. Assess neuromuscular status, including reflexes, muscle strength, and gait.
2. Monitor the client for signs and symptoms of medication overdose (cholinergic crisis) and underdose (myasthenic crisis).
3. Instruct the client to take medications on time to maintain therapeutic blood level, thus preventing weakness, because weakness can impair the client's ability to breathe and swallow.
4. Instruct the client to take the medication with a small amount of food to prevent gastrointestinal symptoms.
5. Instruct the client to eat 45 to 60 minutes after taking medications to decrease the risk for aspiration.
6. Instruct the client to wear a Medic-Alert bracelet.
7. Note that antimyasthenic therapy is lifelong therapy.
8. Evaluate for medication effectiveness, which is based on the improvement of neuromuscular symptoms or strength without cholinergic signs and symptoms.
9. When administering edrophonium chloride, have emergency resuscitation equipment on hand and atropine sulfate available for cholinergic crisis.

E. Tensilon test
1. Edrophonium (Tensilon) is injected intravenously.
2. The **Tensilon test** can cause bronchospasm, laryngospasm, hypotension, bradycardia, and cardiac arrest.
3. Atropine sulfate is the antidote for overdose.
4. Diagnosis of myasthenia gravis: Most myasthenic clients will show a significant improvement in muscle tone within 30 to 60 seconds after injection, and the muscle improvement lasts 4 to 5 minutes.
5. The **Tensilon test** is used to diagnose cholinergic crisis (overdose with anticholinesterase) or myasthenic crisis (undermedication).
   a. In cholinergic crisis, muscle tone does not improve after the administration of Tensilon, and muscle twitching may be noted around the eyes and face.
   b. A Tensilon injection makes the client in cholinergic crisis temporarily worse (negative **Tensilon test**).
   c. A Tensilon injection temporarily improves the condition when the client is in myasthenic crisis (positive **Tensilon test**).

II. ANTIPARKINSONIAN MEDICATIONS

A. Description
1. Antiparkinsonian medications restore the balance of the neurotransmitters acetylcholine and dopamine in the central nervous system (CNS), decreasing the signs and symptoms of Parkinson's disease to maximize the client's functional abilities.
2. These medications include the dopaminergics, which stimulate the dopamine receptors; the anticholinergics, which block the cholinergic receptors; and the catechol-O-methyltransferase inhibitors, which inhibit the metabolism of dopamine in the periphery.
3. Antiparkinsonian medications are also used for Parkinson's disease, in which dopamine-containing neurons in the basal ganglia are destroyed or deficient, which causes loss of fine motor control.

Box 67-1 Antimyasthenic Medications

Ambenonium chloride (Mytelase)
Edrophonium chloride (Tensilon)
Neostigmine bromide (Prostigmin)
Pyridostigmine (Mestinon)

Box 67-2 Signs of Cholinergic Crisis

Abdominal cramps
Nausea, vomiting, and diarrhea
Pupillary miosis
Hypotension and dizziness
Increased bronchial secretions
Increased tearing and salivation
Increased perspiration
Bronchospasm, wheezing, and bradycardia

Box 67-3 Medications to Treat Parkinson's Disease

Medications Affecting the Amount of Dopamine
Amantadine (Symmetrel)
Bromocriptine (Parlodel)
Carbidopa; levodopa (Sinemet)
Levodopa (Larodopa, Dopar)
Pramipexole (Mirapex)
Ropinirole (Requip)
Selegiline hydrochloride (Carbex, Eldepryl)

Anticholinergics
Benztropine mesylate (Cogentin)
Biperiden hydrochloride (Akineton)
Procyclidine hydrochloride (Kemadrin)
Trihexyphenidyl hydrochloride

Catechol-O-Methyltransferase (COMT) Inhibitors
Entacapone (Comtan)
Tolcapone (Tasmar)

B. Dopaminergic medications
   1. Description
      a. Dopaminergic medications stimulate the dopamine receptors and increase the amount of dopamine available in the CNS or enhance neurotransmission of dopamine.
      b. Dopaminergic medications are contraindicated in clients with cardiac, renal, or psychiatric disorders.

⚠ Levodopa taken with a monoamine oxidase inhibitor antidepressant can cause a hypertensive crisis.

   2. Medications (Box 67-3; Fig. 67-1)
   3. Side effects
      a. Dyskinesia
      b. Involuntary body movements
      c. Chest pain
      d. Nausea and vomiting
      e. Urinary retention
      f. Constipation
      g. Sleep disturbances, insomnia or periods of sedation
      h. Orthostatic hypotension and dizziness
      i. Confusion
      j. Mood changes, especially depression
      k. Hallucinations
      l. Dry mouth
   4. Interventions
      a. Assess vital signs.
      b. Assess for risk of injury.
      c. Instruct the client to take the medication with food if nausea or vomiting occurs.
      d. Assess for signs and symptoms of parkinsonism such as rigidity, tremors, akinesia, and bradykinesia, a stooped forward posture, shuffling gait, and masked facies.
      e. Monitor for signs of dyskinesia.
      f. Instruct the client to report side effects and symptoms of dyskinesia.

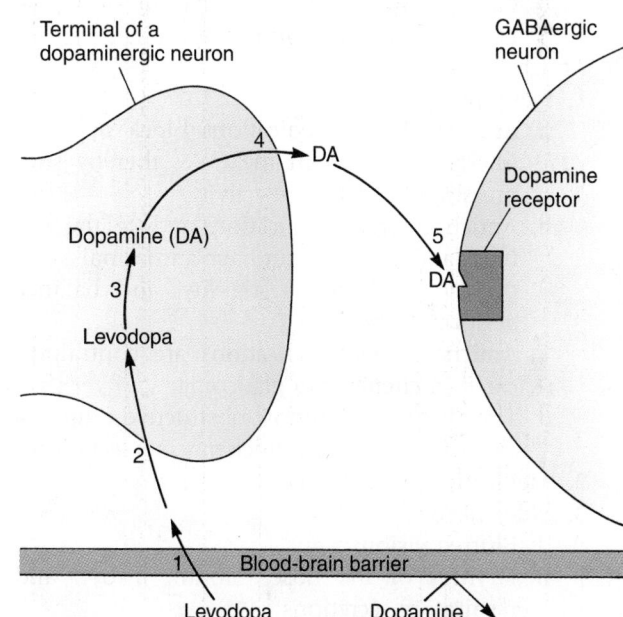

▲ **FIGURE 67-1** Steps leading to alteration of central nervous system function by levodopa. To produce its beneficial effects in Parkinson's disease (PD), levodopa must be (1) transported across the blood-brain barrier; (2) taken up by dopaminergic nerve terminals in the striatum; (3) converted into dopamine (DA); (4) released into the synaptic space; and (5) bound to DA receptors on striatal GABAergic neurons, causing them to fire at a slower rate. Note that DA itself is unable to cross the blood-brain barrier, and hence cannot be used to treat PD. (From Lehne, R. [2010]. *Pharmacology for nursing care* [7th ed.]. St. Louis: Saunders.)

g. Monitor the client for improvement in signs and symptoms of parkinsonism without the development of side effects from the medications.

h. Instruct the client to change positions slowly to minimize orthostatic hypotension.

i. Instruct the client not to discontinue the medication abruptly.

j. Instruct the client to avoid alcohol.

k. Inform the client that urine or perspiration may be discolored and that this is harmless, but may stain the clothing.

l. Advise the client with diabetes mellitus that glucose testing should not be done by urine testing because the results will not be reliable.

m. Instruct the client taking carbidopa-levodopa (Sinemet) to divide the total daily prescribed protein intake among all meals of the day; high-protein diets interfere with medication availability to the CNS.

n. When administering levodopa, instruct the client to avoid excessive vitamin B_6 intake to prevent medication reactions.

C. Anticholinergic medications

1. Description

a. Anticholinergic medications block the cholinergic receptors in the CNS, thereby suppressing acetylcholine activity.

b. Anticholinergic medications reduce the tremors and drooling but have a minimal effect on the bradykinesia, rigidity, and balance abnormalities.

c. Anticholinergic medications are contraindicated in clients with glaucoma.

d. The client with chronic obstructive lung disease can develop dry, thick mucous secretions.

2. Medications (see Box 67-3)

3. Side effects

a. Blurred vision

b. Dryness of the nose, mouth, throat, and respiratory secretions

c. Increased pulse rate, palpitations, and dysrhythmias

d. Constipation

e. Urinary retention

f. Restlessness, confusion, depression, and hallucinations

g. Photophobia

4. Interventions

a. Monitor vital signs.

b. Assess for risk of injury.

c. Monitor the client for improvement in signs and symptoms.

d. Assess the client's bowel and urinary function and monitor for urinary retention, constipation, and paralytic ileus.

e. Monitor for involuntary movements.

f. Encourage the client to avoid alcohol, smoking, caffeine, and aspirin to decrease gastric acidity.

g. Instruct the client to consult with the physician before taking any nonprescription medications.

h. Instruct the client to minimize dry mouth by increasing fluid intake and using ice chips, hard candy, or gum.

i. Instruct the client to prevent constipation by increasing fluids and fiber in the diet.

j. Instruct the client to use sunglasses in direct sunlight because of possible photophobia.

k. Instruct the client to have routine eye examinations to assess intraocular pressure.

⚠ If an anticholinergic medication is discontinued, the signs and symptoms of parkinsonism, such as rigidity, tremors, akinesia, bradykinesia, stooped forward posture, shuffling gait, and masked facies abruptly, may be intensified.

III. ANTICONVULSANT MEDICATIONS

A. Description

1. Anticonvulsant medications are used to depress abnormal neuronal discharges and prevent the spread of seizures to adjacent neurons.

2. Anticonvulsant medications should be used with caution in clients taking anticoagulants, aspirin, sulfonamides, cimetidine (Tagamet), and antipsychotic drugs.

3. Absorption is decreased with the use of antacids, calcium preparations, and antineoplastic medications.

B. Interventions for clients on anticonvulsants

1. Initiate seizure precautions.

2. Monitor urinary output.

3. Monitor liver and renal function tests and medication blood serum levels (Table 67-1)

4. Monitor for signs of medication toxicity, which would include CNS depression, ataxia, nausea, vomiting, drowsiness, dizziness, restlessness, and visual disturbances.

5. If a seizure occurs, assess seizure activity, including location and duration.

6. Protect the client from hazards in the environment during a seizure.

C. Client education (Box 67-4)

D. Hydantoins (Box 67-5)

1. Hydantoins are used to treat partial and generalized tonic-clonic seizures.

2. Phenytoin (Dilantin) also is used to treat dysrhythmias.

3. Side effects

a. Gingival hyperplasia (reddened gums that bleed easily)

b. Slurred speech

TABLE 67-1 Anticonvulsant Medications

Medication	Therapeutic Serum Range
Amobarbital (Amytal)	1-5 mcg/mL
Carbamazepine (Tegretol)	3-14 mcg/mL
Clonazepam (Klonopin)	20-80 ng/mL
Ethosuximide (Zarontin)	40-100 mcg/mL
Ethotoin (Peganone)	10-50 mcg/mL
Lorazepam (Ativan)	50-240 ng/mL
Mephobarbital (Mebaral)	15-40 mcg/mL
Phenobarbital (Luminal)	15-40 mcg/mL
Phenytoin (Dilantin)	10-20 mcg/mL

Box 67-4 Client Education: Anticonvulsants

Take the prescribed medication in the prescribed dose and frequency.

Take anticonvulsants with food to decrease gastrointestinal irritation, but avoid milk and antacids, which impair absorption.

If taking liquid medication, shake well before ingesting.

Do not discontinue the medications.

Avoid alcohol.

Avoid over-the-counter medications.

Wear a Medic-Alert bracelet.

Use caution when driving or performing activities that require alertness.

Maintain good oral hygiene and use a soft toothbrush.

Maintain preventive dental checkups.

Maintain follow-up health care visits with periodic blood studies related to determining toxicity.

Monitor serum glucose levels (diabetes mellitus).

Urine may be a harmless pink-red or red-brown in color.

Report symptoms of sore throat, bruising, and nosebleeds, which may indicate a blood dyscrasia.

Inform the physician if side effects occur, such as bleeding gums, nausea, vomiting, blurred vision, slurred speech, rash, or dizziness.

Box 67-5 Hydantoins

Ethotoin (Peganone)   Phenytoin (Dilantin)
Fosphenytoin (Cerebyx)

Box 67-6 Barbiturates

Amobarbital (Amytal)   Phenobarbital (Luminal)
Mephobarbital (Mebaral)

Box 67-7 Benzodiazepines

Clonazepam (Klonopin)   Diazepam (Valium)
Clorazepate (Tranxene)   Lorazepam (Ativan)

medication; therefore, feedings should be scheduled as far as possible from the time of phenytoin administration.

   b. Monitor therapeutic serum levels to assess for toxicity.

   c. Monitor for signs of toxicity.

   d. When administering phenytoin intravenously, dilute in normal saline because dextrose causes the medication to precipitate.

   e. When administering phenytoin intravenously, infuse no faster than 25 to 50 mg/min; otherwise, hypotension and cardiac dysrhythmias could occur.

   f. Assess for ataxia (staggering gait).

   g. Instruct the client to consult with the physician before taking other medications to ensure compatibility with anticonvulsants.

 Phenytoin decreases the effectiveness of some birth control pills and can have teratogenic effects if taken during pregnancy.

E. Barbiturates (Box 67-6)

  1. Barbiturates are used for tonic-clonic seizures and acute episodes of seizures caused by status epilepticus.

  2. Barbiturates also may be used as adjuncts to anesthesia.

  3. Side effects

   a. Sedation, ataxia, and dizziness during initial treatment

   b. Mood changes

   c. Hypotension

   d. Respiratory depression

   e. Tolerance to the medication

F. Benzodiazepines (Box 67-7)

  1. Benzodiazepines are used to treat absence seizures.

  c. Confusion

  d. Sedation and drowsiness

  e. Nausea and vomiting

  f. Blurred vision and nystagmus

  g. Headaches

  h. Blood dyscrasias: Decreased platelet count and decreased white blood cell count

  i. Elevated blood glucose level

  j. Alopecia or hirsutism

  k. Rash or pruritis

 4. Interventions

  a. Oral tube feedings may interfere with the absorption of orally administered phenytoin and diminish the effectiveness of the

2. Diazepam (Valium) and lorazepam (Ativan) are used to treat status epilepticus, anxiety, and skeletal muscle spasms.
3. Clorazepate (Tranxene) is used as adjunctive therapy for partial seizures.
4. Side effects
   a. Sedation, drowsiness, dizziness, blurred vision
   b. Administer at no more than 5 mg/min intravenously to prevent bradycardia.
   c. Medication tolerance and drug dependency
   d. Blood dyscrasias: Decreased platelet count and decreased white blood cell count
   e. Hepatotoxicity

⚠️ Flumazenil (Romazicon) reverses the effects of benzodiazepines. It should not be administered to clients with increased intracranial pressure or status epilepticus who were treated with benzodiazepines because these problems may recur with reversal.

G. Succinimides (Box 67-8)
   1. Succinimides are used to treat absence seizures.
   2. Side effects
      a. Anorexia, nausea, vomiting
      b. Blood dyscrasias
H. Oxazolidinediones (Box 67-9)
   1. Oxazolidinediones are used for absence seizures.
   2. Side effects
      a. Sedation, drowsiness, fatigue
      b. Headache
      c. Photophobia
      d. Blood dyscrasias
I. Valproates (Box 67-10)
   1. Valproates are used to treat tonic-clonic, partial, and myoclonic seizures.
   2. Side effects
      a. Transient nausea, vomiting, and indigestion
      b. Sedation, drowsiness, and dizziness
      c. Pancreatitis

      d. Blood dyscrasias: Decreased platelet count and decreased white blood cell count
      e. Hepatotoxicity
J. Iminostilbenes
   1. Iminostilbenes are used to treat seizure disorders that have not responded to other anticonvulsants (Box 67-11).
   2. Iminostilbenes are used to treat trigeminal neuralgia.
   3. Side effects
      a. Drowsiness
      b. Dizziness
      c. Nausea and vomiting, dry mouth
      d. Constipation or diarrhea
      e. Rash
      f. Visual abnormalities
      g. Blood dycrasias, agranulocytosis
      h. Headache

IV. CENTRAL NERVOUS SYSTEM STIMULANTS

A. Description
   1. Amphetamines and caffeine stimulate the cerebral cortex of the brain (Box 67-12).
   2. Amphetamines have a high potential for abuse.
   3. Analeptics and caffeine act on the brainstem and medulla to stimulate respiration.
   4. Anorexiants act on the cerebral cortex and hypothalamus to suppress appetite (Box 67-13).
   5. Central nervous system stimulants are used to treat narcolepsy and attention-deficit/hyperactivity disorders.

Box 67-11 Other Anticonvulsants

Carbamazepine (Tegretol)	Pregabalin (Lyrica)
Gabapentin (Neurontin)	Tiagabine (Gabitril Filmtabs)
Lamotrigine (Lamictal)	Topiramate (Topamax)
Levetiracetam (Keppra)	Zonisamide (Zonegran)
Oxcarbazepine (Trileptal)	Vigabatrin (Sabril)

Box 67-8 Succinimides

Ethosuximide (Zarontin)	Methsuximide (Celontin)

Box 67-9 Oxazolidinedione

Trimethadione (Troxidone)

Box 67-10 Valproates

Valproic acid (Depakene, Depacon)
Divalproex sodium (Depakote ER)

Box 67-12 Amphetamines

Amphetamine sulfate
Amphetamine; dextroamphetamine (Adderall)
Atomoxetine (Strattera)
Methylphenidate hydrochloride (Ritalin, Concerta)

Box 67-13 Anorexiants

Benzphetamine hydrochloride (Didrex)
Orlistat (Xenical)
Phendimetrazine (Bontril, Melfiat-105)
Phentermine hydrochloride (Adipex-P, Ionamin)
Sibutramine (Meridia)

6. Central nervous system stimulants are used as adjunctive therapy for exogenous obesity.
7. Other central nervous system stimulants (Box 67-14)

B. Side effects
1. Irritability
2. Restlessness
3. Tremors
4. Insomnia
5. Heart palpitations
6. Tachycardia and dysrhythmias
7. Hypertension
8. Dry mouth
9. Anorexia and weight loss
10. Abdominal cramping
11. Diarrhea or constipation
12. Hepatic failure
13. Psychoses
14. Impotence
15. Dependence and tolerance

C. Interventions
1. Monitor vital signs.
2. Assess mental status.
3. Document the degree of inattention, impulsivity, hyperactivity, and periods of sleepiness.
4. Assess height, weight, and growth of the child.
5. Monitor complete blood count and white blood cell and platelet counts before and during therapy.
6. Monitor for side effects.
7. Monitor sleep patterns.
8. Monitor for withdrawal symptoms such as nausea, vomiting, weakness, and headache.
9. Instruct the client to take the medication before meals.
10. Instruct the client to avoid foods and beverages containing caffeine to prevent additional stimulation.
11. Instruct the client not to chew or crush long-acting forms of the medications.
12. Instruct the client to read labels on over-the-counter products because many contain caffeine.
13. Instruct the client to avoid alcohol.
14. Instruct the client not to discontinue the medication abruptly (can produce extreme fatigue and depression).
15. Instruct the client to take the last daily dose of the CNS stimulant at least 6 hours before bedtime to prevent insomnia.
16. Monitor for drug dependence and abuse with amphetamines.

17. If a child is taking a CNS stimulant, instruct the parents to notify the school nurse.
18. Monitor for calming effects of CNS stimulants within 3 to 4 weeks on children with attention-deficit/hyperactivity disorder.
19. Monitor growth in the child on long-term therapy with methylphenidate hydrochloride (Ritalin) or other medications to treat attention-deficit/hyperactivity disorder.

V. NONOPIOID ANALGESICS

A. Nonsteroidal anti-inflammatory drugs (NSAIDs; Box 67-15)
1. Description
   a. NSAIDs are aspirin and aspirin-like medications that inhibit the synthesis of prostaglandins.
   b. The medications act as an analgesic to relieve pain, antipyretic to reduce body temperature, and anticoagulant to inhibit platelet aggregation.
   c. NSAIDs are used to relieve inflammation and pain and to treat rheumatoid arthritis, bursitis, tendinitis, osteoarthritis, and acute gout.
   d. NSAIDs are contraindicated in clients with hypersensitivity or liver or renal disease.
   e. Clients taking anticoagulants should not take aspirin or NSAIDS.

Box 67-15 Nonopioid Analgesics

Acetaminophen
Acetaminophen (Tylenol)

Aspirin
Aspirin (acetylsalicylic acid; ASA, Aspergum, Bayer Aspirin, Ecotrin)
Aspirin (acetylsalicylic acid), buffered (Alka-Seltzer, Bufferin)

Nonsteroidal Anti-Inflammatory Drugs
Fenoprofen (Nalfon)
Ibuprofen (Motrin, Advil)
Naproxen (Anaprox, Naprosyn, Aleve, Naprelan)
Oxaprozin (Daypro)

Cyclooxygenase-2 (COX-2) Inhibitor
Celecoxib (Celebrex)

Other Nonsteroidal Anti-Inflammatory Drugs
Diclofenac (Voltaren)
Diflunisal (Dolobid)
Etodolac (Lodine)
Indomethacin (Indocin)
Ketorolac
Meclofenamate
Mefenamic acid (Ponstel)
Meloxicam (Mobic)
Piroxicam (Feldene)
Sulindac (Clinoril)

Box 67-14 Other Central Nervous System Stimulants

Doxapram (Dopram)   Theophylline
Theobromine

f. Aspirin and an NSAID should not be taken together because aspirin decreases the blood level and the effectiveness of the NSAID and can increase the risk of bleeding.

g. NSAIDs can increase the effects of warfarin (Coumadin), sulfonamides, cephalosporins, and phenytoin (Dilantin).

h. Hypoglycemia can result if ibuprofen (Motrin) is taken with insulin or an oral hypoglycemic medication.

i. A high risk of toxicity exists if ibuprofen is taken concurrently with calcium blockers.

⚠️ Adolescents and children with flu symptoms, viral illnesses, and varicella should not take aspirin because of the risk of Reye's syndrome.

2. Side effects (Box 67-16)
3. Interventions
   a. Assess client for allergies.
   b. Obtain a medication history on the client.
   c. Assess for history of gastric upset or bleeding or liver or renal disease.
   d. Assess the client for gastrointestinal upset during medication administration.
   e. Monitor for edema.
   f. Monitor the serum salicylate (aspirin) level when the client is taking high doses.
   g. Monitor for signs of bleeding such as tarry stools, bleeding gums, petechiae, ecchymosis, and purpura.
   h. Instruct the client to take the medication with water, milk, or food.
   i. An enteric-coated or buffered form of aspirin can be taken to decrease gastric distress.
   j. Instruct the client that enteric-coated tablets cannot be crushed or broken.
   k. Clients taking aspirin should sit upright for 20 to 30 minutes after taking the dose.
   l. Advise the client to inform other health care professionals if they are taking high doses of aspirin.

m. Note that aspirin should be discontinued 3 to 7 days before surgery to reduce the risk of bleeding.

n. Instruct the client to avoid alcoholic beverages.

B. Acetaminophen (Tylenol)
   1. Description
      a. Acetaminophen inhibits prostaglandin synthesis.
      b. Acetaminophen is used to decrease pain and fever.
   2. Side effects
      a. Anorexia, nausea, vomiting
      b. Rash
      c. Hypoglycemia
      d. Oliguria
      e. Hepatotoxicity
   3. Interventions
      a. Monitor vital signs.
      b. Assess client for history of liver and renal dysfunction, alcoholism, and malnutrition.
      c. Monitor for hepatic damage, which includes nausea, vomiting, diarrhea, and abdominal pain.
      d. Monitor liver enzyme test results.
      e. Instruct the client that self-medication should not be used longer than 10 days for an adult and 5 days for a child.
      f. Note that the antidote for acetaminophen is acetylcysteine (Mucomyst).
      g. Evaluate for the effectiveness of the medication.

⚠️ Acetaminophen is contraindicated in clients with hepatic or renal disease, alcoholism, and/or hypersensitivity.

VI. OPIOID ANALGESICS

A. Description
   1. Opioid analgesics suppress pain impulses but can suppress respiration and coughing by acting on the respiratory and cough center in the medulla of the brainstem.
   2. Opioid analgesics can produce euphoria and sedation and can cause physical dependence.

Box 67-16 Side Effects of Aspirin and Nonsteroidal Anti-Inflammatory Drugs

Aspirin	**Nonsteroidal Anti-Inflammatory Drugs**
Allergic reactions (anaphylaxis, laryngeal edema)	Dysrhythmias
Bleeding (anemia, hemolysis, increased bleeding time)	Blood dyscrasias
Dizziness	Cardiovascular thrombotic events
Drowsiness	Dizziness
Flushing	Gastric irritation
Gastrointestinal symptoms (distress, heartburn, nausea, vomiting)	Hepatotoxicity
Headaches	Hypotension
Decreased renal function	Pruritus
Tinnitus	Decreased renal function
Visual changes	Sodium and water retention
	Tinnitus

3. Opioid analgesics are used for relief of mild, moderate, or severe pain.

B. Medications (Box 67-17)

1. Codeine sulfate
   a. Codeine sulfate also is an effective cough suppressant at low doses.
   b. Codeine sulfate can cause constipation.
2. Hydromorphone hydrochloride (Dilaudid)
   a. Hydromorphone can decrease respirations.
   b. Hydromorphone can cause constipation.
3. Meperidine hydrochloride (Demerol)
   a. Meperidine can cause hypotension, dizziness, urinary retention.
   b. Meperidine may be used for acute pain and as a preoperative medication.
   c. Meperidine may lead to **increased intracranial pressure (ICP)** in clients with head injuries.
   d. Meperidine is contraindicated in clients with head injuries and **increased ICP**, respiratory disorders, hypotension, shock, and severe hepatic and renal disease and in clients taking monoamine oxidase inhibitors.
   e. Meperidine should not be taken with alcohol or a sedative-hypnotic because it may increase the CNS depression.
   f. Meperidine should be used cautiously in children and adults with a seizure disorder or a history of seizures because it decreases the seizure threshold.
4. Morphine sulfate
   a. Morphine can cause respiratory depression, orthostatic hypotension, and constipation.
   b. Morphine may cause nausea and vomiting because of increased vestibular sensitivity.
   c. Morphine is used for acute pain caused by myocardial infarction or cancer, for dyspnea caused by pulmonary edema, for surgery, and as a preoperative medication.
   d. Morphine is contraindicated in clients with severe respiratory disorders; head injuries; increased ICP; severe renal, hepatic, or pulmonary disease; or seizure activity.
   e. Morphine is used with caution in clients with blood loss or shock.

⚠ Respiratory depression is the priority concern with morphine sulfate.

5. Oxycodone with aspirin (Percodan)
   a. Percodan should not be taken by a client allergic to aspirin.
   b. Percodan can cause gastric irritation and should be taken with food or plenty of liquids.
6. Propoxyphene hydrochloride (Darvon) and propoxyphene napsylate (Darvon-N)
   a. Darvon compounds contain aspirin and should not be taken by a client allergic to aspirin.
   b. Darvocet-N contains acetaminophen.
7. Nalbuphine hydrochloride (Nubain) is preferable for treating the pain of a myocardial infarction because it reduces the oxygen needs of the heart without reducing blood pressure.
8. Methadone hydrochloride (Dolophine)
   a. Dilute doses of oral concentrate with at least 90 mL of water.
   b. Dilute dispersible tablets in at least 120 mL of water, orange juice, or acidic fruit beverage.
   c. Methadone is used as a replacement medication for opiate dependence and to facilitate withdrawal.
9. Hydrocodone (Hycodan) frequently is used for cough suppression.

C. Interventions for opioid analgesics
1. Monitor vital signs.
2. Assess the client thoroughly before administering pain medication.
3. Initiate nursing measures such as massage, distraction, deep breathing and relaxation exercises, the application of heat or cold as prescribed, and providing care and comfort before administering the opioid analgesic.

Box 67-17 Opioid Analgesics

Acetaminophen/hydrocodone (Lortab)
Buprenorphine hydrochloride (Buprenex)
Butorphanol tartrate (Stadol)
Codeine sulfate, codeine phosphate
Fentanyl (Duragesic, Sublimaze)
Hydrocodone (Hycodan)
Hydromorphone hydrochloride (Dilaudid)
Levorphanol tartrate (Levo-Dromoran)
Meperidine hydrochloride (Demerol)
Methadone hydrochloride (Dolophine, Methadose)
Morphine sulfate (Duramorph, MS Contin, Kadian, Oramorph SR)

Nalbuphine hydrochloride (Nubain)
Oxycodone (Roxicodone, OxyContin)
Oxycodone hydrochloride; acetaminophen (Percocet)
Oxycodone; aspirin (Percodan)
Oxymorphone hydrochloride (Numorphan)
Pentazocine (Talwin)
Propoxyphene napsylate (Darvon-N)
Remifentanil (Ultiva)
Sufentanil (Sufenta)
Tramadol (Ultram)

4. Administer medications 30 to 60 minutes before painful activities.
5. Monitor respiratory rate and, if the rate is less than 12 breaths/min in an adult, withhold the medication unless ventilatory support is being provided.
6. Monitor pulse and, if bradycardia develops, withhold the dose and notify the physician.
7. Monitor blood pressure for hypotension.
8. Auscultate breath sounds because opioid analgesics suppress the cough reflex.
9. Encourage activities such as turning, deep breathing, and incentive spirometry to prevent atelectasis and pneumonia.
10. Monitor level of consciousness.
11. Initiate safety precautions such as side rails, a night light, and supervised ambulation.
12. Monitor intake and output.
13. Assess for urinary retention.
14. Instruct the client to take oral doses with milk or a snack to reduce gastric irritation.
15. Instruct the client to avoid alcohol.
16. Instruct the client to avoid activities that require alertness.
17. Assess bowel function for constipation, abdominal distention, and decreased peristalsis.
18. Evaluate the effectiveness of medication.
19. Have an opioid antagonist, oxygen, and resuscitation equipment available.

D. Morphine sulfate
1. Side effects
    a. Respiratory depression
    b. Orthostatic hypotension
    c. Urinary retention
    d. Nausea and vomiting
    e. Constipation
    f. Sedation, confusion, and hallucinations
    g. Cough suppression
    h. Reduction in pupillary size
    i. Miosis
2. Interventions
    a. Have naloxone (Narcan) available for overdose.
    b. Assess vital signs and level of consciousness.
    c. Compare rate and depth of respirations to baseline.
    d. Withhold the medication if the respiratory rate is less than 12 breaths/min; respirations of less than 10 breaths/min can indicate respiratory distress.
    e. Monitor urinary output, which should be at least 30 mL/hr.
    f. Monitor bowel sounds for decreased peristalsis because constipation can occur.
    g. Monitor for pupil changes because pinpoint pupils can indicate morphine overdose.
    h. Avoid alcohol or CNS depressants because they can cause respiratory depression.

Box 67-18 Opioid Antagonists

Naloxone hydrochloride (Narcan)
Naltrexone (ReVia)

    i. Instruct the client to report dizziness or difficulty breathing.
    j. If taking sustained-release morphine, the client may need short-acting opioid doses for breakthrough pain.
    k. To administer morphine intravenously, dilute in at least 5 mL of sterile water for injection and administer slowly over 4 to 5 minutes.
    l. Explain to client and family about administration and the sick effects of the medication.

E. Meperidine hydrochloride (Demerol)
1. Side effects
    a. Respiratory depression
    b. Hypotension and dizziness
    c. Tachycardia
    d. Drowsiness and confusion
    e. Constipation
    f. Urinary retention
    g. Nausea and vomiting
    h. Seizures
    i. Tremors
2. Interventions
    a. Monitor vital signs.
    b. Monitor for respiratory depression and hypotension.
    c. Have naloxone available for overdose.
    d. Monitor for urinary retention.
    e. Monitor bowel sounds and for constipation.
    f. To administer meperidine intravenously, dilute in at least 5 mL of sterile water or normal saline for injection and administer the dose over 4 to 5 minutes.

VII. OPIOID ANTAGONISTS

A. Opioid antagonists (Box 67-18) are used to treat respiratory depression from opioid overdose.
B. Interventions
1. Monitor blood pressure, pulse, and respiratory rate every 5 minutes initially, tapering to every 15 minutes, and then every 30 minutes until the client is stable.
2. Place the client on a cardiac monitor and monitor cardiac rhythm.
3. Auscultate breath sounds.
4. Have resuscitation equipment available.
5. Do not leave the client unattended.
6. Monitor the client closely for several hours because when the effects of the antagonist wears off, the client may again display signs of opioid overdose.

Box 67-19 Osmotic Diuretics

Mannitol (Osmitrol)
Urea (Ureaphil)

VIII. OSMOTIC DIURETICS

A. Description
1. Osmotic diuretics (Box 67-19) increase osmotic pressure of the glomerular filtrate, inhibiting reabsorption of water and electrolytes.
2. Osmotic diuretics are used for oliguria and to prevent renal failure, decrease intracranial pressure, and decrease ICP in clients with narrow-angle glaucoma.
3. Mannitol is used with chemotherapy to induce diuresis.

B. Side effects
1. Fluid and electrolyte imbalances
2. Pulmonary edema from the rapid shifts of fluid
3. Nausea and vomiting
4. Headache
5. Tachycardia from the rapid fluid loss
6. Hyponatremia and dehydration

C. Interventions
1. Monitor vital signs.
2. Monitor weight.
3. Monitor urine output.
4. Monitor electrolyte levels.
5. Monitor lungs and heart sounds for signs of pulmonary edema.
6. Monitor for signs of dehydration.
7. Monitor neurological status.
8. Monitor for increased intraocular pressure.
9. Assess for signs of decreasing ICP if appropriate.
10. Change the client's position slowly to prevent orthostatic hypotension.
11. Monitor for crystallization in the vial of mannitol before administering the medication; if crystallization is noted, do not administer the medication from that vial.

🔵 MORE QUESTIONS ON THE CD!

Practice Questions

816. Carbidopa-levodopa (Sinemet) is prescribed for the client with Parkinson's disease. The nurse monitors the client for side effects of the medication. Which of the following would indicate that the client is experiencing a side effect?
1. Pruritus
2. Tachycardia
3. Hypertension
4. Impaired voluntary movements

817. The home health nurse visits a client who is taking phenytoin (Dilantin) for control of seizures. During the assessment, the nurse notes that the client is taking birth control pills. Which of the following information should the nurse include in the teaching plan?
1. Pregnancy should be avoided while taking phenytoin.
2. The client may stop the medication if it is causing severe gastrointestinal effects.
3. There is the potential of decreased effectiveness of birth control pills while taking phenytoin.
4. There is the increased risk of thrombophlebitis while taking phenytoin and birth control pills together.

818. The nurse is caring for a client in the emergency department diagnosed with Bell's palsy. The client has been taking acetaminophen (Tylenol), and acetaminophen overdose is suspected. The nurse anticipates that the antidote to be prescribed is:
1. Pentostatin (Nipent)
2. Auranofin (Ridaura)
3. Fludarabine (Fludara)
4. Acetylcysteine (Mucomyst)

819. The client with trigeminal neuralgia tells the nurse that acetaminophen (Tylenol) is taken daily for the relief of generalized discomfort. Which laboratory value would indicate toxicity associated with the medication?
1. Sodium level of 140 mEq/L
2. Prothrombin time of 12 seconds
3. Direct bilirubin level of 2 mg/dL
4. Platelet count of 400,000/mm^3

820. The client is taking the prescribed dose of phenytoin (Dilantin) to control seizures. Results of a phenytoin blood level study reveal a level of 35 mcg/mL. Which of the following symptoms would be expected as a result of this laboratory result?
1. Hypotension
2. Tachycardia
3. Slurred speech
4. No symptoms, because this is a normal therapeutic level

821. The client arrives at the emergency department complaining of back spasms. The client states, "I have been taking two to three aspirin every 4 hours for the last week, and it hasn't helped my back." Aspirin intoxication is suspected, and the nurse assesses the client for which of the following?
1. Tinnitus
2. Diarrhea

3. Constipation
4. Photosensitivity

822. A client with trigeminal neuralgia is being treated with carbamazepine (Tegretol), 400 mg orally daily. Which of the following indicates that the client is experiencing a side effect to the medication?
1. Uric acid level, 5 mg/dL
2. Sodium level, 140 mEq/L
3. Blood urea nitrogen level, 15 mg/dL
4. White blood cell count, 3000/mm³

823. The nurse is caring for a client with severe back pain. Codeine sulfate has been prescribed for the client. Which of the following does the nurse specifically include in the plan of care while the client is taking this medication?
1. Monitor fluid balance.
2. Monitor bowel activity.
3. Monitor peripheral pulses.
4. Monitor for hypertension.

824. The nurse has given medication instructions to the client receiving phenytoin (Dilantin). The nurse determines that the client has an adequate understanding if the client states that:
1. "Alcohol is not contraindicated while taking this medication."
2. "Good oral hygiene is needed, including brushing and flossing."

3. "The medication dose may be self-adjusted, depending on side effects."
4. "The morning dose of the medication should be taken before a serum drug level is drawn."

825. The client with myasthenia gravis has become increasingly weaker. The physician prepares to identify whether the client is reacting to an over-dose of the medication (cholinergic crisis) or an increasing severity of the disease (myasthenic crisis). An injection of edrophonium (Tensilon) is administered. Which of the following would indicate that the client is in cholinergic crisis?
1. No change in the condition
2. Complaints of muscle spasms
3. An improvement of the weakness
4. A temporary worsening of the condition

Alternate Item Format: Multiple Response

826. Meperidine hydrochloride (Demerol) has been prescribed for a client to treat pain. Select the side effects of this medication. **Select all that apply**.
❏ 1. Diarrhea
❏ 2. Tremors
❏ 3. Drowsiness
❏ 4. Hypotension
❏ 5. Urinary frequency
❏ 6. Increased respiratory rate

ANSWERS

816. 4
Rationale: Dyskinesia and impaired voluntary movement may occur with high levodopa dosages. Nausea, anorexia, dizziness, orthostatic hypotension, bradycardia, and akinesia are frequent side effects of the medication.
Test-Taking Strategy: Use the process of elimination. Options 2 and 3 are comparable or alike and are cardiac-related options, so these options can be eliminated first. Next, focus on the client's diagnosis and select option 4 over option 1 because it is related neurologically. Review the side effects of levodopa if you had difficulty with this question.
Level of Cognitive Ability: Analyzing
Client Needs: Physiological Integrity
Integrated Process: Nursing Process—Analysis
Content Area: Pharmacology
Reference: Hodgson, B., & Kizior, R. (2010). *Saunders nursing drug handbook 2010* (pp. 174–176). St. Louis: Saunders.

817. 3
Rationale: Phenytoin enhances the rate of estrogen metabolism, which can decrease the effectiveness of some birth

control pills. Options 1, 2, and 4 are inappropriate instructions.
Test-Taking Strategy: Use the process of elimination. Option 4 would cause anxiety in the client. A client should not be instructed to stop anticonvulsant medication, as indicated in option 2. Pregnancy does not need to be "avoided." Review medication interactions related to phenytoin if you had difficulty with this question.
Level of Cognitive Ability: Applying
Client Needs: Physiological Integrity
Integrated Process: Teaching and Learning
Content Area: Pharmacology
References: Kee, J., Hayes, E., & McCuistion, L. (2009). *Pharmacology: A nursing process approach* (6th ed., pp. 324, 329). St. Louis: Saunders.
Lehne, R. (2010). *Pharmacology for nursing care* (7th ed., p. 225). St. Louis: Saunders.

818. 4
Rationale: The antidote for acetaminophen is acetylcysteine (Mucomyst). The normal therapeutic serum level of acetaminophen is 10 to 20 mcg/mL. A toxic level is higher than 50 mcg/mL, and levels higher than 200 mcg/mL could

indicate hepatotoxicity. Auranofin (Ridaura) is a gold preparation used to treat rheumatoid arthritis. Fludarabine (Fludara) and pentostatin (Nipent) are antineoplastic agents.
Test-Taking Strategy: Use the process of elimination. Eliminate options 1 and 3 first because they are comparable or alike (antineoplastic agents). Recalling that auranofin is used to treat rheumatoid arthritis will direct you to option 4. Review the antidote for acetaminophen if you had difficulty with this question.
Level of Cognitive Ability: Understanding
Client Needs: Physiological Integrity
Integrated Process: Nursing Process—Planning
Content Area: Pharmacology
Reference: Hodgson, B., & Kizior, R. (2010). *Saunders nursing drug handbook 2010* (p. 11). St. Louis: Saunders.

819. 3
Rationale: In adults, overdose of acetaminophen causes liver damage. Option 3 is an indicator of liver function and is the only option that indicates an abnormal laboratory value. The normal direct bilirubin level is 0 to 0.3 mg/dL. The normal platelet count is 150,000 to 400,000/mm^3. The normal prothrombin time is 10 to 13 seconds. The normal sodium level is 135 to 145 mEq/L.
Test-Taking Strategy: Use the process of elimination. Knowledge that acetaminophen causes liver damage and knowledge of normal laboratory results will assist you in answering this question. Option 3 is the only abnormal value. Also, of all the options, the bilirubin level is the laboratory value most directly related to liver function. Review the effects of toxicity from acetaminophen and normal laboratory values if you had difficulty with this question.
Level of Cognitive Ability: Analyzing
Client Needs: Physiological Integrity
Integrated Process: Nursing Process—Analysis
Content Area: Pharmacology
References: Kee, J., Hayes, E., & McCuistion, L. (2009). *Pharmacology: A nursing process approach* (6th ed., p. 377). St. Louis: Saunders.
Lehne, R. (2010). *Pharmacology for nursing care* (7th ed., p. 845). St. Louis: Saunders.
Pagana, K., & Pagana, T. (2009). *Mosby's diagnostic and laboratory test reference* (9th ed., p. 148). St. Louis: Mosby.

820. 3
Rationale: The therapeutic phenytoin level is 10 to 20 mcg/mL. At a level higher than 20 mcg/mL, involuntary movements of the eyeballs (nystagmus) appears. At a level higher than 30 mcg/mL, ataxia and slurred speech occur.
Test-Taking Strategy: Use the process of elimination and knowledge regarding the therapeutic phenytoin level. From this point, you must know the symptoms that would be noted in the client when the phenytoin level is 35 mcg/mL. Remember that ataxia and slurred speech occur with levels higher than 30 mcg/mL. Review therapeutic levels and associated symptoms if you had difficulty with this question.
Level of Cognitive Ability: Analyzing
Client Needs: Physiological Integrity
Integrated Process: Nursing Process—Assessment
Content Area: Pharmacology

Reference: Hodgson, B., & Kizior, R. (2010). *Saunders nursing drug handbook 2010* (p. 909). St. Louis: Saunders.

821. 1
Rationale: Mild intoxication with acetylsalicylic acid (aspirin) is called salicylism and is experienced commonly when the daily dosage is higher than 4 g. Tinnitus (ringing in the ears) is the most frequent effect noted with intoxication. Hyperventilation may occur because salicylate stimulates the respiratory center. Fever may result, because salicylate interferes with the metabolic pathways coupling oxygen consumption and heat production. Options 2, 3, and 4 are not associated specifically with toxicity.
Test-Taking Strategy: Use the process of elimination. Note that the question refers to aspirin intoxication. Options 2 and 3 relate to gastrointestinal symptoms, are comparable or alike, and are eliminated first. From the remaining options, you must know that tinnitus occurs. If you had difficulty with this question, review aspirin intoxication.
Level of Cognitive Ability: Analyzing
Client Needs: Physiological Integrity
Integrated Process: Nursing Process—Assessment
Content Area: Pharmacology
Reference: Hodgson, B., & Kizior, R. (2010). *Saunders nursing drug handbook 2010* (p. 89). St. Louis: Saunders.

822. 4
Rationale: Adverse effects of carbamazepine appear as blood dyscrasias, including aplastic anemia, agranulocytosis, thrombocytopenia, and leukopenia; cardiovascular disturbances; thrombophlebitis; dysrhythmias; and dermatological effects.
Test-Taking Strategy: Use the process of elimination. If you are familiar with normal laboratory values, you will note that the only option that indicates an abnormal value is option 4. Review the side effects related to this medication if you had difficulty with this question.
Level of Cognitive Ability: Analyzing
Client Needs: Physiological Integrity
Integrated Process: Nursing Process—Analysis
Content Area: Pharmacology
References: Lehne, R. (2010). *Pharmacology for nursing care* (7th ed., p. 237). St. Louis: Saunders.
Pagana, K., & Pagana, T. (2009). *Mosby's diagnostic and laboratory test reference* (9th ed., pp. 998–1000). St. Louis: Mosby.

823. 2
Rationale: While the client is taking codeine sulfate, the nurse would monitor vital signs and assess for hypotension. The nurse also should increase fluid intake, palpate the bladder for urinary retention, auscultate bowel sounds, and monitor the pattern of daily bowel activity and stool consistency. The nurse should monitor respiratory status and initiate deep-breathing and coughing exercises. Additionally, the nurse monitors the effectiveness of the pain medication.
Test-Taking Strategy: Use the process of elimination. Note the strategic word *specifically* and recall that codeine sulfate can cause constipation. If you had difficulty with this question, review nursing measures related to the administration of codeine sulfate.
Level of Cognitive Ability: Applying

Client Needs: Physiological Integrity
Integrated Process: Nursing Process—Planning
Content Area: Pharmacology
Reference: Hodgson, B., & Kizior, R. (2010). *Saunders nursing drug handbook 2010* (p. 267). St. Louis: Saunders.

824. 2

Rationale: Typical anticonvulsant medication instructions include taking the prescribed daily dosage to keep the blood level of the drug constant and having a sample drawn for serum drug level before taking the morning dose. The client is taught not to stop the medication abruptly, avoid alcohol, check with the physician before taking over-the-counter medications, avoid activities in which alertness and coordination are required until medication effects are known, provide good oral hygiene, and obtain regular dental care. The client should also wear a Medic-Alert bracelet.
Test-Taking Strategy: Use the process of elimination. Using knowledge of general principles related to the medication administration will assist you in eliminating options 1 and 3. From the remaining options, recall that medications generally are not taken just before drawing therapeutic serum levels because the results would be artificially high. This leaves oral hygiene as the correct option because of the risk of gingival hyperplasia. Review client education related to phenytoin (Dilantin) if you had difficulty with this question.
Level of Cognitive Ability: Evaluating
Client Needs: Physiological Integrity
Integrated Process: Nursing Process—Evaluation
Content Area: Adult health—Neurological
References: Edmunds, M. (2010). *Introduction to clinical pharmacology* (6th ed., p. 257). St. Louis: Mosby.

Hodgson, B., & Kizior, R. (2010). *Saunders nursing drug handbook 2010* (p. 909). St. Louis: Saunders.

825. 4

Rationale: An edrophonium injection makes the client in cholinergic crisis temporarily worse. An improvement in the weakness indicates myasthenia crisis.

Test-Taking Strategy: Use the process of elimination. Recalling that a cholinergic crisis indicates an overdose of medication, it seems reasonable that a worsening of the condition will occur when medication is administered. Review cholinergic crisis if you had difficulty with this question.
Level of Cognitive Ability: Analyzing
Client Needs: Physiological Integrity
Integrated Process: Nursing Process—Analysis
Content Area: Pharmacology
References: Ignatavicius, D., & Workman, M. (2010). *Medical-surgical nursing: Patient-centered collaborative care* (6th ed., pp. 1017, 1019). St. Louis: Saunders.

Kee, J., Hayes, E., & McCuistion, L. (2009). *Pharmacology: A nursing process approach* (6th ed., pp. 345, 347). St. Louis: Saunders.

Lehne, R. (2010). *Pharmacology for nursing care* (7th ed., pp. 137–138). St. Louis: Saunders.

ALTERNATE ITEM FORMAT: MULTIPLE RESPONSE
826. 2, 3, 4

Rationale: Meperidine hydrochloride is an opioid analgesic. Side effects include respiratory depression, drowsiness, hypotension, constipation, urinary retention, nausea, vomiting, and tremors.
Test-Taking Strategy: Focus on the name of the medication. Recalling that this medication is an opioid analgesic and recalling the effects of an opioid analgesic will assist in identifying the side effects. Review the side effects of this medication if you had difficulty with this question.
Level of Cognitive Ability: Analyzing
Client Needs: Physiological Integrity
Integrated Process: Nursing Process—Assessment
Content Area: Pharmacology
Reference: Hodgson, B., & Kizior, R. (2010). *Saunders nursing drug handbook 2010* (p. 716). St. Louis: Saunders.

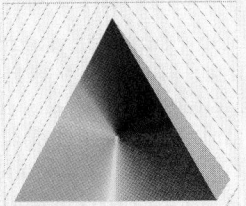

UNIT XVII

The Adult Client With a Musculoskeletal Disorder

PYRAMID TERMS

cast Stiff dressing or casting, made of plaster of Paris or synthetic material, to stabilize a part or parts of the body until healing occurs.

compartment syndrome Condition in which pressure increases in a confined anatomical space, leading to decreased blood flow, ischemia, and dysfunction of these tissues. Initial ischemia with pain, pallor, paresthesia, muscle weakness, and loss of pulses may progress to necrosis and permanent muscle cell dysfunction.

external fixation Stabilization of a fracture by the use of an external frame, with multiple pins applied through the bone.

fat embolism Sudden dislodgment of a fat globule that is freed into the circulation, where it can lodge in a blood vessel and obstruct blood flow to tissue distal to the obstruction.

internal fixation Stabilization of a fracture that involves the application of screws, plates, pins, or nails to hold the fragments in alignment.

reduction Correction or realignment of a bone fracture or joint dislocation.

traction Exertion of a pulling force to a fractured bone or dislocated joint to establish and maintain correct alignment for healing and to decrease muscle spasms and pain.

PYRAMID TO SUCCESS

The Pyramid to Success focuses on the emergency care for a client who sustains a fracture or other musculoskeletal injury, monitoring for complications related to fractures, and carrying out interventions if complications occur. Nursing care related to casts and traction is emphasized. Skill related to instructing the client in the use of an assistive device such as a cane, walker, or crutches is a Pyramid Point. Pyramid Points also include postoperative care following hip surgery or amputation and care of the client with rheumatoid arthritis or osteoporosis. Focus on the points related to the psychosocial effects as a result of the musculoskeletal disorder, such as unexpected body image changes, and the appropriate and available support services needed for the client.

CLIENT NEEDS

Safe and Effective Care Environment

Establishing priorities
Handling hazardous and infectious materials safely
Maintaining asepsis related to wounds
Maintaining confidentiality regarding the disorder and plan of care
Maintaining standard and other precautions
Preventing accidents and injuries
Providing a dietary consultation
Providing informed consent for diagnostic treatments and surgical procedures
Providing physical therapy and occupational therapy referrals
Upholding client rights

Health Promotion and Maintenance

Discussing expected body image changes
Performing physical assessment related to the musculoskeletal system
Promoting health related to diet and activity
Preventing diseases that occur as a result of the aging process

Providing home care instructions regarding care related to a musculoskeletal disorder

Reinforcing the importance of prescribed therapy

Psychosocial Integrity

Assessing available support systems and use of community resources

Assessing the client's ability to cope with feelings of isolation and loss of independence

Considering cultural, religious, and spiritual influences

Discussing grief and loss related to mobility limitations and restrictions

Discussing situational role changes as a result of the musculoskeletal disorder

Identifying unexpected body image changes as a result of injury or disease

Identifying sensory and perceptual alterations

Mobilizing coping mechanisms

Physiological Integrity

Identifying complications of a fracture

Identifying complications related to procedures or injuries

Providing care related to casts and traction

Promoting normal elimination patterns

Promoting self-care measures

Providing emergency care for a fracture or other injury

Providing measures to promote comfort

Teaching about the use of assistive devices for mobility such as canes, walkers, and crutches

Teaching pharmacological therapy

Musculoskeletal System

I. ANATOMY AND PHYSIOLOGY

A. Skeleton
1. Axial portion
   a. Cranium
   b. Vertebrae
   c. Ribs
2. Appendicular portion
   a. Limbs
   b. Shoulders
   c. Hips

B. Types of bones (Box 68-1)
1. Spongy bone
   a. Spongy bone is located in the ends of long bones and the center of flat and irregular bones.
   b. Spongy bone can withstand forces applied in many directions.
2. Dense (compact) bone
   a. Dense bone covers spongy bone.
   b. Forms a cylinder around a central marrow cavity
   c. Better able to withstand longitudinal forces than horizontal forces
3. Characteristics of the bones
   a. Support and protect structures of the body
   b. Provide attachments for muscles, tendons, and ligaments
   c. Contain tissue in the central cavities, which aids in the formation of blood cells
   d. Assist in regulating calcium and phosphate concentrations
4. Bone growth
   a. The length of bone growth results from the ossification of the epiphyseal cartilage at the ends of bones; bone growth stops between the ages of 18 and 25 years.
   b. The width of bone growth results from the activity of osteoblasts; it occurs throughout life but slows down with aging.

⚠ As aging occurs, bone resorption accelerates, decreasing bone mass and predisposing the client to injury.

C. Types of joints (Table 68-1)
1. Characteristics of joints
   a. Allow movement between bones
   b. Formed where two bones join
   c. Surfaces are covered with cartilage.
   d. Enclosed in a capsule (synovial joints)
   e. Contain a cavity filled with synovial fluid (synovial joints)
   f. Ligaments hold the bone and joint in the correct position.
   g. Articulation is the meeting point of two or more bones.
2. Synovial fluid
   a. Found in the synovial joint capsule
   b. Formed by the synovial membrane, which lines the joint capsule
   c. Lubricates the cartilage
   d. Provides a cushion against shocks

D. Muscles
1. Characteristics of muscles
   a. Made up of bundles of muscle fibers
   b. Provide the force to move bones
   c. Assist in maintaining posture
   d. Assist with heat production
2. Process of contraction and relaxation
   a. Muscle contraction and relaxation require large amounts of adenosine triphosphate.
   b. Contraction also requires calcium, which functions as a catalyst.
   c. Acetylcholine released by the motor end plate of the motor neuron initiates an action potential.
   d. Acetylcholine is then destroyed by acetylcholinesterase.
   e. Calcium is required to contract muscle fibers and acts as a catalyst for the enzyme needed for the sliding together action of actin and myosin.
   f. Following contraction, adenosine triphosphate transports calcium out to allow actin and myosin to separate and allow the muscle to relax.
3. Skeletal muscles

Box 68-1 Types of Bones

Long	Flat
Short	Irregular

TABLE 68-1 Types of Joints

Type	Description
Amphiarthrosis	Cartilaginous joint Slightly movable
Condyloid	Freely movable Allows frictionless, painless movement
Diarthrosis	Synovial joint Ball-and-socket joint
Synarthrosis	Fibrous or fixed joint No movement associated with these joints

a. Skeletal muscles are attached to two bones and cross at least one joint.
b. The point of origin is the point of attachment that does not move.
c. The point of insertion is the point of attachment that moves when the muscle contracts.
d. Skeletal muscles act in groups.
e. Prime movers contract to produce movement.
f. Antagonists relax.
g. Synergists contract to stabilize body movement.
h. Nerves activate and control the muscles.

E. Bone healing
1. Description: Bone union or healing is the process that occurs after the integrity of a bone is interrupted.
2. Three stages
   a. The fracture causes soft tissue edema and bleeding because of the vascularity of the bone; this blood solidifies into a hematoma over 48 to 72 hours.
   b. The postinjury blood supply is interrupted, leading to ischemia and necrosis of the bone around the injury site.
   c. Dead cells promote migration of osteoblasts and fibroblasts to the area and healing starts with the formation of fibrocartilage.
   d. Bone union begins as a callus forms with vascular and cellular proliferation surrounding the fracture site; this loose fibrous tissue, or callus, changes into bone over the next 3 to 6 months.
   e. Remodeling occurs as the excess bone tissue of the callus resorbs as time passes and weight-bearing activities are gradually increased; the time required for complete healing varies and is related to factors such as age, bone type, trauma severity, infection, and blood supply.

Box 68-2 Risk Factors Associated With Musculoskeletal Disorders

Autoimmune disorders	Metabolic disorders
Calcium deficiency	Neoplastic disorders
Falls	Obesity
Hyperuricemia	Postmenopausal states
Infection	Trauma and injury
Medications	

II. RISK FACTORS ASSOCIATED WITH MUSCULOSKELETAL DISORDERS (Box 68-2)

III. DIAGNOSTIC TESTS

A. Radiography
1. Description: Radiography is a commonly used procedure to diagnose disorders of the musculoskeletal system.
2. Interventions
   a. Handle injured areas carefully and support extremities above and below the joint.
   b. Administer analgesics as prescribed before the procedure, particularly if the client is in pain.
   c. Remove any radiopaque objects, such as jewelry.
   d. Ask the client if she is pregnant; may be contraindicated in pregnancy.
   e. Shield client's testes, ovaries, or pregnant abdomen.
   f. The client must lie still during a radiographic (x-ray) procedure.
   g. Inform the client that exposure to radiation is minimal and not dangerous.
   h. The health care provider is to wear a lead apron if staying in the room with the client.

B. Arthrocentesis
1. Description: Arthrocentesis is used to diagnose joint inflammation and infection.
   a. Arthrocentesis involves aspirating synovial fluid, blood, or pus via a needle inserted into a joint cavity.
   b. Medication, such as corticosteroids, may be instilled into the joint if necessary to alleviate inflammation.
2. Interventions
   a. Obtain an informed consent.
   b. Apply an elastic compression bandage postprocedure as prescribed.
   c. Use ice to decrease pain and swelling.
   d. Pain may worsen after aspirating fluid from the joint; analgesics may be prescribed.
   e. Pain can continue up to 2 days after administration of corticosteroids into a joint.
   f. Instruct the client to rest the joint for 8 to 24 hours postprocedure.

g. Instruct the client to notify the physician if a fever or swelling of the joint occurs.

C. Arthrography

1. Description: Arthrography is used in unexplained joint pain or inflammation to diagnose trauma to the joint capsule or ligaments.

   a. Arthrography is a radiographic examination of the soft tissues of the joint structures.

   b. A local anesthetic is used for the procedure.

   c. A contrast medium or air is injected into the joint cavity, and the joint is moved through range of motion as a series of x-rays are taken.

2. Interventions

   a. Instruct the client to fast from food and fluids for 8 hours before the procedure as prescribed.

   b. Assess the client for allergies to iodine or shellfish before the procedure.

   c. Obtain an informed consent.

   d. Inform the client of the need to remain as still as possible, except when asked to reposition.

   e. Minimize the use of the joint for 12 hours after the procedure.

   f. Instruct the client that the joint may be edematous and tender for 1 to 2 days after the procedure and may be treated with ice packs and analgesics as prescribed.

   g. Instruct the client that if edema and tenderness last longer than 2 days, the physician should be notified.

   h. If knee arthrography was performed, an elastic compression wrap over the knee may be prescribed for 3 to 4 days and ice applied to decrease pain and swelling.

   i. If air has been used for injection, crepitus may be felt in the joint for up to 2 days.

D. Arthroscopy

1. Description: Arthroscopy is used to diagnose and treat acute and chronic disorders of the joint.

   a. Arthroscopy provides an endoscopic examination of various joints.

   b. Articular cartilage abnormalities can be assessed, loose bodies removed, and the cartilage trimmed.

   c. A biopsy may be performed during the procedure.

2. Interventions

   a. Instruct the client to fast for 8 to 12 hours before the procedure.

   b. Obtain an informed consent.

   c. Administer pain medication as prescribed postprocedure.

   d. Assess the neurovascular status of the affected extremity.

   e. An elastic compression bandage should be worn postprocedure for 2 to 4 days as prescribed.

f. Instruct the client that walking without weight bearing usually is permitted after sensation returns but to limit activity for 1 to 4 days as prescribed following the procedure.

g. Instruct the client to elevate the extremity as often as possible for 2 days following the procedure and to place ice on the site to minimize swelling.

h. Reinforce instructions regarding the use of crutches, which may be used for 5 to 7 days postprocedure for walking.

i. Advise the client to notify the physician if fever or increased knee pain occurs or if edema continues for more than 3 days postprocedure.

E. Bone mineral density measurements

1. Dual-energy x-ray absorptiometry

   a. Dual-energy x-ray absorptiometry measures the bone mass of the spine, wrist and hip bones, and total body.

   b. Radiation exposure is minimal.

   c. Dual-energy x-ray absorptiometry is used to diagnosis metabolic bone disease and to monitor changes in bone density with treatment.

   d. Inform the client that the procedure is painless.

   e. All metallic objects are removed before the test.

2. Quantitative ultrasound

   a. Quantitative ultrasound evaluates strength, density, and elasticity of various bones, using ultrasound rather than radiation.

   b. Inform the client that the procedure is painless.

F. Bone scan

1. Description: A bone scan is used to identify, evaluate, and stage bone cancer before and after treatment; it is also used to detect fractures.

   a. Radioisotope is injected intravenously and will collect in areas that indicate abnormal bone metabolism and some fractures, if they exist.

   b. The isotope is excreted in the urine and feces within 48 hours and is not harmful to others.

2. Interventions

   a. Food and fluids may be withheld, before the procedure.

   b. Obtain an informed consent.

   c. Remove all jewelry and metal objects.

   d. Following the injection of the radioisotope, the client must drink 32 oz of water (if not contraindicated) to promote renal filtering of the excess isotope.

   e. From 1 to 3 hours after the injection, have the client void to clear excess isotope from the bladder before the scanning procedure is completed.

   f. Inform the client of the need to lie supine during the procedure and that the procedure is not painful.

   g. Monitor the injection site for redness and swelling.

   h. Encourage oral fluid intake following the procedure.

⚠ No special precautions are required after a bone scan because a minimal amount of radioactivity exists in the radioisotope used for the procedure.

G. Bone or muscle biopsy

   1. Description: Biopsy may be done during surgery or through aspiration or punch or needle biopsy.

   2. Interventions

     a. Obtain an informed consent.

     b. Monitor for bleeding, swelling, hematoma, or severe pain.

     c. Elevate the site for 24 hours following the procedure to reduce edema.

     d. Apply ice packs as prescribed following the procedure to prevent the development of a hematoma and decrease site discomfort.

     e. Monitor for signs of infection following the procedure.

     f. Inform the client that mild to moderate discomfort is normal following the procedure.

H. Electromyography (EMG)

   1. Description: EMG is used to evaluate muscle weakness.

     a. Electromyography measures electrical potential associated with skeletal muscle contractions.

     b. Needles are inserted into the muscle, and recordings of muscular electrical activity are traced on recording paper through an oscilloscope.

   2. Interventions

     a. Obtain an informed consent.

     b. Instruct the client that the needle insertion is uncomfortable.

     c. Instruct the client not to take any stimulants or sedatives for 24 hours before the procedure.

     d. Inform the client that slight bruising may occur at the needle insertion sites.

     e. Mild analgesics can be used for the pain.

I. Myelography

   1. Description: Myelography requires injection of dye or air into the subarachnoid space followed by radiography to detect abnormalities of the spinal cord and vertebrae.

   2. Preprocedure interventions

     a. Obtain an informed consent.

     b. Provide hydration for at least 12 hours before the test.

     c. Assess client for allergies to iodine or seafood (shellfish).

     d. Premedicate for sedation as prescribed.

   3. Postprocedure interventions

     a. Obtain vital signs and perform neurological assessment frequently as prescribed.

     b. Maintain bedrest as prescribed. The head position varies according to the dye used; the head is usually elevated if an oil-based or water-soluble contrast agent is used and is usually positioned lower than the trunk if air contrast is used.

     c. Encourage fluids and monitor intake and output to validate dye excretion.

     d. If air contrast is used, keep the head lower than the trunk, as prescribed by the physician.

IV. INJURIES

A. Strains

   1. Strains are an excessive stretching of a muscle or tendon.

   2. Management involves cold and heat applications, exercise with activity limitations, anti-inflammatory medications, and muscle relaxants.

   3. Surgical repair may be required for a severe strain (ruptured muscle or tendon).

B. Sprains

   1. Sprains are an excessive stretching of a ligament, usually caused by a twisting motion, such as in a fall or stepping onto an uneven surface.

   2. Sprains are characterized by pain and swelling.

   3. Management involves rest, ice, a compression bandage, and elevation to reduce swelling and provide joint support.

   4. Casting may be required for moderate sprains to allow the tear to heal.

   5. Surgery may be necessary for severe ligament damage.

C. Rotator cuff injuries

   1. The musculotendinous or rotator cuff of the shoulder can sustain a tear, usually as a result of trauma.

   2. Injury is characterized by shoulder pain and the inability to maintain abduction of the arm at the shoulder (drop arm test).

   3. Management involves nonsteroidal anti-inflammatory drugs (NSAIDs), physical therapy, sling support, and ice-heat applications.

   4. Surgery may be required if medical management is unsuccessful or a complete tear is present.

V. FRACTURES

A. Description: A fracture is a break in the continuity of the bone caused by trauma, twisting as a result of muscle spasm or indirect loss of leverage, or bone decalcification and disease that result in osteopenia.

B. Types of fractures (Box 68-3)

C. Assessment of a fracture of an extremity

Box 68-3 Types of Fractures

Closed or simple: Skin over the fractured area remains intact.

Comminuted: The bone is splintered or crushed, creating numerous fragments.

Complete: The bone is separated completely by a break into two parts.

Compression: A fractured bone is compressed by other bone.

Depressed: Bone fragments are driven inward.

Greenstick: One side of the bone is broken and the other is bent; these fractures occur most commonly in children.

Impacted: A part of the fractured bone is driven into another bone.

Incomplete: Fracture line does not extend through the full transverse width of the bone.

Oblique: The fracture line runs at an angle across the axis of the bone.

Open or compound: The bone is exposed to air through a break in the skin, and soft tissue injury and infection are common.

Pathological: The fracture results from weakening of the bone structure by pathological processes such as neoplasia or osteomalacia; also called spontaneous fracture.

Spiral: The break partially encircles bone.

Transverse: The bone is fractured straight across.

Box 68-4 Interventions for a Fracture

Reduction	Traction
Fixation	Cast

1. Pain or tenderness over the involved area
2. Decrease or loss of muscular strength or function
3. Obvious deformity of affected area
4. Crepitation, erythema, edema, or bruising
5. Muscle spasm and neurovascular impairment

D. Initial care of a fracture of an extremity
1. Immobilize affected extremity with cast or splint.
2. Assess neurovascular status of the extremity.
3. Interventions for a fracture (Box 68-4)

⚠ If a compound (open) fracture exists, splint the extremity and cover the wound with a sterile dressing.

E. Reduction restores the bone to proper alignment.
1. Closed **reduction** is a nonsurgical intervention performed by manual manipulation.
   a. Closed **reduction** may be performed under local or general anesthesia.
   b. A **cast** may be applied following **reduction**.
2. Open **reduction** involves a surgical intervention; the fracture may be treated with **internal fixation** devices.

F. Fixation
1. **Internal fixation** follows an open **reduction** (Fig. 68-1).
   a. **Internal fixation** involves the application of screws, plates, pins, or intramedullary rods to hold the fragments in alignment.
   b. **Internal fixation** may involve the removal of damaged bone and replacement with a prosthesis.
   c. **Internal fixation** provides immediate bone strength.
2. **External fixation** is the use of an external frame to stabilize a fracture by attaching skeletal pins

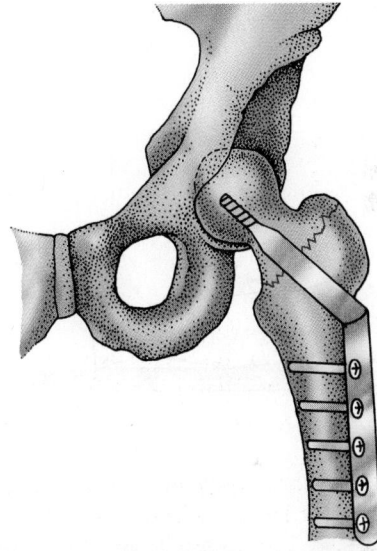

▲ **FIGURE 68-1** A compression hip screw used for open reduction with internal fixation. (From Ignatavicius, D., & Workman, M. [2010]. *Medical-surgical nursing: Patient-centered collaborative care* [6th ed.]. St. Louis: Saunders.)

through bone fragments to a rigid external support (Fig. 68-2)
   a. **External fixation** provides more freedom of movement than with **traction**.
   b. Monitor pin stability and provide pin care to decrease infection risks.
   c. Risk of infection exists with both fixation methods.
   d. **External fixation** is commonly used when massive tissue trauma is present.

G. Traction (Fig. 68-3)
1. Description
   a. **Traction** is the exertion of a pulling force applied in two directions to reduce and immobilize a fracture.
   b. **Traction** provides proper bone alignment and reduces muscle spasms.

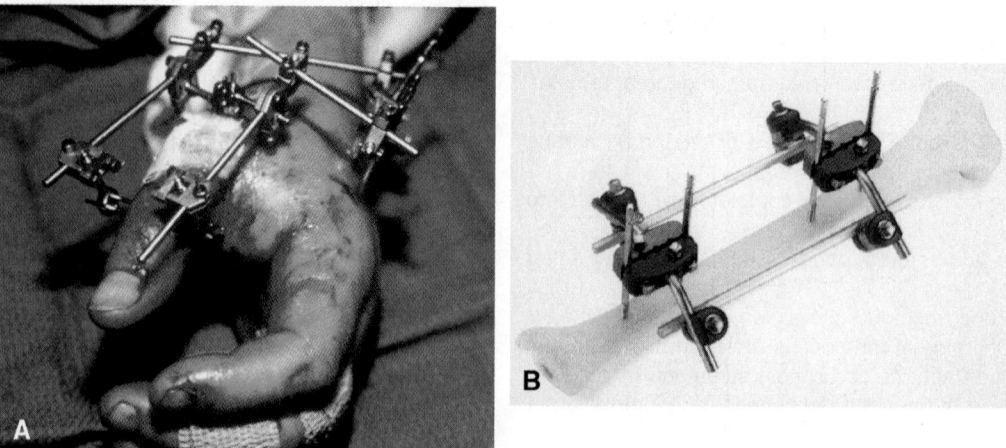

▲ **FIGURE 68-2** External fixators. **A,** Mini-Hoffman system in use on hand. **B,** Hoffman II on the tibia (standard system). (From Lewis, S., Heitkemper, M., Dirksen, S., O'Brien, P., & Bucher, L. [2007]. *Medical-surgical nursing: Assessment and management of clinical problems* [7th ed.]. St. Louis: Mosby.)

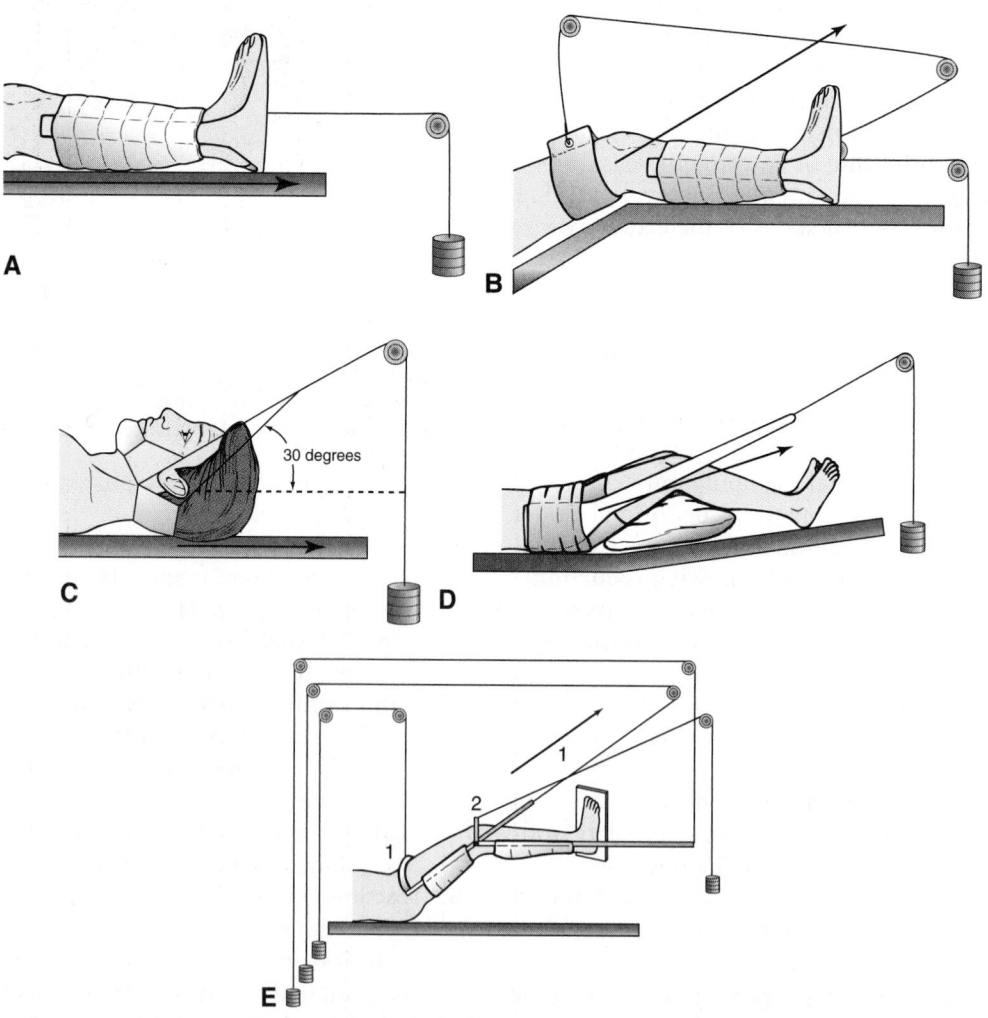

▲ **FIGURE 68-3** Types of traction. **A,** Buck's traction. **B,** Russell's traction. **C,** Head halter traction. **D,** Pelvic traction. **E,** Balanced suspension traction. (From Lewis, S., Heitkemper, M., Dirksen, S., O'Brien, P., & Bucher, L. [2007]. *Medical-surgical nursing: Assessment and management of clinical problems* [7th ed.]. St. Louis: Mosby.)

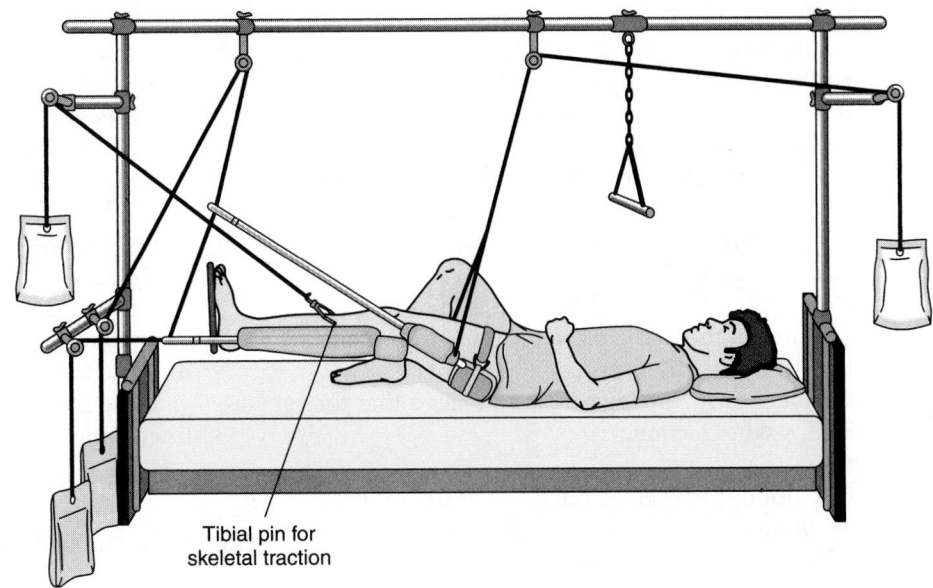

▲ **FIGURE 68-4** Balanced suspension with a Thomas splint and Pearson attachment. The apparatus can be used alone or, as in this case, with skeletal traction. (From Monahan, F., Sands, J., Neighbors, M., Marek, J., & Green, C. [2007]. *Phipps' medical-surgical nursing: Health and illness perspectives* [8th ed.]. St. Louis: Mosby.)

Tibial pin for skeletal traction

2. Interventions
   a. Maintain proper body alignment.
   b. Ensure that the weights hang freely and do not touch the floor.
   c. Do not remove or lift the weights without a physician's prescription.
   d. Ensure that pulleys are not obstructed and that ropes in the pulleys move freely.
   e. Place knots in the ropes to prevent slipping.
   f. Check the ropes for fraying.
H. Skeletal **traction** (Fig. 68-4)
   1. Description
      a. **Traction** is applied mechanically to the bone with pins, wires, or tongs.
      b. Typical weight for skeletal **traction** is 25 to 40 lb.
   2. Interventions
      a. Monitor color, motion, and sensation of the affected extremity.
      b. Monitor the insertion sites for redness, swelling, drainage, or increased pain.
      c. Provide insertion site care as prescribed.
   3. Cervical tongs and a halo fixation device. See Chapter 66 regarding care of the client with these types of devices.
I. Skin **traction** (Box 68-5)
   1. Description: Skin **traction** is applied by using elastic bandages or adhesive, foam boot, or sling.
   2. Cervical skin **traction** relieves muscle spasms and compression in the upper extremities and neck (see Fig. 68-3).
      a. Cervical skin **traction** uses a head halter and chin pad to attach the **traction**.
      b. Use powder to protect the ears from friction rub.
      c. Position the client with the head of the bed elevated 30 to 40 degrees, and attach the weights to a pulley system over the head of the bed.

Box 68-5 Types of Skin Traction

Buck's traction	Pelvic traction
Cervical traction	Russell's traction

3. Buck's (extension) skin **traction** is used to alleviate muscle spasms and immobilize a lower limb by maintaining a straight pull on the limb with the use of weights (see Fig. 68-3).
   a. A boot appliance is applied to attach to the **traction**.
   b. The weights are attached to a pulley; allow the weights to hang freely over the edge of bed.
   c. Not more than 8 to 10 lb of weight should be applied.
   d. Elevate the foot of the bed to provide the **traction**.
4. Russell's skin (sling) **traction**. See Fig 68-3 and Chapter 44 regarding this type of **traction**.
5. Pelvic skin **traction** is used to relieve low back, hip, or leg pain or to reduce muscle spasm (see Fig. 68-3).
   a. Apply the **traction** belt snugly over the pelvis and iliac crest and attach to the weights.
   b. Use measures as prescribed to prevent the client from slipping down in bed.
J. Balanced suspension **traction** (see Fig. 68-3)
   1. Description
      a. Balanced suspension **traction** is used with skin or skeletal **traction**.
      b. Used to approximate fractures of the femur, tibia, or fibula
      c. Balanced suspension **traction** is produced by a counterforce other than client.
   2. Interventions
      a. Position the client in a low Fowler's position on either the side or the back.

b. Maintain a 20-degree angle from the thigh to the bed.

c. Protect the skin from breakdown.

d. Provide pin care if pins are used with the skeletal **traction**.

e. Clean the pin sites with sterile normal saline and hydrogen peroxide or povidone-iodine (Betadine) as prescribed or per agency policy.

K. Dunlop's **traction**

1. Description: Horizontal **traction** is used to align fractures of the humerus; vertical **traction** maintains the forearm in proper alignment.

2. Interventions: Nursing care is similar to that for Buck's skin **traction.**

L. Casts

1. Description: Plaster or fiberglass **casts** are used to immobilize bones and joints into correct alignment after a fracture or injury.

2. Interventions

a. Keep the **cast** and extremity elevated.

b. Allow a wet plaster **cast** 24 to 72 hours to dry (synthetic **casts** dry in 20 minutes).

c. Handle a wet plaster **cast** with the palms of the hands until dry.

d. Turn the extremity every 1 to 2 hours, unless contraindicated, to allow air circulation and promote drying of the **cast.**

e. A hair dryer can be used on a cool setting to dry a plaster **cast** (heat cannot be used on a plaster **cast** because the **cast** heats up and burns the skin).

f. Prepare for bivalving or cutting the **cast** if circulatory impairment occurs.

g. Petal the **cast** or apply moleskin to the edges to protect the client's skin; maintain smooth edges around the **cast** to prevent crumbling of the **cast** material.

h. Monitor for signs of infection such as increased temperature, hot spots on the **cast**, foul odor, or changes in pain.

i. If an open draining area exists on the affected extremity, the physician will make a cutout portion of the **cast** known as a window.

j. Instruct the client not to stick objects inside the **cast.**

k. Teach the client to keep the **cast** clean and dry.

l. Instruct the client in isometric exercises to prevent muscle atrophy.

⚠ Monitor a casted extremity for circulatory impairment such as pain, swelling, discoloration, tingling, numbness, coolness, or diminished pulse. Notify the physician immediately if circulatory compromise occurs.

VI. COMPLICATIONS OF FRACTURES (Box 68-6)

A. Fat embolism

1. Description: A **fat embolism** originates in the bone marrow and occurs after a fracture when a fat globule is released into the bloodstream.

a. Clients with long bone fractures are at the greatest risk for the development of a **fat embolism**.

b. **Fat embolism** can occur within the first 48 to 72 hours following the injury.

2. Assessment: Findings often suggest pulmonary embolism.

a. Restlessness, hypoxemia, or mental status changes

b. Tachycardia and hypotension

c. Dyspnea and tachypnea

d. Petechial rash over the upper chest and neck; these may fade quickly.

3. Interventions (see Priority Nursing Actions)

Box 68-6 Complications of Fractures

Avascular necrosis
Compartment syndrome
Fat embolism
Infection and osteomyelitis
Pulmonary embolism

▬▬▬ PRIORITY NURSING ACTIONS! ▬▬▬

Actions to Take if the Client Develops a Fat Embolism

1. Notify the physician.
2. Administer oxygen .
3. Administer intravenous fluids.
4. Monitor vital signs and respiratory status.
5. Prepare for intubation and mechanical ventilation if necessary.
6. Document the event, actions taken, and the client's response.

A fat embolism originates in the bone marrow and occurs after a fracture when a fat globule is released into the bloodstream. Fat embolism can occur within the first 48 to 72 hours following the injury and clients with long bone fractures are at the greatest risk for the development of a fat embolism. Findings are similar to those noted with pulmonary embolism and include restlessness, hypoxemia, mental status changes, dyspnea, tachypnea, tachycardia, and hypotension. Additionally, a petechial rash may present over the upper chest and neck. The physician is notified immediately while initiating emergency care. The client is maintained on bedrest and is repositioned only as necessary and gently. Oxygen is administered and IV hydration is administered to prevent hypovolemic shock. Vital signs and respiratory status are monitored closely and the client is prepared for intubation and mechanical ventilation if necessary. Corticosteroids may also be prescribed for the client. The nurse then documents the event, actions taken, and the client's response.

Reference: Ignatavicius, D., & Workman, M. (2010). *Medical-surgical nursing: Patient-centered collaborative care* (6th ed., p. 1182). St. Louis: Saunders.

B. Compartment syndrome
1. Description
   a. Tough fascia surrounds muscle groups, forming compartments from which arteries, veins, and nerves enter and exit at opposite ends.
   b. **Compartment syndrome** occurs when pressure increases within one or more compartments, leading to decreased blood flow, tissue ischemia, and neurovascular impairment.
   c. Within 4 to 6 hours after the onset of **compartment syndrome,** neurovascular damage is irreversible if not treated.
2. Assessment
   a. Unrelieved or increased pain in the limb
   b. Tissue that is distal to the involved area becomes pale, dusky, or edematous.
   c. Pain with passive movement
   d. Loss of sensation (paresthesia)
   e. Pulselessness (a late sign)
3. Interventions
   a. Notify the physician immediately and prepare to assist physician.
   b. If severe, assist the physician with fasciotomy to relieve pressure and restore tissue perfusion.
   c. Loosen tight dressings or bivalve restrictive **cast** as prescribed.
C. Infection and osteomyelitis
1. Description: Infection and osteomyelitis (inflammatory response in bone tissue) can be caused by the introduction of organisms into bones leading to localized bone infection.
2. Assessment
   a. Tachycardia and fever (usually above 101° F).
   b. Erythema and pain in the area surrounding the infection
   c. Leukocytosis and elevated erythrocyte sedimentation rate (ESR)
3. Interventions
   a. Notify the physician.
   b. Prepare to initiate aggressive, long-term intravenous antibiotic therapy.
   c. Administer hyperbaric oxygen therapy to promote healing.
   d. Surgery is performed for resistant osteomyelitis with sequestrectomy and/or bone grafts.
D. Avascular necrosis
1. Description: Avascular necrosis occurs when a fracture interrupts the blood supply to a section of bone, leading to bone death.
2. Assessment
   a. Pain
   b. Decreased sensation
3. Interventions
   a. Notify the physician if pain or numbness occurs.
   b. Prepare the client for removal of necrotic tissue because it serves as a focus for infection.

E. Pulmonary embolism
1. Description: Pulmonary embolism is caused by the movement of foreign particles (blood clot, fat, or air) into the pulmonary circulation.
2. Assessment
   a. Restlessness and apprehension
   b. Sudden onset of dyspnea and chest pain
   c. Cough, hemoptysis, hypoxemia, or crackles
3. Interventions
   a. Notify the physician if signs of emboli are present.
   b. Administer oxygen and other prescriptions; IV anticoagulant therapy may be prescribed.

VII. CRUTCH WALKING

A. Description
1. An accurate measurement of the client for crutches is important because an incorrect measurement could damage the brachial plexus.
2. The distance between the axillae and the arm pieces on the crutches should be two to three fingerwidths in the axilla space.
3. The elbows should be slightly flexed, 20 to 30 degrees, when the client is walking.
4. When ambulating with the client, stand on the affected side.
5. Instruct the client never to rest the axillae on the axillary bars.
6. Instruct the client to look up and outward when ambulating and to place the crutches 6 to 10 inches diagonally in front of the foot.
7. Instruct the client to stop ambulation if numbness or tingling in the hands or arms occurs.
B. Crutch gaits (Table 68-2)
C. Assisting the client with crutches to sit and stand
1. Place the unaffected leg against the front of the chair.
2. Move the crutches to the affected side, and grasp the arm of the chair with the hand on the unaffected side.
3. Flex the knee of the unaffected leg to lower self into the chair while placing the affected leg straight out in front.
4. Reverse the steps to move from a sitting to standing position.
D. Going up and down stairs
1. Up the stairs
   a. The client moves the unaffected leg up first.
   b. The client moves the affected leg and the crutches up.
2. Down the stairs
   a. The client moves the crutches and the affected leg down.
   b. The client moves the unaffected leg down.

VIII. CANES AND WALKERS

A. Description: Canes and walkers are made of a lightweight material with a rubber tip at the bottom.
B. Interventions

TABLE 68-2 Crutch Gaits

Type of Gait	Use	Procedure
Two-point gait	Used with partial weight-bearing limitations and with bilateral lower extremity prostheses	The crutch on the affected side and the unaffected foot are advanced at the same time.
Three-point gait	Used for partial weight-bearing or no weight-bearing on the affected leg; requires that the client have strength and balance	Both crutches and the foot of the affected extremity are advanced together, followed by the foot of the unaffected extremity.
Four-point gait	Used if weight-bearing is allowed and one foot can be placed in front of the other	The right crutch is advanced, then the left foot, then the left crutch, and then the right foot.
Swing-to gait	Used when there is adequate muscle power and balance in the arms and legs	Both crutches are advanced together, then both legs are lifted and placed down on a spot behind the crutches. The feet and crutches form a tripod.
Swing-through gait	Used when there is adequate muscle power and balance in the arms and legs.	Both crutches are advanced together; then both legs are lifted through and beyond the crutches and placed down again at a point in front of the crutches.

Modified from Linton, A. (2007). *Introduction to medical-surgical nursing* (4th ed.). St. Louis: Saunders.

1. Stand at the affected side of the client when ambulating; use of a gait or transfer belt may be necessary.
2. The handle should be at the level of the client's greater trochanter.
3. The client's elbow should be flexed at a 15- to 30-degree angle.
4. Instruct the client to hold the cane 4 to 6 inches to the side of the foot.
5. Instruct the client to hold the cane in the hand on the unaffected side so that the cane and weaker leg can work together with each step.
6. Instruct the client to move the cane at the same time as the affected leg.
7. Instruct the client to inspect the rubber tips regularly for worn places.

C. Hemicanes or quadripod canes
1. Hemicanes or quadripod canes are used for clients who have the use of only one upper extremity.
2. Hemicanes provide more security than a quadripod cane; however, both types provide more security than a single-tipped cane.
3. Position the cane at the client's unaffected side, with the straight, nonangled side adjacent to the body.
4. Position the cane 6 inches from client's side, with the hand grip level with the greater trochanter.

D. Walker
1. Stand adjacent to the client on the affected side.
2. Instruct the client to put all four points of the walker flat on the floor before putting weight on the hand pieces.
3. Instruct the client to move the walker forward, followed by the affected or weaker foot and then the unaffected foot.

⚠ Safety is the priority concern when the client uses an assistive device such as a cane, walker, or crutches. Be sure that the client demonstrates correct use of the device.

IX. FRACTURED HIP

A. Types
1. Intracapsular (femoral head is broken within the joint capsule).
   a. Femoral head and neck receive decreased blood supply and heal slowly.
   b. Skin traction is applied preoperatively to reduce fracture and immobilize bone.
   c. Treatment includes a total hip replacement or open **reduction internal fixation** (ORIF) with femoral head replacement (Fig. 68-5).
   d. To prevent hip displacement postoperatively, avoid extreme hip flexion.
2. Extracapsular (fracture is outside the joint capsule)
   a. Fracture can occur at the greater trochanter or can be an intertrochanteric fracture.
   b. Preoperative treatment includes balanced suspension or skin **traction** to relieve muscle spasms and reduce pain.
   c. Surgical treatment includes open **reduction internal fixation** with nail plate, screws, pins, or wires

B. Postoperative interventions
1. Maintain leg and hip in proper alignment and prevent internal or external rotation; avoid extreme hip flexion.
2. Turn client to the unaffected side and only to affected side as prescribed by physician.
3. Elevate the head of the bed 30 to 45 degrees for meals only.

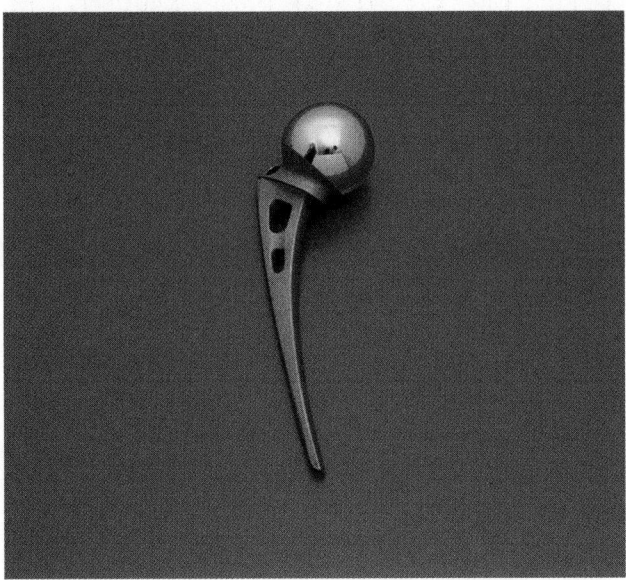

▲ **FIGURE 68-5** Moore prosthesis, used for hip fractures. (From Ignatavicius, D., & Workman, M. [2010]. *Medical-surgical nursing: Patient-centered collaborative care* [6th ed.]. St. Louis: Saunders. Courtesy of Smith & Nephew, Orthopaedics Division, Memphis, TN.)

4. Assist the client to ambulate as prescribed by the physician.
5. Avoid weight bearing on the affected leg as prescribed; instruct the client in the use of a walker to avoid weight bearing.
6. Weight bearing is often restricted after an ORIF and may not be restricted after total hip arthroplasty (THA); always refer to the physician's prescriptions.
7. Keep the operative leg extended, supported, and elevated when getting the client out of bed.
8. Avoid hip flexion greater than 90 degrees and avoid low chairs when out of bed.
9. Monitor for wound infection or hemorrhage.
10. Neurovascular assessment of affected extremity: Check color, pulses, capillary refill, movement, and sensation.
11. Maintain the compression of the Hemovac or Jackson-Pratt drain to facilitate wound drainage.
12. Monitor and record drainage amount, which decreases consistently about 80 mL every 8 hours until 48 hours postoperatively.
13. Carry out postoperative blood salvage to collect, filter, and reinfuse salvaged blood into the client.
14. Use antiembolism stockings or sequential compression stockings; encourage the client to flex and extend the feet to reduce the risk of deep vein thrombosis (DVT).
15. Instruct the client to avoid crossing the legs and activities that require bending over.
16. Physical therapy will be instituted postoperatively with progressive ambulation as prescribed by the physician.

X. TOTAL KNEE REPLACEMENT

A. Description: Total knee replacement is the implantation of a device to substitute for the femoral condyles and tibial joint surfaces.
B. Postoperative interventions
   1. Monitor surgical incision for drainage and infection.
   2. Begin continuous passive motion 24 to 48 hours postoperatively as prescribed to exercise the knee and provide moderate flexion and extension.
   3. Administer analgesics before continuous passive motion to decrease pain.
   4. Prepare the client for out of bed activities as prescribed; have the client avoid leg dangling.
   5. Avoid weight bearing and instruct the client in the use of the prescribed assistive device, such as a walker.
   6. Postoperative blood salvage may be prescribed to collect, filter, and reinfuse salvaged blood into client.

XI. JOINT DISLOCATION AND SUBLUXATION

A. Dislocation: Injury of the ligaments surrounding a joint, which leads to displacement or separating of the articular surfaces of the joint
B. Subluxation: Incomplete displacement of joint surfaces when forces disrupt the soft tissue that surrounds the joints
C. Assessment
   1. Asymmetry of the contour of affected body parts
   2. Pain, tenderness, dysfunction, and swelling
   3. Complications include neurovascular compromise, avascular necrosis, and open joint injuries.
   4. X-rays are taken to determine joint shifting.
D. Interventions
   1. Focus of treatment includes pain relief, joint support, and joint protection.
   2. Immediate treatment is done to reduce the dislocation and realign the dislocated joint.
   3. Open or closed **reduction** is done with a postprocedural joint immobilization.
   4. Intravenous conscious sedation, local, or general anesthesia is used during joint manipulation.
   5. Initial activity restriction is followed by gentle range-of-motion activities and a gradual return of activities to normal levels while supporting the affected joint.
   6. A weakened joint is prone to recurrent dislocation and may require extended activity restriction.

XII. HERNIATION: INTERVERTEBRAL DISK

A. Description: The nucleus of the disk protrudes into the annulus, causing nerve compression.
B. Cervical disk herniation occurs at the C5 to C6 and C6 to C7 interspaces.

1. Cervical disk herniation causes pain radiation to shoulders, arms, hands, scapulae, and pectoral muscles.
2. Motor and sensory deficits can include paresthesia, numbness, and weakness of the upper extremities.
3. Interventions
   a. Conservative management is used unless the client develops signs of neurological deterioration.
   b. Bed rest is prescribed to decrease pressure, inflammation, and pain.
   c. Immobilize the cervical area with cervical collar or brace.
   d. Apply heat to reduce muscle spasms and apply ice to reduce inflammation and swelling.
   e. Maintain head and spine alignment.
   f. Instruct the client in the use of analgesics, sedatives, anti-inflammatory agents, and corticosteroids as prescribed.
   g. Prepare the client for a corticosteroid injection into the epidural space if prescribed.
   h. Assist and instruct the client in the use of a cervical collar or cervical **traction** as prescribed.
4. Cervical collar is used for cervical disk herniation.
   a. A cervical collar limits neck movement and holds the head in a neutral or slightly flexed position.
   b. The cervical collar may be worn intermittently or 24 hours daily.
   c. Inspect the skin under the collar for irritation.
   d. When prescribed and after pain decreases, exercises are prescribed to strengthen the muscles.
5. Client education related to cervical disk conditions
   a. Avoid flexing, extending, and rotating neck.
   b. Avoid the prone position and maintain neck, spine, and hips in a neutral position while sleeping.
   c. Minimize long periods of sitting.
   d. Instruct the client regarding medications such as analgesics, sedatives, anti-inflammatory agents, and corticosteroids.

C. Lumbar disk herniation most often occurs at the L4 to L5 or L5 to S1 interspace.
1. Herniation produces muscle weakness, sensory deficits, and diminished tendon reflexes.
2. The client experiences pain and muscle spasms in the lower back, with radiation of the pain into one hip and down the leg (sciatica).
3. Pain is relieved by bed rest and aggravated by movement, lifting, straining, and coughing.
4. Interventions
   a. Conservative management is indicated unless neurological deterioration or bowel and bladder dysfunction occurs.
   b. Apply heat to decrease muscle spasms and apply ice to decrease inflammation and swelling.

Box 68-7 Types of Disk Surgery

Diskectomy: Removal of herniated disk tissue and related matter
Diskectomy with fusion: Fusion of vertebrae with bone graft
Laminectomy: Excision of part of the vertebrae (lamina) to remove the disk
Laminotomy: Division of the lamina of a vertebra

   c. Instruct the client to sleep on the side, with the knees and hips flexed, and place a pillow between the legs.
   d. Apply pelvic **traction** as prescribed to relieve muscle spasms and decrease pain.
   e. Begin progressive ambulation as inflammation, edema, and pain subside.
5. Client education related to lumbar disk conditions
   a. Instruct the client in the use of prescribed medications such as analgesics, muscle relaxants, anti-inflammatory agents, or corticosteroids.
   b. Instruct the client about application techniques for corsets or braces to maintain immobilization and proper spine alignment.
   c. Instruct the client in correct posture while sitting, standing, walking, and working.
   d. Instruct the client in the correct technique to use when lifting objects such as bending the knees, maintaining a straight back, and avoiding lifting objects above the elbow level.
   e. Instruct in weight control program as prescribed.
   f. Instruct the client in an exercise program to strengthen back and abdominal muscles as prescribed.

D. Disk surgery is used when spinal cord compression is suspected or client's symptoms do not respond to conservative treatment (Box 68-7).
1. Preoperative interventions
   a. Routine preoperative instructions are provided.
   b. Instruct the client about logrolling and range-of-motion exercises.
2. Postoperative interventions: Cervical disk
   a. Monitor for respiratory difficulty from inflammation or hematoma.
   b. Encourage coughing, deep breathing, and early ambulation as prescribed.
   c. Monitor for hoarseness and inability to cough effectively because this may indicate laryngeal nerve damage.
   d. Use throat sprays or lozenges for sore throat, avoiding anesthetic lozenges that may numb the throat and increase choking risks.
   e. Monitor the surgical wound for infection, swelling, redness, drainage, or pain.
   f. Provide a soft diet if the client complains of dysphagia.
   g. Monitor for sudden return of radicular pain, which may indicate cervical spine instability.

3. Postoperative interventions: Lumbar disk
   a. Monitor for wound hemorrhage.
   b. Monitor lower extremities for sensation, movement, color, temperature, and paresthesia.
   c. Monitor for urinary retention, paralytic ileus, and constipation, which can result from decreased movement, opioid administration, or spinal cord compression.
   d. Prevent constipation by encouraging a high-fiber diet, increased fluid intake, and stool softeners as prescribed.
   e. Administer opioids and sedatives as prescribed to relieve pain and anxiety.
   f. Assist and instruct the client to use a prescribed back brace or corset with cotton underwear to prevent skin irritation.
4. Postoperative lumbar disk positioning concerns
   a. In the immediate postoperative period, the client may be expected to lie supine or have other activity restrictions, depending on the specific surgical intervention.
   b. Instruct the client to avoid spinal flexion or twisting and that the spine should be kept aligned.
   c. Instruct the client to minimize sitting, which may place a strain on the surgical site.
   d. When the client is lying supine, place a pillow under the neck and slightly flex the knees.
   e. Avoid extreme hip flexion when lying on side

⚠ Following disk surgery, instruct the client in correct logrolling techniques for turning and repositioning and for getting out of bed.

XIII. AMPUTATION OF A LOWER EXTREMITY

A. Description: Amputation (Fig. 68-6) is the surgical removal of a limb or part of the limb.
B. Postoperative interventions
   1. Monitor vital signs.
   2. Monitor for infection and hemorrhage.
   3. Mark bleeding and drainage on the dressing if it occurs.
   4. Keep a tourniquet at the bedside if prescribed.
   5. Observe for and prevent contractures, which can result from prolonged residual limb elevation.
   6. Monitor for signs of infection, necrosis, and neuroma.
   7. Evaluate for phantom limb sensation and pain; explain sensation and pain to the client, and medicate the client as prescribed.
   8. First 24 hours: Elevate the foot of the bed to reduce edema; then keep the bed flat to prevent hip flexion contractures, if prescribed by the physician.
   9. After 24 to 48 hours postoperatively, position the client prone to stretch the muscles and prevent hip flexion contractures, if prescribed.

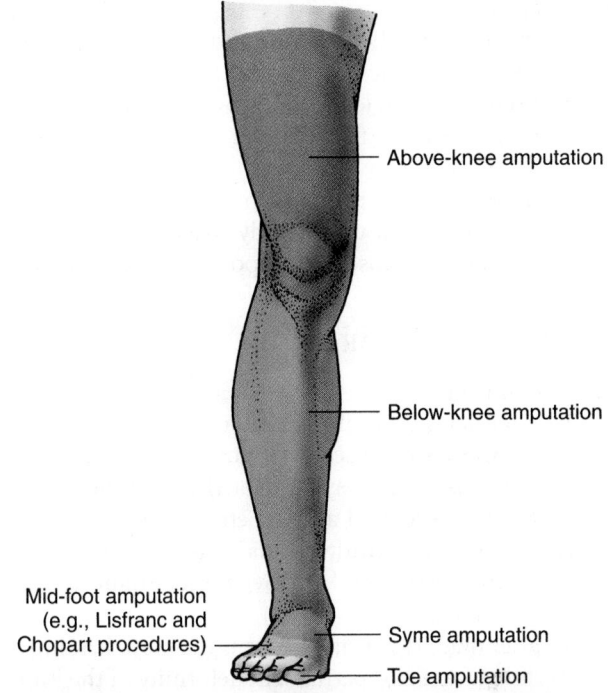

▲ **FIGURE 68-6** Common levels of lower extremity amputation. (From Ignatavicius, D., & Workman, M. [2010]. *Medical-surgical nursing: Patient-centered collaborative care* [6th ed.]. St. Louis: Saunders.)

Labels on figure: Above-knee amputation; Below-knee amputation; Mid-foot amputation (e.g., Lisfranc and Chopart procedures); Syme amputation; Toe amputation

10. To prevent hip flexion contractures, do not elevate the residual limb on a pillow.
11. Maintain surgical application of dressing, elastic compression wrap, or elastic stump (residual limb) shrinker as prescribed to reduce swelling, minimize pain, and mold the residual limb in preparation for prosthesis.
12. As prescribed, wash the residual limb with mild soap and water and dry completely.
13. Massage the skin toward the suture line to mobilize scar and prevent its adherence to underlying bone.
14. Prepare for the prosthesis and instruct the client in progressive resistive techniques by gently pushing the residual limb against pillows and progressing to firmer surfaces.
15. Encourage verbalization regarding loss of the body part, and assist the client to identify coping mechanisms to deal with the loss.

C. Interventions for below-knee amputation
   1. Prevent edema.
   2. Do not allow the residual limb to hang over the edge of the bed.
   3. Discourage long periods of sitting to lessen complications of knee flexion.
D. Interventions for above-knee amputation
   1. Prevent internal or external rotation of the limb.
   2. Place a sandbag, rolled towel, or trochanter roll along the outside of the thigh to prevent external rotation.

E. Rehabilitation
  1. Instruct the client in the use of a mobility aid such as crutches or a walker.
  2. Prepare the residual limb for a prosthesis.
  3. Prepare the client for fitting of the residual limb for a prosthesis.
  4. Instruct the client in exercises to maintain range of motion and upper body strengthening.
  5. Provide psychosocial support to the client.

XIV. RHEUMATOID ARTHRITIS

A. Description
  1. Rheumatoid arthritis is a chronic systemic inflammatory disease (immune complex disorder); the cause may be related to a combination of environmental and genetic factors.
  2. Rheumatoid arthritis leads to destruction of connective tissue and synovial membrane within the joints.
  3. Rheumatoid arthritis weakens the joint, leading to dislocation and permanent deformity of the joint.
  4. Pannus forms at the junction of synovial tissue and articular cartilage and projects into the joint cavity, causing necrosis.
  5. Exacerbations of disease manifestations occur during periods of physical or emotional stress and fatigue.
  6. Vasculitis can impede blood flow, leading to organ or organ system malfunction and failure caused by tissue ischemia.

B. Assessment
  1. Inflammation, tenderness, and stiffness of the joints
  2. Moderate to severe pain with morning stiffness lasting longer than 30 minutes
  3. Joint deformities, muscle atrophy, and decreased range of motion in affected joints
  4. Spongy, soft feeling in the joints
  5. Low-grade temperature, fatigue, and weakness
  6. Anorexia, weight loss, and anemia
  7. Elevated ESR and positive rheumatoid factor
  8. Radiographic study showing joint deterioration
  9. Synovial tissue biopsy reveals inflammation

C. Rheumatoid factor
  1. Blood test used to assist in diagnosing rheumatoid arthritis
  2. Values
     a. Nonreactive: 0 to 39 international units (IU)/mL
     b. Weakly reactive: 40 to 79 IU/mL
     c. Reactive: Higher than 80 IU/mL

D. Medications: Combination of pharmacological therapies includes nonsteroidal anti-inflammatory drugs (NSAIDs), disease-modifying antirheumatic drugs (DMARDs), and glucocorticoids

E. Physical mobility
  1. Preserve joint function.
  2. Provide range-of-motion exercises to maintain joint motion and muscle strengthening.

Box 68-8 Client Education for Rheumatoid Arthritis and Degenerative Joint Disease

Assist the client to identify and correct safety hazards in the home.
Instruct the client in the correct use of assistive or adaptive devices.
Instruct the client in energy conservation measures.
Review the prescribed exercise program.
Instruct the client to sit in a chair with a high straight back.
Instruct the client to use only a small pillow when lying down.
Instruct the client in measures to protect the joints.
Instruct the client regarding the prescribed medications.
Stress the importance of follow-up visits with the health care provider.

  3. Balance rest and activity.
  4. Splints may be used during acute inflammation to prevent deformity.
  5. Prevent flexion contractures.
  6. Apply heat or cold therapy as prescribed to joints.
  7. Apply paraffin baths and massage as prescribed.
  8. Encourage consistency with exercise program.
  9. Use joint-protecting devices.
  10. Avoid weight bearing on inflamed joints.

F. Self-care (Box 68-8)
  1. Assess the need for assistive devices such as raised toilet seats, self-rising chairs, wheelchairs, and scooters to facilitate mobility.
  2. Work with an occupational therapist or health care provider to obtain assistive or adaptive devices.
  3. Instruct the client in alternative strategies for providing activities of daily living.

G. Fatigue
  1. Identify factors that may contribute to fatigue.
  2. Monitor for signs of anemia and administer iron, folic acid, and vitamins as prescribed.
  3. Monitor for medication-related blood loss by testing the stool for occult blood.
  4. Instruct the client in measures to conserve energy, such as pacing activities and obtaining assistance when possible.

H. Disturbed body image
  1. Assess the client's reaction to the body change.
  2. Encourage the client to verbalize feelings.
  3. Assist the client with self-care activities and grooming.
  4. Encourage the client to wear street clothes.

I. Surgical interventions
  1. Synovectomy: Surgical removal of the synovia to help maintain joint function
  2. Arthrodesis: Bony fusion of a joint to regain some mobility
  3. Joint replacement (arthroplasty): Surgical replacement of diseased joints with artificial joints; performed to restore motion to a joint

and function to the muscles, ligaments, and other soft tissue structures that control a joint

XV. OSTEOARTHRITIS (DEGENERATIVE JOINT DISEASE)

A. Description

1. Osteoarthritis is marked by progressive deterioration of the articular cartilage.
2. Osteoarthritis causes bone buildup and the loss of articular cartilage in peripheral and axial joints.
3. Osteoarthritis affects the weight-bearing joints and joints that receive the greatest stress, such as the hips, knees, lower vertebral column, and hands.
4. The cause of primary osteoarthritis is not known. Risk factors include trauma, aging, obesity, genetic changes, and smoking.

B. Assessment

1. Client experiences joint pain that diminishes after rest and intensifies after activity, noted early in the disease process.
2. As the disease progresses, pain occurs with slight motion or even at rest.
3. Symptoms are aggravated by temperature change and climate humidity.
4. Presence of Heberden's nodes or Bouchard's nodes
5. Joint swelling (may be minimal), crepitus, and limited range of motion
6. Difficulty getting up after prolonged sitting
7. Skeletal muscle disuse atrophy
8. Inability to perform activities of daily living
9. Compression of the spine as manifested by radiating pain, stiffness, and muscle spasms in one or both extremities

C. Pain

1. Administer NSAIDs, muscle relaxants, and other medications as prescribed.
2. Prepare the client for corticosteroid injections into joints as prescribed.
3. Position joints in function position and avoid flexion of knees and hips.
4. Immobilize the affected joint with a splint or brace until inflammation subsides.
5. Avoid large pillows under the head or knees.
6. Provide a bed or foot cradle to keep linen off of feet.
7. Instruct the client in the importance of moist heat, hot packs or compresses, and paraffin dips as prescribed.
8. Apply cold applications as prescribed when the joint is acutely inflamed.
9. Encourage adequate rest, recommending 10 hours of sleep at night and a 1- to 2-hour nap in the afternoon.

D. Nutrition

1. Encourage a well-balanced diet.
2. Maintain weight within normal range to decrease stress on the joints.

E. Physical mobility

1. Instruct the client to balance activity with rest and to participate in an exercise program that limits stressing affected joints.
2. Instruct the client that exercises should be active rather than passive and to stop exercise if pain occurs.
3. Instruct the client to limit exercise when joint inflammation is severe.

F. Surgical management

1. Osteotomy: The bone is resected to correct joint deformity, promote realignment, and reduce joint stress.
2. Total joint replacement or arthroplasty
   a. Total joint replacement is performed when all measures of pain relief have failed.
   b. Hips and knees are replaced most commonly.
   c. Total joint replacement is contraindicated in the presence of infection, advanced osteoporosis, or severe joint inflammation.

XVI. OSTEOPOROSIS

A. Description

1. Osteoporosis is a metabolic disease characterized by bone demineralization, with loss of calcium and phosphorus salts leading to fragile bones and the subsequent risk for fractures.
2. Bone resorption accelerates as bone formation slows.
3. Osteoporosis occurs most commonly in the wrist, hip, and vertebral column.
4. Osteoporosis can occur postmenopausally or as a result of a metabolic disorder or calcium deficiency.
5. Client may be asymptomatic until the bones become fragile and a minor injury or movement causes a fracture.
6. Primary osteoporosis
   a. Most often occurs in postmenopausal women; occurs in men with low testosterone levels
   b. Risk factors include decreased calcium intake, deficient estrogen, and sedentary lifestyle.
7. Secondary osteoporosis
   a. Causes include prolonged therapy with corticosteroids, thyroid-reducing medications, aluminum-containing antacids, or anticonvulsants.
   b. Associated with immobility, alcoholism, malnutrition, or malabsorption
8. Risk factors (Box 68-9)

B. Assessment

1. Possibly asymptomatic
2. Back pain occurs after lifting, bending, or stooping.
3. Back pain that increases with palpation
4. Pelvic or hip pain, especially with weight bearing

Box 68-9 Risk Factors for Osteoporosis

Cigarette smoking
Early menopause
Excessive use of alcohol
Family history
Female gender
Increasing age
Insufficient intake of calcium
Sedentary lifestyle
Thin, small frame
White (European descent) or Asian race

5. Problems with balance
6. Decline in height from vertebral compression
7. Kyphosis of the dorsal spine, also known as "dowager's hump"
8. Degeneration of lower thorax and lumbar vertebrae on radiographic studies

⚠ The client with osteoporosis is at risk for pathological fractures.

C. Interventions
1. Assess risk for and prevent injury in client's personal environment.
   a. Assist client to identify and correct hazards in his or her environment.
   b. Position household items and furniture to ensure an unobstructed walkway.
   c. Use side rails to prevent falls.
   d. Instruct in use of assistive devices such as a cane or walker.
   e. Encourage the use of a firm mattress.
2. Provide personal care to client to reduce injuries.
   a. Move the client gently when turning and repositioning.
   b. Assist with ambulation if client is unsteady.
   c. Provide gentle range-of-motion exercises.
   d. Apply a back brace as prescribed during an acute phase to immobilize the spine and provide spinal column support.
3. Provide client instructions to promote optimal level of health and function.
   a. Instruct the client in the use of good body mechanics.
   b. Instruct the client in exercises to strengthen abdominal and back muscles to improve posture and provide support for the spine.
   c. Instruct the client to avoid activities that can cause vertebral compression.
   d. Instruct the client to eat a diet high in protein, calcium, vitamins C and D, and iron.
   e. Instruct the client to avoid alcohol and coffee.
   f. Instruct the client to maintain an adequate fluid intake to prevent renal calculi.

4. Administer medications as prescribed to promote bone strength and decrease pain.

XVII. GOUT

A. Description
1. Gout is a systemic disease in which urate crystals deposit in joints and other body tissues.
2. Gout results from abnormal amounts of uric acid in the body.
3. Primary gout results from a disorder of purine metabolism.
4. Secondary gout involves excessive uric acid in the blood caused by another disease.

B. Phases
1. Asymptomatic: Client has no symptoms but serum uric acid level is elevated.
2. Acute: Client has excruciating pain and inflammation of one or more small joints, especially the great toe.
3. Intermittent: Client has intermittent periods without symptoms between acute attacks.
4. Chronic: Results from repeated episodes of acute gout
   a. Chronic gout results in deposits of urate crystals under the skin.
   b. Chronic gout results in deposits of urate crystals within major organs, such as the kidneys, leading to organ dysfunction.

C. Assessment
1. Swelling and inflammation of the joints, leading to excruciating pain
2. Tophi: Hard, irregularly shaped nodules in the skin containing chalky deposits of sodium urate
3. Low-grade fever, malaise, and headache
4. Pruritis from urate crystals in the skin
5. Presence of renal stones from elevated uric acid levels

D. Interventions
1. Provide a low-purine diet as prescribed, avoiding foods such as organ meats, wines, and aged cheese.
2. Encourage a high fluid intake of 2000 mL/day to prevent stone formation.
3. Encourage weight reduction diet if required.
4. Instruct the client to avoid alcohol and starvation diets because they may precipitate a gout attack.
5. Increase urinary pH (above 6) by eating alkaline ash foods (see Chapter 62).
6. Provide bed rest during the acute attacks with the affected extremity elevated.
7. Monitor joint range-of-motion ability and appearance of joints.
8. Position the joint in mild flexion during acute attack.
9. Protect the affected joint from excessive movement or direct contact with sheets or blankets.

10. Provide heat or cold for local treatments to affected joint as prescribed.
11. Administer medications such as analgesics, anti-inflammatory, and uricosuric agents as prescribed.

 MORE QUESTIONS ON THE CD!

Practice Questions

827. A nurse is conducting health screening for osteoporosis. Which of the following clients is at greatest risk of developing this disorder?
1. A 25-year-old woman who jogs
2. A 36-year-old man who has asthma
3. A 70-year-old man who consumes excess alcohol
4. A sedentary 65-year-old woman who smokes cigarettes

828. A nurse has given instructions to a client returning home after knee arthroscopy. The nurse determines that the client understands the instructions if the client states that he or she will:
1. Resume regular exercise the following day.
2. Stay off the leg entirely for the rest of the day.
3. Report fever or site inflammation to the physician.
4. Refrain from eating food for the remainder of the day.

829. A nurse is one of several persons who witness a vehicle hit a pedestrian at fairly low speed on a small street. The victim is dazed and tries to get up. The leg appears fractured. The nurse would plan to:
1. Try to reduce the fracture manually.
2. Assist the victim to get up and walk to the sidewalk.
3. Leave the victim for a few moments to call an ambulance.
4. Stay with the victim and encourage the person to remain still.

830. A client with a hip fracture asks the nurse why Buck's (extension) traction is being applied before surgery. The nurse's response is based on the understanding that Buck's (extension) traction primarily:
1. Allows bony healing to begin before surgery
2. Provides rigid immobilization of the fracture site
3. Lengthens the fractured leg to prevent severing of blood vessels
4. Provides comfort by reducing muscle spasms and provides fracture immobilization

831. A nurse is evaluating the pin sites of a client in skeletal traction. The nurse would be least concerned with which of the following findings?

1. Inflammation
2. Serous drainage
3. Pain at a pin site
4. Purulent drainage

832. A nurse is assessing the casted extremity of a client. The nurse would assess for which of the following signs and symptoms indicative of infection?
1. Dependent edema
2. Diminished distal pulse
3. Presence of a "hot spot" on the cast
4. Coolness and pallor of the extremity

833. A client has sustained a closed fracture and has just had a cast applied to the affected arm. The client is complaining of intense pain. The nurse elevates the limb, applies an ice bag, and administers an analgesic, with little relief. The nurse interprets that this pain may be caused by:
1. Infection under the cast
2. The anxiety of the client
3. Impaired tissue perfusion
4. The recent occurrence of the fracture

834. A nurse is admitting a client with multiple trauma to the nursing unit. The client has a leg fracture and had a plaster cast applied. In positioning the casted leg, the nurse should:
1. Keep the leg in a level position.
2. Elevate the leg for 3 hours and put it flat for 1 hour.
3. Keep the leg level for 3 hours and elevate it for 1 hour.
4. Elevate the leg on pillows continuously for 24 to 48 hours.

835. A client is being discharged to home after application of a plaster leg cast. The nurse determines that the client understands proper care of the cast if the client states that he or she should:
1. Avoid getting the cast wet.
2. Cover the casted leg with warm blankets.
3. Use the fingertips to lift and move the leg.
4. Use a padded coat hanger end to scratch under the cast.

836. A client being measured for crutches asks the nurse why the crutches cannot rest up underneath the arm for extra support. The nurse's response is based on the understanding that this could most likely result in:
1. A fall and further injury
2. Injury to the brachial plexus nerves
3. Skin breakdown in the area of the axilla
4. Impaired range of motion while the client ambulates

837. A nurse has given a client instructions about crutch safety. The nurse determines that the client needs reinforcement of information if the client states:
1. That he or she will not use someone else's crutches
2. That crutch tips will not slip even when wet
3. The need to have spare crutches and tips available
4. That crutch tips should be inspected periodically for wear

838. A nurse is caring for a client being treated for fat embolus after multiple fractures. Which of the following data would the nurse evaluate as the most favorable indication of resolution of the fat embolus?
1. Minimal dyspnea
2. Clear mentation
3. Oxygen saturation of 85%
4. Arterial oxygen level of 78 mm Hg

839. A nurse has conducted teaching with a client in an arm cast about the signs and symptoms of compartment syndrome. The nurse determines that the client understands the information if the client states that he or she should report which of the following early symptoms of compartment syndrome?
1. Cold, bluish-colored fingers
2. Pain that is out of proportion to the type of injury or condition
3. Pain that increases when the arm is dependent
4. Numbness and tingling in the fingers

840. A client with diabetes mellitus has had a right below-knee amputation. The nurse would assess specifically for which of the following signs because of the history of diabetes?
1. Hemorrhage
2. Edema of the stump
3. Slight redness of the incision
4. Separation of the wound edges

841. A nurse is caring for a client who had an above-knee amputation 2 days ago. The residual limb was wrapped with an elastic compression bandage, which has come off. The nurse immediately:
1. Calls the physician
2. Applies ice to the site
3. Rewraps the stump with an elastic compression bandage

4. Applies a dry sterile dressing and elevates it on one pillow

842. A client is complaining of low back pain that radiates down the left posterior thigh. The nurse further assesses the client to see if the pain is worsened or aggravated by:
1. Bed rest
2. Bending or lifting
3. Ibuprofen (Motrin)
4. Application of heat

843. A nurse is caring for a client who has had spinal fusion, with insertion of hardware. The nurse would be concerned especially with which of the following assessment findings?
1. Temperature of 101.6° F orally
2. Complaints of discomfort during repositioning
3. Old bloody drainage outlined on the surgical dressing
4. Discomfort during coughing and deep-breathing exercises

844. A nurse is caring for a client with a diagnosis of gout. Which of the following laboratory values would the nurse expect to note in the client?
1. Calcium level of 9.0 mg/dL
2. Uric acid level of 8.6 mg/dL
3. Potassium level of 4.1 mEq/L
4. Phosphorus level of 3.1 mg/dL

Alternate Item Format: Multiple Response

845. A nurse is preparing a list of cast care instructions for a client who just had a plaster cast applied to his right forearm. Select all instructions that the nurse would include on the list.
❏ 1. Keep the cast and extremity elevated.
❏ 2. The cast needs to be kept clean and dry.
❏ 3. Allow the wet cast 24 to 72 hours to dry.
❏ 4. Tingling and numbness in the extremity are expected.
❏ 5. Use a hair dryer set on a warm to hot setting to dry the cast.
❏ 6. Use a soft padded object that will fit under the cast to scratch the skin under the cast.

ANSWERS

827. 4
Rationale: Risk factors for osteoporosis include female gender, postmenopausal, advanced age, low-calcium diet, excessive alcohol intake, being sedentary, and smoking cigarettes.

Long-term use of corticosteroids, anticonvulsants, and/or furosemide (Lasix) also increase the risk.
Test-Taking Strategy: Use the process of elimination. Eliminate option 1 first. The 25-year-old woman who jogs (exercises using the long bones) has negligible risk. The 36-year-old man

with asthma is eliminated next because his only risk factor might be long-term corticosteroid use to treat the asthma. Of the two remaining options, the 65-year-old woman has higher risk (age, gender, postmenopausal, sedentary, smoking) than the 70-year-old man (age, alcohol consumption). Review the risk factors associated with osteoporosis if you had difficulty with this question.
Level of Cognitive Ability: Analyzing
Client Needs: Health Promotion and Maintenance
Integrated Process: Nursing Process—Assessment
Content Area: Adult Health—Musculoskeletal
Reference: Ignatavicius, D., & Workman, M. (2010). *Medical-surgical nursing: Patient-centered collaborative care* (6th ed., p. 1153). St. Louis: Saunders.

828. 3
Rationale: After arthroscopy, the client usually can walk carefully on the leg once sensation has returned. The client is instructed to avoid strenuous exercise for at least a few days. The client may resume the usual diet. Signs and symptoms of infection should be reported to the physician.
Test-Taking Strategy: Use the process of elimination. Recalling the general client teaching points related to surgical procedures will direct you to option 3. Review client teaching points following arthroscopy if you had difficulty with this question.
Level of Cognitive Ability: Evaluating
Client Needs: Physiological Integrity
Integrated Process: Nursing Process—Evaluation
Content Area: Adult Health—Musculoskeletal
Reference: Swearingen, P. (2008). *All-in-one care planning resource: Medical-surgical, pediatric, maternity, and psychiatric nursing care plans* (2nd ed., p. 528). St. Louis: Mosby.

829. 4
Rationale: With a suspected fracture, the victim is not moved unless it is dangerous to remain in that spot. The nurse should remain with the victim and have someone else call for emergency help. A fracture is not reduced at the scene. Before the victim is moved, the site of fracture is immobilized to prevent further injury.
Test-Taking Strategy: Use the process of elimination. Eliminate options 1 and 2 first because either of these options could result in further injury to the victim. Of the remaining options, the more prudent action would be for the nurse to remain with the victim and have someone else call for emergency assistance. Review care of the victim with a fracture if you had difficulty with this question.
Level of Cognitive Ability: Applying
Client Needs: Physiological Integrity
Integrated Process: Nursing Process—Implementation
Content Area: Adult Health—Musculoskeletal
Reference: Ignatavicius, D., & Workman, M. (2010). *Medical-surgical nursing: Patient-centered collaborative care* (6th ed., p. 1186). St. Louis: Saunders.

830. 4
Rationale: Buck's (extension) traction is a type of skin traction often applied after hip fracture before the fracture is reduced in surgery. Traction reduces muscle spasms and helps immobilize the fracture. Traction does not lengthen the leg

for the purpose of preventing blood vessel severance. Traction also does not allow for bony healing to begin.
Test-Taking Strategy: Use the process of elimination. Focus on the client's diagnosis, hip fracture. Read each option carefully. Noting the words *provides fracture immobilization* will direct you to option 4. Review the purpose of Buck's (extension) traction if you had difficulty with this question.
Level of Cognitive Ability: Understanding
Client Needs: Physiological Integrity
Integrated Process: Nursing Process—Implementation
Content Area: Adult Health—Musculoskeletal
Reference: Ignatavicius, D., & Workman, M. (2010). *Medical-surgical nursing: Patient-centered collaborative care* (6th ed., p. 1189). St. Louis: Saunders.

831. 2
Rationale: A small amount of serous oozing is expected at pin insertion sites. Signs of infection such as inflammation, purulent drainage, and pain at the pin site are not expected findings and should be reported to the physician.
Test-Taking Strategy: Use the process of elimination. Note the strategic words *least concerned*. Options 1 and 4 seem to indicate an infectious problem and are eliminated first. From the remaining options, note that the complaint of pain is at "a pin site." Also, because serous drainage is an expected finding, select option 2. Review expected findings in the client with skeletal traction if you had difficulty with this question.
Level of Cognitive Ability: Evaluating
Client Needs: Physiological Integrity
Integrated Process: Nursing Process—Evaluation
Content Area: Adult Health—Musculoskeletal
Reference: Ignatavicius, D., & Workman, M. (2010). *Medical-surgical nursing: Patient-centered collaborative care* (6th ed., p. 1191). St. Louis: Saunders.

832. 3
Rationale: Signs and symptoms of infection under a casted area include odor or purulent drainage from the cast or the presence of "hot spots," which are areas of the cast that are warmer than others. The physician should be notified if any of these occur. Signs of impaired circulation in the distal limb include coolness and pallor of the skin, diminished arterial pulse, and edema.
Test-Taking Strategy: Use the process of elimination. Answer this question and think about what you would expect to note with infection—redness, swelling, heat, and purulent drainage. With this in mind, you can eliminate options 2 and 4 easily. From the remaining options, remember that "dependent edema" is not necessarily indicative of infection. Swelling would be continuous. The hot spot on the cast could signify infection underneath that area and is the correct answer to the question. Review signs of infection in an extremity with a cast if you had difficulty with this question.
Level of Cognitive Ability: Analyzing
Client Needs: Physiological Integrity
Integrated Process: Nursing Process—Assessment
Content Area: Adult Health—Musculoskeletal
Reference: Ignatavicius, D., & Workman, M. (2010). *Medical-surgical nursing: Patient-centered collaborative care* (6th ed., p. 1189). St. Louis: Saunders.

833. 3

Rationale: Most pain associated with fractures can be minimized with rest, elevation, application of cold, and administration of analgesics. Pain that is not relieved by these measures should be reported to the physician because the pain unrelieved by medications and other measures may indicate neurovascular compromise. Because this is a new closed fracture and cast, infection would not have had time to set in.

Test-Taking Strategy: Use the process of elimination. Focus on the subject, intense pain. Use of the ABCs—airway, breathing, and circulation—will direct you to option 3. Review care of the client with a fracture and new cast if you had difficulty with this question.

Level of Cognitive Ability: Analyzing
Client Needs: Physiological Integrity
Integrated Process: Nursing Process—Assessment
Content Area: Adult Health—Musculoskeletal
References: Ignatavicius, D., & Workman, M. (2010). *Medical-surgical nursing: Patient-centered collaborative care* (6th ed., pp. 1184–1185). St. Louis: Saunders.

Swearingen, P. (2008). *All-in-one care planning resource: Medical-surgical, pediatric, maternity, and psychiatric nursing care plans* (2nd ed., pp. 516–517). St. Louis: Mosby.

834. 4

Rationale: A casted extremity is elevated continuously for the first 24 to 48 hours to minimize swelling and promote venous drainage. Options 1, 2, and 3 are incorrect.

Test-Taking Strategy: Use the process of elimination. Recalling that edema is a concern and knowledge of the effects of gravity on edema will direct you to option 4. Review care of the client with a new cast if you had difficulty with this question.

Level of Cognitive Ability: Applying
Client Needs: Physiological Integrity
Integrated Process: Nursing Process—Implementation
Content Area: Adult Health—Musculoskeletal
Reference: Ignatavicius, D., & Workman, M. (2010). *Medical-surgical nursing: Patient-centered collaborative care* (6th ed., pp. 1188–1189). St. Louis: Saunders.

835. 1

Rationale: A plaster cast must remain dry to keep its strength. The cast should be handled with the palms of the hands, not the fingertips, until fully dry. Air should circulate freely around the cast to help it dry; the cast also gives off heat as it dries. The client should never scratch under the cast; the client may use a hair dryer on the cool setting to relieve an itch.

Test-Taking Strategy: Use the process of elimination. Knowing that a wet cast can be dented with the fingertips, causing pressure underneath, helps eliminate option 3 first. Knowing that the cast needs to dry helps eliminate option 2 next. Option 4 is dangerous to skin integrity and is also eliminated. Remember that plaster casts, once they have dried after application, should not become wet. Review care of the client with a cast if you had difficulty with this question.

Level of Cognitive Ability: Evaluating
Client Needs: Physiological Integrity
Integrated Process: Nursing Process—Evaluation
Content Area: Adult Health—Musculoskeletal

Reference: Swearingen, P. (2008). *All-in-one care planning resource: Medical-surgical, pediatric, maternity, & psychiatric nursing care plans* (2nd ed., pp. 518–519). St. Louis: Mosby.

836. 2

Rationale: Crutches are measured so that the tops are two to three fingerwidths from the axillae. This ensures that the client's axillae are not resting on the crutch or bearing the weight of the crutch, which could result in injury to the nerves of the brachial plexus.

Test-Taking Strategy: Note the strategic words *most likely*. Recalling the risk associated with brachial nerve plexus injury will direct you to option 2. Review the complications associated with the use of crutches if you had difficulty with this question.

Level of Cognitive Ability: Applying
Client Needs: Physiological Integrity
Integrated Process: Teaching and Learning
Content Area: Adult Health—Musculoskeletal
Reference: Ignatavicius, D., & Workman, M. (2010). *Medical-surgical nursing: Patient-centered collaborative care* (6th ed., p. 1193). St. Louis: Saunders.

837. 2

Rationale: Crutch tips should remain dry. Water could cause the client to slip by decreasing the surface friction of the rubber tip on the floor. If crutch tips get wet, the client should dry them with a cloth or paper towel. The client should use only crutches measured for the client. The tips should be inspected for wear, and spare crutches and tips should be available if needed.

Test-Taking Strategy: Use the process of elimination. Note the strategic words *needs reinforcement of information*. These words indicate a negative event query and ask you to select an option that is incorrect. Remember that crutch tips can slip when they get wet, posing a possible threat to the unsuspecting client. Review client teaching points related to safety and the use of crutches if you had difficulty with this question.

Level of Cognitive Ability: Evaluating
Client Needs: Physiological Integrity
Integrated Process: Teaching and Learning
Content Area: Adult Health—Musculoskeletal
Reference: Potter, P., & Perry, A. (2009) *Fundamentals of nursing* (7th ed., p. 803). St. Louis: Mosby.

838. 2

Rationale: An altered mental state is an early indication of fat emboli; therefore, clear mentation is a good indicator that a fat embolus is resolving. Eupnea, not minimal dyspnea, is a normal sign. Arterial oxygen levels should be 80 to 100 mm Hg. Oxygen saturation should be higher than 95%.

Test-Taking Strategy: Use the process of elimination. Note the strategic words *most favorable indication*. Knowing that the arterial oxygen and oxygen saturation levels are below normal helps eliminate options 3 and 4. Dyspnea, even at a minimal level, is not normal, so eliminate option 1. Review the expected outcomes in a client being treated for fat embolism if you had difficulty with this question.

Level of Cognitive Ability: Evaluating
Client Needs: Physiological Integrity

Integrated Process: Nursing Process—Evaluation
Content Area: Adult Health—Musculoskeletal
References: Ignatavicius, D., & Workman, M. (2010). *Medical-surgical nursing: Patient-centered collaborative care* (6th ed., pp. 1182–1183). St. Louis: Saunders.
   Monahan, F., Sands, J., Marek, J., Neighbors, M., & Green, C. (2007). *Phipps' Medical-surgical nursing: Health and illness perspectives* (8th ed., p. 1538). St. Louis: Mosby.

839. 4
Rationale: The earliest symptom of compartment syndrome is paresthesia (numbness and tingling in the fingers). Other symptoms include pain unrelieved by opioids, pain that increases with limb elevation, and pallor and coolness to the distal limb. Cyanosis is a late sign.
Test-Taking Strategy: Use the process of elimination. Note the strategic word *early*. Knowing that compartment syndrome is characterized by insufficient circulation and ischemia caused by pressure will direct you to option 4. Review the early signs of compartment syndrome if you had difficulty with this question.
Level of Cognitive Ability: Evaluating
Client Needs: Physiological Integrity
Integrated Process: Nursing Process—Evaluation
Content Area: Adult Health—Musculoskeletal
Reference: Ignatavicius, D., & Workman, M. (2010). *Medical-surgical nursing: Patient-centered collaborative care* (6th ed., p. 1181). St. Louis: Saunders.

840. 4
Rationale: Clients with diabetes mellitus are more prone to wound infection and delayed wound healing because of the disease. Postoperative stump edema and hemorrhage are complications in the immediate postoperative period that apply to any client with an amputation. Slight redness of the incision is considered normal, as long as it is dry and intact.
Test-Taking Strategy: Use the process of elimination. Recalling that diabetes mellitus increases the client's chances of developing infection and delayed wound healing will direct you to option 4. Review the complications associated with an amputation in the client with diabetes mellitus if you had difficulty with this question.
Level of Cognitive Ability: Applying
Client Needs: Physiological Integrity
Integrated Process: Nursing Process—Assessment
Content Area: Adult Health—Musculoskeletal
Reference: Black, J., & Hawks, J. (2009). *Medical-surgical nursing: Clinical management for positive outcomes* (8th ed., pp. 1101, 1320–1321). St. Louis: Saunders.

841. 3
Rationale: If the client with an amputation has a cast or elastic compression bandage that slips off, the nurse must wrap the stump immediately with another elastic compression bandage. Otherwise, excessive edema will form rapidly, which could cause a significant delay in rehabilitation. If the client had a cast that slipped off, the nurse would have to call the physician so that a new one could be applied. Elevation on one pillow is not going to impede the development of edema greatly once compression is released. Ice would be of limited value in controlling edema from this cause. If the physician

were called, the prescription likely would be to reapply the compression dressing anyway.
Test-Taking Strategy: Use the process of elimination. Recalling that excessive edema can form rapidly will direct you to option 3. Review care of the client after amputation if you had difficulty with this question.
Level of Cognitive Ability: Applying
Client Needs: Physiological Integrity
Integrated Process: Nursing Process—Implementation
Content Area: Adult Health—Musculoskeletal
Reference: Swearingen, P. (2008). *All-in-one care planning resource: Medical-surgical, pediatric, maternity, and psychiatric nursing care plans* (2nd ed., pp. 512–513). St. Louis: Mosby.

842. 2
Rationale: Low back pain that radiates into one leg (sciatica) is consistent with herniated lumbar disk. The nurse assesses the client to see whether the pain is aggravated by events that increase intraspinal pressure, such as bending, lifting, sneezing, and coughing, or by lifting the leg straight up while supine (straight leg-raising test).
Test-Taking Strategy: Use the process of elimination. Recall that bed rest, heat (or sometimes ice), and nonsteroidal anti-inflammatory drugs usually relieve back pain, whereas bending, lifting, and straining aggravate it. Review the causes of back pain and the factors that alleviate or aggravate pain if you had difficulty with this question.
Level of Cognitive Ability: Applying
Client Needs: Physiological Integrity
Integrated Process: Nursing Process—Assessment
Content Area: Adult Health—Musculoskeletal
Reference: Ignatavicius, D., & Workman, M. (2010). *Medical-surgical nursing: Patient-centered collaborative care* (6th ed., pp. 984–985). St. Louis: Saunders.

843. 1
Rationale: The nursing assessment conducted after spinal surgery is similar to that done after other surgical procedures. For this specific type of surgery, the nurse assesses the neurovascular status of the lower extremities, watches for signs and symptoms of infection, and inspects the surgical site for evidence of cerebrospinal fluid leakage (drainage is clear and tests positive for glucose). A mild temperature is expected after insertion of hardware, but a temperature of 101.6° F should be reported.
Test-Taking Strategy: Use the process of elimination. Note the strategic words *concerned especially*. Thus, you are looking for the option that has the greatest deviation from normal. Options 2 and 4 are expected after surgery and, although the nurse tries to minimize discomfort, the client is likely to have some discomfort, even with proper analgesic use. The words *old* and *outlined* in option 3 indicate that this is not a new occurrence. This leaves the temperature of 101.6° F, which is excessive and should be reported. Review the signs of complications following this surgical procedure if you had difficulty with this question.
Level of Cognitive Ability: Analyzing
Client Needs: Physiological Integrity
Integrated Process: Nursing Process—Assessment
Content Area: Adult Health—Musculoskeletal
Reference: Ignatavicius, D., & Workman, M. (2010). *Medical-surgical nursing: Patient-centered collaborative care* (6th ed., p. 987). St. Louis: Saunders.

844. 2

Rationale: In addition to the presence of clinical manifestations, gout is diagnosed by the presence of persistent hyperuricemia, with a uric acid level higher than 8 mg/dL; a normal value ranges from 2.5 to 8 mg/dL. Options 1, 3, and 4 indicate normal laboratory values. Additionally, the presence of uric acid in an aspirated sample of synovial fluid confirms the diagnosis.

Test-Taking Strategy: Use the process of elimination and knowledge of normal laboratory values. Recalling that increased uric acid levels occur in gout and noting that option 2 is the only abnormal value will assist you in answering the question. Review the manifestations of gout and the normal uric acid level if you had difficulty with this question.

Level of Cognitive Ability: Analyzing
Client Needs: Physiological Integrity
Integrated Process: Nursing Process—Assessment
Content Area: Adult Health—Musculoskeletal
Reference: Ignatavicius, D., & Workman, M. (2010). *Medical-surgical nursing: Patient-centered collaborative care* (6th ed., p. 353). St. Louis: Saunders.

ALTERNATE ITEM FORMAT: MULTIPLE RESPONSE

845. 1, 2, 3

Rationale: A plaster cast takes 24 to 72 hours to dry (synthetic casts dry in 20 minutes). The cast and extremity should be elevated to reduce edema if prescribed. A wet cast is handled with the palms of the hand until it is dry, and the extremity is turned (unless contraindicated) so that all sides of the wet cast will dry. A cool setting on the hair dryer can be used to dry a plaster cast (heat cannot be used on a plaster cast because the cast heats up and burns the skin). The cast needs to be kept clean and dry, and the client is instructed not to stick anything under the cast because of the risk of breaking skin integrity. The client is instructed to monitor the extremity for circulatory impairment, such as pain, swelling, discoloration, tingling, numbness, coolness, or diminished pulse. The physician is notified immediately if circulatory impairment occurs.

Test-Taking Strategy: Focus on the subject, a plaster cast. Recalling that edema occurs following a fracture and recalling the complications associated with a cast will assist you in answering the question. Review cast care instructions if you had difficulty with this question.

Level of Cognitive Ability: Applying
Client Needs: Physiological Integrity
Integrated Process: Teaching and Learning
Content Area: Adult Health—Musculoskeletal
Reference: Ignatavicius, D., & Workman, M. (2010). *Medical-surgical nursing: Patient-centered collaborative care* (6th ed., p. 1184). St. Louis: Saunders.

69

Musculoskeletal Medications

I. SKELETAL MUSCLE RELAXANTS

A. Description

1. Skeletal muscle relaxants (Box 69-1) act directly on the neuromuscular junction or act indirectly on the central nervous system (CNS).
2. Centrally acting muscle relaxants depress neuron activity in the spinal cord or brain.
3. Peripherally acting muscle relaxants act directly on the skeletal muscles, interfering with calcium release from muscle tubules and thus preventing the fibers from contracting.
4. Skeletal muscle relaxants are used to prevent or relieve muscle spasms and treat spasticity associated with spinal cord disease or lesions, acute painful musculoskeletal conditions, and chronic debilitating disorders such as multiple sclerosis, brain attacks (stroke), or cerebral palsy.
5. Skeletal muscle relaxants are contraindicated in clients with severe liver, renal, or heart disease; these medications are often metabolized in the liver or excreted by the kidneys.
6. Skeletal muscle relaxants should not be taken with CNS depressants, such as barbiturates, opioids, alcohol, sedatives, hypnotics, or tricyclic antidepressants, unless specifically prescribed.

B. Side effects

1. Dizziness and hypotension
2. Drowsiness and muscle weakness
3. Dry mouth
4. Gastrointestinal upset
5. Photosensitivity
6. Liver toxicity

C. Interventions

1. Obtain a medical history.
2. Monitor vital signs.
3. Monitor for CNS side effects.
4. Assess for risk of injury.
5. Assess involved joints and muscles for pain and mobility.
6. Monitor renal function studies.
7. Instruct the client to take the medication with food to decrease gastrointestinal upset.

8. Instruct the client to report side effects.
9. Instruct the client to avoid alcohol and CNS depressants.
10. Instruct the client to avoid activities requiring alertness, such as driving or operating equipment.

⚠ Monitor liver function tests when a client is taking a skeletal muscle relaxant because hepatotoxicity can occur.

D. Nursing considerations

1. Baclofen (Lioresal)
   a. Baclofen causes CNS effects such as drowsiness, dizziness, weakness, and fatigue and nausea, constipation, and urinary retention.
   b. Administer with caution in the client with renal or hepatic dysfunction or a seizure disorder.
   c. Baclofen can be administered by the physician through intrathecal infusion using an implantable pump or direct intrathecal administration over 1 minute.
   d. Instruct the client with an implantable pump to maintain medication refill appointments to prevent the pump from emptying and experiencing sudden withdrawal symptoms, which could be life-threatening.
2. Carisoprodol (Soma)
   a. Advise the client to take the medication with food to prevent gastrointestinal upset.
   b. Instruct the client to report any rash or hypersensitivity to the physician.
3. Chlorzoxazone (Paraflex, Parafon Forte, Remular-S)
   a. Monitor the client for hypersensitivity reactions such as urticaria, redness or itching, and possibly angioedema.
   b. Chlorzoxazone may cause malaise and may cause the urine to turn orange or red.
   c. Can cause hepatitis and hepatic necrosis.
4. Cyclobenzaprine (Flexeril)
   a. Cyclobenzaprine is contraindicated in clients who have received monoamine oxidase

Box 69-1 Skeletal Muscle Relaxants

Baclofen (Lioresal)
Carisoprodol (Soma)
Chlorzoxazone (Paraflex, Parafon Forte, Remular-S)
Cyclobenzaprine (Flexeril)
Dantrolene (Dantrium)
Diazepam (Valium)
Metaxalone (Skelaxin)
Methocarbamol (Robaxin)
Orphenadine (Norflex)
Tizanidine (Zanaflex)

Box 69-2 Antigout Medications

Allopurinol (Zyloprim)   Probenecid
Colchicine   Sulfinpyrazone (Anturane)

inhibitors (MAOIs) within 14 days of initiation of cyclobenzaprine therapy and in clients with cardiac disorders.

   b. Cyclobenzaprine has significant anticholinergic (atropine-like) effects and should be used with caution in clients with a history of urinary retention, angle-closure glaucoma, or increased intraocular pressure.

   c. Cyclobenzaprine should be used only for short-term therapy (2 to 3 weeks).

5. Dantrolene (Dantrium)

   a. Dantrolene acts directly on skeletal muscles to relieve spasticity.

   b. Liver damage is the most serious adverse effect.

   c. Liver function values should be monitored before the initiation of treatment and during treatment.

   d. Dantrolene can cause gastrointestinal bleeding, urinary frequency, impotence, photosensitivity, rash, and muscle weakness.

   e. Instruct the client to wear protective clothing when in the sun.

   f. Instruct the client to notify the physician if rash, bloody or tarry stools, or yellow discoloration of the skin or eyes occurs.

6. Diazepam (Valium)

   a. Acts on the CNS to suppress spasticity; does not affect skeletal muscle directly

   b. Sedation is a common side effect.

7. Methocarbamol (Robaxin)

   a. The parenteral form is contraindicated in clients with renal impairment.

   b. The parenteral form can cause hypotension, bradycardia, anaphylaxis, and seizures, especially when the medication is given too rapidly.

   c. Monitor site for extravasation, which can result in thrombophlebitis and tissue sloughing.

   d. Methocarbamol may cause the urine to turn brown, black, or green.

   e. Inform the client to notify the physician if blurred vision, nasal congestion, urticaria, or rash occurs.

8. Tizanidine (Zanaflex) and metaxalone (Skelaxin): Can cause liver damage

9. Orphenadrine (Norflex) has significant anticholinergic (atropine-like) effects and should be used with caution in clients with a history of urinary retention, angle-closure glaucoma, or increased intraocular pressure.

⚠ Safety is a primary concern when the client is taking a skeletal muscle relaxant because these medications cause drowsiness.

II. ANTIGOUT MEDICATIONS

A. Description

1. Antigout medications (Box 69-2) reduce uric acid production and increase uric acid excretion (uricosuric) to prevent or relieve gout or to manage hyperuricemia.

2. Nonsteroidal anti-inflammatory drugs (NSAIDs) are used for their anti-inflammatory effects and to relieve pain during an acute gouty attack (see Chapter 67 for information on NSAIDs).

3. Glucocorticoids may be prescribed to reduce inflammation during an acute gout attack (see Chapter 55 for information on glucocorticoids).

4. Antigout medications should be used cautiously in clients with gastrointestinal, renal, cardiac, or hepatic disease.

B. Side effects

1. Headaches
2. Nausea, vomiting, and diarrhea
3. Blood dyscrasias, such as bone marrow depression
4. Flushed skin and rash
5. Uric acid kidney stones
6. Sore gums
7. Metallic taste

C. Interventions

1. Assess serum uric acid levels.
2. Monitor intake and output.
3. Maintain a fluid intake of at least 2000 to 3000 mL/day to prevent kidney stones.
4. Monitor complete blood cell count and renal and liver function studies.
5. Instruct the client to avoid alcohol and caffeine because these products can increase uric acid levels.
6. Encourage the client to comply with therapy to prevent elevated uric acid levels, which can trigger a gout attack.
7. Instruct the client to avoid foods high in purine as prescribed, such as wine, alcohol, organ meats, sardines, salmon, scallops, and gravy.

8. Instruct the client to take the medication with food to decrease gastric irritation.
9. Instruct the client to report side effects to the physician.
10. Caution the client not to take aspirin with these medications because this could trigger a gout attack.

D. Nursing considerations
1. Allopurinol (Zyloprim)
   a. Can increase the effect of warfarin (Coumadin) and oral hypoglycemic agents
   b. Instruct the client not to take large doses of vitamin C while taking allopurinol because kidney stones may occur.
   c. Hypersensitivity syndrome (rare) can occur, characterized by rash, fever, eosinophilia, and liver and kidney alterations (medication is withheld and the physician is notified).
   d. Advise the client to minimize exposure to sunlight and have an annual eye examination because visual changes can occur from prolonged use of allopurinol.
2. Colchicine
   a Used with caution in older clients, debilitated clients, and clients with cardiac, renal, and/or gastrointestinal disease.
   b. If gastrointestinal symptoms occur (nausea, vomiting, diarrhea, and abdominal pain), the medication is withheld and the physician is notified.
3. Probenecid
   a. Mild gastrointestinal effects can occur and can be reduced by taking the medication with food.
   b. Aspirin and other salicylates interfere with the uricosuric action of the medication.
4. Sulfinpyrazone (Anturane)
   a. Contraindicated in clients with active ulcer disease; used with caution in clients with a history of ulcer disease
   b. Salicylates counteract the uricosuric action of the medication.
   c. Inhibits hepatic metabolism of tolbutamide (Orinase), causing hypoglycemia, and warfarin, causing bleeding tendencies.

⚠ The concurrent use of antigout medications and aspirin causes elevated uric acid levels; the client should be instructed to take acetaminophen (Tylenol) if prescribed rather than aspirin.

III. ANTIARTHRITIC MEDICATIONS (Box 69-3)

A. Description (Fig. 69-1)
1. Rheumatoid arthritis occurs as inflammation progresses into the synovia, cartilage and bone; if this inflammation is not controlled, it will lead to joint destruction, thus affecting client mobility and comfort.

Box 69-3 Antiarthritic Medications

Anakinra (Kineret)
Adalimumab (Humira)
Auranofin (Ridaura)
Aurothioglucose (Solganal)
Azathioprine (Imuran)
Cyclosporine (Neoral)
Etanercept (Enbrel)
Gold sodium thiomalate (Aurolate, Myochrysine)
Leflunomide (Arava)
Methotrexate (Rheumatrex, Trexall)
Penicillamine (Cuprimine)
Infliximab (Remicade)
Sulfasalazine (Azulfidine)

2. The focus of treatment is early diagnosis and aggressive treatment in order to preserve joint function.
3. Medication therapy includes NSAIDs, glucocorticoids, and disease-modifying antirheumatic drugs (DMARDs).
4. Gold salts: Use of gold salts has decreased, but their purpose is to reduce the progression of joint damage caused by arthritic processes. Gold toxicity, characterized by pruritis, rash, metallic taste, stomatitis, and diarrhea, can occur; if toxicity occurs, dimercaprol (BAL in oil) may be prescribed to enhance gold excretion.

B. DMARDs
1. Description
   a. DMARDs are effective antirheumatic medications that are used to slow the degenerative effects of the disorder.
   b. DMARDs are usually prescribed secondary to NSAIDs but are often the first choice in the treatment of severe arthritis.
2. Common side effects of DMARDs include injection site inflammation and pain, ecchymosis, and edema, pancytopenia and infection, fatigue, headache, nausea, vomiting, and flu-like symptoms, and allergic response.
3. Interventions
   a. Instruct the client to monitor for signs of infection and report signs to the physician.
   b. Monitor the injection site for signs of irritation, pain, inflammation, and swelling.
   c. Instruct the client to consult with the physician before receiving live vaccines and to avoid exposure to infections.
   d. Inform the client about the importance of laboratory tests for neutrophil counts, white blood cell counts, and platelet counts before initiation of treatment and during treatment.
4. Anakinra (Kineret): Injection site reactions are common (pruritus, erythema, rash, pain).

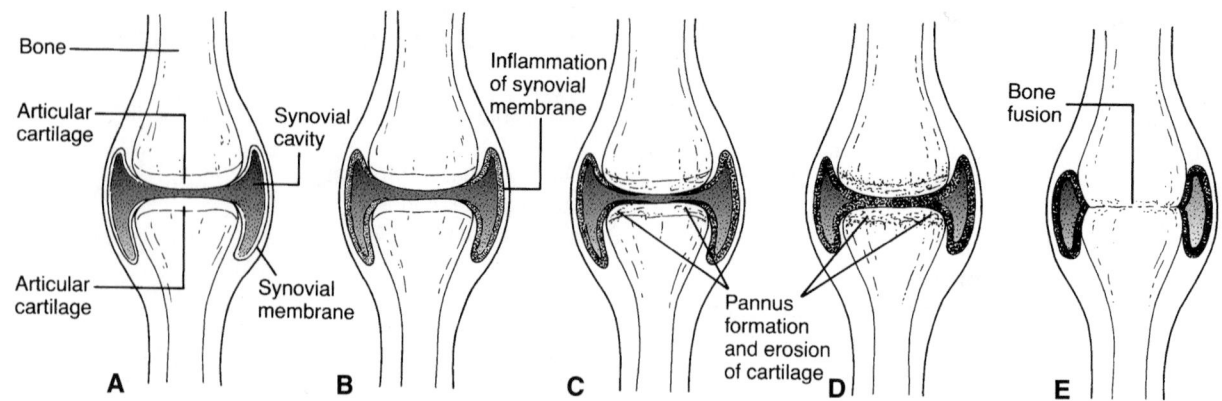

▲ **Figure 69-1** Progressive joint degeneration in rheumatoid arthritis. **A,** Healthy joint. **B,** Inflammation of synovial membrane. **C,** Onset of pannus formation and cartilage erosion. **D,** Pannus formation progresses and cartilage deteriorates further. **E,** Complete destruction of joint cavity, together with fusion of articulating bones. (From Lehne, R. [2010]. *Pharmacology for nursing care* [7th ed.]. St. Louis: Saunders.)

5. Adalimumab (Humira)
   a. Injection site reactions are common.
   b. Has been associated with neurological injury (numbness, tingling, dizziness, visual disturbances, weakness in the legs)
6. Auranofin (Ridaura): Oral gold preparation (not commonly used)
7. Gold sodium thiomalate (Aurolate, Myochrysine), aurothioglucose (Solganal): Intramuscular gold preparations (not commonly used)
8. Azathioprine (Imuran): Immunosuppressive and anti-inflammatory actions; toxic effects include hepatitis and blood dyscrasias.
9. Cyclosporine (Neoral): Immunosuppressive actions; can cause nephrotoxicity
10. Etanercept (Enbrel)
    a. Injection site reactions are common.
    b. Poses a risk for heart failure; has been associated with central nervous system demyelinating disorders and hematological disorders
11. Hydroxychloroquine sulfate (Plaquenil): Associated with retinal damage; inform the client to contact the physician if visual disturbances occur.
12. Leflunomide (Arava): Side effects include diarrhea, respiratory infection, reversible alopecia, rash, and nausea; is hepatotoxic.
13. Methotrexate (Rheumatrex, Trexall): Can cause hepatic fibrosis, bone marrow suppression, gastrointestinal ulceration, and pneumonitis
14. Penicillamine (Cuprimine): Can cause bone marrow suppression and autoimmune disorders
15. Infliximab (Remicade): Can cause infusion reactions (fever, chills, pruritus, urticaria, chest pain); is hepatotoxic
16. Sulfasalazine (Azulfidine): Can cause gastrointestinal and dermatological reactions, bone marrow suppression, hepatitis
C. NSAIDs may be prescribed for their anti-inflammatory and analgesic effects (see Chapter 67 for information on NSAIDs).

D. Glucocorticoids may be prescribed for their anti-inflammatory effects (see Chapter 55 for information on glucocorticoids).

IV. **MEDICATIONS TO PREVENT AND TREAT OSTEOPOROSIS**
A. Description
   1. Osteoporosis is characterized by decreased bone mass and increased bone fragility
   2. Calcium and vitamin D supplementation can reduce the risk of osteoporosis; calcium maximizes bone growth early in life and maintains bone integrity later in life, and vitamin D ensures calcium absorption (see Chapter 55 for information on calcium and vitamin D supplements).
   3. Treatment is aimed at reducing the occurrence of fractures by maintaining or increasing bone strength.
   4. Medications that decrease bone resorption (antiresorptive) and medications that promote bone formation are used.
   5. Antiresorptive medications include raloxifene (Evista), calcitonin, and bisphosphonates.
   6. Teriparatide (Forteo) promotes bone growth.
B. Interventions
   1. Salmon calcitonin (Miacalcin)
      a. Calcitonin is secreted by the thyroid gland and inhibits osteoclastic bone resorption.
      b. Instruct the client how to administer the intranasal or subcutaneous form, depending on the route prescribed.
      c. Intranasal route: Examine the nares for irritation; alternate nostrils for doses.
      d. When calcitonin is taken, it is important to monitor for hypocalcemia.
   2. Bisphosphonates (Box 69-4)
      a. Bisphosphonates inhibit osteoclast-mediated bone resorption, thereby increasing total bone mass.

Box 69-4 Medications to Prevent or Treat Osteoporosis

Calcium and vitamin D	Ibandronate (Boniva)
Alendronate (Fosamax)	Raloxifene (Evista)
Calcitonin, salmon	Risedronate (Actonel)
(Miacalcin)	Teriparatide (Forteo)

b. Bisphosphonates include alendronate (Fosamax), risedronate (Actonel), and ibandronate (Boniva).

c. Contraindicated for clients with esophageal disorders that can impede swallowing and for clients who cannot sit or stand for at least 30 minutes (60 minutes with ibandronate)

d. After taking the medication, the client is instructed to postpone ingesting anything for at least 30 minutes (60 minutes with ibandronate).

e. Adverse effects include esophagitis, muscle pain, and ocular problems; the client is instructed to contact the physician if adverse effects occur.

⚠ Because of the risk of esophagitis, bisphosphonates must be administered in the morning before eating or drinking with a full glass of water; the client must then remain sitting or standing for at least 30 minutes (60 minutes with ibandronate).

3. Raloxifene (Evista)
   a. Antiresorptive medication (nonbisphosphonate)
   b. Contraindicated in clients who have a history of venous thrombotic events
   c. Needs to be discontinued 72 hours prior to prolonged immobilization periods (such as with periods of extended bed rest).
   d. Instruct the client to avoid extended periods of restricted activity (such as when traveling).
4. Teriparatide (Forteo)
   a. Teriparatide stimulates new bone formation, thus increasing bone mass.
   b. Teriparatide is a portion of the human parathyroid hormone and works by increasing the action of osteoblasts.
   c. Reserved for clients at high risk for fractures
   d. Has been associated with the development of bone cancer

💿 MORE QUESTIONS ON THE CD!

Practice Questions

846. The client has been on treatment for rheumatoid arthritis for 3 weeks. During the administration of etanercept (Enbrel), it is most important for the nurse to assess:

1. The injection site for itching and edema
2. The white blood cell counts and platelet counts
3. Whether the client is experiencing fatigue and joint pain
4. A metallic taste in the mouth, with a loss of appetite

847. Allopurinol (Zyloprim) is prescribed for a client and the nurse provides medication instructions to the client. The nurse instructs the client:

1. To drink 3000 mL of fluid a day
2. To take the medication on an empty stomach
3. That the effect of the medication will occur immediately
4. That if swelling of the lips occurs, this is a normal expected response

848. Colchicine is prescribed for a client with a diagnosis of gout. The nurse reviews the client's record, knowing that this medication would be used with caution in which of the following disorders?

1. Myxedema
2. Renal failure
3. Hypothyroidism
4. Diabetes mellitus

849. Alendronate (Fosamax) is prescribed for a client with osteoporosis. The nurse instructs the client to:

1. Take the medication at bedtime.
2. Take the medication in the morning with breakfast.
3. Lie down for 30 minutes after taking the medication.
4. Take the medication with a full glass of water after rising in the morning.

850. A nurse is providing discharge instructions to a client receiving baclofen (Lioresal). Which of the following would be included in the teaching plan?

1. Restrict fluid intake.
2. Avoid the use of alcohol.
3. Notify the physician if fatigue occurs.
4. Stop the medication if diarrhea occurs.

851. A nurse is analyzing the laboratory studies on a client receiving dantrolene sodium (Dantrium). Which of the following laboratory tests would identify an adverse effect associated with the administration of this medication?

1. Creatinine level determination
2. Platelet count determination
3. Blood urea nitrogen level determination
4. Liver function tests

852. Cyclobenzaprine hydrochloride (Flexeril) is prescribed for a client for muscle spasms. The nurse is reviewing the client's record. Which of the following disorders, if noted in the record, would indicate a need to contact the physician about the administration of this medication?
1. Glaucoma
2. Emphysema
3. Hypothyroidism
4. Diabetes mellitus

853. A nurse is administering an intravenous dose of methocarbamol (Robaxin) to a client with multiple sclerosis. For which of the following adverse effects would the nurse monitor?
1. Tachycardia
2. Rapid pulse
3. Bradycardia
4. Hypertension

Alternate Item Format: Multiple Response

854. In monitoring a client's response to disease-modifying antirheumatic drugs (DMARDs), which assessment findings would the nurse consider acceptable responses? **Select all that apply**.
❏ 1. Symptom control during periods of emotional stress
❏ 2. Normal white blood cell, platelet, and neutrophil counts
❏ 3. Radiological findings that show no progression of joint degeneration
❏ 4. An increased range of motion in the affected joints 3 months into therapy
❏ 5. Inflammation and irritation at the injection site 3 days after the injection is given
❏ 6. A low-grade temperature on rising in the morning that remains throughout the day

ANSWERS

846. 2

Rationale: Infection and pancytopenia are side effects of etanercept (Enbrel). Laboratory studies are performed prior to and during medication treatment. The appearance of abnormal white blood cell counts and abnormal platelet counts can alert the nurse to a potentially life-threatening infection. Injection site itching is a common occurrence following administration. A metallic taste with loss of appetite are not common signs of side effects of this medication.
Test-Taking Strategy: Use the process of elimination. Option 4 can be eliminated, because this is not a common side effect. In early treatment, residual fatigue and joint pain may still be apparent. Option 2 monitors for a hematological disorder, which could indicate a reason for discontinuing this medication and should be reported. Review this medication if you had difficulty with this question.
Level of Cognitive Ability: Analyzing
Client Needs: Physiological Integrity
Integrated Process: Nursing Process—Assessment
Content Area: Pharmacology
References: Hodgson, B., & Kizior, R. (2010). *Saunders nursing drug handbook 2010* (p. 440). St. Louis: Saunders.
    Ignatavicius, D., & Workman, M. (2010). *Medical-surgical nursing: Patient-centered collaborative care* (6th ed., p. 343). St. Louis: Saunders.

847. 1

Rationale: Clients taking allopurinol are encouraged to drink 3000 mL of fluid a day. A full therapeutic effect may take 1 week or longer. Allopurinol is to be given with, or immediately after, meals or milk. A client who develops a rash, irritation of the eyes, or swelling of the lips or mouth should contact the physician because this may indicate hypersensitivity.
Test-Taking Strategy: Use the process of elimination. Option 4 can be eliminated easily because it indicates hypersensitivity, which is not a normal expected response. From the remaining options, recalling that this medication is used to treat gout will direct you to option 1. If you had difficulty with this question, review the client instructions related to allopurinol.
Level of Cognitive Ability: Applying
Client Needs: Physiological Integrity
Integrated Process: Teaching and Learning
Content Area: Pharmacology
References: Hodgson, B., & Kizior, R. (2010). *Saunders nursing drug handbook 2010* (p. 35). St. Louis: Saunders.
    Skidmore-Roth, L. (2010). *Mosby's nursing drug reference* (23rd ed., p. 108). St. Louis: Mosby.

848. 2

Rationale: Colchicine is used with caution in older clients, debilitated clients, and clients with cardiac, renal, or gastrointestinal disease. The disorders in options 1, 3, and 4 are not concerns with administration of this medication.
Test-Taking Strategy: Use the process of elimination. Note that options 1, 3, and 4 are endocrine-related disorders. Option 2, the correct option, is different from the others. Review the cautions associated with this medication if you had difficulty with this question.
Level of Cognitive Ability: Analyzing
Client Needs: Physiological Integrity
Integrated Process: Nursing Process—Analysis
Content Area: Pharmacology
Reference: Lehne, R. (2010). *Pharmacology for nursing care* (7th ed., p. 865). St. Louis: Saunders.

849. 4

Rationale: Precautions need to be taken with the administration of alendronate to prevent gastrointestinal side effects (especially esophageal irritation) and to increase absorption of the medication. The medication needs to be taken with a full glass of water after rising in the morning. The client should not eat or drink anything for 30 minutes following administration and should not lie down after taking the medication.

Test-Taking Strategy: Knowledge regarding the administration of alendronate is needed to answer this question. Recalling that this medication can cause esophageal irritation will direct you to option 4. Review this medication if you had difficulty with this question.
Level of Cognitive Ability: Applying
Client Needs: Physiological Integrity
Integrated Process: Teaching and Learning
Content Area: Pharmacology
Reference: Hodgson, B., & Kizior, R. (2010). *Saunders nursing drug handbook 2010* (p. 30). St. Louis: Saunders.

850. 2
Rationale: Baclofen is a skeletal muscle relaxant. The client should be cautioned against the use of alcohol and other central nervous system depressants because baclofen potentiates the depressant activity of these agents. Constipation rather than diarrhea is an adverse effect. Restriction of fluids is not necessary, but the client should be warned that urinary retention can occur. Fatigue is related to a CNS effect that is most intense during the early phase of therapy and diminishes with continued medication use. The client does not need to notify the physician about fatigue.
Test-Taking Strategy: Use the process of elimination. Recalling that baclofen is a skeletal muscle relaxant will direct you easily to option 2. If you were unsure of the correct option, use general principles related to medication administration. Alcohol should be avoided with the use of medications. Review client teaching points related to this medication if you had difficulty with this question.
Level of Cognitive Ability: Applying
Client Needs: Physiological Integrity
Integrated Process: Teaching and Learning
Content Area: Pharmacology
Reference: Lehne, R. (2010). *Pharmacology for nursing care* (7th ed., p. 241). St. Louis: Saunders.

851. 4
Rationale: Dose-related liver damage is the most serious adverse effect of dantrolene. To reduce the risk of liver damage, liver function tests should be performed before treatment and throughout the treatment interval. Dantrolene is administered in the lowest effective dosage for the shortest time necessary.
Test-Taking Strategy: Use the process of elimination. Eliminate options 1 and 3 because these tests assess kidney function and are comparable or alike. From the remaining options, you must recall that this medication affects liver function. Review this medication if you had difficulty with this question.
Level of Cognitive Ability: Analyzing
Client Needs: Physiological Integrity
Integrated Process: Nursing Process—Analysis
Content Area: Pharmacology
Reference: Hodgson, B., & Kizior, R. (2010). *Saunders nursing drug handbook 2010* (pp. 298–300). St. Louis: Saunders.

852. 1
Rationale: Because cyclobenzaprine (Flexeril) has anticholinergic effects, it should be used with caution in clients with a history of urinary retention, glaucoma, and increased intraocular pressure. Cyclobenzaprine should be used only for a short term (2 to 3 weeks).
Test-Taking Strategy: Use the process of elimination. Recalling that this medication has anticholinergic effects will direct you to option 1. If you are unfamiliar with this medication and the contraindications associated with its administration, review this content.
Level of Cognitive Ability: Analyzing
Client Needs: Physiological Integrity
Integrated Process: Nursing Process—Analysis
Content Area: Pharmacology
Reference: Hodgson, B., & Kizior, R. (2010). *Saunders nursing drug handbook 2010* (p. 284). St. Louis: Saunders.

853. 3
Rationale: Intravenous administration of methocarbamol can cause hypotension and bradycardia. The nurse needs to monitor for these side effects. Options 1, 2, and 4 are not a concern with administration of this medication.
Test-Taking Strategy: Use the process of elimination. Eliminate options 1 and 2 first because they are comparable or alike. Knowledge about the specific side effects related to the intravenous use of this medication will direct you to option 3. Remember that hypotension and bradycardia can occur with intravenous administration of methocarbamol. Review this medication if you had difficulty with this question.
Level of Cognitive Ability: Analyzing
Client Needs: Physiological Integrity
Integrated Process: Nursing Process—Assessment
Content Area: Pharmacology
References: Edmunds, M. (2010). *Introduction to clinical pharmacology* (6th ed., pp. 383, 385). St. Louis: Mosby.
　Skidmore-Roth; L. (2010). *Mosby's nursing drug reference* (23rd ed., pp. 699–700). St. Louis: Mosby.

ALTERNATE ITEM FORMAT: MULTIPLE RESPONSE
854. 1, 2, 3, 4
Rationale: Because emotional stress frequently exacerbates the symptoms of rheumatoid arthritis, the absence of symptoms is a positive finding. DMARDs are given to slow the progression of joint degeneration. In addition, the improvement in the range of motion after 3 months of therapy with normal blood work is a positive finding. Temperature elevation and inflammation and irritation at the medication injection site could indicate signs of infection.
Test-Taking Strategy: Use the process of elimination and focus on the subject, acceptable responses to therapy. Recalling that signs of an infection can indicate an unexpected finding will assist in eliminating options 5 and 6. Review the expected effects of this medication if you had difficulty with this question.
Level of Cognitive Ability: Evaluating
Client Needs: Physiological Integrity
Integrated Process: Nursing Process—Assessment
Content Area: Pharmacology
Reference: Lehne, R. (2010). *Pharmacology for nursing care* (7th ed., p. 863). St. Louis: Saunders.

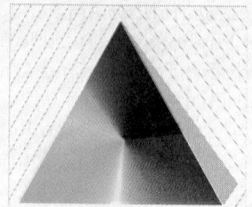

UNIT XVIII

The Adult Client With an Immune Disorder

PYRAMID TERMS

acquired immunity Immunity received passively from the mother's antibodies, animal serum, or antibodies produced in response to a disease. Immunization produces active acquired immunity.

allergy An abnormal, individual response to certain substances that normally do not trigger such an exaggerated reaction.

cellular response A delayed response against slowly developing bacterial infections; also called delayed hypersensitivity.

humoral response An immediate response that provides protection against acute, rapidly developing bacterial and viral infections.

immunodeficiency The absence or inadequate production of immune bodies.

innate immunity Immunity present at birth.

Kaposi's sarcoma Skin lesions that occur in individuals with a compromised immune system.

Lyme disease An infection acquired from a tick bite. Ticks live in wooded areas and survive by attaching to a host.

PYRAMID TO SUCCESS

Pyramid Points focus on the effects of and complications associated with an immune deficiency. Specific focus relates to the nursing care related to the disorder, the impact of the treatment or disorder, and client adaptation. Acquired immunodeficiency syndrome is a pyramid focus, along with protecting the client from infection and preventing the transmission of infection to other individuals. Psychosocial issues relate to social isolation and the body image disturbances that can occur as a result of the immune disorder.

CLIENT NEEDS

Safe and Effective Care Environment

Acting as an advocate related to the client's decisions
Addressing advance directives
Consulting with members of the health care team
Establishing priorities
Handling hazardous and infectious materials safely
Implementing standard and other precautions
Maintaining asepsis
Maintaining confidentiality regarding diagnosis
Obtaining informed consent for treatments and procedures
Preventing infection
Upholding client rights

Health Promotion and Maintenance

Ensuring that the client receives recommended immunizations
Implementing health screening measures
Monitoring for expected body image changes
Preventing disease related to infection
Providing health promotion programs
Respecting client lifestyle choices

Psychosocial Integrity

Assisting in mobilizing appropriate support and resource systems
Assisting the client and family to cope
Assisting the client to cope, adapt, and solve problems during illness or stressful events
Considering religious, spiritual, and cultural preferences

Discussing grief and loss related to death and the dying process

Promoting a positive environment to maintain optimal quality of life

Physiological Integrity

Managing pain
Managing medical emergencies

Monitoring for the expected and unexpected responses to treatments

Promoting nutrition

Protecting the client from infection

Providing basic care and comfort

Reviewing diagnostic test and laboratory test results

70

Immune Disorders

I. FUNCTIONS OF THE IMMUNE SYSTEM

A. The immune system provides protection against invasion by microorganisms from outside the body.

B. The immune system protects the body from internal threats and maintains the internal environment by removing dead or damaged cells.

II. IMMUNE RESPONSE

A. T lymphocytes and B lymphocytes
   1. Lymphocytes migrate to lymphoid tissue where they remain dormant until they need to form sensitized lymphocytes for cellular immunity or antibodies for humoral immunity.
   2. Some B lymphocytes lie dormant until a specific antigen enters the body, at which time they greatly increase in number and are available for defense.
   3. Types of T lymphocytes include helper/inducer, suppressor, and cytotoxic/cytolytic.
   4. T and B lymphocytes are necessary for a normal immune response.

B. Humoral response
   1. **Humoral response** is immediate.
   2. This type of response provides protection against acute, rapidly developing bacterial and viral infections.

C. **Cellular response**
   1. **Cellular response** is delayed; this is also called delayed hypersensitivity.
   2. This type of response is active against slowly developing bacterial infections and is involved in autoimmune responses, some allergic reactions, and rejection of foreign cells.

III. IMMUNITY

A. Natural immunity
   1. Natural immunity is also called native or **innate immunity.**
   2. It is present at birth and includes biochemical, physical, and mechanical barriers of defense, as well as the inflammatory response.

B. **Acquired immunity**
   1. Acquired or adaptive immunity is received passively from the mother's antibodies, animal serum, or antibodies produced in response to a disease.
   2. Immunization produces active **acquired immunity**.

IV. IMMUNIZATIONS (See Chapter 48 for information about immunizations.)

V. LABORATORY STUDIES

A. Antinuclear antibody (ANA) titer determination
   1. The ANA titer determination is a blood test used for the differential diagnosis of rheumatic diseases and for the detection of antinucleoprotein factors and patterns associated with certain autoimmune diseases.
   2. The test is positive at a titer of 1:20 or 1:40, depending on the laboratory.
   3. A positive result does not necessarily confirm a disease.
   4. The ANA titer is positive in most individuals diagnosed with systemic lupus erythematosus (SLE).
   5. An ANA titer result can be false positive in a small proportion of the normal population.

B. Anti-dsDNA antibody test
   1. The anti-dsDNA (double-stranded DNA) antibody test is a blood test done specifically to identify or differentiate DNA antibodies found in SLE.
   2. The test supports a diagnosis, monitors disease activity and response to therapy, and establishes a prognosis for SLE.
   3. Values
      a. Negative: Lower than 70 units by enzyme-linked immunosorbent assay (ELISA)
      b. Borderline: 70 to 200 units
      c. Positive: Higher than 200 units

C. See Chapter 11 for testing related to acquired **immunodeficiency** syndrome (AIDS).

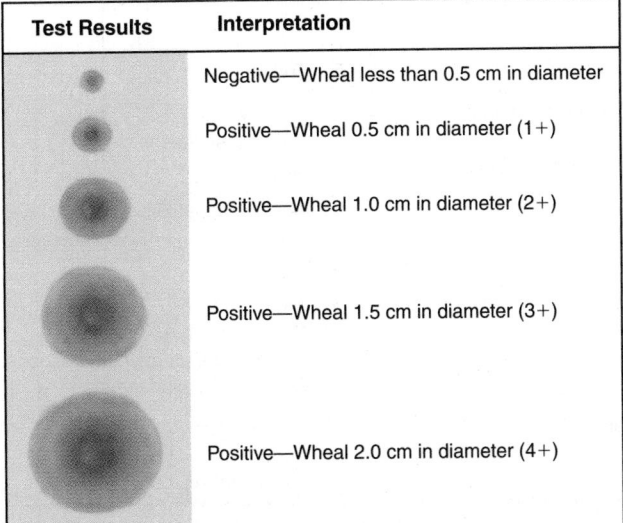

Test Results	Interpretation
	Negative—Wheal less than 0.5 cm in diameter
	Positive—Wheal 0.5 cm in diameter (1+)
	Positive—Wheal 1.0 cm in diameter (2+)
	Positive—Wheal 1.5 cm in diameter (3+)
	Positive—Wheal 2.0 cm in diameter (4+)

▲ **FIGURE 70-1** Interpretation of intradermal test results based on the size of the wheal after 15 to 30 minutes. (From Monahan, F., Sands, J., Neighbors, M., et al. [2007]. *Phipps' medical-surgical nursing: Health and illness perspectives* [8th ed.]. St. Louis: Mosby.)

D. Skin testing
   1. Description
      a. The administration of an allergen to the surface of the skin or into the dermis
      b. Administered by patch, scratch, or intradermal techniques
   2. Preprocedure interventions
      a. Discontinue systemic corticosteroids or antihistamine therapy 5 days before the test as prescribed.
      b. Obtain informed consent.
   3. Postprocedure interventions
      a. Record the site, date, and time of the test.
      b. Record the date and time for follow-up site reading.
      c. Have client remain in waiting room or office for at least 30 minutes after the injection to monitor for adverse effects.
      d. Inspect the site for erythema, papules, vesicles, edema, and wheal (Fig. 70-1).
      e. Measure flare along with the wheal and document the size and other findings.
      f. Provide the client with a list of potential allergens, if identified.

⚠ Have resuscitation equipment available if skin testing is performed because the allergen may induce an anaphylactic reaction.

VI. IMMUNODEFICIENCY

A. Description
   1. **Immunodeficiency** is the absence or inadequate production of immune bodies.
   2. The disorder can be congenital (primary) or acquired (secondary).
   3. Treatment depends on the inadequacy of immune bodies and its primary cause.
B. Assessment
   1. Factors that decrease immune function
   2. Frequent infections
   3. Nutritional status
   4. Medication history, such as use of corticosteroids for long periods
   5. History of alcohol or drug abuse
C. Interventions
   1. Protect the client from infection.
   2. Promote a balanced diet with adequate nutrition.
   3. Use strict aseptic technique for all procedures.
   4. Provide psychosocial care regarding lifestyle changes and role changes.
   5. Instruct the client in measures to prevent infection.
   6. Instruct the client to wear a Medic-Alert bracelet.

⚠ The priority concern for a client with immunodeficiency is infection.

VII. HYPERSENSITIVITY AND ALLERGY

A. Description
   1. An **allergy** is an abnormal, individual response to certain substances that normally do not trigger such an exaggerated reaction.
   2. In some types of allergies, a reaction occurs on a second and subsequent contact with the allergen.
   3. Skin testing may be done to determine the allergen.
   4. Types of hypersensitivity reactions (Table 70-1)
B. Assessment
   1. History of exposure to allergens
   2. Itching, tearing, and burning of eyes and skin
   3. Rashes
   4. Nose twitching, nasal stuffiness
C. Interventions
   1. Identification of the specific allergen
   2. Management of the symptoms with antihistamines, anti-inflammatory agents, or corticosteroids
   3. Ointments, creams, wet compresses, and soothing baths for local reactions
   4. Desensitization programs may be recommended.

VIII. ANAPHYLAXIS

A. Description
   1. Anaphylaxis is a serious and immediate hypersensitivity reaction that releases histamine from the damaged cells.
   2. Anaphylaxis can be systemic or cutaneous (localized).
B. Assessment (Fig. 70-2)
C. Interventions (see Priority Nursing Actions)

TABLE 70-1 Types of Hypersensitivity Reactions

Type	Causative Component	Pathological Process	Reaction
I: Immediate, anaphylactic	IgE	Mast cell degranulation ↓ Histamine and leukotriene release	Anaphylaxis Atopic diseases Skin reactions
II: Cytolytic, cytotoxic	IgG IgM Complement	Complement fixation ↓ Cell lysis	ABO incompatibility Drug-induced hemolytic anemia
III: Immune complex	Antigen-antibody complexes	Deposition in vessels and tissue walls ↓ Inflammation	Arthus reaction Serum sickness Systemic lupus erythematosus Acute glomerulonephritis
IV: Cell-mediated, delayed	Sensitized T cells	Lymphokine release	Tuberculosis Contact dermatitis Transplant rejection

Ig, Immunoglobulin.
From Black, J., & Hawks, J., (2005). *Medical-surgical nursing: Clinical management for positive outcomes* (7th ed.). St. Louis: Saunders.

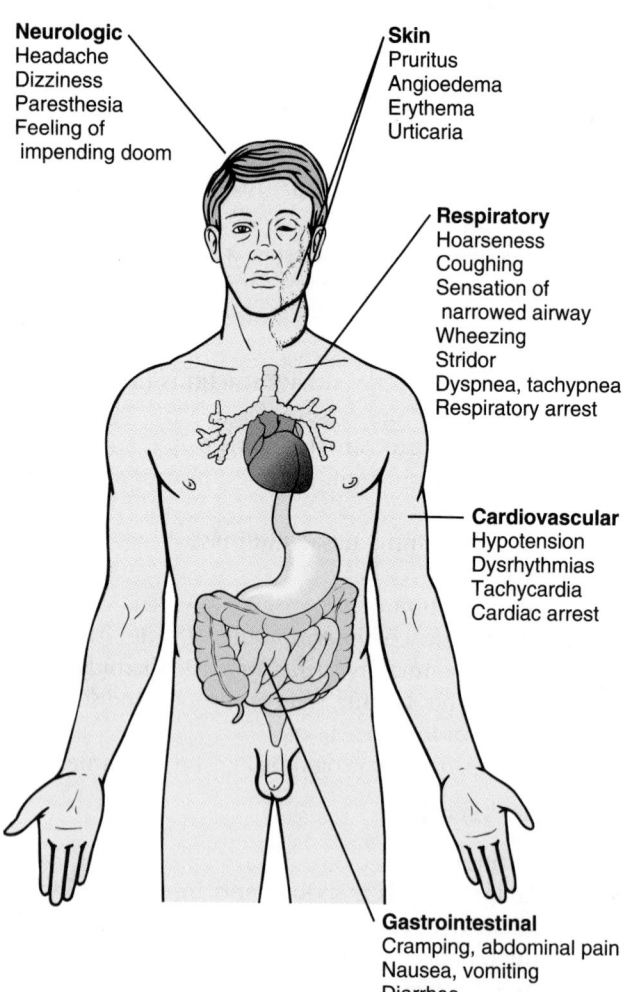

Neurologic
Headache
Dizziness
Paresthesia
Feeling of
 impending doom

Skin
Pruritus
Angioedema
Erythema
Urticaria

Respiratory
Hoarseness
Coughing
Sensation of
 narrowed airway
Wheezing
Stridor
Dyspnea, tachypnea
Respiratory arrest

Cardiovascular
Hypotension
Dysrhythmias
Tachycardia
Cardiac arrest

Gastrointestinal
Cramping, abdominal pain
Nausea, vomiting
Diarrhea

▲ **FIGURE 70-2** Clinical manifestations of a systemic anaphylactic reaction. (From Lewis, S., Heitkemper, M., Dirksen, S., O'Brien, P., & Bucher, L. [2007]. *Medical-surgical nursing: Assessment and management of clinical problems* [7th ed.]. St. Louis: Mosby.)

■■■■ PRIORITY NURSING ACTIONS! ■■■■

Actions to Take if a Client Develops Anaphylaxis
1. Quickly assess respiratory status and maintain a patent airway.
2. Call the physician or Rapid Response Team.
3. Administer oxygen.
4. Start an IV line and infuse normal saline.
5. Prepare to administer diphenhydramine (Benadryl) and epinephrine (adrenalin).
6. Document the event, actions taken, and the client's response.

If the client experiences an anaphylactic reaction, the immediate action would be to assess the respiratory status quickly and maintain a patent airway. The physician or Rapid Response Team is called. In the meantime, the nurse stays with the client and monitors the client's vital signs and for signs of shock. An IV device is inserted if one is not already in place and normal saline is infused. The nurse then prepares for the administration of diphenhydramine and epinephrine and other medications as prescribed. The head of the bed is elevated if the client's blood pressure is normal. The client's feet and legs may be raised. The nurse documents the event, actions taken, and the client's response.

Reference: Black, J., & Hawks, J. (2009). *Medical-surgical nursing: Clinical management for positive outcomes.* (8th ed., pp. 2167-2168). St. Louis: Saunders.

IX. LATEX ALLERGY

A. Description
 1. Latex **allergy** is a hypersensitivity to latex.
 2. The source of the allergic reaction is thought to be the proteins in the natural rubber latex or

Box 70-1 Products That May Contain Natural Rubber Latex

Ace bandages (brown)
Adhesive or elastic bandages
Ambu bag
Balloons
Blood pressure cuff (tubing and bladder)
Catheter leg bag straps
Catheters
Condoms
Diaphragms
Elastic pressure stockings
Electrocardiographic pads
Feminine hygiene pads
Gloves
Intravenous catheters, tubing, and rubber injection ports
Nasogastric tubes
Pads for crutches
Prepackaged enema kits
Rubber stoppers on medication vials
Stethoscopes
Syringes

Note: Health care agencies use as many nonlatex products as possible and have nonlatex supplies available for clients with a latex allergy.

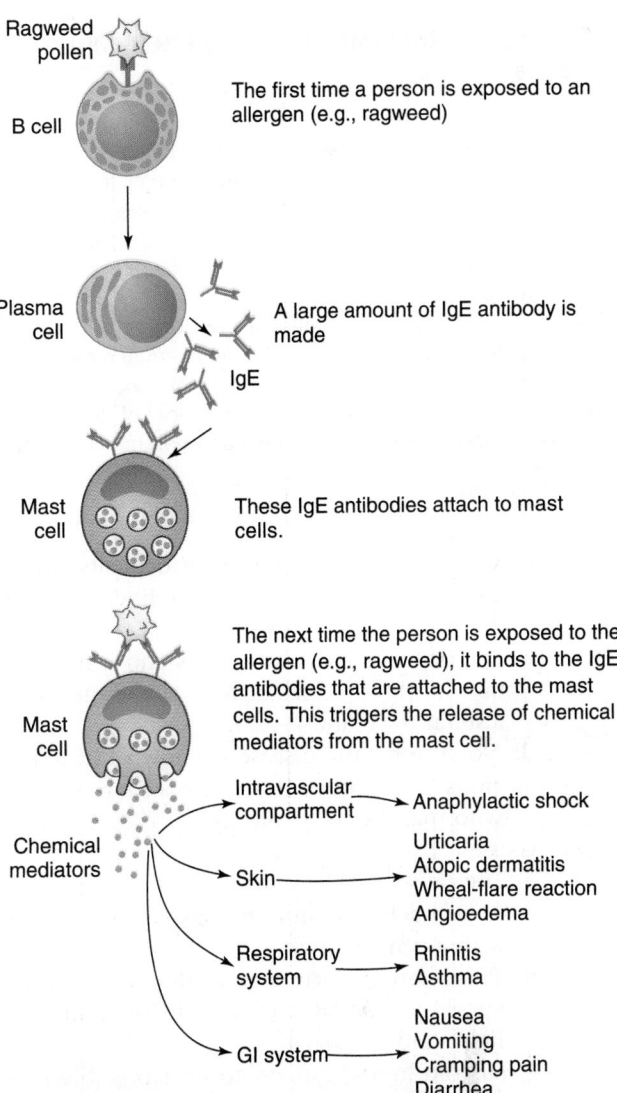

Ragweed pollen

B cell — The first time a person is exposed to an allergen (e.g., ragweed)

Plasma cell — A large amount of IgE antibody is made

IgE

Mast cell — These IgE antibodies attach to mast cells.

Mast cell — The next time the person is exposed to the allergen (e.g., ragweed), it binds to the IgE antibodies that are attached to the mast cells. This triggers the release of chemical mediators from the mast cell.

Chemical mediators

Intravascular compartment → Anaphylactic shock

Skin → Urticaria / Atopic dermatitis / Wheal-flare reaction / Angioedema

Respiratory system → Rhinitis / Asthma

GI system → Nausea / Vomiting / Cramping pain / Diarrhea

▲ **FIGURE 70-3** Steps in a type I allergic reaction. (From Lewis, S., Heitkemper, M., Dirksen, S., O'Brien, P., & Bucher, L. [2007]. *Medical-surgical nursing: Assessment and management of clinical problems* [7th ed.]. St. Louis: Mosby.)

the various chemicals used in the manufacturing process of latex gloves.

3. Symptoms of the **allergy** can range from mild contact dermatitis to moderately severe symptoms of rhinitis, conjunctivitis, urticaria, and bronchospasm to severe life-threatening anaphylaxis.

B. Common routes of exposure (Box 70-1)
1. Cutaneous: Natural latex gloves and latex balloons
2. Percutaneous and parenteral: Intravenous lines and catheters; hemodialysis equipment
3. Mucosal: Use of latex condoms, catheters, airways, and nipples
4. Aerosol: Aerosolization of powder from latex gloves can occur when gloves are dispensed from the box or when gloves are removed from the hands.

C. At-risk individuals
1. Health care workers
2. Individuals who work in the rubber industry
3. Individuals having multiple surgeries
4. Individuals with spina bifida
5. Individuals who wear gloves frequently, such as food handlers, hairdressers, and auto mechanics
6. Individuals allergic to kiwis, bananas, pineapples, tropical fruits, grapes, avocados, potatoes, hazelnuts, and water chestnuts

D. Assessment
1. Anaphylaxis or type I hypersensitivity is a response to natural rubber latex (Fig. 70-3; see Fig. 70-2).
2. A delayed type IV hypersensitivity reaction can occur; symptoms of contact dermatitis include pruritus, edema, erythema, vesicles, papules, and crusting and thickening of the skin and can occur within 6 to 48 hours following exposure.

E. Interventions (Box 70-2)

X. AUTOIMMUNE DISEASE

A. Description
1. Body is unable to recognize its own cells as a part of itself.
2. Autoimmune disease can affect collagenous tissue.

B. Systemic lupus erythematosus (SLE)
1. Description
   a. Chronic, progressive, systemic inflammatory disease that can cause major organs and systems to fail

Box 70-2 Interventions for the Client With a Latex Allergy

Ask the client about a known allergy to latex when performing the initial assessment.
Identify risk factors for a latex allergy in the client.
Use nonlatex gloves and all latex-safe supplies.
Keep a latex-safe supply cart near the client's room.
Apply a cloth barrier to the client's arm under a blood pressure cuff.
Use latex-free syringes, medication containers (glass ampules), and latex-safe intravenous equipment.
Instruct the client to wear a Medic-Alert bracelet.
Instruct the client about the importance of informing health care providers and local and paramedic ambulance companies about the allergy.

  b. Connective tissue and fibrin deposits collect in blood vessels on collagen fibers and on organs.
  c. The deposits lead to necrosis and inflammation in blood vessels, lymph nodes, gastrointestinal tract, and pleura.
  d. No cure for the disease is known but remissions are frequently experienced by clients who manage their care well.
 2. Causes
  a. The cause of SLE is unknown, but is believed to be a defect in immunological mechanisms, with a genetic origin.
  b. Precipitating factors include medications, stress, genetic factors, sunlight or ultraviolet light, and pregnancy.
  c. Discoid lupus erythematosus is possible with some medications but totally disappears after the medication is stopped; the only manifestation is the skin rash that occurs in lupus.
 3. Assessment
  a. Assess for precipitating factors.
  b. Erythema butterfly or rash of the face (malar)
  c. Dry, scaly, raised rash on the face or upper body
  d. Fever
  e. Weakness, malaise, and fatigue
  f. Anorexia
  g. Weight loss
  h. Photosensitivity
  i. Joint pain
  j. Erythema of the palms
  k. Anemia
  l. Positive antinuclear antibody (ANA) test and lupus erythematosus (LE) preparation
  m. Elevated erythrocyte sedimentation rate (ESR) and C-reactive protein level
 4. Interventions
  a. Monitor skin integrity and provide frequent oral care.
  b. Instruct the client to clean the skin with a mild soap, avoiding harsh and perfume substances.
  c. Assist with the use of ointments and creams for the rash as prescribed.
  d. Identify factors contributing to fatigue.
  e. Administer iron, folic acid, or vitamin supplements as prescribed if anemia occurs.
  f. Provide a high-vitamin and high-iron diet.
  g. Provide a high-protein diet if there is no evidence of kidney disease.
  h. Instruct in measures to conserve energy, such as pacing activities and balancing rest with exercise.
  i. Administer topical or systemic corticosteroids, salicylates, and nonsteroidal anti-inflammatory drugs as prescribed for pain and inflammation.
  j. Administer medications to decrease the inflammatory response as prescribed.
  k. Instruct the client to avoid exposure to sunlight and ultraviolet light.
  l. Monitor for proteinuria and red cell casts in the urine.
  m. Monitor for bruising, bleeding, and injury.
  n. Assist with plasmapheresis as prescribed to remove autoantibodies and immune complexes from the blood before organ damage occurs.
  o. Monitor for signs of organ involvement such as pleuritis, nephritis, pericarditis, coronary artery disease, hypertension, neuritis, anemia, and peritonitis.
  p. Note that lupus nephritis occurs early in the disease process.
  q. Provide supportive therapy as major organs become affected.
  r. Provide emotional support and encourage the client to verbalize feelings.
  s. Provide information regarding support groups and encourage the use of community resources.

⚠ For the client with SLE, monitor the blood urea nitrogen and creatinine levels frequently for signs of renal impairment.

 C. Scleroderma (systemic sclerosis)
  1. Description
   a. Scleroderma is a chronic connective tissue disease similar to SLE that is characterized by inflammation, fibrosis, and sclerosis.
   b. This disorder affects the connective tissue throughout the body.
   c. It causes fibrotic changes involving the skin, synovial membranes, esophagus, heart, lungs, kidneys, and gastrointestinal tract.

  d. Treatment is directed toward forcing the disease into remission and slowing its progress.
2. Assessment
   a. Pain
   b. Stiffness and muscle weakness
   c. Pitting edema of the hands and fingers that progresses to the rest of the body
   d. Taut and shiny skin that is free from wrinkles
   e. Skin tissue is tight, hard, and thick, loses its elasticity, and adheres to underlying structures.
   f. Dysphagia
   g. Decreased range of motion
   h. Joint contractures
   i. Inability to perform activities of daily living
3. Interventions
   a. Encourage activity as tolerated.
   b. Maintain a constant room temperature.
   c. Provide small frequent meals, eliminating foods that stimulate gastric secretions, such as spicy foods, caffeine, and alcohol.
   d. Advise the client to sit up for 1 to 2 hours after meals if there is esophageal involvement.
   e. Provide supportive therapy as the major organs become affected.
   f. Administer corticosteroids as prescribed for inflammation.
   g. Provide emotional support and encourage the use of resources as necessary.
D. Polyarteritis nodosa
1. Description
   a. Polyarteritis nodosa is a collagen disease; it is a form of systemic vasculitis that causes inflammation of the arteries in visceral organs, brain, and skin.
   b. Treatment is similar to the treatment for SLE.
   c. Polyarteritis nodosa affects middle-aged men.
   d. The cause is unknown and the prognosis is poor.
   e. Renal disorders and cardiac involvement are the most frequent causes of death.
2. Assessment
   a. Malaise and weakness
   b. Low-grade fever
   c. Severe abdominal pain
   d. Bloody diarrhea
   e. Weight loss
   f. Elevated ESR
3. Interventions
   a. Provide supportive care as required.
   b. Provide a well-balanced diet.
   c. Administer corticosteroids and analgesics to control pain and inflammation.
   d. Provide emotional support and encourage the client to verbalize feelings.
   e. Initiate support services for the client.
E. Pemphigus

1. Description
   a. Pemphigus is a rare autoimmune disease that occurs predominantly between middle and old age.
   b. The cause is unknown, and the disorder is potentially fatal.
   c. Treatment is aimed at suppressing the immune response that causes blister formation.
2. Assessment
   a. Lesions appear as fragile, flaccid bullae.
   b. Partial-thickness lesions bleed, weep, and form crusts when bullae are disrupted.
   c. Debilitation, malaise, and pain
   d. Chewing and swallowing difficulties
   e. Nikolsky's sign: Separation of the epidermis caused by rubbing the skin
   f. Leukocytosis, eosinophilia, foul-smelling discharge from skin
3. Interventions
   a. Provide supportive care.
   b. Provide oral hygiene and increase fluid intake.
   c. Soothe oral lesions.
   d. Assist with oatmeal or potassium permanganate baths, or other soothing baths, as prescribed for relief of symptoms.
   e. Administer topical or systemic antibiotics as prescribed for secondary infections.
   f. Administer corticosteroids and cytotoxic agents as prescribed to bring about remission.

XI. GOODPASTURE'S SYNDROME

A. Description
1. Goodpasture's syndrome is an autoimmune disorder; autoantibodies are made against the glomerular basement membrane and alveolar basement membrane.
2. Goodpasture's syndrome is most common in males and young adults who smoke; the exact cause is unknown.
3. The lungs and the kidneys are affected primarily, and the disorder usually is not diagnosed until significant pulmonary or renal involvement occurs.
B. Assessment
1. Clinical manifestations indicating pulmonary and renal involvement
2. Shortness of breath
3. Hemoptysis
4. Decreased urine output
5. Edema and weight gain
6. Hypertension and tachycardia
C. Interventions
1. Focus on suppressing the autoimmune response with medications such as corticosteroids and plasmapheresis (filtration of the plasma to remove some proteins) to remove the autoantibodies.

2. Provide supportive therapy for pulmonary and renal involvement.

XII. LYME DISEASE

A. Description
 1. **Lyme disease** is an infection caused by the spirochete *Borrelia burgdorferi*, acquired from a tick bite (ticks live in wooded areas and survive by attaching to a host).
 2. Infection with the spirochete stimulates inflammatory cytokines and autoimmune mechanisms.

B. Assessment (Box 70-3; Fig. 70-4)

⚠ The typical ring-shaped rash of Lyme disease does not occur in all clients. Many clients never develop a rash. Additionally, if a rash does occur, it can occur anywhere on the body, not only at the site of the bite.

C. Interventions
 1. Gently remove the tick with tweezers, wash the skin with antiseptic, and dispose of the tick by flushing it down the toilet; the tick may also be placed in a sealed jar so that the health care provider can inspect it and determine its type.
 2. Perform a blood test 4 to 6 weeks after a bite to detect the presence of the disease (testing before this time is not reliable).
 3. Instruct the client in the administration of antibiotics as prescribed; these are initiated immediately (even before the blood testing results are known).
 4. Instruct the client to avoid areas that contain ticks, such as wooded grassy areas, especially in the summer months.
 5. Instruct the client to wear long-sleeved tops, long pants, closed shoes, and hats while outside.

Box 70-3 Assessment and Stages of Lyme Disease

First Stage
Symptoms can occur several days to months following the bite.
A small red pimple develops that may spread into a ring-shaped rash; it may occur anywhere on the body.
Rash may be large or small, or may not occur at all.
Flu-like symptoms occur, such as headaches, stiff neck, muscle aches, and fatigue.

Second Stage
This stage occurs several weeks following the bite.
Joint pain occurs.
Neurological complications occur.
Cardiac complications occur.

Third Stage
Large joints become involved.
Arthritis progresses.

6. Instruct the client to spray the body with tick repellent before going outside.
7. Instruct the client to examine the body when returning inside for the presence of ticks.

XIII. IMMUNODEFICIENCY SYNDROMES

A. Acquired **immunodeficiency** syndrome (AIDS)
 1. AIDS is a viral disease caused by human **immunodeficiency** virus (HIV), which destroys T cells, thereby increasing susceptibility to infection and malignancy (Fig. 70-5).
 2. The syndrome is manifested clinically by opportunistic infection and unusual neoplasms.
 3. AIDS is considered a chronic illness.
 4. The disease has a long incubation period, sometimes 10 years or longer.
 5. Manifestations may not appear until late in the infection.
B. Diagnosis and monitoring the client with AIDS
 1. See Chapter 11 for diagnostic tests.
 2. Refer to Box 70-4 for tests used to evaluate the progression of HIV infection.
C. High-risk groups
 1. Heterosexual or homosexual contact with high-risk individuals
 2. Intravenous drug abusers
 3. Persons receiving blood products
 4. Health care workers
 5. Babies born to infected mothers
D. Assessment
 1. Malaise, fever, anorexia, weight loss, influenza-like symptoms
 2. Lymphadenopathy for at least 3 months
 3. Leukopenia
 4. Diarrhea
 5. Fatigue
 6. Night sweats
 7. Presence of opportunistic infections
 8. Protozoal infections (*Pneumocystis jiroveci* pneumonia, major source of mortality)

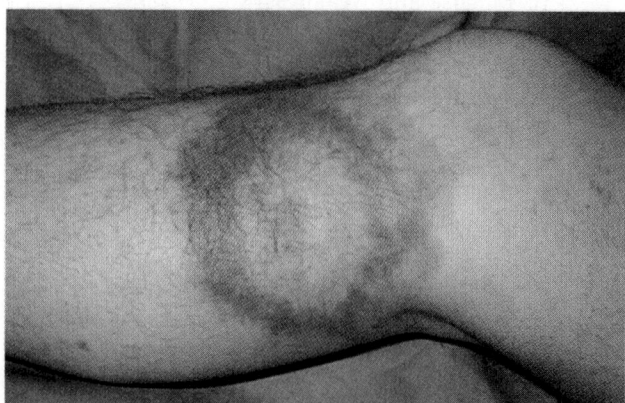

▲ **FIGURE 70-4** Erythema migrans of Lyme disease. (From Swartz, M. [2010]. *Textbook of physical diagnosis: History and examination* [6th ed.]. St. Louis: Saunders.)

9. Neoplasms (**Kaposi's sarcoma**, purplish-red lesions of internal organs and skin, B-cell non-Hodgkin's lymphoma, cervical cancer)
10. Fungal infections (candidiasis, histoplasmosis)
11. Viral infections (cytomegalovirus, herpes simplex)
12. Bacterial infections

E. Interventions
1. Provide respiratory support.
2. Administer oxygen and respiratory treatments as prescribed.
3. Provide psychosocial support as needed.
4. Maintain fluid and electrolyte balance.
5. Monitor for signs of infection.
6. Prevent the spread of infection.
7. Initiate standard and other necessary precautions.
8. Provide comfort as necessary.
9. Provide meticulous skin care.
10. Provide adequate nutritional support as prescribed.
11. See Chapters 25 and 47 for additional information on AIDS.

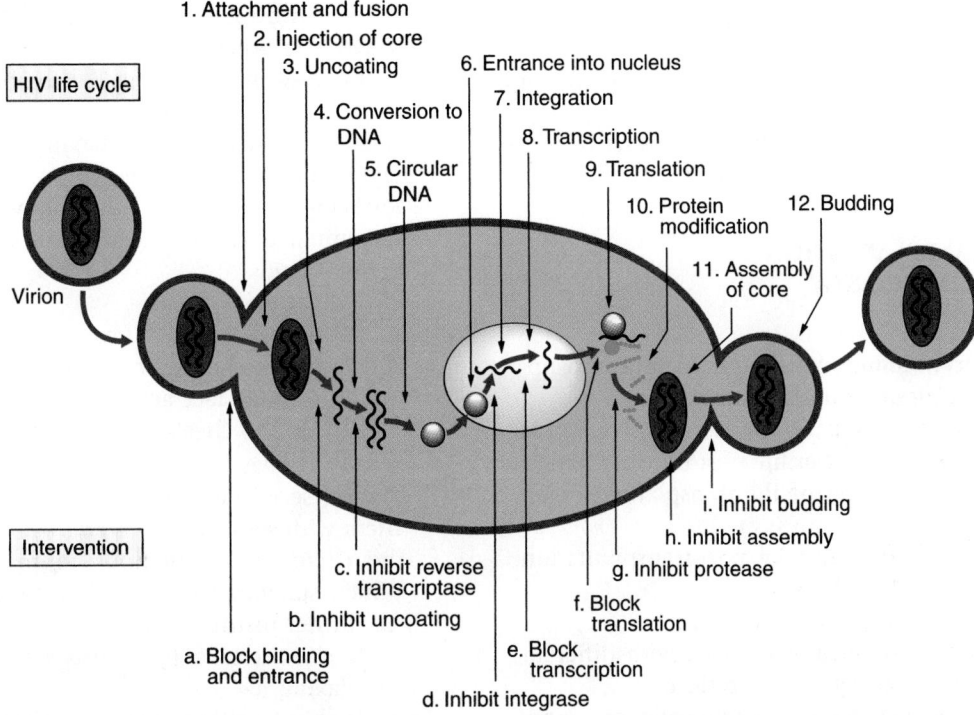

▲ **FIGURE 70-5** The life cycle of HIV. (From Ignatavicius, D., & Workman, M. [2010]. *Medical-surgical nursing: Patient-centered collaborative care* [6th ed.]. St. Louis: Saunders.)

Box 70-4 Tests Used to Evaluate Progression of Human Immunodeficiency Virus (HIV) Infection

Complete Blood Cell Count
White blood cell (WBC) count normal to decreased
Lymphopenia (<30% of the normal number of WBCs)
Thrombocytopenia (decreased platelet count)

Lymphocyte Screen
Reduced CD4+/CD8+ T-cell ratio
CD4+ (helper) lymphocytes decreased
CD8+ lymphocytes increased

Quantitative Immunoglobulin
Immunoglobulin G (IgG) level increased
IgA level frequently increased

Chemistry Panel
Lactate dehydrogenase level increased (all fractions)
Serum albumin level decreased

Total protein increased
Cholesterol level decreased
AST and ALT levels elevated

Anergy Panel
Nonreactive (anergic) or poorly reactive to infectious agents or environmental materials (e.g., pokeweed, phytohemagglutinin mitogens and antigens, mumps, *Candida*)

Hepatitis B Surface Antigen Testing
To detect the presence of hepatitis B

Blood Cultures
To detect septicemia

Chest Radiography
To detect *Pneumocystis jiroveci* infection or tuberculosis

AST, Aspartate aminotransferase; *ALT,* alanine aminotransferase.
From Copstead-Kirkhorn, L., & Banasik, J. (2009). *Pathophysiology* (4th ed.). St. Louis: Mosby.

F. Kaposi's sarcoma

1. Description: Skin lesions that occur primarily in individuals with a compromised immune system

2. Assessment

    a. Kaposi's sarcoma is a slow-growing tumor that appears as raised, oblong, purplish, reddish-brown lesions; may be tender or nontender.

    b. Organ involvement includes the lymph nodes, airways or lungs, or any part of the gastrointestinal tract from the mouth to anus.

3. Interventions

    a. Maintain standard precautions.

    b. Provide protective isolation if the immune system is depressed.

    c. Prepare the client for radiation therapy or chemotherapy as prescribed.

    d. Administer immunotherapy, as prescribed, to stabilize the immune system.

XIV. POST-TRANSPLANTATION IMMUNODEFICIENCY

A. Description

1. Secondary **immunodeficiency** is immunosuppression caused by therapeutic agents.

2. The client must take immunosuppressive agents for the rest of his or her life post-transplantation to decrease rejection of the transplanted organ or tissue.

B. Diagnosis and monitoring of post-transplantation clients

1. Check renal and hepatic function.

2. Monitor the complete cell count with differential to determine signs of infection.

3. Assess all body secretions periodically for blood.

C. High-risk clients

1. Clients with a history of malignancy or premalignancy have an increased susceptibility to malignancy if immunosuppressed.

2. Clients with recent infection or exposure to tuberculosis, herpes zoster, or chickenpox have a high risk for severe generalized disease when on immunosuppressive agents.

D. Assessment

1. Assess for signs of opportunistic infections.

2. Assess nutritional status.

3. Assess for signs of rejection (signs will depend on the organ or tissue transplant).

E. Interventions

1. Strict aseptic technique is necessary.

2. Provide teaching regarding asepsis and the signs of infection and rejection.

3. Provide psychosocial support as needed.

4. Provide client teaching about immunosuppressants.

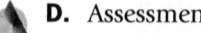 **MORE QUESTIONS ON THE CD!**

Practice Questions

855. The nurse prepares to give a bath and change the bed linens of a client with cutaneous Kaposi's sarcoma lesions. The lesions are open and draining a scant amount of serous fluid. Which of the following would the nurse incorporate into the plan during the bathing of this client?

1. Wearing gloves
2. Wearing a gown and gloves
3. Wearing a gown, gloves, and a mask
4. Wear a gown and gloves to change the bed linens and gloves only for the bath

856. A client is suspected of having systemic lupus erythematous. The nurse monitors the client, knowing that which of the following is one of the initial characteristic signs of systemic lupus erythematous?

1. Weight gain
2. Subnormal temperature
3. Elevated red blood cell count
4. Rash on the face across the bridge of the nose and on the cheeks

857. The nurse provides home care instructions to a client with systemic lupus erythematous and tells the client about methods to manage fatigue. Which statement by the client indicates a need for further instructions?

1. "I should take hot baths because they are relaxing."
2. "I should sit whenever possible to conserve my energy."
3. "I should avoid long periods of rest because it causes joint stiffness."
4. "I should do some exercises, such as walking, when I am not fatigued."

858. A client with pemphigus is being seen in the clinic regularly. The nurse plans care based on which of the following descriptions of this condition?

1. The presence of tiny red vesicles
2. An autoimmune disease that causes blistering in the epidermis
3. The presence of skin vesicles found along the nerve caused by a virus
4. The presence of red, raised papules and large plaques covered by silvery scales

859. The nurse is assisting in planning care for a client with a diagnosis of immunodeficiency. The nurse

would incorporate which of the following as a priority in the plan of care?
1. Protecting the client from infection
2. Providing emotional support to decrease fear
3. Encouraging discussion about lifestyle changes
4. Identifying factors that decreased the immune function

860. A client calls the nurse in the emergency department and tells the nurse that he was just stung by a bumble bee while gardening. The client is afraid of a severe reaction because the client's neighbor experienced such a reaction just 1 week ago. The appropriate nursing action is to:
1. Advise the client to soak the site in hydrogen peroxide.
2. Ask the client if he ever sustained a bee sting in the past.
3. Tell the client to call an ambulance for transport to the emergency department.
4. Tell the client not to worry about the sting unless difficulty with breathing occurs.

861. The community health nurse is conducting a research study and is identifying clients in the community at risk for latex allergy. Which client population is at most risk for developing this type of allergy?
1. Hairdressers
2. The homeless
3. Children in day care centers
4. Individuals living in a group home

862. The home care nurse is performing an assessment on a client who has been diagnosed with an allergy to latex. In determining the client's risk factors associated with the allergy, the nurse questions the client about an allergy to which food item?
1. Eggs
2. Milk
3. Yogurt
4. Bananas

863. The camp nurse prepares to instruct a group of children about Lyme disease. Which of the following information would the nurse include in the instructions?
1. Lyme disease is caused by a tick carried by deer.
2. Lyme disease is caused by contamination from cat feces.
3. Lyme disease can be contagious through skin contact with an infected individual.
4. Lyme disease can be caused by the inhalation of spores from bird droppings.

864. The client is diagnosed with stage I Lyme disease. The nurse assesses the client for which characteristic of this stage?
1. Arthralgias
2. Flu-like symptoms
3. Enlarged and inflamed joints
4. Signs of neurological disorders

865. A female client arrives at the health care clinic and tells the nurse that she was just bitten by a tick and would like to be tested for Lyme disease. The client tells the nurse that she removed the tick and flushed it down the toilet. Which of the following nursing actions is most appropriate?
1. Refer the client for a blood test immediately.
2. Inform the client that there is no test available for Lyme disease.
3. Tell the client that testing is not necessary unless arthralgia develops.
4. Instruct the client to return in 4 to 6 weeks to be tested because testing before this time is not reliable.

866. A Cub Scout leader, who is a nurse preparing a group of Cub Scouts for an overnight camping trip, instructs the scouts about the methods to prevent Lyme disease. Which statement by one of the Cub Scouts indicates a need for further instructions?
1. "I need to bring a hat to wear during the trip."
2. "I should wear long-sleeved tops and long pants."
3. "I should not use insect repellents because it will attract the ticks."
4. "I need to wear closed shoes and socks that can be pulled up over my pants."

867. The client with acquired immunodeficiency syndrome is diagnosed with cutaneous Kaposi's sarcoma. Based on this diagnosis, the nurse understands that this has been confirmed by which of the following?
1. Swelling in the genital area
2. Swelling in the lower extremities
3. Punch biopsy of the cutaneous lesions
4. Appearance of reddish-blue lesions noted on the skin

868. Which of the following individuals is least likely at risk for the development of Kaposi's sarcoma?
1. A kidney transplant client
2. A male with a history of same-gender partners
3. A client receiving antineoplastic medications
4. An individual working in an environment in which he or she is exposed to asbestos

Alternate Item Format: Multiple Response

869. Select the interventions that would apply in the care of a client at high risk for an allergic response to a latex allergy. **Select all that apply.**
   ❑ 1. Use nonlatex gloves.
   ❑ 2. Use medications from glass ampules.
   ❑ 3. Place the client in a private room only.
   ❑ 4. Avoid the use of medication vials that have rubber stoppers.
   ❑ 5. Keep a latex-safe supply cart available in the client's area.
   ❑ 6. Use a blood pressure cuff from an electronic device only to measure the blood pressure.

ANSWERS

855. 2

Rationale: Gowns and gloves are required if the nurse anticipates contact with soiled items such as those with wound drainage or is caring for a client who is incontinent with diarrhea or a client who has an ileostomy or colostomy. Masks are not required unless droplet or airborne precautions are necessary. Regardless of the amount of wound drainage, a gown and gloves must be worn.

Test-Taking Strategy: Use the process of elimination and think about the method of transmission of infection when answering a question of this type. Read the question, noting the task that is presented; in this case, it is bathing and changing linens. Eliminate option 3 because the method of transmission is not respiratory. Eliminate options 1 and 4 because neither provide adequate protection based on the method of transmission. If you had difficulty with this question, review standard and transmission-based precautions.

Level of Cognitive Ability: Applying
Client Needs: Safe and Effective Care Environment
Integrated Process: Nursing Process—Planning
Content Area: Adult Health—Immune
Reference: Potter, P., & Perry, A. (2009). *Fundamentals of nursing* (7th ed., p. 655). St. Louis: Mosby.

856. 4

Rationale: Skin lesions or rash on the face across the bridge of the nose and on the cheeks is an initial characteristic sign of systemic lupus erythematosus (SLE). Fever and weight loss may also occur. Anemia is most likely to occur later in SLE.

Test-Taking Strategy: Use the process of elimination and note the strategic words *characteristic signs.* Recalling the characteristic butterfly rash associated with SLE will direct you to option 4. If you are unfamiliar with this disorder, review this content.

Level of Cognitive Ability: Analyzing
Client Needs: Physiological Integrity
Integrated Process: Nursing Process—Assessment
Content Area: Adult Health—Immune
Reference: Ignatavicius, D., & Workman, M. (2010). *Medical-surgical nursing: Patient-centered collaborative care* (6th ed., pp. 348–349). St. Louis: Saunders.

857. 1

Rationale: To help reduce fatigue in the client with systemic lupus erythematosus, the nurse should instruct the client to sit whenever possible, avoid hot baths (because they exacerbate fatigue), schedule moderate low-impact exercises when not fatigued, and maintain a balanced diet. The client is instructed to avoid long periods of rest because it promotes joint stiffness.

Test-Taking Strategy: Note the strategic words *need for further instructions.* These words indicate a negative event query and the need to select the incorrect client statement. Also, focus on the subject, fatigue. By the process of elimination, you should be directed easily to option 1 as the action that would exacerbate fatigue. If you had difficulty with this question, review measures to prevent fatigue in a client with systemic lupus erythematosus.

Level of Cognitive Ability: Evaluating
Client Needs: Physiological Integrity
Integrated Process: Teaching and Learning
Content Area: Adult Health—Immune
Reference: Black, J., & Hawks, J. (2009). *Medical-surgical nursing: Clinical management for positive outcomes* (8th ed., p. 2071). St. Louis: Saunders.

858. 2

Rationale: Pemphigus is an autoimmune disease that causes blistering in the epidermis. The client has large flaccid blisters (bullae). Because the blisters are in the epidermis, they have a thin covering of skin and break easily, leaving large denuded areas of skin. On initial examination, clients may have crusting areas instead of intact blisters. Option 1 describes eczema, option 3 describes herpes zoster, and option 4 describes psoriasis.

Test-Taking Strategy: Use the process of elimination. Recalling that pemphigus vulgaris is an autoimmune disorder will direct you easily to option 2. If you had difficulty with this question, review the characteristics of this disorder.

Level of Cognitive Ability: Understanding
Client Needs: Physiological Integrity
Integrated Process: Nursing Process—Planning
Content Area: Adult Health—Immune
Reference: Copstead, L., & Banasik, J. (2010). *Pathophysiology* (4th ed., p. 1235). St. Louis: Mosby.

859. 1

Rationale: The client with immunodeficiency has inadequate or absence of immune bodies and is at risk for infection. The priority nursing intervention would be to protect the client from infection. Options 2, 3, and 4 may be components of care but are not the priority.

Test-Taking Strategy: Use Maslow's Hierarchy of Needs theory to answer the question. Remember that physiological needs are the priority. This will direct you to option 1. Review the care of a client with immunodeficiency if you had difficulty with this question.

Level of Cognitive Ability: Applying
Client Needs: Physiological Integrity
Integrated Process: Nursing Process—Planning
Content Area: Adult Health—Immune
Reference: Swearingen, P. (2008). *All-in-one care planning resource: Medical-surgical, pediatric, maternity, and psychiatric nursing care plans* (2nd ed., pp. 15–16). St. Louis: Mosby.

860. 2

Rationale: In some types of allergies, a reaction occurs only on second and subsequent contacts with the allergen. The appropriate action, therefore, would be to ask the client if he ever experienced a bee sting in the past. Option 1 is not appropriate advice. Option 3 is unnecessary. The client should not be told "not to worry."
Test-Taking Strategy: Use the steps of the nursing process to answer the question. Option 2 is the only option that addresses assessment. Review information related to allergic reactions if you had difficulty with this question.
Level of Cognitive Ability: Applying
Client Needs: Physiological Integrity
Integrated Process: Nursing Process—Implementation
Content Area: Adult Health—Immune
Reference: Ignatavicius, D., & Workman, M. (2010). *Medical-surgical nursing: Patient-centered collaborative care* (6th ed., pp. 149–150). St. Louis: Saunders.

861. 1

Rationale: Individuals at risk for developing a latex allergy include health care workers, individuals who work in the rubber industry or those who have had multiple surgeries, have spina bifida, wear gloves frequently, such as food handlers, hairdressers, and auto mechanics, or are allergic to kiwis, bananas, pineapples, tropical fruits, grapes, avocados, potatoes, hazelnuts, or water chestnuts.
Test-Taking Strategy: Focus on the subject, a latex allergy. Recalling the cause and the source of the allergic reaction will direct you easily to option 1. Review the cause of this type of allergy and the individuals at risk if you had difficulty with this question.
Level of Cognitive Ability: Analyzing
Client Needs: Health Promotion and Maintenance
Integrated Process: Nursing Process—Assessment
Content Area: Adult Health—Immune
References: Ignatavicius, D., & Workman, M. (2010). *Medical-surgical nursing: Patient-centered collaborative care* (6th ed., p. 445). St. Louis: Saunders.
   Perry, A., & Potter, P. (2010). *Clinical nursing skills & techniques* (7th ed., p. 197). St. Louis: Mosby.

862. 4

Rationale: Individuals who are allergic to kiwis, bananas, pineapples, tropical fruits, grapes, avocados, potatoes, hazelnuts, or water chestnuts are at risk for developing a latex allergy. This is thought to be the result of a possible cross-reaction between the food and the latex allergen. Options 1, 2, and 3 are unrelated to latex allergy.
Test-Taking Strategy: Use the process of elimination and knowledge regarding the food items related to a latex allergy. Eliminate options 1, 2, and 3 because they are comparable or alike and relate to dairy products. Review the food items associated with a risk for latex allergy if you had difficulty with this question.

Level of Cognitive Ability: Analyzing
Client Needs: Physiological Integrity
Integrated Process: Nursing Process—Assessment
Content Area: Adult Health—Immune
Reference: Ignatavicius, D., & Workman, M. (2010). *Medical-surgical nursing: Patient-centered collaborative care* (6th ed., pp. 394, 445). St. Louis: Saunders.

863. 1

Rationale: Lyme disease is a multisystem infection that results from a bite by a tick carried by several species of deer. Persons bitten by the *Ixodes scapularis* or *I. pacificus* tick can become infected with the spirochete *Borrelia burgdorferi*. Lyme disease cannot be transmitted from one person to another. Histoplasmosis is caused by the inhalation of spores from bat or bird droppings. Toxoplasmosis is caused by the ingestion of cysts from contaminated cat feces.
Test-Taking Strategy: Use the process of elimination. Recalling that this disease is caused by a tick bite will assist in eliminating the incorrect options. If you had difficulty with this question, review the cause of Lyme disease.
Level of Cognitive Ability: Applying
Client Needs: Safe and Effective Care Environment
Integrated Process: Teaching and Learning
Content Area: Adult Health—Immune
Reference: Ignatavicius, D., & Workman, M. (2010). *Medical-surgical nursing: Patient-centered collaborative care* (6th ed., p. 356). St. Louis: Saunders.

864. 2

Rationale: A characteristic of stage I Lyme disease is the development of a rash within 2 to 30 days of infection, generally at the site of the tick bite, but it can be anywhere on the body. However, many individuals may not develop the rash. The rash develops into a concentric ring, giving it a bull's-eye appearance. The lesion enlarges up to 50 to 60 cm, and smaller lesions develop farther away from the original tick bite. In stage I, most infected persons develop flu-like symptoms that last 7 to 10 days; these symptoms may recur later. Neurological deficits occur in stage II. Arthralgias and joint enlargements are most likely to occur in stage III.
Test-Taking Strategy: Use the process of elimination and eliminate options 1 and 3 first because they are comparable or alike. Next, note that the question asks for the characteristic of stage I. From the remaining two options, select the least serious one because the subject of the question relates to stage I. Expect neurological disorders to occur with progression of the disease. If you had difficulty with this question, review the stages of Lyme disease.
Level of Cognitive Ability: Analyzing
Client Needs: Physiological Integrity
Integrated Process: Nursing Process—Assessment
Content Area: Adult Health—Immune
Reference: Ignatavicius, D., & Workman, M. (2010). *Medical-surgical nursing: Patient-centered collaborative care* (6th ed., p. 356). St. Louis: Saunders.

865. 4

Rationale: A blood test is available to detect Lyme disease; however, the test is not reliable if performed before 4 to 6 weeks following the tick bite. Antibody formation takes place in the following manner. Immunoglobulin M is detected 3 to

4 weeks after Lyme disease onset, peaks at 6 to 8 weeks, and then gradually disappears; immunoglobulin G is detected 2 to 3 months after infection and may remain elevated for years. Options 1, 2, and 3 are incorrect.
Test-Taking Strategy: Use the process of elimination. Eliminate option 1 first. The word *immediately* should indicate that this is potentially an incorrect option. A blood test is available; therefore, eliminate option 2. Eliminate option 3 because treatment should begin before the arthralgia develops. If you had difficulty with this question, review the method of diagnosing Lyme disease.
Level of Cognitive Ability: Applying
Client Needs: Physiological Integrity
Integrated Process: Nursing Process—Implementation
Content Area: Adult Health—Immune
Reference: Ignatavicius, D., & Workman, M. (2010). *Medical-surgical nursing: Patient-centered collaborative care* (6th ed., p. 356). St. Louis: Saunders.

866. 3
Rationale: In the prevention of Lyme disease, individuals need to be instructed to use an insect repellent on the skin and clothes when in an area where ticks are likely to be found. Long-sleeved tops and long pants, closed shoes, and a hat or cap should be worn. If possible, heavily wooded areas or areas with thick underbrush should be avoided. Socks can be pulled up and over the pant legs to the prevent ticks from entering under clothing.
Test-Taking Strategy: Use the process of elimination and note the strategic words *need for further instructions*. These words indicate a negative event query and ask you to select an option that is incorrect. Note that option 3 uses the words *should not*. Reading carefully will assist in directing you to this option. If you had difficulty with this question, review the measures to prevent contact with ticks.
Level of Cognitive Ability: Evaluating
Client Needs: Safe and Effective Care Environment
Integrated Process: Teaching and Learning
Content Area: Adult Health—Immune
Reference: Ignatavicius, D., & Workman, M. (2010). *Medical-surgical nursing: Patient-centered collaborative care* (6th ed., p. 356). St. Louis: Saunders.

867. 3
Rationale: Kaposi's sarcoma lesions begin as red, dark blue, or purple macules on the lower legs that change into plaques. These large plaques ulcerate or open and drain. The lesions spread by metastasis through the upper body and then to the face and oral mucosa. They can move to the lymphatic system, lungs, and gastrointestinal tract. Late disease results in swelling and pain in the lower extremities, penis, scrotum, or face. Diagnosis is made by punch biopsy of cutaneous lesions and biopsy of pulmonary and gastrointestinal lesions.
Test-Taking Strategy: Use the process of elimination. Eliminate options 1 and 2 first because these symptoms occur late in the development of Kaposi's sarcoma. From the remaining options, note the strategic word *confirmed*. This strategic word will assist in directing you to the option that will confirm the diagnosis, the biopsy of the lesions. Review diagnostic measures for Kaposi's sarcoma if you had difficulty with this question.
Level of Cognitive Ability: Understanding

Client Needs: Physiological Integrity
Integrated Process: Nursing Process—Assessment
Content Area: Adult Health—Immune
Reference: Ignatavicius, D., & Workman, M. (2010). *Medical-surgical nursing: Patient-centered collaborative care* (6th ed., p. 372). St. Louis: Saunders.

868. 4
Rationale: Kaposi's sarcoma is a vascular malignancy that presents as a skin disorder and is a common AIDS indicator. Malignancy is seen most frequently in men with a history of same-gender partners. Although the cause of Kaposi's sarcoma is not known, it is considered to be caused by an alteration or failure in the immune system. The renal transplant recipient and the client receiving antineoplastic medications are at risk for immunosuppression. Exposure to asbestos is not related to the development of Kaposi's sarcoma.
Test-Taking Strategy: Use the process of elimination. Note the strategic words *least likely at risk*. Option 2 can be eliminated easily. Note that options 1 and 3 are comparable or alike. These clients are at risk for immunosuppression. With this in mind, these options can be eliminated. If you had difficulty with this question, review the risk factors associated with Kaposi's sarcoma.
Level of Cognitive Ability: Analyzing
Client Needs: Health Promotion and Maintenance
Integrated Process: Nursing Process—Assessment
Content Area: Adult Health—Immune
Reference: Black, J., & Hawks, J. (2009). *Medical-surgical nursing: Clinical management for positive outcomes* (8th ed., pp. 2107–2108). St. Louis: Saunders.

ALTERNATE ITEM FORMAT: MULTIPLE RESPONSE
869. 1, 2, 4, 5
Rationale: If a client is allergic to latex and is at high risk for an allergic response, the nurse would use nonlatex gloves and latex-safe supplies, and would keep a latex-safe supply cart available in the client's area. Any supplies or materials that contain latex would be avoided. These include blood pressure cuffs and medication vials with rubber stoppers that require puncture with a needle. It is not necessary to place the client in a private room.
Test-Taking Strategy: Focus on the subject, that the client is at high risk for an allergic response to latex. Recalling that items that contain rubber are likely to contain latex will direct you to the correct interventions. Also, noting the close-ended word *only* in options 3 and 6 will assist in eliminating these options. Review care of the client with a latex allergy if you had difficulty with this question.
Level of Cognitive Ability: Applying
Client Needs: Safe and Effective Care Environment
Integrated Process: Nursing Process—Implementation
Content Area: Adult Health—Immune
References: Black, J., & Hawks, J. (2009). *Medical-surgical nursing: Clinical management for positive outcomes* (8th ed., pp. 2050–2051). St. Louis: Saunders.
Perry, A., & Potter, P. (2010). *Clinical nursing skills & techniques* (7th ed., p. 201). St. Louis: Mosby.

Immunological Medications

I. HUMAN IMMUNODEFICIENCY VIRUS (HIV) AND ACQUIRED IMMUNODEFICIENCY SYNDROME (AIDS)

A. Medications include nucleoside-nucleotide reverse transcriptase inhibitors, non-nucleoside reverse transcriptase inhibitors, protease inhibitors, and fusion inhibitors (Box 71-1; Fig. 71-1).

B. Nucleoside-nucleotide reverse transcriptase inhibitors and non-nucleoside reverse transcriptase inhibitors work by inhibiting the activity of reverse transcriptase.

C. Protease inhibitors work by interfering with the activity of the enzyme protease.

D. Fusion inhibitors work by inhibiting the binding of human **immunodeficiency** virus to cells.

E. Standard treatment consists of using three or four medications in regimens known as highly active antiretroviral therapy (HAART); this therapy is not curative but can delay or reverse loss of immune function, preserve health, and prolong life.

F. Other medications include those that are used to treat complications or opportunistic infections that develop (see Box 71-1).

G. Nucleoside-nucleotide reverse transcriptase inhibitors (NRTIs)

1. Abacavir (Ziagen): Can cause nausea; monitor for hypersensitivity reaction, including fever, nausea, vomiting, diarrhea, lethargy, malaise, sore throat, shortness of breath, cough, and rash.

2. Abacavir; lamivudine (Epzicom): In addition to the effects that can occur from abacavir and lamivudine, hypersensitivity reactions, lactic acidosis, and severe hepatomegaly can occur.

3. Didanosine (Videx): Can cause nausea, diarrhea, peripheral neuropathy, hepatotoxicity, and pancreatitis

4. Emtricitabine (Emtriva): Can cause headache, diarrhea, nausea, rash, hyperpigmentation of the palms and soles, lactic acidosis, and severe hepatomegaly

5. Emtricitabine; tenofovir (Truvada): In addition to the effects that can occur from emtricitabine and tenofovir, lactic acidosis and severe hepatomegaly can occur.

6. Lamivudine (Epivir): Causes nausea and nasal congestion

7. Lamivudine; zidovudine (Combivir): Can cause anemia and neutropenia and lactic acidosis with hepatomegaly

8. Lamivudine; zidovudine; abacavir (Trizivir): In addition to the effects that can occur from lamivudine, zidovudine, and abacavir, hypersensitivity reactions, anemia, neutropenia, lactic acidosis, and severe hepatomegaly can occur.

9. Stavudine (d4t, Zerit): Can cause peripheral neuropathy and pancreatitis

10. Tenofovir (Viread): Can cause nausea and vomiting

11. Zalcitabine (ddC, Hivid) Can cause oral ulcers, peripheral neuropathy, hepatotoxicity, and pancreatitis

12. Zidovudine (Retrovir, azidothymidine, AZT, ZDV): Can cause nausea, vomiting, anemia, leukopenia, myopathy, fatigue, and headache

H. Non-nucleoside reverse transcriptase inhibitors (NNRTIs)

1. Delavirdine (Rescriptor): Can cause rash, liver function changes, and pruritis

2. Efavirenz (Sustiva): Can cause rash, dizziness, confusion, difficulty concentrating, dreams, and encephalopathy

3. Etravirine (Intelence): Can cause rash, gastrointestinal disturbances, headache, hypertension, and peripheral neuropathy

4. Nevirapine (Viramune): Can cause rash, Stevens-Johnson syndrome, hepatitis, and increased transaminase levels

I. Protease inhibitors (PIs)

1. Amprenavir; vitamin E (Agenerase)

   a. Can cause nausea, vomiting, headache, altered taste sensations, perioral paresthesia, rashes, and increased results of liver function studies

   b. Oral solution contains an alcohol that can interact with metronidazole (Flagyl); can cause feelings of inebriation.

2. Atazanavir (Reyataz): Can cause nausea, headache, infection, vomiting, diarrhea, drowsiness,

1025

Box 71-1 Medications for HIV and AIDS

Nucleoside-Nucleotide Reverse Transcriptase Inhibitors (NRTIs)
Abacavir (Ziagen)
Abacavir; lamivudine (Epzicom)
Didanosine (Videx)
Emtricitabine (Emtriva)
Emtricitabine; tenofovir (Truvada)
Emtricitabine; tenofovir; efavirenz (Atripla)
Lamivudine (Epivir)
Lamivudine; zidovudine (Combivir)
Lamivudine; zidovudine; abacavir (Trizivir)
Stavudine (d4t, Zerit)
Tenofovir (Viread)
Zalcitabine (ddC, Hivid)
Zidovudine (Retrovir, azidothymidine, AZT, ZDV)

Non-Nucleoside Reverse Transcriptase Inhibitors (NNRTIs)
Delavirdine (Rescriptor)
Efavirenz (Sustiva)
Etravirine (Intelence)
Nevirapine (Viramune)

Protease Inhibitors (PIs)
Amprenavir; vitamin E (Agenerase)
Atazanavir (Reyataz)
Darunavir (Prezista)
Fosamprenavir (Lexiva)
Indinavir (Crixivan)
Lopinavir; ritonavir (Kaletra)
Nelfinavir (Viracept)

Ritonavir (Norvir)
Saquinavir (Invirase)
Tipranavir (Aptivus)

Integrase Inhibitor
Raltegravir (Isentress)

Fusion Inhibitor
Enfuvirtide (Fuzeon)

CCR5 Antagonist
Maraviroc (Selzentry)

Anti-Inflammatory Medication
Sulfasalazine (Azulfidine)

Anti-Infective Medications
Atovaquone (Mepron)
Metronidazole (Flagyl)
Pentamidine isethionate (Pentam 300)
Sulfamethoxazole; trimethoprim (Bactrim)

Antifungal Medications
Amphotericin B (Fungizone)
Fluconazole (Diflucan)
Ketoconazole (Nizoral)

Antiviral Medications
Acyclovir (Zovirax)
Foscarnet (Foscavir)
Ganciclovir (Cytovene)

insomnia, fever, hyperglycemia, hyperlipidemia, and increased bleeding in clients with hemophilia
3. Fosamprenavir (Lexiva): Similar to amprenavir; can cause nausea, vomiting, headache, altered taste sensations, perioral paresthesia, rashes, and altered liver function
4. Indinavir (Crixivan): Can cause nausea, diarrhea, hyperbilirubinemia, nephritis, and kidney stones
5. Lopinavir-ritonavir combination (Kaletra): Can cause nausea, diarrhea, altered taste sensations, circumoral paresthesia, and hepatitis
6. Nelfinavir (Viracept): Can cause nausea, flatulence, and diarrhea
7. Ritonavir (Norvir): Can cause nausea, vomiting, diarrhea, altered taste sensations, circumoral paresthesia, hepatitis, and increased triglyceride levels
8. Saquinavir (Invirase): Can cause nausea, diarrhea, photosensitivity, and headache
9. Tipranavir (Aptivus): Hepatotoxicity (liver damage); can also cause nausea, vomiting, diarrhea, headache, and fatigue
J. Integrase inhibitor: Raltegravir (Isentress)
   1. Stops HIV replication and is used in combination with other antiretroviral medications

2. Common side effects include nausea, diarrhea, fatigue, headache, and itching.
K. Chemokine receptor 5 (CCR5) antagonist: Maraviroc (Selzentry)
   1. Binds with CCR5 and blocks viral entry
   2. Most common side effects are cough, dizziness, pyrexia, rash, abdominal pain, musculoskeletal symptoms, and upper respiratory tract infections; liver injury, and cardiovascular events have occurred in some clients.
L. Fusion inhibitor: Enfuvirtide (Fuzeon) can cause skin irritation at injection site, fatigue, nausea, insomnia, and peripheral neuropathy.
M. Anti-infective and anti-inflammatory medications: Used to treat opportunistic infections such as *Pneumocystis jiroveci* pneumonia; *Toxoplasma* encephalitis is treated with sulfamethoxazole-trimethoprim (Bactrim; see Box 71-1)
N. Antifungal medications: Used to treat candidiasis, cryptococcal meningitis (see Box 71-1)
O. Antiviral medications: Used to treat cytomegalovirus retinitis, herpes simplex, varicella-zoster virus (see Box 71-1)

⚠️ The client with HIV or AIDS is at high risk for the development of opportunistic infections.

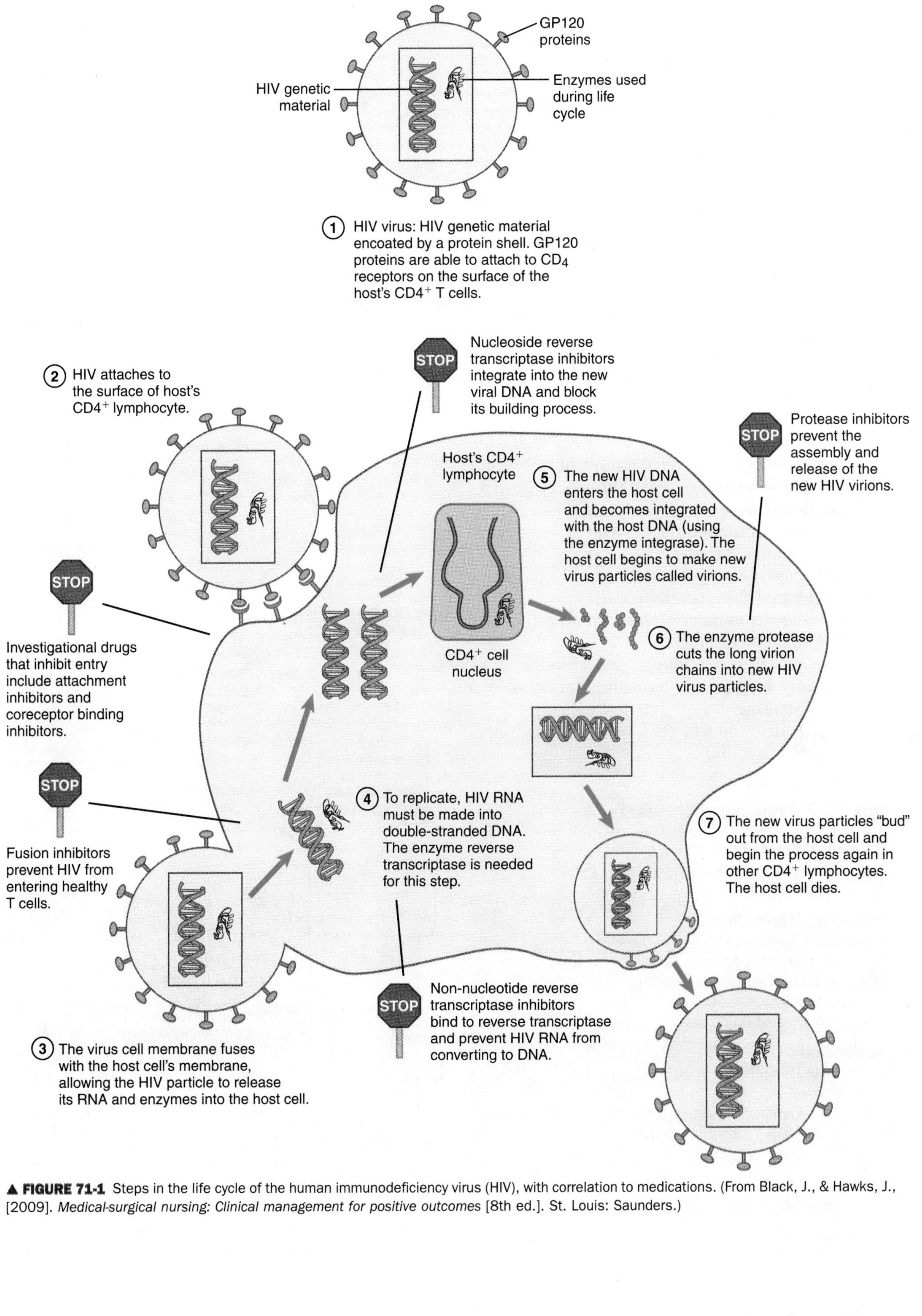

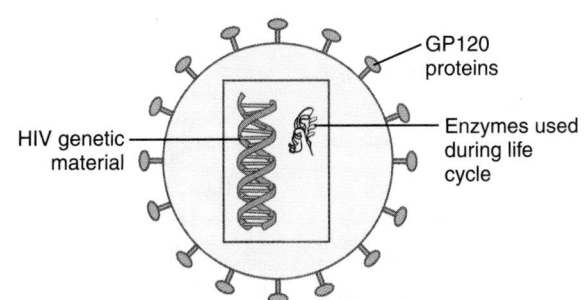

① HIV virus: HIV genetic material encoated by a protein shell. GP120 proteins are able to attach to CD$_4$ receptors on the surface of the host's CD4$^+$ T cells.

GP120 proteins

HIV genetic material

Enzymes used during life cycle

② HIV attaches to the surface of host's CD4$^+$ lymphocyte.

STOP Nucleoside reverse transcriptase inhibitors integrate into the new viral DNA and block its building process.

STOP Protease inhibitors prevent the assembly and release of the new HIV virions.

Host's CD4$^+$ lymphocyte

⑤ The new HIV DNA enters the host cell and becomes integrated with the host DNA (using the enzyme integrase). The host cell begins to make new virus particles called virions.

CD4$^+$ cell nucleus

⑥ The enzyme protease cuts the long virion chains into new HIV virus particles.

STOP Investigational drugs that inhibit entry include attachment inhibitors and coreceptor binding inhibitors.

STOP Fusion inhibitors prevent HIV from entering healthy T cells.

④ To replicate, HIV RNA must be made into double-stranded DNA. The enzyme reverse transcriptase is needed for this step.

⑦ The new virus particles "bud" out from the host cell and begin the process again in other CD4$^+$ lymphocytes. The host cell dies.

③ The virus cell membrane fuses with the host cell's membrane, allowing the HIV particle to release its RNA and enzymes into the host cell.

STOP Non-nucleotide reverse transcriptase inhibitors bind to reverse transcriptase and prevent HIV RNA from converting to DNA.

▲ **FIGURE 71-1** Steps in the life cycle of the human immunodeficiency virus (HIV), with correlation to medications. (From Black, J., & Hawks, J., [2009]. *Medical-surgical nursing: Clinical management for positive outcomes* [8th ed.]. St. Louis: Saunders.)

II. IMMUNOSUPPRESSANTS (Box 71-2; Fig. 71-2)

A. Description: Immunosuppressants are used for transplant recipients to prevent organ or tissue rejection and to treat autoimmune disorders such as systemic lupus erythematosus.

B. Cyclosporine (Sandimmune, Gengraf, Neoral)
1. Used for prevention of rejection following allogenic organ transplantation
2. Usually administered with a glucocorticoid and another immunosuppressant
3. The most common adverse effects are nephrotoxicity, infection, hypertension, and hirsutism.

C. Tacrolimus (Prograf)
1. Used for prevention of rejection following liver or kidney transplantation
2. Adverse effects include nephrotoxicity, neurotoxicity, gastrointestinal effects, hypertension, hyperkalemia, hyperglycemia, hirsutism, and gum hyperplasia.

D. Azathioprine (Imuran)
1. Generally used with renal transplant recipients
2. Can cause neutropenia and thrombocytopenia

E. Cyclophosphamide (Cytoxan, Neosar)
1. Used for its immunosuppressant action to treat autoimmune disorders
2. Can cause neutropenia and hemorrhagic cystitis

F. Methotrexate (Rheumatrex, Trexall)
1. Used for its immunosuppressant action to treat autoimmune disorders
2. Can cause hepatic fibrosis and cirrhosis, bone marrow suppression, ulcerative stomatitis, and renal damage

G. Mycophenolate mofetil (CellCept) and mycophenolic acid (Myfortic)

1. Used to prevent rejection following kidney, heart, and liver transplantation
2. Can cause diarrhea, vomiting, neutropenia, sepsis; increased risk of infection and malignancies, especially lymphomas

H. Basiliximab (Simulect); daclizumab (Zenapax)
1. Used to prevent rejection following kidney transplantation
2. Can cause severe acute hypersensitivity reactions, including anaphylaxis

I. Lymphocyte immune globulin, antithymocyte globulin (equine)
1. Used to prevent rejection following kidney, heart, liver, and bone marrow transplantation
2. Side effects include fever, chills, leukopenia, and skin reactions.
3. Can cause anaphylactoid reactions

Box 71-2 Immunosuppressants

Calcineurin Inhibitors
Cyclosporine (Sandimmune, Gengraf, Neoral)
Tacrolimus (Prograf)

Cytotoxic Medications
Azathioprine (Imuran)
Cyclophosphamide (Cytoxan, Neosar)
Methotrexate (Rheumatrex, Trexall)
Mycophenolate mofetil (CellCept)
Mycophenolic acid (Myfortic)

Antibodies
Basiliximab (Simulect)
Daclizumab (Zenapax)
Lymphocyte immune globulin, antithymocyte globulin (equine)
Muromonab-CD3 (Orthoclone OKT3)
Rho(D) immune globulin (RhoGAM)

Other
Sirolimus (Rapamune)

Glucocorticoids
See Chapter 55.

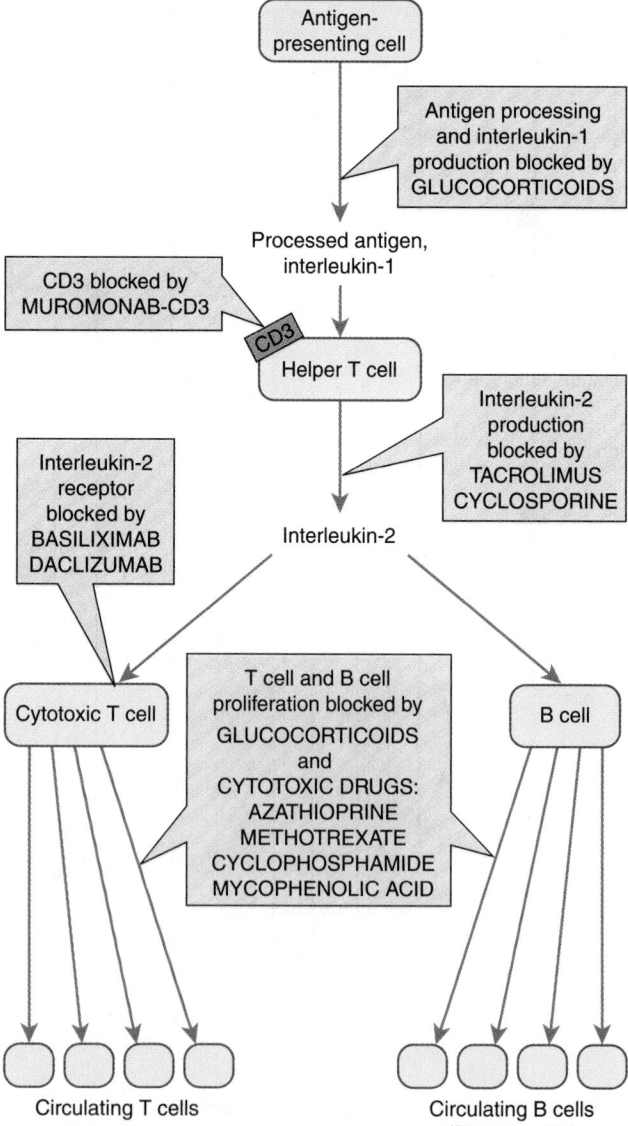

▲ **FIGURE 71-2** Sites of action of immunosuppressant drugs. (From Lehne, R. [2010]. *Pharmacology for nursing care* [7th ed.]. St. Louis: Saunders.)

J. Muromonab-CD3 (Orthoclone OKT3)
1. Used to prevent rejection following kidney, heart, and liver transplantation
2. Side effects include fever, chills, dyspnea, chest pain, nausea, and vomiting.
3. Can cause anaphylactoid reactions

K. Rh₀(D) immune globulin (RhoGAM; see Chapter 31)

L. Sirolimus (Rapamune)
1. Used to prevent renal transplant rejection
2. Increases the risk of infection; raises cholesterol and triglyceride levels; can cause renal injury

3. Other side effects include rash, acne, anemia, thrombocytopenia, joint pain, diarrhea, and hypokalemia.

⚠ Monitor the client taking an immunosuppressant closely for signs of infection.

III. IMMUNIZATIONS (see Chapter 48)

IV. ANTIBIOTICS (Box 71-3)

A. Inhibit the growth of bacteria

Box 71-3 Antibiotics

Aminoglycosides
Amikacin (Amikin)
Gentamicin (Garamycin)
Kanamycin (Kantrex)
Neomycin (Neo-Fradin)
Streptomycin
Tobramycin (Nebcin)

Cephalosporins
Cefaclor (Ceclor)
Cefadroxil (Duricef)
Cefazolin (Ancef, Kefzol)
Cefdinir (Omnicef)
Cefditoren (Spectracef)
Cefepime (Maxipime)
Cefotaxime (Claforan)
Cefotetan (Cefotan)
Cefoxitin (Mefoxin)
Cefpodoxime (Vantin)
Cefprozil (Cefzil)
Ceftazidime (Ceptaz, Fortaz, Tazicef)
Ceftibuten (Cedax)
Ceftizoxime (Cefizox)
Ceftriaxone (Rocephin)
Cefuroxime (Ceftin)
Cephalexin (Keflex)
Loracarbef (Lorabid)

Fluoroquinolones
Ciprofloxacin (Cipro)
Gatifloxacin (Tequin)
Gemifloxacin (Factive)
Levofloxacin (Levaquin)
Lomefloxacin (Maxaquin)
Moxifloxacin (Avelox)
Norfloxacin (Noroxin)
Ofloxacin (Floxin)
Trovafloxacin (Trovan)

Macrolides
Azithromycin (Zithromax)
Clarithromycin (Biaxin)
Dirithromycin (Dynabac)
Erythromycin

Lincosamides
Clindamycin (Cleocin)
Lincomycin (Lincocin)

Monobactam
Aztreonam (Azactam)

Penicillins
Amoxicillin (Amoxil)
Ampicillin (Principen)
Carbenicillin (Geocillin)
Penicillin G (Bicillin L-A, Permapen, Pfizerpen, Wycillin)
Penicillin V (Veetids)
Piperacillin
Ticarcillin (Ticar)

Penicillinase-Resistant Penicillins
Dicloxacillin
Nafcillin
Oxacillin

Sulfonamides
Sulfamethoxazole
Sulfadiazine
Sulfasalazine
Sulfisoxazole
Trimethoprim; sulfamethoxazole (TMP-SMZ; Bactrim, Cotrim, Septra)

Tetracyclines
Demeclocycline (Declomycin)
Doxycycline (Vibramycin)
Minocycline (Minocin)
Oxytetracycline (Terramycin)
Tetracycline (Sumycin)

Antimycobacterials
Antituberculosis agents (see Chapter 59)
Leprostatics: Clofazimine (Lamprene) and dapsone

Antifungal Medications
Amphotericin B (Fungizone)
Fluconazole (Diflucan)
Ketoconazole (Nizoral)

Antiviral Medications
Acyclovir (Zovirax)
Foscarnet (Foscavir)
Ganciclovir (Cytovene)

B. Include medication classifications of aminoglycosides, cephalosporins, fluoroquinolones, macrolides, lincosamides, monobactams, penicillins and penicillinase-resistant penicillins, sulfonamides, tetracyclines, antimycobacterials, and others (see Box 71-3)

C. Adverse effects (Table 71-1)

D. Nursing considerations

  1. Assess for allergies.
  2. Monitor appropriate laboratory values before therapy as appropriate and during therapy to assess for adverse effects.

  3. Monitor for adverse effects and report to physician if any occur.
  4. Determine appropriate method of administration and provide instructions to the client.
  5. Monitor intake and output.
  6. Encourage fluid intake (unless contraindicated).
  7. Initiate safety precautions because of possible central nervous system effects.
  8. Teach client about the medication and how to take the medication; emphasize the importance of completing the full prescribed course.

TABLE 71-1 Antibiotics and their Adverse Effects

Classification	Adverse Effects
Aminoglycosides	Ototoxicity Confusion, disorientation Renal toxicity Gastrointestinal irritation Palpitations, blood pressure changes Hypersensitivity reactions
Cephalosporins	Gastrointestinal disturbances Pseudomembranous colitis Headache, dizziness, lethargy, paresthesias Nephrotoxicity Superinfections
Fluoroquinolones	Headache, dizziness, insomnia, depression Gastrointestinal effects Bone marrow depression Fever, rash, photosensitivity
Macrolides	Gastrointestinal effects Pseudomembranous colitis Confusion, abnormal thinking Superinfections Hypersensitivity reactions
Lincosamides	Gastrointestinal effects Pseudomembranous colitis Bone marrow depression
Monobactams	Gastrointestinal effects Hepatotoxicity Allergic reactions
Penicillins and penicillinase-resistant penicillins	Gastrointestinal effects, including sore mouth and furry tongue Superinfections Hypersensitivity reactions, including anaphylaxis
Sulfonamides	Gastrointestinal effects Hepatotoxicity Nephrotoxicity Bone marrow depression Dermatological effects, including hypersensitivity and photosensitivity Headache, dizziness, vertigo, ataxia, depression, seizures
Tetracyclines	Gastrointestinal effects Hepatotoxicity Teeth (staining) and bone damage Superinfections Dermatological reactions, including rash and photosensitivity Hypersensitivity reactions
Antimycobacterials, leprostatics	Gastrointestinal effects Neuritis, dizziness, headache, malaise, drowsiness, hallucinations

MORE QUESTIONS ON THE CD!

Practice Questions

870. The client with acquired immunodeficiency syndrome and *Pneumocystis jiroveci* infection has been receiving pentamidine (Pentam 300). The client develops a temperature of 101° F. The nurse does further monitoring of the client, knowing that this sign would most likely indicate:
1. That the dose of the medication is too low
2. That the client is experiencing toxic effects of the medication
3. That the client has developed inadequacy of thermoregulation
4. That the client has developed another infection caused by leukopenic effects of the medication

871. Saquinavir (Invirase) is prescribed for the client who is seropositive for human immunodeficiency virus. The nurse provides medication instructions and tells the client to:
1. Avoid sun exposure.
2. Eat low-calorie foods.
3. Eat foods that are low in fat.
4. Take the medication on an empty stomach.

872. The client who is human immunodeficiency virus seropositive has been taking stavudine (d4t, Zerit). The nurse monitors which of the following most closely while the client is taking this medication?
1. Gait
2. Appetite
3. Level of consciousness
4. Gastrointestinal function

873. The client with acquired immunodeficiency syndrome has begun therapy with zidovudine (Retrovir, azidothymidine, AZT, ZDV). The nurse carefully monitors which of the following laboratory results during treatment with this medication?
1. Blood culture
2. Blood glucose level
3. Complete blood count
4. Blood urea nitrogen level

874. The nurse is reviewing the results of serum laboratory studies drawn on a client with acquired immunodeficiency syndrome who is receiving didanosine (Videx). The nurse interprets that the client may have the medication discontinued

by the physician if which of the following significantly elevated results is noted?
1. Serum protein level
2. Blood glucose level
3. Serum amylase level
4. Serum creatinine level

875. The nurse is caring for a post–renal transplantation client taking cyclosporine (Sandimmune, Gengraf, Neoral). The nurse notes an increase in one of the client's vital signs and the client is complaining of a headache. What is the vital sign that is most likely increased?
1. Pulse
2. Respirations
3. Blood pressure
4. Pulse oximetry

876. Amikacin (Amikin) is prescribed for a client with a bacterial infection. The nurse instructs the client to contact the physician immediately if which of the following occurs?
1. Nausea
2. Lethargy
3. Hearing loss
4. Muscle aches

877. The nurse is assigned to care for a client with cytomegalovirus retinitis and acquired immunodeficiency syndrome who is receiving foscarnet (Foscavir), an antiviral. The nurse checks the latest results of which of the following laboratory studies while the client is taking this medication?
1. CD4 cell count
2. Serum albumin level
3. Serum creatinine level
4. Lymphocyte count

Alternate Item Format: Multiple Response

878. Ketoconazole (Nizoral) is prescribed for a client with a diagnosis of candidiasis. Select the interventions that the nurse includes when administering this medication. **Select all that apply**.
- ❑ 1. Restrict fluid intake.
- ❑ 2. Instruct the client to avoid alcohol.
- ❑ 3. Monitor liver function studies.
- ❑ 4. Administer the medication with an antacid.
- ❑ 5. Instruct the client to avoid exposure to the sun.
- ❑ 6. Administer the medication on an empty stomach.

ANSWERS

870. 4
Rationale: Frequent side effects of this medication include leukopenia, thrombocytopenia, and anemia. The client

should be monitored routinely for signs and symptoms of infection. Options 1, 2, and 3 are inaccurate interpretations. *Test-Taking Strategy:* Use the process of elimination, focusing on the strategic words *develops a temperature*. Note the relationship between these strategic words and option 4. Review the side effects of this medication if you had difficulty with this question.

Level of Cognitive Ability: Analyzing
Client Needs: Physiological Integrity
Integrated Process: Nursing Process—Analysis
Content Area: Adult Health—Immune
References: Hodgson, B., & Kizior, R. (2010). *Saunders nursing drug handbook 2010* (p. 897). St. Louis: Saunders.
    Lehne, R. (2010). *Pharmacology for nursing care* (7th ed., p. 1161). St. Louis: Saunders.

871. 1
Rationale: Saquinavir is an antiretroviral (protease inhibitor) used with other antiretroviral medications to manage human immunodeficiency virus infection. Saquinavir is administered with meals and is best absorbed if the client consumes high-calorie, high-fat meals. Saquinavir can cause photosensitivity, and the nurse should instruct the client to avoid sun exposure.
Test-Taking Strategy: Use the process of elimination. Options 2 and 3 can be eliminated first, knowing that these dietary measures likely would not be prescribed for this client. From the remaining options, you must know that this medication can cause photosensitivity. Review this medication if you had difficulty with this question.
Level of Cognitive Ability: Applying
Client Needs: Physiological Integrity
Integrated Process: Teaching and Learning
Content Area: Adult Health—Immune
Reference: Hodgson, B., & Kizior, R. (2010). *Saunders nursing drug handbook 2010* (p. 1023). St. Louis: Saunders.

872. 1
Rationale: Stavudine (d4t, Zerit) is an antiretroviral used to manage human immunodeficiency virus infection in clients who do not respond to or who cannot tolerate conventional therapy. The medication can cause peripheral neuropathy, and the nurse should monitor the client's gait closely and ask the client about paresthesia. Options 2, 3, and 4 are unrelated to this medication.
Test-Taking Strategy: Focus on the name of the medication. Recalling that this medication causes peripheral neuropathy will direct you to option 1. If you are not familiar with this medication and the important assessment measures, review this content.
Level of Cognitive Ability: Analyzing
Client Needs: Physiological Integrity
Integrated Process: Nursing Process—Assessment
Content Area: Adult Health—Immune
References: Hodgson, B., & Kizior, R. (2010). *Saunders nursing drug handbook 2010* (p. 1060). St. Louis: Saunders.
    Lehne, R. (2010). *Pharmacology for nursing care* (7th ed., pp. 1094, 1127). St. Louis: Saunders.

873. 3
Rationale: Common side effects of zidovudine are leukopenia and anemia. The nurse monitors the complete blood count results for these changes. Options 1, 2, and 4 are unrelated to the use of this medication.
Test-Taking Strategy: Focus on the name of the medication. Recalling that zidovudine causes leukopenia will direct you

to option 3. Review this medication if you had difficulty with this question.
Level of Cognitive Ability: Analyzing
Client Needs: Physiological Integrity
Integrated Process: Nursing Process—Assessment
Content Area: Adult Health—Immune
Reference: Hodgson, B., & Kizior, R. (2010). *Saunders nursing drug handbook 2010* (p. 1205). St. Louis: Saunders.

874. 3
Rationale: Didanosine (Videx) can cause pancreatitis. A serum amylase level that is increased to 1.5 to 2 times normal may signify pancreatitis in the client with acquired immunodeficiency syndrome and is potentially fatal. The medication may have to be discontinued. The medication is also hepatotoxic and can result in liver failure.
Test-Taking Strategy: Focus on the name of the medication. Recalling that this medication can cause damage to the pancreas and is hepatotoxic will direct you to the correct option. Review this medication if you had difficulty with this question.
Level of Cognitive Ability: Analyzing
Client Needs: Physiological Integrity
Integrated Process: Nursing Process—Assessment
Content Area: Adult Health—Immune
References: Edmunds, M. (2010). *Introduction to clinical pharmacology* (6th ed., p. 195). St. Louis: Mosby.
    Hodgson, B., & Kizior, R. (2010). *Saunders nursing drug handbook 2010* (p. 343). St. Louis: Saunders.

875. 3
Rationale: Hypertension can occur in a client taking cyclosporine (Sandimmune, Gengraf, Neoral) and, because this client is also complaining of a headache, the blood pressure is the vital sign to be monitored most closely. Other adverse effects include infection, nephrotoxicity, and hirsutism. Options 1, 2, and 4 are unrelated to the use of this medication.
Test-Taking Strategy: Focus on the name of the medication and recall that this medication can cause hypertension. Review the adverse effects of this medication if you had difficulty with this question.
Level of Cognitive Ability: Analyzing
Client Needs: Physiological Integrity
Integrated Process: Nursing Process—Assessment
Content Area: Adult Health—Immune
Reference: Lehne, R. (2010). *Pharmacology for nursing care* (7th ed., p. 815). St. Louis: Saunders.

876. 3
Rationale: Amikacin (Amikin) is an aminoglycoside. Adverse effects of aminoglycosides include ototoxicity (hearing problems) confusion, disorientation, gastrointestinal irritation, palpitations, blood pressure changes, nephrotoxicity, and hypersensitivity. The nurse instructs the client to report hearing loss to the physician immediately. Lethargy and muscle aches are not associated with the use of this medication. It is not necessary to contact the physician immediately if nausea occurs. If nausea persists or results in vomiting, the physician should be notified.
Test-Taking Strategy: Note the strategic words *contact the physician immediately.* Recalling that this medication is an

aminoglycoside (most aminoglycoside medication names end in -*cin*) and that aminoglycosides are ototoxic will direct you to the correct option. Review the adverse effects of aminoglycosides if you had difficulty with this question.
Level of Cognitive Ability: Applying
Client Needs: Physiological Integrity
Integrated Process: Teaching and Learning
Content Area: Adult Health—Immune
Reference: Lehne, R. (2010). *Pharmacology for nursing care* (7th ed., p. 1024). St. Louis: Saunders.

877. 3

Rationale: Foscarnet (Foscavir) is toxic to the kidneys. The serum creatinine level is monitored before therapy, two or three times per week during induction therapy, and at least weekly during maintenance therapy. Foscarnet also may cause decreased levels of calcium, magnesium, phosphorus, and potassium. Thus, these levels also are measured with the same frequency.
Test-Taking Strategy: Use the process of elimination. Recalling that this medication is nephrotoxic will direct you easily to option 3. Review this medication if you are unfamiliar with it.
Level of Cognitive Ability: Analyzing
Client Needs: Physiological Integrity
Integrated Process: Nursing Process—Assessment
Content Area: Adult Health—Immune

Reference: Hodgson, B., & Kizior, R. (2010). *Saunders nursing drug handbook 2010* (p. 504). St. Louis: Saunders.

ALTERNATE ITEM FORMAT: MULTIPLE RESPONSE

878. 2, 3, 5

Rationale: Ketoconazole (Nizoral) is an antifungal medication. It is administered with food (not on an empty stomach) and antacids are avoided for 2 hours after taking the medication to ensure absorption. The medication is hepatotoxic and the nurse monitors liver function. The client is instructed to avoid exposure to the sun because the medication increases photosensitivity. The client is also instructed to avoid alcohol. There is no reason for the client to restrict fluid intake. In fact, this could be harmful to the client.
Test-Taking Strategy: Use general medication guidelines to assist in selecting the correct interventions. Also, remember that this medication is administered with food and that it is hepatotoxic. Review this medication if you had difficulty with this question.
Level of Cognitive Ability: Applying
Client Needs: Physiological Integrity
Integrated Process: Nursing Process—Implementation
Content Area: Adult Health—Immune
Reference: Lehne, R. (2010). *Pharmacology for nursing care* (7th ed., p. 1061). St. Louis: Saunders.

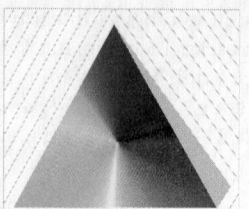

UNIT XIX

The Adult Client With a Mental Health Disorder

PYRAMID TERMS

abuse Act of misuse, deceit, or exploitation; the wrong or improper use or action toward another individual that results in injury, damage, maltreatment, or corruption.

addiction State of dependence or compulsive use. In relation to drug dependence, addiction incorporates the concepts of loss of control with respect to the use of a drug, taking the drug despite related problems and complications, and a tendency to relapse.

coping mechanism Method used to decrease anxiety. The use of a coping mechanism can be conscious, unconscious, constructive, destructive, task-oriented in relation to direct problem solving, or defense-oriented and regulating in response to protect oneself.

crisis Temporary state of disequilibrium in which an individual's usual coping mechanisms or problem-solving methods fail. Crisis can result in personality growth or personality disorganization.

defense mechanism Coping mechanism used in an effort to protect the individual from feelings of anxiety. As anxiety increases and becomes overwhelming, the individual copes by using defense mechanisms to protect the ego and decrease anxiety.

milieu Physical and social environment in which an individual lives. Milieu therapy focuses on positive physical and social environmental manipulation to produce positive change.

restraints (security devices) Physical restraints include any manual method or mechanical device, material, or equipment that inhibits free movement. Chemical restraints include the administration of medications for the specific purpose of inhibiting a specific behavior or movement.

seclusion Placing a client alone in a specially designed room that protects the client and allows for close supervision. Seclusion is the last selected measure in a process to maximize safety to the client and others.

suicide The ultimate act of self-destruction in which an individual purposefully ends his or her own life.

suicide attempt Any willful, self-inflicted, or life-threatening attempt by an individual that has not led to death.

PYRAMID TO SUCCESS

The Pyramid to Success focuses on the therapeutic nurse-client relationship, client rights, hospital admission procedures, the ethical and legal issues related to the care of a client with a mental health disorder, grief and loss, and end-of-life care. Pyramid Points also focus on the use of restraints (security devices), seclusion, and electroconvulsive therapy. Care to a client with an addiction, such as an eating disorder or drug or alcohol disorder is another focus area. Additional areas of focus include anxiety, depression, suicide, abuse and neglect, violence, rape crisis interventions, posttraumatic stress disorders, obsessive-compulsive disorders, schizophrenia, and bipolar disorders. Pyramid Points address the use of medications prescribed for a client with a mental health disorder, particularly lithium carbonate (Lithobid) and the benzodiazepines.

CLIENT NEEDS

Safe and Effective Care Environment

Ensuring client advocacy

Implementing legal responsibilities related to reporting incidences of abuse, neglect, or violence

Maintaining confidentiality

Obtaining informed consent related to treatments, such as restraints (security devices), seclusion, and electroconvulsive therapy

Providing psychiatric consultations and referrals

Providing safety to the client and others

Upholding client rights

Using restraints (security devices) and seclusion appropriately and safely

Health Promotion and Maintenance

Identifying individual lifestyle choices

Performing psychosocial assessment techniques

Providing health promotion programs related to addictions

Identifying community resources for the client

Psychosocial Integrity

Assessing for abuse and neglect situations

Assessing for chemical dependency

Assessing for domestic violence

Addressing grief and loss issues

Providing end-of-life care

Caring for the client who has been sexually abused or raped

Considering religious, cultural, and spiritual influences on health

Developing a therapeutic nurse-client relationship

Identifying appropriate counseling techniques

Identifying coping mechanisms

Identifying support systems

Implementing behavioral interventions

Providing crisis intervention

Providing a therapeutic milieu

Teaching stress-management techniques

Physiological Integrity

Administering medications as prescribed

Assessing for abusive and self-destructive behavior

Monitoring elimination patterns

Monitoring for alterations in body systems related to addictions

Monitoring for expected and untoward effects of medications

Monitoring for potential complications related to medications and treatments, such as electroconvulsive therapy

Monitoring laboratory values related to medication therapy

Monitoring rest and sleep patterns

Providing adequate nutrition

Providing personal hygiene measures

72

Foundations of Psychiatric Mental Health Nursing

 I. NURSE-CLIENT RELATIONSHIP

A. Principles
1. Genuineness, respect, and empathic understanding are characteristics important to the development of a therapeutic nurse-client relationship.
2. The client should be cared for in a holistic manner.
3. The nurse considers the client's cultural beliefs and values in assessing the client's response to the nurse-client relationship and his or her adaptation to stressors.
4. Appropriate limits and boundaries define and facilitate a therapeutic nurse-client relationship.
5. Honest and open communication are important for the development of trust, an underpinning of the therapeutic nurse-client relationship.
6. The nurse uses therapeutic communication techniques to encourage the client to express thoughts and feelings as they address identified problem areas.
7. The nurse respects the client's confidentiality and limits discussion of the client to members of the treatment team.
8. The goal of the nurse-client relationship is to assist the client to develop problem-solving abilities and **coping mechanisms**.

▲ The nurse needs to consider the religious and spiritual practices of the client and whether these practices may give the client hope, comfort, and support while healing.

 B. Phases of a therapeutic nurse-client relationship
1. Preinteraction phase
   a. The preinteraction phase begins before the nurse's first contact with the client.
   b. The nurse's task in the preinteraction phase is to focus on his or her own preconceived ideas, stereotypes, biases, and values that may impinge on the nurse-client relationship.
2. Orientation or introductory phase
   a. Acceptance, trust, and boundaries are established.
   b. Expectations and the time frame of the relationship are identified (establishing a contract).
   c. Client-centered goals are defined.
   d. Termination and separation of the relationship are discussed in anticipation of the time-limited nature of the relationship.
3. Working phase
   a. Exploring, focusing on, and evaluating the client's concerns and problems occurs; an attitude of acceptance and active listening assists the client to express thoughts and feelings.
   b. Encouraging independence in the client facilitates recovery and leads to readiness for termination.
4. Termination or separation phase
   a. Prepare the client for termination and separation on initial contact.
   b. Evaluate progress and achievement of goals.
   c. Identify responses related to termination and separation, such as anger, distancing from the relationship, a return of symptoms, and dependency.
   d. Encourage the client to express feelings about termination.
   e. Identify the client's strengths and anticipated needs for follow-up care.
   f. Refer the client to community resources and other support systems.

II. THERAPEUTIC COMMUNICATION PROCESS

A. Principles
1. Communication includes verbal and nonverbal expression (Fig. 72-1).
2. Successful communication includes appropriateness, efficiency, flexibility, and feedback.
3. Anxiety in the nurse or client impedes communication.
4. Communication needs to be goal-directed within a professional framework.
B. Therapeutic and nontherapeutic communication techniques (Box 72-1)

III. MENTAL HEALTH

A. Mental health is a lifelong process of successful adaptation to changing internal and external environments.

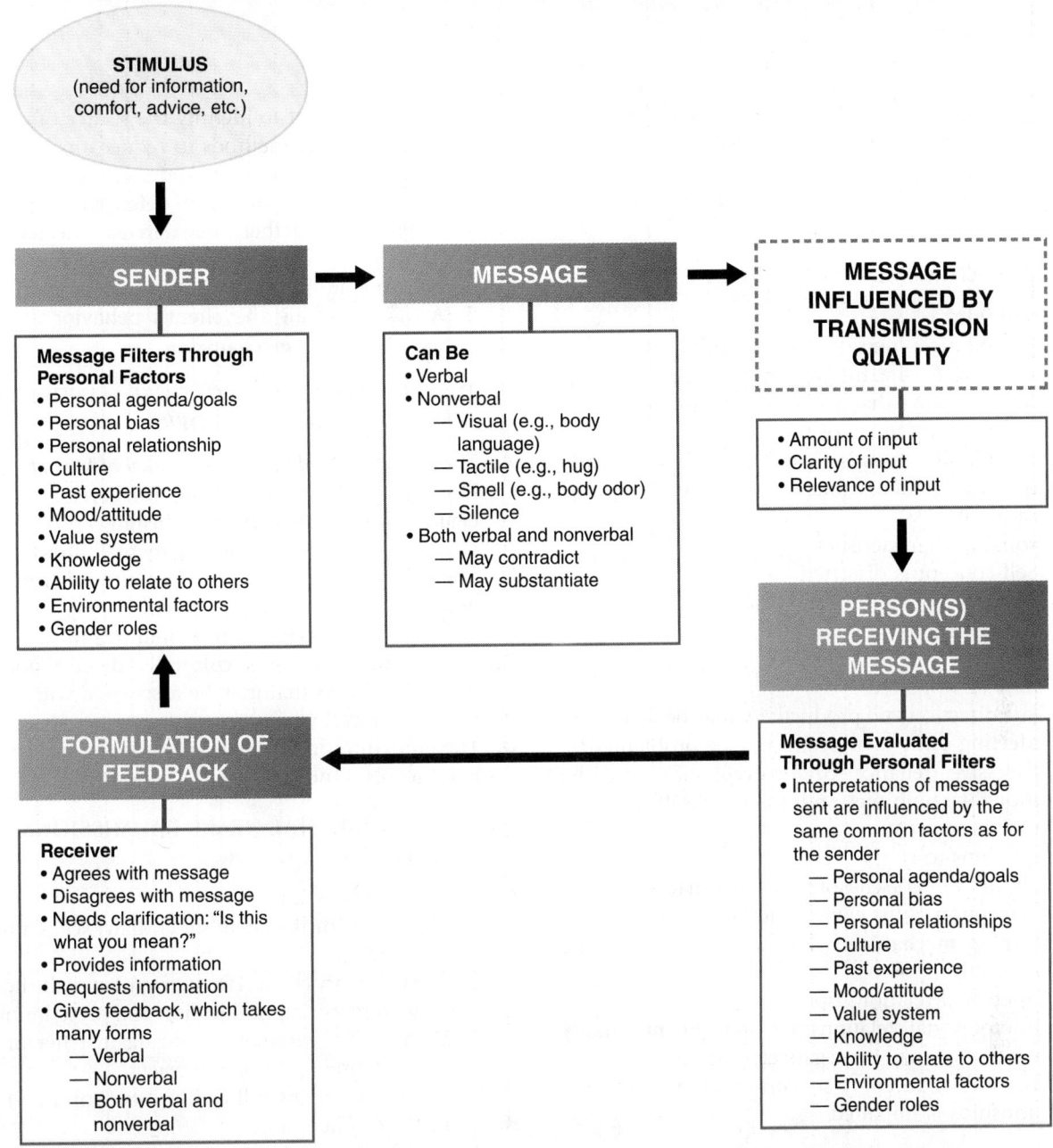

▲ FIGURE 72-1 Operational definition of communication. (Varcarolis, E., Carson, V., & Shoemaker, N. [2010]. *Foundations of psychiatric mental health nursing* [6th ed.]. St. Louis: Saunders.)

Box 72-1 Therapeutic and Nontherapeutic Communication Techniques

Therapeutic Techniques
- Clarifying and validating
- Encouraging formulation of a plan of action
- Focusing and refocusing
- Listening
- Maintaining neutral responses
- Maintaining silence
- Providing acknowledgment and feedback
- Providing information and presenting reality
- Providing nonverbal encouragement
- Reflecting
- Restating
- Sharing perceptions
- Summarizing
- Using broad openings and open-ended questions

Nontherapeutic Techniques
- Asking the client "Why?"
- Being defensive or challenging the client
- Changing the subject
- Giving advice or approval or disapproval
- Making stereotypical comments
- Making value judgments
- Placing the client's feelings on hold
- Providing false reassurance

B. A mentally healthy individual is *in contact with reality*, can relate to people and situations in their environment, and resolve conflicts within a problem-solving framework.

C. A mentally healthy individual has psychobiological resilience.

IV. PSYCHIATRIC–MENTAL HEALTH ILLNESS

A. Description
1. Psychiatric illness is the loss of the ability to respond to the internal and external environment in ways that are in harmony with oneself or the expectations of society.
2. Psychiatric illness is characterized by thought or behavior patterns that impair functioning and cause distress.

B. Personality characteristics
1. Self-concept is distorted.
2. Perception of strengths and weaknesses is unrealistic.
3. Thoughts and perceptions may not be reality-based.
4. The ability to find meaning and purpose in life may be impaired.
5. Life direction and productivity may be disturbed.
6. Meeting one's own needs may be problematic.
7. Excessive reliance or preoccupation on the thoughts, opinions, and actions of self or others may be present.

C. Adaptations to stress
1. The individual's sense of self-control may be affected.
2. Perception of the environment may be distorted.
3. **Coping mechanisms** may not exist or may be ineffective.

D. Interpersonal relationships
1. Interpersonal relationships may be minimally existent or may be negatively affected.
2. The ability to enjoy sustained intimacy in relationships is impaired.

V. COPING AND DEFENSE MECHANISMS

A. **Coping mechanisms**
1. Coping involves any effort to decrease anxiety.
2. **Coping mechanisms** can be constructive or destructive, task-oriented in relation to direct problem solving, or defense-oriented and regulating the response to protect oneself.

B. **Defense mechanisms**
1. As anxiety increases, the individual copes by using **defense mechanisms**.
2. A **defense mechanism** is a **coping mechanism** used in an effort to protect the individual from feelings of anxiety; as anxiety increases and becomes overwhelming, the individual copes by using **defense mechanisms** to protect the ego and decrease anxiety (Box 72-2).

⚠ Coping mechanisms and defense mechanisms are used by the client to decrease anxiety.

C. Interventions
1. Assist the client to identify the source of anxiety and to explore methods to reduce anxiety.
2. Assess the client's use of **defense mechanisms**.
3. Facilitate appropriate use of **defense mechanisms**.
4. Determine whether the **defense mechanisms** used by the client are effective for him or her or create additional distress.
5. Avoid criticizing the client's behavior and the use of **defense mechanisms**.

VI. DIAGNOSTIC AND STATISTICAL MANUAL OF MENTAL HEALTH DISORDERS

A. The *Diagnostic and Statistical Manual of Mental Health Disorders*, published by the American Psychiatric Association, provides guidelines for health care personnel for identifying and categorizing mental illness.

B. The manual is a system used in clinical, research, and educational settings, in which diagnostic criteria are included for each mental health disorder.

C. The manual addresses culturally diverse populations and illness that may be associated with a particular culture.

D. The guidelines in the manual assist the health care team to plan and evaluate the treatment plan.

VII. TYPES OF MENTAL HEALTH ADMISSIONS AND DISCHARGES

A. Voluntary admission
1. The client (or the client's guardian) seeks admission for care.
2. The voluntary client is free to sign out of the hospital with physician notification and prescription.
3. Detaining a voluntary client against her or his will is termed *false imprisonment*.
4. The client retains full civil rights (Box 72-3).

B. Right to confidentiality
1. A client has a right to confidentiality of his or her medical information; the Health Insurance Portability and Accountability Act (HIPAA) of 1996 ensures client confidentiality with regard to the release and electronic transmission of data.
2. Information sometimes must be released in life-threatening situations without the client's consent.
3. In the event of a specific threat against an identified individual, the health care professional has a legal obligation to warn the intended victim of a client's threats of harm.

⚠ Except in an emergency situation, client information can be released only with the client's informed consent, which specifies the information that can be released and the time frame for which the release is valid.

C. Involuntary admission
1. Involuntary admission may be necessary when a person is mentally ill, is a danger to self or

Box 72-2 Types of Defense Mechanisms

Compensation	Putting forth extra effort to achieve in areas where one has a real or imagined deficiency	Projection	Transferring one's internal feelings, thoughts, and unacceptable ideas and traits to someone else
Conversion	Expression of emotional conflicts through physical symptoms	Rationalization	Attempt to make unacceptable feelings and behaviors acceptable by justifying the behavior
Denial	Disowning consciously intolerable thoughts and impulses	Reaction formation	Developing conscious attitudes and behaviors and acting out behaviors opposite to what one really feels
Displacement	Feelings toward one person are directed to another who is less threatening, satisfying an impulse with a substitute object	Regression	Returning to an earlier developmental stage to express an impulse to deal with reality
Dissociation	Blocking of an anxiety-provoking event or period of time from the conscious mind	Repression	Unconscious process in which the client blocks undesirable and unacceptable thoughts from conscious expression
Fantasy	Gratification by imaginary achievements and wishful thinking	Sublimation	Replacement of an unacceptable need, attitude, or emotion with one more socially acceptable
Fixation	Never advancing to the next level of emotional development and organization; persistence in later life of interests and behavior patterns appropriate to an earlier age	Substitution	Replacement of a valued unacceptable object with an object more acceptable to the ego
Identification	Unconscious attempt to change oneself to resemble an admired person	Suppression	Conscious, deliberate forgetting of unacceptable or painful thoughts, ideas, and feelings
Insulation	Withdrawing into passivity and becoming inaccessible so as to avoid further threatening situations	Symbolization	Conscious use of an idea or object to represent another actual event or object; often, the meaning is unclear because the symbol may be representative of something unconscious
Intellectualization	Excessive reasoning to avoid feelings; the thinking is disconnected from feelings, and situations are dealt with at a cognitive level	Undoing	Engaging in behavior considered to be the opposite of a previous unacceptable behavior, thought, or feeling
Introjection	Type of identification in which the individual incorporates the traits or values of another into himself or herself		
Isolation	Response in which a person blocks feelings associated with an unpleasant experience		

Box 72-3 Client Rights

- Right to accessible health care
- Right to coordination and continuity of health care
- Right to courteous and individualized health care
- Right to information about the qualifications, names, and titles of personnel delivering care
- Right to refuse observation by individuals not directly involved in care
- Right to privacy and confidentiality
- Right to informed consent
- Right to treatment and to refuse treatment
- Right to treatment in the least restrictive setting
- Right not to be subjected to unnecessary restraints
- Right to habeas corpus; may request a hearing at any time to be released from the hospital
- Right to information about diagnosis, prognosis, and treatment
- Right to information on the charges of service
- Right to communicate with people outside the hospital through written correspondence, telephone, and personal visits
- Right to keep clothing and personal effects
- Right to be employed
- Right to religious freedom
- Right to execute wills
- Right to retain licenses, privileges, or permits established by the law, such as a driver's or professional license

Modified from Stuart, G. (2009). *Principles and practice of psychiatric nursing* (9th ed.). St. Louis: Mosby.

others, or is in need of psychiatric treatment or physical care.

2. Involuntary admission occurs when a person is admitted or detained involuntarily for mental health treatment because of actual or imminent danger to self or others.

3. A client who is admitted involuntarily retains his or her right for informed consent.

4. The client retains the right to refuse treatments, including medications, unless a separate and specific treatment order is obtained from the court.

5. The client loses the right to refuse treatment when he or she poses an immediate danger to self or others, requiring immediate action by the health care team.

6. An order from a judge is required for involuntary admissions except in the case of emergency, which allows time to obtain the necessary order from a judge; in the case of all involuntary admissions, legal counsel must be provided for the client.

7. A court hearing is held by a judge within a specified time period for a client admitted involuntarily; the specific time period varies by state.

8. In most states, a client can institute a court hearing to seek an expedient judicial discharge (a writ of habeas corpus).

9. At the court hearing, a determination is made as to whether the client may be released from the hospital or detained for further treatment and evaluation or committed to a mental health facility for an undetermined period.

10. A client has the right to treatment in the least restrictive treatment environment; if treatment objectives can be achieved by court-ordered treatment to an outpatient facility as opposed to an inpatient facility, the client has the right to be treated in the outpatient setting.

11. A client is considered legally competent unless he or she has been declared incompetent through a legal hearing separate from the involuntary commitment hearing.

12. In the course of providing nursing care and carrying out medical prescriptions, if the nurse believes that a client lacks competency to make informed decisions, action should be initiated to determine whether a legal guardian needs to be appointed by the court.

D. Release from the hospital
  1. Description
     a. A client may be released voluntarily, against medical advice, or with conditions (conditional release).
     b. A client who has sought voluntary admission has the right to demand and receive release.
  2. Voluntary release
     a. In the absence of an act of self-harm or danger to others, a voluntary client should never be detained.

b. If a voluntary client wishes to be discharged from treatment, but is considered potentially dangerous to self or others, the physician can order the client to be detained while legal proceedings for involuntary status are sought.

c. Some states provide for conditional release of involuntarily hospitalized clients; this enables the treating physician to prescribe continued treatment on an outpatient basis as opposed to discharging the client to follow-up on his or her own initiative.

d. Conditional release usually involves outpatient treatment for a specified period to determine the client's compliance with medication protocol, ability to meet basic needs, and ability to reintegrate into the community.

e. An involuntary client who is released conditionally may be reinstitutionalized while the commitment is still in effect without recommencement of formal admission procedures.

3. Discharge planning and follow-up care
   a. Discharge (unconditional release) is the termination of the client-institution relationship.
   b. This release may be ordered by the psychiatrist, court, or administration for involuntarily admitted clients and may be requested by voluntary clients at any time.
   c. In most states, the client can institute a court hearing to seek an expedient judicial discharge (writ of habeas corpus).
   d. Discharge planning and follow-up care are important for the continued well-being of the client with a mental health disorder.
   e. Aftercare case managers are used to facilitate the client's adaptation back into the community and to provide early referral if the treatment plan is unsuccessful.

🔘 MORE QUESTIONS ON THE CD!

Practice Questions

879. A client with a diagnosis of major depression who has attempted suicide says to a nurse, "I should have died. I've always been a failure. Nothing ever goes right for me." The therapeutic response to the client is:
1. "I don't see you as a failure."
2. "You have everything to live for."
3. "Feeling like this is all part of being ill."
4. "You've been feeling like a failure for a while?"

880. A community health nurse visits a client at home. The client states, "I haven't slept at all the last couple of nights." Which response by the nurse illustrates a therapeutic communication technique for this client?

1. "Go on."
2. "Sleeping?"
3. "You're having difficulty sleeping?"
4. "Sometimes, I have trouble sleeping too."

881. A client admitted to the mental health unit is experiencing disturbed thought processes and believes that the food is being poisoned. Which communication technique would a nurse plan to use to encourage the client to eat?
1. Using open-ended questions and silence
2. Focusing on self-disclosure regarding food preferences
3. List possible reasons in the care plan that the client may not want to eat
4. Offering opinions about the necessity of adequate nutrition

882. A client is admitted to a mental health unit for treatment of psychotic behavior. The client is at the locked exit door and is shouting, "Let me out. There's nothing wrong with me. I don't belong here." A nurse analyzes this behavior as:
1. Denial
2. Projection
3. Regression
4. Rationalization

883. A client says to a nurse, "I'm going to die, and I wish my family would stop hoping for a cure! I get so angry when they carry on like this. After all, I'm the one who's dying." The therapeutic response by the nurse is:
1. "Have you shared your feelings with your family?"
2. "I think we should talk more about your anger with your family."
3. "You're feeling angry that your family continues to hope for you to be cured?"
4. "Well, it sounds like you're being pretty pessimistic. After all, years ago, people died of pneumonia."

884. A nurse employed in a mental health unit is assigned to care for a client admitted to the unit 2 days ago. On review of the client's record, the nurse notes that the admission was a voluntary admission. Based on this type of admission, the nurse anticipates which of the following?
1. The client will resist treatment measures.
2. The client will be angry and will refuse care.
3. The client's family will resist treatment measures.
4. The client will participate in the planning of the care and treatment plan.

885. A nurse enters a client's room, and the client is demanding release from the hospital. The nurse

reviews the client's record and notes that the client was admitted 2 days ago for treatment of an anxiety disorder and that the admission was a voluntary admission. Which of the following actions would the nurse take?
1. Contact the physician.
2. Call the client's family.
3. Persuade the client to stay a few more days.
4. Tell the client that discharge is not possible at this time.

886. A client has been admitted to the mental health unit. On admission assessment, a nurse notes that the client was admitted by involuntary status. Based on this type of admission, the nurse would most likely expect that the client:
1. Presents a harm to self
2. Requested the admission
3. Consented to the admission
4. Provided written application to the facility for admission

887. A nurse is preparing a client for the termination phase of the nurse-client relationship. The nurse prepares to implement which nursing task appropriate for this phase?
1. Planning short-term goals
2. Making appropriate referrals
3. Developing realistic solutions
4. Identifying expected outcomes

888. A nurse is providing care to a client admitted to the hospital with a diagnosis of acute anxiety disorder. The client says to the nurse, "I have a secret that I want to tell you. You won't tell anyone about it, will you?" The appropriate nursing response would be which of the following?
1. "No, I won't tell anyone."
2. "I cannot promise to keep a secret."
3. "If you tell me the secret, I will tell it to your doctor."
4. "If you tell me the secret, I will need to document it in your record."

889. A nurse employed in a mental health clinic is greeted by a neighbor in a local grocery store. The neighbor says to the nurse, "How is Carol doing? She is my best friend and is seen at your clinic every week." The appropriate nursing response is which of the following?
1. "I cannot discuss any client situation with you."
2. "If you want to know about Carol, you need to ask her yourself."
3. "I'm not supposed to discuss this, but because you are my neighbor, I can tell you that she is doing great!"

4. "I'm not supposed to discuss this, but because you are my neighbor, I can tell you that she really has some problems!"

890. A client was admitted involuntarily to the mental health unit because of episodes of extremely violent behavior. The client is demanding to be discharged from the hospital, and a nurse does not allow the client to leave. Which of the following represents the legal ramifications associated with the nurse's behavior?
1. The nurse will be charged with assault.
2. The nurse will be charged with slander.
3. The nurse will be charged with imprisonment.
4. No charge will be made against the nurse because the nurse's actions are reasonable.

891. A nurse is working with a client who has sought counseling after trying to rescue a neighbor involved in a house fire. Despite the client's efforts, the neighbor died. Which action does the nurse engage in with the client during the working phase of the nurse-client relationship?
1. Exploring the client's ability to function
2. Exploring the client's potential for self-harm
3. Inquiring about the client's perception or appraisal of the neighbor's death
4. Inquiring about and examining the client's feelings that may block adaptive coping

892. A client who has just been sexually assaulted is calm and quiet. A nurse analyzes this behavior as indicating which defense mechanism?
1. Denial
2. Projection
3. Rationalization
4. Intellectualization

893. Unresolved feelings related to loss most likely may be recognized during which phase of the therapeutic nurse-client relationship?
1. Working
2. Trusting
3. Orientation
4. Termination

Alternate Item Format: Multiple Response

894. A nurse in the mental health unit reviews therapeutic and nontherapeutic communication techniques with a nursing student. Which of the following are therapeutic communication techniques? **Select all that apply.**
❑ 1. Restating
❑ 2. Listening
❑ 3. Asking the client, "Why?"
❑ 4. Maintaining neutral responses
❑ 5. Giving advice or approval or disapproval
❑ 6. Providing acknowledgment and feedback

ANSWERS

879. 4
Rationale: Responding to the feelings expressed by a client is an effective therapeutic communication technique. The correct option is an example of the use of restating. Options 1, 2, and 3 block communication because they minimize the client's experience and do not facilitate exploration of the client's expressed feelings.
Test-Taking Strategy: Use the process of elimination and knowledge of therapeutic communication techniques to direct you to the option that directly addresses the client's feelings and concerns. Also, option 4 is the only option stated in the form of a question and is open-ended; it will encourage the verbalization of feelings. Review therapeutic communication techniques if you had difficulty with this question.
Level of Cognitive Ability: Applying
Client Needs: Psychosocial Integrity
Integrated Process: Communication and Documentation
Content Area: Mental Health
Reference: Stuart, G. (2009). *Principles and practice of psychiatric nursing* (9th ed., pp. 27–31, 316). St. Louis: Mosby.

880. 3
Rationale: Option 3 uses the therapeutic communication technique of restatement. Although restatement is a technique that has a prompting component to it, it repeats the client's major theme, which assists the nurse to obtain a more

specific perception of the problem from the client. Options 1, 2, and 4 are not therapeutic responses.
Test-Taking Strategy: Use the process of elimination. Option 1 is a general lead and allows the client to direct the discussion. Option 2 uses reflection, which simply repeats a client's words to prompt further discussion. Option 4 focuses on the nurse's problem. Option 3 will provide the perception of the problem from the client's perspective. Review therapeutic communication techniques if you had difficulty with this question.
Level of Cognitive Ability: Applying
Client Needs: Psychosocial Integrity
Integrated Process: Communication and Documentation
Content Area: Mental Health
References: Fortinash, K., & Holoday-Worret, P. (2008). *Psychiatric mental health nursing* (4th ed., p. 417). St. Louis: Mosby.
   Stuart, G. (2009). *Principles and practice of psychiatric nursing* (9th ed., pp. 27–31). St. Louis: Mosby.

881. 1
Rationale: Open-ended questions and silence are strategies used to encourage clients to discuss their problems. Options 3 and 4 are not helpful to the client because they do not encourage the client to express feelings. The nurse should not offer opinions and should encourage the client to identify the reasons for the behavior. Option 2 is not a client-centered intervention.

Test-Taking Strategy: Use the process of elimination. Eliminate options 3 and 4 first because they do not support client expression of feelings. Eliminate option 2 next because it is not a client-centered response. Focusing on the client's feelings will direct you to option 1. Review therapeutic communication techniques if you had difficulty with this question.
Level of Cognitive Ability: Applying
Client Needs: Psychosocial Integrity
Integrated Process: Nursing Process—Planning
Content Area: Mental Health
Reference: Stuart, G. (2009). *Principles and practice of psychiatric nursing* (9th ed., pp. 27–31). St. Louis: Mosby.

882. 1
Rationale: Denial is refusal to admit to a painful reality, which is treated as if it does not exist. In projection, a person unconsciously rejects emotionally unacceptable features and attributes them to other persons, objects, or situations. In regression, the client returns to an earlier, more comforting, although less mature, way of behaving. Rationalization is justifying illogical or unreasonable ideas, actions, or feelings by developing acceptable explanations that satisfy the teller and the listener.
Test-Taking Strategy: Use the process of elimination. The strategic words in the question that should direct you to the correct option are *"There's nothing wrong with me."* Select the option that recognizes the client's attempt to avoid looking at the reality of the situation. If you had difficulty with this question, review defense mechanisms.
Level of Cognitive Ability: Understanding
Client Needs: Psychosocial Integrity
Integrated Process: Nursing Process—Assessment
Content Area: Mental Health
Reference: Varcarolis, E., & Halter, M. (2009). *Essentials of psychiatric mental health nursing: A communication approach to evidence-based care* (pp. 136, 311). St. Louis: Saunders.

883. 3
Rationale: Restating is a therapeutic communication technique in which the nurse repeats what the client says to show understanding and to review what was said. Option 3 uses the therapeutic technique of restating. In option 1, the nurse is attempting to assess the client's ability to discuss feelings openly with family members. In option 2, the nurse attempts to use focusing, but the attempt to discuss central issues is premature. In option 4, the nurse makes a judgment and is nontherapeutic in the one-to-one relationship.
Test-Taking Strategy: Use therapeutic communication techniques to answer the question. Option 3 is the only option that identifies the use of a therapeutic technique and focuses on the client's feelings. Review these techniques if you had difficulty with this question.
Level of Cognitive Ability: Applying
Client Needs: Psychosocial Integrity
Integrated Process: Communication and Documentation
Content Area: Mental Health
Reference: Stuart, G. (2009). *Principles and practice of psychiatric nursing* (9th ed., pp. 27, 32). St. Louis: Mosby.

884. 4
Rationale: Generally, the client seeks voluntary admission. A voluntary admission permits a client to make a written

application for admission. If the client seeks voluntary admission, the most likely expectation is that the client will participate in the treatment program. Options 1, 2, and 3 are not characteristics of this type of admission.
Test-Taking Strategy: Use the process of elimination. Note the strategic words *voluntary admission*. This should direct you to option 4. Additionally, options 1, 2, and 3 are comparable or alike. Review the various types of hospital admission processes if you had difficulty with this question.
Level of Cognitive Ability: Understanding
Client Needs: Psychosocial Integrity
Integrated Process: Nursing Process—Planning
Content Area: Mental Health
Reference: Varcarolis, E., & Halter, M. (2009). *Essentials of psychiatric mental health nursing: A communication approach to evidence-based care* (p. 520). St. Louis: Saunders.

885. 1
Rationale: Generally, the client seeks voluntary admission. Voluntary clients have the right to demand and obtain release. If the client is a minor, the release may be contingent on the consent of a parent or guardian. The nurse needs to be familiar with the state and facility policies and procedures. Many states require that the client submit a written release notice to the facility staff members, who re-evaluate the client's condition for possible conversion to involuntary status if necessary, according to criteria established by laws. The best nursing action is to contact the physician.
Test-Taking Strategy: Use the process of elimination. Noting the type of hospital admission will assist in eliminating option 4. To "persuade" a client to stay in the hospital is inappropriate. Option 2 should be eliminated simply based on the subjects of client rights and confidentiality. Review the various types of hospital admission and discharge processes if you had difficulty with this question.
Level of Cognitive Ability: Applying
Client Needs: Psychosocial Integrity
Integrated Process: Nursing Process—Implementation
Content Area: Leadership and Management—Ethical/Legal
Reference: Stuart, G. (2009). *Principles and practice of psychiatric nursing* (9th ed., pp. 124, 126). St. Louis: Mosby.

886. 1
Rationale: Involuntary admission is made without the client's consent. Involuntary admission is necessary when a person is a danger to self or others or is in need of psychiatric treatment. Options 2, 3, and 4 describe the process of voluntary admission.
Test-Taking Strategy: Use the process of elimination and note the strategic words *involuntary status*. This should direct you easily to option 1. Also, note that options 2, 3, and 4 are comparable or alike. Review the process of involuntary admission if you had difficulty with this question.
Level of Cognitive Ability: Understanding
Client Needs: Psychosocial Integrity
Integrated Process: Nursing Process—Planning
Content Area: Mental Health
References: Stuart, G. (2009). *Principles and practice of psychiatric nursing* (9th ed., p. 124). St. Louis: Mosby.
  Varcarolis, E., & Halter, M. (2009). *Essentials of psychiatric mental health nursing: A communication approach to evidence-based care* (pp. 520–521). St. Louis: Saunders.

887. 2

Rationale: Tasks of the termination phase include evaluating client performance, evaluating achievement of expected outcomes, evaluating future needs, making appropriate referrals, and dealing with the common behaviors associated with termination. Options 1, 3, and 4 identify the tasks of the working phase of the relationship.

Test-Taking Strategy: Use the process of elimination. Noting the strategic words *termination phase* should direct you easily to option 2. If you are unfamiliar with the appropriate tasks of the phases of the nurse-client relationship, review this content.

Level of Cognitive Ability: Applying
Client Needs: Psychosocial Integrity
Integrated Process: Nursing Process—Planning
Content Area: Mental Health
Reference: Stuart, G. (2009). *Principles and practice of psychiatric nursing* (9th ed., pp. 21–22). St. Louis: Mosby.

888. 2

Rationale: The nurse should never promise to keep a secret. Secrets are appropriate in a social relationship, but not in a therapeutic one. The nurse needs to be honest with the client and tell the client that a promise cannot be made to keep the secret. Options 1, 3, and 4 are inappropriate responses.

Test-Taking Strategy: Use the process of elimination. Option 1 can be eliminated easily because it is inappropriate. Options 3 and 4 are not only inappropriate, but are also threatening and may block further communication. Review therapeutic communication techniques and the nurse-client relationship if you had difficulty with this question.

Level of Cognitive Ability: Applying
Client Needs: Psychosocial Integrity
Integrated Process: Communication and Documentation
Content Area: Leadership and Management—Ethical/Legal
References: Fortinash, K., & Holoday-Worret, P. (2008). *Psychiatric mental health nursing* (4th ed., pp. 26–27). St. Louis: Mosby.
 Stuart, G. (2009). *Principles and practice of psychiatric nursing* (9th ed., pp. 27–31, 275). St. Louis: Mosby.

889. 1

Rationale: A nurse is required to maintain confidentiality regarding the client and the client's care. Confidentiality is basic to the therapeutic relationship and is a client's right. The most appropriate response to the neighbor is option 1. Option 2 is a blunt statement and does not acknowledge the issue that the nurse cannot reveal if the named person is or was a client. Options 3 and 4 identify statements that do not maintain client confidentiality. Option 1 is the most direct and correct.

Test-Taking Strategy: Focus on the subject of the question, maintaining confidentiality. This should assist you easily in eliminating options 3 and 4. From the remaining options, select option 1 over option 2 because it is the most direct and correct. Option 2 is a blunt and rude statement. Review confidentiality issues if you had difficulty with this question.

Level of Cognitive Ability: Applying

Client Needs: Safe and Effective Care Environment
Integrated Process: Nursing Process—Implementation
Content Area: Leadership and Management—Ethical/Legal
Reference: Varcarolis, E., & Halter, M. (2009). *Essentials of psychiatric mental health nursing: A communication approach to evidence-based care* (pp. 524–525). St. Louis: Saunders.

890. 4

Rationale: False imprisonment is an act with the intent to confine a person to a specific area. A nurse can be charged with false imprisonment if the nurse prohibits a client from leaving the hospital if the client has been admitted voluntarily and if no agency or legal policies exist for detaining the client. If the client has been admitted involuntarily or had agreed to an evaluation before discharge, the nurse's actions are reasonable.

Test-Taking Strategy: Noting the strategic words *admitted involuntarily* will assist you in eliminating option 3 and direct you to option 4. Options 1 and 2 are unrelated to the subject of the question and can be eliminated easily. Review the subjects related to false imprisonment and hospital admission if you had difficulty with this question.

Level of Cognitive Ability: Understanding
Client Needs: Safe and Effective Care Environment
Integrated Process: Nursing Process—Planning
Content Area: Leadership and Management—Ethical/Legal
Reference: Varcarolis, E., & Halter, M. (2009). *Essentials of psychiatric mental health nursing: A communication approach to evidence-based care* (p. 528). St. Louis: Saunders.

891. 4

Rationale: The client must first deal with feelings and negative responses before the client can work through the meaning of the crisis. Option 4 pertains directly to the client's feelings. Options 1 and 2 do not directly address the client's feelings. Option 3 does not directly focus on the clients's feelings..

Test-Taking Strategy: Focus on the subject of the question, the working phase of the nurse-client relationship. Think about the interventions that occur in this phase. Using the process of elimination, focus on this subject and on the option that focuses on the feelings of the client. This will direct you to option 4. Review the phases of the nurse-client relationship if you had difficulty with this question.

Level of Cognitive Ability: Applying
Client Needs: Psychosocial Integrity
Integrated Process: Caring
Content Area: Mental Health
Reference: Stuart, G. (2009). *Principles and practice of psychiatric nursing* (9th ed., pp. 190–191). St. Louis: Mosby.

892. 1

Rationale: Denial is refusal to admit to a painful reality and may be a response by a victim of sexual abuse. Projection is transferring one's internal feelings, thoughts, and unacceptable ideas and traits to someone else. Rationalization is justifying the unacceptable attributes about oneself. Intellectualization is the excessive use of abstract thinking or generalizations to decrease painful thinking.

Test-Taking Strategy: Use the process of elimination and note the strategic words *calm* and *quiet*. These behaviors indicate denial in a sexually abused victim. If you had difficulty with this question, review content related to the sexually abused victim and defense mechanisms.
Level of Cognitive Ability: Understanding
Client Needs: Psychosocial Integrity
Integrated Process: Nursing Process—Assessment
Content Area: Mental Health
References: Stuart, G. (2009). *Principles and practice of psychiatric nursing* (9th ed., p. 722). St. Louis: Mosby.
Varcarolis, E., & Halter, M. (2009). *Essentials of psychiatric mental health nursing: A communication approach to evidence-based care* (pp. 136, 311). St. Louis: Saunders.

893. 4
Rationale: In the termination phase, the relationship comes to a close. Ending treatment sometimes may be traumatic for clients who have come to value the relationship and the help. Because loss is an issue, any unresolved feelings related to loss may resurface during this phase. Options 1, 2, and 3 are incorrect.
Test-Taking Strategy: Note the strategic words *unresolved, loss,* and *recognized* in the question. Considering the phases of the therapeutic nurse-client relationship will direct you to option 4. Review these phases and the nursing implications if you had difficulty with this question.
Level of Cognitive Ability: Understanding
Client Needs: Psychosocial Integrity
Integrated Process: Caring

Content Area: Mental Health
References: Stuart, G. (2009). *Principles and practice of psychiatric nursing* (9th ed., p. 560). St. Louis: Mosby.
Varcarolis, E., & Halter, M. (2009). *Essentials of psychiatric mental health nursing: A communication approach to evidence-based care* (pp. 113–114). St. Louis: Saunders.

ALTERNATE ITEM FORMAT: MULTIPLE RESPONSE
894. 1, 2, 4, 6
Rationale: Therapeutic communication techniques include listening, maintaining silence, maintaining neutral responses, using broad openings and open-ended questions, focusing and refocusing, restating, clarifying and validating, sharing perceptions, reflecting, providing acknowledgment and feedback, giving information, presenting reality, encouraging formulation of a plan of action, providing nonverbal encouragement, and summarizing.
Test-Taking Strategy: Focus on the subject, therapeutic communication techniques. This will assist you in selecting the correct answers. Review therapeutic and nontherapeutic techniques if you had difficulty with this question.
Level of Cognitive Ability: Understanding
Client Needs: Psychosocial Integrity
Integrated Process: Teaching and Learning
Content Area: Mental Health
Reference: Stuart, G. (2009). *Principles and practice of psychiatric nursing* (9th ed., pp. 27–31). St. Louis: Mosby.

Models of Care

73

I. MILIEU THERAPY

A. Description
1. The **milieu** refers to the physical and social environment in which an individual is receiving treatment.
2. **Milieu** therapy uses a safe environment to meet the individual client's treatment needs.
3. Safety is the most important priority in managing the **milieu**.
4. **Milieu** therapy is staffed by persons educated to provide support, understanding, and individual attention; all encounters with the client have the goal of being "therapeutic."
5. All members of the treatment team contribute to the planning and functioning of the **milieu**; the team generally includes a registered nurse, social worker, exercise therapist, recreational therapist, psychologist, psychiatrist, occupational therapist, and clinical nurse specialist or nurse practitioner.
6. All members of the treatment team are viewed as significant and valuable to the client's successful treatment outcomes.

B. Focus of **milieu** therapy
1. The physical and social environment is used to effect a positive change directed toward accomplishing the client's treatment goals.
2. Community meetings, activity groups, social skills groups, and physical exercise programs are used to accomplish treatment goals.
3. One-to-one relationships with staff are used to examine client behaviors, feelings, and interactions within the context of the therapeutic group activities.

⚠ The focus of milieu therapy is to empower the client through involvement in setting his or her own goals and to develop purposeful relationships with the staff to assist in meeting these goals.

II. INTERPERSONAL PSYCHOTHERAPY

A. Description
1. A treatment modality that uses a therapeutic relationship to modify the client's feelings, attitudes, and behaviors

2. Therapeutic communication forms the foundation of the therapist-client relationship.

B. Focus of interpersonal psychotherapy
1. To establish a contract, clarify roles, and work within an agreed-on time frame to help meet the client's goals
2. The therapist-client relationship is used as a way for the client to examine other relationships in his or her life.

C. Levels of psychotherapy (Box 73-1)
1. Supportive therapy
   a. Allows the client to express feelings, explore alternatives, and make decisions in a safe, caring environment
   b. May be needed briefly or over a period of years
   c. No plan exists to introduce new methods of coping; instead, the therapist reinforces the client's existing **coping mechanisms**.
2. Re-educative therapy
   a. Involves learning new ways of perceiving and behaving
   b. The client explores alternatives in a planned, systematic way; this requires a longer period of therapy than supportive therapy.
   c. The client enters into a contract that specifies desired changes of behavior.
   d. Techniques may include short-term psychotherapy, reality therapy, cognitive restructuring, behavior modification, and development of coping skills
3. Reconstructive therapy
   a. Psychotherapy or psychoanalysis is used to make major changes in the client's life.
   b. Several years of therapy may be required, and focus is on all aspects of the client's life.
   c. Emotional and cognitive restructuring of self takes place.
   d. Positive outcomes include a greater understanding of self and others, more emotional freedom, and the development of potential abilities.

III. BEHAVIOR THERAPY

A. Treatment approach that uses the principles of Skinnerian (operant conditioning) or Pavlovian

Box 73-1 Levels of Psychotherapy

- Supportive therapy
- Re-educative therapy
- Reconstructive therapy

Box 73-2 Stages of Group Development

- Initial stage
- Working stage
- Termination stage

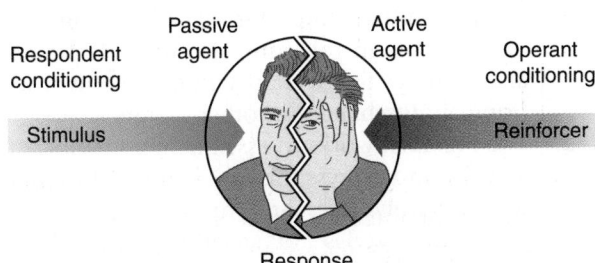

Passive agent — Active agent

Respondent conditioning — Operant conditioning

Stimulus — Reinforcer

Response

▲ **FIGURE 73-1** Respondent versus operant conditioning. (From Varcarolis, E., Carson, V., & Shoemaker, N. [2010]. *Foundations of psychiatric mental health nursing* [6th ed.]. St. Louis: Saunders.)

(classical conditioning) behavior theory to bring about behavioral change

B. The belief is that most behaviors are learned.

C. Operant conditioning refers to the manipulation of selected reinforcers to elicit and strengthen desired behavioral responses; the reinforcer refers to the consequence of the behavior, which is defined as anything that increases the occurrence of a behavior (Fig. 73-1).

D. In classical conditioning (respondent conditioning), the individual responds to a stimulus, but is basically a passive agent (see Fig. 73-1).

E. Desensitization is a form of behavior therapy whereby exposure to increasing increments of a feared stimulus is paired with increasing levels of relaxation, which helps reduce the intensity of fear to a more tolerable level.

F. Aversion therapy is a form of behavior therapy whereby negative reinforcement is used to change behavior; a stimulus *attractive* to the client is paired with an *unpleasant* event in hopes of endowing the stimulus with negative properties and dissuading the behavior.

G. Modeling is behavioral therapy whereby the therapist acts as a role model for specific identified behaviors so that the client learns through imitation.

IV. COGNITIVE THERAPY

A. An active, directive, time-limited, structured approach used to treat a variety of disorders, including anxiety, depression, and phobias

B. It is based on the principle that how individuals feel and behave is determined by how they think about the world and their place in it; their cognitions are based on the attitudes or assumptions developed from previous experiences.

C. Therapeutic techniques are designed to identify, reality-test, and correct distorted conceptualizations

and the dysfunctional beliefs underlying these cognitions.

D. The therapist helps the individual change the way he or she thinks, relieving symptoms.

V. GROUP DEVELOPMENT AND GROUP THERAPY

A. Description: Group therapy involves a therapist and, ideally, five to eight members working on his or her individual goals within the context of a group, which presumably increases the opportunity for feedback and support.

B. Stages of group development (Box 73-2)

1. Initial stage
   a. During this stage, group development involves superficial rather than open and trusting communication.
   b. Members become acquainted with each other and search for similarities between themselves and other group members.
   c. Members may be unclear about the purpose or goals of the group.
   d. Group norms, roles, and responsibilities are established.

2. Working stage
   a. During this stage, the real work of the group is accomplished.
   b. Members are familiar with each other, the group leader, and the group roles and feel free to address and attempt to solve their problems.
   c. Conflict and cooperation surface during the group's work as the members learn to work with each other.

3. Termination stage
   a. Members' feelings are explored regarding their accomplishments and the impending termination of the group.
   b. The termination stage provides an opportunity for members to learn to deal more realistically and comfortably with this normal part of human experience.

C. Group therapy models (*Note:* These models apply to individual or group psychotherapy.)

1. Psychoanalytical group psychotherapy
   a. The therapist holds a main position.
   b. Each client in the group has a relationship with the therapist.
   c. Communication is focused on three levels— unconscious, semiconscious, and conscious information.

2. Transactional analysis
   a. The three ego states of the individual are examined.
   b. The goal is for individuals in the group to communicate from the proper ego states for the situation and responses of others, lessening conflict and promoting mature relationships.
3. Rational emotive therapy is a type of cognitive therapy in which the therapist focuses on how irrational beliefs and thoughts contribute to psychological distress.
4. Rogerian therapy
   a. The therapist's goal is to help the members express their feelings toward one another during group sessions.
   b. The therapist's role is one of encouraging the expression of feelings, clarifying these feelings with clients, and accepting clients and their feelings nonjudgmentally.
5. Gestalt therapy
   a. Emphasis is on the "here and now."
   b. Emphasizes self-expression, self-exploration, and self-awareness in the present
   c. The client and therapist focus on everyday problems and try to solve them.
   d. The individual becomes aware of the total self and the surrounding environment.
   e. Awareness of the problem renders the client capable of change.
   f. The therapist's role is to help the members express their feelings and grow from their experiences.
6. Interpersonal group therapy: Promotes the individual's comfort with others in the group, which then transfers to other relationships
7. Self-help or support groups (Box 73-3)

Box 73-3 Self-Help and Support Groups

- Adult Children of Alcoholics
- Al-Anon
- Alcoholics Anonymous
- Co-Dependents Anonymous
- Gamblers Anonymous
- Narcotics Anonymous
- Overeaters Anonymous
- Parents Without Partners
- Bereavement groups
- Cancer support groups
- Groups to help deal with unexpected body image changes, such as mastectomy or colostomy
- Mental illness support groups
- Recovery groups, such as for individuals who have experienced trauma
- Smoking cessation groups

⚠ Support groups are based on the premise that individuals who have experienced a problem are able to help others who have a similar problem.

VI. FAMILY THERAPY

1. Family therapy is a specific intervention mode based on the premise that the member with the presenting symptoms signals the presence of problems in the entire family; this premise also assumes that a change in one member will bring about changes in other members.
2. The therapist works to assist family members to identify and express their thoughts and feelings; define family roles and rules; try new, more productive styles of relating; and restore strength to the family.

🖸 MORE QUESTIONS ON THE CD!

Practice Questions

895. A nurse employed in a mental health unit of a hospital is the leader of a group psychotherapy session. The nurse's role in the termination stage of group development is to:
   1. Encourage problem solving.
   2. Encourage accomplishment of the group's work.
   3. Acknowledge the contributions of each group member.
   4. Encourage members to become acquainted with one another.

896. All treatment team members are seen as equally important in helping clients meet their treatment goals. This type of therapy approach is:
   1. Milieu therapy
   2. Interpersonal therapy
   3. Behavior modification
   4. Rational emotive therapy

897. An 18-year-old woman is admitted to an inpatient mental health unit with the diagnosis of anorexia nervosa. A cognitive behavioral approach is used as part of her treatment plan. A nurse understands that the purpose of this approach is to:
   1. Provide a supportive environment.
   2. Examine intrapsychic conflicts and past issues.
   3. Emphasize social interaction with clients who withdraw.
   4. Help the client identify and examine dysfunctional thoughts and beliefs.

898. A client with major depression is considering cognitive therapy. The client asks a nurse, "How does this treatment work?" The nurse tells the client that:

1. "This type of treatment will help you relax and develop new coping skills."
2. "This type of treatment helps you confront your fears by gradually exposing you to them."
3. "This type of treatment helps you examine how your past life has contributed to your problems."
4. "This type of treatment helps you examine how your thoughts and feelings contribute to your difficulties."

899. A client is preparing to attend a Gambler's Anonymous meeting for the first time. The prototype used by this group is the 12-step program developed by Alcoholics Anonymous. A nurse tells the client that the first step in the 12-step program is which of the following?
1. Admitting to having a problem
2. Substituting other activities for gambling
3. Stating that the gambling will be stopped
4. Discontinuing relationships with friends who are gamblers

900. A client asks a nurse about milieu therapy. The nurse responds, knowing that the primary focus of milieu therapy can best be described as which of the following?
1. A form of behavior modification therapy
2. A cognitive approach to changing behavior
3. A living, learning, or working environment
4. A behavioral approach to changing behavior

901. A nurse is caring for a client with a phobia who is being treated for the condition. The client is introduced to short periods of exposure to the phobic object while in a relaxed state. The nurse understands that this form of behavior modification can best be described as:
1. Milieu therapy
2. Aversion therapy
3. Self-control therapy
4. Systematic desensitization

902. A client with an eating disorder is planning to attend group meetings with Overeaters Anonymous, and a nurse describes this group to the client. The nurse determines that the client needs additional information if the client states which of the following about this self-help group?
1. "The leader is a nurse or psychiatrist."
2. "The members provide support to each other."
3. "People who have a similar problem are able to help others."
4. "It is designed to serve people who have a common problem."

903. A nurse is conducting a group therapy session, and a client with a manic disorder is monopolizing the group. The appropriate nursing action is which of the following?
1. Ask the client to leave.
2. Refer the client to another group.
3. Tell the client to stop monopolizing.
4. Thank the client for the contribution and tell him or her to allow others a chance to contribute.

Alternate Item Format: Multiple Response

904. Select the characteristics of the termination stage of group development. **Select all that apply.**
- ❑ 1. The group evaluates the experience.
- ❑ 2. The real work of the group is accomplished.
- ❑ 3. Group interaction involves superficial conversation.
- ❑ 4. Group members become acquainted with each other.
- ❑ 5. Some structuring of group norms, roles, and responsibilities takes place.
- ❑ 6. The group explores members' feelings about the group and the impending separation.

ANSWERS
895. 3

Rationale: In the termination stage, the group leader's task is to acknowledge the contributions of each member and the experience of the group as a whole. In this stage, the group members prepare for separation and assist each other to prepare for the future. Options 1 and 2 identify the tasks of the working stage. Option 4 identifies the orientation stage.

Test-Taking Strategy: Use the process of elimination. Eliminate options 1 and 2 first because they are comparable or alike. From the remaining options, note the relationship between the words *termination stage* in the question and option 3. Review the stages of group development if you had difficulty with this question.

Level of Cognitive Ability: Applying
Client Needs: Psychosocial Integrity
Integrated Process: Nursing Process—Implementation
Content Area: Mental Health
References: Stuart, G. (2009). *Principles and practice of psychiatric nursing* (9th ed., p. 601). St. Louis: Mosby.

Varcarolis, E., & Halter, M. (2009). *Essentials of psychiatric mental health nursing: A communication approach to evidence-based care* (pp. 113–114). St. Louis: Saunders.

896. 1

Rationale: All treatment team members are viewed as significant and valuable to the client's successful treatment outcomes in milieu therapy. Behavior modification is based on rewards and punishment. Rational emotive therapy deals with the correction of distorted thinking. Interpersonal therapy is based on a one-to-one or group therapy approach in which the therapist-client relationship is often used as a way for the client to examine other relationships in his or her life.

Test-Taking Strategy: Focus on the subject. Note the relationship between the words *helping clients to meet their treatment goals* and option 1. Review the types of therapy noted in the options if you had difficulty with this question.

Level of Cognitive Ability: Understanding
Client Needs: Psychosocial Integrity
Integrated Process: Nursing Process—Implementation
Content Area: Mental Health
References: Fortinash, K., & Holoday-Worret, P. (2008). *Psychiatric mental health nursing* (4th ed., p. 521). St. Louis: Mosby.

Stuart, G. (2009). *Principles and practice of psychiatric nursing* (9th ed., p. 157). St. Louis: Mosby.

897. 4

Rationale: Cognitive behavioral therapy is used to help the client identify and examine dysfunctional thoughts and to identify and examine values and beliefs that maintain these thoughts. Options 1, 2, and 3 are incorrect.

Test-Taking Strategy: Use the process of elimination and note the strategic words *cognitive behavioral*. Focusing on these words will direct you to option 4. If you are unfamiliar with this type of therapy and its purpose, review this content.

Level of Cognitive Ability: Understanding
Client Needs: Psychosocial Integrity
Integrated Process: Nursing Process—Planning
Content Area: Mental Health
References: Fortinash, K., & Holoday-Worret, P. (2008). *Psychiatric mental health nursing* (4th ed., pp. 517–518). St. Louis: Mosby.

Stuart, G. (2009). *Principles and practice of psychiatric nursing* (9th ed., p. 474). St. Louis: Mosby.

898. 4

Rationale: Cognitive therapy frequently is used for clients with depression. This type of therapy is based on exploring the client's subjective experience. Cognitive therapy includes examining the client's thoughts and feelings about situations and how these thoughts and feelings contribute to and perpetuate the client's difficulties and mood.

Test-Taking Strategy: Focusing on the word *cognitive* will assist you in selecting the correct option. Look for a similar word used in the question and repeated in one of the options. Note the relationship of the word *cognitive* in the question and *thoughts* in option 4. Review this form of therapy if you had difficulty with this question.

Level of Cognitive Ability: Applying
Client Needs: Psychosocial Integrity
Integrated Process: Nursing Process—Implementation
Content Area: Mental Health
Reference: Stuart, G. (2009). *Principles and practice of psychiatric nursing* (9th ed., pp. 305, 562–563). St. Louis: Mosby.

899. 1

Rationale: The first step in the 12-step program is to admit that a problem exists. Options 3 and 4 are unrealistic as a first step in the process to recovery. Although option 2 may be a strategy, it is not the first step.

Test-Taking Strategy: Use the process of elimination and note the strategic words *first step* in the question. This will assist in directing you to option 1. If you are unfamiliar with the 12-step program, review this content.

Level of Cognitive Ability: Applying
Client Needs: Psychosocial Integrity
Integrated Process: Nursing Process—Implementation
Content Area: Mental Health
References: Stuart, G. (2009). *Principles and practice of psychiatric nursing* (9th ed., pp. 416, 450). St. Louis: Mosby.

Varcarolis, E., & Halter, M. (2009). *Essentials of psychiatric mental health nursing: A communication approach to evidence-based care* (pp. 353–354). St. Louis: Saunders.

900. 3

Rationale: Milieu therapy, or "therapeutic community," has as its focus a living, learning, or working environment. Such therapy may be based on numerous therapeutic modalities ranging from structured behavioral therapy to spontaneous, humanistically oriented approaches. Although milieu may include behavioral approaches, option 3 describes its primary focus.

Test-Taking Strategy: Use the process of elimination. Note that options 1, 2, and 4 are comparable or alike and that option 3 identifies a comprehensive description. Review milieu therapy if you had difficulty with this question.

Level of Cognitive Ability: Understanding
Client Needs: Psychosocial Integrity
Integrated Process: Nursing Process—Implementation
Content Area: Mental Health
Reference: Stuart, G. (2009). *Principles and practice of psychiatric nursing* (9th ed., p. 157). St. Louis: Mosby.

901. 4

Rationale: Systematic desensitization is a form of therapy used when the client is introduced to short periods of exposure to the phobic object while in a relaxed state. Exposure is gradually increased until the anxiety about or fear of the object or situation has ceased. Options 1, 2, and 3 are incorrect.

Test-Taking Strategy: Use the process of elimination. Focus on the strategic words *introduced to short periods of exposure*. This will direct you to the correct option. If you had difficulty with this question, review systematic desensitization.

Level of Cognitive Ability: Understanding
Client Needs: Psychosocial Integrity
Integrated Process: Nursing Process—Implementation
Content Area: Mental Health
References: Fortinash, K., & Holoday-Worret, P. (2008). *Psychiatric mental health nursing* (4th ed., p. 180). St. Louis: Mosby.

Stuart, G. (2009). *Principles and practice of psychiatric nursing* (9th ed., p. 567). St. Louis: Mosby.

902. 1

Rationale: The sponsor of a self-help group is an experienced member of the group. A nurse or psychiatrist may be asked by the group to serve as a resource, but would not be the leader of the group. Options 2, 3, and 4 are characteristics of a self-help group.

Test-Taking Strategy: Use the process of elimination and focus on the subject, self-help group. Note the strategic words *needs additional information* in the question. Note that options 2, 3, and 4 are comparable or alike. This will direct you easily to option 1, the correct option. Review the characteristics of a self-help group if you had difficulty with this question.

Level of Cognitive Ability: Evaluating
Client Needs: Psychosocial Integrity
Integrated Process: Teaching and Learning
Content Area: Mental Health
Reference: Stuart, G. (2009). *Principles and practice of psychiatric nursing* (9th ed., p. 602). St. Louis: Mosby.

903. 4

Rationale: If a client is monopolizing the group, the nurse must be direct and decisive. The best action is to thank the client and suggest that the client stop talking and try listening to others. Although option 3 may be a direct response, option 4 is a more specific and direct statement. Options 1 and 2 are inappropriate.

Test-Taking Strategy: Use the process of elimination. Eliminate options 1 and 2 first because they are comparable or alike. Use therapeutic communication techniques to assist in directing you to option 4. If you had difficulty with this question, review therapeutic communication techniques for the client with a manic disorder.

Level of Cognitive Ability: Applying
Client Needs: Psychosocial Integrity
Integrated Process: Nursing Process—Implementation

Content Area: Mental Health
Reference: Stuart, G. (2009). *Principles and practice of psychiatric nursing* (9th ed., pp. 27–31, 287, 521, 602). St. Louis: Mosby.

ALTERNATE ITEM FORMAT: MULTIPLE RESPONSE
904. 1, 6

Rationale: The stages of group development include the initial stage, the working stage, and the termination stage. During the initial stage, the group members become acquainted with each other, and some structuring of group norms, roles, and responsibilities takes place. During the initial stage, group interaction involves superficial conversation During the working stage, the real work of the group is accomplished. During the termination stage, the group evaluates the experience and explores members' feelings about the group and the impending separation.

Test-Taking Strategy: Focus on the subject, the termination stage. Reading each item presented and recalling the stages of group development will assist you in answering this question. Review these stages if you had difficulty with this question.

Level of Cognitive Ability: Understanding
Client Needs: Psychosocial Integrity
Integrated Process: Nursing Process—Planning
Content Area: Mental Health
Reference: Varcarolis, E., & Halter, M. (2009). *Essentials of psychiatric mental health nursing: A communication approach to evidence-based care* (pp. 113–114). St. Louis: Saunders.

74

Mental Health Disorders

I. ANXIETY

A. Description
1. Anxiety is a normal response to stress.
2. It is a subjective experience that includes feelings of apprehension, uneasiness, uncertainty, or dread.
3. Anxiety occurs as a result of a threat that may be misperceived or misinterpreted or of a threat to identity or self-esteem.
4. Anxiety may result when values are threatened or preceding new experiences.

B. Types of anxiety
1. Normal: A healthy type of anxiety
2. Acute: Precipitated by imminent loss or change that threatens one's sense of security
3. Chronic: Anxiety that persists as a characteristic response to daily activities

C. Levels of anxiety
1. Mild
   a. Mild anxiety is associated with the tension of everyday life.
   b. The individual is alert.
   c. The perceptual field is increased.
   d. Mild anxiety can be motivating, produce growth, enhance creativity, and increase learning.
2. Moderate
   a. The focus is on immediate concerns.
   b. Moderate anxiety narrows the perceptual field.
   c. Selective inattentiveness occurs.
   d. Learning and problem solving still occur.
3. Severe
   a. Severe anxiety is a feeling that something bad is about to happen.
   b. A significant narrowing in the perceptual field occurs.
   c. Focus is on minute or scattered details.
   d. All behavior is aimed at relieving the anxiety.
   e. Learning and problem solving are impossible.
   f. The individual needs direction to focus.
4. Panic
   a. Panic is associated with dread and terror and a sense of impending doom.
   b. The personality is disorganized.
   c. The individual is unable to communicate or function effectively.
   d. Increased motor activity occurs.
   e. Loss of rational thoughts with distorted perception occurs.
   f. Inability to concentrate occurs.
   g. If prolonged, panic can lead to exhaustion and death.

D. Interventions: General nursing measures (see Priority Nursing Actions)

■■■ PRIORITY NURSING ACTIONS! ■■■

Actions to Take for a Client Experiencing Anxiety
1. Provide a calm environment, decrease environmental stimuli, and stay with the client.
2. Ask the client to identify what and how he or she feels.
3. Encourage the client to describe and discuss his or her feelings.
4. Help the client to identify the causes of the feelings if he or she is having difficulty doing so.
5. Listen to the client for expressions of helplessness and hopelessness.
6. Document the event, significant information, actions taken and follow-up actions, and the client's response.

If a client experiences anxiety, immediate actions are to provide a calm environment, decrease environmental stimuli, and stay with the client. Excess stimulation would escalate the anxiety. Next, asking the client to identify what and how he or she feels and helping the client to identify the causes of the feelings help to increase the client's awareness of the connection between behaviors and feelings. This awareness helps to decrease the anxiety. While listening to the client, the nurse observes for expressions of helplessness and hopelessness that could indicate self-harm intentions. The nurse provides follow-up care as needed based on observations and assessments. Finally, the nurse documents the event, significant information, actions taken and follow-up actions, and the client's response.

Reference: Varcarolis, E., & Halter, M. (2009). *Essentials of psychiatric mental health nursing: A communication approach to evidence-based care* (p. 132). St. Louis: Saunders.

1. Recognize the anxiety.
2. Establish trust.
3. Protect the client.
4. Do not criticize **coping mechanisms**.
5. Do not force the client into situations that provoke anxiety.
6. Decrease stimulation in the environment.
7. Modify the environment by setting limits or limiting interaction with others.
8. Provide creative outlets.
9. Provide activities that limit the amount of time for destructive behavior.
10. Promote relaxation techniques, such as breathing exercises or guided imagery.
11. Monitor vital signs, and administer antianxiety medications as prescribed.

⚠ The immediate nursing action for a client with anxiety is to decrease stimuli in the environment and provide a calm and quiet environment.

E. Interventions: Mild to moderate levels
1. Help the client identify the anxiety.
2. Encourage the client to talk about feelings and concerns.
3. Help the client identify thoughts and feelings that occurred before the onset of anxiety.
4. Encourage problem solving.
5. Encourage gross motor exercise.
F. Interventions: Severe to panic levels
1. Reduce the anxiety quickly.
2. Use a calm manner.
3. Always remain with the client.
4. Minimize environmental stimuli.
5. Provide clear, simple statements.
6. Use a low-pitched voice.
7. Attend to the physical needs of the client.
8. Provide gross motor activity.
9. Administer antianxiety medications as prescribed.

II. GENERALIZED ANXIETY DISORDER

A. Description
1. Generalized anxiety disorder is an unrealistic anxiety about everyday worries that persists over time and is not associated with another psychiatric or medical disorder.
2. Physical symptoms occur.
B. Assessment
1. Restlessness and inability to relax
2. Episodes of trembling and shakiness
3. Chronic muscular tension
4. Dizziness
5. Inability to concentrate
6. Chronic fatigue and sleep problems
7. Inability to recognize the connection between the anxiety and physical symptoms
8. Client is focused on the physical discomfort.

C. Panic disorder
1. Description
   a. Panic disorder produces a sudden onset of feelings of intense apprehension and dread.
   b. The cause usually cannot be identified.
   c. Severe, recurrent, intermittent anxiety attacks lasting 5 to 30 minutes occur.
2. Assessment
   a. Choking sensation
   b. Labored breathing
   c. Pounding heart
   d. Chest pain
   e. Dizziness
   f. Nausea
   g. Blurred vision
   h. Numbness or tingling of the extremities
   i. Sense of unreality and helplessness
   j. Fear of being trapped
   k. Fear of dying
3. Interventions
   a. Remain with the client.
   b. Attend to physical symptoms.
   c. Assist the client to identify the thoughts that aroused the anxiety and identify the basis for these thoughts.
   d. Assist the client to change the unrealistic thoughts to more realistic thoughts.
   e. Use cognitive restructuring to replace distorted thinking.
   f. Administer antianxiety medications if prescribed.

III. POSTTRAUMATIC STRESS DISORDER

A. Description: After experiencing a psychologically traumatic event, the individual is prone to re-experience the event and have recurrent and intrusive dreams or flashbacks.
B. Stressors
1. Natural disaster
2. Terrorist attack
3. Combat experiences
4. Accidents
5. Rape
6. Crime or violence
7. Sexual, physical, and emotional **abuse**
8. Re-experiencing the event as flashbacks
C. Assessment
1. Emotional numbness
2. Detachment
3. Depression
4. Anxiety
5. Sleep disturbances and nightmares
6. Flashbacks of event
7. Hypervigilance
8. Guilt about surviving the event
9. Poor concentration and avoidance of activities that trigger the memory of the event
D. Interventions (Box 74-1)

IV. PHOBIAS

A. Description
1. Irrational fear of an object or situation that persists, although the person may recognize it as unreasonable
2. Associated with panic level anxiety if the object, situation, or activity cannot be avoided
3. **Defense mechanisms** commonly used include repression and displacement.
B. Types (Box 74-2)
C. Interventions
1. Identify the basis of the anxiety.
2. Allow the client to verbalize feelings about the anxiety-producing object or situation; frequently talking about the feared object is the first step in the desensitization process.

Box 74-1 Interventions for Posttraumatic Stress Disorder

Be nonjudgmental and supportive.
Assure client that his or her feelings and behaviors are normal reactions.
Assist client to recognize the association between his or her feelings and behaviors and the trauma experience.
Encourage client to express his or her feelings; provide individual therapy that addresses loss of control or anger issues.
Assist client to develop adaptive coping mechanisms and to use relaxation techniques.
Encourage use of support groups
Facilitate a progressive review of the trauma experience.
Encourage client to establish and re-establish relationships.
Inform client that hypnotherapy or systematic desensitization may be used as a form of treatment.

Box 74-2 Types of Phobias

Acrophobia	Fear of heights
Agoraphobia	Fear of open spaces
Astraphobia	Fear of electrical storms
Claustrophobia	Fear of closed spaces
Hematophobia	Fear of blood
Hydrophobia	Fear of water
Monophobia	Fear of being alone
Mysophobia	Fear of dirt or germs
Nyctophobia	Fear of darkness
Pyrophobia	Fear of fires
Social phobia	Fear of situations in which one might be embarrassed or criticized; fear of making a fool of oneself
Xenophobia	Fear of strangers
Zoophobia	Fear of animals

---

3. Teach relaxation techniques, such as breathing exercises, muscle relaxation exercises, and visualization of pleasant situations.
4. Promote desensitization by gradually introducing the individual to the feared object or situation in small doses.

⚠ Always stay with the client experiencing anxiety to promote safety and security. Never force the client to have contact with the phobic object or situation.

V. OBSESSIVE-COMPULSIVE DISORDER

A. Obsessions: Preoccupation with persistently intrusive thoughts and ideas
B. Compulsions
1. A compulsion is the performance of rituals or repetitive behaviors designed to prevent some event, divert unacceptable thoughts, and decrease anxiety.
2. Obsessions and compulsions often occur together and can disrupt normal daily activities.
3. Anxiety occurs when one resists obsessions or compulsions and from being powerless to resist the thoughts or rituals.
4. Obsessive thoughts can involve issues of violence, aggression, sexual behavior, orderliness, or religion and uncontrollably can interrupt conscious thoughts and the ability to function.
C. Compulsive behavior patterns (behaviors or rituals)
1. Compulsive behavior patterns decrease the anxiety.
2. The patterns are associated with the obsessive thoughts.
3. The patterns neutralize the thought.
4. During stressful times, the ritualistic behavior increases.
5. **Defense mechanisms** include repression, displacement, and undoing.
D. Interventions (Box 74-3)

Box 74-3 Interventions for Obsessive-Compulsive Disorder

Ensure that basic needs (food, rest, grooming) are met.
Identify situations that precipitate compulsive behavior; encourage client to verbalize concerns and feelings.
Be empathetic toward client and aware of his or her need to perform the compulsive behavior.
Do not interrupt compulsive behaviors unless they jeopardize the safety of client or others (provide for client safety related to the behavior).
Allow time for client to perform the compulsive behavior, but set limits on behaviors that may interfere with client's physical well-being to protect client from physical harm.
Implement a schedule for client that distracts from the behaviors (structure simple activities, games, or tasks for client).
Establish a written contract that assists client to decrease the frequency of compulsive behaviors gradually.
Recognize and reinforce positive nonritualistic behaviors.

VI. SOMATOFORM DISORDERS

A. Description (Box 74-4)

1. Somatoform disorders are characterized by persistent worry or complaints regarding physical illness without supportive physical findings.
2. The client focuses on the physical signs and symptoms and is unable to control the signs and symptoms.
3. The physical signs and symptoms increase with psychosocial stressors.
4. The anxiety is redirected into a somatic concern.
5. The client may unconsciously use somatization for secondary gains, such as increased attention and decreased responsibilities.

B. Conversion disorder

1. Description
   a. A physical symptom or a deficit suggesting loss or altered body function related to psychological conflict or a neurological disorder.
   b. Conversion disorder is an expression of a psychological conflict or need.
   c. The most common conversion symptoms are blindness, deafness, paralysis, and the inability to talk.
   d. Conversion disorder has no organic cause.
   e. Symptoms are beyond the conscious control of the client and are directly related to conflict.
   f. The development of physical symptoms reduces anxiety.
2. Assessment
   a. "*La belle indifference*": Unconcerned with symptoms
   b. Physical limitation or disability
   c. Feelings of guilt, anxiety, or frustration
   d. Low self-esteem and feelings of inadequacy
   e. Unexpressed anger or conflict
   f. Secondary gain

C. Hypochondriasis

1. Description
   a. Preoccupation with fears of having a serious disease
   b. No evidence of physical illness exists.
   c. Hypochondriasis significantly impairs social and occupational functioning.
2. Assessment
   a. Preoccupation with physical functioning
   b. Frequent somatic complaints
   c. Complaints of fatigue and insomnia
   d. Anxiety
   e. Difficulty expressing feelings
   f. Extensive use of home remedies or nonprescription medications

Box 74-4 Types of Somatoform Disorders

Conversion disorder	Somatization disorder
Hypochondriasis	

g. Repeatedly visiting a physician despite repeated reassurance and normal test results
   h. Secondary gain

D. Somatization disorder

1. Description
   a. The client has multiple physical complaints involving numerous body systems.
   b. The cause of these complaints is presumed to be psychological.
2. Assessment
   a. Physical complaints of pain; denial of emotional problems; and signs of anxiety, fear, and low self-esteem may be present.
   b. Secondary gain: The client may unconsciously use somatization for secondary gains, such as increased attention and decreased responsibilities.

E. Interventions

1. Obtain a nursing history and assess for physical problems.
2. Explore the needs being met by the physical symptoms with the client.
3. Assist the client to identify alternative ways of meeting needs.
4. Assist the client to relate feelings and conflicts to the physical symptoms.
5. Convey understanding that the physical symptoms are real to the client.
6. Assure the client that physical illness has been ruled out.
7. Explore the source of anxiety and stimulate verbalization of anxiety.
8. Encourage the use of relaxation techniques as the anxiety increases.
9. Use a pain assessment scale if the client complains of pain, and implement pain reduction measures as required.
10. Report and assess any new physical complaint.
11. Encourage diversional activities.
12. Provide positive feedback.
13. Assist the client in recognizing his or her own feelings and emotions.
14. Administer antianxiety medications if prescribed.

⚠ For a client with a somatoform disorder, allow a specific time period for the client to discuss physical complaints because the client will feel less threatened if this behavior is limited rather than stopped completely. Avoid responding with positive reinforcement about the physical complaints.

VII. DISSOCIATIVE DISORDER

A. Description

1. Dissociative disorder is a disruption in integrative functions of memory, consciousness, or identity.
2. Dissociative disorder is associated with exposure to an extremely traumatic event.

B. Dissociative identity disorder (multiple personality)

1. Description
   a. Two or more fully developed, distinct and unique personalities exist within the client.
   b. The host is the primary personality, and the other personalities are referred to as *alters*.
   c. Alter personalities may take full control of the client, one at a time, and may or may not be aware of each other.
   d. The alters may be aware of the host, but the host is not usually aware of the alters.
2. Assessment
   a. The client may have an inability to recall important information (unrelated to ordinary forgetfulness).
   b. Transition from one personality to the other is related to stress or a traumatic event and is sudden.
   c. Dissociation is used as a method of distancing and defending one's self from anxiety and traumatizing experiences.

C. Dissociative amnesia
1. Description
   a. Inability to recall important personal information because it provokes anxiety
   b. Memory impairment may range from partial to almost complete.
2. Assessment
   a. Localized: The client blocks out all memories about a specified period.
   b. Selective: The client recalls some but not all memories about a specified period.
   c. Generalized: The client has a loss of all memory about past life.

D. Dissociative fugue
1. Description

   a. The client assumes a new identity in a new environment.
   b. The disorder may occur suddenly.
2. Assessment
   a. The client may drift from place to place.
   b. The client develops few social relationships.
   c. When the fugue lifts, the client returns home and is unable to recall the fugue state.

E. Depersonalization disorder
1. Description: An altered self-perception in which one's own reality is temporarily lost or changed
2. Assessment
   a. Feelings of detachment
   b. Intact reality testing

F. Interventions
1. Develop a trusting relationship with the client.
2. Encourage verbal expression of painful experiences, anxieties, and concerns.
3. Explore methods of coping.
4. Identify sources of conflict.
5. Focus on the client's strengths and skills.
6. Orient the client.
7. Provide nondemanding simple routines.
8. Allow the client to progress at his or her own pace.
9. Implement stress reduction techniques.
10. Plan for individual, group, or family psychotherapy to integrate dissociated aspects of personality or memory and to expand self-awareness.

VIII. MOOD DISORDERS

A. Bipolar disorder
1. Description (Box 74-5)
   a. Bipolar disorder is characterized by episodes of mania and depression with periods of normal mood and activity in between.

Box 74-5 Assessment of Bipolar Disorder

Mania	**Depression**
Becomes angry quickly	Increased or decreased appetite
Delusional self-confidence	Decrease in activities of daily living
Distracted by environmental stimuli	Decreased emotion and physical activity
Extroverted personality	Easily fatigued
Flight of ideas	Inability to make decisions
Grandiose and persecutory delusions	Poor concentration
High and unstable affect	Internalizing hostility
Significant decrease in appetite	Introverted personality
Inability to eat or sleep because of involvement in more important things	Social isolation and withdrawn from groups
Inability to sleep yet still active	Lack of energy
Unlimited energy	Lack of initiative
Inappropriate affect	Lack of self-confidence and low self-esteem
Inappropriate dress	Lack of sexual interest
Initiation of activity	Psychomotor retardation
Pressured speech	Suicidal thinking
Restlessness	
Sexually promiscuous	
Urgent motor activity	

Box 74-6 Dealing With Inappropriate Behaviors Associated With Bipolar Disorder

Aggressive Behavior

Assist client in identifying feelings of frustration and aggression.

Encourage client to talk out instead of acting out feelings of frustration.

Assist client in identifying precipitating events or situations that lead to aggressive behavior.

Describe the consequences of the behavior on self and others.

Assist in identifying previous coping mechanisms.

Assist client in problem-solving techniques to cope with frustration or aggression.

De-escalation Techniques

Maintain safety for client, other clients, and self.

Maintain large personal space and use a nonaggressive posture.

Use a calm approach and communicate with a calm, clear tone of voice (be assertive, not aggressive).

Determine what client considers to be his or her need.

Avoid verbal struggles.

Provide client with clear options that deal with client's behavior.

Assist client with problem solving and decision making regarding options.

Manipulative Behavior

Set clear, consistent, realistic, and enforceable limits, and communicate expected behaviors.

Be clear about consequences associated with exceeding set limits and follow through with consequences in a nonpunitive manner, if necessary.

Discuss client's behavior in a nonjudgmental and nonthreatening manner.

Avoid power struggles with client (avoid arguing with client).

Assist client in developing means of setting limits on own behavior.

---

b. The medication of choice has traditionally been lithium carbonate, which can be toxic and requires regular monitoring of serum lithium levels.

c. Other medications such as divalproex (Valproate) or olanzapine (Zyprexa) may be prescribed; carbamazepine (Tegretol) may also be prescribed to reduce the symptoms of acute bipolar manic episodes.

2. Interventions for mania (Box 74-6)

a. Remove hazardous objects from the environment.

b. Assess the client closely for fatigue.

c. Use comfort measures to promote sleep.

d. Provide frequent rest periods.

e. Monitor the client's sleep patterns.

f. Provide a private room if possible.

g. Administer a hypnotic or sedative medication as prescribed.

h. Encourage the client to ventilate feelings.

i. Use calm, slow interactions.

j. Help the client focus on one topic during the conversation.

k. Ignore or distract the client from grandiose thinking.

l. Present reality to the client.

m. Do not argue with the client.

n. Limit group activities and assess the client's tolerance level; solitary activities may be necessary.

o. Provide high-calorie finger foods and fluids.

p. Supervise the client's choice of clothing.

q. Reduce environmental stimuli.

r. Set limits on inappropriate behaviors.

s. Provide physical activities and outlets for tension.

t. Avoid competitive games.

u. Provide gross motor activities such as walking.

v. Provide structured activities or one-to-one activities with the nurse.

Box 74-7 Interventions for Depressed Clients

Assess for homicidal and suicidal ideation.

Provide safety from suicidal actions.

Assist with activities of daily living.

Use gentle encouragement to participate in activities of daily living and unit therapies.

Do not push decision making or making complex choices or decisions that client is not ready to make.

Monitor sleep patterns.

Monitor nutritional intake and weight.

Monitor for general hygiene and self-care deficits; deficits may indicate worsening depression.

Provide achievable activities in which client can achieve success (focus on strengths).

Remind client of times when he or she felt better and was successful.

Spend time with client to communicate client's value.

Respond to anger therapeutically.

---

w. Provide simple and direct explanations for routine procedures.

x. Supervise the administration of medication.

3. Major depressive disorder

a. Assessment (see Box 74-5)

b. Interventions for depressed clients (Box 74-7)

⚠ Monitor a depressed client closely for signs of suicidal ideation. If the client presents with increased energy, monitor closely because it could mean that the client now has the energy to perform the suicide act.

IX. SCHIZOPHRENIA

A. Description

1. Schizophrenia is a group of mental disorders characterized by psychotic features (hallucinations and

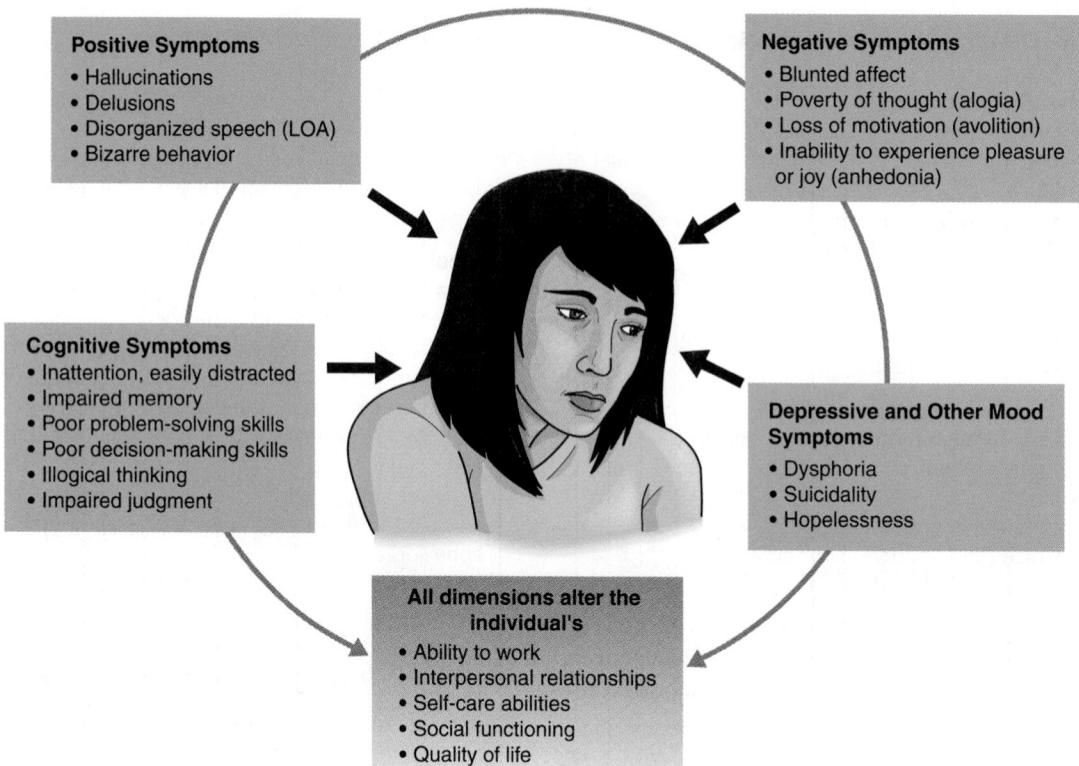

Positive Symptoms
- Hallucinations
- Delusions
- Disorganized speech (LOA)
- Bizarre behavior

Negative Symptoms
- Blunted affect
- Poverty of thought (alogia)
- Loss of motivation (avolition)
- Inability to experience pleasure or joy (anhedonia)

Cognitive Symptoms
- Inattention, easily distracted
- Impaired memory
- Poor problem-solving skills
- Poor decision-making skills
- Illogical thinking
- Impaired judgment

Depressive and Other Mood Symptoms
- Dysphoria
- Suicidality
- Hopelessness

All dimensions alter the individual's
- Ability to work
- Interpersonal relationships
- Self-care abilities
- Social functioning
- Quality of life

▲ **FIGURE 74-1** Treatment-relevant dimensions of schizophrenia. *LOA*, looseness of association. (From Varcarolis, E., Carson, V., Shoemaker, N. [2010]. *Foundations of psychiatric mental health nursing* [6th ed.]. St. Louis: Saunders.)

delusions), disordered thought processes, and disrupted interpersonal relationships.

2. Disturbances in affect, mood, behavior, and thought processes occur.

B. Assessment (Fig. 74-1)

1. Physical characteristics
   a. Unkempt appearance
   b. Body image distortions
   c. May be preoccupied with somatic complaints
   d. May neglect hygiene, eating, sleeping, and elimination
2. Motor activity (Box 74-8)
   a. Catatonic posturing: Holding bizarre postures for long periods
   b. Catatonic excitement: Moving excitedly, with no environmental stimuli present
   c. Possible total immobilization
   d. Inability to respond to commands or responding only to commands
   e. Waxy flexibility
   f. Repetitive or stereotyped movements
   g. Motor activity that may be increased, as evidenced by agitation, pacing, inability to sleep, loss of appetite and weight, and impulsiveness
   h. Possible inability to initiate activity (anergia)
3. Emotional characteristics
   a. Mistrust
   b. View of the world as threatening and unsafe

Box 74-8 Abnormal Motor Behaviors

Description
Abnormal motor behavior or activity displayed by mentally ill client that occurs as a result of a psychiatric disorder

Types
Echolalia
Repeating the speech of another person
Echopraxia
Repeating the movements of another person
Waxy flexibility
Having one's arms or legs placed in a certain position and holding that same position for hours

   c. Affect blunted, flat, or inappropriate
   d. May display feelings of ambivalence, helplessness, anxiety, anger, guilt, or depression in response to hallucinations or delusions or as a result of grief related to losses imposed by the illness
4. Compulsive rituals: Constant repetitive activity performed as an attempt to solve conflicting feelings
5. Overcompliance: Attempt to deny responsibility for any action by doing only what another person instructs exactly

Box 74-9 Abnormal Thought Processes

Description
Abnormal thought processes displayed by mentally ill client that occur as a result of a psychiatric disorder

Types
Circumstantiality
Before getting to the point or answering a question, client gets caught up in countless details and explanations
Confabulation
Filling a memory gap with detailed fantasy believed by the teller; the purpose of confabulation is to maintain self-esteem; seen in organic conditions such as Korsakoff's psychosis
Flight of ideas
Constant flow of speech in which client jumps from one topic to another in rapid succession; a connection between topics exists, although it is sometimes difficult to identify; seen in manic states
Looseness of association
Haphazard, illogical, and confused thinking and interrupted connections in thought; seen mostly in schizophrenic disorders
Neologisms
Client makes up words that have meaning only for the individual; often part of a delusional system
Thought blocking
Sudden cessation of a thought in the middle of a sentence; client is unable to continue the train of thought; often, sudden new thoughts come up unrelated to the topic
Word salad
Mixture of words and phrases that has no meaning

Box 74-10 Delusions

Description
A false belief held to be true, even when there is evidence to the contrary

Types
Grandeur
False belief that one is a powerful and important person
Jealousy
False belief that one's partner or mate is going out with other persons
Persecution
Thought that one is being singled out for harm by others

Interventions
Ask client to describe the delusion.
Be open and honest in interactions to reduce suspiciousness.
Focus conversation on reality-based topics, rather than on the delusion.
Encourage client to express feelings and focus on feelings that the delusions generate.
If client obsesses on the delusion, set firm limits on the amount of time for talking about the delusion.
Do not argue with client or try to convince client that the delusions are false.
Validate if part of the delusion is real.

6. Affective disturbances
   a. Flat or incongruent affect or inappropriate affect
   b. Altered thought processes
7. Abnormal thought processes (Box 74-9)
   a. Impaired reality testing
   b. Fragmentation of thoughts
   c. Thought blocking
   d. Loose associations
   e. Echolalia
   f. Distorted perception of the environment
   g. Neologisms
   h. Magical thinking
   i. Inability to conceptualize meaning in words or thoughts
   j. Inability to organize facts logically
   k. Delusions associated with thought processes or content
8. Types of delusions (Box 74-10)
   a. Loss of reference, in which the client believes that certain events, situations, or interactions are related directly to self
   b. Delusions of persecution, in which the client believes that he or she is being harassed, threatened, or persecuted by some powerful force
   c. Delusions of grandeur, in which the client attaches special significance to self in relation to others or the universe and has an exaggerated sense of self that has no basis in reality
   d. Somatic delusions, in which the client believes that his or her body is changing or responding in an unusual way, which has no basis in reality
9. Perceptual distortions
   a. Illusions, which may be brief experiences with a misinterpretation or misperception of reality
   b. Hallucinations (five senses) with no basis in reality (Box 74-11), such as perceiving objects, sensations, or images
10. Language and communication disturbances (Box 74-12)
    a. Related to disorders in thought process
    b. Inability to organize language
    c. Difficulty communicating clearly
    d. Inappropriate responses to a situation
    e. A single word or phrase may represent the whole meaning of the conversation such that the client may feel that he or she has communicated adequately.
    f. Development of a private language
C. Types of schizophrenia (Box 74-13)
   1. Catatonic schizophrenia
      a. Psychomotor disturbances
      b. Immobility

Box 74-11 Hallucinations

Description

Sense perception (occurs with one of the five senses) for which no external stimuli exist; can have an organic or functional cause

Types

Auditory
Hearing voices when none are present
Gustatory
Experiencing taste in the absence of stimuli
Olfactory
Smelling smells that do not exist
Tactile
Feeling touch sensations in the absence of stimuli
Visual
Seeing things that are not there

Interventions

Ask client directly about hallucination.
Avoid reacting to hallucination as if it were real.
Decrease stimuli or move client to another area.
Do not negate client's experience.
Focus on reality-based topics.
Attempt to engage client's attention through a concrete activity.
Respond verbally to anything real that client talks about.
Avoid touching client.
Monitor for signs of increasing anxiety or agitation, which may indicate that hallucinations are increasing.

Box 74-12 Language and Communication Disturbances

Clang association
Repetition of words or phrases that are similar in sound but in no other way
Echolalia
Repetition of words or phrases heard from another person
Mutism
Absence of verbal speech
Neologism
A new word devised that has special meaning only to the client
Pressured speech
Speaking as if the words are being forced out quickly
Verbigeration
Purposeless repetition of words or phrases
Word salad
Form of speech in which words or phrases are connected meaninglessly

Box 74-13 Types of Schizophrenia

Catatonic	Residual
Disorganized	Undifferentiated
Paranoid	

    h. Stereotyped or repetitive behavior
  2. Disorganized schizophrenia
    a. Extreme social withdrawal
    b. Disorganized speech or behavior
    c. Flat or inappropriate affect
    d. Silliness unrelated to speech
    e. Stereotyped behaviors
    f. Grimacing mannerisms
    g. Inability to perform activities of daily living
  3. Paranoid schizophrenia
    a. Suspiciousness
    b. Hostility
    c. Delusions
    d. Auditory hallucinations
    e. Anxiety and anger
    f. Aloofness
    g. Persecutory themes
    h. Violence
  4. Residual schizophrenia
    a. Diagnosed as schizophrenic in the past
    b. Time limited between attacks, but may last for many years
    c. The client exhibits considerable social isolation and withdrawal and impaired role functioning.
  5. Undifferentiated schizophrenia
    a. Undifferentiated schizophrenia does not meet the criteria for paranoid, disorganized, or catatonic schizophrenia.
    b. Delusions and hallucinations
    c. Disorganized speech
    d. Disorganized or catatonic behavior
    e. Flat affect
    f. Social withdrawal
D. Interventions (Box 74-14)
E. Interventions: Active hallucinations
  1. Monitor for hallucination cues and assess content of hallucinations.
  2. Intervene with one-on-one contact.
  3. Decrease stimuli or move the client to another area.
  4. Avoid conveying to the client that others also are experiencing the hallucination.
  5. Respond verbally to anything real that the client talks about.
  6. Avoid touching the client.
  7. Encourage the client to express feelings.
  8. During a hallucination, attempt to engage the client's attention through a concrete activity.
  9. Accept and do not joke about or judge the client's behavior.

    c. Stupor
    d. Waxy flexibility
    e. Excessive purposeless motor activity
    f. Echolalia
    g. Automatic obedience

Box 74-14 Interventions for Schizophrenia

Assess client's physical needs.

Set limits on client's behavior when it interferes with others and becomes disruptive.

Maintain a safe environment.

Initiate one-on-one interaction and progress to small groups as tolerated.

Spend time with client, even if client is unable to respond.

Monitor for altered thought processes.

Maintain ego boundaries and avoid touching client.

Limit the time of interaction with client.

Avoid an overly warm approach; a neutral approach is less threatening.

Do not make promises to client that cannot be kept.

Establish daily routines.

Assist client to improve grooming and accept responsibility for personal care.

Sit with client in silence if necessary.

Provide brief, frequent contact with client.

Tell client when you are leaving.

Tell client when you do not understand.

Do not "go along" with client's delusions or hallucinations.

Provide simple concrete activities, such as puzzles or word games.

Reorient client as necessary.

Help client establish what is real and unreal.

Stay with client if he or she is frightened.

Speak to client in a simple, direct, and concise manner.

Reassure client that the environment is safe.

Remove client from group situations if client's behavior is too bizarre, disturbing, or dangerous to others.

Set realistic goals.

Initially, do not offer choices to client, and gradually assist client in making his or her own decisions.

Use canned or packaged food, especially with a paranoid schizophrenic client.

Provide a radio or tape player at night for insomnia.

Explain to client everything that is being done.

Set limits on client's behavior if client is unable to do so.

Decrease excessive stimuli in the environment.

Monitor for suicide risk.

Assist client to use alternative means to express feelings, such as through music or art therapy or writing.

10. Provide easy activities and a structured environment with routine activities of daily living.
11. Monitor for signs of increasing fear, anxiety, or agitation.
12. Decrease stimuli as needed.
13. Administer medications as prescribed.

⚠ For a client with hallucinations, safety is the first priority—ensure that the client does not have an auditory command telling him or her to harm self or others.

F. Interventions: Delusions
   1. Interact based on reality.
   2. Encourage the client to express feelings.
   3. Do not dispute the client or try to convince the client that delusions are false.
   4. Initiate activities on a one-on-one basis.
   5. Alter hospital routines as necessary, such as using canned or packaged food or food from home.
   6. Recognize accomplishments and provide positive feedback for successes.

X. PARANOID DISORDERS

A. Description
   1. Paranoid disorder is a concrete, pervasive delusional system characterized by persecutory and grandiose beliefs.
   2. The client exhibits suspiciousness and mistrust of others.
   3. The client often is viewed by others as hostile, stubborn, and defensive.

B. Behaviors

1. Suspicious and mistrustful
2. Emotionally distant
3. Distortion of reality
4. Poor insight and poor judgments
5. Hypervigilance
6. Low self-esteem
7. Highly sensitive, difficulty in admitting own error, and taking pride in being correct
8. Hypercritical and intolerant of others
9. Hostile, aggressive, and quarrelsome
10. Evasive
11. Concrete thinking

C. Delusions
   1. Delusions serve a purpose in establishing identity and self-esteem.
   2. The client may have grandiose and persecutory delusions.
   3. Process of delusion includes denial, projection, and rationalization.
   4. As trust in others increases, the need for delusions decreases.

D. Types of paranoid disorders (Box 74-15)
   1. Paranoid personality disorder (see later)
      a. Suspicious
      b. Nonpsychotic
      c. No hallucinations or delusions
      d. No symptoms of schizophrenia
   2. Paranoia-induced state
      a. Abrupt onset in response to stress; subsides when stress decreases
      b. No hallucinations, but experiences paranoid delusions
      c. May be sensitive and suspicious before the development of delusions

   d. No symptoms of schizophrenia
3. Paranoia
   a. Exhibits an organized delusional system
   b. No hallucinations
   c. Reserved and sensitive before onset
   d. Psychotic state
   e. No symptoms of schizophrenia
4. Paranoid schizophrenia
   a. Before the onset, the client becomes cold, withdrawn, distrustful, resentful, argumentative, sarcastic, and defiant.
   b. Bizarre, numerous, and changeable delusions occur.
   c. Delusions become less logical as the client becomes more disorganized.
   d. Persecutory hallucinations occur.
   e. Psychotic state ensues.
   f. All symptoms of schizophrenia are present.
E. Interventions (Box 74-16)

⚠ Do not whisper or laugh in front of a client with a paranoid disorder because the client will think that you are talking about or laughing at him or her; this increases the paranoia.

XI. PERSONALITY DISORDERS

A. Description
   1. Personality disorders include various inflexible maladaptive behavior patterns or traits that may impair functioning and relationships.
   2. The client usually remains in touch with reality and typically has a lack of insight into his or her behavior.

3. Stress exacerbates manifestations of the personality disorder.
4. In severe cases, the personality disorder may deteriorate to a psychotic state.

B. Characteristics
1. Poor impulse control
   a. Acting out to manage internal pain
   b. Forms of acting out include physical and verbal attacks, such as yelling and swearing, and self-injurious behaviors, such as cutting own skin, banging the head, punching self, manipulation, substance **abuse**, promiscuous sexual behaviors, and **suicide attempts**.
   c. The client may be preoccupied with self, religion, or sex.
2. Mood characteristics
   a. May experience abandonment and depression
   b. Moods may include rage, guilt, fear, and emptiness.
3. Impaired judgment
   a. Difficulty with problem solving
   b. Inability to perceive the consequences of behavior
4. Impaired reality testing: Distortion of reality and often projection of own feelings onto others
5. Impaired object relations: Rigid and inflexible, with difficulty in intimate relationships
6. Impaired self-perception: Distorted self-perception and experience of self-hate or self-idealization
7. Impaired thought processes
   a. Concrete or diffuse thinking
   b. Difficulty concentrating
   c. Impaired memory
8. Impaired stimulus barrier
   a. Inability to regulate incoming sensory stimuli
   b. Increased excitability
   c. Excessive response to noise and light
   d. Poor attention span
   e. Agitated
   f. Insomnia

Box 74-15 Types of Paranoid Disorders

Paranoid personality	Paranoia
Paranoid state	Paranoid schizophrenia

Box 74-16 Interventions for Paranoid Disorders

Assess for suicide risk.	Refocus conversation to reality-based topics.
Diminish suspicious behavior.	Use role playing to help client identify thoughts and feelings.
Avoid direct eye contact.	
Establish a trusting relationship.	Provide positive reinforcement for successes.
Promote increased self-esteem.	Do not argue with delusions.
Remain calm, nonthreatening, and nonjudgmental.	Use concrete, specific words.
Provide continuity of care.	Do not be secretive with client.
Respond honestly to client.	Do not whisper in client's presence.
Follow through on commitments made to client.	Assure client that he or she will be safe.
Acknowledge client's feelings, but tell client that you do not share his or her interpretation of an event.	Involve client in noncompetitive tasks.
	Provide client with the opportunity to complete small tasks.
Provide a daily schedule of activities.	Monitor eating, drinking, sleeping, and elimination patterns.
Assist client to identify diversionary activities.	Limit physical contact.
Gradually introduce client to groups.	Monitor for agitation, and decrease stimuli as needed.

C. Cluster A personality disorder types include the odd, eccentric types—schizoid, schizotypal, and paranoid.
1. Schizoid personality disorder is characterized by an inability to form warm, close social relationships.
   a. Social detachment and lack of close relationships
   b. Interest in solitary activities
   c. Aloof and indifferent
   d. Restricted expression of emotions
   e. Lack of interest in others
2. Schizotypal personality disorder is characterized by the display of abnormal or highly unusual thoughts, perceptions, speech, and behavior patterns.
   a. Suspicious
   b. Paranoia
   c. Magical thinking
   d. Odd thinking and speech
   e. Relationship deficits
3. Paranoid personality disorder is characterized by suspiciousness and mistrust of others (paranoia).
   a. May be suspicious and distrusting
   b. May be argumentative
   c. May be hostile, aloof
   d. May be rigid, critical, and controlling of others
   e. May have thoughts of grandiosity

D. Cluster B personality disorders include the over-emotional, erratic types—histrionic, narcissistic, antisocial, and borderline.
1. Histrionic personality disorder is characterized by overly dramatic and intensely expressive behavior.
   a. Lively and dramatic and enjoys being the center of attention
   b. Has poor and shallow interpersonal relations
   c. May be sexually seductive or provocative
   d. Dramatizes his or her life and may appear theatrical
   e. Overly concerned with appearance
   f. Easily bored
2. Narcissistic personality disorder is characterized by an increased sense of self-importance and preoccupation with fantasies and unlimited success.
   a. Need for admiration and inflation of accomplishments
   b. Overestimation of abilities and underestimation of contributions of others
   c. Lack of empathy and sensitivity to needs of others
3. Antisocial personality disorder comprises a pattern of irresponsible and antisocial behavior, selfishness, an inability to maintain lasting relationships, poor sexual adjustment, a failure to accept social norms, and a tendency toward irritability and aggressiveness.
   a. Perceives the world as hostile
   b. Superficial charm and hostility
   c. No shame or guilt
   d. Self-centered
   e. Unreliable
   f. Easily bored
   g. Poor work history
   h. Inability to tolerate frustration
   i. View others as objects to be manipulated
   j. Poor judgment
   k. Impulsive
4. Borderline personality disorder is characterized by instability in interpersonal relationships, unstable mood and self-image, and impulsive and unpredictable behavior.
   a. Unclear identity
   b. Unstable and intense
   c. Extreme shifts in mood
   d. Easily angered
   e. Easily bored
   f. Argumentative
   g. Depression
   h. Self-destructive behavior
   i. Manipulation
   j. Inability to tolerate anxiety
   k. Chronic feelings of emptiness and fear of being alone
   l. Splitting—sees others as all good or all bad; creates conflict between individuals by playing one person against another

E. Cluster C personality disorders include the anxious, fearful types of personality disorders—obsessive-compulsive personality, avoidant, and dependent.
1. Obsessive-compulsive personality disorder is characterized by difficulty expressing warm and tender emotions, perfectionism, stubbornness, the need to control others, and a devotion to work.
   a. Overly conscientious
   b. Inflexible and preoccupied with details and rules
   c. Extremely devoted to work to the exclusion of leisure activities and friendships
   d. Miserly and stubborn
   e. Hoarding behavior
   f. Engages in rituals
2. Avoidant personality disorder is characterized by social withdrawal and extreme sensitivity to potential rejection.
   a. Feelings of inadequacy
   b. Hypersensitive to reactions of others and poor reaction to criticism
   c. Social isolation
   d. Lack of support system
3. Dependent personality disorder is characterized by an intense lack of self-confidence, low self-esteem, and inability to function independently,

such that the individual passively allows others to make decisions and assume responsibility for major areas in the person's life; the dependent client has great difficulty making decisions.

F. General interventions for a client with a personality disorder

1. Maintain safety against self-destructive behaviors.
2. Allow the client to make choices and be as independent as possible.
3. Encourage the client to discuss feelings rather than act them out.
4. Provide consistency in response to the client's acting-out behaviors.
5. Discuss expectations and responsibilities with the client.
6. Discuss the consequences that will follow certain behaviors.
7. Inform the client that harm to self, others, and property is unacceptable.
8. Identify splitting behavior.
9. Assist the client to deal directly with anger.
10. Develop a written safety or behavioral contract with the client.
11. Encourage the client to keep a journal recording daily feelings.
12. Encourage the client to participate in group activities, and praise nonmanipulative behavior.
13. Set and maintain limits to decrease manipulative behavior.
14. Remove the client from group situations in which attention-seeking behaviors occur.
15. Provide realistic praise for positive behaviors in social situations.

XII. COGNITIVE IMPAIRMENT DISORDERS

A. Autism: See Chapter 36.
B. Attention-deficit/hyperactivity disorder: See Chapter 36.
C. Dementia and Alzheimer's disease
1. Dementia
   a. Dementia is a syndrome with progressive deterioration in intellectual functioning secondary to structural or functional changes.
   b. Long-term and short-term memory loss occur, with impairment in judgment, abstract thinking, problem-solving ability, and behavior.
   c. Dementia results in a self-care deficit.
   d. The most common type of dementia is Alzheimer's disease.
2. Alzheimer's disease (Box 74-17)
   a. Alzheimer's disease is an irreversible form of senile dementia caused by nerve cell deterioration.
   b. Individuals with Alzheimer's disease experience cognitive deterioration and progressive loss of ability to carry out activities of daily living.

Box 74-17 Alzheimer's Disease

Agnosia
Failure to recognize or identify familiar objects despite intact sensory function
Amnesia
Loss of memory caused by brain degeneration
Aphasia
Language disturbance in understanding and expressing spoken words
Apraxia
Inability to perform motor activities, despite intact motor function

---

   c. The client experiences a steady decline in physical and mental functioning and usually requires long-term care in a specialized facility in the final stages of the illness.
3. Interventions
   a. Identify and reinforce retained skills.
   b. Provide continuity of care.
   c. Orient the client to the environment.
   d. Furnish the environment with familiar possessions.
   e. Acknowledge the client's feelings.
   f. Assist the client and family members to manage memory deficits and behavior changes.
   g. Encourage family members to express feelings about caregiving.
   h. Provide the caregiver with support and identify the resources and support groups available.
   i. Monitor the client's activities of daily living.
   j. Remind the client how to perform self-care activities.
   k. Help the client maintain independence.
   l. Provide the client with consistent routines.
   m. Provide the client with exercise, such as walking with an escort.
   n. Avoid activities that tax the memory.
   o. Allow the client plenty of time to complete a task.
   p. Use constant encouragement with the client with a simple step-by-step approach.
   q. Provide the client with activities that distract and occupy time, such as listening to music, coloring, and watching television.
   r. Provide the client with mental stimulation with simple games or activities.
4. Wandering
   a. Provide the client with a safe environment.
   b. Prevent unsafe wandering.
   c. Provide the client with close supervision.
   d. Close and secure doors.
   e. Use identification bracelets and electronic surveillance.

 Providing a safe environment is a priority in the care of a client with Alzheimer's disease.

5. Communication
   a. Adapt to the communication level of the client.
   b. Use a firm volume and a low-pitched voice to communicate.
   c. Stand directly in front of the client and maintain eye contact.
   d. Call the client by name and identify self; wait for a response.
   e. Use a calm and reassuring voice.
   f. Use pantomime gestures if the client is unable to understand spoken words.
   g. Speak slowly and clearly, using short words and simple sentences.
   h. Ask only one question at a time and give one direction at a time.
   i. Repeat questions if necessary, but do not rephrase.
6. Impaired judgment
   a. Remove throw rugs, toxic substances, and dangerous electrical appliances from the environment.
   b. Reduce hot water heater temperature.
7. Altered thought processes
   a. Call the client by name.
   b. Orient the client frequently.
   c. Use familiar objects in the room.
   d. Place a calendar and clock in a visible place.
   e. Maintain familiar routines.
   f. Allow the client to reminisce.
   g. Make tasks simple.
   h. Allow time for the client to complete a task.
   i. Provide positive reinforcement for positive behaviors.
8. Altered sleep patterns
   a. Allow the client to wander in a safe place until he or she becomes tired.
   b. Prevent shadows in the room by using indirect light.
   c. Avoid the use of hypnotics because they cause confusion and aggravate the sundown effect.
9. Agitation
   a. Assess the precipitant of the agitation.
   b. Reassure the client.
   c. Remove items that can be hazardous when the client is agitated.
   d. Approach the client slowly and calmly from the front, and speak, gesture, and move slowly.
   e. Remove the client to a less stressful environment; decrease excess stimuli.
   f. Use touch gently.
   g. Do not argue with or force the client.

XIII. PSYCHOSEXUAL ALTERATIONS

A. Sexuality
   1. One's sense of being a sexual individual
   2. Includes how one looks, behaves, and relates to others

Box 74-18 Sexual Expression

Bisexuality
Sexual attraction to and activity with both genders
Heterosexuality
Male-female sexual relationships
Homosexuality
Sexual attraction to a member of the same gender
Transvestism
Obsession with wearing clothing of the opposite gender

B. Sexual expression (Box 74-18)
C. Alterations in sexual behavior
   1. Transsexualism: Feeling that one's gender is inappropriate and desiring to acquire sexual characteristics of the opposite gender
   2. Exhibitionism: Sexual urges and fantasies that result in exposure of genitals to strangers to bring sexual gratification or arousal
   3. Fetishism: Using nonliving objects for sexual gratification
   4. Pedophilia: Desiring sexual activity with a child younger than 13 years of age
   5. Sexual masochism: Sexual gratification that involves receiving pain
   6. Sexual sadism: Sexual gratification that involves inflicting pain
   7. Voyeurism: Sexual gratification through observing others disrobing or engaging in sexual activity
   8. Zoophilia: Intense sexual arousal or desire for sexual contact with animals
   9. Frotteurism: Intense sexual arousal or desire when rubbing against a nonconsenting person
D. Interventions
   1. Assess sexual history, history of trauma or **abuse**, and precipitating event for the sexual disorder.
   2. Encourage the client to explore personal beliefs.
   3. Provide a nonjudgmental attitude.
   4. Provide supportive psychotherapy.

MORE QUESTIONS ON THE CD!

Practice Questions

905. A client who is delusional says to a nurse, "The federal guards were sent to kill me." The nurse's best response is:
   1. "I don't believe this is true."
   2. "The guards are not out to kill you."
   3. "What makes you think the guards were sent to hurt you?"
   4. "I don't know anything about the guards. Do you feel afraid that people are trying to hurt you?"

906. A male client with delirium becomes disoriented and confused in his room at night. The best initial nursing intervention is to:
1. Move the client next to the nurse's station.
2. Use an indirect light source and turn off the television.
3. Keep the television and a soft light on during the night.
4. Play soft music during the night, and maintain a well-lit room.

907. A client is admitted to the mental health unit with a diagnosis of depression. A nurse develops a plan of care for the client and includes which appropriate activity in the plan?
1. Reading and writing most of the day
2. Several activities from which the client can choose
3. Nothing, until the client asks to participate in milieu
4. A structured program of activities in which the client can participate

908. When planning the discharge of a client with chronic anxiety, a nurse directs the goals at promoting a safe environment at home. The appropriate maintenance goal should focus on which of the following?
1. Ignoring feelings of anxiety
2. Identifying anxiety-producing situations
3. Continued contact with a crisis counselor
4. Eliminating all anxiety from daily situations

909. A client is unwilling to go out of the house for fear of "doing something crazy in public." Because of this fear, the client remains homebound except when accompanied outside by the spouse. Based on these data, a nurse determines that the client is experiencing:
1. Agoraphobia
2. Social phobia
3. Claustrophobia
4. Hypochondriasis

910. A nurse is conducting a group therapy session. During the session, a client with mania consistently talks and dominates the group session, and this behavior is disrupting group interactions. The nurse would initially:
1. Ask the client to leave the group session.
2. Ask another nurse to escort the client out of the group session.
3. Tell the client that she will not be able to attend any future group sessions.
4. Tell the client that she needs to allow other clients in the group time to talk.

911. A client is admitted to a medical nursing unit with a diagnosis of acute blindness. Many tests are performed, and there seems to be no organic reason why this client cannot see. The client became blind after witnessing a hit-and-run car accident, when a family of three was killed. A nurse suspects that the client may be experiencing a:
1. Psychosis
2. Repression
3. Conversion disorder
4. Dissociative disorder

912. A manic client announces to everyone in the dayroom that a stripper is coming to perform this evening. When a nurse firmly states that this is inappropriate and will not happen, the client becomes verbally abusive and threatens physical violence to the nurse. Based on the analysis of this situation, the nurse determines that the appropriate action would be to:
1. Orient the client to time, person, and place.
2. Tell the client that the behavior is inappropriate.
3. Escort the manic client to her room, with assistance.
4. Tell the client that smoking privileges are revoked for 24 hours.

913. A nurse is planning activities for a client who has bipolar disorder with aggressive social behavior. Which of the following activities would be most appropriate for this client?
1. Chess
2. Writing
3. Ping pong
4. Basketball

914. A nurse observes that a client is pacing, agitated, and presenting aggressive gestures. The client's speech pattern is rapid, and affect is belligerent. Based on these observations, the nurse's immediate priority of care is to:
1. Provide safety for the client and other clients on the unit.
2. Provide the clients on the unit with a sense of comfort and safety.
3. Assist the staff in caring for the client in a controlled environment.
4. Offer the client a less stimulated area to calm down and gain control.

915. A nurse is discharging a client with a history of command hallucinations to harm self or others. The nurse provides instructions to the client about interventions for hallucinations and anxiety and determines that the client understands the instructions if the client states:

1. "My medications won't make me anxious."
2. "I'll go to support group and talk so that I don't hurt anyone."
3. "I won't get anxious or hear things if I get enough sleep and eat well."
4. "I can call my therapist when I'm hallucinating so that I can talk about my feelings and plans and not hurt anyone."

916. A nurse is caring for a male client diagnosed with catatonic stupor. The client is lying on the bed with his body pulled into a fetal position. The appropriate nursing intervention is which of the following?

1. Ask direct questions to encourage talking.
2. Leave the client alone and intermittently check on him.
3. Sit beside the client in silence with occasional open-ended questions.
4. Take the client into the dayroom with other clients so that they can help watch him.

917. A client is admitted to the mental health unit with a diagnosis of schizophrenia. A nursing diagnosis formulated for the client is *disturbed thought processes related to paranoia*. In formulating nursing interventions with the members of the health care team, a nurse provides instructions to:

1. Increase socialization of the client with peers.
2. Avoid laughing or whispering in front of the client.
3. Begin to educate the client about social supports in the community.
4. Have the client sign a release of information to appropriate parties so that adequate data can be obtained for assessment purposes.

Alternate Item Format:
Multiple Response

918. Select the nursing interventions for a hospitalized client with mania who is exhibiting manipulative behavior. **Select all that apply**.

- ❑ 1. Communicate expected behaviors to the client.
- ❑ 2. Ensure that the client knows that he or she is not in charge of the nursing unit.
- ❑ 3. Assist the client in identifying ways of setting limits on personal behaviors.
- ❑ 4. Follow through about the consequences of behavior in a nonpunitive manner.
- ❑ 5. Enforce rules and inform the client that he or she will not be allowed to attend therapy groups.
- ❑ 6. Be clear with the client regarding the consequences of exceeding limits that have been set regarding behavior.

ANSWERS
905. 4
Rationale: It is most therapeutic for the nurse to empathize with the client's experience. Disagreeing with delusions may make the client more defensive, and the client may cling to the delusions even more. Encouraging discussion regarding the delusion is inappropriate.
Test-Taking Strategy: Use therapeutic communication techniques. Eliminate options 1 and 2 because they are comparable or alike and are statements that disagree with the client. Option 3 encourages discussion regarding the delusion. Review communication techniques with a client experiencing delusions if you had difficulty with this question.
Level of Cognitive Ability: Applying
Client Needs: Psychosocial Integrity
Integrated Process: Communication and Documentation
Content Area: Mental Health
Reference: Stuart, G. (2009). *Principles and practice of psychiatric nursing* (9th ed., pp. 27–31, 339–340). St. Louis: Mosby.

906. 2
Rationale: Provision of a consistent daily routine and a low stimulating environment is important when a client is disoriented. Noise, including radio and television, may add to the confusion and disorientation. Moving the client next to the nurses' station is not the initial action.

Test-Taking Strategy: Use the process of elimination and note the strategic word *initial* in the question. Eliminate options 3 and 4 first because they are comparable or alike. Focusing on the strategic word will direct you easily to option 2. Review measures related to a client who is disoriented and confused if you had difficulty with this question.
Level of Cognitive Ability: Applying
Client Needs: Psychosocial Integrity
Integrated Process: Nursing Process—Implementation
Content Area: Mental Health
Reference: Varcarolis, E., & Halter, M. (2009). *Essentials of psychiatric mental health nursing: A communication approach to evidence-based care* (p. 312). St. Louis: Saunders.

907. 4
Rationale: A client with depression often has a depressed mood and is withdrawn. The client also experiences difficulty concentrating, loss of interest or pleasure, low energy, fatigue, and feelings of worthlessness and poor self-esteem. The plan of care needs to provide successful experiences in a stimulating yet structured environment. Options 1, 2, and 3 are too "restrictive" and offer little or no structure and stimulation.
Test-Taking Strategy: Use the process of elimination. Recall that a depressed client requires a structured and stimulating program in a safe environment. Option 4 is the only option that will provide a safe and effective environment. Review

care of the client with depression if you had difficulty with this question.
Level of Cognitive Ability: Applying
Client Needs: Psychosocial Integrity
Integrated Process: Nursing Process—Planning
Content Area: Mental Health
Reference: Stuart, G. (2009). *Principles and practice of psychiatric nursing* (9th ed., p. 307). St. Louis: Mosby.

908. 2
Rationale: Recognizing situations that produce anxiety allows the client to prepare to cope with anxiety or avoid a specific stimulus. Counselors will not be available for all anxiety-producing situations, and this option does not encourage the development of internal strengths. Ignoring feelings will not resolve anxiety. Elimination of all anxiety from life is impossible.
Test-Taking Strategy: Use the process of elimination. Eliminate option 4 first because of the word *all*. Eliminate option 1 next because feelings should not be ignored. From the remaining options, select option 2 because this option is more client-centered and helps prepare the client to deal with anxiety should it occur. Review home care planning for a client with chronic anxiety if you had difficulty with this question.
Level of Cognitive Ability: Applying
Client Needs: Safe and Effective Care Environment
Integrated Process: Nursing Process—Planning
Content Area: Mental Health
Reference: Fortinash, K., & Holoday-Worret, P. (2008). *Psychiatric mental health nursing* (4th ed., p. 189). St. Louis: Mosby.

909. 1
Rationale: Agoraphobia is a fear of open spaces and the fear of being trapped in a situation from which there may not be an escape. Agoraphobia includes the possibility of experiencing a sense of helplessness or embarrassment if an attack occurs. Avoidance of such situations usually results in reduction of social and professional interactions. Social phobia focuses more on specific situations, such as the fear of speaking, performing, or eating in public. Claustrophobia is a fear of closed places. Clients with hypochondriacal symptoms focus their anxiety on physical complaints and are preoccupied with their health.
Test-Taking Strategy: Use the process of elimination. Focusing on the strategic words *remains homebound* will direct you to option 1. If you had difficulty with this question, review phobia types and associated client behaviors.
Level of Cognitive Ability: Understanding
Client Needs: Psychosocial Integrity
Integrated Process: Nursing Process—Assessment
Content Area: Mental Health
Reference: Varcarolis, E., & Halter, M. (2009). *Essentials of psychiatric mental health nursing: A communication approach to evidence-based care* (pp. 137–138). St. Louis: Saunders.

910. 4
Rationale: Manic clients may be talkative and can dominate group meetings or therapy sessions by their excessive talking. If this occurs, the nurse initially would set limits on the client's behavior. Initially, asking the client to leave the session or asking another person to escort the client out of the session

is inappropriate. This may agitate the client and escalate the client's behavior further. Option 3 is also an inappropriate initial action because it violates the client's right to receive treatment and is a threatening action.
Test-Taking Strategy: Use the process of elimination and note the strategic word *initially*. Eliminate options 1 and 2 first because they are comparable or alike. Next, eliminate option 3 because it violates the client's right to receive treatment and is a threatening action. Remember that setting firm limits with the client initially is best. Review care of a client with mania if you had difficulty with this question.
Level of Cognitive Ability: Applying
Client Needs: Psychosocial Integrity
Integrated Process: Nursing Process—Implementation
Content Area: Mental Health
Reference: Stuart, G. (2009). *Principles and practice of psychiatric nursing* (9th ed., pp. 287, 521). St. Louis: Mosby.

911. 3
Rationale: A conversion disorder is the alteration or loss of a physical function that cannot be explained by any known pathophysiological mechanism. A conversion disorder is thought to be an expression of a psychological need or conflict. In this situation, the client witnessed an accident that was so psychologically painful that the client became blind. A dissociative disorder is a disturbance or alteration in the normally integrative functions of identity, memory, or consciousness. Psychosis is a state in which a person's mental capacity to recognize reality, communicate, and relate to others is impaired, interfering with the person's ability to deal with life's demands. Repression is a coping mechanism in which unacceptable feelings are kept out of awareness.
Test-Taking Strategy: Use the process of elimination. The key to the correct option lies in the fact that the client presents no organic reason to account for the blindness—hence, a conversion disorder. If you had difficulty with this question, review defense mechanisms and the concepts associated with a conversion disorder.
Level of Cognitive Ability: Understanding
Client Needs: Psychosocial Integrity
Integrated Process: Nursing Process—Assessment
Content Area: Mental Health
References: Stuart, G. (2009). *Principles and practice of psychiatric nursing* (9th ed., pp. 251, 243). St. Louis: Mosby.
Varcarolis, E., & Halter, M. (2009). *Essentials of psychiatric mental health nursing: A communication approach to evidence-based care* (pp. 157–158). St. Louis: Saunders.

912. 3
Rationale: The client is at risk for injury to self and others and should be escorted out of the dayroom. Option 4 may increase the agitation that already exists in this client. Orientation will not halt the behavior. Telling the client that the behavior is inappropriate already has been attempted by the nurse.
Test-Taking Strategy: Use the process of elimination and Maslow's Hierarchy of Needs theory to answer the question. Look for the option that promotes safety of the client, other clients, and staff. If you had difficulty with this question, review the appropriate interventions when dealing with a manic client.

Level of Cognitive Ability: Applying
Client Needs: Safe and Effective Care Environment
Integrated Process: Nursing Process—Implementation
Content Area: Mental Health
References: Fortinash, K., & Holoday-Worret, P. (2008). *Psychiatric mental health nursing* (4th ed., pp. 221, 230). St. Louis: Mosby.

Varcarolis, E., & Halter, M. (2009). *Essentials of psychiatric mental health nursing: A communication approach to evidence-based care* (p. 259). St. Louis: Saunders.

913. 2

Rationale: Solitary activities that require a short attention span with mild physical exertion are the most appropriate activities for a client who is exhibiting aggressive behavior. Writing (journaling), walks with staff, and finger painting are activities that minimize stimuli and provide a constructive release for tension. Competitive games should be avoided because they can stimulate aggression and increase psychomotor activity.
Test-Taking Strategy: Use the process of elimination. Options 1, 3, and 4 are comparable or alike in that they are activities that the client cannot do alone. Option 2 identifies a solitary activity. Review care of a client with aggressive social behavior if you had difficulty with this question.
Level of Cognitive Ability: Applying
Client Needs: Physiological Integrity
Integrated Process: Nursing Process—Planning
Content Area: Mental Health
References: Stuart, G. (2009). *Principles and practice of psychiatric nursing* (9th ed., p. 233). St. Louis: Mosby.

Varcarolis, E., & Halter, M. (2009). *Essentials of psychiatric mental health nursing: A communication approach to evidence-based care* (p. 36). St. Louis: Saunders.

914. 1

Rationale: Safety of the client and other clients is the priority. Option 1 is the only option that addresses the safety needs of the client and other clients. Option 2 addresses other clients' needs only. Option 3 is not client-centered. Option 4 addresses the client's needs only.
Test-Taking Strategy: Note the strategic words *immediate priority* and use Maslow's Hierarchy of Needs theory to prioritize. Note the words *agitated, aggressive,* and *belligerent.* Safety is the strategic priority focus. Option 1 is the umbrella option and addresses the safety of all. Review nursing interventions to provide safety to clients if you had difficulty with this question.
Level of Cognitive Ability: Applying
Client Needs: Safe and Effective Care Environment
Integrated Process: Nursing Process—Implementation
Content Area: Leadership and Management—Delegating/ Prioritizing
Reference: Fortinash, K., & Holoday-Worret, P. (2008). *Psychiatric mental health nursing* (4th ed., p. 521). St. Louis: Mosby.

915. 4

Rationale: The risk for impulsive and aggressive behavior may increase if a client is receiving command hallucinations to harm self or others. The nurse should ask the client whether he or she has intentions to hurt himself or herself or others. Talking about auditory hallucinations can interfere with subvocal muscular activity associated with a hallucination. Options 1, 2, and 3 will aid in wellness, but are not specific interventions for hallucinations, if they occur.
Test-Taking Strategy: Use the process of elimination. Options 1, 2, and 3 are interventions that a client can carry out to aid wellness. Option 4 is a specific agreement to seek help and evidences self-responsible commitment and control over one's own behavior. Review teaching points for a client with a history of hallucinations if you had difficulty with this question.
Level of Cognitive Ability: Evaluating
Client Needs: Psychosocial Integrity
Integrated Process: Nursing Process—Evaluation
Content Area: Mental Health
Reference: Fortinash, K., & Holoday-Worret, P. (2008). *Psychiatric mental health nursing* (4th ed., p. 269). St. Louis: Mosby.

916. 3

Rationale: Clients who are withdrawn may be immobile and mute and may require consistent, repeated approaches. Communication with withdrawn clients requires much patience from the nurse. Interventions include the establishment of interpersonal contact. The nurse facilitates communication with the client by sitting in silence, asking open-ended questions, and pausing to provide opportunities for the client to respond.
Test-Taking Strategy: Eliminate option 2 because the client would not be left alone. Option 4 relies on other clients to care for this client, which is an inappropriate expectation. Asking direct questions of this client is not therapeutic. Option 3 provides for client supervision and communication as appropriate. Review care of a client with catatonic stupor if this question was difficult.
Level of Cognitive Ability: Applying
Client Needs: Psychosocial Integrity
Integrated Process: Nursing Process—Implementation
Content Area: Mental Health
References: Fortinash, K., & Holoday-Worret, P. (2008). *Psychiatric mental health nursing* (4th ed., pp. 259–260). St. Louis: Mosby.

Varcarolis, E., & Halter, M. (2009). *Essentials of psychiatric mental health nursing: A communication approach to evidence-based care* (p. 277). St. Louis: Saunders.

917. 2

Rationale: Disturbed thought process related to paranoia is the client's problem, and the plan of care must address this problem. The client is experiencing paranoia and is distrustful and suspicious of others. The members of the health care team need to establish a rapport and trust with the client. Laughing or whispering in front of the client would be counterproductive. Options 1, 3, and 4 ask the client to trust on a multitude of levels. These options are actions that are too intrusive for a client who is paranoid.
Test-Taking Strategy: Use the process of elimination and knowledge regarding this disorder to answer the question. Noting that the client has paranoia will direct you to option 2. Review this disorder if you had difficulty with this question.
Level of Cognitive Ability: Applying
Client Needs: Psychosocial Integrity
Integrated Process: Nursing Process—Implementation

Content Area: Mental Health
Reference: Stuart, G. (2009). *Principles and practice of psychiatric nursing* (9th ed., p. 355). St. Louis: Mosby.

ALTERNATE ITEM FORMAT: MULTIPLE RESPONSE
918. 1, 3, 4, 6
Rationale: Interventions for dealing with the client exhibiting manipulative behavior include setting clear, consistent, and enforceable limits on manipulative behaviors; being clear with the client regarding the consequences of exceeding limits set; following through with the consequences in a nonpunitive manner; and assisting the client in identifying means of setting limits on personal behaviors. Enforcing rules and informing the client that he or she will not be allowed to attend therapy groups is a violation of a client's rights.

Ensuring that the client knows that he or she is not in charge of the nursing unit is inappropriate; power struggles need to be avoided.
Test-Taking Strategy: Focus on the subject, manipulative behavior. Recalling clients' rights and that power struggles need to be avoided will assist in selecting the correct interventions. Review care of the client with manipulative behavior if you had difficulty with this question.
Level of Cognitive Ability: Applying
Client Needs: Psychosocial Integrity
Integrated Process: Nursing Process—Implementation
Content Area: Mental Health
References: Stuart, G. (2009). *Principles and practice of psychiatric nursing* (9th ed., p. 385). St. Louis: Mosby.

Varcarolis, E., & Halter, M. (2009). *Essentials of psychiatric mental health nursing: A communication approach to evidence-based care* (p. 259). St. Louis: Saunders.

I. EATING DISORDERS

A. Description: Eating disorders are characterized by uncertain self-identification and grossly disturbed eating habits (Fig. 75-1).

B. Compulsive overeating
  1. Compulsive overeating is binge-like overeating without purging.
  2. Food consumption is out of the individual's control and occurs in a stereotyped fashion.
  3. The client may be repulsed by eating, and the eating relieves tension but does not produce pleasure.
  4. The client is aware that eating patterns are abnormal and feels depressed after eating.
  5. The client eats secretly during a binge and consumes high-calorie and easily digestible food.
  6. The client repeatedly tries to diet, but without success.
  7. The client feels helpless and hopeless about weight.
  8. When experiencing guilt, anger, depression, boredom, loneliness, inadequacy, or ambivalence, the client responds by eating.

C. Anorexia nervosa
  1. Description
     a. Onset often is associated with a stressful life event.
     b. The client intensely fears obesity.
     c. Body image is distorted, and the client has a disturbed self-concept.
     d. The client is preoccupied with foods that prevent weight gain and has a phobia against foods that produce weight gain.
     e. The eating disorder can be life-threatening.
     f. Death can occur from starvation, **suicide**, cardiomyopathies, or electrolyte imbalance.
  2. Assessment
     a. Refusal to eat and appetite loss
     b. Appetite denial
     c. Feelings of lack of control
     d. Self-induced vomiting and self-administered enemas
     e. Compulsive exercising

  f. Overachiever and perfectionist
  g. Decreased temperature, pulse, and blood pressure
  h. Weight loss
  i. Gastrointestinal disturbances
  j. Constipation
  k. Electrolyte imbalances
  l. Scaly, dry skin
  m. Presence of lanugo on extremities
  n. Sleep disturbances
  o. Hormone deficiencies
  p. Amenorrhea for at least three consecutive menstrual periods
  q. Teeth and gum deterioration
  r. Cyanosis and numbness of extremities
  s. Esophageal varices from vomiting
  t. Bone degeneration

⚠ The client with an eating disorder experiences an altered body image.

D. Bulimia nervosa
  1. Description
     a. The client indulges in eating binges followed by purging behaviors.
     b. Most clients remain within a normal weight range, but think that their lives are dominated by the eating-related conflict.
  2. Assessment
     a. Preoccupied with body shape and weight
     b. Consumption of high-calorie food in secret; guilt about secretive eating
     c. Binge-purge syndrome
     d. Attempts to lose weight through diets, vomiting, enemas, cathartics, and amphetamines or diuretics
     e. Has a need to control, yet experiences feelings of powerlessness or loss of control
     f. Low self-esteem
     g. Poor interpersonal relationships
     h. Decreased or absence of interest in sex
     i. Mood swings
     j. Electrolyte imbalances

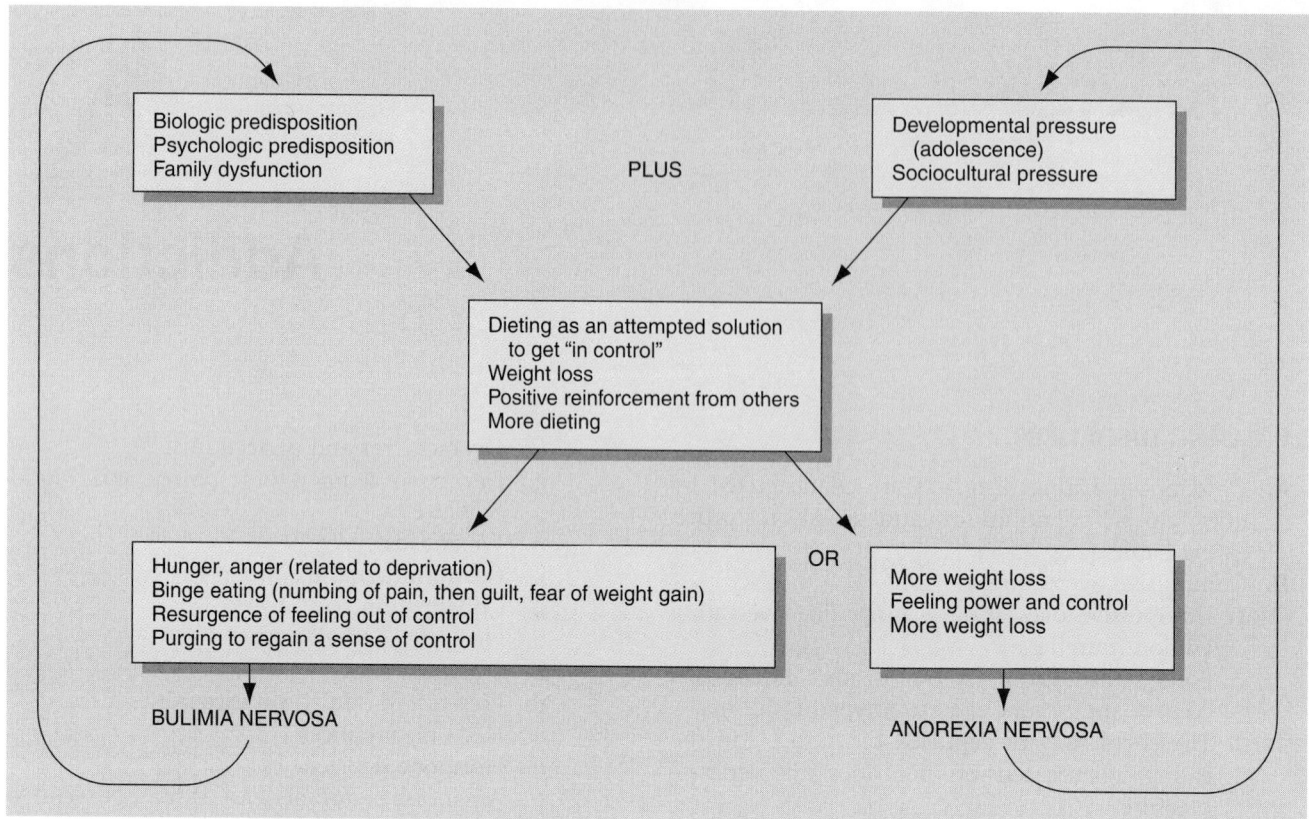

▲ **FIGURE 75-1** Cycle of eating disorders. (From Fortinash, K., & Holoday-Worret, P. [2008]. *Psychiatric mental health nursing* [4th ed.]. St. Louis: Mosby.)

k. Loss of tooth enamel and dental decay
l. Stomach ulcers and rectal bleeding
m. Esophageal varices from vomiting
n. Cardiac disease and hypertension

E. Interventions: Clients with an eating disorder

1. Assess the client's nutritional status and the severity of any medical problems.
2. Establish a one-to-one therapeutic relationship with the client; the nurse needs to establish trust and recognize any client reluctance to establish a relationship.
3. Establish a contract with the client concerning the nutritional plan for the day.
4. Assist the client to identify precipitants to the eating disorder.
5. Encourage the client to express feelings about the eating behavior and about how the client feels about his or her body.
6. Be accepting and nonjudgmental.
7. Work with the client on exploring self-concept and establishing identity
8. Implement behavior modification techniques.
9. Supervise the client during mealtimes and for a specified period after meals.
10. Set a time limit for each meal.
11. Provide a pleasant, relaxed environment for eating.

12. Monitor for signs of physical complications related to the eating disorder.
13. Record intake and output.
14. Weigh the client daily at the same time, using the same scale, after the client voids.
15. When weighing the client, ensure that the client is wearing the same clothing as when the previous weight was taken.
16. Monitor and restore fluid and electrolyte balance.
17. Monitor elimination patterns.
18. Assess and limit the client's activity level.
19. Encourage the client to participate in diversional activities.
20. Assess the client's suicidal potential.
21. Administer antidepressant medication if prescribed.
22. Encourage psychotherapy.
23. Refer the client to support groups.

II. SUBSTANCE ABUSE DISORDERS

A. Description: Substance **abuse** disorders cause behavioral and physiological changes (Box 75-1).
B. Substance dependence
1. Substance dependence is a pattern of repeated use of a substance, which usually results in tolerance, withdrawal, and compulsive drug-taking behavior.

Box 75-1 CAGE Screening Questionnaire

C Have you ever felt the need to cut down on your drinking/drug use?

A Have you ever been annoyed at criticism of your drinking/drug use?

G Have you ever felt guilty about something that you have done when you have been drinking or taking drugs?

E Have you ever had an eye opener—drinking or taking drugs first thing in the morning to get going or to avoid withdrawal symptoms?

2. The client takes substances in larger amounts and over longer periods than was intended.
3. The client has the desire to cut down, but efforts to decrease or discontinue use are unsuccessful.
4. Daily activities revolve around the use of a substance.

⚠ Screening tools are available to assess a substance abuse disorder, including Michigan Alcohol Screening Test (MAST), Drug Abuse Screening Test (DAST), and CAGE screening questionnaire.

C. Substance tolerance is the need for increased amounts of the substance to achieve the desired effect.
D. Substance **abuse**
   1. The client recurrently uses substances.
   2. The client experiences recurrent, significant harmful consequences related to the use of substances.
   3. The client may have legal issues to resolve, and involvement with the legal system is common.
E. Substance withdrawal
   1. Physiological and substance-specific cognitive symptoms occur.
   2. Substance withdrawal occurs when an individual experiences a decrease in blood levels of a substance to which the individual is physiologically dependent.
F. Other factors to consider in a client with a substance-related disorder
   1. Rebellion and peer group pressure in adolescence may contribute to the onset of substance use.
   2. Substance use may become a coping mechanism for decreasing physical and emotional pain.
   3. Depression may precede or occur as a result of or in association with substance use.
   4. Grief and loss may be associated with substance use.
G. Dysfunctional behaviors related to substance **abuse**
   1. Preoccupation with obtaining and using substance
   2. Manipulation to avoid consequences of behavior
   3. Impulsiveness
   4. Anger, including physical and verbal **abuse**

5. Avoidance of relationships
6. Sense of self-importance and requiring special treatment
7. Denial—blaming everything but the substance use for problems
8. Use of rationalization and projection to justify unacceptable behavior
9. Likely to be involved in codependent relationships whereby a significant other also unknowingly serves as a significant enabler
10. Low self-esteem
11. Depression

III. ALCOHOL ABUSE

A. Description
   1. Alcohol is a central nervous system (CNS) depressant affecting all body tissues.
   2. Physical dependence is a biological need for alcohol to avoid physical withdrawal symptoms, whereas psychological dependence refers to craving for the subjective effect of alcohol.
B. Risk factors
   1. Biological predisposition; genetic and familial predisposition may also be a risk factor.
   2. Depressed and highly anxious characteristics
   3. Low self-esteem
   4. Poor self-control
   5. History of rebelliousness, poor school performance, delinquency
   6. Poor parental relationships
C. Assessment
   1. Slurred speech
   2. Uncoordinated movements
   3. Unsteady gait
   4. Restlessness
   5. Belligerence
   6. Confusion
   7. Sneaking drinks, drinking in the morning, experiencing blackouts
   8. Binge drinking
   9. Arguments about drinking
   10. Missing work
   11. Increased tolerance to alcohol
   12. Intoxication, with blood alcohol levels of 0.1% (100 mg alcohol/dL blood) or greater

⚠ Part of the assessment should include the type of alcohol, how much consumed, and for how many years.

D. Psychological symptoms
   1. Depression
   2. Hostility
   3. Suspiciousness
   4. Rationalization
   5. Irritability
   6. Isolation

7. Decrease in inhibitions
8. Decrease in self-esteem
9. Denial that a problem exists
E. Complications associated with chronic alcohol use
   1. Vitamin deficiencies
      a. Vitamin B deficiency causing peripheral neuropathies
      b. Thiamine deficiency, causing Korsakoff's syndrome
   2. Alcohol-induced persistent amnesic disorder, causing severe memory problems
   3. Wernicke's encephalopathy, causing confusion, ataxia, and abnormal eye movements
   4. Hepatitis; cirrhosis of the liver
   5. Esophagitis and gastritis
   6. Pancreatitis
   7. Anemias
   8. Immune system dysfunctions
   9. Brain damage
   10. Peripheral neuropathy
   11. Cardiac disorders

IV. ALCOHOL WITHDRAWAL

A. Description
   1. Early signs develop within a few hours after cessation of alcohol intake.
   2. These signs peak after 24 to 48 hours and then rapidly disappear, unless the withdrawal progresses to alcohol withdrawal delirium.
   3. At the onset of withdrawal (Box 75-2), follow agency protocol using specified withdrawal assessment scales as indicated by unit or agency policy.
   4. Chlordiazepoxide (Librium) is the most commonly prescribed medication for acute alcohol withdrawal and is usually given orally, unless a more immediate onset is required (any benzodiazepine would decrease the withdrawal symptoms because of cross-tolerance; see Chapter 77 for a list of benzodiazepines).

Box 75-2 Early Signs of Alcohol Withdrawal

Anorexia (nausea and vomiting may occur)
Anxiety
Easily startled
Hyperalertness
Hypertension
Insomnia
Irritability
Jerky movements
Possibly experiences hallucinations, illusions, delusions, or vivid nightmares
Possibly reports a feeling of "shaking inside"
Seizures (usually appear 7 to 48 hours after cessation of alcohol)
Tachycardia
Tremors

---

5. An intramuscular injection of vitamin B$_1$ (thiamine) followed by several days of oral administration is administered to prevent Wernicke' encephalopathy.
B. Withdrawal (see Box 75-2)
C. Withdrawal delirium: The state of delirium usually peaks 48 to 72 hours after cessation or reduction of intake (although can occur later) and lasts 2 to 3 days (Box 75-3).

⚠ Withdrawal delirium is a medical emergency. Death can occur from myocardial infarction, fat emboli, peripheral vascular collapse, electrolyte imbalance, aspiration pneumonia, or suicide.

D. Interventions
   1. Provide care in a nonjudgmental manner.
   2. Check the client frequently.
   3. Monitor vital signs and neurological signs (every 15 minutes) and provide one-to-one supervision.
   4. Provide a quiet, nonstimulating environment; encourage a family member (one at a time) to stay with the client to minimize anxiety.
   5. Orient the client frequently.
   6. Explain all treatments and procedures in a quiet and simple manner.
   7. Initiate seizure precautions.
   8. Administer sedating or anticonvulsant medication as prescribed.
   9. Provide small, frequent, high-carbohydrate foods (administer antiemetic before meals as needed).
   10. Monitor intake and output.
   11. Administer vitamins (multivitamin, vitamin B complex including thiamine, and vitamin C)
   12. Assist client with activities of daily living and assist with ambulation if stable.
   13. Allow client to express fears.
E. Disulfiram (Antabuse) therapy
   1. Description
      a. Disulfiram is an alcohol deterrent that may be prescribed for alcoholic dependence.

Box 75-3 Manifestations of Alcohol Withdrawal Delirium

Agitation
Anorexia
Anxiety
Delirium
Diaphoresis
Disorientation with fluctuating levels of consciousness
Fever (temperature 100° F to 103° F)
Hallucinations and delusions
Insomnia
Tachycardia and hypertension

b. The medication sensitizes the client to alcohol, so a disulfiram-alcohol reaction occurs if alcohol is ingested.

c. The client must abstain from alcohol for at least 12 hours before the initial dose is administered.

d. Adverse effects usually begin within several minutes to ½ half after consuming alcohol and may last ½ to 2 hours.

e. The client must avoid drinking alcohol for 14 days after disulfiram therapy has been discontinued; otherwise, the client is at risk for a disulfiram-alcohol reaction.

2. Adverse reactions
   a. Facial flushing
   b. Sweating
   c. Throbbing headache
   d. Neck pain
   e. Nausea and vomiting
   f. Hypotension
   g. Tachycardia
   h. Respiratory distress

3. Client education
   a. Educate about the effects of the medication.
   b. Ensure that the client agrees to abstain from alcohol and any alcohol-containing substances.
   c. Instruct the client that the effects of the medication may occur for several days after discontinuance.
   d. Other medications used to assist with cravings include acamprosate calcium (Campral) and naltrexone (ReVia)

F. Dealing with the client who **abuses** alcohol (Boxes 75-4 and 75-5)

⚠ Instruct the client who is on disulfiram (Antabuse) therapy to avoid the use of substances that contain alcohol, such as cough medicines, rubbing compounds, vinegar, mouthwashes, and aftershave lotions. The client needs to read the labels of all products.

Box 75-4 Dealing With the Client Who Abuses Alcohol

Direct the client's focus to the substance abuse problem.
Identify situations that precipitate angry feelings with the client.
Set limits on manipulative behavior and verbal and physical abuse.
Hold the client firmly to reasonable limits, consistently reinforcing rules, with reasonable consequences for breaking rules.
Hold the client accountable for all behaviors.
Assist the client to explore strengths and weaknesses.
Encourage the client to focus on strengths if the client is losing control.
Encourage the client to participate in group therapy and support groups.

V. DRUG DEPENDENCY

A. CNS depressants
   1. CNS depressants include alcohol, benzodiazepines, and barbiturates and act as a depressant, sedative, or hypnotic.
   2. Intoxication (Box 75-6)
   3. Overdose can produce cardiovascular or respiratory depression, coma, shock, seizures, and death.
   4. Overdose: If the client is awake, vomiting is induced and activated charcoal is administered; if the client is comatose, establishment and maintenance of an airway and gastric lavage with activated charcoal are the priorities; seizure precautions are indicated.
   5. Flumazenil (Romazicon) intravenously may be used for benzodiazepine overdose to reverse the effects.
   6. Withdrawal effects include nausea, vomiting, tachycardia, diaphoresis, irritability, tremors, insomnia, and seizures; withdrawal must be treated with a carefully titrated similar drug (abrupt withdrawal can lead to death).
   7. Withdrawal from CNS depressants such as barbiturates is generally treated with a barbiturate such as phenobarbital or a long-acting benzodiazepine.

B. CNS stimulants
   1. CNS stimulants include substances such as amphetamines, cocaine, and crack.
   2. Intoxication (Box 75-7)

Box 75-5 Therapies for Clients With Substance Abuse and Their Families

Behavior therapy, aversion conditioning with disulfiram (Antabuse) or another medication
Hospitalization
Psychotherapy (individual, group, family)
Support groups such as Alcoholics Anonymous; Narcotics Anonymous; Pills Anonymous; Al-Anon, Al-a-Teen, or Narc-Anon (for family members and friends of alcoholics or addicts); and Adult Children of Alcoholics
Transitional living programs (halfway houses)

Box 75-6 Intoxication: Central Nervous System Depressants

Drowsiness
Hypotension
Impairment of memory, attention, judgment, and social or occupational functioning
Incoordination and unsteady gait
Irritability
Slurred speech

Box 75-7 Intoxication: Central Nervous System Stimulants

Dilated pupils
Euphoria
Hypertension
Impairment of judgment and social or occupational functioning
Insomnia
Nausea and vomiting
Paranoia, delusions, hallucinations
Potential for violence
Tachycardia

Box 75-8 Intoxication: Opioids

Constricted pupils
Decreased respirations
Drowsiness
Euphoria
Hypotension
Impairment of memory, attention, and judgment
Psychomotor retardation
Slurred speech

Box 75-9 Intoxication: Hallucinogens

Agitation and belligerence
Anxiety and depression
Bizarre behavior, regressive behavior, or violent behavior
Blank stare
Diaphoresis
Dilated pupils
Elevated vital signs including blood pressure
Hallucinations
Impairment of judgment and social and occupational functioning
Incoordination
Muscular rigidity and chronic jerking
Paranoia
Seizures
Tachycardia
Tremors

---

3. Overdose can produce respiratory distress, ataxia, hyperpyrexia, seizures, coma, stroke, myocardial infarction, and death.
4. Overdose is treated with antipsychotics and management of associated effects.
5. Withdrawal effects include fatigue, depression, agitation, apathy, anxiety, insomnia, disorientation, lethargy, and craving.
6. Withdrawal is treated with antidepressants, a dopamine agonist, or bromocriptine (Parlodel); withdrawal is primarily supportive, particularly when dealing with the severe depression and suicidal ideation that accompanies stimulant withdrawal.

C. Opioids
1. Opioids include substances such as opium, heroin, meperidine (Demerol), morphine sulfate, codeine sulfate, methadone (Dolophine), hydromorphone (Dilaudid), OxyContin (oxycodone), hydrocodone (Lortab), and fentanyl (Sublimaze).
2. Intoxication (Box 75-8)
3. Overdose can produce respiratory depression, shock, coma, seizures, and death.
4. Overdose is treated with an opioid antagonist such as naloxone (Narcan).
5. Withdrawal effects include yawning, insomnia, irritability, rhinorrhea, diaphoresis, cramps, nausea and vomiting, muscle aches, chills, fever, lacrimation, and diarrhea.
6. Withdrawal may be treated by methadone detoxification or tapering dosage with other opioids.

7. Clonidine (Catapres), an α-adrenergic blocker, assists in reducing the severity of sympathetic nervous system–generated withdrawal discomfort.
8. Specific measures for symptom management may also be used, such as bismuth subsalicylate (Kaopectate) for diarrhea and acetaminophen (Tylenol) for muscle aches.

D. Hallucinogens
1. Hallucinogens include substances such as lysergic acid diethylamide (LSD), mescaline (peyote), psilocybin (mushrooms), and phencyclidine (PCP).
2. Intoxication (Box 75-9)
3. Overdose effects of LSD, peyote, and psilocybin include psychosis, brain damage, and death; effects of PCP include psychosis, hypertensive **crisis**, hyperthermia, seizures, and respiratory arrest.
4. Treatment (LSD, peyote, psilocybin) involves low environmental stimuli (speak slowly, clearly, and in a low voice) and medications to treat anxiety.
5. Treatment (PCP) involves possible gastric lavage (if alert); treatment to acidify the urine to assist in excreting drug; and interventions to treat behavioral disturbances, hyperthermia, hypertension, and respiratory distress.
6. Withdrawal is primarily supportive and may include medications to target particular problem behaviors, such as agitation.

E. Inhalants
1. Inhalants include gases or liquids such as butane, paint thinner, paint and wax removers, airplane glue, nail polish remover, and nitrous oxide.
2. Intoxication (Box 75-10)
3. Overdose can cause damage to the nervous system and death.
4. Management of withdrawal is mainly supportive including treating affected body systems.

Box 75-10 Intoxication: Inhalants

Enhancement of sexual pleasure

Euphoria

Excitation followed by drowsiness, lightheadedness, disinhibition, and agitation

Giggling and laughter

Box 75-11 Withdrawal: Nursing Care

Obtain information regarding the type of drug and amount consumed.

Assess vital signs.

Remove unnecessary objects from the environment.

Provide one-to-one supervision if necessary.

Provide a quiet, calm environment with minimal stimuli.

Maintain client orientation.

Ensure client's safety by implementing seizure precautions.

Use security devices if necessary and prescribed to prevent client from harming self and others.

Provide for physical needs.

Provide food and fluids as tolerated.

Administer medications as prescribed to decrease withdrawal symptoms.

Collect blood and urine samples for drug screening.

F. Marijuana (*Cannabis sativa*)

1. Marijuana generally is smoked, but can be ingested.
2. Marijuana causes euphoria, detachment, relaxation, talkativeness, slowed perception of time, anxiety, and paranoia.
3. Long-term dependence can result in lethargy, difficulty concentrating, memory loss, and possibly chronic respiratory disorders.
4. Withdrawal management is mainly supportive.

G. Other recreational and club drugs

1. Methylenedioxymethamphetamine (MDMA, ecstasy), gamma hydroxybutyrate (GHB), methamphetamine (crank, meth, crystal meth), and ketamine (special K)
2. Effects include euphoria, increased energy, increased self-confidence, and increased sociability.
3. Adverse effects include hyperthermia, rhabdomyolysis, renal failure, hepatotoxicity, depression, panic attacks, psychosis, cardiovascular collapse, and death.
4. The use of over-the-counter medications containing ephedrine or pseudoephedrine to manufacture illegal supplies of methamphetamine has led many states to adopt laws requiring limited sales and signatures for the purchase of these medications.
5. Programs for **addiction** also address nicotine withdrawal and the pharmacological and psychotherapeutic interventions for this problem, such as nicotine patches, nicotine inhalers, and bupropion (Zyban) for the reduction of withdrawal and cravings.
6. Anabolic steroids have also gained increased attention as increasingly adverse events, including death, have become more widely publicized.

H. Interventions: Withdrawal (Box 75-11)

1. Initiate seizure precautions.
2. Hydrate the client.
3. Monitor vital signs every hour.
4. Monitor intake and output.
5. Orient the client frequently.
6. Maintain minimal stimuli.
7. Approach the client in an accepting and nonjudgmental manner.
8. Direct the client's focus to the substance **abuse** problem.
9. Assist the client with identifying situations that precipitate angry feelings.
10. Assist the client to deal with emotions.
11. Limit the client's placing blame or rationalizing to explain the substance **abuse** problem.
12. Assist the client to use assertive techniques rather than manipulation to meet needs.
13. Set limits on manipulative behavior and verbal and physical **abuse**.
14. Maintain firm and reasonable limits, consistently reinforcing rules, with reasonable consequences for breaking rules.
15. Hold the client accountable for all behaviors.
16. Assist the client to explore strengths and weaknesses.
17. Encourage the client to focus on strengths if the client is losing control.
18. Encourage the client to participate in unit activities.
19. Encourage the client to participate in group therapy and support groups.

I. Dual diagnoses

1. Sometimes the use of alcohol and drugs masks underlying psychiatric pathology.
2. Psychiatric pathology may also be precipitated by substance use and **abuse**.
3. When psychiatric disorders and substance **abuse** are present together, it is often referred to as dual diagnosis.
4. Separating psychiatric diagnosis from substance dependence can be done only over time after a sustained period of abstinence.

J. **Addiction** and **abuse** in health care professionals: Suspicious signs

1. Frequently reporting that drugs have been wasted without being witnessed by another nurse

2. Administering maximum dosages of controlled substances when other nurses do not

3. A variance in usual pain relief in the absence of a change in dosage or frequency in their clients

4. Work patterns include the following: Always volunteering to carry narcotic (opioids) keys; choosing shifts in which less supervision is present; choosing work areas where the use of controlled substances is high, such as critical care units, operating room, anesthesia, and trauma units.

5. Nurses have a professional and ethical obligation to report impaired coworkers.

6. Most impaired nurses are able to return to work through the State Board of Nursing assistance and monitoring programs; such programs usually require strict adherence to clearly stated rules and regular reports and drug screens.

K. Codependency issues

1. Codependency refers to the presence of coexisting behaviors present in a significant other, which serves to enable the addict or alcoholic to continue the irresponsible patterns of use without experiencing consequences.

2. Examples of codependency: Paying bills for which the addict or alcoholic is responsible, bailing the addict or alcoholic out of jail, helping the addict or alcoholic to call in sick.

3. It is important to address codependency issues with the family to maximize the chance for recovery of the client with the **addiction** and the person with the codependent behaviors.

 MORE QUESTIONS ON THE CD!

Practice Questions

919. A home health nurse visits a client at home and determines that the client is dependent on drugs. Which of the following assessment questions would assist the nurse to provide appropriate nursing care?
1. "Why did you get started on these drugs?"
2. "How much do you use and what effect does it have on you?"
3. "How long did you think you could take these drugs without someone finding out?"
4. The nurse does not ask any questions for fear that the client is in denial and will throw the nurse out of the home.

920. A female client with anorexia nervosa is a member of a predischarge support group. The client verbalizes that she would like to buy some new clothes, but her finances are limited. Group members have brought some used clothes to the client to replace the client's old clothes. The client believes that the new clothes were much too tight and has reduced her calorie intake to 800 calories daily. A nurse evaluates this behavior as:
1. Normal behavior
2. Evidence of the client's disturbed body image
3. Regression as the client is moving toward the community
4. Indicative of the client's ambivalence about hospital discharge

921. A nurse determines that the wife of an alcoholic client is benefiting from attending an Al-Anon group when the nurse hears the wife say:
1. "I no longer feel that I deserve the beatings my husband inflicts on me."
2. "My attendance at the meetings has helped me to see that I provoke my husband's violence."
3. "I enjoy attending the meetings because they get me out of the house and away from my husband."
4. "I can tolerate my husband's destructive behaviors now that I know they are common with alcoholics."

922. A hospitalized client with a history of alcohol abuse tells a nurse, "I am leaving now. I have to go. I don't want any more treatment. I have things that I have to do right away." The client has not been discharged. The client is scheduled for an important diagnostic test to be performed in 1 hour. After the nurse discusses the client's concerns with the client, the client dresses and begins to walk out of the hospital room. The appropriate nursing action is to:
1. Call the nursing supervisor.
2. Call security to block all exit areas.
3. Restrain the client until the physician can be reached.
4. Tell the client that the client cannot return to this hospital again if the client leaves now.

923. A nurse is preparing to perform an admission assessment on a client with a diagnosis of bulimia nervosa, and a nursing student will be observing the nurse. The nurse asks the student about the expected assessment findings and determines that the student needs to research the disorder further if the student states that which of the following is a characteristic finding?
1. Dental decay
2. Loss of tooth enamel
3. Electrolyte imbalances
4. Body weight well below ideal range

924. A nurse is caring for a female client who was admitted to the mental health unit recently for anorexia nervosa. The nurse enters the client's room and notes that the client is engaged in rigorous push-ups. Which nursing action is appropriate?
  1. Interrupt the client and weigh her immediately.
  2. Interrupt the client and offer to take her for a walk.
  3. Allow the client to complete her exercise program.
  4. Tell the client that she is not allowed to exercise rigorously.

925. A client with a diagnosis of anorexia nervosa, who is in a state of starvation, is in a two-bed room. A newly admitted client will be assigned to this client's room. Which of the following clients would be an appropriate choice as this client's roommate?
  1. A client with pneumonia
  2. A client receiving diagnostic tests
  3. A client who thrives on managing others
  4. A client who could benefit from the client's assistance at mealtime

926. A nurse is monitoring a client who abuses alcohol for signs of alcohol withdrawal. Which of the following would alert the nurse to the potential for withdrawal delirium?

  1. Hypotension, ataxia, hunger
  2. Stupor, agitation, muscular rigidity
  3. Hypotension, coarse hand tremors, agitation
  4. Hypertension, changes in level of consciousness, hallucinations

927. The spouse of a client admitted to the mental health unit for alcohol withdrawal says to a nurse, "I should get out of this bad situation." The most helpful response by the nurse would be:
  1. "Why don't you tell your husband about this?"
  2. "What do you find difficult about this situation?"
  3. "This is not the best time to make that decision."
  4. "I agree with you. You should get out of this situation."

Alternate Item Format: Multiple Response

928. Select the appropriate interventions for caring for a client in alcohol withdrawal. **Select all that apply.**
  ❑ 1. Monitor vital signs.
  ❑ 2. Maintain NPO status.
  ❑ 3. Provide a safe environment.
  ❑ 4. Address hallucinations therapeutically.
  ❑ 5. Provide stimulation in the environment.
  ❑ 6. Provide reality orientation as appropriate.

ANSWERS
919. 2
Rationale: Whenever the nurse carries out an assessment for a client who is dependent on drugs, it is best for the nurse to attempt to elicit information by being nonjudgmental and direct. Option 1 is incorrect because it is judgmental and off focus and reflects the nurse's bias. Option 3 is incorrect because it is judgmental, insensitive, and aggressive, which is nontherapeutic. Option 4 is incorrect because it indicates passivity on the nurse's part and uses rationalization to avoid the therapeutic nursing intervention.
Test-Taking Strategy: Use the process of elimination and therapeutic communication techniques to answer the question. Also, focus on the subject, provide appropriate nursing care. Review assessment of a client who is a substance abuser if you had difficulty with this question.
Level of Cognitive Ability: Analyzing
Client Needs: Psychosocial Integrity
Integrated Process: Nursing Process—Assessment
Content Area: Mental Health
Reference: Fortinash, K., & Holoday-Worret, P. (2008). *Psychiatric mental health nursing* (4th ed., pp. 316–317). St. Louis: Mosby.

920. 2
Rationale: Disturbed body image is a concern with clients with anorexia nervosa. Although the client may struggle with ambivalence and show regressed behavior, the client's coping pattern relates to the basic issue of disturbed body image. The nurse should address this need in the support group.
Test-Taking Strategy: Use the process of elimination, focusing on the information provided in the question, which is related directly to an altered body image. This should direct you to the correct option. Review the needs of a client with anorexia nervosa if you had difficulty with this question.
Level of Cognitive Ability: Evaluating
Client Needs: Psychosocial Integrity
Integrated Process: Nursing Process—Evaluation
Content Area: Mental Health
Reference: Stuart, G. (2009). *Principles and practice of psychiatric nursing* (9th ed., pp. 466, 472). St. Louis: Mosby.

921. 1
Rationale: Al-Anon support groups are a protected, supportive opportunity for spouses and significant others to learn what to expect and to obtain excellent pointers about successful behavioral changes. Option 1 is the healthiest response because it exemplifies an understanding that the alcoholic

partner is responsible for his behavior and cannot be allowed to blame family members for loss of control. In option 2, the nonalcoholic partner should not feel responsible when the spouse loses control. Option 4 indicates that the wife remains codependent. Option 3 indicates that the group is viewed as an escape, not a place to work on issues.

Test-Taking Strategy: Use the process of elimination. Note the strategic words *benefiting from attending an Al-Anon group.* This will direct you to option 1. Review the purpose of this group if you had difficulty with this question.

Level of Cognitive Ability: Evaluating
Client Needs: Psychosocial Integrity
Integrated Process: Nursing Process—Evaluation
Content Area: Mental Health
Reference: Stuart, G. (2009). *Principles and practice of psychiatric nursing* (9th ed., pp. 431, 449). St. Louis: Mosby.

922. 1

Rationale: A nurse can be charged with false imprisonment if a client is made to believe wrongfully that he or she cannot leave the hospital. Most health care facilities have documents that the client is asked to sign relating to the client's responsibilities when the client leaves against medical advice. The client should be asked to sign this document before leaving. The nurse should request that the client wait to speak to the physician before leaving, but if the client refuses to do so, the nurse cannot hold the client against the client's will. Restraining the client and calling security to block exits constitutes false imprisonment. All clients have a right to health care and cannot be told otherwise.

Test-Taking Strategy: Use the process of elimination. Keeping the concept of false imprisonment in mind, eliminate options 2 and 3 because they are comparable or alike. Eliminate option 4, knowing that all clients have a right to health care. From the options presented, the best action is option 1. Review the points related to false imprisonment if you had difficulty with this question.

Level of Cognitive Ability: Applying
Client Needs: Safe and Effective Care Environment
Integrated Process: Nursing Process—Implementation
Content Area: Mental Health
Reference: Varcarolis, E., & Halter, M. (2009). *Essentials of psychiatric mental health nursing: A communication approach to evidence-based care* (p. 528). St. Louis: Saunders.

923. 4

Rationale: Clients with bulimia nervosa initially may not appear to be physically or emotionally ill. They are often at or slightly below ideal body weight. On further inspection, a client exhibits dental decay and loss of tooth enamel if the client has been inducing vomiting. Electrolyte imbalances are present.

Test-Taking Strategy: Focus on the subject, bulimia nervosa, and note the strategic words *needs to research.* Eliminate options 1 and 2 because they are comparable or alike. From the remaining options, recall that in anorexia nervosa the body weight is normally well below ideal body weight. Option 4 is a characteristic sign of anorexia nervosa, not bulimia nervosa. Review the characteristics of these disorders if you had difficulty with this question.

Level of Cognitive Ability: Evaluating

Client Needs: Psychosocial Integrity
Integrated Process: Teaching and Learning
Content Area: Mental Health
References: Fortinash, K., & Holoday-Worret, P. (2008). *Psychiatric mental health nursing* (4th ed., p. 397). St. Louis: Mosby.
   Varcarolis, E., & Halter, M. (2009). *Essentials of psychiatric mental health nursing: A communication approach to evidence-based care* (p. 200). St. Louis: Saunders.

924. 2

Rationale: Clients with anorexia nervosa frequently are preoccupied with rigorous exercise and push themselves beyond normal limits to work off caloric intake. The nurse must provide for appropriate exercise and place limits on rigorous activities. Options 1, 3, and 4 are inappropriate nursing actions.

Test-Taking Strategy: Use the process of elimination and focus on the client's diagnosis. Also, focus on the need for the nurse to set firm limits with clients who have this disorder. If you had difficulty with this question, review interventions for the client with anorexia nervosa.

Level of Cognitive Ability: Applying
Client Needs: Physiological Integrity
Integrated Process: Nursing Process—Implementation
Content Area: Mental Health
Reference: Stuart, G. (2009). *Principles and practice of psychiatric nursing* (9th ed., p. 470). St. Louis: Mosby.

925. 2

Rationale: The client undergoing diagnostic tests is an acceptable roommate. The client with anorexia nervosa is most likely experiencing hematological complications, such as leukopenia. Having a roommate with pneumonia would place the client with anorexia nervosa at risk for infection. The client with anorexia nervosa should not be put in a situation in which the client can focus on the nutritional needs of others or being managed by others because this may contribute to sublimation and suppression of personal hunger.

Test-Taking Strategy: Use the process of elimination and note the strategic words, *in a state of starvation.* Recalling the characteristics associated with anorexia nervosa will direct you to option 2. Review care of the client with anorexia nervosa if you had difficulty with this question.

Level of Cognitive Ability: Analyzing
Client Needs: Safe and Effective Care Environment
Integrated Process: Nursing Process—Planning
Content Area: Mental Health
References: Stuart, G. (2009). *Principles and practice of psychiatric nursing* (9th ed., pp. 461–462). St. Louis: Mosby.
   Varcarolis, E., & Halter, M. (2009). *Essentials of psychiatric mental health nursing: A communication approach to evidence-based care* (p. 199). St. Louis: Saunders.

926. 4

Rationale: Symptoms associated with withdrawal delirium typically include anxiety, insomnia, anorexia, hypertension, disorientation, hallucinations, changes in level of consciousness, agitation, fever, and delusions.

Test-Taking Strategy: Use the process of elimination. Review each option carefully to ensure that all the symptoms in the option are correct. Eliminate options 1 and 3 first, knowing

that hypertension rather than hypotension occurs. From the remaining options, recalling that the client who is stuporous is not likely to exhibit withdrawal delirium will direct you to option 4. Review these symptoms if you had difficulty with this question.
Level of Cognitive Ability: Analyzing
Client Needs: Physiological Integrity
Integrated Process: Nursing Process—Assessment
Content Area: Mental Health
Reference: Stuart, G. (2009). *Principles and practice of psychiatric nursing* (9th ed., pp. 434–435). St. Louis: Mosby.

927. 2
Rationale: The most helpful response is one that encourages the client to solve problems. Giving advice implies that the nurse knows what is best and can foster dependency. The nurse should not agree with the client, and the nurse should not request that the client provide explanations.
Test-Taking Strategy: Use therapeutic communication techniques. Eliminate option 1 because of the word *why*, which should be avoided in communication. Eliminate option 4 because the nurse is agreeing with the client. Eliminate option 3 because this option places the client's feelings on hold. Option 2 is the only option that addresses the client's feelings. Review therapeutic communication techniques if you had difficulty with this question.
Level of Cognitive Ability: Applying
Client Needs: Psychosocial Integrity
Integrated Process: Communication and Documentation
Content Area: Mental Health

Reference: Stuart, G. (2009). *Principles and practice of psychiatric nursing* (9th ed., pp. 27–31, 189). St. Louis: Mosby.

ALTERNATE ITEM FORMAT: MULTIPLE RESPONSE
928. 1, 3, 4, 6
Rationale: When the client is experiencing withdrawal from alcohol, the priority for care is to prevent the client from harming self or others. The nurse would provide a low stimulation environment to maintain the client in as calm a state as possible. The nurse would monitor the vital signs closely and report abnormal findings. The nurse would reorient the client to reality frequently and would address hallucinations therapeutically. Adequate nutritional and fluid intake need to be maintained.
Test-Taking Strategy: Use therapeutic communication techniques to assist in selecting the correct interventions. Also, recalling the characteristics associated with alcohol withdrawal will assist in answering correctly. Review these interventions if you had difficulty with this question.
Level of Cognitive Ability: Applying
Client Needs: Psychosocial Integrity
Integrated Process: Nursing Process—Implementation
Content Area: Mental Health
Reference: Fortinash, K., & Holoday-Worret, P. (2008). *Psychiatric mental health nursing* (4th ed., p. 392). St. Louis: Mosby.

76 Crisis Theory and Intervention

I. CRISIS INTERVENTION

A. Description
1. **Crisis** is a temporary state of severe emotional disorganization caused by failure of **coping mechanisms** and lack of support.
2. The ability for decision making and problem solving is inadequate.
3. Treatment is aimed at assisting the client and the family through the stressful situation.

B. Phases of a **crisis**
1. Phase 1: External precipitating event
2. Phase 2
   a. Perception of the threat
   b. Increase in anxiety
   c. Client may cope or resolve the **crisis**.
3. Phase 3
   a. Failure of coping
   b. Increasing disorganization
   c. Emergence of physical symptoms
   d. Relationship problems
4. Phase 4
   a. Mobilization of internal and external resources
   b. Goal is to return the client to at least a precrisis level of functioning.

C. Types of crises (Box 76-1)

D. **Crisis** intervention
1. Treatment is immediate, supportive, and directly responsive to the immediate **crisis**.
2. Interventions are goal-directed.
3. Feelings of the client are acknowledged.
4. Intervention provides opportunities for expression and validation of feelings.
5. Connections are made between the meaning of the event and the **crisis**.
6. The client explores alternative **coping mechanisms** and tries out new behaviors.

II. GRIEF

A. Grief is a natural emotional response to loss that individuals must experience as they attempt to accept the loss.

B. Grief usually involves moving through a series of stages or tasks to help resolve the grief (Box 76-2).

C. Feelings associated with grief include anger, frustration, loneliness, sadness, guilt, regret, and peace.

D. Healing can occur when the pain of the loss has lessened and the survivor has adapted to life without the deceased; the survivor continues to experience memories of the deceased.

E. Types of grief
1. Normal grief: Physical, emotional, cognitive, or behavioral reactions can occur; the process of resolution can take months to years.
2. Anticipatory grief occurs before the loss and is associated with an acute, chronic, or terminal illness.
3. Disenfranchised grief occurs when a loss is experienced and cannot be acknowledged openly (societal norms do not define the loss as a loss within its traditional definition).
4. Dysfunctional grief occurs with prolonged emotional instability and a lack of progression to successful coping with the loss.
5. Grief in children is based on the developmental level of the child (Box 76-3).

III. LOSS

A. Loss is the absence of something desired or previously thought to be available.

B. Actual loss can be identified by others and can arise in response to or in anticipation of a situation.

C. Perceived loss is experienced by one person and cannot be verified by others.

D. Anticipatory loss is experienced before the loss occurs.

E. Mourning
1. Mourning is the outward and social expression of loss.
2. Mourning may be dictated by cultural and religious beliefs.

F. Bereavement
1. Bereavement includes the inner feelings and the outward reactions of the survivor.
2. Bereavement includes grief and mourning.

IV. NURSE'S ROLE: GRIEF AND LOSS (Box 76-4)

A. Allow ongoing opportunities for fully informed choices.

Box 76-1 Types of Crises

Maturational
Relates to developmental stages and associated role changes; examples include marriage, birth of a child, and retirement

Situational
Arises from an external source, is often unanticipated, and is associated with a life event that upsets an individual's or group's psychological equilibrium; examples include loss of a job or a change in job, change in financial status, death of a loved one, divorce, abortion, and severe physical or mental illness

Adventitious
Relates to a crisis of disaster or an event that is not a part of everyday life and is unplanned and accidental; this type of crisis may result from a natural disaster or catastrophic event, such as a flood, earthquake, hurricane, fire, tornado, war, riots, or act of terrorism, or a crime of violence, such as rape, assault, murder, or spousal or child abuse

Box 76-2 The Grief Response

Stage 1: Shock and Disbelief
Survivor may have feelings of numbness, difficulties with decision making, emotional outbursts, denial, and isolation.

Stage 2: Experiencing the Loss
Survivor may feel angry at the loved one who died or may feel guilt about the death.
Bargaining or depression or both also may occur in this stage.

Stage 3: Reintegration
Survivor begins to reorganize his or her life and accepts the reality of the loss.

B. Facilitate the grief process; assess the survivor's grief, and assist the survivor to feel the loss and complete the tasks of the grief process.
C. Grief affects survivors physically, psychologically, socially, and spiritually; a multidisciplinary team approach, including a bereavement specialist, facilitates the grief process.

⚠ The nurse's role in the grief and loss process includes communicating with the client, family members, and significant other. The nurse must consider the survivor's culture, religion, family structure, individual life experiences, coping skills, and support systems.

V. END-OF-LIFE ISSUES

A. Description: End-of-life issues are related to death and dying.
B. Cultural and religious issues (see Chapter 6 and Box 6-4 for information regarding cultural and religious issues)

Box 76-3 Grief in Children

Birth to 1 Year
Infant has no concept of death.
Infant reacts to the loss of mother or caregiver.

1 to 2 Years
Toddler may see death as reversible.
Grief response occurs only to the death of the significant person in the toddler's life.
Toddler may scream, withdraw, or become disinterested in the environment.

2 to 5 Years
Child may see death as reversible.
Child has a sense of loss and is concerned about who will provide care.
Regressive or aggressive behavior may occur.

5 to 9 Years
Child begins to see death as permanent.
Child may feel responsible for the occurrence.
Child has difficulty concentrating.

Preadolescent Through Adolescent
Adolescent sees death as permanent.
Adolescent experiences a strong emotional reaction.
Adolescent may regress.

Box 76-4 Communication Process

Determine how much the client and family want to know.
Determine whether there is a spokesperson for the family.
Be aware of cultural and religious beliefs and how they may affect the communication process; consider personal space issues, eye contact, and touch.
Obtain an interpreter, if necessary.
Allow opportunity for informed choices.
Assist with the decision-making process if asked; use problem solving to assist in decision making, and avoid interjecting personal views or opinions.
Encourage expression of feelings, concerns, and fears.
Be honest, and let the client and family know that you will not abandon them.
Ask the client and family about their expectations and needs.
Be a sensitive listener; sit in silence if necessary and appropriate.
Extend touch and hold the client's or family member's hand if appropriate.
Encourage reminiscing.
If you do not know what to do in a particular situation, seek assistance.
If you do not know what to say to a client or family who is talking about death, listen attentively and use therapeutic communication techniques, such as open-ended questions or reflection.
Acknowledge your own feelings; let the client and family know that the topic of conversation is a difficult one and that you do not know what to say.
Realize that it is acceptable to cry with the client and family during the grief process.

C. Legal and ethical issues
1. Outcomes related to care during illness and the dying experience should be based on the client's wishes.
2. Issues for consideration may include organ and tissue donations, advance directives or other legal documents, withholding or withdrawing treatment, and cardiopulmonary resuscitation.

D. Palliative care
1. Palliative care focuses on caring interventions and symptom management rather than cure for diseases that no longer respond to treatment.
2. Pain and symptoms are controlled; the dying client should be as pain-free and as comfortable as possible.
3. Hospice care provides support and care for clients in the last phases of incurable diseases so that they might live as fully and as comfortably as possible; client and family needs are the focus of any intervention.

E. Near-death physiological manifestations
1. As death approaches, metabolism is reduced, and the body gradually slows down until all function ends.
2. Sensory: The client experiences blurred vision, decreased sense of taste and smell, decreased pain and touch perception, and loss of blink reflex and appears to stare (hearing is believed to be the last sense lost).
3. Respirations
   a. Respirations may be rapid, slow, shallow, and irregular.
   b. Respirations may be noisy and wet sounding (death rattle).
   c. Cheyne-Stokes respiration is alternating periods of apnea and deep, rapid breathing.
4. Circulation
   a. Heart rate slows, and blood pressure falls progressively.
   b. Skin is cool to touch, and the extremities become pale, mottled, and cyanotic.
   c. Skin is wax-like very near death.
5. Urinary output gradually decreases; incontinence may occur.
6. Gastrointestinal motility and peristalsis diminish, leading to constipation, gas accumulation, and distention; a bowel movement may occur before death or at the time of death.
7. Musculoskeletal system: The client gradually loses ability to move, has difficulty speaking and swallowing, and loses the gag reflex.

F. Death
1. Death occurs when all vital organs and body systems cease to function.
2. Generally, respirations cease first, and then the heartbeat stops a few minutes thereafter.

G. Brain death occurs when the cerebral cortex stops functioning or is irreversibly damaged.

H. Nursing care
1. Frequency of assessment depends on the client's stability (at least every 8 hours); as changes occur, assessment needs to be done more frequently.
2. Physical care (Box 76-5)

⚠ Avoid repeated, unnecessary assessments on a dying client. Assessment should be limited to obtaining essential data.

Box 76-5 Physical Care of the Dying Client

Pain
Administer pain medication.
Do not delay or deny pain medication.

Dyspnea
Elevate the head of the bed or position the client on his or her side.
Administer supplemental oxygen.
Suction fluids from the airway as needed.

Skin
Assess color and temperature.
Assess for breakdown.
Implement measures to prevent breakdown.

Dehydration
Maintain regular oral care.
Encourage taking ice chips and sips of fluid.
Do not force the client to eat or drink.
Use moist cloths to provide moisture to the mouth.
Apply lubricant to the lips and oral mucous membranes.

Anorexia, Nausea, and Vomiting
Provide antiemetics before meals.
Have family members provide the client's favorite foods.
Provide frequent small portions of favorite foods.

Elimination
Monitor urinary and bowel elimination.
Place absorbent pads under the client and check frequently.

Weakness and Fatigue
Provide rest periods.
Assess tolerance for activities.
Provide assistance and support as needed for maintaining bed or chair positions.

Restlessness
Maintain a calm soothing environment.
Do not restrain.
Limit the number of visitors at the client's bedside (consider cultural practices).
Allow a family member to stay with the client.

3. Psychosocial care
   a. Monitor for anxiety and depression.
   b. Monitor for fear (Box 76-6).
   c. Encourage the client and family to express feelings.
   d. Provide support and advocacy for the client and family.
   e. Provide privacy for the client and family.
   f. Provide a private room for the client.
4. Postmortem care (Box 76-7)
   a. Maintain respect and dignity for the client.
   b. Determine whether the client is an organ donor; if so, follow appropriate procedures related to the donation.
   c. Consider cultural rituals, state laws, and agency procedures when performing postmortem care.
   d. Prepare the body for immediate viewing by the family.
   e. Provide privacy and time for the family to be with the deceased person.

VI. DEPRESSION

A. Description (see Chapter 74)
   1. Depression affects feelings, thoughts, and behaviors.
   2. It can occur after a loss, including loss of self-esteem, the end of a significant relationship, the death of a loved one, or a traumatic event.

Box 76-6 Fear Associated With Dying

Fear of Pain
Fear of pain may occur based on anxieties related to dying. Do not delay or deny pain relief measures to a terminally ill client.

Fear of Loneliness and Abandonment
Allow family members to stay with the client.
Holding hands, touching (if culturally acceptable), and listening to the client are important.

Fear of Being Meaningless
Client may feel hopeless and powerless.
Encourage life reviews and focus on the positive aspects of the client's life.

Modified from Lewis, S., Heitkemper, M., & Dirksen, S. (2007). *Medical-surgical nursing: Assessment and management of clinical problems* (7th ed.). St. Louis: Mosby.

Box 76-7 General Postmortem Procedures

Close the client's eyes.
Replace dentures.
Wash the body.
Place pads under the perineum.
Remove tubes and dressings.
Straighten the body and place a pillow under the head in preparation for family viewing.

---

3. The loss is followed by grief and mourning; if this process does not resolve, depression results.
4. Depression may be mild, moderate, or severe.
5. Treatment includes counseling, antidepressant medication, and electroconvulsive therapy (ECT).

B. Mild depression
   1. Mild depression is triggered by an external event and follows the normal grief reaction.
   2. Mild depression lasts less than 2 weeks.
   3. Feeling sad
   4. Feeling let down or disappointed
   5. Mild alterations in sleep patterns
   6. Feeling less alert
   7. Irritability
   8. Disinterested in spending time with others
   9. Increased use of alcohol or drugs

C. Moderate depression
   1. Moderate depression persists over time.
   2. The person experiences a sense of change and often seeks help.
   3. Despondent and gloomy
   4. Dejected
   5. Low self-esteem
   6. Helplessness and powerlessness
   7. May experience intense anxiety and anger
   8. Diurnal variation: The person may feel better at a certain time of the day, such as in the morning.
   9. Slow thought processes and difficulty in concentrating
   10. Rumination: Persistent thinking about and discussion of a particular subject
   11. Negative thinking and suicidal thoughts
   12. Sleep disturbances
   13. Social withdrawal
   14. Anorexia, weight loss, and fatigue
   15. Somatic complaints
   16. Menstrual changes
   17. Increased use of alcohol or drugs

D. Severe depression
   1. Intense and pervasive
   2. Despair and hopelessness
   3. Guilt and worthlessness
   4. Flat affect
   5. May show agitation and pace about
   6. Poor posture and unkempt appearance
   7. Decreased speech
   8. Self-destructive thoughts; however, the person may lack energy to act on the thought
   9. Social withdrawal
   10. Poor concentration and overwhelmed by simple tasks
   11. Severe psychomotor retardation
   12. Anorexia and considerable weight loss
   13. Constipation and urinary retention
   14. Lack of sexual interest
   15. Terminal insomnia

16. Diurnal variation: The person feels worse in the morning and better as the day goes on.
17. Delusions and hallucinations

E. Interventions
1. Altered thought processes
   a. Encourage the client to discuss losses or changes in the life situation.
   b. Encourage the client to express sadness or anger and allow adequate time for verbal responses.
   c. Assist the client in developing short-term goals.
   d. Encourage the use of problem solving and positive thinking.
   e. Limit decision making.
   f. Spend short periods of time throughout the day with the client.
   g. Be on time when a schedule is planned with the client.
   h. Sit in silence with a client who is not verbalizing.
   i. Use simple, concrete words when communicating.
   j. Avoid a cheerful attitude.
2. Risk for self-harm
   a. Assess for **suicide** clues and intervene to provide safety precautions as necessary.
   b. Assess lethality of plans.
   c. Do not leave the client alone for extended periods.
   d. If the client has a suicidal plan, place on one-to-one supervision.
   e. Form a suicidal contract with the client.

⚠ For a client at risk for self-harm, ask the client directly, "Have you thought of hurting yourself?"

3. Activity intolerance
   a. Encourage daily exercise.
   b. Assist with activities of daily living if the client is unable to perform them.
   c. Begin with one-to-one activities.
   d. Provide activities for easy mastery to increase self-esteem and help in alleviating guilt feelings.
   e. Provide activities that do not require a great deal of concentration (simple card games, drawing).
   f. Engage in gross motor activities (walking).
   g. Eventually bring the client into small group activities and then large groups.
4. Altered nutrition
   a. Ensure adequate nutrition.
   b. Offer small, high-calorie, high-protein snacks and fluids throughout the day.
   c. Stay with the client during meals.
   d. Weigh the client weekly.
   e. Assess bowel patterns for constipation.

5. Sleep pattern disturbance
   a. Ensure adequate sleep.
   b. Provide rest periods after activities.
   c. Encourage the client to dress and stay out of bed during the day.
   d. Provide relaxation measures at bedtime.
   e. Decrease environmental stimuli at bedtime.
   f. Spend time with the client before bedtime.

VII. ELECTROCONVULSIVE THERAPY (ECT)

A. Description
1. ECT is an effective treatment for depression that consists of inducing a tonic-clonic seizure by passing an electrical current through electrodes attached to the temples.
2. The administration of a muscle relaxant minimizes seizure activity, preventing damage to long bones and cervical vertebrae.
3. The usual course is 6 to 12 treatments given 2 to 3 times per week.
4. Maintenance ECT once a month may help decrease the relapse rate for a client with recurrent depression.
5. ECT is not a permanent cure.
6. ECT is not always effective in clients with dysthymic depression, depression and personality disorders, drug dependence, or depression secondary to situational or social difficulties.
7. At-risk clients include clients with recent myocardial infarction, brain attack (stroke), or intracranial mass lesions.

B. Uses
1. Clients with major depressive and bipolar depressive disorders, especially when psychotic symptoms are present, such as delusions of guilt, somatic delusions, and delusions of infidelity
2. Clients who have depression with marked psychomotor retardation and stupor
3. Manic clients whose conditions are resistant to lithium and antipsychotic medications and clients who are rapid cyclers (a client with a bipolar disorder who has many episodes of mood swings close together)
4. Clients with schizophrenia (especially catatonia), clients with schizoaffective syndromes, and psychotic clients

C. Indications for use (Box 76-8)
D. Preprocedure
1. Explain the procedure to the client.
2. Encourage the client to discuss feelings, including myths regarding ECT.
3. Teach the client and family what to expect.
4. Informed consent must be obtained when voluntary clients are being treated.
5. For involuntary clients, when informed consent cannot be obtained, permission may be obtained from the next of kin, although in

Box 76-8 Electroconvulsive Therapy (ECT): Indications for Use

When antidepressant medications have no effect
When there is a need for a rapid definitive response, such as when a client is suicidal or homicidal
When the client is in extreme agitation or stupor
When the risks of other treatments outweigh the risk of ECT
When the client has a history of poor medication response, a history of good ECT response, or both
When the client prefers ECT as a treatment

Box 76-9 Suicidal Clues

Giving away personal, special, and prized possessions
Canceling social engagements
Making out or changing a will
Taking out or changing insurance policies
Positive or negative changes in behavior
Poor appetite
Sleeping difficulties
Feelings of hopelessness
Difficulty in concentrating
Loss of interest in activities
Client statements indicating an intent to attempt suicide
Sudden calmness or improvement in a depressed client
Client inquiries about poisons, guns, or other lethal objects

some states the permission for ECT must be obtained from the court.
6. Maintain NPO status after midnight or at least 4 hours before treatment.
7. Baseline vital signs are taken.
8. The client is requested to void.
9. Hairpins, contact lenses, and dentures are removed.
10. Administer preoperative medication if prescribed; glycopyrrolate (Robinul) or atropine sulfate may be prescribed to prevent the potential for aspiration and to minimize bradydysrhythmias in response to electrical stimulus.
E. During the procedure
1. Place a blood pressure cuff on one of the client's arms.
2. As the intravenous line is inserted, electroencephalographic and electrocardiographic electrodes are attached.
3. A pulse oximeter is placed on the client's finger.
4. Blood pressure is monitored throughout the treatment.
5. Medications administered may include a short-acting anesthetic such as methohexital sodium (Brevital Sodium), thiopental sodium (Pentothal), and a muscle relaxant such as succinylcholine (Anectine).
6. Throughout the procedure, 100% oxygen by mask via positive pressure is administered.
7. An airway or bite-block is placed to prevent biting the tongue.
8. An electrical stimulus is administered; the seizure should last 30 to 60 seconds.
F. Postprocedure
1. The client is transported to a recovery room with the blood pressure cuff and oximeter in place, where oxygen, suction, and other emergency equipment are available.
2. When the client is awake, talk to the client and take vital signs.
3. The client may be confused; provide frequent orientation (brief, distinct, and simple) and reassurance.

4. The client returns to the nursing unit when at least a 90% oxygen saturation level is maintained, vital signs are stable, and mental status is satisfactory.
5. Assess the gag reflex before giving the client fluids, food, or medication.
G. Potential side effects
1. Major side effects include confusion, disorientation, and short-term memory loss.
2. The client may be confused and disoriented on awakening.
3. Memory deficits may occur, but memory usually recovers completely, although some clients have memory loss lasting 6 months.

VIII. SUICIDAL BEHAVIOR

A. Description
1. Suicidal clients characteristically have feelings of worthlessness, guilt, and hopelessness that are so overwhelming that they feel unable to go on with life and feel unfit to live.
2. The nurse caring for a depressed client always considers the possibility of **suicide**.
B. High-risk groups
1. Clients with a history of previous **suicide attempts**
2. Family history of **suicide attempts**
3. Adolescents
4. Older adults
5. Disabled or terminally ill clients
6. Clients with personality disorders
7. Clients with organic brain syndrome or dementia
8. Depressed or psychotic clients
9. Substance abusers
C. Clues (Box 76-9)
D. Assessment (Box 76-10)
E. Interventions
1. Initiate **suicide** precautions.
2. Remove harmful objects.
3. Do not leave the client alone.
4. Provide a nonjudgmental, caring attitude.

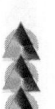
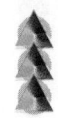
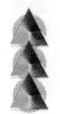

Box 76-10 Suicidal Client: Assessment

Plan

Does the client have a plan?

What is the plan, how lethal is the plan, and how likely is death to occur?

Does the client have the means to carry out the plan?

Client History of Attempts

What suicide attempts occurred in the past and what harm occurred?

Was the client accidentally rescued?

Have the past attempts and methods been the same, or have methods increased in lethality?

Psychosocial Factors

Is client alone or alienated from others?

Is hostility or depression present?

Do hallucinations exist?

Is substance abuse present?

Has client had any recent losses or physical illness?

Has client had any environmental or lifestyle changes?

5. Develop a contract that is written, dated, and signed and that indicates alternative behavior at times of suicidal thoughts.

6. Encourage the client to talk about feelings and to identify positive aspects about self.

7. Encourage active participation in own care.

8. Keep the client active by assigning achievable tasks.

9. Check that visitors do not leave harmful objects in the client's room.

10. Identify support systems.

11. Do not allow the client to leave the unit unless accompanied by a staff member.

12. Continue to assess the client's **suicide** potential.

⚠ Provide one-to-one supervision at all times for the client at risk for suicide.

IX. ABUSIVE BEHAVIORS

A. Anger
1. Anger is a feeling of annoyance that may be displaced onto an object or person.
2. Anger is used to avoid anxiety and gives a feeling of power in situations in which the person feels out of control.

B. Aggression can be harmful and destructive when not controlled.

C. Violence is physical force that is threatening to the safety of self and others.

D. Assessment
1. History of violence or self-harm
2. Poor impulse control and low tolerance of frustration
3. Defiant and argumentative
4. Raising of voice

5. Making verbal threats
6. Pacing and agitation
7. Muscle rigidity
8. Flushed face
9. Glaring at others

E. Interventions
1. Maintain safety.
2. Use a calm approach and communicate with a calm, clear tone of voice (be assertive, not aggressive, and avoid verbal struggles).
3. Maintain a large personal space and use a non-aggressive posture.
4. Listen actively and acknowledge the client's anger.
5. Determine what the client considers to be his or her need.
6. Provide the client with clear options that deal with the client's behavior, set limits on behavior, and make the client aware of the consequences of anger and violence.
7. Discuss the use of **restraints** or **seclusion** if the client is unable to control angry behavior that may lead to violence.
8. Assist the client with problem solving and decision making regarding the options.

F. **Restraints** and **seclusion**
1. Description
   a. Physical **restraints**: Any manual method or mechanical device, material, or equipment that inhibits free movement
   b. **Seclusion**: A process in which a client is placed alone in a specially designed room for protection and close supervision
   c. Chemical **restraints**: Medications given for a specific purpose of inhibiting a specific behavior or movement and that have an impact on the client's ability to relate to the environment
2. Use of **restraints** and **seclusion**

⚠ Restraints require a written prescription by a physician, which must be reviewed and renewed every 24 hours; the prescription must specify the type of restraint to be used, the duration of the restraint or seclusion, and the criteria for release (agency policy and procedures need to be followed).

   a. **Restraints** and **seclusion** should never be used as punishment or for the convenience of the health care staff.
   b. **Restraints** and **seclusion** are used when behavior is physically harmful to the client or others and when alternative or less restrictive measures are insufficient in protecting the client or others from harm.
   c. The nurse must document the behavior leading to the use of **restraints** or **seclusion**.

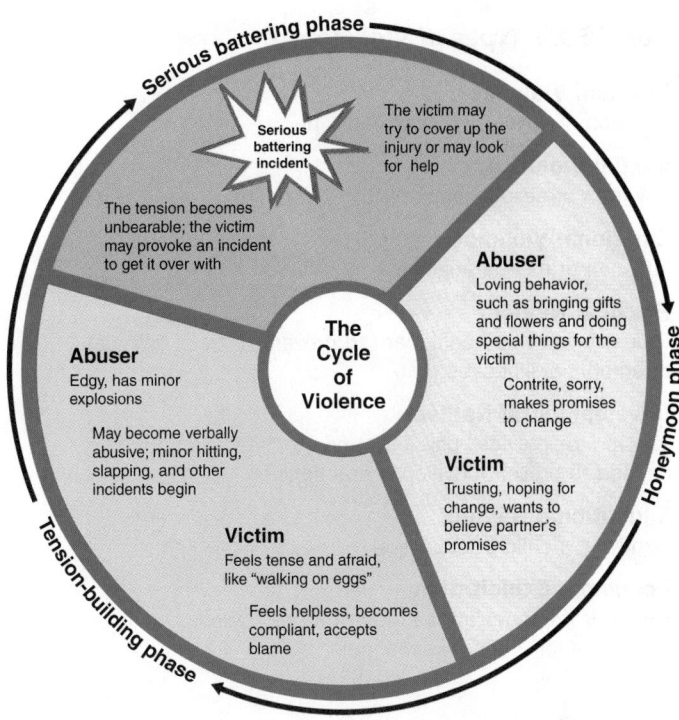

▲ **FIGURE 76-1** The cycle of violence. (From Varcarolis, E., Carson, V., & Shoemaker, N. [2010]. *Foundations of psychiatric mental health nursing* [6th ed.]. St. Louis: Saunders.)

  d. **Restraints** and **seclusion** are used when the client anticipates that a controlled environment would be helpful and requests **seclusion**.
  e. In an emergency, a qualified nurse may place a client in **restraints** or **seclusion** and obtain a written or verbal prescription as soon as possible thereafter.
  f. Within 1 hour of the initiation of **restraints** or **seclusion**, the psychiatrist must make a face-to-face assessment and evaluation of the client and must continuously re-evaluate the need for continued **restraints** or **seclusion**.
  g. While in **restraints** or **seclusion**, the client must be protected from all sources of harm by having one-to-one supervision with a staff member within an arm's length of the client.
  h. The client in **restraints** or **seclusion** needs constant one-to-one supervision; physical, safety, and comfort needs must be assessed every 15 to 30 minutes, and these observations are also documented (e.g., food, fluids, bathroom needs, range-of-motion exercise, and ambulation).

X. FAMILY VIOLENCE

A. Description (Fig. 76-1)
  1. Violence begins with threats or verbal or physical minor assaults (tension building), and the victim attempts to comply with the requests of the abuser.
  2. The abuser loses control and becomes destructive and harmful (acute battering), while the victim attempts to protect himself or herself.

  3. After the battering, the abuser becomes loving and attempts to make peace (calmness and defusion of tension).
  4. The abuser justifies that violence is normal and the victim is responsible for the **abuse**.
  5. Outsiders are usually unaware of what is happening in the family.
  6. Family members are isolated socially and lack autonomy and trust among each other; caring and intimacy in the family are absent.
  7. Family members expect other members of the family to meet their needs, but none are able to do so.
  8. The abuser threatens to abandon the family.
B. Types of violence (Box 76-11)
C. The vulnerable person
  1. The vulnerable person is the one in the family unit against whom violence is perpetrated.
  2. The most vulnerable individuals are children and older adults.
  3. The perpetrator of violence and the person targeted by the violence can be male or female.
  4. Battering is a crime.
D. Characteristics of abusers
  1. Impaired self-esteem
  2. Strong dependency needs
  3. Narcissistic and suspicious
  4. History of **abuse** during childhood
  5. Perceive victims as their property and believe that they are entitled to **abuse** them
E. Characteristics of victims
  1. Victims feel trapped, dependent, helpless, and powerless.

Box 76-11 Types of Violence

Physical Violence
Infliction of physical pain or bodily harm

Sexual Violence
Any form of sexual contact without consent

Emotional Violence
Infliction of mental anguish

Physical Neglect
Failure to provide health care to prevent or treat physical or emotional illnesses

Developmental Neglect
Failure to provide physical and cognitive stimulation needed to prevent developmental deficits

Educational Neglect
Depriving a child of education

Economic Exploitation
Illegal or improper exploitation of money, funds, or other resources for one's personal gain

Box 76-12 Assessment Questions for Violence and Abuse

"Has anyone ever touched you in a way that made you uncomfortable?"
"Is anyone hurting you now?
"How do you and your partner deal with anger (or disagreement)?"
"Has your partner ever hit you?"
"Have you ever been threatened by _____"
"Does your partner prevent you from seeing family or friends"
"Does your partner ever use the children to manipulate you?"
"Did (or does) anyone in your family deal with anger by hitting?"
"Who do you play with most often? Is there anyone you do not like playing with? Are there games you don't like playing?"

2. Victims of **abuse** may become depressed as they are trapped in the abusers' power and control cycle (see Fig. 76-1).
3. As victims' self-esteem becomes diminished with chronic **abuse**, they may blame themselves for the violence and be unable to see a way out of the situation.

F. Interventions
1. Report suspected or actual cases of child **abuse** or **abuse** of an older adult to appropriate authorities (follow state and agency guidelines).
2. Assess for evidence of physical injuries.
3. Ensure privacy and confidentiality during the assessment, and provide a nonjudgmental and empathetic approach to foster trust; reassure the victim that he or she has not done anything wrong. Box 76-12 lists sample assessment questions.
4. Assist the victim to develop self-protective and other problem-solving abilities.
5. Even if the victim is not ready to leave the situation, encourage the victim to develop a specific safety plan (a fast escape if the violence returns) and where to obtain help (hotlines, safe houses, and shelters); an abused person is usually reluctant to call the police.
6. Assess suicidal potential of the victim.
7. Assess the potential for homicide.
8. Assess for the use of drugs and alcohol.
9. Determine family coping patterns and support systems.
10. Provide support and assistance in coping with contacting the legal system.
11. Assist in resolving family dysfunction with prescribed therapies.

12. Encourage individual therapy for the victim that promotes coping with the trauma and prevents further psychological conflict.
13. Encourage individual therapy for the abuser that focuses on preventing violent behavior and repairing relationships.
14. Encourage psychotherapy, counseling, group therapy, and support groups to assist family members to develop coping strategies.
15. Assist the family to identify an access to community and personal resources.
16. Maintain accurate and thorough medical health records.

XI. **CHILD ABUSE** (see Chapter 36)
A. Description: Child **abuse** involves physical, emotional, or sexual **abuse** and neglect.
B. Assessment
1. Physical **abuse**
a. Unexplained bruises, burns, or fractures
b. Bald spots on the scalp
c. Apprehensiveness in the child
d. Extreme aggressiveness or withdrawal
e. Fear of parents
f. Lack of crying when approached by a stranger
2. Physical neglect
a. Inadequate weight gain
b. Poor hygiene
c. Consistent hunger (begs or steals food)
d. Inconsistent school attendance
e. Constant fatigue
f. Reports of lack of child supervision
g. Delinquency
3. Emotional **abuse**
a. Speech disorders
b. Habit disorders, such as sucking, biting, rocking
c. Learning disorders
d. Self-harm behaviors

4. Sexual **abuse**
   a. Difficulty walking or sitting
   b. Torn, stained, or bloody underclothing
   c. Pain, swelling, or itching of the genitals
   d. Bruises, bleeding, or lacerations in the genital or anal area
   e. Poor peer relations
   f. Delinquency
   g. Changes in sleep patterns
   h. Self-harm behaviors
5. Shaken baby syndrome
   a. **Abuse** can cause intracranial hemorrhage, leading to cerebral edema and death.
   b. The infant often has respiratory problems.
   c. The nurse would note full bulging fontanels and a head circumference greater than expected.
6. Child abduction
   a. Many cases involve abduction by a family member (usually a parent) who takes or keeps the child and violates a custody order.
   b. Children younger than 6 years of age are most vulnerable to abduction.
   c. Parents more likely to abduct their child include parents who have made a prior threat of intent, parents who suspect **abuse** of the child, parents wanting the child to grow up in their country of origin, and parents with a mental illness (especially sociopaths).

C. Interventions
1. Assess injuries; support the child during a thorough physical assessment.
2. The child is likely to be removed from the abusive environment to a safe place to prevent further injury while the case is being investigated.
3. Move slowly and avoid any loud noises when near the child.
4. Communicate with the child at the child's eye level.
5. Reassure the child that he or she is not "bad" and is not responsible for the abuser's behavior.
6. Document accurately and completely all information related to the suspected **abuse**.
7. When working with parents in follow-up care or counseling, assist the parents in identifying stressors and alternative ways to express feelings.
8. Provide education to the parents, and refer parents to **crisis** hotlines and community support systems such as Parents Anonymous (a group for parents who have been abused or fear that they may **abuse** their child physically) or Parents United International (a group devoted to helping sexually abused families).

⚠ Report cases of suspected abuse of a child or older adult to appropriate authorities (follow state and agency guidelines); reporting is mandated by federal law.

XII. ABUSE OF THE OLDER ADULT

A. Description
1. **Abuse** of an older adult involves physical, emotional, or sexual **abuse**; neglect; and economic exploitation.
2. Older adults at most risk include individuals who are dependent because of illness, immobility, or altered mental status.
3. Factors that contribute to **abuse** and neglect include long-standing family violence, caregiver stress, and the older adult's increasing dependence on others.
4. Victims may attempt to dismiss injuries as accidental, and abusers may prevent victims from receiving proper medical care to avoid discovery.
5. Victims often are isolated socially by their abusers.

B. Assessment
1. Physical **abuse**
   a. Sprains, dislocations, or fractures
   b. Abrasions, bruises, or lacerations
   c. Pressure sores
   d. Puncture wounds
   e. Burns
   f. Skin tears
2. Sexual **abuse**
   a. Torn or stained underclothing
   b. Discomfort or bleeding in the genital area
   c. Difficulty in walking or sitting
   d. Unexplained genital infections or disease
3. Emotional **abuse**
   a. Confusion
   b. Fearful and agitated
   c. Changes in appetite and weight
   d. Withdrawn and loss of interest in self and social activities
4. Neglect
   a. Disheveled appearance
   b. Dressed inadequately or inappropriately
   c. Dehydration and malnutrition
   d. Lacking physical needs, such as glasses, hearing aids, and dentures
5. Signs of medication overdose
6. Economic exploitation
   a. Inability to pay bills and fearful when discussing finances
   b. Confused, inaccurate, or no knowledge of finances

C. Interventions
1. Assess for physical injuries and treat physical injuries.
2. Report cases of suspected **abuse** to appropriate authorities (follow state and agency guidelines).
3. Separate the older adult from the abusive environment, if possible, and contact adult protective services for assistance in placement while the **abuse** is being investigated.
4. Explore alternative living arrangements that are least restrictive and disruptive to the victim.

▬▬▬ PRIORITY NURSING ACTIONS! ▬▬▬

Actions to Take When an Older Client Is Physically Abused

1. Assess and treat the wounds.
2. Remove the victim from immediate danger.
3. Adhere to mandatory abuse reporting laws.
4. Notify the caseworker of the family situation.
5. Document the occurrence, findings, actions taken, and the victim's response.

When a victim is abused, the priority is to assess and treat any physical injuries. The nurse stays with the victim and provides comfort and support. After physical injuries are treated, the nurse ensures that the client is safe and is removed from the threatening environment. Elder abuse needs to be reported, so the nurse would adhere to the mandatory abuse reporting laws of the state. The nurse also contacts the caseworker of the family situation so that the incident is reported and follow-up with the family can occur. If there is no caseworker, the nurse contacts social services or the appropriate service to initiate this process. Finally, the nurse documents the occurrence, findings, actions taken, and the victim's response.

References: Fortinash, K., & Holoday-Worret, P. (2008). *Psychiatric mental health nursing* (4th ed., pp. 491-492). St. Louis: Mosby. Stuart, G. (2009). *Principles and practice of psychiatric nursing* (9th ed., p. 328). St. Louis: Mosby.

---

5. The older adult who has been abused may need assistance for financial or legal matters.
6. Provide referrals to emergency community resources.
7. When working with caregivers, assess the need for respite care or counseling if needed to deal with caregiver stress (see Priority Nursing Actions).

▲ **XIII. RAPE AND SEXUAL ASSAULT**

A. Description
1. Rape is engaging another person in a sexual act or sexual intercourse through the use of force and without the consent of the sexual partner.
2. The victim is not required by law to report the rape or assault.
3. Often, the victim is blamed by others and receives no support from significant others.
4. Acquaintance rape involves someone known to the victim.
5. Statutory rape is the act of sexual intercourse with a person younger than the age of legal consent, even if the minor consents.
6. Marital rape
   a. The belief that marriage bestows rights to sex whenever wanted and without consent of the partner contributes to the occurrence of marital rape.

b. Victims of marital rape describe being forced to perform acts they did not wish to perform and being physically abused during sex.

B. Assessment
1. Female client
   a. Obtain the date of the last menstrual period.
   b. Determine the form of birth control used and the last act of intercourse before rape.
   c. Determine the duration of intercourse, orifices violated, and whether penile penetration occurred.
   d. Determine whether a condom was used by the perpetrator.
2. Shame, embarrassment, and humiliation
3. Anger and revenge
4. Afraid to tell others because of fear of not being believed

C. Males may be sexually abused as children and as adults and are the usual targeted victim of pedophiles; males may have more difficulty with disclosing their **abuse**.

D. Rape trauma syndrome
1. Sleep disturbances, nightmares
2. Loss of appetite
3. Fears, anxiety, phobias, suspicion
4. Decrease in activities and motivation
5. Disruptions in relationships with partner, family, friends
6. Self-blame, guilt, shame
7. Lowered self-esteem, feelings of worthlessness
8. Somatic complaints

E. Interventions
1. Perform the assessment in a quiet, private area.
2. Stay with the victim.
3. Assess the victim's stress level before performing treatments and procedures.
4. Victim should not shower, bathe, douche (female), or change clothing until an examination is performed.
5. Obtain written consent for the examination, photographs, laboratory tests, release of information, and laboratory samples.
6. Assist with the female pelvic examination and obtain specimens to detect semen (the pelvic examination may trigger a flashback of the attack); a shower and fresh clothing should be made available to the client after the examination.
7. Preserve any evidence.
8. Treat physical injuries and provide client safety.
9. Document all events in the care of the victim.
10. Reinforce to the victim that surviving the assault is most important; if the victim survived the rape, he or she did exactly what was necessary to stay alive.
11. Refer the victim to **crisis** intervention and support groups.

MORE QUESTIONS ON THE CD!

Practice Questions

929. A nurse in the emergency department is caring for a young female victim of sexual assault. The client's physical assessment is complete, and physical evidence has been collected. The nurse notes that the client is withdrawn, confused, and at times physically immobile. These behaviors are interpreted by the nurse as:
1. Signs of depression
2. Normal reactions to a devastating event
3. Evidence that the client is a high suicide risk
4. Indicative of the need for hospital admission

930. A nurse is reviewing the assessment data of a client admitted to the mental health unit. The nurse notes that the admission nurse documented that the client is experiencing anxiety as a result of a situational crisis. The nurse determines that this type of crisis could be caused by:
1. Witnessing a murder
2. The death of a loved one
3. A fire that destroyed the client's home
4. A recent rape episode experienced by the client

931. A nurse is conducting an initial assessment on a client in crisis. When assessing the client's perception of the precipitating event that led to the crisis, the appropriate question to ask is:
1. "With whom do you live?"
2. "Who is available to help you?"
3. "What leads you to seek help now?"
4. "What do you usually do to feel better?"

932. A nurse is developing a plan of care for a client in a crisis state. When developing the plan, the nurse considers which of the following?
1. A crisis state indicates that the client has a mental illness.
2. A crisis state indicates that the client has an emotional illness.
3. Presenting symptoms in a crisis situation are similar for all clients experiencing a crisis.
4. A client's response to a crisis is individualized and what constitutes a crisis for one client may not constitute a crisis for another client.

933. A nurse observes that a client with a potential for violence is agitated, pacing up and down the hallway, and is making aggressive and belligerent gestures at other clients. Which statement would be appropriate to make to this client?
1. "You need to stop that behavior now."
2. "You will need to be placed in seclusion."
3. "You seem restless; tell me what is happening."

4. "You will need to be restrained if you do not change your behavior."

934. A depressed client on an inpatient unit says to a nurse, "My family would be better off without me." The nurse's best response is:
1. "Have you talked to your family about this?"
2. "Everyone feels this way when they are depressed."
3. "You will feel better once your medication begins to work."
4. "You sound very upset. Are you thinking of hurting yourself?"

935. A nurse has been observing a client closely who has been displaying aggressive behaviors. The nurse observes that the behavior displayed by the client is escalating. Which nursing intervention is least helpful to this client at this time?
1. Initiate confinement measures.
2. Acknowledge the client's behavior.
3. Assist the client to an area that is quiet.
4. Maintain a safe distance with the client.

936. Which behavior observed by a nurse indicates a suspicion that a depressed adolescent client may be suicidal?
1. The client runs out of the therapy group, swearing at the group leader, and runs to her room.
2. The client gives away a prized CD and a cherished autographed picture of the performer.
3. The client becomes angry while speaking on the telephone and slams down the receiver.
4. The client gets angry with her roommate when the roommate borrows the client's clothes without asking.

937. A client is admitted to the mental health unit after an attempt of suicide by hanging. A nurse's most important aspect of care is to maintain client safety. This is accomplished best by:
1. Requesting that a peer remain with the client at all times
2. Removing the client's clothing and placing the client in a hospital gown
3. Assigning a staff member to the client who will remain with the client at all times
4. Admitting the client to a seclusion room where all potentially dangerous articles are removed

938. The police arrive at the emergency department with a client who has seriously lacerated both wrists. The initial nursing action is to:
1. Administer an antianxiety agent.
2. Examine and treat the wound sites.

3. Secure and record a detailed history.
4. Encourage and assist the client to ventilate feelings.

939. A moderately depressed client who was hospitalized 2 days ago suddenly begins smiling and reporting that the crisis is over. The client says to a nurse, "I'm finally cured." The nurse interprets this behavior as a cue to modify the treatment plan by:
1. Suggesting a reduction of medication
2. Allowing increased "in-room" activities
3. Increasing the level of suicide precautions
4. Allowing the client off-unit privileges as needed

940. A nurse is planning care for a client being admitted to the nursing unit who attempted suicide. Which of the following priority nursing interventions would the nurse include in the plan of care?
1. One-to-one suicide precautions
2. Suicide precautions with 30-minute checks
3. Checking the whereabouts of the client every 15 minutes
4. Asking the client to report suicidal thoughts immediately

941. An emergency department nurse is caring for an adult client who is a victim of family violence. Which priority instruction would be included in the discharge instructions?
1. Information regarding shelters
2. Instructions regarding calling the police
3. Instructions regarding self-defense classes
4. Explaining the importance of leaving the violent situation

942. A female victim of a sexual assault is being seen in the crisis center. The client states that she still feels "as though the rape just happened yesterday," even though it has been a few months since the incident. The appropriate nursing response is which of the following?
1. "You need to try to be realistic. The rape did not just occur."
2. "It will take some time to get over these feelings about your rape."
3. "Tell me more about the incident that causes you to feel like the rape just occurred."
4. "What do you think that you can do to alleviate some of your fears about being raped again"?

Alternate Item Format: Multiple Response

943. A nurse is preparing to care for a dying client, and several family members are at the client's bedside. Select the therapeutic techniques that the nurse would use when communicating with the family. **Select all that apply.**
❑ 1. Discourage reminiscing.
❑ 2. Make the decisions for the family.
❑ 3. Encourage expression of feelings, concerns, and fears.
❑ 4. Explain everything that is happening to all family members.
❑ 5. Touch and hold the client's or family member's hand if appropriate.
❑ 6. Be honest and let the client and family know that they will not be abandoned by the nurse.

ANSWERS

929. 2
Rationale: During the acute phase of the rape crisis, the client can display a wide range of emotional and somatic responses. The symptoms noted indicate a normal reaction. Options 1, 3, and 4 are incorrect interpretations.
Test-Taking Strategy: Use the process of elimination and knowledge regarding client responses to devastating events to answer the question. Focus on the symptoms noted in the question to direct you to option 2. If you had difficulty with this question, review normal and abnormal client responses to dealing with devastating crisis events.
Level of Cognitive Ability: Analyzing
Client Needs: Psychosocial Integrity
Integrated Process: Nursing Process—Assessment
Content Area: Mental Health
Reference: Fortinash, K., & Holoday-Worret, P. (2008). *Psychiatric mental health nursing* (4th ed., pp. 507–508). St. Louis: Mosby.

930. 2
Rationale: A situational crisis arises from external rather than internal sources. External situations that could precipitate a crisis include loss of or change of a job, the death of a loved one, abortion, change in financial status, divorce, addition of new family members, pregnancy, and severe illness. Options 1, 3, and 4 identify adventitious crises. An adventitious crisis refers to a crisis of disaster; it is unplanned or accidental.
Test-Taking Strategy: Use the process of elimination. Eliminate options 1, 3, and 4 because they are comparable or alike types of occurrences. If you had difficulty with this question, review the types of crisis.
Level of Cognitive Ability: Understanding
Client Needs: Psychosocial Integrity
Integrated Process: Nursing Process—Analysis
Content Area: Mental Health
Reference: Stuart, G. (2009). *Principles and practice of psychiatric nursing* (9th ed., pp. 186–187). St. Louis: Mosby.

931. 3

Rationale: A nurse's initial task when assessing a client in crisis is to assess the individual or family and the problem. The more clearly the problem can be defined, the better the chance a solution can be found. Option 3 would assist in determining data related to the precipitating event that led to the crisis. Options 1 and 2 assess situational supports. Option 4 assesses personal coping skills.

Test-Taking Strategy: Use the process of elimination and note the strategic words *precipitating event*. Focus on these strategic words when selecting the correct option. Eliminate options 1 and 2 because these data would determine support systems. Eliminate option 4 because this question would be asked when determining coping skills. Review assessment techniques for the client in crisis if you had difficulty with this question.

Level of Cognitive Ability: Applying
Client Needs: Psychosocial Integrity
Integrated Process: Nursing Process—Assessment
Content Area: Mental Health
Reference: Fortinash, K., & Holoday-Worret, P. (2008). *Psychiatric mental health nursing* (4th ed., p. 456). St. Louis: Mosby.

932. 4

Rationale: Although each crisis response can be described in similar terms as far as presenting symptoms are concerned, what constitutes a crisis for one client may not constitute a crisis for another client because each is a unique individual. Being in the crisis state does not mean that the client has an emotional or mental illness.

Test-Taking Strategy: Use the process of elimination. Eliminate option 3 because of the word *all*. Next, eliminate options 1 and 2 because a crisis does not indicate "illness." Review the characteristics of a crisis state if you had difficulty with this question.

Level of Cognitive Ability: Understanding
Client Needs: Psychosocial Integrity
Integrated Process: Nursing Process—Planning
Content Area: Mental Health
Reference: Stuart, G. (2009). *Principles and practice of psychiatric nursing* (9th ed., p. 190). St. Louis: Mosby.

933. 3

Rationale: The best statement is to ask the client what is causing the agitation. This will assist the client to become aware of the behavior and may assist the nurse in planning appropriate interventions for the client. Option 1 is demanding behavior that could cause increased agitation in the client. Options 2 and 4 are threats to the client and are inappropriate.

Test-Taking Strategy: Use the process of elimination. Eliminate option 1 because of the demand that it places on the client. Eliminate options 2 and 4 because they indicate threats to the client. Review appropriate nursing actions for the agitated client if you had difficulty with this question.

Level of Cognitive Ability: Applying
Client Needs: Psychosocial Integrity
Integrated Process: Communication and Documentation
Content Area: Mental Health
Reference: Stuart, G. (2009). *Principles and practice of psychiatric nursing* (9th ed., pp. 27–31, 342). St. Louis: Mosby.

934. 4

Rationale: Clients who are depressed may be at risk for suicide. It is critical for the nurse to assess suicidal ideation and plan. The nurse should ask the client directly whether a plan for self-harm exists. Options 1, 2, and 3 do not deal directly with the client's feelings.

Test-Taking Strategy: Using therapeutic communication techniques will assist in directing you to the correct option. Option 4 is the only option that deals directly with the client's feelings. Additionally, clients at risk for suicide need to be assessed directly regarding the potential for self-harm. Review care of the client at risk for suicide if you had difficulty with this question.

Level of Cognitive Ability: Applying
Client Needs: Psychosocial Integrity
Integrated Process: Communication and Documentation
Content Area: Mental Health
Reference: Stuart, G. (2009). *Principles and practice of psychiatric nursing* (9th ed., pp. 27–31, 296). St. Louis: Mosby.

935. 1

Rationale: During the escalation period, the client's behavior is moving toward loss of control. Nursing actions include taking control, maintaining a safe distance, acknowledging behavior, moving the client to a quiet area, and medicating the client if appropriate. To initiate confinement measures during this period is inappropriate. Initiation of confinement measures is most appropriate during the crisis period.

Test-Taking Strategy: Note the strategic words *behavior, escalating,* and *least helpful*. Recalling that the least restrictive measures should be used will direct you to option 1. Review care of the client with aggressive behavior if you had difficulty with this question.

Level of Cognitive Ability: Applying
Client Needs: Psychosocial Integrity
Integrated Process: Nursing Process—Implementation
Content Area: Mental Health
Reference: Varcarolis, E., & Halter, M. (2009). *Essentials of psychiatric mental health nursing: A communication approach to evidence-based care* (pp. 428–431). St. Louis: Saunders.

936. 2

Rationale: A depressed suicidal client often gives away that which is of value as a way of saying goodbye and wanting to be remembered. Options 1, 3, and 4 deal with anger and acting-out behaviors that are often typical of any adolescent.

Test-Taking Strategy: Use the process of elimination. Eliminate options 1, 3, and 4 because they are comparable or alike. Option 2 is different and is an action that could indicate that the client may be "saying goodbye." Review behaviors that indicate a suicide intent if you had difficulty with this question.

Level of Cognitive Ability: Analyzing
Client Needs: Psychosocial Integrity
Integrated Process: Nursing Process—Assessment
Content Area: Mental Health
Reference: Stuart, G. (2009). *Principles and practice of psychiatric nursing* (9th ed., p. 316). St. Louis: Mosby.

937. 3
Rationale: Hanging is a serious suicide attempt. The plan of care must reflect action that ensures the client's safety. Constant observation status (one-to-one) with a staff member who is never less than an arm's length away is the best choice. Seclusion should not be the initial intervention, and the least restrictive measure should be used. Placing the client in a hospital gown and requesting that a peer remain with the client would not ensure a safe environment.
Test-Taking Strategy: Use the process of elimination. Eliminate option 4 because seclusion should not be the initial intervention. Eliminate option 1 next because the responsibility to safeguard a client is not the peer's responsibility. Eliminate option 2 because removing one's clothing would not maximize all possible safety strategies. Review nursing interventions for the client at risk for suicide if you had difficulty with this question.
Level of Cognitive Ability: Applying
Client Needs: Safe and Effective Care Environment
Integrated Process: Nursing Process—Implementation
Content Area: Mental Health
Reference: Stuart, G. (2009). *Principles and practice of psychiatric nursing* (9th ed., p. 327). St. Louis: Mosby.

938. 2
Rationale: The initial nursing action is to assess and treat the self-inflicted injuries. Injuries from lacerated wrists can lead to a life-threatening situation. Other interventions, such as options 1, 3, and 4, may follow after the client has been treated medically.
Test-Taking Strategy: Note the strategic word *initial.* Use Maslow's Hierarchy of Needs theory to prioritize. Physiological needs come first. Option 2 addresses the physiological need. Review care of the client who attempted suicide if you had difficulty with this question.
Level of Cognitive Ability: Applying
Client Needs: Physiological Integrity
Integrated Process: Nursing Process—Implementation
Content Area: Leadership and Management—Delegating/Prioritizing
References: Fortinash, K., & Holoday-Worret, P. (2008). *Psychiatric mental health nursing* (4th ed., p. 473). St. Louis: Mosby.
  Stuart, G. (2009). *Principles and practice of psychiatric nursing* (9th ed., p. 316). St. Louis: Mosby.

939. 3
Rationale: A client who is moderately depressed and has only been in the hospital 2 days is unlikely to have such a dramatic cure. When a depression suddenly lifts, it is likely that the client may have made the decision to harm himself or herself. Suicide precautions are necessary to keep the client safe.
Test-Taking Strategy: Use the process of elimination. Options 1 and 4 support the client's notion that a cure has occurred. Option 2 allows the client to increase isolation and would present a threat to the client's safety. Safety is of the utmost importance; option 3 is the correct option. Review care of the client with depression if you had difficulty with this question.
Level of Cognitive Ability: Analyzing
Client Needs: Safe and Effective Care Environment

Integrated Process: Nursing Process—Planning
Content Area: Mental Health
Reference: Stuart, G. (2009). *Principles and practice of psychiatric nursing* (9th ed., pp. 287, 301). St. Louis: Mosby.

940. 1
Rationale: One-to-one suicide precautions are required for a client who has attempted suicide. Options 2 and 3 may be appropriate, but not at the present time, considering the situation. Option 4 also may be an appropriate nursing intervention, but the priority is identified in option 1. The best intervention is constant supervision so that the nurse may intervene as needed if the client attempts to harm himself or herself.
Test-Taking Strategy: Use the process of elimination, noting the strategic words *attempted suicide.* Option 1 is the only option that provides a safe environment. Review interventions for the suicidal client if you had difficulty with this question.
Level of Cognitive Ability: Applying
Client Needs: Safe and Effective Care Environment
Integrated Process: Nursing Process—Implementation
Content Area: Mental Health
References: Stuart, G. (2009). *Principles and practice of psychiatric nursing* (9th ed., p. 327). St. Louis: Mosby.
  Varcarolis, E., & Halter, M. (2009). *Essentials of psychiatric mental health nursing: A communication approach to evidence-based care* (p. 417). St. Louis: Saunders.

941. 1
Rationale: Tertiary prevention of family violence includes assisting the victim after the abuse has already occurred. The nurse should provide the client with information regarding where to obtain help, including a specific plan for removing the self from the abuser and information regarding escape, hotlines, and the location of shelters. An abused person is usually reluctant to call the police. Teaching the victim to fight back is not the appropriate action for the victim when dealing with a violent person.
Test-Taking Strategy: Note the strategic word *priority.* Focus on the subject of the question, which relates to providing the client with a safe environment. Use Maslow's Hierarchy of Needs theory to assist in directing you to option 1. If you had difficulty with this question, review the nursing measures for caring for a victim of family violence.
Level of Cognitive Ability: Applying
Client Needs: Safe and Effective Care Environment
Integrated Process: Nursing Process—Implementation
Content Area: Mental Health
Reference: Fortinash, K., & Holoday-Worret, P. (2008). *Psychiatric mental health nursing* (4th ed., pp. 491–492). St. Louis: Mosby.

942. 3
Rationale: Option 3 allows the client to express her ideas and feelings more fully and portrays a nonhurried, nonjudgmental, supportive attitude on the part of the nurse. Clients need to be reassured that their feelings are normal and that they may express their concerns freely in a safe, caring environment. Option 4 places the problem solving totally on the client. Option 2 places the client's feelings on hold. Option 1 immediately blocks communication.

Test-Taking Strategy: Use the process of elimination. Option 3 is the only option that addresses the client's feelings. Always address the client's feelings first. Review therapeutic communication techniques if you had difficulty with this question.
Level of Cognitive Ability: Applying
Client Needs: Psychosocial Integrity
Integrated Process: Caring
Content Area: Mental Health
Reference: Stuart, G. (2009). *Principles and practice of psychiatric nursing* (9th ed., pp. 27–31, 722). St. Louis: Mosby.

ALTERNATE ITEM FORMAT: MULTIPLE RESPONSE
943. 3, 5, 6
Rationale: The nurse must determine whether there is a spokesperson for the family and how much the client and family want to know. The nurse needs to allow the family and client the opportunity for informed choices and assist with the decision-making process if asked. The nurse should encourage expression of feelings, concerns, and fears and reminiscing. The nurse needs to be honest and let the client and family know that they will not be abandoned. The nurse should touch and hold the client's or family member's hand, if appropriate.
Test-Taking Strategy: Recalling therapeutic communication techniques and client and family rights will assist you in answering this question. Review these techniques and care of the dying client if you had difficulty with this question.
Level of Cognitive Ability: Applying
Client Needs: Psychosocial Integrity
Integrated Process: Caring
Content Area: Mental Health
Reference: Potter, P., & Perry, A. (2009). *Fundamentals of nursing* (7th ed., pp. 473–477). St. Louis: Mosby.

Psychiatric Medications

I. SELECTIVE SEROTONIN REUPTAKE INHIBITORS (SSRIs) (Box 77-1)

A. Description
1. Inhibit serotonin uptake and elicit an antidepressant response
2. The potential for medication interactions is high, and complete medication assessments must be obtained and evaluated; inquire about the use of herbal therapies, especially St. John's wort.

B. Side effects
1. Nausea, vomiting, cramping, and diarrhea
2. Dry mouth
3. Central nervous system (CNS) stimulation, including akathisia (restlessness, agitation)
4. Blood pressure changes
5. Photosensitivity
6. Insomnia, somnolence (sleepy, drowsy), apathy
7. Nervousness
8. Headache, dizziness
9. Seizure activity
10. Weight loss or gain
11. Decreased libido
12. Apathy
13. Tremors
14. Increased sweating

C. Interventions
1. SSRIs interact with numerous medications.
2. Monitor vital signs because SSRIs can potentially lower or elevate blood pressure.
3. Monitor weight.
4. Initiate safety precautions, particularly if dizziness occurs.
5. Instruct the client to avoid alcohol.
6. Administer with a snack or meal to reduce the risk of dizziness and lightheadedness.
7. Monitor the suicidal client, especially during improved mood and increased energy levels.
8. Instruct the client taking fluoxetine (Prozac) or bupropion (Wellbutrin) to take the medication early in the day to prevent interference with sleep.
9. For the client on long-term therapy, monitor liver and renal function test results; altered values may occur requiring dosage adjustments.
10. Monitor white blood cell and neutrophil counts; the medication may be discontinued if levels decrease below normal.
11. If priapism (painful, prolonged penile erection) occurs, the medication is withheld and the physician is notified.
12. Inform the client about the possibility of decreased libido.
13. Instruct the client to change positions slowly to avoid a hypotensive effect.
14. Instruct the client to report any visual changes to the physician.
15. Educate the client about the potential for discontinuation syndrome if medication is stopped abruptly rather than tapered; the syndrome is characterized by gastrointestinal distress, behavioral or perceptual oddities, movement problems, and sleep disturbances.
16. Be aware of the potential for serotonin syndrome, characterized by elevated temperature, muscle rigidity, and elevated creatine phosphokinase levels; this risk is greatly increased when SSRIs are given with monoamine oxidase inhibitors (MAOIs). This medication combination needs to be avoided.
17. Instruct the client that over-the-counter (OTC) cold medicines can increase the likelihood of serotonin syndrome.
18. In pregnancy, consultation with an obstetrician is recommended regarding taking these medications.
19. Monitor the medication response in children, adolescents, and older adults because the response may be different than in an adult client.
20. Encourage psychotherapy.

II. TRICYCLIC ANTIDEPRESSANTS (Box 77-2)

A. Description
1. Block the reuptake of norepinephrine (and serotonin) at the presynaptic neuron; used to treat depression
2. May reduce seizure threshold
3. May reduce effectiveness of antihypertensive agents
4. Concurrent use with alcohol or antihistamines can cause CNS depression.

5. Concurrent use with MAOIs can cause hypertensive **crisis**.
6. Cardiac toxicity can occur, and all clients should receive an electrocardiogram (ECG) before treatment and periodically thereafter.
7. Overdose is life-threatening, necessitating immediate treatment (see Priority Nursing Actions).

Box 77-1 Reuptake Inhibitors

Selective Serotonin Reuptake Inhibitors
Citalopram (Celexa)
Escitalopram (Lexapro)
Fluoxetine (Prozac)
Fluvoxamine (Luvox)
Paroxetine (Paxil, Pexeva)
Sertraline (Zoloft)

Serotonin-Norepinephrine Reuptake Inhibitors
Venlafaxine (Effexor)
Duloxetine (Cymbalta)
Desvenlafaxine (Pristiq)

Atypical Antidepressants
Amoxapine
Bupropion (Wellbutrin)
Mirtazapine (Remeron)
Nefazodone
Trazodone (Desyrel)

▬▬▬ PRIORITY NURSING ACTIONS! ▬▬▬

Actions to Take for a Tricyclic Antidepressant Overdose

1. Check airway and maintain a patent airway.
2. Administer oxygen.
3. Check vital signs.
4. Obtain an electrocardiogram.
5. Prepare for gastric lavage with activated charcoal.
6. Prepare to administer physostigmine (a cholinesterase inhibitor) and antidysrhythmic medications.
7. Document the event, actions taken, and the client's response.

A tricyclic antidepressant overdose can be life-threatening. Signs and symptoms include dysrhythmias, including tachycardia, intraventricular blocks, complete atrioventricular block, and ventricular fibrillation; hypothermia; flushing; dry mouth; dilation of the pupils; confusion, agitation, and hallucinations; and seizures followed by coma. The immediate action is to check the airway and institute measures such as oxygen to maintain a patent airway. Vital signs are checked and monitored, and an electrocardiogram is obtained to check for dysrhythmias. Gastric lavage with activated charcoal is done to prevent further absorption of the medication. Physostigmine (a cholinesterase inhibitor) is given to counteract anticholinergic effects, and antidysrhythmics are administered as needed. The nurse documents the event, actions taken, and the client's response.

Reference: Lehne, R. (2010). *Pharmacology for nursing care* (7th ed., p. 342). St. Louis: Saunders.

---

8. The tricyclic antidepressant clomipramine (Anafranil) may be used to treat obsessive-compulsive disorder.

B. Side effects
1. Anticholinergic effects: Dry mouth, difficulty voiding, dilated pupils and blurred vision, decreased gastrointestinal motility, constipation
2. Photosensitivity
3. Cardiovascular disturbances such as tachycardia or dysrhythmias; orthostatic hypotension
4. Sedation
5. Seizures (with bupropion)
6. Weight gain
7. Anxiety, restlessness, irritability
8. Decreased or increased libido with ejaculatory and erection disturbances

C. Interventions
1. Monitor the suicidal client, especially during improved mood and increased energy levels.
2. Instruct the client to change positions slowly to avoid a hypotensive effect.
3. Monitor pattern of daily bowel activity.
4. Assess for urinary retention.
5. For the client on long-term therapy, monitor liver and renal function test results.
6. Administer with food or milk if gastrointestinal distress occurs.
7. Administer the entire daily oral dose at one time, preferably at bedtime.
8. Instruct the client to avoid alcohol and nonprescription medications to prevent adverse medication interactions.
9. Instruct the client to avoid driving and other activities requiring alertness until the response is known; sedation is expected in early therapy and may subside with time.
10. When the medication is discontinued by the physician, it should be tapered gradually.
11. The potential for medication interactions with OTC cold medication exists.
12. Caution the client about photosensitivity and to take measures to prevent exposure to sunlight.
13. Encourage oral hygiene and the use of hard candies and mouth rinses to relieve dry mouth.
14. Encourage psychotherapy.

Box 77-2 Tricyclic Antidepressants

Amitriptyline	Nortriptyline (Aventyl HCl,
Clomipramine (Anafranil)	Pamelor)
Desipramine (Norpramin)	Protriptyline (Vivactil)
Doxepin (Sinequan)	Trimipramine (Surmontil)
Imipramine (Tofranil)	

Box 77-3 Monoamine Oxidase Inhibitors

| Isocarboxazid (Marplan) | Tranylcypromine (Parnate) |
| Phenelzine (Nardil) | Selegiline (Emsam) |

⚠ Inform the client that antidepressant medication may take several weeks to produce the desired effect (client response may not occur until 2 to 4 weeks after the first dose).

III. MONOAMINE OXIDASE INHIBITORS (MAOIs) (Box 77-3)

A. Description
1. Inhibit the enzyme monoamine oxidase, which is present in the brain, blood platelets, liver, spleen, and kidneys
2. Monoamine oxidase metabolizes amines, norepinephrine, and serotonin, so the concentration of these amines increases with MAOIs.
3. Clients who have depression and have not responded to other antidepressant therapies, including electroconvulsive therapy, are given MAOIs.
4. Concurrent use with amphetamines, antidepressants, dopamine, epinephrine, guanethidine, levodopa, methyldopa, nasal decongestants, norepinephrine, reserpine, tyramine-containing foods, or vasoconstrictors may cause hypertensive **crisis**.
5. Concurrent use with opioid analgesics may cause hypertension or hypotension, coma, or seizures.

B. Side effects
1. Orthostatic hypotension
2. Restlessness
3. Insomnia
4. Dizziness
5. Weakness, lethargy
6. Gastrointestinal upset
7. Dry mouth
8. Weight gain
9. Peripheral edema
10. Anticholinergic effects
11. CNS stimulation (anxiety, agitation, mania)
12. Delay in ejaculation

C. Hypertensive crisis
1. Hypertension
2. Occipital headache radiating frontally
3. Neck stiffness and soreness
4. Nausea and vomiting
5. Sweating
6. Fever and chills
7. Clammy skin
8. Dilated pupils
9. Palpitations, tachycardia, or bradycardia
10. Constricting chest pain
11. Antidote for hypertensive **crisis**: phentolamine by intravenous injection

D. Interventions
1. Monitor blood pressure frequently for hypertension.
2. Monitor for signs of hypertensive **crisis**.
3. If palpitations or frequent headaches occur, withhold the medication and notify the physician.
4. Administer with food if gastrointestinal distress occurs.
5. Instruct the client that the medication effect may be noted during the first week of therapy, but maximum benefit may take 3 weeks.
6. Instruct the client to report headache, neck stiffness, or neck soreness immediately.
7. Instruct the client to change positions slowly to prevent orthostatic hypotension.
8. Instruct the client to avoid caffeine or OTC preparations such as weight-reducing pills or medications for hay fever and colds.
9. Monitor for client compliance with medication administration.
10. Instruct the client to carry a Medic-Alert card indicating that an MAOI medication is being taken.
11. Avoid administering the medication in the evening because insomnia may result.
12. When the medication is discontinued by the physician, it should be discontinued gradually.
13. Instruct the client to avoid foods that require bacteria or molds for their preparation or preservation and foods that contain tyramine (Fig. 77-1; Box 77-4).

⚠ Teach the client about foods that contain tyramine. Consuming tyramine-containing foods when taking an MAOI can cause hypertensive crisis.

IV. MOOD STABILIZERS (Box 77-5)

A. Description: Affect cellular transport mechanism and enhance serotonin or γ-aminobutyric acid (GABA) function, or both, which are associated with mood

B. Lithium
1. Concurrent use with diuretics, fluoxetine (Prozac), methyldopa, or nonsteroidal anti-inflammatory drugs increases lithium reabsorption by the kidney or inhibits lithium excretion, either of which increases the risk of lithium toxicity.
2. Acetazolamide (Diamox), aminophylline, phenothiazines, or sodium bicarbonate may increase renal excretion of lithium, reducing its effectiveness.
3. The therapeutic dose is only slightly less than the amount producing toxicity.
4. The therapeutic drug serum level of lithium is 0.6 to 1.2 mEq/L; the actual dose at which the therapeutic effect is achieved and the levels at which toxicity occurs is highly variable among individual clients.

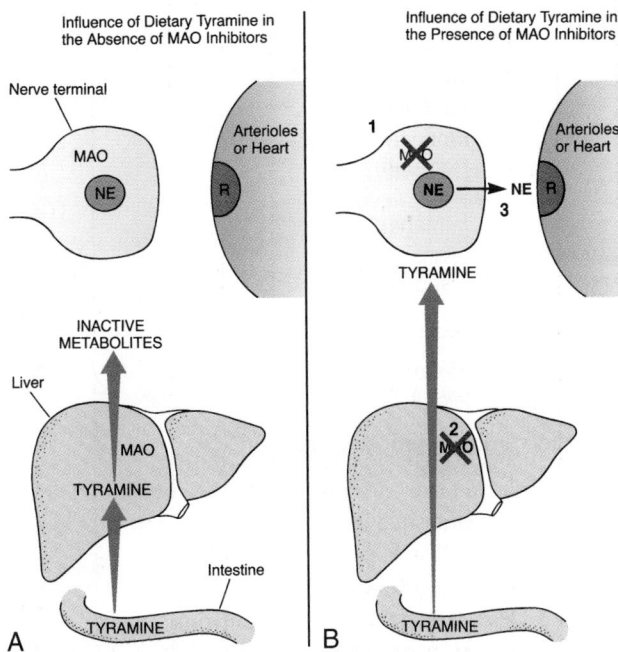

▲ **FIGURE 77-1** Interaction between dietary tyramine and monoamine oxidase inhibitors (MAOIs). **A,** In the absence of MAOIs, dietary tyramine is absorbed from the intestine, transported to the liver, and immediately activated by monoamine oxidase (MAO). No tyramine reaches the general circulation. **B,** Three events occur in the presence of MAOIs: (1) inhibition of neuronal MAO increases levels of norepinephrine (NE) in sympathetic nerve terminals; (2) inhibition of hepatic MAO allows dietary tyramine to pass through the liver and enter the systemic circulation intact; (3) on reaching peripheral sympathetic nerve terminals, tyramine promotes the release of accumulated NE stores, causing massive vasoconstriction and excessive stimulation of the heart. *R,* receptor for NE. (From Lehne, R. [2010]. *Pharmacology for nursing care* [7th ed.]. St. Louis: Saunders.)

Box 77-4 Foods to Avoid That Contain Tyramine

Avocados
Bananas
Beef or chicken liver
Brewer's yeast
Broad beans
Caffeine, such as in coffee, tea, or chocolate
Cheese, especially aged, except cottage cheese
Figs
Meat extracts and tenderizers
Overripe fruit
Papaya
Pickled herring
Raisins
Red wine, beer, sherry
Sausage, bologna, pepperoni, salami
Sour cream
Soy sauce
Yogurt

Box 77-5 Mood Stabilizers

Lithium Preparations
Lithium carbonate (Lithobid)
Lithium citrate

Other Mood Stabilizers
Aripiprazole (Abilify)
Carbamazepine (Tegretol)
Gabapentin (Neurontin)
Lamotrigine (Lamictal)
Olanzapine (Zyprexa)
Olanzapine/fluoxetine (Symbyax)
Oxcarbazepine (Trileptal)
Quetiapine (Seroquel)
Risperidone (Risperdal)
Valproate sodium (Depacon), valproic acid (Depakene), divalproex sodium (Depakote)
Ziprasidone (Geodon)

---

5. The causes of an increase in the lithium level include decreased sodium intake; fluid and electrolyte loss associated with excessive sweating, dehydration, diarrhea, or diuretic therapy; and illness or overdose.
6. Serum lithium levels should be checked every 1 to 2 months or whenever any behavioral change suggests an altered serum level.
7. Blood samples to check serum lithium levels should be drawn in the morning, 12 hours after the last dose was taken.

C. Side effects
1. Polyuria
2. Polydipsia
3. Anorexia, nausea
4. Dry mouth
5. Mild thirst
6. Weight gain
7. Abdominal bloating
8. Soft stools or diarrhea
9. Fine hand tremors
10. Inability to concentrate
11. Muscle weakness
12. Lethargy
13. Fatigue
14. Headache
15. Hair loss
16. Hypothyroidism

D. Interventions
1. Monitor the suicidal client, especially during improved mood and increased energy levels.
2. Administer the medication with food to minimize gastrointestinal irritation.
3. Instruct the client to avoid excessive amounts of coffee, tea, or cola, which have a diuretic effect.
4. Do not administer diuretics while the client is taking lithium.

5. Instruct the client to avoid alcohol.
6. Instruct the client to avoid OTC medications.
7. Instruct the client that he or she may take a missed dose within 2 hours of the scheduled time; otherwise, the client should skip the missed dose and take the next dose at the scheduled time.
8. Instruct the client not to adjust the dosage without consulting the physician because lithium should be tapered and not discontinued abruptly.
9. Instruct the client about the signs and symptoms of lithium toxicity.
10. Instruct the client to notify the physician if polyuria, prolonged vomiting, diarrhea, or fever occurs.
11. Instruct the client that the therapeutic response to the medication is noted in 1 to 3 weeks.
12. Monitor the ECG, renal function tests, and thyroid tests (ensure that these tests are performed before the start of therapy).
13. Instruct the client to take the medication with food or milk to decrease gastrointestinal upset.
14. Monitor weight.

⚠️ Instruct the client taking lithium (Lithobid) to maintain a fluid intake of six to eight glasses of water a day and an adequate salt intake to prevent lithium toxicity.

E. Lithium toxicity
   1. Description
      a. Occurs when ingested lithium cannot be detoxified and excreted by the kidneys
      b. Symptoms of toxicity begin to appear when the serum lithium level is 1.5 to 2 mEq/L.
   2. Mild toxicity
      a. Serum lithium level is 1.5 mEq/L.
      b. Apathy
      c. Lethargy
      d. Diminished concentration
      e. Mild ataxia
      f. Coarse hand tremors
      g. Slight muscle weakness
   3. Moderate toxicity
      a. Serum lithium level 1.5 to 2.5 mEq/L
      b. Nausea, vomiting
      c. Severe diarrhea
      d. Mild to moderate ataxia and incoordination
      e. Slurred speech
      f. Tinnitus
      g. Blurred vision
      h. Muscle twitching
      i. Irregular tremor
   4. Severe toxicity
      a. Serum lithium level greater than 2.5 mEq/L
      b. Nystagmus
      c. Muscle fasciculations

Box 77-6 Benzodiazepines

Alprazolam (Xanax, Niravam)
Chlordiazepoxide (Librium)
Clonazepam (Klonopin)
Clorazepate (Tranxene)
Diazepam (Valium)
Flurazepam (Dalmane)
Lorazepam (Ativan)
Midazolam (Versed)
Oxazepam (Serax)
Quazepam (Doral)
Temazepam (Restoril)
Triazolam (Halcion)

Nonbenzodiazepine Anxiolytic
Buspirone (BuSpar)

      d. Deep tendon hyperreflexia
      e. Visual or tactile hallucinations
      f. Oliguria or anuria
      g. Impaired level of consciousness
      h. Tonic-clonic seizures or coma, leading to death
   5. Interventions for lithium toxicity
      a. Withhold lithium and notify the physician.
      b. Monitor vital signs and level of consciousness.
      c. Monitor cardiac status.
      d. Prepare to obtain samples monitoring lithium, electrolyte, blood urea nitrogen, and creatinine levels and complete blood cell count.
      e. Monitor for suicidal tendencies and institute suicide precautions.

V. ANTIANXIETY OR ANXIOLYTIC MEDICATIONS

A. Description
   1. Antianxiety medications depress the CNS, increasing the effects of GABA, which produces relaxation and may depress the limbic system.
   2. Benzodiazepines have anxiety-reducing (anxiolytic), sedative-hypnotic, muscle-relaxing, and anticonvulsant actions (Box 77-6).
   3. Benzodiazepines are contraindicated in clients with acute narrow-angle glaucoma and should be used cautiously in children and older adults.
   4. Benzodiazepines interact with other CNS medications, producing an additive effect.
   5. Abrupt withdrawal of benzodiazepines can be potentially life-threatening, and withdrawal should occur only under medical supervision.

B. Side effects
   1. Daytime sedation
   2. Ataxia
   3. Dizziness
   4. Headaches
   5. Blurred or double vision
   6. Hypotension

7. Tremor
8. Amnesia
9. Slurred speech
10. Urinary incontinence
11. Constipation
12. Paradoxical CNS excitement
13. Lethargy
14. Behavioral change
C. Acute toxicity
1. Somnolence
2. Confusion
3. Diminished reflexes and coma
4. Flumazenil (Romazicon), a benzodiazepine antagonist administered intravenously, reverses benzodiazepine intoxication in 5 minutes.
5. A client being treated for an overdose of a benzodiazepine may experience agitation, restlessness, discomfort, and anxiety.
D. Interventions
1. Monitor for motor responses such as agitation, trembling, and tension.
2. Monitor for autonomic responses such as cold clammy hands and sweating.
3. Monitor for paradoxical CNS excitement during early therapy, particularly in older adults and debilitated clients.
4. Monitor for visual disturbances because the medications can worsen glaucoma.
5. Monitor liver and renal function test results and complete blood cell counts.
6. Reduce the medication dose as prescribed for the older adult client and for the client with impaired liver function.
7. Initiate safety precautions because the older adult client is at risk for falling when taking the medication for sleep or anxiety.
8. Assist with ambulation if drowsiness or lightheadedness occurs.
9. Instruct the client that drowsiness usually disappears during continued therapy.
10. Instruct the client to avoid tasks that require alertness until the response to the medication is established.
11. Instruct the client to avoid alcohol.
12. Instruct the client not to take other medications without consulting the physician.
13. Instruct the client not to stop the medication abruptly (can result in seizure activity).
E. Withdrawal
1. To lessen withdrawal symptoms, the dosage of a benzodiazepine should be tapered gradually over 2 to 6 weeks.
2. Abrupt or too rapid withdrawal results in the following:
   a. Restlessness
   b. Irritability
   c. Insomnia
   d. Hand tremors
   e. Abdominal or muscle cramps
   f. Sweating
   g. Vomiting
   h. Seizures

Box 77-7 Barbiturates and Sedative-Hypnotics

Barbiturates
Amobarbital sodium (Amytal Sodium)
Butabarbital sodium (Butisol Sodium)
Pentobarbital sodium (Nembutal Sodium)
Phenobarbital sodium (Luminal Sodium)
Secobarbital sodium (Seconal Sodium)

Sedative-Hypnotics
Chloral hydrate (Aquachloral Supprettes, Somnote)
Eszopiclone (Lunesta)
Meprobamate (Miltown)
Ramelteon (Rozerem)
Zaleplon (Sonata)
Zolpidem (Ambien)

VI. BARBITURATES AND SEDATIVE-HYPNOTICS (Box 77-7)

A. Description
1. Depress the reticular activating system by promoting the inhibitory synaptic action of the neurotransmitter GABA
2. Used for short-term treatment of insomnia or for sedation to relieve anxiety, tension, and apprehension
B. Side effects
1. Dizziness and drowsiness
2. Confusion
3. Irritability
4. Allergic reactions
5. Agranulocytosis
6. Thrombocytopenic purpura
7. Megaloblastic anemia
C. Overdose
1. Tachycardia
2. Hypotension
3. Cold and clammy skin
4. Dilated pupils
5. Weak and rapid pulse
6. Signs of shock
7. Depressed respirations
8. Absent reflexes
9. Coma and death may result from respiratory and cardiovascular collapse.
D. Withdrawal
1. Severe withdrawal symptoms begin within 24 hours after the medication is discontinued in an individual with severe medication dependence.
2. Gradual withdrawal is used to detoxify a dependent client.

3. Anxiety
4. Insomnia
5. Nightmares
6. Daytime agitation
7. Tremors
8. Delirium
9. Seizures
10. Behavioral changes

E. Interventions
1. Administer lower doses as prescribed for the older client.
2. Medications should be used with caution in the client who has suicidal tendencies or has a history of drug **addiction**.
3. Maintain safety by supervising ambulation and using side rails at night.
4. Instruct the client to take the medication as directed.
5. Instruct the client to avoid driving or operating hazardous equipment if drowsiness, dizziness, or unsteadiness occurs.
6. Instruct the client to avoid alcohol.
7. For insomnia, instruct the client to take the medication 30 minutes before bedtime; avoid taking with a large amount of food to help absorption.
8. Instruct the client that a hangover effect may occur in the morning.
9. Instruct the client not to discontinue the medication abruptly.
10. Instruct the client taking chloral hydrate to take the medication with food and a full glass of water, fruit juice, or ginger ale to prevent gastric irritation.

VII. ANTIPSYCHOTIC MEDICATIONS (Box 77-8)

A. Description
1. Improve the thought processes and the behavior of the client with psychotic symptoms, especially clients with schizophrenia

Box 77-8 Antipsychotic Medications

Typical Antipsychotics
Chlorpromazine (Thorazine)
Fluphenazine decanoate (Prolixin Decanoate)
Haloperidol
Loxapine (Loxitane)
Molindone (Moban)
Pimozide (Orap)
Thiothixene (Navane)
Trifluoperazine

Atypical Antipsychotics
Aripiprazole (Abilify)
Clozapine (Clozaril)
Olanzapine (Zyprexa)
Quetiapine (Seroquel)
Risperidone (Risperdal)
Ziprasidone (Geodon)

2. Affect dopamine receptors in the brain, reducing the psychotic symptoms
3. Typical antipsychotics are more effective for positive symptoms of schizophrenia, such as hallucinations, aggression, and delusions; typical antipsychotic medications also block the chemoreceptor trigger zone and vomiting center in the brain, producing an antiemetic effect.
4. Atypical antipsychotics are more effective for the negative symptoms of schizophrenia, such as avolition, apathy, and alogia.
5. The effects of antipsychotic medications are potentiated when given with other medications acting on the CNS.

B. Side effects (Box 77-9)

Box 77-9 Side Effects of Antipsychotic Medications

Anticholinergic Effects
Dry mouth
Increased heart rate
Urinary retention
Constipation
Hypotension

Extrapyramidal Side Effects
Parkinsonism
Tremors
Mask-like facies
Rigidity
Shuffling gait
Dysphagia
Drooling

Dystonias
Abnormal or involuntary eye movements, including oculogyric crisis
Facial grimacing
Twisting of the torso or other muscle groups

Akathisia
Restlessness
Constant moving about

Tardive Dyskinesia
Protrusion of the tongue
Chewing motion
Involuntary movements of the body and extremities

Other Side Effects
Drowsiness
Blood dyscrasias
Pruritus
Photosensitivity
Elevated blood glucose level
Increased weight
Impaired body temperature regulation
Gynecomastia
Lactation

C. Extrapyramidal syndrome
 1. Parkinsonism
   a. Tremors
   b. Mask-like facies
   c. Dysphagia, drooling
   d. Rigidity, shuffling gait
 2. Dystonia
   a. Facial grimacing
   b. Abnormal or involuntary eye movements
 3. Akathisia
   a. Restlessness
   b. Constant moving about
 4. Tardive dyskinesia
   a. Protrusion of the tongue
   b. Chewing motions
   c. Involuntary movements of the body and extremities
D. Interventions
 1. Monitor vital signs.
 2. Monitor for symptoms of neuroleptic malignant syndrome (can occur with antipsychotic medications).
 3. Monitor urine output.
 4. Monitor serum glucose level.
 5. The client taking an antipsychotic medication may require long-term medication for parkinsonian symptoms.
 6. Administer the medication with food or milk to decrease gastric irritation.
 7. For oral use, the liquid form might be preferred because some clients hide tablets in their mouths to avoid taking them.
 8. The absorption rate is faster with the liquid form of oral medication.
 9. Avoid skin contact with the liquid concentrate to prevent contact dermatitis.
 10. Protect the liquid concentrate from light.
 11. Dilute the liquid concentrate with fruit juice.
 12. Inform the client that a full therapeutic effect of the medication may not be evident for 3 to 6 weeks after initiation of therapy; however, an observable therapeutic response may be apparent after 7 to 10 days.
 13. Inform the client that some medications may cause a harmless change in urine color to pinkish to red-brown.
 14. Instruct the client to use sunscreen, hats, and protective clothing when outdoors.
 15. Instruct the client to avoid alcohol or other CNS depressants.
 16. Instruct the client to change positions slowly to avoid orthostatic hypotension.
 17. Instruct the client to report signs of agranulocytosis, including sore throat, fever, and malaise.
 18. Instruct the client to report signs of liver dysfunction, including jaundice, malaise, fever, and right upper abdominal pain.

 19. When discontinuing antipsychotics, the medication dosage should be reduced gradually to avoid sudden recurrence of psychotic symptoms.

⚠ Monitor for extrapyramidal side effects in the client taking an antipsychotic medication.

VIII. NEUROLEPTIC MALIGNANT SYNDROME

A. Description
 1. Neuroleptic malignant syndrome is a potentially fatal syndrome that may occur at any time during therapy with neuroleptic (antipsychotic) medications.
 2. Although rare, neuroleptic malignant syndrome more commonly occurs at the initiation of therapy, after the client has changed from one medication to another, after a dosage increase, or when a combination of medications is used.
B. Assessment
 1. Dyspnea or tachypnea
 2. Tachycardia or irregular pulse rate
 3. Fever
 4. High or low blood pressure
 5. Increased sweating
 6. Loss of bladder control
 7. Skeletal muscle rigidity
 8. Pale skin
 9. Excessive weakness or fatigue
 10. Altered level of consciousness
 11. Seizures
 12. Severe extrapyramidal side effects
 13. Difficulty swallowing
 14. Excessive salivation
 15. Oculogyric **crisis**
 16. Dyskinesia
 17. Elevated white blood cell count, liver function results, and creatine phosphokinase level
C. Interventions
 1. Notify the physician.
 2. Monitor vital signs.
 3. Initiate safety and seizure precautions.
 4. Prepare to discontinue the medication.
 5. Monitor level of consciousness.
 6. Administer antipyretics as prescribed.
 7. Use a cooling blanket to lower the body temperature.
 8. Monitor electrolyte levels and administer fluids intravenously as prescribed.

IX. MEDICATIONS TO TREAT ATTENTION-DEFICIT/ HYPERACTIVITY DISORDER (Box 77-10)

A. Children with attention-deficit/hyperactivity disorder may require medication to reduce hyperactive behavior and lengthen attention span.
B. Medications that are most effective in controlling this disorder are CNS stimulants.

Box 77-10 Medications to Treat Attention-Deficit/Hyperactivity Disorder

Amphetamine
Atomoxetine (Strattera)
Dexmethylphenidate (Focalin)
Dextroamphetamine (Dexedrine)
Dextroamphetamine and amphetamine (Adderall XR)
Methamphetamine (Desoxyn)
Methylphenidate (Ritalin, Concerta, Metadate CD, Methylin)

Box 77-11 Medications to Treat Alzheimer's Disease

Donepezil (Aricept)   Rivastigmine (Exelon)
Galantamine (Razadyne)   Tacrine (Cognex)
Memantine (Namenda)

C. CNS stimulants, which increase agitation and activity in adults, have a calming effect on children with attention-deficit/hyperactivity disorder and increase alertness and sensitivity to stimuli.

D. Side effects
   1. Tachycardia
   2. Anorexia and weight loss
   3. Elevated blood pressure
   4. Dizziness
   5. Agitation

E. Interventions
   1. Monitor for CNS side effects.
   2. Obtain a baseline ECG.
   3. Monitor the blood pressure
   4. Instruct the child and parents that OTC medications need to be avoided.
   5. Instruct the child and parents that the last dose of the day should be taken at least 6 hours before bedtime (14 hours for extended-release forms) to prevent insomnia.
   6. Monitor height and weight (particularly in children).
   7. Reinforce that several weeks of therapy may be necessary before the therapeutic effect is noted.
   8. Instruct the client and parents that a drug-free period may be prescribed to allow growth of the child if the medication has caused growth retardation.

X. **MEDICATIONS TO TREAT ALZHEIMER'S DISEASE** (Box 77-11)

A. Acetylcholinesterase inhibitors may be used in clients with Alzheimer's disease to improve cognitive functions in the early stages.

B. Donepezil (Aricept)
   1. An inhibitor of acetylcholinesterase used to treat mild to moderate dementia of Alzheimer's disease

   2. Side effects include nausea and diarrhea.
   3. Donepezil can slow the heart rate through its vagotonic effect.

C. Galantamine (Razadyne)
   1. An inhibitor of cholinesterase used to treat mild to moderate dementia of Alzheimer's disease.
   2. Side effects include nausea, vomiting, diarrhea, anorexia, and weight loss.
   3. Galantamine can cause bronchoconstriction; it should be used with caution in clients with asthma and chronic obstructive pulmonary disease.

D. Memantine (Namenda)
   1. N-methyl-D-aspartate (NMDA) receptor antagonist indicated for treatment of moderate to severe dementia of Alzheimer's disease
   2. Side effects include dizziness, headache, confusion, and constipation.
   3. Memantine should not be used in combination with other NMDA antagonists such as amantadine (Symmetrel) or ketamine (Ketalar); such combinations produce undesirable additive effects.
   4. Sodium bicarbonate and other medications that alkalinize the urine can decrease renal excretion of memantine; accumulation to toxic levels can result.

E. Rivastigmine (Exelon)
   1. Cholinesterase inhibitor used to treat mild to moderate dementia of Alzheimer's disease
   2. Side effects include nausea, vomiting, diarrhea, abdominal pain, and anorexia.
   3. Rivastigmine should be used with caution in clients with peptic ulcer disease, bradycardia, sick sinus syndrome, urinary obstruction, and lung disease because it enhances cholinergic transmission, intensifying symptoms of these disorders.

F. Tacrine (Cognex)
   1. A centrally acting cholinesterase inhibitor used to treat mild to moderate dementia of Alzheimer's disease
   2. Side effects include ataxia, loss of appetite, nausea, vomiting, and diarrhea.
   3. An adverse effect is hepatotoxicity; liver function studies need to be monitored.

💿 MORE QUESTIONS ON THE CD!

Practice Questions

944. A client's medication sheet contains a prescription for sertraline (Zoloft). To ensure safe administration of the medication, a nurse would administer the dose:
   1. On an empty stomach
   2. At the same time each evening
   3. Evenly spaced around the clock
   4. As needed when the client complains of depression

945. A client with schizophrenia has been started on medication therapy with clozapine (Clozaril). A nurse assesses the results of which laboratory study to monitor for adverse effects from this medication?
1. Platelet count
2. Blood glucose level
3. White blood cell count
4. Liver function studies

946. A client is scheduled for discharge and will be taking phenobarbital (Luminal) for an extended period. A nurse would place highest priority on teaching the client which of the following points that directly relates to client safety?
1. Take the medication only with meals.
2. Take the medication at the same time each day.
3. Use a dose container to help prevent missed doses.
4. Avoid drinking alcohol while taking this medication.

947. A nurse is describing the medication side effects to a client who is taking oxazepam (Serax). The nurse incorporates in discussions with the client the need to:
1. Consume a low-fiber diet.
2. Increase fluids and bulk in the diet.
3. Rest if the heart begins to beat rapidly.
4. Take antidiarrheal agents if diarrhea occurs.

948. A nurse is administering risperidone (Risperdal) to a client who is scheduled to be discharged. Before discharge, which of the following should the nurse teach the client?
1. Get adequate sunlight.
2. Avoid foods rich in potassium.
3. Continue driving as usual.
4. Get up slowly when changing positions.

949. A nurse is teaching a client who is being started on imipramine (Tofranil) about the medication. The nurse informs the client that the maximum desired effects may:
1. Start during the first week of administration
2. Not occur for 2 to 3 weeks of administration
3. Start during the second week of administration
4. Not occur until after 2 months of administration

950. A client receiving tricyclic antidepressants arrives at the mental health clinic. Which observation would indicate that the client is following the medication plan correctly?
1. Client reports not going to work for this past week.
2. Client arrives at the clinic neat and appropriate in appearance.

3. Client complains of not being able to "do anything" anymore.
4. Client reports sleeping 12 hours per night and 3 to 4 hours during the day.

951. A nurse notes that a client with schizophrenia and receiving an antipsychotic medication is moving her mouth, protruding her tongue, and grimacing as she watches television. The nurse determines that the client is experiencing:
1. Parkinsonism
2. Tardive dyskinesia
3. Hypertensive crisis
4. Neuroleptic malignant syndrome

952. A nurse is performing a follow-up teaching session with a client discharged 1 month ago. The client is taking fluoxetine (Prozac). What information would be important for the nurse to obtain during this client visit regarding the side effects of the medication?
1. Cardiovascular symptoms
2. Gastrointestinal dysfunctions
3. Problems with mouth dryness
4. Problems with excessive sweating

953. A client who has been taking buspirone (BuSpar) for 1 month returns to the clinic for a follow-up assessment. A nurse determines that the medication is effective if the absence of which manifestation has occurred?
1. Paranoid thought process
2. Rapid heartbeat or anxiety
3. Alcohol withdrawal symptoms
4. Thought broadcasting or delusions

954. A client taking lithium carbonate (Lithobid) reports vomiting, abdominal pain, diarrhea, blurred vision, tinnitus, and tremors. The lithium level is 2.5 mEq/L. The nurse interprets this level as:
1. Toxic
2. Normal
3. Slightly above normal
4. Excessively below normal

955. A home health nurse visits a client. The client gives the nurse a bottle of clomipramine (Anafranil). The nurse notes that the medication has not been taken by the client in 2 months. What behaviors observed in the client would validate noncompliance with this medication?
1. Complaints of insomnia
2. Complaints of hunger and fatigue
3. A pulse rate less than 60 beats/min
4. Frequent handwashing with hot soapy water

956. A hospitalized client has begun taking bupropion (Wellbutrin) as an antidepressant agent. A nurse monitors this client for which side effect indicating that the client is taking an excessive amount of medication?
1. Constipation
2. Seizure activity
3. Increased weight
4. Dizziness when getting upright

Alternate Item Format: Multiple Response

957. A hospitalized client is started on phenelzine (Nardil) for the treatment of depression. A nurse instructs the client to avoid consuming which foods while taking this medication? **Select all that apply.**
❑ 1. Figs
❑ 2. Yogurt
❑ 3. Crackers
❑ 4. Aged cheese
❑ 5. Tossed salad
❑ 6. Oatmeal cookies

ANSWERS

944. 2

Rationale: Sertraline (Zoloft) is classified as an antidepressant. Sertraline generally is administered once every 24 hours. It may be administered in the morning or evening, but evening administration may be preferable because drowsiness is a side effect. The medication may be administered without food or with food if gastrointestinal distress occurs. Sertraline is not prescribed for use as needed.

Test-Taking Strategy: Use the process of elimination. Recalling that this medication is an antidepressant administered daily will direct you to option 2. Review this medication if you had difficulty with this question.

Level of Cognitive Ability: Applying
Client Needs: Physiological Integrity
Integrated Process: Nursing Process—Implementation
Content Area: Pharmacology
References: Kee, J., Hayes, E., & McCuistion, L. (2009). *Pharmacology: A nursing process approach* (6th ed., p. 417). St. Louis: Saunders.

Lehne, R. (2010). *Pharmacology for nursing care* (7th ed., p. 356). St. Louis: Saunders.

Varcarolis, E., & Halter, M. (2009). *Essentials of psychiatric mental health nursing: A communication approach to evidence-based care* (p. 233). St. Louis: Saunders.

945. 3

Rationale: A client taking clozapine (Clozaril) may experience agranulocytosis, which is monitored by reviewing the results of the white blood cell count. Treatment is interrupted if the white blood cell count decreases to less than 3000 cells/mm^3. Agranulocytosis could be fatal if undetected and untreated. The other options are not related specifically to the use of this medication.

Test-Taking Strategy: Use the process of elimination. Recalling that this medication causes agranulocytosis will direct you to option 3. Review the adverse effects of this medication if you had difficulty with this question

Level of Cognitive Ability: Analyzing
Client Needs: Physiological Integrity
Integrated Process: Nursing Process—Assessment
Content Area: Pharmacology
Reference: Hodgson, B., & Kizior, R. (2010). *Saunders nursing drug handbook 2010* (p. 267). St. Louis: Saunders.

946. 4

Rationale: Phenobarbital (Luminal) is an anticonvulsant and hypnotic agent. The client should avoid taking any other CNS depressants such as alcohol while taking this medication. The medication may be given without regard to meals. Taking the medication at the same time each day enhances compliance and maintains more stable blood levels of the medication. Using a dose container or "pillbox" may be helpful for some clients.

Test-Taking Strategy: Use the process of elimination. Focus on the subject, client safety, and note the strategic words *highest priority*. This tells you that more than one or all the options may be partially or totally correct and that you must prioritize your answer. Remember that alcohol should not be consumed when a hypnotic is taken. Review client teaching points related to this medication if you had difficulty with this question.

Level of Cognitive Ability: Applying
Client Needs: Safe and Effective Care Environment
Integrated Process: Teaching and Learning
Content Area: Pharmacology
Reference: Hodgson, B., & Kizior, R. (2010). *Saunders nursing drug handbook 2010* (p. 902). St. Louis: Saunders.

947. 2

Rationale: Oxazepam (Serax) causes constipation, and the client is instructed to increase fluid intake and bulk (high fiber) in the diet. If the heart begins to beat fast, the physician is notified because this could indicate overdose. Additionally, diarrhea could indicate an incomplete intestinal obstruction and, if this occurs, the physician is notified.

Test-Taking Strategy: Use the process of elimination. Recalling that constipation is a side effect of this medication will direct you to option 2. Review the side effects and adverse effects of oxazepam if you had difficulty with this question.

Level of Cognitive Ability: Applying
Client Needs: Physiological Integrity
Integrated Process: Teaching and Learning
Content Area: Pharmacology
Reference: Stuart, G. (2009). *Principles and practice of psychiatric nursing* (9th ed., p. 518). St. Louis: Mosby.

948. 4

Rationale: Risperidone (Risperdal) can cause orthostatic hypotension. Sunlight should be avoided by the client taking this medication. Food interaction is not a concern. With any

psychotropic medication, caution needs to be taken until the individual can determine whether his or her level of alertness is affected.
Test-Taking Strategy: Knowledge regarding the nursing considerations related to the administration of risperidone is required to answer this question. Remember that risperidone can cause orthostatic hypotension. Review this medication if you had difficulty with this question.
Level of Cognitive Ability: Applying
Client Needs: Physiological Integrity
Integrated Process: Teaching and Learning
Content Area: Pharmacology
Reference: Hodgson, B., & Kizior, R. (2010). *Saunders nursing drug handbook 2010* (p. 1005). St. Louis: Saunders.

949. 2
Rationale: The maximum therapeutic effects of imipramine (Tofranil) may not occur for 2 to 3 weeks after antidepressant therapy has been initiated. Options 1, 3, and 4 are incorrect.
Test-Taking Strategy: Focus on the strategic word *maximum*. Recalling that it takes 2 to 3 weeks for a maximum therapeutic effect to occur with most antidepressants will direct you to option 2. Review this medication if you had difficulty with this question.
Level of Cognitive Ability: Applying
Client Needs: Physiological Integrity
Integrated Process: Teaching and Learning
Content Area: Pharmacology
Reference: Hodgson, B., & Kizior, R. (2010). *Saunders nursing drug handbook 2010* (p. 589). St. Louis: Saunders.

950. 2
Rationale: Depressed individuals sleep for long periods, are unable to go to work, and feel as if they cannot "do anything." When these clients have had some therapeutic effect from their medication, they report resolution of many of these complaints and exhibit an improvement in their appearance.
Test-Taking Strategy: Use the process of elimination. The client's behaviors or reports identified in options 1, 3, and 4 are symptoms of depression. The improvement in appearance indicates a therapeutic response to the medication, indicating compliance with the medication regimen. Review the expected effect of a tricyclic antidepressant if you had difficulty with this question.
Level of Cognitive Ability: Evaluating
Client Needs: Physiological Integrity
Integrated Process: Nursing Process—Evaluation
Content Area: Pharmacology
References: Kee, J., Hayes, E., & McCuistion, L. (2009). *Pharmacology: A nursing process approach* (6th ed., p. 410). St. Louis: Saunders.
Varcarolis, E., & Halter, M. (2009). *Essentials of psychiatric mental health nursing: A communication approach to evidence-based care* (p. 231). St. Louis: Saunders.

951. 2
Rationale: Tardive dyskinesia is a reaction that can occur from antipsychotic medication. It is characterized by uncontrollable involuntary movements of the body and extremities, particularly the tongue. Parkinsonism is characterized by tremors, mask-like facies, rigidity, and a shuffling gait. Hypertensive crisis can occur from the use of monoamine oxidase inhibitors and is characterized by hypertension, occipital headache radiating frontally, neck stiffness and soreness, nausea, and vomiting. Neuroleptic malignant syndrome is a potentially fatal syndrome that may occur at any time during therapy with neuroleptic (antipsychotic) medications. It is characterized by dyspnea or tachypnea, tachycardia or irregular pulse rate, fever, blood pressure changes, increased sweating, loss of bladder control, and skeletal muscle rigidity.
Test-Taking Strategy: Focus on the data in the question. Remember that tardive dyskinesia is characterized by uncontrollable involuntary movements of the body and extremities, particularly the tongue. Review the side effects and extrapyramidal side effects of antipsychotic medications if you had difficulty with this question.
Level of Cognitive Ability: Analyzing
Client Needs: Physiological Integrity
Integrated Process: Nursing Process—Assessment
Content Area: Pharmacology
References: Stuart, G. (2009). *Principles and practice of psychiatric nursing* (9th ed., p. 528). St. Louis: Mosby.
Varcarolis, E., & Halter, M. (2009). *Essentials of psychiatric mental health nursing: A communication approach to evidence-based care* (pp. 294, 298). St. Louis: Saunders.

952. 2
Rationale: The most common side effects related to this medication include central nervous system and gastrointestinal system dysfunction. Fluoxetine (Prozac) affects the gastrointestinal system by causing nausea and vomiting, cramping, and diarrhea. Excessive sweating, dry mouth, and cardiovascular symptoms are not side effects associated with this medication.
Test-Taking Strategy: Use the process of elimination. Recalling that this medication causes gastrointestinal problems will direct you to option 2. Review the side effects related to this medication if you had difficulty with this question.
Level of Cognitive Ability: Analyzing
Client Needs: Physiological Integrity
Integrated Process: Nursing Process—Assessment
Content Area: Pharmacology
References: Edmunds, M. (2010). *Introduction to clinical pharmacology* (6th ed., p. 276). St. Louis: Mosby.
Lehne, R. (2010). *Pharmacology for nursing care* (7th ed., pp. 356–357). St. Louis: Saunders.

953. 2
Rationale: Buspirone (BuSpar) is not recommended for the treatment of drug or alcohol withdrawal, thought disorders, or schizophrenia. Buspirone most often is indicated for the treatment of anxiety.
Test-Taking Strategy: Note the strategic words *absence of which manifestation*. Recalling that buspirone is an antianxiety medication will direct you to the correct option. Review the action and use of this medication if you had difficulty with this question.
Level of Cognitive Ability: Evaluating
Client Needs: Physiological Integrity
Integrated Process: Nursing Process—Evaluation
Content Area: Pharmacology

References: Hodgson, B., & Kizior, R. (2010). *Saunders nursing drug handbook 2010* (pp. 154–155). St. Louis: Saunders.

Varcarolis, E., & Halter, M. (2009). *Essentials of psychiatric mental health nursing: A communication approach to evidence-based care* (p. 146). St. Louis: Saunders.

954. 1

Rationale: Maintenance serum levels of lithium are 0.6 to 1.2 mEq/L. Symptoms of toxicity begin to appear at levels of 1.5 to 2 mEq/L. Lithium toxicity requires immediate medical attention with lavage and possible peritoneal dialysis or hemodialysis.

Test-Taking Strategy: Use the process of elimination. Recalling that the high end of the maintenance level is 1.2 mEq/L will direct you to option 1. Review the maintenance level and signs of toxicity if you had difficulty with this question.

Level of Cognitive Ability: Understanding
Client Needs: Physiological Integrity
Integrated Process: Nursing Process—Assessment
Content Area: Pharmacology
Reference: Hodgson, B., & Kizior, R. (2010). *Saunders nursing drug handbook 2010* (p. 683). St. Louis: Saunders.

955. 4

Rationale: Clomipramine (Anafranil) is a tricyclic antidepressant used to treat obsessive-compulsive disorder. Weight gain and tachycardia are side effects of this medication. Sedation sometimes occurs. Insomnia seldom is a side effect.

Test-Taking Strategy: Recalling that this medication is a tricyclic antidepressant used to treat obsessive-compulsive disorder will direct you to option 4. Review the purpose and use of this medication if you had difficulty with this question.

Level of Cognitive Ability: Evaluating
Client Needs: Physiological Integrity
Integrated Process: Nursing Process—Evaluation
Content Area: Pharmacology
References: Kee, J., Hayes, E., & McCuistion, L. (2009). *Pharmacology: A nursing process approach* (6th ed., p. 416). St. Louis: Saunders.

Lehne, R. (2010). *Pharmacology for nursing care* (7th ed., p. 388). St. Louis: Saunders.

Varcarolis, E., & Halter, M. (2009). *Essentials of psychiatric mental health nursing: A communication approach to evidence-based care* (p. 149). St. Louis: Saunders.

956. 2

Rationale: The nurse monitors for signs of toxicity. Seizure activity is common in bupropion dosages greater than 450 mg daily. This medication does not cause significant orthostatic blood pressure changes. Weight gain is an occasional side effect, whereas constipation is a common side effect of this medication.

Test-Taking Strategy: Use the process of elimination and note the strategic words *side effect* and *excessive amount*. These strategic words will direct you to option 2. Review this medication if you had difficulty with this question.

Level of Cognitive Ability: Analyzing
Client Needs: Physiological Integrity
Integrated Process: Nursing Process—Assessment
Content Area: Pharmacology
Reference: Hodgson, B., & Kizior, R. (2010). *Saunders nursing drug handbook 2010* (p. 154). St. Louis: Saunders.

ALTERNATE ITEM FORMAT: MULTIPLE RESPONSE
957. 1, 2, 4

Rationale: Phenelzine (Nardil) is a monoamine oxidase inhibitor (MAOI). The client should avoid ingesting foods that are high in tyramine. Ingestion of these foods could trigger a potentially fatal hypertensive crisis. Foods to avoid include yogurt; aged cheeses; smoked or processed meats; red wines; and fruits such as avocados, raisins, or figs.

Test-Taking Strategy: Recall that phenelzine is an MAOI and that foods high in tyramine needed to be avoided. Next, from the food items listed in the question, identify the foods that contain tyramine. Review the food items to avoid with MAOIs if you had difficulty with this question.

Level of Cognitive Ability: Applying
Client Needs: Physiological Integrity
Integrated Process: Nursing Process—Implementation
Content Area: Pharmacology
Reference: Varcarolis, E., & Halter, M. (2009). *Essentials of psychiatric mental health nursing: A communication approach to evidence-based care* (p. 237). St. Louis: Saunders.

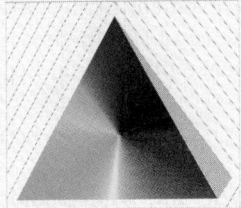

Comprehensive Test

958. An emergency department nurse is caring for a client who has been identified as a victim of physical abuse. In planning care for the client, which of the following is the priority nursing action?
1. Adhering to the mandatory abuse reporting laws
2. Notifying the case worker of the family situation
3. Removing the client from any immediate danger
4. Obtaining treatment for the abusing family member

959. A nurse assesses a client with the admitting diagnosis of bipolar affective disorder, mania. The symptom presented by the client that requires the nurse's immediate intervention is the client's:
1. Outlandish behaviors and inappropriate dress
2. Nonstop physical activity and poor nutritional intake
3. Grandiose delusions of being a royal descendent of King Arthur
4. Constant, incessant talking that includes sexual innuendoes and teasing the staff

960. A nurse is caring for a client who is scheduled for electroconvulsive therapy. The nurse notes that an informed consent has not been obtained for the procedure. On review of the record, the nurse notes that the admission was an involuntary hospitalization. Based on this information, the nurse determines:
1. That the physician will provide the informed consent
2. That an informed consent does not need to be obtained
3. That an informed consent should be obtained from the family
4. That an informed consent needs to be obtained from the client

961. A client newly diagnosed with diabetes mellitus is instructed by the physician to obtain glucagon for emergency home use. The client asks a home care nurse about the purpose of the medication. The nurse instructs the client that the purpose of the medication is to treat:
1. Hypoglycemia from insulin overdose
2. Hyperglycemia from insufficient insulin
3. Lipoatrophy from insulin injections
4. Lipohypertrophy from inadequate insulin absorption

962. A nurse is providing care to a Puerto Rican–American client who is terminally ill. Numerous family members are present most of the time, and many of the family members are very emotional. The appropriate action is to:
1. Restrict the number of family members visiting at one time.
2. Inform the family that emotional outbursts are to be avoided.
3. Request permission to move the client to a private room and allow the family members to visit.
4. Contact the physician to speak to the family regarding their behaviors.

963. A client presents to the emergency department with upper gastrointestinal bleeding and is in moderate distress. In planning care, which nursing action would be the first priority for this client?
1. Thorough investigation of precipitating events
2. Insertion of a nasogastric tube and Hematest of emesis
3. Complete abdominal examination
4. Assessment of vital signs

964. A nurse is performing an assessment on a client with dementia. Which data gathered during the assessment indicate a manifestation associated with dementia?
1. Confabulation
2. Improvement in sleeping
3. Absence of sundown syndrome
4. Presence of personal hygienic care

965. A nurse is caring for a client with anorexia nervosa. The nurse is monitoring the behavior of the client and understands that a client with anorexia nervosa manages anxiety by:
1. Engaging in immoral acts
2. Always reinforcing self-approval
3. Observing rigid rules and regulations
4. Having the need always to make the right decision

966. A nurse provides instructions to a malnourished client regarding iron supplementation during pregnancy. Which statement, if made by the client, would indicate an understanding of the instructions?
1. "The iron is best absorbed if taken on an empty stomach."
2. "Meat does not provide iron and should be avoided."
3. "Iron supplements will give me diarrhea."
4. "My body has all the iron it needs and I don't need to take supplements."

967. Levothyroxine (Synthroid) is prescribed for a client diagnosed with hypothyroidism. A nurse reviews the client's record and notes that the client is presently taking warfarin (Coumadin). The nurse contacts the physician, anticipating that the physician will prescribe which of the following?
1. An increased dosage of Coumadin
2. A decreased dosage of Coumadin
3. An increased dosage of Synthroid
4. A decreased dosage of Synthroid

968. A nurse is teaching a client with emphysema about positions that help breathing during dyspneic episodes. The nurse instructs the client to avoid which of the following positions that would aggravate breathing?
1. Sitting up with the elbows resting on knees
2. Standing and leaning against a wall
3. Lying on the back in a low-Fowler's position
4. Sitting up and leaning on a table

969. A client is about to undergo a lumbar puncture. A nurse describes to the client that which of the following positions will be used during the procedure?

1. Side-lying with the legs pulled up and the head bent down onto the chest
2. Side-lying with a pillow under the hip
3. Prone with a pillow under the abdomen
4. Prone in slight Trendelenburg's position

970. A nurse recognizes that which of the following interventions is unlikely to facilitate effective communication between a dying client and family?
1. The nurse encourages the client and family to identify and discuss feelings openly.
2. The nurse makes decisions for the client and family to relieve them of unnecessary demands.
3. The nurse assists the client and family in carrying out spiritually meaningful practices.
4. The nurse maintains a calm attitude and one of acceptance when the family or client expresses anger.

971. A depressed client verbalizes feelings of low self-esteem and self-worth typified by statements such as "I'm such a failure. I can't do anything right." The best nursing response would be to:
1. Tell the client that this is not true, that we all have a purpose in life.
2. Identify recent behaviors or accomplishments that demonstrate the client's skills.
3. Reassure the client that you know how the client is feeling and that things will get better.
4. Remain with the client and sit in silence; this will encourage the client to verbalize feelings.

972. A nurse has just admitted to the nursing unit a client with a basilar skull fracture who is at risk for increased intracranial pressure. Pending specific physician prescriptions, the nurse would safely place the client in which positions? **Select all that apply.**
☐ 1. Neck in neutral position
☐ 2. Head of bed elevated 30 to 45 degrees
☐ 3. Flat, with head turned to the side
☐ 4. Head midline
☐ 5. Neck in a flexed position

973. A nurse reviews the arterial blood gas results of an assigned client and notes that the laboratory report indicates a pH of 7.30, Pco_2 of 58 mm Hg, Po_2 of 80 mm Hg, and HCO_3 of 27 mEq/L. The nurse interprets that the client has which acid-base disturbance?
1. Metabolic acidosis
2. Metabolic alkalosis
3. Respiratory acidosis
4. Respiratory alkalosis

974. A nurse has admitted a client to the clinical nursing unit after a modified right radical mastectomy for the treatment of breast cancer. The nurse plans to place the right arm in which of the following positions?
1. Elevated above shoulder level
2. Elevated on a pillow
3. Level with the right atrium
4. Dependent to the right atrium

975. On the second postpartum day, a client complains of burning on urination, urgency, and frequency of urination. A urinalysis indicates the presence of a urinary tract infection. A nurse instructs the client regarding measures to take for the treatment of the infection. Which of the following statements, if made by the client, would indicate a need for further instructions?
1. "The prescribed medication must be taken until it is finished."
2. "My fluid intake should be increased to at least 3000 mL daily."
3. "I need to urinate frequently throughout the day."
4. "Foods and fluids that will increase urine alkalinity should be consumed."

976. A client received 20 units of Humulin NPH insulin subcutaneously at 8:00 AM. A nurse should assess the client for a hypoglycemic reaction at:
1. 10:00 AM
2. 11:00 AM
3. 5:00 PM
4. 11:00 PM

977. A community health nurse is working with disaster relief in a local community after a hurricane that destroyed many homes in the community. The nurse is working to find housing for the survivors and is organizing counseling services. The nurse's actions represent which type of level of prevention?
1. Primary
2. Secondary
3. Tertiary
4. Fourth

978. A pregnant woman in her second trimester calls a prenatal clinic nurse to report a recent exposure to a child with rubella. Which of the following responses by the nurse would be appropriate and supportive to the woman?
1. "There is no need to be concerned if you don't have a fever or rash within the next 2 days."
2. "Be sure to tell the physician on your next prenatal visit, but there is little risk in the second trimester."

3. "You should avoid all school-age children during pregnancy."
4. "You were wise to call. I will check your rubella titer screening results, and we can immediately identify if future interventions are needed."

979. A breast-feeding mother of an infant with lactose intolerance asks a nurse about dietary measures. The nurse tells the mother to avoid:
1. Hard cheeses
2. Green leafy vegetables
3. Dried beans
4. Egg yolk

980. A client with diabetes mellitus is told that amputation of the leg is necessary to sustain life. The client is very upset and tells a nurse, "This is all the doctor's fault. I have done everything that the doctor has asked me to do!" The nurse interprets the client's statement as:
1. An expected coping mechanism
2. A need to notify the hospital lawyer
3. An expression of guilt on the part of the client
4. An ineffective coping mechanism

981. A client brought to the emergency department is dead on arrival (DOA). The family of the client tells the physician that the client had a terminal cancer. The emergency department physician examines the client and asks a nurse to contact the medical examiner regarding an autopsy. The family of the client tells the nurse that they do not want an autopsy performed. Which of the following responses to the family is appropriate?
1. "It is required by federal law. Why don't we talk about it and why don't you tell me why you don't want the autopsy done?"
2. "The decision is made by the medical examiner."
3. "I will contact the medical examiner regarding your request."
4. "An autopsy is mandatory for any client who is DOA."

982. A client who is positive for human immunodeficiency virus (HIV) delivers a newborn infant. A nurse provides instructions to help the client regarding care of her infant. Which statement by the client indicates the need for further instructions?
1. "I will be sure to wash my hands before and after bathroom use."
2. "Support groups are available to assist me with understanding my diagnosis of HIV."
3. "I need to breast-feed, especially for the first 6 weeks postpartum."
4. "My newborn infant should be on antiviral medications for the first 6 weeks after delivery."

983. An adolescent client is diagnosed with conjunctivitis, and a nurse provides information to the client about the use of contact lenses. Which statement by the client indicates the need for further information?
1. "My contact lenses can be worn if they are cleaned as directed."
2. "I should not wear my contact lenses."
3. "I should obtain new contact lenses."
4. "My old contact lenses should be discarded."

984. A client with diabetes mellitus is self-administering NPH insulin from a vial that is kept at room temperature. The client asks a nurse about the length of time an unrefrigerated vial of insulin will maintain its potency. The appropriate response to the client is which of the following?
1. 2 weeks
2. 1 month
3. 2 months
4. 6 months

985. A nurse is caring for a client scheduled for a transsphenoidal hypophysectomy. The preoperative teaching instructions should include which most important statement?
1. "Your hair will need to be shaved."
2. "Deep breathing and coughing will be needed after surgery."
3. "Brushing your teeth will not be permitted for at least 2 weeks after surgery."
4. "You will receive spinal anesthesia."

986. During a routine prenatal visit, a client complains of gums that bleed easily with brushing. A nurse performs an assessment and teaches the client about proper nutrition to minimize this problem. Which statement, if made by the client, indicates an understanding of the proper nutrition to minimize this problem?
1. "I will eat three servings of cracked wheat bread each day."
2. "I will eat fresh fruits and vegetables for snacks and for dessert each day."
3. "I will drink 8 oz of water with each meal."
4. "I will eat two saltine crackers before I get up each morning."

987. A 6-year-old child has just been diagnosed with localized Hodgkin's disease, and chemotherapy is planned to begin immediately. The mother of the child asks a nurse why radiation therapy was not prescribed as a part of the treatment. The appropriate and supportive response to the mother is:
1. "I'm not sure. I'll discuss it with the physician."
2. "The child is too young to have radiation therapy."

3. "It's very costly, and chemotherapy works just as well."
4. "The physician would prefer that you discuss treatment options with the oncologist."

988. A nurse is preparing to care for a newborn who will be returning from surgery with a colostomy that was created for imperforate anus. When the infant returns from surgery, the nurse assesses the stoma and notes that it is red and edematous. Which of the following is the appropriate nursing intervention?
1. Call the physician.
2. Document the findings.
3. Apply ice immediately.
4. Elevate the buttocks.

989. A nurse in the labor room is performing an initial assessment on a newborn infant. On assessment of the infant's head, the nurse notes that the ears are low-set. Which of the following nursing actions would be most appropriate?
1. Cover the ears with gauze pads.
2. Document the findings.
3. Arrange for hearing testing.
4. Notify the physician.

990. A clinic nurse is assessing jaundice in a child with hepatitis. Which anatomical area would provide the best data regarding the presence of jaundice?
1. The nail beds
2. The skin in the abdominal area
3. The skin in the sacral area
4. The membranes in the ear canal

991. A nurse is assigned to care for a client who is in traction. The nurse prepares a plan of care for the client and includes which nursing action in the plan?
1. Monitor the weights to ensure that they are resting on a firm surface.
2. Check the weights to ensure that they are off of the floor.
3. Ensure that the knots are at the pulleys.
4. Ensure the head of the bed is kept at a 45- to 90-degree angle.

992. A nurse is setting up the physical environment for an interview with a client and plans to obtain subjective data regarding the client's health. Which interventions are appropriate? **Select all that apply.**
❑ 1. Set the room temperature at a comfortable level.
❑ 2. Provide seating for the client so that the client faces a strong light.
❑ 3. Ensure that the distance between the client and nurse is at least 6 feet.
❑ 4. Place a chair for the client across from the nurse's desk.

❑ 5. Remove distracting objects from the inter-viewing area.

❑ 6. Ensure comfortable seating at eye level for the client and nurse.

993. A nurse is caring for an older adult who has been placed in Buck's extension traction after a hip fracture. On assessment of the client, the nurse notes that the client is disoriented. The appropriate nursing intervention is to:
1. Ask the family to stay with the client.
2. Apply restraints to the client.
3. Ask the laboratory to perform electrolyte studies.
4. Reorient the client frequently and place a clock and calendar in the client's room.

994. A nurse is preparing a plan of care for a client in skin traction. The nurse includes in the plan that a priority intervention is to assess the client frequently for:
1. The presence of bowel sounds
2. Signs of infection around the pin sites
3. Signs of skin breakdown
4. Urinary incontinence

995. A home care nurse is visiting a client who is in a body cast. While performing an assessment, the nurse evaluates the psychosocial adjustment of the client to the cast. The nurse would most appropriately assess:
1. The type of transportation available for follow-up care
2. The ability to perform activities of daily living
3. The need for sensory stimulation
4. The amount of home care support available

996. When counseling a female Amish client, a nurse should:
1. Speak only to the husband.
2. Use complex medical terminology.
3. Avoid using scientific or medical jargon.
4. Stand close to the client and speak loudly.

997. A client has refused to eat more than a few spoonfuls of breakfast. The physician has prescribed that tube feedings be initiated if the client fails to eat at least half of a meal because the client had been losing weight for the prior 2 months. A nurse enters the room, looks at the tray, and states, "If you don't eat any more than that, I'm going to have to put a tube down your throat and get a feeding in that way." The client begins crying and tries to eat more. Based on the nurse's actions, the nurse may also be accused of a tort known as which of the following?
1. Assault
2. Battery

3. Slander
4. Invasion of privacy

998. A registered nurse (RN) is planning assignments for the clients on a nursing unit. The RN needs to assign four clients and has one RN, a licensed practical (vocational) nurse, and two nursing assistants on a nursing team. Which of the following clients would the RN most appropriately assign to the licensed practical (vocational) nurse?
1. A client who requires a 24-hour urine collection
2. An older adult requiring assistance with a bed bath and frequent ambulation
3. A client on a mechanical ventilator requiring frequent assessment and suctioning
4. A client with an abdominal wound requiring frequent wound irrigations and dressing changes

999. To perform cardiopulmonary resuscitation (CPR), a nurse would use this method to open the airway in which of the following situations?

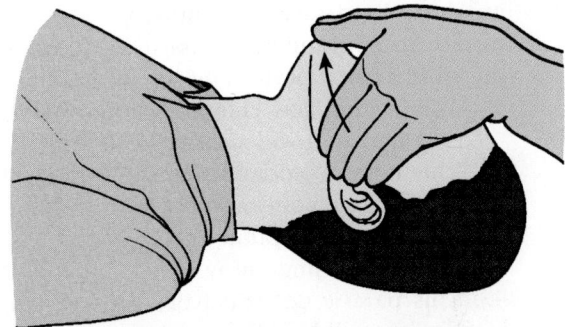

From Harkreader, H., Hogan, M.A., & Thobaben, M. [2007]. *Fundamentals of nursing: Caring and clinical judgment* [3rd ed., p. 968]. St. Louis: Saunders.

1. In all situations requiring CPR
2. If neck trauma is suspected
3. If the client has a history of seizures
4. If the client has a history of headaches

1000. A nurse teaches skin care to a client receiving external radiation therapy. Which of the following statements, if made by the client, would indicate the need for further instruction?
1. "I will handle the area gently."
2. "I will avoid the use of deodorants."
3. "I will limit sun exposure to 1 hour daily."
4. "I will wear loose-fitting clothing."

1001. A physician's prescription reads levothyroxine (Synthroid), 150 mcg orally daily. The medication label reads Synthroid, 0.1 mg per tablet. A nurse administers how many tablet(s) to the client?
_____ tablet(s)

1002. Metformin (Glucophage) is prescribed for a client with type 2 diabetes mellitus. A nurse tells the client that the most common side effect of the medication is:
1. Hypoglycemia
2. Gastrointestinal disturbances
3. Weight gain
4. Flushing and palpitations

1003. Which interventions apply to the care of a child who is having a seizure? **Select all that apply.**
❑ 1. Insert an oral airway.
❑ 2. Place the child in a supine position.
❑ 3. Loosen clothing around the child's neck.
❑ 4. Restrain the child.
❑ 5. Time the seizure.
❑ 6. Stay with the child.

1004. A 13-year-old child is diagnosed with Ewing's sarcoma of the femur. After a course of radiation and chemotherapy, it has been decided that leg amputation is necessary. After the amputation, the child becomes very frightened because of aching and cramping felt in the missing limb. Which nursing statement would be appropriate to assist in alleviating the child's fear?
1. "This aching and cramping is normal and temporary and will subside."
2. "This normally occurs after the surgery and we will teach you ways to deal with it."
3. "The pain medication that I give you will take these feelings away."
4. "This pain is not real pain, and relaxation exercises will help it go away."

1005. A nursing instructor asks a nursing student to identify the priorities of care for an assigned client. The student correctly identifies the client needs that are the priority by telling the nursing instructor that:
1. Actual or life-threatening concerns are the priority.
2. Time constraints related to the client's needs are the priority.
3. Obtaining needed supplies to care for the client is the priority.
4. Completing care in a reasonable time frame is the priority.

1006. A client arrives at the clinic complaining of fatigue, lack of energy, constipation, and depression. Hypothyroidism is diagnosed, and levothyroxine (Synthroid) is prescribed. A nurse instructs the client that the expected outcome of the medication is to:
1. Increase energy levels.

2. Achieve normal thyroid hormone levels.
3. Increase blood glucose levels.
4. Alleviate depression.

1007. A community health nurse is preparing a poster for an educational session for a group of women and will be discussing the risk factors associated with breast cancer. Which risk factors for breast cancer should the nurse list on the poster? Select all that apply.
❑ 1. Family history of breast cancer
❑ 2. Early menarche
❑ 3. Early menopause
❑ 4. Previous cancer of the breast, uterus, or ovaries
❑ 5. Multiparity
❑ 6. High-dose radiation exposure to chest

1008. A nurse is caring for a client with acute pancreatitis and is monitoring the client for paralytic ileus. Which assessment data would alert the nurse to this occurrence?
1. Firm, nontender mass palpable at the lower right costal margin
2. Severe, constant pain with rapid onset
3. Inability to pass flatus
4. Loss of anal sphincter control

1009. A nurse inspects the color of the drainage from a nasogastric tube on a postoperative client approximately 24 hours after gastric surgery. Which of the following findings indicate the need to notify the physician?
1. Light yellowish brown drainage
2. Dark red drainage
3. Dark brown drainage
4. Green-tinged drainage

1010. A nurse is preparing to discontinue a client's nasogastric tube. The client is positioned properly, and the tube has been flushed with 15 mL of air to clear secretions. Before removing the tube, the nurse makes which statement to the client?
1. "Take a deep breath when I tell you and breathe normally while I remove the tube."
2. "Take a deep breath when I tell you and bear down while I remove the tube."
3. "Take a deep breath when I tell you and slowly exhale while I remove the tube."
4. "Take a deep breath when I tell you and hold it while I remove the tube."

1011. A client with a history of lung disease is at risk for developing respiratory acidosis. A nurse assesses this client for which signs and symptoms characteristic of this disorder?

1. Bradycardia and hyperactivity
2. Decreased respiratory rate and depth
3. Headache, restlessness, and confusion
4. Bradypnea, dizziness, and paresthesias

1012. A nurse is caring for a client with a resolved intestinal obstruction who has a nasogastric tube in place. The client has tolerated the tube being clamped every 2 hours for 1 hour. The physician has now prescribed the nasogastric tube to be removed. Before removing the tube, the nurse assesses for:
1. Proper nasogastric tube placement
2. Normal serum electrolyte levels
3. The presence of bowel sounds in all four quadrants
4. Normal pH of the gastric aspirate

1013. A nurse has administered approximately half of an enema solution to a preoperative client when the client complains of pain and cramping. Which nursing action is the most appropriate?
1. Raise the enema bag so that the solution can be instilled quickly.
2. Clamp the tubing for 30 seconds and restart the flow at a slower rate.
3. Reassure the client and continue the flow.
4. Discontinue the enema and notify the physician.

1014. A client experiencing a great deal of stress and anxiety is being taught to use self-control therapy. Which statement by the client indicates a need for further teaching about the therapy?
1. "An advantage of this technique is that change is likely to last."
2. "This form of therapy can be applied to new situations."
3. "Talking to oneself is a basic component of this form of therapy."
4. "It provides a negative reinforcement when the stimulus is produced."

1015. A nurse is preparing a list of home care instructions regarding stoma and laryngectomy care to a client who had a laryngectomy. Which instructions that would be included in the list? **Select all that apply**.
❏ 1. Avoid swimming and use care when showering.
❏ 2. Keep the humidity in the home low.
❏ 3. Avoid exposure to people with infections.
❏ 4. Restrict fluid intake.
❏ 5. Obtain a Medic-Alert bracelet.
❏ 6. Prevent debris from entering the stoma.

1016. A physician prescribes 2000 mL of 5% dextrose and half-normal saline to infuse over 24 hours. The drop factor is 15 drops (gtt)/1 mL. A nurse sets the flow rate at how many drops per minute? (Round to the nearest whole number.)
_____ gtt/min

1017. A client is returned to the nursing unit after thoracic surgery with chest tubes in place. During the first few hours postoperatively, a nurse assesses for drainage and expects to note that it is:
1. Serous
2. Serosanguineous
3. Bloody
4. Bloody, with frequent small clots

1018. A client has had radical neck dissection and begins to hemorrhage at the incision site. A nurse should take which actions in this situation? **Select all that apply**.
❏ 1. Lower the head of the bed to a flat position.
❏ 2. Apply manual pressure over the site.
❏ 3. Monitor the client's airway.
❏ 4. Call the physician immediately.
❏ 5. Monitor vital signs.

1019. A sexually active 20-year-old client has developed viral hepatitis. Which of the following statements, if made by the client, would indicate a need for further teaching?
1. "A condom should be used for sexual intercourse."
2. "I can never drink alcohol again."
3. "I won't go back to work right away."
4. "My close friends should get the vaccine."

1020. A nurse would include which interventions in the plan of care for a client with hypothyroidism? **Select all that apply**.
❏ 1. Instruct the client about thyroid replacement therapy.
❏ 2. Encourage the client to consume fluids and high-fiber foods in the diet.
❏ 3. Provide a cool environment for the client.
❏ 4. Instruct the client to consume a high-fat diet.
❏ 5. Instruct the client to contact the physician if episodes of chest pain occur.
❏ 6. Inform the client that iodine preparations will be prescribed to treat the disorder.

1021. A nurse is preparing to care for a client who will be weaned from a cuffed tracheostomy tube. The nurse is planning to use a tracheostomy plug and plans to insert it into the opening in the outer cannula. Which of the following nursing interventions are required before plugging the tube?

1. Place the inner cannula into the tube.
2. Deflate the cuff on the tube.
3. Ensure that the client is able to swallow.
4. Ensure that the client is able to speak.

1022. A client is diagnosed with glaucoma. Which of the following assessment data gathered by a nurse identifies a risk factor associated with this eye disorder?
1. A history of migraine headaches
2. Frequent urinary tract infections
3. Cardiovascular disease
4. Frequent upper respiratory infections

1023. A client with retinal detachment is admitted to the nursing unit in preparation for a scleral buckling procedure. Which of the following would a nurse anticipate to be prescribed?
1. Bathroom privileges only
2. Elevating the head of the bed to 45 degrees
3. Placing an eye patch over the client's affected eye
4. Wearing dark glasses to read or watch television

1024. A nurse is caring for a client who is on strict bedrest. The nurse develops a plan of care with goals related to the prevention of deep vein thrombosis and pulmonary emboli. Which of the following nursing actions would be most helpful to prevent these disorders from developing?
1. Applying a heating pad to the lower extremities
2. Encouraging active range-of-motion exercises
3. Placing a pillow under the knees
4. Restricting fluids

1025. A nurse is caring for a suicidal client. The appropriate nursing intervention in dealing with this client is to:
1. Demonstrate confidence in the client's ability to deal with stressors.
2. Provide hope and reassurance that the problems will resolve themselves.
3. Display an attitude of detachment, confrontation, and efficiency.
4. Provide authority, action, and participation.

1026. A client with tuberculosis whose status is being monitored in an ambulatory care clinic asks a nurse when it is permissible to return to work. The nurse replies that the client may resume employment when:
1. Three sputum cultures are negative.
2. Five sputum cultures are negative.

3. A sputum culture and a chest x-ray are negative.
4. A sputum culture and a Mantoux test are negative.

1027. A client comes to the emergency department after an assault and is extremely agitated, trembling, and hyperventilating. The appropriate initial nursing action would be to:
1. Encourage the client to discuss the assault.
2. Place the client in a quiet room alone to decrease stimulation.
3. Remain with the client until the anxiety decreases.
4. Begin to teach relaxation techniques.

1028. A nurse is caring for a client admitted to the hospital with a suspected diagnosis of acute appendicitis. Which of the following laboratory results would the nurse expect to note if the client does have appendicitis?
1. Leukopenia with a shift to the right
2. Leukocytosis with a shift to the right
3. Leukocytosis with a shift to the left
4. Leukopenia with a shift to the left

1029. A nurse is developing a plan of care for a client experiencing anxiety after the loss of a job. The client is verbalizing concerns regarding the ability to meet role expectations and financial obligations. The appropriate nursing diagnosis for this client is:
1. *Dysfunctional family process*
2. *Disturbed thought process*
3. *Risk for anxiety*
4. *Ineffective coping*

1030. A nurse is monitoring the chest tube drainage system in a client with a chest tube. The nurse notes intermittent bubbling in the water seal chamber. Which of the following is the appropriate action?
1. Change the chest tube drainage system.
2. Document the findings.
3. Check for an air leak.
4. Notify the physician.

1031. A client arrives in the emergency department in a crisis state. The client shows signs of profound anxiety and is unable to focus on anything but the object of the crisis and the impact on self. The initial nursing assessment would focus on:
1. The object of the crisis
2. The presence of support systems
3. The physical condition of the client
4. The client's coping mechanisms

1032. After performing an initial abdominal assessment on a client with a diagnosis of cholelithiasis, a nurse documents that the bowel sounds are normal. Which of the following descriptions best describes "normal bowel sounds"?
1. Waves of loud gurgles auscultated in all four quadrants
2. Very high-pitched loud rushes auscultated especially in one or two quadrants
3. Relatively high-pitched clicks or gurgles auscultated in all four quadrants
4. Low-pitched swishing auscultated in one or two quadrants

ANSWERS
958. 3
Rationale: Whenever an abused client remains in the abusive environment, priority must be placed on ascertaining whether the client is in any immediate danger. If so, emergency action must be taken to remove the client from the abusing situation. Options 1, 2, and 4 may be appropriate interventions, but are not the priority.
Test-Taking Strategy: Use Maslow's Hierarchy of Needs theory, remembering that if a physiological need is not present, safety is the priority. This will direct you to option 3, the only option that directly addresses client safety. Review care of a client who is a victim of physical abuse if you had difficulty with this question.
Level of Cognitive Ability: Applying
Client Needs: Safe and Effective Care Environment
Integrated Process: Nursing Process—Planning
Content Area: Mental Health
Reference: Fortinash, K., & Holoday-Worret, P. (2008). *Psychiatric mental health nursing* (4th ed., pp. 491-492). St. Louis: Mosby.

959. 2
Rationale: Mania is a mood characterized by excitement, euphoria, hyperactivity, excessive energy, decreased need for sleep, and impaired ability to concentrate or complete a single train of thought. Mania is a period when the mood is predominantly elevated, expansive, or irritable. All options reflect a client's possible symptoms. Option 2 clearly presents a problem, however, that compromises physiological integrity and needs to be addressed immediately.
Test-Taking Strategy: Note the strategic word *immediate* and use Maslow's Hierarchy of Needs theory to assist you in answering the question. Option 2 is the only option that reflects a physiological need. Review care of a client with mania if you had difficulty with this question.
Level of Cognitive Ability: Analyzing
Client Needs: Physiological Integrity
Integrated Process: Nursing Process—Assessment
Content Area: Mental Health
Reference: Stuart, G. (2009). *Principles and practice of psychiatric nursing* (9th ed., pp. 287, 521). St. Louis: Mosby.

960. 4
Rationale: Clients who are admitted involuntarily do not lose their right to informed consent. Clients must be considered legally competent until they have been declared incompetent through a legal proceeding. The informed consent needs to be obtained from the client.
Test-Taking Strategy: Knowledge regarding the hospital admission processes and client's rights is necessary to answer this question. If you had difficulty with this question, focus on the subject of client rights to direct you to option 4. Review client rights if you had difficulty with this question.
Level of Cognitive Ability: Understanding
Client Needs: Safe and Effective Care Environment
Integrated Process: Nursing Process—Planning
Content Area: Leadership and Management—Ethical/Legal
Reference: Stuart, G. (2009). *Principles and practice of psychiatric nursing* (9th ed., p. 538). St. Louis: Mosby.

961. 1
Rationale: Glucagon is used to treat hypoglycemia resulting from insulin overdose. The family of the client is instructed in how to administer the medication. In an unconscious client, arousal usually occurs within 20 minutes of glucagon injection. When consciousness has been regained, oral carbohydrates should be given. Lipoatrophy and lipohypertrophy result from insulin injections.
Test-Taking Strategy: Use the process of elimination. Noting the word *glucagon* will assist in determining that the medication contains some form of glucose. This relationship will direct you to option 1. Review the purpose of this medication if you are unfamiliar with it.
Level of Cognitive Ability: Applying
Client Needs: Physiological Integrity
Integrated Process: Teaching and Learning
Content Area: Pharmacology
Reference: Kee, J., Hayes, E., & McCuistion, L. (2009). *Pharmacology: A nursing process approach* (6th ed., p. 803). St. Louis: Saunders.

962. 3
Rationale: In the Puerto Rican–American culture, loud crying and other physical manifestations of grief are considered socially acceptable. Of the options provided, option 3 is the only one that identifies a culturally sensitive approach on the part of the nurse. Options 1, 2, and 4 are inappropriate nursing interventions.
Test-Taking Strategy: Focus on the clients of the question, the family members. Use the process of elimination and therapeutic nursing interventions, recalling the characteristics of the culture and the importance of cultural sensitivity. This will direct you to option 3. If you had difficulty with this question, review the characteristics of this culture.
Level of Cognitive Ability: Applying
Client Needs: Psychosocial Integrity
Integrated Process: Nursing Process—Implementation
Content Area: Fundamental Skills—Cultural Diversity

References: Black, J., & Hawks, J. (2009). *Medical-surgical nursing: Clinical management for positive outcomes* (8th ed., p. 82). St. Louis: Saunders.

Giger, J., & Davidhizar, R. (2008) *Transcultural nursing assessment and intervention* (5th ed. p. 679). St. Louis: Mosby.

963. 4

Rationale: The priority nursing action is to assess the vital signs. This would indicate the amount of blood loss that has occurred and provides a baseline by which to monitor the progress of treatment. The client may be unable to provide subjective data until the immediate physical needs are met. Although an abdominal examination and an assessment of the precipitating events may be necessary, these actions are not the priority.

Test-Taking Strategy: Note the strategic words *first priority*. Use the process of elimination and the ABCs—airway, breathing, and circulation. This will direct you to option 4. Review care of a client with a gastrointestinal bleed if you had difficulty with this question.

Level of Cognitive Ability: Applying
Client Needs: Physiological Integrity
Integrated Process: Nursing Process—Implementation
Content Area: Adult Health—Gastrointestinal
Reference: Ignatavicius, D., & Workman, M. (2010). *Medical-surgical nursing: Patient-centered collaborative care* (6th ed., pp. 709, 1223). St. Louis: Saunders.

964. 1

Rationale: The clinical picture of dementia ranges from mild cognitive deficits to severe, life-threatening alterations in neurological functioning. For the client to use confabulation or the fabrication of events or experiences to fill in memory gaps is not unusual. Often, lack of inhibitions on the part of the client may constitute the first indication of something being "wrong" to the client's significant others (e.g., the client may undress in front of others, or the formerly well-mannered client may exhibit slovenly table manners). As the dementia progresses, the client will have episodes of wandering or sundowning.

Test-Taking Strategy: Use the process of elimination and focus on the client's diagnosis. Noting the subject, a manifestation, will direct you to option 1. If you had difficulty with this question, review the manifestations associated with dementia.

Level of Cognitive Ability: Analyzing
Client Needs: Psychosocial Integrity
Integrated Process: Nursing Process—Assessment
Content Area: Mental Health
References: Stuart, G. (2009). *Principles and practice of psychiatric nursing* (9th ed., p. 394). St. Louis: Mosby.

Varcarolis, E., & Halter, M. (2009). *Essentials of psychiatric mental health nursing: A communication approach to evidence-based care* (p. 311). St. Louis: Saunders.

965. 3

Rationale: Clients with anorexia nervosa have the desire to please others. Their need to be correct or perfect interferes with rational decision-making processes. These clients are moralistic. Rules and rituals help these clients manage their anxiety.

Test-Taking Strategy: Use the process of elimination and focus on the subject, managing anxiety. Eliminate options 2 and 4 because of the close-ended word *always*. Option 1 is not characteristic of a client with anorexia. Review the characteristics associated with this disorder if you had difficulty with this question.

Level of Cognitive Ability: Understanding
Client Needs: Psychosocial Integrity
Integrated Process: Nursing Process—Assessment
Content Area: Mental Health
References: Fortinash, K., & Holoday-Worret, P. (2008). *Psychiatric mental health nursing* (4th ed., p. 400). St. Louis: Mosby.

Varcarolis, E., & Halter, M. (2009). *Essentials of psychiatric mental health nursing: A communication approach to evidence-based care* (p. 199). St. Louis: Saunders.

966. 1

Rationale: Iron is needed to allow for transfer of adequate iron to the fetus and to permit expansion of the maternal red blood cell mass. During pregnancy, the relative excess of plasma causes a decrease in the hemoglobin concentration and hematocrit, known as physiological anemia of pregnancy. This is a normal adaptation during pregnancy. Meats are an excellent source of iron. Iron supplements usually cause constipation. Iron is best absorbed if taken on an empty stomach.

Test-Taking Strategy: Use the process of elimination, focusing on the strategic words *understanding of the instructions*. Knowledge of basic principles related to nutrition during pregnancy will assist in eliminating options 2 and 4. From the remaining options, remember that iron causes constipation. Review client teaching points related to iron supplementation if you had difficulty with this question.

Level of Cognitive Ability: Evaluating
Client Needs: Physiological Integrity
Integrated Process: Nursing Process—Evaluation
Content Area: Maternity—Antepartum
Reference: McKinney, E., James, S., Murray, S., & Ashwill, J. (2009). *Maternal-child nursing* (3rd ed., pp. 304). St. Louis: Saunders.

967. 2

Rationale: Levothyroxine (Synthroid) accelerates the degradation of vitamin K–dependent clotting factors. As a result, the effects of warfarin (Coumadin) are enhanced. If thyroid hormone replacement therapy is instituted in a client who has been taking warfarin, the dosage of warfarin should be reduced.

Test-Taking Strategy: Use the process of elimination. Recalling that levothyroxine enhances the effects of warfarin will direct you to the correct option. Review these medication interactions if you had difficulty with this question.

Level of Cognitive Ability: Analyzing
Client Needs: Physiological Integrity
Integrated Process: Nursing Process—Analysis
Content Area: Pharmacology
Reference: Lehne, R. (2010). *Pharmacology for nursing care* (7th ed., p. 694). St. Louis: Saunders.

968. 3

Rationale: The client should use the positions outlined in options 1, 2, and 4. These allow for maximal chest expansion.

The client should not lie on the back because it reduces movement of a large area of the client's chest wall. Sitting is better than standing, whenever possible. If no chair is available, leaning against a wall while standing allows accessory muscles to be used for breathing and not posture control.

Test-Taking Strategy: Use the process of elimination, noting the strategic words *dyspneic episodes* and *avoid*. Also, note that options 1, 2, and 4 are comparable or alike in that they all address upright positions. If you had difficulty with this question, review client teaching points related to emphysema.

Level of Cognitive Ability: Applying
Client Needs: Physiological Integrity
Integrated Process: Teaching and Learning
Content Area: Adult Health—Respiratory
Reference: Ignatavicius, D., & Workman, M. (2010). *Medical-surgical nursing: Patient-centered collaborative care* (6th ed., p. 624). St. Louis: Saunders.

969. 1
Rationale: A client undergoing lumbar puncture is positioned lying on the side, with the legs pulled up to the abdomen and the head bent down onto the chest. This position helps open the spaces between the vertebrae and allows for easier needle insertion by the physician. The nurse remains with the client during the procedure to help the client maintain this position. The other options identify incorrect positions for this procedure.

Test-Taking Strategy: Use the process of elimination. Recalling that a lumbar puncture is the introduction of a needle into the subarachnoid space will direct you to option 1. It is reasonable that the position of the client must facilitate this, and the correct option is the only position that flexes the vertebrae and widens the spaces between them. Review care of a client undergoing a lumbar puncture if you had difficulty with this question.

Level of Cognitive Ability: Applying
Client Needs: Physiological Integrity
Integrated Process: Nursing Process—Implementation
Content Area: Adult Health—Neurological
Reference: Pagana, K., & Pagana, T. (2009). *Mosby's diagnostic and laboratory test reference* (9th ed., p. 615). St. Louis: Mosby.

970. 2
Rationale: Maintaining effective and open communication among family members affected by death and grief is of the greatest importance. Option 1 describes encouraging discussion of feelings and is likely to enhance communications. Option 3 is also an effective intervention because spiritual practices give meaning to life and have an impact on how people react to crisis. Option 4 is also an effective technique because the client and family need to know that someone will be there who is supportive and nonjudgmental. Option 2 describes the nurse removing autonomy and decision making from the client and family, who are already experiencing feelings of loss of control in that they cannot change the process of dying. This is an ineffective intervention, which could impair communication further.

Test-Taking Strategy: Use the process of elimination, noting the strategic words *unlikely to facilitate*. Understanding that

people in crisis usually feel helpless and unable to control their circumstances can assist in identifying option 2 as a response that further removes control. Review these therapeutic interventions if you had difficulty with this question.

Level of Cognitive Ability: Understanding
Client Needs: Psychosocial Integrity
Integrated Process: Caring
Content Area: Fundamental Skills—End-of-Life Care
References: Potter, P., & Perry, A. (2009) *Fundamentals of nursing* (7th ed., p. 478). St. Louis: Mosby.
 Swearingen, P. (2008). *All-in-one care planning resource: Medical-surgical, pediatric, maternity, & psychiatric nursing care plans* (2nd ed., p. 113). St. Louis: Mosby.

971. 2
Rationale: Feelings of low self-esteem and worthlessness are common symptoms of a depressed client. An effective plan of care to enhance the client's personal self-esteem is to provide experiences for the client that are challenging, but that will not be met with failure. Reminders of the client's past accomplishments or personal successes are ways to interrupt the client's negative self-talk and distorted cognitive view of self. Silence may be interpreted as agreement. Options 1 and 3 give advice and devalue the client's feelings.

Test-Taking Strategy: Use the process of elimination and therapeutic communication techniques. Focus on the client's diagnosis. You can eliminate options 1 and 3 easily. From the remaining options, focusing on the client's diagnosis will direct you to option 2. Review care of a client with depression if you had difficulty with this question.

Level of Cognitive Ability: Applying
Client Needs: Psychosocial Integrity
Integrated Process: Nursing Process—Implementation
Content Area: Mental Health
Reference: Stuart, G. (2009). *Principles and practice of psychiatric nursing* (9th ed., pp. 286, 289). St. Louis: Mosby.

972. 1, 2, 4
Rationale: The head of the client at risk for or with increased intracranial pressure should be positioned so that the head is in a neutral, midline position. The nurse should avoid flexing or extending the neck or turning the head side to side. The head of the bed should be raised to 30 to 45 degrees. Use of proper positions promotes venous drainage from the cranium to keep intracranial pressure from elevating.

Test-Taking Strategy: Use the process of elimination, noting the strategic words *at risk for increased intracranial pressure*. Visualize each of the positions identified in the options and identify those that will increased intracranial pressure. Review care of a client at risk for or with increased intracranial pressure if you had difficulty with this question.

Level of Cognitive Ability: Applying
Client Needs: Physiological Integrity
Integrated Process: Nursing Process—Implementation
Content Area: Adult Health—Neurological
Reference: Black, J., & Hawks, J. (2009). *Medical-surgical nursing: Clinical management for positive outcomes* (8th ed., pp. 1932, 1942). St. Louis: Saunders.

973. 3
Rationale: The normal pH is 7.35 to 7.45. Normal P_{CO_2} is 35 to 45 mm Hg. In respiratory acidosis, the pH is low and P_{CO_2} is elevated. Options 1, 2, and 4 are incorrect interpretations of the values identified in the question.
Test-Taking Strategy: Remember that in a respiratory imbalance you will find an opposite response between the pH and P_{CO_2}. Also, remember that the pH is low in an acidotic condition. Recalling this information will allow you to eliminate each of the incorrect options. Review interpretation of arterial blood gas results if you had difficulty with this question.
Level of Cognitive Ability: Analyzing
Client Needs: Physiological Integrity
Integrated Process: Nursing Process—Analysis
Content Area: Fundamental Skills—Fluids & Electrolytes/Acid-Base
Reference: Ignatavicius, D., & Workman, M. (2010). *Medical-surgical nursing: Patient-centered collaborative care* (6th ed., pp. 204-206). St. Louis: Saunders.

974. 2
Rationale: The client's operative arm should be positioned so that it is elevated on a pillow and not exceeding shoulder elevation. This position promotes optimal drainage from the limb, without impairing the circulation to the arm. If the arm is positioned flat (option 3) or dependent (option 4), this could increase the edema in the arm, which is contraindicated because of lymphatic disruption caused by surgery.
Test-Taking Strategy: Use the process of elimination. Read each option carefully and attempt to visualize the position identified in the option. Using the principles of circulation and gravity will direct you to option 2. Option 2 avoids the two extremes of height in positioning the limb affected by surgery. Review care of a client after mastectomy if you had difficulty with this question.
Level of Cognitive Ability: Applying
Client Needs: Physiological Integrity
Integrated Process: Nursing Process—Planning
Content Area: Adult Health—Oncology
Reference: Ignatavicius, D., & Workman, M. (2010). *Medical-surgical nursing: Patient-centered collaborative care* (6th ed., p. 1674). St. Louis: Saunders.

975. 4
Rationale: A client with a urinary tract infection must be encouraged to take the medication for the entire time it is prescribed. The client should also be instructed to drink at least 3000 mL of fluid each day to flush the infection from the bladder and to urinate frequently throughout the day. Foods and fluids that acidify the urine need to be encouraged.
Test-Taking Strategy: Use the process of elimination. Note the strategic words *indicate a need for further instructions*. These words indicate a negative event query and ask you to select an option that is incorrect. Recall that foods and fluids that acidify the urine should be consumed, rather than foods and fluids that cause urine alkalinity. If you had difficulty with this question, review nursing considerations for a client with a urinary tract infection.
Level of Cognitive Ability: Evaluating
Client Needs: Physiological Integrity
Integrated Process: Teaching and Learning

Content Area: Maternity—Postpartum
Reference: McKinney, E., James, S., Murray, S., & Ashwill, J. (2009). *Maternal-child nursing* (3rd ed., p. 707). St. Louis: Saunders.

976. 3
Rationale: NPH is an intermediate-acting insulin. The onset of action is 1.5 hours, it peaks in 4 to 12 hours, and the duration of action is 16 to 24 hours. Hypoglycemic reactions most likely occur during peak time.
Test-Taking Strategy: Use the process of elimination and knowledge regarding the onset, peak, and duration of action for NPH insulin. Recalling that peak action is between 4 and 12 hours will direct you to option 3. Review the characteristics of NPH insulin if you had difficulty with this question.
Level of Cognitive Ability: Applying
Client Needs: Physiological Integrity
Integrated Process: Nursing Process—Assessment
Content Area: Adult Health—Endocrine
Reference: Ignatavicius, D., & Workman, M. (2010). *Medical-surgical nursing: Patient-centered collaborative care* (6th ed., p. 1485). St. Louis: Saunders.

977. 3
Rationale: Tertiary prevention involves the reduction of the amount and degree of disability, injury, and damage after a crisis. Primary prevention means keeping the crisis from occurring, and secondary prevention focuses on reducing the intensity and duration of the crisis during the crisis itself. There is no known fourth care prevention level.
Test-Taking Strategy: Identify the scenario in the question and the role of the nurse in the question. Focus on these nursing roles and use knowledge regarding the various levels of prevention to answer the question. If you had difficulty with this question, review the levels of prevention.
Level of Cognitive Ability: Understanding
Client Needs: Safe and Effective Care Environment
Integrated Process: Nursing Process—Implementation
Content Area: Fundamental Skills—Safety/Infection Control
References: Ignatavicius, D., & Workman, M. (2010). *Medical-surgical nursing: Patient-centered collaborative care.* (6th ed., pp. 163-164). St. Louis: Saunders.
    Maurer, F., & Smith, C. (2009). *Community/public health nursing practices: Health for families and populations* (4th ed., pp. 574-576). St. Louis: Saunders.

978. 4
Rationale: Rubella virus is spread by aerosol droplet transmission through the upper respiratory tract and has an incubation period of 14 to 21 days. The risks of maternal and subsequent fetal infection during the second trimester include hearing loss and congenital anomalies. Rubella titer determination is a standard antenatal test for pregnant women during their initial screening and entry into the health care delivery system. Option 4 helps clarify maternal concerns with accurate information based on the acquisition of rubella infection and potential fetal side effects.
Test-Taking Strategy: Use the process of elimination and knowledge regarding the transmission of rubella virus to the fetus. Also, use of therapeutic communication techniques will

direct you to option 4. Option 4 addresses the client's concerns. Review concepts related to exposure to rubella during pregnancy if you had difficulty with this question.
Level of Cognitive Ability: Applying
Client Needs: Psychosocial Integrity
Integrated Process: Caring
Content Area: Maternity—Antepartum
Reference: McKinney, E., James, S., Murray, S., & Ashwill, J. (2009). *Maternal-child nursing* (3rd ed., pp. 177-178). St. Louis: Saunders.

979. 1
Rationale: Breast-feeding mothers with lactose-intolerant infants need to be encouraged to limit dairy products. Cheese is a dairy product. Alternative calcium sources that can be consumed by the mother include egg yolk, green leafy vegetables, dried beans, cauliflower, and molasses.
Test-Taking Strategy: Use the process of elimination. Note the strategic word *avoid* in the question. Knowledge that lactose is the sugar found in dairy products will easily direct you to option 1. Review the dietary management for an infant with lactose intolerance if you had difficulty with this question.
Level of Cognitive Ability: Applying
Client Needs: Physiological Integrity
Integrated Process: Teaching and Learning
Content Area: Fundamental Skills—Nutrition
Reference: Nix, S. (2009). *Williams' basic nutrition and diet therapy* (13th ed., p. 77). St. Louis: Mosby.

980. 1
Rationale: The nurse needs to be aware of the effective and ineffective coping mechanisms that can occur in a client when loss is anticipated. The expression of anger is known to be a normal response to impending loss, and the anger may be directed toward the self, God or other spiritual being, or caregivers. Notifying the hospital lawyer is inappropriate. Guilt may or may not be a component of the client's feelings, and the data in the question do not indicate that guilt is present.
Test-Taking Strategy: Focus on the data provided in the question. Note that options 1 and 4 address coping mechanisms. This provides you with the clue that one of these options may be the correct response. Additionally, knowledge of the stages of grief associated with loss will direct you to option 1. Review these stages and expected client responses if you had difficulty with this question.
Level of Cognitive Ability: Analyzing
Client Needs: Psychosocial Integrity
Integrated Process: Nursing Process—Analysis
Content Area: Mental Health
Reference: Ignatavicius, D., & Workman, M. (2010). *Medical-surgical nursing: Patient-centered collaborative care* (6th ed., pp. 1200, 1202-1203). St. Louis: Saunders.

981. 3
Rationale: An autopsy is required by state law in certain circumstances, including the sudden death of a client and a death that occurs under suspicious circumstances. A client may have provided oral or written instructions regarding an autopsy after death. If an autopsy is not required by law, these oral or written requests will be granted. If no oral or written

instructions were provided, state law determines who has the authority to consent for an autopsy. Most often, the decision rests with the surviving relative or next of kin.
Test-Taking Strategy: Use knowledge regarding the laws and issues surrounding autopsy and therapeutic communication techniques to answer the question. Eliminate options 1 and 4 because these statements are not completely accurate. From the remaining options, option 3 is the therapeutic and appropriate response to the family. Review the issues and laws surrounding autopsy if you had difficulty with this question.
Level of Cognitive Ability: Applying
Client Needs: Psychosocial Integrity
Integrated Process: Caring
Content Area: Fundamental Skills—End-of-Life Care
Reference: Potter, P., & Perry, A. (2009) *Fundamentals of nursing* (7th ed., p. 479). St. Louis: Mosby.

982. 3
Rationale: The mode of perinatal transmission of human immunodeficiency virus (HIV) to the fetus or neonate of an HIV-positive woman can occur during the antenatal, intrapartal, or postpartum period. HIV transmission can occur during breast-feeding. HIV-positive clients should be encouraged to bottle-feed their infants. Frequent handwashing is encouraged. Support groups and community agencies can be identified to assist the parents with the newborn infant's home care, the impact of the diagnosis of HIV infection, and available financial resources. It is recommended that infants of HIV-positive clients receive antiviral medications for the first 6 weeks of life.
Test-Taking Strategy: Use the process of elimination. Note the strategic words *need for further instructions* in the question. These words indicate a negative event query and ask you to select an option that is incorrect. Recalling that breast-feeding is discouraged in the HIV-positive woman will direct you to the correct option. Review home care measures for the HIV-positive client if you had difficulty with this question.
Level of Cognitive Ability: Evaluating
Client Needs: Safe and Effective Care Environment
Integrated Process: Teaching and Learning
Content Area: Maternity—Postpartum
Reference: McKinney, E., James, S., Murray, S., & Ashwill, J. (2009). *Maternal-child nursing* (3rd ed., pp. 88, 657). St. Louis: Saunders.

983. 1
Rationale: If the client wears contact lenses, he or she should be instructed to discontinue wearing them until the infection has cleared completely. Obtaining new contact lenses would eliminate the chance of reinfection from contaminated contact lenses and would lessen the risk of a corneal ulceration.
Test-Taking Strategy: Use the process of elimination. Note the strategic words *need for further information* in the question. These words indicate a negative event query and ask you to select an option that is incorrect. Options 2, 3, and 4 are comparable or alike in that they relate to avoiding the use of contact lenses during infection. If you had difficulty with this question, review treatment measures for conjunctivitis.
Level of Cognitive Ability: Evaluating
Client Needs: Safe and Effective Care Environment
Integrated Process: Teaching and Learning

Content Area: Child Health—Eye/Ear/Throat/Respiratory/Cardiovascular
Reference: McKinney, E., James, S., Murray, S., & Ashwill, J. (2009). *Maternal-child nursing* (3rd ed., p. 1563). St. Louis: Saunders.

984. 2
Rationale: An insulin vial in current use can be kept at room temperature for 1 month without significant loss of activity. Direct sunlight and heat must be avoided.
Test-Taking Strategy: Use the process of elimination. Note the strategic word *unrefrigerated* in the question. This word will assist in directing you to the correct option. If you are unfamiliar with the concepts related to insulin stability, review this information.
Level of Cognitive Ability: Applying
Client Needs: Physiological Integrity
Integrated Process: Teaching and Learning
Content Area: Pharmacology
Reference: Kee, J., Hayes, E., & McCuistion, L. (2009). *Pharmacology: A nursing process approach* (6th ed., p. 793). St. Louis: Saunders.

985. 3
Rationale: Based on the location of the surgical procedure, spinal anesthesia would not be used. Additionally, the hair would not be shaved. Although coughing and deep breathing are important, specific to this procedure is avoiding brushing the teeth to prevent disruption of the surgical site.
Test-Taking Strategy: Consider the anatomical location and the surgical procedure itself to eliminate options 1 and 4. Although you may be tempted to select option 2, note the strategic words *most important*. Because of the anatomical location of the surgery, option 3 is most important. Review this surgical procedure if you had difficulty with this question.
Level of Cognitive Ability: Applying
Client Needs: Physiological Integrity
Integrated Process: Teaching and Learning
Content Area: Adult Health—Endocrine
Reference: Ignatavicius, D., & Workman, M. (2010). *Medical-surgical nursing: Patient-centered collaborative care* (6th ed., p. 1432). St. Louis: Saunders.

986. 2
Rationale: Fresh fruits and vegetables provide vitamins and minerals needed for healthy gums. Cracked wheat bread may abrade the tender gums. Drinking water with meals has no direct effect on gums. Eating saltine crackers before arising helps decrease nausea.
Test-Taking Strategy: Use the process of elimination and focus on the subject of the question. Eliminate options 1 and 4 first because these measures could irritate fragile gums. From the remaining options, eliminate option 3, remembering that drinking water with meals has no direct effect on gums. Review measures that promote dental health during pregnancy if you had difficulty with this question.
Level of Cognitive Ability: Evaluating
Client Needs: Physiological Integrity
Integrated Process: Nursing Process—Evaluation
Content Area: Maternity—Antepartum

Reference: Nix, S. (2009). *Williams' basic nutrition and diet therapy* (13th ed., pp. 18-19). St. Louis: Mosby.

987. 2
Rationale: Radiation therapy is usually delayed until a child is 8 years old, whenever possible, to prevent retardation of bone growth and soft tissue development. Options 1, 3, and 4 are inappropriate responses to the mother.
Test-Taking Strategy: Note the age of the child in the question. Additionally, use therapeutic communication techniques and knowledge regarding the effects of radiation to answer this question. Options 1 and 4 are nontherapeutic and place the mother's inquiry on hold. From the remaining options, use the child's age as a guide in directing you to option 2. Review the effects of radiation therapy if you had difficulty with this question.
Level of Cognitive Ability: Applying
Client Needs: Physiological Integrity
Integrated Process: Nursing Process—Implementation
Content Area: Child Health—Hematological/Oncological
Reference: McKinney, E., James, S., Murray, S., & Ashwill, J. (2009). *Maternal-child nursing* (3rd ed., p. 1310). St. Louis: Saunders.

988. 2
Rationale: A fresh colostomy stoma would be red and edematous, but this would decrease with time. The colostomy site then becomes pink without evidence of abnormal drainage, swelling, or skin breakdown. The nurse would document these findings because this is a normal expectation. Options 1, 3, and 4 are inappropriate interventions.
Test-Taking Strategy: Use the process of elimination. Note the strategic words *returns from surgery*. You would expect redness and edema at this time. Review postoperative colostomy assessment if you had difficulty with this question.
Level of Cognitive Ability: Applying
Client Needs: Physiological Integrity
Integrated Process: Nursing Process—Implementation
Content Area: Child Health—Gastrointestinal/Renal
Reference: McKinney, E., James, S., Murray, S., & Ashwill, J. (2009). *Maternal-child nursing* (3rd ed., p. 1126). St. Louis: Saunders.

989. 4
Rationale: Low or oddly placed ears are associated with various congenital defects and should be reported immediately. Although the findings would be documented, the most appropriate action would be to notify the physician. Options 1, 2, and 3 are inaccurate and inappropriate nursing actions.
Test-Taking Strategy: Use the process of elimination. Knowledge regarding the normal assessment findings in a newborn infant is required to answer this question. Recalling that low-set ears is an abnormal finding will direct you to option 4. Review normal assessment findings in a newborn if you had difficulty with this question.
Level of Cognitive Ability: Applying
Client Needs: Physiological Integrity
Integrated Process: Nursing Process—Implementation
Content Area: Maternity—Postpartum

Reference: McKinney, E., James, S., Murray, S., & Ashwill, J. (2009). *Maternal-child nursing* (3rd ed., p. 508). St. Louis: Saunders.

990. 1

Rationale: Jaundice, if present, is best assessed in the sclera, nail beds, and mucous membranes. Generalized jaundice appears in the skin throughout the body. Option 4 is an inappropriate area to assess for the presence of jaundice.

Test-Taking Strategy: Use the process of elimination. Note the strategic word *best* in the question. Options 2 and 3 can be eliminated first because jaundice present in the skin is generalized. From the remaining options, recalling that skin discoloration can best be assessed in the nail beds will direct you to option 1. Review assessment findings related to jaundice if you had difficulty with this question.

Level of Cognitive Ability: Analyzing
Client Needs: Health Promotion and Maintenance
Integrated Process: Nursing Process—Assessment
Content Area: Child Health—Gastrointestinal/Renal
Reference: McKinney, E., James, S., Murray, S., & Ashwill, J. (2009). *Maternal-child nursing* (3rd ed., p. 1133). St. Louis: Saunders.

991. 2

Rationale: To achieve proper traction, weights need to be free-hanging, with knots kept away from the pulleys. Weights should not be kept resting on a firm surface. The head of the bed is usually kept low to provide countertraction.

Test-Taking Strategy: Use the process of elimination. Attempt to visualize the traction, recalling that there must be weight to exert the pull from the traction setup. This concept will assist in eliminating options 1 and 3. Recalling that countertraction is needed will assist in eliminating option 4. Review care of a client in traction if you had difficulty with this question.

Level of Cognitive Ability: Applying
Client Needs: Physiological Integrity
Integrated Process: Nursing Process—Planning
Content Area: Adult Health—Musculoskeletal
References: Black, J., & Hawks, J. (2009). *Medical-surgical nursing: Clinical management for positive outcomes* (8th ed., p. 525). St. Louis: Saunders.
   Ignatavicius, D., & Workman, M. (2010). *Medical-surgical nursing: Patient-centered collaborative care* (6th ed., p. 1189). St. Louis: Saunders.

992. 1, 5, 6

Rationale: When preparing the physical environment for an interview, the nurse would set the room temperature at a comfortable level. The nurse would provide sufficient lighting for the client and nurse to see each other. The nurse would avoid having the client face a strong light because the client would have to squint into the full light. Distracting objects and equipment should be removed from the interview area. The nurse should arrange seating so that the nurse and client are seated comfortably at eye level, and the nurse avoids facing the client across a desk or table because this creates a barrier. The distance between the nurse and the client should be set by the nurse at 4 to 5 feet. If the nurse places the client any closer, the nurse will be invading the client's private space and

may create anxiety in the client. If the nurse places the client farther away, the nurse may be seen as distant and aloof by the client.

Test-Taking Strategy: Read each intervention carefully. Use the guidelines for preparing the physical environment for conducting an interview to select the appropriate interventions. Review these guidelines if you had difficulty with this question.

Level of Cognitive Ability: Applying
Client Needs: Health Promotion and Maintenance
Integrated Process: Nursing Process—Planning
Content Area: Adult Health—Health Assessment/Physical Exam
Reference: Jarvis, C. (2008). *Physical examination and health assessment* (5th ed, pp. 57-58). St. Louis: Saunders.

993. 4

Rationale: An inactive older adult may become disoriented because of lack of sensory stimulation. The most appropriate nursing intervention would be to reorient the client frequently and to place objects such as a clock and a calendar in the client's room to maintain orientation. The family can assist with orientation of the client, but it is inappropriate to ask the family to stay with the client. It is not the within the scope of nursing practice to prescribe laboratory studies. Restraints may cause further disorientation and should not be applied unless specifically prescribed; agency policies and procedures should be followed before the application of restraints.

Test-Taking Strategy: Use the process of elimination. Eliminate option 3 first because it is not within the realm of nursing practice to prescribe laboratory studies. Next, eliminate option 2 because restraints may add to the disorientation that the client is experiencing. It is inappropriate to place the responsibility of the client on the family, so eliminate option 1. Note the relationship between the words *disoriented* in the question and *reorient* in the correct option. Review the measures related to caring for a client who is disoriented if you had difficulty with this question.

Level of Cognitive Ability: Applying
Client Needs: Psychosocial Integrity
Integrated Process: Nursing Process—Implementation
Content Area: Adult Health—Musculoskeletal
Reference: Swearingen, P. (2008). *All-in-one care planning resource: Medical-surgical, pediatric, maternity, & psychiatric nursing care plans* (2nd ed., p. 755). St. Louis: Mosby.

994. 3

Rationale: Skin traction is achieved by Ace wraps, boots, and slings that apply a direct force on the client's skin. Traction is maintained with 5 to 8 lb of weight, and this type of traction can cause skin breakdown. There are no pin sites with skin traction. Urinary incontinence is not related to the use of skin traction. Although constipation can occur as a result of immobility and monitoring bowel sounds may be a component of the assessment, this intervention is not the priority assessment.

Test-Taking Strategy: Use the process of elimination. Note the strategic word *priority* in the question. Eliminate option 2 first because there are no pin sites with skin traction. Visualizing the traction setup and knowledge of the complications

associated with this type of traction will direct you to option 3. Review the complications associated with skin traction and the priority nursing interventions if you had difficulty with this question.
Level of Cognitive Ability: Applying
Client Needs: Physiological Integrity
Integrated Process: Nursing Process—Planning
Content Area: Adult Health—Musculoskeletal
Reference: Black, J., & Hawks, J. (2009). *Medical-surgical nursing: Clinical management for positive outcomes* (8th ed., p. 515). St. Louis: Saunders.

995. 3
Rationale: A psychosocial assessment of a client who is immobilized would most appropriately include the need for sensory stimulation. This assessment should also include such factors as body image, past and present coping skills, and coping methods used during the period of immobilization. Although transportation, home care support, and the ability to perform activities of daily living are components of an assessment, they are not as specifically related to psychosocial adjustment as is the need for sensory stimulation.
Test-Taking Strategy: Use the process of elimination and focus on the strategic words *psychosocial* and *most appropriately*. Option 2 can be eliminated first because it relates to physiological integrity rather than psychosocial integrity. Next, eliminate options 1 and 4 because they are most closely related to physical supports, rather than psychosocial needs of the client. Review the components of a psychosocial assessment if you had difficulty with this question.
Level of Cognitive Ability: Applying
Client Needs: Psychosocial Integrity
Integrated Process: Nursing Process—Assessment
Content Area: Adult Health—Musculoskeletal
Reference: Potter, P., & Perry, A. (2009) *Fundamentals of nursing* (7th ed., pp. 1348-1349). St. Louis: Mosby.

996. 3
Rationale: Complex scientific or medical terminology should be avoided when counseling an Amish client (or any client). When counseling a female Amish client, most often the husband and wife will want to discuss health care options together. Standing close and speaking loudly is inappropriate in most counseling situations.
Test-Taking Strategy: Use knowledge of the Amish society and therapeutic communication techniques to answer this question. Options 2 and 4 can be eliminated first because option 4 is inappropriate and option 2 is not a therapeutic intervention. Option 1 can be eliminated because of Amish cultural habits. Review Amish society and cultural beliefs if you had difficulty with this question.
Level of Cognitive Ability: Applying
Client Needs: Psychosocial Integrity
Integrated Process: Communication and Documentation
Content Area: Fundamental Skills—Cultural Diversity
Reference: Maurer, F., & Smith, C. (2009). *Community/public health nursing practices: Health for families and populations* (4th ed., pp. 278-281, 294). St. Louis: Saunders.

997. 1
Rationale: Assault occurs when a person puts another person in fear of harmful or offensive contact and the victim fears and believes that harm will result as a result of the threat. In this situation, the nurse could be accused of the tort of assault. Battery is the intentional touching of another's body without the person's consent. Slander is verbal communication that is false and harms the reputation of another. Invasion of privacy is committed when the nurse intrudes into the client's personal affairs or violates confidentiality.
Test-Taking Strategy: Use the process of elimination. Focusing on the words used by the nurse and noting that the nurse threatens the client will direct you to option 1. Review the descriptions in each option if you had difficulty with this question.
Level of Cognitive Ability: Understanding
Client Needs: Physiological Integrity
Integrated Process: Nursing Process—Implementation
Content Area: Leadership and Management—Ethical/Legal
Reference: Potter, P., & Perry, A. (2009) *Fundamentals of nursing* (7th ed., p. 331). St. Louis: Mosby.

998. 4
Rationale: When delegating nursing assignments, the nurse needs to consider the skills and educational level of the nursing staff. Collecting a 24-hour urine sample and frequent ambulation can most appropriately be provided by the nursing assistant, considering the clients identified in each option. The client on the mechanical ventilator requiring frequent assessment and suctioning should most appropriately be cared for by the registered nurse. The licensed practical (vocational) nurse is skilled in wound irrigation and dressing changes, so this client would be assigned to this staff member.
Test-Taking Strategy: Use the principles related to delegations and assignments, and consider the education and job position as described by the nurse practice act and employee guidelines. Note the strategic word *assessment* in option 3. This should alert you that this client should be assigned to the registered nurse. Options 1 and 2 can be eliminated because a nursing assistant can easily perform these tasks. This will assist in directing you to option 4. If you had difficulty with this question, review the principles related to a delegation and assignment making.
Level of Cognitive Ability: Applying
Client Needs: Safe and Effective Care Environment
Integrated Process: Nursing Process—Planning
Content Area: Leadership and Management—Delegating/Prioritizing
Reference: Cherry, B., & Jacob, S. (2008). *Contemporary nursing: Issues, trends, & management* (4th ed., pp. 406-407). St. Louis: Mosby.

999. 2
Rationale: The jaw thrust without the head tilt maneuver is used when head or neck trauma is suspected. This maneuver opens the airway while maintaining proper head and neck alignment, reducing the risk of further damage to the neck. Options 1, 3, and 4 are incorrect. Additionally, it is unlikely that the nurse would be able to obtain data about the client's history.

Test-Taking Strategy: Focus on the data in the question. Eliminate option 1 because of the close-ended word *all*. Noting that the client requires CPR will assist in eliminating options 3 and 4. Review CPR guidelines and the various test-taking strategies if you had difficulty with this question.
Level of Cognitive Ability: Applying
Client Needs: Physiological Integrity
Integrated Process: Nursing Process—Implementation
Content Area: Critical Care
References: Black, J., & Hawks, J. (2009). *Medical-surgical nursing: Clinical management for positive outcomes* (8th ed., p. 2197). St. Louis: Saunders.
  Perry, A., & Potter, P. (2010). *Clinical nursing skills & techniques* (7th ed., pp. 732-733). St. Louis: Mosby.

1000. 3
Rationale: The client needs to be instructed to avoid exposure to the sun. Options 1, 2, and 4 are accurate measures in the care of a client receiving external radiation therapy.
Test-Taking Strategy: Use the process of elimination. Note the strategic words *need for further instruction*. These words indicate a negative event query and ask you to select an option that is an incorrect statement. Eliminate option 1 because of the word *gently* and option 4 because of the word *loose*. From the remaining options, recalling that sun exposure is to be avoided will assist in answering the question. Review skin care measures for a client receiving external radiation if you had difficulty with this question.
Level of Cognitive Ability: Evaluating
Client Needs: Physiological Integrity
Integrated Process: Teaching and Learning
Content Area: Adult Health—Oncology
Reference: Ignatavicius, D., & Workman, M. (2010). *Medical-surgical nursing: Patient-centered collaborative care* (6th ed., p. 420). St. Louis: Saunders.

1001. 1.5
Rationale: It is necessary to convert 150 mcg to mg. In the metric system, to convert smaller to larger, divide by 1000 or move the decimal three places to the left: 150 mcg = 0.15 mg. Next, use the formula to calculate the correct dose.

Formula:

$$\frac{\text{Desired}}{\text{Available}} \times \text{Tablet} = \text{Tablets per dose}$$

$$\frac{0.15\,\text{mg}}{0.1\,\text{mg}} \times 1\,\text{tablet} = 1.5\,\text{tablets}$$

Test-Taking Strategy: In this medication calculation problem, it is necessary first to convert micrograms to milligrams. Next, follow the formula for the calculation of the correct dose. Label each figure, including the answer. Recheck your work, and make sure that the answer makes sense. If you had difficulty with this question, review medication calculation problems.
Level of Cognitive Ability: Applying
Client Needs: Physiological Integrity
Integrated Process: Nursing Process—Implementation
Content Area: Fundamental Skills—Medications/Blood & IV Therapy

Reference: Kee, J., & Marshall, S. (2009). *Clinical calculations: With applications to general and specialty areas* (6th ed., p. 86). St. Louis: Saunders.

1002. 2
Rationale: The most common side effect of metformin (Glucophage) is gastrointestinal disturbances, including decreased appetite, nausea, and diarrhea. These generally subside over time. This medication does not cause weight gain; clients lose an average of 7 to 8 lb because the medication causes nausea and decreased appetite. Although hypoglycemia can occur, it is not the most common side effect.
Test-Taking Strategy: Use the process of elimination, noting the strategic words *most common side effect*. Remember that the most common side effect of metformin is gastrointestinal disturbances. Review these side effects if you had difficulty with this question.
Level of Cognitive Ability: Applying
Client Needs: Physiological Integrity
Integrated Process: Nursing Process—Implementation
Content Area: Pharmacology
Reference: Hodgson, B., & Kizior, R. (2010). *Saunders nursing drug handbook 2010* (p. 726). St. Louis: Saunders.

1003. 3, 5, 6
Rationale: During a seizure, the child is placed on his or her side in a lateral position. Positioning on the side prevents aspiration because saliva drains out the corner of the child's mouth. The child is not restrained because this could cause injury to the child. The nurse would loosen clothing around the child's neck and ensure a patent airway. Nothing is placed in the child's mouth during a seizure because this could injure the child's mouth, gums, or teeth. The nurse would stay with the child to reduce the risk of injury and allow for observation and timing of the seizure.
Test-Taking Strategy: Visualize this clinical situation. Recalling that airway patency and safety is the priority will assist in determining the appropriate interventions. Review care of a child experiencing a seizure if you had difficulty with this question.
Level of Cognitive Ability: Applying
Client Needs: Physiological Integrity
Integrated Process: Nursing Process—Implementation
Content Area: Child Health—Neurological/Musculoskeletal
Reference: Hockenberry, M., & Wilson, D. (2009). *Wong's essentials of pediatric nursing* (8th ed., p. 1012). St. Louis: Mosby.

1004. 1
Rationale: After amputation, phantom limb pain is a temporary condition that some children may experience. This sensation of burning, aching, or cramping in the missing limb is most distressing to the child. The child needs to be reassured that the condition is normal and only temporary. Options 2, 3, and 4 are inappropriate responses to the child.
Test-Taking Strategy: Use therapeutic communication techniques. Note that the subject of the question relates to alleviating the child's fear. Option 1 is the only option that would alleviate fear. Options 2, 3, and 4 imply that this pain may be permanent. Review care of a child after amputation if you had difficulty with this question.
Level of Cognitive Ability: Applying
Client Needs: Psychosocial Integrity
Integrated Process: Caring

Content Area: Child Health—Hematological/Oncological
Reference: Hockenberry, M., & Wilson, D. (2009). *Wong's essentials of pediatric nursing* (8th ed., pp. 1121-1122). St. Louis: Mosby.

1005. 1

Rationale: Setting priorities means deciding which client needs or problems require immediate action and which can be delayed until a later time because they are not urgent. Client problems that involve actual or life-threatening concerns are always considered first. Although time constraints, obtaining needed supplies, and completing care in a reasonable time frame are components of time management, these items are not the priority in planning care for the client, based on the options provided.
Test-Taking Strategy: Use the process of elimination and principles related to prioritizing to answer the question. Noting the strategic words *life-threatening* in option 1 will assist in directing you to this option. Review the principles related to prioritizing if you had difficulty with this question.
Level of Cognitive Ability: Applying
Client Needs: Safe and Effective Care Environment
Integrated Process: Nursing Process—Planning
Content Area: Leadership and Management—Delegating/Prioritizing
Reference: Potter, P., & Perry, A. (2009) *Fundamentals of nursing* (7th ed., pp. 262-263). St. Louis: Mosby.

1006. 2

Rationale: Laboratory determinations of serum thyroid-stimulating hormone (TSH) level are an important means of evaluation. Successful therapy causes elevated TSH levels to decline. These levels begin their decline within hours of the onset of therapy and continue to decrease as plasma levels of thyroid hormone build up. If an adequate dosage is administered, TSH levels remain suppressed for the duration of therapy.
Test-Taking Strategy: Use the process of elimination. Note the strategic words *expected outcome*. Relate the diagnosis hypo*thyroid*ism with *thyroid* hormone levels in the correct option. If you had difficulty with this question, review the therapeutic effects of levothyroxine (Synthroid).
Level of Cognitive Ability: Applying
Client Needs: Physiological Integrity
Integrated Process: Teaching and Learning
Content Area: Pharmacology
Reference: Lehne, R. (2010). *Pharmacology for nursing care* (7th ed., pp. 693-694, 699). St. Louis: Saunders.

1007. 1, 2, 4, 6

Rationale: Risk factors for breast cancer include family history of breast cancer; age older than 40 years; early menarche; late menopause; previous cancer of the breast, uterus, or ovaries; nulliparity or first child born after age 30 years; and high-dose radiation exposure to chest.
Test-Taking Strategy: Focus on the subject, the risk factors associated with breast cancer. Thinking about the physiology associated with the reproductive system and the most common causes of cancer will assist in answering the question. Review these risk factors if you had difficulty with this question.
Level of Cognitive Ability: Analyzing
Client Needs: Health Promotion and Maintenance

Integrated Process: Nursing Process—Assessment
Content Area: Adult Health—Oncology
Reference: Ignatavicius, D., & Workman, M. (2010). *Medical-surgical nursing: Patient-centered collaborative care* (6th ed., p. 1665). St. Louis: Saunders.

1008. 3

Rationale: An inflammatory reaction such as acute pancreatitis can cause paralytic ileus, the most common form of non-mechanical obstruction. Inability to pass flatus is a clinical manifestation of paralytic ileus. Option 1 is the description of the physical finding of liver enlargement. The liver is usually enlarged in cases of cirrhosis or hepatitis. Although this client may have an enlarged liver, an enlarged liver is not a sign of paralytic ileus or intestinal obstruction. Pain is associated with paralytic ileus, but the pain usually manifests as a more constant generalized discomfort. Pain that is severe, constant, and rapid in onset is more likely caused by strangulation of the bowel. Loss of sphincter control is not a sign of paralytic ileus.
Test-Taking Strategy: Use the process of elimination. Noting the word *paralytic* will assist in directing you to option 3. Review the clinical manifestations of paralytic ileus if you had difficulty with this question.
Level of Cognitive Ability: Analyzing
Client Needs: Physiological Integrity
Integrated Process: Nursing Process—Assessment
Content Area: Adult Health—Gastrointestinal
Reference: Ignatavicius, D., & Workman, M. (2010). *Medical-surgical nursing: Patient-centered collaborative care* (6th ed., p. 1303). St. Louis: Saunders.

1009. 2

Rationale: For the first 12 hours after gastric surgery, the nasogastric tube drainage may be dark brown to dark red. Later, the drainage should change to a light yellowish brown color. The presence of bile may cause a green tinge. The physician should be notified if dark red drainage is noted 24 hours postoperatively.
Test-Taking Strategy: Focus on the subject, need to notify the physician. Use the process of elimination and recall that bleeding is a concern in the postoperative client. This concept will direct you to option 2. Review the signs of postoperative complications after gastric surgery if you had difficulty with this question.
Level of Cognitive Ability: Analyzing
Client Needs: Physiological Integrity
Integrated Process: Nursing Process—Analysis
Content Area: Adult Health—Gastrointestinal
Reference: Ignatavicius, D., & Workman, M. (2010). *Medical-surgical nursing: Patient-centered collaborative care* (6th ed., p. 291). St. Louis: Saunders.

1010. 3

Rationale: The client should take a deep breath because the client's airway will be temporarily obstructed during tube removal. The client is then told to exhale slowly and the tube is withdrawn during exhalation. Bearing down could inhibit the removal of the tube. Breathing normally could result in aspiration of gastric secretions during inhalation. Holding the breath does not facilitate tube removal.

Test-Taking Strategy: Use the process of elimination and attempt to visualize the process of tube removal to direct you to option 3. Remember, exhaling slowly facilitates the process of removal. Review the procedure for removal of a nasogastric tube if you had difficulty with this question.
Level of Cognitive Ability: Applying
Client Needs: Physiological Integrity
Integrated Process: Nursing Process—Implementation
Content Area: Adult Health—Gastrointestinal
Reference: Potter, P., & Perry, A. (2009). *Fundamentals of nursing* (7th ed., p. 1209). St. Louis: Mosby.

1011. 3
Rationale: When a client is experiencing respiratory acidosis, the respiratory rate and depth increase in an attempt to compensate. The client also experiences headache; restlessness; mental status changes, such as drowsiness and confusion; visual disturbances; diaphoresis; cyanosis as the hypoxia becomes more acute; hyperkalemia; rapid, irregular pulse; and dysrhythmias.
Test-Taking Strategy: Use the process of elimination and knowledge of the signs and symptoms of respiratory acidosis to answer this question. Remember that restlessness and confusion occur in respiratory acidosis. If this question was difficult, review the clinical manifestations associated with respiratory acidosis.
Level of Cognitive Ability: Analyzing
Client Needs: Physiological Integrity
Integrated Process: Nursing Process—Assessment
Content Area: Fundamental Skills—Fluids & Electrolytes/Acid-Base
Reference: Ignatavicius, D., & Workman, M. (2010). *Medical-surgical nursing: Patient-centered collaborative care* (6th ed., p. 206). St. Louis: Saunders.

1012. 3
Rationale: Distention, vomiting, and abdominal pain are a few of the symptoms associated with intestinal obstruction. Nasogastric tubes may be used to remove gas and fluid from the stomach, relieving distention and vomiting. Bowel sounds return to normal as the obstruction is resolved and normal bowel function is restored. Discontinuing the nasogastric tube before normal bowel function may result in a return of the symptoms, necessitating reinsertion of the nasogastric tube. Serum electrolyte levels, tube placement, and pH of the gastric aspirate are important assessments for the client with a nasogastric tube in place, but would not assist in determining the readiness for removing the nasogastric tube.
Test-Taking Strategy: Use the process of elimination. Eliminate options 1 and 4 first because they are comparable or alike. Assessing the pH of the gastric aspirate is one method of assessing tube placement. From the remaining options, focus on the subject and the client's diagnosis to direct you to option 3. Review abdominal assessment in a client with an intestinal obstruction if you had difficulty with this question.
Level of Cognitive Ability: Analyzing
Client Needs: Physiological Integrity
Integrated Process: Nursing Process—Assessment
Content Area: Adult Health—Gastrointestinal

Reference: Potter, P., & Perry, A. (2009). *Fundamentals of nursing* (7th ed., p. 1208). St. Louis: Mosby.

1013. 2
Rationale: The enema fluid should be administered slowly. If the client complains of fullness or pain, the flow is stopped for 30 seconds and restarted at a slower rate. Slow enema administration and stopping the flow temporarily, if necessary, decrease the likelihood of intestinal spasm and premature ejection of the solution. The higher the solution container is held above the rectum, the faster the flow and the greater the force in the rectum. There is no need to discontinue the enema and notify the physician at this time. Although client reassurance is important, continuing the flow is inappropriate.
Test-Taking Strategy: Use the process of elimination. Eliminate options 1 and 3 first because they are comparable or alike. From the remaining options, focusing on the subject will direct you to option 2. Review the procedure for administering an enema if you had difficulty with this question.
Level of Cognitive Ability: Applying
Client Needs: Physiological Integrity
Integrated Process: Nursing Process—Implementation
Content Area: Fundamental Skills—Perioperative Care
Reference: Perry, A., & Potter, P. (2010). *Clinical nursing skills & techniques* (7th ed., pp. 912-913). St. Louis: Mosby.

1014. 4
Rationale: Option 4 describes aversion therapy. Options 1, 2, and 3 are characteristics of self-control therapy.
Test-Taking Strategy: Use the process of elimination. Note the strategic words *need for further teaching* in the question. These words indicate a negative event query and ask you to select an option that is incorrect. Think about the subject, self-control. This subject will direct you to option 4. If you are unfamiliar with self-control therapy, review this content.
Level of Cognitive Ability: Evaluating
Client Needs: Psychosocial Integrity
Integrated Process: Teaching and Learning
Content Area: Mental Health
Reference: Varcarolis, E., & Halter, M. (2009). *Essentials of psychiatric mental health nursing: A communication approach to evidence-based care* (p. 30). St. Louis: Saunders.

1015. 1, 3, 5, 6
Rationale: The nurse would teach the client how to care for the stoma, depending on the type of laryngectomy performed. Most interventions focus on protection of the stoma and the prevention of infection. Interventions include to avoid swimming, use care when showering, avoid exposure to people with infections, prevent debris from entering the stoma, and obtain a Medic-Alert bracelet. Additional interventions include wearing a stoma guard or high-collared clothing to cover the stoma, increasing the humidity in the home, and increasing fluid intake to 3000 mL/day to keep the secretions thin.
Test-Taking Strategy: Recalling that most interventions focus on protection of the stoma and the prevention of infection will assist in identifying the client instructions for home care. Review stoma and laryngeal care instructions if you had difficulty with this question.

Level of Cognitive Ability: Applying
Client Needs: Physiological Integrity
Integrated Process: Teaching and Learning
Content Area: Adult Health—Oncology
Reference: Ignatavicius, D., & Workman, M. (2010). *Medical-surgical nursing: Patient-centered collaborative care* (6th ed., pp. 605-606). St. Louis: Saunders.

1016. 21
Rationale: Use the intravenous flow rate formula.
Formula:

$$\frac{\text{Total volume} \times \text{Drop factor}}{\text{Time in minutes}} \times = \text{Drops per minute}$$

$$\frac{2000\,\text{mL} \times 15\,\text{gtt}}{1440\,\text{minutes}} = \frac{30,000}{1440} = 20.8, \text{or } 21\,\text{gtt/min}$$

Test-Taking Strategy: Use the formula for calculating intravenous flow rates when answering the question. Verify the answer using a calculator. Review intravenous infusion rates if you had difficulty with this question.
Level of Cognitive Ability: Applying
Client Needs: Physiological Integrity
Integrated Process: Nursing Process—Implementation
Content Area: Fundamental Skills—Medications/Blood & IV Therapy
Reference: Kee, J., & Marshall, S. (2009). *Clinical calculations: With applications to general and specialty areas* (6th ed., p. 223). St. Louis: Saunders.

1017. 3
Rationale: In the first few hours after surgery, the drainage from the chest tube is bloody. After several hours, it becomes serosanguineous. The client should not experience frequent clotting. Proper chest tube function should allow for drainage of blood before it has the chance to clot in the chest or the tubing.
Test-Taking Strategy: Recall that after thoracic surgery, there may be considerable capillary oozing for hours in the postoperative period. This will lead you to choose the bloody drainage over serous or serosanguineous. Knowing that patent chest tubes do not allow blood to collect in the pleural space eliminates the option of blood with clots. If you had difficulty with this question, review the assessment measures required for the care of a client with a chest tube.
Level of Cognitive Ability: Analyzing
Client Needs: Physiological Integrity
Integrated Process: Nursing Process—Assessment
Content Area: Adult Health—Respiratory
References: Black, J., & Hawks, J. (2009). *Medical-surgical nursing: Clinical management for positive outcomes* (8th ed., p. 1617). St. Louis: Saunders.

Ignatavicius, D., & Workman, M. (2010). *Medical-surgical nursing: Patient-centered collaborative care* (6th ed., pp. 646, 648). St. Louis: Saunders.

1018. 2, 3, 4, 5
Rationale: If the client begins to hemorrhage from the surgical site after radical neck dissection, the nurse elevates the head of the bed to maintain airway patency and prevent aspiration. The nurse applies pressure over the bleeding site and calls the physician immediately. The nurse monitors the client's airway and vital signs.

Test-Taking Strategy: Focus on the client situation. Options 2 and 3 are indicated if the client is hemorrhaging. Calling the physician is also indicated immediately, but lowering the head of bed does not help with airway maintenance. If you had difficulty with this question, review nursing actions if a client begins to hemorrhage.
Level of Cognitive Ability: Applying
Client Needs: Physiological Integrity
Integrated Process: Nursing Process—Implementation
Content Area: Adult Health—Respiratory
Reference: Black, J., & Hawks, J. (2009). *Medical-surgical nursing: Clinical management for positive outcomes* (8th ed., p. 1561). St. Louis: Saunders.

1019. 2
Rationale: To prevent transmission of hepatitis, a condom is advised during sexual intercourse and vaccination of the partner. Alcohol should be avoided because it is detoxified in the liver and may interfere with recovery. Rest is especially important until laboratory studies show that liver function has returned to normal. The client's activity is increased gradually.
Test-Taking Strategy: Use the process of elimination, focusing on the strategic words *need for further teaching*. These words indicate a negative event query and ask you to select an option that is incorrect. Noting the strategic word *never* in option 2 will direct you to this option. Review client instructions regarding hepatitis if you had difficulty with this question.
Level of Cognitive Ability: Evaluating
Client Needs: Physiological Integrity
Integrated Process: Teaching and Learning
Content Area: Adult Health—Gastrointestinal
Reference: Ignatavicius, D., & Workman, M. (2010). *Medical-surgical nursing: Patient-centered collaborative care* (6th ed., p. 1358). St. Louis: Saunders.

1020. 1, 2, 5
Rationale: The clinical manifestations of hypothyroidism are the result of decreased metabolism from low levels of thyroid hormone. Interventions are aimed at replacement of the hormones and providing measures to support the signs and symptoms related to a decreased metabolism. The nurse encourages the client to consume a well-balanced diet that is low in fat for weight reduction and high in fluids and high-fiber foods to prevent constipation. The client often has cold intolerance and requires a warm environment. The client would notify the physician if chest pain occurs because it could be an indication of overreplacement of thyroid hormone. Iodine preparations may be used to treat hyperthyroidism. These medications decrease blood flow through the thyroid gland and reduce the production and release of thyroid hormone.
Test-Taking Strategy: Focus on the client's diagnosis, hypothyroidism. Recalling that in this disorder the client has a decreased metabolic rate will assist in determining the appropriate interventions. Review interventions for the client with hypothyroidism and hyperthyroidism if you had difficulty with this question.
Level of Cognitive Ability: Applying
Client Needs: Physiological Integrity
Integrated Process: Nursing Process—Implementation
Content Area: Adult Health—Endocrine

References: Black, J., & Hawks, J. (2009). *Medical-surgical nursing: Clinical management for positive outcomes* (8th ed., p. 1023). St. Louis: Saunders.

Ignatavicius, D., & Workman, M. (2010). *Medical-surgical nursing: Patient-centered collaborative care* (6th ed., p. 1458). St. Louis: Saunders.

1021. 2
Rationale: Plugging a tracheostomy tube is usually done by inserting the tracheostomy plug (decannulation stopper) into the opening of the outer cannula. This closes off the tracheostomy, and airflow and respiration occur normally through the nose and mouth. When plugging a cuffed tracheostomy tube, the cuff must be deflated. If it remains inflated, ventilation cannot occur, and respiratory arrest could result. The ability to swallow or speak is unrelated to weaning and plugging the tube.
Test-Taking Strategy: Note the strategic word *required* in the question. This should assist in directing you to the option that addresses a priority physiological need. Use the process of elimination to direct you to option 2 because an inflated cuff would cause airway obstruction. Review this procedure if you had difficulty with this question.
Level of Cognitive Ability: Applying
Client Needs: Physiological Integrity
Integrated Process: Nursing Process—Implementation
Content Area: Adult Health—Respiratory
Reference: Black, J., & Hawks, J. (2009). *Medical-surgical nursing: Clinical management for positive outcomes* (8th ed., pp. 1546-1547). St. Louis: Saunders.

1022. 3
Rationale: Hypertension, cardiovascular disease, diabetes mellitus, and obesity are associated with the development of glaucoma. Options 1, 2, and 4 do not identify risk factors associated with this eye disorder.
Test-Taking Strategy: Use the process of elimination. Focusing on the subject, a risk factor associated with glaucoma, will direct you to option 3. If you had difficulty with this question, review the risk factors associated with this disorder.
Level of Cognitive Ability: Analyzing
Client Needs: Physiological Integrity
Integrated Process: Nursing Process—Assessment
Content Area: Adult Health—Eye
Reference: Black, J., & Hawks, J. (2009). *Medical-surgical nursing: Clinical management for positive outcomes* (8th ed., p. 1700). St. Louis: Saunders.

1023. 3
Rationale: The nurse places an eye patch over the client's affected eye to reduce eye movement. Some clients may need bilateral patching. Depending on the location and size of the retinal break, activity restrictions may be needed immediately. These restrictions are necessary to prevent further tearing or detachment and to promote drainage of any subretinal fluid. The nurse positions the client as prescribed by the physician.
Test-Taking Strategy: Use the process of elimination. Remember that the eye needs to be protected and rested. This should direct you to option 3. If you had difficulty with this question, review care of a client with retinal detachment.
Level of Cognitive Ability: Analyzing

Client Needs: Physiological Integrity
Integrated Process: Nursing Process—Planning
Content Area: Adult Health—Eye
Reference: Ignatavicius, D., & Workman, M. (2010). *Medical-surgical nursing: Patient-centered collaborative care* (6th ed., p. 1101). St. Louis: Saunders.

1024. 2
Rationale: Clients at greatest risk for pulmonary emboli are immobilized clients. Basic preventive measures include early ambulation, leg elevation, active leg exercises, elastic stockings, and intermittent pneumatic calf compression. Keeping the client well hydrated is essential because dehydration predisposes to clotting. A pillow under the knees may cause venous stasis. Heat should not be applied without a physician's prescription.
Test-Taking Strategy: Use the process of elimination and basic principles related to the care of the immobile client to answer this question. If you are unfamiliar with these basic measures, review this content.
Level of Cognitive Ability: Applying
Client Needs: Physiological Integrity
Integrated Process: Nursing Process—Planning
Content Area: Adult Health—Respiratory
Reference: Ignatavicius, D., & Workman, M. (2010). *Medical-surgical nursing: Patient-centered collaborative care* (6th ed., p. 678). St. Louis: Saunders.

1025. 4
Rationale: A crisis is an acute, time-limited state of disequilibrium resulting from situational, developmental, or societal sources of stress. A person in this state is temporarily unable to cope with or adapt to the stressor by using previous coping mechanisms. The person who intervenes in this situation (the nurse) "takes over" for the client who is not in control and devises a plan (action) to secure and maintain the client's safety. When this has occurred, the nurse works collaboratively with the client (participates) in developing new coping and problem-solving strategies.
Test-Taking Strategy: Use the process of elimination. A client who experiences a suicidal crisis is in a state of acute disequilibrium. Remember that in a crisis an authority figure must emerge to take action. Review care of the client in crisis if you had difficulty with this question.
Level of Cognitive Ability: Applying
Client Needs: Psychosocial Integrity
Integrated Process: Nursing Process—Implementation
Content Area: Mental Health
Reference: Varcarolis, E., & Halter, M. (2009). *Essentials of psychiatric mental health nursing: A communication approach to evidence-based care* (p. 371). St. Louis: Saunders.

1026. 1
Rationale: The client must have sputum cultures performed every 2 to 4 weeks after initiation of antituberculosis drug therapy. The client may return to work when the results of three sputum cultures are negative because the client is considered noninfectious at that point.
Test-Taking Strategy: Use the process of elimination. Knowing that a positive Mantoux test never reverts to negative helps you eliminate option 4. From the remaining options, it is necessary to know that three negative sputum cultures are

required. If this question was difficult, review these concepts related to tuberculosis.
Level of Cognitive Ability: Applying
Client Needs: Safe and Effective Care Environment
Integrated Process: Teaching and Learning
Content Area: Adult Health—Respiratory
Reference: Ignatavicius, D., & Workman, M. (2010). *Medical-surgical nursing: Patient-centered collaborative care* (6th ed., p. 670). St. Louis: Saunders.

1027. 3
Rationale: This client is in a severe state of anxiety. When a client is in a severe or panic state of anxiety, it is crucial for the nurse to remain with the client. Processing the anxiety at this point would increase the client's level of anxiety further. The client in a severe state of anxiety would be unable to learn relaxation techniques.
Test-Taking Strategy: Use the process of elimination and note the strategic words *appropriate initial*. The best action in this situation is to remain with the client. If you are unfamiliar with the symptoms of the different levels of anxiety and the interventions that are indicated, review this information.
Level of Cognitive Ability: Applying
Client Needs: Safe and Effective Care Environment
Integrated Process: Nursing Process—Implementation
Content Area: Mental Health
Reference: Varcarolis, E., & Halter, M. (2009). *Essentials of psychiatric mental health nursing: A communication approach to evidence-based care* (p. 132). St. Louis: Saunders.

1028. 3
Rationale: Laboratory findings do not establish the diagnosis of appendicitis, but there is often an elevation of the white blood cell count (leukocytosis) with a shift to the left (an increased number of immature white blood cells).
Test-Taking Strategy: Use the process of elimination. Knowledge that an inflammatory process causes an increase in the white blood cell count will assist in eliminating options 1 and 4. From the remaining options, it is necessary to understand the significance of a shift to the left. If you are unfamiliar with the meaning of shift to the left, review this content.
Level of Cognitive Ability: Analyzing
Client Needs: Physiological Integrity
Integrated Process: Nursing Process—Assessment
Content Area: Adult Health—Gastrointestinal
Reference: Ignatavicius, D., & Workman, M. (2010). *Medical-surgical nursing: Patient-centered collaborative care* (6th ed., p. 1316). St. Louis: Saunders.

1029. 4
Rationale: Ineffective coping may be evidenced by inability to meet basic needs, inability to meet role expectations, alteration in social participation, use of inappropriate defense mechanisms, or impairment of usual patterns of communication. Disturbed thought processes are evidenced by altered attention span; distractibility; and disorientation to time, place, person, and events. A dysfunctional family process may exist when the family has difficulty adapting or responding to the changes or traumatic experience of the member in crisis.
Test-Taking Strategy: Use the data presented in the question to direct you to the correct option. Option 3 can be

eliminated because the client is presently experiencing anxiety. Eliminate option 1 because there are no data in the question that address the family. Similarly, there are no data to suggest disturbed thought processes, so this option can be eliminated, leaving option 4 as the correct option. Review nursing diagnoses for a client experiencing anxiety if you had difficulty with this question.
Level of Cognitive Ability: Analyzing
Client Needs: Psychosocial Integrity
Integrated Process: Nursing Process—Analysis
Content Area: Mental Health
Reference: Stuart, G. (2009). *Principles and practice of psychiatric nursing* (9th ed., pp. 228-229, 231). St. Louis: Mosby.

1030. 2
Rationale: Bubbling in the water seal chamber is caused by air passing out of the pleural space into the fluid in the chamber. Intermittent bubbling is normal. It indicates that the system is accomplishing one of its purposes, removing air from the pleural space. Continuous bubbling during inspiration and expiration indicates that an air leak exists. If this occurs, it must be corrected.
Test-Taking Strategy: Focus on the strategic words *intermittent bubbling* and *water seal chamber*. Recalling that intermittent bubbling is normal will direct you to option 2. If you are unfamiliar with chest tube drainage systems, review this content.
Level of Cognitive Ability: Applying
Client Needs: Physiological Integrity
Integrated Process: Nursing Process—Implementation
Content Area: Adult Health—Respiratory
Reference: Black, J., & Hawks, J. (2009). *Medical-surgical nursing: Clinical management for positive outcomes* (8th ed., p. 1622). St. Louis: Saunders.

1031. 3
Rationale: The initial nursing assessment of a client in a crisis state is to evaluate the physical condition of the client, the potential for self-harm, and the potential for harm to others. After this has been determined and appropriate interventions have been initiated, the nurse proceeds with the mental health interview.
Test-Taking Strategy: Use Maslow's Hierarchy of Needs theory to answer the question. Physiological needs take priority over other needs. Option 3 is the only option that addresses a physiological need. Review care of a client in crisis if you had difficulty with this question.
Level of Cognitive Ability: Analyzing
Client Needs: Physiological Integrity
Integrated Process: Nursing Process—Assessment
Content Area: Mental Health
Reference: Varcarolis, E., & Halter, M. (2009). *Essentials of psychiatric mental health nursing: A communication approach to evidence-based care* (p. 371). St. Louis: Saunders.

1032. 3
Rationale: Although frequency and intensity of bowel sounds vary depending on the phase of digestion, normal bowel sounds are relatively high-pitched clicks or gurgles. Loud gurgles (borborygmi) indicate hyperperistalsis. Bowel sounds are more high-pitched and louder (hyperresonance) when the intestines are under tension, such as in intestinal obstruction.

A swishing or buzzing sound represents turbulent blood flow associated with a bruit. Bruits are not normal sounds.

Test-Taking Strategy: Use the process of elimination. Normally, bowel sounds are audible in all four quadrants, so options 2 and 4 can be eliminated. From the remaining options, use knowledge regarding normal findings to direct you to option 3. Review abdominal assessment if you had difficulty with this question.

Level of Cognitive Ability: Understanding
Client Needs: Physiological Integrity
Integrated Process: Nursing Process—Assessment
Content Area: Adult Health—Gastrointestinal
Reference: Jarvis, C. (2008) *Physical examination and health assessment* (5th ed, p. 570). St. Louis: Saunders.

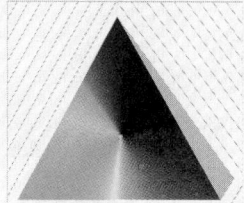

Reference List

Ackley, B., Ladwig, G., Swan, B., & Tucker, S. (2008). *Evidence-based nursing care guidelines: Medical-surgical interventions.* St. Louis: Mosby.

Alexander, M., Corrigan, A., Gorski, L., Hankins, J., & Perucca, R. (2010). *Infusion nursing: An evidence-based approach* (3rd ed.). St. Louis: Saunders.

American Heart Association. (Winter 2005–2006). Highlights of the 2005 American Heart Association guidelines for cardiopulmonary resuscitation and emergency cardiovascular care. *Currents in Emergency Cardiac Care, 16*(4), 7–11.

American Heart Association. (1992). Guidelines for cardiopulmonary resuscitation and emergency cardiac care: An international consensus on science and circulation. *Circulation, 102*(Suppl.), 217–222.

American Heart Association. Emergency Cardiac Care Committee and Subcommittees. (1992). Guidelines for cardiopulmonary resuscitation and emergency cardiac care. Part VIII: Ethical consideration in resuscitation. *Journal of the American Medical Association, 268* (16), 2282–2288.

American Heart Association. Web site at www.americanheart.org.

American Hospital Association. (1992). *A patient's bill of rights.* Available at: http://www.patienttalk.info/AHA-Patient_Bill_of_ Rights. htm. Retrieved February, 2, 2010.

American Nurses Association. (2001). *Code of ethics for nurses with interpretive statements.* Washington, DC: American Nurses Publishing. Available at: http://nursingworld.org/MainMenuCategories/ ThePracticeofProfessionalNursing/EthicsStandards/CodeofEthics. aspx. Retrieved February 2, 2010.

Association of Women's Health Obstetrics, Mattson, S., & Smith, J. (2004). *Core curriculum for maternal-newborn nursing* (3rd ed.). St. Louis: Saunders.

Behrman, R., Kliegman, R., & Jenson, H. (2004). *Nelson textbook of pediatrics* (17th ed.). St. Louis: Saunders.

Betz, C., & Sowden, L. (2004). *Pediatric nursing reference* (5th ed.). St. Louis: Mosby.

Black, J., & Hawks, J. (2005). *Medical-surgical nursing: Clinical management for positive outcomes* (7th ed.). St. Louis: Saunders.

Black, J., & Hawks, J. (2009). *Medical-surgical nursing: Clinical management for positive outcomes* (8th ed.). St. Louis: Saunders.

Bryant, R., & Nix, D. (2007). *Acute & chronic wounds: Current management concepts* (3rd ed.). St. Louis: Mosby.

Callen, N., & Schutze, G. (n.d.). *Immunizations for children with HIV/ AIDS.* Available at: http://www.bayloraids.org/curriculum/files/ 20.pdf. Retrieved January 15, 2010.

Centers for Disease Control and Prevention (CDC). (2010). *Contraindications to vaccines chart.* Available at: http://www.cdc.gov/vaccines/recs/ vac-admin/contraindications-vacc.htm. Retrieved January 10, 2010.

Centers for Disease Control and Prevention (CDC). (2010). *Recommended immunization schedules for persons aged 0 through 18 years— United States, 2010.* Available at: http://www.immunize.org/CDC/ schedules/. Retrieved January 12, 2010.

Chernecky, C., & Berger, B. (2004). *Laboratory tests and diagnostic procedures* (4th ed.). St. Louis: Saunders.

Chernecky, C., & Berger, B. (2008). *Laboratory tests and diagnostic procedures* (5th ed.). St. Louis: Saunders.

Cherry, B., & Jacob, S. (2008). *Contemporary nursing: Issues, trends & management* (4th ed.). St. Louis: Mosby.

Christensen, B., & Kockrow, E. (2006). *Foundations of nursing* (5th ed.). St. Louis: Mosby.

Clark, J., Queener, S., & Karb, V. (2000). *Pharmacologic basis of nursing practice* (6th ed.). St. Louis: Mosby.

Commission on Graduates of Foreign Nursing Schools (CGFNS). Available at: http://www.cgfns.org. Retrieved July 12, 2010.

Copstead-Kirkhorn, L., & Banasik, J. (2010). *Pathophysiology* (4th ed.). St. Louis: Mosby.

D'Avanzo, C. (2008). *Pocket guide to cultural health assessment* (4th ed.). St. Louis: Mosby.

Ebersole, P., Hess, P., & Luggen, A. (2004). *Toward healthy aging* (6th ed.). St. Louis: Mosby.

Ebersole, P., Hess, P., Touhy, T., Jett, K., & Luggen, A. (2008). *Toward healthy aging* (7th ed.). St. Louis: Mosby.

Edmunds, M. (2010). *Introduction to clinical pharmacology* (6th ed.). St. Louis: Mosby.

Elkin, M., Perry, A., & Potter, P. (2007). *Nursing interventions and clinical skills* (4th ed.). St. Louis: Mosby.

Exubera (insulin human [rDNA origin]). (2008). Available at: http:// www.drugs.com/pro/exubera.html. Retrieved August 12, 2010.

Fortinash, K., & Holoday-Worret, P. (2008). *Psychiatric mental health nursing* (4th ed.). St. Louis: Mosby.

Gahart, B., & Nazareno, A. (2009). *2009 Intravenous medications* (25th ed.). St. Louis: Mosby.

Gahart, B., & Nazareno, A. (2010). *2010 Intravenous medications* (26th ed.). St. Louis: Mosby.

Geissler, C., & Powers, H. (2009). *Fundamentals of human nutrition for students and practitioners in health sciences.* St. Louis: Churchill Livingstone.

Giger, J., & Davidhizar, R. (2008). *Transcultural nursing assessment & intervention* (5th ed.). St. Louis: Mosby.

Harkreader, H., Hogan, M. A., & Thobaben, M. (2007). *Fundamentals of nursing: Caring and clinical judgment* (3rd ed.). St. Louis: Saunders.

Hockenberry, M. (2004). *Wong's clinical manual of pediatric nursing* (6th ed.). St. Louis: Mosby.

Hockenberry, M., & Wilson, D. (2007). *Wong's nursing care of infants and children* (8th ed). St. Louis: Mosby.

Hockenberry, M., & Wilson, D. (2009). *Wong's essentials of pediatric nursing* (8th ed.). St. Louis: Mosby.

Hockenberry, M., Wilson, D., & Winkelstein, M. (2005). *Wong's essentials of pediatric nursing* (7th ed.). St. Louis: Mosby.

Hockenberry, M., Wilson, D., Winkelstein, M., & Kline, N. (2003). *Wong's nursing care of infants and children* (7th ed.). St. Louis: Mosby.

Hodgson, B., & Kizior, R. (2009). *Saunders nursing drug handbook 2009.* St. Louis: Saunders.

Hodgson, B., & Kizior, R. (2010). *Saunders nursing drug handbook 2010*. St. Louis: Saunders.

Huber, D. (2010). *Leadership and nursing care management* (4th ed.). St. Louis: Saunders.

Ignatavicius, D., & Workman, M. (2010). *Medical-surgical nursing: Patient-centered collaborative care* (6th ed.). St. Louis: Saunders.

Jarvis, C. (2008). *Physical examination and health assessment* (5th ed.). St. Louis: Saunders.

Jarvis, C. (2008). Physical Examination and Health Assessment DVD series, DVD 8: *Abdomen*, Version 2. St. Louis: Saunders.

Johnstone, M. (2009). *Bioethics: A nursing perspective* (5th ed.). St. Louis: Churchill Livingstone.

Kee, J., Hayes, E., & McCuiston, L. (2009). *Pharmoclogy: A nursing process approach* (6th ed.). St. Louis: Saunders.

Kee, J., & Marshall, S. (2009). *Clinical calculations: With applications to general and specialty areas* (6th ed.). St. Louis: Saunders.

Kuebler, K., Heidrich, D., & Esper, P. (2007). *Palliative end-of-life care: Clinical practice guidelines* (2nd ed.). St. Louis: Saunders.

Lehne, R. (2010). *Pharmacology for nursing care* (7th ed.). St. Louis: Saunders.

Lewis, S., Heitkemper, M., Dirksen, S., O'Brien, P., & Bucher, L. (2007). *Medical-surgical nursing: Assessment and management of clinical problems* (7th ed.). St. Louis: Mosby.

Lowdermilk, D., & Perry, S. (2006). *Maternity nursing* (7th ed.). St. Louis: Mosby.

Lowdermilk, D., & Perry, S. (2007). *Maternity & women's health care* (9th ed.). St. Louis: Mosby.

Lowdermilk, D., Perry, S., & Cashion, M. C. (2010). *Maternity nursing* (8th ed.). St. Louis: Mosby.

Marriner-Tomey, A. (2009). *Guide to nursing management and leadership* (8th ed.). St. Louis: Mosby.

Maurer, F., & Smith, C. (2009). *Community/public health nursing practices: Health for families and populations* (4th ed.). St. Louis: Saunders.

McEwen, M., & Pullis, B. (2009). *Community-based nursing: An introduction* (3rd ed.). St. Louis: Saunders.

McKinney, E., James, S., Murray, S., & Ashwill, J. (2009). *Maternal-child nursing* (3rd ed.). St. Louis: Saunders.

Meiner, S., & Lueckenotte, A. (2006). *Gerontologic nursing* (3rd ed.). St. Louis: Mosby.

Monahan, F., Sands, J., Neighbors, M., Marek, J., & Green, C. (2007). *Phipps' medical-surgical nursing: Health and illness perspectives* (8th ed.). St. Louis: Mosby.

Morse, S., Ballard, R., Holmes, K., & Moreland, A. (2003). *Atlas of sexually transmitted diseases and AIDS* (3rd ed.). London: Mosby.

Mosby's dictionary of medicine, nursing & health professions (8th ed.). (2009). St. Louis: Mosby.

Mosby's nursing video skills. (2008). *Basic skills: Nutrition & fluids: Taking aspiration precautions*. St. Louis: Mosby.

Mosby's nursing video skills. (2008). *Basic skills: Restraints and alternatives: Applying restraints*. St. Louis: Mosby.

Mosby's nursing video skills. (2008). *Basic skills: Vital signs: Assessing pain*. St. Louis: Mosby.

Mosby's nursing video skills. (2008). *Intermediate skills: Pressure ulcers and wound care: Irrigating wounds*. St. Louis: Mosby.

Mulholland, J. M. (2007). *The nurse, the math, the meds: Drug calculations using dimensional analysis*. St. Louis: Mosby.

Murray, S., & McKinney, E. (2006). *Foundations of maternal-newborn nursing* (4th ed.). St. Louis: Saunders.

National Council of State Boards of Nursing (Eds.). (2010). *2010 NCLEX-RN® detailed test plan*. Chicago: Author.

National Council of State Boards of Nursing. Web site: http://www.ncsbn.org.

Newell, R., & Gournay, K. (2009). *Mental health nursing: An evidence-based approach* (2nd ed.). St. Louis: Churchill Livingstone.

Nix, S. (2009). *Williams' basic nutrition and diet therapy* (13th ed.). St. Louis: Mosby.

Office of U.S. Citizenship and Immigration Services (USCIS) Web site: uscis.gov/graphics/howdoi/Health_Cert.htm.

Pagana, K., & Pagana, T. (2009). *Mosby's diagnostic and laboratory test reference* (9th ed.). St. Louis: Mosby.

Pearson Professional Center Web site: http://www.pearsonvue.com/nclex.

Peckenpaugh, N. (2010). *Nutrition essentials and diet therapy* (11th ed.). St. Louis: Saunders.

Perry, A., & Potter, P. (2010). *Clinical nursing skills & techniques* (7th ed.). St. Louis: Mosby.

Perry, S., Hockenberry, M., Lowdermilk, D., & Wilson, D. (2010). *Maternal child nursing care* (4th ed.). St. Louis: Mosby.

Potter, P., & Perry, A. (2009). *Fundamentals of nursing* (7th ed.). St. Louis: Mosby.

Proehl, J. (2009). *Emergency nursing procedures* (4th ed.). St. Louis: Saunders.

Skidmore-Roth, L. (2009). *Mosby's drug guide for nurses* (8th ed.). St. Louis: Mosby.

Skidmore-Roth, L. (2010). *Mosby's nursing drug reference* (23rd ed.). St. Louis: Mosby.

Stanhope, M., & Lancaster, J. (2008). *Public health nursing: Population-centered health care in the community* (7th ed.). St. Louis: Mosby.

Stuart, G. (2009). *Principles and practice of psychiatric nursing* (9th ed.). St. Louis: Mosby.

Swartz, M. (2006). *Textbook of physical diagnosis: History and examination* (5th ed.). St. Louis: Saunders.

Swearingen, P. (2008). *All-in-one care planning resource: Medical-surgical, pediatric, maternity, & psychiatric nursing care plans* (2nd ed.). St. Louis: Mosby.

The Diabetes Monitor. (2007). *Exenatide (Byetta)*. Available at: http://www.diabetesmonitor.com/byetta.htm. Retrieved February 2, 2010.

Thibodeau, G. A., & Patton, K. T. (2010). *The human body in health and disease* (5th ed.). St. Louis: Mosby.

Touhy, T., & Jett, K. (2010). *Ebersole and Hess' gerontological nursing & healthy aging* (3rd ed.). St. Louis: Mosby.

Tucker, S. (2004). *Pocket guide to fetal monitoring assessment* (5th ed.). St. Louis: Mosby.

U.S. Department of Agriculture. (2010). *MyPyramid*. Available at: http://www.mypyramid.gov. Retrieved February 2, 2010.

U.S. Department of Health and Human Services. (n.d.). *Health information privacy*. Available at: http://www.hhs.gov/ocr/privacy/hipaa/understanding/consumers/index.html. Retrieved July 12, 2010.

Varcarolis, E. (2006). *Foundations of psychiatric mental health nursing* (5th ed.). St. Louis: Saunders.

Varcarolis, E., & Halter, M. (2009). *Essentials of psychiatric mental health nursing: A communication approach to evidence-based care*. St. Louis: Saunders.

Wikipedia. (n.d.). *Amish*. Available at: http://en.wiktionary.org/wiki/Amish. Retrieved February 2, 2010.

Wikipedia. (n.d.). *Hispanic and Latino Americans*. Available at: http://en.wikipedia.org/wiki/Hispanic-American. Retrieved February 2, 2010.

Wikipedia. (n.d.). *Indigenous peoples of the Americas*. Available at: http://en.wikipedia.org/wiki/Native-American. Retrieved February 2, 2010.

Wikipedia. (n.d.). *White American*. Available at: http://en.wikipedia.org/wiki/White_American. Retrieved February 2, 2010.

Wilson, S., & Giddens, J. (2005). *Health assessment for nursing practice*. (3rd ed., CD). St. Louis: Mosby.

Wilson, S., & Giddens, J. (2009). *Health assessment for nursing practice* (4th ed.). St. Louis: Mosby.

Winters, V. (1984). Implantable vascular access devices. *Oncology Nursing Forum, 11*(6), 25–30.

Wong, D., Perry, S., Hockenberry, M., Lowdermilk, D., & Wilson, D. (2006). *Maternal child nursing care* (3rd ed.). St. Louis: Mosby.

Zerwekh, J., & Claborn, J. (2009). *Nursing today: Transition and trends* (6th ed). St. Louis: Saunders.

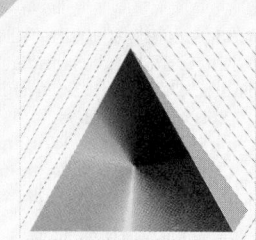

Index

A

Abbreviations
    laboratory measurement, 115b
    medication dosage-related, 560b
ABCDs; *See* cardiopulmonary resuscitation (CPR)
ABCs
    assessing in burn victims, 505b
    using during prioritizing, 69, 69b
    using during test-taking, 27, 28b
Abdomen
    assessment of, 402
    measuring girth of, 704f
    normal newborn, 340
Abdominal aneurysm resection, 229
Abdominal thrust maneuver, 200, 205b, 206f, 207
Abdominal ultrasound, 272
Abdominal wall defects
    in children, 475
ABO blood groups, 167, 168
Abortions, 280, 280b
Abruptio placentae, 315, 315f
Absence seizures, 952b
Absorption
    defining digested nutrient, 130, 130
    fats enhancing vitamin, 130, 131b
Abuse
    behaviors associated with, 1088
    child, 422, 422b, 1088–1089
    cycle of violence, 1089, 1089f
    defining, 368, 1034–1035
    elder, 414, 1091, 1092b
    fetus injuries from physical, 263
    nurse's responsibility to report, 58, 414
    and posttraumatic stress disorder, 1053, 1054b
    screening questions to determine, 392, 1090b
Acceleration/deceleration patterns, 301, 302b, 302f
Accidents
    increases with aging, 181, 181b
    safety measures to prevent, 181, 181b
Accommodation
    of conflict, 70
    vision/eye, 395b, 898, 905
Accountability
    definition of, 64, 66
    with delegation, 72
    lacking in functional nursing, 66
Acculturation, 35, 39
Accutane, 594b, 595
Acetaminophen
    description and side effects of, 971b, 972
    poisoning, 480
Acid-ash diet, 876b
Acid-base balance
    arterial blood gases, 108, 108b, 109, 109b, 109t
    components of, 103
    hydrogen ion regulation in blood, 103, 103b, 103f
    illustration of healthy, 103f
    imbalances, 109b, 109t
    and kidney function, 851
    metabolic acidosis, 106, 107, 107b, 107t
    metabolic alkalosis, 107t, 108, 108b
    pyramid study points, 102–109, 731–732
    respiratory acidosis, 104, 105b, 105f, 106t
    respiratory alkalosis, 106, 106b, 107t, 109t

Acidity (pH)
    homeostasis, 852
    and kidney function, 851
    values with acidosis and alkalosis, 109t
Acidosis
    clinical manifestations of, 106t
    diagram illustrating, 105f
Acids, 103
Acitretin, 593, 593b
Acne vulgaris, 572, 594, 594b, 595f
Acoustic neuroma, 917
Acquired immunity, 1010–1011, 1012
Acquired immunodeficiency syndrome (AIDS)
    cancer incidence higher with, 602
    CD T-cell counts, 124
    in children, 538, 539b, 539f, 540b, 540t
        antiretroviral medications for, 538, 540b
        common infections and conditions with, 539b
    description and treatment, 1018
    high risk groups, 1018
    life cycle correlation with medications, 1027f
    medications, 1025, 1027f
    during pregnancy, 285, 285b
    tests to evaluate progression of, 1019b
Acrocyanosis, 340, 343f
Actinic keratosis, 571, 591, 592b
Active transport, 86
Acuity tests, 901
Acute lymphocytic leukemia, 607, 608b
    in children, 527, 527b
Acute myelogenous leukemia, 607, 608b
    in children, 527, 527b
Acute renal failure (ARF)
    definition of, 849–850
    description and causes of, 855, 857b
    phases and signs of, 855, 857b
Acute respiratory distress syndrome, 746
Acute respiratory failure, 745
Adapalene, 594b, 595
Addictions
    defining, 1034–1035
    eating disorders, 1071, 1072f
    in newborns, 351f, 350, 351
    substance abuse disorders
        alcohol abuse, 1073, 1075b
        alcohol withdrawal, 1074, 1074b
        defining, 1072
        drug dependency, 1075, 1075b, 1076b, 1077b
        screening tools, 1073, 1073b
Addisonian crisis
    definition of, 646, 653, 653b, 653t
Addison's disease, 646, 653, 653b, 653t
Adenocarcinomas
    definition of, 600–601
    prostate cancer, 619
Adenoiditis, 434, 434f
Administration
    of blood transfusions, 167–177, 169, 171b
    of intravenous therapy, 156
    of medications
        calculating dosages, 193, 194b
        Celsius and Fahrenheit conversion, 191, 191b
        drug measurement systems/conversions, 190, 190b, 191, 191b
        infusions by unit dosage per hour, 195, 195b
        intravenous flow rates, 194, 194b

Administration (*Continued*)
        labels, 191
        metric system conversion, 190, 190b, 191b
        oral medications, 192
        parenteral medications, 192, 192f, 193f
        percentage and ratio solutions, 191b, 194
        in powder form, 193, 194b
        prescriptions, 191, 191b
        Pyramid terms and study points, 189–195
    of parenteral nutrition, 141–146, 142f
    types of gastrointestinal tube feedings, 237, 237b
    of vaccines, 551b
Administrative staff
    roles of, 71
Admission agreements, 54b
Adolescents
    characteristics of hospitalized, 378
    communication approaches with, 379
    developmental characteristics of, 385
    as maternal risk factor, 262
    medication administration considerations in, 562b
    risky behaviors by, 385
Adrenal cortex
    disorders of, 653, 653b, 653t
    function and location of, 648, 649b
    hormones of, 650b
Adrenal glands
    disorders of, 653, 653b, 653t, 654f, 655b
    function and location of, 648, 649b
    renal function of, 852
Adrenal medulla
    disorders of, 653, 653b, 653t
    function and location of, 648, 649b
Adrenalectomy, 646, 655, 655b
Adrenergic agonists, 842, 842b
Adrenergic blockers, 837, 837b, 928
Adrenocorticotropic hormone (ACTH), 649b, 650f, 651, 654
Advance directives
    definition of, 48
    do not resuscitate (DNR) orders, 58
    nurse's role in, 58
    for organ donation and transplantation, 53
    Patient Self-Determination Act, 58
Adventitious sounds, 400t
Advocacy
    definition of, 48
    principles of ethical, 49
Aerosol masks, 741
Afterbirth pain, 325
Afterload, 782
Against Medical Advice forms, 52
Aging
    and accidents, 181, 181b
    cancer risks with, 602
    cardiovascular system changes with, 411
    cataract development with, 904, 904f, 905b
    defined, 411
    and elder abuse, 414, 1091, 1092b
    eye changes with, 412
    hearing loss with, 912, 912b
    and infections, 413, 413b
    as maternal risk factor, 262
    medication issues with, 413
    mental health concerns with, 412, 413b

Foreign body airway obstruction (FBAO)
  abdominal thrust maneuver, 200, 205*b*, 206*f*
Foreign-educated nurses
  credentialing agencies, 15
  documents needed, 14, 15*b*
  licensure requirements, 14, 15*b*
  state requirements, 14, 15, 15*b*
  VisaScreen certificates, 15–16
  work visas, 15
Formal organizations; *See* organizations
Formula feeding, 345
Four P's
  of labor, 298, 298*b*
Fowler's position, 225–234, 225, 226*f*
Fractures, 984
  in children, 514, 514*b*
  description of, 984
  hip, 990, 991*f*
  interventions, 985, 985*b*, 985*f*, 986*f*, 987*b*, 987*f*
  rib, 744
  traction, reduction or fixation, 985, 985*b*, 985*f*, 986*f*, 987*b*, 987*f*
  types of, 985*b*
Fraud, 52
Fresh-frozen plasma, 167, 168
Freud, Sigmund
  psychosexual theory, 371, 372*b*, 374*b*
Friedman curve, 303, 304*f*
Frontline managers, 67
Frostbite, 571
Fructose, 131*b*
Full liquid diet, 134
Full-thickness burn injuries
  defining, 565–566
  description and illustration of, 577, 577*f*, 578*f*
Functional nursing, 66
Fundal height, 262, 262*b*, 262*f*
Fundus
  flaccid or tender, 323, 323*f*
  massage for uterine atony, 331
Fusion inhibitors, 1026, 1026*b*

G
Gag reflex, 340, 691, 941*b*
Gait
  assessment of, 402
  changes with aging, 411
Gallbladder
  anatomy and physiology of, 693
  cholecystitis, 701
Gastrectomy, 698
Gastric analysis, 693, 693*b*
Gastric bypass surgery, 700, 700*f*, 701*b*
Gastric cancer, 615, 615*b*
Gastric protectants, 722, 724*b*
Gastric resection, 698
Gastric surgery, 698
Gastric tubes, 236*f*, 239
Gastric ulcers, 697, 698*b*, 723*f*
Gastritis, 697, 697*b*
Gastroduodenostomy, 615*b*, 698
Gastroesophageal reflux disease (GERD)
  in adults, 697
  in children, 470, 470*b*
  positioning patient with, 228
Gastrointestinal bleeding
  with renal failure, 858
Gastrointestinal studies
  serum tests, 119
  types of, 693, 693*b*
Gastrointestinal system
  anatomy and physiology of, 692
  anthrax transmission through, 184, 184*b*, 184*f*
  assessing newborn's, 342
  bariatric surgery, 700, 700*b*, 700*f*
  cancer compromising functions of, 602
  changes with aging, 411
  diagnostic procedures, 693, 693*b*
  disorders (*See* gastrointestinal disorders)
  fluid volume deficit and excess affecting, 87*t*
  hypocalcemia and hypercalcemia affecting, 93*t*
  hypokalemia and hyperkalemia affecting, 91*t*
  hyponatremia and hypernatremia affecting, 89*t*
  maternal effects during pregnancy, 267
  medications (*See* gastrointestinal medications)
  organs and functions of, 692
  postoperative assessment of, 215
  postpartum changes in, 324
  pyramid terms and study points regarding, 690–691

Gastrointestinal system disorders
  appendicitis, 712
  bariatric surgery, 700, 700*f*, 701*b*
  Billroth I and II procedures, 690, 698, 698*f*, 699*f*
  bowel perforation signs, 694, 694*b*
  in children (*See* gastrointestinal disorders [pediatric])
  cholecystitis, 690, 701, 702*b*
  cirrhosis, 690, 702, 702*b*, 703*f*, 704*f*
  colostomy irrigation, 710, 712*b*
  Crohn's disease, 690, 711
  diverticulosis and diverticulitis, 690, 694*b*, 712
  dumping syndrome, 690, 699, 699*b*
  duodenal ulcers, 698*b*, 699
  esophageal varices, 690, 704, 705*f*
  gastric cancer, 615, 615*b*
  gastric ulcers, 697, 698*b*
  gastritis, 697, 697*b*
  gastroesophageal reflux disease (GERD), 697
  hemorrhoids, 713
  hepatitis, 690, 705, 706, 706*b*, 707, 708, 708*b*
  hiatal hernia, 690, 701
  medications (*See* gastrointestinal system medications)
  pancreatitis, 691, 708
  patient education regarding, 690–691
  peptic ulcer disease, 697, 698*f*, 699*f*
  peritonitis, 694, 694*b*
  positioning clients with, 228, 228*b*
  risk factors, 693*b*
  surgical interventions, 698, 700, 701, 704, 710, 712, 713
  tubes (*See* gastrointestinal tubes)
  ulcerative colitis, 691, 709, 710*f*, 711*f*, 712*b*
  vitamin B$_{12}$ deficiency, 699, 700*b*
Gastrointestinal system disorders (pediatric)
  abdominal wall defects, 475
  appendicitis, 473
  celiac disease, 472, 473*b*
  cleft lip and palate, 468, 468*f*
  constipation and encopresis, 476, 477*b*
  diarrhea, 467
  esophageal atresia, 469, 469*f*
  gastroesophageal reflux disease, 470, 470*b*
  gastroschisis, 476
  hepatitis, 478, 478*b*
  Hirschsprung's disease, 474, 474*f*
  hypertrophic pyloric stenosis, 471, 472*f*
  imperforate anus, 477, 477*b*
  intestinal parasites, 481
  intussusception, 475, 475*f*
  irritable bowel syndrome, 477
  lactose intolerance, 472
  lead poisoning, 479, 480*t*
  omphalocele, 475
  poison ingestion, 479, 479*b*, 480*t*
  pyloromyotomy, 472
  tracheoesophageal fistula, 469, 469*f*
  umbilical hernia, 476
  vomiting and nausea, 467
Gastrointestinal system medications
  antacids, 722, 723*f*, 723*t*
  antiemetics, 726, 726*b*
  bile acid sequestrants, 724, 724*b*
  for Crohn's disease, 725, 725*b*
  for diarrhea, 727
  gastric protectants, 722, 724*b*
  for *Helicobacter Pylori* infections, 724, 724*b*
  for hepatic encephalopathy, 724
  histamine 2 (H$_2$) -receptor antagonists, 722, 724*b*
  for inflammatory bowel disease, 725, 725*b*
  for irritable bowel syndrome (IBS), 725
  laxatives, 726, 726*b*
  muscarinic antagonists, 722
  pancreatic enzyme replacements, 725, 725*b*
  prokinetic agents, 724
  proton pump inhibitors, 724, 724*b*
  for ulcerative colitis, 725, 725*b*
Gastrointestinal tubes, 228, 236, 236*f*, 237, 239*b*
Gastrojejunostomy, 615*b*, 616, 698
Gastronomy tubes, 237, 237*b*, 238, 239*b*
Gastroschisis, 476
Gemcitabine, 641
Generalized anxiety disorder, 1053
Generic names, 189, 191
Genetic abnormalities, 263
Genitalia
  assessment of, 405, 406
  normal newborn, 341

Genitourinary system
  changes in older adults, 181*b*
German measles, 263, 289, 545, 546*f*
Germinal tumors, 611*b*
Gestalt therapy, 1048
Gestation period, 261
Gestational diabetes mellitus, 282
Gestational hypertension, 287, 287*t*
Giardiasis, 481
Giger and Davidhizar's Transcultural Assessment Model, 35, 36*f*
Glasgow Coma Scale, 934–935, 941, 941*b*
Glaucoma
  definition of, 898
  description and types of, 905
  medications, 924, 925*f*, 927*b*
  tonometry, 903
  treatments for, 905
Gliptins, 682, 682*b*
Glomerulonephritis, 494, 495*b*, 873
Glomerulus, 851
Gloves
  and hospital-acquired infections, 182, 182*b*
Glucagon, 685
Glucocorticoids, 593, 593*b*, 650*b*, 678, 678*b*, 726*b*, 765, 765*b*, 767*b*
  for arthritis and gout, 1004, 1004*b*
  for preventing organ rejection, 891, 891*b*
  topical for skin disorders, 591
Gluconeogenesis, 663*f*
Glucose
  food sources of, 131*b*
  to treat hypoglycemia, 663*b*
Glucose studies
  diabetes mellitus autoantibody panel, 121*t*, 122
  fasting blood glucose, 121, 121*t*
  glucose tolerance test, 121*t*, 122
  glycosylated hemoglobin, 121*t*, 122
  glycosylated serum albumin, 121*t*, 122
Glucose tolerance test, 121*t*, 122, 650, 651*b*
Gluten-free diets, 472, 473*b*
Glycogenolysis, 663*f*
Glycosuria, 272
Glycosylated hemoglobin, 121*t*, 122, 650
Glycosylated serum albumin, 121*t*, 122, 651
Goals
  from a graduate's perspective, 22, 23
Goiter, 656
Gonadotropic hormones, 254*b*, 649*b*, 650*f*
Gonorrhea, 263, 271*t*, 291, 350
Good Samaritan laws, 52
Goodell's sign, 262
Goodpasture's syndrome, 1017
Gout
  antigout medications, 1004, 1004*b*
  description of, 996
  low-purine diet for, 137
  nonsteroidal antiinflammatory drugs (NSAIDs), 1004, 1004*b*
Graafian follicle, 254*b*
Grafts
  types of wound, 583*b*
Graft-*versus*-host disease, 607
Granulocyte colony-stimulating factors, 640, 640*b*
Granulocyte-macrophage colony-stimulating factors, 640, 640*b*
Graphic option questions
  description and example of, 10, 10*b*
Grave's disease, 646, 656, 657*f*
Gravida, 261, 261*b*
Grief
  in children, 1083*b*
  definition and types of, 1082, 1083*b*
  nurse's role in, 1082
  in older clients, 412, 413*b*
Grooming, 392
Group B streptococcus (GBS), 290
Group development
  and group therapy, 1047, 1047*b*
Growth and development
  developmental stages
    hospitalized adolescents, 378
    hospitalized infants and toddlers, 377
    hospitalized preschoolers, 377
    hospitalized school-age children, 378
  NCLEX-RN study points, 435, 436
  pyramid terms regarding, 368–369
  theories of
    cognitive development theory, 370
    Erikson's theory, 370, 371*t*